MEMORY CHIPS FOR DRUG PROTOTYPES

PHYSIOLOGY FEATURES

(*continued on inside back cover*)

Drug Therapy in Nursing

Drug Therapy in Nursing

Diane S. Aschenbrenner, RN, CS, MS
Course Coordinator
Johns Hopkins University
School of Nursing
Baltimore, Maryland

Leah Wilder Cleveland, RN, EdD, CDE, CNS
Clinical Faculty, Undergraduate Nursing
Azusa Pacific University
Azusa, California

Assistant Clinical Director
Kaiser Permanente Medical Center
Bellflower, California

Samantha J. Venable, RN, MS, FNP
Professor
Saddleback College
Mission Viejo, California

LIPPINCOTT WILLIAMS & WILKINS
A Wolters Kluwer Company
Philadelphia • Baltimore • New York • London
Buenos Aires • Hong Kong • Sydney • Tokyo

Acquisitions Editor: Margaret Zuccarini
Managing Editor/Development: Lisa Popeck
Developmental Editors: Danielle DiPalma and Renee Gagliardi
Editorial Assistant: Helen Kogut
Senior Project Editor: Erika Kors
Senior Production Manager: Helen Ewan
Managing Editor/Production: Barbara Ryalls
Art Director: Carolyn O'Brien
Design: Holly Reid McLaughlin
Manufacturing Manager: William Alberti
Indexer: Michael Ferreira
Compositor: Circle Graphics
Printer: Quebecor

9 8 7 6 5 4 3 2 1

Library of Congress Cataloging-in-Publication Data

Aschenbrenner, Diane S.
Drug therapy in nursing / Diane S. Aschenbrenner, Leah Wilder Cleveland, Samantha J. Venable.
p. ; cm.
Rev. ed. of: Nursing management in drug therapy / Leah Cleveland . . . [et al.], © 1999.
Includes bibliographical references and index.
ISBN 0-7817-3269-7 (alk. paper)
1. Chemotherapy. 2. Pharmacology. 3. Nursing. I. Cleveland, Leah. II. Venable, Samantha J. III. Nursing management in drug therapy. IV. Title.
[DNLM: 1. Drug Therapy—Nurses' Instruction. 2. Pharmacology—Nurses' Instruction. WB 330 A813d 2002]
RM125 .N83 2002
615.5'8—dc21

2001050546

To my children, John, Emily, and Allison for their continuing patience,
and to my students for all that they have taught me.

D.S.A.

It is my pleasure and privilege to dedicate this volume to my family, friends, nursing professionals, faculty colleagues, and my students both current and former, all of whom were enthusiastic, excited, and very supportive throughout this extraordinary and challenging professional and personal project.

L.W.C.

Dedicated to my husband, Ben, for his unconditional love, support, and encouragement and to my parents John and Mary Gelrud for teaching me that anything is possible.

S.J.V.

CONTRIBUTORS

Delia Baquiran, RN, MSN, MSB
Chemotherapy Course Trainer, Oncology Nursing Society
Oncology Projects Consultant
New York, New York

Kathy Shane, BSN, OCN, RN
Shift Coordinator
Johns Hopkins Oncology Center
Baltimore, Maryland

Brenda K. Shelton, RN, MS, CCRN, AOCN
Critical Care Clinical Nurse Specialist
Johns Hopkins Oncology Center
Baltimore, Maryland

REVIEWERS

Judy K. Anderson, MSN, CCRN
Assistant Professor
Viterbo College
LaCrosse, Wisconsin

Kim Baily, RN, PhD
Assistant Professor, Department of Nursing
Cerritos College
Norwalk, California

Jean Krajicek Bartek, RN, PhD, CCRN
Associate Professor
University of Nebraska Medical Center
College of Nursing and Medicine
Omaha, Nebraska

Susan Buchholz, RN, BSN, MSN
Assistant Professor, Nursing Department
Georgia Perimeter College
Clarkston, Georgia

Brenda M. Cherry, MSN, BSN, AD, FNP-C
Assistant Professor of Nursing
Georgia Perimeter College
Clarkston, Georgia

Tanya Drake, MSN, RN
Professor, Department of Nursing
Rockland Community College
Suffern, New York

Sharon Dublin, BSc, BN, MN, RN
Assistant Professor
Department of Nursing
St. Francis Xavier University
Antigonish, Nova Scotia
Canada

Mary Elliott, RN, BScN, MEd
Professor
Humber College of Applied Arts & Technology
Etobicoke, Ontario
Canada

Heidi Francen
Student
Texas Christian University
Fort Worth, Texas

Colleen Glavinspiehs, BS, MSN, DNS
Professor of Nursing
Burlington County College
Pemberton, New Jersey

MaryLynn Youngwerth Gonsalves, BSN, MPH
Graduate Student
Johns Hopkins University
Baltimore, Maryland

Janet Gysi, MA, ARNP-C
Family Nurse Practitioner
Private Practice
Panama City, Florida

Amy M. Hall, RN, MS
Assistant Professor
Saint Francis Medical Center College of Nursing
Peoria, Illinois

Leland Hall
Student
Mount Royal College
Calgary, Alberta
Canada

Kathryn Henley Haugh, RN, MSN
Assistant Professor
University of Virginia
School of Nursing
Charlottesville, Virginia

Deborah Huntley, MS, RN, CS
Assistant Professor
Georgia Perimeter College
Clarkston, Georgia

Geraldine K. Jackson, RN, MSN
Associate Professor of Nursing
Rockland Community College
Suffern, New York

Peggy Jenkins, MS, BS, CCRN
Associate Professor of Nursing
Hartwick College
Onconta, New York

Shirley L. King, RN, BN, MN
Coordinator, Nursing
Mount Royal College
Calgary, Alberta
Canada

Carly Kotelko
Student
University of Calgary
Calgary, Alberta
Canada

Juliette Kruse, RN, BSN, MSN
Lecturer
San Francisco State University
San Francisco, California

Jane A. Madden, MSN, RN
Assistant Professor
Deaconess College of Nursing
St. Louis, Missouri

Linda McIntosh, RN, LPC, MSN, MS
Clinical Instructor, School of Nursing
North Carolina A & T State University
Greensboro, North Carolina

Brenda Schyf, RN, BN, BA, MEd
Health Sciences Coordinator
University of New Brunswick at Saint John
Department of Nursing
Saint John, New Brunswick
Canada

Marsha K. Sharp, RN, MSN
Assistant Professor
Elizabethtown Community College
Elizabethtown, Kentucky

Matthew Simmonds, BSc
Student
Mount Royal College
Calgary, Alberta
Canada

Teresa Stewart
Student
Gateway Community College
Phoenix, Arizona

Diane M. Tomasic, RN, MSEd, MN, EdD
Professor of Nursing
West Liberty State College
West Liberty, West Virginia

Emily Triebwasser, BSc
Student
University of Calgary
Calgary, Alberta
Canada

Karen S. Webber, RN, MN
Assistant Professor
School of Nursing
Memorial University of Newfoundland
St. John's, Newfoundland

JoNell Wells, PhD, RN, OCN
Assistant Professor
Texas Christian University
Harris College of Nursing
Fort Worth, Texas

Craig A. Wyman, BSN, MSN, MA
Associate Professor
Clinton Community College
Plattsburgh, New York

ACKNOWLEDGMENTS

The author team would like to acknowledge all of the numerous people at Lippincott Williams & Wilkins whose hard work has helped to bring this text to production. Special thanks to team members Lisa Popeck, for coordinating the project; Danielle Dipalma, for editing; Erika Kors, for production editing; Helen Kogut, for overall assistance; and Doris Wray, for ancillaries production. The author team is especially grateful to Margaret Zuccarini for her continued faith in this book and in us.

Leah Wilder Cleveland, RN, EdD, CDE, CNS was a founding member for *Nursing Management in Drug Therapy* and assisted in developing the vision for the second edition of this important textbook, now known as *Drug Therapy in Nursing*. Her hard work and dedicated efforts are appreciated as being an important driving force throughout this revision process.

PREFACE

"How will I ever learn all of this?" and "Where do I begin?" are questions that nursing students frequently ask themselves and their faculty when beginning to study pharmacology. The subject is indeed vast for novices in the profession who lack the skills to organize drug information appropriately. Students feel overwhelmed by all of the isolated pieces of drug information they must learn. Consequently, they lose sight of "the forest for the trees."

Prototype Approach

For years, many pharmacology faculty have favored a prototype approach to teaching pharmacology. This method encourages identification of "the trees" and facilitates recognition of "the forest." Use of a prototype, a drug that is representative of a class (or group) of drugs, helps students because it offers a systematic approach to grouping drug data, while beginning to recognize individual drug names. It gives students a "method" of learning and organizing large amounts of information. *Drug Therapy in Nursing* is designed and written by faculty who themselves teach nursing pharmacology using the prototype approach. At last, nursing pharmacology faculty have a text that matches the way they teach. *Drug Therapy in Nursing* is that text!

Clinical Judgment and Clinical Application

Drug Therapy In Nursing is unique in that it presents a totally nursing-focused framework to support the teaching and learning of nursing pharmacology. Learning the pharmacology facts about different drug prototypes is only half of the knowledge nursing students need. Because they are learning to be nurses, they must understand how to apply this knowledge to patient care. Nurses must learn to think critically, evaluate information, and make decisions. However, this essential aspect of knowledge application has never been thoroughly addressed in nursing pharmacology texts. Frequently, students view the *nursing application* of drug knowledge as less important than learning the hard drug facts. This thinking is fostered when the pharmacology textbooks they use present the nursing process after or apart from drug knowledge in a brief paragraph or chart. *Drug Therapy in Nursing* fully integrates core drug knowledge with core patient information, appropriately stressing, as no other text does, the relationship between the two bodies of information.

As with all other factual, scientific, or medical information used by nurses, students must learn to integrate this knowledge into their practice and apply it to patient care. Applying drug information to patient care may overwhelm students because every patient is different, with different responses, positive or negative, to the same drug therapy. If the student sees each patient situation as an isolated case, learning is again hampered. This text provides a systematic framework for assessing and evaluating patient responses that change in accord with health, age, gender, lifestyle, and other factors. This important *patient focus* is strengthened by use of the nursing process framework. Pharmacologic facts are integrated into nursing to help the student apply knowledge to practice, safely administer drugs, educate patients, and begin to make the journey from novice to expert.

Use of a Systematic Framework

The authors of *Drug Therapy In Nursing* present a systematic framework for drug therapy with every prototype drug. The framework consists of two basic areas of information—first, core drug knowledge and core patient variables—and second, actions of the nurse using this knowledge.

Core Drug Knowledge highlights the important drug facts about a prototype drug. Core drug knowledge includes pharmacotherapeutics, pharmacokinetics, pharmacodynamics, contraindications and precautions, adverse effects, and drug interactions.

Core Patient Variables identify the major factors that should be assessed in every patient to determine special considerations that need to be taken into account when administering a drug to that patient. Core patient variables include health status; lifespan and gender; lifestyle, diet, and habits; environment; and culture. The relevant variables for each particular prototype are presented in the text.

The nurse utilizes knowledge about the drug and knowledge about the patient to maximize the therapeutic effects of the drug, minimize the adverse effects of the drug, and provide patient and family education. The authors of this text call what the nurse does with knowledge about the drug and the individual patient "nursing management in drug therapy."

Organization

Drug Therapy in Nursing has thirteen units and ten appendices. The first three units address the principles and process of nursing management in drug therapy, and the basics of core drug knowledge and patient-related variables. The next ten units present the nursing management of drugs affecting various body systems and disease states. The text concludes with ten appendices.

Unit I, Principles and Process of Nursing Management in Drug Therapy, consists of three chapters. Chapter 1 explains the framework of the text and how this framework relates to the application of drug knowledge to clinical practice. This is a crucial chapter for students to read so that they best understand the content in the rest of the text. The remaining chapters address safeguards in drug development and delivery, the variety of drug preparations, and modes of administration.

Unit II, Core Drug Knowledge, includes three chapters that present the basics of pharmacology: pharmacotherapeutics, pharmacokinetics, pharmacodynamics, adverse effects, and drug interactions.

Unit III, Core Patient Variables, includes seven chapters that highlight information pertinent to patient assessment relevant to drug therapy. This is not an exhaustive list of every aspect that can be considered by these variables. The topics include lifespan issues (children, pregnant or breast-feeding women, and older adults); lifestyle, diet, and habits issues (substance abuse and dietary considerations); environment (influences on drug therapy); and culture (influences on drug therapy). The core patient variable of health status is not presented, as this includes all physiology, pathophysiology, and disease states.

Units IV through XIII present drugs affecting the various body systems and drugs used to treat diseases and their symptoms.

Appendices present essential information on Canadian drug information, diagnostic and imaging agents, enzymes and debridement therapy, enteral nutrition, parenteral nutrition, antidotes, immunizations, antiemetic drugs, therapeutic and toxic levels of selected drugs, and drugs causing photosensitivity. Emphasis is given in the appendices to the nursing management of these drug therapies.

Pedagogy

- **Learning Objectives** identify key content within chapters to help direct student learning.
- **Key Terms** identify terms that are key to understanding each chapter's contents.
- **Chapter Summaries** highlight the most important information presented in each chapter.
- **Questions for Study and Review** encourage the student to reflect on the important aspects of chapters. Answers are provided in the back of the text.

New Features With This Edition

- More **physiology and pathophysiology information** relevant to drug therapy to assist with understanding and critical thinking
- **Focus on Research boxes** highlighting current research in pharmacology. The implications for nursing practice are addressed for each article.
- **Separate chapters on men's and women's health and sexuality**
- **Hard cover,** to address students' concern that paper cover gets dog-eared, tattered, or torn easily

Key Features

- **Concept Maps** introduce the student to all drugs that are discussed in the chapter. Each map identifies the drug class, its prototype, and drugs in the class that are similar to or different from the prototype.
- **Physiology Figures** illustrate physiologic processes relevant to the drug class and link drug actions to physiology.
- **Memory Chips** assist students in studying and preparing for clinical practice, providing a quick reference of key points for each prototype drug.
- **Community-Based Concerns** highlight nursing issues related to drug therapy carried out in patients' homes and communities.
- **Critical Thinking Scenarios** challenge students to develop critical thinking skills for applying pharmacology knowledge to patient care. Answers are provided on "connection" (web link: http://connection.LWW.com/go/aschenbrenner) for this text.
- **Drug Summary Tables** relate pharmacotherapeutics and general dosage data to pharmacokinetic parameters.
- **Drug Interaction Tables** highlight known drug-drug and drug-food interactions. When diagnostic and laboratory test values are affected by drug use, this information is pointed out as well.

Ancillary Package

These excellent ancillary materials make teaching and learning even easier!

Faculty Resource Package

This useful package will help you design lectures, interact with your students online, and develop tests to assess your students' progress. Includes . . .

- **Connection companion web site** provides a convenient source to discuss teaching strategies with your peers, as well as all of the answers to the critical thinking scenarios found throughout the text and communication tools to use in your classroom. In addition, the complete Instructor's Manual will be located on **Connection.** Log on to http://connection.LWW.com/go/aschenbrenner to learn more.
- **Instructor's resource CD-ROM** provides one convenient source for all of the materials you need to develop a well-rounded course, including the Instructor's Manual, Testbank, Image Bank, and PowerPoint® slides.

Student Resource Package

Ease the learning process for your students with this complete package developed just for them. Includes . . .

- **Study Guide with student study CD-ROM** helps students review all the key material from *Drug Therapy in Nursing*. Includes a CD-ROM with student learning exercises and over 300 NCLEX-style review questions.
- **Connection companion web site** presents hotlinks to drug updates, case studies, guidelines to critical thinking questions, chapter study outlines and much more to develop students' knowledge about drug therapy.

The author team is excited to present *Drug Therapy In Nursing* in this dramatic new format that captures what experienced nurses have known for a long time—nurses must be able to apply drug knowledge to clinical practice to meet the individual needs of their patients. We believe that this text introduces students to the intricacies and challenges presented by nursing pharmacology and provides them with the tools to become clinically effective professional nurses and critical thinkers in the 21st century.

Diane S. Aschenbrenner, RN, CS, MS, Lead Author
Leah Wilder Cleveland, RN, EdD, CDE, CNS
Samantha J. Venable, RN, MS, FNP

CONTENTS

Unit V
Central Nervous System Drugs

Unit VI
Drugs Used to Control Pain and Inflammation

Unit VII
Cardiovascular and Renal System Drugs

Unit VIII
Blood and Immune System Drugs

Unit IX
Respiratory System Drugs

Unit X
Gastrointestinal System Drugs

Unit XI
Endocrine System Drugs

Unit XII
Antineoplastic Drugs

Unit XIII
Antimicrobial Drugs

Appendices

Unit I

Principles and Process of Nursing Management in Drug Therapy

Chapter 1

NURSING MANAGEMENT IN DRUG THERAPY

KEY TERMS

adverse effects
contraindications and precautions
core drug knowledge
core patient variables
culture
drug interactions
drug response
environment
health status
life span and gender
lifestyle, diet, and habits
nursing management in drug therapy
pharmacodynamics
pharmacokinetics
pharmacotherapeutics
prototype approach
prototype drug

Learning Objectives

At the completion of this chapter the student will:

1. Identify the defining components of core drug knowledge.
2. Identify the defining components of core patient variables.
3. Define nursing management of drug therapy.
4. Describe how the prototype approach to drugs is a helpful learning tool.
5. Differentiate the three main sources of data used in assessment of core drug variables.
6. Describe how core drug knowledge and core patient variables are used in nursing management in drug therapy.
7. Explain general strategies for maximizing the therapeutic effects of drug therapy.
8. Explain general strategies for minimizing adverse effects of drug therapy.
9. Identify the importance of patient and family education in drug therapy.
10. Discuss how to evaluate drug therapy and its nursing management.
11. Describe the varied settings in which nurses use nursing management techniques to assist patients receiving drug therapy.

Nurses have a vital role in managing drug therapy of individuals with medical conditions. Nurses use pharmacology (i.e., the scientific body of drug knowledge) and apply it to meeting the assessed care needs of the patient. The pharmacologic facts relevant to each drug, termed **core drug knowledge,** are:

- **Pharmacotherapeutics:** the desired, therapeutic effect of the drug
- **Pharmacokinetics:** the changes that occur to the drug when it is inside the body
- **Pharmacodynamics:** the effects of the drug on the body
- **Contraindications and precautions:** when the drug should not be used or must be used carefully with monitoring
- **Adverse effects:** unintended and usually undesired effects that may occur with the drug
- **Drug interactions:** effects that may occur when the drug is given along with another drug, food, or substance

These components of core drug knowledge are discussed in more depth later in the text.

Nurses assess the individual for factors that may or will interact with drug therapy. These areas of assessment, termed **core patient variables,** are:

- **Health status:** the presence of disease, illness, and allergy; chronic conditions causing system or organ dysfunction or diminished memory or mental capacity
- **Life span and gender:** age, physiologic development, reproductive stage, ability to read and write, and gender
- **Lifestyle, diet, and habits:** amount of activity and exercise; sleep-wake patterns; occupation; financial resources and/or access to health insurance coverage to offset the cost of the drug; eating preferences and patterns; use or abuse of substances (e.g., nicotine, alcohol, and illegal drugs); use of over-the-counter (OTC) drugs; and use of alternative health practices (e.g., herbal medicine, folk remedies)
- **Environment:** location in which the drug therapy will be administered, such as hospital, home, or long-term care facility; the physical environment that may influence aspects of drug therapy; exposure to potentially harmful substances; sun exposure that may affect the drug or cause an effect in the person receiving the drug
- **Culture:** religious and ethnic backgrounds that may alter the pharmaceutical effect of the drug or reduce the individual's receptiveness to drug therapy

The nurse considers the assessed data from the core drug knowledge and the core patient variable categories and determines significant interactions between them. A significant interaction is an area in which key elements of the drug overlap—or potentially may overlap—with specific patient factors, thus requiring nursing management. **Nursing management in drug therapy** is the planning and implementing of actions to maximize the therapeutic effects and minimize the adverse effects of a drug. The nurse also considers these significant interactions in planning and providing patient and family education relevant to the drug therapy. Finally, the nurse evaluates both the effectiveness of the drug therapy and the nursing interventions. Thus, the nurse applies knowledge in an individualized manner to meet the care needs of a particular patient receiving a particular drug therapy.

Nursing management in drug therapy helps ensure quality and comprehensive nursing care. It occurs in all settings, including hospitals, long-term care facilities, outpatient centers and clinics, health care providers' offices, and patients' homes. Some aspects of nursing management are more relevant to a particular setting. For example, it is more important for the nurse to consider the patient's lifestyle when drug therapy occurs in the home.

The term *patient* is used in this text to identify the person who is taking the drug. It should not be interpreted to mean that drug therapy or the nursing management involved occurs solely in an acute, inpatient setting. More drug therapy now occurs outside of a hospital.

THE DRUG PROTOTYPE

Currently, about 2,000 single-ingredient prescription drugs; 10,000 combination prescription drugs; 1,000 nonprescription, OTC, single-ingredient drugs; and 350,000 combination OTC drugs are listed in the *United States Pharmacopeia.* New drugs are added every year. The sheer volume of drug forms makes it impossible for the nurse to memorize up-to-date information regarding nursing management of every drug. Therefore, a method of learning and remembering more of the vast information about drugs is to use a **prototype approach.** A **prototype drug** is typical of a group of drugs within a drug class. For example, hydrochlorothiazide is a prototype drug that represents all of the thiazide diuretics. By learning the core drug knowledge about the prototype, the nurse then knows something about related drugs.

MANAGING DRUG THERAPY THROUGH THE NURSING PROCESS

The nurse uses the nursing process when managing the care of a patient receiving drug therapy. Figure 1-1 shows how the nursing process corresponds to the phases of nursing management in drug therapy. The nursing process is a series of steps in which the nurse assesses and identifies a patient's response to health-related problems, and then plans and implements interventions to manage the problem and promote a healthful outcome. The six steps of the nursing process are assessment, diagnosis, outcome identification, planning, intervention, and evaluation.

ASSESSMENT OF CORE DRUG KNOWLEDGE

Nurses need to know about all drugs a patient is taking, including prescribed and OTC drugs. The first step for a nurse is to identify the core drug knowledge relevant to a patient's

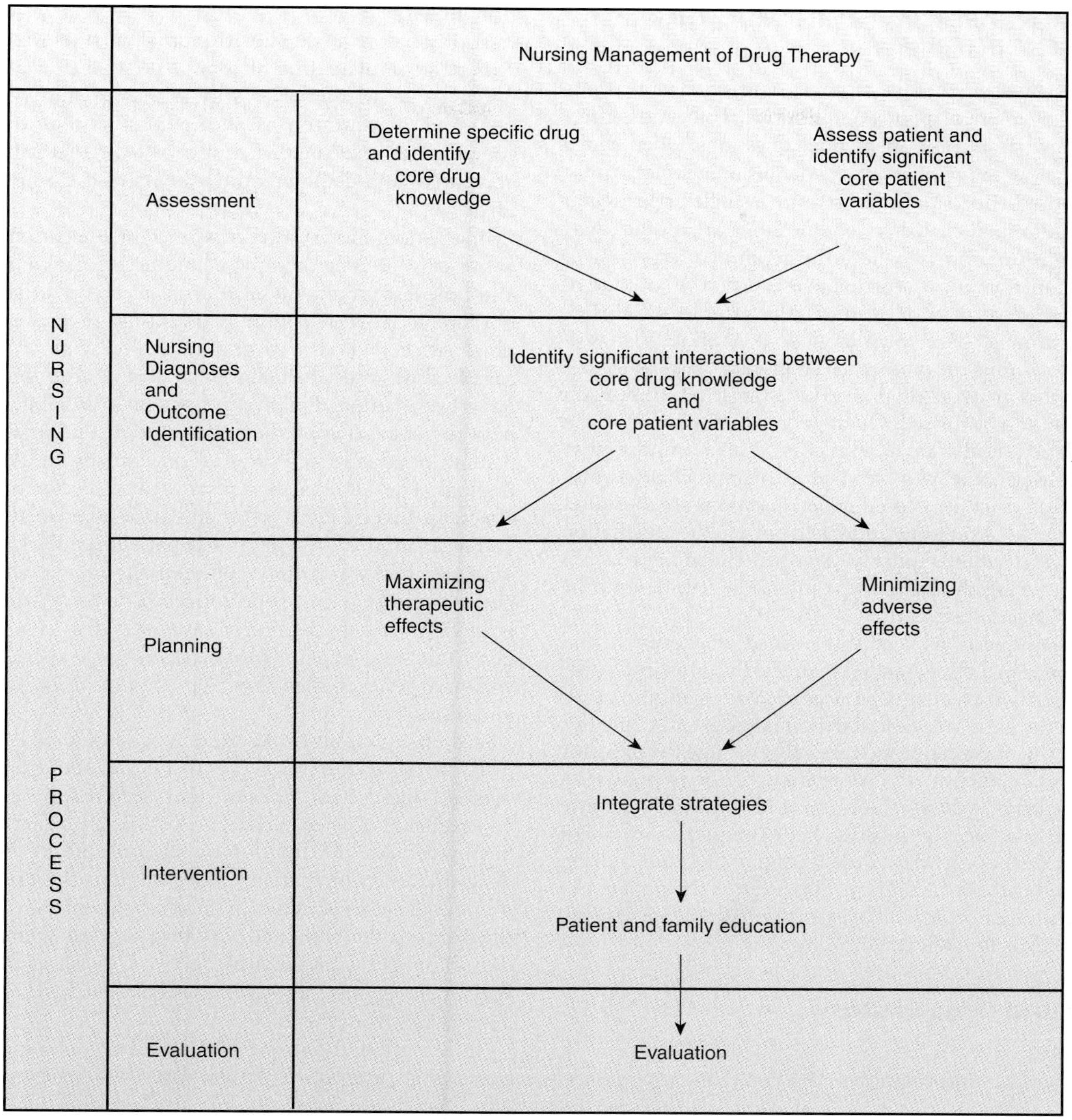

Figure 1-1. Relationship of nursing management in drug therapy to the nursing process.

drug therapy. The nurse needs to be familiar with the core drug knowledge of every drug the patient is taking to determine whether interactions with core patient variables are likely to occur and what nursing management is required. Although it would be difficult, if not impossible, to memorize information on every available drug, the nurse is responsible for using available, current drug references to review unfamiliar data prior to administering the drug or instructing the patient to self-administer the drug.

In the assessment phase, the nurse identifies the drug to be administered and its prototype, which requires the ability to discriminate among the therapeutic uses of the prototype and determine for which use it was chosen for this patient at this time. The various other pharmacologic facts must be assessed to determine the core drug knowledge for the drug prototype.

ASSESSMENT OF CORE PATIENT VARIABLES

In drug therapy, the nurse assesses the current health status of the patient and gathers data on other core patient variables to identify those that are relevant to the individual patient. Assessment of the core patient variables allows the nurse to predict (to some degree) the future needs of the patient. Data for this assessment come from three sources: 1) the patient interview and history, 2) the physical examination, and 3) the medical record, which includes current laboratory and other diagnostic findings. Pertinent findings are then assimilated to form a current, accurate picture of the patient's needs regarding drug therapy. These facts establish a baseline for the patient's treatment and care.

ASSESSMENT APPROACHES IN DRUG THERAPY: THE PATIENT INTERVIEW

Most assessment data come from an assessment interview, in which the patient responds to questions. To be most effective, the nurse should ask open-ended questions. Open-ended questions allow the patient to give details and explanations, whereas closed-ended questions require a single or particular response. Although closed-ended questions are a quick way to obtain information, they limit the depth of a response.

An example of an open-ended question is, "What kind of drug allergies do you have, if any?" An example of a closed-ended question is, "Are you allergic to penicillin?" The second question limits the patient's response to "Yes" or "No." Although this answers the immediate question, important information can be missed. Open-ended questions may elicit that the patient is allergic to ampicillin. This is important to know because people who are allergic to ampicillin may also be allergic to penicillin. Closed-ended questions are most useful in emergency situations and when particular information needs to be determined quickly. An open-ended approach is preferable during the assessment interview if time and the patient's physical state permit.

Follow-up questions need to be asked whenever the patient responds in a closed-ended manner. If, for example, the patient identifies an allergy to a particular drug, the nurse should ask the patient to describe the allergic event. Using this technique, the nurse can more carefully evaluate the patient's response. The patient may believe an event or response is a sign of an allergy, when in fact it may be a normal response to or an adverse effect of the drug. For example, if the patient describes a rash occurring on the third day of taking a drug, this may indicate a true allergy. However, if the patient describes a rash that occurred 6 weeks after completing a drug, a drug allergy is unlikely.

Health and Drug History

Health Status

The nurse gathers information about core patient variables, such as health status, from the patient interview or history component of the assessment for drug therapy. A patient's health status includes information about illnesses, diseases, chronic conditions, and allergies. This information allows the nurse to assess functioning of body systems and organs. Impaired functioning may interact with or alter the action of a drug. Pharmacotherapeutics, pharmacokinetics, and pharmacodynamics may all be affected. For example, if the patient has kidney disease and the drug is excreted through the renal system, the drug will not be eliminated as rapidly as it would in someone with normal kidney function. Because the drug is not eliminated as quickly, the drug levels may remain higher than normally expected. The patient may then exhibit increased therapeutic effect from the drug or be at increased risk for adverse effects. Patients with impaired functioning of a body system or organ may have special educational needs regarding drug therapy. For example, patients with impaired vision, hearing, or dexterity or those with decreased memory or mental capacity need special nursing considerations to meet their educational needs.

Drug History

In addition to assessing health status, the nurse explores the patient's complete drug history. A complete drug history is necessary to adequately assess the health status of the patient and to accurately assess a patient's needs and knowledge regarding current or proposed drug regimens (see the accompanying display, Components of a Complete Drug History).

In the drug history interview, the nurse seeks information about current drug therapy, including the drug name, dose, and time last given. Any new drugs to be prescribed should not interact adversely with a current drug regimen. In addition, patients who are to be admitted to acute or long-term care facilities must be maintained on the drug therapy they have been taking. Finally, the patient's drug therapy may have direct bearing on the understanding and interpretation of data obtained from physical assessment and laboratory findings. The data may be a result of an expected therapeutic effect, an adverse effect, or an interaction between drugs.

For example, knowing that a patient regularly takes the anticoagulant warfarin (Coumadin) would explain why the patient's clotting time is prolonged. Knowing that a patient is currently taking digoxin (Lanoxin), a drug that slows the heart rate, may explain why that person is experiencing adverse drug effects, such as extreme bradycardia with nausea and weakness.

Asking a patient to describe why he or she is taking the drug provides a great deal of information about the learning needs of that patient. The nurse may find that the patient has an excellent knowledge base, or, conversely, that the patient has inadequate information or misconceptions concerning drug therapy. One patient may state that the drug is a diuretic to treat hypertension; another patient may state that the drug is a fluid pill; and another patient may have no understanding of what the drug does or why it was prescribed. Patients have different learning needs that require different approaches from the nurse.

Information about recently used drugs is important because some drugs have long-lasting effects that may interact with a newly administered drug. A patient may have stopped

Components of a Complete Drug History

- Currently prescribed medications
- Prescribed dosages and routes of the medications
- When each medication was last taken
- Patient's description of why the medication was prescribed
- Other prescribed medications taken in the recent past but not currently
- Reason the medications were stopped
- Known drug allergies
- When allergic effect occurred
- Description of specific allergic effects that occurred
- Known food or environmental allergies
- Over-the-counter (OTC) medications used, such as cough and cold remedies, vitamins and minerals, and headache remedies
- Frequency of OTC drug use
- Last time the OTC medications were used

taking a drug for a variety of reasons. The patient may no longer have a medical indication for the drug, or the patient may have had an adverse reaction. The drug may have been discontinued on the advice of the prescriber, or the patient may have discontinued it independently. People may stop taking a drug for various reasons: they think they no longer need it, they think it is not effective, they are experiencing unpleasant adverse effects, or they cannot afford the drug.

Allergies need to be correctly identified and documented carefully in the medical record. Drug, food, and environmental allergies should be noted. Although allergies are an individual aspect of the health status, they are usually considered part of the complete drug history, so they are discussed as part of the drug history rather than as a separate element. Health care providers need to know the patient's allergies so that they do not prescribe or administer drugs to which the individual is allergic. Ask the patient to describe the symptoms of the allergic reaction and note these in the appropriate area of the patient's record. True allergic reactions include formation of rash or hives, itching, redness, swelling, difficulty breathing, and anaphylactic shock. Descriptions of nausea or vomiting, however, are adverse effects to drug therapy. Food or environmental allergies need to be identified and documented in addition to drug allergies. Elements of some foods are found in some drugs; for example, iodine is an element of many contrast media used in radiologic studies. Environmental allergens, if present, may complicate the health status of the individual. The nurse should also gather data about the patient's use of OTC drugs; these preparations may interact with prescribed drugs and alter their effect or produce adverse effects.

Life Span and Gender

The assessment interview allows the nurse to gather information about the core patient variables of life span and gender. Information should be sought on several topics during the assessment interview (see the accompanying display, Additional Components of the Patient Interview). Again, the goal is to determine which core patient variables are relevant to the drug therapy.

During assessment, the nurse should determine the patient's developmental level, ability to read and write, and ability to understand directions. This information is needed to plan patient education on drug therapy, including the nurse's approach and teaching methods.

It is important to determine the stage of the reproductive cycle for female patients. Certain drugs may cross the placenta, impacting fetal growth and development and sometimes causing birth defects or teratogenic effects. If a drug is extremely toxic to the fetus, women need to be cautioned not to become pregnant while taking the drug. If the woman is already pregnant, alternative drug therapy is usually indicated. If a woman is past childbearing age (postmenopausal), a drug that is toxic to a fetus may be used. Additionally, assessment for breast-feeding is important, because some drugs cross into breast milk and will have some effect on the infant and the mother.

Additional Components of the Patient Interview

General Function and Activity Level

- Developmental level
- Ability to see, read, and write
- Ability to hear and understand spoken instruction
- Occupation
- Activity and exercise patterns
- Sleep and rest patterns
- Dietary patterns: frequency of meals and snacks, foods usually eaten, foods avoided, medical dietary supplements, including vitamins, minerals, and herbal or folk remedies
- Female patients: reproductive status (e.g., pregnant or planning pregnancy, lactating), premenopausal, postmenopausal

Lifestyle-Drug Use

- Insurance and other economic resources to pay for drug therapy
- Street (illegal) drugs used: frequency and route of street drugs, last time street drugs were used
- Alcohol used: amount of alcohol consumed daily, last time alcohol consumed
- Cigarettes or other nicotine-containing products used: amount used daily
- Caffeine used: amount of daily caffeine consumption

Environment

- Description of home setting or living accommodations
- Location of home (city, industrial, suburban, rural)

Culture

- Religious beliefs
- Ethnic practices

Lifestyle, Diet, and Habits

The nurse should ask questions about a patient's lifestyle because of its potential effect on drug therapy. For example, the patient's levels of exercise and general activity may influence drug effect. Patients who are very active and who exercise are more likely to have better circulatory systems than those who are inactive. This will have an impact on the distribution of drugs within the body. People who are very active may also be more likely to incur accidental injury than others and therefore will be at greater risk for adverse drug effects, such as prolonged bleeding with warfarin, an anticoagulant.

The patient's use of street drugs, alcohol, cigarettes, and caffeine must be determined, because these substances can affect some drug actions or alter the health or physiologic functioning of the patient. For example, cigarette smoking may have caused respiratory disease.

Information on normal dietary intake is useful, because food or food elements interact with certain drugs. For example, monoamine oxidase inhibitors (an antidepressant) interact with tyramine-rich foods (e.g., aged cheese, red wine) and can induce a hypertensive crisis. Some foods affect the absorption and action of a drug; for example, milk interferes with the absorption of tetracycline. Because instructions for taking many drugs include whether they should be taken with food, the nurse needs to know how frequently and regularly the patient eats. If a drug is to be taken three times a day with food and the patient eats three meals a day, the patient may be instructed to take the drug with meals. However, if the patient normally only eats one or two meals a day or eats five or six meals a day and this was not assessed, the patient will not receive the correct dosage if the instruction to take with meals is followed. Many drugs can increase or decrease appetite or alter taste sensations. The nurse needs to assess the patient for these potential effects.

Sleep and rest patterns and occupation are important to assess, because they also have a bearing on drug therapy. People who work nights and sleep during the day will need a variation in the timing of their drug dosages, which are usually recommended to be given on a daytime schedule to allow for uninterrupted sleep at night. Knowledge of the patient's customary rest patterns provides a baseline to determine whether drug therapy is therapeutic (e.g., a drug given to induce sleep) or whether an adverse drug effect (e.g., insomnia) is occurring. Certain occupations may place the patient more at risk for injury and therefore more prone to adverse effects from some drugs.

Economic factors may determine whether the patient will adhere to prescribed drug therapy and, therefore, should be assessed. If the drug is very expensive and the patient cannot afford the drug or health insurance to offset or defray drug costs, the patient's inability to purchase the drug may preclude his or her adherence to therapy.

Environment

The home setting or living environment should be assessed, because it may give clues to the patient's adherence to the drug regimen or to potential risks from the therapy. For example, if a patient is receiving a drug that causes dizziness as an adverse effect, stairs in the house may pose a risk for falls. If the home does not have running water, a patient may be unable to adhere to handwashing instructions that precede self-injection of insulin. General factors to assess include cleanliness, lighting, adequate heat, water, and refrigeration. A home visit by a visiting or home health nurse may be the most accurate way to obtain this information.

Environmental factors outside of the home may also affect drug therapy. Environmental elements or substances in the environment may predispose the patient to adverse drug effects. Direct sunlight, for example, may cause a sunburn when the patient is prone to photosensitivity from tetracycline, an antibiotic. The nurse needs to determine the environment in which the drug will be administered. Some drug therapy occurs only in certain environments or settings (e.g., general anesthetics are only given in an operating room). Other drugs, such as oral antibiotics, may be used in all health care settings, including the patient's home. Selection of strategies to maximize therapeutic effect or minimize adverse effects may depend on the drug administration environment. Materials selected for patient and family teaching may also depend on the environment in which drug therapy occurs.

Patients may start drug therapy in one environment and continue therapy in another—for example, the hospital and then the home—or therapy may be lifelong, as with antidiabetic agents. The patient may begin taking a drug in a hospital and continue taking it in a subacute care center before concluding therapy in the center or continuing therapy at home. Planning for discharge of a patient from an acute care setting begins the day of admission. Therefore, during assessment, the nurse must gather data that will be important in meeting the goals of drug therapy once the patient is discharged. Where the patient will go after discharge will alter the education required. If the patient will receive drug therapy at home, the nurse needs to assess the home as previously described.

Some home drug therapies, such as intravenous (IV) therapy, may require special equipment, technologies, or skills. In these cases, the nurse assesses the ability of the patient or responsible caregiver to administer drug therapy safely and effectively. Additional assessments are made about the ability to take appropriate actions if a problem occurs. For example, the nurse needs to know whether the patient or caregiver can describe the actions he or she would take if an infection occurred as a result of IV therapy. The nurse can assess this information by asking hypothetical questions about typically encountered problems and having the patient or caregiver describe how to handle the problem described.

Culture

Culture is the last core patient variable to include in the health history and drug assessment. Religious restrictions or cultural practices may affect the patient's acceptance of prescribed drug therapy. Christian Scientists, for example, who believe in healing through prayer, may not accept drug therapy to manage hypertension. Patients with some ethnic backgrounds may have altered responses to particular drug therapies. African Americans, for example, exhibit a diminished therapeutic response to antihypertensive agents, such as angiotensin-converting enzyme inhibitors.

PHYSICAL EXAMINATION

After completing the health history interview, the nurse performs the second part of the assessment—the physical examination.

Core Patient Variables

The physical examination—also focused on the core patient variables of general status, life span, and gender—should be comprehensive. The patient's history and present complaints (the main reason for seeking health care) usually dictate which body systems require in-depth assessment. General observation will provide some information on health status. Physical assessment of the systems (e.g., the respiratory system) will provide information about disease or illness. Approximate age and, depending on the stage, pregnancy, can be determined by general observation. Baseline data, such as vital signs, height, and weight, must be measured. Ideally, the height and weight are taken directly by the nurse or someone delegated by the nurse (as opposed to asking the patient for this information). An accurate measurement of body size is an important factor in computing the correct dose of many drugs. During emergencies, this information may be estimated.

The nurse should closely inspect the skin of all patients for rashes and document their appearance and location. Failure to do so could result in the rash's being misinterpreted as a drug reaction. Other areas to inspect closely are the peripheral blood vessels if IV drugs may be ordered. If a history of IV drug abuse is reported, scarring or inflammation of the vessels may be present. In such cases, potential problems with IVs may be anticipated.

All gathered data must be analyzed in terms of the specific current and proposed drugs, identifying any actual and potential problems related to providing drug therapy.

SUPPORTIVE STUDIES: MEDICAL RECORD AND DIAGNOSTIC FINDINGS

In addition to drug history and physical examination, complete assessment data for the core patient variables are also derived from a review of the patient's medical record and test results. The medical record provides information about the patient's health status, lifestyle, diet, habits, and environment.

Areas of the medical record that are specifically important include laboratory and other diagnostic test results. For drug therapy, pertinent findings may include blood levels of a drug or test results related to drug action. For example, blood glucose levels are pertinent findings in diabetic patients receiving insulin to control hyperglycemia. A computed tomography scan report indicating the tumor burden of a patient receiving chemotherapy is also a relevant finding. The nurse should review all diagnostic findings, paying special attention to those findings relevant to body systems at risk for adverse effects from currently used drugs (Table 1-1).

Past medical records may be used to verify the patient's drug history. Moreover, they may provide details relevant to the patient's current treatment. Patients may forget previous drug reactions, past illnesses, family histories, and other essential baseline information, but these data may be available in previous medical records. Review of the medical record is important regardless of whether the drug is administered in a hospital, extended care facility, outpatient center, or the patient's home. This part of the assessment can be done either before or after the interview and physical examination.

See the accompanying display, Identifying Core Patient Variables, for a critical thinking approach to the identification of the core patient variables discussed in the previous sections.

TABLE 1-1 General* Laboratory Test Values: Normal Ranges

System Tested	Diagnostic Test	Normal Values
Hepatic	Bilirubin (total)	0.3–1.0 mg/dL
	Indirect unconjugated bilirubin	0.2–0.7 mg/dL
	Direct conjugated bilirubin	0.1–0.4 mg/dL
	AST (formerly SGOT)	7–27 U/L
	ALT (formerly SGPT)	1–21 U/L
	PTT	20–30 s
	PT	12–14 s
Renal	BUN	8–25 mg/dL
	Serum creatinine	0.6–1.5 mg/dL
	Creatinine clearance	Women: 120–180 L/d Men: 140–200 L/d
Hematologic	Hct	Women: 36%–48% Men: 42%–52%
	Hgb	Women: 12–16 g/dL Men: 14–18 g/dL
	WBC count	5,000–10,000/mm^3
	Platelets	150,000–400,000/mm^3

*Ranges for normal laboratory test values may vary according to health care setting, the laboratory performing the test, and the testing equipment. This information should be considered a basic guide. Nurses need to be familiar with normal ranges used in the facility or agency in which they work.

IDENTIFYING SIGNIFICANT INTERACTIONS: NURSING DIAGNOSES AND OUTCOMES

Data that have been gathered throughout the assessment are interpreted by the nurse as to their relevance in drug therapy for a patient. The nurse reviews the core drug knowledge and the core patient variables from which significant interactions may be generated. The nursing diagnoses and patient outcomes are names or labels given to these interactions.

Nursing diagnoses are based on classifications proposed by the North American Nursing Diagnosis Association. The diagnosis may reflect a current, actual problem or the risk of a problem's developing related to drug therapy. A patient may be receiving a drug that addresses a current problem, yet its use may put the patient at risk for developing other problems. For example, a patient has a nursing diagnosis of Chronic Pain related to cancer. If the patient is taking morphine

Critical Thinking Scenario

Identifying core patient variables

1. Propose questions to ask patients who tell you that they are allergic to a drug.
2. Your patient, a 75-year-old man living on a fixed income from a social security pension, is to be discharged on a new drug for hypertension. In assessing core drug knowledge for the patient's drug therapy, you identify adverse effects of dizziness and dry mouth. Identify the core patient variables that you would evaluate most carefully for relevance to this patient's drug therapy.

to control the pain, the diagnoses related to the drug therapy would be Risk for Injury related to sedation from narcotic drug use and Constipation related to adverse effects of morphine (see the accompanying display, Selected Nursing Diagnoses Pertaining to Drug Effects).

In addition to diagnoses that reflect current or potential problems from effects of drugs, many other types of drug-related diagnoses may be appropriate. The diagnosis of Deficient Knowledge may be appropriate if a new drug has been prescribed. Ineffective Therapeutic Regimen Management may be appropriate if the individual has not been taking drug therapy as prescribed due to a misunderstanding of the directions. Ineffective Coping may be a nursing diagnosis for a patient who continually forgets to take a prescribed drug for a chronic condition (e.g., insulin for diabetes). Nursing diagnoses are highly individualized and cannot be predicted from prescribed drug therapy alone. Reputable textbooks devoted specifically to nursing diagnosis contain additional information.

The next phase of the nursing process is outcome identification—that is, the determination of the desired results of nursing interventions. Outcomes develop from the data gained in assessment and the diagnosis selected. A plan for a patient receiving drug therapy would identify outcomes related to the patient's specific drug regimen.

PLANNING AND INTERVENTION

Once the significant interactions between the core drug knowledge and the core patient variables have been identified, the nurse devises strategies to maximize the therapeutic effects and minimize the adverse effects of the drug therapy. The nursing process step of planning is used.

Planning begins with identifying interventions necessary to reach the desired outcome. Planning continues by defining what needs to be done to achieve the identified outcomes. Performance of the plan is intervention, the next phase of the nursing process. With intervention, the nurse integrates the devised strategies into the nursing plan of care for the patient receiving drug therapy. These strategies are relevant to the physical act of drug administration in addition to patient and family education pertaining to drug therapy.

Selected Nursing Diagnoses Pertaining to Drug Effects

- Constipation
- Diarrhea
- Acute Pain
- Chronic Pain
- Fatigue
- Risk for Infection
- Risk for Injury
- Disturbed Sensory Perception
- Ineffective Sexuality Patterns
- Disturbed Sleep Pattern
- Disturbed Thought Processes
- Interrupted Breast-feeding
- Acute Confusion
- Deficient Fluid Volume
- Excess Fluid Volume
- Imbalanced Nutrition: More than body requirements
- Imbalanced Nutrition: Less than body requirements
- Impaired Urinary Elimination
- Urinary Retention

MAXIMIZING THERAPEUTIC EFFECTS

To maximize the therapeutic effects of any given drug therapy, the nurse must know what the desired therapeutic effects are and how they are achieved. Strategies appropriate for the patient are then used to promote these effects. Although these strategies are drug specific, a few general principles exist:

- Administer the drug in a manner that will promote its absorption. A drug administered orally may be given with meals or on an empty stomach, depending on the drug. When giving a drug parenterally, use the appropriate administration technique for the desired route. A route different from that prescribed may alter absorption and the desired effect. For example, if an intramuscular injection is accidentally given subcutaneously, absorption will be slower and the onset of the therapeutic effect delayed.
- Administer the drug at the appropriate time. This will maintain blood levels of the drug to promote therapeutic effects.
- Monitor laboratory values, when appropriate, to determine that the prescribed dose achieves a therapeutic drug level.

MINIMIZING ADVERSE EFFECTS

Many of the nursing care strategies are directed at minimizing the adverse effects of drug therapy. Again, the strategies are specific to the drug, but there are some common to all drug therapy:

- Before initiating drug therapy, verify that the patient is not allergic to the drug or whether the drug is contraindicated for this patient for some reason.
- Administer the drug in a manner consistent with standard safety protocols. For example, some drugs need to be administered IV at a regular, steady rate, and the use of an IV infusion controller, or pump, is considered standard for these drugs.
- Monitor the patient and relevant laboratory findings closely for evidence of known adverse effects from drug therapy. Patients at high risk for developing a particular adverse effect should be monitored especially carefully.
- Discontinue or withhold a drug's administration if warranted by the laboratory findings. Notify the prescriber of the findings and your actions.
- Report evidence of adverse effects to the prescriber as soon as possible.
- Modify administration techniques, when appropriate, to decrease the incidence of adverse effects. For example, if the drug causes the patient gastrointestinal distress on an empty stomach, administer the drug with food.

- Implement special techniques for certain drugs to detect the onset of adverse effects. For example, monitor blood pressure before administering each dose of an antihypertensive drug to determine whether the blood pressure has decreased too much to administer the drug.

PATIENT AND FAMILY EDUCATION

An essential part of implementing any therapeutic plan is patient and family education. The nurse integrates the recognized interactions of the core drug knowledge and the core patient variables into patient and family education on drug therapy. Thus, the education is specific to the drug therapy and specific to the patient's needs.

Core Drug Knowledge

The nurse has a crucial role in educating patients and their families about drug therapy. The goal of patient education is for the individual patient to understand the drug and its effects well enough to self-medicate safely and effectively and to monitor the **drug response** (i.e., the anticipated therapeutic and adverse effects). Basic drug therapy education should include the name of the drug, the reason the drug was prescribed (pharmacotherapeutics), the intended effect of the drug (pharmacodynamics), and important adverse effects that may occur and should be reported to the nurse or health care provider. If the patient will be taking the drug at home, he or she also needs to know when to take it, how frequently and for how long, how to store it, and what to do if a dose is missed. In addition, the patient must be aware of any special concerns regarding other drugs or foods taken (drug interactions), and trained in any special techniques needed for self-administration of the drug to maximize therapeutic or minimize adverse effects. This information is obtained from the health care prescriber's prescription of the drug in addition to the core drug knowledge of pharmacokinetics and pharmacodynamics.

Core Patient Variables

Any or all of the core patient variables may have a bearing on the educational needs of the patient or the family. Patient variables may affect which educational materials need to be provided and the format or method of presentation.

Health Status

Education related to the core patient variable of health status includes those activities that need to be performed while the patient receives the drug to maintain health or to detect early changes in health that are related to adverse effects of the drug. For example, there may be a need for periodic laboratory tests, such as monitoring levels of theophylline (a bronchodilator) or monitoring bleeding time in a patient receiving an anticoagulant. There may also be a need for periodic examination or assessment by a health care provider, for example to monitor blood pressure when the patient is receiving antihypertensives.

The current health status of the patient must also be considered. The following are questions a nurse should consider when designing a patient education program for drug therapy:

- Has any current disease or condition impaired any organ or system functioning, leaving the patient at higher risk for certain adverse effects? If so, information on these adverse effects may need to be emphasized more during educational sessions than with other patients.
- Does the patient have impaired vision, which may prohibit reading drug labels or contribute to making errors, such as misreading the number "3" as a "5" in the instruction, "Take 3 times a day"? A vision problem may also indicate that educational material cannot be presented in written form to this patient.
- Does the patient have a hearing loss that may interfere with the comprehension of oral teaching?
- Does the patient have difficulty with small motor movements, perhaps due to arthritis in the hands? If so, difficulty in opening drug bottles may be a problem.
- Does the patient remember spoken conversations well? If not, written education may be more effective. If memory loss is severe, adherence to the prescribed drug regimen may be difficult to achieve, and memory aids about drugs and their dosing may be indicated.
- Does the patient have the mental capacity to understand the information presented on drug therapy? If not, another person may need to be responsible for administering the drug to the patient.

Life Span and Gender

The life span variable becomes important when a drug therapy produces adverse effects on a developing fetus. Women of childbearing age need to be educated not to become pregnant while taking certain drugs. Age is also an important consideration when determining a patient education approach. For example, drug education for a preschooler will most likely be directed to the parents, whereas education for an adolescent is directed so that the adolescent becomes an active partner in the educational process.

Lifestyle, Diet, and Habits

It is important to consider lifestyle and behavioral changes the patient may need to make during drug therapy because of the action or adverse effect of the drug. For example, a patient taking narcotics for pain will be drowsy because the drug depresses the central nervous system. This patient should be cautioned not to drive a car or operate potentially hazardous machinery while taking the drug. A patient receiving an antihistamine for an allergic reaction may also experience drowsiness as an adverse drug effect and should be similarly cautioned. Other lifestyle changes may be indicated, such as avoiding alcohol or cigarettes, because they may alter a drug's effect. For example, cimetidine has reduced effectiveness in decreasing gastric acid production in a patient who smokes cigarettes while taking this drug.

The patient's lifestyle determines the value placed on patient education. The patient education information may be considered important by the nurse, but the patient may not share this view; thus, the educational process will not be very effective. The nurse needs to determine what the patient wants to know about the drug and what the patient believes has the most significance for him or her. Ideally, the educational process should begin at this point, even if it is not the point that the nurse believes is most important. Meeting the needs of the patient will increase the effectiveness of the education and promote receptivity to additional teaching at a later time.

Learning Style and Literacy Level

Consider the patient's learning style when selecting an approach to patient education. Some people are more visual learners, and the use of videotapes may be a better teaching medium for them than printed information. Other people need to be physically involved in their learning and role playing or demonstration and return demonstration may be better educational techniques for them.

When using written educational materials, take into consideration the patient's literacy level: Can he or she read and write in the language used in those materials? Written materials are appropriate for individuals who can read. However, they must be at the patient's reading level. If appropriate, standardized drug information sheets may be used. Many health care settings distribute these for patient use. Additionally, some drug references are available that are designed to be photocopied and given to patients. If a standard information sheet is unavailable, the nurse can create one or simply write down instructions for taking the drugs along with a dosage schedule (see the accompanying display, Patient Education Guidelines).

Environment

Environment is an important consideration when educating a patient and family about drug therapy. The extent of teaching will vary, depending on the environment in which the patient will receive the drug. Although some education is required regardless of the setting, more information is necessary if the patient will be taking the drug at home. These patients must know about all aspects of the drug so that its administration can be safely and effectively self-managed. If another person—family member or someone else—will be responsible for the patient's drug therapy at home, that person needs to be included in the educational process.

The physical properties of the home may also affect the patient education required; the home setup may increase the risk of injury or adverse effects from a drug. For example, if the home has scatter rugs, the patient needs to be educated about the increased risk for falls while receiving drug therapy that may cause an unsteady gait. (For more information see the accompanying display, General Considerations for Home- or Community-Based Drug Therapy.)

Culture

When educating the patient and family about drug therapy, the nurse needs to be sensitive to the patient's cultural frame of reference. A person's religious and ethnic background influences his or her beliefs about health, wellness, and the role of drug therapy in maintaining or restoring health. Cultural background may also influence communication patterns and determine who in the family is the appropriate member to be involved in educational sessions. Depending on the culture, this may or may not be the patient. The patient's cultural background is neither right nor wrong. To provide effective education, the nurse must consider cultural issues and modify content or presentation accordingly. The nurse must adapt to meet the patient's needs.

Patient Education Guidelines

When preparing educational materials for patients receiving drug therapy, the nurse includes guidelines on the following:

- ❑ Drug name: generic and trade names
- ❑ Purpose of the drug
- ❑ Contraindication to taking the drug
- ❑ When to take the drug (time, frequency)
- ❑ Duration of treatment
- ❑ How to take the drug
- ❑ What to do if a dose is forgotten
- ❑ Special instructions related to lifestyle changes while on the drug
- ❑ Hazardous activities to avoid while on the drug
- ❑ Any dietary restrictions or additions
- ❑ Drug-food interactions
- ❑ Drug-drug interactions, including those that may result from over-the-counter drugs
- ❑ Adverse effects and instructions on what to do about them
- ❑ Special storage needs if applicable
- ❑ Special directions for drug disposal
- ❑ Therapeutic monitoring needed while taking the drug
- ❑ Periodic laboratory tests needed while taking the drug
- ❑ Precautions related to pregnancy or lactation
- ❑ Health care providers who should be notified about the drug therapy (e.g., dentist by patient taking an anticoagulant)
- ❑ Advisability of carrying or wearing a drug alert card or medical identification
- ❑ Period of time drug remains active after discontinuing therapy

EVALUATION

Like the nursing process, nursing management in drug therapy ends with evaluation. At the end of the established time frame for achieving an expected outcome, the nurse measures the patient's progress. Was the outcome or goal achieved? Was the nursing management effective? These two measurements are not the same. An outcome can be achieved despite an ineffective plan. For example, a patient may not have adverse effects from drug therapy despite the nurse's not thoroughly identifying actions to minimize adverse effects. Or the management may have been appropriate, although the goal was not achieved. For example, the patient may experience an adverse drug effect even though the nurse appropriately identified and implemented strategies to minimize adverse effects. In evaluating the effectiveness of drug therapy, one of the most important aspects to consider is whether the drug

General Considerations for Home- or Community-Based Drug Therapy

The nurse needs to explore considerations, such as those below, when assessing the ability of the patient or responsible others to self-manage drug therapy safely at home:

Patient Considerations

- Ability to see and read labels
- Ability to remember dosage schedule
- Ability to open medication containers
- Ability to perform any special techniques required for drug administration

Home Considerations

- Safe storage areas for keeping medications out of the reach of small children who may live in or visit the patient's home
- Adequate refrigeration if the medication needs to be chilled
- Convenient and safe storage areas for equipment, particularly the equipment needed to administer medication (e.g., intravenous (IV) pumps and controllers, nebulizers)
- Adequate and secure disposal containers for medication or equipment

Educational Considerations and Aids

- Thorough, clear, written instructions for medication administration
- Memory aids, such as a calendar, dosage chart, or a clock-faced picture with the appropriate medication doses identified at the correct times
- Organized, convenient system for accessing medication such as
  - Keeping all medication containers in a bowl, small box, or on a special shelf
  - Dispensing one day's medication in a pill box or commercially available organizer or the individual compartments of an empty egg carton
- Numbering or color coding drug containers if the patient has a reading or language problem
- Organized, convenient system for drug delivery equipment (syringes, alcohol wipes, transdermal patches, drug pumps, IV tubing, and so forth), such as a box, a plastic storage container with a snap-on lid, or clean, dry glass jars with screw tops
- Impervious, puncture-proof containers with properly fitting lids, such as coffee cans or plastic milk jugs, for disposing of needles, syringes, and other equipment

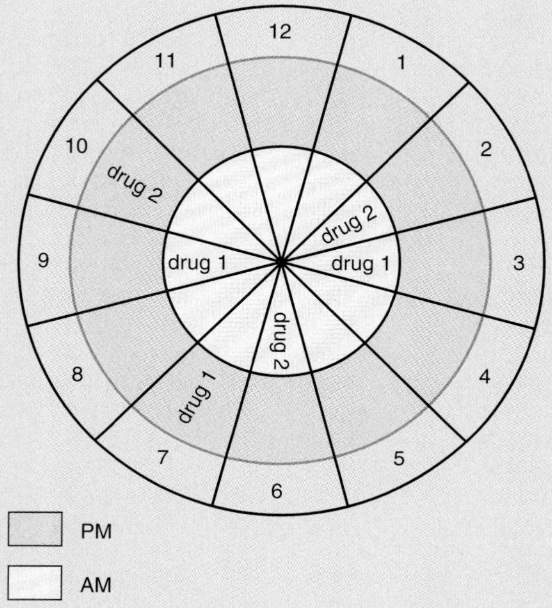

achieved the desired effect. For example, an antihypertensive drug is given to lower blood pressure. Did the blood pressure drop to a safe and normal range? If so, then the evaluation shows that drug therapy was effective.

If the patient does not achieve the expected outcomes, the nurse must reassess to identify the barriers to success. Perhaps the nurse missed an important interaction between the core drug knowledge and the core patient variables. Perhaps the nurse did not identify a core patient variable. Perhaps the teaching strategies used were not effective for this patient, and a different approach should be attempted. Perhaps the identified outcome is not appropriate for this patient, or the outcome may be appropriate but the time frame inadequate. Evaluation is not merely determining if the goals were achieved or the management was effective. The reason behind any treatment failure must be identified and steps taken to achieve desired results effectively.

CLINICAL PATHWAYS

Nursing management in drug therapy may be used in clinical pathways (also known as critical pathways). A clinical pathway is an interdisciplinary approach to care that establishes common protocols for patients with the same medical diagnoses. These pathways specify the responsibilities, actions, and time frame required of each discipline (e.g., nursing, medicine, physical therapy, pharmacy, respiratory therapy) to meet the objectives needed to complete the care plan.

Clinical pathways provide a standard of care for all patients with the same diagnosis. The pathway accounts for the drugs ordered as a treatment for or response to a specific condition. For example, the clinical pathway for a patient with deep vein thrombosis usually has drug therapy beginning with the anticoagulant heparin. After 3 to 4 days, the patient usually receives an oral anticoagulant, such as warfarin sodium. When the patient's blood tests indicate that the oral anticoagulant is at a therapeutic level, heparin therapy stops. If the patient meets the requirements of the pathway in the time specified, the therapy is evaluated as effective.

Nursing management in drug therapy still occurs with the use of the clinical pathway. Clinical pathways are not substitutes for nursing assessment and judgment. Assessment of core drug knowledge and core patient variables, identification of their significant interactions, the development of strategies to maximize therapeutic effects and minimize adverse effects, and patient and family education not only form the basis of astute nursing care but also contribute to early identification of a patient at risk of "falling off" the pathway. Early identification of the patient at risk alters plans of care, prevents complications, and minimizes additional inpatient days.

CHAPTER SUMMARY

- Core drug knowledge consists of basic pharmacologic facts about each drug. It is composed of pharmacotherapeutics, pharmacokinetics, pharmacodynamics, contraindications and precautions, adverse effects, and drug interactions.
- Core patient variables are features that make a patient unique at any given time.
- The nurse determines which of the patient's core patient variables are significant for a particular drug therapy. They include health status; life span and gender; lifestyle, diet, and habits; environment; and culture.
- The nurse determines which significant interactions will occur between the core drug knowledge and the core patient variables. Based on the determined interactions, the nurse then recommends strategies to maximize the therapeutic effect and minimize the adverse effects of drug therapy. The nurse integrates these strategies into a nursing plan of care. Patient and family education is also based on the interactions between core drug knowledge and core patient variables. This is nursing management in drug therapy.
- A prototype drug is a drug that is representative of a class of drugs. Learning the core drug knowledge about the prototype provides the nurse with information about several other drugs in the same class as the prototype drug. It is a way to organize and simplify learning.
- In providing nursing management of drug therapy, the steps of the nursing process are used. Nursing management of drug therapy occurs in all health care environments, including acute care, long-term care, and home and community settings.
- A thorough drug assessment provides the baseline information needed for effective nursing management of drug therapy. It includes the patient history, physical assessment, and examination of the medical record.
- Nursing diagnoses and outcomes are labels given to the identified interactions between core drug knowledge and core patient variables.
- Nursing diagnoses for patients receiving drug therapy reflect current or potential problems relevant to the therapy.
- Expected outcomes define the units of measure by which to gauge the effectiveness of drug therapy.
- Patient and family education is a crucial aspect of nursing management in drug therapy. Individualized education proceeds from the baseline core drug knowledge and core patient variables.
- Drug therapy is evaluated as effective if the desired effect of the drug occurs. The nurse also evaluates whether the management plan was effective. If conclusions drawn from the evaluation show that the drug effect or the management plan was not achieved, the nurse must determine why and then respond accordingly.
- An important goal of home-based drug therapy is for patients and caregivers to acquire the knowledge and skills needed to implement drug therapy safely and effectively. The nursing management of drug therapy must take the home setting into consideration. Education should be structured so that patients and caregivers can assume maximal responsibility for administering and monitoring drug therapy safely and effectively.

QUESTIONS FOR STUDY AND REVIEW

1. How does the nurse assess core patient variables?
2. Why does the nurse need to assess the core drug knowledge of each drug a patient receives?
3. How does learning core drug knowledge about prototype drugs help the nurse?

NEED MORE HELP?

? Chapter 1 of the study guide for *Drug Therapy in Nursing* contains exercises and activities to reinforce your understanding of the concepts presented in this chapter. For additional information see the text's accompanying web site at *http://www.connection.lww.com.*

REFERENCES AND BIBLIOGRAPHY

Bakker, D. A., Blais, D., Reed, E., Vaillancourt, C., Gervais, S., & Beaulieu, P. (1999). Descriptive study to compare patient recall of information: Nurse-taught versus video supplement. *Canadian Oncology Nursing Journal, 9*(3), 115–120.

Bates, B. (1999). *A guide to physical examination and history taking* (7th ed.). Philadelphia: Lippincott Williams & Wilkins.

Carpenito, L. J. (2000). *Nursing diagnosis: Application to clinical practice* (8th ed.). Philadelphia: Lippincott Williams & Wilkins.

DeSales, T., Wellard, S., & Bethune, E. (1999). Registered nurses' perceptions of teaching: Constraints to the teaching moment. *International Journal of Nursing Practice, 5*(1), 14–20.

Fischbach, F. T. (2000). *A manual of laboratory and diagnostic tests* (6th ed.). Philadelphia: Lippincott Williams & Wilkins.

Frauman, A. C., & Skelly, A. H. (1999). Evolution of the nursing process. *Clinical Excellence in Nurse Practitioners, 3*(4), 238–244.

Fulmer, T. T., Feldman, P. H., Kim, T. S., Carty, B., Beers, M., Molina, M., & Putnam, M. (1999). An intervention study to enhance medication compliance in community-dwelling elderly individuals. *Journal of Gerontological Nursing, 25*(8), 6–14.

Harkleroad, A., Schirf, D., Volpe, J., & Holm, M. B. (2000). Critical pathway development: An integrative literature review. *American Journal of Occupational Therapy, 54*(2), 148–154.

Harper, P. J. (1999). The placebo effect and the hidden benefits of oral medications. *British Journal of Nursing, 8*(9), 589–592.

Herring, L. (1999). Critical pathways: An efficient way to manage care. *Nursing Standard, 13*(47), 36–37.

Payne, J. (2000). The nursing interventions classification: A language to define nursing. *Oncology Nursing Forum, 27*(1), 99–103.

Redman, B. (1997). *The practice of patient education* (8th ed.). St. Louis: Mosby-Year Book.

Ward-Griffin, C., & McKeever, P. (2000). Relationships between nurses and family caregivers: Partners in care? *ANS Advanced Nursing Science. 22*(3), 89–103.

Chapter 2

PHARMACEUTICALS: DEVELOPMENT, SAFEGUARDS, AND DELIVERY

KEY TERMS

Canadian Food and Drugs Act
chemical classification
chemical name
clinical trials
controlled substance
drug classification
Federal Food, Drug, and Cosmetics Act of 1938
generic name
legend drugs
National Formulary
pharmacodynamics
pharmacogenetics
pharmacognosy
pharmacokinetics
pharmacology
pharmacotherapeutics
physiologic classification
placebo response
Practitioners Reporting Network
Pure Food and Drug Act of 1906
therapeutic classification
toxicology
trade name
United States Adopted Names Council
United States Pharmacopeia

Learning Objectives

At the completion of this chapter the student will:

1. Identify key concepts relevant to nursing management in pharmacotherapy.
2. Name four main sources of drugs and biologic products.
3. Describe the differences in the ways that drugs are named.
4. Explain the significance of drug classifications.
5. Identify sources of drug information.
6. Describe the scope of nursing responsibilities related to pharmacology.
7. Discuss the application of the nursing process related to pharmacology.
8. Describe the intent, scope, and benefits of drug standards and legislation.
9. Identify several references and resources that list standards regulating drug development, distribution, and use.
10. Explain new drug development and the role of nurses in clinical trials.
11. Differentiate between over-the-counter and legend (prescription) drugs.
12. Discuss the significance of the 1970 Controlled Substance Act and its relationship to nursing practice.
13. Compare drug legislation in the United States with drug legislation in Canada.

Pharmacology, one of the most dynamic and basic aspects of nursing, draws on and incorporates information from various disciplines, including anatomy, chemistry, microbiology, physiology, and psychology. Pharmacology is the study of drugs and their interaction—at any cellular level—with the body's components. The study of pharmacology also includes how the drug is transformed within the body.

The science of pharmacology consists of several branches: **pharmacogenetics, pharmacognosy** (the study of natural elements as drug sources), **pharmacodynamics, pharmacokinetics, pharmacotherapeutics,** and **toxicology.**

Drugs used today have controlled, and in some cases cured, a variety of health problems ranging from hypertension and heart disease to cancer, pneumonia, and mental health disorders. A comprehensive view of pharmacology accounts for not only prescribed drugs, but also for nonprescription, over-the-counter drugs; social drugs (alcohol, caffeine, nicotine, and tobacco); illegal or illicit drugs; and environmental drugs, such as toxins in the air and workplace.

PHARMACOLOGY AND NURSING MANAGEMENT

A thorough understanding of pharmacology is only one part of a nurse's role relative to drug therapy. Today, nurses face increased responsibility and involvement with every aspect of drug therapy, primarily because of public concern about drug effects as well as current trends in health care.

Nurses often have the most contact with patients and their families; they often coordinate the patient care activities of the other health care team members, and they assume a major role in educating the patient and family about drug use and drug combinations relative to potential interactions. Having a thorough and up-to-date core drug knowledge and developing a firm grasp of core patient variables are key responsibilities of the nurse administering drug therapy. Accurate and appropriate nursing assessment and planning based on nursing diagnosis, anticipated outcomes, intervention, and evaluation techniques are necessary to administer drug therapy safely. Additionally, nurses are increasingly more responsible for administering complex drugs by newer and potentially more dangerous routes.

Administration of drugs is only one aspect of pharmacology. Other elements focus on ethics and the law. Nurses have an ethical and legal obligation to assist patients in achieving optimal health by providing instruction, sharing information with them and their families, and involving them in health care decisions and activities. To do all of this successfully, the nurse must possess a thorough knowledge of pharmacology and related areas, such as pathophysiology, nutrition, and psychology.

SCOPE OF PHARMACOLOGY

Pharmacology includes the study of drugs in terms of their medicinal purposes, chemicals with toxic characteristics, and chemicals used for mind-altering (psychotropic) or social purposes. The scope of pharmacology includes pharmacotherapeutics, pharmacokinetics, pharmacodynamics, as well as adverse effects, toxicities, and interactions. A currently evolving branch of pharmacology, known as clinical pharmacology, studies the potential uses of a drug for human beings. Clinical pharmacology research is directed at discovering new uses for known and established drugs and identifying possibilities for new chemicals.

PHARMACOTHERAPEUTICS

Pharmacotherapeutics is the use of medicinal agents (drug therapy) for preventing, managing, and curing illness and disease. During the 20th century, pharmacotherapeutics expanded to include pharmacologic agents used in diagnosing disease (e.g., radioisotopes). The 20th century also saw the evolution of comparative pharmacology (the study of the effects of drugs on various animals and humans). Comparative pharmacology studies how the human response to a drug is different from an animal response. Beginning in the 20th century in the United States, all new drugs were tested extensively on animals before testing and use in humans.

PHARMACOKINETICS

Pharmacokinetics refers to the absorption, distribution, metabolism, and excretion of a drug in a living organism (Fig. 2-1). Pharmacokinetics is the fate of a drug as it moves through the body and how the body influences drug concentrations. Once considered a feature of pharmacodynamics, scientists now recognize it as a separate function. Pharmacokinetics focuses on the rates at which drugs are absorbed and on factors that affect absorption. It also considers the elements of distribution, storage, metabolism (also referred to as breakdown or biotransformation), and excretion.

PHARMACODYNAMICS

It is critical for nurses to understand the mechanisms of drug action. When the study of pharmacodynamics was first developed in the late 19th century, it focused on the physical effects of drugs and the mechanisms of drug actions in living

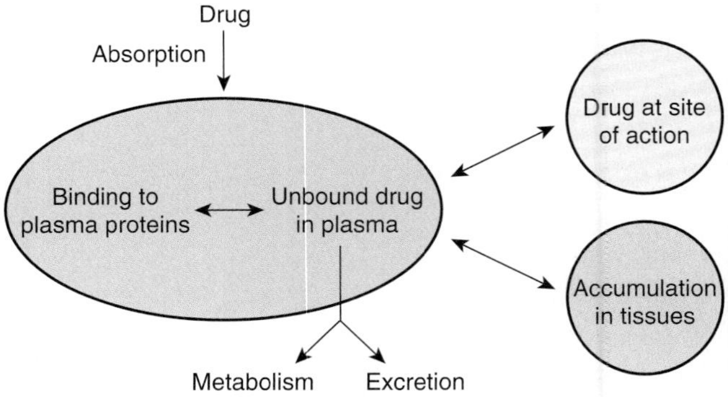

Figure 2-1. Absorption, distribution, metabolism, and excretion characteristics of a drug. (Reproduced with permission from Gossel, T. A. [May, 1999]. Pharmacology: A profile on pharmacokinetics. *U.S. Pharmacist.*)

organisms. Today, pharmacodynamics includes the study of biochemical and physiologic actions of drugs and the changes that drugs undergo from absorption to excretion. By studying the interrelationships between the physical and chemical properties of drugs and the living cells and tissues responding to them, researchers have developed synthetic drugs, learned how to alter chemical structures of existing drugs and their action(s) to enhance therapeutic effects and reduce adverse reactions, and are able to predict pharmacologic and toxicologic potential.

PHARMACOGENETICS

Pharmacogenetics is the study of genetically inherited conditions that 1) affect the way drugs act on the body and 2) modify the way the body acts on drugs. Pharmacogenetic responses differ from adverse or toxic effects of drugs; they result in unanticipated drug response because of differences in drug action based on heredity. These genetic differences modify the manner in which an organism metabolizes the drug. Consequently, pharmacogenetic factors may produce either a diminished or an enhanced response to a drug.

ADVERSE EFFECTS AND TOXICITY

Some of the most common problems of therapeutic drug use are adverse effects, such as toxicity (i.e., poisonous level of a drug in the body). Another branch of pharmacology—toxicology—focuses on the study of poisons.

HISTORICAL PERSPECTIVES OF DRUG DEVELOPMENT

Throughout history, humankind has been interested in the treatment and prevention of disease. Early civilizations viewed disease with great superstition, and treatments were often directed toward driving away evil spirits and invoking religious and mystical powers. Pharmacologic knowledge up to the 19th century was derived empirically (from observation and practical experience). During the 19th century, however, pharmacology evolved into a highly specialized science, and the branch of pharmaceutical chemistry developed. The ability to isolate active components of drugs for study under controlled conditions facilitated the scientific method of inquiry; medicine based on reason and theory began to replace empirical medicine.

The emerging sciences of botany and physiology, quantitative chemistry, and systematic biology enabled modern pharmacology to emerge. Pharmacologists could study the action of pure drugs in the body and discover new active drugs in the plant world. Today, researchers examine rain forests and jungles for new natural drugs to treat diseases. Scientists of the 21st century expect to develop new drugs through chemical synthesis, manipulation of enzymes and hormones, and genetic engineering, making pharmacology a complex science with a vast drug-manufacturing component. Highlights of advancements in pharmacology during the 20th century include computer technology, which facilitates rational drug design and replaces some animal studies. Biotechnology permits targeting specific drug action and expands drug development procedures. Receptor isolation expands the potential for developing drugs with greater selectivity and reduced toxicity. New drug classes result in novel means to treat and manage disease. Cell culture techniques permit the study of drug action at cellular and molecular levels. Immunochemistry leads to diagnosis that is more accurate and treatment of formerly untreatable diseases. Gene therapy treats a number of currently untreatable diseases. (For more information see the accompanying display, Pharmacology Across the Ages.)

Pharmacology Across the Ages

- **Prehistory** (before written language). Archeological findings (some before 4000 B.C.) suggest tribal beliefs that evil spirits caused illness. Magical spells and potions of elemental substances (plants, animals, waters) used by tribal healers exorcised the evil spirits.
- **2700 B.C., China.** First pharmacology "textbook" documents medicinal use of natural substances (e.g., laxative properties of rhubarb and senna).
- **2100 B.C., Sumeria (Iraq).** Earliest prescriptions of medicinal mixtures are recorded.
- **2000 B.C., Babylon; North and South America.** Hammurabi's Code of Law provides protection from unskilled physicians (medical malpractice) and rewards for successful treatment of illness.
  - North American Iroquois Indians use herbs to stimulate taste.
  - South American Peruvian Incas use herbs as diuretics and respiratory stimulants.
- **1500 B.C., Egypt, Israel.** Early Egyptian scrolls record observations, diagnoses, remedies (e.g., aloe, castor oil, honey, opium, peppermint, vinegar), and medical data describing drug forms (gargles, poultices, powders); this is the beginning of polypharmacy.
  - Hebrew teacher-physicians use wine, fig poultices, and vinegar for medicine; Talmud records health practices and taboos.
  - The Mosaic Health Code records hygienic and sanitary practices.
- **400 B.C., Greece.** Writings of Hippocrates (father of medicine) identify more than 400 drugs and treatment methods (diet, exercise, lifestyle).
- **200 B.C., India.** Hindu priests record using colchicum, gentian, castor beans, and digitalis for medicinal purposes.
- **100 A.D., Greece.** Dioscorides writes *De Materia Medica,* a medical textbook, discussing drugs and their uses.
- **200 A.D., Greece.** Galen advocates medicinal use of vegetable preparations.
- **500–1500 A.D., Arab settlements; monastic gardeners of Europe.** Compendium of drugs (e.g., borax, ergot, cinnabar) and drug uses develops as Arabs practice pharmacy separately from medicine. The compilation systematizes the preparation of medicinal compounds and serves as the first set of drug standards.
  - Herbs such as clover, primrose, and belladonna were cultivated for medicinal purposes, although folk remedies and superstition still dominated pharmacology in Europe.

(continued)

Pharmacology Across the Ages (Continued)

- **1500–1700 A.D., Europe and the Americas.** Interest in pharmacology and chemistry is renewed during the Renaissance. Spices are studied for medicinal properties.
  - In the Americas, Aztec and other Native American cultures record use of herbs and plants (e.g., balsam, chili, sarsaparilla, tobacco, cihuapatli [an oxytocic], and peyote [a hallucinogen]).
- **1700 A.D.–present, scientists worldwide.** Pharmacologic advances (e.g., antibiotics, enzymes, hormones, vaccines) are spurred by technology.

Historically, drug development has long followed an almost exclusive male model—an exception being a therapeutic need distinctive to women—and extrapolated results of research on male subjects to women. Thus, drugs were prescribed for women despite their never having been evaluated in women. A 1993 U.S. Food and Drug Administration (FDA) guideline called for both sexes to be included in drug development and evaluation. It emphasized checking for pharmacokinetic differences between men and women, between pre- and postmenopausal women, and in different phases of the menstrual cycle. Attention was directed to evaluating potential drug-drug interactions, especially those involving contraceptive steroids, with a possible reduction or loss of their effectiveness.

SOURCES OF DRUGS

Plants, animals, synthetic chemicals, and genetically engineered chemicals are four sources of current drug products.

PLANTS

Drug sources from the plant world date to primitive times. Common drugs from plants include digitalis (purple foxglove), morphine (opium poppy), and vincristine (periwinkle). Drugs that come from plants are classified according to their physical and chemical properties:

- Alkaloids (alkaline substances) react with body acids to form a salt, which is readily soluble in body fluids.
- Glycosides contain a carbohydrate or sugar molecule.
- Gums are mucilaginous secretions—usually polysaccharides—with the ability to attract and hold water.
- Oils are water insoluble and are classified as volatile or fixed. Volatile oils, which are derived strictly from plants, evaporate when exposed to air. Fixed oils, also known as fatty oils, are derived from both animals and plants; their consistency varies with temperature.
- Resins are water insoluble, solid or semisolid organic substances of vegetable origin and are commonly used as laxative or caustic agents.

ANIMALS

Traditionally, drugs from animal sources include agents such as insulin, pituitary hormones, some vitamins, antibiotics, and biologic agents (e.g., vaccines, immune serums). Today, genetically engineered hormones (e.g., insulin, pituitary hormone, erythropoietin) are rapidly replacing animal-based drugs. The advantage of genetically engineered drugs is their purity. Because no foreign proteins are involved, they do not induce antibody production.

SYNTHETIC AGENTS

Most drugs used today are either partially or wholly synthetic chemical compounds that have been produced in a laboratory. A partially synthetic agent contains a derivative of a natural substance combined with a pure chemical. An example is penicillin V, known as Pen-Vee K. The penicillin molecule, which is unstable in gastric acid, is modified so that it can be given orally.

An advantage of synthetic drugs is that they are pure chemicals and, unlike drugs from a natural source, are unaffected by pharmacodynamic changes—namely, deterioration in potency and stability. Another advantage of synthetic agents is their economy; they are usually less expensive to produce. Pharmacologic chemistry has become so sophisticated that a minor alteration in a known chemical drug structure can create a completely new drug—ideally, a drug with greater therapeutic effects and fewer adverse effects. The computer age allows pharmaceutical companies to design new agents by compiling existing information about established drugs and then manipulating the chemical formulas of these drugs electronically. Obviously, this technique will facilitate research and development of new pharmaceutical agents.

DRUG NOMENCLATURE

All drugs are known by at least three names: a **chemical name,** a **generic name** (sometimes called the official name), and a **trade name** (Fig. 2-2).

The chemical name of a drug precisely describes the drug's atomic and molecular structure using exact chemical nomenclature (language) and terminology. The chemical name, which is usually long and complex, is not practical for everyday use but is useful to chemists and biochemists.

The generic name of a drug is also known as its nonproprietary name. Each drug has only one generic name, which identifies the drug's active ingredient. As a general rule, generic names are less complicated than the chemical names from which they are derived, but they are more complicated than trade names, which may be easier to remember. Generic names are easily recognizable because the first letter of the name is typically not capitalized.

The United States Adopted Name Council assigns an official name to each drug as mandated by the United States government in 1962. These names are published in the **United States Pharmacopeia** and the **National Formulary.** The official name for a drug is most often its generic name.

The trade name, also known as brand or proprietary name, is given to a drug by the drug manufacturer. Trade names, which are usually easy to say and remember, are protected by trademark. The symbol ™ or ® after the trade name indicates that the drug molecule and name are registered by

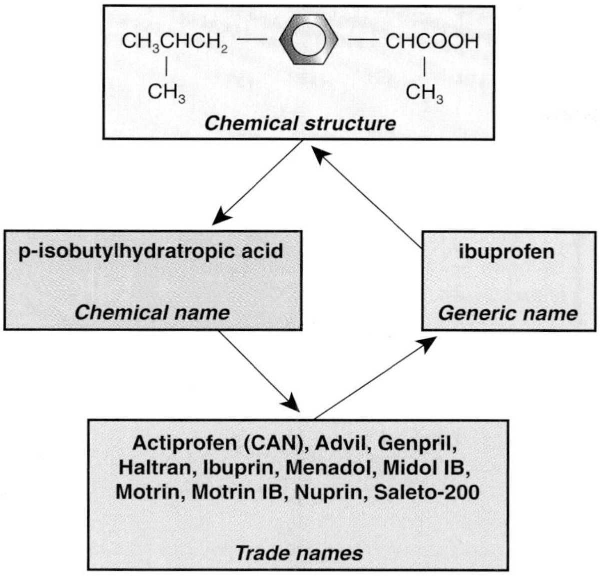

Figure 2-2. A drug called by another name may still be the same drug. Nomenclature is a core feature of pharmacology. The four configurations illustrate various names for the same drug.

the drug manufacturer, and the use of the drug and its name are restricted to the drug's manufacturer. The manufacturer receives a 17-year patent on the drug, which provides an opportunity to recover part of the costs used in research, development, and testing of the drug. The trade name is easily recognizable because the first letter is capitalized and the ™ or ® symbol may be present. Unless governed by patent protection, any drug can be marketed in different formulations and by multiple drug companies. Consequently, the number of trade names a drug has can be extensive.

IMPLICATIONS FOR NURSES

Name recognition is important in drug therapy. The nurse has the responsibility of accurately transcribing drug orders, administering the drugs correctly, and documenting the patient's response. Usually a drug is ordered by the generic or the brand name, and numerous brand names may exist for the same drug. Health care practitioners and prescribers typically order drugs by generic names to avoid confusion between brand names that look and sound alike.

To prevent an error when administering any drug, the nurse should check the drug name at least three times—before, during, and after selecting the drug. If the names used for the order and those on the drug label are different (e.g., trade name and generic equivalent), the nurse must verify that the two names constitute the same drug before administering the drug.

As a rule, generic formulations and trade name formulations are therapeutically equivalent. The House of Representatives legislation (H.R. 1685) "Generic Drug Access Act of 2001" requires therapeutic equivalence for generic drugs. A distinct advantage of generic drugs is their lower cost to the patient.

DRUG CLASSIFICATIONS (FAMILIES)

Drugs that share similar characteristics are grouped together as a pharmacologic group or family. Because thousands of drugs are available today, studying them as individual agents would be an overwhelming task. Fortunately, drugs can be systematically classified into a reasonable number of drug groups known as a **drug classification** (or drug class).

DESCRIPTIVE CATEGORIES

There are several ways to classify drugs that share similar characteristics, namely, by chemical composition, physiologic effect (on body systems), and therapeutic uses or actions (clinical indications). For example, the **chemical classification** of a drug such as morphine sulfate describes its chemical base of opium. Morphine sulfate, therefore, is classified as an opiate or opioid. The **physiologic classification** of morphine sulfate describes its effects on body systems; therefore, morphine sulfate is classified as a central nervous system depressant. The **therapeutic classification** of morphine sulfate describes the drug by its use in therapy; therefore, morphine sulfate is also known as an opioid narcotic analgesic. It should be readily apparent that any one drug may belong to more than one drug class (family) depending on the classification system being used.

Information about a drug prototype covers core drug knowledge representative of the drug class. Data include the prototype's pharmacotherapeutics, pharmacokinetics, pharmacodynamics, contraindications and precautions for use, major adverse effects and other side effects, and significant drug interactions, such as those occurring between the drug and other drugs or foods and those affecting laboratory test results.

However, even though a particular drug may be described as the prototype, there may be a new drug in that class that is clinically superior. As an example, digitalis is the prototype in the cardiac glycoside class (classification based on chemical characteristics); however, a newer drug, digoxin, is more clinically significant. Also, drug characteristics and administration concerns assigned to the prototype are general. They may or may not always apply to the other drugs in the class.

SOURCES OF DRUG INFORMATION

Because pharmacology is a dynamic science, new drugs are continually being developed, and new uses for existing drugs are frequently discovered. Nurses need reliable and up-to-date drug reference information. Awareness of reliable available resources and the specific type of information provided in those resources enables the nurse to be efficiently and completely informed about safe drug administration and new therapeutic developments. Many drug-oriented publications help fill the need of nurses, health care providers, pharmacists, and others for current and detailed drug information. To be fully informed, the nurse in a clinical situation may have to consult several references (Table 2-1).

TABLE 2-1 Sources of Drug Information

Resource	Features	Evaluation and Commentary
Official Pharmacopeiae		
The United States Pharmacopeia (USP) and National Formulary (NF)	Drugs listed by official name Primary focus on sources, chemistry, physical properties of drugs; tests for identity, purity, and assay (measurement); and official storage requirements	• Federal Pure Food and Drug Act (1906) adopted USP and NF as official pharmacopeiae • Published every 5 y with periodic supplements • Formerly listed drugs deleted and replaced by newer or better drugs, or drug listing removed after high incidence of toxicity reported • More useful as a drug reference to the pharmaceutical industry than to the nursing profession
The British Pharmacopeia (BP)	Similar to USP and NF	• Adopted by Parliament (1968 Medical Act) for use in the United Kingdom • Published every 5 y
The International Pharmacopeia (2nd ed.)	Latin drug nomenclature	• Published by the United Nations • Used to encourage worldwide pharmacopeiae development and drug standardization • Official status conferred when adopted by individual nations • Published in English, French, and Spanish
Unofficial Compendia		
American Hospital Formulary Service (AHFS) Drug Information '97, '98, '99, etc.	Includes extensive drug information, particularly on drug classes Presents objective overviews of individual preparations of drugs available in the United States	• Published annually and updated with periodic supplements • Highly regarded drug reference
The British National Formulary (BNF)	Provides detailed descriptions of currently used preparations in medical practice	• Published by the British Medical Association and the Pharmaceutical Society of Great Britain
Facts and Comparisons	Provides concise but thorough monographs organized by drug class Begins each class section with a therapeutic overview followed by additional sections organized by chemical classifications Offers comparisons of drugs (including over-the-counter [OTC] products)	• Updated monthly with supplemental entries • Available in print or CD-ROM • Generally more usable than the Physicians Desk Reference (PDR) • Published by Facts and Comparisons, St. Louis, MO
Food and Drug Administration (FDA) Drug Bulletin	Offers recent FDA reviews of various drugs (usually common ones) and new clinical findings	• Free, quarterly newsletter • Includes a MedWatch form for reporting unusual clinical experiences with drugs to the FDA
USP Dispensing Information (USPDI)	Covers drug categories, prescribing precautions and considerations, side effects, drug actions, and impact on lifestyle, dosage forms, and labeling data	• Written in nontechnical language • A major advantage, the presentation of side effect potential (rare to common) • Clearly identifies side effects to be reported to the health care provider • Highly valuable reference for nurses • Published annually and updated bimonthly
American Medical Association Drug Evaluations	Presents information about specific drugs, including those that are being used for valid, though unlabeled, clinical applications	• Compiled by the American Medical Association's Department of Drugs • Published by W. B. Saunders, Philadelphia, PA

(*continued*)

TABLE 2-1 Sources of Drug Information (Continued)

Resource	Features	Evaluation and Commentary
Pharmaceutical Package Inserts	Constitutes a concise compilation of specific drug information relative to clinical indications, safe dosage ranges, and unranked secondary (side) effects	• Manufacturer's leaflet enclosed with a drug product as it leaves the pharmaceutical distributor • Of limited value to the nursing process
Physician's Desk Reference (PDR)	Provides concise monograph of drug information similar to the manufacturer's package inserts	• Commonly consulted in clinical settings • Written by pharmaceutical company that manufactures the drug
PDR for Nonprescription Drugs	Besides concise monograph of OTC drug information, includes photographs of the drugs and a section on self-care of minor health problems	• Format similar to the PDR • First published in 1980 in response to the rapid growth and availability of OTC drugs and the general public's increasing health awareness and interest in managing self-care
Drug Interactions and Updates Quarterly	Presents drug interactions grouped together by drug class Rates drug-drug interactions according to clinical significance (e.g., minor, moderate, major)	• Fills needs emanating from constantly changing and increasing knowledge and experience with established and newly developed drugs • Covers changes in drug treatments and therapeutic regimens
Electronic Databases		
FDA web page, Medline, PharmInfoNet Web Page, Toxline, and others	Current drug-related information	• Available through the National Library of Medicine's on-line services
Cumulative Index to Nursing and Allied Health Literature (CINAHL)	Represents publications of major health care journals Abstracts available for many articles listed	• Available through private on-line services (e.g., Compuserve) • Libraries and schools have access through CD-ROM disks • Access through personal computers
Journals (selected)		
Journal of the American Pharmaceutical Association	Monthly publication that identifies newly approved or marketed drugs and new FDA-approved indications for existing drugs	• More current than PDR
American Journal of Nursing	General and specific drug information in a nursing frame of reference and with a nursing perspective	• Usually includes a section on new drugs • Information on drugs (new or old) and their clinical considerations provided in intermittent articles
Textbooks (selected)		
Goodman and Gilman's The Pharmacological Basis of Therapeutics	Complete and thorough Recognized leader of pharmacology textbooks	• Excellent, thorough reference text • Considered to be an authoritative source for those learning or working with pharmacology • Does not address nursing-related pharmacotherapeutic issues

SAFEGUARDS IN DRUG DEVELOPMENT AND DELIVERY

Most nurses administer drug therapy as part of their daily routine, and advanced practice nurses (e.g., nurse practitioners) may prescribe and dispense medications as well. Every state has its own nurse practice act that fully describes nursing activities involving drug therapy. Practicing nurses should be familiar with the nurse practice act in their state because these acts define nurses' roles and responsibilities. Similarly, familiarity with governmental safeguards that promote drug safety, reliability, and uniformity help nurses administer drug therapy safely and appropriately. These regulations help to ensure that commercially available drugs are safe and effective.

New drugs are being developed at an unprecedented rate. Any new drug that comes to market undergoes years of testing to determine the drug' pharmacologic properties and its potential for toxicity.

STANDARDS FOR DRUG PURITY AND CONTENT

Since 1820, the United States Pharmacopeia (U.S.P.) has been the source for standards of strength, quality, purity, and preparation of medicinal compounds. In 1888, the American Pharmaceutical Association began publishing another resource, the National Formulary (NF), which expanded this effort to set national standards for drug quality. Before that time, there was little need for standard resources because of the scarcity of effective drugs. In 1906, the Pure Food and Drug Act was passed, and these compendiums became the official drug standards in the United States. Passage of the pure food, drug, and cosmetic acts protected the public from adulterated or mislabeled drugs and empowered the federal government to enforce these standards. In addition, the legislation required drug manufacturers to follow these standards to ensure that drugs were uniform, pure, and reliable. Later, amendments (1941–1945) to the 1906 Pure Food and Drug Act required that biologic products used as drugs (e.g., insulin, antibiotics) be certified on a batch-by-batch basis by a government agency.

The U.S.P. is the current authoritative source for drug standards and is revised every 5 years by a group of experts in chemistry, microbiology, nursing, pharmaceutics, and pharmacology. Drugs are deleted when their clinical use shows unacceptably high toxicity or when newer, more effective agents are developed. Originally, the U.S.P. restricted its data to single drugs, and the NF was a reference for mixtures and formulas. Gradually, both reference books were expanded to include single- and multiple-drug mixtures, and the two books have since been combined; the reference is now called the *United States Pharmacopeia-National Formulary.*

LEGISLATION FOR DRUG SAFETY AND EFFICACY

Federal legislation protects the public from drugs that are impure, toxic, ineffective, or not tested prior to marketing. The primary purpose of federal legislation is to ensure safety.

Pure Food and Drug Acts

The history of drug regulation reflects several medical and public health events. The **Pure Food and Drug Act of 1906** became law mostly because of revelations of unsanitary and unethical practices in the meatpacking industry and because of the many potent and dangerous drugs on the market. Although these products contained opioids (e.g., opium, morphine, or heroin), no law required the manufacturer to list the ingredients on the product label.

In addition, the Pure Food and Drug Act designated the U.S.P. and NF as the official standards and empowered the federal government to enforce those standards. The **Federal Food, Drug, and Cosmetics Act of 1938** (FFDCA) was enacted largely in response to a considerable number of deaths (more than 100) caused by the marketing of a drug called elixir of sulfanilamide, which was combined with the solvent diethylene glycol (investigations revealed this to be a nephrotoxic compound) and not adequately tested for safety before marketing. The FFDCA also established the FDA as the agency for monitoring and controlling drug manufacture and marketing.

An important area of focus of the 1938 FFDCA was the drug label. The act stipulated that the drug label must contain the following:

- No false or misleading statements
- The suggested dose and frequency of use
- The name and business address of the manufacturer/packer or distributor
- The amount of all dependency-producing drugs in a product and the statement, "Warning: May Be Habit Forming"
- The kind, quantity, and percentage of certain specified ingredients that could be harmful (e.g., drugs containing alcohol, atropine, digitalis)
- Complete, understandable directions for safe use and warnings against unsafe use by children, pregnant women, and people with contraindicating pathologic conditions

In addition, the law allowed the FDA to prohibit the marketing of any drug judged to be incompletely tested or dangerous.

In the early 1960s, a drug-related tragedy altered drug testing methods and expanded the scope of drug-regulating legislation. Based on results of animal testing, thalidomide, a sedative drug, was marketed across Europe as a nontoxic hypnotic. Hundreds of pregnant women who took the drug gave birth to infants with phocomelia, a condition characterized by severely shortened, deformed, or missing limbs. Thalidomide was not a widespread problem in the United States because the drug had been withheld by the FDA. However, babies with thalidomide-associated deformities were born in the United States, particularly to women who traveled outside the country and obtained and used the drug. Today, the Public Health Service (PHS) is responsible for maintaining basic research programs through the National Institutes of Health. Biologicals used as drugs are also certified by the PHS.

Kefauver-Harris Amendment

The thalidomide tragedy was one of the events that led to requirements of more extensive testing of new drugs for teratogenic effects, stipulations that manufacturers prove both drug safety and efficacy, and passage of the 1962 Kefauver-Harris Amendment to the 1938 FFDCA. This amendment authorized the FDA to establish official names for drugs, and in the early 1960s, the **United States Adopted Names Council** was established to ensure uniform drug nomenclature.

The Kefauver-Harris Amendment also tightened controls on drug safety, especially experimental drugs, stating that adverse reactions and contraindications must be cited and included in the literature. Additionally, the amendment ordered evaluation of the testing methods used by manufacturers, specified the process for withdrawal of approved drugs when safety and effectiveness were in doubt, and mandated the establishment of the clinical efficacy of new drugs before marketing. The law applied to both new and existing drugs. Furthermore, all drugs marketed between 1938 and 1962 were required to be tested for effectiveness to remain on the market.

CLINICAL TRIALS

The first step in the development of a new drug is in the discovery or synthesis of a potential new drug molecule. Years of research and millions of dollars go into the development of a new drug. When searching for new agents, a variety of methods may be used to identify potentially useful compounds. For example, manufacturers may start with known, active compounds and modify their chemical structure to alter pharmacokinetic or pharmacodynamic actions. It is expected that burgeoning technology and scientific advances will significantly increase the success of drug development by using robotics and improved scientific methods. As a result, pharmaceutical companies will be able to find much better compounds by being more selective, including screening out toxic compounds, and decrease the average of time testing investigational drugs and getting them to market. Currently, only about 10% of new drugs that begin **clinical trials** now prove safe and effective enough to win regulatory approval.

Preclinical Testing

Once a new drug is developed, pharmaceutical manufacturers must establish the drug's pharmacologic activity, safety, and toxicity profiles before it can be tested in humans. Some of these tests investigate the potential for the drug to cause cancer or birth defects. Long-term administration of the drug to animal subjects is usually needed to produce reliable results. Other tests determine the amount of the drug needed to produce either clinical or toxic actions. The most useful drugs usually show a large differential (margin of safety) between these dosages. The results of the animal studies are the basis for studying the drug in humans. Preclinical trials are designed to provide basic safety, bioavailability, pharmacokinetic, and initial efficacy data.

Phases of a Clinical Trial

After preclinical testing concludes, the drug manufacturer submits the safety and effectiveness data from animal studies to the FDA in what is known as an investigational new drug (IND) application. The IND includes the following:

- All known information regarding the biologic, chemical, pharmacologic, and toxicologic properties of the new agent
- Precise details of how the drug is manufactured and storage requirements to preserve its stability
- Name and qualifications of each investigator who will participate in the clinical trial
- A signed affidavit by each investigator attesting that the study will be adequately supervised and that study volunteers have given informed consent
- Study protocols (guidelines) that clearly define how the drug is to be administered to study subjects (e.g., dose, route, duration) and what specific observations will be made during the clinical trial

If approved, the IND undergoes a clinical trial in humans. Clinical trials occur in four phases (I–IV) and may require from 5 to 9 years for completion (Fig. 2-3). Phases I through III take place before a new drug is marketed. Phase IV testing is completed after marketing begins. Recently, the FDA has changed its policy to include women in early clinical trials (phases I and II), to determine whether gender differences and female physiology (e.g., menstrual cycle, menopause) influence pharmacotherapeutics, pharmacodynamics, and pharmacokinetics.

Phase I

Healthy human volunteers are given the drug, after which blood, urine, and other appropriate samples are taken to monitor drug metabolism. All pharmacologic and biologic effects of the drug are carefully noted. This information is useful in determining the potential of future testing. If the drug is expected to have significant toxicity, as is usually the case in cancer and acquired immunodeficiency syndrome (AIDS) therapy, volunteers with the disease are used in phase I testing rather than healthy volunteers (Katzung, 1998).

Phase II

Assuming no adverse effects are identified in the phase I trial, small numbers of people (10–200) with the disease the drug is intended to treat are given various dosages of the test compound and studied in great detail. Dose response, toxicity, and pharmacotherapeutic effectiveness are carefully monitored and dosage guidelines are usually determined in this phase. Results from the long-term animal studies are reviewed and compared with the human results—especially concerning the effects, if any, on fertility and reproduction.

Phase III

Assuming no serious problems are uncovered in phase II, phase III trials involve testing the drug on a larger scale. Most of the risks associated with the new drug therapy are identified at this time. These widespread tests are also intended to uncover some less frequent or even rare adverse effects that sometimes affect only a small portion of the population. Double-blind studies (studies in which neither the patient nor the researcher knows whether the drug or a placebo was given) and crossover design studies (studies comparing the study drug with an existing drug) are frequently used during this phase. Nurses are generally most involved in this phase of clinical trials and may be responsible for administering investigational drugs to patients.

Individual personal responses to an investigational drug may vary considerably (see the accompanying display, Candidate for a New Drug). Some patients taking an investigational drug may believe that it is better than existing forms of therapy because it is new. These patients may have unrealistic expectations regarding the drug's usefulness or actions. Others may be more reluctant to participate in the study because they feel like "guinea pigs." Most patients, however, tend to respond in a positive way to any therapeutic intervention by interested and caring health care personnel. This positive result is called the **placebo response** and may involve objective, physiologic, and biochemical changes and changes in subjective complaints (e.g., stomach upset, insomnia, sedation) associated with the disorder being treated.

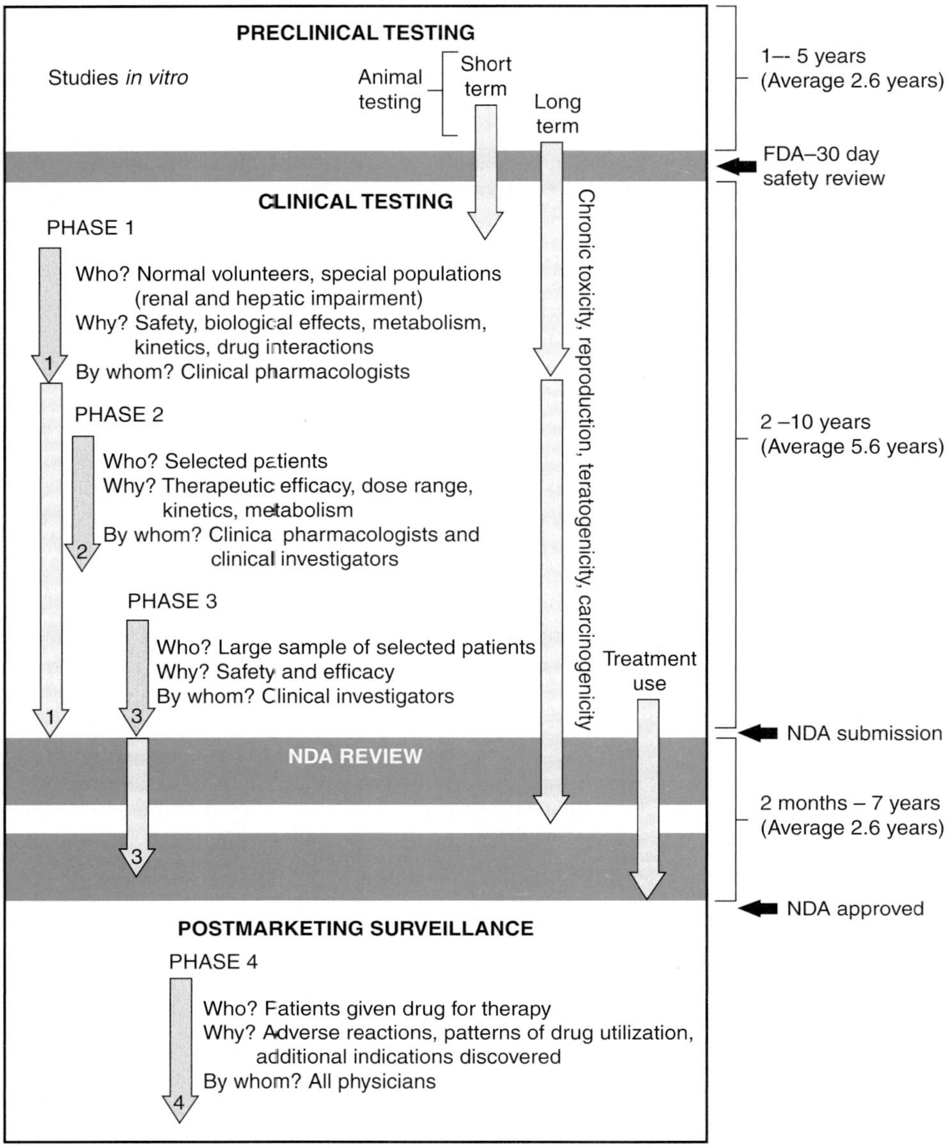

Figure 2-3. Phases of drug development in the United States. (Reproduced with permission from Hardman, J. G., et al. [1996]. *Goodman and Gilman's The Pharmacological Basis of Therapeutics* [9th ed.]. New York: McGraw-Hill.) FDA, Food and Drug Administration; NDA, New Drug Application.

The placebo response occurs relatively consistently in 20 to 40% of patients in almost all studies.

Patients must be fully informed about the potential risks and benefits associated with the intended study. One of the nurse's roles is to assist patients with their feelings regarding the clinical trial because these feelings may affect the quality and integrity of the investigation.

If the drug proves safe and effective through the first three phases of the clinical trial, the manufacturer may then apply for a new drug application (NDA). Again, all preclinical and clinical data are reviewed by the FDA. Approval of the NDA means that the drug may be marketed. The FDA now requires analysis by gender in almost all new applications for new drugs. Because the distribution patterns of fat differ in men and women, many dosing schedules have been found to be excessive, and even harmful, in women.

Critical Thinking Scenario

Candidate for a new drug

Steve Smith has been diagnosed as having AIDS. He is being considered for treatment with a new drug during phase III clinical trials. Steve expresses concern about taking a new drug, especially in view of his declining health status and what he has heard about a shortened clinical evaluation process for AIDS drugs; he asks you, "What does the term 'new drug' mean?" What is your response?

Phase IV

Postmarketing surveillance of the drug enables the FDA to monitor the drug while it is in widespread distribution. The pharmaceutical company that markets the drug keeps careful records on the results of therapy and must advise the FDA of any adverse effects and other effects on therapy. Occasionally, reports of toxicity occur with enough frequency that precautions for use are expanded and emphasized (e.g., aplastic anemia with felbamate [Felbatol]) or a drug may be removed from the market (e.g., terfenadine [Seldane]) because of serious side effects.

Another area of considerable interest in this phase is the effect of the drug on elderly patients and children because, heretofore, these groups have usually been excluded from early clinical trials. Once a drug goes on the market, the FDA continues to monitor it for safety. If safety problems appear, the agency limits the uses the drug is approved for or pulls the drug from the market.

The Approval Process

The Prescription Drug User Free Act is legislation that Congress passed in 1992. Under pressure from both the pharmaceutical industry and AIDS activists, this Act was passed, which allows the FDA to charge drug manufacturers for the FDA drug approval process. This influx of money allowed the FDA to hire additional reviewers, which reduced approval times from an average of 3 years to an average of 12 months. Five drugs—an unprecedented number—were taken off the market between September 1997 and September 1998. A sixth drug—troglitazone (Rezulin)—was removed in March 2000. Prior to that, the most recent drug withdrawal was in 1992 and withdrawals were rare overall. The FDA maintains that the change in approval times did not represent a lowering of its standards and reviewed the 1997 to 1998 withdrawals for any correlation between the withdrawals and the decreased approval time. Friedman et al. concluded that "there was no obvious thread linking these five drug withdrawals to any fundamental problem with the FDA review process itself, including increased review speeds."

Approving a drug for therapeutic use involves a long, complex, and expensive process. On average, it takes 12 years for a new drug to be approved. The preclinical, clinical, and FDA review processes may be accelerated when an urgent need is perceived (e.g., AIDS, cancer therapy). In recent years, certain laws and protocols have been initiated to speed the drug approval process. For example, the Drug Regulation and Reform Act of 1978 allows a shorter period of time for new drug investigative efforts, thus speeding the ability to get new drugs to the public (see the accompanying display, Streamlining the Drug Approval Process).

Some drugs that may be useful for treating rare diseases never reach the market because manufacturers cannot hope to recover the huge amounts of money spent on drug research and development. These drugs are called orphan drugs. The 1983 Orphan Drug Act offers substantial tax credits to pharmaceutical companies to develop drugs that have a limited market or that treat rare diseases or conditions.

Streamlining the Drug Approval Process

Because of the high cost of research and development, many new and promising drugs never become available for consumers, primarily because of money: Manufacturers project that not enough revenue will be generated by drug sales to cover the cost of drug development.

Orphan Drugs

This is particularly true of drugs that have limited use, such as those used to treat rare or unusual diseases. These drugs are known as "orphans" because no pharmaceutical manufacturer is willing to assume the risk and expense of commercial development.

To meet the need of an individual who may benefit from an esoteric drug, the Orphan Drug Act of 1983 was enacted. The act provides certain tax benefits to companies that invest in drugs useful in the diagnosis, treatment, or prevention of rare diseases. Other legislation defined these rare diseases as those affecting fewer than 1 of every 200,000 people in the United States or diseases that may affect more than 1 of every 200,000 people but with no reasonable expectation that the company will recover development costs from sales within the United States.

Compassionate Use

Another recent development that helps to streamline the drug approval process is the compassionate use protocol, whereby certain drugs are made available to patients without complete Food and Drug Administration (FDA) approval. Since 1988, these protocols have enabled patients with life-threatening diseases to obtain investigational drugs without requiring them to enroll in a full clinical trial.

Expedited Process

All investigational new drugs (INDs) undergo the four phases of clinical evaluation; treatment INDs shorten this process, however. For example, acquired immunodeficiency syndrome (AIDS) poses a public health threat. Drug companies with AIDS drugs in phase II or III clinical trials may apply for FDA approval to use the drugs in patients who meet appropriate criteria.

ADDITIONAL SAFEGUARDS

In recent years, the FDA and the U.S.P. have begun several programs to ensure adequate postmarketing surveillance of drugs. These programs rely heavily on health care practitioners, including nurses, pharmacists, and physicians, to report problems or suspected problems with drug products to the FDA or U.S.P.

MedWatch

The MedWatch program, sponsored by the FDA, encourages voluntary reporting from health professionals and consumers about adverse effects from drug products or medical devices directly to the FDA by mail, electronic mail (www.fda.gov/medwatch), or fax. MedWatch's goals are to increase awareness of serious reactions caused by drugs or medical devices, to facilitate the reporting of adverse reactions, and to provide the health community with regular feedback about product safety issues. An FDA task force report recommends the FDA, health care practitioners, the pharmaceutical industry, and consumers work together to deal with the growing issues involving the actions and interactions of drugs that are used by the American public.

Suspicion that a medical product may be related to a serious event is sufficient cause for a health professional to submit a MedWatch report. About 6% of reports of suspected drug-related adverse events to the FDA's Center for Drug Evaluation and Research came through the MedWatch program (1998 data; 232,470 total reports). Years after marketing, an evolving safety profile and new information about a drug or device may affect its clinical use (Fig. 2-4).

Practitioners Reporting Network

The **Practitioners Reporting Network** sponsored by the U.S.P. involves four coordinated reporting programs:

- The U.S.P. Drug Product Problem Reporting Program specifically targets drug packaging and is dedicated to reporting problems with unclear labeling, defective packaging, poor product quality, suspected counterfeiting, or product tampering.
- The U.S.P. Drug Product Problem Reporting Program for Radiopharmaceuticals targets problems with adverse effects or quality of radioactive drugs.
- The Medication Errors Reporting Program looks for actual or potential medication errors that may involve labeling, packaging, miscalculations, misinterpretation, or other problems in drug nomenclature, marketing, advertising, or use of abbreviations.
- The Medical Device and Laboratory Product Problem Reporting Program looks at quality, performance, and safety of medical devices.

Medication Error Index

To rank medication errors according to severity, the National Coordinating Council for Medication Error Reporting and Prevention developed the Medication Error Index to assist health care professionals in evaluating the extent of harm caused by an error (see the accompanying display, Medication Error Index).

LEGISLATION TO PROMOTE TRUTH IN ADVERTISING

In 1912, Congress passed the Sherley Amendment to the 1906 Federal Pure Food and Drug Act, which prohibited drug manufacturers from making fraudulent therapeutic claims about their products. The FFDCA of 1938 bolstered this amendment that, for the first time, provided labeling requirements. Manufacturers were required to use standard drug nomenclature, and the presence and amount of certain potentially toxic drugs (including atropine, alcohol, or opiates) had to be disclosed. Directions for safe use and dosage had to be listed, and the manufacturer's or distributor's name needed to be clearly marked. False or misleading statements were prohibited from appearing on the label.

Today, the Federal Trade Commission regulates the advertisement of medications aimed at the general public. The FDA regulates advertising of medications to medical personnel and relies on reports from practitioners and its own investigators to uncover abuses and fraud. Drug companies can be sanctioned for promoting the use of drugs in a manner that is not consistent with the agency-approved package insert.

The stated intent of the FDA is not to regulate medical practice, but to guarantee the safety, purity, effectiveness, and reliability of drugs sold in the United States. However, the agency does intend to prevent manufacturers from promoting so-called off-label or unlabeled uses of drugs to encourage the development of proper safety and efficacy data. Sanctions may also be imposed if a manufacturer advertises greater efficacy or fewer adverse effects in its product, unless there is a substantial body of evidence to support these claims.

Many people believe that a pill can cure every symptom or condition that develops. Indeed, many conditions are controlled or cured with the help of drugs, and there is a definite role for drugs in contemporary medicine. However, some conditions may be better treated with alternative forms of therapy, such as biofeedback, diet, exercise, stress reduction, guided imagery, and meditation. As every nurse knows, television and radio commercials and the news media often contribute to the public's perspective on drugs. Consequently, society is increasingly drug oriented. Pharmaceuticals and drugs are a multimillion-dollar business that grows each year. Hundreds of millions of dollars are spent annually to promote the sale of prescription and nonprescription drugs.

LEGISLATION REGARDING CONTROLLED SUBSTANCES

The Harrison Narcotic Law of 1914 legally defined the term *narcotic* and provided the first effective regulation regarding the manufacture and distribution of certain drugs known for their abuse potential, including cocaine, marijuana, and opium. The 1970 Comprehensive Drug Abuse Prevention and Control Act (also called the Controlled Substances Act, or CSA) established the Drug Enforcement Agency (DEA), formerly known as the Bureau of Narcotics and Dangerous Drugs (BNDD) of the United States Department of Justice, as the regulatory body responsible for the safe distribution and control of potentially addictive drugs. This act, which was designed to remedy the escalating problem of drug abuse, categorized and controlled drugs according to their abuse potential and medical usefulness on a scale of I to V, hence the term **controlled substance.** This act also defined the terms drug dependency and drug addiction and established education and treatment programs for drug abuse.

Under the CSA, five categories, known as schedules, were established, and controls (relative to health care facilities) were placed on prescribing, dispensing, and storing drugs according to the scheduled category (Table 2-2).

- Schedule I. C-I drugs, such as the opioid heroin, the hallucinogens lysergic acid diethylamide (LSD) and mescaline, the "date-rape drug" gamma-hydroxybutyrate (GHB), and the central nervous system (CNS) depressant methaqualone (Quaalude), have high potential for abuse and no accepted medical use. To prescribe a schedule I drug, a

MEDWATCH

THE FDA MEDICAL PRODUCTS REPORTING PROGRAM

For VOLUNTARY reporting by health professionals of adverse events and product problems

Forum Approved OMB No. 0910-0291 Expires 12/31/94
See OMB statement on reverse

FDA Use Only [DAVIS]

Triage unit sequence #

Page _____ of _____

A. Patient information

1. Patient identifier — In confidence
2. Age at time of event: or Date of birth:
3. Sex — ☐ female ☐ male
4. Weight — _____ lbs or _____ kgs

B. Adverse event or product problem

1. ☐ Adverse event and/or ☐ Product problem (e.g., defects/malfunctions)

2. Outcomes attributed to adverse event (check all that apply)
- ☐ death _____ (mo day yr)
- ☐ life-threatening
- ☐ hospitalization- initial or prolonged
- ☐ disability
- ☐ congenital anomaly
- ☐ required intervention to prevent permanent impairment/damage
- ☐ other: _____

3. Date of event (mo day yr)
4. Date of this report (mo day yr)
5. Describe event or problem
6. Relevant tests/laboratory data, including dates
7. Other relevant history, including preexisting medical conditions (e.g., allergies, race, pregnancy, smoking and alcohol use, hepatic/renal dysfunction, etc)

PLEASE TYPE OR USE BLACK INK

C. Suspect medication(s)

1. Name (give labeled strength & mfr/labeler, if known) #1 #2
2. Dose, frequency & route used #1 #2
3. Therapy dates (if known, give duration) from-to (or best estimates) #1 #2
4. Diagnosis for use (indication) #1 #2
5. Event abated after use stopped or dose reduced — #1 ☐yes ☐no ☐doesn't apply; #2 ☐yes ☐no ☐doesn't apply
6. Lot # (if known)) #1 #2
7. Exp. date (if known) #1 #2
8. Event reappeared after reintroduction — #1 ☐yes ☐no ☐doesn't apply; #2 ☐yes ☐no ☐doesn't apply
9. NDC # (for product problems only)
10. Concomitant medical products and therapy dates (exclude treatment of event)

D. Suspect medical device

1. Brand name
2. Type of device
3. Manufacturer name & address
4. Operator of device — ☐ health professional ☐ lay user/patient ☐ other: _____
5. Expiration date (mo day yr)
6. model # _____ catalog # _____ serial # _____ lot # _____ other #
7. If implanted, give date (mo day yr)
8. If explanted, give date (mo day yr)
9. Device available for evaluation? (Do not send to FDA) ☐ yes ☐ no ☐ returned to manufacturer on _____ (mo day yr)
10. Concomitant medical products and therapy dates (exclude treatment of event)

E. Reporter (see confidentiality section on back)

1. Name, address & phone #
2. Health professional? ☐ yes ☐ no
3. Occupation
4. Also reported to — ☐ manufacturer ☐ user facility ☐ distributor
5. If you do NOT want your identity disclosed to the manufacturer, place an "X" in this box. ☐

FDA

Mail to: MEDWATCH
5600 Fishers lane
Rockville, MD 20852-9787

or FAX to:
1-800-FDA-0178

FDA Form 3500 (6/93)

Submission of a report does not constitute an admission that medical personnel or the product caused or contributed to the event.

Figure 2-4. Example of a MedWatch form for reporting an adverse effect to the Food and Drug Administration (FDA). FDA authorities define a serious event as any occurrence that is fatal, life-threatening, permanently or significantly disabling, requires or prolongs hospitalization, results in a congenital anomaly, or requires intervention to prevent permanent impairment or damage.

Medication Error Index

Category A	No error, although the circumstances or events may have resulted in an error.

Medication Errors Without Harm

Category B	Error occurred but did not reach patient.
Category C	Error occurred and reached patient but did not cause harm.
Category D	Error occurred that reached patient, resulting in need for patient monitoring. No patient harm.

Medication Errors Causing Harm

Category E	Error occurred, resulting in need for treatment or medical intervention. It caused temporary patient harm.
Category F	Error occurred, resulting in hospitalization (initial or prolonged). Caused temporary patient harm.
Category G	Error occurred, causing permanent patient harm.
Category H	Error occurred, causing a neardeath experience (anaphylaxis, cardiac or respiratory arrest, etc.).

Medication Error Resulting in Death

Category I	Error resulted in patient death.

Developed by The National Coordinating Council for Medication Error Reporting and Prevention

physician must obtain special clearance from the FDA. C-I drugs are generally restricted to research.

- Schedule II. C-II drugs, such as the opioids morphine, meperidine (Demerol), methadone (Dolophine), and codeine; CNS stimulants, such as amphetamines and methylphenidate (Ritalin); and CNS depressants, such as pentobarbital (Nembutal) and secobarbital (Seconal) have acceptable medical uses. A prescription written in triplicate form—with one copy being forwarded to the DEA—is required to obtain these drugs. In extreme emergencies, however, a C-II substance may be ordered over the telephone. This order must be signed by the prescriber within 48 hours. Refills require a new prescription.
- Schedule III. C-III drugs, such as codeine-combination products, hydrocodone tablets (Vicodin), or opium solutions (found in low concentrations in cough suppressants); certain CNS stimulants, such as the anorexiant benzphetamine (Didrex); and anabolic steroids have a lower abuse/dependence potential. A written or telephone order may be acceptable, and the order may be refilled five times within 6 months of the date of issue. The prescription must be rewritten after 6 months or five refills.
- Schedule IV. C-IV drugs, such as the benzodiazepine anxiolytics, anticonvulsants, muscle-relaxants, and sedatives; the nonbenzodiazepine hypnotics zolpidem (Ambien) and chloral hydrate (Aquachloral Suprettes); the intermediate-acting sedative barbiturate butabarbital (Butisol); the opioid analgesics propoxyphene (Darvon) or pentazocine (Talwin), present a very low risk for abuse or dependence. As with C-III drugs, prescriptions for C-IV drugs must be rewritten after 6 months or five refills.
- Schedule V. C-V drugs, such as the antidiarrheal preparations diphenoxylate (Lomotil) and loperamide (Imodium), which contain dilute solutions of codeine (no more than 2 mg/mL) or opium (no more than 1 mg/mL), pose the lowest risk for abuse and dependence. Many of these drugs may be obtained without a prescription.

Drugs may be moved from one schedule category to another. For example, propoxyphene, which was originally assigned a C-V rank, was reassigned to the more restrictive C-IV category because of its popularity for misuse, abuse, and overdose. Tetrahydrocannabinol (THC, the active ingredient in marijuana)—ranked in the C-I category for many years—was moved to C-II because of its legitimate clinical use as a powerful antiemetic to relieve the adverse effects of cancer chemotherapy.

TABLE 2-2 Schedule of Controlled Substances*

Scheduled Category	Abuse Potential	Example
C-I	High abuse potential	No accepted medical use (heroin, hashish, LSD, GHB)
C-II	High abuse potential Severe dependence liability	Amphetamines, some opioid narcotics (e.g., morphine sulfate, meperidine), dronabinol, short-acting barbiturates (e.g., pentobarbital, secobarbital)
C-III	Less abuse potential than C-II drugs Moderate dependence liability	Nonbarbiturate sedatives (e.g., benzodiazepines), some opioid narcotics (e.g., codeine combinations) nonamphetamine stimulants (e.g., pemoline)
C-IV	Less abuse potential than C-III drugs Limited dependence liability	Anxiolytics (e.g., intermediate-acting barbiturates), benzodiazepine anticonvulsants (e.g., clonazepam), some narcotic analgesics (e.g., propoxyphene), nonbarbiturate sedatives (e.g., chloral hydrate)
C-V	Limited abuse potential	Small amounts of narcotics (e.g., codeine) used as antitussives or antidiarrheals

*Drugs under the jurisdiction of the Controlled Substances Act are divided into five schedules based on their potential for abuse and physical and psychological dependence.

LSD, lysergic acid diethylamide; GHB, gamma-hydroxybutyrate

Nursing Management of Controlled Substances

The prescribing, dispensing, and storing of controlled substances are subject to considerably greater governmental control than the use of conventional prescription drugs. Procedures to follow in virtually every step from manufacture to administration to wasting or discarding are precisely defined by law. Whenever a nurse administers a controlled substance, the following must be recorded on the narcotic log sheet:

- Date and time of administration
- Drug name and dose
- Patient's name
- Prescriber's name
- Administering nurse's name

In the health care facility, stock supplies of narcotics must be kept in double-locked storage cabinets. Keys to the cabinet are restricted to licensed nurses, who are also responsible for the accurate accounting of all narcotics. The nurse finishing a shift and the nurse beginning a shift generally perform the narcotic count together. The handling of controlled substances is a nursing responsibility that should never be taken lightly. Transfer of a C-II, C-III, or C-IV drug to anyone other than the person for whom it is prescribed is a crime. Violation of the CSA can result in a fine, imprisonment, or both. Any nurse who violates the CSA is also subject to loss of the nursing license and the right to practice nursing.

LEGISLATION REGARDING DRUG DISTRIBUTION

The Durham-Humphrey amendments (1952) to the 1938 FFDCA separated drugs for the first time into two major classifications: nonprescription drugs and legend (prescription) drugs.

Prescription drugs must be identified by the legend (inscription) on the container: "Caution: Federal law prohibits dispensing without a prescription." Containers of controlled substances must also display an additional warning label: "Caution: Federal law prohibits the transfer of this drug to any person other than the patient for whom it was prescribed." Common prescription drugs include hypnotic, narcotic, or other drugs with abuse potential and potentially toxic drugs that may be unsafe if used without the supervision of a licensed practitioner (nurse practitioner, physician, dentist). The Durham-Humphrey amendment further specifies procedures for the distribution of **legend drugs.** A prescription from a licensed practitioner is required before the drug can be dispensed, and refills are not permitted without authorization of the prescriber.

Labeling, according to the U.S.P., is the written, printed, or graphic matter affixed to an immediate container, package, or wrapper in which the medication is enclosed. Things that are not attached (e.g., patient information/instruction sheets) are not considered part of the label. The prescription label remains a primary source of information to patients about the proper use of their medications. Cautions regarding use and storage are usually on auxiliary labels and some medications require their use. The following are examples of auxiliary labels:

- Avoid prolonged or excessive exposure to sunlight or sunlamp while taking this medication.
- Avoid the use of grapefruit juice with this product.
- Avoid the use of laxatives with this product.
- Do not take this drug if you are pregnant or suspect that you may be pregnant.
- Do not take with dairy products or antacids, or within 1 hour before or 2 hours after taking this medication.
- Do not use past the expiration date.
- May cause drowsiness. Alcohol may intensify this effect. Use care when operating a car or dangerous machinery.
- Must be refrigerated/do not freeze.
- Take all of this medication/complete the full course of therapy.
- Take on empty stomach, at least 1 hour before or 2 hours after meals.
- Take with full glass of water.

Online Pharmacies

Resolution 2763 (Internet Pharmacy Consumer Protection Act of 1999) was introduced into the House of Representatives. This would amend the FFDCA with respect to the sale of prescription drugs through the Internet and would require an Internet pharmacy page to provide:

- Name, address, and telephone number of the individual(s)' principal place of business
- A listing of the state(s) in which the individual is authorized by law to dispense prescription drugs
- Name of each individual who serves as a pharmacist for purposes of the site and each state in which the individual is authorized by law to dispense prescription drugs
- Names of all individuals (and their respective license numbers) who provide medical consultations through the site for purposes of providing prescriptions

Other pending legislation with an indirect affect on online pharmacies includes House Resolution 237 (Consumer Internet Privacy Enhancement Act of 2001), and House Resolution 809 (Online Privacy Protection Act of 2001). These bills would require every web site to indicate how personal identifiable information is used and would also require similar notice if this information is made available to third parties.

SAFEGUARDS THAT PROTECT THE UNBORN

The FDA has established five categories (categories A, B, C, D, and X) to rank the potential for a systemically absorbed drug to cause birth defects. The effects of drugs assigned to pregnancy risk category A have been studied in animals and found to be relatively safe for the fetus during pregnancy. Animal studies, however, cannot be true predictors of teratogenicity because of wide inter- and intraspecies variations in the pharmacokinetic properties of drugs, including placental transfer. Drugs in risk category B may impose adverse effects on the fetus, although studies are inadequate to confirm the risk. Drugs in risk category C pose potential risks to the fetus, but the benefits of use during pregnancy outweigh the risks. Drugs in category D have been proved to cause fetal harm, but their benefits to the woman may outweigh potential risks. Drugs in category X are proven harmful to the fetus, and the potential for fetal harm outweighs any benefit from their use.

Several factors determine the effects teratogenic drugs may have on the fetus during pregnancy. One important factor is the dose reaching the fetus. Most drugs cross the placenta by simple diffusion. Many drugs reach 50% to 100% of the concentration in fetal blood as that in maternal blood (Gurnee & Sylvestri, 1998). Other determining factors are that point in fetal development when the drug exposure occurs, the duration of the exposure, environmental factors (occurring simultaneously with drug exposure), and the susceptibility (or resistance) of the fetus itself to teratogenesis. Gestational weeks 4 to 10 constitute the most vulnerable window of risk for major congenital malformations (Gurnee & Sylvestri, 1998). For more information, refer to Chapter 8, Life Span: Pregnant or Breast-feeding Women.

NONGOVERNMENTAL INSTITUTIONAL CONTROLS

Health care institutions, such as hospitals and skilled nursing facilities, may adopt additional regulations to ensure safe drug therapy and drug distribution. The Joint Commission for Accreditation of Hospitals and Healthcare Organizations (JCAHO) is a watchdog group that provides the impetus for this. JCAHO sets the standards for quality of patient care and accreditation of health care institutions.

Generally, drug-related regulations to meet these standards of care vary greatly among institutions, but most guarantee that the drug therapy that has been prescribed for any patient is continually reviewed for appropriateness, safety, and efficacy. Examples of these regulations include automatic discontinuation of antibiotic orders after 7 to 10 days of treatment or automatic discontinuation of narcotic or controlled substance orders after 48 to 72 hours. Institutional regulations exist to prevent prolonged, costly, and sometimes inappropriate administration of drugs. Development and implementation of such policies usually require a cooperative collaborative effort among the nursing, pharmacy, and medical staffs.

CANADIAN LEGISLATION REGARDING DRUG SAFETY AND EFFICACY

Canadian drug laws are similar to those in the United States, and the Health Protection Branch of the Department of National Health and Welfare is responsible for maintaining quality and safety of drug development, manufacture, and distribution. The Health Protection Branch is also responsible for the administration and enforcement of the **Canadian Food and Drugs Act,** the Canadian Narcotic Control Act, and the Proprietary or Patent Medicine Act. These acts are designed to protect the consumer from health hazards and fraud or deception in the sale and use of cosmetics, drugs, foods, and medical devices.

CANADIAN FOOD AND DRUGS ACT

In 1953, the Canadian Food and Drugs Act established standards for labeling, packaging, manufacture, quality, and advertising. The act is amended yearly. Schedule A of this act lists diseases (e.g., alcoholism, arteriosclerosis, cancer) for which no cosmetic, drug, food, or device may be advertised or sold to the general public as a treatment, prevention, or cure. Schedule B of this act requires that drugs comply with certain standards as set forth in recognized compendiums (e.g., USSP-NF, British Pharmacopoeia, Canadian Formulary, British Pharmaceutical Codex, Compendium of Pharmaceuticals and Specialties). Manufacturing premises, processes, and conditions must be approved before Schedule B medicines may be marketed. Moreover, safety testing is required for batches of certain types of drugs. For example, sales of insulin preparations, radioactive isotopes, antibiotics for parenteral use, serums, and live vaccines depend on approval by the Minister of National Health and Welfare. The legend "Canadian Standard Drug" must appear on the inner and outer labels of a drug to signify that it meets the standards prescribed for it. Drugs contained in Schedules C and D must list location, process, and condition of manufacturing.

CONTROLS ON PRESCRIBING

Schedule F of the Canadian Food and Drugs Act also defines prescription drugs, including antibiotics, hormones, and tranquilizers. The label on prescription drugs must show directions for use and the symbol "Pr" indicating that a prescription is required. Advertisement of prescription drugs to the general public is restricted. Only licensed practitioners may prescribe prescription drugs, and refills are limited to a period of 6 months in an amount specified by the prescriber.

CONTROLLED SUBSTANCES

Schedule G of the Canadian Food and Drugs Act identifies the controlled substances (e.g., amphetamines, barbiturates). The container of a controlled substance must be marked with Ⓒ symbol. Prescriptions for controlled substances cannot be refilled unless the original prescription specifies the number of refills allowed with dates for refills or intervals between refills.

Restricted drugs, such as LSD and dimethoxyamphetamine, are listed in Schedule H. Sale of these drugs is prohibited because they have no recognized medical use, although the Minister of National Health and Welfare may authorize access to these drugs by qualified investigators for the purposes of research.

In 1961, the Canadian Narcotics Control Act provided regulations regarding the manufacture, sale, distribution, and possession of narcotics and other drugs of abuse. This act has been amended a number of times. The most recent Canadian drug legislation is the 1982 Narcotic Control Act. This law is similar in scope to the 1970 United States Comprehensive Drug Abuse Prevention and Control Act. Drugs are placed into categories depending on their potential for abuse. CNS stimulants, barbiturates, and other drugs affecting the CNS are placed in Schedule G of their categorization system. Canada, like the United States, has strict requirements for nurses who must account for all narcotic drugs used within a health care institution or agency. Narcotics are dispensed only with a written prescription and "N" must appear on the label.

IMPACT OF LEGAL AND INSTITUTIONAL CONTROLS ON NURSING MANAGEMENT

Nurses need to be familiar not only with institutional protocols for safe and effective drug administration, but also with official and professional regulations and laws. Drug laws and nurse practice acts vary from state to state, and these regulations define nursing responsibilities related to drug safety and effectiveness in patient care. Nurses must be familiar with the current regulations in their states and in their nursing practice settings. Nurses can stay up-to-date by regularly consulting with representatives of regulatory bodies, arranging in-service training and information sessions, and understanding the policies of their own agencies.

In professional practice, nurses must adhere to and obey established drug control laws and protocols. They must avoid advising patients on the use of drugs, and they cannot provide drug therapy without proper authorization. Within the institution, nurses are responsible not only for drug security (to prevent unauthorized use or accidental loss) but also for safely administering drugs. Infraction of the laws and protocols to protect and promote patient safety may result in the loss of one's nursing license.

PATIENT EDUCATION AS A SAFEGUARD IN DRUG THERAPY

Educating patients is well documented as a key safeguard in drug therapy. Educating patients about drug therapy improves adherence to drug therapy and promotes therapeutic outcomes. In other words, patients who understand the prescribed drug regimen have the best chance of achieving the maximum benefit from it.

Patient education requires a nurse to have skills in gathering data, individualizing instructions, prompting and supporting the patient, and assessing and evaluating the pharmacotherapeutic response for determining patient outcomes. An effective patient teaching program parallels the nursing process—the nurse assesses the patient's learning needs, formulates a diagnosis, identifies a desired outcome, develops and implements a teaching plan, and evaluates the teaching and learning that has occurred (see the accompanying display, Strategies for Enhancing Patient Education).

CONSUMER DRUG INFORMATION ON THE INTERNET

The explosive growth of the Internet has created countless opportunities for patients to access health-related information, products, and services. It has forever changed the way many consumers obtain prescription drugs and health information. Opting for the convenience and privacy of the information-rich Internet, consumers have increasingly gone on line for information on medications.

The quality of information provided on these sites has become a concern for health care providers, though. One study evaluated selected sites on the quality of information for 30 commonly prescribed drugs. The sites were evaluated according to sponsorships, references cited, frequency of updates, ease of use, and organization of the web page, as well as the quality and quantity of information provided. One consistent weakness of all the sites was a lack of regular updates. The author concluded that these sites provided useful consumer drug information, but failed to meet the standards set for an ideal website (Buck, 1999).

Consumers have also gone online for their prescription drug needs. A combination of high-profile congressional hearings, sensational cases, anecdotal reporting by the media, and recently published scientific studies raises legitimate concerns about the potential for illegitimate Internet sites to put consumers' health at risk by selling prescription drugs without a valid physician-patient relationship with sales oftentimes from offshore locations.

PATIENT LEARNING NEEDS

Learning needs for drug education vary among patients, as does their adherence to the prescribed treatment regimen. Some variations result from clinical factors, such as the nurse-patient relationship. Others variations are related to the scope or complexity of drug therapy in relation to pharmacotherapeutic, pharmacokinetic, and pharmacodynamic parameters; contraindications, precautions, and adverse effects of therapy; and the potential for drug interactions with undesired effects.

Variations may also relate to core patient variables: health status; life span and gender; lifestyle, diet, and habits; environment; and culture (see Chapter 1; also see the accompanying display, Assessment: Another Safeguard).

Strategies for Enhancing Patient Education

- Avoid jargon; communicate in short words and sentences.
- Include written information using diagrams and illustrations.
- Promote understanding with repetition and reinforcement.
- Relate new information to the patient's existing knowledge and previous experiences.
- Highlight and recap important information. Ask the patient to repeat the instructions or demonstrate new techniques.

Assessment: Another Safeguard

To ensure the patient's safe adherence to drug therapy and to formulate an effective, relevant drug teaching plan, the nurse needs not only to assess the patient's learning needs, but also the patient's health history, asking about the following:

- Allergies or idiosyncratic reactions to drugs or foods
- Chronic conditions
- Drugs and other medications currently used (including vitamins, other supplements, and over-the-counter drugs)
- Pregnancy status now and future plans (for women of childbearing age)
- Use of alcohol, caffeine, nicotine, or illicit substances

TEACHING FOCUS AND CONTENT

Because each patient processes information differently, the nurse should attempt to individualize and communicate information so that the patient or the caregiver can understand it and act on it appropriately. If possible, the nurse should prepare written or audiovisual materials for the patient to consult as needed. Basic patient education in drug therapy should begin with an assessment of the patient's health history as it relates to drug therapy (see the Patient Education Guidelines display in Chapter 1).

EVALUATING AND DOCUMENTING EDUCATIONAL OUTCOMES

Evaluation and documentation of patient education should include time of teaching, content of teaching, the patient's response to the teaching session, an evaluation of the patient's grasp of the subject matter, and an assessment of unmet or future learning needs. Like documentation of drug therapy and other nursing care, documentation of patient education activities becomes part of the clinical and legal record, serving as a reference for other health care professionals and helping to guide future drug therapy.

IMPORTANCE OF NURSING MANAGEMENT

Pharmacotherapy, the use of drugs in treating and preventing disease, is one of the most common medical treatment modalities. Over the years, consequently, counseling and teaching patients about their drug regimens have become increasingly significant aspects of nursing practice. Nursing functions in regard to drug therapy are largely educational, particularly as use of community-based health care escalates.

The importance of pharmacotherapy in nursing practice continues to grow. Nurses are legally responsible for the drugs they administer and for safe drug administration. When caring for patients with acute health problems, the nurse is the health care provider who usually administers drugs. This function becomes significantly more demanding as more new drugs entering the marketplace, multiple-drug therapies grow more complex, and drug delivery systems become more sophisticated. This requires a thorough understanding of therapeutic drug actions and adverse drug reactions.

In some clinical settings, however, nurses are allowed to modify drug regimens according to specifically designed protocols, and almost all states now allow advanced practice nurses to prescribe drugs. Future nursing practice will likely involve the prescribing of selected drugs.

Application of the nursing process to the pharmacologic aspects of patient care is especially important because long-term use of drug therapy is frequently necessary to control chronic disease processes. Nursing management in drug therapy may be considered an applied science because it relies on knowledge and principles from many different disciplines, such as anatomy and physiology, anthropology, biochemistry, mathematics, microbiology, organic chemistry, psychology, and sociology.

CHAPTER SUMMARY

- Sources of drugs include plants, animals and humans, minerals, and chemical substances.
- Each drug is identified by at least three names. They include the chemical name; the generic (nonproprietary) name, which is a contraction or shortening of the chemical name; and the trade or brand (proprietary) name. In the United States, official names are assigned by the government and are usually the same as the generic name.
- There are several ways to classify drugs that share similar characteristics, namely, by clinical indications, effects on body systems, or chemical composition. Drug classifications (also known as families) emphasize common characteristics of each grouping, usually identify a prototype drug, and facilitate the association of new drugs within an established family as new drugs become available.
- Sources of drug information include pharmacopoeias, which are official sources; compendiums, which are unofficial sources; product-insert literature from pharmaceutical firms; published reports; and findings in journals and electronic databases.
- The FFDCA (1938), an amendment to the 1906 Pure Food and Drug Act, established the FDA, required government approval prior to marketing a drug, and established the elements of drug labeling. In addition to directions for use and recommended dosages, labels had to include a warning about the presence of any habit-forming drugs in the product and their effects.
- The Kefauver-Harris Amendment (1962) to the FFDCA required manufacturers to provide evidence of efficacy and safety before marketing a product and gave the FDA a central role in the conduct of clinical research.
- Legislation aimed at curbing drug abuse, the Comprehensive Drug Abuse Prevention and Control Act (1970), aided drug education, research, treatment, and enforcement. The Controlled Substances Act classified and controlled drugs according to their potential and liability for abuse. This act further mandated the appropriate procedures for dispensing, storage, record keeping, and destruction of all controlled substances.
- The approval process for a new drug is lengthy and expensive. First the FDA approves an IND application. Following animal studies, phases I through IV involve testing the drug on various populations of human volunteers. Phase III uses research methods to identify infrequent or rare adverse reactions. The FDA approves an NDA if study results are satisfactory.
- The FDA program, MedWatch, takes reports from health professionals and consumers about adverse reactions and disseminates information about those reactions, as well as labeling changes, and other safety issues.

QUESTIONS FOR STUDY AND REVIEW

1. What is the purpose of the U.S.P. and the NF?
2. How is an understanding of pharmacokinetics and pharmacodynamics helpful to the nurse in the clinical application of drug therapy?
3. Explain the ways in which drugs are named.
4. How are drugs classified? What is the purpose of placing drugs in classifications?
5. Discuss the purpose and intent of government regulations, such as the Food, Drug, and Cosmetics Act, the Durham-Humphrey amendments, or the Canadian Narcotics Control Act. What safeguards do these laws provide?
6. Explain the purpose and extent of clinical trials. Identify some advantages and disadvantages to clinical trials.
7. What are controlled substances? What are some nursing implications related to administering a controlled substance? What special precautions are required for handling controlled substances?
8. Explain the purpose of the FDA pregnancy categories.
9. Identify some points about safe drug use that should be taught to all patients.
10. What kinds of information about drugs should be included in the patient teaching plan?

NEED MORE HELP?

? Chapter 2 of the study guide for *Drug Therapy in Nursing* contains exercises and activities to reinforce your understanding of the concepts presented in this chapter. For additional information see the text's accompanying web site at *http://www.connection.lww.com*.

REFERENCES AND BIBLIOGRAPHY

Alastair, J. J. (1999). The safety of new medicines: The importance of asking the right questions. *Journal of the American Medical Association, 281*(18), 1735–1739.

Anonymous. (2000). Online pharmacies—take heed! *Drug Benefit Trends, 12*(1), 21–22.

Anonymous. (1999). Update on the increasing regulation of Internet and online pharmacies. *Drug Benefit Trends, 11*(9), 27–28.

Anonymous. (1994). FDA launches MEDWATCH program: Monitoring adverse drug reactions. Food and Drug Administration (FDA). *NP News, 2*, 1, 4.

Buck, M. S. (1999). Recent actions by the Food and Drug Administration (FDA). *Pediatric Pharmacotherapy, 5*(12), 5–12.

Cardinale, V. (1998). Consumers looking for more answers, clearer directions. *Drug Topics Supplement, 142*(11), 23s.

Drug facts and comparisons. (2000). St. Louis: Facts and Comparisons.

Friedman, M. A., Woodcock, J., Lumpkin, M. M., Shuren, J. E., Hass, A. E., & Thompson, L. J. (1999). The safety of newly approved medicines: Do recent market removals mean there is a problem? *Journal of the American Medical Association, 281*(18), 1728–1734.

Gossel, T. A. (1998). Exploring pharmacology. *U.S. Pharmacist, 23*(9), 96–103.

Gossel, T. A. (1998). Pharmacology: Back to basics. *U.S. Pharmacist, 23*(11), 96–103.

Gossel, T. A. (1999). Pharmacology: A profile on pharmacokinetics. *U.S. Pharmacist, 24*(5), 71–77.

Gossel, T. A. (1999). Pharmacodynamics: How drugs act. *U.S. Pharmacist, 24*(9), 101–108.

Gurnee, M., & Sylvestri, M. (1998). Teratogenicity of drugs. *U.S. Pharmacist, 23*(9), 70–77.

Hansten, P. D., Horn, J. R., Koda-Kimble, M. A., & Young, L. L. Y. (1997). Drug interactions and updates. *Drug Interactions and Updates Quarterly, 15*, 879.

Hardman, J. G., Limbird, L. E., Molinoff, P. B., Ruddon, R. W., & Gilman, A. G. (Eds.). (1997). *Goodman and Gilman's the pharmacological basis of therapeutics* (9th ed.). New York: McGraw-Hill.

Isselbachter, K. J., Braunwald, E., Wilson, J. D., Martin, J. B., Fauci, A. S., & Kasper, D. L. (Eds.). (1994). *Harrison's principles of internal medicine* (13th ed.). New York: McGraw-Hill.

Katzung, B. C. (Ed.). (2000). *Basic and clinical pharmacology* (8th ed.). New York: McGraw-Hill.

Leake, C. D. (1975). *An historical account of pharmacology to the twentieth century.* Springfield, IL: Charles C Thomas Press.

McEvoy, G. K., Litvak, K., & Welsh, O. H., Jr. (Eds.). (2000). *Drug information.* Bethesda: American Hospital Formulary Service.

Padron, V. A., Hospodka, R. J., DeSimone, E. M., Keefner, K. R., & Baker, K. R. (1998). What the prescription label should tell the patient. *U.S. Pharmacist, 23*(1), 58–75.

Sonnedecker, G. (1976). *Kremers and Urdang's history of pharmacy* (4th ed.). Philadelphia: JB Lippincott.

Tone, B. (1999). Rushing through? Questioning the safety of drug approvals. *Nurseweek, 1222*(12), 1,15.

U.S. Department of Health and Human Services, Food and Drug Administration. (1999). Task force report: Managing the risks from medical product use: creating a risk management framework. Washington, D. C.: U.S. Government Printing Office.

Wagner, E. H. (1997). Preventing decline in function. Evidence from randomized trials around the world. *Western Journal of Medicine, 167*(4), 295–298.

Chapter 3

DRUG PREPARATIONS AND ADMINISTRATION

KEY TERMS

buccal
capsules
elixir
emulsion
enteral route
enteric coating
intra-arterial
intra-articular
intradermal
intramuscular
intrathecal
intravenous
intravenous piggyback
intravenous push
local effect
parenteral route
subcutaneous
sublingual
suspension
sustained-release
syrup
systemic effect
tablet
topical route
troches

Learning Objectives

At the completion of this chapter the student will:

1. Describe the three routes for administering drugs.
2. Differentiate systemic and local effects related to the various routes of drug administration.
3. Describe the variety of oral forms of enteral drugs.
4. Differentiate the three main methods of parenteral drug administration.
5. Describe the methods of topical administration.
6. Describe how the route of administration interacts with core drug knowledge.
7. Describe how the route of administration interacts with the core patient variables.
8. Describe nursing interventions to maximize therapeutic and minimize adverse effects based on drug administration route.

Drug therapy can be administered by several different routes or methods. These routes of administration require different preparations or forms of a drug. Most drugs are available from the drug manufacturer in multiple forms. The selection of the route and form is based on the interaction between core drug knowledge and core patient variables. In managing drug therapy, nurses use this information to assess patient needs, plan care, administer drugs, and evaluate the effectiveness of therapy. This chapter describes the different routes of drug administration, explains the different forms of drug preparations, and shows how the route and drug form interact with the core drug knowledge and the core patient variables.

DRUG ADMINISTRATION ROUTES: GENERAL CONSIDERATIONS

The three basic routes of drug administration are enteral, parenteral, and topical. (Some authorities place topical in the parenteral category.)

The **enteral route** uses the gastrointestinal (GI) tract for the ingestion and absorption of drugs. The most common method of administering drugs through the enteral route is orally. The enteral route also includes drugs that are administered through a nasogastric (NG) or a gastrostomy (G) tube.

The **parenteral route** avoids or circumvents the GI tract and is associated with all forms of injections: intramuscular (IM), subcutaneous (SC, or SQ), and intravenous (IV). Less commonly used parenteral routes are intradermal (into the dermis), intrathecal (into the cerebrospinal fluid), intra-articular (into a joint), and intra-arterial (into an artery).

The **topical route** is technically another parenteral route because it also bypasses the GI tract. Drugs administered topically are applied to the skin or mucous membranes, including those of the eyes, ears, nose, vagina, rectum, and lungs.

Drugs are administered for their local or systemic effects. For example, most drugs applied topically to the skin or mucous membranes exert their effect at that site, which is a **local effect.** However, certain drugs given topically are absorbed by the skin and distributed throughout the body systems to produce a **systemic effect.** Drugs given for a systemic effect by any route must be capable of being transported into the blood and distributed through the body to a location distant from the administration site.

Drugs administered by a route other than the enteral route have the advantage of avoiding the first-pass metabolism in the liver. Drugs administered enterally are absorbed from the stomach and small intestine. However, they first pass through the liver, the primary organ for drug metabolism, before being distributed throughout the body. Drugs administered parenterally and even some topical drugs are transported directly into the blood, thereby bypassing the liver. (See Chapter 4 for a complete discussion of the first-pass effect and the processes of pharmacokinetics.)

ENTERAL ROUTE AND FORMS

The enteral route involves using the GI tract for the administration, absorption, and use of drugs. Enteral drugs, particularly oral drugs, are manufactured and prepared in a variety of forms, including solid tablets and capsules and liquid elixirs and syrups. Because the oral route of administration is the most common enteral route, oral dosage forms are the most common preparations. They are convenient, economical, and easy to use.

Some oral drugs, such as antacids and laxatives, are given for the local effect in the GI tract, but most are given to achieve a systemic effect. In most cases, patients can reliably self-medicate with oral drug forms.

ORAL DRUG FORMS

Tablets

A **tablet** is a solid dosage form that is prepared by compressing or molding a drug into various sizes and shapes. In many cases, tablets are scored; that is, designed to be easily broken at a point so that one-half or one-quarter of the dose may be given. Unless a tablet is scored, it should never be broken because this could result in inaccurate dosage.

The active ingredients in tablets are commonly mixed with lactose or other sugars, binding agents, or other inert material to facilitate manufacturing and ensure stability of the preparation. When the patient swallows the tablet, it is propelled to the stomach, where it dissolves and releases the drug into the gastric contents.

Drugs that are appropriate for use in tablet form have some limitations. First, the drug must be stable in gastric contents. Because gastric juices may be highly acidic, drugs that rapidly degrade in acid environments may not be administered using conventional tablets. An additional consideration is flavor, because the tablet will begin to dissolve as soon as it is placed in the mouth. Bitter, irritating, or unpleasant tasting drugs are not usually administered in conventional tablet form. These limitations may be overcome by using a special coating on the tablet.

An **enteric coating** is a waxlike layer that is used over some tablets. This layer resists the acid environment of the stomach but dissolves in areas in which the local pH is neutral or slightly alkaline (e.g., the small intestine). Enteric coatings may be used to protect acid-labile drugs, to provide a sustained-release dose, or to guard against local adverse effects from a drug. Other types of commonly used coatings include film or sugar. Both of these coatings are used to protect the patient from bitter or unpleasant tasting drugs. These coatings do not impart any time-release characteristics.

Sustained-release (also called controlled-, timed-, extended-, or prolonged-release) tablets are formulated to release a drug slowly over an extended period, rather than rapidly like conventional tablets. Sustained release occurs by several methods:

- Layers of enteric coatings may be applied, and the drug is released in response to changes in the surrounding pH of the GI fluid.

- The tablet may be formulated to release the drug in a steady, controlled manner.
- The tablet may be formulated to release the drug in a series of pulsations.

In most cases, the total dose of drug in a sustained-release preparation is higher than that found in a regular tablet. Regardless, the patient may safely take the higher dose because it is released in a controlled fashion, thereby preventing any adverse effects from overdosage.

Sublingual and Buccal Tablets

Sublingual and buccal preparations are less commonly used tablet forms. These small, hard, compressed tablets are designed to dissolve rapidly in the vascular mucous membranes of the mouth. **Buccal** tablets are placed in the buccal pouch (between the cheek and gum), and **sublingual** tablets are placed under the tongue. Because these areas are highly vascular, drugs are quickly absorbed into the bloodstream, and a rapid onset of drug effect occurs. At the same time, drugs administered in this way avoid the first-pass phenomenon because they are not ingested into the GI tract.

Sublingual and buccal tablets must be relatively nonirritating, flavorless, and highly water soluble. Although typically considered oral forms because they are placed in the mouth, some experts think of the sublingual and buccal forms as parenteral preparations because they are not absorbed in the GI tract. Others consider them a variation of the topical route.

Troches

Troches, also called pastilles or lozenges, are commonly used for a local effect in the mouth or pharynx (throat). The drug is embedded in hard candy or another suitably flavored vehicle that the patient holds within the mouth, where it slowly dissolves. Antitussives, anti-infectives, local anesthetics, antihistamines, or analgesics are administered this way.

Capsules

Capsules are solid dosage forms in which the drug is usually encased in a shell of hard or soft gelatin. Because the active ingredients are enclosed in gelatin, foul-tasting drugs can be easily administered in capsules. Another advantage is that many patients find gelatin capsules easier to swallow than tablets. Unlike tablets, capsules cannot be easily divided or broken into equal pieces, so one disadvantage is that dosage may not be as flexible. When the patient swallows the capsule, the drug is carried to the stomach where the gelatin capsule quickly dissolves and releases the drug into the gastric contents.

The most common capsules encase a powdered drug. Soft, elastic capsules are somewhat thicker and may be used to encase a drug paste, semiliquid, or liquid (provided the drug itself does not dissolve the capsule). In addition, the contents may be altered in one of several ways to produce a sustained-release dosage form as follows:

- Layers of enteric coatings may be applied to the drug particles, producing what is commonly known as microencapsulation. The drug is released in response to changes in the surrounding pH of the GI fluid. The rate of release is controlled by varying the thickness of the layers around the drug particles.
- The capsule may be formulated to release the drug in a steady, controlled manner from a matrix of drug encased in a slowly dissolving substance, such as wax.
- The drug is bound to ion-exchange resins, chemical compounds that form insoluble complexes within the capsule. Changes in the local environment, such as altered electrolyte content or pH, cause the drug to be released slowly from the resin matrix.

Like their tablet counterparts, sustained-release capsules may contain higher doses than those found in regular-release forms, but the patient may safely take the higher dose because the drug is released in a controlled fashion.

Syrups

A concentrated solution of sugar, such as sucrose, in water is known as a **syrup.** Most syrups that contain 65% or more sucrose are also resistant to mold, yeasts, and other microorganisms, and they have a reasonable shelf life with no need for refrigeration. Occasionally, sucrose may crystallize out of solution, clouding the syrup or giving it the appearance of particulate matter.

Elixirs

An **elixir** is a clear hydroalcoholic mixture that is usually sweetened or otherwise pleasantly flavored. Most elixirs contain ethanol and water, but glycerin, sorbitol, propylene glycol, flavoring agents, aspartase, and even syrups may also be found in elixirs. The alcohol content of elixirs varies greatly and can exceed 25%. Elixirs are stored at room temperature, and the alcohol content usually prevents the growth of any mold or other microorganisms. Elixirs should always be clear. Cloudiness indicates contamination.

Emulsions and Suspensions

Many drug preparations use mixtures of two chemically incompatible substances. These preparations may be administered orally. Rarely, they may be used topically.

An **emulsion** is created when two liquids that do not mix well are combined, and one liquid distributes uniformly through the other. Because these mixtures tend to separate rapidly, it is important to remember to shake the preparation well immediately before measuring a dose, and to administer the dose soon after pouring and measuring. To enhance the stability of the mixture, an emulsifying agent is added. Most emulsions consist of a nonaqueous agent (oil or lipid phase) dispersed with an aqueous (water) agent. In general, nothing should be added to emulsions because additives may adversely effect the stability of the mixture.

A **suspension** is a drug preparation consisting of two agents: a finely divided solid dispersed within a liquid. The stability of the preparation depends on the ability of the dispersing medium to wet the solid particles. Surface-active agents may be used.

NASOGASTRIC OR GASTROSTOMY TUBE FORMS

Patients who cannot swallow but who have a functioning GI tract may have an NG or G tube in place. An NG tube is a soft, flexible tube that is advanced through a nostril and into the stomach for administering food, fluids, and drugs, usually for a short time. There is a risk of aspiration from gastric reflux with an NG tube because the tube prevents closure of the gastroesophageal sphincter. A G tube is surgically inserted into the stomach for administering food, fluids, and drugs to patients needing long-term care. Providing drugs and foods through a G tube is preferred over an NG tube because the G tube method leaves the gastroesophageal sphincter intact. Regurgitation is less likely with a G tube than with an NG tube. Drugs should be either liquid or crushed and in a liquid vehicle when administering through a tube. A liquid drug form is preferred because research has shown that this form causes less clotting of tubes than crushed and dissolved drugs. Remember that sustained-release or enteric-coated tablets should never be crushed. Not only does this alter the pharmacokinetics of the drug but it is likely to cause obstruction when administered through a tube (Belknap, Seifer, & Petermann, 1997).

NURSING MANAGEMENT IN ENTERAL DRUG ADMINISTRATION

Core Drug Knowledge

Although the oral method of drug delivery is most common, not all drugs can be administered orally. Gastric acids and enzymes destroy many drugs; others simply may not be absorbed.

Absorption may begin in the stomach, but most absorption of orally administered drugs occurs in the small intestine. Food may interfere with the dissolution and absorption of certain drugs, especially enteric-coated drugs, because of the considerable variation in individual gastric emptying times and therefore in the length of time a drug spends in the stomach.

Assessment of Relevant Core Patient Variables

Health Status

A primary consideration for administering an oral drug is the patient's condition. Can the patient tolerate an oral drug? Patients who are vomiting, uncooperative, or unconscious or whose condition requires that they receive nothing by mouth (i.e., no oral food or fluid) are not suited for oral drug therapy. Alternate routes should be used. If the patient cannot swallow at all but has a working GI system, the drug may be given through an NG or a G tube. Drugs administered through tubes must be given in a liquid form. Drugs can be crushed and dissolved in water for instillation, except for sustained-release or enteric-coated drugs.

If patients can take oral drugs but have difficulty swallowing tablets, pills, and capsules, the drugs may be crushed and mixed in a few milliliters of water or liquid or in a tablespoon of jelly, applesauce, or pudding. Large volumes of fluid or food should be avoided because the patient must consume the full volume to receive the full drug dose. Alternately, a liquid drug form may be substituted. Sublingual drugs may be administered even to unconscious patients because these drug forms are so rapidly absorbed by the vasculature.

Life Span and Gender

The high sugar content of syrups can mask unpleasant drug flavors, making them useful vehicles for administering drugs orally to both adults and children. Because they usually contain little or no alcohol, syrups are especially good vehicles for drugs administered to children. Because of the potentially high alcohol content, elixirs are usually not used in children or in adults who should avoid ethanol.

Environment

Oral drug forms are easily self-administered by patients and can be used in home environments and acute or long-term care settings.

Planning and Intervention

Maximizing Therapeutic Effects

Capsules with sustained-release pellets in them can be opened and the pellets sprinkled on food or mixed with a liquid; the patient must eat or drink all the food or fluid. Because emulsions and suspensions have a tendency to separate, they should be shaken well immediately before measuring a dose and then administered promptly.

Drugs administered through an NG or a G tube should be instilled slowly without excessive force. Some may be allowed to flow in by gravity. The tube should be flushed with 10 to 30 mL of water before and after drug administration to ensure that the patient receives the full dose and to maintain the patency of the tube.

Minimizing Adverse Effects

Drugs that have enteric coatings and drugs in sustained-release form should never be chewed, crushed, or broken. Doing so increases the risk of adverse effects, including toxicity, because more drug is available all at once.

Repeated doses of sucrose-containing syrups may increase the risk of gingivitis or dental caries. Good oral hygiene should accompany the use of syrups. Also, diabetic patients may need to monitor their glucose levels closely if they are receiving large doses of drugs in syrups.

Before administering a drug through an NG or a G tube, the nurse must verify that the tube is in the stomach by checking for residual gastric contents. In addition, the head of the patient's bed should be elevated to help prevent aspiration from reflux. If the patient is also receiving tube feedings, the nurse should review information on the specific drug because some drugs are not absorbed well with tube feeding formulas.

To ensure safety, the nurse must closely follow the cardinal rules of drug administration. Historically known as five rights, a recent sixth right (i.e., documentation) has been added by some authors (see the accompanying display, Six Rights of Drug Administration).

To administer a drug at the "right time" using the "right route," the nurse must be able to read and interpret the medication order correctly. Standard abbreviations are frequently used in medication orders. The nurse needs to be knowledgeable about these abbreviations (Table 3-1). To administer the "right dose," dosage calculation is often necessary. The reader is referred to any drug dosage calculation book for all of the specific information needed. Information on calculating pediatric doses is provided in Chapter 7. Occasionally, the nurse may need to convert the unit of measurement for the drug to another unit of measurement (Table 3-2). ■

TABLE 3-1 Abbreviations Related to Medication Administration

Abbreviation	Meaning
a.c.	before meals
p.c.	after meals
qd	every day
qod	every other day
qhs	every night at hour of sleep
qam	every morning
bid	twice a day
tid	three times a day (usually limited to hours awake)
qid	four times a day (usually limited to hours awake)
q4h	every four hours
q6h	every six hours
qh	every hour
prn	as needed
ad lib	as desired
IM	intramuscularly
IV	intravenously
SQ or SC	subcutaneous
PO	by mouth
SL	sublinguinal
OD	right eye
OS	left eye
OU	both eyes
STAT	immediately

PARENTERAL ROUTE

The parenteral route is associated with all forms of drugs administered by a syringe, needle, or catheter. The three most commonly used parenteral routes are IM, SC, and IV.

INTRAMUSCULAR ADMINISTRATION

The **intramuscular** technique involves injecting drugs into certain muscles. This method requires specific knowledge of anatomy and aseptic technique. Because muscles have a good blood supply, drugs that are injected into a muscle will move directly into the bloodstream without having to be broken down and absorbed as are oral drugs processed by the GI tract. Thus, the onset of action is faster with IM injections. Muscles have more blood vessels than the SC tissue; therefore, the onset of action after IM injection occurs at a more rapid rate than after drugs injected subcutaneously.

Six Rights of Drug Administration

In managing drug therapy safely and effectively, the nurse must heed the six rights of drug administration:

right	Patient
right	Drug
right	Time
right	Dose
right	Route
right	Documentation

Drugs given IM can be administered in solutions or suspensions, such as oils or irritating chemicals. Many injectable drugs are dry powders and must be reconstituted before administration, possibly requiring a specific amount of diluent. Thin and watery solutions given IM move promptly into the blood vessels. Because suspensions or drugs with an oil base are thicker or more viscous, they move more slowly into the blood vessels. A deposit of the drug is formed within the muscle that is slowly moved into the bloodstream.

The most common sites for IM injection are the deltoid, dorsogluteal, ventrogluteal, rectus femoris, and vastus lateralis muscles. Students should refer to their nursing practice

TABLE 3-2 Measurement Equivalents

Metric	Household
1 milliliter or 1 cubic centimeter	
5 milliliters	1 teaspoon
15 milliliters	1 tablespoon
30 milliliters	2 tablespoons or 1 ounce
500 milliliters	1 pint
1,000 milliliters or 1 Liter	1 quart or 2 pints
1 gram or 1,000 milligrams or 10,000 micrograms	
1 kilogram or 1,000 grams	2.2 pounds

textbooks for more information on the specific techniques used for administering IM injections. Figure 3-1 shows the anatomic landmarks and identifies the injection sites for these muscles.

SUBCUTANEOUS ADMINISTRATION

Subcutaneous drugs are administered under the skin into fat and connective tissue. These drugs must be highly soluble, low volume (less than 2 mL in a good-sized adult), and nonirritating (to prevent tissue damage, tissue necrosis, and sterile abscess formation). Distribution of the drug is through the capillaries and is less rapid than by the IM route. Distribution slows if the patient has inadequate peripheral circulation or if the drug is administered into scar tissue, which is avascular; onset will therefore be delayed.

The SC route may be used for vaccines, insulin, heparin, and narcotics. The sites used for this route are the upper, lateral arm; anterior thigh; abdomen; and midback above the scapula. The size of the individual determines the angle of injection. Students should refer to nursing practice textbooks to review SC injection techniques. Figure 3-2 shows how to identify anatomic landmarks and sites for SC injections.

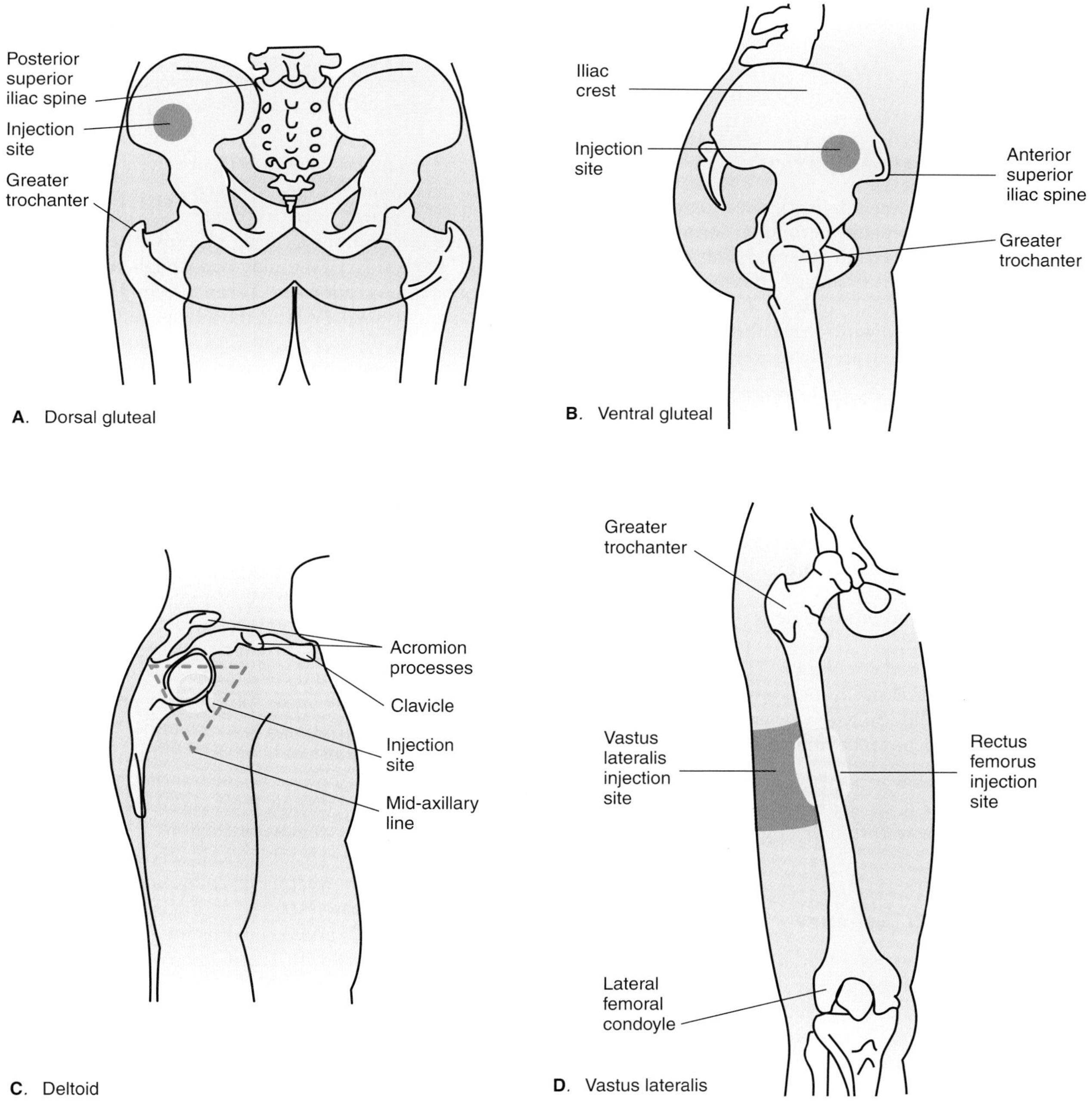

Figure 3-1. Anatomic landmarks and intramuscular (IM) injection sites: (**A**) dorsal gluteal; (**B**) ventral gluteal; (**C**) deltoid; (**D**) vastus lateralis and rectus femoris.

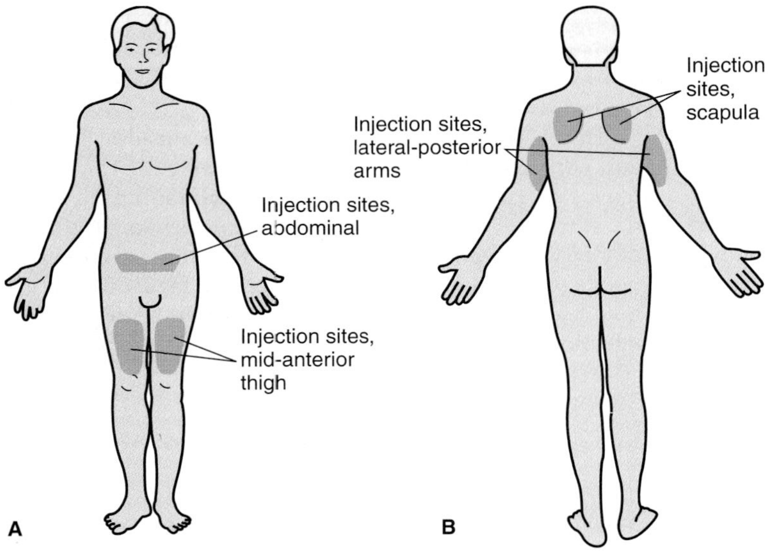

Figure 3-2. Subcutaneous (SC) injection sites: (**A**) anterior view: abdominal, mid-anterior thigh; (**B**) posterior view: scapula, lateral-posterior arms.

INTRAVENOUS ADMINISTRATION

The **intravenous** technique administers a drug directly into the bloodstream, bypassing the need for absorption from the GI tract or transportation from other parts of the body, such as muscle or subcutaneous tissue. IV administration ensures prompt, sometimes immediate, onset of action and eliminates the uncertainty associated with varied absorption rates from other routes. The following are advantages of the IV route:

- Has immediate effect (e.g., nitroprusside for a patient in hypertensive crisis)
- Allows administration of a large volume of drug (e.g., with certain antibiotics, such as cefoxitin)
- Avoids tissue irritation or injury resulting from IM or SC administration (e.g., with chemotherapeutic drugs, vasopressors, such as norepinephrine (Levophed), or cardiac glycosides, such as digoxin (Lanoxin), because the blood buffers the drug)
- Is acceptable when no other route is possible (e.g., in an unconscious patient)
- Circumvents impaired circulation
- Has potential for prolonged, continuous administration of solutions, such as lidocaine (Xylocaine) or aminophylline (Truphylline), which can be titrated for the desired effect

The IV route, however, is also one of the most dangerous routes. Once the drug is given, it cannot be readily retrieved, nor can its distribution through the body be slowed or stopped.

Peripheral Drug Delivery

A peripheral vascular access device, usually an angiocatheter or a butterfly set, is placed to give drugs intravenously. IV drug solutions may be run through tubing into the access device, either continually or intermittently.

Prescribed drugs may be given by continuous IV infusion to maintain a certain blood level of the drug. They are ordered either in volume (mL) per hour or strength (milligram [mg] or micrograms [μg]) per hour. Aminophylline, lidocaine, and heparin are examples of drugs that are given continuously to achieve maximum therapeutic effect.

When the patient receives continuous IV fluids and is also to receive intermittent IV drug therapy, the drug is given through a secondary IV tubing or through volumetric dose chamber administration sets. When a secondary IV tubing is used to administer an IV drug, the tubing is added to the main line tubing, usually at a Y port. This is called "piggybacking" because the tubing with the drug rides on top of the primary fluid tubing. Antibiotics are frequently given intermittently by **intravenous piggyback** (IV piggyback). Such drugs are diluted in a small volume of IV solution (usually 50–100 mL of sterile normal saline solution or 5% dextrose in water for an adult) and infused over 30 to 90 minutes (according to the specific drug). The main IV infusion then resumes at the original preset rate.

Volumetric chamber administration sets connect to the main bag of IV fluid and have IV tubing connected that attaches to the peripheral venous access device. They can be run as continuous infusions, in which fluid leaves the chamber and is replaced with fluid from the IV bag, or they can infuse only what is currently inside the chamber until manually refilled. When drugs are added to the chamber for infusion, the set is adjusted to infuse only what is in the chamber. When the drug is infused the set may be returned to a continuous infusion, or refilled with only the main IV solution. These sets are primarily used when fluid restrictions are important, such as with pediatric, elderly, or critically ill patients.

Certain IV drugs, whether given by piggyback or through a metered dose infusion set, may be incompatible with an existing continuous IV infusion. If this situation arises, the tubing should be flushed with 10 mL of an appropriate solution (usually sterile normal saline) before and after administration of the drug.

If intravenous drugs are prescribed intermittently, and other fluids are not running constantly, the access device is capped to prevent blood from coming out and bacteria from entering the body. This cap may be permanently attached to a small extension tubing set. This tubing is secured to the peripheral device. When an access device is equipped this way it is referred to as being "locked" or that the patient has a "lock" in place.

Drug infusion locks are used for patients who require intermittent IV drugs but who do not need continuous IV fluid administration. As with piggybacks, the drug is usually diluted in 50 to 100 mL of solution. When the drug infusion is complete the tubing is disconnected from the lock, allowing the patient more ease of movement. The lock is kept patent (open, without blood clotting occurring) with small volumes of either normal saline (0.9% sodium chloride) solution or heparin pushed through the lock on a routine basis, usually every 8 hours. Depending on the solution that is used for flushing, the lock device is commonly referred to as a saline lock or a heparin lock. Saline locks are flushed with 0.5 to 2 mL of sterile normal saline solution. Heparin locks are flushed with 10 to 100-U heparin. The nurse should be familiar with established institution protocols regarding the exact method for flushing drug infusion locks.

Direct administration into a vein or an established drug infusion lock of a concentrated drug in a very small amount of solution (usually 1–2 mL) is called an **intravenous push** (IVP or IV push). The drug is pushed into the vein very slowly over at least 1 minute. The exact amount of time depends on the drug and the dose. Drugs given by IVP may be used for intermittent dosing or for treating emergencies, such as cardiac arrest.

Central Access

Certain patients may require IV access for a prolonged time, or they may not be able to have peripheral vascular access devices inserted. Devices used for these patients include single or multilumen central venous catheters and implantable venous access ports. A central venous catheter is inserted by the health care provider into a vein (jugular or subclavian) near the heart. The catheter may have as many as three lumens to allow the administration of various solutions and drugs. Peripherally inserted central lines (PIC) or peripherally inserted midlines can be inserted by nurses specially skilled in the technique. These lines may also be multilumened, and drugs may be delivered continuously, intermittently, or by IVP.

An implantable vascular access port (VAP) is surgically implanted under the skin with the distal end inserted into a large central vein. A special needle (a Huber needle) is used to suffuse the drug into the port. These ports are used for intermittent infusions of, for example, antineoplastic drugs. Use of a VAP requires advanced skills and expertise on the part of the nurse.

OTHER PARENTERAL DELIVERY ROUTES

Other parenteral routes are intradermal, intra-articular, intra-arterial, and intrathecal, although these are not as common as IM, SC, and IV.

Intradermal injections are made into the dermis just below the epidermis. This technique is used primarily for local anesthesia and for sensitivity tests, such as allergy and tuberculin tests. A small needle (25-Ga or 27-Ga) and small-volume syringes (less than 1 mL) are used for intradermal injections. The most common sites for intradermal injections are the medial forearm and the back over the scapula because the skin is thinner there.

An **intra-articular** injection is performed only by a skilled practitioner and involves injecting a drug into a joint. Corticosteroids are typically administered by intra-articular injection to relieve pain in an acutely inflamed joint. The effect is local.

Intra-arterial drug administration requires a surgeon to insert a catheter into an artery leading directly to the targeted treatment area. The drug is delivered under positive pressure through the catheter. The positive pressure overcomes the pressure within the arterial system. For example, powerful undiluted chemotherapeutic agents can be delivered directly to a tumor by way of the artery that feeds it. Intra-arterial ports can also be implanted by a surgeon.

In **intrathecal** administration, a drug is delivered into the cerebrospinal fluid. It may be administered directly into the spinal subarachnoid space (a spinal) or outside the subarachnoid space (an epidural). Drugs are introduced into these areas by a catheter placed by specially trained health care providers. The drugs most commonly used are local anesthetics, antibiotics, and radiographic contrast media. This route is commonly used to deliver an anesthetic during labor and delivery. Pain relief can also be achieved with drugs given over this route by the nurse or by the patient using a patient-controlled analgesia device.

NURSING MANAGEMENT IN PARENTERAL DRUG ADMINISTRATION

Parenteral administration may be selected for a variety of reasons. This route allows drugs to be distributed directly to the vascular system without having to be absorbed by the GI tract and sent to the liver before circulating. The erratic absorption associated with the movement of the drug through the GI tract is avoided. Drugs that are highly metabolized by the first-pass mechanism can be given in smaller doses when given parenterally rather than orally as more drug is presented to the vascular system initially. Some drugs are almost completely metabolized during the first pass, so the parenteral route for these drugs is chosen exclusively. Moreover, drugs that are rapidly destroyed by GI secretions can be given parenterally to promote their effectiveness. Parenteral routes may also be necessary because of the GI irritant nature of the drug. Drugs administered by the parenteral routes have a faster onset of action than those administered orally or topically.

Assessment of Relevant Core Patient Variables

Health Status

A parenteral route may be chosen because the patient cannot tolerate oral drugs, cannot swallow, or has a condition that warrants resting the GI tract or keeping it empty. Muscle mass needs to be sufficient for the volume of drug if given intramuscularly. The gluteal muscle mass can deteriorate if the person does not walk (e.g., because of paralysis), and in such cases may need to be avoided as a site for IM injections. The patient's veins must be able to accept a venous access device if drugs are to be given intravenously. When peripheral access devices cannot be inserted, central venous access devices may be used.

Life Span and Gender

Infants have small muscle mass. The largest muscle mass at birth is the vastus lateralis. This is the preferred site for IM injections in infants, although the rectus femoris may also be used. The deltoid is never used for IM injections in infants. The gluteal muscles develop with walking and usually are not used for injections until the child has been walking for 1 year. Elderly people have decreased muscle mass overall and decreased tissue elasticity, which may result in drugs oozing from injection sites. Muscle mass needs to be determined prior to IM injections.

Lifestyle, Diet, and Habits

Parenteral forms of drugs are more expensive than oral forms. Parenteral administration requires specialized skills, equipment, and education. Placement of IV access devices into peripheral veins may be difficult for patients who are IV substance abusers.

Environment

Patients, particularly diabetic patients who receive insulin, can be taught to give themselves SC injections at home. The techniques for IM injections can also be taught to patients and their families for home use, although this is not as common. IV administration of drugs is usually done in an acute or a long-term care setting; however, it can also be done in the home setting with a home health nurse administering the drug therapy.

Planning and Intervention

Maximizing Therapeutic Effects

Selecting the appropriate-sized syringe and needle is key to administering an IM or SC injection in the desired location. Selection is based on the patient, the type of required injection, the administration site, and characteristics of the drug (how viscous, how irritating, and how much volume).

A continuous IV infusion should be monitored to ensure that therapeutic blood levels are achieved and that drug therapy is effective. After administration of an intermittent IV drug, the lock needs to be flushed to maintain patency. If heparin is used to keep the lock patent, it is normally necessary to flush the lock prior to drug infusion with sterile normal saline solution, and then again after the infusion before flushing with the heparin. This is because many drugs are incompatible with heparin.

Minimizing Adverse Effects

To prevent infections, the drug, all parts of the syringe that have come into contact with the drug, and the shaft of the needle that enters the patient's body must be sterile. Meticulous administration technique is needed because most parenteral drugs enter the bloodstream readily, quickly spreading any organisms introduced with the injection.

Site selection is important because incorrect placement of the needle may damage blood vessels or nerves. Knowledge of the muscles, visible or palpable anatomic landmarks, and location of major nerves and blood vessels in the underlying tissue is an absolute necessity for safe administration.

The oils and irritating chemicals found in the solutions or suspensions of some parenteral drugs may be dangerous if given IV. Care must be taken by careful site selection and aspiration before injection to prevent the inadvertent administration of an IM drug into a blood vessel.

To prevent bacterial growth, reconstituted drugs usually require refrigeration if they are not completely used after dilution. The reconstituted drug container needs to be labeled with the patient's name, dilution date, and volume and type of diluent used.

When administering drugs that are very irritating to the tissues, the nurse may use an injection technique known as the Z-track method to prevent the drug from seeping up from the muscle into the SC tissue. SC tissue is displaced to one side prior to inserting the needle into the muscle. The drug is then injected, the needle withdrawn, and the SC tissue allowed to go back into place. Students are referred to their nursing practice texts for more detailed information.

Patients receiving drugs such as aminophylline, dopamine, and heparin by continuous IV infusion need to be closely monitored. These drugs have powerful effects on the body, and their adverse effects can be serious or life threatening. The rate of administration of drugs such as these should be regulated carefully by using an IV pump or controller. Because the drug enters the bloodstream directly, blood levels of the drug can rise above desired therapeutic levels quickly. Blood levels, therefore, should be closely monitored.

See the accompanying display, Choosing the Right Drug Administration Site, for a critical thinking approach to choosing an administration route. ■

TOPICAL ROUTE AND FORMS

The topical route of drug administration involves applying drug preparations to the skin or mucous membranes, including the eyes, ears, nose, rectum, vagina, and lungs. The pri-

Critical Thinking Scenario

Choosing the right drug administration site

Georgia Govans, 79 years old, is admitted with osteomyelitis of the hip, a severe infection, after a recent repair of a hip fracture. She has a temperature of 101°F on admission and a history of severe peripheral vascular disease.

1. Consider which route will most likely be chosen to administer antibiotics to this patient.
2. Select and support a choice of drug delivery method based on the patient's history and her drug requirements.

mary advantage is that topical drugs usually act locally, although some can have systemic effects. A disadvantage of topical drugs is that most are intended for only one specific site. For example, ophthalmic drugs are only used in the eyes, and dermatologic drugs are only used on the skin. Drugs that can be administered in topical forms include antibiotics, antiseptics, antifungals, anti-inflammatory agents, antipyretics, vasodilators, hormones, antismoking agents, analgesics, antiemetics, and débriding agents.

The most common and widely used topical agents are applied to the skin. Dermatologic preparations come in several forms: lotion, creams, liquids, ointments, and emollients. Emollients are applied liberally to dry skin. Most drugs applied to the intact skin have primarily local effects because little drug is absorbed through the outer epidermis. Absorption increases under the following circumstances:

- The skin is abraded or denuded.
- The drug is added to a specific solvent because only lipid-soluble substances are absorbed through the intact skin.
- The medicated skin is covered by an occlusive dressing (e.g., in treatment for psoriasis).

Most dermatologic drugs are applied in a thin layer or in a measured amount (topical nitroglycerin is applied in inches). Single-dose, adhesive-backed drug applications, called transcutaneous or transdermal drug delivery systems, are currently available. Some examples of the transdermal drug delivery route include nitroglycerin (Nitro-Dur) for patients with coronary artery disease, scopolamine (Transderm-Scop) for patients who suffer from motion sickness, and fentanyl (Duragesic) for patients with severe pain. Although this drug form can be expensive, its ability to avoid first-pass effects is an advantage. The transdermal system usually requires less frequent application and is convenient.

Drugs administered to the eye take the form of drops or ointments that are applied to the rim of the lower lid. Drugs administered in the ear are in the form of drops. Drugs administered through the rectum are either in suppositories (waxy, bullet-shaped systems that dissolve in the body from body heat) or ointments. Drugs administered into the vagina are in the form of suppositories, creams, foams, liquids, or tablets (moistened prior to insertion to promote dissolving inside the body).

Drugs given into the nose are either in liquid sprays, drops, or aerosol preparations. Inhalers, another form of aerosolized therapy, are used for respiratory conditions and have an effect on the lungs but are inhaled through mouth breathing. Patients should shake the inhaler well, exhale fully, and then inhale while pushing down on the inhaler to activate it. They should breathe in the puff of drug and hold the breath for several seconds before exhaling. The timing of this is difficult for many patients. The use of a spacer, which acts as a reservoir for the drug, is helpful for many patients. The patient activates the inhaler, and the drug enters the spacer. The patient then breathes in from the spacer. If multiple puffs of the inhaler are ordered, the patient should wait 1 to 2 minutes between puffs. The inhaler and the patient's mouth should be rinsed after drug administration.

NURSING MANAGEMENT IN TOPICAL DRUG ADMINISTRATION

Assessment of Relevant Core Patient Variables

For the most part, assessment involves inspecting the skin for integrity. If the skin is not intact, aseptic technique becomes an important factor in infection control.

Planning and Intervention

To maximize therapeutic effects and minimize adverse effects, the nurse should wear gloves or use an applicator when administering dermatologic drugs to avoid infecting the patient and to protect his or her own skin from the drug. If the skin is broken, the nurse needs to use sterile technique when applying a dermatologic drug to prevent introducing bacteria and other organisms into the body. If an adverse effect occurs with drugs given by a transdermal system, removing the patch usually relieves the symptoms.

To ensure safety when administering all forms of topical drugs, the nurse must again observe the six rights of drug administration. ■

CHAPTER SUMMARY

- The three routes of drug administration are enteral, parenteral, and topical.
- The drug route may produce systemic effects, local effects, or both.
- Oral drugs may also be in sustained-release or enteric-coated form to delay onset of action of the drug.
- Food, fluids, and other drugs may alter the absorption of enteric drugs.
- The parenteral route avoids the GI tract and the irregularities of absorption, including the first-pass effect. The most common methods of parenteral drug administration are the IM, SC, and IV routes.
- Onset of drug action is more rapid with the parenteral than with the enteral route.
- Patient characteristics (age, weight, muscle mass) and drug characteristics (volume, viscosity, irritability) are considered when selecting a site for IM drug administration.

- Administration of IV drugs may be through continuous drip, intermittent infusion, or IVP methods into peripheral or central venous access devices.
- Topical drugs include those that are applied to the skin and mucous membranes of the eyes, ears, nose, rectum, and vagina.

QUESTIONS FOR STUDY AND REVIEW

1. Which route of drug administration is most frequently used?
2. What is the advantage of an enteric-coated tablet?
3. Why might a parenteral route of a drug be prescribed instead of an enteral route?
4. Which parenteral technique poses the greatest risk for rapid drug toxicity to a patient?

NEED MORE HELP?

Chapter 3 of the study guide for *Drug Therapy in Nursing* contains exercises and activities to reinforce your understanding of the concepts presented in this chapter. For additional information see the text's accompanying web site at *http://www.connection.lww.com*.

REFERENCES AND BIBLIOGRAPHY

Anderson, R. P. (1998). Alternative routes of opioid administration in palliative care: Pharmacologic and clinical concerns. *Journal of Pharmaceutical Care in Pain & Symptom Control, 6*(1), 5–21.

Anonymous. (1997). Position statement. Insulin administration. *Diabetes Care, 20*(Suppl. 1), 546–549.

Basskin, L. E. (1999). New pharmacotherapy. Oral transmucosal fentanyl citrate: A new dosage form for breakthrough malignant pain. *American Journal of Pain Management, 9*(4), 129–138.

Belknap, D. C., Seifer, C. F., & Petermann, M. (1997). Administration of medications through enteral feeding catheters. *American Journal of Critical Care, 6*(5), 382–392.

Grond, S., Radbruch, L., & Lehmann, K. A. (2000). Clinical pharmacokinetics of transdermal opioids: focus on transdermal fentanyl. *Clinical Pharmacokinetics, 38*(1), 59–89.

McConnell, E. A. (1997). Clinical do's and don'ts. Using transdermal medication patches. *Nursing, 27*(7), 18.

Naysmith, M. R., & Nicholson, J. (1998) Nasogastric drug administration. *Professional Nurse, 13*(7), 424–427.

Roger, M. A., & King, L. (2000). Drawing up and administering intramuscular injections: A review of the literature. *Journal of Advanced Nursing, 31*(3), 574–582.

Sharar, S. R., Bratton, S. L., Carrougher, G. J., Edwards, W. T., Summer, G., Levy, F. H., & Cortiella, J. (1998). A comparison of oral transmucosal fentanyl citrate and oral hydromorphone for inpatient pediatric burn wound care analgesia. *Journal of Burn Care and Rehabilitation, 19*(6), 516–521.

Starr, C. (2000). Innovations in drug delivery. *Patient Care, 34*(1), 107–108, 113–114, 117–121.

Unit II

Core Drug Knowledge

Chapter 4

PHARMACOTHERAPEUTICS AND PHARMACOKINETICS

KEY TERMS

absorption
active transport
bioavailability
biotransformation
blood-brain barrier
clearance
competitive binding
distribution
enterohepatic cycling
excretion
filtration
first-pass phenomenon
half-life
metabolism
metabolites
nonspecific binding
passive diffusion
pharmacokinetics
pharmacotherapeutics
pinocytosis
placental barrier
plasma-protein binding
solubility
steady state

Learning Objectives

At the completion of this chapter the student will:

1. Define pharmacotherapeutics and pharmacokinetics.
2. Describe how drug administration routes and dosage forms affect drug absorption.
3. Identify factors that affect absorption of drug molecules.
4. Identify the ways that drugs cross cell membranes.
5. Describe factors that influence the distribution of drug molecules.
6. Discuss factors that may alter the biotransformation process.
7. Explain how decreased plasma protein binding may cause an excess of free drug in the body.
8. Identify how drug molecules are excreted from the body.

As health care delivery settings, policies, and personnel evolve and change, today's nurse must focus more than ever on ensuring safe and effective patient care, especially in drug therapy. The nurse must be knowledgeable in administering drugs and determining the patient's actual response to drug therapy, as well as in anticipating, interpreting, and reporting drug actions and interactions. To carry out these responsibilities, the nurse needs a solid understanding of pharmacotherapeutics and pharmacokinetics.

PHARMACOTHERAPEUTICS

Pharmacotherapeutics is the reason why the drug is prescribed and the clinical indication for its use. Pharmacotherapeutics directly relates to core drug knowledge and core patient variables such as life span and gender (see the accompanying display, Gender-Related Differences in Pharmacotherapeutics). In pharmacotherapy, drugs are used to prevent, diagnose, relieve, treat, or cure disease because a drug is a substance that interacts with a living organism to produce a biologic response. This is termed the therapeutic use of a drug. Typically, a response to a drug results from a biochemical or physiologic interaction between the drug and a cellular component (receptor) to which a drug binds to produce its effects. Exceptions to this include antacids, free radicals, osmotic diuretics, and chelators of heavy metals.

DOSE-RESPONSE RELATIONSHIP

The dose required to produce a desired therapeutic response can vary substantially among patients. The dose-response curve describes the relationship between the dose of a drug administered and the response it produces. The curve is determined by plotting the observed clinical response on a linear scale against a logarithmic scale of the drug dose used to gain that response.

A drug that produces a greater effect at a lower dose than another drug is considered to have a greater potency. Potency—the product of a drug's affinity and efficacy—reflects its overall ability as an agonist to stimulate a receptor. The dose-response curve illustrates two important points: first, each drug-induced response has a threshold; second, this response will reach a plateau rather than increase indefinitely. Drugs produce multiple predictable biologic effects. Each effect has its own distinctive dose-response relationship, and a curve may be drawn for each one of them. The safety of a drug is partly indicated by its dose-response curve. A gradual slope indicates that a relatively large change in dose will produce a relatively small change in effect. Conversely, a steep slope means that a small change in dose will produce very large changes in drug response. The drug with a steep dose-response curve will be difficult to administer safely.

Each drug has its own characteristic rates of absorption, distribution, metabolism, and excretion. The relationship between the plasma concentrations of the drug and the level of therapeutic effectiveness is demonstrated by the anticonvulsant drug, phenytoin (Dilantin). If indicated, monitoring the plasma level of a compound yields information about the efficacy and safety of a drug and allows it to be more closely controlled in terms of dosage, scheduling, and route of administration.

Gender-Related Differences in Pharmacotherapeutics

- Men appear less affected than women by nicotine and components of tobacco smoke that adversely affect the cardiovascular system.
- Women demonstrate a greater response to antihypertensive drug therapy.
- Gender response to thrombolytic and oral anticoagulant treatment following myocardial infarction is unequal with women showing less benefit and greater incidences of bleeding.
- Prophylactic low-dose aspirin therapy (325 mg/day) is equally beneficial, although there is unequal benefit in decreasing the risk of cerebral vascular accident.
- The female myocardium is smaller and appears to have electrophysiologic differences; women may be more prone to suffer sudden death during therapy with an antiarrhythmic agent.
- Women demonstrate a greater frequency of autoimmune diseases because of their stronger antibody reaction. Autoimmune diseases showing sex-dependent incidence (ratio of female: male cases) are thyroid disease (15:1), multiple sclerosis (2:1), osteoporosis (4:1), scleroderma (4:1), systemic lupus erythematosus (9:1). (Davis, 1998; Lewis, 2000).

PHARMACOKINETICS

Pharmacokinetics, which refers to the ways in which the body processes drugs, is a mathematical science. The four basic components of pharmacokinetics are absorption, distribution, metabolism, and excretion (abbreviated as ADME) (see Figure 2-1). These components describe the quantitative and time-dependent changes of the drug in both the plasma drug concentration and the total amount of the drug in the body.

Absorption is the process by which a drug moves from its site of administration into the venous or lymphatic circulation. Any drug (except those injected IV) must first be absorbed before it can produce an action within the body. Absorption is described in terms of rate and extent. As a general rule, some drug is lost during the absorption process, so that only a portion of the drug administered is available to produce a pharmacologic effect. **Bioavailability** is the term used to describe the fraction of the administered dose that reaches the systemic circulation and produces effects.

Distribution is the delivery of the drug into any and all body compartments it can penetrate. Distribution delivers the drug from the bloodstream to its site(s) of action (e.g., interstitial and cellular fluids) as well as sites where no effects are produced (e.g., sites where storage or inactivation occurs). Finally, the drug must be eliminated. Drug elimination usually begins with hepatic metabolism and is followed with renal excretion.

Metabolism (also known as biotransformation) is the alteration or changing of a drug to more ionized or water-soluble and less lipid-soluble forms called **metabolites.** Drug excretion usually finishes through renal excretion; most drugs are renally eliminated either as drug metabolites or unchanged drug molecules.

ADME processes are interrelated and involve drug passage across cell membranes.

ABSORPTION

Absorption is the movement of a drug from its site of administration to the bloodstream. The rate, extent, and efficiency of absorption depend on both the dosage form of the drug and the route of administration. Therefore, selection of the drug preparation and administration route may depend on the unique properties of the drug or how rapidly the therapeutic objective is desired. Drugs reach the systemic circulation enterally (i.e., through the gastrointestinal [GI] tract) or by routes that bypass the GI tract (e.g., parenteral or topical routes). The dosage form of a drug and its route of drug administration have important consequences for the pharmacokinetic processes. Additional factors influencing drug absorption include drug solubility and ionization of drug solution.

Drug Dosage Forms

Drug formulations in a liquid (e.g., elixir, suspension, etc.) are immediately available for absorption, because the drug is already in solution. Drugs administered in a semisolid or solid form must first disintegrate and dissolve into a solution before absorption can occur. Enteric coating of capsules or tablets delays disintegration; these forms are formulated specifically to disintegrate in the alkaline environment of the small intestine.

Routes of Drug Administration

The route of administration for a drug is primarily determined by its chemical properties (e.g., solubility in water or lipids) and the therapeutic or treatment objective (e.g., rapid onset of action, localized effect) for its use. Two major routes of drug administration are enteral and parenteral. Table 4-1

TABLE 4-1 Absorption Characteristics Related to Common Drug Administration Routes

Route	Pattern of Absorption	Advantages	Limitations and Precautions
IV	No absorption occurs. Effects are immediate.	Ideal for emergency use Accommodates large doses Suitable for irritating substances (which must be diluted)	Increased risk for adverse reactions Should be injected slowly (few exceptions) Unsuitable for oily solutions or insoluble substances Risk of infection Not suitable for routine self-administration
SC	Aqueous solution promotes prompt absorption. Depot preparations (oily) promote slow or sustained absorption. Absorption depends on local blood flow.	Suitable for implantation of solid pellets Suitable for some insoluble suspensions	Unsuitable for large volumes Irritating substances—possibility of pain or tissue necrosis
IM	Aqueous solution promotes prompt absorption. Depot preparations (oily) exhibit slow or sustained absorption. Absorption depends on local blood flow.	Suitable for moderate volumes, oily preparations, and some irritating substances	Contraindicated with anticoagulants Increases creatine phosphokinase (CPK), a benchmark for MI and muscle damage, and may interfere with diagnostic values and interpretation Injection possibly painful
PO	Absorption is highly dependent on many variables.	Convenient Economical Relatively safe	Requires patient adherence Bioavailability potentially erratic because of many variables Unsuitable for patients with dysphagia
Topical	Absorption is incomplete, erratic, unless drug is specifically formulated for this route. Absorption is slow.	High patient acceptability Convenient and easy to use	Few drugs available in topical formulations Possible systemic absorption from applications to damaged skin
Inhalation	Absorption is rapid.	Aerosol forms readily available Convenient and easy to use	Requires patient instruction to use nebulizer correctly May cause coughing or wheezing
Rectal	Absorption may be erratic.	Useful for small children or unconscious patients May provide local or systemic effect	May be uncomfortable for conscious patients Systemic effect possible from absorption

describes absorption characteristics related to various drug administration routes.

Enteral Drug Administration

Drugs administered enterally can be absorbed in the oral or gastric mucosa, or in the small or large intestines. This route is also routinely associated with the administration of fluids and nutrients (e.g., tube feedings).

Oral Route. Administering drugs by mouth (PO, abbreviation for the Latin *per ora*) is the most common route of enteral drug administration. It is convenient, inexpensive, and relatively safe and simple. However, this route involves one of the most complicated pathways to the tissues. Although some drugs are absorbed from the stomach, most drugs are absorbed from the duodenum by a passive process. Drugs entering the body by the enteral route first go through the portal circulation to the liver before reaching the general circulation; this process is known as the first-pass phenomenon (or effect). First-pass metabolism may significantly limit a drug's effectiveness by extensively breaking down the drug before it ever reaches the general circulation. For example, more than 90% of nitroglycerin is eliminated by the hepatic first-pass phenomenon. Drugs that are highly metabolized during the first-pass effect will lose much of their active dose before ever entering the general circulation. In contrast, drugs that are not highly metabolized will lose little of their active dose, with most of the drug dose entering the general circulation.

Sublingual and Buccal Drugs. Sublingual and buccal drugs have a distinct advantage over oral drugs that are swallowed. Placement under the tongue or in the cheek allows the drug to diffuse directly into the capillary network and enter the general circulation, bypassing the first-pass phenomenon.

Parenteral Drug Administration

Drugs administered parenterally bypass the GI tract. The parenteral route is used for drugs requiring rapid onset of action, for patients who are unconscious, for drugs that are completely inactivated by the first-pass phenomenon, and for drugs that are unstable, unpredictable, and poorly absorbed within the GI tract. Parenteral drug administration provides the greatest control over the actual dose delivered.

Parenteral routes include intravenous (IV), intramuscular (IM), subcutaneous (SC), intradermal (ID), and intra-articular (IA) and intrathecal. All nurses may use the IV, IM, SC, and ID routes; advanced practice nurses may use the IA and intrathecal routes as well. A distinct advantage to parenteral drugs is that they present fewer barriers between the sites of drug administration and drug action. They must still be absorbed, however, to exert a pharmacologic effect on the system.

Intravenous Route. The most common parenteral route is IV; using this route, the drug bypasses the hepatic first-pass phenomenon. Injected directly into a vein, absorption is instantaneous and complete. Infusion times may be rapid—seconds to minutes—when the drug is injected as a bolus (a single, relatively large quantity of a substance intended for therapeutic use). Infusion times may be hours when the drug is administered through an intermittent or continuous IV drip.

Intramuscular Route. Intramuscular injection is a common route of parenteral drug administration. Absorption of parenterally administered drugs depends on the type of solution. For example, a water-based aqueous solution is absorbed rapidly. Some drug formulations (e.g., emulsions, suspensions) are slow in dissolving to delay absorption and to prolong systemic effects. Other factors that influence absorption are the size of the muscle and circulation to the muscle.

Subcutaneous Route. The SC route carries drugs into the region just below the epidermis. After an SC injection, drug diffusion into the capillary network injection occurs at a somewhat slower rate than that following IM injection and much faster than the intradermal route. From a pharmacokinetic perspective (ADME characteristics), however, the SC and IM routes are considered nearly identical.

Intradermal Route. The ID route involves administering a substance just between the skin layers. Drugs administered in this manner diffuse slowly into the local microcapillary system. Generally, this route is used for instilling substances of various strengths during allergy testing.

Intra-articular and Intrathecal Routes. A drug is delivered directly into the synovial fluid of the joint with IA administration; anti-inflammatory and local anesthetic drugs are routinely administered by this route for a localized effect. With this method, systemic drug absorption is negligible.

Intrathecal administration places the drug directly into the subarachnoid or subdural space; this method is indicated when it is impossible to achieve sufficient plasma levels for diffusion into the cerebrospinal fluid. Examples of drugs administered by the intrathecal route are epidural anesthetics and analgesics and some antineoplastics. Because this method bypasses the blood–brain barrier, the drug is absorbed directly into the central nervous system target.

Other Routes of Drug Administration

Topical Route. The topical route involves applying specific drug formulations (e.g., creams, gels, liquids, ointments, solutions) to the cornea, skin, or mucous membranes of the eye, mouth, nose, oropharynx, rectum, urethra, and vagina. This route is used for localized or systemic effects through transdermal or transmucosal effects. Topical drug preparations have anesthetic, antiinflammatory, antimicrobial, antiseptic, astringent, bacteriostatic, cleansing, emollient, or fungicidal effects. Advantages to topical drug administration are that absorption through mucous membranes occurs readily, drugs quickly enter the vascular system, and GI secretions do not destroy them.

Inhalation or Intranasal Route. The lungs serve as a major site of administration for a number of agents. Inhalation drugs vaporize easily or can be dispersed as a gas (e.g., anesthetics or breathing treatment) or by an aerosol device. They are readily and rapidly absorbed because of the large surface area of the alveolar membrane and the micron-sized drug particles. They may provide a local effect (e.g., bronchodilation), or a systemic effect (e.g., vasopressin for antidiuretic effect, cromolyn for prophylactic antiallergic effects).

Rectal Route. Drugs absorbed from suppositories in the lower rectum enter vessels that drain into the inferior vena cava, thus bypassing the liver. The rectal route prevents decreased stomach pH, intestinal enzymes, or the hepatic first-pass phenomenon from completely inactivating or destroying a drug.

The rate and extent of rectal drug absorption are slower compared with oral absorption, although this does not correlate to serum levels. Studies show that serum levels for some rectally administered drugs exceed serum levels found after oral administration.

Suppositories tend to move upward in the rectum into a region where veins that lead to the liver (e.g., superior hemorrhoidal vein) predominate. Consequently, only about 50% of a rectal dose can be assumed to bypass the liver (Katzung, 1998). Like the sublingual route, the rectal route facilitates drug absorption with drugs that produce nausea or vomiting in a patient who is already vomiting. It is a suitable route for patients who cannot take oral drugs or who are unconscious.

Transdermal Route. Transdermal drug delivery systems are small, drug-impregnated patches, which when applied to the skin, provide continuous and sustained drug delivery for a constant, steady drug-blood concentration level. The epidermis of intact skin acts as a lipid barrier, allowing absorption of only lipid-soluble substances.

Ophthalmic and Otic Routes. Ophthalmic and otic preparations are used primarily for local effects. Ophthalmic preparations in solution form are absorbed rapidly and more slowly in ointment form. A conjunctival sac insert (sometimes called a membrane-controlled drug delivery system) provides a sustained-release preparation. Drainage through the nasolacrimal canal, however, does allow some absorption, and some systemic effects may occur. This systemic absorption avoids the hepatic first-pass phenomenon. Conversely, otic drugs have a negligible systemic absorption.

Drug Solubility

Solubility refers to the ability of a drug to dissolve and form a solution. Two primary factors in drug absorption are drug solubility and ability of the drug to move through cell membranes. Water solubility is important for a solid drug that is given orally because the drug must first disintegrate and dissolve in the aqueous fluids of the GI tract. Drugs already in liquid form (e.g., solutions, emulsions, suspensions) bypass this process. Typically, a drug already in solution will be absorbed faster than the same drug in a solid form, which must first disintegrate and dissolve.

Lipid solubility is essential for any drug that must diffuse across the cell membrane because the membrane is partially composed of lipids. Lipid solubility depends on the drug's chemical structure and is influenced by the cellular environment at the absorptive site. Many drugs are lipid soluble as well as water soluble and can dissolve in body fluids and pass through cell membranes. In this case, the administration route is unimportant.

Generally, the faster and more completely a drug dissolves at its absorptive site, the more rapidly it will be absorbed and therapeutic effects occur.

Ionization

Ionization has an important influence on how effectively absorption occurs. A molecule dissociates into ions when it dissolves in water or other liquids. In dissociating, the molecule gives up or accepts a proton, thus converting some molecules into charged particles (i.e., ions). Ionized drugs are poorly absorbed, because they do not diffuse easily across lipid membranes. Conversely, nonionized drug molecules are lipid soluble and easily pass through lipid membranes. Rarely are drugs all ionized or nonionized; usually there is an equilibrium between the two.

Whether ionization occurs is largely determined by the pH of the surrounding medium. Typically, the pH of the absorptive environment determines the extent to which a molecule will ionize. For example, an acidic drug (e.g., aspirin) would remain nonionized and be well absorbed within the acidic environment of the stomach. Conversely, an alkaline drug would ionize in the stomach's acidic environment and not be absorbed in the stomach but instead be absorbed within the alkaline environment of the small intestine. This is the rationale for enteric-coated or timed-release drug formulations.

Processes of Drug Absorption

Depending on their chemical properties, drugs may be absorbed from the GI tract by one of several different passive or active methods. Figure 4-1 illustrates some of these methods.

Passive Processes

Passive processes of drug absorption include diffusion, facilitated diffusion, and filtration.

Diffusion. Diffusion is the process by which gas and liquid molecules move from an area of higher concentration to an area of lower concentration to become equally distributed across the cell membrane. Lipid-soluble molecules (e.g., alcohol, carbon dioxide, fatty acids, oxygen) readily move across most biologic membranes after dissolving in the lipid matrix of the membrane. Water-soluble drugs penetrate the cell membrane through aqueous channels. Most drugs are distributed through diffusion.

Facilitated Diffusion. In facilitated diffusion, a carrier system transports substances across the cell membrane without energy expenditure. Some substances (e.g., glucose) are too large to pass through the pores and are unable to dissolve in lipids. At the membrane's outer surface, these substances combine with a special lipid-soluble carrier that then transports them across the cell membrane. Molecular movement

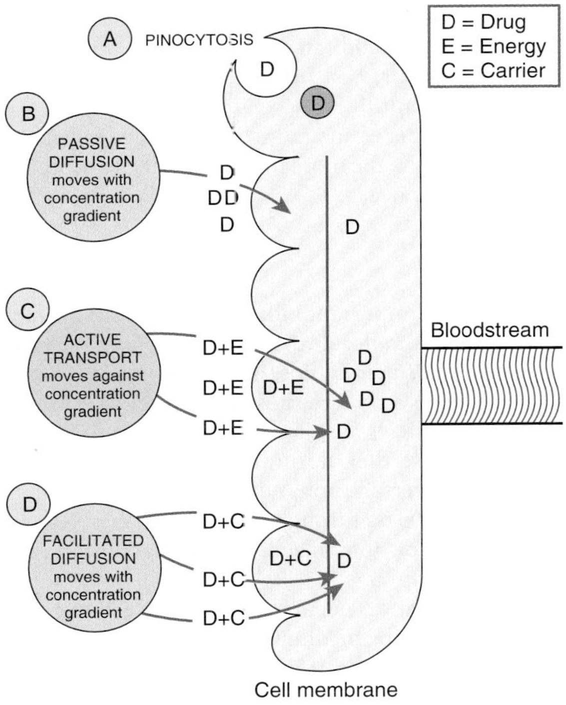

Figure 4-1. Medications move across the cell membrane by passive diffusion (i.e., moving with concentration gradient), active transport (i.e., moving against a concentration gradient so that energy is required), and facilitated diffusion (i.e., moving with concentration gradient but a carrier is needed). (Adapted from Kuhn, Merrily [1998]. *Pharmacotherapeutics: A Nursing Process Approach.* Philadelphia: F. A. Davis.)

in facilitated diffusion is similar to that of passive diffusion—substances move from areas of higher concentrations to areas of lower concentration. A carrier is needed to cross the cell membrane, but energy is not required because the drug does not move across a concentration gradient. The rate of movement depends on three factors:

1. The differences in drug concentrations
2. The amount of readily available carrier
3. The speed at which the carrier binds and releases the transported substance

Insulin is an example of a drug distributed by facilitated diffusion.

Filtration. **Filtration** is the passage of a drug through the pores of a semipermeable membrane. This type of transport is regulated by the concentration of osmotically active particles on either side of the membrane. To achieve balance (equal dilution of solute particles on either side of the cell membrane), osmotic or hydrostatic pressure drives the molecules down a concentration gradient. Although filtration has a minor role in drug absorption, it is an important and essential component in the excretion of many drugs.

Active Processes

Active processes of drug absorption include active transport and pinocytosis.

Active Transport. **Active transport** is similar to facilitated diffusion, except that an energy source is required to move molecules across the cell membrane because this movement takes place against a concentration gradient (from an area of lower to an area of higher concentration) or an electrochemical gradient (e.g., "sodium-potassium pump"). Generally, active transport is more rapid than passive diffusion.

Pinocytosis. During **pinocytosis** the cell membrane surrounds and engulfs a substance on its outer surface, forms a membrane-covered vesicle, and carries it inside the cell.

Pinocytosis is important in the transport of proteins and strong electrolyte solutions. Cells commonly use pinocytosis to transport fat-soluble vitamins (i.e., A, D, E, and K).

Bioavailability

Bioavailability is the fraction of administered drug that reaches the systemic circulation. For example, if 100 mg of a drug is administered orally and 70 mg of the drug is absorbed unchanged, the bioavailability is 70%. Bioavailability is determined by comparing a drug's peak plasma level after a particular mode of administration (e.g., oral) with peak plasma drug levels following IV injection, in which the entire drug dosage enters the circulation. The extent of drug absorption may be calculated by plotting plasma concentrations of the drug versus time and measured by the area under the curve (AUC). The curve reflects the extent of drug absorption.

Figure 4-2 illustrates the bioavailability of a drug administered both IV and PO. Factors that influence bioavailability are first-pass hepatic metabolism, solubility of the drug, chemical instability in gastric pH, and drug formulation.

Drug Absorption and Core Patient Variables

The general health status of the patient, influenced by certain core patient variables, has a direct bearing on drug absorption (see the accompanying display, Drug Absorption and Core Patient Variables).

$$\text{Bioavailability} = \frac{\text{AUC oral}}{\text{AUC injected}} \times 100$$

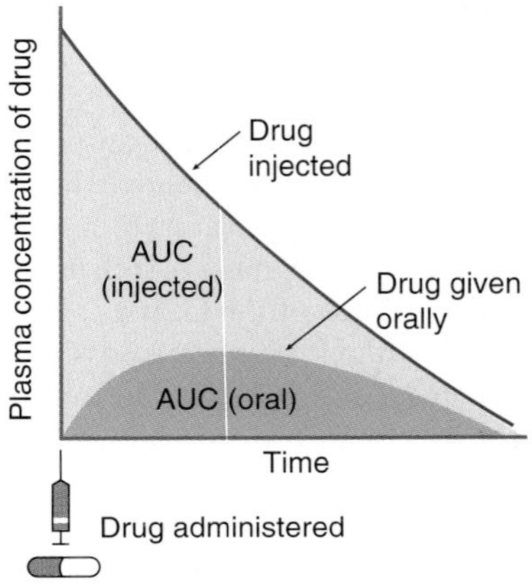

Figure 4-2. Determination of the bioavailability of a drug. AUC = area under curve.

Drug Absorption and Core Patient Variables

1. **Health status.** Any change in health status related to circulation, condition of the GI tract, or pH of body fluids (e.g., disease, trauma, strenuous physical exercise, or drug therapy) can reduce drug absorption. The condition of the gastric and intestinal surfaces affects oral drug absorption.
2. **Contact time, surface area of contact, and the condition of the absorptive surface** may increase or decrease the amount of drug absorbed.
   - For example: Large surfaces (e.g., pulmonary alveolar epithelium, gastric and intestinal mucosa) absorb drugs rapidly.
   - Decreased absorptive surface from damage (e.g., radiation), disease (e.g., inflammatory bowel disease) or surgery (e.g., surgically shortened intestine) lessens drug absorption.
3. Absorption from the GI tract depends on factors such as **gastric volume, GI pH, gastric emptying time, intestinal transit rate, gastric motility, and GI enzyme levels.**
   - Delayed transport from the stomach to the intestine (e.g., food in the stomach) will dilute the drug and increase the contact time by slowing gastric emptying.
   - Decreased GI motility (e.g., constipation) permits increased drug contact time with the GI mucosa, allowing extra time for absorption, which may lead to increased drug effects and toxicity.
   - Increased intestinal motility may enhance drug dissolution and absorption; a patient with increased intestinal motility (e.g., diarrhea), will move a drug very quickly through the GI tract, reducing the amount of time the drug remains in contact with the GI mucosa and impairing drug absorption.
4. **Life span and gender.** There are gender-related variations that alter absorption.
   - For example, ingested solids versus liquids empty more slowly from women's stomachs, gastric acidity is lower in women, and women have lower gastric levels of alcohol dehydrogenase.
5. **Lifestyle, diet, and habits**
   - Diet may stimulate digestive enzymes and alter the gastric and intestinal mucosa. Generally, drugs ingested with food are slower absorbed than drugs taken on an empty stomach. Some drugs and food form complexes that cannot pass through the mucosal lining of the GI tract (e.g., tetracycline antimicrobials that bind with calcium, magnesium, iron, aluminum), and thus effective blood levels may not be reached. Some drugs are destroyed by the high acidity and peptic activity of gastric digestive enzymes.
   - The quality of blood flow to the site of absorption affects how much of the drug is absorbed. For example: Increased blood flow (e.g., application of heat or massage) enhances drug absorption because of the resulting increase in circulation. Similarly, absorption slows when blood flow decreases (e.g., shock or vasoconstriction). Some muscles normally have greater blood supply; for example, a drug injected into the deltoid muscle will be absorbed faster than one injected into the gluteus muscle because of the greater blood flow to the deltoid muscle.

Overall, it is important for the nurse to consider health status; life span and gender; lifestyle, diet, and habits; environment; and culture as factors that may influence all four components of pharmacokinetics (see, for instance, the accompanying displays, Pharmacokinetics: Age-Related Changes and How Food Alters Pharmacokinetics.)

Pharmacokinetics: Age-Related Changes

- Age-related changes that slow drug absorption
  Decreased intracellular fluid
  Increased gastric pH
  Decreased gastric blood flow and motility
  Reduced cardiac output and circulation
  Slower metabolism
- Age-related changes that alter drug distribution
  Increased adipose tissue and decreased lean muscle mass (women more than men)
  Decreased cardiac output
  Hypoalbuminemia
  Dehydration
- Age-related changes that alter drug metabolism
  Decreased hepatic efficiency
  Decreased enzymatic activity
- Age-related changes that alter drug excretion
  Decreased nephron efficiency
  Reduced glomerular filtration rate

DISTRIBUTION

Distribution describes the process by which drug molecules leave the blood stream and are transported by body fluids to sites of action (e.g., extracellular fluid and/or the cells of the target tissue) where the drug produces its effects. The drug is also distributed to body tissues where no effects are produced (e.g., storage sites, sites of inactivation and excretion).

Several factors influence the distribution of drugs—the volume of distribution, cardiac output, regional blood flow and capillary permeability, degree of plasma protein

How Food Alters Pharmacokinetics

Food alters drug absorption:
- Changes the acidity of the GI tract
- Stimulates secretion of digestive juices
- Alters motility of the digestive tract
- Binds to drugs
- Competes for absorption sites

Food alters drug metabolism:
- Interferes with drug action
- Contributes pharmacologically active substances
- Changes the components of the diet (raising or lowering protein or carbohydrate levels; e.g., diets deficient in fat decrease activity of microsomal enzymes)
- Interrupts oxidizing and drug metabolizing enzyme activity
- Alters the rate of metabolism, as in vitamin (A, C, E, and riboflavin) and mineral (zinc, iodine, magnesium, and potassium) deficiencies. (Mineral deficiencies have reportedly decreased drug oxidation and drug clearance.)

Food alters excretion:
- Changes the acidity of the urine. Urinary pH normally ranges between 6 and 7 and an acidic shift can be made by ingesting vitamin C. For example, manipulation of urine's pH can alter the extent of reabsorption and the amount of renal excretion of acidic and basic drugs.

binding and drug reservoirs or storage sites, drug concentration, tissue affinity, and physiologic barriers.

Volume of Distribution

Following PO or parenteral administration, a dose of a drug is distributed into all the body compartments and tissues that it is physically able to penetrate. This is termed volume of distribution (Vd). The time it takes for this to occur is called the distribution phase, and this phase is usually relatively rapid. Vd has little to do with the process of distribution; a drug's Vd is the mathematically determined hypothetical volume of blood, fat, and total body water into which the drug appears distributed. Vd is one of the determinants of drug dose. An altered Vd requires adjustment of drug dosage to achieve minimum effective concentration in a target tissue or organ. Drugs that are highly water soluble have a low Vd and reach high concentrations in serum; conversely, drugs that are highly lipid soluble and highly tissue bound have a high Vd and therefore a lower serum level.

There are gender differences to consider with Vd. On average, women have a higher percentage of body fat than men, causing women to have a greater Vd for highly lipophilic drugs (e.g., diazepam, trazodone). This results in a lower peak plasma level but a longer half-life. Conversely, women have a lower Vd for highly hydrophilic agents (e.g., alcohol, aminoglycoside antibiotics). In the case of ethanol, this means that an equal amount per kg of body weight will produce higher levels in body fluids, delivering higher ethanol levels to brain cells and thereby producing greater intoxication.

Blood Flow and Capillary Permeability

Initially, drug distribution depends on cardiac output, regional blood flow, and capillary permeability. There is a wide variability in blood flow to tissues and capillary beds as a result of unequal distribution of cardiac output to various organs. For example, blood flow to the brain, liver, and kidney is greater than that of the skeletal muscles followed by adipose tissue. The quantity of drug that enters the tissue is directly proportional to the perfusion of that tissue.

Plasma Protein Binding

One mechanism of drug distribution is **plasma protein binding**; drugs circulate in the plasma either bound or unbound to plasma protein, usually albumin. Bound drug molecules are pharmacologically inactive and they remain that way until released from the protein. Only the unbound portion of the drug is available to cross membranes and produce an effect. Drugs vary in their ratio of bound to unbound (free) molecules. The binding is reversible; for example, when the concentration of the free drug decreases due to metabolism and excretion, the bound drug becomes unbound and pharmacologically available to exert an effect by dissociating from the plasma protein. Thus, the free drug concentration is maintained as a constant fraction of the total drug in the plasma.The rates of association with and dissociation from the proteins are so fast, the bound and unbound drug fractions are always in a state of dynamic equilibrium. In most cases, the degree of binding is fairly constant across the therapeutic concentration range.

Binding of Drugs to Plasma Proteins

Albumin is the most abundant plasma protein; acidic drugs bind strongly to albumin. The large size of plasma proteins (molecular weight about 68,000) keeps it within the bloodstream, and therefore bound drug molecules cannot leave the bloodstream to reach sites of action or to undergo metabolism and excretion. Consequently, plasma proteins serve as reservoirs for drugs. Other plasma proteins that may serve as drug reservoirs are alpha-1 acid glycoproteins (AAG) and lipoproteins. Basic drugs as well as the protease inhibitors have a high affinity for AAG.

Plasma protein binding depends mainly on the blood level of albumin because many acidic drugs are bound to albumin and many alkaline drugs are bound to AAG. There is significantly less binding to other plasma proteins.

Plasma protein binding is expressed as a percentage. This percentage represents the amount of the total drug that is bound and depends largely on the chemical structure of the drug. Changes in binding are important for drugs that are normally highly bound in the plasma (more than 90%). A small alteration in the extent of a drug's binding may produce a large change in the amount of unbound and pharmacologically active drug. For example, hypoalbuminemia may alter the level of free drug. Examples of tightly bound drugs are warfarin and propranolol (90% and 93%, respectively). The fraction of total molecules that may be bound varies significantly. The percentages of loosely protein-bound drugs usually range between 10% and 35%.

Competition for Protein Binding Sites. If two drugs are given and each drug has a high affinity for albumin, they will compete for the available binding sites. Competitive binding is a property that accounts for clinically important drug interactions. Two drugs competing for the same protein sites will displace each other—in some cases, with serious consequences (Fig. 4-3). A weakly bound drug will offer little competition; however, if the drugs have relatively equal binding capabilities, the drug molecule with the greatest affinity will be the one most extensively bound. For example, the nonnarcotic analgesic aspirin and the anticoagulant warfarin compete for the same protein-binding sites. It is likely that aspirin will displace warfarin, thereby increasing free warfarin and possibly causing bleeding tendencies.

Other Drug Reservoirs

In addition to plasma protein binding, drugs may be distributed to bone, fat, plasma proteins, or other tissues for storage. Once bound, these storage areas can serve as drug reservoirs for prolonged periods of time. Fat-soluble drugs (lipophilic drugs) have a high affinity for adipose tissue. Drugs that accumulate in fat tend to remain there for long periods of time because adipose tissue is characterized by a relatively low blood flow. They are usually released slowly into the bloodstream only after the drug administration stops.

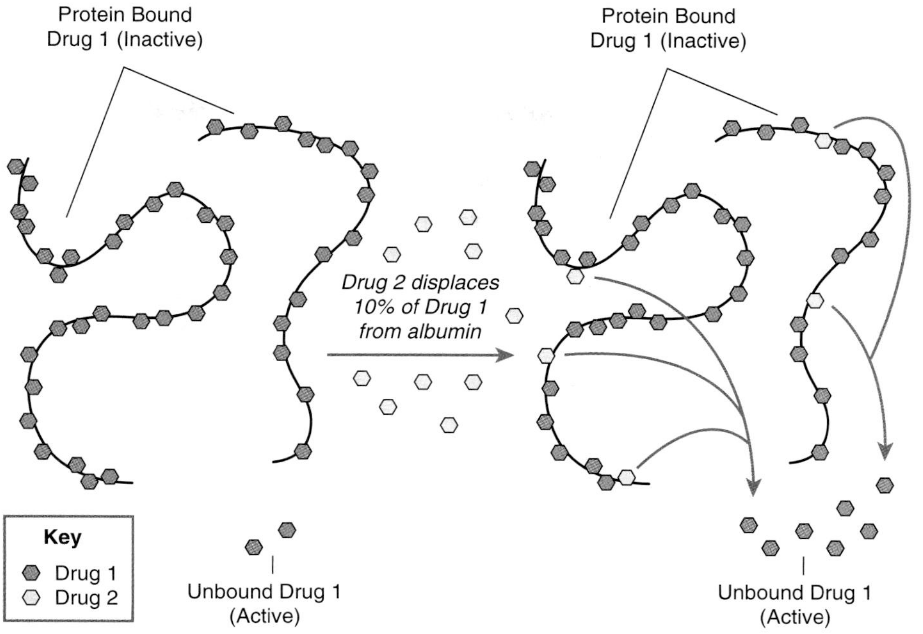

Figure 4-3. Consequence of drug displacement from albumin and other plasma proteins. Some drugs (e.g., "Drug 1" in figure) are greater than 90% bound to plasma proteins. The "free" (unbound) drug molecules, but not the bound molecules, are available to act at receptors. In the figure, Drug 2 displaces only 5 molecules of Drug 1, which more than triples the serum concentration of free (active) Drug 1. This could be fatal if Drug 1 has a narrow margin of safety. Displacement of drugs which are less-highly protein bound is less significant. For example, if Drug 1 were 50% bound and 50% free, displacement of 10% of the bound fraction would increase the free fraction from 50% to 55%. This small increment is unlikely to be clinically relevant.

Drug Concentration

The level of drug concentration, which may be adversely affected by some body processes and structures, is another concern related to health status and drug distribution. Alterations in the drug concentration level may complicate therapeutic objectives. For example, antibiotics are not typically distributed to abscesses and exudates, glands (e.g., prostate) tend to be impermeable to most antibiotics, and drug distribution to tumors tends to be unpredictable.

Tissue Affinity

Differences in drug concentration levels in the tissues may result from tissue affinity for the drug, blood flow, and protein or tissue binding. Some tissues and organs, for example, have an affinity for certain drugs (e.g., barbiturates are fat soluble). Affinity is the chemical force that drives certain atoms to unite with certain others to form compounds and attract molecules to specific sites. These sites serve as storage reservoirs that allow a drug to accumulate, pooling the drug by binding it to various tissues.

Physiologic Barriers

Some organs have specialized capillary networks that prevent drug distribution by preventing (in various degrees) the drug from leaving the vascular system.

With its unique anatomy, the **blood–brain barrier** is a selective mechanism that opposes the passage of most ions and large molecular compounds from the blood to the brain tissue. This structure of capillaries is characterized by very tight junctions through which most drugs cannot pass. Consequently, drugs must be lipid soluble or have a transport system to leave the bloodstream and reach a site of action within the brain. There are special transport mechanisms present in the brain capillaries for glucose, amino acids, amines, purines, nucleosides, and organic acids. Examples of drugs that can pass the blood–brain barrier include anesthetic gases, ethanol, some steroids, and some sedative-hypnotic agents.

Another barrier is the **placental barrier**, although in this sense the term barrier is technically inaccurate. The thick membranes of the placenta do not create an absolute barrier to the passage of drugs from mother to fetus. More accurately, the placental barrier is more like a placental passage because the fetus is exposed to all drugs taken by the mother to some extent. Many drugs and substances that may cross the placenta may cause teratogenic effects (birth defects) or fetal toxicity. Lipid-soluble molecules, for example, preferentially diffuse across the placenta. The same factors that determine a drug's movement across other membranes also determine a drug's movement across the placenta. Steroids, narcotics, anesthetics, and some antibiotics are easily transported across the placental membrane, producing their effects in the fetus.

Drug Distribution and Core Patient Variables

Distribution may be influenced by certain core patient variables (e.g., health status, life span and gender) (see the accompanying display, Drug Distribution and Core Patient Variables).

METABOLISM

Metabolism is the process by which the body changes the chemical structure of a drug. The liver is the major site for drug metabolism, although every tissue has some ability to metabolize drugs. Tissues with considerable activity include the GI tract, lungs, skin, and kidneys.

Drug Distribution and Core Patient Variables

Health Status

1. Hepatic dysfunction alters the manufacture of albumin. For example, an alteration of health status (e.g., hepatic impairment), diet (e.g., malnutrition), and habits (e.g., ethanol consumption, smoking) directly affect the liver.
2. Conditions such as hypoalbuminemia, hepatic disease, and renal disease can decrease the extent of drug binding, particularly of acidic and neutral drugs. A diseased liver cannot synthesize the protein building blocks needed for albumin production. Thus, there is a greater concentration of free drug and a greater risk of increased drug response and toxicity.

Life Span and Gender

1. At birth, the blood–brain barrier is not fully developed; this causes an increased vulnerability of the infant to CNS poisons and greater sensitivity to drugs that act on the brain in comparison with older children and adults.
2. In pregnant women and fetuses, some drugs may be distributed to and bind with receptor sites in such a way that tissues may be adversely affected. For instance, bones and teeth, which contain calcium, can accumulate substances that bind with calcium (e.g., tetracycline antibiotics).
3. Blood albumins are not thought to possess a gender-dependent predilection, although levels of some globulin proteins (e.g., corticosteroid-binding and sex-hormone binding) are lower in women. Although the small differences in protein levels between the genders are unlikely to be clinically significant, lower blood albumin levels may increase the effect of drugs that are normally highly protein bound.

Xenobiotic (i.e., foreign nonfood) substances or chemicals (e.g., most drugs, environmental pollutants, food additives, fillers, dyes, contaminants) initiate the process of metabolism because they are foreign or alien to the organism. Through the process of metabolism, the body attempts to neutralize or detoxify the substance and eliminate it. The resulting metabolic actions may effect many changes on the original molecule before its secretion or excretion.

Biotransformation is the outcome of these metabolic processes. From metabolism and biotransformation, a drug (or chemical) is converted into another chemical, called a metabolite. Sometimes the metabolites are also pharmacologically active. Other times drugs may be administered initially as inert or inactive compounds—known as prodrugs—and they must be metabolized to their active forms. Enzymes break down drugs and their resulting metabolites. Enzymatic transformation of drugs serves to enhance the renal excretion of ingested xenobiotic substances and as well as some endogenous compounds (e.g., steroids, vitamins, fatty acids). The liver contains millions of cells in the parenchyma (hepatocytes); hepatocytes contain the enzymes that transform or convert drugs.

Drugs may require a one- or two-phase set of hepatic (liver) transformations before they can be excreted. Phase I reactions most frequently involve the cytochrome P-450 system (also called microsomal mixed function oxidase). Phase I reactions are oxidation reactions and usually convert the parent drug to a metabolite sufficiently polar so it can then be renally excreted. Phase II reactions are conjugation reactions and considered synthetic. They involve the combination of a drug or its metabolite with an equal portion of an endogenous water-soluble substance (e.g., glucuronic acid). These conjugates are highly polar and rapidly excreted in the urine and feces. Other metabolic sites exist (e.g., GI mucosa, kidney, lung, brain, skin) where different metabolic enzymes carry out biotransformation phases I and II (Katzung, 2000).

Hepatic First-Pass Phenomenon

Orally administered drugs are first absorbed through the walls of the small intestine and initially travel through the portal vein to the liver, where they undergo metabolism before reaching the systemic circulation. Furthermore, the liver can excrete the drug into the bile. Any of these sites can contribute to this reduction in bioavailability and this process is known as the **first-pass phenomenon** (or effect) (Fig 4-4). When this process is so complete that it prevents the drug from reaching a serum concentration sufficient to exert a pharmacologic effect, the drug is described as having experienced an **extensive first-pass effect.** For these types of drugs, the first-pass effects must be overcome. This is accomplished either by changing the chemical formulation of the drug, manipulating the dose, or by administering the drug in a way that bypasses the GI tract.

Cytochrome P-450 Enzymes and Isoenzymes

The hepatic microsomal enzyme system is responsible for metabolizing and biotransforming drugs. This enzyme system is known as the cytochrome P-450 (CYP-450) system. This system is important for the metabolism of many endogenous compounds (e.g., steroids, lipids) and for the detoxification of exogenous substances (e.g., drugs, chemicals). The CYP-450 system contains 12 identified families of heme-containing isoenzymes; they occur in packets—known as microsomes—and are localized in the endoplasmic reticulum (or microsomal fraction) of numerous cells in the liver, intestine, and throughout the body. Hence, the term microsomal enzyme system; this enzyme system commonly carries out drug-metabolizing activity.

A number indicates the family name; it is followed by a capital letter for the subfamily (e.g., CYP3A). Another number is added to indicate the specific isoenzyme (CYP3A4). Although there are 12 identified CYP gene families, CYP 1, 2, and 3 families encode the enzymes involved in the majority of all drug biotransformations. Each of the isoenzymes has a broad and overlapping specificity.

Some drugs can either induce or inhibit the synthesis of different isoenzymes. Thus, drug clearance may be accelerated or diminished. The interplay of these processes is responsible for many drug-drug interactions. For example, CYP3A4 is the most abundant of all isoenzymes (20% to 60% of total) and it has the broadest substrate (substance acted upon and changed by an enzyme) of any known iso-

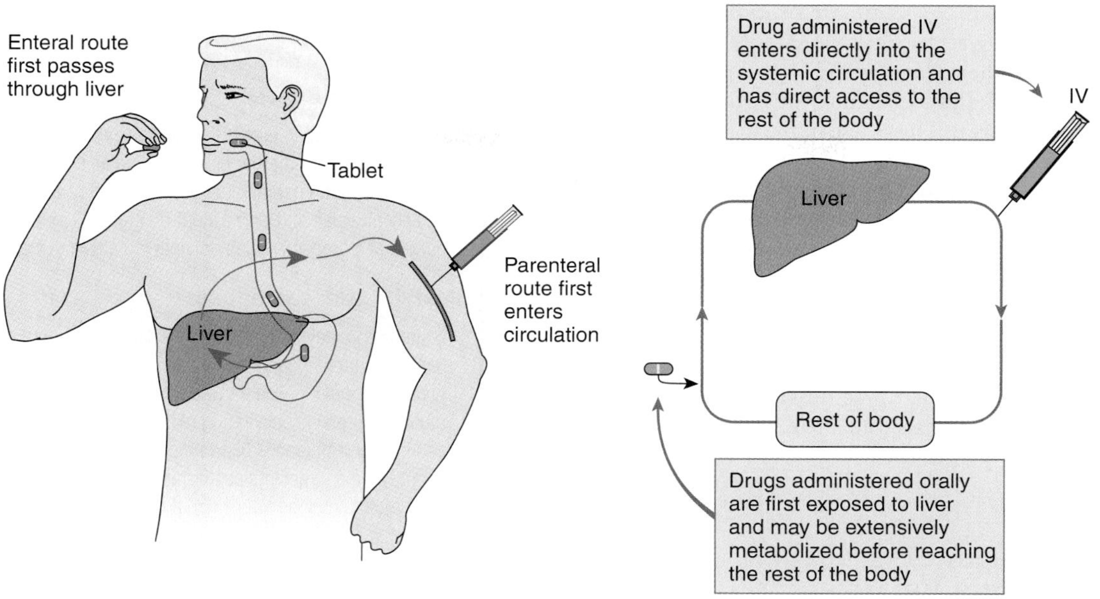

Figure 4-4. First-pass phenomenon. A drug administered by the enteral route passes through the liver, where the drug is metabolized and transformed by a process known as first-pass phenomenon, or first-pass effect, before circulating in the bloodstream. In contrast, a drug administered by the parenteral route enters the circulation directly.

enzyme. It is considered responsible for the metabolism of more than 50% of the drugs currently in therapeutic use. Extensive metabolism by CYP3A4 in the GI tract is a significant factor contributing to the poor oral bioavailability of some drugs.

CYP-450 Isoenzyme Inducers and Inhibitors

Most drugs are metabolized by at least one CYP isoenzyme (e.g., 1A2, 2C9, 2C19, 2D6, or 3A4). Drugs that are metabolized by a specific isoenzyme are called substrates of that isoenzyme.

A drug that is described as a CYP inducer increases the amount of the isoenzyme. By increasing its activity (usually accomplished by stimulating its synthesis) metabolism of that isoenzyme's substrates are also altered. For example, an inducer of CYP3A4 isoenzyme (e.g., carbamazepine, phenobarbital, phenytoin) may cause a significant decrease in the blood level of CYP3A4 substrate drugs (e.g., alprazolam, fentanyl, midazolam). Although metabolism returns to normal after the inducing drug is gone, induction persists for several days.

A drug that is described as a CYP inhibitor decreases the isoenzyme and, consequently, decreases the metabolism of isoenzyme's substrates. Thus, a marked increase in the blood level and pharmacologic action of the drug may occur. For example, concomitant administration of a CYP2D6 isoenzyme inhibitor (e.g., cimetidine, fluoxetine, paroxetine) may cause a distinct elevation of a CYP2D6 drug (e.g., amitriptyline, desipramine, haloperidol). This process is usually competitive and reversible with normal metabolism occurring once the inhibitor is gone. A drug may be a CYP inhibitor without being a substrate. An example of this is fluconazole, which is not a CYP substrate, but is a moderate inhibitor (Olin, Beltran, Blasing, & Goldberg, 2000).

Enterohepatic Cycling

Drugs that enter the GI system or are stored in bile are absorbed and carried through the portal system to the liver. Here the drug or its active metabolites may be secreted into bile; the bile is then excreted into the small intestine. Circadian reabsorption of 70% to 80% of the bile may cause the drug or its metabolites to be returned to the systemic circulation. This process, known as **enterohepatic cycling**, may prolong the biologic activity and delay the eventual disposition of the drug.

This phenomenon of enterohepatic cycling may be associated with a delayed elimination of drug from the body and a prolongation of its biologic effect (Hardman, Limbird, Molinof, Ruddon, & Gilman, 1996).

Pathologic and Other Processes Affecting Hepatic Metabolism

Hepatic metabolism may be altered or faulty in patients with liver damage (e.g., secondary to alcoholism, polydrug use, or overdose) or compromised from systemic disease (e.g., cancer, surgery, immunosuppression).

Any drug that can cause hepatotoxicity has the potential to prolong a person's metabolic response to any other drug. Such an interaction is known as metabolic inhibition. It results from the inhibition or poisoning of the microsomal enzymes that play a role in biotransformation. When a drug's metabolism has been inhibited, circulating drug levels will increase. The patient may, therefore, exhibit more of the therapeutic effect or be more prone to adverse effects. Numerous drugs and drug classes can cause hepatic dysfunction, necrosis, injury, and hepatotoxicity (e.g., anticonvulsants, nonsteroidal antiinflammatory drugs [NSAIDs], and antibiotics).

In contrast, some drugs stimulate or induce the hepatic microsomal enzyme system. This increases the liver's capacity to metabolize other drugs, which may lead to an interaction known as stimulation. Some drugs can enhance their own rates of metabolism. This is one of the ways in which tolerance develops. Examples of drugs known as "self-inducers" include alcohol, carbamazepine, phenobarbital, phenytoin, and rifampin. When a drug is known to be a metabolic inducer, the metabolism of any concurrent drugs may be affected. Typically, dosage adjustments may be required to offset the enhanced metabolism of the affected drug. This is usually determined by careful therapeutic monitoring of both interacting drugs. Should the original inducing drug be reduced or discontinued, the nurse must watch for signs of increased toxicity of the second drug, because the levels may increase quickly once the hepatic enzyme levels return to normal.

Drug Metabolism and Core Patient Variables

See the accompanying display, Drug Metabolism and Core Patient Variables, for coverage of this topic.

> **Drug Metabolism and Core Patient Variables**
>
> **Life Span and Gender**
>
> 1. Drug metabolism in patients whose enzymatic metabolic systems are either immature or functioning less efficiently (e.g., neonates, children, and older adults) is highly variable but is usually diminished. Decreased drug metabolism places the patient at increased risk of adverse effects from the drug.
>
> **Lifestyle, Diet, and Habits**
>
> 1. Malnutrition may prolong drug effects as a result of poor hepatic microsomal metabolism.
> 2. In obese people, phase II transformations tend to occur more rapidly, thereby necessitating higher drug dosages. Obesity significantly influences distribution in drugs that are highly lipophilic (e.g., anesthetics, barbiturates).
> 3. Drug effects may be intensified if the specific drug places the person at nutritional risk by producing anorexia, increased appetite, nausea and vomiting, nutritional deficiencies, stomatitis, or toxic reactions, for example.
> 4. Diet may contribute to individual variations in drug metabolism. Charcoal-broiled foods and cruciferous vegetables induce one CYP isoenzyme, whereas grapefruit juice inhibits one.
> 5. Exposure to cigarette smoke and pesticides may cause a more rapid metabolism of some drugs because of enzyme induction.
>
> **Environment**
>
> 1. Reduced partial pressure of oxygen at higher altitudes may affect enzymatic reduction systems.
> 2. Environmental pollutants may affect induction or inhibition of hepatic enzymes (Fauci, Braunwald, Wilson, Martin, Hauser, Longo, et al., 2000).
> 3. Light is a key modulator in the regulation of metabolic pathways and in specific settings may affect drug response (e.g., intensive care units that commonly remain constantly lit) (Wetterberg, 1994).

EXCRETION

The term **excretion** refers to removal of a drug (or its metabolites) from the body. Although some drugs are excreted from the body essentially unchanged, most drugs have only a small part of their dose removed unchanged. Drug excretion occurs mainly through the kidneys into the urine, although various other body organs and mechanisms have vital roles in drug excretion; among them are the hepatic, respiratory, and biliary systems, the GI tract, and the extrahepatic structures (sweat, salivary glands, skin). The most important processes of renal excretion are glomerular filtration, tubular secretion, and tubular reabsorption.

One of the most important terms used in applied pharmacokinetics, **clearance** is the rate of disappearance of the drug molecules from the circulation. Clearance of a drug relates to its removal from the blood by clearing processes (e.g., hepatic metabolism, renal excretion).

Drugs with a slow clearance rate are removed more slowly, increasing the circulating blood levels as half-life is increased. Drugs with a high clearance rate are removed quickly; therefore, they produce lower circulating blood levels. Protein binding capacity and body weight may affect drug clearance rates. Patients with renal, cardiac, or hepatic compromise or dysfunction will have decreased clearance, giving them greater exposure to both the therapeutic effects of the drug and its adverse or toxic effects. Some drugs (e.g., aminoglycosides, some analgesics) exhibit nephrotoxicity and therefore may affect the renal clearance of all other drugs.

Renal Excretion

Renal clearance is governed by the processes of filtration, secretion, and reabsorption (Brody, Larner, and Minneman, 1998) (Fig. 4-5).

Glomerular Filtration

Most drugs or their metabolites are efficiently excreted in the urine by glomerular filtration. The glomerular filtration rate (GFR = 125 mL/min) is normally about 20% of the renal plasma flow (600 mL/min). Low-molecular-weight molecules (i.e., less than 15 angstroms) readily pass through the glomeruli and, along with water, become the glomerular filtrate. Any free drugs will appear in the filtrate, whereas protein-bound drugs will remain with the unfiltered serum proteins. Drug molecules bound to protein and large molecular weight molecules—because of their size—are not filtered out and excreted. These are retained in the blood that leaves the efferent arteriole by way of the glomerulus (Brody et al., 1998).

Tubular Secretion

Tubular secretion is an active process that occurs in the proximal tubule. Compounds that are secreted usually also undergo glomerular filtration, and therefore renal clearance is

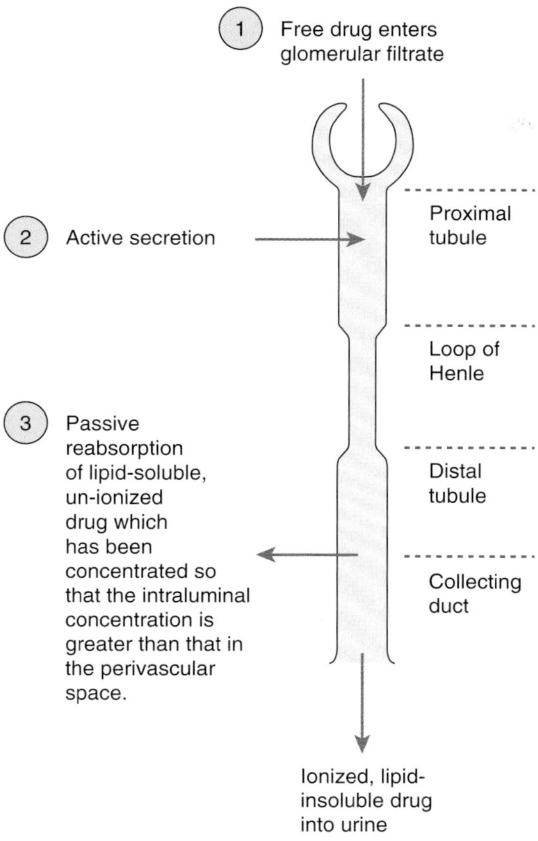

Figure 4-5. Renal drug elimination.

the sum of both routes. Acids and bases are secreted through the proximal tubules, with their rate of excretion being dependent on their plasma concentration. Tubular secretion is dependent on active carriers. In contrast to glomerular filtration in which the volume of plasma cleared is independent of plasma drug concentration, the volume of plasma that can be cleared by tubular secretion correlates with the plasma concentration of the drug. When plasma-drug concentration is low, tubular secretion may increase to approximately 650 mL/min. Conversely, if the tubular secretion is saturated (active transport has a limited number of carrier molecules), the rate of clearance may decrease dramatically (Brody et al., 1998).

Tubular Reabsorption

As the filtrate moves through the renal tubule, two types of reabsorption may occur, namely active or passive. In active reabsorption, a carrier mechanism is involved, energy is consumed, and the drug or metabolite may be moved from a high concentration in the filtrate to a low concentration in the efferent arteriolar blood. In passive reabsorption, lipid-soluble drugs and some water-soluble drugs diffuse down a concentration gradient back into the blood.

Drugs or metabolites that are weak bases or weak acids are influenced by the health status variable of urinary pH. Excretion of these substances may be enhanced or diminished therapeutically by manipulating the pH of urine; making the urine alkaline increases renal clearance of weak acid drugs (e.g., probenecid, salicylic acid). As a result, more of the acid will exist in ionized form and not be reabsorbed. Urine may be made more alkaline using thiazide diuretics or antacids. Similarly, weak bases (e.g., amphetamine, morphine) will be excreted more efficiently when the urine is acidified. Ascorbic acid may be used to acidify the urine.

Other Methods of Excretion

Hepatic excretion of drugs and metabolites occurs through concentration in bile with bile being lost into the small intestine. Most drugs are eliminated from the body through the liver or kidney and when the patient has liver damage, some impairment of hepatic excretion may be expected. Some drugs are eliminated in other ways and this is termed extrahepatic excretion. For example, macromolecules (e.g., heparin, amphotericin B) are engulfed and digested by phagocytic cells (e.g., hepatic Kupffer cells). This is termed reticuloendothelial system clearance. Volatile and gaseous drugs (e.g., alcohol, anesthetics, solvents) may be excreted unchanged by the lungs through respiration or excreted through the skin. Patients with compromised pulmonary status will not eliminate drugs as quickly through the lungs. Although few studies exist, these routes of clearance are not known to be involved in clinically significant drug interactions.

Drug Excretion and Core Patient Variables

See the accompanying display, Drug Excretion and Core Patient Variables, for coverage of this topic.

STEADY STATE AND DRUG PLASMA LEVELS

STEADY STATE AND HALF-LIFE

The full therapeutic effect of a drug dose can usually be seen when steady state has been achieved. **Steady state**, which is the evenly distributed concentration of a drug, occurs when the administration rate equals the rate of drug elimination. Achievement of steady state is independent of a drug's dosing (i.e., intervals between administration of a drug). This means that more frequent dosing of a drug (i.e., giving the drug every hour instead of every 8 hours) does not create steady state. Steady state is dependent on the half-life of the drug. **Half-life** (abbreviated $t_{1/2}$) is the time needed for the plasma concentration of a drug to be reduced by 50%; plasma concentrations are reduced by the pharmacokinetic processes of metabolism and excretion. Steady state is achieved in approximately five half-lives. Drugs with short half-lives are rapidly cleared from the body; drugs with longer half-lives stay in the body for a longer duration of time.

Drug Excretion and Core Patient Variables

Health Status

1. Renal impairment or renal failure decreases a drug's elimination from the body. If renal excretion is an important route of its elimination and the drug is given on a regular dosing schedule, its slowed removal from the body will produce a greater accumulation of drug in the body with an increased the likelihood of additional therapeutic and adverse effects.
2. If cardiac output is decreased, the kidney may not be perfused adequately, decreasing glomerular filtration rate as well as excretion of drugs.
3. Hepatic compromise or dysfunction will also decrease the elimination of drugs.
4. Drug therapy may produce nephrotoxicity as an adverse effect. Therefore, the renal elimination of all other drugs may be decreased.

Life Span and Gender

1. In elderly patients, the rate of drug clearance is reduced.
2. Clinical studies demonstrate that there are gender differences in the major modes of clearance. Some drugs in which gender demonstrates a faster clearance are:

   Antimicrobial agents—females: erythromycin; males: cefotaxime

   Cardiovascular agents—females: verapamil; males: digoxin, lidocaine, procainamide

   CNS drugs—females: alprazolam, diazepam, midazolam; males: clozapine, desipramine, fluphenazine, oxazepam, thiothixene

   Immunosuppressants—females: cyclosporine, methylprednisolone, prednisolone

   NSAID analgesics—females: naproxen, salicylic acid

   The clinical implications of these statistically significant deviations are unknown (Davis, 1998).

CHAPTER SUMMARY

- Drug plasma (or serum) levels are affected by the pharmacokinetic processes of absorption, distribution, storage in inactive tissue depots, metabolism and biotransformation, and excretion. A variation in the rates of these processes accounts for the changing tissue concentrations of drugs within a group of individuals and within the same individual at different times. Pharmacokinetic processes are influenced by health status; life span (age, pregnancy, and breastfeeding) and gender; lifestyle, diet, and habits; and environment. Onset of action, peak concentration level, and duration of action are additional factors that help determine a drug's pharmacokinetic profile. These factors are determined by the drug's bioavailability and blood concentration level.
- Absorption represents the stage from the time the drug enters the body until it enters the venous or lymphatic circulation. Drug absorption depends on variables that influence drug movement into the circulation. These variables include dosage form, site and route of administration, and such physicochemical factors as passive diffusion, active transport, and pinocytosis. Blood flow to the absorptive site, surface area of the absorptive site, pain, stress, hepatic first-pass phenomenon, enterohepatic recycling, dosage form, drug solubility, GI motility, and drug interactions are additional variables influencing drug absorption.
- Bioavailability refers to the extent of drug absorption and its distribution of to the site of action.
- Distribution describes the process by which drug solutions are transported by body fluids to sites of action. Blood flow, whether a drug is hydrophilic or hydrophobic, and the extent of the drug's protein-binding capacity all influence drug distribution within the body. Drugs typically bind to plasma proteins (primarily albumin) for distribution throughout the body. The extent of protein binding may be affected by the patient's health status.
- The volume of distribution refers to the size of a compartment that would be filled with a drug in the same concentrations as those found in the body's plasma or blood. It represents the body compartments where drugs distribute and act. A high volume of distribution indicates a lower blood concentration level, whereas a low volume of distribution reflects a higher concentration level.
- Drug metabolism (or biotransformation) changes the drug from its pharmacologically active form to a more water-soluble molecule that can be excreted readily from the renal and hepatobiliary systems. This process usually reduces the amount of active drug in the body. Drug metabolites, however, may exhibit pharmacologic activity. The patient's health status can affect drug metabolism.
- Drug excretion describes the movement of drugs or drug metabolites from the tissues into the organs of excretion. Excretion of metabolized drugs typically occurs through the kidney. Other routes of excretion include the exocrine (sweat and salivary) glands, GI tract, liver, lungs, and skin.
- Drug plasma levels and the intensity and length of pharmacologic action are regulated by the processes of biotransformation and excretion.

QUESTIONS FOR STUDY AND REVIEW

1. What factors may influence absorption?
2. What is meant by the first-pass phenomenon?
3. What is biotransformation?
4. What are some of the possible reasons for the observed differences in individual drug responses?
5. How is drug elimination likely to be different in elderly patients? In patients with chronic illness?

NEED MORE HELP?

Chapter 4 of the study guide for *Drug Therapy in Nursing* contains exercises and activities to reinforce your understanding of the concepts presented in this chapter. For additional information see the text's accompanying website at *http://www.connection.lww.com.*

REFERENCES AND BIBLIOGRAPHY

Brody, T. M., Larner, J., Minneman, K. P. (Eds.). (1998). *Human pharmacology* (2nd ed.). St. Louis: Mosby.

Davis, M. W. (1998). Impact of gender on drug responses. *Drug Topics, 142*(9), 91–100.

Drug facts and comparisons. (2000). St. Louis: Facts and Comparisons.

Fauci, A., Braunwald, E., Wilson, J. D., Martin, J. B., Hauser, S. L., Longo, D. L., Kasper, D. L., Isselbachter, K. J. (Eds.). (1999). *Harrison's online.* New York: McGraw-Hill.

Fletcher, C. V., Acosta, E. P., & Strykowski, J. M. (1994). Gender differences in human pharmacokinetics and pharmacodynamics. *Journal of Adolescent Health, 15,* 619–629.
Gossel, T. A. (1998). Exploring pharmacology. *U.S. Pharmacist, 23*(9), 96–103.
Gossel, T. A. (1998). Pharmacology: Back to basics. *U.S. Pharmacist, 23*(11), 96–103.
Gossel, T. A. (1999). Pharmacology: A profile on pharmacokinetics. *U.S. Pharmacist, 24*(5), 71–77.
Gossel, T. A. (1999). Pharmacodynamics: How drugs act. *U.S. Pharmacist, 24*(9), 101–108.
Hardman, J. G., Limbird, L. E., Molinof, P. B., Ruddon, R. W., & Gilman, A. (Eds.). (1997). *Goodman and Gilman's pharmacological basis of therapeutics* (9th ed.). New York: McGraw-Hill.
Katzung, B. C. (Ed.) (2000). *Basic and clinical pharmacology.* (8th ed.). New York: McGraw Hill.
Lewis, J. F. & Mensah, G. A. (2000). Ethnic and gender disparities in cardiovascular mortality . . . The scientific basis, mechanisms, and strategies for closing the gap in the new millennium. Anaheim, CA: Joint Symposium: Association of Black Cardiologists/American College of Cardiology, Scientific Session.
Silverstein, H. (1999). Use of a new device to deliver medication to the inner ear. *Ear, Nose and Throat Journal 78*(8), 595–600.
Tyson, S. R. (1999). *Gerontological nursing care.* Philadelphia: W. B. Saunders.
Wetterburg, L. (1994). Light and biological rhythms. [Review]. *Journal of Internal Medicine, 235,* 5–19.

Chapter 5

PHARMACODYNAMICS

KEY TERMS

affinity
agonist
antagonist
antimetabolites
competitive antagonist
dose-response curve
drug action
drug effects
drug efficacy
drug potency
drug-enzyme interaction
drug-receptor interaction
efficacy
loading dose
maintenance dose
mixed agonist
noncompetitive antagonist
potency
receptor

Learning Objectives

At the completion of this chapter the student will:

1. Define pharmacodynamics.
2. Define drug effects.
3. Explain specific pharmacodynamic concepts, including drug-receptor activity, drug-enzyme interaction, agonist and antagonist actions, dose-response curve, and therapeutic index.

Pharmacodynamics is the effect of what a drug actually does to the body. It represents the study of the processes by which a drug alters the physiology of the cell. These processes include uptake, movement, binding, and interactions of pharmacologically active molecules at their tissue site(s) of action.

Drugs commonly bind to one of four primary protein target sites: carrier molecules, enzymes, ion channels, or receptors. Exceptions to this include the general anesthetics, which bind to membrane lipids, and a number of antimicrobial, antitumor, carcinogenic, and mutagenic agents that act directly on DNA.

DRUG CHARACTERISTICS

In general, drugs have several common characteristics:

- *Drugs do not create responses.* Drugs actually modify existing responses by some physiologic interaction. For example, the drug atropine decreases salivary secretions and the drug bisacodyl speeds evacuation of the large intestine.
- *Drugs exert multiple rather than single effects on the body.* Drugs cause more than one physiochemical effect in the body. For example, metaproterenol dilates the bronchial passages; it may produce tachycardia or palpitations as adverse effects.
- *Drug action results from a physicochemical interaction between the drug and a functionally important molecule or structure in the body.* For example, a nonsystemic antacid, such as magnesium hydroxide, interacts with gastric acid to neutralize the acid; an antiemetic drug, such as prochlorperazine, interferes with neurotransmission in brain structures to relieve nausea.

DRUG EFFECTS

Body responses that result from drug action represent **drug effects.** Drug effects are dose related. To produce a therapeutic or intended effect, a drug must be present in appropriate concentrations at its site of action. Although the amount of drug administered is an obvious variable for concentration levels, there are specific phases of drug activity that influence the drug concentration that is achieved.

The pharmaceutical phase of drug action includes the actual drug preparations and dosage forms and focuses on how the drug dissolves and gets into solution. The pharmacokinetic phase consists of the ways in which the body affects the drug; it involves how the body processes the drug for absorption, distribution, metabolism, and excretion (see Chapter 4). The pharmacodynamic phase consists of the ways in which the drug affects the body. This involves drug uptake, movement, binding, and the interaction of pharmacologically active molecules at the drug-receptor site.

Some drugs produce their effects in a nonspecific manner by producing a biochemical or physical alteration of the cell's external or internal environment. Thus, they are considered to be structurally nonspecific. For example, the effectiveness of emollient stool softeners is based on their ability to reduce the surface tension of fecal material to allow greater absorption of water; the active ingredients in antacids alter the pH of body fluids, and osmotic diuretics alter the composition of body fluid by increasing the osmolarity of plasma, glomerular, and tubular fluid, resulting in a decreased reabsorption of fluid and electrolytes.

Drugs that produce their effects through enzyme interactions or combination with receptors are considered to be structurally specific. Most drugs produce their effects by combining with receptors.

In addition to therapeutic or intended effects, drugs may produce nontherapeutic and undesired effects, also known as adverse effects. Adverse effects causing serious harm or threat to life are referred to as toxicities (see Chapter 6).

THEORIES OF DRUG-RECEPTOR ACTIVITY

A **receptor** is a specialized area on the cell wall or within the cellular cytoplasm. Receptors may be considered special body "chemicals" and are usually cellular proteins or nucleic acids, but they can also be enzymes and lipids. Because drugs are chemicals, they exert their effects by interacting with other chemicals. Receptors do not stimulate actions that the cell is normally unable to perform; rather they have a regulatory action on normal function. Interactions between drugs and their receptors can be summed up in a general equation:

$$\text{Drug} + \text{Receptor} \rightarrow \text{Drug-receptor (binding)} = \text{Response}$$

This combination functions to alter cellular components and cellular activity. The outcome may be either agonistic (activation) or antagonistic (blockade).

An **agonist** is a drug that has the ability to initiate the desired therapeutic effect by binding to a receptor. This attraction, however, is not permanent. Rather, it seems to be related to the number of receptors occupied, and it is a brief, dynamic, reversible process involving weak ionic bonds between the agonist molecule and the receptor structures. A drug receptor occupied by an agonist molecule cannot respond to any other molecule.

An **antagonist** is a drug that has an affinity for the same receptor sites as an agonist. Antagonist drugs attach to cell receptors by affinity; they do not achieve a response (known as efficacy), however. Antagonistic drugs prevent receptor stimulation from another molecule. Antagonistic drugs may also be called receptor blockers because they "block" the receptor from binding to agonist molecules. An automobile in a parking space may be used as an analogy; the parked car is doing nothing, but it prevents another car from parking in that particular spot.

The therapeutic value of many agents results from their ability to act as receptor antagonists. For example, used as antidotes for drug toxicity or poisoning, antihistamines reduce allergic symptoms by binding to histamine receptors (H1) and preventing them from being stimulated by the histamine released in allergic response. An opioid antagonist (e.g., naloxone) completely reverses symptoms of opioid overdose by blocking the opioid receptors in the central nervous system (CNS). Beta-adrenergic antagonists (selective and nonselective) are used to treat a variety of cardiovascular disorders. Antagonistic drugs are subdivided into two major classes: competitive antagonists and noncompetitive antagonists.

Competitive antagonists have a reversible receptor binding; that is, they produce a receptor blockade by competing with agonist molecules for that same receptor. If their affinities are equivalent, the molecule that will become bound is the one present in greatest numbers. Virtually all available drugs that function as antagonists exist in the competitive class.

Noncompetitive antagonists, in contrast, exhibit irreversible receptor binding. This irreversible mechanism reduces the total number of receptors available for an agonistic action. Because the intensity of an agonistic response depends on (and is proportional to) the number of receptors occupied, irreversible receptor binding decreases the number of receptors available and thereby reduces the maximal effect of the agonist. Irreversible binding does not last forever, however. As cells break down their "old" receptors and synthesize new ones, the effects of noncompetitive binding eventually subside. Few noncompetitive antagonist drugs are used clinically due to their irreversible binding, which can extend drug effects excessively (several days or longer).

Some substances that bind with receptors are called **mixed agonists** or partial antagonists. The narcotic agonist-antagonist analgesics are good examples of a mixed agonist. These drugs compete with other substances at the opioid mu receptor. The mu receptors mediate morphine-like effects. The narcotic agonist-antagonist drugs may be partially agonistic or antagonistic at the mu receptor. They are potent analgesic agents with a lower abuse potential than pure narcotic agonists because of their mixture of activities. When given to someone with opiate dependence, their narcotic antagonistic activity may precipitate withdrawal symptoms.

SINGLE OCCUPANCY AND MODIFIED OCCUPANCY THEORIES

Single occupancy and modified occupancy are two theoretical models of drug-receptor activity.

Single occupancy hypothesizes that the intensity of a drug response is proportional to the number of receptors occupied by the drug, and that a maximal drug response will occur when all of the available receptors have been occupied. Further assumptions are that all drugs binding at a particular receptor have an identical ability to bind and to influence that receptor. Some phenomena, however, cannot be explained by single occupancy (i.e., how one drug can be more potent or more effective than another). Modified occupancy explains these phenomena by affinity.

Affinity is the term used to describe the tendency of a drug to be at a given receptor site. Drugs with high affinities have a high attraction to a receptor site. In turn, this drug-receptor affinity reflects **potency**, or the power of a compound or drug to produce a therapeutic response. Drugs may be compared with each other to establish potency. For example, the narcotic analgesic, morphine sulfate, is often used to evaluate the potency of other narcotics.

A drug's intrinsic activity reflects its efficacy (effectiveness). **Efficacy** is the term used to describe the drug's ability to initiate a biologic activity and its maximum therapeutic ability. Occasionally, the terms intrinsic activity and efficacy are used interchangeably.

Most drugs produce their effects in one of three ways: by drug-receptor interaction, by drug-enzyme interaction, or by nonspecific drug interactions.

Drug-Receptor Interaction

The action of many drugs is produced by its interaction with a specialized area of the cell called a **receptor**. Although numerous receptors exist—each cell membrane may have tens of thousands of receptors—individual receptors participate in regulating only a few processes. Although receptors may vary in their selectivity—in a number of instances similar chemical compounds can occupy the same receptor—many different kinds of receptors are needed to regulate the body's various physiologic activities. For example, each neurotransmitter (e.g., acetylcholine, dopamine, norepinephrine), each hormone (e.g., estrogen, insulin, thyrotropin), and each of the other assorted molecules (e.g., histamine, prostaglandins) has its own receptors.

Receptors may have shapes that are specific for particular drugs. Often, the analogy of a lock and key is used to describe the cellular attraction between a receptor site and a drug molecule (Fig. 5-1). The drug represents the key that fits into the lock (receptor). This concept helps to explain how a drug interacts with one receptor type and not with others.

Some receptors have subtypes, and these are usually indicated with a number or a Greek letter. These subtypes may have shapes that are slightly different. Scientists have identified at least three receptor subtypes for a neurotransmitter, acetylcholine, and at least six receptor subtypes for the adrenal hormone, epinephrine. This subtle difference in shape helps explain more selective or more specific drug-receptor complexes. Drug development toward existing receptor subtypes enables agonist or antagonist drug actions to be very specific in terms of stimulating or blocking only one or a few of the subtypes.

Drug-Enzyme Interaction

The second way in which drugs exert their effects is by an interaction with an enzyme. Enzymes control all biochemical cellular reactions. Enzymatic inhibition by a drug will alter the physiologic response. The neurologic disorder myasthenia gravis, for example, is characterized by pro-

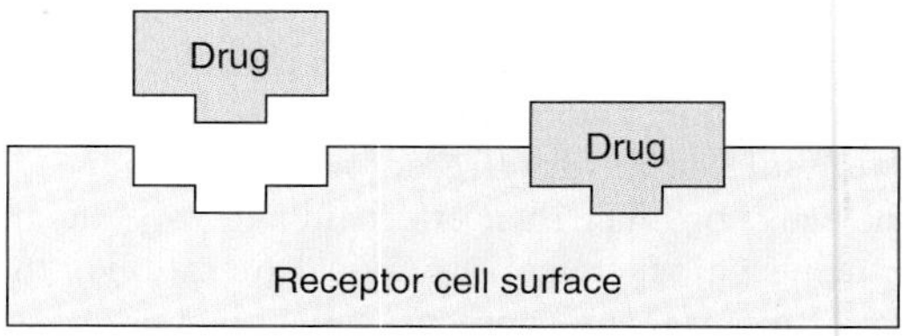

Figure 5-1. Receptor site and drug molecule.

found muscle weakness due to acetylcholine deficiency. To treat the disease symptoms, the cholinergic drug, neostigmine, is used to interfere with inactivation of acetylcholine by acetylcholinesterase at the neuromuscular junction.

Nonspecific Drug Interaction

The action of most drugs involves receptors; however, some drugs exert their effects by a nonspecific interaction rather than binding to a receptor. Drug effects may occur, for example, through an alteration of normal metabolic pathways, a chemical action, or a physical action on the cell (Table 5-1).

VARIABLES THAT INFLUENCE THE DOSE OF A DRUG

LOADING AND MAINTENANCE DOSES

Sometimes a faster therapeutic effect is desired than what can be achieved with steady state. This is accomplished by using a **loading dose**, which is higher than the usual amount of drug needed to sustain a therapeutic effect (e.g., maintenance dose). The loading dose may be divided to minimize the possibility of toxic adverse effects. During the five half-lives of the loading dose, the drug level remains at or above the therapeutic range. After the loading dose, the standard size dose is administered to maintain the drug in therapeutic range.

A prime example of the use of loading and maintenance dosing is the cardiac glycoside, digoxin. Digoxin has a long half-life (1.4 days) and it takes more than a week to reach steady-state tissue/serum concentrations with the usual maintenance dosage. In acute situations when a therapeutic effect is needed more quickly, a loading dose is given. For example, the total loading dose for digoxin is between 0.75 and 1.5 mg. For a total dose of 1.5 mg, half of the total loading dose (0.75 mg) is administered initially. Between 8 and 12 hours later, 25% of the total dose (0.375 mg) is given, with the final 25% (0.375 mg) given again 8 to 12 hours later. The subsequent maintenance dose (0.125 to 0.50 mg/day) is calculated from estimates of digoxin loss and is lower than the loading dose.

THERAPEUTIC INDEX

Two factors predict the quantitative aspect of a drug's margin of relative safety. These factors are known as the effective dose 50% (ED_{50}) and lethal dose 50% (LD_{50}). The ratio of effective dose : lethal dose is called the therapeutic index (TI).

$$TI = LD_{50}/ED_{50}$$

ED_{50} identifies the dose that is required to produce a therapeutic effect in 50% of the drug-tested populations. LD_{50} is the dose that kills 50% of the drug-tested populations.

TABLE 5-1 Mechanisms of Action of Nonspecific Drugs

Drug Class	Drug Example(s)	Probable Mechanism(s) of Action
Antimetabolites (chemotherapy)	fluorouracil (5-FU)	Replaces uracil in messenger RNA synthesis Cancer cells ultimately composed of nonfunctional proteins
Antidepressants Monoamine oxidase inhibitors	phenelzine (Nardil)	Inhibits metabolic catabolism of norepinephrine released from nerve endings
Antiparkinson drugs	levodopa (Dopar)	Can cross blood-brain barrier Synthesized to neurotransmitter dopamine in brain
Drugs Acting Through Chemical Actions on Other Cells or Other Chemicals		
Antacids	sodium bicarbonate	Chemically neutralizes gastric acid
Anticoagulants	heparin	Inhibits conversion of prothrombin to thrombin by inactivating factor Xa
Chelating agents Antidotes for heavy metal (lead, iron, mercury, arsenic) poisoning	deferoxamine (Desferal), dimercaprol (BAL in Oil), EDTA	Chemically binds (chelates) heavy metal ions
Skin antiseptics and disinfectants	alcohol	Destroys protein on bacterial cell walls
Drugs Acting Through Physical Actions on Cells		
General anesthetics	fluothane, halothane	Possibly alters physicochemical characteristics of nerve cell membranes
Osmotic diuretics	mannitol (Osmitrol)	Increases urine production by increasing urinary osmotic pressure Reduces H^+ reabsorption
Saline cathartics	magnesium hydroxide (Milk of Magnesia)	Increases osmotic pressure in GI tract Pulls water into intestines Increases evacuation of GI contents

A wide TI means the drug is relatively safe. These drugs may be dosed without undue concern, because the size of the dose is unlikely to harm the patient. A narrow TI requires that doses or plasma concentrations be carefully adjusted, because the safe dose is not greatly different from a dangerous dose. The danger involved in administration of a drug increases as the TI approaches 1, meaning that the effective dose is the same as the lethal dose.

TOLERANCE

Drug tolerance occurs when a fixed dose of a drug can no longer produce its effect and when successively larger doses of a drug are required to maintain the same level of effect. This may occur because of receptor tolerance or metabolic tolerance. In receptor tolerance, receptor response is a function of the concentration of the drug. Large concentrations of the drug may produce receptor downregulation, and the drug effect diminishes.

In metabolic tolerance, successive doses of a drug are met with diminishing effect as a result of the induction of degradative enzymes. The length of exposure relates to metabolic tolerance. Tolerance is a significant issue in pain control achieved by narcotic analgesics, whereby chronic pain becomes less responsive to the dose and type of analgesic. This necessitates frequent adjustment of doses and switching or supplementation of analgesics. Tachyphylaxis is the rapid appearance of progressive decrease in response following repetitive administration of a pharmacologically or physiologically active substance; increasing dosages cannot overcome the tolerance. This occurs with CNS agents (e.g., stimulants, such as dextroamphetamine) and with some bronchodilators and vasodilators.

Pharmacodynamics: Age-Related Changes

- Increased myocardial sensitivity to anesthesia
- Increased analgesic effect from opioids (or other CNS depressants)
- Increased sedative effect from benzodiazepines (or other CNS depressants)
- Increased anticoagulant effect from anticoagulant therapy
- Exaggerated responses to cardiovascular drugs (normal homeostatic responsiveness is altered)

Note: When administering drug therapy to an elderly patient, the nurse should be alert to the possibility of moderate reductions in drug clearance and the potential for exaggerated pharmacodynamic responsiveness.

IMPLICATIONS FOR NURSING MANAGEMENT

Nursing management in drug therapy requires the nurse to integrate core drug knowledge, including information on basic pharmacokinetics and pharmacodynamics with data from the assessment of core patient variables.

MAXIMIZING THERAPEUTIC EFFECTS

To promote effective drug therapy, the nurse must understand the principles of pharmacotherapeutics, pharmacokinetics, and pharmacodynamics and how core patient variables interact with these principles. Assessments of core patient variables should help predict whether the drug will act typically. If drug action is judged to be typical, the nurse then ensures that administration, dosing, and patient and family education are based on the core drug knowledge and assessment findings.

Assessing the patient's status for the appropriateness of the therapeutic regimen is crucial because circumstances change and patients may respond differently to a drug than was intended. For example, a patient's age plays a role in pharmacodynamics (see the accompanying display, Pharmacodynamics: Age-Related Changes). Because drug action depends on drug absorption, the nurse must also assess the appropriateness of the administration site and route and the probable effect. For instance, a patient with impaired swallowing may be unable to take drugs by the oral route; IM or SC drug administration may be unsuitable for a patient with impaired circulation or lipodystrophy.

MINIMIZING ADVERSE EFFECTS

If atypical drug action or effect is likely to occur, the nurse can make appropriate modifications in managing drug therapy to promote an effective outcome. For example, a patient with liver failure is more likely to develop adverse effects or toxicities. In such a case, drug dosage may need to be modified or the intervals between doses changed. Minimally, drug levels need to be monitored and the patient carefully assessed for early signs of adverse effects.

CHAPTER SUMMARY

- No drug has a single action. Drug action occurs by a change in cellular environment or by an alteration in the rate of cellular function. Drugs do not create responses; they simply modify existing responses. Changes in cellular environment are brought about by physical or chemical reactions; a drug may have one or both actions.
- Receptors—cellular proteins or nucleic acids—are specialized cellular structures with which many drugs react. Agonist substances—occurring internally or administered to the patient—directly alter the receptor's functional properties. Antagonist drugs inhibit the action of an agonist.
- Drug potency refers to the relative amount of a drug required to produce a response.

QUESTIONS FOR STUDY AND REVIEW

1. What are the three general mechanisms by which drugs interact with the body to produce a biologic effect?
2. What is meant by the terms *drug agonist* and *drug antagonist*?

NEED MORE HELP?

Chapter 5 of the study guide for *Drug Therapy in Nursing* contains exercises and activities to reinforce your understanding of the concepts presented in this chapter. For additional information see the text's accompanying website at *http://www.connection.lww.com.*

REFERENCES AND BIBLIOGRAPHY

Bullock, D. L. (1999). Viewpoint–Pharmacogenetics and its impact on drug development. *Drug Benefit Trends, 11*(1), 53–54.

Carrico, J. M. (2000). Human genome project and pharmacogenomics: Implications for pharmacy. *Journal of the American Pharmaceutical Association, 40*(1), 115–116.

Fauci, A., Braunwald, E., Wilson, J. D., Martin, J. B., Hauser, S. L., Longo, D. L., Kasper, D. L., Isselbachter, K. J. (Eds.). (1999). *Harrison's Online.* New York: McGraw-Hill.

Fletcher, C. V., Acosta, E. P., & Strykowski, J. M. (1994). Gender differences in human pharmacokinetics and pharmacodynamics. *Journal of Adolescent Health, 15,* 619–629.

Gossel, T. A. (1998). Exploring pharmacology. *U.S. Pharmacist, 23*(9), 96–103.

Gossel, T. A. (1998). Pharmacology: Back to basics. *U.S. Pharmacist, 23*(11), 96–103.

Gossel, T. A. (1999). Pharmacodynamics: How drugs act. *U.S. Pharmacist, 24*(9), 101–108.

Hardman, J. G., Limbird, L. E., Molinof, P. B., Ruddon, R. W., Gilman, A. (Eds.). (1997). *Goodman and Gilman's pharmacological basis of therapeutics* (9th ed.). New York: McGraw-Hill.

Kroetz, D. L. (2000). Genomics and proteomics in drug discovery and development. Presented at the Millennial World Congress of Pharmaceutical Sciences, San Francisco, California, April 16–20.

Lewis, J. F., & Mensah, G. A. (2000). Ethnic and gender disparities in cardiovascular mortality. . .The scientific basis, mechanisms, and strategies for closing the gap in the new millennium. Anaheim, CA: Joint Symposium of the Association of Black Cardiologists/American College of Cardiology, Scientific Session.

Chapter 6

ADVERSE EFFECTS AND DRUG INTERACTIONS

KEY TERMS

additive effect
adverse effect
allergic reaction
anaphylaxis
antagonistic drug interaction
chelation
drug interaction
drug toxicity
idiosyncratic drug response
neurotoxicity
object drug
potentiation
precipitant drug
radiopharmaceutical
side effect
synergistic effect
toxic effect

Learning Objectives

At the completion of this chapter the student will:

1. Identify the core drug knowledge of adverse effects and drug interactions.
2. Name and explain the major toxicities that may occur from drug therapy.
3. Identify core patient variables related to adverse effects and drug interactions.
4. Relate the interaction of core drug knowledge to core patient variables for adverse effects and drug interactions.
5. Describe how alcohol and nicotine affect drug disposition and action.
6. Describe how interactions between drugs and food can produce alterations in the drug's therapeutic effect or in the use of nutrients.
7. Generate a nursing plan of care from the interactions between core drug knowledge and core patient variables for adverse effects and drug interactions.
8. Describe nursing interventions to maximize therapeutic effects and minimize adverse effects in drug therapy.
9. Determine key points for patient and family education about adverse effects and drug interactions.

As drug therapy becomes more complex, the number of significant adverse reactions and drug interactions will grow and pose potentially serious problems. The administration of more than one drug is common. As the number of drugs a patient receives increases, so does the probability of a drug interaction. Just like the principles that govern the behavior of drugs in the body, the administration of one drug may influence the pharmacodynamics, pharmacokinetics, and pharmacotherapeutics of another drug.

An **adverse effect** of drug therapy is an effect—other than the desired therapeutic effect—that may occur during drug therapy. The effect may result from too much of a therapeutic effect (e.g., hypotension may result from antihypertensive drug therapy) or from other pharmacodynamic effects of the drug (e.g., beta blockers are given for their effect on the heart but they also have an effect on the bronchial tree). These effects are usually dose dependent and predictable. Adverse effects may also result from an allergic or idiosyncratic reaction. These effects may or may not be dose related, and are usually unpredictable. They also tend to be more serious adverse effects.

Historically, different terms were used to differentiate mild from serious, nontherapeutic drug effects. A **side effect** usually refers to a minor effect, such as nausea, whereas a **toxic effect** usually refers to a more serious effect, such as impaired renal function. A side effect may be uncomfortable or undesirable but not significant enough to warrant discontinuing therapy. A toxic effect, conversely, may cause significant impairment, tissue or organ damage, or death. In reality, the distinction among terms is blurry, and classification as to one or the other is somewhat arbitrary. The term adverse effect encompasses all nontherapeutic responses to drug therapy and is used throughout this text.

A **drug interaction** occurs when one drug and a second drug or element (e.g., food) have an effect on each other. This effect, or interaction, may increase or decrease the therapeutic effect on one or both of the drugs, create a new effect, or increase the incidence of an adverse effect.

To maximize therapeutic effect, minimize adverse effects, and plan for appropriate patient and family education, nurses need to understand these aspects of core drug knowledge (adverse effects and drug interactions) in their management of drug therapy.

ADVERSE EFFECTS

Every drug can produce adverse effects. Adverse effects most commonly are mild and perhaps only bothersome to the patient (such as nausea). They may also be serious or even life threatening (such as liver failure). Serious adverse effects lead to a small number of drugs withdrawn from the market yearly. The reason for this is not because the drug was approved without testing. Clinical studies are done on all drugs under development and all adverse effects in the study participants are identified. Sometimes, complete knowledge of adverse effects cannot occur until the drug has been used for a longer period of time than the length of the trial. Sometimes adverse effects can only be identified when used more extensively by certain patient populations, such as older adults, or patients with a certain disease process (i.e. renal disease). These patients may not have been adequately represented in the study population. It is important for nurses and other health care professionals to be alert for adverse effects from drug therapy. Adverse effects may be mistaken for aging or disease pathology. For example, slight memory loss may be attributed to changes with aging, or hyperglycemia may be attributed to uncontrolled diabetes rather than to an adverse effect.

ALLERGIC REACTIONS

Allergic reactions account for up to 10% of all adverse effects. Frequently, the terms hypersensitivity and drug allergy are used to indicate the same type of drug response, although this is not entirely correct. A hypersensitivity reaction is marked by abnormal sensitivity or an exaggerated response by the body to the stimulus of a foreign agent. A drug allergy, or **allergic reaction**, is marked by increasing reactivity on subsequent exposures to the foreign agent.

The allergic response represents an altered physiologic reaction to a drug because a prior exposure to the drug stimulated the immune system to develop antibodies. Subsequent exposure to the drug produces an antigen-antibody response, prompting the release of histamine, which damages body tissues. Allergic reactions vary widely in terms of type, onset, extent, and severity. They are not predictable from the drug therapy, nor are they dose related. Common allergic reactions include rash, hives, redness, swelling, and itching (Table 6-2).

Antibiotics (penicillin), diagnostic agents (iodine-based contrast media), biologicals (antitoxins, vaccines, enzymes), and miscellaneous drugs (aspirin, gold salts, iron dextran, phenothiazines, topical anesthetics, and tranquilizers) are frequently implicated in allergic reactions. An individual demonstrating a mild allergic response, such as a rash, to a particular drug should avoid reexposure to that drug because reexposure to a chemical antigen may cause anaphylaxis.

Anaphylaxis is a systemic reaction caused by contraction of smooth muscles and increased vascular permeability. It is characterized by dyspnea, bronchospasm, laryngeal edema, cardiac dysrhythmias, and occasionally seizures, hypotension, and acute cardiovascular collapse. Anaphylaxis is a medical emergency and is treated by IV administration of epinephrine, antihistamines (usually diphenhydramine), and bronchodilators (usually aminophylline). Anaphylaxis is the most serious of allergic reactions.

IDIOSYNCRATIC RESPONSES

An **idiosyncratic drug response** is an unusual, abnormal, or peculiar response to a drug (e.g., an exaggerated or diminished response to the drug's effects or an unanticipated, unexplainable response to a drug, such as excitability after administration of a sedative). Sometimes an idiosyncratic response is referred to as a paradoxical response. Idiosyncratic responses are thought to occur because of genetic enzymatic deficiencies that alter the drug's metabolism. For example, individuals with decreased production of G6PD-glucose-6-phosphate dehydrogenase deficiency (about 10% of African-American males) will develop a serious hemolytic anemia when given the antimalarial agent primaquine. Symptoms of

TABLE 6-1 Influence of Adverse Effects on Body Systems

Body System	Adverse Effects	Common Drug Causes
Central nervous system	*Delirium, disorientation,* lethargy, psychomotor retardation, subjective feelings of loss and sadness	Antidepressants, corticosteroids, hypnotics, indomethacin, methyldopa, reserpine, sedatives
Cardiovascular	*Arrhythmias,* heart failure, *hypotension, fluid and electrolyte imbalances*	Beta-adrenergic blockers (e.g., propranolol), corticosteroids, diuretics
Respiratory	Asthma, respiratory depression	Opioids, propranolol
Eye, ear, nose, and throat	Blurred vision, *blindness, cataract development, corneal and retinal changes* *Deafness,* dizziness, vertigo, tinnitus	Aminoglycoside antimicrobials, chloroquine, corticosteroids, phenothiazines, quinine, salicylates
Gastrointestinal	Nausea and vomiting, anorexia, thirst, constipation, diarrhea, flatus, abdominal pain/cramping *Hepatitis, biliary obstruction, hepatic necrosis*	Acetaminophen, halothane, tetracycline
Genitourinary	Urinary frequency or retention, impotence, *glomerulonephritis, acute or chronic renal failure*	Aminoglycoside antimicrobials, aspirin, histamine-2-receptor blockers, nonsteroidal anti-inflammatory drugs
Hematopoietic	*Hemolytic anemia, thrombocytopenia, agranulocytosis*	Antineoplastic drugs, chlorpromazine, meprobamate, phenylbutazone, quinidine
Integumentary	Alopecia, rashes, skin pigmentation changes	Antiepileptic drugs (phenytoin, carbamazepine), antineoplastic drugs, barbiturates, sulfonamides
Reproductive	*Teratogenic effects, fetal and neonatal functional abnormalities*	Antineoplastic drugs, isotretinoin, narcotics

Note: Serious adverse effects are italicized.

systemic lupus erythematosus (SLE) associated with procainamide and malignant hyperthermia associated with the general anesthetic halothane are also considered to be idiosyncratic drug responses. Idiosyncratic responses are not considered allergic reactions.

DRUG TOXICITY

Drugs accumulate in the body whenever the dosage exceeds the amount the body can eliminate through metabolism and excretion. A drug accumulation that causes problems (e.g.,

TABLE 6-2 Allergic Reactions to Drugs

Type of Reaction	Response and Symptoms	Possible Causes
Type I: Involves IgE antibodies	Immediate tissue reactions; angioedema (giant wheals)	Insect bites
	Urticaria (hives), *anaphylaxis (shock),* asthma, rhinitis	Antibiotics, nonsteroidal anti-inflammatory drugs
Type II: Involves IgG and IgM antibodies	Drug-induced autoimmune disorders, such as *systemic lupus erythematosus*	Hydralazine
	Granulocytopenia (decreased granulocytes, a blood abnormality)	Methyldopa, penicillin, procainamide, sulfonamide
	Thrombocytopenia purpura	Quinidine
Type III: Involves formation of antigen—antibody complexes with the blood vessels	Antigen–antibody tissue responses; arthralgia, *drug fever,* lymphadenopathy, urticaria (hives) and other skin eruptions Serum sickness (delayed response occurring 6–14 d after drug exposure) Stevens-Johnson syndrome	Iodides, penicillin, sulfonamides, succinimide
Type IV: Involves cell-mediated response	Contact dermatitis, such as poison ivy	Reexposure to antigen Products containing topical benzene and phenol

Note: Major adverse effects are italicized.

poisoning, blood abnormalities, coma) is known as **drug toxicity**. Several factors may be responsible for this. The drug may have a narrow therapeutic margin of safety (e.g., digitalis, insulin), the drug may be taken for a long time (e.g., phenytoin, lithium, theophylline), or drug-drug interactions may alter the usual pharmacokinetics of each drug. Effects of drug toxicity occur because of high doses, accumulation of the drug, or the individual's hyperresponsiveness to the drug. The likelihood of toxicity is inversely proportional to the margin of safety, although no drug is completely lacking in toxic potential. Serious drug toxicities can cause cellular death, which can lead to failure of the organ.

How severely drug or chemical toxicity will impair organ function depends on the organ's reserve capacities and regeneration capabilities. For example, more than 80% of renal function must be lost before impairment is suspected or detected on a routine examination. Injuries to a tissue with a high capacity for regeneration (e.g., liver) are usually reversible unless there is repeated exposure to the toxic chemical (e.g., alcohol) resulting in cirrhosis and permanent scarring. Among the most serious toxicities are neurotoxicity, also known as central nervous system (CNS) toxicity, hepatotoxicity, cardiotoxicity, nephrotoxicity, and ototoxicity.

Neurotoxicity

Injury to the CNS is largely irreversible because the highly differentiated neurons of the brain cannot divide and regenerate. **Neurotoxicity** can occur after exposure to drugs and other chemicals and gases (e.g., alcohol, solvents, insecticides, industrial vapors, and pollutants). The extreme susceptibility of neural tissue to toxicants is largely due to its high metabolic rate, high lipid content, and high circulatory requirement (14% of cardiac output to approximately 20% of body mass). Immature nervous systems (e.g., fetal and neonatal nervous systems) are also characterized by extreme susceptibility to neurotoxicants.

Manifestations of CNS toxicity include structural damage, such as that associated with lead-induced encephalopathy; molecular-level damage, such as cyanide-induced enzyme inhibition; or functional-level damage, such as behavioral dysfunction. Signs and symptoms of neurotoxicity include drowsiness, auditory and visual disturbances, restlessness, nystagmus (oscillating eyeballs), and tonic-clonic (grand mal) seizures.

Hepatotoxicity

Hepatic anatomy and hepatic function both contribute significantly to the high susceptibility of the liver to toxicants. The liver (5% of body mass) receives approximately 30% of the cardiac output. Blood draining from the stomach and small intestines is delivered directly to the liver by the hepatic portal vein. As a result, the liver is exposed first to relatively large concentrations of ingested drugs or other potential toxicants. Hepatic exposure to toxicants can be significant because the highest activity of cytochrome P450-mixed function oxidase enzymes and most biotransformations occur within this system. Manifestations of hepatotoxicity include hepatitis, jaundice, elevated liver enzyme levels, and fatty infiltration of the liver.

Nephrotoxicity

The renal system is similar to the hepatic system in that it is susceptible to poisoning because of its extensive vascularity. The kidneys receive a large portion of the cardiac output (25%) in relation to their mass (0.5%). The largest concentration of cytochrome P-450 is found in the cells of the proximal tubule and, generally, this is the site of nephrotoxicity. The cells within the proximal tubule are responsible for filtering, concentrating, and eliminating toxicants. As water is reabsorbed, the concentration of chemicals in the tubule can rise to toxic levels, thereby increasing the potential for damage. Chemically induced kidney damage is typically manifested as acute tubular necrosis.

Immunotoxicity

A wide variety of drugs can affect the immune system. Some may cause immunosuppression, whereas others may directly destroy immune system components. For example, the effect of immunosuppression may be an increased incidence of bacterial, viral, and parasitic infections, and theoretically, immunosuppression may interfere with the immune system's protective, or surveillance, function, resulting in an increased incidence of carcinogenesis. Benzene (a highly toxic hydrocarbon used as a solvent) causes lymphocytopenia and affects other bone marrow elements, resulting in a deficiency in cell-mediated immunity. Numerous other chemicals and drugs (e.g., penicillins, sulfonamides, preservative sulfites, polyvinyl chloride fumes) can induce immunologically mediated respiratory and hypersensitivity diseases.

Cardiotoxicity

Irregularities in cardiac rhythms and conduction and possibly heart damage may result from an adverse effect known as cardiotoxicity. Drugs associated with cardiotoxicity include the antineoplastics doxorubicin and daunorubicin. Why they are cardiotoxic is unknown, but the effect is more dramatic in elderly patients and children younger than 2 years. Characteristics of cardiotoxicity include transient cardiac arrhythmias and depression of myocardial function. Congestive heart failure, which responds poorly to the standard treatment of digitalization and diuresis, also may occur.

Ototoxicity

Many drugs can produce ototoxicity, which affects the eighth cranial nerve and results in inner ear or auditory nerve damage. Structures of the inner ear that may be affected include the cochlea (responsible for hearing sound) and the vestibule and semicircular canals (responsible for balance). Ototoxicity may or may not be reversible.

Signs and symptoms of ototoxicity include tinnitus, which is a buzzing or ringing sound in the ear, and sensorineural hearing loss. Also called nerve deafness, sensorineural hearing loss usually begins with high-frequency sound and may worsen until low-frequency sound is difficult to hear. Drugs closely associated with ototoxicity include aspirin and other salicylates, loop diuretics, quinidine, quinine, and aminoglycosides. Other signs and symptoms, particularly of vestibular toxicity, include light-headedness, vertigo, a spinning sensation from a seated position, and nausea and vomiting.

DRUG INTERACTIONS AND INTERACTION MECHANISMS

Just as various kinds of adverse effects can occur, so can various kinds of drug interactions. Drug interactions may involve changes in drug absorption, protein binding, biotransformation, and excretion. Drug interactions may occur among drugs administered concurrently or between drugs and foods. They may also cause false results in various laboratory and diagnostic tests.

PHARMACOKINETIC INTERACTIONS

Interactions Involving Gastrointestinal Absorption

There are several mechanisms by which one drug may affect the gastrointestinal (GI) absorption of another. These mechanisms include drug binding in the GI tract; alterations in GI motility, gastric pH, and intestinal flora; and drug metabolism within the walls of the intestine, including the intestinal mucosa (Fig. 6-1). For many GI absorption interactions, however, the mechanism is unknown.

Drug Binding in the GI Tract

Drug binding in the GI tract occurs by several mechanisms. An agent with a large surface area can use its surface to absorb another drug and prevent it from passing across the intestinal wall. This is the case with activated charcoal, antacids, and kaolin-pectin mixtures. This binding in the GI tract reduces the pharmacotherapeutic effects of the **object**

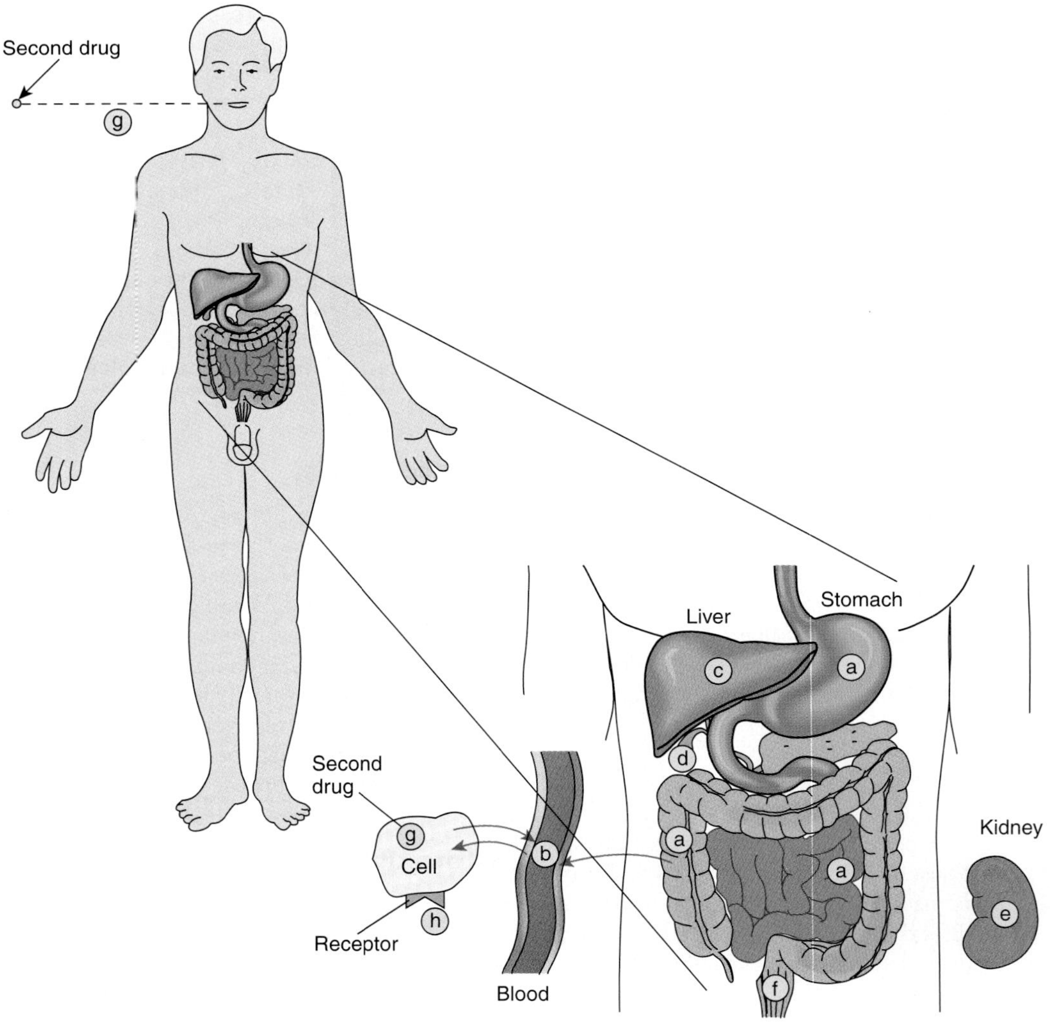

Figure 6-1. Drug interaction sites within the body. Drug interactions can occur in numerous body sites. Absorption can be enhanced or reduced in the gut (**a**); protein binding can be affected within the vasculature (**b**); metabolism can be affected in the liver (**c**); excretion can be affected either through bile (**d**); the kidney (**e**), or in feces (**f**); tissue binding of one drug can be affected by another (**g**); and finally, drugs may have an effect through action on specific receptors (**h**).

drug (i.e., the one affected by the interaction). The use of activated charcoal in treating a drug overdose takes advantage of this interaction.

In another kind of interaction, an object drug is rendered inactive as the result of **chelation**, whereby an agent binds with the object drug, removing it from circulation or keeping it from accumulating in areas where it does not belong. Other object drugs form insoluble, nonabsorbable complexes; for example, antacids and sucralfate reduce the GI absorption of the anti-infective quinolones, and metals (aluminum, calcium) or iron salts significantly inhibit the GI absorption of most tetracyclines, methyldopa, and levodopa.

Bile-binding resins (e.g., cholestyramine, colestipol) can also bind drugs and will inhibit the GI absorption of thiazide diuretics, thyroxine, warfarin, and acidic nonsteroidal anti-inflammatory drugs.

Alterations in Motility

Most orally administered drugs are absorbed in the small intestine. In some cases, a drug's rate of absorption is affected by the rate of gastric emptying. Anticholinergic drugs, for example, slow gastric emptying time, thereby slowing absorption (e.g., of acetaminophen); whereas metoclopramide hastens absorption by speeding the rate of gastric emptying.

GI motility may also influence the extent of absorption. For example, a slowing of GI motility will allow drugs that dissolve slowly or poorly in GI fluids additional time to dissolve before reaching their absorptive sites in the small intestine, thereby increasing bioavailability. Conversely, however, some drugs are degraded to inactive substances in the stomach; in this situation, the small intestine would receive more intact drug for absorption if the gastric emptying rate were increased. The bioavailability of levodopa, for example, is enhanced with antacid-induced accelerated gastric emptying.

Alterations in pH

The effects of GI pH on drug absorption can be complex because the effects of nonionized drug forms depend on dissolution. Some drugs manifest pH-dependent degradation, and pH may affect GI motility. Predicting the effect that pH changes will have on the absorption of a particular drug is usually difficult. Ketoconazole, for example, demonstrates the importance of pH on drug dissolution. To dissolve adequately enough to be absorbed, ketoconazole requires an acid medium; therefore, its bioavailability would be markedly reduced by administering a drug that decreases gastric acidity, such as a histamine-2-receptor antagonist.

Alterations in Intestinal Flora

In contrast to the large bowel, where many bacterial flora are present, the stomach, duodenum, jejunum, and upper ileum are relatively uncolonized by bacteria. Drugs that are well absorbed from the small intestine are insignificantly affected by changes in the GI tract flora. Conversely, changes in intestinal flora adversely affect drugs that are not well absorbed by the small intestine or those that are secreted back into the intestine after absorption.

In some individuals, a substantial amount of digoxin, a drug used to treat congestive heart failure, is degraded by intestinal flora. Administration of an antibiotic to these individuals may substantially increase plasma digoxin concentrations because of the reduced bacterial inactivation of digoxin. This would place the patient at risk for developing adverse effects from the drug therapy.

Another example of changes in bacterial flora affecting pharmacotherapeutic effects is the interaction between oral contraceptives and oral antibiotics. Several cases of unintended pregnancy have occurred in women who also received antibiotic therapy (most often implicated are the penicillins and tetracycline).

Interactions Involving Enzyme Induction

The primary function of drug-metabolizing enzymes is to transform lipid-soluble drugs into more water-soluble metabolites. This promotes their excretion through the urine and bile. Some drugs increase the synthesis of the hepatic drug-metabolizing enzymes, and this process is called enzyme induction. When other drugs that are ordinarily metabolized by enzyme induction are concurrently given, they will demonstrate a decrease in pharmacotherapeutic and pharmacologic effects because of their increased metabolism (Fig. 6-2). Some drugs induce their own metabolism (e.g., carbamazepine and phenobarbital). Some drugs, particularly those known as social drugs, may induce hepatic metabolizing enzymes.

Most of the enzyme-inducing drugs are the CNS depressant anticonvulsants (e.g., carbamazepine, phenobarbital, phenytoin), although one antimicrobial drug, rifampin, demonstrates enzyme-inducing characteristics. Phenobarbital is considered to be the classic enzyme-inducer; it stimulates the liver to increase production of microsomal enzymes,

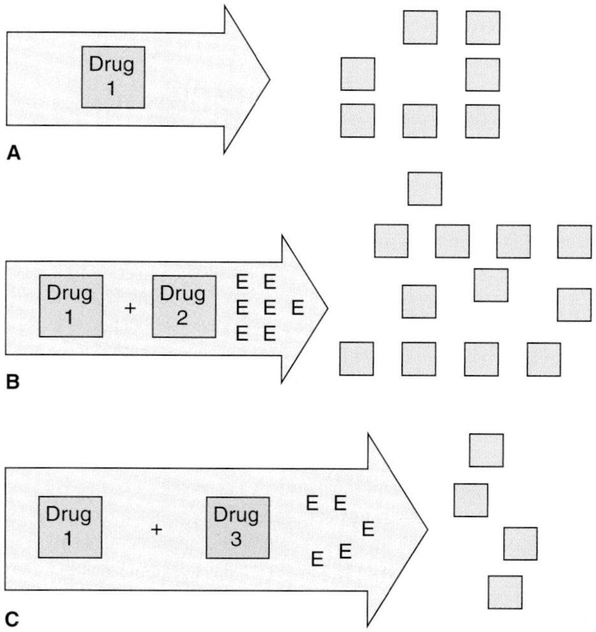

Figure 6-2. Normal drug metabolism is shown in (**A**). In some drug-drug interactions involving enzyme activity, drug metabolism will be increased (**B**) or decreased (**C**) by the addition of another drug that induces or inhibits the hepatic microsomal enzyme system.

which leads to an increased biotransformation of a wide variety of drugs and consequently reduces their plasma concentrations. Enzyme induction involves the synthesis of new enzyme and is a relatively slow, gradual process; its appearance takes several days, and its maximum effect is not apparent for as long as several weeks.

Another CNS depressant associated with enzyme induction is alcohol. Chronic alcohol ingestion increases the metabolism and reduces the activity of isoniazid, phenytoin, tolbutamide, and warfarin. Nicotine may also induce drug metabolizing enzymes. For more information, see the accompanying display, Smoking and Enzyme Induction.

Interactions Involving Enzyme Inhibition

One drug can interfere with the metabolism of another drug, thereby increasing the pharmacotherapeutic effect of one of the drugs. For example, many commonly used drugs, such as alcohol, cimetidine, erythromycin, fluoxetine, and propoxyphene, may inhibit the activity of hepatic enzymes used in drug metabolism. This is known as enzyme inhibition. Some enzyme-inhibiting drugs, such as verapamil, inhibit their own metabolism and that of other drugs.

Drug interactions that cause enzyme inhibition are not clinically noticeable if the drug that inhibits metabolism is started first. When the second drug is added, it will be titrated until serum levels are appropriate or the desired therapeutic response is obtained. Problems will be evident, however, if the drug that inhibits metabolism is started after the other drug or drugs. Drug levels of the first drug will then decrease, and the therapeutic effect will also decrease. If the drug causing metabolic inhibition is stopped first, drug levels of the other drug will increase, causing additional therapeutic effects and possibly adverse effects.

Inhibited drug metabolism is one of the most common causes of drug interaction. The clinical significance of an enzyme-inhibition interaction depends on core patient variables, such health status (e.g., concurrent drug therapy with enzyme inhibitors or inducers, hepatic dysfunction), life span (particularly age) and gender, and culture (genetic differences).

Smoking and Enzyme Induction

Smoking tends to alter the disposition and action of many drugs. A very important effect is the reduction of the drug level in the blood and the subsequent decrease of drug effect primarily as a result of enzyme induction. Following is a list of examples of potential drug interactions caused by smoking:

- Smokers taking benzodiazepine may require higher doses to achieve equivalent sedative effects to those of nonsmokers.
- In smokers taking heparin, the drug half-life is shorter and elimination is greater than in nonsmokers.
- Patients with diabetes who are heavy smokers may have insulin requirements almost one third higher than nonsmokers.
- Considerable epidemiologic evidence correlates smoking with increased risk of adverse cardiovascular effects (cardiovascular accident, myocardial infarction, thromboembolism).
- Smokers who receive the narcotic analgesics pentazocine or propoxyphene need significantly increased dosage to experience the same effect as nonsmokers.
- In patients who smoke and who take propranolol for angina pectoris, smoking reduces serum drug concentrations, increases drug clearance, and inhibits the expected therapeutic effect.

Interactions Involving Renal Excretion

Drugs are either eliminated unchanged, or as metabolites, or in both ways. Most interactions involving drug excretion occur in the kidney, but the liver and GI tract are occasional sites of drug excretion interactions. Most decreases in glomerular filtration occur because of changes in the filtration pressure, which may be altered by changes in the systemic blood pressure or by changes in the glomerular hydrostatic pressure (both of which are alterations in health status). When a patient's glomerular filtration rate decreases, drugs primarily eliminated by glomerular filtration accumulate and possibly result in drug toxicity.

Drug interactions may result from altered renal tubular secretion. The active process of tubular secretion occurs in the proximal portion of the renal tubule. To be secreted, a drug molecule must pass from the blood through the basolateral membrane and into the proximal tubular cell cytoplasm.

Distinct and unique systems are used for organic, ionic transport. These transport systems are a series of proteins located on the basolateral membrane, and each protein has a unique affinity for anion or cation transport. Generally, substances that are excreted by one system of proteins do not compete for excretion with the other system (e.g., organic anion system). Instead, drugs sharing a similar transport system commonly interact with each other by competitive inhibition. An example of this is the interaction between probenecid (Benemid) and the penicillins. Probenecid reduces the renal excretion of penicillins (also the cephalosporins), and this interaction is commonly used to enhance the pharmacotherapeutic effect of the penicillins.

Interactions Involving Radiopharmaceuticals

Interactions involving a therapeutic drug or contrast agent and a **radiopharmaceutical** (i.e., a radioactive compound used in diagnosis and treatment) are pharmacokinetic, because the interaction alters or modifies drug distribution. (Because radiopharmaceutical compounds do not exert any pharmacologic activity, the possibility of a pharmacodynamic interaction does not exist.) See the accompanying display, Mechanisms of Radiopharmaceutical Drug Interactions.

PHARMACODYNAMIC INTERACTIONS

Many drugs are capable of interacting with each other. Pharmacodynamic interactions may occur when drugs with similar actions or adverse effects are administered simultaneously. Just because there are known interactions between drugs in certain combinations does not necessarily mean that they cannot be given together. Sometimes drug interactions are actively sought as part of a therapeutic objective. For example,

Mechanisms of Radiopharmaceutical Drug Interactions

How an organ system handles a radiopharmaceutical may be altered by pharmacotherapeutics or pharmacodynamics of a drug:

- Patients medicated with an opioid before radionuclide hepatobiliary imaging may exhibit clinical signs of cholelithiasis—or other nonspecific gallbladder disease—because the narcotic analgesic prevents the radiopharmaceutical from emptying into the duodenum.
- The toxic effect of a therapeutic drug or contrast agent (drug-induced disease) may alter the way an organ system handles a radiopharmaceutical. For example, gallium-67 is useful in detecting lymphomas and many inflammatory disorders. Some drugs (e.g., amiodarone, nitrofurantoin, bleomycin) can cause pulmonary interstitial pneumonitis or fibrosis, which can easily be confused with other forms of diffuse pulmonary disease not related to drug therapy.
- Competition between a therapeutic medication and a radiopharmaceutical (contrast agent) for receptor binding sites or elimination pathways may alter the way the body handles the radiopharmaceutical. For example, a radioactive iodine uptake study is frequently used as a diagnostic tool for thyroid function. Iodine-123 or iodine-131 is given orally, and uptake measurements are usually made at 4 hours and 24 hours. If the patient is taking certain expectorants, vitamins, or even topical medications containing iodine salts, test results may be normal. In such instances, the false-negative results occur because the iodine-containing compounds may compete with the radioactive iodine for uptake binding sites in the thyroid gland. As a result, the radioiodine uptake in the gland is reduced to a normal range, and patients who actually have hyperthyroidism will appear to have a normal or balanced thyroid status (euthyroid). Conversely, a drug-induced reduction of thyroid uptake may result in a diagnosis of hypothyroidism (a false-positive study result) in euthyroid patients.
- A physiochemical attraction or interaction between a therapeutic medication and a radiopharmaceutical or a drug-induced change in the environment in which the radiopharmaceutical exists may alter the way the body handles the radiopharmaceutical. For example, administration of iron dextran physiochemically alters the distribution of the bone-seeking radiotracer technetium-99 (Tc99). Resulting images may reveal a decreased skeletal uptake of Tc-99.

in the treatment of chronic moderate hypertension, several antihypertensive drugs may be administered; their combined effects may be additive or synergistic.

Additive Effect

An **additive effect** occurs when two or more "like" (in terms of effects) drugs are combined, and the result is the sum of the individual drug's effects. For example, 1 (drug A) + 1 (drug B) = 2. This additive effect may be purposeful or harmful. For example, combining two analgesic drugs (e.g., codeine and acetaminophen) is a purposeful additive drug interaction that controls pain better than either drug alone. An example of a harmful additive drug interaction is combining alcohol with a salicylate; the incidence of GI bleeding is greatly increased because each agent independently can cause GI bleeding.

Synergistic Effect

A **synergistic effect** occurs when two or more "unlike" drugs are used together to produce a combined effect, and the outcome is a drug effect greater than any of either drug's activity alone. For example, 1 (drug A) + 1 (drug B) = 3.

Just like an additive interaction, a synergistic interaction may be purposeful or harmful. A beneficial synergistic effect occurs with the combination of penicillin G and an aminoglycoside antibiotic in the treatment of subacute bacterial endocarditis. A harmful synergy is represented by the interaction between the hypnotic drugs and alcohol; this interaction causes a prolonged hypnotic effect that may be fatal.

Another type of synergistic interaction may be used to achieve a therapeutic objective; this occurs when two or more "like" drugs in terms of effects, but different in terms of site or mechanism of action, are used together. For example, combining an alpha-adrenergic blocker (vasodilator), a beta-adrenergic blocker (sympatholytic), and a diuretic (which lowers blood volume) achieves antihypertensive effects better than any single drug alone.

Potentiation

The pharmacodynamic interaction of **potentiation** is sometimes used to mean synergism. This is not entirely correct. Potentiation best describes a particular type of synergistic interaction in which the effect of only one of the two drugs is increased. In other words, a drug that has a mild effect enhances the effect of a second drug. For example, 1/2 (drug A) + 1 (drug B) = 2.

Antagonistic Interactions

An **antagonistic drug interaction** is the opposite of synergism. It results in a therapeutic effect that is less than the effect of either drug alone because the second drug either diminishes or cancels the effects of the first drug. For example, 1 (drug A) + 1 (drug B) = 0. This effect is seen with the combination of the heparin antagonist protamine sulfate (a strong basic anticoagulant) given as an antidote for heparin (a strong acidic anticoagulant)-induced bleeding; a stable salt forms, resulting in a loss of anticoagulant activity of both drugs.

TOXIC EFFECTS OF DRUG INTERACTIONS

A toxic effect occurs when a drug's effect exceeds its therapeutic level. Toxic effects may be additive or synergistic. Combining drugs that possess a potentially ototoxic effect (e.g., furosemide, aminoglycoside antibiotics) may result in a combined effect of damage to the eighth cranial nerve and deafness (ototoxicity). The negative side of drug interactions is that the expected therapeutic effect of a drug may be greatly distorted by the interacting **precipitant drug.**

DRUG INCOMPATIBILITIES

Drug incompatibilities are similar to drug-drug interactions in that a chemical inactivation or physical reaction occurs. This reaction may involve two or more drugs, inside or outside the body, ultimately affecting a drug's action. For more information, see the accompanying display, Drug Incompatibilities and Drug Administration.

DRUG-FOOD INTERACTIONS

Food and drugs may interact to alter the effect of pharmacotherapy. Drug efficacy may be either diminished or enhanced nutritionally by changes in drug absorption, drug metabolism, and drug excretion. The absorption of orally administered drugs is by far the most common cause of changes in drug efficacy (Table 6-3).

Food stimulates physiologic changes in the GI tract that may increase, decrease, delay, or prevent the absorption of drugs. For instance, pectin food fibers delay food's entry from the stomach to the duodenum, thus increasing the time for orally administered drugs to be absorbed from the intestine. The amount of bile released and the pH of the intestinal contents are affected by the type of foods consumed and their transit times. These considerations and others become especially important if absorption time or rate affect the efficacy of drug therapy.

A few drugs are better absorbed or better tolerated by the patient when taken with food; however, absorption occurs more slowly and less completely when most drugs are taken with food.

DRUG-NUTRIENT INTERACTIONS

Drug interactions may also result from nutrients interacting with drugs. Although drug-nutrient interactions are not as common as drug-drug or drug-food interactions, they can have an impact on therapeutic outcome. Drugs can affect nutritional status by altering nutrient absorption, metabolism, use, or excretion. Minerals in foods can combine or compete with drugs or alter the GI environment to affect the normal absorption processes of drugs and minerals. There are three types of drug-mineral interactions:

1. Malabsorption of the mineral or drug
2. Mineral depletion or retention
3. Drug-mineral interactions induced by simultaneous antacid ingestion

Drug Incompatibilities and Drug Administration

When administering drugs parenterally (IV, IM, SC), the nurse must be especially alert to the possibility of drug incompatibilities and drug interactions. The most common kinds of incompatibilities are chemical and physical.

Chemical Incompatibilities

Chemical incompatibilities between drugs change both the drug's molecular structure and its pharmacologic properties. The alteration may be beneficial. For example, heparin and protamine sulfate (a heparin antagonist) form an ionic bond lacking any anticoagulant activity. Conversely, the chemical incompatibility may also be harmful; for example, combining multivitamins and antibiotics in the same IV solution changes the solution's pH and inactivates the antibiotic.

Physical Incompatibilities

Physical incompatibilities occur when two drugs are mixed together. The mixture results in the formation of a precipitate. Phenytoin and a diluent containing dextrose, for example, produce a cloudy, white precipitate. This kind of reaction usually interferes with the pharmacologic activity of one or both drugs. This is one of the reasons that manufacturers provide specific instructions for preparation, dilution, and addition of drugs to other solutions. These instructions should be followed carefully.

EFFECTS OF DRUG INTERACTIONS ON LABORATORY TEST RESULTS

Many drugs can alter the results of standard laboratory tests. For example, amphotericin B, most diuretics, and the corticosteroids frequently suppress serum potassium levels. Adrenergic agents, estrogen, and nicotine increase serum cortisol. Serum prolactin levels are reduced by bromocriptine and levodopa. Some of the cephalosporins artificially elevate creatinine levels and may cause the dosage to be unnecessarily readjusted to a subtherapeutic level. The cardiac-depressant antiarrhythmic drugs (quinidine, procainamide, and disopyramide) produce visible electrocardiographic changes and may cause the electrocardiogram to be misinterpreted.

NURSING MANAGEMENT OF ADVERSE EFFECTS AND DRUG INTERACTIONS

When administering drug therapy, the nurse's main concerns focus on ensuring a beneficial outcome by maximizing therapeutic effects, minimizing adverse effects and drug interactions, and providing appropriate drug education for the patient and family. This is accomplished by relating core drug knowledge and core patient variables across the nursing process.

Understanding the interrelationship of core drug knowledge and core patient variables is important because health-related physiologic and emotional changes (e.g., sickness or pregnancy); lifestyle (active or inactive, body rhythms or metabolism), diet, and habits (use of alcohol, caffeine, tobacco); extremes of age; environment; and cultural influences (e.g., genetic and ethnic variations, attitudes, and temperament) may interact and predispose the patient to adverse effects from drug therapy.

Assessment of Core Patient Variables

Health Status

Some patients are at increased risk for adverse effects and drug interactions because of their health conditions and the drugs that they must take to control these conditions. The following are among the diseases and dis-

TABLE 6-3 Selected Drug-Food Interactions That Affect Efficacy

Object Drug	Interactants	Effect
tetracycline	Antacids, sodium bicarbonate, milk, milk products, iron	Decreased efficacy due to chelation of tetracycline
erythromycin preparations, penicillin G	Fruit, fruit juices, tomato, vegetable juices	Decreased efficacy due to faster intestinal hydrolysis
monoamine oxidase inhibitors	Tyramine-rich foods (avocados, beer, broad beans, Chianti, fermented foods, pickled fish, sour cream, yeast, yogurt)	Increased efficacy resulting in acute hypertension, headache, palpitations, nausea, vomiting, occasional cardiovascular accident
levodopa	High-protein foods (eggs, meat, protein supplements)	Impaired absorption of levodopa
	Pyridoxine (vitamin B_6)	Enhances peripheral conversion of levodopa to dopamine
digoxin	Chocolate, oxalic acid (spinach), phytic acid (cereal grains, nuts, legumes), bran	Decreases calcium absorption and decreases digoxin absorption (therefore, decreases drug efficacy)
calcium-channel blockers	Grapefruit juice	Enhances drug absorption
quinolones	Antacids	Alters absorption and decreases drug efficacy because of drug binding

orders that are associated with extensive drug therapy or organ impairment:

- Cardiovascular diseases: congestive heart failure, arrhythmias, hypertension, and hyperlipidemia
- Connective tissues diseases: SLE and rheumatoid arthritis
- Endocrine disorders: diabetes mellitus
- GI disease: peptic ulcer disease, Crohn disease
- Hepatic disease: cirrhosis, cancer
- Mental and emotional disorders: major depression, bipolar disorder
- Chronic respiratory disease: asthma, emphysema
- Seizure disorders

Other health-related factors that contribute to adverse effects include the incidence of chronic or multiple diseases in a patient, polypharmacy (multiple drugs for multiple disorders), incorrect self-administration of drugs, omission (i.e., not taking) of drug therapy, taking someone else's drugs, and use of over-the-counter drugs.

Lifestyle, Diet, and Habits

How patients conduct their lives, what and when they eat, and their various habits and choices may influence the effects of drug therapy. Because certain foods, beverages, and mineral or vitamin supplements can affect the absorption and effectiveness of some drugs, the nurse should remember to ask patients about their diet and other habits. In this way, the nurse can inform patients about possible interactions between a prescribed drug and foods, nutrients, or other substances, such as alcohol or tobacco (see Chapter 10, Lifestyle: Substance Abuse). For example, hypophosphatemia has been observed with dextrose feeding solutions and sucralfate, an ulcer therapy containing aluminum. Nutritional support (e.g., partial parenteral nutrition, total parenteral nutrition) is associated with metabolic complications (e.g., imbalances in sodium, potassium, and phosphate levels). Aluminum absorption is greatly enhanced by orange juice; milk, however, has no effect. Absorption of the calcium-channel blockers is greatly enhanced by grapefruit juice. Some combinations, therefore, should be avoided and some promoted. Understanding these interactions may contribute to therapeutic outcomes.

Exploring various habits with patients is another way to promote a therapeutic outcome. For instance, smoking tobacco and marijuana, the so-called social drugs, is known to increase the metabolism of theophylline. The effect that smoking has on inducing drug metabolism occurs primarily in young to middle-aged smokers. Older smokers are relatively resistant. Smoking-induced enzyme induction may persist in the patient for months even after the patient stops smoking. Many of the drug interactions connected with smoking directly correlate with the amount of smoking. Heavy smokers (more than 20 cigarettes/day) are more likely to experience interactions with drugs than light to moderate smokers (20 or fewer cigarettes/day). The enzyme induction is thought to result from polycyclic hydrocarbons in the smoke. Therefore, patients who use smokeless (chewing) tobacco do not experience the same interactions. They would, however, be at risk for drug interactions occurring when nicotine is the interactant (e.g., nicotine gum and nicotine patches used in smoking-cessation programs).

Another habit, alcohol use—particularly alcoholism (see the accompanying display, Drug Interactions and

Critical Thinking Scenario

Drug interactions and drug metabolism

Your patient, Jason P., is a patient with long-term alcoholism who now has tuberculosis. He is to begin isoniazid therapy. In light of Mr. P.'s alcohol consumption, propose modifications that may be needed in this therapy.

Drug Metabolism) has significant adverse effects on drug therapy in the following ways:

- Chronic alcoholism promotes enzyme induction.
- Acute alcohol intoxication tends to inhibit drug metabolism (whether or not the drinker is suffers from alcoholism).
- Severe alcohol-induced hepatic dysfunction may inhibit the ability to metabolize drugs.
- Disulfiram (Antabuse) and disulfiram-like reactions may occur with certain drug combinations.
- Additive CNS depression occurs from using alcohol concurrently with other CNS depressant drugs.

Life Span and Gender

The nurse must keep in mind that adverse effects are more likely to occur in the very young because of immature physiologic and metabolic enzyme systems and in the very old because of the physiologic and metabolic changes that occur with aging. In elderly patients, for example, the most common adverse effects are predictable, dose-dependent exaggerations of the normal drug response. Many older adults take at least one drug-drug or drug-alcohol combination to manage one or more chronic conditions.

Environment

Most drugs are sensitive to the environment because pharmacokinetic and pharmacodynamic properties may be adversely affected by the manner in which drugs are stored. Excessive heat or extreme temperature changes, light, and moisture affect drug stability. When administering drug therapy and teaching patients, the nurse needs to emphasize the importance of following the manufacturer's recommendations for drug storage.

The patient also may be adversely affected by the environment while taking certain drugs. For instance, some drugs (e.g., sulfonamide antimicrobials, sulfonylurea hypoglycemics, tricyclic antidepressants) can cause the adverse effect of photosensitivity. These drugs make the skin extremely sensitive to sunlight or strong ultraviolet light. Even brief exposure can cause a severe sunburn, hives, or a rash. Other drugs (e.g., anticholinergics, belladonna alkaloids) reduce the body's tolerance to heat or inhibit the body's ability to reduce temperature by perspiration. These types of drugs may make the individual vulnerable to heat stroke in hot weather or during exercise.

Culture

In the relatively new field of pharmacoanthropology, researchers study variant responses to drugs and other chemicals in ethnically and racially distinct groups (see Chapter 13). Differences in rates of drug metabolism and drug response may result from a genetic inability to eliminate a drug in the expected manner, structural variations in the binding receptor sites, and coexisting environmental variables, such as general health status, nutritional status, and use of alcohol or caffeine.

Nursing Diagnoses and Outcomes

Nursing diagnoses are related to specific adverse effects of the ordered drug therapy and to drug interactions. Outcomes are directed at preventing or minimizing either occurrence without harm to the patient. Some examples include the following:

- Risk for Infection related to drug-induced myelosuppression
  Desired outcome: The patient will not develop infection while on drug therapy.
- Altered Nutrition: Less than Body Requirements related to drug-induced nausea, vomiting, anorexia, stomatitis
  Desired outcome: Despite adverse effects, the patient will receive enough nourishment to meet physiologic needs.
- Risk for Poisoning (toxicity) related to use of drug with a narrow therapeutic margin
  Desired outcome: The patient will receive drug therapy without harmful or poisonous effects.

Planning and Intervention

Maximizing Therapeutic Effects

When drug interactions are intentional and desirable, the nurse needs to give the drugs at the prescribed time intervals. They should be administered at the same time if this is necessary to achieve the interaction. When drug interactions are not desired but both drugs are needed for therapy, the doses must be administered at different times to promote therapeutic effect of each drug.

Minimizing Adverse Effects

To help protect the patient from serious adverse effects and drug interactions, the nurse must obtain a drug history from the patient, beginning with a list of all drugs that the patient has taken. Drug monographs and other reliable references may then be consulted for complete descriptions of known or suspected drug interactions.

If a patient is currently taking a drug that may interact with another drug in the current regimen, the drugs should not be coadministered. The nurse can either stagger drug administration times, if this is sufficient to minimize an interaction, or contact the prescriber about changing one of the ordered drugs. If the interaction is potentially serious, the prescriber should be consulted before the nurse or patient begins administering the new drug. In general, when unexpected effects occur during drug therapy, a drug interaction should be suspected and investigated fully.

Throughout therapy, the patient should be monitored for signs and symptoms of interactions and adverse effects and for alterations in health status that increase the risk for adverse effects. In addition, serum drug levels should be monitored, when appropriate, to detect changes that forewarn of impending toxicity.

Patient and Family Education

Before and throughout drug therapy, the nurse needs to inform and instruct the patient and family about adverse effects and drug interactions. Initial instruction includes teaching the patient how to minimize the occurrence of these effects and how to cope with them. In addition, the nurse must teach the patient which effects to expect, which to report to the prescriber, and which effects require immediate medical attention.

Ongoing Assessment and Evaluation

During drug therapy, the nurse continues to monitor for adverse effects and drug interactions and consider the possibility of a drug interaction each time a new drug is added to the treatment plan. Next, the nurse should determine whether the patient is experiencing drug effects other than the intended therapeutic effects. These may include adverse effects, drug allergies, or an idiosyncratic effect. Other concerns include whether the patient may be experiencing a drug-drug or drug-food interaction. These effects may result either from one drug enhancing the action of the other drug to the degree that a toxic drug level occurs or from one drug negating the effect of the other drug by antagonizing (inactivating) the drug's therapeutic action. If none of these effects occurs and the therapeutic effect has been achieved, drug therapy is evaluated as successful. ■

CHAPTER SUMMARY

- Adverse drug effects are undesirable patient responses to a specific drug therapy. They may be minor (i.e., annoying) to the patient or serious (i.e., life threatening). Serious adverse effects are known as toxicities.
- Some adverse effects are predictable, anticipated, dose related, and cause little harm to the patient. Others are unpredictable and may be patient sensitivity related or represent a drug-drug or drug-food interaction. The significance of these effects may vary.
- Some adverse effects may be induced accidentally as drug or food interactions; others may result from toxic drug levels for various reasons. Patient sensitivity reactions are due either to allergic or idiosyncratic responses.
- Core patient variables influence a patient's adverse responses to drug therapy.
- Core patient variables that predispose patients to adverse effects include physiologic and psychological changes associated with health (e.g., disease or pregnancy), temperament and attitudes toward drug therapy, extremes of age, extremes of body weight, diet, habits, circadian and diurnal rhythms, environment, and culture (e.g., genetic and ethnic variations).
- Core drug processes that predispose patients to adverse effects include drug bioavailability, drug additives, drug degradation, dosage, route of administration, and the number of drugs administered concurrently.
- When unexpected effects occur, a drug interaction should be suspected.
- Careful drug histories should be taken at every initial health assessment.

QUESTIONS FOR STUDY AND REVIEW

1. In what ways can drugs interact with other drugs?
2. What symptoms may occur if a patient develops an allergy to a particular drug?
3. Define ototoxicity.

NEED MORE HELP?

Chapter 6 of the study guide for *Drug Therapy in Nursing* contains exercises and activities to reinforce your understanding of the concepts presented in this chapter. For additional information see the text's accompanying website at *http://www.connection.lww.com.*

REFERENCES AND BIBLIOGRAPHY

Anonymous. (1994). FDA launches MEDWATCH program: Monitoring adverse drug reactions. Food and Drug Administration (FDA). *NP News, 2,* 1, 4.

Berger, B. (1999). Effective patient counseling. *U.S. Pharmacist, 24*(2), 64–73.

Brody, T. M., Larner, J., Minneman, K. P. (Eds.). (1998). *Human pharmacology* (2nd ed.). St. Louis: Mosby.

Brown, C. H. (2000). Overview of drug interactions. *U.S. Pharmacist (Health System edition), 25*(5), H53–H530. http:\\www.uspharmacist.com/newlook/displayarticle.cfm?item_num=522.

DeBisschop, M., & Oliphant, C. M. (1999). Medication use and falls in elderly patients. *U.S. Pharmacist, 24*(11), 98–103.

Fauci, A., Braunwald, E., Wilson, J. D., Martin, J. B., Hauser, S. L., Longo, D. L., Kasper, D. L., Isselbachter, K. J. (Eds.). (1999). *Harrison's Online.* New York: McGraw-Hill.

Gebhart, F. (2000). Is standard dosing to blame for adverse reactions? *Drug Topics, 144*(2), 34.

Gianni, L., & Dreitlein, W. B. (1998). Some popular OTC herbals can interact with anticoagulant therapy. *U.S. Pharmacist, 23*(5), 80–86.

Hansten, P. D., Horn, J. R., Koda-Kimble, M. A., & Young, L. L. Y. (1997). Drug interactions and updates. *Drug Interactions and Updates Quarterly, 15,* 879.

Hardman, J. G., Limbird, L. E., Molinof, P. B., Ruddon, R. W., & Gilman, A. G. (Eds.). (1997). *Goodman and Gilman's pharmacological basis of therapeutics* (9th ed.). New York: McGraw-Hill.

Kirk, J. K., Lightfoot, S. M., & Conner, S. L. (1998). Some clinically important drug interactions. *Drug Topics, 64*(7), 79–92.

Mancano, M. (1999). Drugs and grapefruit juice interactions: Part 2. *Pharmacy Times, 65*(10), 38–41.

Mancano, M. A. (2000). Drug interactions with levothyroxine. *Pharmacy Times, 66*(3), 24–26.

Mancano, M. (2000). Drug interactions with oral contraceptives. *Pharmacy Times, 66*(2), 24–26.

Mancano, M. (1999). Drug interactions: What pharmacists need to know. *Pharmacy Times, 65*(5), 42–44.

McEvoy, G. K., Litvak, K., & Welsh Jr., O. H. (Eds.). (2000). *Drug information.* Bethesda, MD: American Hospital Formulary Service.

O'Brien, D., & Haddad, A. R. (1997). Counseling patients on drug-food interactions. *U.S. Pharmacist, 22*(6), 62–75.

Ryan-Haddad, A., & Wegner, A. (1998). Drug-alcohol interactions in elderly patients. *U.S. Pharmacist, 23*(2), 98–109.

Ryan-Haddad, A., Bramble, J. C., Lee, B., Mucker, A., & Kellner, V. (2000). OTC product labels and older patients. *U.S. Pharmacist, 25*(1), 38–47.

Smith, M. C. (1998). Rx-to-OTC switches: Reflections and projections. *Drug Topics, 142*(14), 70–79.

White-Sax, B. (1999). What you should know about generic drugs. *Pharmacy Times Supplement, 65*(2), 25–26.

Unit III

Core Patient Variables

Chapter 7

LIFE SPAN: CHILDREN

KEY TERMS

body surface area
kernicterus
nomogram
pediatric patient
play therapy

Learning Objectives

At the completion of this chapter the student will:

1. Identify key areas of core drug knowledge for children that differ from key areas of core drug knowledge for adults.
2. Explain why calculating drug dosages for children is different from calculating drug dosages for adults.
3. Describe methods for calculating dosages for children of different ages.
4. Identify key core patient variables for children and explain how they differ from those of adults when considering drug therapy.
5. Discuss key developmental variables for each of the pediatric age groups (infant, toddler, preschooler, school-aged, and adolescent) that affect how the nurse administers drug therapy.
6. Propose some common nursing diagnoses related to drug therapy in children.
7. Describe key nursing interventions to promote maximal therapeutic effects and minimal adverse effects during pediatric drug therapy.
8. Identify key points to include in educating patients and families about pediatric drug therapy.

When implementing pediatric drug therapy, the nurse must remember that children are different from adults in many ways. Although some drugs and administration routes are similar in adults and children, the nursing management of drug therapy varies greatly. For example, physiologic differences in children, the child's immature body systems, greater fluid composition, and smaller size all affect the core drug knowledge. These differences can exaggerate or diminish the pediatric patient's response to drug therapy, making some drug actions and outcomes less predictable in the child than in the adult.

Additionally, in children, core patient variables are different from adult patients and from child to child because of the different developmental stages of childhood. The **pediatric patient** is usually defined as younger than 16 years and weighing less than 50 kilograms.

This chapter focuses on core drug knowledge that is relevant and unique to pediatric patients and core patient variables that emphasize children's needs according to developmental changes. Special issues in managing pediatric drug therapy are explored; these issues include maximizing therapeutic effects, minimizing adverse effects, and educating patients and families.

NURSING MANAGEMENT OF THE PEDIATRIC PATIENT

Core Drug Knowledge Related to Children

Pharmacotherapeutics

Therapeutic indications and effects of drug therapy are similar for children and adults. The major difference is in the drug dosage. Unlike most adult drug dosages, almost all pediatric drug dosages are based on the weight of the child in kilograms. Dosage is usually specified in terms of milligrams of drug per kilogram of body weight (mg/kg). The correct drug dosage is crucial in pediatric drug therapy. The child's small and immature body systems make overdosages potentially lethal.

Dosage Calculations

It is difficult and unnecessary to commit drug dosages to memory because each child is a different weight. Most pediatric dosage calculations are based on the child's body surface area or weight in kilograms. The **body surface area** is the external surface of the body expressed in square meters. The ratio of body surface area to weight is inversely proportional to length; therefore, the infant or young child who is shorter and weighs less than the adult has relatively greater surface area than would be expected from the weight. Body surface area is calculated using a standard formula (see the accompanying display, Calculating Pediatric Drug Dosages).

Body surface area can be determined by using a nomogram (Fig. 7-1). A **nomogram** is a measuring device, such as a chart or a graph, that shows relationships between numerical variables. A representative nomogram used to estimate body surface area in children may have several columns of calibrated measures representing height, surface area, and weight. Body surface area is calculated by drawing a line across the columns to connect the patient's height with the patient's weight. The numeral at which the line intersects the central surface area column is the patient's estimated body surface area.

Once body surface area is determined, the dosage can be computed using the formula in the display entitled Calculating Pediatric Drug Dosages. A child's drug dosage may also be determined by comparing the child's weight to the recommended dose per kilograms of weight.

Pharmacodynamics

The mechanism of action of a drug is the same in all individuals at all ages. However, what distinguishes individual responses is the ability of the organ systems to function fully and appropriately. In very young children, the immaturity of the organ systems may cause them to have less than optimal functioning. This may necessitate increasing or decreasing drug doses to prevent toxicity and to achieve a therapeutic drug level.

Pharmacokinetics

A child's age, growth, and maturation can affect how the body absorbs, distributes, metabolizes, and excretes a drug. By understanding how drugs affect pediatric patients differently from adult patients, the nurse can help maximize the therapeutic effects of drug therapy and minimize adverse effects. Dosages must often be lowered to account for immature body systems or impaired systems in neonates and infants.

Absorption

Absorption of a drug depends on various factors. In the pediatric patient, age, disease process, dosage form, route of administration, and foods and drugs present in the child's body have an effect on drug absorption.

The infant's gastrointestinal (GI) tract is less acidic and has a higher pH value than that of an adult. This is especially true in the premature infant whose immature GI tract secretes less acid than the full-term newborn or older child. As the GI tract matures, the gastric pH decreases and the GI tract becomes more acidic, reaching adult values at approximately 1 year of age. These differences in pH affect drug absorption. For example, a drug such as digoxin is very well absorbed in an acidic environment. Therefore, less digoxin would be absorbed from the premature infant's GI tract than the older child or adult's GI tract.

Drug route also affects absorption. Drugs administered intramuscularly (IM) or subcutaneously (SC) are affected by age and disease-related circumstances. The rate of absorption may be decreased in the infant or child because of erratic blood flow from the immature peripheral circulation. The neonate's blood flow is particularly

Calculating Pediatric Drug Dosages

Body Surface Area Method

Step 1. Determine the body surface area (BSA) of the child. It is measured in meters squared. A standard formula is used. Computations should be made with a calculator.

$$BSA = \sqrt{\frac{\text{Weight in kg} \times \text{Height in cm}}{3,600}}$$

Example: Child weighs 10 kg and is 45 cm tall

1. Multiply weight in kilograms by height in centimeters.

$$BSA = \frac{10 \times 45}{3,600}$$

2. Divide product by 3600.

$$= \frac{450}{3,600}$$

3. Enter square root sign on calculator.

$$= \sqrt{0.125}$$

4. Round the BSA to the nearest hundredth.

$$= 0.35\ m^2$$

Step 2. Determine dose using the computed BSA and this formula:

$$\frac{\text{Child's BSA}}{1.7\ m^2\ (\text{average adult BSA})} \times \text{Usual adult dose} =$$

Child's dose

Example: Child's BSA = 0.35 m², and usual adult dose is 100 mg.

$$= \frac{0.35\ m^2}{1.7\ m^2} \times 100$$

$$= 20.588\,(20.59)\ \text{mg is child's dose.}$$

Body Weight Method

Usual dose: 1 kg :: × dose : weight of child in kg

Example: Usual dose is 10 mg/1 kg and child weighs 18 kg

10 mg : 1 kg :: × mg : 18 kg

× = 180 mg

slow and erratic. Increased absorption of topical drugs is common in pediatric patients, especially infants. Compared with adults, infants and children have a greater body surface area. The infant's skin exhibits greater permeability as well. An increased body surface area combined with increased permeability results in increased absorption of topical agents. Increased absorption may result in adverse effects that usually do not occur in the adult patient.

Distribution

In a pediatric patient, factors that differentiate drug distribution processes from those in an adult include differences in body water and fat, immature liver function, and an immature blood–brain barrier.

Differences in Body Water and Fat. A drug's distribution is affected by the water and fat content of the body. Children, especially infants, have a higher concentration of water in their bodies and a lower concentration of fat. Newborns have the greatest proportional water content, followed by infants, children, and then adults (Table 7-1). Assessing the amount of water in the body of an infant or child is an important activity prior to administering water-soluble drugs. Because infants and children have a greater proportion of body water, water-soluble drugs are diluted to a greater degree. The drug moves to areas of water throughout the body, not just in the blood. This results in lower concentrations of the drug in the blood. With drugs such as gentamicin, proportionately increased dosages may be required to achieve or maintain therapeutic levels.

To a lesser degree, fat-soluble drugs are affected by the proportionately lower fat in the infant and child. Because fat distribution increases with age, fat-soluble drugs are distributed to a greater degree in the adult. Because fat-soluble drugs are not widely distributed in the infant's and child's body, greater blood concentrations may result, leading to toxicity.

Immature Liver Function. In the infant and especially in the neonate, immature liver function affects drug distribution. The neonate's immature liver produces fewer plasma proteins, especially albumin, with which drugs bind. Pharmacologic effects of drugs result from unbound (i.e., free) drug. In the neonate and infant, more free drug is available because less drug is bound to the fewer plasma proteins. This results in increased blood levels of drugs, which can cause greater adverse effects

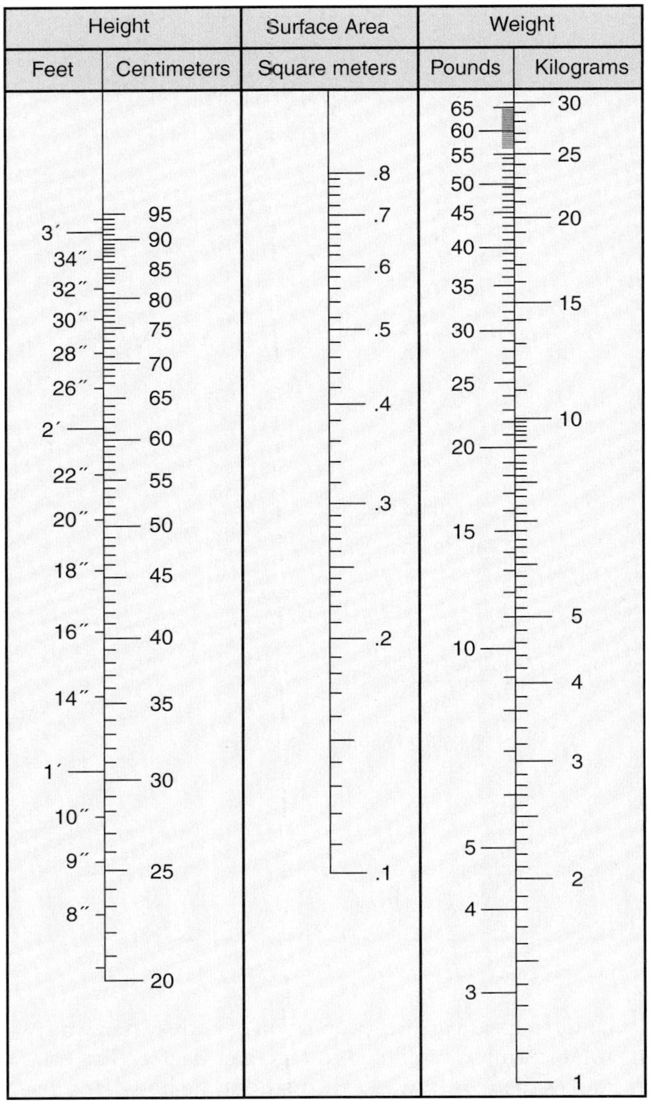

Figure 7-1. A pediatric nomogram is a device for estimating body surface area in children. To use it, draw a line from the child's height to the child's weight. The point at which this line intersects the surface area in the middle is the child's estimated body surface area.

and toxicity in infants. Drug binding to serum proteins reaches adult levels by 6 months of age.

Multiple drugs administered to an infant may compete for the same binding sites, resulting in either higher blood concentrations of both drugs or of the drug with less affinity for the binding site. Other naturally occurring substances found in the body can also compete for fewer binding sites in the pediatric patient's body. For example, bilirubin, which may increase during the neonatal period, binds with plasma proteins. When a drug such as sulfa is administered to the neonate who has an increased bilirubin level, sulfa competes with bilirubin for binding sites. This leaves more bilirubin free in the blood. Although rare, the bilirubin level can increase to a dangerous level, resulting in accumulation of bilirubin

TABLE 7-1 Proportional Water Content Across the Life Span

Age	Percentage of Body Water
Newborn	75%–85%
Infant	Approximately 85%
One-year-old	65%
Two-year-old	60%
Adult	50%–60%

in the central nervous system (CNS), a life-threatening condition called **kernicterus.**

Immature Blood–Brain Barrier. At birth, the blood–brain barrier is not fully developed. The blood–brain barrier prevents drugs in general circulation from passing to the circulation of the brain, thereby protecting the brain from toxic substances. Therefore, newborns are particularly vulnerable to CNS toxicity. The effect of drugs that affect the CNS (e.g., phenobarbital and morphine) will be intensified. In addition, infants will experience exaggerated CNS responses to other drugs targeted for other body systems.

Metabolism

The liver metabolizes most drugs. The immaturity of the neonatal and infant liver results in decreased or incomplete metabolism of many drugs. This may necessitate lower drug dosages or an increased interval between doses to achieve appropriate blood levels. In children with liver disease, drug metabolism is further complicated by the liver's inability to detoxify drugs. A child with an immature liver or compromised liver function is at risk for drug toxicity.

Drugs requiring oxidation for metabolism are frequently more rapidly metabolized in children than in adults because children have a faster resting respiratory rate. These drugs include phenobarbital, phenytoin, and the methylxanthines (e.g., theophylline and caffeine). With these types of drugs, children may require higher dosages or more frequent administration schedules than do adults to maintain therapeutic blood levels.

Excretion

Most drugs are eliminated from the body through the urine. This requires a functioning renal system. Drug elimination depends on glomerular filtration rate, tubular reabsorption, and maturity. In children with impaired renal function, drug dosages need to be altered to achieve and maintain therapeutic drug levels.

The neonate, especially the preterm infant, has immature kidneys, and renal excretion of drugs is slow. Drug dosages and therapeutic drug levels, therefore, must be monitored closely to prevent toxicity. In addition, the reduced glomerular filtration rate and decreased tubular secretion and reabsorption for the first 6 months of life extends the half-life of many drugs (e.g., penicillin, sulfonamide, and cephalosporin). Drugs with a narrow margin between effective and toxic doses must be administered at longer dosage intervals to prevent toxicity. At about 3 months of age, the infant's kidneys can concentrate urine at the adult level, but urinary excretion remains low until the child is about 30 months old, when the kidneys become functionally mature.

A few drugs are excreted through the biliary tree into the intestinal tract. Biliary blood flow is decreased during the first few days of life; therefore, careful monitoring of drug levels and signs and symptoms of toxicity is imperative.

Contraindications and Precautions

Not all drugs that are safe for adults are safe for children, partly because not all drugs have been adequately tested in clinical trials on pediatric patients. Because the full therapeutic and adverse effects of drugs prescribed for children are unknown, cautious administration and careful, frequent assessments are advised. Some drugs are known to be dangerous in children, and these drugs are contraindicated. The core drug knowledge must be determined for each drug before administering it to a child.

Adverse Effects and Drug Interactions

Adverse effects of some drugs are more severe and more likely to occur in children due to their immature body systems. Alternatively, some adverse effects affect the body systems only at specific phases of development. For example, tetracycline administered to a child between the age of 4 months and 8 years will stain the permanent teeth. Glucocorticoids given to a child of any age will suppress growth if the child has not matured to full adult size. Drug receptor sensitivity varies with age; it may be increased or decreased for certain drugs. This may promote adverse effects and necessitate lower or higher drug dosages than would normally be expected (see Chapter 6).

Drug interactions in children are similar to those occurring in adults. See the accompanying display, Calling on Core Drug Knowledge for Children.

Assessment of Core Patient Variables Related to Children

Health Status

A child's disease process can affect absorption of drugs from the GI tract. Diarrhea, for example, decreases intestinal transit time and therefore decreases the time available for a drug to be absorbed. Children with hepatic or renal disease cannot metabolize or excrete drugs as easily and are more prone to adverse effects from drugs than other children. As with adults, any chronic disease or condition may alter the effects of certain drugs and must be seriously considered in drug therapy.

Life Span and Gender

The nurse must always consider the developmental stage of the pediatric patient. In planning appropriate drug administration methods, the nurse needs to explain the treatment and enlist the child's cooperation. If this is not possible, the nurse must seek appropriate assistance to administer the drug therapy safely. Developmental considerations are especially important when the nurse communicates with the child. To elicit cooperation and obtain necessary information, the nurse must communicate at an appropriate level of understanding for the child. The following are age-appropriate considerations in administering drugs to infants and children.

Infants (Birth–12 Months)

Some infants with a well-developed sucking reflex may willingly swallow a pleasant-tasting liquid drug through a bottle nipple. Preliminary field testing of a new device, the Rx Medibottle, in which liquid medication is mixed with 1 ounce of formula or apple juice and then "fed" to the baby demonstrated high infant acceptance of this technique (Kraus, Stohlmeyer, & Hannon, 1999). Other babies may spit out oral medicine, making it difficult for the nurse to administer a full dose. Infant drops may be administered by gently squeezing the child's cheeks to open the mouth, and then placing the drops in the buccal pouch to ensure they will be swallowed. Drugs in rectal suppository form may be given to infants if necessary. To avoid expulsion of the suppository before the drug is absorbed, however, the nurse may need to hold the child's buttocks together for a short time.

If the IM route must be used, the nurse should choose the smallest gauge needle appropriate for the drug. The preferred injection site for infants and children up to age 3 years is the vastus lateralis. This muscle is in the side of the thigh in the upper outer quadrant of the area between the greater trochanter and the knee. The vastus lateralis has few nerves and blood vessels and forms the largest muscle mass in this age group.

Normally, a ⅜-inch needle is used for the vastus lateralis in infants; if this is not available a ⅝-inch or less needle should be used. The angle of injection should be modified from the usual 90 degrees to 45 degrees toward the frontal plane of the knee. The 45-degree angle ensures that the needle does not transverse the blood vessel.

The rectus femoris is another possible injection site. This muscle is located near the vastus lateralis but is anterior midthigh; the needle should be injected at a 90-degree angle.

In infants, neither the deltoid nor the dorsogluteal muscle sites are used because the muscle masses are

Critical Thinking Scenario

Calling on core drug knowledge for children

You are caring for a premature newborn in the nursery. The newborn is receiving intravenous antibiotic therapy to treat an infection. Which specific aspects of core drug knowledge do you think will most help you anticipate any adverse effects of drug therapy?

too small and undeveloped. The ventrogluteal muscle site, which is large at birth, is not recommended for use in infants because problems encountered in positioning the child make it difficult to locate the muscle site accurately.

Drugs may be administered intravenously (IV) to the infant through a peripheral site. These IV sites differ from those used for adults. Ideally, the nurse selects a site that is easy to access and that poses the least risk to the patient. In the neonate and infant, the scalp's many superficial veins offer easy access. The superficial temporal vein just in front of the pinna of the ear and the metopic vein in the middle of the forehead are relatively easy to find and are less risky for patients (Fig. 7-2). Other suitable IV sites for infants and older children include the vessels in the nondominant hand, forearm, upper arm, feet, and antecubital fossa. Distal IV sites are used first and are moved proximally as necessary. The feet provide good IV sites and are used in infants.

Toddlers (13 Months–3 Years)

Developmentally, toddlers can swallow liquid forms of drugs, and older toddlers can chew oral drugs. Because toddlers experience anxiety when separated from their parents, having a parent nearby usually helps the child's cooperation during drug therapy. The nurse should attempt to elicit cooperation from the toddler but should be prepared for the toddler to resist. A toddler's resistance may be associated with a past experience, such as unpleasantly flavored drugs or a painful injection.

Toddlers are also likely to be anxious or uncooperative during administration of rectal suppositories because of their experiences with toilet training and sphincter control. Toddlers have vivid imaginations but limited understanding of how the body works. A common fear is that important body contents will leak out from an injection site. As with infants, the vastus lateralis and rectus femoris remain the IM injection sites of choice for toddlers.

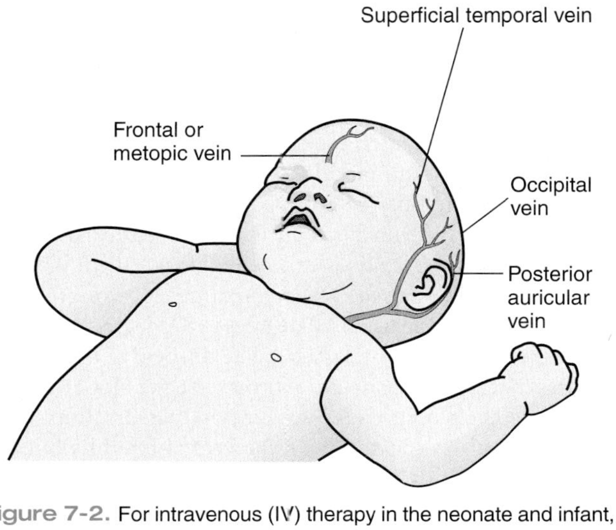

Figure 7-2. For intravenous (IV) therapy in the neonate and infant, the scalp is an excellent site. The superficial temporal vein and the metopic vein in the central forehead are the preferred sites because they are easy to find and reasonably safe.

When IV drug therapy is necessary for toddlers, the scalp veins are still appropriate and can be used up to age 18 months. By this time, hair follicles mature and skin layers thicken, making IV access more difficult (Weinstein, 2000). Although the scalp provides excellent IV access, it is not the first choice because of the anxiety it causes parents. Parents feel uneasy because of the scalp's close proximity to the brain and because the area must be shaved at the IV site. If a scalp vein must be used and the site shaved, the nurse should ask the parents whether they would like to save the hair, and collect it for them if desired. Saving their child's hair makes the procedure less distressing to some parents. For toddlers, as for infants, other peripheral IV sites are also used. If possible, the nurse tries to avoid using the foot so as not to impede the toddler's mobility or cause undue frustration. The foot veins are used, however, in children who need to be immobile.

Preschoolers (3–5 Years)

Preschoolers are often uncooperative during drug administration. Strategies for enlisting cooperation include offering choices (e.g., between liquid medicines or chewable tablets) when feasible. Heightened awareness and the fear of punishment or body mutilation in this age group may influence their perception of and cooperation with drug therapy. Nurses (and parents) should always reassure preschoolers that the drug is to help them feel better and keep them healthy.

Several sites may be used for IM injections in preschoolers, most commonly the vastus lateralis, rectus femoris, and ventrogluteal sites. The ventrogluteal site is free of major nerves and blood vessels and is characterized by deep muscle mass. It is located between the anterior superior iliac spine, above the greater trochanter, and the posterior iliac crest. The drug is injected into the gluteus medius muscle, which is in the ventrogluteal site. Injection in the gluteus medius is less painful than injection in the vastus lateralis.

The dorsogluteal site can be used if necessary but only in children who have been walking for at least 1 year, because the gluteus maximus muscle at this site is developed by walking. By 3 years (with the exception of developmentally delayed children), almost all preschoolers have been walking for at least 1 year. The dorsogluteal site is located by drawing an imaginary line from the head of the femur to the posterior superior iliac spine. The injection is then delivered into the gluteus maximus at the upper outer portion above the line.

When IV drug therapy is necessary, peripheral sites are selected for the preschooler. Scalp veins are no longer used.

School-Aged Children (6–12 Years)

The school-aged child is often very cooperative. As with the preschooler, the nurse offers choices to help the school-aged patient exercise control. The school-aged child's greatest fears of drug therapy are usually related to negative past experiences. School-aged children can tolerate warning of drug therapy without fears and anxiety escalating. The school-aged child takes pride in accomplishments.

Oral drugs may still be provided in liquid form or chewable tablets. Many school-aged children can now swallow pills, and these may be provided as well. Generally, if rectal drug forms must be used, the school-aged child will feel embarrassment. School-aged and older children, like adults, must be ensured privacy at all times throughout the procedure.

The ventrogluteal site is recommended for an IM injection in the school-aged child, but the vastus lateralis, rectus femoris, and dorsogluteal sites may also be used in this age group. Although it is not the preferred administration site, the deltoid muscle may also be used for small volumes of drugs (0.5 mL) or vaccines.

Adolescents (13–16 Years)

An adolescent's ability to cooperate is highly developed, much like an adult's. The nurse offers adolescents control whenever possible and lets them make choices. The nurse also offers support and encouragement without treating adolescents like children. Adolescents are more likely to cooperate and participate in drug therapy treatment when they have a complete understanding of the treatment regimen. Adolescents are particularly sensitive about their bodies and their independence. Thus, privacy and control are important issues to consider when administering drug therapy to this age group.

Routes of administration are similar to those for adults. Oral forms of drug therapy include tablets or pills. Suppositories can be used, but the adolescent is likely to be embarrassed. IM injection sites are usually the same as for adults unless the adolescent is particularly small. Careful examination is necessary to be sure that adequate muscle mass is available for IM injection. Site selection for IV therapy in adolescents is the same as for adults.

Lifestyle, Diet, and Habits

The infant's primary food intake is milk and formula. These substances decrease acidity and increase gastric pH. Drug absorption is usually affected by acidity and pH levels; therefore, food and drug interactions are a primary concern when administering oral drug therapy to infants.

Use and abuse of some substances, such as caffeine, alcohol, tobacco, and street drugs, will cause the same complications in children as in adults during drug therapy. Therefore, use of these substances by school-aged children and adolescents should be explored. Adolescence is a time of experimentation, which includes experimentation with legal and illegal substances, such as cigarettes, alcohol, and street drugs. School-aged children and preadolescents may also experiment with these substances. Nurses must try to elicit this information for all school-aged or adolescent patients throughout drug therapy, because potential adverse effects or interactions of these substances may cause serious complications. Regardless of the patient's age and appearance, the nurse should never assume that the child does or does not use or abuse certain substances. Questions regarding substance use should be posed in the health assessment interview in a nonjudgmental, matter-of-fact manner.

The economic circumstances of the patient and family should also be considered. Can the family pay for the child's drug therapy? Are insurance and other resources available?

Environment

Children may receive drug therapy in any setting, although some types of drugs may be administered primarily in one setting or another, just as in the adult population. Children receiving drug therapy at home need to have a parent or guardian responsible for ensuring that the child receives the prescribed therapy. General considerations about the home need to be assessed just as they are assessed for adults. Does the home have electricity, running water, a refrigerator, indoor plumbing, and a safe place to store prescription and nonprescription drugs away from children?

Culture

The beliefs of the family will greatly affect a child's attitude and adherence to the therapeutic regimen. Questions to consider and assessment concerns include the following: Does the child's cultural background suggest suspicions about or taboos against drug therapy? Do health practices in the child's family rely on other forms of healing, such as using herbal or natural medicines, acupuncture, prayer, or mysticism? Do family religious beliefs directly conflict with the use of drug therapy? The child's cultural background and heritage must be considered quite seriously when planning drug therapy (see Chapter 13).

Nursing Diagnoses and Outcomes

Nursing diagnoses and outcomes related to specific drug therapy for children are much the same as they are for adults. However, many drug therapies are burdensome for families to maintain or pose special concerns or risks to a child's normal growth and development. Common nursing diagnoses and outcomes may include the following:

- Delayed Growth and Development
  Desired outcome: The patient will achieve normal growth and development during drug therapy.
- Ineffective Family Therapeutic Regimen Management
  Desired outcome: Family members will master effective management strategies of the patient's drug regimen.
- Caregiver Role Strain
  Desired outcome: The patient and family will develop effective coping skills to avoid, reduce, or relieve stress on family caregivers.

Planning and Intervention

Maximizing Therapeutic Effects

To administer drugs safely and effectively to children, the nurse must understand pediatric anatomy and physiology, the patient's developmental and cognitive levels, and the child's diagnosis and prognosis. The nurse must use this knowledge to select appropriate drug administration sites, equipment, and administration techniques.

Oral Drug Therapy

Although usually not painful, administration of oral medications can be traumatic, especially when the drug flavor is foul and the child protests. Many pediatric drugs come in liquid form and should be drawn up into a syringe (without a needle) for accurate measurement. The drug can then be transferred to a medicine cup for older cooperative children who prefer this.

If the patient cannot swallow pills, some pills can be crushed and dissolved in a liquid or soft food that masks the flavor of the drug. Another method to mask unpleasant tasting drugs for children is to offer a flavored ice pop or ice chips to help numb the taste buds and promote cooperation. When a tablet is crushed and diluted in a liquid or soft food, such as applesauce, gelatin, or ice cream, the nurse should dilute the drug in the smallest amount of liquid or food possible to ensure that the child receives the full dose and does not leave any in the residue.

The nurse should work carefully with the child to ensure that all of the drug is taken. If the child drools or spits out some of the drug, the nurse should calculate the amount of drug lost. If the total is significant, the nurse should report the estimated amount lost to the prescriber and obtain an order for a replacement dose. For drugs that pose a high toxicity risk, another dose is unlikely to be ordered. For example, when digoxin (which slows the heart) is given to children with congestive heart failure, an overdose can be lethal.

Parenteral Drug Therapy

To ensure accurate parenteral drug delivery, the nurse must choose age-appropriate equipment. For example, the length and gauge of a needle must be suited to the child's age and growth level. A needle that is too long for the child's size will deliver a drug into the muscle rather than into the subcutaneous tissue; this would speed the rate of absorption.

When offering a child choices to gain his or her cooperation during drug administration, the nurse should present only those choices that truly exist. For example, the nurse should not ask a preschooler if he or she would like to take medicine now if the child does not really have the choice to refuse. Instead, the nurse should ask which drug the child wants to take first or how many bandages the child would like to apply after an injection.

Rectal Drug Therapy

The nurse always gives a full explanation to the patient and family regarding the need to administer a drug rectally and asks the child to attempt to retain the drug for as long as possible. The developmental level of the child, as always, is taken into consideration with the administration of rectal drugs. Young children should be dissuaded from going to the bathroom and encouraged to participate in a quiet activity. This will allow time for the drug to be absorbed. Older children and adolescents need to have their privacy maintained during the administration of rectal suppositories.

Minimizing Adverse Effects

Calculating Drug Dosages Accurately

When determining a drug dosage, the nurse must remember that pediatric muscle mass, body water, fat content, gastric pH levels, and liver functioning vary greatly from the adult's. These variations affect the rate of absorption, making it vital that dosage calculations be correct.

The nurse is responsible for ensuring the accuracy of a prescribed drug dose prior to administration. Research has shown that, when math calculations are required to determine the correct dose, prescribing errors are more likely to occur in children than in adults (Lesar, 1998). (For more information see the accompanying display, Medication Administration Errors.)

Overdosage of many drugs can cause serious or even fatal effects in children. Because pediatric dosages are small in volume, even a little error may produce serious adverse effects. The nurse must remember that the pediatric drug dosage is not merely a reduced adult dosage; rather, it is calculated by specific equations adjusted to the child's weight and body surface area (see the display, Calculating Pediatric Drug Dosages).

Focus on Research

Medication administration errors

Lesar, T. S. (1998). Errors in the use of medication dosage equations. *Archives of Pediatric and Adolescent Medicine, 152*(4):340–344.

The Study

An analysis was done of 200 consecutive prescribing errors made in a tertiary-care teaching hospital. The prescribing errors had occurred in pediatric and adult patients; all involved dosage calculation. All of the errors had potentially adverse outcomes. A significantly greater number of errors occurred with the pediatric patients (4.94 errors/1,000 patient days vs 0.13 errors for adults). Over half (56.1%) of the pediatric errors would have resulted in an overdose if the error had not been detected before drug administration. The most frequent type of dosing error was decimal point misplacement (in 27.9% of the pediatric errors). The next most frequent error type was failure to divide the total daily dose into individual doses (16.3% of errors).

Nursing Implications

Nurses need to be able to calculate drug dosages accurately. This is especially important for pediatric drug doses. The nurse provides the final check, after the physician and pharmacist, for the accuracy of the calculated dose. Every drug dose should be checked prior to administration to prevent medication errors and maximize patient safety.

Special Precautions for Pediatric Drug Routes

One way for nurses to promote a good outcome when administering drug therapy is to call on their knowledge of normal growth and development in children and their knowledge of safe administration techniques for specific routes.

Oral Route

- Drug volume should not exceed that which can be swallowed by a very small mouth. The drug dose should be mixed in a small amount of liquid so all of the dose is taken.
- Avoid adding a drug dose to formula. The infant may refuse future feedings because of the foul taste.
- Balance dosage schedules with feeding schedules. Consider whether the drug should be given with meals or on an empty stomach. Check for the possibility of a food-drug interaction.

Intramuscular Route

- Assess whether a less painful route is possible.
- If the IM route is unavoidable, apply a topical, local anesthetic, such as a lidocaine and prilocaine combination (EMLA cream), to numb the injection site.
- Locate anatomic landmarks and boundaries of injection sites.
- Evaluate muscle mass, skin condition, and potential complications related to the child's diagnosis.
- Rotate injection sites as needed, and use appropriate equipment and techniques.
- Seek help to hold the child still while administering the IM injection.

Intravenous Route

- Minimize initial pain on starting the IV by applying a topical anesthetic.
- Check the IV insertion site hourly for infiltration in infants and children.
- Monitor fluid status for signs of overload (risk is greatest in neonates and young infants because of their immature kidney function).
- Control the IV infusion rate by using volumetric pumps and microdrip calibrated chambers.
- Supply no more than 1 hour's worth of fluid when administering a continuous IV drip with an infusion pump (in case the pump malfunctions).
- Engage the lock feature on a volumetric pump to prevent unauthorized changes in the drip rate.

Although many nursing drug references give dosage ranges for children, they do not include dosages specific to preterm and full-term neonates. Nurses administering drugs to these young patients should use a pediatric drug guide that gives ranges of pediatric dosages in mg/kg of body weight or by dose for all children.

To prevent mathematical errors, drug dosage calculations should always be double-checked by another nurse before administering any dose to a child. Even a simple mathematical error can be disastrous. For example, merely misplacing a decimal point could result in a child's receiving 10 times the appropriate amount of drug (see the accompanying display, Special Precautions for Pediatric Drug Routes).

Reducing Psychological Stress and Anxiety

Some adverse effects in pediatric drug therapy involve psychological distress of the child or parent. The nurse who understands age-related emotional needs can use appropriate communication techniques to help allay anxiety and negative, stress-provoking feelings regarding drug therapy. For school-aged children and adolescents, questions and feelings should be discussed and answered as simply and honestly as possible.

Although infants do not converse, they do communicate nonverbally. Parents are also helpful in providing a history of the infant's experiences, behaviors, and schedule. They can also provide an interpretation of the infant's nonverbal cues. Infants are very much in tune with their parents and can sense their feelings. If the parents are anxious, the infant is likely to be anxious as well. Therefore, parents should be offered reassurance and full explanations regarding procedures and rationales. During therapy, the parents may comfort the infant by maintaining eye contact, gently stroking the head, or talking in soothing tones. Parents should not be asked to restrain the infant but should be at hand to comfort the child. After administering drug therapy, they should cuddle and comfort the child.

Because toddlers need to view drug therapy as positively as possible, they should be comforted and praised after receiving a drug regardless of whether they were cooperative or uncooperative. Whatever their behavior, they should never be referred to as a "bad boy" or "bad girl." Toddlers take pride in their accomplishments, and positive feedback and praise enhance their sense of self-esteem.

Play therapy is a useful activity for reducing a child's anxiety and promoting understanding of drug therapy. To familiarize the child with an administration procedure, the nurse should encourage role play with dolls and appropriate medical equipment. During role play, the nurse can further encourage the child to express feelings of anxiety or anger.

For preschoolers and school-aged children, care should be taken to explore the child's experiences with the health care delivery system, because these experiences strongly influence their behavior, which, like toddlers' behaviors, should be accepted without value judgments. Similarly, the nurse should take advantage of opportunities to provide positive feedback and avoid negativity.

Providing Patient and Family Education

A crucial step in administering pediatric drug therapy is educating the child, the parents, and significant others. Providing honest and detailed explanations and rationales helps reassure the family and other caregivers. Patient and family education is especially important if drug therapy continues when the child returns home. It is important to include the child in drug education. Children have a right to appropriate information regarding any medicine they take. The nurse should provide age-appropriate explanations. Including children in drug education, starting at an early age, helps them to grow into the role of informed consumers. The position paper, *Ten Guiding Principles for Teaching Children and Adolescents about Medicines,* issued by the United States Pharmacopeia supports the inclusion of children in patient education on drug therapy.

For toddlers, the rationale for drug therapy and type of administration should be fully explained to the parents in private, away from the toddler. Toddlers should receive a very brief, straightforward, honest explanation before receiving drug therapy and especially before an invasive procedure. Otherwise, their fears and anxiety will escalate.

Preschoolers require simple explanations. They often understand more than they can articulate. The information on the drug therapy should be accurate but brief. Giving preschoolers a simple description of the medication administration procedure and calmly informing them, for example, telling them that they might feel a momentary "pinch" or "stick," is generally sufficient to prepare them. The information should be supplied just before a procedure so that there is little time for their fears and anxiety to escalate. Parents or primary caretakers are usually provided the opportunity to be with the child during the procedure.

The school-aged child can understand somewhat more in-depth explanations and will ask many specific questions regarding drug therapy. Answers and explanations should be honest and as detailed as necessary for the patient and parents. Information should be provided on what the child wants to know, not just what the health care provider believes the child should know.

Adolescents should be treated like adults in regard to full explanations and rationale for drug therapy. The nurse should invite adolescents to be involved in these discussions and encourage them to express their questions and feelings. Nurses should stress the importance of therapeutic adherence because adolescents are at the age when they assume more responsibility for their own health and well-being. Many adolescents take responsibility for scheduling and administering their own drug therapy.

At the least, initial education for school-aged children, adolescents, and parents should include the following:

- Generic and trade names of drugs
- Rationale for drug therapy
- What the therapeutic drug effect should be
- Route by which drug will be administered
- When drug should be administered and over what period of time
- Potential adverse effects
- Special drug-related precautions or restrictions (e.g., exercise, diet)

In addition, the nurse should educate as many family members or other caregivers as possible. Doing so promotes accurate and safe drug administration to the child at home and ensures that sources of information about the child's drug history are easily obtained, especially in an emergency.

School-aged children and adolescents typically require instruction in proper techniques for self-administering drug therapy. For example, children with diabetes need to learn how to select injection sites and administer injections. Children with asthma need instruction in using respiratory inhalers. Other patients may need instruction in how to mix, shake, or otherwise prepare drugs before measuring the dose.

Parents and pediatric patients should be given as much opportunity to practice drug administration techniques as possible while the nurse observes and offers feedback and supervision. For example, techniques should be reevaluated frequently during admissions to the hospital or at scheduled medical visits, because problems related to poor technique frequently arise. In one study of over-the-counter drug use, only 30% of the parents could state the correct dose for their child and measure it correctly (Simon and Weinkle, 1997).

However, another study (McMahon, Rimsza, & Bay, 1997) shows that effective teaching helps parents learn to give the correct amount of a drug. Parents in this study who were most successful in administering a correct dose had been given a syringe with a line marked at the correct dose and a demonstration of measuring the dose. They were asked to provide a return demonstration. One month later, 100% of these parents could measure a correct dose, compared with 37% of parents who had only received verbal instructions on administering the drug.

The importance of administering a drug at the appropriate times and continuing therapy for the full course of treatment must be emphasized to parents and children. Sometimes parents will stop administering a drug once the child no longer exhibits signs or symptoms of an illness. This is especially true if the child protests or has difficulty taking the drug. Nurses should stress that interrupting drug therapy before the full course of treatment may result in recurrence of an infection or development of a drug-resistant infection.

Preventing illness and injury helps eliminate the need for many types of drug therapy and the subsequent risk of adverse effects. The importance of education and health promotion in pediatric drug therapy cannot be overemphasized. Some therapy-related issues to include in health education are highlighted in the accompanying display, Health Education to Minimize Drug Therapy Use and Adverse Effects in Children.

Ongoing Assessment and Evaluation

Nursing management of drug therapy in children is considered effective when the developmental needs of the patient have been met, the care has been family oriented, and the drug has achieved its therapeutic effect without adverse effect to the child. Children who are receiving drug therapy for chronic conditions need to be reassessed and evaluated frequently and during regular yearly pediatric checkups to ensure that they are safely adhering to prescribed drug therapy, self-administering drug therapy as indicated, and growing and developing normally while undergoing drug therapy. ■

COMMUNITY-BASED CONCERNS

Health Education to Minimize Drug Therapy Use and Adverse Effects in Children

- Explain the role of childhood immunizations in maintaining health, the need to identify the recommended schedule of immunizations, the importance of receiving all recommended immunizations; and the potential adverse effects that may follow the immunization.
- Show the family and child how to perform frequent, thorough hand washing. Explain how this prevents the spread of infections, including cold and influenza viruses.
- Teach families the importance of the regular use of sunscreen with children to prevent sunburn resulting from drug-induced photosensitivity and to protect the child against skin cancer later in life.
- Caution families to avoid accidental overdosage and poisonings by keeping all drugs (prescription and over-the-counter products) out of the reach of children, by insisting on childproof caps for drug containers, and by installing child-resistant latches on cupboards where drugs and other dangerous products are stored. Instruct family members never to describe drugs as "candy."
- Assist patients and families to develop hygienic practices that will prevent or minimize transmitting parasitic infections by fecal-oral contamination (from not washing hands after using the toilet or touching soiled diapers) or by sharing hairbrushes or hats contaminated by lice.
- Demonstrate how to use car seats appropriately for children of different ages and sizes to prevent injury in car accidents.

CHAPTER SUMMARY

- Children are different from adults both physically and emotionally, and these differences seriously impact the planning of safe and effective drug therapy.
- A child's age, growth, and development are crucial aspects in relating core drug knowledge with core patient variables in drug therapy.
- A child's age, weight, body surface area, water content, and fat content must be considered when determining the proper dose of a drug. Drug dosage is calculated for each child using mathematical formulas.
- It is vital that pediatric dosages are accurate because even small errors can cause adverse effects, toxicity, or death. All dosage calculations should be verified by a second nurse.
- To maximize the therapeutic effect of any drug therapy, the nurse must ensure that all of the appropriate dose was administered by the desired route.
- Many of the adverse effects of drug therapy can be avoided or minimized when the nurse ensures that the child receives the appropriate drug dosage calculated specifically for each child. Nurses should have access to a pediatric drug reference or guide that gives the pediatric ranges for drug doses, including those for preterm and full-term neonates.
- One of the adverse effects in pediatric drug administration is psychological distress in the child or parent. The nurse using knowledge of age-related emotional needs and communication techniques can greatly help relieve this emotional distress and enhance drug therapy compliance.
- Patient and family education regarding drug therapy should include information needed to help the child receive the drug safely and effectively. Teaching involves giving honest and straightforward explanations about drug therapy, answering questions and allaying patient and family anxiety, and emphasizing the importance of drug compliance.

QUESTIONS FOR STUDY AND REVIEW

1. How does the neonate's and infant's liver functioning affect drug distribution?
2. What is body surface area?
3. What dose adjustment might be expected when a water-soluble drug is given to an infant?
4. Are all drugs that are safe for adults also safe for children?
5. What is the appropriate site of an IM injection for an infant?
6. Why is it important to assess the preschool or school-aged child's past experience with health care providers and drug therapy? Why is patient and family education important with pediatric patients?

NEED MORE HELP?

Chapter 7 of the study guide for *Drug Therapy in Nursing* contains exercises and activities to reinforce your understanding of the concepts presented in this chapter. For additional information see the text's accompanying web site at *http://www.connection.lww.com.*

REFERENCES AND BIBLIOGRAPHY

Arrowsmith, J., & Campbell, C. (2000). A comparison of local anaesthetics for venipuncture. *Archives of Disease in Childhood, 82*(4), 309–310.

Buck, M. L. Preventing medication errors in children. http://nurses.medscape.com/UVA/PedPharm/1999/v05.n10/pp0510.buck/pp0510.buck-02.html.

Day, M. W. (2000). Using intraosseous access in children. *Nursing 2000, 30*(1), 68.

Essink-Tjebbes, C. M., Hekster, Y. A., Liem, K. D., & van Dongen, R. T. (1999). *Pharmacy World and Science, 21*(4), 173–176.

Jacobson, A. F. (1997). Research for practice. Pediatric IM injections: One site does not fit all. *American Journal of Nursing 97* (11; *Nurse Practitioner Extra Ed.), 20,* 22.

Kraus, D. M., Stohlmeyer, L. A., & Hannon, P. R. (1999). Infant acceptance and effectiveness of a new oral liquid medication delivery system. *American Journal of Health System Pharmacy, 56*(11), 1094–1101.

Lesar, T. S. (1998). Errors in the use of medication dosage equations. *Archives of Pediatric and Adolescent Medicine, 152*(4), 340–344.

May, K., Britt, R., & Newman, N. M. (1999). Pediatric registered nurse usage and perception of EMLA. *Journal of the Society of Pediatric Nursing, 4(3),* 105–112.

McMahon, S. R., Rimsza, M. E., & Bay, R. C. (1997). Parents can dose liquid medication accurately. *Pediatrics. 100*(3 Pt 1), 330–333.

National Institute of Allergy and Infectious Diseases. (1997). Nasal spray flu vaccine proves effective in children. *Healthline, 16(10),* 8–9.

Simon, H. K., & Weinkle, D. A. (1997). Over the counter medications. Do parents give what they intend to give? *Archives of Pediatric and Adolescent Medicine, 151*(7), 654–656.

Squire, S. J., Kirchhoff, K. T, & Hissong, K. (2000). Comparing two methods of topical anesthesia used before intravenous cannulation in pediatric patients. *Journal of Pediatric Health Care, 14*(2), 68–72.

Stevens, B., Johnston, C., Taddio, A., Jack, A., Narciso, J., Stremler, R., Koren, G., & Aranda, J. (1999). Management of pain from heel lance with lidocaine- prilocaine (EMLA) cream: Is it safe and efficacious in preterm infants? *Journal of Developmental and Behavioral Pediatrics. 20*(4), 216–221.

Stovroff, M., & Teague, W. G. (1998). Intravenous access in infants and children. *Pediatric Clinics of North America. 45*(6), 1373–93, viii.

Tulga, F., & Mutlu, Z. (1999). Four types of topical anaesthetic agents: Evaluation of clinical effectiveness. *Journal of Clinical Pediatric Dentistry, 23*(3), 217–220.

United States Pharmacopeia. (1999). Position Statement. Ten guiding principles for teaching children and adolescents about medicines. http://www.usp.org/frameset.htm?http://www.usp.org/information.

Weinstein, S. (2000). *Plumer's principles and practice of intravenous therapy* (7th ed.). Philadelphia: Lippincott Williams & Wilkins.

Chapter 8

LIFE SPAN: PREGNANT OR BREAST-FEEDING WOMEN

KEY TERMS

eclampsia
fetal alcohol syndrome
fetal hydantoin syndrome
gestational diabetes
hyperemesis gravidarum
lactation
organogenesis
preeclampsia
teratogenic

Learning Objectives

At the completion of this chapter the student will:

1. Identify how core drug knowledge of drug therapy in pregnant or breast-feeding patients may vary from core drug knowledge in other life span groups.
2. Identify how normal physiologic changes with pregnancy alter pharmacokinetics of drug therapy.
3. Define teratogenic effect and its relevance in managing drug therapy in the pregnant patient.
4. Differentiate the classifications of drugs for use in pregnancy.
5. Describe why adverse effects of drug therapy may be overlooked in pregnant patients.
6. Identify how the pregnant or breast-feeding patient's core patient variables in drug therapy may vary from the core patient variables of other life span groups.
7. Relate the interaction of core drug knowledge to core patient variables when providing drug therapy in pregnant or breast-feeding patients.
8. Generate a nursing plan of care from the interactions between core drug knowledge and core patient variables for drug therapy in pregnant or breast-feeding patients.
9. Describe nursing interventions to maximize therapeutic and minimize adverse effects in drug therapy in pregnant and breast-feeding patients.
10. Determine key points for patient and family education in drug therapy for pregnant or breast-feeding patients.

Although prevalence varies, drug therapy during pregnancy is common. In studies done in different parts of the world from the 1970s to the 1990s, the percentage of pregnant women who reported using prescription medicines ranged from 6% to 97% (Gilstrap & Little, 1998). Nursing management of drug therapy for pregnant women is challenging for several reasons. Nursing care is needed for both the patient and the fetus because most drugs pass, usually by diffusion, through the placental membrane to the fetus or through breast milk to the infant.

Drug therapy in pregnant women is used primarily for two reasons: to treat a preexisting medical condition or to treat complications that arise during pregnancy. Although drug therapy may be indicated during pregnancy or during **lactation** (the secretion of breast milk), nursing management must focus on both the therapeutic effects on the patient and the adverse effects on the developing fetus or infant being breast-fed.

The nurse must know about the physiologic changes that occur during pregnancy and how they may alter the patient's response to a drug. The nurse must also understand the adverse effects of certain drugs on the developing fetus. Although adverse effects of drug therapy to the breast-fed infant are generally less severe than those to the fetus during pregnancy, the nurse must be familiar with the potential adverse effects from drug therapy during lactation.

This chapter presents core drug knowledge and core patient variables that pertain to pregnancy and lactation. In addition, some general guidelines are presented for maximizing therapeutic effects, minimizing adverse effects, and providing patient and family education for any drug therapy.

NURSING MANAGEMENT OF THE PREGNANT OR BREAST-FEEDING PATIENT

Core Drug Knowledge

Pharmacotherapeutics

The pharmacotherapeutics of drug therapy are no different in a pregnant woman than in a nonpregnant woman. The important consideration in drug therapy for pregnant women is the potential adverse effects on the developing fetus. There should always be a clear clinical indication for drug therapy before a drug is prescribed or self-administered. Although the range for most drug dosages remains the same for the pregnant patient, the nurse must always consider the risk of fetal effects. The lowest therapeutic dose of a drug should be administered to the pregnant woman to help minimize fetal effects.

Some health problems occur secondary to pregnancy and require drug therapy. These problems include **preeclampsia** (a serious hypertensive condition that develops during pregnancy) or **eclampsia** (a life-threatening condition resulting from uncontrolled preeclampsia, involving cerebral edema and convulsions). **Gestational diabetes,** a form of diabetes that develops during pregnancy, may also occur. Occasionally, if the fetus has a health problem, drugs are administered to the pregnant woman with the intent of treating the fetus as the drug passes through the placenta. For example, digoxin is used to treat fetal tachycardia and congestive heart failure; the drug is administered to the mother to treat the fetus.

Pharmacokinetics

Several physiologic and anatomic changes occur during pregnancy. They can alter the pharmacokinetics of drugs and involve the endocrine, gastrointestinal (GI), cardiovascular, circulatory, and renal systems.

Absorption

Changes in the GI system are influenced by pregnancy hormones and mechanical pressure from the growing uterus. Progesterone decreases gastric tone and motility and prolongs stomach emptying time. The pharmacokinetics of orally administered drugs may be altered, although this has not been demonstrated clinically. During pregnancy, progesterone promotes functional respiratory system changes. Tidal volume increases 30% to 40%, with a 50% increase in minute volume by term. These increases, along with pulmonary vasodilation, which also occurs during pregnancy, enhance the absorption of inhalable drugs.

Distribution and Metabolism

Hemodynamic changes in the cardiovascular system alter heart rate, cardiac output, venous and arterial blood pressures, blood volume, circulation, and coagulation. The heart rate increases about 10 to 15 beats per minute (bpm) above baseline as a result of a 40% increase in blood volume. A 50% increase in plasma volume causes a hemodilution of plasma albumin, which potentiates changes in drug distribution. Plasma lipid levels increase throughout pregnancy as a result of the more complete absorption and decreased elimination of fats during pregnancy. These changes in lipid levels may alter drug transport mechanisms and drug distribution.

Drugs are distributed by the circulatory system to the fetus by passing, usually by diffusion, through the placenta. Drugs competing with the hormones of pregnancy for albumin binding sites may result in a larger amount of unbound (or free) drug in circulation, leaving the drug available to cross the placental membrane and enter the fetal circulation. Drugs that are lipophilic (fat soluble) and not protein bound pass easily through the placenta's lipid membrane.

Drugs are also distributed into breast milk. Drugs that are widely distributed throughout the mother's body are usually minimally passed into breast milk, producing low drug concentrations in the breast milk. Other drugs, such as those with increased lipid solubility and low protein binding (such as central nervous system [CNS] agents) pass more easily and may produce high drug concentrations in the breast milk. Lipophilic drugs pass easily because breast milk contains a high percentage of fat. Drugs that are not highly protein bound have more active, free drug molecules in the bloodstream, which diffuse into breast milk. Other drugs that are more likely to diffuse into breast milk include drugs with lower molecular weights and those with organic bases; these drugs may become "trapped" in the breast milk because of its low pH, producing high drug concentrations.

Not all drugs present in breast milk are well absorbed by the neonate. Drugs with poor bioavailability usually do not achieve high concentrations in the neonate's circulation. This is because breast milk drug levels are not equivalent to blood drug levels in the mother. A breast-feeding infant usually ingests less than 2% of the mother's total dose.

Drug metabolism is not altered by pregnancy or breast-feeding.

Excretion

Changes in renal function during pregnancy result from changes in the renal plasma flow, glomerular filtration rates, and renal tubular reabsorption. By the third trimester, the renal blood flow has increased 40% to 50% from the prepregnant level. Increases in renal plasma flow cause greater capillary pressures, requiring an increase in filtration through the glomerulus. The glomerular filtration rate increases about 50% and contributes to increased excretion rates. Therefore, drug excretion rates may be increased during pregnancy.

Pharmacodynamics

There are two dramatic physical changes that occur in the mother during pregnancy: by 32 weeks' gestation, there is a 50% increase in cardiac output, and during the second trimester there is decreased arterial blood pressure that continues throughout the rest of the pregnancy. These conditions necessitate careful evaluation of a drug's pharmacodynamics.

Contraindications and Precautions

Some drugs are contraindicated during pregnancy, and others should be given with caution if they pose a threat to the developing fetus by passing through the placenta. Some drugs can cause **teratogenic** effects (i.e., physical defects) in the developing fetus. Hence, potential fetal risks are always a serious consideration, and the benefits of maternal drug therapy during pregnancy must be weighed against the risks to the fetus. The identification of a drug as a teratogen is traditionally based on the findings of animal teratology studies. This method is problematic, because animal models are frequently poor predictors of whether a drug is a human teratogen. Nonhuman primates are good predictors of human teratogenicity, because they are the most genetically similar to humans; however, nonhuman primates are rarely used in experiments because of the expense. Rodents are used most frequently in teratology studies. Unfortunately, rodents are very dissimilar to humans in terms of their physiology, metabolism, and ontogenetic development. Although animal studies do not provide all of the information in determining teratogenicity of a drug, they have an important role in screening drugs for their potential to cause human birth defects. The ultimate assessment of drug safety during pregnancy, unfortunately, comes from the use of the drugs in humans. Human teratogens are identified by examination of data reported in the literature by astute health care providers and in epidemiologic studies.

Pregnancy Categories

In 1980, the U.S. Food and Drug Administration (FDA) developed a categorical ranking based on research findings to help classify drugs by the risks posed to the fetus weighed against the potential benefits to the pregnant woman. The categories are A, B, C, D, and X (see the accompanying display, FDA Pregnancy Categories). Categories A and B (and to some extent C) are generally based on increasing risk. Categories D and X (and to some extent C) are based on risk versus potential benefit. Drug manufacturers are required by law to state these pregnancy categories in all printed drug reference material and package inserts to inform health care providers making drug administration decisions. Recently, the FDA has received comments that the categories do not supply enough information for providers and consumers to make informed decisions about drug therapy. Additional criticism is that the FDA, in trying to keep the categories simple, has grouped drugs together that do not have identical risks. Based on these concerns, the FDA Pregnancy Labeling Task Force has proposed revising the current pregnancy labeling. The recommendations for revisions include replacing the current letter category and text description with a narrative text that is more informative (FDA, 1999).

Lactation Categories

In 1994, the American Academy of Pediatrics Committee on Drugs published its recommendations on drugs

FDA Pregnancy Categories

Category A: Controlled human studies in pregnant women fail to demonstrate a risk to the fetus.

Category B: Animal studies fail to demonstrate fetal risk, but there are no controlled human studies in pregnant women; or animal studies demonstrate fetal risk that was not confirmed in controlled human studies in pregnant women.

Category C: Animal studies demonstrate fetal risk, and there are no controlled human studies in pregnant women to rule out fetal risk, or there are no animal or human studies. Drugs are given if the benefit justifies risk.

Category D: Controlled human studies demonstrate positive evidence of fetal risk. In life-threatening situations, the benefit may be acceptable despite the risk.

Category X: Controlled human studies demonstrate fetal risk. The fetal risk outweighs any possible benefit. Use in pregnant or potentially pregnant women is contraindicated.

and breast-feeding. The report identified several categories rating the risk factors:

- Drugs that are contraindicated
- Drugs that require temporary cessation
- Drugs with unknown effects on breast-feeding infants but that may be of concern
- Drugs that are associated with significant effects on some breast-feeding infants and that should be given with caution
- Drugs that are usually compatible with breast-feeding

All contraindicated drugs have been reported to cause signs and symptoms in the infant or produce an adverse effect on lactation. The American Academy of Pediatrics states that this list is not complete and recommends that all drugs of abuse should be avoided by lactating women, even though reports of neonatal adverse effects are not found in the literature.

Breast-feeding should stop if the woman is receiving any radioactive compounds, such as those used for treating malignant tumors or an overactive thyroid gland. The patient should pump her breasts during the time that breast milk is radioactive and discard that milk in a biohazard container designed for radioactive materials. Breast-feeding can resume when the drug is stopped and breast milk contains no radioactivity. Drugs with unknown effects on the neonate that may be of concern include psychotropic drugs and several anti-infectives, such as chloramphenicol (Chloromycetin), metoclopramide (Reglan), and metronidazole (Flagyl).

Drugs that are associated with significant neonatal effects after breast-feeding and that should be used with caution include aspirin, clemastine (Tavist), 5-aminosalicylic acid (Paser Granules), phenobarbital, primidone (Mysoline), and sulfasalazine (Azulfidine). Most reported effects for these drugs include sedation and diarrhea. Often the drugs identified as being compatible with breast-feeding are not part of large research studies. Rather, information is obtained from single case reports or small series of reports.

Adverse Effects

There are two major considerations when evaluating adverse effects of drug therapy in pregnant women. One concerns the common discomforts or side effects of pregnancy, such as nausea and vomiting, light-headedness or hypotension, constipation, heartburn, urinary frequency, heart palpitations, and fatigue. These symptoms may mask the adverse effects of drug therapy in pregnant patients, making adverse effects more difficult to assess.

The other major concern is the adverse effect that maternal drug therapy can have on the developing fetus. Several factors are important when considering the effects of drugs on the fetus. The timing of the drug exposure is critical because of the constant changes during fetal development. Before implantation, the fertilized ovum may not be affected by maternal drug use, although some drugs, such as alcohol, produce a hostile intrauterine environment, thereby preventing implantation and causing a spontaneous abortion. The period from conception to implantation is theorized to be the "protected period"; that is, without a vascular interface between the mother and the conceptus, it is believed that drugs in the mother's circulation cannot pass to the conceptus and have an effect on it.

After implantation, up to day 58 or 60 after conception, is the critical period of **organogenesis.** During this period, the major fetal organ systems are forming. When drugs that cause teratogenic effects are administered during this period, major malformations of fetal organ systems may result (Table 8-1). Malformations that are lethal to the embryo will result in spontaneous abortions. Drug therapy should be delayed until after this period, if possible. Unfortunately, most women do not realize they are pregnant or seek prenatal care until after this time period, so accidental exposure to teratogens may occur.

After 60 days, the embryonic phase is complete and the fetal phase begins. This phase continues throughout the remainder of the pregnancy. Exposure to drugs during the remainder of pregnancy continues to have the potential for harming the fetus. The fetal effects that may occur are of four primary types:

- Damage to structures or organs that were formed normally during organogenesis
- Damage to systems undergoing tissue development
- Growth retardation
- Fetal death or stillbirth

TABLE 8-1 Prescription Drugs with Known Human Teratogenicity and Their Therapeutic Indication

Teratogenic Drug or Drug Class	Indication
aminopterin, methylaminopter, busulfan, cyclophosphamide, thalidomide*	Antineoplastic
androgenic hormones, diethylstilbestrol	Hormone replacement
coumarin	Anticoagulant
etretinate	Psoriasis
isotretinoin	Recalcitrant cystic acne
lithium	Antimanic
methimazole	Antithyroid
penicillamine	Cystinuria and rheumatoid arthritis
phenytoin, trimethadione, valproic acid	Anticonvulsant
tetracycline	Antibiotic

*Originally used as a tranquilizer and sedative; also currently used as an antiinfective for leprosy.

Combinations of these damages may also occur. Fetal effects may be caused by a teratogen but may also be caused by agents that have no apparent potential to produce abnormal embryonic development. An example is coumarin derivatives, used as anticoagulants, which may produce eye and brain defects from hemorrhagic accidents in the fetus. Fetal growth retardation is the most common fetal effect. However, it is difficult to determine whether this effect is caused by the drug therapy or the primary condition for which the drug therapy is prescribed. For example, the antihypertensive drug propranolol is associated with fetal growth retardation; however, untreated hypertension is also associated with this condition.

Additionally, there are some drugs that create adverse neonatal effects (Table 8-2). These agents are not normally related to teratogenic effects but instead create a situation that makes it difficult for the neonate to adapt to life outside the uterus. Examples are floppy infant syndrome from the use of benzodiazepines (antianxiety agents, sedatives) near the time of delivery, and premature closing of the ductus arteriosus from the use of prostaglandin synthetase inhibitors (i.e., nonsteroidal anti-inflammatory drugs, such as aspirin or indomethacin [Indocin]).

The list of known human teratogenic drugs is surprisingly small (see Table 8-1 for a sampling). However, there are other drugs suspected of human teratogenicity from animal studies. Teratogens cause specific patterns of adverse effects in the developing fetus. For example, the most commonly prescribed anticonvulsant, phenytoin (Dilantin) (a hydantoin), has been found to cause **fetal hydantoin syndrome.** This syndrome is characterized by craniofacial abnormalities, limb defects, growth deficiency, and mental deficiency (Hansen & Smith, 1975). It is believed that these abnormalities occur because of phenytoin's competition for folic acid binding sites.

TABLE 8-2 Selected Nonteratogenic Drugs with Adverse Fetal Effects

Nonteratogenic Drug	Adverse Fetal Effects
acetaminophen	Renal failure
adrenocortical hormones	Adrenocortical suppression, electrolyte imbalance
amphetamines	Withdrawal
cocaine	Vascular disruption, withdrawal, intrauterine growth retardation
meperidine	Neonatal depression
phenobarbital (excess)	Neonatal bleeding, death
cigarette smoking	Premature births, intrauterine growth retardation
thiazide diuretics	Thrombocytopenia, salt and water depletion, possible neonatal death

Other anticonvulsants have since been found to produce fetal abnormalities. Most are classified as pregnancy category D drugs, although carbamazepine (Tegretol) is classified as a pregnancy category C drug.

The risks for adverse effects of drug therapy on the breast-feeding infant are not as great as the risks of drug therapy during pregnancy, because the breast-feeding infant usually ingests less than 2% of the total dose of the drug given to the mother. The risk for adverse effects is still possible; therefore, breast-feeding is a precaution in the case of many drug therapies and a contraindication for others. The United States National Health Promotion and Disease Prevention objectives targeted the year 2000 as the year for increasing the percentage of mothers who breast-feed in the early postpartum period; the objective aim was to increase the then current level of approximately 60% to a projected level of 75%.

As more women breast-feed, nurses need to know more about whether the administration of a particular drug poses a risk to the breast-feeding infant.

Drug Interactions

Drug interactions are unchanged during pregnancy and breast-feeding.

Assessment of Relevant Core Patient Variables Related to Pregnancy and Breast-Feeding

Health Status

There are several considerations when assessing health status during pregnancy. First, if the patient has a preexisting condition that requires drug therapy, the health care providers must consider whether the prescribed drug therapy will have adverse effects on the fetus. Second, it must be determined whether the pregnancy will have any adverse effects on the mother's health that will require changes in drug therapy. Third, if the pregnancy induces changes in health status that require new drug therapy, any adverse effects of this drug therapy on the fetus will have to be determined.

The pregnant woman must be assessed for preexisting conditions and particularly those being treated with drug therapy. Special attention should be given to any cardiovascular problems, because the cardiovascular system undergoes many changes and stresses during pregnancy. Drug selection may need to be altered, or dosage changes may be necessary because of the pregnancy.

Seizure disorder is a condition that is important to consider during pregnancy. A woman with a seizure disorder who is planning a pregnancy must first seriously consider how anticonvulsant drug therapy will affect the fetus. Anticonvulsants may be continued throughout pregnancy if necessary to prevent seizures; seizures in a pregnant woman may cause fetal hypoxia, leading to CNS damage. If anticonvulsants must be continued during pregnancy, drug selection is important. Some anticonvulsants (e.g., trimethadione [Tridione], and valproic acid [Depakote]) are recommended to be avoided.

Only drugs with pregnancy class X are strictly contraindicated. The decision to maintain therapy with drugs having a class D or even a class C rating needs to be made based on the ratio of risk to benefit; these are relative contraindications. Anticonvulsants may be discontinued for select patients on medical consultation. Specific monitoring to detect abnormalities should be done.

Diabetes is another important preexisting condition to consider, although it may also develop during pregnancy. Between 1% and 5% of women have diabetes before pregnancy. Another 2% to 3% of pregnant women develop gestational diabetes, in which the secretion of placental hormones (human placental lactogen, cortisol, progesterone, and catecholamines) causes the pregnant woman to develop an insulin resistance as the pregnancy progresses. Hyperglycemia may result and require either an increase in insulin therapy or, in the case of gestational diabetes, initiation of insulin therapy. Because hyperglycemia is believed to increase the incidence of congenital anomalies (particularly during the first trimester), a primary goal for the pregnant patient is to maintain normal blood glucose levels (euglycemia). Insulin is the drug of choice for controlling blood glucose levels because, unlike oral hypoglycemic drugs, it does not cross the placenta. After the neonate is delivered, maternal insulin needs should return to baseline levels, and insulin therapy is usually no longer necessary.

Another alteration of health status that may occur during pregnancy is **hyperemesis gravidarum,** commonly referred to as pernicious vomiting of pregnancy. When hyperemesis gravidarum is severe, antiemetic drug therapy is needed to control the vomiting. Currently, antiemetic drug therapy consists of administering drugs from the piperazine class (e.g., meclizine [Antivert] and cyclizine [Marezine]) and the phenothiazine class (e.g., chlorpromazine [Thorazine], prochlorperazine [Compazine], and promethazine [Phenergan]). The piperazines have not been found to be teratogenic. The phenothiazines are generally considered safe with low and infrequent usage, although some studies show that animal or infant malformations can occur. However, when using antiemetics, the risk for adverse fetal effects, especially during the first trimester, must be considered.

Preeclampsia is another serious condition that can develop and require drug therapy during pregnancy. Preeclampsia, a hypertensive condition of pregnancy, typically develops after the 24th gestational week. It is characterized by a triad of symptoms: hypertension, edema, and proteinuria. Uncontrolled preeclampsia may lead to eclampsia, a condition characterized by cerebral edema and convulsions. The primary goal of preeclampsia treatment is prevention of eclampsia and the stabilization of the patient until the fetus reaches maturity. Treatment for preeclampsia is aimed at decreasing CNS irritability and reducing maternal blood pressure to enhance placental and maternal circulation to the organs. Drug therapy for preeclampsia includes magnesium sulfate, which is the drug of choice for preventing convulsions (see Chapter 44), and hydralazine, which is the drug of choice for treating hypertension (see Chapter 30). Other drugs used in treating hypertension in preeclampsia include diazoxide (Hyperstat IV), nifedipine (Procardia), and labetalol (Trandate).

Another condition that may occur secondary to pregnancy is thrombus formation. The decreased venous return and increased clotting factors and fibrinogen levels that are characteristic in pregnancy produce a state of hypercoagulation, which increases the risk of clot formation. Pregnant women who develop thrombosis are treated with heparin.

Lifestyle, Diet, and Habits

Lifestyle, diet, and habits of pregnant or breast-feeding women can have a serious impact on the course of the pregnancy and the development of the fetus or infant. For example, alcohol is a known human teratogen. **Fetal alcohol syndrome** is a serious pattern of teratogenic effects seen in infants born to women who may have consumed alcohol chronically during pregnancy. Fetal alcohol syndrome is marked by certain physical malformations at birth and severe growth retardation, mental retardation, and microcephaly. Cocaine abuse is known to cause adverse fetal effects and is suspected to be a human teratogen. Opiate abuse does not appear to significantly increase the risk of congenital anomalies, but other adverse outcomes are associated with their use. These include abruptio placentae, neonatal withdrawal, preterm birth, and fetal growth retardation. Smoking tobacco has also been found to have adverse fetal effects, most notably fetal growth retardation.

Environment

Although some health alterations occurring in pregnancy require drug therapy that is administered in the hospital setting, such as magnesium sulfate for preeclampsia, most drug therapy given during pregnancy or breast-feeding will be administered in the patient's home.

Culture

Cultural beliefs may effect whether a woman is accepting of certain drug therapies while she is pregnant or breast-feeding. Assess for these beliefs when managing drug therapy in the pregnant or breast-feeding woman.

Nursing Diagnoses and Outcomes

Nursing diagnoses formulated for the pregnant or breast-feeding patient receiving drug therapy will be similar to diagnoses made for patients with other life span concerns. The main difference is that for the pregnant or breast-feeding woman, the nursing diagnosis must address the needs of the patient and her child. Relevant nursing diagnoses may include the following:

- Risk for Injury to the fetus related to adverse effects of maternal drug therapy

  Desired outcome: *The patient will demonstrate therapeutic drug effects with minimal adverse effect to the fetus or infant by avoiding unnecessary drugs* *throughout pregnancy and lactation and by using nonpharmacologic measures to relieve common discomforts of pregnancy.*

- Anxiety related to perceived danger of drug therapy to fetus or infant

  Desired outcome: The patient's anxiety will be minimal during drug therapy.
- Risk for Injury to the patient related to failure to receive needed drug therapy because of its potential adverse effects on the fetus or infant

  Desired outcome: The patient will not sustain an injury from choices made about receiving drug therapy.

Planning and Intervention

The nurse and other health care providers have a responsibility to the pregnant patient to consider the benefit:risk ratio of drug therapy, to educate the childbearing patient regarding possible teratogenic effects, and to support the patient's decision regarding accepting or refusing drug therapy.

Maximizing Therapeutic Effects

If a prescribed drug therapy does not have adverse effects for the developing fetus or the child of the breast-feeding woman, this should be emphasized when teaching patients. Women may be reluctant to take needed drug therapy if they believe it may be harmful to the fetus.

Minimizing Adverse Effects

No drug can be considered absolutely safe when administered during pregnancy, although general guidelines can assist the health care provider with drug therapy decisions. Women of childbearing age should always be assessed regarding pregnancy before any drug therapy is initiated. During pregnancy, nonpharmacologic alternatives to drug therapy should be used if possible. This is especially true for common discomforts of pregnancy, such as nausea and vomiting, light-headedness or hypotension, constipation, heartburn, urinary frequency, heart palpitations, and fatigue. Limiting drug use in pregnancy decreases maternal and fetal adverse effects. If drug therapy is required, the nurse should first check the drug's FDA pregnancy category to determine safety. An evaluation of the risk versus the benefits should show justification for administering a drug. When a drug is to be administered, the nurse should consult with the prescriber so that the minimum therapeutic dose is used for as short a time as possible. Drug therapy should be delayed, if possible, until after the first trimester of pregnancy, when all major fetal organ systems are forming, especially if the drug has the potential for causing teratogenic effects.

The pregnant patient and fetus need to be monitored for both therapeutic and adverse effects of drug therapy. If prolonged drug use is necessary and this poses risk to the woman or the fetus, serum levels should be monitored to detect elevations that may lead to adverse effects. Dosage adjustments or discontinuation of the drug may be needed to reverse adverse effects or prevent toxicity. When complications of pregnancy occur, only drugs that are absolutely necessary should be administered to reduce risks of adverse effects. The nurse must be careful to distinguish discomforts of pregnancy (e.g., nausea, vomiting, heartburn, light-headedness, urinary frequency, heart palpitations) from possible adverse drug effects when evaluating a patient. In addition, the pediatrician should be informed about maternal drug therapy. Knowledge of fetal exposure to drugs assists the pediatrician in making appropriate health care decisions regarding the neonate.

When questions and concerns arise regarding drug therapy and breast-feeding, the same strategies are used to prevent adverse effects. They include using nonpharmacologic remedies, determining the safest drug possible based on how the amount of drug transferred to breast milk and the possible neonatal effects, and assessing blood concentrations of the drug in the breast-feeding infant (if adverse effects are possible). Each drug administered to the lactating patient should be evaluated individually for its neonatal adverse effects. When managing drug therapy in a lactating patient, the nurse should also assess the infant for adverse effects of the drug. Other methods used to reduce neonatal drug exposure include scheduling drug therapy just after breast-feeding or before the infant is going to sleep for a lengthy period. Some drugs, such as antineoplastic drugs and drugs of abuse, are contraindicated during lactation. If the patient is taking these drugs, breast-feeding should be discontinued. Agents such as general anesthetics, sedatives, and radioactive compounds required for a short-term diagnostic test should be cleared from the patient's circulation before breast-feeding resumes. The nurse must know the half-life and the duration of action of the drug to determine when breast-feeding should be re-initiated. The risks to the developing neonate must be balanced against the advantages of the drug to the woman. See the accompanying display, Ensuring Drug Safety During Lactation.

Providing Patient and Family Education

The nurse's role in counseling about pregnancy and fetal drug effects ideally begins before pregnancy. This will assist women in making informed choices regarding drug therapy and help minimize the risk of accidental exposure to teratogens in the early stages of pregnancy (from conception to day 60). Informing women of childbearing

Critical Thinking Scenario

Ensuring drug safety during lactation

Your patient, a breast-feeding mother, tells you that she frequently gets stress headaches and takes aspirin for them. She would like the aspirin to have as little effect on the baby as possible. What advice can you offer her?

age about fetal drug effects provides them with information useful in making decisions about when to plan pregnancy and what actions to take when pregnancy occurs.

Patient and family education during pregnancy and breast-feeding is primarily focused on adverse effects to the fetus and infant. If the woman is exposed to a drug prior to learning that she is pregnant she will need information regarding what degree of risk to the fetus has occurred, if any. Each pregnant patient should be given information on the drug's effects, both therapeutic and adverse, and should be permitted to make an informed decision as to whether or not to receive the drug therapy.

The pregnant patient should also be instructed about adverse effects of drug therapy so that she can anticipate them and distinguish them from normal pregnancy-related problems. The nurse should instruct the patient to notify the health care provider if adverse drug effects occur. The woman who is lactating should also be informed of possible adverse effects of drug therapy on the infant and be instructed to report those findings immediately to the health care provider.

To help relieve typical discomforts of pregnancy, the nurse should teach the patient how to use nonpharmacologic strategies, such as eating dry crackers first thing in the morning to prevent nausea.

Ongoing Assessment and Evaluation

Nursing management of drug therapy during pregnancy and lactation is considered effective when maternal therapeutic needs have been met without harm to the fetus or the breast-feeding infant. Other measures of effective drug therapy include patient- and family-oriented drug education and assessment findings indicating that mother and child are not experiencing adverse drug effects. ■

CHAPTER SUMMARY

- Drug therapy may be indicated for pregnant or lactating women to manage preexisting or newly developed conditions. Although therapeutic effects may be achieved in the woman, drug therapy may adversely affect the fetus or infant.
- The physiologic changes that occur during pregnancy may alter drug absorption, distribution, and elimination.
- Pregnancy is a contraindication for using some drugs and a precaution for using others because drugs may pass through the placenta to the fetus and may cause teratogenic effects. The potential fetal risks must be compared with maternal benefits when drug therapy is required.
- Drugs may also be excreted into breast milk, although the total is a small percentage of the maternal dose. Based on potential risks to the infant during breast-feeding, drugs have been classified as contraindicated, requiring temporary cessation, having unknown effects, cautioned, and compatible with breast-feeding. The nurse should be familiar with the prescribed drugs and the substances of abuse that are contraindicated during breast-feeding.
- Symptoms of pregnancy may mask adverse effects of drug therapy in the mother. Discomforts commonly associated with pregnancy, such as nausea and vomiting, light-headedness or hypotension, constipation, heartburn, urinary frequency, heart palpitations, and fatigue, are also frequent adverse drug effects.
- Limiting drug use during pregnancy and lactation decreases maternal and fetal adverse effects. Nonpharmacologic alternatives to drug therapy should be used if possible, particularly when treating the common discomforts of pregnancy.
- Substances of abuse are contraindicated during pregnancy and lactation because they can cause serious teratogenic effects, such as fetal alcohol syndrome, in the fetus and infant.
- The minimum therapeutic dose should be used for as short a time as possible during pregnancy. If possible, drug therapy should be delayed until after the first trimester of pregnancy, during which the fetal organ systems are forming.
- Both the pregnant patient and fetus and the lactating patient and breast-feeding infant should be monitored for therapeutic and adverse effects of drug therapy.

QUESTIONS FOR STUDY AND REVIEW

1. Which FDA pregnancy category rating includes the criterion, "The fetal risk outweighs any possible benefit," and what does that mean?
2. Explain what types of drugs are more easily transferred across the placenta to the fetus.
3. Explain why gestational weeks 3 through 8 are considered critical when drug administration is considered during pregnancy.
4. Describe the physiologic changes in the renal system that increase drug excretion rates.
5. Why are drugs that are lipophilic more likely to enter breast milk?

NEED MORE HELP?

Chapter 8 of the study guide for *Drug Therapy in Nursing* contains exercises and activities to reinforce your understanding of the concepts presented in this chapter. For additional information see the text's accompanying web site at *http://www.connection.lww.com.*

REFERENCES AND BIBLIOGRAPHY

American Academy of Pediatrics. (1994). The transfer of drugs and other chemicals into human milk. *Pediatrics, 93*(1), 137–150.

Fisher, G., Johnson, R. E., Eder, H., Jagsch, R., Peternell, A., Weninger, M., Langer, M., & Aschauer, H. N. (2000). Treatment of opioid-dependent pregnant women with buprenorphine. *Addiction, 95*(2), 239–244.

Food and Drug Administration. (1999). Concept paper on pregnancy labeling summary of comments from a public hearing and model pregnancy labeling based on recommendations. May 20.www.fda.gov/help.html.

Folsom Obstetrics and Gynecology Medical Group, P.C. (2000) Drugs in pregnancy and lactation. http://folsomobgyn.com/drugs_in_pregnancy_and_lactation.htm.

Gilstrap III, L. C., Little, B. B. (Eds.). (1998). *Drugs and pregnancy,* 2nd edition. New York: Chapman and Hall.

Hansen, J. W., & Smith, D. W. (1975). The fetal hydantoin syndrome. *Journal of Pediatrics, 87,* 285–287.

Larimore, W. L., & Petrie, K. A. (2000). Drug use during pregnancy and lactation. *Primary Care, 27*(1), 35–53.

Pregnancy and epilepsy. http://www.medscape.com/adis/DTP/2000/v15.n04/dtp1504.02/dtp1504.02-01.html.

Stevenson, A. M. (1998) Issues in pharmacology. Teratogens. *American Journal of Maternal/Child Nursing, 23*(6), 333.

U.S. Department of Health and Human Services. Centers for Disease Control and Prevention. (2000) Accutane-exposed pregnancies. *MMWR Morbidity and Mortality Weekly Report, 49*(2), 28–31.

Chapter 9

LIFE SPAN: OLDER ADULTS

KEY TERMS

benefit:risk ratio
frail elderly
geriatric patient
nonadherence
older adult
paradoxical excitement
polypharmacy

Learning Objectives

At the completion of this chapter the student will:

1. Identify how core drug knowledge of drug therapy in older adults may vary from core drug knowledge in younger adults.
2. Identify how normal physiologic changes with aging alters pharmacokinetics of drug therapy.
3. Define polypharmacy and its relevance in managing drug therapy in the older adult.
4. Describe why adverse effects of drug therapy may be overlooked in older adults.
5. Identify how the older adult's core patient variables in drug therapy may vary from the younger adult's core patient variables.
6. Relate the interaction of core drug knowledge to core patient variables when providing drug therapy in older adults.
7. Generate a nursing plan of care based on the interactions between core drug knowledge and core patient variables for drug therapy in older adults.
8. Describe nursing interventions to maximize therapeutic and minimize adverse effects in drug therapy in older adults.
9. Determine key points for patient and family education in drug therapy for older adults.

Many physiologic changes occur with normal aging.

Metabolism

The efficiency of the liver's metabolism of substances gradually declines throughout the aging process. In the older adult, three major physiologic changes greatly affect the efficiency of the liver. First, the size of the liver changes, and the number of metabolically active hepatocytes may decrease as much as 50%. The most changes occur when adults are in their 60s or 70s. Second, because cardiac output declines in general with age, blood flow to the liver declines as well. With less oxygen available, the liver's capacity to remove many metabolic byproducts is reduced. Third, the overall efficiency of the liver to metabolize drugs and other chemicals is reduced.

Normal hepatic metabolism of substances occurs in two major phases. Phase I metabolic reactions include oxidation, reduction, and hydrolysis of drug molecules. During phase I, the liver creates metabolites that may retain some degree of pharmacologic activity. Phase II reactions combine the drug or other metabolite produced in phase I with highly water-soluble forms of acetate, glucuronic acid, sulfate, or an amino acid. This produces an inactive metabolized form of the drug that is excreted in the urine or feces. Ultimately, most phase I and II reactions make drugs more water soluble, which restricts their access to the tissues, promotes removal from the body, and thereby terminates pharmacologic activity.

Aging affects the efficiency of both phases of metabolic activity but tends to alter phase I more than phase II reactions. Because drug metabolism is slowed by reduced oxidation in phase I, drug blood levels are higher and drug half-lives are extended in older adults. This usually alters the appropriate dose and dosing interval and the duration of side effects. For example, when elderly adults receive a benzodiazepine (e.g., to relieve anxiety or promote sleep), they may experience associated cognitive impairments, such as sedation, confusion, and decreased mental alertness for a longer time than normal after drug therapy ceases. Often, standard half-life parameters are inaccurate for the elderly patient. Nurses should obtain age-related drug half-life information to evaluate drug responses accurately in older patients. Nurses who are unfamiliar with age-related differences may mistakenly interpret an older patient's altered cognitive function as a normal sign of aging rather than as a residual drug effect.

Excretion

Efficient renal function is a crucial factor in ensuring drug clearance from the blood and excretion from the body and in terminating drug action. Aging can significantly decrease renal efficiency by altering the two main processes by which the kidneys remove drugs from the blood: glomerular filtration and renal tubular secretion. Both of these processes decline in efficiency with age and ultimately result in slower drug excretion and altered drug half-life.

One of the standard markers for renal function is the serum creatinine concentration, which reflects creatinine clearance from the blood by way of glomerular filtration. Despite the decline in the efficiency of glomerular filtration in the older patient, serum creatinine levels often remain in the normal range (Table 9-2). This is because creatinine production declines in the older patient as muscle mass decreases; hence, there is less overall creatinine in the older adult to be filtered. These so-called normal creatinine levels can be misleading and should not be interpreted as an indication of normal renal function in elderly patients.

Pharmacodynamics

Decreased organ efficiency in the older adult alters pharmacodynamic responses. Because absorption is prolonged in the older adult, there is commonly a significantly delayed response to single doses of drugs. For example, the older adult taking aspirin for intermittent joint pain usually experiences a longer onset of action. This delayed onset is not experienced for drugs that the older adult takes on a regular basis because steady blood levels are maintained when doses are taken at regular intervals.

Most drug responses are based on the drug-receptor interaction. A patient's response to a particular drug depends on how efficiently that receptor system operates or on the number of available receptors for that drug. An example of this is the elderly patient and the beta-adrenergic receptor system. As a result of aging, the beta-adrenergic receptor system seems to operate less efficiently and possibly with fewer receptors. This explains why the older adult is typically less responsive to beta-adrenergic agonists (stimulants), such as isoproterenol (Isuprel), yet shows enhanced sensitivity to beta-adrenergic antagonists (beta-blockers), such as propranolol (Inderal). Age-related changes affect the parasympathetic muscarinic-receptor system as well. Generally, the older adult has an increased response to anticholinergic drugs, such as atropine, and to the anticholinergic effects of drugs such as the tricyclic antidepressants.

TABLE 9-2 Age-Related Differences in Creatinine in Men

Age (Yr)	Creatinine Clearance Levels*	Serum Creatinine
17–24	140	0.808
25–34	140	0.808
35–44	133	0.813
45–54	127	0.829
55–60	119	0.837
65–74	109	0.825
75–84	96	0.843

*Ccl_{cr} = (140 – age) (weight)/(72) (serum creatinine)

NOTE: Women also demonstrate a similar decline in Ccl_{cr} with age. Ccl_{cr} for women is about 85% of values in men.

Decreases in the number of receptors are also associated with decreases in the respective neurotransmitter(s) themselves. Older patients, for example, have decreased amounts of the neurotransmitters dopamine and acetylcholine.

Contraindications and Precautions

Drug contraindications are generally similar for older adults as for younger adults. Some diseases or conditions that may contraindicate certain drug therapies are more likely to occur in older adults. Moreover, because of the older adult's decreased renal function and possibly metabolic function, many drugs should be used with caution. Some drugs or drug classes cause substantially more adverse effects in older adults than in other age populations and are generally considered inappropriate for older adults, although with proper clinical management, monitoring, and dose limitations these drugs may be used. Use of inappropriate drugs may be a significant problem in the current health care system, however. In one study of more than 2,000 older adults who are nursing home-eligible but homebound, almost 10% of them received prescriptions that were deemed inappropriate (Golden, Preston, Barnett, Liorente, Hamdan, & Silverman, 1999).

The nurse needs to work closely with physicians, nurse practitioners, and pharmacists to minimize the use of drugs that are generally contraindicated in older adults by seeking safer alternative drug therapy. Simultaneously, the nurse must realize that there will be occasions when an "inappropriate" drug will be used because it is the best therapy to treat the older adult. During these occasions, the nurse will need to work closely with the rest of the health care team, providing clinical care to minimize potential adverse outcomes to the patient.

Adverse Effects

Although the same adverse effects from any given drug therapy will occur in older adults as in other age groups, physiologic changes in older adults place them at greater risk for certain adverse effects. Adverse drug effects are an important cause of hospital admissions in older adults (Mannesse, Derkx, de Ridder, Man in 't Veldt, & van der Cammen (a), 2000).

Due to the less effective blood–brain barrier, older adults may be more vulnerable to CNS side effects, such as increased depressant or sedative activity of drugs. In addition, decreased dopamine concentrations in the brains of older adults render them more susceptible to parkinsonian effects of dopamine antagonists, such as the phenothiazine antipsychotics and metoclopramide (see Chapter 19 for details). Older adults are also more responsive to anticholinergic drugs and drugs with anticholinergic adverse effects (see Chapter 15). Depending on the severity of these adverse responses, drug dosages may be limited or may be contraindicated for a particular patient.

Drug-induced behavioral changes often affect the older adult. Sometimes they occur unexpectedly. For example, when beginning drug therapy with a sedative or a benzodiazepine to treat anxiety, the older patient may experience an effect that is the opposite to the intended effect. This is known as **paradoxical excitement,** whereby the patient is wide awake and hyperactive rather than calm and relaxed.

Determining whether an older patient is experiencing an adverse effect or a normal age-related health problem is difficult. Age-related health problems often mimic the adverse effects of drug therapy. For example, hearing loss can be a sign of aging or it can be a serious adverse effect of some antimicrobial drugs (e.g., gentamicin). Loss of balance and unsteadiness while walking are often experienced by older patients and may be confused with the adverse effects of some drugs that cause dizziness or light-headedness. Clearly, the nurse needs to distinguish between these two conditions.

Drug Interactions

Drug interactions are the same for older adults as for other populations, but because older adults tend to take more drugs, they are at higher risk for more drug interactions. It is not uncommon for older adults to be taking between 8 and 12 prescribed and OTC drugs to treat a variety of diseases. Often the combination of so many different drugs causes serious drug interactions. For example, a patient who is taking a total of 10 different prescriptions and OTC drugs risks 45 different two-drug combinations that could interact to produce an adverse effect. In one study of nursing home patients, two thirds of the residents experienced an average of 2 probable adverse drug reactions over 4 years; two thirds of the adverse effects were attributed to polypharmacy (Cooper, 2000) (see the accompanying display, Adverse Drug Reactions in Nursing Facility Residents).

Assessment of Relevant Core Patient Variables Related to Older Adults

Health Status

Aging is associated with a decline in normal bodily maintenance and function. The major organ systems (cardiovascular, respiratory, GI, genitourinary, endocrine, and others) all decline significantly with advancing age and cause a multitude of health problems that often require drug therapy. When assessing the older patient's health status, several areas concern nurses: polypharmacy, for example, has the potential for causing serious drug interactions and adverse reactions. The compromised health status of the older adult can further alter the pharmacokinetics of certain drugs and is of equal concern. In such cases, the nurse needs to assess the functional ability of the older adult's body systems and determine if the patient has any diseases that may affect prescribed drug

ever, because of older patients' age-related health prob-

the nurse should verify that the patient can remember to

Cooper, J. W. (1996). Probable adverse drug reactions in a rural geriatric nursing home population: a four-year study. *Journal of American Geriatric Society, 44*(2), 194–197.

Cooper, J. W. (1999). Adverse drug reaction-related hospitalizations of nursing facility patients: A 4-year study. *Southern Medical Journal, 92*(5), 485–490.

Cooper, J. W. (2000). Adverse drug reactions in geriatric nursing facility residents. Medscape Pharmacology. *Medscape 2000,* http://www.medscape.com/Medscape/p_2.n01/mp0118.coop/mp0118.coop.html.

Flaherty, J. H. (1998). Psychotherapeutic agents in older adults. Commonly prescribed and over-the-counter remedies: causes of confusion. *Clinics in Geriatric Medicine, 14*(1), 101–127.

Fulmer, T. T., Feldman, P. H., Kim, T. S., Carty, B., Beers, M., Molina, M., & Putnam, M. (1999). An intervention study to enhance medication compliance in community-dwelling elderly individuals. *Journal of Gerontological Nursing, 25*(8), 6–14.

Golden, A. G., Preston, R. A., Barnett, S. D., Liorente, M., Hamdan, K., & Silverman, M. A. (1999). Inappropriate mediation prescribing in homebound older adults. *Journal of American Geriatric Society, 47*(8), 948–953.

Hanlon, J. T., Schmader, K. E., Koronkowski, M. J., Weinberger, M., Landsman, P. B., Samsa, G. P., & Lewis, I. K. (1998). Adverse drug events in high risk older outpatients. *Journal of the American Geriatrics Society, 45*(8), 945–948.

Jones, B. A. (1997). Decreasing polypharmacy in clients most at risk. *AACN Clinical Issues, 8*(4), 627–634.

Mannesse, C. K., Derkx, F. H., de Ridder, M. A., Man in 't Veld, A. J., & van der Cammen, T. J. (2000). Contribution of adverse drug reactions to hospital admission of older patients. *Age and Aging, 29*(1), 35–39.

Mannesse, C. K., Derkx, F. H., de Ridder, M. A., Man in 't Veld, A. J., & van der Cammen, T. J. (2000). Do older hospital patients recognize adverse drug reactions? *Age and Aging, 29*(1), 79–81.

Monane, M., Monane, S., & Semla, T. (1997). Optimal medication use in elders. Key to successful aging. *Western Journal of Medicine, 167*(4), 233–237.

Resnick, N. M., & Marcantonio, E. R. (1997). How should clinical care of the aged differ? *The Lancet, 350*(9085), 1157–1158.

Roberts, S. L., Johnson, L. H., & Keely, B. (1999). Fostering hope in the elderly congestive heart failure patient in critical care. *Geriatric Nursing, 20*(4), 195–199.

Vestal, R. E. (1997). Aging and pharmacology. *Cancer, 80*(7), 1302–1310.

Ward-Griffin, C., & McKeever, P. (2000). Relationships between nurses and family caregivers: partners in care? ANS. *Advances in Nursing Science, 22*(3), 89–103.

Chapter 10

LIFESTYLE: SUBSTANCE ABUSE

KEY TERMS

abstinence syndrome
addiction
habituation
psychedelic
psychoactive
psychological dependence
substance abuse
tissue dependence
tolerance

Learning Objectives

At the completion of this chapter the student will:

1. Describe the scope of substance abuse in the United States.
2. Identify etiologic factors associated with substance abuse.
3. Identify frequently abused drugs and list common medical problems associated with their abuse.
4. Describe the pharmacologic basis for physical and psychological drug dependence, tolerance, and addiction.
5. Explain the adverse effects associated with chronic abuse of alcohol, cocaine, marijuana, and opioids.
6. Discuss the nursing management of patients who abuse substances, including alcohol, cocaine, marijuana, hallucinogenics, and opioids.

Lifestyle, diet, and habits is a core patient variable that exerts one of the most significant effects on a patient's response to drug therapy. The use of substances such as alcohol, tobacco products, and "street" (or illicit) drugs can seriously complicate drug therapy as well as the patient's general condition. Substance use and abuse interacts with drug therapy in several ways: chronic abuse may create health problems that require treatment with drug therapy; treatment or prevention of withdrawal from a substance may require drug therapy; and concurrent use of a substance may interact with drug therapy prescribed for a physiologic problem.

Substance abuse is the inappropriate and usually excessive self-administration of a drug substance for nonmedical purposes. Drugs with a high abuse potential have the ability to stimulate compulsive drug-seeking behavior. Contemporary substance abuse has pervasive economic, legal, medical, moral, psychological, religious, and social implications. In the United States, the combined yearly medical and social costs of drug abuse are believed to exceed $240 billion (see the accompanying display, How Many Substance Abusers?).

Substance abuse occurs throughout the life span and cuts across all racial, socioeconomic, ethnic, and cultural groups. Furthermore, factors in the patient's environment, family, or community can influence susceptibility to substance abuse and lead to addiction.

Drug **addiction** is a complex process involving interactions among the drug (availability, cost, pharmacology, toxicology), the user (personal resources, psychiatric profile, temperament), and society (family and peer influences, positive versus negative advertising, social attitudes).

COMMUNITY-BASED CONCERNS

How Many Substance Abusers?

The most commonly abused substances in the United States are alcohol, amphetamines, anabolic-androgenic steroids, barbiturates, benzodiazepines, caffeine, cocaine, hallucinogens, inhalant chemicals, marijuana, nicotine, opiates/opioids, and sedative-hypnotic drugs. Statistics from 1998 National Household Survey on Drug Abuse* indicate the following:

- Cocaine use: 3–5 million (age 12 and older)
- Alcohol use: 113 million (10.5 million are youths aged 12–20†)
- Illicit drug use: 13.6 million
- Inhalant use: 3 million
- Marijuana use: 10 million
- Tobacco use: 60 million (4.1 million are youths aged 12–17‡)
- Cigar use: 2 million (age 12 and older)

*Annual survey conducted by Substance Abuse and Mental health Services Administration. An estimated 4.1 million people met the diagnostic criteria for dependence on illicit drugs (including 1.1 million youths ages 12–17).

†33 million are binge drinkers (>5 on any one occasion); 5.1 million youths engaged in binge drinking; 12 million are heavy drinkers (>5 drinks on >5 days/month); 2.3 million youths may be classified as heavy drinkers.

‡Youths (ages 12–17) currently smoking cigarettes are significantly more likely to use illicit drugs and drink heavily than nonsmoking youths.

The three components of drug addiction are psychological dependence, physical dependence, and tolerance. Psychological dependence, thought by some experts to be the most important factor in addiction, involves the compulsive use of and craving for a drug. This chapter discusses various factors involved in substance abuse, several commonly abused drug categories and how they affect the body, and nursing management of substance-abusing patients.

CAUSES OF SUBSTANCE ABUSE

DOPAMINE HYPOTHESIS

Scientists are becoming increasingly convinced that there is a link between the neurotransmitter dopamine and drugs of abuse, and that dopamine plays a key role in a wide range of addictions. Research studies have demonstrated that in dopamine-rich areas of the brain, nicotine behaves in a manner remarkably similar to that of cocaine; the surge of dopamine in an addict's brain essentially triggers a cocaine high. Brain imaging technology can track the increase of dopamine and link it to feelings of euphoria. Dopamine is associated with feelings of pleasure and elation. Dopamine levels can be elevated by a hug or kiss, a word of praise, a winning poker hand, or the effects of a drug. This dopamine hypothesis—although controversial and incomplete—gives way to the recognition that there may be a clear biologic basis for drug dependence; addiction may be a disorder of the brain no different from other forms of mental illness.

The major drugs of abuse mimic the structure of neurotransmitters. Neurotransmitters serve as a basis for every thought and emotion, for memory, and for learning; they carry the signals between all the neurons (nerve cells) in the brain. At a purely chemical level, every enjoyable experience amounts to an explosion of dopamine in the brain.

Several other factors play a role in determining why some people abuse substances (see the accompanying display, Who's at Risk for Substance Abuse?). These include physiologic, genetic, developmental, and environmental factors.

Who's at Risk for Substance Abuse?

- Individuals with chronic pain (e.g., back, joint, musculoskeletal disorders) who may occasionally misuse or abuse their prescribed drugs (Fauci, et al., 1999)
- Teenagers—especially if they are dealing with self-esteem issues
- The socioeconomically disadvantaged—may be desperate to "escape their world" selling and using drugs to survive
- Health care professionals (e.g., physicians, nurses, pharmacists) who have easy access to drugs and may begin using drugs or substances to promote sleep or arousal, decrease physical discomfort, and manage stress and anxiety
- Individuals with a family history of substance abuse, including alcoholism
- Individuals with a history of child abuse or sexual assault

PHYSIOLOGY

The physiologic effects of drugs with a high potential for abuse (e.g., narcotics) involve the body's adaptation to the toxic effects of the drugs at the biochemical and cellular level. Four physiologic changes characterize this process: tolerance, tissue dependence, withdrawal, and psychological dependence.

With drug use over time, tolerance develops. **Tolerance** occurs when the body develops a natural resistance to the drug's physical or euphoric effects, making it necessary to take increasing doses more frequently to achieve the desired effect. The actual changes in liver cells, which occur as a result of drug use, help the body to metabolize drugs more rapidly.

Tissue dependence occurs when actual changes in body cells, secondary to the physical dependency (tolerance), cause the body to "need" the drug for homeostasis. Withdrawal will occur when the drug is stopped. Dependency alone does not define addiction. A patient may be physically dependent on a drug without showing behavior patterns associated with addiction.

Abstinence syndrome, typically called withdrawal, develops when excessive drug use is stopped or interrupted. This interruption results in physical signs and symptoms of withdrawal as the body tries to return to "normal." Caffeine-withdrawal headache, heroin-withdrawal myalgia and diaphoresis, and barbiturate-withdrawal seizures are examples of abstinence syndrome. **Psychological dependence** (craving) results from the direct influence of drugs on brain chemistry. The drug causes an altered state of consciousness and distorted perceptions that are pleasurable and satisfying to the user. The recollection of these pleasurable feelings, along with the physiologic changes due to tolerance and the fear of withdrawal symptoms, reinforce continued use of the drug.

GENETICS

Genetic factors also play an important role in drug dependence, and this genetic vulnerability varies. For example, certain genes may predispose an individual to or protect the person from alcoholism.

Several studies emphasize the effects of heredity and maintain that the disease of addiction—a chronic, progressive, recurrent, incurable, and potentially fatal condition—is a consequence of genetic deficiencies in brain tissues or neurotransmitters. For example, a vast body of evidence from studies of alcoholism suggests that genetic factors are more influential than environmental factors and that alcoholism is a multifactorial disorder in which biologic and genetic factors interact. These conclusions are supported by animal research (breeding of "alcoholic" rats) and studies of twins (alcohol metabolism, alcohol drinking patterns, each twin's response to alcohol), and studies of adoptees whose biologic parents suffered from alcoholism (Fauci, Braunwald, Wilson, Martin, Hanser, Long, et al., 1999).

DEVELOPMENT AND ENVIRONMENT

Developmental and environmental influences can trigger changes in brain hormones. For example, chronic stress can decrease brain levels of neurotransmitters, such as metenkephalin, dopamine, norepinephrine, and serotonin. Many sociologic studies suggest that physical or emotional stress caused by abuse, anger, peer pressure, and other environmental stressors causes individuals to seek and sustain use of mind-altering drugs, leading to drug dependence. Several kinds of developmental and environmental factors may influence a person's substance abuse, including personality traits, mood disorders, availability of drugs, cultural attitudes, and socioeconomic circumstances (e.g., affluence, boredom).

Personality Traits

No absolute addictive personality has been identified, and the ability to respond to stress and peer pressure varies among individuals. However, substance abusers are frequently described as having a low tolerance for frustration, being impulsive and manipulative, and experiencing fears of failure. Feelings of inadequacy, resentment, hostility, and anger are other common characteristic descriptions thought to predispose a person to substance abuse. People with one or several of these personality traits may use substances to escape from reality or to relieve emotional discomfort.

Mood Disorders

The literature and clinical findings provide evidence that mood disorders have a major impact on health status, quality of life, and likelihood of substance abuse. About 32% of all patients with mood disorders (e.g., depression and anxiety, dependent personality, antisocial personality) are substance dependent or substance abusers at some time in their lifetime (Fauci, et al., 1999).

Patients who have depression or anxiety and who cannot cope with life's daily pressures and problems may try to escape from a mental or physical environment perceived as anxiety ridden, bleak, and joyless. People with a dependency disorder are unable to face everyday experiences independently. Instead, they use something (e.g., other people, drugs, the sick role) to help them feel powerful and secure. Often, this behavior pattern becomes a vicious cycle. Larger or stronger amounts of drug may be needed to resolve the discomfort. People who have an antisocial personality may initially use substances to help them relate socially and to relieve their loneliness. The effects of alcohol and drugs provide the courage to be social and have fun.

Availability of Drugs and Drug Diversion

Availability of a drug is a significant factor in developing and maintaining abuse. Drugs are readily available in hospitals and clinics, which helps explain, in part, the unusually high incidence of drug abuse in health care providers, nurses, and pharmacists (see the accompanying display, Considering Substance Abuse Among Professionals).

Diversion of prescription drugs (and prescription drug abuse) is relatively small compared to the overall drug abuse problem nationwide. Regardless, the Drug Enforcement Administration (DEA) estimates that drug diversion is a $25 billion-a-year industry. There are two types of diverting individuals: the "doctor shopper," who is often well educated, well dressed, and convincing, and the chemically dependent patient. They visit different health care practitioners, emergency departments, 24-hour clinics, urgent care centers, or pharmacies and presents with various subjective problems (e.g., cannot be measured by laboratory test or radiograph) that are usually treated with a controlled substance. A doctor shopper can earn a living by obtaining controlled substances and selling them on the street, usually keeping a supply for personal use. The chemically dependent patients are less likely to sell drugs on the street; they are compulsive users of controlled substances and will often hoard a supply for fear of running out and experiencing withdrawal.

The most commonly diverted prescription medications are scheduled controlled substances/stimulants (e.g., methylphenidate, phentermine), narcotic analgesics (e.g., hydrocodone products) and depressants (benzodiazepines). Cariso- prodol (a centrally acting muscle relaxant) is the most abused, nonscheduled drug in the United States. Carisprodol is metabolized to meprobamate—a C-IV antianxiety agent, and several states have scheduled carisprodol as a C-IV narcotic (Weathermon, 1999). Illicit uses of carisprodol include taking it with diphenhydramine, hydrocodone, or methadone; the combination of these drugs produces a heroin-type high.

Cimetidine is readily available because of its over-the-counter (OTC) status and is involved with drug diversion. Cimetidine is available by itself as an antacid. Cimetidine, through an effect on several microtonal enzyme systems, reduces hepatic drug metabolism thereby delaying elimination and increasing the bioavailability of abused drugs. Cimetidine taken prior to using crack, methadone, or alcohol will achieve a stronger or prolonged response.

Clonidine is a drug used to treat alcohol and opioid withdrawal symptoms. The abuser will take clonidine as a means to get through the shakiness associated with withdrawal until the next dose of abused drug can be obtained.

Critical Thinking Scenario

Considering substance abuse among professionals

As a nursing student, you may become aware of health care professionals who jeopardize their careers and their patients' safety by using drugs inappropriately. Propose some reasons why you think this may happen.

Cultural Attitudes

Culture plays a complex role in the development of drug use and abuse. A corresponding change in rates of substance abuse rapidly develops when people move from one culture to another (Coleman, 1993). Four attitudes have been identified and described as having an influential effect on substance use:

1. Complete abstinence (e.g., Church of Jesus Christ of the Latter Day Saints [Mormon], Muslim cultures)
2. Ritualistic or ceremonial use (e.g., African, South American cultures)
3. Sociable/convivial use (e.g., French, Italian, Mediterranean cultures) in which substance use is closely tied to social situations
4. Functional/utilitarian use (e.g., Holland, United States) in which society allows people to use substances according to their own personal needs

Socioeconomic Circumstances

The lure of easy money has made drug abuse a major problem in many cities and towns across the United States. Some individuals may use or traffic drugs to escape harsh surroundings of poverty and illiteracy and change the perception of reality. Those who are not economically disadvantaged may use psychoactive drugs as a form of recreation and relaxation or for a variety of other reasons (e.g., to alter a mood, explore feelings, promote social interaction, escape boredom, stimulate creativity, improve physical performance, or enhance the senses).

SUBSTANCE ABUSE AND THE CENTRAL NERVOUS SYSTEM

Virtually all abused drugs have some effect on the central nervous system (CNS) and, with continued use, result in a physiologic or a psychological dependence otherwise known as **habituation** and addiction. However, used with medical supervision, many drugs that affect the CNS have a therapeutic influence. These drugs are invaluable therapeutically because of the very specific physiologic and behavioral changes that result. Drugs selectively affecting the CNS may be used for analgesic, anticonvulsant, antipyretic, antiemetic, or anorectic purposes or to suppress movement disorders. These drugs can also be used without altering consciousness to treat mood (anxiety, depression, mania) and thought (schizophrenia) disorders. Socially acceptable stimulants (amphetamines), depressants (alcohol), and anxiolytics (benzodiazepines) that produce stability, relief, and pleasure illustrate the nonmedical, self-use of CNS drugs.

The excessive use of these drugs, however, can have adverse effects when their use leads to dependence. In combination with alcohol, additive pharmacologic effects may occur after administration of all antihistamines, anxiolytics, CNS depressants, and narcotics. Commonly abused drugs that affect the CNS are classified into three main categories:

1. CNS stimulants (**psychoactive** drugs)
2. CNS depressants
3. Hallucinogens (**psychedelic** drugs).

A miscellaneous category of abused substances includes inhalants (e.g., airplane or model glue, gasoline, nitrous oxide), designer drugs (e.g., analogues of fentanyl), antipsychotic drugs (e.g., lithium), anabolic or androgenic steroids (e.g., testosterone analogues), and over-the-counter (OTC) drugs containing caffeine and phenylpropanolamine (e.g., diet pills, antihistamines). For a visual depiction of selected drugs of abuse, see Figure 10-1.

CNS STIMULANTS

The most commonly abused CNS stimulants include cocaine and the amphetamines. These CNS stimulants initially increase heart rate and blood pressure. The more potent stimulants energize muscles, decrease appetite, cause some degree of mental and physical alertness, give a feeling of self-confidence, and induce some degree of euphoria. Psychoactive drugs (particularly cocaine and methamphetamine) affect nerve impulses by disrupting the normal functioning of stimulatory neurotransmitters—dopamine, norepinephrine, and serotonin. The body responds to more frequent and higher doses of the drug by releasing smaller quantities of these neurotransmitters. Excess amounts can cause insomnia, hypertension, and cardiovascular problems—especially if the individual has a sensitivity to the drug. Intoxication with amphetamines, cocaine, hallucinogens, and marijuana may cause panic attacks. Prolonged use may lead to anxiety, confusion, dependency, depression, exhaustion, anhedonia (inability to experience normal pleasure), irritability, paranoia, and violence as the neurotransmitters are depleted. Synthesis of the depleted neurotransmitters may take months to occur after chronic, heavy use.

The CNS stimulants have a wide range of effects that increase their potential for abuse. Caffeine, nicotine, amphetamines, and cocaine increase alertness and energy, lessen drowsiness and fatigue, increase concentration and thinking, alleviate moodiness, and impart a "high" or happy feeling. All stimulant drugs pose a risk for both physical and psychological dependence.

Caffeine is categorized as a mild CNS stimulant. It is found in coffee, tea, cocoa, colas and other soft drinks, and in chocolate. It is also found in many OTC products, such as analgesics and weight control products.

Nicotine is the drug in tobacco products (cigarettes, cigars, pipe tobacco, snuff), and it is highly addictive. Tobacco use is the principal cause of preventable morbidity, disability, and premature death in the United States. Nicotine gum and transdermal patches are available by prescription or OTC to facilitate withdrawal.

Amphetamines (amphetamine sulfate, dextroamphetamine, and methamphetamine) are anorexiants used medically in short-term use for treating obesity, narcolepsy (a chronic disorder characterized by recurrent attacks of drowsiness and sleep during daytime), and attention deficit hyperactivity disorder (ADHD). These drugs may be taken by some individuals (e.g., health care professionals and others) to increase alertness and decrease fatigue. This type of use is dangerous but not always labeled abusive. Drug abusers typically take

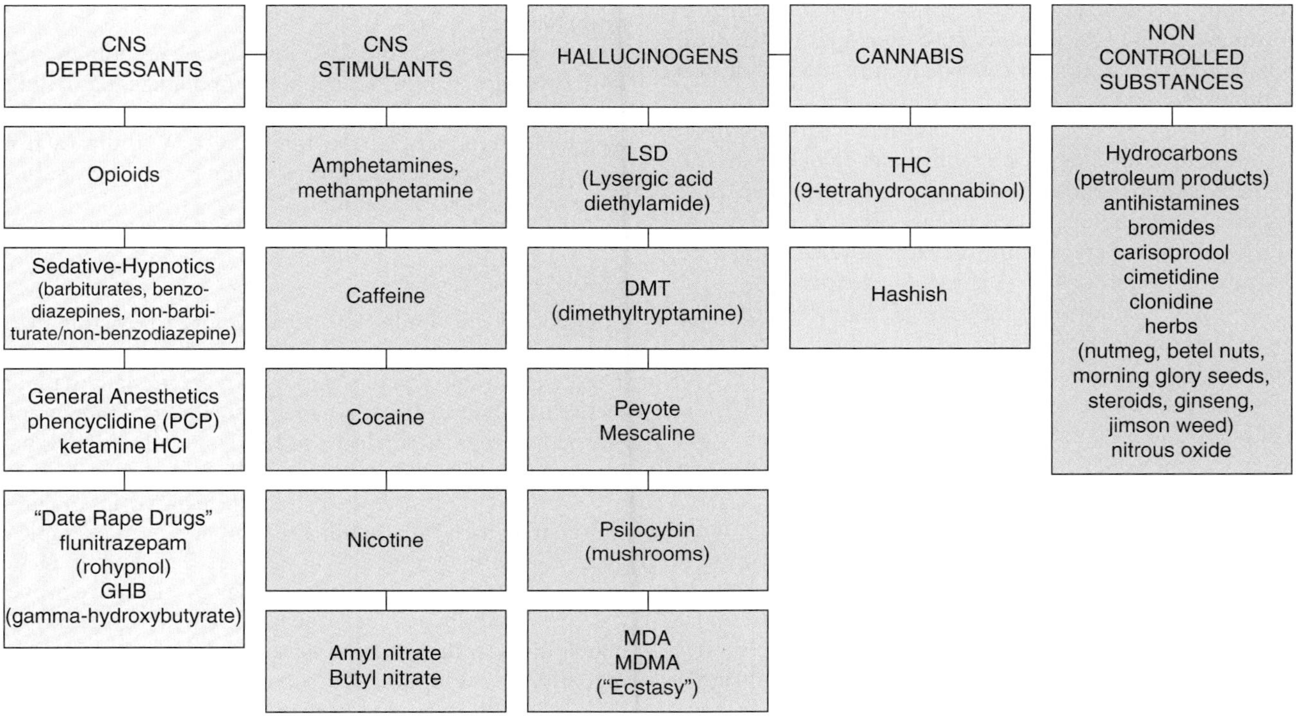

Figure 10-1. Selected drugs of abuse.

large oral doses or inject amphetamine—known as "speed"—for an intense rush effect that lasts only a short time. A recent study demonstrated that abnormal brain chemistry associated with methamphetamine abuse is evident months after the drug abuse has stopped. Brain scans showed a reduction of *N*-acetyl-aspartate compounds in the basal ganglia. Reduced *N*-acetyl-aspartate levels are associated with a variety of diseases, including dementias, epilepsy, multiple sclerosis, brain tumors, and cerebral infarction. The researchers noted that methamphetamine apparently does not cause neurotoxicity when given in low doses to children with ADHD.

Cocaine, another popular drug of abuse, produces a powerful but short-acting effect. Cocaine is not only psychologically addicting, it is also physically addicting because of its effect on neurotransmitters. The life-controlling effect of cocaine can lead an addict to exclusion of all other aspects of existence. A cocaine habit can cost an addict thousands of dollars a week to maintain.

Inhalants such as the aromatic hydrocarbons (i.e., paint thinner, lighter fluid, glue) produce an excitatory effect when inhaled.

As a general rule, withdrawal symptoms are not as dangerous with the stimulants as they are with the sedative-hypnotic drugs. The symptoms, which occur within 24 hours and can last up to a week or more, cause fatigue, severe depression, and occasionally seizures.

CNS DEPRESSANTS

Small doses of CNS depressants decrease heart rate, respiration, and reaction time, although initially they induce some euphoria. They relax the muscles, suppress physical and mental pain, diminish inhibitions, and promote sedation. CNS depressants, such as the opioids, can also decrease muscular coordination and energy and cause constipation, depression, nausea, vomiting, physical dependence, and withdrawal symptoms if used to excess.

Commonly abused CNS depressants include sedative-hypnotics, the most common of which are alcohol, barbiturates, and benzodiazepines. Sedative-hypnotic drugs can cause physical and psychological dependence. Regular use of these drugs over a long period leads to drug tolerance and a need for larger and larger doses to achieve the desired effect.

Alcohol is the number one drug problem in America. Because of its complex nature, alcoholism is difficult to define. Generally, individuals are considered alcoholics if their lifestyle is dominated by the acquisition and consumption of alcoholic beverages and when this behavior interferes adversely with personal, professional, social or family responsibilities and relationships.

Barbiturates, once the mainstay of sedative-hypnotic drugs, are also used as anesthetics and anticonvulsants. Many barbiturates are short-acting drugs, which helps explain the problem with abuse, that is, the person needs to use more drug to sustain the desired effect. Examples of barbiturates used habitually include pentobarbital, secobarbital, and amobarbital. Methaqualone has been withdrawn from the market and is no longer legally manufactured.

Benzodiazepines, which were initially developed as an alternative to the highly dependency-producing barbiturates, are longer-acting drugs. However, they still are characterized by a physical and psychological dependence if taken regularly over a prolonged period. Benzodiazepines, which are used primarily to relieve anxiety and to provide a hypnotic, or sedative, effect, are widely prescribed and therefore readily available. Some common benzodiazepines used habitually are diazepam, alprazolam, clorazepate, and lorazepam.

Abrupt withdrawal from sedative-hypnotic drugs (i.e., going "cold turkey") should never be attempted, because withdrawal symptoms are serious and potentially fatal. Withdrawal symptoms include agitation, dysphoria, insomnia, vomiting, diarrhea, ataxia, hallucinations, acute psychosis, muscle and abdominal cramps, anorexia, and seizures. These symptoms may occur 12 to 72 hours after the last use of the drug and may last up to 14 days. Withdrawal from alcohol, opioids, and sedative hypnotics can also induce panic symptoms and panic attacks.

OPIOIDS

Opioids (also known as narcotic analgesics) are commonly used medically to relieve pain, suppress coughing, enhance anesthetic effect for surgery, and relieve severe diarrhea. These narcotic drugs have a high potential for abuse and are extremely addicting both physically and psychologically. Frequently used and abused opioids include heroin, opium (paregoric), morphine, meperidine (Demerol), codeine, pentazocine (Talwin), and propoxyphene (Darvon). Administered orally, heroin and morphine undergo first-pass metabolism and have only one third to one sixth the effect of heroin or morphine administered parenterally. Therefore, abusers of these drugs usually administer them by injection or inhalation.

All opioids affect the CNS and cause cerebral changes, mood changes, confusion, euphoria, and analgesia. Regular use of narcotics over an extended time (several weeks) usually results in tolerance to the drug's effects. Withdrawal from narcotic use produces symptoms within 8 to 12 hours; these symptoms can remain for up to 10 days.

DESIGNER DRUGS

These drugs are similar in their structure to existing drugs and are developed with relative ease in illegal laboratories. They are extremely potent and used recreationally with addictive capabilities greater than existing drugs. For example, alpha, 3-methyl fentanyl (the street version of fentanyl) may be represented as "China White" (heroin) and is 35 times more potent than heroin. Fentanyl, a narcotic analgesic legitimately used during and after surgery, is an example of an existing drug "designed" into others. These analogues of existing substances, which offer similar psychoactive properties, are primarily designed to bypass federal regulation and control due to their different chemical formulations. Two meperidine analogues that have appeared on the street include MPPP (1-methyl-4-phenyl-4-propionoxypiperidine and PEPAP (1-[2-phenylethyl]-4-acetyloxypiperidine). They are often marketed as "new heroin." MPPP is popular among drug abusers because when it is injected, it produces a euphoria similar to that produced by heroin. An impurity formed during the illicit manufacture of MPPP, called MPTP (1-methyl-4-phenyl-1,2,3,6-tetrahydro-pyridine), destroys brain cells and much of the voluntary muscular movement. MPTP produces a crippling condition that closely resembles Parkinson disease.

TRANQUILIZERS

Certain tranquilizing drugs, known as "date rape" drugs, have made headlines. They are Rohypnol ("roofies") and gamma-hydroxybutyrate (GHB, "liquid X"). Rohypnol is the trade name for flunitrazepam—a sedative-hypnotic benzodiazepine that produces muscle relaxation and amnesia, as well. Rohypnol is not approved for use in the United States. These drugs are odorless and nearly tasteless and can easily be slipped into a beverage. They quickly depress the CNS and respiratory systems, especially when mixed with alcohol. The resulting hypoxemia triggers loss of consciousness and memory. There is a very narrow margin between GHB's anesthetic dose and lethal dose. GHB's popularity stems from its ease of manufacture (e.g., home chemistry kits and instructions on the Internet). Because of concern about Rohypnol, GHB, and other similarly abused sedative-hypnotics, Congress passed the Drug-Induced Rape Prevention and Punishment Act of 1996 in October, 1996. This legislation increased Federal penalties for use of any controlled substance to aid in sexual assault.

HALLUCINOGENS

Hallucinogenic drugs have pronounced mental and emotional effects because they distort the way the brain interprets sensory information. They can also mimic certain mental illnesses (e.g., thought disorders, schizophrenia). Included in this category are the naturally occurring substances (marijuana, mescaline, and psilocybin) and the synthetic substances (lysergic acid diethylamide [LSD], dimethyltryptamine, and phencyclidine hydrochloride [PCP]). Psychedelic drugs are, with the exception of marijuana, not used medically. Psychedelics do not cause physical dependence, and only marijuana has been shown to produce psychological dependence.

Relatively new amphetamine-derivative drugs with special stimulatory effects on the brain are termed hallucinogenic amphetamines (e.g., 3,4-methylenedioxymethamphetamine [MDMA], "ecstasy"). These drugs can be inhaled, injected, or swallowed. They cause a long-lasting reduction in the brain's supply of serotonin and produce powerful psychic changes.

Another drug, ketamine, an anesthetic used in animals, replaced PCP as an anesthetic for use in humans. It produces some emergent hallucinogenic effects (hallucinations and sensory distortion) that immobilize and detach the user from reality. Ketamine does not depress the circulatory or respiratory systems. Its effects are equivalent to those of being severely inebriated.

ANABOLIC-ANDROGENIC STEROIDS

These drugs are synthetic formulations of the male hormone testosterone. The abuse of these drugs in men and women to increase strength and enhance athletic performance is widespread. Anabolic-androgenic steroids (AAS) also have a dramatic effect on emotions and make the user feel more confident and aggressive. Continued use of AAS may lead to emotional instability, rage, depression, or psychosis. A number of athletic organizations have banned these substances. Serious health problems are associated with both short- and long-term use of AAS. These problems include sex hormone imbalances (i.e., amenorrhea, erectile dysfunction), changes in secondary sexual characteristics (i.e., gynecomastia, hypomastia, testicular atrophy, ovarian atrophy), permanent sterility, hepatic cancer, and myocardial infarction.

COMMONLY ABUSED DRUGS

Of the most commonly abused drugs, alcohol, cocaine, heroin, and marijuana appear to receive the most publicity and are among the most dramatic abuse situations encountered in clinical practice.

The drugs discussed in this chapter are commonly abused drugs that have little, if any, therapeutic medical use. The drugs discussed in this section are not legal, with the exception of alcohol and, in some instances, marijuana.

NURSING MANAGEMENT IN COMMONLY ABUSED DRUGS

The nurse's role in substance abuse involves understanding of core knowledge related to specific drugs, prevention, assessment of potential or actual abuse, and formulation of nursing diagnoses related to the assessment findings. Once the nurse has gathered the data and created nursing diagnoses, outcome criteria can be identified and interventions implemented. Finally, the nurse should evaluate whether the outcome criteria have been met and what further work with the patient is needed.

Core Drug Knowledge in Alcohol Abuse

Pharmacokinetics

Alcohol, known clinically as ethanol (ETOH), does not require digestion before absorption. It is completely absorbed by the stomach and small intestine within 2 hours after ingestion. However, food in the stomach decreases the effects of alcohol, delays gastric emptying time, and retards absorption from the small intestine. Once in systemic circulation, alcohol is immediately distributed to the rest of the body at a rate proportional to blood flow and water content. Consequently, high concentrations in the brain, liver, lung, and kidney develop rapidly. After completion of absorption, brain and blood alcohol levels are very similar.

The liver metabolizes alcohol by two different pathways—using the enzyme alcohol dehydrogenase and the microsomal ethanol oxidizing system (MEOS). In the average adult, 90% to 98% of an ingested dose of alcohol is converted to acetaldehyde by alcohol dehydrogenase. This is then oxidized to acetate by aldehyde dehydrogenase. The acetate is finally oxidized in the liver to carbon dioxide and water. These actions primarily take place in the cytoplasm and mitochondria of the hepatocyte. The remaining 2% to 10% is excreted unchanged in the urine and expired air. The average rate of metabolism of alcohol by nontolerant individuals is 100 mg/kg of body weight per hour (or 7 g per hour in a person who weighs 70 kg).

People with chronic alcoholism metabolize alcohol by way of the MEOS, which occurs primarily in the endoplasmic reticulum. Metabolism of ethanol by this pathway produces an end product of acetaldehyde and free radicals, both of which damage liver cells. Metabolism by this pathway is also dangerous because cytochrome P-450, an enzyme that is integral to the pathway, is required by the liver to transform toxins, drugs, and excess fat-soluble vitamins. If P-450 is being used to metabolize alcohol, it cannot perform its other tasks. The result is susceptibility to organ damage from other toxins, drugs, and vitamins. Alcohol is excreted in urine by the kidneys, in the breath by the respiratory system, and in sweat by the skin.

Pharmacodynamics

Alcohol affects many body systems (see the accompanying display, Health Problems Related to Alcohol and Other Substances). Alcohol is thought to interfere with the transmission of nerve impulses at synaptic junctions, although this exact mechanism is unclear. It is similar in action to that of general anesthetics and probably exerts its action on the brain by dissolving in neuronal plasma membranes rather than by acting on a specific receptor.

Like the general anesthetics, alcohol sequentially depresses the CNS (i.e., the cerebrum, cerebellum, spinal cord, medulla). However, the excitatory stage of alcohol is longer, and the anesthetic stage is equivalent to toxicity. There is a very narrow therapeutic margin between alcohol's anesthetic dose and lethal dose.

Adverse Effects

Alcohol depresses the CNS. However, the depressant effects may appear to be stimulatory because alcohol depresses the higher centers of the brain, causing individuals to shed behavioral and social inhibitions. The degree of depression produced is directly proportional to the quantity of alcohol consumed (Table 10-1).

Awareness of these two effects may depend on the excitability of the CNS at the time of drug administration, which is influenced by the environmental setting in which the drug is used and the personality of the user. For example, in a quiet, nonsocial environment, the excitatory influence may be impaired, and the drug's CNS depressant effects of sedation and drowsiness dominate. In a social setting, where there is increased sensory input, the effects of low doses of alcohol may be perceived as stimulation because the drinker may demonstrate talkativeness, increased self-confidence, and a release of usual inhibitions.

Alcohol impairs muscular coordination. It increases the heart rate and dilates the blood vessels, causing body heat loss and, in low doses, lowers the blood pressure, which is thought to reduce the risk of myocardial infarction in patients with higher levels of high-density lipoproteins. With large doses of alcohol, however, dangerous levels of cardiovascular depression can occur. Prolonged alcohol use causes hypertension and cardiovascular damage (i.e., alcoholic cardiomyopathy).

Alcohol irritates the gastrointestinal (GI) tract by causing an increase in digestive enzymes. Ulceration of the gastric mucosa is a serious complication of excessive alcohol consumption. Alcohol also causes altered bowel function (constipation or diarrhea). The risk of developing alcoholic liver disease is related to the quantity

Health Problems Related to Alcohol and Other Substances

Abscess at injection site*
Amenorrhea
Bacterial endocarditis*
Cardiac arrhythmias and cardiomyopathy†
Cancers of the upper GI tract, liver†
Cellulitis
Cirrhosis of the liver†
Constipation
Dental caries; tooth loss
Fluid and electrolyte imbalances
Gastritis and GI bleeding†
Hepatic dysfunction and hepatitis*
HIV and AIDS*
Impotence†
Malnutrition and vitamin deficiencies
Increased incidence of peptic ulcer disease†
Overdosage*
Pancreatitis†
Peripheral neuritis
Pneumonia* and other respiratory infections
Pregnancy complications and neonatal drug dependency*
Pulmonary embolism (PE) and septic PE*
Seizures
Skin abscesses
Tetanus*
Thrombophlebitis*
Tuberculosis*
Wernicke-Korsakoff syndrome†

*Most likely associated with opioid abuse
†Most likely associated with alcohol abuse

TABLE 10-1 Blood Alcohol Levels and Stages of Intoxication

Blood Alcohol Level (mg/dL)	Physical and Behavioral Effects
<50	Body sway, euphoria, excitement, impaired judgment, incoordination, increased sociability, loss of inhibitions
50–100	Disturbed gait, impaired ability to operate machinery (e.g., motor vehicles), increased reaction time, increasingly impaired judgment, distractibility, slurred speech
100–140	Ataxia, increasingly impaired mental and motor skills, impaired short-term memory
140–200	Inability to operate a motor vehicle, staggering gait
200–300	Blackouts; in combination with other CNS depressants, death secondary to additive effects
>300	Severe respiratory and cardiovascular depression, coma, death

and duration of alcohol consumption. Excessive alcohol consumption causes fatty deposits in the liver. This can damage and scar the liver (cirrhosis) and lead to complications, such as ascites, esophageal varices, and portal hypertension. Excess alcohol consumption inhibits antidiuretic hormone and therefore increases urine production. Finally, alcohol disrupts endocrine functions, causing alterations and fluctuations in blood glucose, catecholamine, and aldosterone levels. Alcoholics are frequently immunologically compromised with an increased risk for mortality resulting from cancers of the upper GI tract and liver.

Drug Interactions

Alcohol has no nutritional value, and it interferes with the absorption of vitamins and minerals. Alcohol can affect iron absorption, folate activities, and platelets. These harmful effects can result in a variety of anemias. See Table 10-2 for more information regarding drug interactions with alcohol.

Core Drug Knowledge in Cocaine Abuse

Cocaine is derived from the leaves of *Erythroxylon coca*. It is available in two forms: crystalline cocaine hydrochloride and highly purified cocaine alkaloid. Cocaine hydrochloride is usually administered orally, IV, or by nasal insufflation because it is water soluble and unstable when exposed to heat. The alkaloid form of cocaine—called "crack" because of the popping sound it makes when the crystals are heated—is stable on exposure to heat but is water insoluble so it is usually administered by smoking (inhalation). On the street, pure cocaine is diluted or "cut" with other substances to increase its quantity and thereby increase profits to the sellers.

Freebasing consists of converting the cocaine alkaloid to a freebase rock form using a solvent (e.g., diethyl ether). This rock is then heated, and the fumes are inhaled. Potentially dangerous because the fumes are potent and diethyl ether is flammable, many users report being hooked after only one use. Treatment for cocaine addiction is difficult because of the high physical and psychological dependence associated with its use.

Pharmacokinetics

Cocaine is rapidly absorbed into the bloodstream regardless whether it is snorted, inhaled, or injected. Cocaine has a 1- to 2-minute onset of action and a 30-minute duration of action after smoking or IV injection; peak effects after inhaling cocaine occur in 30 to 60 minutes with a duration of action of several hours. There is only a 30% to 40% bioavailability after oral administration, and GI absorption may continue for several hours. Orally administered cocaine has a slower onset of action, approximately 1 hour.

Cocaine is extensively metabolized in the liver and the blood. Metabolites may be detected in the urine for 2 or more days. Because cocaine is so rapidly metabolized in the liver, the user must inhale, inject, or smoke the drug approximately every 30 minutes to maintain the high. Cocaine is characterized by tachyphylaxis (rapid appearance of a progressive decrease in response following repetitive administration); thus, its psychoactive effects rapidly diminish despite its continued presence in the plasma.

The elimination half-life for cocaine is similar for all forms of administration–about 50 minutes for the oral route, 80 minutes for the intranasal route, and 60 minutes for the IV route.

Pharmacodynamics

Cocaine has pronounced effects on the CNS and peripheral nervous systems. It impairs the uptake of norepinephrine and epinephrine by presynaptic nerve endings, thus activating the adrenergic systems and causing hypertension, tachycardia, and vasoconstriction. Cocaine interferes with serotonin uptake, causing dramatic alterations in the sleep-wake cycle and

TABLE 10-2 Agents That Interact With Alcohol

Interactants	Effect and Significance	Nursing Management
Analgesics (e.g., aspirin)	Combination may cause severe stomach irritation	Monitor for upper or lower GI bleeding.
Anesthetics*	Potentiation of the anesthetic effect	Observe during patient's recovery from anesthetic effects. Recovery may be prolonged.
Anticoagulants	Potentiation of the anticoagulant effect, leading to possible hemorrhage	Observe for signs of bleeding: bruising, black tarry stools.
Anticonvulsants	Accelerated anticonvulsant drug metabolism	Monitor for poor seizure control. Also monitor for seizures and provide for patient safety.
Antidiabetics, hypoglycemics	Unpredictable; rise or fall of blood glucose level	Monitor blood glucose levels regularly.
Antihistamines	Additive sedative effects; increased incidence of accidents due to drowsiness and increased response time	Caution patient that drinking and driving do not mix.
Antihypertensives	Additive hypotensive effects	Monitor blood pressure. Explain strategies for coping with orthostatic hypotension.
Antipsychotics* (e.g., phenothiazines)	Significant respiratory depression	Monitor breathing. Provide respiratory assistance if needed.
Barbiturates	Significant synergistic effects with alcohol	Monitor for severe respiratory depression.
Diuretics	Significant increased hypotensive effects due to antidiuretic hormone and diuresis	Monitor fluid and electrolyte levels. Caution patient about orthostatic hypotension.
Narcotics*	Synergistic, intensified CNS depressant effects	Provide respiratory support if significant respiratory depression occurs.
Sedative-hypnotics*	Additive effects; adverse effects on alertness and performance	Caution patient that sedative drugs and alcohol should not be consumed together.
Vitamins	Continuous alcohol use interferes with vitamin absorption and synthesis	Monitor for nutritional deficiencies (thiamine, folate, B_{12}) and paresthesias.

*These are potentially hazardous when ingested by a heavy drinker, patient with long-term alcoholism, or patient recovering from alcoholism.

feelings of intense energy. It also impairs dopamine reuptake, thus activating the dopaminergic system and causing euphoria as well as the strong reinforcing properties of the drug. With long-term use, dopamine becomes progressively depleted from nerve endings, causing the dysphoria that is so prominent during withdrawal. This frequently leads to drug craving and the very high rate of relapse. Cocaine also interferes with sodium ion activity in peripheral nerves causing local anesthetic actions.

Adverse Effects

Adverse reactions to cocaine include:

- CNS stimulation, including severe agitation, anxiety, excitement, paranoid psychosis
- Cardiovascular effects, including atrioventricular arrhythmias, severe hypertension, cardiomyopathy, coronary/peripheral vasoconstriction, myocardial infarction, intestinal/renal ischemia
- Pulmonary complications, including pneumothorax, pulmonary edema, respiratory arrest
- Metabolic complications, including disseminated intravascular coagulation, hepatotoxicity, hyperthermia, renal failure, rhabdomyolysis
- Complications of nasal inhalation, including anosmia, nasal mucosal atrophy, nasal septal necrosis, rhinorrhea

High doses of pure cocaine in freebase form (crack) can overtax the cardiovascular system and cause sudden death from acute myocardial infarction or rupture of the aorta. Cocaine sensitizes cardiac cells and causes an increase in contractility. Corresponding high levels of epinephrine secondary to excitement from cocaine cause the individual to be particularly susceptible to cardiac arrest.

Core Drug Knowledge in Opioid Abuse

Heroin is a synthetically manufactured opioid that possesses morphine-like pharmacologic activity. Heroin is the most abused opioid in the United States (Kinney, 1996). Heroin has a poor oral availability. Abusers often begin by smoking or subcutaneously injecting the drug. Eventually they resort to administration by IV injection. Pure heroin is very expensive and dangerously powerful. For these reasons, street heroin is usually mixed with fillers, such as sugars, starches, or quinine. The mixed substance contains only 1% to 10% heroin.

Pharmacokinetics

The rate of heroin's absorption by the bloodstream depends on the method of administration. Absorption increases in speed from oral use to IV injection. Typically, effects are felt within about 30 minutes after oral administration and with a range of 5 to 15 minutes after smoking or injecting. Depending on the dose, the effects of injected heroin persist approximately 4 to 6 hours. Most heroin is converted to morphine and excreted by the kidneys. Insignificant quantities of unconverted heroin may be found in urine and feces.

Pharmacodynamics

Heroin acts on the body in a manner similar to that of other opioids. An intense rush follows IV administration of heroin. This rush subsides in a few minutes, and the effects resemble those following oral dosing. The abuser feels relaxed, carefree, somewhat dreamy, but able to carry on with many normal activities. Taking daily doses of heroin (at least 24 mg) usually results in a clinically significant dependence in a few weeks.

Adverse Effects

The pathophysiologic effects of heroin are also similar to those of the other opioids (see Chapter 24). However, the degree of some effects is greater. An overdose of heroin may result in severe respiratory depression, pulmonary edema, coma, and possibly death. Some pathophysiologic effects specific to IV heroin use include infections with human immunodeficiency virus or hepatitis from contaminated needles, toxic reactions to contaminants injected along with the heroin, vasculitis, and thromboembolic complications (see the accompanying display, Highs and Lows of Selected Substance Use, and Table 10-3.)

Core Drug Knowledge in Marijuana Abuse

The most commonly abused psychedelic drug is marijuana, which is derived from the hemp species, *Cannabis sativa*. Marijuana refers to the entire plant chopped and dried; the more potent hashish is the dried resinous exudate of the flowering tops.

The major ingredient of marijuana is 9-tetrahydrocannabinol (THC). The THC concentration in the average marijuana cigarette has significantly increased over the last 3 decades. A typical marijuana cigarette delivers a dose of THC ranging from 2.5 to 5 mg.

Pharmacotherapeutics

An oral form of marijuana, dronabinol, is now used in the United States to treat anorexia in AIDS patients and for reducing nausea and vomiting in cancer patients undergoing chemotherapy. Studies are ongoing related to its effectiveness in reducing intraocular pressure associated with glaucoma.

Highs and Lows of Selected Substance Use

The following signs and symptoms of intoxication and withdrawal can be used as a guide to assessing stages of substance use in patients with suspected or confirmed problems.

Signs and Symptoms of Alcohol Intoxication

Ataxia and nystagmus
Facial flushing and increased blood pressure
Mood swings and irritability
Slurred speech and sedation

Signs and Symptoms of Alcohol Withdrawal

Anxiety, hallucinations
Nausea and vomiting, tremors, seizures
Hyperthermia, diaphoresis
Labile blood pressure, tachycardia

Signs and Symptoms of Cocaine Intoxication

Elation and euphoria, grandiosity
Hypervigilance
Motor agitation, pupillary dilation
Tachycardia

Signs and Symptoms of Cocaine Withdrawal

Depression
Polyphagia
Fatigue, nightmares, sleep disturbance

Signs and Symptoms of Opioid Intoxication

Apathy, attention impairment, dysphoria
Euphoria
Motor retardation, sedation, slurred speech

Signs and Symptoms of Opioid Withdrawal

Fever, diaphoresis, myalgia, tremors
Diarrhea, lacrimation, rhinorrhea
Insomnia, mydriasis, piloerection, yawning

Signs and Symptoms of Inhalant Intoxication

Almost immediate euphoria and grandiosity, distorted perceptions, possible hallucinations, light-headedness

Pharmacokinetics

The systemic availability of THC after smoking is about 25%, with a peak plasma concentration occurring after 10 to 30 minutes. The duration of the entire effect is about 2 to 3 hours. The effectiveness of THC after oral ingestion is less than after smoking it: systemic availability is less (6% to 20%), onset of CNS effects is 30 to 60 minutes, peak plasma concentrations are reached within 2 to 3 hours, and the duration of effect is about 4 to 6 hours for psychoactive effects and more than 24 hours for appetite stimulant effects.

The THC is converted quite rapidly to a pharmacologically active metabolite, 11-hydroxy-9-THC. Further metabolism yields an inactive metabolite (11-nor-9-carboxy-9-THC), which is excreted in the urine. Plasma half-life of THC is approximately 13 days, and the urinary elimination half-life for 11-nor-9-carboxy-9-THC is approximately 10 days. The concentrations of these metabolites, however, do not correlate well with THC's clinical effects and are poor predictors of behavioral impairment or intoxication. The slow urinary elimination is an ideal marker for detecting marijuana use (Craig & Stitzel, 1994).

Pharmacodynamics

The mechanism of action of THC is unknown. However, antiemetic and other pharmacologic effects occur within minutes of use. THC produces minor psychic effects, such as an altered sense of time, a period of euphoria followed by sedation, less discriminate hearing, and enhanced visual stimuli.

Adverse Effects

Some of the adverse effects of THC include decreased myocardial oxygen supply, a dose-related increase in heart rate (20 to 50 bpm after one or two marijuana cigarettes), and impaired fertility. Cannabinoid receptors are concentrated most heavily in the cerebellum, the part of the brain that controls motor coordination, and in the hippocampus, which governs learning and memory. Large numbers are also found in the cerebral cortex, the seat of higher thinking, and lesser numbers are scattered in the immune system. They are largely absent from the brain-stem regions that govern heartbeat and respiration. At high levels of intake, a cannabis psychosis may occur, and regular heavy cannabis users may suffer repeated psychotic episodes and personality changes. Chronic use of THC appears to cause permanent brain damage as evidenced by loss of short-term memory, decreased motivation, impaired performance of simple and complex motor tasks, development of acute anxiety that may reach panic proportions, and severe psychological dependence.

Although smoking marijuana is often thought to be relatively safe compared with smoking tobacco, the smoke is virtually identical in both cases. Smoking marijuana involves inhaling larger volumes of smoke and holding the breath as much as four times longer than with tobacco, which ultimately makes smoking three to four marijuana joints a day equivalent to smoking 1 pack of tobacco cigarettes a day and a "possible causal role for marijuana in the pathogenesis of . . . bullous emphysema" (Johnson, 2000).

Tolerance to the effects of marijuana develops quite slowly. Evidence that marijuana is addictive has been obscured due partly to the fact that THC is readily stored in body fat and marijuana users who quit are often "weaned" off the drug slowly as small amounts continue to filter into the bloodstream. Several studies, however, have shown that there is a "flu-like" withdrawal syndrome from marijuana. The National Institute of Drug Abuse (which funds most of the marijuana research in the United States) estimates that 100,000 people seek treatment every year for marijuana dependency.

Core Drug Knowledge in Hallucinogen Abuse

Although often associated with the 1960s, LSD and PCP are still used. LSD is taken orally, and PCP can be taken orally, smoked, or injected. Tolerance develops with continued use of these drugs. However, psychological dependence is rare, and physical dependence does not occur. In addition, there is no specific withdrawal syndrome associated with these drugs. LSD and PCP have no accepted medical use and are classified as schedule I drugs.

Pharmacokinetics

The effects of LSD and PCP usually occur 30 to 90 minutes after ingestion or inhalation and can last between 8 and 12 hours. The effects depend on the amount taken, the user's personality, the user's mood and expectations, and the setting in which the drug is used.

PCP is rapidly metabolized in the liver to inactive metabolites. Larger doses of PCP may result in accumulation of large amounts of nonmetabolized PCP in the urine. PCP has a half-life of 30 minutes to 1 hour in small amounts, and 1 to 4 days in large doses.

Pharmacodynamics

The mechanism of action is unclear, although some experts think serotonin-antagonistic activity within the brain is responsible for its hallucinogenic properties. Alterations in sensory perception, distortions of size, body image distortions, and surreal feelings of separation of body parts are prominent features of LSD. Sensory input is also enhanced, which creates vivid visual illusions, hallucinations, and intensely colored visual images.

Adverse Effects

Subjective effects and mood changes are quite variable with LSD. A dream-like state with feelings of good humor, euphoria, relaxation, and a sense of wonderment may predominate. Conversely, "bad trips" may occur. These consist of dysphoria, nervousness, anxiety, disorientation, hallucinations, panic attacks, and a severe psychotic attack. LSD produces adrenergic effects, most notably, hypertension, hyperpnea, tachycardia, hyperthermia, pupillary dilation, and hyperreflexia. Diaphoresis, salivation, lacrimation, nausea, and vomiting may also occur.

Dopaminergic and anticholinergic effects on the body occur with PCP use. In addition, it shares some of the dysphoric properties of the opioids. After low doses, the user has a sense of thinking and acting swiftly. Moods may range from euphoria and a sense of "bouncing" to depression. Larger doses cause changes in mood that are quite unpredictable and labile. A sense of unreality

TABLE 10-3 Characteristics of Substance Abuse

Substance	Nystagmus	Pulse	Pupil Size/ Reaction	Possible Effects	Duration of Effects	Methods of Ingestion	Symptoms of Overdose
Alcohol	Possible if BA high	Possible increase	Near normal/slow	Bloodshot, watery eyes Alcohol breath odor Motor incoordination Slurred speech Elevated BP	Rapid absorption Metabolism: 0.2 BA reduction per hour	Oral	Coma Cold, clammy skin Rapid, weak pulse Respiratory depression
CNS depressants	Possible with high dose	Decrease	Near normal/slow	Similar to alcohol; odor absent Drowsiness	barbiturates: 1–16 h tranquilizers: 4–8 h chloral hydrate: 5–8 h	Oral Injected	Similar to alcohol
Narcotic analgesics (opioids)	None	Decrease	Constriction/very slight visible reaction	Ptosis Muscle relaxation Skin cool to touch Pruritus/itching Dry mouth Euphoria Constipation	heroin: 4–6 h demerol: 3–4 h codeine: 3–4 h propoxyphene: 6–12 h fentanyl: 5–21 min methadone: 22–25 h	Injected Oral Snorted Smoked	Shallow breathing Cold, clammy skin Rapid, weak pulse Respiratory depression Death
CNS stimulants (cocaine)	None	Increase	Dilation/slowed	Restlessness Talkativeness Hyperreflexia Dry mouth Body tremors Anorexia Paranoia	cocaine: 15–90 min (depends on ingestion method) methamphetamine: 4–8 h	Oral Smoked Snorted Injected	Agitation Paranoia Acute psychosis Seizures

Inhalants	Depends on substance	Increase	Depends on substance/near normal	Substance odor Confusion Reddened nasal passages Watery eyes Sneezing, coughing	Variable Depends on substance	Inhaled	Loss of consciousness Coma Death
Phencyclidine	None	Increase	Near normal/near normal	Slow speech Memory loss Agitation Blank stare Noncommunicative rigidity Gait ataxia Cyclic behavior	Onset: 1–5 min Peak: 15–30 min $t_{1/2}$: 4–6 h Duration: 24–48 h	Oral Smoked Injected Absorbed Inhaled	Violent behavior Paranoia Seizures Acute psychosis Heart failure Death
Cannabis	None	Increase	Slight dilation/near normal	Reddening of conjunctivae Lack of inhibitions Body tremors Disorientation Lack of attention	Onset: minutes Peak: 20–30 min $t_{1/2}$: 1–3 h Duration variable due to fat solubility	Smoked Oral	Fatigue Paranoia Acute psychosis
Hallucinogens	Depends on substance	Increase	Dilation/slowed	Hallucinations Tremors Distorted perceptions Piloerection (LSD) Flashbacks	Variable Depends on substance	Oral Smoked Inhaled Injected Absorbed	Acute psychosis Death (often from trauma)

BA = blood alcohol level; BP = blood pressure.

predominates. Under the influence of PCP, an individual may experience a "bad trip" and become irrational, extremely combative, and violent. The lack of pain secondary to its anesthetic effect and use seems to exaggerate the individual's strength. In some cases, PCP can cause severe psychoses, seizures, respiratory depression, intracerebral hemorrhage, hyperpyrexia, and death.

Flashbacks—hallucinatory episodes that occur days to years after taking the drug—occur with LSD and PCP use. Prolonged psychotic episodes (lasting several days to several months) with visual hallucinations have been precipitated by LSD or PCP.

Core Drug Knowledge in Inhalant Abuse

Inhalants, another kind of psychedelic drugs, are volatile chemicals and gases that produce behavioral effects and are subject to abuse. Commonly abused inhalants include model glue, spray paint and hair spray propellants, cleaning solvents, gasoline, and kerosene. Nonmedical nitrous oxide is another popular inhalant. These substances are generally sniffed from rags, paper or plastic bags, gauze, or ampules. Long-term inhalant abuse can cause permanent CNS, hepatic, renal, and bone marrow damage and greatly reduced mental and physical abilities.

Pharmacokinetics

Inhalants are rapid-acting substances. Their effects are almost immediate. The duration of the effect depends on the substance used. For example, effects of glue, paint, or gasoline usually last several or more hours, whereas the effects of nitrous oxide typically last less than 5 minutes. The effects of amyl nitrate (or butyl nitrate) last from a few seconds to several minutes.

Pharmacodynamics

Inhalation of volatile chemicals and gases produces a short-lived mild intoxication that typifies the early stages of anesthesia. These agents produce a sense of exhilaration and light-headedness. Judgment, vision, memory, and perception of reality are impaired. These substances are slightly hallucinogenic and cause a CNS depression because of the hypoxia they induce. Abusive, violent behavior has also been known to occur in people who abuse inhalants.

Adverse Effects

Psychological dependence can develop, but physical dependence is rare. Development of tolerance to the substance occurs, and more of the substance is needed over time.

Toxicities depend on the properties of the individual solvents. The consequences of inhaling these substances can be severe. Abuse of inhalants has been implicated in severe brain damage, cancer, neuropathies, kidney failure, liver damage, respiratory failure, and cardiac arrest.

Assessment of Core Patient Variables in Substance Abuse

Health Status

When the nurse suspects that a patient may be abusing substances, a physical, psychological, and functional health assessment should be performed. The assessment should focus on several key areas (see the accompanying display, Assessment Checklist for Suspected or Confirmed Substance Abuse).

Substance abuse screening may be easily incorporated into a health habits survey with questions moving from legal and less stigmatized substances, such as caffeine, nicotine, alcohol, to inquiries about street drugs. Questions about drug use or abuse should cover lifetime experience because recovering users remain at risk for relapse. In addition, a complete health and drug history should be taken. During this time, the nurse should try to obtain as much information regarding legal and illegal drug use as possible. When providing this information, the patient may use street names to refer to particular drugs or drug classes. Therefore, the nurse must be familiar with commonly used street names for legal and illicit drugs (Table 10-4).

The nurse can also ask the patient about any family history of substance abuse at this time. During the physical assessment, the nurse conveys a nonjudgmental attitude, which may encourage the patient to communicate. Anyone is more likely to open up to someone who is on his or her side. The nurse also should not assume someone is or is not a drug user. There is no stereotypical drug user. People who abuse drugs are from all socioeconomic and cultural backgrounds.

Life Span and Gender

Substance abuse throughout the life span poses serious problems for patients, families, and the community.

Maternal Substance Abuse

It is estimated that 10% of infants may have been exposed to illicit drugs during the gestational period. When alcohol, caffeine, and nicotine are considered, some researchers report as many as 33% of all pregnant women have used a psychoactive drug during pregnancy.

Alcohol use during pregnancy increases the number of spontaneous abortions, incidence of fetal demise, problematic pregnancies, and neonates who are lower in birth weight and slower in postnatal growth. Specific toxic effects of alcohol on the developing fetus are known as fetal alcohol syndrome (FAS). The incidence of FAS in some parts of the United States is estimated to be as high as 1 in 300 births. It is a common cause of a birth defect that is preventable. There appears to be no established safe amount of alcohol or a safe time to drink it during pregnancy or lactation. Alcohol is teratogenic, but unlike other teratogens, alcohol does not uniformly affect all exposed to it. FAS causes growth deficiency, CNS dysfunction, craniofacial abnormalities, microcephaly, and other major organ defects.

Assessment Checklist for Suspected or Confirmed Substance Abuse

Physical Status

General Appearance
- ❑ Clean or neat
- ❑ Dirty or disheveled

Speech
- ❑ Normal
- ❑ Rapid
- ❑ Slow
- ❑ Slurred
- ❑ Incoherent

Eyes

Pupils
- ❑ Normal and reactive to light
- ❑ Normal (slow or fixed)
- ❑ Dilated
- ❑ Pinpoint and reactive to light
- ❑ Pinpoint (slow or fixed)

Vision
- ❑ Normal
- ❑ Nystagmus
- ❑ Blurred

Nose
- ❑ Normal
- ❑ Nasal membranes ulcerated
- ❑ Nasal septum perforated
- ❑ Excessive secretions

Mouth
- ❑ Breath odor: (describe)

Skin
- ❑ Normal
- ❑ Bruised
- ❑ Cuts and abrasions
- ❑ Needle marks or scars
- ❑ Sores, signs of infection
- ❑ Color: normal, pale, cyanotic, flushed
- ❑ Turgor: normal, dry, moist, perspiring

Neurologic

Muscular
- ❑ No symptoms
- ❑ Tremors
- ❑ Negative or depressed tendon reflexes
- ❑ Motor incoordination

Level of Consciousness
- ❑ Awake, stuporous, semicomatose, comatose

Vital Signs

Respirations
- ❑ Normal
- ❑ Rapid
- ❑ Shallow
- ❑ Depressed

Pulse
- ❑ Rate
- ❑ Rhythm (specify)

Blood Pressure
- ❑ Normal range
- ❑ Hypotensive
- ❑ Hypertensive

Temperature
- ❑ Normal
- ❑ Subnormal
- ❑ Elevated

Psychological/Emotional Status

Sensorium
- ❑ Clear, clouded, disoriented, visual or auditory hallucinations or both

Memory
- ❑ Evidence of memory loss

General Behavior
- ❑ Passive
- ❑ Aggressive
- ❑ Agitated
- ❑ Hyperactive
- ❑ Euphoric
- ❑ Combative
- ❑ Uncooperative

Functional Status

Nutritional/Metabolic Findings
- ❑ Malnourished
- ❑ Skin lesions
- ❑ Condition of hair
- ❑ GI complaints (specify)

Roles and Relationships
- ❑ Marital or significant other problems
- ❑ Unemployment or underemployment
- ❑ Excessive absenteeism at work or school

Coping Strategies and Stress Tolerance
- ❑ Binge drinking
- ❑ Drug behaviors of lying, denial, and blame
- ❑ Paranoia
- ❑ Frequent complaints of stress and anxiety
- ❑ Suicidal ideation or attempts

TABLE 10-4 Identifying Drug Street Names

Substance	Generic or Brand Names (or Active Ingredients)	Selected Street Names
CNS depressant: barbiturates	amobarbital, pentobarbital, secobarbital	Downers, reds, red devils, R.D.s, yellows, blues, rainbows, Christmas trees
CNS depressant: benzodiazepines	alprazolam, chlordiazepoxide, diazepam, flunitrazepam, flurazepam, lorazepam	In general: coral, idiot pills, M&Ms, tranq, Uncle Milty, ups & downs For chlordiazepoxide: green and whites, libs, roaches For diazepam: V, Vals For flunitrazepam: roofies, rophies, rope
CNS depressant: nonbenzodiazepine	chloral hydrate, gamma hydroxybutyrate (GHB), meprobamate	In general: ludes, Qs, 714s, vitamin Q For GHB: easy lay, G, grievous bodily harm, liquid X
CNS depressant: opioids	codeine, propoxyphene, fentanyl, heroin, hydrocodone, hydromorphone, meperidine, methadone, morphine, opium, oxycodone, oxymorphone, pentazocine	For fentanyl: China white, king ivory, dance fever, jackpot For heroin: China white, smack, horse, junk, H, hard stuff, Mexican brown, gumball, schoolboy, downtown For hydromorphone: drug stores, heroin For methadone: dolls, dollies For morphine: Miss Emma, morf, M
CNS stimulant: amphetamines	amphetamines, benzedrine, biphetamine, cocaine, desoxyn, dextroamphetamine, methamphetamine	For amphetamines: uppers, whites, mini-bennies, hearts, dexies, black beauties For cocaine: snow, flake, blow, rock, whiff, cola, oca, toot, nose candy, girl, crack, uptown For methamphetamine: meth, speed, crystal, crank
CNS stimulant: inhalants	aerosols, amyl nitrate, butyl nitrate, chloroform, ether, freon, gasoline, nitrous oxide, paint, paint thinner, toluene	Glue, locker room, rush, laughing gas, poppers, snappers, kick
Cannabis	dronabinol (Marinol), hashish, hash oil, marijuana, Thai stick	For marijuana: pot, grass, weed, Colombian, Jamaican red, Mexican commercial, sensemilla, kona gold, joint, roach, honey, reefer, ganja, mota
Hallucinogens	DET (diethyltryptamine), DMT (dimethyltryptamine), DOM (4-methyl 2,4-dimethoxyamphetamine), LSD, mescaline, peyote, psilocybin, STP, MDA/MDMA/MMDA (all variations of 3,4-methylenedioxyamphetamine)	For LSD: acid, L, microdots, sunshine, windowpane, paper acid, blotter acid For MDA, etc.: ecstasy, love drug, rave, XTC For peyote/Mescaline: buttons, mesc, mescal button, cactus For psilocybin: shrooms, magic mushrooms
PCP (phencyclidine)	ketamine, ketalar, sernyl	In general: angel dust, peace pill, elephant tranquilizer, rocket fuel, shermans, kools, zombie, tictac For ketamine: special K, super K, super acid, vitamin K

Fetal physiology differs from neonatal and adult physiology. These differences suggest that maternal ingestion of psychoactive substances may produce a more dramatic effect in the fetus.

Fetal nourishment occurs through the placenta. To reach the fetus, drugs in the maternal environment must cross over the continuous lipid membrane of the placenta. Substances with a molecular weight of less than 600 (e.g., alcohol, cocaine) cross over easily. Drug effects may persist for a greater length of time in the fetal environment because fetal blood is moderately acidotic, there are fewer protein-binding sites, and undeveloped hepatic function decreases the ability to metabolize and excrete the substance. Although excretion occurs through the placenta, recirculation throughout the amniotic fluid may occur prior to drug excretion.

The effects of opioid abuse during pregnancy include preterm birth, intrauterine growth retardation, and low birth weight. Cocaine use during pregnancy has disastrous effects on the fetus; it causes potent vasoconstriction that reduces placental blood flow by about 50% (Cold & Marshall, 1994). This results in fetal hypoxia and alters the maternal-fetal nutrient exchange. Fetal effects of maternal cocaine and methamphetamine use include abruptio placentae, preterm labor and delivery, intrauterine growth retardation, microcephaly (decrease in head circumference), low birth weight, and cerebral infarction. Fetal exposure may be recognized in a neonatal withdrawal syndrome characterized by tremor, poor feeding, increased muscle tone, abnormal sleep patterns, and high-pitched crying.

Women who use these drugs should be counseled to avoid breast-feeding because these drugs are concentrated in breast milk.

Effects in Infancy

Opioid-exposed infants experience several common complications: hypoglycemia, septicemia, and hyperbilirubinemia. In addition to metabolic problems, term infants are at risk for pneumonia and meconium aspiration. Preterm and full-term infants will experience withdrawal symptoms. Narcotic abstinence syndrome, which contributes significantly to neonatal morbidity, is characterized by CNS hyperirritability, GI dysfunction, increased muscle tone, respiratory distress, tremor, and vague autonomic symptoms (e.g., fever, skin mottling, sneezing, yawning). Initially, some infants may require drug therapy and treatment in the neonatal intensive care unit. Some symptoms may persist for 3 or 4 months or more.

Effects in Childhood

Children of alcoholics (COAs) face a broad range of problems that vary in severity and are associated with all phases of the life span. They are at risk for a range of cognitive deficits, especially those related to verbal ability, attention deficit hyperactivity disorder, antisocial personality disorder, anxiety, and depression. The prevalence of alcoholism is higher in all first-degree relatives of patients with alcoholism, and on average, COAs are three to five times more likely to develop alcoholism than non-COAs (Kinney, 1996).

Effects in Adolescence

The greatest physical and emotional changes occur during adolescence. The struggle toward independence is a time of great conflict, and rebellion is common during this period. Common forms of rebellion include style of dress and appearance, although rebellion can take destructive forms, such as illicit drug use and excessive alcohol drinking.

Several risk factors have been identified for adolescent substance abuse:

- Family constitution and stressful family events
- Poor parent-child relationships
- Low self-esteem
- Psychological disturbances, such as depression
- Low academic motivation
- Other problem behaviors
- Absence of religion
- High experience-seeking behavior
- High family and peer substance use
- Early tobacco use

Effects in Older Adults

In the United States, adults who are 65 and older are the fastest-growing segment of the population (Kinney, 1996). Retirement often brings changes in the older person's societal role as well as a decrease in social and financial status. Losses (e.g., declining health, financial problems, illness and death of family and friends) are a common experience of aging. Depressive symptoms related to these losses are common in older people. For some, alcohol or drug use becomes a way of coping with age-related changes, which normally cause physiologic changes (lean body tissue and total body water decreases; body fat increases). These changes have an important effect on how the body metabolizes drugs. Reductions in blood flow with age may result in an inability of the liver and kidneys to process drugs as efficiently as in youth; benzodiazepines, for example, are metabolized at about half the rate seen in a younger individual, making these drugs more difficult to use in the older population. One study indicated that 2.5 million older adults and 21% of all hospitalized patients over the age of 65 have alcohol-related problems (Hays, Oslin, & Blow, 1999).

Alcohol- and drug-related medical problems may not be recognized because multiple medical problems are common in the elderly, and they may be mistaken for age-related problems. The following are examples: confusion, depression, falls and other accidents, idiosyncratic reaction to prescribed drugs, inattention to self-care, incontinence, labile moods, or malnutrition.

Environment

As with other chronic drug use, heavy and chronic use of cocaine and methamphetamine, especially, is accompanied by dysphoria and anhedonia. Former substance abusers are at risk for relapse, because the perceived cure for the dysphoria is more drug use. Recurrence of symptoms and intense drug craving may occur even after long abstinence. Environmental triggers may produce intense desire for the drug even after years of recovery.

Culture

Some populations, most notably East Asians and American Indians, exhibit an unusual response of facial flushing, vasodilation, and tachycardia after consuming ethanol. These individuals have a genetic deficiency in the enzyme aldehyde dehydrogenase, which leads to an accumulation of acetaldehyde even after consuming relatively small amounts of ethanol.

Nursing Diagnoses and Outcomes

A comprehensive nursing assessment yields subjective and objective data helpful in formulating nursing diagnoses and desired outcomes relevant to short- or long-term drug history and actual or potential health problems related to substance abuse. Nursing diagnoses may vary according to which substances are used and what symptoms appear. In addition to Deficient Knowledge, Disturbed Sensory Perception (Visual and Auditory), and Risk for Poisoning, additional typical nursing diagnoses and outcomes may include the following:

- Ineffective Denial related to impaired ability to accept consequences of behavior
  Desired outcome: The patient will acknowledge an alcohol and/or substance abuse problem; explain the psychological and physiologic effects of alcohol or drug use; abstain from alcohol and drug use; state recognition of the need for continued treatment; express a sense of hope; use alternative coping mechanisms to cope with stress; and have a plan for high-risk situations for relapse.
- Risk for Other-Directed Violence related to drug or alcohol abuse
  Desired outcome: The patient will demonstrate control of behavior with assistance from others; have a decreased number of violent responses; and describe causation and possible preventive measures.
- Ineffective Health Maintenance related to substance abuse
  Desired outcome: The patient will identify barriers to health maintenance and verbalize an intent to or engage in health maintenance behaviors, including abstinence and sobriety.
- Self-Concept Disturbance related to self-destructive behavior (substance abuse)
  Desired outcome: The patient will appraise self-situations in a realistic manner without distortions; verbalize and demonstrate increased positive feelings; and demonstrate healthy adaptation and coping skills.

Planning and Intervention

In general, nursing interventions involve maximizing the therapeutic effects of the treatment plan, minimizing factors that may contribute to resumption of substance abuse, and providing patient education to help the patient cope with denial and recognize the significance of his or her substance abuse problem.

Maximizing Recovery

Initial nursing interventions in acutely intoxicated patients are generally directed toward preventing life-threatening or debilitating effects from the substance itself or its withdrawal. These nursing interventions evolve from the specific physiologic and psychological effects of the particular substance. For example, if the patient is experiencing hallucinogen and CNS-stimulant intoxication or withdrawal, the nurse needs to monitor vital signs and mental status and provide a quiet, dim, nonstimulating, nonthreatening environment. Additional monitoring focuses on emotional status and possible seizure activity.

Because physical or psychological withdrawal symptoms may follow abrupt cessation of a substance, the first intervention is medical detoxification if the person entering treatment is currently under the influence of drugs. Physiologic symptoms associated with drug withdrawal may be treated with various pharmacotherapies. For example, diazepam or lorazepam are used to modify the symptoms of alcohol withdrawal and prevent the seizures it can precipitate. Clonidine (Catapres) is frequently used to manage the symptoms of opioid and cocaine withdrawal.

Minimizing Relapse

For alcohol, cocaine, or narcotic abusers, treatment is lifelong, and relapses do occur. However, several therapies may promote motivation to remain substance free and increase the patient's chances for success. They include psychotherapy and support groups and administration of withdrawal and anticraving drugs. The various methods used in treating alcoholism are discussed in the accompanying display, Nursing Management Strategies in Alcoholism.

Some patients who have withdrawn from alcohol and who desire to achieve continued sobriety may elect to take the drug disulfiram (Antabuse). Its effects rely on a

Nursing Management Strategies in Alcoholism

Nursing interventions are modified according to the problems and complications encountered in patients with alcoholism. Some general interventions follow.

Acute Alcohol Intoxication

- Maintain an open and adequate airway.
- Support respiration and blood pressure.
- Alleviate hypoglycemia, ketoacidosis, dehydration, and neurologic deficit by administering glucose and IV fluids containing potassium, magnesium, phosphate, and vitamins (thiamine, pyridoxine, and folic acid).

Alcohol Withdrawal Syndrome

- Administer drug therapy as prescribed (e.g., primarily benzodiazepines chlordiazepoxide or lorazepam, to suppress the withdrawal syndrome.

Chronic Alcoholism

- Inform the patient of the necessity for complete abstinence from alcohol use, including alcohol in "benign" products such as cough syrups and food flavoring (vanilla extract).
- Refer the patient and family to social and environmental support groups, such as Alcoholics Anonymous, Alateen, Al-Anon.
- Teach about preventive medical and pharmacologic treatments, such as aversion therapy with disulfiram (Antabuse), hypnotherapy, psychotherapy, and treatment programs in private or public clinics outside of a hospital setting.

drug interaction (between ethanol and disulfiram) to produce unpleasant and undesirable symptoms as a deterrent to alcohol ingestion. The very unpleasant symptoms of a disulfiram-alcohol reaction include facial flushing, throbbing headache, hyperventilation, tachycardia, palpitations, nausea and copious vomiting (within 60 minutes after alcohol ingestion), hypotension, shortness of breath, vertigo, syncope, confusion, and profuse diaphoresis. In very severe reactions, myocardial infarction, cardiovascular collapse, unconsciousness, convulsions, and even death may occur.

Patients withdrawing from cocaine addiction may be treated with amantadine (Symmetrel), bromocriptine (Parlodel), buprenorphine (Buprenex), carbamazepine (Tegretol), desipramine (Norpramin), and lithium. These drugs have been used clinically with varying degrees of success.

Treatment for heroin addicts is possible. However, the process is slow, and some methods used are somewhat controversial (see the accompanying display, Treating Heroin Addiction Pharmacologically).

Treatment for marijuana abuse consists mainly of nonpharmacologic interventions combined with an exercise program to help deal with withdrawal symptoms and cravings for the drug.

Because no addiction results from LSD or PCP use, no withdrawal syndrome results, and no treatment is required. Treatment for LSD and PCP is necessary only when the user experiences a "bad trip" (see the accompanying display, Intervening on a "Bad Trip").

Treatment for acute inhalant intoxication is similar to that for CNS depressant overdosage. Patients need oxygen and other respiratory assistance. They should not receive any vasopressive therapy, such as injected epinephrine, because the interaction between a vasopressor and an inhalant will trigger serious arrhythmias.

Providing Patient and Family Education

After identifying a substance-abuse problem, the nurse can intervene by assisting the patient and family to develop ways to prevent substance abuse; communicating and reinforcing healthy coping strategies and stress-reduction behaviors; recognizing the patient's values, beliefs, and support systems; and identifying and encouraging contact with self-help groups, community resources, rehabilitative organizations, and support groups.

The nurse can help family members identify their feelings and responses to the substance-abuse problem and cope with these feelings. Family members can be referred to counseling services and emotional support groups. Entry into substance abuse treatment programs is frequently through an evaluation and referral center. This is also an opportune time for the nurse to teach the family more about the hazards of substance abuse. The

Treating Heroin Addiction Pharmacologically

For many substance abusers, overcoming heroin or other opioid addiction is a long and difficult process. Over the years, many treatment interventions have been proposed and used with varying degrees of success, failure, and controversy.

Methadone

Oral methadone is substituted for heroin at a dose sufficient to suppress opioid withdrawal and then, theoretically, reduced by 50% every other day. This treatment effectively suppresses withdrawal symptoms and has a long duration of action (24 hours). About 1 mg of methadone is equivalent to 1.5 mg heroin.

However, methadone is a long-acting narcotic analgesic and only needs to be administered once or twice a day. Therefore, drug-seeking activity and drug focus can often be eliminated during therapy and rehabilitation. Moreover, methadone can be decreased gradually. Theoretically, the patient can be weaned from drug use entirely.

This kind of treatment, however, is controversial for several reasons: some practitioners argue that methadone therapy simply substitutes one addicting substance for another. Additionally, illicit methadone markets have developed because of the widespread use of methadone programs and the fact that patients are allowed to take larger quantities home and make fewer clinic visits.

Clonidine

Clonidine (Catapres), an adrenergic agonist and anti-hypertensive drug, is useful in treating mild heroin dependence and withdrawal. It suppresses the sensory nervous system and the hyperactivity that accompanies withdrawal. Clonidine facilitates withdrawal in two ways: it may be substituted for methadone (after methadone facilitates withdrawal) and then withdrawn, or it may be used with the long-acting, opioid antagonist, naltrexone (Trexan) as a substitute for methadone. Ultimately, the clonidine is withdrawn, leaving the patient solely on naltrexone.

Naltrexone

A recent treatment option for heroin addiction is long-term naltrexone (Trexan, ReVia). Naltrexone is a long-acting narcotic antagonist. An oral dose of 50 mg effectively blocks the receptors for 24 hours so that heroin has no effect and the patient experiences no real pleasure from taking the drug. The decision to "do drugs" must be made a day in advance.

Other Pharmacotherapies

ORLAAM (L-acetylmethadol, methadyl acetate), a long-acting opioid is active for up to 72 hours after oral administration.

Psychiatric Treatment and Support Programs

Traditional psychiatric treatment has been relatively ineffective for heroin and other opioid addicts. Therapeutic communities (e.g., Synanon) led by health care professionals and ex-addicts appear to be somewhat more effective in the treatment of recently detoxified users. These organizations help restructure the addict's lifestyle and orientation through leadership, group help, and self-help.

Intervening on a "Bad Trip"

Nursing interventions for managing the terrifying perceptions and hallucinations or "bad trips" resulting from LSD or PCP use rely on decreasing sensory stimuli and providing comfort and support. Some guidelines follow:

LSD

- Place patients in a quiet room to decrease sensory stimuli.
- Remain with patients, and help them calm down by talking to them while panic and agitation is at a peak. This will help to alleviate fear and anxiety.
- Administer tranquilizers, barbiturates or benzodiazepines, or nicotinic acid as prescribed to counteract the chemical effects of LSD. Do not administer phenothiazines. They may induce hypotension, confusion, and an increased panic reaction because of their influence on the anticholinergic-like effects of LSD.

Ketamine (or PCP)

- Put the patient in a dark, quiet room, and closely observe him or her.
- Avoid verbal communication because any sensory stimuli may cause further reaction and agitation.
- If pharmacologic therapy is prescribed (e.g., benzodiazepines), administer as directed. As in association with bad LSD trips, phenothiazines should be avoided because of their addictive anticholinergic effects.

nurse can also explain that relapses may occur and that support groups (e.g., Alcoholics Anonymous, Alateen, Narcotics Anonymous) exist for helping the patient and family members deal with relapses and work through new problems related to recovery and altered relationships. The goal of treatment is stressed as being longer and longer periods of abstinence and sobriety. Relapse prevention includes teaching patients to identify and manage feelings, recognize high-risk situations, and develop effective coping strategies.

Ongoing Assessment and Evaluation

Health consequences of substance abuse are usually manifested by changes in physiologic and behavioral functioning; therefore, evaluative guidelines related to detoxification, withdrawal, and rehabilitation will correspond to signs that the patient has returned to normal physiologic and psychological functioning.

Nurses and other health care professionals have a community responsibility to provide information regarding substance abuse. Meeting this responsibility may involve providing information and counseling or referring patients, friends, and neighbors to treatment resources. The nurse should be familiar with the community resources and keep up-to-date on common drug abuse problems and their treatment.

Recovery is lifelong and requires total abstinence from the abused substance. The recovering person can never return to controlled use without rekindling the addiction problem. ■

CHAPTER SUMMARY

- Substance abuse is a significant problem nationwide and worldwide.
- Strong evidence supports a dopamine hypothesis toward drug abuse/addiction and a biologically inherited tendency toward alcoholism.
- Peer pressure, alienation, hedonism, mass media and advertising, affluence, and boredom are among the factors frequently cited as those leading to the misuse or abuse of drugs by adolescents. Many of these same factors apply to adults.
- Any substance causing acute CNS depression (e.g., narcotic analgesics and opioids) is capable of producing psychological or physical dependence during chronic use.
- Drug abuse is a complex biopsychosocial problem that does not lend itself to simple solutions; no drugs are likely to be effective outside of a standard comprehensive treatment and rehabilitation program. Entry into drug treatment frequently occurs through an evaluation and referral center; medical detoxification may be necessary.
- Substance abuse shows no favoritism within economic categories, ethnic backgrounds, social classes, or races.
- Long-term excessive alcohol use has the greatest scope of effect on all body systems; the pathophysiologic changes are most evident within the cardiovascular, CNS, and GI systems and significantly contribute to morbidity and mortality.
- Pharmacotherapies for opioid and stimulant abuse (drugs such as nicotine patches, naloxone, naltrexone) are simply adjuncts to psychosocial, rehabilitative, and educational interventions.
- Disulfiram (Antabuse) is one method to help prevent alcoholism relapse by creating unpleasant side effects if alcohol is used while the patient is on disulfiram therapy.
- Methadone maintenance for heroin addiction stabilizes the individual on a regular daily oral dose of methadone, preferably in conjunction with supportive psychological or psychiatric counseling. Regular administration of methadone exerts its antiwithdrawal effects by development of tolerance to methadone and cross-tolerance to heroin. An alternative approach to opioid withdrawal is the administration of narcotic antagonists to extinguish drug-seeking behavior by blocking the euphoric effects of heroin.
- The signs and symptoms of barbiturate and alcohol intoxication are strikingly similar; additive CNS depressant effects from alcohol, barbiturates, and opioids in combination may result in unpredictably abrupt and severe impairment.
- Accidents and unintentional overdose are common causes of death from all classes of drugs and occur according to systemic drug action (e.g., respiratory depression).
- Nurses practicing in all specialties and settings need to be knowledgeable about drugs of abuse, patterns of abuse, detection of abuse and dependence, and intervention in acute and chronic illnesses resulting from substance abuse.

QUESTIONS FOR STUDY AND REVIEW

1. What adverse effects can occur if alcohol is taken concurrently with barbiturates, benzodiazepines, or other CNS depressants?

2. Define the following: drug abuse, drug misuse, addiction, physical dependence, and psychological dependence.
3. Explain the use of disulfiram (Antabuse).
4. What factors place an individual at high risk for substance abuse?
5. Name some health problems related to alcohol and other substance abuse.
6. Methadone maintenance for opioid addiction is controversial. Why is this so?
7. Describe nursing interventions for an individual experiencing a hallucinogenic "bad trip."
8. Name several drugs that are frequently associated with abuse, and propose some reasons for their abuse.

NEED MORE HELP?

Chapter 10 of the study guide for *Drug Therapy in Nursing* contains exercises and activities to reinforce your understanding of the concepts presented in this chapter. For additional information see the text's accompanying website at *http://www.connection.lww.com.*

REFERENCES AND BIBLIOGRAPHY

Bergman, H. D. (1996). Alcoholism: An update for the pharmacist. *Community Pharmacist, 56,* 45–49.

Brody, T. M., Larner, J., Minneman, K. P. (Eds.). (1998). *Human pharmacology* (2nd ed.). St. Louis: Mosby.

Burnham, T. H., & Short, R. M. (Eds.). (2000). *Drug facts and comparisons.* St. Louis: Facts and Comparisons.

Cold, J. A., & Marshall, L. (1994). Maternal substance abuse: The neonate. *U.S. Pharmacist, 19,* H4–H18.

Coleman (1993). Overview of substance abuse. *Primary Care 20*, 1–18.

Craig, C. R., & Stitzel, R. E. (Eds.). (1994). *Modern pharmacology* (4th ed.). Boston: Little, Brown and Company.

Ernst, T. (2000). Neuronal damage from methamphetamine use persists despite long-term abstinence. *Neurology, 54,* 1344–1349.

Fauci, A., Braunwald, E., Wilson, J. D., Martin, J. B., Hauser, S. L., Longo, D. L., Kasper, D. L., & Isselbachter, K. J. (Eds.). (1999). *Harrison's online.* New York: McGraw-Hill.

Ferrell, D. (December 16, 1996). Scientists unlocking secrets of marijuana's effects. *Los Angeles Times,* A1, A20.

Gennaro, A., Chase, G., Marderosian, A. D., Harvey, S., Hussar, D., Medwick, T., Rippie, E. G., Schwartz, J. B., Swinyard, E. A., & Zink, G. L. (Eds.). (1995). *Remington's pharmaceutical sciences* (19th ed.). Philadelphia: Philadelphia College of Pharmacy and Science.

Hansten, P. D., Horn, J. R., Koda-Kimble, M. A., & Young, L. L. Y. (1997). Drug interactions and updates. *Drug Interactions and Updates Quarterly, 16,* 879.

Hardman, J. G., Limbird, L. E., Molinof, P. B., Ruddon, R. W., Gilman, A. G. (Eds.). (1997). *Goodman and Gilman's pharmacological basis of therapeutics* (9th ed.). New York: McGraw-Hill.

Hays, L., Oslin, D., & Blow, F. (December 1999). Substance use disorders in the elderly: Prevalence, special considerations and treatment. Symposium: American Academy of Addiction Psychiatry.

Holmquist, G. L. (1999). The appropriate use of opioids in the management of chronic pain: A pharmacist's perspective. *Pharmacy Times, 65,* (Supplement), 2–11.

Johnson, M. K. (2000). Marijuana may cause emphysema. *Thorax, 55,* 340–342.

Kinney, J. (1996). *Clinical manual of substance abuse* (2nd ed). St. Louis: Mosby-Year Book.

Kirn, W. (1998). Crank. *Time, 151*(24), 24–32.

Kujdyck, N. (1997). Stress, substance abuse and sanity among pharmacists. *Drug Topics, 141,* 134–143.

McEvoy, G. K., Litvak, K., & Welsh, O. H., Jr. (Eds.). (1997). *Drug information.* Bethesda: American Hospital Formulary Service.

Nash, J. M. (1997). Addicted. *Time, 14*(18), 68–76.

Setter, S., & Johnson, M. (1997). Smoking cessation and drug therapy. *U.S. Pharmacist, 22,* 91–100.

Substance Abuse and Mental Health Services Administration. (1998). *The 1998 national household survey on drug abuse.* [On-line]. Available: http://www.nidh.nih.gov/.

Weathermon, R. A. (1999). Controlled substances diversion: Who attempts it and how. *U.S. Pharmacist, 24*(12), 32–47.

Chapter 11

LIFESTYLE, DIET, AND HABITS: NUTRITIONAL CONSIDERATIONS

KEY TERMS

alternative therapy
botanical preparations
complementary therapy
herbal preparations
mineral cations
phytomedicines
trace elements
vitamins

Learning Objectives

At the completion of this chapter the student will:

1. Discuss the role of nutrition in health maintenance.
2. Identify common nutritional factors affecting drug efficacy.
3. Identify common ways that drug therapy may alter nutritional status.
4. Differentiate prescribed uses of vitamins and herbal and botanical preparations from unprescribed uses.
5. Identify core patient variables that increase the risk for the occurrence of drug-nutrient interactions.
6. Identify key aspects of nursing management to maximize therapeutic effect and minimize adverse effects from drug interactions with diet, diet supplements, and herbal and botanical preparations.

The core patient variable lifestyle, diet, and habits represents the entirety of how a person lives his life and the choices he or she makes to accept or reject behaviors that influence health. In drug therapy, this variable is assessed relative to how these factors interact with the prescribed drug therapy. Previously, this text has examined an unhealthy lifestyle choice (the use and abuse of substances) and how it relates to drug therapy. In this chapter a different lifestyle choice, normal dietary habits, and the use of herbal, botanical, and nutritional supplements are discussed.

The core patient variable of diet interacts with the patient's health in several ways. First, a well-balanced diet may prevent chronic illness, and therefore indirectly decrease the need for drug therapy. Second, nutritional supplements and herbal and botanical preparations may be given to treat deficiencies that occur with some types of chronic illness, or those that are adverse effects of drug therapy. Nutritional supplements and herbal and botanical preparations may also be taken to increase wellness or to meet normal nutritional needs. Additionally, certain foods, beverages, dietary supplements, and herbal and botanical preparations can affect the absorption and effectiveness of some drugs or produce an adverse effect. These points are discussed in this chapter.

Nutritional supplements such as vitamins and herbs are now commonly used by many people in the United States. The selection and use of a particular supplement is made independently by the individual without supervision or consultation with a health care provider. Although these practices may have a positive effect on health, they may also interact with prescribed drug therapy, producing an adverse effect. These interactions with drug therapy will be briefly discussed in this chapter.

DIETARY FACTORS AFFECTING DRUG EFFICACY

Health status in general has a nutritional base. A proper well-balanced diet provides a healthy person with an adequate supply of nutrients. The expected drug response in the body is based on the body having the normal balance of elements, including dietary factors. When dietary factors are altered, drug therapy may produce different effects in the body than would normally occur.

Several factors related to malnutrition have been suggested to alter drug disposition (see the accompanying display, Pharmacokinetic and Nutrient Interactions). Protein levels are one significant factor. Diminished protein status results in lower amounts of plasma proteins and can significantly increase the concentration of free drug available. As only free drug is active, this increase in free drug will increase the drug's pharmacologic effect and the risk for adverse effects. This is especially important for drugs that are normally highly protein bound. Albumin is the most important protein, in terms of drug action, because most protein binding by drugs occurs with albumin molecules (see Chap. 4). Drug binding to albumin is also affected by high fat meals and fasting. Both of these situations lead to high serum levels of free fatty acids that compete with the drug for albumin-binding sites. Additionally, a diet poor in proteins may inhibit the biotransformation of drugs as protein deficiency may make drug-metabolizing systems less effective. See the accompanying display, Malnutrition and Drug Action.

Malnourished individuals exhibit decreased oxidative metabolism and reduced glomerular filtration rate, potentially

Pharmacokinetic and Nutrient Interactions

Absorption

- Changing the acidity of the digestive tract (rapid-acting carbohydrates (e.g., candy) causing sustained/timed release medication to dissolve too quickly
- Stimulating secretion of digestive enzymes (e.g., griseofulvin is absorbed better when taken with foods—especially fat—that stimulate the release of digestive enzymes)
- Altering the rate of absorption (e.g., acidic foods/beverages interfere with nicotine absorption from nicotine gum used for smoking cessation; aspirin is more slowly absorbed when taken with food)
- Binding to drugs (e.g., calcium binds to tetracycline, limiting drug absorption)
- Competing for absorption sites in the intestines (e.g., dietary amino acids interfere with levodopa absorption)

Distribution

- Changing binding of drug allows more free drug in blood stream (low protein)

Metabolism

- Acting as structural analogues (e.g., anticoagulants and vitamin K)
- Competition for metabolic enzyme systems (e.g., phenobarbital and folate)
- Altering enzyme activity and contributing pharmacologically active substances (e.g., monoamine-oxidase inhibitors and tyramine)

Excretion

- Changing the acidity of the urine (e.g., vitamin C can alter urinary pH and limit the excretion of aspirin)

Critical Thinking Scenario

Malnutrition and drug action

Larry Willis, a 35-year-old homeless man, is brought to the emergency department by the police who found him collapsed and having a seizure on the street. He is malnourished. He is admitted to the hospital and started on a standard dose of phenytoin, a drug used to prevent seizures in epilepsy, which is a highly protein-bound drug. He is showing signs of adverse effects from the phenytoin. Use your knowledge of the effect of diet on drug actions to determine why this has occurred.

*Parts of this chapter are based on material provided by Leah Wilder Cleveland.

increasing blood concentrations of the drug or an active metabolite. This increases the effect of the drug, both its therapeutic and adverse effects.

Dietary factors that promote obesity have an indirect effect on drug therapy. Body composition is an important consideration in determining drug response. For example, distribution of fat-soluble drugs is increased in the obese and the elderly because of the increased proportion of adipose tissue to lean body mass (see Chap. 9).

Excessive intake of vitamins may also adversely affect the action of some drugs; for example, increased pyridoxine intake may adversely affect the therapeutic effect of levodopa by increasing its metabolism. Increased or decreased intake of some elements may alter the absorption or reabsorption of a drug. For example, changes in the dietary intake of sodium will alter the reabsorption of lithium in the renal tubule. Significant decreases in dietary sodium will result in extra lithium's being reabsorbed, higher circulating levels of lithium, and potential drug toxicity from elevated lithium levels.

Food and nutrient intake can affect drug excretion by changing the urinary pH. For example, acidic drugs are more rapidly excreted in alkaline urine. A diet rich in meat or in vegetables may also influence the urine pH—either acidic or basic—and in this way the renal excretion of drugs may be changed considerably because drugs are generally either weak organic acid or bases. Conversely, drugs may also interfere with the availability and utilization of certain nutrients (e.g., vitamins, electrolytes, or trace elements); this interaction may occur with the long-term administration of certain drugs (e.g., antibiotics, oral contraceptives, anticonvulsants, laxatives) or the chronic consumption of alcohol. Deficiency of certain nutritional factors or even diseases can then be the consequence of such interactions.

A particular food or the manner in which food is prepared can also affect drug disposition. Cruciferous vegetables markedly induce chemical oxidations when added to the diet and increase drug metabolism (Mahan & Escott-Stump, 2000). The polycyclic hydrocarbons—similar to those found in cigarette smoke—generated from charcoal broiling of foods—may increase drug metabolism. An increased drug metabolism will lower circulating levels of the drug. This is known to be true with the methylxanthines, such as theophylline.

Finally, the timing of when food and beverages are consumed in relation to when drug therapy is taken may alter the effectiveness of the drug therapy. Some drugs need to be taken on an empty stomach to promote absorption, some drugs will bind with certain types of foods, which prevents drug absorption, and some drugs need to be taken with food for best results. See Chapter 4 for further discussion.

DRUG THERAPY AND NUTRITIONAL STATUS

Drugs potentially affect the status of almost every nutrient; particularly important to consider are folate, pyridoxine (both B vitamins), and vitamin A because their intake is often marginal and many commonly used drugs affect them (Table 11-1). Some drugs affect nutrient metabolism and excretion by an "antivitamin" process. They inhibit the synthesis of specific enzymes through competing for the vitamins or vitamin metabolites necessary to their structure. For example, the antineoplastic drug methotrexate is a folic-acid antagonist; without folic acid, synthesis of deoxyribonucleic acid (DNA) is inhibited, cell replication ceases, and cell death results. A drug may also form a complex with a nutrient, thus making it unavailable for use by the body. For example, the anti-tuberculosis drug isoniazid forms a complex with pyridoxine, interfering with its metabolism resulting in vitamin B_6 deficiency.

Other "antivitamin" drugs include hydralazine and L-dopa (which affect levels of vitamin B_6) and the coumarin anticoagulants as intentional vitamin K antagonists (which block the action of vitamin K to prolong bleeding time).

Some commonly used drugs have nutrition-related actions. For example, chronic phenytoin therapy is associated with folate deficiency and megaloblastic anemia. Folic acid and phenytoin are structurally similar and are thought to compete with each other for the same surface receptors. Diuretic drugs increase the excretion of nutrients by interfering with reabsorption in the renal tubules. Chronic use may result in depletion of potassium, magnesium, and zinc because renal excretion of these minerals is increased.

COMPLEMENTARY NUTRITIONAL THERAPIES

The use of nutritional supplements and herbal and botanical preparations is often considered as an **alternative therapy** for health. Although these choices have been traditional in some non-Western cultures, they are now being used more frequently in Western cultures, where they have come to be viewed less as alternative practices to Western medicine and more as augmentations or supplements to health care. The term **complementary therapy** is now often used for these choices. Complementary nutritional therapies include supplements of basic food elements, vitamins, and minerals, as well as the use of herbs and botanicals.

NUTRITIONAL SUPPLEMENTS

If patients do not have enough of a nutrient, oral supplements of that nutrient may be prescribed as adjuncts to drug therapy.

Protein

Protein is one of the most important and abundant substrates in the body and contains 4 kcal/g. The body may draw on dietary or tissue protein to obtain needed energy when the supply from carbohydrates and fats is inadequate. Proteins are polymers of essential and/or nonessential amino acids. Although animal proteins generally contain sufficient essential amino acids, many plant proteins do not and vegetarians may not eat a wide enough variety of plants to en-

TABLE 11-1 Adverse Drug Effects on Nutrients

Classifications and Selected Drugs	Nutrients Affected (Likely Depleted)
Anti-gout: colchicine	Beta-carotene, sodium, vitamin B_{12}
Anti-hypertensive agents	
Vasodilators: hydralazine	Vitamin B_6
ACE inhibitors	Zinc
Anti-infective agents	
Aminoglycosides: neomycin (PO)	Iron, magnesium, nitrogen, potassium, sodium, vitamins A, B_{12}, K
Amoxicillin	Biotin, vitamin K (possibly other B vitamins)
Anti-tuberculosis agents: isoniazid	Calcium, niacin, vitamins B_6, D, E
Sulfa: co-trimoxazole	Folic acid
Tetracyclines	Calcium, magnesium, vitamin B_6, zinc
Trimethoprim	Folic acid
Anti-inflammatory agents: Aspirin, other NSAIDS (e.g., ibuprofen, indomethacin, naproxen)	Folic acid, iron, vitamins C (and possibly B_{12}), zinc
Anti-secretory agent: omeprazole	Calcium, magnesium, vitamin B_{12},
Beta-adrenergic blocking agents	
Beta-1 atenolol, metoprolol, propranolol, timolol	Coenzyme Q-10, potassium
Beta-2 albuterol	Calcium, magnesium
Bile acid sequestrants: cholestyramine, clofibrate	Beta-carotene, fat, folic acid, iron, vitamins A, B_{12}, D, E, K
Cardiovascular agent: digoxin	Calcium, magnesium, thiamine
Corticosteroids: cortisone, dexamethasone, methylprednisolone, prednisone	Calcium, potassium, selenium, vitamin D, zinc
Diuretic agents	
Loop: bumetanide, ethacrynic acid, furosemide	Magnesium, potassium, Vitamins B_1, B_6, zinc
Potassium-sparing: spironolactone, triamterene	Coenzyme Q-10
Thiazide: hydrochlorothiazide	Magnesium, potassium, sodium, thiamine, zinc
Estrogen replacement: Estratab, Premarin, Prempro	Folic acid, niacin, vitamins B_6, C
HMG-CoA reductase: atorvastatin, lovastatin, pravastatin, simvastatin	Coenzyme Q-10
Minerals	
Magnesium and aluminum antacids	Calcium, copper, iron, phosphate, potassium, zinc
Potassium supplements	Vitamin B_{12}
Oral contraceptives	Vitamins B_2, B_6, B_{12}, C
Sodium bicarbonate: Alka Seltzer	Folic acid, magnesium, potassium, protein/amino acids
Sulfonylureas: glipizide, glyburide (second generation); chlorpropamide, tolazamide, tolbutamide (first generation)	Folic acid, vitamin B_{12}
Thyroid hormone replacement: levothyroxine	Calcium

sure an adequate supply. Quality protein should provide approximately 15% to 20% of a healthy person's well-balanced diet.

Individuals wishing to build muscle mass may take amino acid supplements and eat excess protein in the belief that increased protein intake facilitates the deposition of protein into muscles. Ingested amounts exceeding those needed to replace body losses, however, are simply converted into fat and stored. Some amino acids (e.g., L-carnitine) have gained popularity as preventive or therapeutic agents and are taken as dietary supplements. Their use may be hazardous in that there may be competition for transport with other amino acids into cells or the central nervous system (CNS). The research supporting their use is considered to be nonexistent or marginal by many nutritional experts. Essential amino acids, lysines, and arginine, promoted as regulators of body composition and muscle growth because they stimulate growth hormone secretion, have been disproved clinically to have these effects. Tryptophan has been used to enhance brain serotonin concentrations as a sleep inducer and in conjunction with weight loss regimens.

Carbohydrates

Carbohydrates (CHOs)—especially sugars and starches—are the most common dietary component; they contain 4 kcal/g and provide the body's primary source of fuel for heat and energy. A well-balanced diet for a healthy person supplies approximately 50% to 60% of the total kilocalories from CHOs. Simple sugars (e.g., fructose, sucrose) are refined sugars used primarily in soft drinks and baked goods that may cause an increase in serum insulin and triglyceride concentrations due to their rapid absorption. Conversely, starches are complex CHOs that must be digested; thus causing a slower absorption of glucose and lower serum levels of glucose, insulin, and triglycerides. Complex CHOs are useful in the dietary therapy of types 1 and 2 diabetes mellitus and individuals with atherosclerotic vascular disease or hyperlipidemia and would be adjuncts to drug therapy for these conditions.

Fat

Dietary fats from animal and plant sources provide the body's alternate or storage form of heat and energy. Fat—a more concentrated fuel—supplies 9 kcal/g. Fat should supply no more than 25% to 30% of the total intake of a well-balanced diet in a healthy person. Triglycerides are the predominant dietary lipids. Other important natural and dietary lipids include cholesterol and its esters and phospholipids. Cholesterol is an important component of cell membranes and a precursor of steroid hormones. Phospholipids, like cholesterol, are important components of cellular membranes and intracellular organelles. Although the body is able to synthesize adequate amounts of phospholipids, phospholipid compounds are marketed over-the-counter as health aids (e.g., lecithin) for the treatment or prevention of aging, cancer, heart disease, and obesity to name a few. Data to support these claims are limited or nonexistent.

Essential fatty acids—linolenic (omega-3; derived from corn, peanuts, soybeans) and linoleic acids (omega-6; derived from halibut, salmon) must be supplied in the diet. Patients who are receiving all of their nutrition parenterally will need to have fats administered to meet all their nutritional needs.

Dietary Fiber

Dietary fiber—a group of plant substances resistant to human digestion—is categorized by the food industry as soluble (which dissolves in neutral or acid detergent) or insoluble (which does not dissolve). Important characteristics of fiber are its water retention ability, cation exchange properties, and antioxidant actions. Fiber may be recommended to be added to the diet to treat or prevent constipation, which can be an adverse effect of some drug therapies. If the patient cannot consume sufficient oral, dietary fiber, drug therapies of bulk-producing laxatives, such as psyllium, may be prescribed.

Vitamins

Vitamins are a chemically diverse group of organic compounds needed by the body to maintain health by regulating metabolism and assisting in the biochemistry of food digestion as cofactors for enzymes. Small quantities of each necessary vitamin must be obtained exogenously, either because the vitamin cannot be synthesized in humans or because its rate of synthesis is too slow to produce sufficient quantities. The Food and Drug Administration considers the vast majority of vitamin products to be dietary supplements and their control falls under the Dietary Health and Supplement Education Act. Vitamins are generally classified as water soluble or lipid soluble; there are 13 vitamins—A, D, E, K (lipid-soluble), and vitamin C as well as 8 B-complex vitamins (water-soluble). Water-soluble vitamins are stored in the body only to a limited extent, and frequent consumption of these compounds is needed to maintain adequate body levels. Conversely, lipid-soluble vitamins are maintained in the body much longer, do not require such frequent ingestion, and have a greater potential for toxicity.

Recommended dietary allowances (RDA), established by the federal government, were designed to serve as dietary guidelines based on the idea that people would obtain essential and nonessential nutrients from a variety of foodstuffs. People's eating habits vary widely, however. Thus, a major industry supplying vitamin and mineral products has developed, which focuses on these "missing" nutrients. A significant percentage of the U.S. population takes some form of vitamin or mineral supplement daily; many take doses far in excess of the RDA and what is needed for optimal health. Vitamins may be prescribed when general nutritional status is poor, oral intake is insufficient, or the body has additional demands for a vitamin, such as Vitamin C to promote wound healing. Information on vitamins' effects on the body and potential drug interactions are shown in Table 11-2. Vitamin supplements may also be prescribed to correct for general malnutrition to

TABLE 11-2 Vitamins: Actions and Drug Interactions

Vitamin	Action	Interaction with Drug Therapy
Thiamine (vitamin B_1)	Absorbed in the small intestine Converts carbohydrates into energy Needed for neuromuscular transmission and for maintaining the structure of nervous system membranes	Antacids and other medicines (e.g., H_2 receptor antagonists) that reduce stomach acid or destroy it
Riboflavin (vitamin B_2)	Absorbed in the small intestine Needed for the metabolism of amino acids and the conversion of dietary vitamin B_6 to its active form	Antipsychotics and tricyclic antidepressants contribute to riboflavin deficiency.
Pyridoxine (vitamin B_6)	Absorbed in the small intestine Is active in the metabolism of amino acids and neurotransmitters Essential to many enzyme reactions Synthesized by intestinal bacteria	Isoniazid contributes to deficiency.

(continued)

TABLE 11-2 Vitamins: Actions and Drug Interactions (Continued)

Vitamin	Action	Interaction with Drug Therapy
Vitamin B_{12} (Cobalamin)	Absorbed through the intrinsic factor in the small intestine Required by all DNA-synthesizing cells to facilitate folic acid metabolism	Alcohol interferes with the normal absorption of vitamin B_{12}.
Folic acid	Is one of a family of compounds called folates Necessary for making red blood cells and neurologic function Need for folate is increased in severe infection, cancer, and pregnancy	Drugs that contribute to folate deficiency include zidovudine, barbiturates, methotrexate, phenytoin, and trimethoprim. Alcohol blocks folate absorption.
Niacin (vitamin B_3)	Needed for the metabolism of proteins, carbohydrates, and fats Large doses (up to 2 g/d) have beneficial lowering effects on cholesterol and triglyceride levels Synthesized by intestinal bacteria	Deficiency of niacin may affect drug absorption, metabolism or excretion.
Pantothenic acid (vitam n B_5)	Contributes to the metabolism of carbohydrates and fats and the synthesis of steroids	Drugs whose effects depend on the metabolism of fatty acids, amino acids, carbohydrates, or the acetylation of proteins may be adversely affected by deficiency.
Vitamin C (ascorbic acid)	Best-known antioxidant vitamin Readily absorbed from the small intestine; when supplies are low, the kidney reabsorbs it from the urine Vitamin C is effective in wound healing through its role in collagen formation Involved in the manufacture of hormones, steroids, and neurotransmitters Necessary for the conversion of folate into its active form and the absorption of iron Increases the net antioxidant action of vitamin E	May impair excretion of some drugs.
Vitamin A	Essential for normal growth, development and maintenance of epithelial tissue Essential to the integrity of night vision Helps in normal bone development and tooth formation Functions as an antioxidant	Chronic use of mineral oil as a laxative may cause deficiency.
Vitamin D (Calciferol)	Available in the diet, but the major portion is produced from synthesis in the skin It is important for calcium and phosphate metabolism Appears to have metabolic roles in tissues not central to overall calcium homeostasis	Not applicable
Vitamin E (Tocopherol)	Absorbed in and with fat, and requires pancreatic and biliary enzymes for absorption Its antioxidant properties protect and stabilize cell membranes	Anticoagulant effects of coumarin drugs are increased with regular daily intake of 1200 IU of vitamin E.
Vitamin K	Occurs in two forms—one from dietary sources of leafy green vegetables and liver and a second, less active form from synthesis by intestinal bacteria Essential role in blood clotting; aids in production of prothrombin Involved in bone formation	Anticoagulant effects of coumarin drugs are decreased by consumption of vitamin K.

achieve optimal health; and maximize the therapeutic effects and minimize the adverse effects from drug therapy.

Minerals

Major Mineral Cations

Major **mineral cations** include calcium, magnesium, potassium, and sodium. Their movement across cell membranes is highly regulated; they function in energy metabolism, membrane transport, and maintenance of membrane potential.

No RDA for potassium and sodium has been established. Potassium is the principal intracellular cation in body tissues. It has an important role in many physiologic processes including transmission of nerve impulses, contraction of cardiac, skeletal, and smooth muscle; acid base balance, and the maintenance of normal renal function. Sodium functions to maintain the body's balance of calcium and potassium. It has an important effect in cardiac function, regulating osmotic pressure in the cells and fluids, acting as an ion balance in the tissues, producing a buffering action in the blood, and guarding against excessive loss of water from the tissues. Calcium is a critical component of the skeleton and is vital to neuromuscular transmission, cellular signaling, and blood clotting. The adult RDA is 800 mg. Menopausal women especially at risk for osteoporosis are recommended to consume 1,500 mg daily. Magnesium is involved in a great number of enzymatic reactions. Deficiency produces osteomalacia, neuromuscular disorders, seizures, and cardiac dysrhythmias. The adult RDA is 280 to 350 mg daily. Excess magnesium may cause CNS changes, hypotension, and cardiac toxicity including cardiac arrest.

If a patient is severely deficient in one or more of these electrolytes, IV replacement will be used to prevent serious complications; oral replacements may be ordered to treat less severe deficits. Electrolyte imbalances may increase the risk for adverse effects from some drug therapies (i.e., low potassium increases risk of arrhythmias from digoxin). Electrolyte imbalances may also occur as an adverse effect from some drug therapies (i.e., low potassium from diuretics). Supplements are often used as adjuncts to drug therapy for these reasons.

Trace Elements

There are a number of essential **trace elements**, also known as microminerals. The most important of these include chromium, copper, iron, selenium, and zinc. Trace elements are present in minute amounts in body tissues and are essential to optimal growth, health, and development. Seafood is usually rich in nearly all micronutrients except manganese, which is readily available from plant sources.

Chromium improves insulin action; deficiency may cause elevated levels of blood sugar, cholesterol and triglycerides. Copper is used in making blood cells and is active in the metabolism of iron. Copper-containing enzymes are involved in immune functions. Severe illness, high-dose zinc supplementation, and antacids can reduce absorption of copper; supplementation may be necessary with total parenteral nutrition and zidovudine treatment, because zidovudine reduces copper levels.

Iron is an essential nutrient. It is needed to make red blood cells and deficiency results in anemia. Iron participates in oxidation and reduction reactions. It must be tightly bound to serum proteins to prevent potentially destructive oxidant effects. Bound to serum proteins, it is first stored and then distributed throughout the body.

Selenium is an especially important antioxidant. Its levels correlate with immune function—specifically, albumin levels, lean body mass, and total lymphocyte count. Deficiency occurs in infection and increased metabolic rates; deficiency is associated with heart disease and anemia. Zinc is absorbed in the small intestine; high-fiber diets limit its absorption. Zinc promotes wound healing and functions in antibody production. Deficiency impairs protein metabolism and the immune response.

The trace minerals may be administered if dietary intake is low or the patient is malnourished. They are usually included in a multivitamin formula. Correction of generalized malnourishment is often an adjunct to drug therapy to achieve maximum therapeutic effect from the drug or to prevent adverse effects from drug therapy.

HERBAL AND BOTANICAL PREPARATIONS

Herbal and **botanical preparations** are those substances derived from a plant source used as a dietary supplement or as a medication. Although herbal and botanical preparations have been traditional in some non-Western cultures, they are now being used more frequently in Western cultures as augmentations or supplements to health care. For example, recent Gallup surveys report more than 28 million Americans taking one or more herbal supplements (Oldendick, Coker, Wieland, Raymond, Probst, Schell, et al., 2000). This revival of interest in herbal, botanical, and dietary supplements in the United States during the past two decades can be attributed to an aging population with a large number of chronic diseases for which there are no satisfactory conventional medical treatments or the conventional treatment for which involves severely limiting adverse effects. It can also be attributed to a pervasive "back to nature" movement in a society increasingly attracted to good nutrition, exercise, and preventive health care as a means of remaining young and active.

Plants have historically been used for medicinal purposes. Many drugs used today are derived from plants. Therapeutic agents derived from plants or the preparations made from them are called **phytomedicines**. Aspirin, for example, comes from the bark of the willow tree, and digoxin is derived from digitalis or purple foxglove. The difference today is that many herbs and other plant substances are being sold over the counter. Many of the most popular herbal, botanical, and dietary preparations are marketed as a means of preventing aging-associated disorders, providing energy enhancement and a feeling of well-being, and assisting with weight loss, as well as for more traditional therapeutic uses. Their regulation may be limited because they are considered food sources rather than drug therapies. The bioavailability, or activity, of a preparation may vary widely between manufacturers. Consumers tend to think of these substances as harmless because they are sold over the counter. In actuality, they may cause significant adverse effects (just as prescription drugs may) (see the accompanying display, Herbal and Botanical Preparations and Potential Adverse Effects). Furthermore, they may

Herbal and Botanical Preparations and Potential Adverse Effects

Borage: possible hepatotoxicity from toxic alkaloids
Calamus: nephrotoxicity and seizures
Chaparral: acute hepatitis, hepatic failure, and renal failure
Coltsfoot: hepatotoxicity, photosensitivity, and possible carcinogenicity
Comfrey: hepatotoxicity, possible carcinogenicity
Ephedra/ephedrine (*ma huang*): arrhythmias, cerebrovascular accident, heart failure, hypertension, myocardial infarction, nephrolithiasis, psychosis, and seizures
Germander: hepatitis and hepatic cell necrosis
Hemlock: seizures and respiratory failure
Kava: oculogyric crisis and exacerbation of Parkinson disease
Life root: venoocclusive disease
Lily of the valley: digitalis-like toxicity
Pennyroyal: abortifacient and hepatic failure
Sassafras: hallucinations, hepatotoxicity, and possible carcinogenic activity
Senna: syncope, loss of bowel function and death from cardiac dysrhythmias
Willowbark: Reye syndrome

interact with prescribed drugs in ways that affect their therapeutic response (Table 11-3).

Secondary to the increased over-the-counter use of herbs and botanicals, Western medicine has recently examined many of these substances in clinical studies. Some findings support the use of these substances in the treatment or management of disease or altered physiology. Therefore, an herb or botanical may be prescribed for a patient (e.g., St. John's wort for depression and saw palmetto for benign prostatic hypertrophy).

NURSING MANAGEMENT OF THE PATIENT WITH DIETARY CONSIDERATIONS

Assessment of Relevant Core Patient Variables

Abnormal dietary intake and the use of herbs and nutritional supplements may have a bearing on drug therapy, so the nurse should question the patient during an initial drug assessment to uncover relevant information.

TABLE 11-3 Selected Reported Uses of Herbs and Botanicals and Possible Drug Interactions

Name	Reported Uses (By System)	Possible Drug Interactions
Bromelian (*Ananas comosus*)	Immune: reduces pain, bruising, and swelling from trauma (e.g., sports injuries) or surgery and speeds healing Skin: healing minor burns GI: relieves symptoms of GI upset, healing gastric ulcers, digestive enzyme for pancreatic insufficiency CV: angina, thrombosis, thrombophlebitis, varicose veins Musculoskeletal: reduces joint inflammation in rheumatoid, arthritis, osteoarthritis, sciatica, bursitis, tendinitis, and scleroderma Respiratory: suppresses cough, decreases bronchial secretions, increases lung function in patients with upper respiratory tract infections, sinusitis GU: prevents the thickening of the fibrous connective tissue in the penis associated with Peyronie disease Adjunct treatment in cancer with chemotherapy to prevent metastasis, increases therapeutic effect of chemotherapy drugs and antibiotics Adjunct AIDS treatment as an antiviral agent	Bromelian can increase the risk of bleeding if taken along with anticoagulants and will increase the effects of antibiotics if taken concurrently.
Chamomile (*Chamaemelum nobile*) (English, German)	Tea: stops pains from gas, heartburn, and ulcers Cream or ointment: reduces symptoms of psoriasis, eczema, or radiation burns from cancer therapies	Concomitant use of chamomile while taking anticoagulant medications should be avoided because excessive anticoagulation may occur.

(*continued*)

TABLE 11-3 Selected Reported Uses of Herbs and Botanicals and Possible Drug Interactions (Continued)

Name	Reported Uses (By System)	Possible Drug Interactions
	Solutions or tinctures in bath water: helps heal skin problems and hemorrhoids Inhaled vapor: soothes lungs and decreases cough	
Cranberry (Other names—marsh apple, mountain cranberry) (*Vaccinium macrocarpon*)	Prevents urinary tract infections (UTI) Possible antitumor effects	May enhance the elimination of some drugs normally excreted in the urine.
Echinacea (Other names—American cone flower, hedgehog, snakeroot) (*Echinacea purpurea*)	Immune system: stimulates system to prevent illness or speed recovery from illness	May interfere or counteract immunosuppressant therapy.
Ephedrine (Other names—*ma huang*, Chinese ephedra, Natural ecstasy, Teamster's tea)	CNS stimulant Increases metabolism and promotes weight loss Appetite suppressant Aphrodisiac	May increase CNS stimulation and adverse effects from caffeine, decongestants, sympathomimetics, bronchodilators, and CNS stimulants.
Evening primrose oil (*Oenothera biennis*)	Corrects deficiency of essential fatty acids Treats skin rashes Reduces inflammation Decreases breast pain, premenstrual symptoms	May interact with certain types of antipsychotic drugs (e.g., phenothiazines) and put the individual at risk for temporal lobe epilepsy.
Garlic (Other names—Allium, Stinking rose, Camphor of the poor) (*Allium sativum*)	Controls diabetes Treats infections CV: atherosclerosis, elevated cholesterol, hypertension, thrombosis, prevents age-dependent vascular changes	May interfere with existing hypoglycemic therapy. May potentiate the antithrombotic effects of anti-inflammatory drugs. Bleeding times with concomitant antiplatelet or anticoagulant therapy may increase.
Ginger root (Other names—Zingiber) (*Zingiber officinale*)	Emesis Inflammation Cancerous tumors Infections Antioxidant agent Antitumor agent Antimicrobial agent	Excessive consumption of ginger (dosage unknown) may interfere with cardiac, antidiabetic, or anticoagulant therapy.
Ginseng (*Panax*) (Other names—Asian ginseng, Western ginseng, five fingers, tartar root, seng and sang)	Depression and stress Improves concentration and work efficiency Aphrodisiac Insomnia	May increase the effect of monoamine oxidase inhibitors (e.g., phenelzine, selegeline, St. John's wort), antihypertensives, and hypoglycemics. May interfere with the action of steroids. Red ginseng may increase the CNS stimulant effects of coffee or tea.
Green tea (Other names—*matsu-cha*)	CV: atherosclerosis, elevated cholesterol levels Infections Cancer prevention Fluid retention	Antitumor activity of doxorubicin may be enhanced.
Hawthorn (Other names—bread and cheese tree, gazels, hagthorn, haw hazels, mayblossom, quick, thorn, whitehorn) (*Crataegus laevigata, C. oxyacantha, C. monogyna, C. pentagyna*).	CV: Angina, arteriosclerosis, hyperlipidemia, hypertension, narrowed coronary vessels	Can potentiate the cardiac glycoside actions of digitalis.

(*continued*)

TABLE 11-3 Selected Reported Uses of Herbs and Botanicals and Possible Drug Interactions (Continued)

Name	Reported Uses (By System)	Possible Drug Interactions
Kava (Other names—wa, kawa, kava-kava, onga) (*Piper methysticom*)	Anxiety Insomnia Jet lag Pain and stiffness Uncontrolled epilepsy	May intensify the effects of barbiturates and alcohol.
Licorice (*Glycyrrhiza glabra*)	Respiratory: coughs, bronchitis Infections: (*Staphylococcus*, *Streptococcus*, HIV, hepatitis A, herpes virus, *Candida*) GI: gastric ulcers, chronic gastritis, constipation Cancerous tumors Musculoskeletal: arthritis, rheumatism, spasms Primary adrenocortical insufficiency	Increased risk of hypokalemia when given with thiazide diuretics.
Passion flower (Other names—passion fruit, granadilla, water lemon, maypop) (*Passiflora incarnata*)	Anxiety Insomnia Nervous gastrointestinal conditions Seizures	Excessive dosing may enhance the action of antidepressants.
Psyllium (*Plantago afra*)	GI: constipation, irritable bowel syndrome, Crohn disease, hemorrhoids; reduces risk of colon cancer Obesity CV: hypertension, heart disease	Can interfere with drug absorption if taken within 1 hour of the time other medications are taken.
Saw palmetto (Other names—sabal, American dwarf palm tree, *serenoa repens*)	Benign prostatic hypertrophy	May change the effects of contraceptive pills and patches and of hormone replacement therapy.
St. John's wort Other names—*Hypericum*, amber, Devil's scourge, goat weed)	Mild to moderate depression Seasonal affective disorder and other mood problems Insomnia and hypersomnia Wounds and burns HIV infection and AIDS Hemorrhoids	Serotonin syndrome may occur when this herb is used with other serotonergic drugs (e.g., SSRIs, trazodone, tricyclic antidepressants, amphetamines). May produce increased drug effect when given with other antidepressants.
Valerian (*Valeriana officinalis*)	Anxiety, insomnia, and nervous irritability. GI: colic, diarrhea, stomach cramps, irritable bowel syndrome Dysmenorrhea, PMS	May potentiate CNS depression from sedatives.

If the assessment reveals an abnormal dietary intake, such as low protein or malnutrition, the deficiency must be corrected in some way. The nurse should determine why the patient is malnourished. Does the patient make poor choices as to what to eat, or is there a lack of money to buy food? Is there insufficient knowledge about what types of food should be in a balanced diet? Is the patient unable to feed himself because of muscle weakness? Is impaired cognition causing the patient to forget to eat? Does the patient have nausea or loss of appetite either from a disease process or as an adverse effect of drug therapy?

To assess the use of herbs and nutritional supplements, the nurse should focus data collection on the substances that the patient takes (e.g., drugs, nutritional supplements, herbs, and other preparations); why the patient takes them; which brands are used; and who recommended their use. This information is important and will help the nurse determine whether the desired effect of self-administered drug therapy is based on fact, fad, or tradition.

The nurse should also document the patient's age and life span status, because many of these therapies are not recommended for use with children, during pregnancy, or during lactation. The nurse should also carefully assess older adults, those who are chronically ill, those with a history of marginal or inadequate nutritional intake, and anyone receiving multidrug therapy over a period of time because such patients are likely to have drug-induced nutritional deficiencies. Because the effects of drug therapy can be altered by specific foods, the time that a patient normally consumes food and beverages prior to self-administering drug therapy at home should be determined.

Nursing Diagnoses and Outcomes

Nursing diagnoses and outcomes related to nutritional considerations will vary depending on the dietary factor and the drug therapy that the patient is receiving. Some potential general diagnoses include:

- Risk for Injury related to low protein levels and malnutrition

  Desired outcome: Protein levels and malnutrition will be corrected to prevent adverse effects from drug therapy.
- Risk for Injury related to adverse effects from excessive use of vitamins or herbs

  Desired outcome: The patient will not develop any adverse effects while using nutritional supplements.
- Risk for Injury related to drug interactions of vitamins, herbs, or food intake with prescribed drug therapy.

  Desired outcome: Drug interactions will be prevented in the patient while on drug therapy.
- Deficient Knowledge related to interactions of vitamins or herbs with drug therapy

  Desired outcome: The patient will obtain sufficient knowledge to make knowledgeable choices regarding the use of vitamins and herbs while on drug therapy.
- Health Seeking Behaviors related to the use of nutritional supplements

  Desired outcome: The patient will effectively use nutritional supplements to complement drug therapy to increase health.

Planning and Intervention

Maximizing Therapeutic Effects and Minimizing Adverse Effects

If the patient has been assessed to have low protein levels the nurse should consult with the physician or nurse practitioner about protein replacement. Oral protein supplements or a high protein diet may be ordered. If levels are significantly below normal, intravenous infusions of albumin may be indicated. If the patient is generally malnourished but eating, a well-balanced diet should be encouraged. The nurse should verify that the patient is capable of feeding himself and offer appropriate assistance if needed. The nurse should work with the physician or nurse practitioner to alleviate nausea, vomiting, or loss of appetite related to disease process or drug therapy that prevents sufficient oral intake.

If the patient cannot take in enough food orally, vitamins or other nutritional supplements may be ordered. In some cases enteral nutrition (i.e., tube feedings) or total parenteral nutrition may be necessary to correct the imbalances.

If the assessment reveals that the patient is at risk for an interaction among a prescribed drug and foods, nutrients, herbs or nutritional supplements,the nurse can discuss with the patient the many ways that these interactions affect nutritional status and drug therapy effectiveness. The nurse may also need to discuss these findings with the prescriber of drug therapy.

Many of the nurse's actions to maximize the therapeutic effect or minimize the adverse effect of drug therapy, in relation to dietary factors, are centered around patient education.

Providing Patient and Family Education

- Teach the patient about the potential interactions of food, nutrients, and complementary nutritional therapies with prescribed drug therapy.
- Emphasize to the patient and family the importance of being well nourished while receiving prescribed drug therapy.
- Teach when the patient should take the prescribed drug in relation to meals if this is relevant for the particular drug (for example—should the drug be taken on an empty stomach to promote absorption).
- Encourage the patient to inform all of their health care providers about all dietary supplements used.
- Teach that botanical supplements as treatment for serious health conditions should be used only on the advice and supervision of a qualified health practitioner.
- Instruct the parents of children, pregnant women, or breast-feeding mothers not to use botanical products unless advised to do so by a qualified health practitioner, particularly if their use is associated with toxicity or drug and food interactions.
- Counsel the patient about the variable quality of nutritional products.
- Advise the patient to watch for any unusual reactions to any medication and to report them to the health care provider.

Ongoing Assessment and Evaluation

The nurse should assess for potential drug interactions when a patient is taking any dietary supplement or herbal preparation in addition to prescribed drug therapy. These interactions may present a less therapeutic effect of the prescribed drug than anticipated, or adverse effects of either the prescribed drug or the supplemental therapy. Drug therapy can be evaluated as effective if dietary factors have not impaired drug action or produced adverse effects. Dietary treatments may be evaluated as effective if they return the patient to a normal physiologic status, or they work efficiently as adjuncts to drug therapy. ■

CHAPTER SUMMARY

- Numerous medications and nutrients interact, which can lead to imbalances or interfere with drug effectiveness.
- Supplementary use of vitamins, herbals, and botanicals may be prescribed by a health care provider to meet normal nutritional needs or to treat diseases or pathologies. The use of these nutritional supplements may also be self prescribed by the patient.
- Foods and nutrients can alter the absorption, distribution, metabolism, and excretion of medications.
- Adverse drug-nutrient interactions are most likely to occur with medications taken for chronic conditions, if several medications are taken, or if nutrition status is poor or deteriorating.
- When assessing for the extent of drug-nutrient interactions, it is important for the nurse to consider the patient's age, drug dose, and duration of therapy for medications known to have an adverse effect on nutrients.
- Patients may not recognize the importance of mentioning their use of dietary supplements or their normal dietary patterns during a drug history. Nurses need to be aware of this and routinely ask patients about this information.

QUESTIONS FOR STUDY AND REVIEW

1. What factors in a patient's drug history suggest a likelihood of drug-nutrient interactions?
2. Describe how drugs and nutrients can interact and alter metabolism.
3. Describe how foods can alter drug absorption.
4. Why is it important for the nurse to routinely assess patients for their use of dietary supplements or herbal preparations?

NEED MORE HELP?

Chapter 11 of the study guide for *Drug Therapy in Nursing* contains exercises and activities to reinforce your understanding of the concepts presented in this chapter. For additional information see the text's accompanying website at *http://www.connection.lww.com.*

REFERENCES AND BIBLIOGRAPHY

Brown, C. H. (2000). Overview of drug interactions. *US Pharmacist: Health System Edition, 25*(5). HS3–HS30.

Caron, M. F., & White, C. M. (2001). Evaluation of the antihyperlipidemic properties of dietary supplements. *Pharmacotherapy, 21*(4), 481–487.

Crone, C., Gabriel, G., & Wise, T. N. (2001). Non-herbal nutritional supplements—the next wave: A comprehensive review of risks and benefits for the C-L psychiatrist. *Psychosomatics, 42*(4), 285–299.

Delzenne, N. M., & Verbeek, R. K. (2001). Interactions of food and drug metabolism [article in French]. *Journal de Pharmacie de Belgique, 56*(2), 33–37.

Elvin-Lewis, M. (2001). Should we be concerned about herbal remedies? *Journal of Ethnopharmacology, 75*(2–3), 141–164.

Loke, Y. K., & Derry, S. (2001). Reporting of adverse drug reactions in randomized controlled trials—a systematic survey. *BMC Clinical Pharmacology, 1*(1), 3.

Maka, D. A., & Murphy, L. K. (2000). Drug-nutrient interactions: A review. *AACN Clinical Issues, 11*(4), 580–589.

Rogers, E. A., Gough, J. E., & Brewster, K. L. (2001). Are emergency department patients at risk for herb–drug interactions? *Academic Emergency Medicine, 8*(9), 932–934.

Shelton, M. J., Wynn, H. E., Hewitt, R. G., & Di Francesco, R. (2001). Effects of grapefruit juice on pharmacokinetic exposure to indinavir in HIV-positive subjects. *Journal of Clinical Pharmacology, 41*(4), 435–442.

Wilder, B. J., Leppik, I., Heitpas, T. J., Cloyd, J. C., Raninitis, E. J., & Cook, J. (2001). Effect of food on absorption of Dilantin Kapseals and Mylan extended phenytoin sodium capsules. *Neurology, 57*(4), 582–589.

Chapter 12

ENVIRONMENT: INFLUENCES ON DRUG THERAPY

KEY TERMS

carcinogens
environment
hepatic drug-metabolizing enzymes
industrial chemicals
pollutants

Learning Objectives

At the completion of this chapter the student will:

1. Identify environmental settings appropriate for pharmacotherapy.
2. Identify limitations for drug therapy for each specific environmental setting.
3. Discuss environmental influences on drug stability and effectiveness.
4. Discuss environmental influences on adverse effects of drug therapy.
5. Identify the relationship between environment and occupation.
6. Discuss the influence of environment on the acquisition of disease states.
7. Identify the role of the nurse regarding environmental influences on drug therapy.

The core patient variable of environment also has relevance to drug therapy. **Environment** refers to the physical setting in which the drug is administered as well as to factors in the environment that may increase the risk for adverse effects, injury, or toxicity from drug therapy.

Many factors influence the physical setting in which a particular drug or class of drugs may be administered safely. Environmental factors inside the patient's home or community may affect drug therapy and predispose the patient to noncompliance or adverse drug effects. Environmental influences such as heat or cold may affect the stability or effects of certain drugs or drug classes. The physical environment of the home may predispose the patient to harm. Certain occupations make particular adverse effects more dangerous. These interactions of environment on drug therapy are discussed in this chapter, as well as environmental influences on the development of disease and the nurse's role regarding environment and pharmacotherapy.

PHYSICAL SETTINGS FOR DRUG THERAPY

Drug therapy may be administered in a variety of settings. These include acute care hospitals, acute rehabilitative units, transitional care units, outpatient units, long-term care facilities, and the home or community environment.

ACUTE CARE HOSPITALS

Even in the acute care hospital setting, certain drugs or drug classes cannot be administered everywhere in the hospital. For instance, the patient receiving IV digoxin needs to be placed on a continuous heart monitor. This necessitates the drug being administered in a critical care unit, or step-down unit, both of which have the ability to monitor the patient safely.

Surgical patients receive inhaled anesthetics such as tubocurarine only in the surgical suite where the anesthesiologist or nurse anesthetist monitors the patient. Patients in active labor or immediately after delivery receive drugs such as oxytocin in the delivery suite or postpartum unit. In an emergency, oxytocin may also be administered in the emergency department.

Most oncology drugs such as 5-fluorouracil (5-FU) may be given on any medical unit; however, administration of oncologic drugs requires specially trained nursing staff. These nurses must understand specifics about handling chemotherapeutic drugs, recognizing and administering rapid treatment of severe adverse effects, and properly disposing of oncologic drugs (see Chapter 45).

ACUTE REHABILITATIVE UNITS

Acute rehabilitative units (ARUs) may be located in a portion of the acute care facility or another site off the main campus of the hospital. Although these units are able to administer most routes of drugs, including IV drugs, they are developed to focus on the physical rehabilitation of the patient. Thus, if the patient needs medication that requires close monitoring, or equipment such as heart monitors, the patient is generally moved back into the acute care hospital.

TRANSITIONAL CARE UNITS

Transitional care units (TCUs) have been developed to bridge the care of patients who are well enough to be discharged from the acute care facility but may not be eligible for a long-term facility because of the need for IV drug therapy or intense physical therapy. Like an ARU, these units may be in a portion of the acute care facility or in a totally different location. Because the patient:nurse ratio is higher in the TCU, drug therapy that requires close monitoring or equipment such as heart monitors limits the type of pharmacotherapy administered in this type of unit.

OUTPATIENT UNITS

In the acute care facility, the term outpatient refers to the patient who arrives in the morning for a procedure with the expectation of returning home after the procedure is completed. Occasionally, the patient has a complication that requires that she or he be admitted to the acute care facility after the procedure.

In the community, outpatient refers to the delivery of health care in an environment other than the acute care setting. This may include urgent care centers, doctor offices, mental health clinics, or outpatient surgical suites,

Most pharmacotherapy may be administered in outpatient units as long as the individual site has the ability to monitor the patient closely and has life-saving equipment and drugs readily available. In some cases, laboratory testing on-site may also be required. For instance, prior to administration of IM gold salts, a complete blood count and urinalysis must be performed.

Outpatient chemotherapy is done routinely. The limitation in the acute care setting is also pertinent in the outpatient setting—the need for specialized personnel. Additionally, disposal of chemotherapeutic agents needs to be addressed carefully in this setting.

LONG-TERM CARE FACILITIES

Long-term care facilities generally admit patients who do not require intense observation. These patients range from trauma patients to the elderly who will live out the remainder of their lives in the facility. Long-term care facilities may have a very limited scope of care or a much broader scope, depending on the philosophy of the institution. Most facilities are capable of administering IV medications, but do not if the particular medication also requires special monitoring equipment. Some of the facilities have acute long-term care, including the use of ventilators. Medication administration will be dependent on the scope of the individual facility and their ability to monitor patients closely. Additionally, certain drugs also require the ability to intervene with life-saving equipment and drugs.

HOME ENVIRONMENT

Most drug routes are safe to use for administering medication in the home environment. Limiting factors include close monitoring of the patient and need for special monitoring equipment. Although some patients receive pharmacotherapy from a home health nurse, many other patients are taught to self-administer medications or family members and friends are taught to safely deliver the drugs.

The decision to teach the patient or family to administer drugs is made after a careful evaluation of the home environment by the home health nurse. Assessment of the patient's environment may give important clues to its potential influence on therapeutic effectiveness, the patient's adherence to the drug regimen, and the potential risks from drug therapy itself. For example, if a patient is receiving a drug that causes dizziness as an adverse effect, stairs in the home may pose a risk for falls or injury.

General factors to consider in the home include cleanliness, lighting, adequate heat, water, refrigeration and walkways in and around the house that are found to be unobstructed and in good repair. The nurse also needs to determine whether the patient lives alone or with other family members or caregivers who can help with the responsibilities of health care and assist with obtaining and administering drug therapy if needed.

The nurse must assess whether the patient has the required financial resources, transportation, and knowledge to obtain the drugs. Additionally, the nurse must assess for the correct equipment for measuring dosages and administration of the drug. Finally, the nurse must assess the patient's ability to monitor therapeutic effects and recognize any adverse drug effects.

ENVIRONMENTAL INFLUENCES ON DRUG STABILITY AND EFFECTS

Many drugs are sensitive to the physical environment. For example, excess heat, light, or moisture or sudden temperature changes can affect the stability of a drug and many drugs lose their potency when exposed to these elements. Interactions between drugs and the environment may involve storage of the drug or the impact of the environment on the drug's pharmacokinetic and pharmacodynamic processes. The nurse should determine where and how the patient's drugs are stored, because some individuals do not leave their drugs in the original containers.

The environment can also modify drug effects. For example, temperature affects drug activity. Heat relaxes peripheral vessels, accelerates the circulation, and thus intensifies the actions of some drugs such as vasodilators; cold has the opposite effect—it retards drug action by constricting the blood vessels and slowing circulation. High altitude puts the body under stress and relative oxygen deprivation at high altitudes may make some drugs ineffective whereas it will increase the sensitivity to others, such as alcohol and central nervous system depressants.

In some cases, environmental influences can actually abate the action of certain drugs. For instance, nitroglycerin, a drug used for acute anginal pain, is affected by air, light, and moisture. Because of these environmental interactions, the drug needs to remain in its original container and to be replaced frequently.

It is important to remember that environmental influences can affect pharmacotherapy in any environmental setting, not just the home environment. For instance, some intravenous drugs that are administered in the acute hospital setting, such as nitroprusside and amphotericin-B, must be covered in aluminum foil or with a brown bag during administration to avoid light sensitivity.

ENVIRONMENTAL INFLUENCES ON ADVERSE EFFECTS AND INJURY

Environmental chemicals are increasingly being recognized as agents that cause significant drug interactions in some individuals. For example, polychlorinated biphenyls (found in industrial solvents or used as flame retardant), polycyclic aromatic hydrocarbons (caused by incomplete combustion of organic materials and found in cigarette smoke), chlorinated hydrocarbons (found in pesticides), and consumption of ethanol are active inducers of **hepatic drug-metabolizing enzymes**. People chronically exposed to these chemicals metabolize some drugs (e.g., cimetidine, theophylline) more rapidly than normal.

A patient's environment may also influence the relationship between physiologic function, drug effects and adverse effects or injury. Alcohol, tobacco, or pesticides may alter the pharmacokinetics of certain drugs and increase the patient's risk of adverse drug effects. For example, benzodiazepines such as lorazepam, in combination with alcohol, may increase the adverse effect of respiratory depression to such an extent that death may occur. Another example is heat and antihypertensive drugs. Almost all of the antihypertensive drugs may cause the adverse effect of orthostatic hypotension. Combine pharmacotherapy for hypertension with patients who enjoy soaking in a spa or hot-tub and the outcome may be syncope. Photosensitivity is another potentially adverse effect that is associated with many different types of drugs. The nurse must assess the patient's environment for potential exposure to sunlight while taking these drugs and emphasize ways to minimize this potential adverse effect.

We previously mentioned that the role of the home health nurse is to assess the physical environment of the patient to determine the limitations for home pharmacotherapy. Now let us extend that assessment to include finding ways to decrease the potential for injury related to pharmacotherapy. For example, many patients receive narcotic analgesics to control pain when they return home. Some of the most frequent adverse effects to narcotic analgesics are sedation and dizziness. In the home environment, it is important for the home health nurse to assess potential hazards such as stairs and loose rugs to emphasize teaching the patient of these potential hazards to avoid when feeling sedated or dizzy.

It is also important to remember that simple things done on an everyday basis may be affected by environmental influences of pharmacotherapy. For instance, the patient who is a stay-at-home mother may not recognize that the heat of her home can increase the adverse effects of sedation and weakness when taking certain drugs. When she attempts to make dinner, a simple task such as cutting up vegetables may become hazardous.

ENVIRONMENTAL INFLUENCES AND OCCUPATION

In the broad context of environmental influences, the patient's occupation must also be considered. There are certain types of adverse effects such as sedation and dizziness that are enhanced by environmental influences and can lead to serious or deadly harm to patients with certain occupations. For instance, sedation or dizziness in a patient who works as a taxicab driver may lead to accident and injury to the patient as well as others in his cab. Drugs that cause photosensitivity may actually cause partial thickness burns to a patient who works as a lifeguard. The nurse must evaluate the patient's risk for adverse events based on his or her occupation prior to discharge from the hospital.

Patients who work in an environment that exposes them to **industrial chemicals** and pesticides have the highest risk for adverse effects and drug toxicity, because these environmental **pollutants** affect drug biotransformation. These factors have been thought to be responsible for decreased efficacy, prolonged pharmacologic effects, and increased toxicity (Hardman, Limbird, Molinoff, Ruddon, & Gilman, 1997). Individuals are chronically exposed to numerous environmental compounds and conditions that can induce or inhibit the activity of hepatic mixed-function oxidases. Some chemicals can induce the hepatic drug-metabolizing activity. These chemicals include polychlorinated biphenyls (PCBs; historically used in industry as insulators), polycyclic aromatic hydrocarbons (PAHs), and cigarette smoke.

There is, overall, a host of factors that can influence drug handling in an individual patient. It is recognized that a variety of human diseases may develop from chronic exposure to certain chemicals. A large number of drugs and chemicals, environmental pollutants, and endogenous substances are extensively metabolized in the liver before excretion from the body. The environment can influence the metabolism of these substances. A variety of factors in the environment can influence the metabolism of chemicals by CYP450 dependent enzymes. These include concurrent drug treatment, cigarette smoking, and exposure to occupational and environmental pollutants.

ENVIRONMENTAL INFLUENCES ON THE DEVELOPMENT OF DISEASE

The development of disease frequently results in the need for pharmacotherapy. The environments in which individuals live and work can have a profound impact on their quality of life, health, and incidence and management of disease. Agents in the environment and work setting that can be toxic or hazardous to human tissues enter the body by inhalation, percutaneous absorption, ingestion, and sensory organs. Each agent can produce an impact on human health, leading to acute conditions such as accidents, poisoning, respiratory or skin diseases, or chronic health conditions such as cancer and cardiovascular, genetic, respiratory, or neurologic diseases. Because chemical toxicants alter physiologic function, the resulting health problems may be considered drug-induced diseases. There is strong circumstantial evidence for the importance of environmental factors as **carcinogens**. Smoking and diet (see Chapter 11) are by far the largest contributors, although a wide variety of industrial carcinogens have also been positively identified. A number of chemicals in the environment and workplace (e.g., polycyclic hydrocarbons, aromatic amines) are known to be carcinogenic. For example, the most common tumors in developed countries (e.g., lung, breast, GI, prostate) are rare in many developing countries. There are at present stringent laws to safeguard workers in those occupations in which a high incidence of cancer has been associated with particular chemicals (Fig. 12-1).

THE NURSE'S ROLE

The nurse's role is extending more frequently beyond inpatient hospital settings to homes, schools, and industry. The nurse's role now includes the expanded range of health care concerns of health education, home health care, hospice, and public health, as individuals are now being discharged from health care institutions at earlier and earlier stages in their treatment. Nurses monitor drug response and provide patient education regarding medication in a variety of patient care environments.

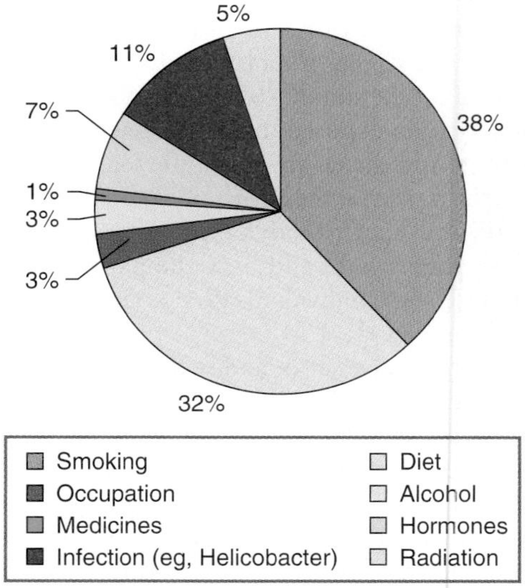

Figure 12-1. Environmental factors in cancer etiology. Adapted from Greene, R. J., & Harris, N. D. (2000). *Pathology and therapeutics for pharmacists.* (4th ed.). London: Pharmaceutical Press.

NURSING MANAGEMENT OF THE PATIENT WITH ENVIRONMENTAL CONSIDERATIONS

Assessment

Drug action is not exclusively a biologic phenomenon. Environment is an important determinant of drug response. A number of components of the institutional environment are under the control of nursing. In the hospital it is important for the nurse to assess factors that influence drug outcome, such as new or strange environment; unfamiliar people, noises and equipment or procedures; and lack of physical activity. All of these factors may increase the need for some medications, such as analgesics, laxatives, and sedative-hypnotics. For example, providing a quiet, cool environment and reducing external stimuli to decrease tension and stimulation will enhance the anxiolytic effects of sedative drugs.

Controlling the environment after discharge is a much more difficult task for the nurse. It is important that the nurse determine the environment in which the drug will be administered because drug therapies may occur in multiple environments. For example, patients may start chemotherapy or antidiabetic therapy in one environment, such as the acute care hospital, and continue therapy in the home environment.

Individuals may not realize that environmental factors may have an adverse effect on their prescribed drug therapy. With that in mind and to safeguard the patient, the nurse needs to conduct a complete drug assessment focusing on environmental and occupational influences.

Nursing Diagnoses and Outcomes

- Risk for Injury related to environmental hazards such as falls from stairs or loose rugs

  Desired outcome: The patient will remain without a fall.
- Risk for Injury related to decreased drug stability due to environmental factors

  Desired outcome: The patient will store drugs as directed.
- Impaired Skin Integrity related to environmental exposure to sunlight

  Desired outcome: The patient will take measures to control the amount of direct sunlight to exposed skin and use sunscreen at all times.

Planning and Intervention

The planning and intervention phases of the nursing process contain short- and long-term goals. Often these are modified as therapy proceeds. When working with patients to blend the element of environment into a regime that promotes health maintenance and disease prevention, the nurse's role may be broad and include elements of advocacy, education, referral, consultation, clinical care, management, organization, research, and evaluation. At this stage of the nursing process, however, the nurse's primary role usually focuses on patient education.

The rapport established early in the nurse-patient relationship provides the basis for the trust that is needed as the nurse continues to collaborate with the patient. To maximize the benefits of drug therapy as it is affected or changed by environment, the nurse needs to teach the patient about safe therapy and promote collaboration among health care providers and the patient. It may be necessary for the nurse to teach patients how to evaluate their personal and occupational environments for hazardous chemicals and, if appropriate, suggest the wearing or use of protective equipment. Another interesting aspect of patient education is to teach the patient about discarding medications. Therapeutic drugs can contaminate the environment because of metabolic excretion, improper disposal, or industrial waste.

It is vital for the nurse to consider the patient's learning style when selecting an approach to patient education. Some people are more visual learners, and the use of pictures or audiovisual materials may be more suitable for them than printed information. Other people need to be physically involved in their learning, making role-playing or demonstration and return demonstration more effective educational techniques for them. When using written educational materials, it is important for the nurse to assess whether the patient can read. Additionally, the materials used should be designed in the patient's mother language. Written materials are appropriate for individuals who can read; however, they must be at the patient's reading level. The extent of teaching will vary, depending on the environment in which the patient will receive the drug (e.g., home, clinic, group home, hospice). Although some education is required whatever the setting, more information is necessary if the patient will be taking the drug at home than if the patient receives the drug than in a rehabilitation center or other facility. The patient must be knowledgeable about all aspects of the drug regimen so that its administration can be safely and effectively self-managed. If another person—a family member or someone else—will be responsible for the patient's drug therapy at home, that person needs to be included in the educational process.

Ongoing Assessment and Evaluation

The nurse should evaluate the patient for increased or decreased drug effectiveness related to environmental stimuli. The nurse should also assess the patient for signs of adverse effects that may have been induced by environmental factors. The nurse should review measures to control environmental factors with the patient at each clinic visit.

CHAPTER SUMMARY

- Environmental settings include acute care hospitals, acute rehabilitative units, transitional care units, outpatient units, home and community.
- Limitations of pharmacotherapy for any setting include need for close monitoring of the patient, need for specialized equipment, need for life-saving equipment and drugs, and need for specialized personnel.
- Environmental influences can affect the stability of a drug.
- Environmental influences can affect the effectiveness of a drug.
- Environmental influences can increase the risk for adverse effects, toxicity, and patient injury.
- Environmental influences can increase the risk for injury to specific occupations.
- The nurse's role is to identify possible environmental influences to pharmacotherapy and institute appropriate patient education.

QUESTIONS FOR STUDY AND REVIEW

1. Identify elements of the environment essential for the nurse to assess regarding drug therapy.
2. How can smoking, alcohol, or environmental chemical exposures influence the response of a patient's drug response?
3. What is the nurse's role in managing the patient with environmental considerations?

NEED MORE HELP?

Chapter 12 of the study guide for *Drug Therapy in Nursing* contains exercises and activities to reinforce your understanding of the concepts presented in this chapter. For additional information see the text's accompanying website at *http://www.connection.lww.com.*

REFERENCES AND BIBLIOGRAPHY

Fauci, A., Braunwald, E., Wilson, J. D., Martin, J. B., Hauser, S. L., Longo, D. L., Kasper, D. L., Isselbachter, K. J. (Eds.). (1999). *Harrison's online.* New York: McGraw-Hill.

Katzung, B. C. (Ed.). (2000). *Basic and clinical pharmacology.* (8th ed.). New York: McGraw-Hill.

Greene, R. J., & Harris, N. D. (2000). *Pathology and therapeutics for pharmacists* (4th ed.). London: Pharmaceutical Press.

Hardman, J. G., Limbird, L. E., Molinoff, P. B., Ruddon, R. W., & Gilman, A. G. (Eds.). (1997). *Goodman & Gilman's pharmacological basis of therapeutics.* (9th ed.). New York: McGraw-Hill Health Professions Division.

Levine, R. R., Walsh, C. T., & Schwartz-Bloom, R. D. (2000). Pharmacology: Drug actions and reactions (6th ed.). New York: The Parthenon Publishing Group.

Chapter 13

CULTURE: CONSIDERATIONS IN DRUG THERAPY

KEY TERMS

biocultural ecology
cultural blindness
cultural competence
culture
ethnicity
ethnocentrism
stereotyping

Learning Objectives

At the completion of this chapter the student will:

1. Identify the influences that culture and ethnicity have on health and illness.
2. Recognize similarities and differences among the five major ethnic groups in the United States.
3. Describe why it is important to assess a patient's culture when managing his or her drug therapy.
4. Describe techniques that can be used in nursing management in drug therapy when working with patients and families of different cultures.

North America has been called a "melting pot." A better term of description might be "cultural mosaic," because this signifies that individuals who emigrate to North America blend into society while retaining their individuality in terms of their culture. **Culture** is the shared customs and traditions, norms and values, institutions, arts, history, and folklore of a group. Similarly, **ethnicity** refers to a group that shares a common cultural heritage and that is linked by race, nationality, or language. An ethnic group is part of a larger social group.

The United States is becoming an increasingly multicultural society. In terms of nursing management and drug therapy, this means that a patient's basic beliefs about health and disease may vary based on his or her cultural heritage. American society is primarily composed of five major ethnic population subgroups: whites, blacks, Asians/Pacific Islanders, Hispanics, and Native Americans. Each native and immigrant group has special cultural attitudes to contribute in terms of health, illness, and health care practices. Within each group, cultural attitudes, customs, and values may also vary widely (i.e., not all members of a culture have identical beliefs and practices). There is also a tendency for members of minority cultures to assume some or all of the practices and beliefs of the majority. Some aspects of minority cultures also become consumed into the practices of the majority, producing a blend of cultural beliefs and attitudes.

Nurses today are being challenged to learn more about how cultural differences affect health, influence health-seeking behaviors, influence a patient's adherence or nonadherence to treatment regimens, and alter their responses to drug therapy. Nurses already know that language and economics continue to be the main barriers to appropriate health care for many culturally diverse populations.

As patient populations become more culturally diverse, cultural competence becomes another feature of skillful nursing. **Cultural competence** is an awareness of one's own values and beliefs without letting them have undue influence on those of other backgrounds, a demonstration of knowledge and understanding of another's culture, acceptance of and respect for cultural differences, and adoption of care in consideration of a patient's culture.

Nurses must be aware that patients with various cultural and ethnic backgrounds may have beliefs and practices that differ from their own. These beliefs and practices are not wrong or inferior, merely different. Regardless of the patient's ethnicity or cultural background, nurses must be mindful of patients' beliefs and practices and consider them respectfully when managing drug therapy.

Ethnic groups share similarities in biologic and cultural characteristics. The term **biocultural ecology** (Purnell & Paulanka, 1998) refers to specific physical, biologic, and psychological variations in ethnic and racial groups. These variations include skin color; physical body differences; genetic, hereditary, endemic, and topographic diseases; individual psychological makeup; and biologic differences that affect the ways drugs are metabolized.

Recent pharmaceutical research has revealed that there are some differences in drug metabolism, dosing requirements, therapeutic response, and adverse effects among racial and ethnic groups. For the purposes of this text, the core patient variable of culture is to be interpreted broadly. In this text, the term *culture* includes religious practices and beliefs, the use of medical or other health practices, ethnicity, and genetic variations—all of which may influence a patient's behavior in health and in illness.

WORLD VIEW

Culture represents a way of perceiving, behaving in, and evaluating the world. A person's cultural identify influences his or her perception of the environment. Beliefs about the causes and effects of illness, health practices, and health-seeking behaviors are all influenced by a person's or group's perception of the environment—the world view. Three kinds of world-view health beliefs have been identified. These perspectives are known as biomedical health beliefs, magicoreligious health beliefs, and holistic health beliefs.

BIOMEDICAL VIEW

In general, North Americans describe health from the scientific point of view. Scientific thinking underlies the biomedical view of health, in which life and life processes are controlled by physical and biochemical processes that can be manipulated by humans. For example, specific causes (bacteria, viruses) for an illness can be identified and a specific treatment (drug therapy, surgery) can be developed to effect a cure.

MAGICORELIGIOUS VIEW

Predominant themes of magicoreligious health beliefs among some cultural groups focus on the concept of supernatural forces controlling health and illness as well as illness's being the result of "being bad" or "opposing God's will." Those who ascribe to these views perceive health as a gift from God and illness as an opportunity to realign with God. Prayer to God is used to cope with disease and to seek intervention for healing. Some cultures (e.g., West Indian) believe that magic, voodoo, or a hex or spell by a sorcerer or witch can cause illness. Some Mexican-American and other Latin-American groups believe that illness results from selection by the evil eye, or *mal ojo*. In these cases, the person will seek treatment from a traditional or folk healer, perhaps in addition to scientific therapies. The person's subscription to magicoreligious health beliefs influences his or her approach to health care.

HOLISTIC VIEW

A harmonious balance of the forces of nature is the basis of the holistic health belief view. According to this view, everything in the universe has a place and a function to perform according to natural laws that maintain order. Disturbance of these laws creates imbalance, chaos, and disease. Four facets of the individual's nature—physical, mental, emotional, and spiritual—must be in balance and harmony for the individual to be healthy.

Traditional Native-American and Chinese-American cultures have a holistic belief system. Disease occurs when an imbalance exists in the individual's nature. An example of holistic health beliefs among Chinese-American groups is the yin and yang theory of health and illness; among Mexican-American and other Hispanic groups, it is the hot and cold theory of illness. Therapies that may be used to restore a state of balance may include exercise, herbal remedies, meditation, and nutritional or dietary changes.

For example, within the biomedical worldview of health, tuberculosis is clearly defined as an infection caused by *Mycobacteria*. According to a holistic world view, however, in which disease results from multiple environmental "hot" interactions, tuberculosis is caused by the interrelationships of poverty, malnutrition, overcrowding, and mycobacteria.

IMPACT OF CULTURAL DIVERSITY ON HEALTH CARE

PURNELL'S MODEL FOR CULTURAL COMPETENCE

To understand any culture thoroughly, it is helpful to examine it with the use of a conceptual framework. Purnell and Paulanka's evolving model for cultural competence (Purnell & Paulanka, 1998) is an example of a conceptual framework that is geared specifically to health care providers. This model identifies 12 aspects (or domains) of every culture that health care providers should consider. The domains are:

1. Overview (heritage and residence)
2. Communication
3. Family roles and organization
4. Workforce issues
5. Biocultural ecology
6. High-risk health behaviors
7. Nutrition
8. Pregnancy and child-bearing practices
9. Death rituals
10. Spirituality
11. Health care practices
12. Health care practitioners

This text does not intend to present comprehensive descriptions of every culture in the United States, nor does it provide instructions for performing a comprehensive cultural assessment. For this text, the intention is to provide general knowledge of cultural concerns relevant to nursing management in drug therapy. With that intent, a brief description of the factors related to nursing management in drug therapy and the five most common cultures in the United States are presented. Although Purnell and Paulanka's model is evolving, certain domains are easily applicable to nursing management in drug therapy. These aspects are overview (heritage and residence), communication, family roles and organization, spirituality, health care practices, and biocultural ecology.

According to Purnell and Paulanka's model, heritage describes where a people come from and residence describes where they currently live. Heritage and residence are important factors to consider because they provides clues about potential illnesses or conditions that may be present in the patient and require drug therapy. For example, new immigrants to the United States who have lived in areas where malaria is prevalent (e.g., Egypt, Italy, Turkey, Vietnam) may need to be screened for malaria, and if they test positive, to receive drug treatment. Another example: patients who currently live in crowded, poor, urban areas may need to be screened for tuberculosis.

Communication is an important part of culture for the nurse to assess. Communication includes verbal language (including dominant language, dialects, contextual use of words, and paralanguage variations such as voice volume, tone, and inflection) and nonverbal language (e.g., eye contact, facial expression, use of touch, and temporality of world view). Temporal relationships are defined according to whether a culture is oriented to the past, present, or the future (Purnell & Paulanka, 1998). Past-oriented cultures (e.g., German) may value the importance of providing historical background before presenting new information. Present-oriented cultures (e.g., Chinese) place more importance on the "here and now" than on the past or future. Future-oriented cultures (e.g., white American, Europeans) believe it is important to prepare for what lies ahead. Punctuality is also part of temporal relationships; some cultures see promptness as important for all aspects of life, whereas others may be more relaxed about time, especially in social situations. The nurse needs to be mindful of all of these issues when working with patients. The ability to communicate effectively with a patient will have a major impact on assessment, teaching, and the entire nurse—patient relationship.

The domain of family roles and organization defines the relationships among those inside and outside the family. Family roles and organization include head of household and gender roles; family goals and priorities; developmental tasks of children and adolescents; roles of the aged and extended family; social status; and acceptance or nonacceptance of nontraditional lifestyles (e.g., divorce, single parenting, same-sex relationships). This information is important for the nurse to consider when providing teaching to the patient and family. For example, some Middle Eastern men may feel that the health care provider does not respect them as the head of the family if patient education is directed toward a female family member (even if the woman is the patient).

Spirituality includes all formal religious beliefs and the use of prayer. It also includes all behaviors that provide meaning to life and strength to the individual. Spirituality may influence nutrition, health care practices, and the other cultural domains. Identifying sources of strength and comfort for patients is important because these resources assist in promoting health and higher-level wellness. The nurse should consider spirituality to treat the patient holistically.

Health care practices include the focus of typical care (acute or preventive); the basis for health care (traditional, magicoreligious, or biomedical); beliefs regarding individual responsibility for health; self-medicating practices; views about mental illness, chronic illness, rehabilitation, organ donation, and transplantation; and responses to pain and the sick role. These practices not only influence how a patient re-

For example, alpha thalassemia, an inherited disorder of hemoglobin metabolism, affects Chinese Americans with greater frequency than other cultural groups (except those of Mediterranean origin), placing them at greater risk for anemia. In addition, a sex-linked genetic disease—a deficiency of glucose-6-dehydrogenase (G6PD)—is common in the Chinese American (Gaspard, 1994). This disease is characterized by a lack of the G6PD enzyme and results in anemia. Chinese-American populations also have an increased incidence of lactose intolerance, which leads to gastric symptoms, such as diarrhea, when milk or other dairy products are consumed. Certain drugs are metabolized differently and have different effects in Chinese Americans (Levy, 1993). Among these drugs are mephenytoin (Mesantoin), diazepam (Valium) (poorly metabolized in 15% to 20% of Chinese Americans); beta blockers, atropine (Sal-Tropin), and alcohol (increased sensitivity); antidepressants and neuroleptics (increased responses at lower doses) and analgesics (decreased sensitivity, but increased gastrointestinal [GI] adverse effects). Specific variations of drug metabolism among Chinese Americans is difficult to determine because most clinical drug studies have not differentiated them from other Asians.

Some variation of drug response by Chinese Americans is not related to differences in drug metabolism. Lithium carbonate (Eskalith), used in managing bipolar disorder, is a drug that is not metabolized but has a different effect in Chinese Americans than in Europeans and whites. Chinese Americans require lower levels of lithium to have a therapeutic response. Part of the explanation for the differences in drug response lies in the number and type of drug receptors. Just as different drugs can be metabolized only by specific liver enzymes, receptors are custom designed to accept only certain drug configurations. As with enzymes, the number and type of receptors are influenced by genetics. Chinese Americans, and other Chinese people, appear to have a greater number of lithium-activated receptors.

Hispanic Americans

Hispanic Americans are a large minority in the United States because of birth rates and immigration. Members of the Hispanic-American community have their origins primarily in Puerto Rico, and in Mexico, Cuba, and other Latin American countries. For discussion here, the culture of Mexican Americans will be presented.

Mexican Americans may speak either Spanish or English as their primary language. They may also be bilingual. Historically, Mexican Americans were more present oriented than future oriented. Because time is viewed as relative, punctuality is relaxed, especially in social situations, although in modern society, the trend is toward greater punctuality. Mexican-American families tend to be patriarchal with the male head of the household as the primary decision maker. These roles too are changing, with greater responsibility being shared with female family members.

Although some Mexican Americans tend to view life as chance, believing that health is purely the result of good luck (if one's good luck changes, so does one's good health), others have a dominant fatalism and hold the opinion that God is responsible for delivering health or illness and that good health should not be taken for granted. Still others are deeply involved in formal religions, primarily Catholicism but also with the Church of Jesus Christ of Latter Day Saints (LDS), Jehovah's Witnesses, Seventh Day Adventists, Presbyterians, and Baptists. In this context, appropriate ways of preventing ill health involve using herbs and spices, praying and wearing religious artifacts, and maintaining a balanced diet and physical activity. Socioeconomic and educational backgrounds will influence the beliefs held by the individual Mexican American.

Individuals are expected to maintain equilibrium by eating and working properly. Good health exists when the biologic, psychosocial, and spiritual natures are holistically balanced in relation to the environment. The more serious physical and mental-emotional illnesses are brought to the male *curandero* or female *curandera*, who is a holistic healer in the community. The use of herbs (commonly in the form of teas and poultices) is a popular treatment offered by folk healers. Western medicine is also used.

As with other cultural groups, Mexican Americans believe that disease occurs when there is an imbalance between opposing life forces. For Mexican Americans, these forces are perceived as hot, cold, wet, and dry. The body is composed of four kinds of fluids (also known as humors), which may vary in temperature and moisture content. They are blood (hot and wet), yellow bile (hot and dry), phlegm (cold and wet), and black bile (cold and dry). Imbalances may exist among these fluids, and these imbalances are manifested as illness. Maintaining a balance between these is important to promote wellness. When the four humors are balanced, the body is healthy.

These concepts provide a way of determining the remedy for a particular illness. Illness is thought to be caused by prolonged exposure to hot or cold; to cure the illness, the opposite quality of the etiologic agent is applied to absorb the hot or cold. For example, a cold substance is used to treat a hot illness. Hot conditions include constipation, diarrhea, fever, infections, kidney problems, liver problems, rashes, skin ailments, sore throat, and ulcers. Cold foods include barley water, chicken, fish, dairy products, fresh vegetables, goat meat, honey, raisins, and tropical fruits. Cold herbs and medicines include linden, milk of magnesia, orange-flower water, sage, and sodium bicarbonate.

Conversely, hot substances are used to treat cold conditions. Cold conditions include cancer, colds, dysmenorrhea, earache, headache, joint pains, malaria, paralysis, pneumonia, rheumatism, stomach cramps, teething pain, and tuberculosis. Hot foods include aromatic beverages, beef, cheese, chili peppers, chocolate, eggs, pork, liquor, goat milk, onions, peas, temperate-zone fruits, and whole grains (except barley). Hot herbs and medicines include anise, aspirin, cinnamon, castor oil, cod-liver oil, iron preparations, garlic, ginger, penicillin, tobacco, and vitamin preparations.

It is important to remember that hot and cold do not refer to temperature but are descriptive of the nature of a particular substance. Food, beverages, animals, and people possess the characteristics of hot and cold in varying degrees. Other

Hispanic groups also consider items as hot or cold, but different substances are classified into these categories.

Few clinical drug studies have separated Mexican Americans from other Hispanics, so information regarding variations in drug metabolism must be generalized from findings related to Hispanics. There have been some studies that show that Hispanics may metabolize some drugs differently from other cultural groups. For example, studies indicate that Hispanics need lower doses of antidepressants and experience greater adverse effects from these drugs. Further complicating the issue is the fact that many Mexican Americans have mixed heritage. Thus, generalizations may not be accurate for all Mexican Americans. See the accompanying display, Diversity, Drug Therapy, and Implications for Teaching.

Native Americans

The Native-American population in the United States consists of more than 500 federally recognized tribes as well as many others that are not so recognized. Native Americans (or American Indians) are the original inhabitants of North America, and each tribal community is unique in its cultural beliefs. The Navajo Indians are the largest tribe that requires that the person have at least one-quarter Navajo blood to be considered part of the tribe. The Navajo Indians will be presented as the example of Native Americans.

The Navajo tribe lives in a large reservation that consists of portions of Arizona, Utah, and New Mexico. In New Mexico, they are more scattered and live with Zuñi Indians and settlers from the LDS church. A nomadic people, the Navajo will travel great distances searching for adequate grazing grounds for their sheep. Navajo Indians speak Navajo, which until the 1970s was only a spoken language. A few older Navajo people will speak some English or Spanish; younger Navajo are usually bilingual and speak Navajo and English. The Navajo and Apache have similar languages but their dialects are different. Minor variations in the pronunciation of Navajo words may change the meaning of the word or phrase spoken. Navajo Indians believe that silence is an appropriate way to communicate nonverbally and feel comfortable even during long silences. Navajos, especially older people, take their time to respond carefully and thoughtfully to what is said to them.

In contrast to whites, who view time in a present-future-past sequence, Navajo Indians view time in a present-past-future sequence. This means that Native Americans attach little value to planning for the future, often considering it foolish. Time has little meaning or importance. Activities begin when people or members of a group gather.

Navajo, like most other Native Americans, are matrilineal. Men are important, but grandmothers and mothers are the center of society. No decisions are made unless the appropriate older woman is present.

Native-American religion predominates among the Navajo, although some have been converted to Christian religions, such as the LDS church, Jehovah's Witnesses, and some evangelical groups. The Navajo Indians view spirituality as being in a state of harmony with one's surroundings. Prayer is important. Spirituality cannot be separated from healing and is important in healing ceremonies. Illnesses result from not being in harmony with nature, from the spirits of an evil person, such as a witch, or from violating tribal taboos. Healing ceremonies restore mental, physical, and spiritual balance. The Navajo may use Western medicine in addition to healing from tribal ceremonies.

Type 2 diabetes is very common among Navajo, as it is among all Native Americans. Other health problems common to the Navajo are severe combined immunodeficiency syndrome (failure of antibody response and cell-mediated immunity, not related to AIDS), Navajo neuropathy (an inherited condition in which there is complete absence of myelinated fibers and death occurs before age 24), albinism, and genetic blindness. Although little research has been conducted on variation in drug metabolism in Navajos, or other Native Americans, it is known that Navajo can have increased adverse effects to some medications. For example, adverse reactions to lidocaine (Xylocaine), an anesthetic and antiarrhythmic, occur in 29% of Navajos but only in 11% to 15% of whites.

Critical Thinking Scenario

Diversity, drug therapy, and implications for teaching

Forty-nine-year-old Maria Alvarez is a bilingual Mexican American. She is newly diagnosed with type 2 diabetes with prescribed "diabetic teaching" related to insulin administration. The nurse reviews cultural phenomena affecting health and health care among Mexican Americans and adult teaching-learning principles before working with Mrs. Alvarez.

1. What are some of the most significant considerations for the nurse to explore prior to teaching Mrs. Alvarez?
2. During one of the teaching sessions, the nurse plans to use pamphlets to teach Mrs. Alvarez about insulin. What may be a limitation of printed material?

NURSING MANAGEMENT OF CULTURALLY DIVERSE GROUPS

In administering drug therapy to culturally diverse patient populations, the nurse needs to respect each patient's cultural heritage, beliefs, and practices. A health care provider not fully aware of a patient's background may be unable to understand many of the patient's health beliefs and practices. Lack of knowledge or misunderstanding may unintentionally turn what should be a therapeutic experience into a degrading and humiliating experience for patients of other cultures. If possible, every effort should be made to accommodate the patient's traditional practices with standard drug therapy while providing nursing care to maximize therapeutic effects, minimize adverse effects, and promote health and safety for the patient and the family.

When caring for patients, the nurse should be conscious of ethnocentrism, stereotyping, and cultural blindness. Because culture influences individuals so strongly in the way they feel, think, act, and judge the world, it is not atypical for individuals to subconsciously restrict their view of the world to the point of being unable to accept other cultures. This is called ethnocentrism. Health care providers exhibit ethnocentricity if they act from the mistaken belief that only their own cultural and ethnic beliefs are normal, superior, or right. **Ethnocentrism** inhibits acceptance of others and may lead to a clash of values and poor communication. **Stereotyping** means making the assumption that all patients of a particular culture or ethnic group will have the same response.

Health care providers may exhibit **cultural blindness** if they proceed as if differences do not exist. Because the American health care system is based on the dominant pattern of Western scientific health beliefs and practices, it is not uncommon for health care providers to dismiss any deviations from the established pattern. The implication of all this is clear: throughout care, nurses must remember to be nonjudgmental and to convey respect.

Nursing Diagnoses and Outcomes

When developing nursing diagnoses, the nurse needs to be aware of cultural beliefs, values, and behaviors that may influence the patient's situation. Although all nursing diagnoses may have related cultural factors, some can be specifically identified as having strong cultural implications (see the accompanying display, Nursing Diagnoses and Outcomes Related to Drug Therapy and Cultural Diversity).

Nursing Diagnoses and Outcomes Related to Drug Therapy and Cultural Diversity

Impaired Verbal Communication

Desired outcome: Effective communication about drug therapy will be established among the patient, patient's family, and health care providers, despite possible language differences.

Anxiety related to new drug treatment

Desired outcome: Patient will recognize and express feelings of anxiety and will identify potential and actual sources of anxiety when health care practices during drug therapy interfere with cultural habits and health practices.

Fear of Health Seeking Behaviors related to barriers to health care (e.g., caregiver's judgments of nonadherence or deviant behaviors) or fear of being criticized for traditional practices and inability to communicate these needs effectively in the English language

Desired outcome: Patient will recognize and express feelings of spiritual distress when health care practices, such as drug therapy, interfere with spiritual beliefs.

Ineffective Health Maintenance

Desired outcome: Patient (and family) will verbalize an understanding of beneficial, neutral, and harmful cultural health practices as they relate to drug therapy.

Ineffective Coping or Disabled Family Coping

Desired outcome: Individual (or family) will more effectively deal with stress after talking with health care provider who explains the reason for expected outcome of planned drug therapy as it relates to cultural beliefs and practices.

Spiritual Distress

Desired outcome: Patient will recognize feelings of spiritual distress when health care practices, such as drug therapy, interfere with traditional beliefs and habits.

Planning and Intervention

After the beliefs of the patient and family about health and disease, drugs and drug therapy, personal health habits, and chronic illness are assessed, planning and implementation may proceed.

Maximizing Therapeutic Effects

When drug therapy is recommended, the nurse must make an effort to determine whether prescribed therapies are consistent with the patients' physical needs, cultural backgrounds, religious preferences, dietary preferences, and self-care practices. The nurse can then incorporate them into nursing practice whenever possible and when not contraindicated for health reasons.

Minimizing Adverse Effects

Nurses and patients need to be aware that certain cultural practices (e.g., using herbal preparations in addition to conventional drug therapy) may create drug toxicity or herb-drug interactions. Conventional prescribed drugs may have similar or antagonistic actions to an herb or herbal product. For example, overmedication may result when ginseng (a tonic stimulant and an antihypertensive) is taken in combination with an antihypertensive drug (Spector, 1996). Some foods may also interact with some drug therapies; normal dietary patterns need to be assessed to help prevent this (see Chapter 11).

Providing Patient and Family Education

The communication style of the patient should be considered when preparing to provide patient education. The reasons for a treatment plan must be shared with patients and families and explained in language and at levels they can understand. When planning educational materials for patients whose primary language is not English, nurses should make every effort to obtain interpreters or translations of written materials. Interpreters are preferred to translators because an interpreter will make sure that the meaning behind the message is the same; translators merely change the words from one language to another (see the accompanying display,

Communicating With Patients Who Speak Another Language). Pictures that reinforce the content of the verbal and written instructions are also helpful. Many computer systems are available that can automatically translate instructions into other languages (e.g., Spanish). Computer programs can also alter the level of language to be appropriate for the patient's educational background. Nurses should compile and maintain a listing of community resources that are available to assist patients of different cultures.

If the patient is present-time oriented, his or her understanding of acute and chronic illness may be affected by the perception of time. In such cases, the nurse teaching a patient about drugs for a chronic disease (e.g., hypertension) may be more successful emphasizing short-term problems (e.g., what may happen if the drug is not taken on time) than long-term problems, such as stroke and myocardial infarction.

The nurse should also consider gender roles and the importance of various family relationships to the patient when teaching about drug therapy. Be certain that the appropriate person is present before you begin. For example, this might be the grandmother of a Navajo Indian patient or the husband of a Mexican-American woman.

Ongoing Assessment and Evaluation

To evaluate the effectiveness of nursing care for a patient of another culture, the nurse determines the extent to which the goals have been met by comparing the patient's current status with the identified outcome criteria. ■

Communicating With Patients Who Speak Another Language

Use an interpreter (preferably) or a translator. Use dialect-specific interpreters (if possible) trained in health care. If possible, use an interpreter of the same age and same gender as the patient.

- Look at the patient when you speak, not at the interpreter.
- Speak slowly.
- Do not raise your voice or exaggerate your mouth movements.
- Provide time for interpretation or translation.
- Allow time for the patient to think before he or she responds.
- Avoid using relatives and children as interpreters; they may not be objective and the patient or relative may be embarrassed by the content of the discussion.
- Listen attentively.

If interpreter or translator is not available:

- Remember that patients often understand more language than they can speak.
- Limit the number of words you use, and include as many words of the patient's language as possible.
- Speak slowly, but not loudly.
- Use nonverbal language.

CHAPTER SUMMARY

- Many cultural groups in North America embrace both their original culture and the dominant North American culture.
- Although generalizations may be made regarding the beliefs of different cultural groups, these statements cannot be applied to all individuals sharing a cultural background. Every individual must be assessed for his or her unique beliefs.
- Individual health-seeking behaviors and health practices exist and differ, sometimes markedly, among the major cultural groups in the United States.
- Medicinal plants and symbolic rituals play significant roles in the health practices of many cultural groups.
- Patients should be advised of the potential for chemical interactions between folk medicine or herbal remedies and traditional (Western) drug therapy.
- Factors related to communication, time, and environmental control influence the relationship between the nurse and the patient whose backgrounds are culturally different.
- Individual variation in response to the effects of drugs and pharmacokinetic drug differences may occur because of biologic and genetic differences among individuals. For example, some patients may metabolize certain drugs more slowly because of a genetically induced enzyme deficiency.
- Nursing management should emphasize a thorough assessment of a patient's health beliefs, traditional practices, and cultural influences, so that the nurse and other health care providers may implement interventions that complement the patient's values. Therapeutic regimens that accommodate a patient's cultural values (and traditional rituals) are more likely to foster adherence to drug therapy and discourage alienation from the health care system.
- Cultural, ethnic, and environmental influences add complex issues to pharmacotherapy.

QUESTIONS FOR STUDY AND REVIEW

1. How does culture differ from ethnic group?
2. How is an awareness of cultural differences helpful when providing nursing management in drug therapy?
3. Describe strategies that can be used when your patient does not speak the same language as you.
4. Explain how an individual's concept of time will influence patient teaching about drug therapy.
5. Why are clinical drug studies that describe a drug's altered pharmacokinetic process in Hispanics not always very applicable to Mexican Americans?

NEED MORE HELP?

Chapter 13 of the study guide for *Drug Therapy in Nursing* contains exercises and activities to reinforce your understanding of the concepts presented in this chapter. For additional information see the text's accompanying website at *http://www.connection.lww.com.*

REFERENCES AND BIBLIOGRAPHY

Andrews, M. M., & Boyle, J. S. (1995). *Transcultural concepts in nursing care* (2nd ed.). Philadelphia: J. B. Lippincott.

Caraco, Y., Sheller, J., & Wood, A. J. (1999). Impact of ethnic origin and quinidine coadministration on codeine's disposition and pharmacodynamics effects. *Journal of Pharmacology and Experimental Therapeutics, 290*(1), 413–422.

Ding, P. Y., Hu, O.,Y., Pool, P. E., & Liao, W. (2000). Does Chinese ethnicity affect the pharmacokinetics and pharmacodynamics of angiotensin-converting enzyme inhibitors? *Journal of Human Hypertension, 14*(3), 163–170.

Ergul, A., Tackett, R. L., & Puett, D. (1999). Distribution of endothelin receptors in saphenous veins of African Americans: Implications of racial differences. *Journal of Cardiovascular Pharmacology, 34*(3), 327–332.

Gaspard, K. J. (1994). The red blood cell and alterations in oxygen transport. In C. M. Porth (Ed.). *Pathophysiology: Concepts of altered states* (4th ed., pp. 323–339). Philadelphia: J. B. Lippincott.

Johnson, J. A. (2000). Predictability of the effects of race or ethnicity on pharmacokinetics of drugs. *International Journal of Clinical Pharmacology and Therapeutics, 38*(2), 53–60.

Jones, J., Ritenbaugh, C., Spence, M., & Hayward, A. (1991). Severe combined immunodeficiency among the Navajo: Characterization of phenotypes, epidemiology and population genetics. *Human Biology, 63*(5), 669–682.

Kalow, W. (1984). Pharmaco-anthropology outline: Problems and nature of case history. *Federation Proceedings, 43*(8), 2314–2318.

Leininger, M. (1995). *Transcultural nursing: Concepts, theories, research and practice* (2nd ed.). New York & Columbus, OH: McGraw-Hill and Greyden Press.

Levy, R. (1993). Ethnic and racial differences in response to medicines: Preserving individualized therapy in managed pharmaceutical programs. *Pharmaceutical Medicine, 7*, 139–165.

Purnell, L. D., & Paulanka, B. J. (1998). *Transcultural health care.* Philadelphia: F. A. Davis.

Strickland, T. L., Ranganath, V., Lin, K-M., Poland, R. E., Mendoza, R., & Smith, M. W. (1991). Psychopharmacologic considerations in the treatment of black American populations. *Psychopharmacology Bulletin, 27*(4), 441–448.

Unit IV

Peripheral Nervous System Drugs

Chapter 14

DRUGS AFFECTING ADRENERGIC FUNCTION

KEY TERMS

adrenergic nervous system
agonists
antagonists
autonomic nervous system
central nervous system
neurotransmitters
nonselective-acting drugs
parasympathetic nervous system
peripheral nervous system
selective-acting drugs
sympathetic nervous system
synaptic transmission

Learning Objectives

At the completion of this chapter the student will:

1. Describe the anatomy and physiology of the adrenergic nervous system.
2. Describe synaptic transmission.
3. Describe the role of adrenergic agonists and antagonists in a variety of therapeutic uses.
4. Identify core drug knowledge about drugs that act as adrenergic agonists or antagonists.
5. Identify core patient variables relevant to drugs that act as adrenergic agonists or antagonists.
6. Relate the interaction of core drug knowledge to core patient variables for drugs that act as adrenergic agonists or antagonists.
7. Generate a nursing plan of care from the interactions between core drug knowledge and core patient variables for drugs that act as adrenergic agonists or antagonists.
8. Describe nursing interventions to maximize therapeutic and minimize adverse affects for drugs that act as adrenergic agonists or antagonists.
9. Determine key points for patient and family education for drugs that act as adrenergic agonists or antagonists.

Adrenergic agonists

Nonselective adrenergic agonists
- **epinephrine**
- ephedrine
- norepinephrine

Alpha-1 adrenergic agonists
- **phenylephrine**
- methoxamine

Alpha-2 adrenergic agonists
- clonidine

Beta adrenergic agonists
- **isoproterenol**
- dopamine
- dobutamine
- respiratory agents

Adrenergic antagonists

Alpha adrenergic antagonists
- **prazosin**
- doxazosin
- terazosin
- phentolamine
- phenoxybenzamine

Beta adrenergic antagonists
- **propranolol**
- atenolol
- metoprolol
- pindolol
- nadolol
- timolol
- carvedilol
- labetalol
- sotalol

The symbol (C) indicates the **drug class**.
Drugs in bold type marked with the symbol (P) are **prototypes**.
Drugs in blue type with no symbol are **closely related** to the prototype.
Drugs in **red** type with no symbol are **significantly different** from the prototype.
Drugs in **black** type with no symbol are **also used in drug therapy**; no prototype.

The nervous system is divided into two main branches: the **central nervous system** (CNS) and the **peripheral nervous system** (PNS) (Fig. 14-1). The CNS is composed of the brain and spinal cord. The PNS consists of all neurons that are found outside the brain and spinal cord. The PNS is further subdivided into two major divisions: efferent and afferent. The efferent division has neurons that carry signals away from the brain and spinal cord to the periphery, whereas the afferent division contains neurons that carry impulses from the periphery to the CNS. The efferent division may be further subdivided into the somatic nervous system and the **autonomic nervous system** (ANS). The ANS is further subdivided into the **sympathetic nervous system** (SNS) and the **parasympathetic nervous system** (PSNS).

This chapter focuses on drugs that affect the **adrenergic nervous system** (ANS). These drugs include adrenergic **agonists** (stimulators) and adrenergic **antagonists** (blockers). The prototype nonselective adrenergic agonist is epinephrine. The prototype alpha-1 agonist is phenylephrine, and the prototype alpha-2 agonist is clonidine. The prototype nonselective beta agonist is isoproterenol. The adrenergic antagonists are categorized similarly. Phentolamine is the prototype nonselective alpha antagonist, whereas the prototype nonselective beta-adrenergic antagonist (more commonly referred to as a beta-adrenergic blocker) is propranolol. Prazosin is the prototype alpha-1 adrenergic antagonist.

PHYSIOLOGY

FUNCTION OF THE AUTONOMIC NERVOUS SYSTEM

The ANS has been identified as an involuntary system responsible for the control of smooth muscle (e.g., bronchi, blood vessels, and gastrointestinal [GI] tract), cardiac muscle, and exocrine glands (e.g., gastric, sweat, and salivary glands). These regulatory functions of the body are monitored by both the SNS and PSNS.

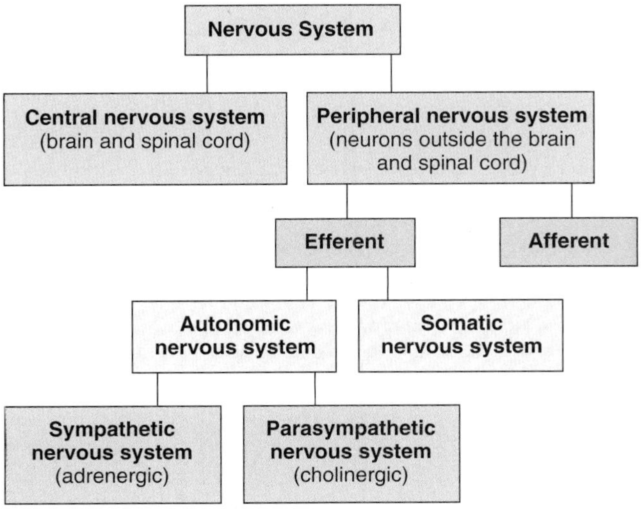

Figure 14-1. The human nervous system.

REGULATION OF PHYSIOLOGIC PROCESSES

Organs and tissues in the body may be stimulated by the SNS or PSNS. Some organs and tissues are regulated by both. When both the SNS and PSNS stimulate a particular organ or tissue, the action may be oppositional or complementary. Figure 14-2 presents the major effects of the SNS and PSNS on the body.

SYNAPTIC TRANSMISSION

The actual connection between neurons and effector organs or tissues relies on **neurotransmitters** and **synaptic transmission**. The neurotransmitters in the ANS include acetylcholine (ACh), norepinephrine (NE), and epinephrine (Epi). The major neurotransmitter SNS is ACh. Synaptic transmission initially involves the synthesis of neurotransmitters in the nerve terminal with subsequent storage of the neurotransmitter awaiting an action potential that allows the neurotransmitter to be released. After release, the neurotransmitter diffuses across the synaptic gap and reversibly binds to a receptor on the postsynaptic cell. After binding and exerting an effect, the neurotransmitter is dissociated from its binding site by a variety of mechanisms that then allow the neurotransmitter to be degraded or "reuptaked" for reuse (Fig. 14-3). To effect an action, the neurotransmitter needs to bind with an appropriate receptor site on the effector organ or tissue. This simple statement reflects the entire concept of neuropharmacologic drug therapy.

In the SNS, preganglionic transmission is mediated by ACh, whereas postganglionic transmission is mediated by NE. ACh also stimulates the adrenal medulla to release Epi (Fig. 14-4). Once the postganglionic neurons transmit their impulse to the effector organs or tissues through their neurotransmitters, several events may occur. For example, beta-1 stimulation by NE increases the heart rate, while at the same time beta-2 stimulation induces bronchodilation.

NEUROTRANSMITTERS

Acetylcholine

The precursors to ACh are choline and acetyl-coenzyme A. After formation and storage, ACh is released in response to an action potential, then binds to cholinergic receptors on the target organs or tissues. After dissociation, ACh is degraded into two inactive products, acetate and choline, by acetylcholinesterase (AchE).

Norepinephrine

There are several precursors to NE including phenylalanine, tyrosine, dopa, and dopamine as the final step. NE is produced and stored in the presynaptic nerve terminals of the SNS. As with ACh, it responds to an action potential. NE may bind to presynaptic alpha-2 receptors or postsynaptic alpha-1- and beta-adrenergic receptors. Transmission is terminated by reuptake of NE back to the nerve terminal where it can be restored for further use or degraded by monamine oxidase.

Physiology

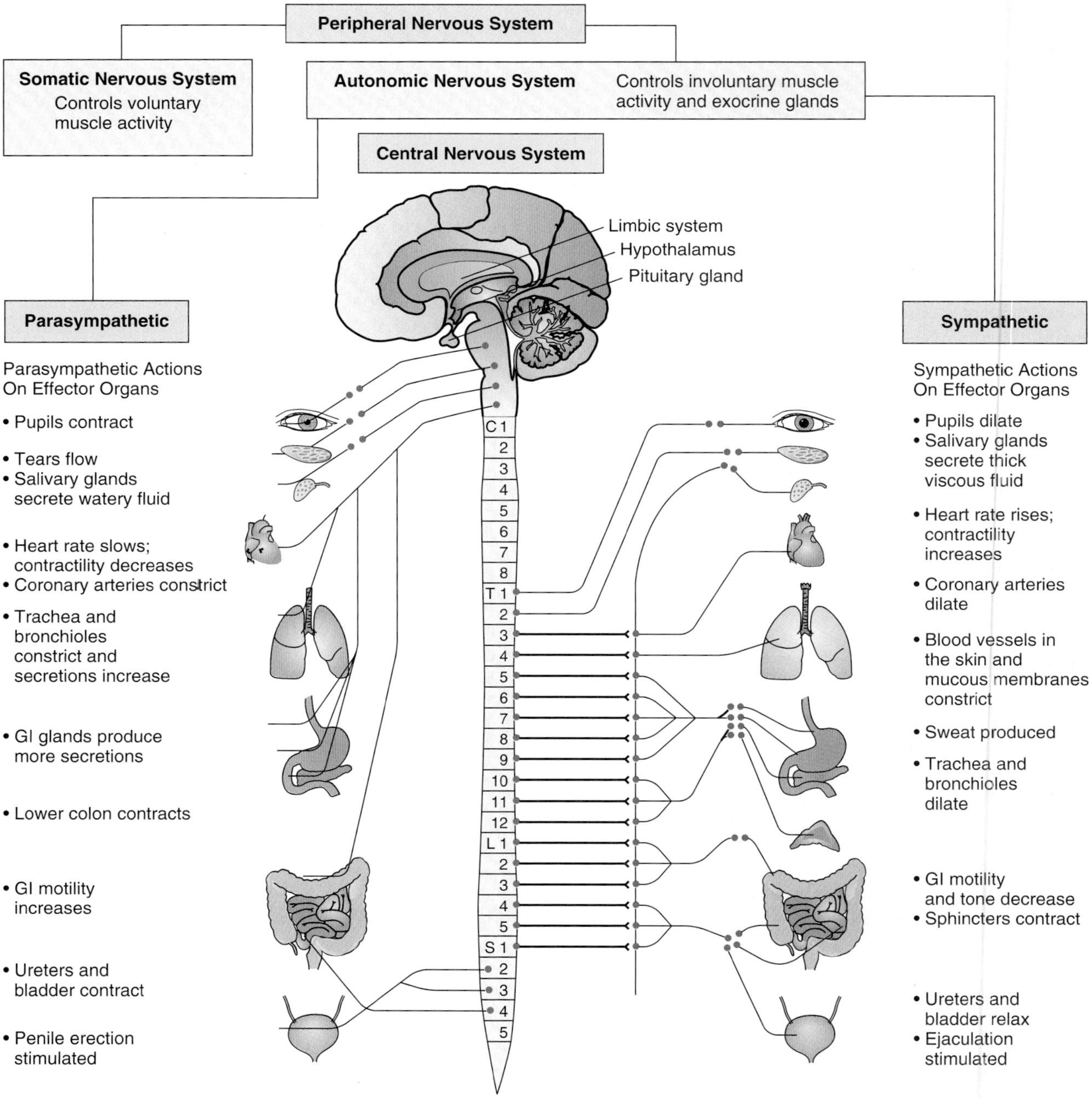
Peripheral Nervous System
Somatic Nervous System
Controls voluntary muscle activity
Autonomic Nervous System
Controls involuntary muscle activity and exocrine glands
Central Nervous System
Limbic system
Hypothalamus
Pituitary gland
Parasympathetic
Sympathetic
Parasympathetic Actions On Effector Organs
• Pupils contract
• Tears flow
• Salivary glands secrete watery fluid
• Heart rate slows; contractility decreases
• Coronary arteries constrict
• Trachea and bronchioles constrict and secretions increase
• GI glands produce more secretions
• Lower colon contracts
• GI motility increases
• Ureters and bladder contract
• Penile erection stimulated
Sympathetic Actions On Effector Organs
• Pupils dilate
• Salivary glands secrete thick viscous fluid
• Heart rate rises; contractility increases
• Coronary arteries dilate
• Blood vessels in the skin and mucous membranes constrict
• Sweat produced
• Trachea and bronchioles dilate
• GI motility and tone decrease
• Sphincters contract
• Ureters and bladder relax
• Ejaculation stimulated
C 1
2
3
4
5
6
7
8
T 1
2
3
4
5
6
7
8
9
10
11
12
L 1
2
3
4
5
S 1
2
3
4
5

Figure 14-2. Actions of the nervous system. While the brain and spinal cord make up the central nervous system (CNS), the neurons found outside the CNS make up the peripheral nervous system, which carries nerve impulses to and from the CNS over afferent (to the brain and spinal cord) and efferent (from the brain and spinal cord) pathways. The efferent pathways, which make up the autonomic nervous system, regulate voluntary and involuntary activities of the smooth muscles and glands. The autonomic nervous system is in charge of the parasympathetic and sympathetic nervous systems. The parasympathetic nerves govern craniosacral impulses, whereas the sympathetic nerves govern impulses associated with the thoracolumbar region. The parasympathetic nervous system is associated with decreased exocrine gland activity (tearing and salivation) and increased gastrointestinal activity (motility, secretion, and contraction). Drugs that affect parasympathetic function are known as cholinergic drugs. Those that stimulate parasympathetic activity are called cholinergic agonists; those that inhibit or block parasympathetic activity are called cholinergic antagonists or anticholinergic drugs.

Physiology

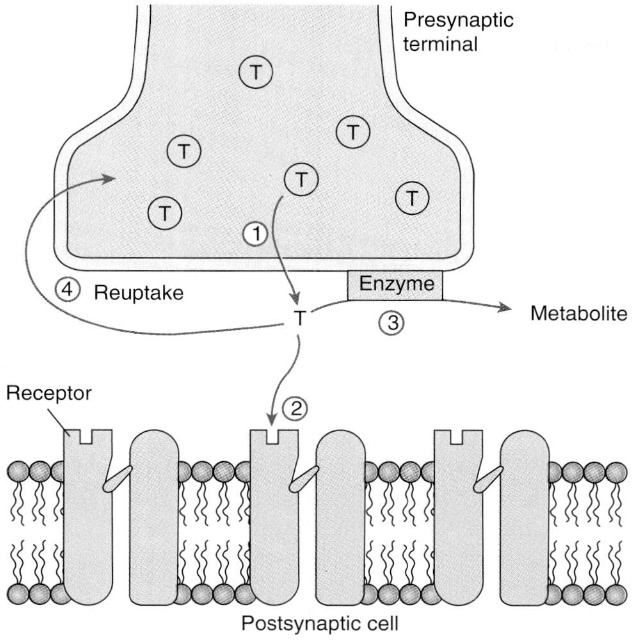

Figure 14-3. Synaptic transmission. (1) Neurotransmitter (T) release. (2) Transmitter binds to receptor. (3) Degradation of transmitter. (4) Reuptake of transmitter.

Epinephrine

Epinephrine is converted enzymatically from NE in the adrenal medulla. It is stored in the adrenal medulla and, like other neurotransmitters, responds to an action potential. It then travels through the bloodstream throughout the body to target organs. Its termination occurs through hepatic metabolism.

RECEPTORS

Receptors are either adrenergic or cholinergic. In the SNS, there are several types of adrenergic receptors, including alpha-adrenergic and beta-adrenergic receptors. Another type of receptor, the dopaminergic receptor, is related to adrenergic receptors in that dopamine is the precursor to NE. As such, it can activate both alpha- and beta-adrenergic receptors.

There are also subtypes of alpha- and beta-adrenergic receptors. The current significant adrenergic subtypes are alpha-1, alpha-2, beta-1, and beta-2 receptors. Dopaminergic receptors are known to exist as subtypes, and at least five have been identified.

Alpha-1 receptors are located in the eyes, blood vessels, bladder, male sex organs, and the prostatic capsule. Alpha-2 receptors are located in presynaptic nerve terminals. Beta-1 receptors are found primarily in the heart, but also in the kidney. Beta-2 receptors are located in the arterioles of the heart, lung, and skeletal muscles, as well as in the bronchi, uterus, liver, and skeletal muscle.

The subtypes respond to stimulation by one or more neurotransmitters. Alpha-1 and beta-1 receptors respond to all three sympathetic neurotransmitters (Epi, NE, and dopamine). Alpha-2 receptors respond to Epi and NE, whereas beta-2 receptors respond only to Epi. In addition to alpha-1 and beta-1 receptors, dopamine also affects dopaminergic receptors (Table 14-1). The relative selectivity of various adrenergic agonists can be used to therapeutic benefit in determining which effector organs or tissues should be targeted.

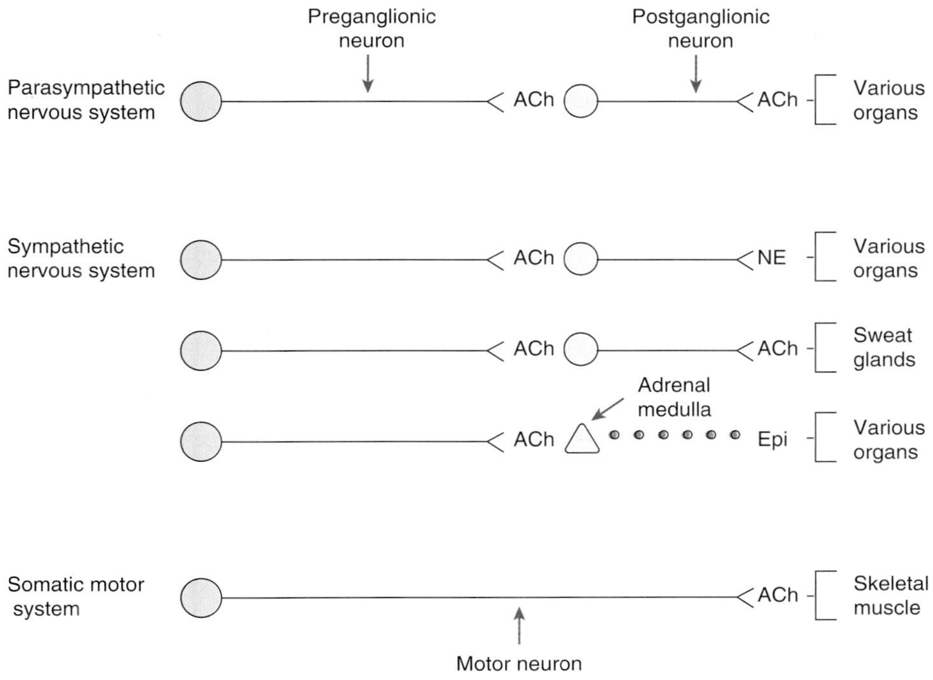

Figure 14-4. Neurotransmitters in the ANS.

TABLE 14-1 Receptor Specificity of Adrenergic Neurotransmitters

	Alpha-1	Alpha-2	Beta-1	Beta-2	Dopamine
Epinephrine	Yes	Yes	Yes	Yes	No
Norepinephrine	Yes	Yes	Yes	No	No
Dopamine	Yes	No	Yes	No	Yes

PATHOPHYSIOLOGY

The various tissues and organs that are innervated by the ANS are diverse, and few discrete disorders are directly related to compromise of the SNS. Instead, the therapeutic uses of sympathetic drugs are related to providing extra-adrenergic stimulation or blockade to that which is seen in normal ANS functioning. Because adrenergic receptors are distributed throughout the body and because adrenergically innervated organs and tissues show a predominance of one type of receptor over another, it is important to examine the major effects mediated by the different types of receptors to understand the implications of drug treatment in differing pathologic states (Table 14-2).

TABLE 14-2 Adrenergic Receptor Subtypes' Location and Action

Location	Response to Stimulation
Alpha-1	
Eye	Mydriasis (dilation) of the pupil
Arterioles	Constriction
Veins	Constriction
Male sex organs	Ejaculation
Bladder neck	Contraction
Prostatic capsule	Contraction
Alpha-2	
Presynaptic nerve terminal	Inhibition of norepinephrine release
Beta-1	
Heart	Increased rate Increased force of contraction Increased atrioventricular conduction
Kidney	Release of renin
Beta-2	
Arterioles (heart, lung, skeletal muscle)	Dilation
Bronchi	Dilation
Uterus	Relaxation
Liver	Glycogenolysis
Skeletal muscle	Contraction, glycogenolysis
Dopamine	
Kidney	Kidney vasculature dilation

ADRENERGIC AGONISTS

Adrenergic agonists are drugs that mimic the action of the SNS; thus, they are also known as sympathomimetic agents. They exert their effects by direct stimulation of adrenergic receptors or by indirect stimulation. Indirect mechanisms include increasing the transmission of NE, inhibiting NE reuptake, or inhibiting monoamine oxidase. (Remember, the last two are related to the dissociation and termination of NE binding to adrenergic receptors, thus inhibiting these processes will result in continuation of NE's effects.)

These drugs are generally divided into two groups: catecholamines and noncatecholamines. Catecholamines receive their name because of a similar chemical structure they possess (Table 14-3). Because of this chemical similarity, they also possess three similar characteristics. First, they have a short duration of action; this results in their need to be administered in a continuous fashion (e.g., IV infusion). Second, they cannot be given orally. As oral agents, they could not be given continuously and there are substances in the body that would instantaneously degrade them. Third, they do not cross the blood-brain barrier. Noncatecholamines have directly opposite characteristics. They have a longer duration of action, may be given orally, and do cross the blood–brain barrier.

Adrenergic agonists are also classified according to their selectivity. Agents that stimulate multiple adrenergic subtype receptors are called **nonselective-acting drugs**. Nonselective adrenergic agonists stimulate both alpha and beta receptors. Agents that target a specific subtype receptor are called **selective-acting drugs**. To maximize therapeutic effects and minimize adverse effects, selective drugs are used more frequently. It is important to remember that selectivity is not exclusive. Although a selective drug is preferential to a given subtype receptor, given in higher doses it may also stimulate other subtype receptors.

TABLE 14-3 Catecholamines

Catecholamines
dobutamine
dopamine
epinephrine
isoproterenol
norepinephrine

NONSELECTIVE ADRENERGIC AGONISTS

Nonselective adrenergic agonists stimulate most receptors; thus, they have a multitude of uses. It is important to remember that all of the subtypes are stimulated, regardless of which subtype would be most helpful for a specific pathology.

The prototype for nonselective adrenergic agonists is epinephrine. This drug stimulates alpha-1, alpha-2, and beta-1 and beta-2 receptors. The only adrenergic receptor subtype it does not stimulate is dopamine receptors.

NURSING MANAGEMENT OF THE PATIENT RECEIVING EPINEPHRINE

Core Drug Knowledge

Pharmacotherapeutics

Epinephrine has a wide variety of indications, including in anaphylactic shock, asthma, cardiopulmonary resuscitation, simple glaucoma, as an adjunct in topical anesthesia, ventricular fibrillation, cataracts, chloroquine poisoning, cluster headaches, croup, gastrointestinal (GI) hemorrhage, herpes simplex infection, hyperkalemia, hypothermia, mastocytosis, obstetric analgesia, open heart surgery, priapism, septic shock, and wheezing in infants.

Pharmacokinetics

Epinephrine may be administered parenterally, topically, or by inhalation. Depending on the administration method, Epi exerts its effects very quickly and is metabolized rapidly. It is well absorbed following IM or SC injection. Its duration of action ranges between 1 and 4 hours. It is metabolized in the liver and excreted through the kidneys (Table 14-4).

Pharmacodynamics

Epinephrine is a potent sympathomimetic drug with profound effects on a variety of organ systems. It stim-

TABLE 14-4 Summary of Selected Adrenergic Agonists

Drug (Trade) Name	Selected Indications	Route and Dosage Range	Pharmacokinetics
Nonselective Adrenergic Agonists			
epinephrine (Adrenalin, Epinephrine)	Anaphylactic shock, asthma, cardiopulmonary resuscitation, glaucoma, adjunct in topical anesthesia, ventricular fibrillation, cataracts, chloroquine poisoning, cluster headaches, croup, gastrointestinal hemorrhage, herpes simplex, hyperkalemia, hypothermia, mastocytosis, obstetric analgesia, open heart surgery, priapism, septic shock, wheezing in infants	*Adult:* IV, 1–4 μg/min of 4 μg/mL [15–60 mL/h]; other special dosages for ICU use *Child:* SC (asthma), 0.01 mL/kg/dose (1 : 1000), with maximum of 0.4–0.5 mL, repeated every 15–20 min for three to four doses or q4h if needed; IM/SC (anaphylaxis), 0.01 mL/kg, with maximum 0.3 mL of 1:1,000 solution; if response inadequate, IV 0.1 mL/kg of 1 : 10,000 solution every 5–10 min; inhalation, 0.05 mL/kg to a max of 0.5 mL/dose of 2.25% solution	*Onset:* IV, instant; SC > 1 h *Duration:* 20–30 min; SC, 4 h $t_{1/2}$: NA
ephedrine (*Canadian:* Omni-Tuss)	Asthma, enuresis, nasal congestion, rhinorrhea, sinusitis Hypotension	*Adult:* PO, 25–50 mg q3–4h *Adult:* IM, 25–50 mg; IV, 10–25 mg IV slow push	*Onset:* PO, 15–60 min; IM, 10–20 min; IV, instant *Duration:* PO, 3–5 h; IM/IV, 1 h $t_{1/2}$: 3–6 h
norepinephrine (Levophed)	Hypotension, shock, GI bleeding, glaucoma, hypothermia, ventricular fibrillation	*Adult:* IV, 8–12 μg/min at 2–3 mL/min	*Onset:* 1–2 min *Duration:* 1–2 min $t_{1/2}$: 7–18 h
Alpha-1 Adrenergic Agonists			
phenylephrine (Dristan, Dimetapp, Neo-Synephrine, others); *Canadian:* Dionephrine	Nasal congestion, common cold, glaucoma, shock, hypotensive crisis, anesthetic adjunct, PSVT	*Adult:* Topical, 1–2 sprays of 0.25%–1% solution q3–4h; IM, 2–5 mg; IV, 0.2–0.5 mg (IM/IV adjusted for indication)	*Onset:* IM, 10–15 min; IV, immediate *Duration:* IM 30–120 min; IV, 15–20 min $t_{1/2}$: 2–3 h

(*continued*)

TABLE 14-4 Summary of Selected Adrenergic Agonists (Continued)

Drug (Trade) Name	Selected Indications	Route and Dosage Range	Pharmacokinetics
methoxamine (Vasoxyl)	Hypotension, blood pressure maintenance during anesthesia, shock, SVT	*Adult:* IM, 10–15 mg; IV, 3–10 mg by slow push depending on condition	*Onset:* 30–120 s *Duration:* 60 min $t_{1/2}$: NA
Alpha-2 Adrenergic Agonists			
clonidine (Catapres; *Canadian:* Apo-Clonidine) (see Chapter 26)	Cancer pain (epidural), antihypertensive, alcohol withdrawal, diabetic diarrhea, menopausal flushing, opiate detoxification, herpetic neuralgia, ulcerative colitis	*Adult:* PO, 100–300 µg bid; IM/IV, 150 µg; epidural, 75–150 µg	*Onset:* 30–60 min *Duration:* 24 h $t_{1/2}$: 12–16 h
Beta-Adrenergic Agonists			
isoproterenol (Isuprel)	Asthma, CPR, COLD, MI, cerebral vasospasm, status asthmaticus, torsades de pointes, hypothermia, poisoning, AV block, bradycardia	*Adult:* SL, 10–20 mg up to tid for asthma; IM, 0.2 mg followed by 0.02–1.0 mg contingent on response; IV, 2–10 µg/min until response	*Onset:* Rapid *Duration:* 2 h $t_{1/2}$: Unknown
dobutamine (Dobutrex)	Cardiac surgery, CHF, inotropic support, low-output syndrome, myocardial revascularization, hypothermia, shock	*Adult:* IV, 2.5–10 µg/kg/min adjusted to response in cardiac output	*Onset:* 1–2 min *Duration:* Length of infusion $t_{1/2}$: 2 min
dopamine (Intropin; *Canadian:* Revimine)	Hemodynamic stabilization, heart failure, shock	*Adults:* low dose, 2–5 µg/kg/min; moderate dose, 5–10 µg/kg/min; high dose, 20–50 µg/kg/min	*Onset:* 1–2 min *Duration:* length of infusion $t_{1/2}$: 2 min

ulates all adrenergic receptors and causes the greatest adverse effects in the cardiovascular system and CNS. It acts directly on the postsynaptic adrenergic receptors.

Following activation of the receptor, Epi is metabolized and inactivated by catechol-O-methyltransferase (COMT) or monoamine oxidase. Depending on the location and distribution of receptors, Epi exerts a variety of responses in different effector organs tissues. In the cardiovascular system, Epi exerts positive inotropic and chronotropic effects on the myocardium by stimulating beta-1-adrenergic receptors. In the skin and viscera, Epi stimulates alpha-adrenergic receptors, causing vasoconstriction and vasodilation in skeletal muscle vessels. The overall effect is to increase systolic pressure and slightly decrease diastolic pressure. In the respiratory system, Epi causes bronchodilation by stimulation of beta-2 adrenergic receptors and is used for this purpose to treat patients with asthma or to manage anaphylactic shock.

Contraindications and Precautions

Absolute contraindications to Epi include hypersensitivity, closed angle glaucoma, during labor, in patients receiving cyclopropane, chloroform, or trichloroethylene general anesthesia, patients with severe organic cardiac disease, and in shock states other than anaphylactic shock. The action of Epi can exacerbate the symptoms of closed angle glaucoma. As a beta-2 agonist, Epi administered during labor can delay progression to the second stage. In patients receiving general anesthetic agents, Epi may induce myocardial sensitization to catecholamines, resulting in cardiac irritability. The cardiovascular effects of Epi, such as increased myocardial oxygen demand, increased heart rate, vasoactivity, and potential to induce arrhythmias, may be detrimental to patients with severe cardiac disorders. These same cardiovascular effects may worsen shock states, although Epi is used to manage anaphylactic shock and ventricular fibrillation.

Relative contraindications include cerebrovascular disease, such as cerebral arteriosclerosis or organic brain syndrome. The alpha effects of Epi has the potential to induce cerebrovascular hemorrhage with these disease states, especially when Epi is administered IV. Another relative contraindication is hypertension, because the vascular effects of Epi can worsen this condition. Patients with hyperthyroidism may become more sensitive to catecholamines, resulting in cardiotoxic symptoms. Epi also increases glycogenolysis in the liver. Patients with diabetes mellitus should be monitored for hyperglycemia.

Adverse Effects

Adverse effects are frequent because of Epi's ability to stimulate the four major adrenergic subtypes. Potential severe adverse effects include hypertensive crisis, angina, cerebral hemorrhage, and cardiac arrhythmias. If extravasation occurs during parenteral administration, necrosis may result because of its potent vasoconstrictive properties.

Patients with hyperthyroidism or hypertension are more susceptible to headaches, anxiety, fear, and palpitations after taking Epi. In others, the main adverse effects are tremor, weakness, dizziness, anxiety, pallor, palpitations, apprehensiveness, sweating, nausea, and vomiting.

In patients with diabetes, Epi may increase blood glucose levels. This increase is caused by the breakdown on glycogen that was stimulated in response to Epi's effect on beta-2 receptors in the liver and in skeletal muscle.

Drug Interactions

Epinephrine interacts with a variety of different classes of compounds, including tricyclic antidepressants, oxytocics, halogenated anesthetics, beta blockers, and blood glucose measurements (Table 14-5). Epi increases blood glucose levels and promotes hepatic glycogenolysis. Therefore, it may interfere with blood glucose determinations.

Assessment of Relevant Core Patient Variables

Health Status

The nurse should document preadministration vital signs. If Epi is being given for respiratory distress, the nurse should auscultate and document the patient's lung sounds. In patients diabetes, the nurse should obtain a baseline glucose level.

Before administering Epi in a nonemergency situation, the nurse should evaluate for diseases, disorders, or medications that contraindicate the safe use of Epi or require special monitoring. It is also important to evaluate the use of over-the-counter (OTC) or herbal medications, because these agents may contain sympathomimetic ingredients. When Epi is administered during an emergency, the potential benefits always outweigh the risks associated with Epi.

Life Span and Gender

The nurse should document the age and gender of the patient. The nurse should assess women of child-bearing age for pregnancy and lactation. Epi must be administered carefully to very young (infants and small children) and very old patients, because adverse drug effects may be more pronounced in these age groups. In children with asthma, Epi may produce hypotension and syncope. Epi is in Food and Drug Administration (FDA) pregnancy risk category C. Its use should be avoided in pregnant or lactating women.

Lifestyle, Diet, and Habits

The nurse should document the patient's occupation and activities of daily living. Patients treated with Epi for glaucoma may develop corneal pigmentation, which may impair their vision. This may have a significant impact on people working in transportation (e.g., airline flight crew, truck drivers) and those working at night in low light conditions.

Patients with diabetes receiving Epi for chronic conditions (e.g., asthma) should monitor blood glucose closely. Insulin dosages may need to be adjusted.

Environment

The nurse should be aware of the environment in which the drug will be administered and assess the home or living environment if appropriate. Epi when administered IV is given in a hospital setting, or possibly by trained emergency personnel in the community. It may be administered by other routes in any setting.

Nursing Diagnoses and Outcomes

- Imbalanced Nutrition: Less Than Body Requirements related to drug-induced anorexia or nausea
  Desired outcome: The patient will maintain adequate nutrition by learning how to cope with adverse effects or use an antiemetic agent if recommended.
- Disturbed Sleep Pattern, Insomnia, related to CNS excitation secondary to adrenergic drug therapy
  Desired outcome: The patient will learn about and practice sleep hygiene or take bedtime sedatives

TABLE 14-5 Agents That Interact With P Epinephrine

Interactants	Effect and Significance	Nursing Management
tricyclic antidepressants	Potentiation of epinephrine's vasopressor effect	Consult prescriber about adjusting epinephrine dosage.
oxytocic drugs used in labor and delivery	Synergistic vasoconstriction, resulting in hypertension (when epinephrine is administered to correct hypotension)	Monitor patient's blood pressure and vital signs carefully.
beta blockers	Hypertension resulting from beta-agonist action of epinephrine	Monitor blood pressure; avoid concurrent use if possible.
halogenated anesthetics	Arrhythmias resulting from sensitization of the myocardium to catecholamines	Monitor patient's cardiovascular status and ECG carefully during and after anesthesia.

TABLE 14-6 Agents That Interact With Phenylephrine

Interactants	Effect and Significance	Nursing Management
monoamine oxidase inhibitors	Increased amount of norepinephrine available for release, resulting in headache, hypertension, hyperpyrexia, and possibly in hypertensive crisis	Avoid concurrent use if possible.
tricyclic antidepressants	Inhibition of reuptake of norepinephrine in the neuron and diminished pressor effect of phenylephrine	Anticipate dosage adjustment of phenylephrine. Monitor patient carefully for hypertension and cardiac arrhythmias.
oxytocics	Synergistic vasoconstriction, resulting in hypertension (when epinephrine is administered to correct hypotension)	Monitor patient's blood pressure and vital signs carefully.

fore should only be given if absolutely necessary. The nurse should also assess for recent use of prescription drugs (e.g., tricyclic antidepressants, MAOIs). Positive findings should be communicated to the health care provider in nonemergency situations prior to administration of phenylephrine. Because parenteral phenylephrine is not a first-line drug in the management of shock states, its use in an emergency would outweigh the potential risks.

The nurse should obtain pretreatment vital signs to establish a baseline for therapeutic monitoring and detecting potential adverse effects. During therapy, the nurse needs to monitor therapeutic effects to evaluate the decrease in frequency or severity of target symptoms or the resumption of functions that were previously changed.

Life Span and Gender

The nurse should document the age and gender of the patient. The nurse should assess women of child-bearing age for pregnancy and lactation. During pregnancy, phenylephrine is used only if absolutely necessary because it is not known whether phenylephrine causes fetal abnormalities. If the patient is breast-feeding, the infant should be monitored for adrenergic stimulation. If this occurs, the drug may need to be discontinued.

Elderly patients may be at higher risk due to blurring of vision from mydriasis. The topical 10% ophthalmic phenylephrine solution should be avoided in infants and used cautiously with the elderly, because there is an increased risk of systemic absorption.

Lifestyle, Diet, and Habits

The nurse should document the patient's occupation and activities of daily living. The nurse should advise the patient to exercise caution when driving or operating machinery at night or under very bright light, because mydriasis may cause temporary blindness. Additionally, the nurse should ask the patient about use of OTC cough, cold, or herbal remedies containing sympathomimetic ingredients, which will intensify the effects of phenylephrine.

Environment

The nurse should be aware of the environment in which the drug will be administered and assess the home or living environment, if appropriate. Phenylephrine is administered in the hospital for treatment of hypotension and shock. For other uses, it may be self-administered by the patient in any environment.

Nursing Diagnoses and Outcomes

- Impaired Gas Exchange related to bronchoconstriction or bronchospasm
  Desired outcome: Gas exchange will remain unimpaired by coughing or drug-induced bronchoconstriction.
- Imbalanced Nutrition: Less Than Body Requirements related to anorexia or nausea secondary to use of an adrenergic drug
  Desired outcome: The patient will take sufficient nourishment, manage diet adequately, and use antiemetics if necessary.
- Disturbed Sleep Pattern, insomnia, related to CNS excitation secondary to phenylephrine use
  Desired outcome: The patient will maintain normal sleep patterns by practicing sleep hygiene measures and using a sedative at bedtime if necessary.

Planning and Intervention

Maximizing Therapeutic Effects

Blood loss or volume deficits should be replaced prior to the use of IV phenylephrine to treat hypotension. It may be used concurrently with replacement therapy if necessary to prevent cerebral or coronary artery ischemia. For topical use, the following factors should be considered:

- To produce optimal mydriasis, the nurse must be careful to instill the ophthalmic form of phenylephrine into the conjunctival cul-de-sac.
- If the phenylephrine is in nasal spray form, the nurse should demonstrate the proper way to administer the spray. The patient can then perform a repeat demonstration.

- The patient should be encouraged to use phenylephrine exactly as prescribed and at the required dosage frequency to enhance therapeutic effects.

Minimizing Adverse Effects

IV phenylephrine should be administered through a large vein, preferably in the antecubital space, when given to treat hypotension. This will help prevent extravasation, which may cause necrosis as a result of vasoconstriction. The IV site should be checked frequently for patency. If extravasation does occur, the antidote is phentolamine (Regitine), a potent alpha blocker. Inject the phentolamine SC into the affected tissue with a fine-gauge needle.

During topical drug therapy, the following are strategies to teach the patient to minimize adverse effects:

- Avoid night-time driving because blurred vision can be hazardous. Wearing sunglasses, however, may relieve the glare of bright lights and reduce photophobia.
- Time doses to prevent disrupting sleep, and use effective sleep hygiene measures (dimmed lights, reduced noise, soothing music).
- Avoid OTC drugs that contain sympathomimetic ingredients that potentiate the effect of phenylephrine.

Providing Patient and Family Education

- The nurse should stress the hazards associated with driving and operating heavy or dangerous machinery until the effects of the drug are known.
- Patients should be taught about drug interactions and advised not to use phenylephrine if they are taking MAOIs, tricyclic antidepressants, or drugs that treat glaucoma.
- The nurse should teach the patient to recognize and report signs and symptoms of adverse effects requiring medical attention, such as a fast, pounding, or irregular heartbeat; chest pain that lasts longer than 5 minutes; trouble breathing; or tingling in the hands or feet.

Ongoing Assessment and Evaluation

Measuring goal attainment is relatively straightforward for patients taking phenylephrine and other adrenergic drugs. Assessing lifestyle and occupation and recognizing and managing adverse effects are important. Because the contraindications and precautions for phenylephrine are many, it is important to complete a detailed and thorough history and physical examination on any patient anticipating long-term adrenergic drug therapy. ■

MEMORY CHIP

Phenylephrine

- Alpha-adrenergic agonist and vasopressor (constricts blood vessels, raises blood pressure)
- Treats hypotension, shock related to vascular failure, nasal congestion; also used during anesthesia
- Significant contraindications: hypersensitivity, severe hypertension, ventricular tachycardia, and closed angle glaucoma
- Most common adverse effects: hypertension, headache, sleep disturbances
- Most serious adverse effect: reflex bradycardia
- Important drug–drug interaction: possible life-threatening interaction with monoamine oxidase inhibitors
- Maximizing therapeutic effects: instill eye drops in conjunctival cul-de-sac
- Minimizing adverse effects: avoid situations that increase blurred vision
- Most significant patient education: stress safety related to blurred vision

DRUG CLOSELY RELATED TO PHENYLEPHRINE

Methoxamine (Vasoxyl) is a parenteral vasopressor agent used for blood pressure support during surgery and for terminating some supraventricular tachycardias. It increases blood pressure by increasing peripheral resistance through the alpha receptors.

Methoxamine is contraindicated for use in patients with severe hypertension, hyperthyroidism, bradycardia, partial atrioventricular block, myocardial disease, severe arteriosclerosis, or sulfite hypersensitivity.

Like phenylephrine, methoxamine may interact with MAOIs, tricyclic antidepressants, and oxytocics. In addition, methoxamine may interact with bretylium, which results in arrhythmias. It may partially or fully reverse the antihypertensive effects of guanethidine. Lastly, use with halogenated hydrocarbon anesthetics can sensitize the myocardium to the effects of catecholamines.

Potential adverse effects include hypertension, ventricular ectopic beats, nausea and vomiting, headache, anxiety, sweating, pilomotor response, uterine hypertonus, fetal bradycardia, and urinary urgency.

ALPHA-2 ADRENERGIC AGONISTS

Alpha-2 adrenergic agonists, such as clonidine, have a narrow range of specific clinical indications. They are primarily used as antihypertensives. For a full discussion of alpha-2 adrenergic agonists, particularly clonidine, see Chapter 30. Clonidine is also presented in Table 14-4.

BETA-ADRENERGIC AGONISTS

Beta-adrenergic agonists also mimic the action of the SNS; thus they are also also known as sympathomimetic agents. They exert their effects by stimulation of one or both beta-adrenergic receptors. Like the alpha-adrenergic drugs, they are classified as either a catecholamine or noncatecholamine.

Beta-adrenergic agonists are also labeled according to their selectivity. Drugs that stimulate both beta-1 and beta-2 receptors are nonselective. Those that target either beta-1 or beta-2 are selective. To maximize therapeutic effects and minimize adverse effects, selective drugs are used most frequently. Again, as with alpha-adrenergic drugs, selectivity is preferential but not exclusive. A prototypical beta-adrenergic agonist is the relatively nonselective isoproterenol. In contrast to the selective beta-adrenergic agonists, such as the beta-1 agonist dobutamine and the beta-2 agonist albuterol, isoproterenol can stimulate both subclasses with approximately equal potency. The specific receptor agonists for beta-1 and beta-2 receptors are summarized in Table 14-4 along with ephedrine, which is an indirect-acting beta-adrenergic agonist.

NURSING MANAGEMENT OF THE PATIENT RECEIVING P ISOPROTERENOL

Core Drug Knowledge

Pharmacotherapeutics

Pharmacotherapeutics for isoproterenol include both emergency and chronic conditions (e.g., chronic airway limitation). In an emergency, isoproterenol is used for treating hypovolemic, cardiogenic, and septic shock, low cardiac output (hypoperfusion), and congestive heart failure (CHF). Its use is as an adjunct to fluid and electrolyte replacement therapy and other drugs and treatments medically necessary to maintain basic functions in these conditions. Isoproterenol is also used in treating mild or transient episodes of heart block that do not require electric shock or pacemaker therapy. It is also used in serious episodes of heart block and Adams-Stokes attacks, except when these are caused by ventricular tachycardia or fibrillation. Isoproterenol is also used in cardiac arrest until electric shock or pacemaker therapies are available. Although isoproterenol is approved for these uses, it is generally not the drug of choice, because of its potential adverse effects on the cardiac system. It can also be used to treat bronchospasms that occur during anesthesia.

Isoproterenol is used in respiratory drugs used to manage asthma, bronchitis, or emphysema.

Pharmacokinetics

Poorly absorbed after oral administration, isoproterenol is usually administered by inhaler or by parenteral means. Sublingual or rectal routes are occasionally used. If given IV, the onset is rapid with a duration of about 8 to 50 minutes, depending on the dose. Using an inhaler, peak bronchodilation occurs within 15 to 30 minutes. Duration of action ranges from 1.5 to 3 hours. The drug is metabolized in the lungs and liver by COMT and then conjugated and excreted mainly through urine. The half-life is biphasic with a rapid half-life of 2.5 to 5 minutes and a slower one of 3 to 7 hours (see Table 14-4).

Pharmacodynamics

As a beta stimulator, isoproterenol stimulates both beta-1 and beta-2 sites. Stimulation of beta-1 sites increases contractility (positive inotropic effect) and increases the heart rate (positive chronotropic effect). Stimulation of beta-2 receptor sites produces vasodilation. This effect is most pronounced in the bronchi, skeletal muscle and vasculature, and GI tract. The effect of these actions is that cardiac output is increased, while total peripheral resistance is reduced. The systolic blood pressure will increase, whereas the diastolic blood pressure will decrease. Renal perfusion will increase in patients experiencing cardiogenic or septicemic shock, although it may decrease in normotensive patients.

Contraindications and Precautions

Isoproterenol is contraindicated in tachyarrhythmias, tachycardia or heart block caused by digitalis intoxication, ventricular arrhythmias that require inotropic therapy, and angina. The use of isoproterenol is not a substitute for replacement of blood, plasma, fluids, and electrolytes; these therapies should precede use of isoproterenol. Caution should be used in patients with coronary artery disease, coronary insufficiency, diabetes, and hyperthyroidism and in patients sensitive to the sympathomimetic effects of isoproterenol. If the heart rate becomes greater than 110 bpm, the rate of infusion should be decreased or temporarily stopped. If doses are given that bring the heart rate to more than 130 bpm, ventricular arrhythmias may develop. Such an elevated rate also places more stress on the heart, increasing the cardiac workload and the oxygen needs of the heart. Therefore, it can have a negative effect on the injured or failing heart; caution must be used in these conditions. If angina or precordial distress develops, the infusion is stopped immediately.

Some products of isoproterenol contain sulfites, which may cause allergic-type reactions in susceptible patients. The reactions may include anaphylactic symptoms and asthmatic episodes, including life-threatening episodes.

Isoproterenol is a pregnancy category C drug. It is not known whether it is excreted in breast milk.

Adverse Effects

Adverse effects are generally related to too much sympathetic stimulation. Cardiovascular effects are tachycardia, palpitations, hypertension, hypotension, ventricular arrhythmias, tachyarrhythmias, precordial distress, and angina. CNS effects include flushing, sweating, mild tremors, nervousness, headache, dizziness, and weakness. GI effects of nausea and vomiting can also occur. Overdosage produces the effects of tachycardia or other arrhythmias, palpitations, angina, hypotension, or hypertension.

Drug Interactions

The profile of drug interactions is similar to that for alpha-adrenergic agonists. Isoproterenol also interacts with oxytocics and tricyclic antidepressants (Table 14-7).

TABLE 14-7 Agents That Interact With Isoproterenol

Interactants	Effect and Significance	Nursing Management
tricyclic antidepressants	Potentiates hypertensive effects of both drugs	Anticipate dosage adjustment of isoproterenol. Monitor blood pressure and cardiac rhythm.
oxytocics used in obstetrics	Synergistic vasoconstriction, resulting in hypertension	Monitor patient's blood pressure and vital signs carefully.
halogenated anesthetics	Cardiac arrhythmias resulting from sensitization of the myocardium to catecholamines	Monitor cardiac rhythm before, during, and after general anesthesia.

Assessment of Relevant Core Patient Variables

Health Status

The patient should have received blood, plasma, fluids, and electrolytes prior to receiving isoproterenol. It is important to determine whether the patient has tachyarrhythmias, tachycardia or heart block caused by digitalis toxicity, ventricular arrhythmias requiring inotropic therapy, or angina, because these are contraindications for its use. It is also important to determine whether the patient is receiving any drugs that might interact with the isoproterenol.

Pretreatment physical assessment should include measurements such as blood pressure, electrocardiogram (ECG), and auscultation of heart and lung sounds. During therapy, monitoring the therapeutic drug effect should show whether the frequency and severity of target symptoms decrease or resume.

Life Span and Gender

The nurse should document the age and gender of the patient. The nurse should assess women of childbearing age for pregnancy and lactation. If the patient is pregnant, isoproterenol should be used only if absolutely necessary because it is not known whether isoproterenol causes fetal abnormalities. The drug is in Food and Drug Administration pregnancy risk category C. If the patient is breast-feeding, the infant should be monitored for evidence of adrenergic stimulation, such as tachycardia. If this occurs, isoproterenol may need to be discontinued. Elderly patients may be at higher risk of injury due to blurring of vision.

Lifestyle, Diet, and Habits

The nurse should document the patient's occupation and activities of daily living. Because of possible blurred vision, the nurse should advise the patient to exercise caution when driving or operating machinery. This is particularly important for patients with a hazardous occupation.

Environment

The nurse should be aware of the environment in which the drug will be administered and assess the home or living environment, if appropriate. Isoproterenol, when used parenterally to treat shock, is administered in a controlled environment within the hospital. Isoproterenol may be used in any environment when used for its respiratory effects.

Nursing Diagnoses and Outcomes

- Anxiety related to stimulation of the SNS
  Desired outcome: The patient will employ strategies to compensate for sympathetic stimulation.
- Imbalanced Nutrition: Less Than Body Requirements related to anorexia or nausea secondary to isoproterenol use
  Desired outcome: The patient's nutritional status will be adequately maintained through appropriate dietary management and use of antiemetics, if needed.
- Risk for Injury related to blurred vision
  Desired outcome: The patient will remain without injury.
- Disturbed Sleep Pattern, insomnia, related to CNS excitation secondary to isoproterenol
  Desired outcome: Normal sleep patterns will prevail by implementing sleep hygiene measures and bedtime sedation as needed.

Planning and Intervention

Maximizing Therapeutic Effects

When administering parenteral isoproterenol, the nurse should verify that the patient has received volume replacements prior to beginning isoproterenol to treat shock. For nonemergencies, the nurse should encourage the patient to take the isoproterenol exactly as prescribed and at the required dosage frequency to enhance therapeutic potential. The nurse may also need to instruct the patient in the correct use of a metered dose inhaler.

Minimizing Adverse Effects

When isoproterenol is given parenterally, it is important to start with a small dose and gradually increase the administration rate. The patient's heart rate, blood pressure, and ECG are monitored carefully and continuously throughout therapy. Additionally, the nurse should monitor the patient's intake and output, because kidney output is indicative of kidney function. If the cardiac output decreases, the kidneys will not be adequately perfused. The central venous pressure is monitored by the use of a Swan-Ganz pulmonary artery catheter. The patient's overall response to therapy is carefully monitored.

Isoproterenol is administered only through a large-gauge IV catheter in the antecubital or central vein, because absorption is unpredictable. Administration through small catheters in the extremities is unsafe and unpredictable for vasopressor therapy; tissue necrosis may result. The nurse should carefully assess the IV site frequently for extravasation. An IV pump is always used to regulate the flow of the drug.

Acute tolerance can develop during continuous IV administration. The drug is mixed in a small volume of solution so that the concentration is high. It is important to run fluid replacements separately from drug therapy to allow for maximum dosing flexibility. (Dosage and fluid rate can be adjusted independently.) This helps to prevent tolerance.

The nurse should monitor the patient for acidosis because this lessens the response to vasopressors and must be corrected if it exists or develops during therapy.

The nurse should also promote sleep hygiene to overcome drug-induced CNS stimulation and plan meals to promote appetite and counterbalance drug-induced anorexia.

For patients with cardiovascular problems, key interventions involve identifying adverse effects, such as anginal pain and irregular rhythms. For patients with asthma, key interventions involve monitoring lung sounds and assessing respiratory function. The nurse should emphasize the importance of adhering to the prescribed frequency of inhaled isoproterenol to avoid rebound bronchoconstriction.

Providing Patient and Family Education

Patient and family education is limited because of the emergency nature of treatment of shock.

- The nurse should teach the patient and family that the purpose of this drug is to treat shock and to help raise the blood pressure, and that heart rate, blood pressure, and ECG will be constantly monitored to determine both the therapeutic effects and any adverse effects of drug therapy.
- Chronic airway limitation (CAL) patients using isoproterenol should be taught how to used a metered-dose inhaler or nebulizer. (Note: CAL is a new term for COPD or COLD. All three mean the same thing.)

Ongoing Assessment and Evaluation

The pulse rate, blood pressure, and ECG of the patient on parenteral isoproterenol will be monitored constantly to assess for evidence of recovery from shock or deepening shock. Drug therapy is effective when the patient recovers from shock without serious adverse effects.

For patients receiving long-term therapy for respiratory effects, the nurse should monitor the efficacy of treatment. Advise the patient to contact the health care provider if the nebulizer or metered-dose inhaler is needed daily because the patient should receive adjunctive drugs to stabilize her or his respiratory status. The nurse should also arrange for periodic evaluation of blood pressure and pulse to assess for potential adverse effects. ■

MEMORY CHIP

Isoproterenol

- Treats hypovolemic and septic shock, CHF, asthma, and ophthalmologic disorders such as glaucoma
- Potent bronchodilator
- Significant contraindications: tachyarrhythmias, tachycardia, heart block, or angina
- Most common adverse effects: tachycardia, palpitations, hypertension, angina, tremors, headache
- Most serious adverse effect: ventricular dysrhythmias
- Maximizing therapeutic effects: best administered and absorbed parenterally or by inhalation
- Minimizing adverse effects: use the drug exactly as prescribed to avoid rebound symptoms
- Most significant patient education: use of inhaler or nebulizer

DRUGS CLOSELY RELATED TO ISOPROTERENOL

Dopamine

Dopamine (Intropin) is a parenteral adrenergic agonist that mimics the actions of the endogenous neurotransmitter dopamine. Dopamine stimulates dopamine, alpha-1, and beta-1 receptors. Unlike isoproterenol, it does not affect alpha-2 or beta-2 receptors. At low doses, dopamine stimulates the dopamine receptors resulting in increased renal perfusion. At moderate doses, dopamine stimulates both dopamine and beta-1 receptors, resulting in a positive inotropic action on the heart. At high doses, stimulation of alpha-1 receptors results in vasoconstriction and decreased renal perfusion. Dopamine is discussed in depth in Chapter 29.

Dobutamine

Dobutamine (Dobutrex) is a parenteral inotropic agent. It is a synthetic compound structurally similar to dopamine and other catecholamines. Dobutamine primarily stimulates beta-1 receptors, but it also has minor affects on alpha-1 and beta-2 receptors. Stimulation of beta-1 receptors increases myocardial contractility and stroke volume with minor chronotropic effects, resulting in increased cardiac output. Systolic blood pressure is generally elevated as a consequence of increased stroke volume, although diastolic blood pressure and mean arterial pressure are usually unchanged with normal doses in normotensive patients. Increased myocardial contractility results in increased coronary blood flow and myocardial oxygen consumption. Unlike dopamine, dobutamine does not affect dopaminergic receptors, nor does it cause release of NE from sympathetic nerve endings. Dobutamine is used for patients with heart failure and cardiogenic shock. It is discussed in more detail in Chapter 29.

Respiratory Beta Agonists

There are many drugs used in the management of CAL diseases. They may be given orally, parenterally, nebulized, or by metered-dose inhalers. These drugs may be nonselective or selective of beta-2 receptors. To minimize adverse effects, use of beta-2 selective drugs has become the community standard. Beta-2 respiratory agonists differ from each other in the way they are delivered, as well as their onset and duration of action. These drugs are discussed in Chapter 35.

ADRENERGIC ANTAGONISTS

ALPHA-ADRENERGIC ANTAGONISTS

Alpha-adrenergic antagonists block the stimulation of alpha receptors. Clinically relevant drugs in current use block alpha-1 receptors in the vasculature. There are no therapeutic agents approved by the FDA for alpha-1 blockade for receptors located in the eye nor for alpha-2 blockade. The prototype for alpha-adrenergic antagonists is prazosin (Minipress).

NURSING MANAGEMENT OF THE PATIENT RECEIVING PRAZOSIN

Core Drug Knowledge

Pharmacotherapeutics

Prazosin is used in the management of refractory CHF, Raynaud vasospasm, and treatment of prostatic outflow obstruction. It is frequently used in treating hypertension alone or in combination with other drugs.

Pharmacokinetics

Prazosin is given orally and is metabolized in the liver and excreted in the bile, feces, and urine. It crosses the placenta and may enter breast milk. A single oral dose has a duration of action of 10 hours and a half-life of 2 to 4 hours (Table 14-8).

TABLE 14-8 Summary of Selected Adrenergic Antagonists

Drug (Trade) Name	Selected Indications	Route and Dosage Range	Pharmacokinetics
Alpha-Adrenergic Antagonists			
prazosin (Minipress; *Canadian:* Alti-Prozosin)	Hypertension, angina, CHF, BPH, Raynaud vasospasm	*Adult:* PO 3–20 mg daily in divided doses (initial dose 0.5–1 mg to minimize hypotension syncope	*Onset:* Varies *Duration:* 10 h $t_{1/2}$: 2–3 h
doxazosin (Cardura)	Hypertension, BPH	*Adult:* PO 1–16 mg daily according to individual response	*Onset:* 2 h *Duration:* 24 h $t_{1/2}$: 22 h
terazosin (Hytrin; *Canadian:* Alti-Terazosin)	Hypertension BPH	*Adult:* PO 1–5 mg per day PO 10–20 mg per day	*Onset:* 1–2 h *Duration:* Unknown $t_{1/2}$: 12 h
phentolamine (Regitine; *Canadian:* Rogitine)	Drug infiltration Pheochromocytoma-induced hypertension (HTN) and sweating, micturitional disorders, Raynaud vasospasm, impotence	Infiltrate area with small amount of solution made by diluting 5–10 mg in 10-mL 0.9% sodium chloride *Adult:* 2.5–5 mg IV *Child:* 0.05–0.1 mg/kg IV	*Onset:* 15–20 min IV immediate *Duration:* IM; 30–45 min; 15–30 min $t_{1/2}$: 19 min
phenoxybenzamine (Dibenzyline)	Pheochromocytoma-induced HTN and sweating, micturitional disorders, Raynaud vasospasm, impotence	*Adult:* PO 20–30 mg bid; can be given IV, but not IM or SC, because drug is an irritant	*Onset:* 2 h *Duration:* 3–4 d $t_{1/2}$: 24 h
Beta-Adrenergic Antagonists			
propranolol (Inderal; *Canadian:* Apo-Propanolol)	Cardiac arrhythmias, MI, hypertrophic asubaortic stenosis, HTN, pheochromocytoma, prophylaxis of migraine, angina, essential tremor	*Adult:* PO, 80–320 mg/d in divided doses; IV, 1–3 mg at 1 mg/min with monitoring	*Onset:* PO, 20–30 min, IV, immediate *Duration:* PO, 6–12 h; IV, 4–6h $t_{1/2}$: 3–5 h
atenolol (Tenormin; *Canadian:* Tenolin	Angina, HTN, post-MI, arrhythmias, CHF, anxiety, irritable bowel syndrome, alcohol withdrawal	*Adult:* PO, 50–100 mg daily	*Onset:* PO, varies *Duration:* 24 h $t_{1/2}$: 6–7 h

(*continued*)

TABLE 14-8 Summary of Selected Adrenergic Antagonists (Continued)

Drug (Trade) Name	Selected Indications	Route and Dosage Range	Pharmacokinetics
acebutolol (Sectral; *Canadian:* Apo-Acebutolol)	Ventricular arrhythmias, angina, HTN	*Adult:* PO, 200 mg bid *Adult:* PO, 400–800 mg/d using graded dosages until blood pressure is controlled	*Onset:* Varies *Duration:* 6–8 h $t_{1/2}$: 3–4 h
metoprolol (Betaloc, Lopressor, Toprol XL; *Canadian:* Apo-Metoprolol)	Angina, HTN, post-MI	*Adult:* PO, 12.5–400 mg/d depending on patient's condition and response; IV, 2–20 mg titrated to response	*Onset:* PO, 15 min; IV, immediate *Duration:* 15–19 h $t_{1/2}$: 3–4 h
pindolol (Visken; *Canadian:* Apo-Pindolol)	HTN	*Adult:* PO, 5 mg bid	*Onset:* Varies *Duration:* Unknown $t_{1/2}$: 3–4 h
	Angina	*Adult:* PO, 2.5–5.0 mg/d up to 40 mg/d	*Onset:* Varies *Duration:* Unknown $t_{1/2}$: 3–4 h
penbutolol (Levatol)	HTN	*Adult:* PO, 10–40 mg/d	*Onset:* Varies *Duration:* 20 h $t_{1/2}$: 5 h
betaxolol (Betopic, Kerlone)	HTN, cardiovascular disorders	*Adult:* PO, 10–40 mg/d	*Onset:* 30–60 min *Duration:* 12–15 h $t_{1/2}$: 14–22 h
	Glaucoma	*Adult:* topical, 1 drop 0.5% solution in affected eye(s) bid	*Onset:* Unknown *Duration:* Unknown $t_{1/2}$: 14–22 h
metipranolol (OptiPranolol)	Glaucoma Ocular HTN	*Adult:* topical, 1 drop 0.3% solution in affected eye(s) bid *Adult:* PO, 10–40 mg bid	*Onset:* 0.5–3 h *Duration:* <24 h $t_{1/2}$: 3 h
sotalol (Betapace; *Canadian:* Alti-Sotalol)	Ventricular arrhythmias, angina, HTN	*Adult:* PO, 80–320 mg daily in divided doses; IV, 0.2–1.5 mg/kg over 5 min with monitoring	*Onset:* 2–3 h *Duration:* 24 h $t_{1/2}$: 7–18 h
nadolol (Corgard; *Canadian.* Apo-Nadol)	Angina, HTN, cardiovascular disorders	*Adult:* PO, 40–160 mg daily; IV, 0.01–0.05 mg/kg at 1 mg/min to 10 mg maximum	*Onset:* Varies *Duration:* 17–24 h $t_{1/2}$: 20–24 h
timolol (Blocadren; *Canadian:* Gen-Timolol)	HTN, angina, arrhythmias, post-MI, prophylaxis of migraine	*Adult:* PO, 10–60 mg daily or bid in divided doses; IV, 0.5 followed by oral dosing	*Onset:* 0.5–3 h *Duration:* NA $t_{1/2}$: NA
	Glaucoma	*Adult:* topical, 1 drop of 0.25% solution in affected dyes bid	*Onset:* 15–20 min *Duration:* NA $t_{1/2}$: NA
Alpha/beta Adrenergic Antagonists			
labetalol (Normodyne)	HTN	*Adult:* 100 mg bid; maintenance, 200–400 mg qd *Child:* 4 mg/kg d in two divided doses	*Onset:* PO, 20 min; IV, 2–5 min *Duration:* PO, 8–24 h; IV, 2–4 h $t_{1/2}$: 2.5–8 h
carvedilol (Coreg)	HTN	*Adult:* 6.25 mg PO bid 7–10 d, then increase to 12.5 mg PO bid, maximum 25 mg PO bid *Child:* Not approved	*Onset:* 1–2 h *Duration:* Unknown $t_{1/2}$: 7–10 h
	heart failure	*Adult:* 3.125 mg PO bid × 2 wk; then 6.25 mg PO bid; maximum 25 mg PO bid *Child:* Not approved.	
	Static angina	*Adult:* 25–50 mg PO bid	
	Post-MI	*Adult:* 2.5 mg IV followed by 12.5–25 mg/PO bid × 6 mo.	

Pharmacodynamics

Prazosin selectively blocks postsynaptic alpha-1 adrenergic receptors, decreasing sympathetic tone of the vasculature, dilating arterioles and veins, and lowering supine and standing blood pressure.

Contraindications and Precautions

The main contraindication to prazosin use is hypersensitivity. Prazosin should be used with caution in patients with angina pectoris because severe hypotension may cause or worsen angina. Prazosin is also used cautiously in patients with CHF, renal failure, or pregnancy.

Adverse Effects

The most common adverse effects of prazosin are lightheadedness, dizziness, headache, drowsiness, weakness, lethargy, nausea, and palpitations. These effects may spontaneously resolve or be alleviated with a decreased dosage. Other common adverse effects include reflex tachycardia, orthostatic hypotension, nasal congestion, and inhibition of ejaculation.

Prazosin is well known for causing "first-dose syncope." This may be avoided by administering a lower first dose with food. Prazosin-induced syncope is unpredictable and does not correlate with serum prazosin levels. Syncope may be preceded by tachycardia (120 to 160 bpm) and occurs more frequently with dosage increases alone or combined with the adjunctive use of other antihypertensive agents.

Prazosin may cause adverse effects in practically any body system. These include edema, dyspnea, and angina. Prazosin therapy may also induce rash, pruritus, priapism, urinary frequency, incontinence, blurred vision, dry mouth, pancreatitis, liver function test abnormalities, diaphoresis, fever, arthralgia, positive ANA titer, and mental depression.

Drug Interactions

Concomitant administration of prazosin with other antihypertensive agents will increase the hypotensive effect of both agents. This can be therapeutically advantageous, but it may also induce orthostatic hypotension. Patients receiving more than one antihypertensive agent should be instructed in strategies to reduce the incidence of orthostatic hypotension and their blood pressure should be closely monitored.

Assessment of Relevant Core Patient Variables

Health Status

The nurse should assess the patient's history for diseases or disorders that may contradict the use of prazosin. Positive findings should be communicated to the provider prior to administration. Before and throughout therapy the nurse should closely monitor the patient's heart rate and blood pressure and assist the patient with position changes and ambulation.

Life Span and Gender

The nurse should document the age and gender of the patient. The nurse should assess women of child-bearing age for pregnancy and lactation. Elderly patients are more likely to be affected by postural hypotension and the possibility of syncope. If it is determined that the patient is pregnant, prazosin must be used cautiously, if at all, because it is in FDA pregnancy risk category C. Safety and efficacy have not been established in pediatric patients.

Lifestyle, Diet, and Habits

The nurse should document the patient's occupation and activities of daily living. Patients should be cautious when operating machinery, exercising, driving, changing positions, or climbing stairs.

Environment

The nurse should be aware of the environment in which the drug will be administered and assess the home or living environment, if appropriate. Prazosin may be administered in any setting by health care providers, nurses, or patient themselves.

Nursing Diagnoses and Outcomes

- Ineffective Tissue Perfusion, decreased, related to prazosin-induced hypotension
  Desired outcome: Adequate tissue perfusion will be maintained despite hypotension.
- Imbalanced Nutrition: Less Than Body Requirements related to nausea secondary to prazosin use
  Desired outcome: The patient will receive adequate nourishment by practicing appropriate dietary management.
- Risk for Injury related to orthostatic hypotension
  Desired outcome: The patient will remain free of injury.

Planning and Intervention

Maximizing Therapeutic Effects

The nurse should emphasize the importance of taking the prescribed dose on a daily basis at the prescribed dosage. The nurse should explain the importance of refraining from OTC drug use because many OTC drugs contain ingredients that decrease the effectiveness of prazosin.

Minimizing Adverse Effects

Nursing strategies to minimize adverse effects include having the patient take the first dose just before bedtime, lie down if syncope occurs, monitor weight, and check for edema. The nurse should explain the importance of changing position slowly to avoid orthostatic hypotension.

Providing Patient and Family Education

- Patients should be advised to take the drug as prescribed and to avoid operating machinery or driving for about 4 hours after the first dose.

- The nurse should teach the patient about additional adverse effects, such as dizziness and weakness (after changing position rapidly, in hot weather, after exercising, and after drinking alcohol). To avoid injury from these effects, the patient may need to avoid driving or engaging in tasks that require alertness until the body adjusts to the drug, to change positions slowly, to use caution when climbing stairs, to cool down when exercising, and to avoid consuming alcoholic beverages.
- The nurse should highlight those symptoms that should be reported to the provider should they occur. These symptoms include blurred vision, difficulty breathing, fainting spells, light-headedness, irregular heartbeat, palpitations or chest pain, mental depression, prolonged painful erections, swelling of the legs and ankles, and protracted vomiting.

Ongoing Assessment and Evaluation

It is important for the nurse to monitor blood pressure, heart and lung sounds, and edema. It is important to determine whether any other drugs are being taken concurrently with prazosin to identify significant potential drug interactions. ■

DRUGS CLOSELY RELATED TO PRAZOSIN

Doxazosin

Like prazosin, doxazosin (Cardura) is an oral, alpha-adrenergic blocking agent used in the treatment of hypertension and for benign prostatic hyperplasia. It is pharmacologically similar to prazosin and terazosin but has the longest duration of action of agents in the group. Because of its duration, it may be dosed once daily.

MEMORY CHIP

Prazosin

- Vasodilator
- Treats refractory CHF, hypertension, Raynaud vasospasm, prostatic obstruction
- Significant contraindication: hypersensitivity
- Most common adverse effects: light-headedness, dizziness, headache, drowsiness, weakness, lethargy, nausea, and palpitations
- Most serious adverse effect: "first dose syncope"
- Maximizing therapeutic effects: refrain from administering any OTC drug in combination with prazosin
- Minimizing adverse effects: stress safety issues regarding CNS effects
- Most significant patient education: safe ways to cope with postural hypotension

Doxazosin is highly metabolized in the liver, with the majority of an oral dose being eliminated in feces, suggesting enterohepatic recycling, and the remainder excreted in urine. Neither advanced age nor renal failure significantly alters the elimination half-life.

Doxazosin interacts with more drugs than prazosin does but has minimal adverse reactions. Drug interactions include other antihypertensive agents, dopamine, Epi, estrogens, metaraminol, methoxamine, nonsteroidal antiinflammatory agents (NSAIDs), and phenylephrine.

Terazosin

Like prasozin and doxazosin, terazosin (Hytrin) is an alpha-adrenergic blocking agent used in the treatment of hypertension and benign prostatic hypertrophy (BPH). The duration of action of terazosin is longer than that of prazosin but shorter than that of doxazosin. In a head-to-head comparison with finasteride (Proscar), terazosin achieved superior results in the management of BPH. In addition to its alpha-1 blockade, terazosin also alters lipid metabolism, decreasing the levels of total cholesterol, low-density lipoprotein (LDL) cholesterol, and very low-density lipoprotein (VLDL) cholesterol.

Antihypertensive effects are seen within 15 minutes, and peak plasma levels are observed approximately 1 hour after administration. The plasma half-life is about 12 hours. Excretion of terazosin occurs as both unchanged drug and metabolites in the urine and in the feces. Only 10% of the terazosin dose is excreted renally as unchanged drug; therefore, impaired renal function has no significant effect on the elimination of terazosin.

Contraindications/precautions, drug interactions and adverse effects are almost identical to those of prazosin.

DRUGS SIGNIFICANTLY DIFFERENT FROM PRAZOSIN

Phentolamine

Unlike prazosin, phentolamine (Regitine) blocks both alpha-1 and alpha-2 receptors. It is used in the management of tissue necrosis caused by extravasation of parenterally administered drugs and the management of symptoms from a pheochromocytoma, an adrenaline secreting tumor. It may induce similar adverse effects to prazosin, but it more likely to cause reflex tachycardia because of its ability to block alpha-2.

Phentolamine is contraindicated in patients with a known hypersensitivity. It is also contraindicated for use in patients with a history of acute myocardial infarction or any evidence of coronary artery disease because of its cardiac stimulating effects and resultant increase in myocardial oxygen demand. Reflex tachycardia can exacerbate angina. It is used with caution in patients with gastric and duodenal ulcers because the drug has a histamine-like effect. Phentolamine can stimulate secretion of gastric acid and pepsin in the stomach, which can aggravate peptic ulcer disease.

Phentolamine should not be used in conjunction with Epi. Phentolamine can antagonize its alpha-receptor-mediated actions and exaggerate its beta-adrenergic responses, resulting in hypotension, vasodilation, and tachycardia. Potential adverse reactions are similar to those of prazosin.

Phenoxybenzamine

Like phentolamine, phenoxybenzamine (Dibenzyline) blocks both alpha-1 and alpha-2 receptors. It is useful in the treatment of sweating and hypertension associated with pheochromocytoma, urinary symptoms of BPH, and symptoms of certain peripheral vasospastic conditions such as acrocyanosis, Raynaud phenomenon, and frostbite. The effects of phenoxybenzamine are similar to those of phentolamine. Phenoxybenzamine has a slower onset of action (effects begin in several hours) and a longer duration of action (effects of a single dose may last 3 to 4 days).

BETA-ADRENERGIC ANTAGONISTS

Beta-adrenergic antagonists are frequently and more commonly called beta-blockers. These comprise a significant group of drugs that can be grouped according to their specificity of action at the beta-1 and beta-2 receptors. If the predominant actions of stimulation of each of the two groups of beta-adrenergic receptors is considered, it follows that sometimes a therapeutic effect will require stimulation of beta-1 only (tachycardia, increased lipolysis, inotropy) or sometimes of both beta-1 and beta-2 (vasodilation, decreased peripheral resistance, bronchodilation) receptors.

Beta-1 blockade is effected by atenolol, acebutolol, alprenolol, metoprolol, betaxolol, and esmolol; beta-2 blockade has only one specific drug that triggers vasodilation, bronchodilation, and peripheral vascular resistance, namely butoxamine, which has no significant clinical application. The nonselective beta-blockers include propranolol, metipranolol, nadolol, penbutolol, pindolol, timolol, carteolol, and sotalol. Propranolol is the prototype nonselective beta-blocker.

NURSING MANAGEMENT OF THE PATIENT RECEIVING PROPRANOLOL

Core Drug Knowledge

Pharmacotherapeutics

Propranolol is used in the treatment of hypertension, angina, irregular cardiac rhythms, paroxysmal atrial tachycardias, ventricular tachycardias, digitalis intoxication, myocardial infarction, pheochromocytoma, migraine, hypertrophic subaortic stenosis, and essential tremor. It has been used to treat a wide variety of other disorders, including situational anxiety and substance withdrawal.

Pharmacokinetics

Propranolol is well absorbed following oral administration, and peak serum levels are observed within 2 to 6 hours of ingestion; however, hypotensive stability may not occur for 2 to 3 weeks. Beta blockade may occur within 1 to 2 hours. Parenteral dosing shifts the onset and duration to much lower times. Much of an ingested dose is subjected to first-pass metabolism in the liver. Metabolites are excreted through urine. Propranolol crosses the placenta and is excreted into breast milk. It has a half-life of 3 to 5 hours (longer with the sustained-release formulation). With IV dosing, half-life is shorter (see Table 14-8).

Pharmacodynamics

Propranolol is a noncardioselective beta-blocking drug that has similar effects on beta-1 (cardiac) and beta-2 (bronchial, vascular smooth muscle) receptors. Beta-1 blockade decreases heart rate and myocardial contractility during periods of high sympathetic activity (e.g., physical exercise). This results in a decreased cardiac output. As cardiac output decreases, so does blood pressure. In cardiac conduction tissue, beta blockade results in slowing of atrioventricular conduction and suppression of automaticity. These actions result in a decreased oxygen demand, thus suggesting its use as an antianginal agent. Propranolol also blocks beta-1 receptors in the kidneys. This action decreases the release of renin, which will result in a decreased blood pressure. Many of the adverse effects of propranolol are due to its overlapping beta-2 blockade. These include bronchospasm, hypoglycemia, and peripheral vasoconstriction. Although its role in reducing hypertension is complex, propranolol is an effective antihypertensive.

Contraindications and Precautions

The main contraindications for propranolol include severe bradycardia, complete heart block, cardiogenic shock, uncompensated cardiac failure, airway diseases, Raynaud syndrome, and in patients receiving antidepressant drugs. The action of propranolol depresses conduction through the atrioventricular node and decreases contractility. These actions can exacerbate cardiac disorders. Beta blockade results in bronchoconstriction, which exacerbates symptoms of chronic airway disorders. In Raynaud disease, symptoms can be exacerbated secondary to a reduced cardiac output and a relative increased alpha stimulation. Propranolol has been associated with major depression, although the mechanism is unclear. Abrupt discontinuation of propranolol in patients with hyperthyroidism may induce a thyroid storm.

Caution is used in patients with pheochromocytoma and vasospastic angina because unopposed alpha stimulation may result in hypertension. Propranolol should be used cautiously in patients with diabetes because beta blockade can mask the signs of hypoglycemia, especially palpitations, tachycardia, and tremors. Patients receiving propranolol should be monitored closely with surgery because of the cardiodepressant effects of general anesthetics. Patients with renal and hepatic diseases also require close monitoring to ensure clearance of the drug from the body. Other conditions that may be exacerbated by propranolol therapy include myasthenia gravis and psoriasis. Propranolol is secreted in breast milk, thus women who are breast-feeding should not take this drug.

Adverse Effects

If propranolol or a similar beta blocker is withdrawn abruptly, myocardial ischemia, infarction, ventricular arrhythmias, severe hypertension, or angina may occur. In the CNS, propranolol may cause cognitive dysfunction in the elderly or depression. Hallucinations and psychosis have been reported with high doses of the drug. These effects resolve after discontinuation. The drug predisposes to hypoglycemia in patients with type 1 diabetes and may trigger hyperthyroidism in susceptible individuals. In the GI system, diarrhea is common and may be severe enough to require discontinuation. With long-term therapy, weight gain is common.

Drug Interactions

Beta antagonists have many interactions with other drugs. Some of the more significant interactions include those with clonidine, Epi, verapamil, aminophylline, barbiturates, phenothiazines, cimetidine, ergot derivatives, hydralazine, NSAIDs, insulin, lidocaine, prazosin, quinidine, and rifampin (Table 14-9).

Elevated bilirubin levels may occur in patients who have chronic renal failure and who are taking propranolol, because its metabolites interfere with the bilirubin analysis. In addition, food enhances the bioavailability of propranolol, which may account for slight fluctuations in beta blockade or adverse effects (depending on dose scheduling).

Assessment of Relevant Core Patient Variables

Health Status

The nurse should assess for conditions for which the drug is contraindicated or for which special precautions might be necessary (e.g., uncontrolled asthma or chronic obstructive lung disease, severe sinus bradycardia, right ventricular hypertrophy or failure secondary to pulmonary hypertension, second- or third-degree atrioventricular block, cardiac failure, or cardiogenic shock). It is also important to determine whether any other drugs are being taken concurrently to identify significant potential drug interactions.

Because propranolol is used mainly to treat angina, cardiac arrhythmias, migraine headaches, hypertension, and tremors, the physical assessment should include blood pressure, ECG, cardiovascular status, genitourinary function, and mental and neurologic status. Heart and lung sounds should be auscultated as well.

Life Span and Gender

The nurse should document the age and gender of the patient. The nurse should assess women of child-bearing age for pregnancy and lactation. If the patient is pregnant, propranolol should be administered only if necessary. This drug is has an FDA pregnancy risk category C, and the possibility for inducing fetal abnormalities is unestablished. If the patient is breast-feeding, the infant should be monitored for adrenergic blockade. If this occurs, the administration may need to be discontinued. Elderly patients may be at risk for injury due to blurred vision resulting from propranolol use.

Lifestyle, Diet, and Habits

The nurse should document the patient's occupation and activities of daily living. Patients, particularly those in hazardous occupations, should be advised to exercise caution when driving or operating machinery at night or in bright light conditions. Mydriasis may cause temporary night blindness, which may prove perilous.

Environment

The nurse should be aware of the environment in which the drug will be administered and assess the home or living environment, if appropriate. Propranolol may be administered in any setting by health care providers, nurses, or patients themselves.

Nursing Diagnoses and Outcomes

- Sexual Dysfunction related to decreased libido or erectile dysfunction secondary to beta blockade
  Desired outcome: The patient will adapt to altered sexual functioning and understand that decreased libido or erectile dysfunction will be reversible on cessation of therapy.
- Risk for Injury related to dizziness secondary to beta blockade
  Desired outcome: The patient will not sustain injury and will learn safe methods for dealing with dizziness and postural hypotension.
- Disturbed Sleep Pattern, Insomnia and Drowsiness, secondary to beta blockade
  Desired outcome: The patient will sleep normally and awaken rested.
- Activity Intolerance related to lethargy and weakness secondary to beta blockade
  Desired outcome: The patient will maintain a satisfactory activity level.
- Risk for Deficient Fluid Volume related to drug-induced diarrhea
  Desired outcome: The patient will remain adequately hydrated and nourished despite adverse GI effects. The patient will report any intolerable GI effects.

Planning and Intervention

Maximizing Therapeutic Effects

The nurse should instruct the patient to take propranolol exactly as prescribed and at the required dosage frequency to enhance the therapeutic potential. Patients

TABLE 14-9 Agents That Interact With Propranolol

Interactants	Effect and Significance	Nursing Management
clonidine	Life-threatening increases in blood pressure after discontinuation of clonidine therapy	When clonidine is to be withdrawn from concomitant therapy with a beta blocker, discontinue the beta blocker first, and monitor blood pressure carefully.
epinephrine	Initial hypertension followed by bradycardia	Consult with prescriber: Labetalol (alpha/beta blocker) or alpha blockers (e.g., prazosin, doxazosin) may prevent rebound hypertension.
verapamil	Increased hypotensive effects of both drugs	Monitor blood pressure carefully for serious hypotension.
aminophylline	Reduced elimination of theophylline	Monitor for signs and symptoms of theophylline toxicity.
barbiturates	Decreased propranol levels resulting from barbiturate induction	Monitor for increased blood pressure. Monitor respiration.
phenothiazines	Increased levels of both drugs; phenothiazines inhibit first-pass metabolism of propranolol	Administer concomitant therapy with caution. Monitor phenothiazine level, and decrease dosage if prescribed.
cimetidine	May increase propranolol level twofold	Monitor cardiac function carefully (i.e., blood pressure, heart rate), and lower dosage of propranolol as prescribed.
ergot derivatives	Peripheral ischemia and cold extremities	If used together, monitor for peripheral ischemic effects (i.e., cold extremities), and substitute a selective beta blocker (e.g., atenolol) if ischemia occurs.
hydralazine	Increased levels of both drugs	If concurrent therapy is required, administer with food or switch to a sustained-release beta blocker. Monitor blood pressure carefully.
nonsteroidal anti-inflammatory drugs	Decreased propranolol level	Monitor blood pressure.
insulin	Prolonged hypoglycemia with masking of symptoms	Monitor blood glucose level regularly. Anticipate adjustment in drug dosages. Consult prescriber about lowering propranolol dosage, and monitor impact on blood glucose level.
lidocaine	Increased, potentially toxic lidocaine level	Consult prescriber about lower lidocaine dosage. Monitor for enhanced inotropic effect of propranolol.
prazosin	Increased postural hypotension from prazosin	Monitor blood pressure. Caution patient to rise slowly from seated position and use hand railings, particularly on stairs.
quinidine	Moderate increase in drug levels	Use caution with concomitant administration. Monitor for hypotension, bradycardia, arrhythmias, and heart failure.
alcohol	Decreased absorption and increased elimination of propranolol, resulting in tachycardia and possible increase in hypertension	Advise patient to avoid ethanol. Monitor blood pressure and heart rhythm.
rifampin	Rifampin-induced enzymes that decrease beta blocker levels by increasing metabolism and clearance	If concurrent therapy is required, monitor blood pressure carefully. A higher dose of propranolol may be required in patients receiving rifampin for longer than 1 to 2 wk. Or the prescriber may substitute atenolol or nadolol for propranolol.

taking propranolol in sustained-release form should be advised to swallow the whole drug and not to chew, crush, or break it. Patients may also take the drug with food to increase the drug's bioavailability and to avoid possible GI upset (e.g., diarrhea).

Patients should be informed about missing a dose and advised to take the dose as soon as possible unless it is within 4 hours of the next dose (8 hours for sustained-release forms). In such cases, they should skip the missed dose and return to the regular schedule.

Minimizing Adverse Effects

Some standards of care relating to beta-adrenergic antagonists, such as propranolol, are concerned with safety and require the nurse to perform certain interventions. First, the nurse should check the apical and peripheral pulses before giving propranolol. If the pulse is irregular or if there is bradycardia, the drug should be withheld and the prescriber notified, because these may be early signs of adverse or cardiotoxic effects.

Next, bronchoconstriction and altered cardiac output may result from adrenergic blockade. Therefore, the nurse should monitor cardiac rhythm and conduction (by ECG), blood pressure, and pulmonary wedge pressure, particularly when adrenergic antagonists, such as propranolol, are administered intravenously.

Third, in patients with angina, the nurse should monitor the frequency of anginal pain episodes and tolerance to activity.

Next, in patients with hypertension, the nurse should assess drug effectiveness by monitoring blood pressure and comparing the findings with baseline measurements.

Finally, in patients with impaired renal or hepatic function, the nurse should monitor for signs of drug accumulation and potential toxicity. See the accompanying display, Thinking Critically About Beta Blocker Therapy.

Providing Patient and Family Education

- Sympatholytic drugs interfere with compensatory and homeostatic mechanisms regulated by the normal functioning of the SNS, particularly in response to stress. Therefore, it is crucial to identify and monitor environmental stressors for patients receiving adrenergic antagonists, such as propranolol.
- Careful teaching about adverse effects is important. This includes teaching patients how to take their own pulses and detect irregular rhythms or bradycardias.
- Therapeutic adherence is promoted by reminding patients and their family members that drug therapy is meant to control certain life-threatening or debilitating conditions and should be taken even when the patient is feeling well and has no symptoms.
- If drug therapy is being discontinued, it is important to stress tapering or gradual withdrawal to prevent rebound symptoms and to adjust the activity levels to suit the reduced blockade.
- Another safety factor: the patient should be taught to change position slowly to reduce dizziness and light-headedness and to avoid operating machinery or driving until full adaptation to side effects has occurred. Factors known to enhance postural hypotension (e.g., heat, exercise, alcohol consumption) should be avoided.

Ongoing Assessment and Evaluation

The same assessment focus is used for adrenergic antagonists as for the adrenergic agonists. All patients with cardiovascular disorders are considered worthy of extra attention when taking an adrenergic antagonist, such as propranolol. When evaluating the success of nursing management in propranolol therapy, the nurse anticipates the absence of signs and symptoms for the condition being treated and minimal adverse effects.

If propranolol is being given for angina or hypertension, blood pressure should be within normal limits, and there should be a reduced frequency of anginal attacks and tolerance to reasonable activity. For antiarrhythmic indications, no arrhythmias should be evident on ECG findings. Moreover, the patient should be free from injury resulting from postural hypotension or dizziness. The patient may report sexual adjustment. Ideally, the patient and family can understand, recognize, and cope with adverse effects. ■

Critical Thinking Scenario

Thinking critically about beta blocker therapy

Mr. DiGiovanni is a 65-year-old man with hypertension and angina. His health care provider recently increased his propranolol dosage from 40 mg qid to 60 mg qid. He complaints to you that he is experiencing erectile dysfunction.

1. Discuss what you know about the effects of propranolol on sexual performance.
2. Choose elements related to propranolol therapy to include in a teaching plan for Mr. DiGiovanni, and provide rationale for your choices.
3. What other health care professionals may work with the nurse to provide the best care for Mr. DiGiovanni?

MEMORY CHIP

Propranolol

- Beta blocker
- Treats hypertension, angina, cardiac arrhythmias, migraine
- Decreases heart rate and contractility, slows conduction, suppresses automaticity
- Significant contraindications: bradycardia, complete heart block, cardiogenic shock, uncompensated cardiac failure, reactive airway diseases, and Raynaud disease
- Most common adverse effects: postural hypotension, bronchospasm
- Most serious adverse effect: myocardial infarction
- Maximizing therapeutic effects: take the medication exactly as prescribed, never double a dose
- Minimizing adverse effects: minimize situational and environmental stressors, stress safety issues
- Most significant patient education: self-monitoring techniques for pulse rate and heartbeat, safe mobility related to postural hypotension, and never abruptly stop taking the medication

DRUGS CLOSELY RELATED TO PROPRANOLOL

Atenolol

Atenolol (Tenormin) is a competitive, beta-1 selective adrenergic antagonist, similar to metoprolol. It may be administered orally or parenterally. Atenolol has a longer plasma half-life than metoprolol does, reducing the frequency of administration. As with all selective beta-blockers, high doses result in attenuated or lost selectivity for the beta-1 receptor. Atenolol does not possess membrane-stabilizing activity as pindolol and propranolol do. In addition, atenolol has the lowest lipid solubility within the class, which affects its route of elimination and, theoretically, its potential for causing CNS side effects.

Metoprolol

Metoprolol (Lopressor) is a competitive, beta-1 selective adrenergic antagonist, similar to atenolol. It is only administered orally. Metoprolol does not have intrinsic sympathomimetic activity and does not exhibit membrane-stabilizing activities. Metoprolol is more lipid soluble than atenolol, but less than propranolol. Metoprolol has one of the shortest plasma half-lives of the orally administered cardioselective beta-blockers.

Pindolol

Pindolol (Viskin) is an oral, nonselective, beta-receptor antagonist with intrinsic sympathomimetic activity (ISA). This means that it has partial agonist activity. Pindolol is the beta-blocker with the highest degree of ISA and nonselective antagonist qualities. The effect of ISA, as with beta blockade in general, can be selective or nonselective in nature. The partial agonist potential of pindolol is greater for beta-2 than beta-1 receptors, resulting in the ability to be partially vasodilatory.

Nadolol

Nadolol (Corgard) is an oral, nonselective, beta-adrenergic receptor antagonist similar to propranolol. Nadolol does not demonstrate appreciable intrinsic sympathomimetic or membrane-stabilizing activities. Unlike propranolol, nadolol possesses a low degree of lipid solubility and has the longest plasma half-life of all the beta-adrenergic blocking agents.

Timolol

Timolol (Blockadren) is a nonselective beta-adrenergic receptor antagonist, similar to propranolol and nadolol. Timolol does not demonstrate appreciable intrinsic sympathomimetic or membrane-stabilizing activities. Like propranolol, timolol possesses a relatively high degree of lipid solubility and is subject to first-pass metabolism by the liver. Timolol is available for both oral ophthalmic use.

DRUGS SIGNIFICANTLY DIFFERENT FROM PROPRANOLOL

Carvedilol

Carvedilol (Coreg) is a combined alpha- and nonselective beta-blocker. Although it has some pharmacologic similarities to labetalol, the ratio of beta-1 to alpha-1 effects is much greater for carvedilol than for labetalol. Carvedilol also possesses antioxidant properties (an effect not shared by other beta-blockers). Carvedilol has multiple actions that make it a useful cardiovascular drug. Similar to labetalol, carvedilol antagonizes both alpha-1 and beta receptors. However, the ratio of beta-blockade to alpha-1 blockade for carvedilol is approximately 10 to 100:1. The ratio for labetalol is 1.5:1. Carvedilol is indicated for the management of hypertension, heart failure, stable angina, and as postmyocardial infarction prophylaxis. It is frequently administered with other antihypertensive agents to gain additive therapeutic effects.

When initiating carvedilol therapy, the patient should have a standing blood pressure measurement 1 hour after dosing. An initial dose of 6.25 mg should be maintained for 7 to 14 days; then, the patient should be evaluated for the effectiveness of the dose. If further control of diastolic blood pressure is needed, the dosage may be increased to 12.5 mg orally twice daily for an additional 7 to 14 days. If needed, the dosage may be further increased to the maximum recommended dosage of 25 mg orally twice daily if tolerated. If the pulse rate drops below 55 bpm, the dosage of carvedilol should be reduced. Doses should be taken with food to slow the rate of absorption and reduce the risk of orthostatic hypotension.

Labetalol

Labetalol (Normodyne) is an oral and parenteral competitive nonselective beta-adrenergic and selective postsynaptic alpha-1 adrenergic receptor blocker. Labetalol blocks beta-1 receptors in the heart, beta-2 receptors in bronchial and vascular smooth muscle, and alpha-1 receptors in vascular smooth muscle. The beta-blocking activity is 3 to 7 times as potent as the alpha-blocking ability. The result of labetalol's actions at alpha and beta receptors leads to vasodilation and decreased total peripheral resistance, which results in decreased blood pressure without a substantial decrease in resting heart rate, cardiac output, or stroke volume.

Sotalol

Sotalol (Betapace) is an oral, nonselective beta-adrenergic blocking agent. Unlike other beta-blockers, sotalol has no sympathomimetic activity or membrane-stabilizing effects but does possess class III antiarrhythmic properties similar to those of amiodarone. As a result, sotalol is used as an antiarrhythmic. It is primarily used in the management of ventricular arrhythmias and angina.

CHAPTER SUMMARY

- Regulation of physiologic processes in the ANS is managed by oppositional or complementary stimulation by the adrenergic and cholinergic nervous systems.
- To effect an action, a neurotransmitter needs to bind with an appropriate receptor site on the effector organ or tissue.
- Alpha-1 adrenergic agonists, such as phenylephrine, stimulate alpha-1 receptors directly. They are most commonly used as nasal decongestants and in ophthalmology to achieve mydriasis. They may also be used as vasopressors to treat vascular failure and related shock.
- Nonselective adrenergic agonists, such as Epi, are used to treat anaphylactic shock, asthma, hemorrhage, and ventricular fibrillation. The nonselective activity stimulates all four adrenergic subtypes.
- Alpha-adrenergic antagonists, such as prazosin, are used to treat hypertension and BPH.
- Beta-adrenergic antagonists, such as propranolol, are used to treat hypertension, angina, and cardiac arrhythmias.
- Alpha- and beta-adrenergic antagonists, such as labetalol, are used to treat hypertension and heart failure.

QUESTIONS FOR STUDY AND REVIEW

1. You have been assigned to a cardiac care unit and are particularly interested in patients with angina. Which parameters are key to your predrug therapy assessments for a patient about to receive beta blockers?
2. When working with patients with angina, which factors are most important to you during therapeutic monitoring?
3. How will you recognize impending toxicity in a patient receiving propranolol?
4. What will you do if it appears that the patient is showing cardiotoxic effects from propranolol?
5. You are assisting in the care of a patient in cardiogenic shock and have been asked to prepare an IV solution of isoproterenol in dextrose 5% in lactated Ringer solution. After hanging the IV drug container and starting the infusion, how long do you expect the infusion to last?
6. What initial change in the above patient's status are you likely to see first, and how long will these effects last?
7. Why are the rest of the nurses concerned about uncorrected hypovolemia?

NEED MORE HELP?

Chapter 14 of the study guide for *Drug Therapy in Nursing* contains exercises and activities to reinforce your understanding of the concepts presented in this chapter. For additional information see the text's accompanying website at *http://www.connection.lww.com.*

REFERENCES AND BIBLIOGRAPHY

Bennett, M. R. (1999). One hundred years of adrenaline: The discovery of autoreceptors, *Clinical Autonomic Research, 9*(3), 145–159.

CCIS System. (2001). *Computerized Clinical Information System.* Denver, CO: Micromedex.

Clinical Drug Monographs [CDRom]. (2001). Gold Standard Media.

Drug Facts and Comparisons. (2000). St. Louis: Facts and Comparisons Division.

Hardman, J. G., Limbird, L. E., Molinof, P. B., Ruddon, R. W., & Gilman, A. (Eds.). (1997). *Goodman and Gilman's pharmacological basis of therapeutics* (9th ed.). New York: McGraw-Hill.

Karch, A. (2001). *2001 Lippincott's nursing drug guide.* Philadelphia: Lippincott Williams & Wilkins

Katzung, B. C. (2000). *Basic and clinical pharmacology* (8th ed.), New York: McGraw-Hill.

Pepper, G. A. (1999). Pharmacology of antihypertensive drugs. *Journal of Obstetric, Gynecological, and Neonatal Nursing, 28*(6), 649–659.

Pepper, G. S., & Lee, R. W. (1999). Sympathetic activation in heart failure and its treatment with beta-blockade. *Archives of Internal Medicine, 159*(3), 225–234.

Porth, C. (1998). *Pathophysiology: Concepts of altered health states* (5th ed.). Philadelphia: Lippincott Williams & Wilkins.

Sever, P. S. (1999). Alpha 1-blockers in hypertension. *Current Medical Research and Opinions, 15*(2), 95–103.

Shuster, J. (1998). Combining nonprescription medications. *Nursing, 28*(6), 77.

Tatro, D. (Ed.). (2000). *Drug interaction facts* (6th ed.). St. Louis: Facts and Comparisons.

Vansal, S. S., & Feller, D. R. (1999). Direct effects of ephedrine isomers on human beta-adrenergic receptor subtypes. *Biochemical Pharmacology, 58*(5), 807–810.

Watson, A. (1998). Alpha adrenergic blockers and adrenaline. A mysterious collapse. *Australian Family Physician, 27*(8), 714–715.

White, M., et al. (1999). Effects of age and hypertension on cardiac responses to the alpha$_1$ agonist phenylephrine in humans. *American Journal of Hypertension, 12*(2 Pt. 1), 151–158.

Chapter 15

DRUGS AFFECTING CHOLINERGIC FUNCTION

KEY TERMS

autonomic nervous system
cholinergic agonists
cholinergic antagonists
cholinergic crisis
miosis
muscarinic receptor
nicotinic receptor
parasympathetic nervous system
sympathetic nervous system

Learning Objectives

At the completion of this chapter the student will:

1. Describe the anatomy and physiology of the cholinergic nervous system.
2. Describe synaptic transmission.
3. Describe the role of cholinergic agonists and antagonists in a variety of therapeutic uses.
4. Identify core drug knowledge about drugs that act as cholinergic agonists or antagonists.
5. Identify core patient variables relevant to drugs that act as agonists or cholinergic antagonists.
6. Relate the interaction of core drug knowledge to core patient variables for drugs that act as cholinergic agonists or antagonists.
7. Generate a nursing plan of care from the interactions between core drug knowledge and core patient variables for drugs that act as cholinergic agonists or antagonists.
8. Describe nursing interventions to maximize therapeutic and minimize adverse affects for drugs that act as cholinergic agonists or antagonists.
9. Determine key points for patient and family education for drugs that act as cholinergic agonists or antagonists.

Cholinergic agonists

Direct-acting muscarinic agonists

pilocarpine
bethanechol
acetylcholine
carbachol
methacholine

Direct-acting nicotinic agonists

nicotine

Indirect-acting cholinergic agonists

neostigmine
edrophonium
ambenonium
physostigmine
pyridostigmine
tacrine
irreversible cholinesterase inhibitors

Cholinergic antagonists

atropine
antisecretory anticholinergics
benztropine
hyoscyamine
ipratropium
scopolamine
trihexyphenidyl

The symbol (C) indicates the **drug class**.

Drugs in bold type marked with the symbol (P) are **prototypes**.

Drugs in blue type with no symbol are **closely related** to the prototype.

Drugs in red type with no symbol are **significantly different** from the prototype.

Drugs in **black** type with no symbol are **also used in drug therapy**; no prototype.

As described in Chapter 14, the **autonomic nervous system** (ANS) is divided into the adrenergic (sympathetic) and cholinergic (parasympathetic) nervous systems. These systems work in combination or opposition to maintain homeostasis within the body. This chapter identifies drugs used to treat the major disorders that are affected by deficiencies or excesses in cholinergic neurotransmission. It also discusses the wide range of therapeutic uses of cholinergic drugs. This chapter presents the cholinergic drugs that are categorized into cholinergic stimulants, called **cholinergic agonists** or parasympathomimetics, and cholinergic blockers, known as **cholinergic antagonists**, anticholinergics, or parasympatholytics.

The cholinergic drugs are also categorized by the type of cholinergic receptor they affect. For example, pilocarpine (Akarpine) is the prototype direct-acting muscarinic agonist, whereas nicotine (Nicotrol, Prostep) is the prototype direct-acting nicotinic agonist. Neostigmine (Prostigmin) is the prototype indirect-acting cholinergic agonist, also known as an anticholinesterase or cholinesterase inhibitor. The prototype representing the cholinergic antagonists is atropine (Atropine Sulfate).

PHYSIOLOGY

FUNCTION OF THE AUTONOMIC NERVOUS SYSTEM

As mentioned in Chapter 14, the ANS is an involuntary system responsible for the control of smooth muscle, cardiac muscle, and exocrine glands. These regulatory functions of the body are monitored by both the **sympathetic** and **parasympathetic nervous systems.** The sympathetic and parasympathetic nervous systems either work as complementary or oppositional systems to maintain involuntary function of the body. The reader is referred to Chapter 14 for discussion of synaptic transmission, neurotransmitters, and regulation of physiologic processes.

CHOLINERGIC RECEPTORS

There are three types of cholinergic receptors: nicotinic$_N$, nicotinic$_M$, and muscarinic (Fig. 15-1). Activation of nicotinic$_N$ receptors promotes ganglionic transmission in both the sympathetic and parasympathetic nervous systems as well as release of epinephrine from the adrenal medulla. Conversely, antagonists of nicotinic$_N$ block ganglionic transmission and release of epinephrine. Activation of nicotinic$_M$ receptors causes contraction of skeletal muscle. Activation of muscarinic receptors results in a variety of actions based on the parasympathetic target organ involved (Table 15-1).

Nicotinic receptors have a high affinity for responding to nicotine, a plant alkaloid, and will also respond to acetylcholine. They have a very low affinity for response to muscarine. Muscarinic receptors respond to acetylcholine, and also bind muscarine, an alkaloid substance isolated from mushrooms.

PATHOPHYSIOLOGY

The various tissues and organs that are innervated by the ANS are diverse, and few discrete disorders are directly related to compromise of the parasympathetic nervous system. Instead, the therapeutic uses of parasympathetic drugs are related to providing extra cholinergic stimulation or blockade to normal ANS functioning. Any disorders of the

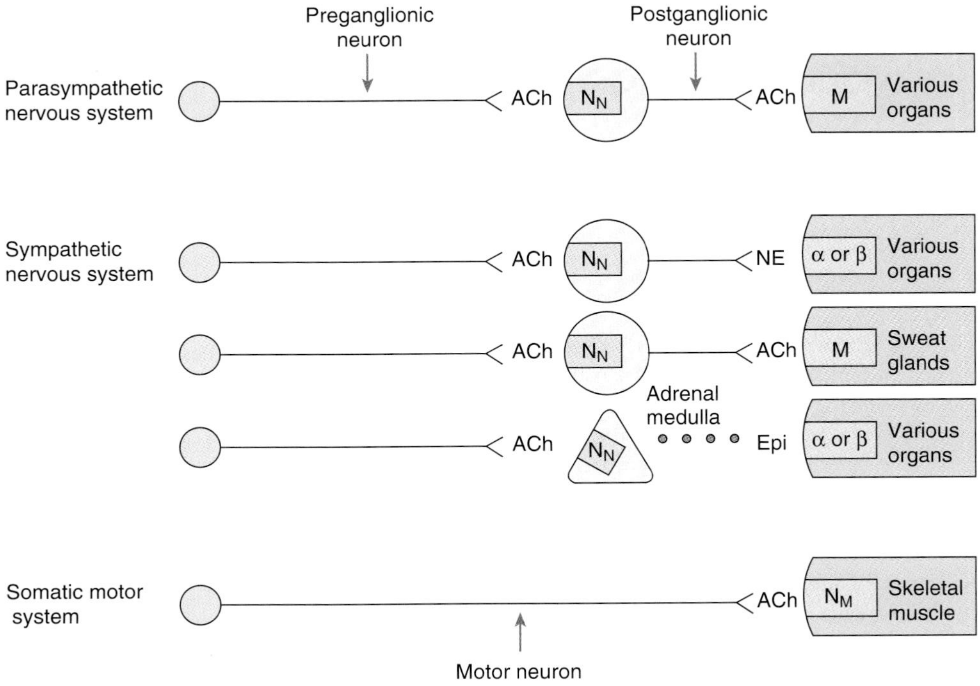

Figure 15-1. Cholinergic receptor subtypes: N_N = nicotinic$_N$; N_M=nicotinic$_M$; M = muscarinic. Adrenergic receptor subtypes: α = alpha; β = beta.

TABLE 15-1 Cholinergic Receptor Subtypes' Location and Action

Location	Response to Stimulation
Nicotinic$_N$	
All autonomic nervous system ganglia	Stimulation of sympathetic and parasympathetic *post-ganglionic* transmission
Adrenal medulla	Release of epinephrine
Nicotinic$_M$	
Neuromuscular junction	Contraction of skeletal muscle
Muscarinic	
Eye	Miosis (pupillary constriction) Contraction of the ciliary muscle
Heart	Decreased rate
Lung	Bronchoconstriction Increased bronchial secretions
Blood vessels	Vasodilation Hypotension
GU system	Micturition
GI tract	Increased salivation Increased intestinal tone and motility Increased gastric secretions Defecation
Sweat glands	Increased sweating
Sex organs	Erection

bronchi, cardiovascular system, gastrointestinal or genitourinary tracts, skeletal muscle, eyes, and many glands may respond to cholinergic stimulation through their muscarinic and nicotinic receptors.

CHOLINERGIC AGONISTS

Cholinergic agonists include direct-acting muscarinic agonists, direct-acting nicotinic agonists, and indirect-acting cholinergic agonists.

DIRECT-ACTING MUSCARINIC AGONISTS

Direct-acting muscarinic agonists are drugs that bind to the muscarinic receptors located in various tissues and organs throughout the body. Their activation elicits a response that resembles the action of the parasympathetic nervous system; thus, they are also called parasympathomimetic agents. The muscarinic drugs are the choline esters, such as acetylcholine (Miochol), bethanechol (Urecholine), carbachol (Isopto Carbachol), and methacholine (Provocholine), and the alkaloids (e.g., muscarine, pilocarpine). Although pilocarpine has limited therapeutic scope, it is the ideal prototype for the direct-acting muscarinic agonists.

NURSING MANAGEMENT OF THE PATIENT RECEIVING PILOCARPINE

Core Drug Knowledge

Pharmacotherapeutics

Pilocarpine is a direct-acting cholinergic agonist with ophthalmic uses. The major indications for pilocarpine are open-angle glaucoma, acute treatment of angle-closure glaucoma, miosis induction to counteract mydriatic effects of sympathomimetics used in surgery, and miosis induction following ophthalmoscopy to counteract the effects of cycloplegics and mydriatics. Oral pilocarpine is used in the treatment of xerostomia (dry mouth) caused by hypofunction of the salivary gland due to radiotherapy for cancer of the head or neck.

Pharmacokinetics

Pilocarpine may be applied topically by solution or an ocular system that allows sustained-release over 7 days. With topical administration, **miosis** (pupillary constriction) occurs within 10 to 30 minutes and a maximal decrease in intraocular pressure (IOP) occurs within 2 to 4 hours (Table 15-2). As an oral agent, peak effects are achieved in about 1 hour. Peak effects may take longer if the drug is taken with food. The mechanism for inactivation of pilocarpine is not clear but is thought to occur at the neuronal synapses and in plasma. Pilocarpine and its degradation products are excreted in the urine.

Pharmacodynamics

Pilocarpine directly stimulates cholinergic receptors. It produces miosis by contracting the iris sphincter. In open-angle glaucoma, pilocarpine contracts the ciliary muscle, increasing the outflow of aqueous humor, which reduces IOP. In closed-angle glaucoma, pilocarpine-induced miosis opens the angle of the anterior chamber of the eye, allowing the aqueous humor to exit. Pilocarpine also counteracts the mydriatic effects of sympathomimetic agents used in ophthalmologic examinations. When administered orally, pilocarpine stimulates secretions of the exocrine glands. All secretory glands may be affected, including an increase in salivary flow.

Contraindications and Precautions

It is important to note that some contraindications may not be applicable to ophthalmic use and that others are not applicable to oral use. Hypersensitivity is a contraindication regardless of the formulation utilized.

Ophthalmic pilocarpine is contraindicated for use in patients with a history of retinal detachment. Miotics can precipitate detachment of the retina, resulting in a sudden drop in IOP. Ophthalmic pilocarpine is also contraindicated for use in patients with acute iritis or other conditions that would be exacerbated by pupillary constriction.

TABLE 15-2 Summary of Selected Cholinergic Agonists

Drug (Trade) Name	Selected Indications	Route and Dosage Range	Pharmacokinetics
Direct-Acting Muscarinic Agonists			
pilocarpine (Akarpine)	Dry mouth from chemotherapy Open-angle glaucoma, changes in intraocular pressure, reversal of mydriasis	*Adult:* PO, 5 mg tid for chemotherapy-induced dry mouth (xerostomia) *Adult:* intraocular, 1 drop of 1%–2% solution q6–8 h or 20–40 μg/h by intraocular delivery device (Ocusert)	*Onset:* 10–30 min *Duration:* 4–8 h $t_{1/2}$: 3/4–1-1/2 h
acetylcholine (Miochol)	Cataract extraction, iridectomy, iris incarceration, keratoplasties, ophthalmic surgery, peripheral iridectomy, parotitis, renal failure, respiratory distress syndrome	*Adult:* intraocular, 5–20 mg intraocular as 0.5–2.0 mL solution	*Onset:* 10–30 min *Duration:* 10 min $t_{1/2}$: Minutes
bethanechol (Bethanechol Chloride; *Canadian:* Duvoid)	Decompensated bladder, lower motor neuron lesions, neurogenic bladder, postpartum urinary retention, urinary retention, postoperative urinary retention, atonies, sexual dysfunction, bladder dysfunction, parotitis, motion sickness	*Adult:* PO, 10–50 mg tid or qid	*Onset:* 30–90 min *Duration:* 1–6 h $t_{1/2}$: Variable
carbachol (Isopto Carbachol)	Glaucoma	*Adult:* topical, 2 drops of 0.75%–3.0% solution tid for glaucoma	*Onset:* 10–20 min *Duration:* 8 h $t_{1/2}$: Minutes
Methacholine (Provocholine)	Diagnosis of bronchial airway hyperactivity	Individualized	*Onset:* Rapid *Duration:* 15–75 m $t_{1/2}$: Unknown
Direct-Acting Nicotinic Agonist			
nicotine (Nicotrol, Prostep)	Smoking cessation	*Adult:* PO, 2 mg chewing gum prn; transdermal, 5–22 mg daily depending on number of weeks without cigarettes	*Onset:* Transdermal 1–2 h *Duration:* 2–24 h $t_{1/2}$: 3–4 h
Indirect-Acting Cholinergic Agonists			
neostigmine (Neostigmine Methylsulfate, Prostigmin; *Canadian:* PMS Neostigmine Methylsulfate)	Myasthenia gravis (MG) Neuromuscular blockade reversal Paralytic ileus and urinary retention	*Adult:* PO, 150 mg/d *Adult:* SC/IM, 0.5 mg *Adult:* 0.5 mg, then 0.5 mg q3h up to five times	*Onset:* PO, 2–4; SC/IM, 20–30 min; IV, 60 s *Duration:* PO, 2.5–4 h; IV 1–2 h $t_{1/2}$: 50–90 min
edrophonium (Tensilon)	Diagnosis of MG, differentiation between cholinergic and myasthenic crises, antagonism of neuromuscular blockade, parotitis, supraventricular tachycardia, Eaton-Lambert syndrome	*Adult:* IV, 1–10 mg depending on the indication	*Onset:* IV, 30–60 s *Duration:* IV 5–10 min $t_{1/2}$: 5–10 min
ambenonium (Mytelase)	MG, parotitis	*Adult:* PO, 5–25 mg tid or qid	*Onset:* 20–30 min *Duration:* 3–8 h $t_{1/2}$: Unknown

(*continued*)

TABLE 15-2 Summary of Selected Cholinergic Agonists (Continued)

Drug (Trade) Name	Selected Indications	Route and Dosage Range	Pharmacokinetics
physostigmine (Antilirium, Isopto Eserine, prazosin hydrochloride)	Alzheimer's disease Antidote for anticholinergic overdose Glaucoma, parotitis, acute myelogenous leukemia, chronic pain	*Adult:* PO 6–18 mg in four to nine divided doses daily *Adult:* IV, 2 mg slow push over 2 min or more *Adult:* 0.25% or 0.5%, 1 drop up to four times daily or 1 cm 0.25% ointment one to three times daily	*Onset:* IV, 3–5 min *Duration:* 30–60 min $t_{1/2}$: 15–40 min
pyridostigmine (Mestinon, Regonol)	Motion sickness MG Reversal of nondepolarizing neuromuscular blockade	*Adult:* PO, 30 mg tid *Adult:* PO, 600 mg paced throughout the day *Adult:* IV, 0.1–0.25 mg/kg	*Onset:* PO, 35–45 min; IV, 5 min *Duration:* 3–6 h $t_{1/2}$: 1.9–3.7 h
tacrine (Cognex)	Alzheimer disease, AIDS dementia, tardive dyskinesia, anticholinergic overdose	*Adult:* PO, 10 mg qid increasing by 40 mg/d every 6 wk; IV slow push, 0.25–0.5 mg/kg	*Onset:* Varies *Duration:* Unknown $t_{1/2}$: 2–4 h

Because of its systemic effects, oral pilocarpine has more contraindications and precautions. These contraindications and precautions occur because of pilocarpine's ability to mimic the effects of the parasympathetic nervous system. For example, patients with asthma, chronic bronchitis, or chronic airway limitation (CAL) may have exacerbations of these conditions because pilocarpine stimulates the mucous cells of the respiratory tract and increases bronchial smooth muscle tone and airway resistance. Pilocarpine causes contractions of the gallbladder or biliary smooth muscle, possibly resulting in biliary obstruction, cholangitis, or cholecystitis. Patients with cardiac disease may not be able to compensate for the transient changes in heart rhythm or hemodynamics caused by oral pilocarpine. Pilocarpine increases ureteral smooth muscle tone and may precipitate renal colic, especially in patients with nephrolithiasis. Oral pilocarpine may induce dose-related central nervous system (CNS) effects that could exacerbate conditions of psychiatric disturbances or cognitive disturbances.

Pilocarpine is classified as a pregnancy category C drug. The oral dosage form should only be used if the benefits outweigh the risks to the fetus.

Finally, patients using pilocarpine ophthalmic or oral preparations should be cautioned about night-time driving, particularly the elderly and those with opaque lenses. Loss of visual acuity and accommodation is greater in poor light.

Adverse Effects

The ophthalmic adverse effects of pilocarpine include transient stinging and burning, tearing, and ciliary spasm. The ocular system (Ocusert) may cause conjunctival irritation. Systemic adverse effects include hypertension, tachycardia, bronchiolar spasm, pulmonary edema, salivation and sweating, and nausea and vomiting. When systemic effects occur with other cholinergic agonists, there is a possibility of a **cholinergic crisis**, which needs to be recognized quickly and managed effectively. The crisis is caused by cholinergic toxicity and results in medullary paralysis (central respiratory paralysis), peripheral respiratory paralysis, excessive tracheobronchial and salivary secretions, bronchospasm, and laryngospasm. These effects may cause respiratory failure, which can be reversed with the maintenance of a patent airway. Muscle twitching, fasciculations, and paralysis may also occur. All symptoms of cholinergic crisis may be reversed with atropine, an anticholinergic drug.

Drug Interactions

There are no known significant interactions between pilocarpine and other drugs, although other cholinergic agonists or blockers may enhance or antagonize its effects (Table 15-3).

Assessment of Relevant Core Patient Variables

Health Status

Cholinergic agonists, such as pilocarpine, do not have a wide range of therapeutic uses, but when they are used, they may cause systemic side effects and interact with preexisting disorders in life-threatening ways. A careful history and physical assessment will identify contraindications and precautions necessary for the person taking pilocarpine.

The nurse needs to determine whether the patient has uncontrolled asthma or acute iritis, because these are contraindications to pilocarpine therapy. Patients should be assessed for significant cardiovascular disease because they may be unable to compensate for transient changes in hemodynamics or rhythm induced by pilocarpine. Pilocarpine should be used cautiously in patients with chronic bronchitis or CAL because it may increase airway resistance, bronchial smooth muscle tone, and bronchial

TABLE 15-3 Agents That Interact With Pilocarpine

Interactants	Effect and Significance	Nursing Management
cholinergic drugs	Enhanced cholinergic effect	Monitor increased and prolonged cholinergic stimulation.
anticholinergic drugs	Decreased cholinergic effect	Keep in mind that a dosage adjustment may be needed.

secretions. Patients with a history of biliary disease or nephrolithiasis should also be closely monitored.

Life Span and Gender

The nurse should document the age and gender of the patient. The nurse should assess women of child-bearing age for pregnancy and lactation. If the patient is pregnant, this drug should be used only if necessary, because it is not known if pilocarpine causes fetal abnormalities. If the patient is breast-feeding, the infant should be monitored for cholinergic stimulation; if this occurs, the drug may need to be discontinued. Elderly patients may be at higher risk of injury because of blurred vision.

Lifestyle, Diet, and Habits

The nurse should document the patient's occupation and activities of daily living. Patients should be advised to exercise caution when driving or operating machinery at night or in low light, because miosis causes difficulty in dark adaptation.

Environment

The nurse should be aware of the environment in which the drug will be administered and assess the home or living environment if appropriate. Pilocarpine may be administered in any setting by a health care provider, nurse, or the patient.

Nursing Diagnoses and Outcomes

- Risk for Injury related to blurred vision
  Desired outcome: The patient will remain free of injury.
- Disturbed Sensory Perception (Visual) secondary to instillation of topical miotic.
  Desired outcome: The patient will adapt to blurring and adapt activity accordingly.
- Acute Pain related to local corneal irritation by miotic instillate
  Desired outcome: The patient will remain free from irritation.

Planning and Intervention

Maximizing Therapeutic Effects

Because pilocarpine is usually instilled, the nurse should demonstrate how to instill drops into the conjunctival sac. To obtain the optimal intraocular hypotensive effect using the Ocusert system, the nurse must also demonstrate the placement and insertion of the system into the inferior conjunctival sac.

If both the solution and gel are used, the solution should be applied first, then the gel is applied 5 minutes later. Following administration of the solution, finger pressure should be applied on the lacrimal sac for 1 to 2 minutes.

Oral pilocarpine should be administered at regular intervals throughout the day.

Minimizing Adverse Effects

As with all cholinergic agonists, the use of pilocarpine requires the availability of an antidote in case of systemic overdose or cholinergic crisis. Atropine is the usual agent for this purpose. For patients with known allergies or suspected hypersensitivity, life support measures need to be available in case of bronchial spasm or allergic reactions. Systemic side effects include stimulation of sphincters, so patients may need access to a bedpan or urinal.

Contact lenses should be removed before ophthalmic treatment. If pilocarpine drops are applied to the eyes when soft contact lenses are in place, the lenses can deteriorate or absorb the drug. It also is possible that hard contact lenses can cause corneal abrasion or roughening of the corneal surface. Corneal abrasion can increase systemic absorption, possibly causing toxicity.

Providing Patient and Family Education

- Patients should be cautioned about blurred vision and how this may be hazardous.
- Patients should be taught to recognize systemic adverse effects and how to manage them.
- Patients using the Ocusert system need instruction for inserting and removing the ocular device safely and antiseptically.

Ongoing Assessment and Evaluation

During therapy, monitoring of therapeutic effects should reveal the decrease in frequency or severity of target symptoms or the resumption of the problem for which pilocarpine was prescribed. Nurses familiar with ophthalmic surgery and conditions will be adept at continuous assessment and evaluation of changes in IOP. Moreover, they can use a tonometer to gauge significant changes in IOP. Other evaluations would include the effectiveness of minimizing adverse side effects. ■

MEMORY CHIP

Pilocarpine

- A direct-acting muscarinic agonist used for simple and acute glaucoma, preoperative and postoperative intraocular tension, mydriasis, and xerostomia
- Significant contraindications (ophthalmic): hypersensitivity, history of retinal detachment, and acute iritis
- Significant contraindications (oral): hypersensitivity, severe respiratory diseases
- Most common adverse effects: blurred vision, myopia
- Most serious adverse effects: cholinergic crisis, bronchospasm
- Maximizing therapeutic effects: administer ophthalmic solution into the conjunctival cul-de-sac
- Minimizing adverse effects: availability of antidote, aseptic technique for ophthalmic administration
- Most significant patient education: symptoms of cholinergic crisis and need for immediate medical attention

DRUGS CLOSELY RELATED TO PILOCARPINE

Bethanechol

Bethanechol (Urecholine) is a synthetic muscarinic stimulant with primary effects on the urinary and GI tracts. Its effect on the bladder results from stimulation of muscarinic receptors in the detrusor muscle. As the detrusor contracts, the bladder capacity decreases, resulting in micturition. Bethanechol also stimulates ureteral peristalsis and relaxes the trigone and external sphincter. Because bethanechol is a direct-acting agonist, spinal cord injury will not compromise its actions. Stimulation of muscarinic receptors in the GI tract restores peristalsis, increases motility, and increases the resting lower esophageal sphincter pressure. Bethanechol also stimulates the lower GI tract, resulting in defecation. It is the preferred drug in the treatment of postpartum and postoperative nonobstructive urinary retention. It is also used in the management of urinary retention related to phenothiazine or tricyclic antidepressant therapy.

As an oral agent, bethanechol may induce systemic adverse effects similar to those of pilocarpine. Like pilocarpine, drug interactions include other cholinergic or anticholinergic drugs. In addition, bethanechol in conjunction with ganglionic blocking agents may result in a critical decrease in blood pressure.

Acetylcholine

As a drug, acetylcholine (Miochol) is limited to use in the management of ophthalmologic surgery. It produces complete miosis in cataract surgery, keratoplasty, iridectomy, and other anterior segment surgery in which rapid miosis is required. Because it is given topically, systemic adverse effects rarely occur. However, it may induce problems for patients with acute cardiac failure, bronchial asthma, peptic ulcer, hyperthyroidism, GI spasms (cramps), urinary tract obstruction, and Parkinson disease. It is contraindicated for use in patients with acute iritis and acute inflammatory disease of the anterior chamber of the eye.

Carbachol

Carbachol (Isopto Carbachol) is used in the management of glaucoma. It is administered as a ophthalmologic solution up to 3 times daily. Like pilocarpine, it works by direct stimulation of the muscarinic cholinergic receptors in the eye. Contraindications and adverse effects are similar to pilocarpine.

Methacholine

Methacholine (Provocholine) is a parasympathomimetic inhalation agent used to assist in the diagnosis of bronchial airway hyperreactivity in patients who do not have clinically apparent asthma. Methacholine induces bronchoconstriction in asthmatic patients more readily than in nonasthmatic patients.

Contraindications and precautions include hypersensitivity to parasympathomimetic agents, concurrent beta-antagonist therapy, epilepsy, cardiovascular disease characterized by bradycardia, peptic ulcer disease, thyroid disease, urinary tract obstruction, or patients with clinically apparent asthma, wheezing, or very low baseline pulmonary function test results.

Women of child-bearing age should be given this diagnostic test within 10 days of the first day of their menses or within 2 weeks following a negative pregnancy test result. Methacholine should not be administered to women who breast-feed because it is unknown whether the drug is excreted in breast milk. When given to patients receiving beta-blockers, the effects of methacholine can be exaggerated or prolonged. Common adverse effects include headache, throat irritation, light-headedness, and pruritus. Because acute respiratory distress may occur, emergency equipment and medications should be at the bedside during this diagnostic test.

DIRECT-ACTING NICOTINIC AGONISTS

The direct-acting nicotinic agonists are drugs that stimulate nicotinic receptors directly. The two significant classes of nicotinic stimulants are the ganglionic stimulants (e.g., nicotine) and the neuromuscular nicotinic stimulants that are discussed in Chapter 16.

Nicotine is an important drug, although its selection as a prototype may be considered controversial by some. However, because of its significant abuse potential in smoking and chewing tobacco and its therapeutic uses in smoking cessation, it is presented as the prototype for direct-acting nicotinic agonists.

NURSING MANAGEMENT OF THE PATIENT RECEIVING NICOTINE

Core Drug Knowledge

Pharmacotherapeutics

Nicotine replacement is used as an adjunct to smoking cessation programs. Various formulations are available, such as gum, transdermal patches, and nasal spray. The nicotine gum and transdermal patches are available over the counter (OTC) in the United States. The patches are preferred for maintenance therapy during smoking cessation programs, unless the patient is allergic to the patches. Gum or nasal spray may be useful for episodic or bolus effects of nicotine and in institutional settings in which smoking is not allowed (see Table 15-2).

Pharmacokinetics

When delivered as a chewing gum, nicotine is readily absorbed through the buccal mucosa when the gum is chewed. However, the amount of nicotine absorbed depends on how long the saliva remains in the mouth. Very little nicotine is absorbed from the GI tract due to extensive first-pass metabolism through the liver. Regular use of the gum provides steady-state blood levels of nicotine similar to those achieved by smokers. However, peak plasma levels occur much more slowly than inhaling tobacco smoke. Nicotine levels reach the brain within 7 seconds after a single puff on a cigarette, but peak concentrations of the gum can take 15 to 20 minutes; the transdermal patch can require as long as 4 hours to reach peak concentrations.

Nicotine is widely distributed in the body tissues, particularly the CNS. It crosses the placenta and is secreted in milk. The concentrations of nicotine in amniotic fluid and fetal serum exceed those in maternal serum. Detectable amounts also appear in the serum and urine of infants of nursing mothers who smoke.

Nicotine is metabolized in the liver by oxidation and excreted by the kidneys as unchanged nicotine and metabolites.

Pharmacodynamics

Nicotine is a potent ganglionic and CNS stimulant, with actions that are mediated through specific nicotine receptors. In small doses, all autonomic ganglia are stimulated; in larger doses, initial stimulation is followed by blockade. The dependency potential of nicotine is based mostly on its CNS stimulant effects.

Contraindications and Precautions

Nicotine in any dosage form should not be used in patients immediately after myocardial infarction, with life-threatening arrhythmias, or with severe or worsening angina pectoris. It should not be used in patients who have allergies to any of the components of the delivery system, including gum, nasal spray, and transdermal patches. Smoking should be avoided during nicotine therapy because of the potential for overdose and toxicity (e.g., dizziness, nausea, and headache).

Adverse Effects

The adverse effects of nicotine in the cardiovascular system include peripheral vasoconstriction and tachycardia. In the CNS, the effects may include headache, paresthesias, tiredness, insomnia, nervousness, nausea, hot flashes, and nightmares. Diarrhea, dry mouth, nausea, and dyspepsia are adverse effects on the GI system. Use of Nicotrol spray may cause nasal irritation, lacrimation, throat irritation, sneezing, and coughing. The transdermal patches may cause erythema, pruritus, edema, or rash at the site of administration.

The nicotine transdermal system and nasal spray are classified as FDA pregnancy category D, although the benefits of nicotine replacement therapy during pregnancy appear to outweigh the risks of continued smoking during pregnancy.

Drug Interactions

Adenosine and lithium carbonate interact with nicotine (Table 15-4).

Assessment of Relevant Core Patient Variables

Health Status

A careful history and physical examination will identify contraindications and precautions necessary for the person beginning nicotine replacement therapy. The patient's desire to cease smoking or the requirement not to smoke usually prompts nicotine replacement therapy. Before therapy begins, the nurse needs to ensure that the patient is neither in the immediate postmyocardial infarction period nor a victim of significant cardiovascular disease (e.g., arrhythmias, angina pectoris) because these are contraindications to therapy. Prior to application of transdermal nicotine patches, skin test results should be reviewed to determine sensitivity to the drug.

Life Span and Gender

The nurse should document the age and gender of the patient as well as assess women of child-bearing age for pregnancy and lactation. If the patient is pregnant, nicotine therapy should be used only if necessary, particularly in cases in which the benefits of smoking cessation are important. If the patient is breast-feeding, the infant should be monitored for respiratory or CNS stimulation. If this occurs, the timing of breast-feeding or the administration of the nicotine may need to be staggered to minimize adverse effects. Older adults undergoing nicotine therapy may be at higher risk for dizziness and sleep disturbances resulting from CNS stimulation.

TABLE 15-4 Agents That Interact With Nicotine

Interactants	Effect and Significance	Nursing Management
adenosine	Enhanced cardiovascular effects of adenosine	Advise patients undergoing stress tests to avoid chewing nicotine gum or reduce adenosine dosage to avoid angina.
lithium	Potentiates effects of nicotine	Monitor for increased effect.

Lifestyle, Diet, and Habits

The nurse should document the patient's occupation and activities of daily living. Patients should be advised not to smoke during nicotine therapy to avoid overdosage and adverse effects. Patients whose job requires shift work should be aware that sleep disturbances may disrupt their rest. The nurse should inspect the patient's oral cavity for dentures and other significant dental work. Nicotine gum is heavier and stickier than regular gum and may affect artificial teeth or other dental work.

Environment

The nurse should be aware of the environment in which the drug will be administered. Nicotine in any of its dosage forms may be administered in any setting by health care providers, nurses, or patients themselves. In institutional or other smoke-free settings, nicotine replacement therapy may be almost obligatory.

Culture

The nurse should explore the patient's underlying cultural beliefs and values regarding smoking. In many cultural groups, such as Japanese-American, Austrian, Polish immigrant, and highly acculturated Latino, smoking tobacco is popular and widely sanctioned. It is important to recognize that some patients may have more difficulty giving up smoking than others because of cultural influences.

Nursing Diagnoses and Outcomes

- Risk for Injury to mouth or teeth or dental work related to gum viscosity, sore throat or mouth related to use of the intranasal spray

  Desired outcome: The patient will remain free of injury or problems related to adverse effects of therapy.
- Disturbed Sleep Pattern related to drug-induced insomnia

  Desired outcome: The patient will experience undisturbed sleep.

Planning and Intervention

Maximizing Therapeutic Effects

The following interventions by the nurse may help to maximize the therapeutic effects of nicotine therapy:

- The patient should be encouraged to adhere to the recommended dosage schedule because this is most likely to reduce craving.
- Because nicotine replacement therapy is an adjunctive measure in smoking cessation programs, all other program measures should be promoted and encouraged.
- Because craving is substantially increased when patients are exposed to others who smoke (promoting effects from secondary smoke inhalation, reinforcing old habits, and recalling pleasurable sociocultural influences), the nurse should encourage the patient to minimize exposure to these influences initially.

Minimizing Adverse Effects

Overstimulation of the CNS may be counteracted by promoting good sleep hygiene and adjusting the dosage and timing of the last nicotine dose of the day. Other adverse effects may require the episodic use of analgesics for headaches.

Avoiding GI effects requires good mouth care, particularly for the patient using nicotine gum, or antiemetics for nausea and antidiarrheals, as needed. For patients using the transdermal nicotine patches, good skin care and rotation of patch sites will help to minimize skin reactions. Upper respiratory tract effects may be counteracted with a room humidifier. Adverse effects that cannot be managed and that may be specific to the delivery system warrant a change to a different system on a trial basis.

Providing Patient and Family Education

- The nurse should caution patients receiving nicotine replacement therapy about adverse effects and the possibility of overdosing by resumption of tobacco smoking during therapy.
- The nurse should watch the patient demonstrate the correct use of sprays or transdermal patches to ensure safe, optimal self-dosing.
- The nurse should instruct the patient how to manage adverse effects and encourage the patient to contact the health care provider if self-management is ineffective or if serious or persistent adverse effects continue.
- If toxicity or overdosing is suspected, the therapy must be discontinued until the effects abate and then a decreased dosage or frequency of dosing can be reintroduced.

- The nurse should encourage the patient to avoid other stimulants during nicotine therapy, including caffeine-containing beverages, because these may lead to exaggerated CNS stimulation experienced as irritability and nervousness.
- The nurse should caution the patient and family to keep nicotine out of the reach of children.
- The nurse should incorporate all other smoking cessation program measures in the teaching because replacement therapy is a short-term adjunct measure only.

Ongoing Assessment and Evaluation

During therapy, symptoms of tobacco craving should gradually subside. Throughout therapy the nurse should be alert for signs and symptoms of overdosing, because this usually means that the patient is "cheating" and smoking tobacco while taking the nicotine replacement. Dizziness, nausea, and headaches may result and promote nonadherence to the therapeutic use of nicotine. Other evaluative measures include assessing the quantitative decrease of adverse effects and promoting therapeutic adherence. ■

INDIRECT-ACTING CHOLINERGIC AGONISTS

Chapter 14 discusses synaptic transmission of neurotransmitters. As a quick review, the final step of synaptic transmission is termination. After the neurotransmitter crosses the synaptic gap and binds to a receptor, the neurotransmitter is cleared from the synaptic gap by either enzymatic degradation, reuptake, or diffusion. Acetylcholine, the neurotransmitter of the cholinergic nervous system, is cleared from the synaptic gap by acetylcholinesterase, also known as cholinesterase. Any drug that inhibits cholinesterase will be the functional equivalent of a cholinergic receptor stimulant—or agonist—because of its ability to prolong the activity of acetylcholine at the synapse. Because of this, some indirect-acting cholinergic agonists are also known as cholinesterase inhibitors or anticholinesterase agents. It is important to remember that acetylcholine stimulates both nicotinic and muscarinic receptor sites; thus, cholinesterase inhibitors prolong the action of acetylcholine throughout the body.

There are two major groups of indirect-acting cholinergic receptor stimulants, the reversible and "irreversible" cholinesterase inhibitors. Neostigmine (Prostigmin) is the prototype for reversible cholinesterase inhibitors.

> **MEMORY CHIP**
>
> **Nicotine**
>
> - A direct-acting nicotinic agonist used as an adjunct to smoking cessation programs
> - Significant contraindications: immediately post MI, life-threatening dysrhythmias, severe angina
> - Most common adverse effects: erythema, pruritus, burning, headache, insomnia
> - Most serious adverse effect: vasculitis
> - Maximizing therapeutic effects: adherence to the recommended dosing
> - Minimizing adverse effects: limit timing of last dose to promote rest and sleep
> - Most significant patient education: correct use of multiple administration routes, avoidance of other stimulants

NURSING MANAGEMENT OF THE PATIENT RECEIVING NEOSTIGMINE

Core Drug Knowledge

Pharmacotherapeutics

The most significant indication for neostigmine therapy is myasthenia gravis. In this disease, the neuromuscular junction is affected by an autoimmune process that diminishes the number of functional nicotinic receptors at the junction. This gives rise to the characteristic weakness and fatigue that accompany exercise in people with this disease. The use of neostigmine effectively increases the amount of acetylcholine available at the myoneural junction, resulting in enhanced strength of muscle contraction.

Other clinical indications include urinary retention and paralytic ileus. Neostigmine is also used as an antidote for nondepolarizing neuromuscular blocking agents.

Pharmacokinetics

Neostigmine is may be administered both orally and parenterally. It is poorly absorbed when given orally. Onset of action occurs from 2 to 4 hours when taken orally, and 10 to 30 minutes when given parenterally. The drug is metabolized by microsomal liver enzymes and hydrolyzed by cholinesterases. Duration of effect varies considerably among patients. Approximately 80% of neostigmine is excreted in the urine within 24 hours as unaltered drug and metabolites (see Table 15-2).

Pharmacodynamics

Neostigmine is a reversible inhibitor of postsynaptic cholinesterase and therefore acts as a cholinergic agent by increasing the synaptic presence of acetylcholine.

Contraindications and Precautions

Neostigmine is absolutely contraindicated in patients with GI obstruction or ileus and urinary tract obstruction because it increases contractions of smooth muscle. It should not be used in patients with peritonitis because it increases GI motility, which would exacerbate the disorder. Neostigmine should be used with caution in patients with peptic ulcer disease because it stimulates gastric acid secretion, again inducing an exacerbation of the disorder. The CNS stimulation induced by neostigmine may exacerbate hyperthyroidism or seizure disorders.

Neostigmine should be used cautiously in patients with hypotension and bradycardia because it can further decrease the blood pressure and heart rate by increasing vagal tone. Neostigmine also has direct stimulatory effects on the myocardium, which can increase oxygen demand. This can be dangerous for patients with cardiac disease, particularly coronary artery disease alone or in association with cardiac arrhythmias. In the respiratory system, neostigmine may induce bronchoconstriction; thus, it should be used cautiously in patients with asthma, chronic bronchitis, or CAL.

Adverse Effects

The most serious adverse effects result in a cholinergic crisis, which may be life threatening.

Symptoms include nausea and vomiting, diarrhea, salivation, sweating, peripheral vasodilation, bronchial constriction, and respiratory arrest. In patients with myasthenia gravis, it is sometimes necessary to distinguish between a cholinergic crisis and a myasthenic crisis. In the case of a cholinergic crisis, it is likely that too much anticholinesterase has been given, whereas a myasthenic crisis may be the result of inadequate dosages failing to control myasthenic symptoms. A challenge dose of edrophonium (Tensilon) will differentiate the two states. If there is no relief or an increase in muscle weakness, then the patient is receiving too much anticholinesterase. If there is an improvement with edrophonium, then an increase in cholinesterase inhibitor dosage is indicated.

The most common unwanted effects of neostigmine's cholinergic stimulation of end organs are nausea and vomiting, diarrhea, abdominal pain, miosis, salivation, diaphoresis, sinus bradycardia, bronchospasm, and increased bronchial secretions.

Drug Interactions

Neostigmine and the anticholinesterase drugs in general interact with steroids, aminoglycoside antibiotics, depolarizing muscle relaxants, local and some general anesthetics, and magnesium, all of which have an influence on the neuromuscular junction (Table 15-5). Steroids may decrease the anticholinesterase effects of neostigmine with the clinical result being a worsening of the myasthenic condition. This may require an increased dose of the latter or alternate dosing of each class of agent. Some of the aminoglycosides cause a mild neuromuscular blockade, which may antagonize the effects of neostigmine. For the depolarizing muscle relaxants, such as succinylcholine, neostigmine may increase the length of neuromuscular blockade, so concurrent usage in people with myasthenia is contraindicated.

Assessment of Relevant Core Patient Variables

Health Status

Prior to administration, the nurse should perform a baseline physical assessment to document the current status of the patient, especially respiratory status and muscle strength. Myasthenia affects the muscles of respiration and other muscle groups, so respiratory function may be further compromised in the presence of upper respiratory tract infections or allergies. This is of particular concern because undertreatment or overtreatment can lead to life-threatening crises.

The nurse should also assess for a history of diseases or disorders that contraindicate the use of neostigmine. Positive finding should be communicated to the health care provider prior to administration of neostigmine.

Life Span and Gender

The nurse should document the age and gender of the patient. Because of lower body mass and decreased renal functioning, elderly patients may be more prone

TABLE 15-5 Agents That Interact With Neostigmine

Interactants	Effect and Significance	Nursing Management
aminoglycoside antibiotics (neomycin, streptomycin, kanamycin)	Mild nondepolarizing blocking action	Monitor for increased neuromuscular blockade.
corticosteroids	Decreases effect of anticholinesterase therapy in myasthenia gravis	Ensure respiratory support if needed.
depolarizing muscle relaxants (succinylcholine) and mivacurium	Increased, prolonged neuromuscular blockade	Avoid use if possible. If not, administer these drugs only as directed and only if indicated. Provide emergency respiratory support.
magnesium	Antagonizes and counteracts beneficial effects of neostigmine	Avoid magnesium-containing drugs and foods.
anticholinesterase drugs	Excessive GI stimulation and symptoms of cholinergic crisis or underdosage in patients with myasthenia gravis	Have antidote (atropine or belladonna) available to treat overdosage.

to the psychotogenic effects of cholinergic overdose, including restlessness, anxiety, and agitation. The nurse should also determine whether the patient is pregnant or breast-feeding because these patients should avoid neostigmine.

Lifestyle, Diet, and Habits

The nurse should document the patient's occupation, activities of daily living, and rest and exercise patterns. Patients taking neostigmine for myasthenia gravis may need to pace their daily activities to allow the peak and duration effects of neostigmine dosing to support their muscular and respiratory work.

Environment

The nurse should be aware of the environment in which the drug will be administered and assess the home or living environment, if appropriate. Neostigmine in its oral form may be administered in any setting by health care providers, nurses, or the patient and family members.

Nursing Diagnoses and Outcomes

- Impaired Gas Exchange related to drug-induced bronchospasm, increased secretions, or respiratory paralysis
  Desired outcome: The patient will maintain effective gas exchange.
- Ineffective Airway Clearance
  Desired outcome: The patient will maintain effective airway clearance.
- Ineffective Breathing Pattern related to drug dosage
  Desired outcome: The patient will maintain effective breathing patterns.
- Self-Care Deficit (Feeding, Bathing/Hygiene, Dressing/Grooming, Toileting) related to the impact of neuromuscular weakness secondary to overdose
  Desired outcome: The patient will seek assistance in carrying out self-care as needed.

Planning and Intervention

Maximizing Therapeutic Effects

The nurse should administer neostigmine at regular intervals throughout the day to ensure effective blood levels. If the patient has difficulty swallowing or breathing, the parenteral form of neostigmine should be administered until oral therapy can be tolerated.

Minimizing Adverse Effects

As with other cholinergic stimulants, the use of neostigmine requires the availability of an antidote in case of systemic overdose or cholinergic crisis. Atropine is the usual antidote. For patients with known allergies or suspected hypersensitivity, life-support measures need to be available in case of bronchial spasm or hypersensitivity reactions. Because adverse systemic effects include stimulation of sphincters, patients may need access to a bedpan or urinal in case of rapid responses.

If the patient has a history of allergies or asthma or chronic obstructive lung disease, careful monitoring of the first few doses of neostigmine is required to ensure that respiratory difficulties do not occur.

Providing Patient and Family Education

The key aspects for patient and family education include managing serious adverse effects and recognizing crisis states that may require prompt and expert intervention:

- It is usually productive to explore aspects of long-term therapy that sometimes escape the attention or resources of acute care staff, such as decreased libido.
- Patients and their families may need assistance in understanding how to recognize myasthenic crisis (undermedication) and distinguish it from cholinergic crisis (overmedication) and how to respond to either situation. In myasthenic crisis due to undermedication, muscle weakness becomes pronounced and may cause quadriparesis, quadriplegia, shortness of breath, respiratory insufficiency, and difficulty in swallowing. Conversely, in a cholinergic crisis due to overmedication, there is an increase in GI motility with diarrhea and cramping, bradycardia, muscle fasciculation, pupillary constriction, and increased salivation and sweating (see the accompanying display, Considerations Pertaining to Neostigmine Therapy). The nurse should advise the patient and family to seek immediate care should any of these symptoms occur.

Ongoing Assessment and Evaluation

The nurse should be familiar with procedures for detecting and managing myasthenic or cholinergic crises. The achievement of therapeutic goals is assessed and relates to detailed therapeutic monitoring of neuromuscular

Critical Thinking Scenario

Considerations pertaining to neostigmine therapy

Amy Rose, a 27-year-old legal assistant, has been admitted to your unit with a diagnosis of myasthenia gravis. She has been started on neostigmine therapy, and you are wondering how to differentiate between undermedication and the possibility of a myasthenic crisis, and overmedication and the possibility of a cholinergic crisis.

1. Explain the key differences between the two situations, and propose a nursing management strategy that you could use for either situation.
2. Discuss the implications of a health care provider–ordered edrophonium test. Why do you think this test would be ordered?

functioning, vital signs, respiratory rate and capacity, mobility, self-care levels, and self-esteem.

An important component of the ongoing assessment is the patient's neuromuscular status. This would focus on vital capacity (respiratory status), presence of ptosis, diplopia, ability to chew and swallow, strength of hand grip bilaterally, and gait if the patient is ambulatory. Acute care settings often provide a detailed assessment sheet designed specifically for the person with myasthenia gravis. Other data should include baseline and ongoing blood pressure and pulse and respiratory rates. ■

DRUGS CLOSELY RELATED TO P NEOSTIGMINE

Edrophonium

Edrophonium (Tensilon) is a rapid-acting, short-duration, parenteral cholinesterase inhibitor. It is the drug of choice for diagnosing myasthenia gravis because of its rapid onset of action and reversibility. Other uses include assessing cholinesterase inhibitor therapy, differentiating cholinergic and myasthenic crises, and reversing the effects of nondepolarizing neuromuscular blockers after surgery.

Ambenonium Chloride

Ambenonium chloride (Mytelase) is an oral, slowly reversible anticholinesterase agent. It is indicated for use in patients with myasthenia gravis to improve muscle strength. Ambenonium chloride's actions are similar to those of pyridostigmine, but it tends to produce more muscarinic side effects. Contraindications, adverse effects, and drug interactions are similar to those of neostigmine.

MEMORY CHIP

P Neostigmine

- An indirect-acting cholinoceptor stimulant used in the management of myasthenia gravis
- Significant contraindications: GI obstruction or ileus, urinary tract obstruction, peritonitis
- Most common adverse effects: nausea or vomiting, diarrhea, abdominal pain, miosis, salivation, diaphoresis, sinus bradycardia
- Most serious adverse effects: cholinergic crisis, cardiac arrest
- Maximizing therapeutic effects: administer at regular intervals throughout the day to ensure adequate blood levels
- Minimizing adverse effects: availability of atropine, the antidote for cholinergic crisis
- Most significant nursing responsibility: differentiate between cholinergic crisis and myasthenic crisis
- Most significant patient education: symptoms of cholinergic crisis and need for immediate medical attention

Physostigmine

Physostigmine (Antilirium) is a parenteral and ophthalmic cholinesterase inhibitor. The difference between physostigmine and neostigmine is that it is a tertiary amine, whereas neostigmine is a quaternary amine. This causes an increased activity of physostigmine in the CNS. Physostigmine most commonly is used as an ophthalmic agent in the treatment of open-angle glaucoma. It also is used to counteract toxic anticholinergic effects (both central and peripheral) of other drugs, particularly in overdose situations. In the past it was used to treat tricyclic antidepressant (TCA) overdose, but has lost favor for this use due to its own potentially harmful effects. It has also been used to treat Alzheimer disease and hereditary ataxias.

Pyridostigmine

Pyridostigmine (Mestinon) is an oral cholinesterase inhibitor. It is somewhat longer acting than neostigmine and also possesses fewer muscarinic effects. Pyridostigmine is marketed in both regular and sustained-release tablets and is the most commonly used agent of the group for oral treatment of myasthenia gravis. It is also used to reverse the actions of nondepolarizing neuromuscular blockers after surgery.

Tacrine

Tacrine hydrochloride (Cognex) is another oral cholinesterase inhibitor. It is the first drug approved for improving cognitive symptoms, such as memory, attention, reason, language, and the ability to perform simple tasks associated with Alzheimer disease. It is thought that elevated levels of acetylcholine in the cerebral cortex are believed to be responsible for improvement in cognition. This mechanism requires that intact cholinergic neurons are present. As dementia progresses, fewer intact cholinergic neurons remain, and tacrine becomes less effective. There is no evidence that tacrine alters the underlying pathologic processes of dementia.

DRUGS SIGNIFICANTLY DIFFERENT FROM P NEOSTIGMINE

Most of the irreversible cholinesterase inhibitors are in the organophosphate category. Because of the phosphate element of these drugs, they are highly lipid soluble and are easily absorbed from any administration site. Their ease of absorption, coupled with their potential toxicity, is the basis for their use as insecticides and chemical warfare agents.

There are a few therapeutically useful irreversible inhibitors, such as echothiophate and isoflurophate (Floropryl), which are used for glaucoma that is refractory to the usual miotics.

Overdose or accidental overexposure to irreversible anticholinesterase drugs is characterized by cholinergic crisis. The antidote of choice is pralidoxime (Protopam, PAM). Pralidoxime is not effective in reversing overdose of reversible anticholinesterase drugs. It works best when given immediately after the exposure. It does not cross the blood-brain barrier and thus is ineffective in reversing anticholinesterase in the CNS.

CHOLINERGIC ANTAGONISTS

The cholinergic antagonists are drugs that antagonize, or block, muscarinic or nicotinic receptors directly. They may be clustered into three categories: antimuscarinic drugs (the largest group), antinicotinic drugs (with two subcategories: ganglionic blockers and neuromuscular blockers), and cholinesterase regenerators.

The ganglionic blockers include mecamylamine (Inversine) and trimethaphan (Arfonad). Their clinical significance is to decrease blood pressure in critical situations; thus, they are covered in Chapter 30. The neuromuscular blockers, which are covered in Chapter 16, include succinylcholine and the curare derivatives. The antimuscarinic drugs of clinical significance include atropine, anisotropine, benztropine, scopolamine, propantheline, ipratropium, and hyoscyamine. Atropine is the ideal prototype for the antimuscarinic group of cholinergic antagonists.

NURSING MANAGEMENT OF THE PATIENT RECEIVING ATROPINE

Core Drug Knowledge

Pharmacotherapeutics

Atropine has a multitude of therapeutic uses. It is used in emergency situations, such as symptomatic bradycardia, pulseless electrical activity, ventricular asystole, or cardiopulmonary resuscitation. Preoperatively, it is used to decrease respiratory secretions and block cardiovagal reflexes and succinylcholine-induced arrhythmias during surgery. Other uses include reversal of organophosphate insecticide toxicity or neuromuscular blockade, mydriasis or cycloplegia induction, treatment of iritis or uveitis, or management of traveler's diarrhea. It is also used as adjunctive treatment of GI disorders, such as duodenal ulcer, irritable bowel syndrome, or GI hypermotility caused by cholinergic stimulation.

Pharmacokinetics

Following intramuscular administration, onset of effect is usually rapid, peaking at 30 minutes and lasting up to 5 hours (Table 15-6). Topical administration to the eyes may take 30 to 40 minutes to produce cycloplegia (paralysis of ciliary muscles), whereas IV administration produces rapid effects. Atropine is partially metabolized in the liver with about 60% of a dose eliminated unchanged through the kidneys.

Pharmacodynamics

Atropine is a competitive inhibitor at autonomic postganglionic cholinergic receptors. These include receptors found in GI and pulmonary smooth muscle, exocrine glands, the heart, and the eye. The principal actions of atropine are a reduction in salivary, bronchial, and sweat gland secretions; mydriasis; cycloplegia; changes in heart rate; contraction of the bladder detrusor muscle and of the GI smooth muscle; decreased gastric secretion; and decreased GI motility.

It is important to note that the action of atropine on the heart rate is dose dependent. In doses of 0.4 to 0.6 mg, atropine causes a slight sinus bradycardia due to vagal stimulation. In larger doses (1 to 2 mg), it causes sinus tachycardia secondary to inhibition of vagal control of the sinoatrial node in the heart.

Contraindications and Precautions

Contraindications to atropine use include hypersensitivity to anticholinergics or sulfites. Atropine is contraindicated in myasthenia gravis, because the drug competes with the small amount of acetylcholine that has potential to act in the body. Atropine is relatively contraindicated in acute myocardial infarction, because the drug can potentiate arrhythmias. In addition, the increase in heart rate caused by atropine increases the oxygen demand on the heart and can exacerbate myocardial ischemia. Precautions should be observed with patients who drive or perform hazardous tasks for a living (due to the adverse effects of drowsiness and blurred vision). Precautions are also needed for the elderly as well as those with glaucoma, severe forms of hepatic disease, ulcerative colitis, renal disease, prostatic hypertrophy, coronary artery disease, congestive heart failure, arrhythmias, tachycardia, hypertension, asthma, and allergies. Finally, precautions are needed with anyone with increased sensitivity (e.g., infants, small children) and with patients with brain damage, hyperthyroidism, and hyperthermia. All of these circumstances may be exacerbated with atropine and other anticholinergics.

Adverse Effects

The most common adverse effects of atropine are blurred vision, dry mouth, constipation, and urinary retention. The most serious potential adverse effect is an anticholinergic overdose. This is characterized by the hallmarks of "mad as a hatter (CNS psychotic effect), dry as a bone (salivary), red as a beet (peripheral vasodilation), and blind as a bat (mydriasis)."

In the CNS, the predominant effect is drowsiness, sometimes with confusion, especially in the elderly. Other potential adverse effects include elevation of IOP, decreased ability to sweat, and tachycardia. Although anticholinergic drugs are used in the management of asthma, the drying of respiratory secretions may induce mucus plugs that may actually induce bronchospasm and asthma attacks.

Atropine is an FDA pregnancy category C drug and should be avoided by pregnant or lactating women.

Drug Interactions

Atropine interacts with phenothiazine antipsychotics and with haloperidol (Table 15-7). Cardiac status as measured by electrocardiography (ECG) may be affected by

TABLE 15-6 Summary of Selected Cholinergic Antagonists

Drug (Trade) Name	Selected Indications	Route and Dosage Range	Pharmacokinetics
atropine (Atropine Sulfate; *Canadian:* Apo-Benztropine)	Anesthesia induction, premedication for surgery Bradycardia Biliary spasm, GI radiography, irritable bowel syndrome, peptic ulcers, urinary incontinence, asthma, bronchitis, reversal of bronchospasm, hiccups, organophosphate poisoning, arrhythmias (e.g., angiography induced, post-myocardial infarction, succinylcholine induced), myelodysplasia, neuromuscular blockade reversal, hyperhidrosis, hypothermia, rhinorrhea, tetanus asystole, dental procedures	*Adult:* SC, IM, or IV, 0.3–0.6 mg 60 min before inducing anesthesia *Adult:* IV, 0.5–2.0 mg *Adult:* 0.3–1.2 mg q4–6h any route for GI or anticholinergic uses	*Onset:* SC, varies; IM, 10–15 min; IV, immediate *Duration:* 4 h $t_{1/2}$: 2.5 h
benztropine (Benztropine Mesylate, Cogentin)	Drug-induced extrapyramidal symptoms, akathisia, dystonic reactions, haloperidol-induced acute dystonic reaction, parkinsonism, drooling, myoclonus, priapism	*Adult:* PO, IM, IV, 1–4 mg daily or bid	*Onset:* PO, 1 h; IM, IV, 15 min *Duration:* PO, IM, IV 6–10 h $t_{1/2}$: 4–8 h
hyoscyamine (Cystospaz)	Abdominal cramps, anticholinesterase poisoning, biliary disorders, colic, diverticulitis, dysentery, enterocolitis, GI disorders, irritable bowel syndrome, neurogenic bowel disturbances, Parkinson disease, peptic ulcer, pylorospasm, spastic colon, splenic flexure syndrome, pancreatitis, rhinitis	*Adult:* PO, 0.125–0.25 mg q4h, PO (sustained-release product), 375–0.75 mg q12h; SC, IM, IV push, 0.25–0.5 mg	*Onset:* PO, 5–20 min; IV, 2 min *Duration:* 4–12 h $t_{1/2}$: Not applicable
ipratropium (Atrovent; *Canadian:* Alti-Ipratropium)	Asthma, chronic bronchitis, chronic obstructive lung disease, rhinorrhea	*Adult:* inhaler, 36 μg qid	*Onset:* 15 min *Duration:* 3–4 h $t_{1/2}$: 1.6 h
pralidoxime (Protopam)	Anticholinesterase or organophosphate poisoning	*Adult:* IV initially, 1–2 g/100 mL in normal saline solution over 30 min, then PO, 1–3 g repeated in 5 h	*Onset:* IV, rapid *Duration:* Not applicable $t_{1/2}$: 0.8–2.7 h
propantheline (Pro-Banthine, Propantheline Bromide; *Canadian:* Propanthel)	Duodenal ulcer, GI spasmolytic, hyperhidrosis, sialorrhea, urinary incontinence	*Adult:* PO, 15–30 mg 30 min before meals and 30 mg at bedtime or 15–30 mg q4–6h	*Onset:* 30–60 min *Duration:* 6 h $t_{1/2}$: 3–4 h
scopolamine (Scopolamine Hydrobromide, Hyoscine Hydrobromide)	Motion sickness Preanesthetic premedication, obstetric amnesia, antidelirium Glaucoma, ophthalmology, uveitis	*Adult:* PO or transdermal patch, 0.6–1.0 mg *Adult:* PO, 1 mg 1–4 h before anesthesia; IM, 0.4–0.6 mg 45–60 min before anesthesia *Adult:* topical, 1–2 drops of 0.25% solution in eye 1 h before refraction; 1–2 drops up to four times daily for uveitis	*Onset:* PO/IM, 30 min *Duration:* 4–6 h $t_{1/2}$: 8 h

TABLE 15-7 Agents That Interact With Atropine

Interactants	Effect and Significance	Nursing Management
phenothiazines	Decreased antipsychotic efficacy of phenothiazines	Adjust phenothiazine dosage.
haloperidol	Decreased serum haloperidol levels, worsening of symptoms, onset of tardive dyskinesia	Avoid concurrent atropine or lower haloperidol dosage; monitor carefully.

atropine. Atropine may interfere with ECG measurements through its cardiovascular effects and result in spurious cardiac findings. The ECG interpretation should note the atropine therapy.

Assessment of Relevant Core Patient Variables

Health Status

Because of its many actions on the body, the nurse must carefully assess the patient for contraindications or precautions to its use prior to administration. It is important to determine whether the patient has acute angle-closure glaucoma, obstructive disease of the GI tract, paralytic ileus, obstructive uropathy, intestinal atony (particularly in elderly or debilitated patients), megacolon complicating ulcerative colitis, unstable cardiovascular status in acute hemorrhage, tachycardia secondary to cardiac insufficiency of thyrotoxicosis, myasthenia gravis, toxemia of pregnancy, or previous exposure to high temperatures.

Positive finding should be communicated to the health care provider. The nurse should also determine if the patient has chronic obstructive lung disease, severe heart disease, hypertension, ulcerative colitis, ileus, chronic lung disease, hyperthyroidism, autonomic neuropathy, hepatic or renal disease or prostatic hypertrophy, esophageal reflux, or hiatal hernia. Because these conditions may be exacerbated with atropine therapy, the nurse should provide close monitoring of these patients. The nurse should also assess the patient's use of OTC or herbal medications. These drugs frequently contain atropine-like ingredients that may induce severe adverse effects.

Life Span and Gender

The nurse should document the age of the patient. Atropine must be used carefully with infants, young children, and anyone older than 40 years because the adverse effects may be more pronounced in these age groups.

Environment

The nurse should document the patient's occupation and activities of daily living. People treated with atropine may experience mydriasis and hence difficulties adjusting to changing light intensities. This may have a significant impact on people working in transportation (airline flight crew, drivers) and those working at night (photophobia and temporary blindness in response to bright lights).

Nursing Diagnoses and Outcomes

- Urinary Retention related to adverse effects of drug
  Desired outcome: The patient will eliminate without difficulty.
- Constipation related to adverse effects of drug
  Desired outcome: The patient will continue baseline elimination pattern.
- Risk for Injury related to drug-induced drowsiness and blurred vision
  Desired outcome: The patient will understand adverse effects and develop a repertoire of strategies for their management.
- Ineffective Sexuality Patterns or Sexual Dysfunction related to anticholinergic impact on erection and ejaculation in men and vaginal secretions in women
  Desired outcome: The patient and partner will adjust sexual functioning and develop a repertoire of strategies to maintain satisfaction level.

Planning and Intervention

Maximizing Therapeutic Effects

Two factors should be considered for the person receiving atropine because they arise directly from consideration of the interactions between core drug knowledge and core patient variables. First, patients taking atropine for peptic ulcer disease should adhere to dietary restrictions established to prevent exacerbations of the disease, thereby allowing the therapeutic potential of the atropine to be achieved. The nurse may suggest administering the larger dose at bedtime to decrease sleep-disturbing pain. Second, patients need to be encouraged to take their atropine exactly as prescribed and at the required dosage frequency to enhance therapeutic potential.

Minimizing Adverse Effects

Because a prominent anticholinergic effect is dry mouth, good oral hygiene is important. Dryness may be relieved with hard candies, chewing gum, or lip gloss. Blurred vision and mydriasis can be hazardous for drivers, particularly at night, so these activities are best avoided. Bright lights and photophobia may be counteracted with sunglasses. For patients with a complaint of dry eyes, administer artificial tears.

Atropine alters the body's ability to regulate temperature, so extremes of heat and strenuous exercise should be minimized, along with adequate if not aggressive hydration. Constipation is a troubling adverse effect that may be managed by adding fiber to the diet, promoting hydration, and exercising moderately.

In longer term therapy, the nurse needs to stress the importance of mouth care and monitor the need for urinary catheterization or measures to relieve constipation and abdominal distention. A distressing adverse effect for many patients relates to their preferred modes of sexual expression, which may be dramatically changed with anticholinergic drugs. If appropriate, supportive counseling may be useful or directive teaching about alternatives to intercourse, although many of these issues are better managed by a sex therapist.

Providing Patient and Family Education

Important aspects of patient and family teaching include recognizing and managing adverse effects:

- Older men should be informed of the need to report any changes in urinary stream because this may be a prodromal symptom of prostatic hypertrophy.
- Aids to elimination should be suggested, including adequate exercise, dietary fiber, and increased fluid intake.
- It is particularly important to stress the hazards associated with driving, especially at night, because night vision may be altered significantly by atropine.
- The nurse should remind the patient to avoid all OTC or herbal medications without the direct approval of the health care provider. As previously mentioned, these medications frequently contain atropine-like ingredients.

Ongoing Assessment and Evaluation

Assessment of goal attainment is relatively straightforward for patients receiving anticholinergic therapy with atropine. Ongoing assessment will include data about elimination patterns, sexual functioning and adjustment, and recognition and management of side effects. The ongoing assessments may be tailored to the clinical indications for which atropine or other anticholinergics are prescribed but should include any concurrent drug therapy to rule out the possibility of drug interactions. Vital signs measured at onset of therapy should be compared with vital signs throughout therapy and used to monitor and detect adverse effects.

Bowel and bladder function should be assessed on an ongoing basis because of the profound impact that drug therapy may have on elimination. Because of the potential for confusion, anyone at risk for adverse CNS effects should have a mental status assessment. ■

DRUGS CLOSELY RELATED TO ATROPINE

Antisecretory Anticholinergics

There are many anticholinergic drugs used to decrease the secretion of gastric acids. These include anisotropine (Valpin), clidinium (Quarzan), glycopyrrolate (Robinul), hexocyclium (Tral Filmtabs), isopropamide (Darbid), mepenzolate (Cantil), methantheline (Banthine), methscopolamine (Pamine), oxyphencyclimine (Daricon), propantheline (Pro-Banthine), and tridihexethyl chloride (Panthilon). All are oral agents; however, glycopyrrolate may also be given parenterally. Since the advent of histamine-2 blockers and proton pump inhibitors, these drugs have fallen out of favor because they induce a myriad of adverse effects. However, for patients unresponsive to histamine-2 blockers or proton pump inhibitors, these drugs may be effective.

Benztropine

Benztropine (Cogentin) is an oral and parenteral synthetic muscarinic-receptor antagonist that is structurally similar to atropine. It is used adjunctively with other agents to treat all types of parkinsonian syndromes including antipsychotic-induced extrapyramidal symptoms. It produces less CNS stimulation than does trihexyphenidyl, another commonly used anticholinergic drug used in the management of Parkinson disease. The drug may be helpful in geriatric patients who cannot tolerate cerebral-stimulating agents. Therapeutic effects may take 2 to 3 days. Adverse effects are similar to atropine.

MEMORY CHIP

Atropine

- An antimuscarinic drug that is commonly given preoperatively to reduce postoperative secretions; the drug of choice for cholinergic crisis
- Significant contraindications: hypersensitivity to sulfites, myasthenia gravis, acute myocardial infarction
- Most common adverse effects: blurred vision, constipation, dry mouth, urinary retention
- Most serious adverse effect: severe bradycardia
- Maximizing therapeutic effects: take the medication exactly as prescribed and the required dosage
- Minimizing adverse effects: good oral hygiene, fluid replacement
- Most significant patient education: safety issues for blurred vision, avoid OTC and herbal medications without the direct approval of the health care provider

Hyoscyamine

Hyoscyamine (Cytospaz) relaxes smooth muscle spasm resulting from parasympathetic stimulation. It inhibits GI propulsive motility and decreases gastric acid secretion. It also controls excessive pharyngeal, tracheal, and bronchial secretions. It requires only half the dose of atropine; therefore, it has a lower potential to induce adverse effects.

Ipratropium

Ipratropium bromide (Atrovent) is a synthetic anticholinergic agent that is structurally very similar to atropine. It may be administered by oral or nasal inhalation. The actions of ipratropium parallel those of atropine on the bronchial smooth muscle, salivary glands, GI tract, and heart when administered by the intravenous route. When administered by oral inhalation, however, ipratropium exhibits greater antimuscarinic activity on the bronchial smooth muscle and systemic effects are minimal. Compared with atropine, ipratropium is roughly twice as potent as a bronchodilator, and it exhibits a more bronchodilation than inhibition of salivary secretion.

Intranasal administration of ipratropium produces a localized parasympatholytic effect. This action reduces watery hypersecretion from mucosal glands of the nose thereby relieving rhinorrhea associated with the common cold or allergic or nonallergic perennial rhinitis.

Although ipratropium may be used for the management of asthma, it is more commonly used for cholinergic-mediated bronchospasm associated with chronic obstructive pulmonary disease.

Scopolamine

Scopolamine (Isopto Hyoscine) is a naturally occurring anticholinergic agent found in belladonna leaf. Compared with atropine, scopolamine is more potent in its anticholinergic effects on the iris, ciliary body, and salivary, bronchial, and sweat glands. It is less potent than atropine on the heart and on bronchial and GI smooth muscle. In contrast to atropine, scopolamine at therapeutic doses produces CNS depression characterized by drowsiness, euphoria, amnesia, fatigue, and dreamless sleep resulting from decreased periods of rapid eye movement. Paradoxical CNS excitation such as restlessness, hallucinations, or delirium can occur, especially when the patient is experiencing severe pain. Scopolamine is very effective for the prevention of motion sickness and this indication represents the most common clinical use. Other uses for scopolamine include treatment of iritis, uveitis, and Parkinson disease.

Trihexyphenidyl

Trihexyphenidyl (Artane) is used adjunctively to treat all types of parkinsonian syndromes including antipsychotic-induced extrapyramidal symptoms. This drug is frequently used in combination with other antiparkinsonian agents, and it is effective in from 50% to 75% of patients. In general, anticholinergic agents can help control tremor but are less effective for treating bradykinesia or rigidity. Additionally, trihexyphenidyl can block dopamine reuptake, thus prolonging dopamine's effects. Tolerance to the effects of trihexyphenidyl can occur with prolonged use.

CHAPTER SUMMARY

- Parasympathetic or cholinergic drugs can be stimulating or blocking in their action. The cholinergic stimulating drugs are known as cholinergic agonists, and the cholinergic blocking agents are known as cholinergic antagonists or anticholinergics.
- Drugs that interfere with acetylcholinesterase's breakdown of acetylcholine are known as anticholinesterase agents.
- In the parasympathetic system, the transmitter is acetylcholine, and the receptors may be muscarinic or nicotinic.
- Therapeutic uses of cholinergic drugs are varied and related to providing extra cholinergic stimulation or blockage to normal ANS functioning.
- A prototype of a direct-acting muscarinic agonist is pilocarpine, which is used for simple and acute glaucoma, preoperative and postoperative intraocular tension, and mydriasis.
- A prototype direct-acting nicotinic agonist is nicotine, which is used as an adjunct to smoking cessation programs.
- A prototype indirect-acting cholinergic receptor stimulant is neostigmine, which is used to control the symptoms of myasthenia gravis. As with any of the cholinergic drugs, adverse effects involve many of the major organ systems.
- Atropine is the prototype of the antimuscarinic anticholinergic drugs. It is most commonly used preoperatively to dry postoperative secretions.

QUESTIONS FOR STUDY AND REVIEW

1. After abdominal surgery, a common postoperative drug order is for bethanechol. Why is this ordered, and how would you know whether it has been effective? If the patient becomes short of breath after a few doses of bethanechol, what would you do?
2. If you administer a cholinergic drug, why would you assess your patient for flushing of the skin, a headache, a sudden drop of blood pressure, and decreased pulse rate?
3. How would you respond to and manage a cholinergic crisis?
4. You may have encountered a way of remembering anticholinergic poisoning through the terms "mad as a hatter, blind as a bat, red as a beet, and dry as a bone." How does "dry as a bone" relate to adverse anticholinergic effects?

NEED MORE HELP?

? Chapter 15 of the study guide for *Drug Therapy in Nursing* contains exercises and activities to reinforce your understanding of the concepts presented in this chapter. For additional information see the text's accompanying website at *http://www.connection.lww.com.*

REFERENCES AND BIBLIOGRAPHY

Cazzola, M., Centanni, S., & Donner, C. F. (1998). Anticholinergic agents. *Pulmonary Pharmacologic Therapy, 11*(5–6), 381–392.

CCIS System. (2001). *Computerized Clinical Information System.* Denver, CO: Micromedex.

Clinical Drug Monographs [CDRom]. (2001). Gold Standard Media.

Drug Facts and Comparisons. (2000). St. Louis: Facts and Comparisons Division

Hardman, J. G., Limbird, L. E., Molinof, P. B., Ruddon, R. W., & Gilman, A. (Eds.). (1997). *Goodman and Gilman's pharmacological basis of therapeutics* (9th ed.). New York: McGraw-Hill.

Ikeda, A., Nishimura, K., & Izumi, T. (1998). Pharmacological treatment in acute exacerbations of chronic obstructive pulmonary disease. *Drugs Aging, 12*(2), 129–137.

Karch, A. (2001). *2001 Lippincott's nursing drug guide.* Philadelphia: Lippincott Williams & Wilkins

Katzung, B. (1998). *Basic and clinical pharmacology* (7th ed.). Stamford: Appleton & Lange

Porth, C. (1998). *Pathophysiology: Concepts of altered health states* (5th ed.), Philadelphia: Lippincott Williams & Wilkins.

Sullivan, J., & Abrams, P. (1999). Pharmacological management of incontinence. *European Urology, 36,* (Suppl. 1), 89–95.

Tatro, D. (Ed.). (2000). *Drug interaction facts* (6th ed.). St. Louis: Facts and Comparisons.

Wein, A. J. (1998). Pharmacologic options for the overactive bladder. *Urology, 51,* (2A Suppl.), 43–47.

Unit **V**

Central Nervous System Drugs

Chapter **16**

DRUGS PRODUCING ANESTHESIA AND NEUROMUSCULAR BLOCKING

KEY TERMS

anesthesia
balanced anesthesia
depolarizing drugs
dissociative anesthesia
end plate
general anesthetic
local anesthetic
narcoanalysis
neuroleptanesthesia
nondepolarizing drugs
paralysis

Learning Objectives

At the completion of this chapter the student will:

1. Describe the physiology of the central nervous system (CNS) as it relates to anesthesia and neuromuscular blocking.
2. Identify observable changes in stages of anesthesia and neuromuscular blockade.
3. Identify risk and disease factors that may influence a patient's response to anesthetics and neuromuscular blocking agents.
4. Identify core drug knowledge about anesthetic and neuromuscular blocking agents.
5. Identify core patient variables related to anesthetic and neuromuscular blocking agents.
6. Relate the interaction of core drug knowledge to core patient variable for anesthetic and neuromuscular blocking agents.
7. Generate a nursing plan of care based on the interactions between core drug knowledge and core patient variables for anesthetic and neuromuscular blocking agents.
8. Describe nursing interventions to maximize therapeutic and minimize adverse effects for anesthetic and neuromuscular blocking agents.
9. Determine key points for patient and family education for anesthetic and neuromuscular blocking agents.

General anesthetic agents

Inhalant agents

- **isoflurane**
- desflurane
- enflurane
- halofIurane
- sevoflurane
- nitrous oxide

Parenteral agents

- **propofol**
- thiopental
- etomidate
- ketamine
- fentanyl
- benzodiazepines

Local anesthetic agents

- **lidocaine**
- bupivacaine
- etidocaine
- mepivacaine
- prilocaine
- procaine
- topical anesthetics

Neuromuscular blocking agents

Nondepolarizing agents

- **tubocurarine**
- pancuronium bromide
- pipecuronium
- vecuronium

Depolarizing agents

- **succinylcholine**

The symbol C indicates the **drug class**.

Drugs in bold type marked with the symbol P are **prototypes**.

Drugs in blue type with no symbol are **closely related** to the prototype.

Drugs in **red** type with no symbol are **significantly different** from the prototype.

Drugs in **black** type with no symbol are **also used in drug therapy**; no prototype.

Anesthesia produces a loss of feeling or sensation. It is used to permit the performance of surgical or other painful procedures. Anesthetics are classified as general or local agents. **General anesthesia** is characterized by a state of unconsciousness, analgesia, and amnesia, with skeletal muscle relaxation and loss of reflexes. General anesthetic drugs are subdivided into inhaled agents and parenteral agents. **Local anesthesia** is the condition that results when sensory transmission from a local area of the body to the central nervous system (CNS) is blocked. Neuromuscular blocking agents are used to cause **paralysis** (i.e., loss of function) for surgical procedures or to facilitate mechanical ventilation; these agents are subdivided into nondepolarizing and depolarizing agents.

This chapter discusses drugs used to induce anesthesia and skeletal muscle paralysis. Inhaled anesthetics are represented by the prototype drug isoflurane (Forane). Parenteral anesthetics are represented by the prototype drug propofil (Diprivan). Local anesthetics are represented by the prototype drug lidocaine (Xylocaine). Nondepolarizing neuromuscular junction (NMJ) blockers are represented by the prototype drug tubocurarine (Tubarine). Depolarizing NMJ blockers are represented by the prototype drug succinylcholine (Anectine).

PHYSIOLOGY

CNS ANESTHESIA

The CNS is responsible for providing control systems and surveillance for many vegetative and conscious functions, including appetite, satiety, attention, arousal, and activity. Various sleep and arousal mechanisms are linked to the brain, particularly the raphe nuclei and locus ceruleus in the pons and other parts of the reticular activating system (RAS). Therefore, if a patient experiences sensations of pain, disruptions in the usually smooth regulation of arousal and activity may result.

At a synaptic level in the CNS, normal arousal mechanisms are affected through presynaptic release of neurotransmitters, such as norepinephrine, serotonin, and dopamine. These transmitters diffuse across the synaptic cleft to the postsynaptic effector membrane, which is usually another neuron. The postsynaptic membrane contains receptors for the transmitters.

In normal arousal, the transient combination of the transmitter with the receptor causes membrane changes, leading to propagation of the action potential. An action potential is the brief reversal of electrical polarization of a nerve or muscle cell membrane. In the neuron, the action potential constitutes the nerve impulse. The transmitter can be metabolized by postsynaptic enzymes (e.g., monoamine oxidase) or removed from further activity through reuptake into the presynaptic storage vesicles. Anesthetics may provoke a decreased release of neurotransmitters or an increased reuptake and inhibition of the postsynaptic enzymes. The result is a diminished postsynaptic response, leading to decreased arousal, decreased sensation (including pain), and loss of consciousness.

LOCAL ANESTHESIA

Nerve impulses depend on the flow of ion currents through channels in the cell's membrane. Nerve cells are negatively polarized at rest and this is maintained by active Na+/K+ exchange. When a cell is stimulated, it becomes depolarized and an action potential occurs. Local anesthetics reversibly block all nerve impulses by disrupting permeability to sodium during an action potential.

NEUROMUSCULAR BLOCKADE

Muscle relaxation and paralysis can occur through disturbances at a variety of sites. These sites include the CNS, somatic nerves, motor nerve terminals, acetylcholine receptor sites, the motor end plate, the muscle membrane, or the internal contractile units. Normal muscle function involves the arrival of a nerve impulse at the motor nerve terminal followed by the release of acetylcholine into the synaptic cleft. Neuromuscular blockade occurs at acetylcholine receptor sites where the neurotransmitter acetylcholine reacts with the muscle cell membrane, causing depolarization and subsequent muscle relaxation.

Nondepolarizing drugs prevent neural communication by depolarizing the muscle; in other words, the muscle remains in a relaxed state. Depolarizing drugs cause muscle depolarization and prevent repolarization; that is, the muscle experiences rapid contractions followed by flaccid paralysis and is unable to receive further neurocommunication.

PATHOPHYSIOLOGY

Anesthetics are functional drugs because they are not used to treat a pathologic disease or disorder. However, patients have a variety of conditions that require anesthesia. General anesthetics are used to induce and maintain anesthesia during surgery, **narcoanalysis** (the use of sedating drugs to help uncover unconscious material during psychoanalysis), electroconvulsive therapy, **dissociative anesthesia** (a loss of perception of certain stimuli whereas that of others remains intact) and **neuroleptanesthesia** (also called conscious sedation).

Neuromuscular blocking agents are used in conjunction with inhalation or parenteral anesthetics during surgical procedures or to facilitate induction and maintenance of mechanical ventilation.

GENERAL ANESTHETIC AGENTS

Anesthesia is used to avoid sensations, especially pain, and memories associated with surgery and diagnostic procedures. Anesthetic agents are subdivided into general and local anesthetics. General anesthetics are discussed here and local anesthetics are discussed later in this chapter.

The action of general anesthetics produces a state of unconsciousness and whole body anesthesia. After administration of a general anesthetic, loss of consciousness and sensation usually follows increasing levels or stages of CNS depression. Slower-acting anesthetics allow some differentiation, whereas faster-acting anesthetics do not show precise delineation of stages. Classic studies with early anesthetics indicate the presence of four stages, which are differentiated through increasing influence on reflex activity, muscle tone, and respiration. Stages I and II constitute anesthetic induction; keeping the patient at stage III is anesthetic maintenance. Reversal of the stages to the conscious state is the process of recovery.

- Stage I, analgesia: the patient remains conscious, may be able to converse, and experiences some analgesia as the anesthetic reduces sensory transmission in the spinothalamic tract.
- Stage II, excitement: systolic pressure rises, and the patient may experience excitation and restlessness along with an increased respiratory rate. In addition, the patient may experience delirium. Stage II is usually circumvented by administering a short-acting IV barbiturate beforehand.
- Stage III, surgical anesthesia: stage III may have four planes, or levels, characterized by differential responses of the ocular muscles, eye reflexes, and pupil size. It begins in plane I with the resumption of regular respiration and the beginning of muscle relaxation. By plane IV, spontaneous respiration ceases. Most surgery occurs when the patient is in planes II and III.
- Stage IV, medullary depression: once respirations cease, the patient enters stage IV in which the respiratory and vasomotor centers are depressed. Unless rapid intervention and support occur, coma and death follow.

It is not always desirable to produce general anesthesia with a single agent, because too deep a level of unconsciousness may ensue. To overcome this, a process called **balanced anesthesia** is used. Balanced anesthesia relies on a combination of drugs to produce loss of consciousness, analgesia, and muscle relaxation, while producing and maintaining a lighter stage of anesthesia. Drugs used in balanced anesthesia include inhaled or parenteral anesthetics, ultrashort-acting barbiturates, neuromuscular blocking agents, benzodiazepines, and opioid analgesics. The minute-to-minute maintenance of anesthesia is sensitively adjusted with the inhalational drug.

As previously mentioned, general anesthetics are subdivided into inhaled and parenteral agents.

C INHALANT ANESTHETIC AGENTS

Inhalant anesthetic agents include isoflurane (Forane), desflurane (Suprane), enflurane (Ethrane), halofluorane, sevoflurane (Ultane), and nitrous oxide. The inhalant anesthetics are typified by isoflurane (Forane), a halogenated ether that is the prototype for this group.

NURSING MANAGEMENT OF THE PATIENT RECEIVING P ISOFLURANE

Core Drug Knowledge

Pharmacotherapeutics

Isoflurane is used to induce and maintain anesthesia and is typically part of balanced anesthesia. It is used in intensive care units for sedation, in obstetrics for analgesia, and in ocular surgical procedures (e.g., cataract removal, lens implantation, reconstructions) because it lowers intraocular pressure.

Pharmacokinetics

Isoflurane produces surgical anesthesia within 7 to 10 minutes and is usually administered with 50% to 70% nitrous oxide. It is administered slowly because its pungent odor would otherwise tend to cause breath holding or coughing. It is absorbed through the alveoli and is minimally biotransformed. A tiny fraction of the inhaled dose is transformed in the liver into trifluoroacetic acid and excreted in the urine as fluoride ion. The majority of isoflurane is excreted unchanged through expired air. Table 16-1 provides a comparison of the pharmacokinetic properties of halogenated general anesthetics.

Pharmacodynamics

The exact mechanism of action of isoflurane is unknown. Several theories have been postulated (Fig. 16-1). The minimum alveolar concentration (MAC) of isoflurane is 1.15% for adults. However, it decreases to 0.5% when administered with 70% nitrous oxide. MAC is a measure of potency and is the concentration of anesthetic gas required to eliminate movement in 50% of patients challenged by a standardized skin incision. The smaller the MAC, the more potent the agent is. The exact mechanism of the inhalational anesthetics is not known. However, it is likely that the effects are mediated through physicochemical properties of the gases, rather than through specific binding with receptors or through potentiation or inhibition of specific neurotransmitters.

Contraindications and Precautions

The main contraindications to isoflurane are hypersensitivity to halogenated compounds and predisposition to malignant hyperthermia, which is often determined from the individual or family history. In patients with increased intracranial pressure (ICP), isoflurane will increase cerebral blood flow, which may lead to exacerbation of the increased ICP.

Isoflurane may cause intraoperative hyperglycemia and leukocytosis, which may be of concern for patients with diabetes. Isoflurane is assigned to pregnancy category C and should be used in pregnant women only when the benefits outweigh the risks. Use of isoflurane in patients with myasthenia gravis can cause an increase in muscular weakness due to the neuromuscular blocking effects of anesthetics.

Adverse Effects

With many anesthetics, blood pressure drops during induction and returns following surgical stimulation. Prolonged hypotension may occur with isoflurane, but otherwise the myocardium appears stable with this agent. Malignant hyperthermia, characterized by a sudden temperature spike, is a possibility with this agent, although the reported incidence is low. Like other anesthetics,

TABLE 16-1 Summary of Selected Inhalant Anesthetic Agents

Drug (Trade) Name	Selected Indications	Route and Dosage Range	Pharmacokinetics
isoflurane (Forane)	Anesthesia: induction, maintenance	*Adult:* 1.5%–3% in oxygen or in oxygen/nitrous oxide for induction, 1%–2.5% for maintenance	*Onset:* 7–10 min *Duration:* 7–19 min $t_{1/2}$: minimal biotransformation
desflurane (Suprane)	Anesthesia: induction, maintenance	*Adult:* 3%–11% in oxygen or in oxygen/nitrous oxide (monitored anesthesia care 2.8%–7.5%)	*Onset:* 2–2.6 min *Duration:* 5–7 min $t_{1/2}$: 2.5 min
enflurane (Ethrane)	Anesthesia, patient-controlled obstetric analgesia	*Adult:* 2%–4.5% in oxygen or in oxygen/nitrous oxide for induction, 0.5–3% for maintenance	*Onset:* 2.3 min *Duration:* 5 min $t_{1/2}$: 2–3 min
sevoflurane (Ultane)	Anesthesia: induction, maintenance	*Adult:* 1.8%–5% in oxygen or in oxygen/nitrous oxide for induction, 0.75%–3% for maintenance	*Onset:* 1–2 min *Duration:* 4–14 min $t_{1/2}$: 2–3 min

isoflurane depresses renal function. However, it is not generally nephrotoxic, and it has a higher cardiovascular and respiratory margin of safety than halothane, desflurane, or enflurane. Respiratory depression occurs with all inhaled anesthetics, resulting in the need for mechanical ventilation throughout surgery. Rarely, postanesthesia respiratory depression may occur, especially in obese patients. Tremor and shivering may occur in response to a decreased body temperature, but these adverse effects are generally self limiting. Nausea and vomiting may also occur. During surgery, the airway is protected by the endotracheal tube. Should vomiting occur postsurgery, aspiration is another potential adverse effect. During labor and obstetric delivery, isoflurane can produce uterine relaxation, which can delay delivery and increase postpartum hemorrhage.

Chronic accidental exposure, which can occur in operating room personnel, may increase the incidence of spontaneous abortions, birth defects, and stillbirths. Isoflurane has been observed to react with dry adsorbents in anesthetic circle systems to form carbon monoxide and cause carboxyhemoglobinemia. To avoid this adverse effect, adsorbants should be changed prior to use.

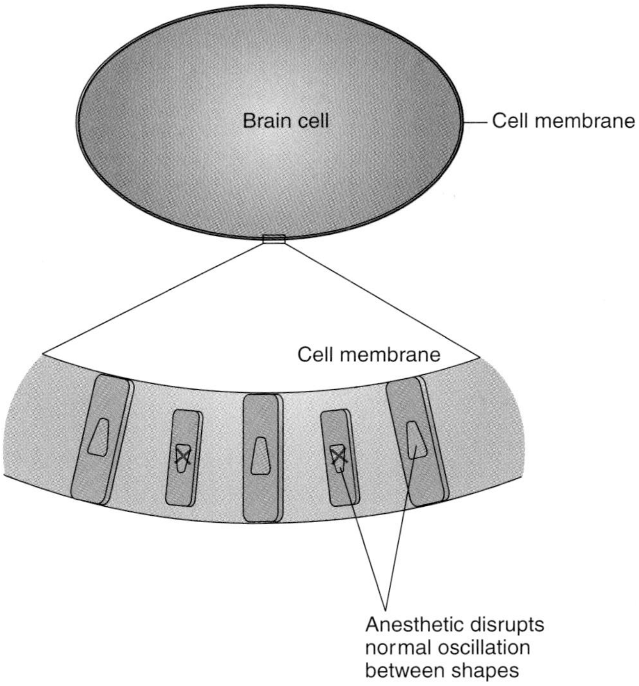

Figure 16-1. New theories of the mechanism of anesthesia. Older theories of anesthetic mechanisms of action suggest that anesthetics bind to or dissolve in the lipid layers of cell membranes, causing swelling, disruption, and loss of feeling. A newer theory suggests that multiple mechanisms may be at play. These mechanisms involve the cell membrane proteins, which are thought to oscillate between two shapes. Now it is thought that anesthetics disrupt this oscillation.

Drug Interactions

If isoflurane is administered to a patient receiving labetalol, there is a synergistic hypotensive effect. Combined use of these drugs increases the time to the resumption of spontaneous respirations. In addition, extra caution is needed when caring for these patients during postanesthesia recovery. Additional interactions are identified in Table 16-2.

Assessment of Relevant Core Patient Variables

Health Status

The nurse should take a careful health history. Many factors influence the process of anesthetic induction, maintenance, and recovery, including lung conditions, cardiovascular status, obesity, previous drug history, and comorbidity. Inhalation anesthetics are administered through the lungs and absorbed across alveolar surfaces. Therefore, lung condition may have a profound

TABLE 16-2 Agents That Interact With P Isoflurane

Interactants	Effect and Significance	Nursing Management
nondepolarizing muscle relaxants, such as atracurium, doxacurium, gallamine, metocurine, mivacurium, pancuronium, pipercuronium, tubocurarine, vecuronium	Potentiates effects of neuromuscular blockers and prolongs blockade	Monitor respiratory function (dosage may need to be reduced). Prepare to provide ventilatory support.
alfentanil	Prolongs respiratory depression and increases incidence of bradycardia	Monitor respiratory and cardiac function. Provide ventilatory support.
labetalol	Additive hypotensive effects and decreased cardiac output	Monitor cardiac function. Use extra caution if interaction is anticipated.

impact on the efficacy and nature of anesthesia. Patients with chronic obstructive lung disease, asthma, and a history of cigarette smoking all present potential problems in anesthesia based on changes in lung compliance, bronchoconstriction, and ventilation:perfusion ratios. This results in a significantly increased rate of postoperative complications in patients with compromised pulmonary function. Similar issues arise for patients with cardiovascular compromise or disease, because absorption, distribution, metabolism, and excretion of inhalant anesthetics are all affected by blood flow through the lungs and the rest of the body.

Life Span and Gender

The nurse should document the age of the patient. Special challenges with isoflurane administration become evident depending on the age group. In neonates and infants, the size of the airway and larynx may contribute to difficulties with intubation. In addition, immature hepatic and renal function, higher metabolic rate, and a greater proportion of body tissue being water all contribute to the need to adjust dosages of drugs and IV fluids using body surface area nomograms. As patients age and organ systems start to fail, similar difficulties may occur in detoxification and excretion of administered anesthetic agents. This may lead to increased intensity and duration of drug effects, including toxic effects.

The nurse should assess women of child-bearing age for pregnancy. The pregnant woman presents unique challenges during obstetric or other surgery because the fetus has to be considered, both in terms of placental drug flow and in the transplacental transfer of drugs. Isoflurane has a low pregnancy safety rating (pregnancy category C), and its use in pregnant women is determined by the balance between therapeutic benefit and potential harm to the fetus and woman.

Lifestyle, Diet, and Habits

The nurse should measure the patient's height and weight. The patient who suffers from morbid obesity and requires anesthesia may experience problems with isoflurane administration. The obese patient may be particularly prone to longer recovery times and a greater incidence of adverse effects with fat-soluble anesthetics, such as isoflurane and methoxyflurane. Compounding these difficulties, obese patients often present with other comorbid conditions, such as hypertension, cardiac insufficiency, respiratory difficulties, and diabetes, all of which can generate their own special anesthetic challenges.

One other significant category of anesthetic challenge is drug abusers; drugs commonly abused are often found in conjunction with disease states that require special attention during anesthesia. For example, with alcohol abuse, there is often an elevated level of hepatic enzymes, which may increase the requirement for anesthetic drugs. In addition, liver dysfunction may lead to changes in metabolism of such agents. With drug dependency, the postanesthetic period may require more careful monitoring than usual in case abstinence syndromes develop. The nurse should take a careful drug history to reveal previous use or abuse of drugs that have the potential to cause significant interactions with isoflurane and other anesthetic agents.

Environment

The nurse should be aware of the environment in which the drug will be administered. Isoflurane and other general anesthetics may be administered in special settings by anesthesiologists (a type of specialist physician) and nurse anesthetists (advanced practice nurses trained in anesthesiology). Administration usually only occurs in settings that allow for postanesthetic recovery and full life support.

Nursing Diagnoses and Outcomes

- Ineffective Airway Clearance related to suppressed cough reflex and the presence of secretions

  Desired outcome: The patient will maintain effective airway clearance by being suctioned as necessary and through undergoing deep breathing and coughing exercises as appropriate.
- Ineffective Breathing Pattern related to respiratory depression secondary to drugs used during anesthesia

Desired outcome: The patient will maintain effective breathing despite respiratory depression by administration of oxygen as appropriate.

- Risk for Aspiration related to drug-induced nausea and vomiting, gastrointestinal (GI) distention, hypoxia, and stimulation of the vomiting center

  Desired outcome: *The patient's nausea and vomiting will be minimized by preanesthetic administration with anticholinergic agents to reduce the risk of aspiration and nausea.*
- Ineffective Thermoregulation related to CNS depression secondary to drugs used during anesthesia

  Desired outcome: *The patient will be warmed as necessary during the postanesthetic disturbance of thermoregulation.*
- Disturbed Sensory Perception, varied, related to CNS depression secondary to drugs used during anesthesia

  Desired outcome: *The patient will remain free of sensory or perceptual alterations through careful reorientation, repeated as necessary.*

Planning and Intervention

Maximizing Therapeutic Effects

Preinduction and induction should be carried out in a low stimulus environment; that is, environmental stimuli, particularly noise, are kept to a minimum. It is important to teach the patient preoperatively to anticipate induction procedures and measures useful for promoting uncomplicated recovery. The nurse should give preoperative support and reasonable reassurance to voiced concerns. In addition, the nurse should advise patients scheduled for surgery to avoid stressors and aim for a good night's sleep the evening before surgery, if at home, or promote sleep preoperatively if the patient is already in the hospital.

Minimizing Adverse Effects

After anesthesia, it is important to monitor blood pressure and temperature to detect residual hypotension and the possibility of malignant hyperthermia. Because gaseous or volatile inhalational agents (e.g., isoflurane) are expired quickly through the lungs, the recovery phase is often short. However, there is a potentially greater need for postoperative analgesia; the nurse should administer this and then follow up with an accurate pain assessment. Shivering and tremors are common following anesthesia, which the nurse can manage with blankets. It is important to maintain adequate respiratory support until normal respiration is resumed. This may include administering oxygen and asking the patient to perform deep breathing exercises, cough, or change position.

Recovering patients need to be in a room in which the air supply is continually replaced and exhaled gases are carried out through exhaust vents. The nurse may prevent aspiration by assisting the patient into a side-lying position and by administering antiemetic drugs. It is important to monitor vital signs frequently to prevent complications, such as shock. When the patient returns to the room or unit from the postanesthesia care unit (PACU), the nurse should continue monitoring vital signs, bowel sounds, and urine output, because these are specifically related to the effects of isoflurane.

Providing Patient and Family Education

Family and patient education falls into preoperative and postoperative categories:

- The nurse should provide preoperative teaching to allow patients to anticipate the surgery and anesthesia without excessive fear and to assimilate routines designed to assist in postoperative recovery.
- Postoperatively, the nurse should instruct patients to avoid nonprescribed CNS depressants or herbal agents until approved by the health care provider.
- For outpatient surgeries, the nurse should discharge the patient into the care of a responsible adult and instruct the patient not to drive or engage in any hazardous activities requiring full alertness or coordination.

Ongoing Assessment and Evaluation

The evaluation of progress in the postanesthesia recovery phase is often carried out in two stages. In both stages, the degree to which specified outcomes have been obtained will determine what happens next.

Initially, the unconscious patient may be transferred to a postanesthetic recovery area. The patient should regain consciousness, orientation, some stability of vital signs, and an ability to cooperate with instructions during this stage. At this point, the patient can be transferred back to a room or unit, and a less stringent postoperative protocol may be followed. Once the immediate postsurgical, postanesthetic goals have been reached, longer term goals may be set. Other assessments related to the procedure or surgery itself are distinct from those required by the postanesthetic state. When the patient returns to the room or unit, the nurse will continue to monitor vital signs, bowel sounds, and urine output, because these are specifically related to the use of isoflurane. ■

DRUGS CLOSELY RELATED TO P ISOFLURANE

Desflurane

Desflurane (Suprane) is an inhalation volatile liquid general anesthetic with a MAC of 7.0. It is used for induction or maintenance of anesthesia during surgery for adults. It is not recommended for use in children because of the high incidence of cough and laryngospasm. In addition to use in children, desflurane is contraindicated for used in patients with coronary artery disease, increased heart rate, or hypertension.

MEMORY CHIP

Isoflurane

- A potent inhalation anesthetic
- Significant contraindications: hypersensitivity to halogenated compounds, predisposition to malignant hyperthermia
- Most common adverse effects: hypotension, hypothermia, nausea, or vomiting
- Most serious adverse effect: respiratory depression
- Maximizing therapeutic effects: low stimulus environment, preoperative teaching regarding anesthetic induction
- Minimizing adverse effects: monitor need of respiratory support
- Most significant patient education: preoperative teaching regarding anesthesia and surgical procedures

Enflurane

Enflurane (Ethrane) is a halogenated inhalational anesthetic used for general anesthesia. Both onset of action and recovery from anesthesia are rapid with a MAC of 1.70. As with most inhalational anesthetics, enflurane is typically used with adjunctive medications such as narcotics and nitrous oxide, and it can be given in low doses to provide analgesia for procedures not requiring loss of consciousness. Enflurane is an excellent muscle relaxant, providing enough relaxation for intraabdominal surgery. Contraindications, precautions, and adverse effects are similar to those of isoflurane.

Haloflurane

Haloflurane is used less often in North America because of the availability of agents with less severe adverse effects. Hepatotoxicity occurs in 1:10,000 adults but is rare in children. Therefore, halothane is used mainly for pediatric anesthesia. Haloflurane has a MAC of 0.78.

Sevoflurane

A newer inhalational agent, sevoflurane (Ultane), although expensive, appears to offer advantages above and beyond others in its class. In comparison, adjustment of depth of anesthesia is easier with sevoflurane than with either enflurane, halothane, or isoflurane. Induction and recovery from anesthesia are rapid and cardiorespiratory depression is minimal, which makes it generally safe in patients with coronary artery disease. Additionally, because of its low tissue solubility and nonirritating odor, sevoflurane is an appropriate agent for pediatric patients.

DRUG SIGNIFICANTLY DIFFERENT FROM ISOFLURANE

Nitrous oxide is a colorless, odorless, tasteless, nonflammable, nonirritating, inorganic gas, rather than a halogenated ether. It is used commonly as an adjunct in balanced anesthesia to decrease the MAC of halogenated agents. It is a powerful analgesic, but a relatively weak inhalational anesthetic. Nitrous oxide is also used in low doses to provide analgesia in obstetrics and during procedures that do not require unconsciousness, as well as dental procedures.

Nitrous oxide is readily absorbed into the blood through the pulmonary capillary system. It has a relatively low solubility in blood and a MAC of 100%. Nitrous oxide is rapidly eliminated in the expired breath, essentially unchanged, with minimal diffusion through the skin.

Benefits must outweigh the risk for use during pregnancy because animal studies reveal nitrous oxide can cause fetal death, growth retardation, and skeletal anomalies. Prolonged administration of nitrous oxide can cause inactivation of methionine synthase, a vitamin B12-dependent enzyme, resulting in leukopenia and anemia. This does not occur within the time frame of clinical surgery but poses a potential problem for providers who are chronically exposed to nitrous oxide.

PARENTERAL ANESTHETIC AGENTS

Parenteral anesthetics are also known as induction agents. There are several classes of drugs that are used as a parenteral anesthetics in balanced anesthesia. These include barbiturates, benzodiazepines, opioid analgesics, and nonbarbiturate hypnotic agents. Parenteral anesthetics that will be discussed include propofol (Diprivan), thiopental (Pentothal), etomidate (Amidate), ketamine (Ketalar), fentanyl (Sublimaze), and the benzodiazepines.

Propofol (Diprivan), a nonbarbiturate hypnotic agent, is the prototype for parenteral anesthetics (Table 16-3). Propofol appears as a milky white solution because it is formulated in a solution with soybean oil, glycerol, and egg phospholipids–thus the nickname "the milk of anesthesia."

NURSING MANAGEMENT OF THE PATIENT RECEIVING PROPOFOL

Core Drug Knowledge

Pharmacotherapeutics

Propofol may be used for general anesthesia, sedation induction and maintenance, and status epilepticus.

Pharmacokinetics

Propofol is administered IV and is rapidly distributed to all tissues in the body. Loss of consciousness usually occurs within 40 seconds. The duration of a bolus injection is 3 to 5 minutes.

Propofol crosses the placenta and is distributed into breast milk. Propofol is metabolized in the liver but extrahepatic routes of metabolism also occur. Recovery from anesthesia is rapid and is associated with minimal psychomotor impairment. The kinetics of propofol do not appear to be affected by chronic hepatic or renal disease.

TABLE 16-3 Summary of Selected Parenteral Anesthetic Agents

Drug (Trade) Name	Selected Indications	Route and Dosage Range	Pharmacokinetics
propofol (Diprivan)	Anesthesia induction and maintenance, monitored anesthesia care (MAC), sedation for diagnostic and surgical procedures, continuous sedation in intensive care unit.	*Adult:* IV, 5 μg/kg/min for 5 min for sedation, 2–2.5 mg/kg for induction, 6–12 mg/kg/h for maintenance, 0.5 mg/kg over 3–5 min for MAC initiation, 1.5–4.5 mg/kg/h for maintenance	*Onset:* 30 sec *Duration:* 3–10 min $t_{1/2}$: biphasic initial: 40 min; terminal: 1–3 d
droperidol (inapsine, innovar)	Tranquilization and antinauseant/antiemetic in surgical and diagnostic procedures; premedication; induction and adjunct in general and regional anesthesia; neuroleptanalgesia	*Adult:* IM, 2.5–10 mg 30–60 min preop	*Onset:* 3–10 min *Duration:* 2–4 h $t_{1/2}$: 2.2 h
etomidate (Amidate)	Anesthetic induction or adjunct, cardioversion, status epilepticus, head injury	*Adult:* 0.3 mg/kg IV over 15–60 s or 10–20 μg/kg/min for maintenance	*Onset:* 20 s *Duration:* 4–10 min $t_{1/2}$: 1.5–4 min (serum); 2.6 h (elimination)
ketamine (Ketalar)	Anesthesia for short surgical or diagnostic procedures not requiring skeletal muscle relaxation	*Adult:* IM, 5–10 mg/kg for induction, 2–4 mg/kg for sedation; IV, 1–2 mg/kg over 60 s for induction and 0.1–0.5 mg/min for maintenance	*Onset:* IM, 3–4 min; IV, 30 s *Duration:* IM, IV, 5–10 min $t_{1/2}$: 10–15 min (initially), 2.5 h
midazolam (Versed)	Anesthesia induction, cardiac catheterization, conscious sedation, endoscopy, gastroscopy, premedication	IM, IV, titrated	*Onset:* IM, 15 min; IV, 3–5 min *Duration:* 30–60 min $t_{1/2}$: 1.2–12.3 h

Pharmacodynamics

The cellular mechanism of anesthesia for propofol is unclear. However, the clinical response is clear: anesthesia is immediate and short-lived. Cardiorespiratory depression occurs. Apnea and significant hypotension are possible and may be dose related. Decreased cerebral blood flow and intraocular pressure are also noted. Propofol is a weak analgesic agent and is generally administered with analgesics. Concomitant use of opiates may intensify cardiorespiratory depression.

Contraindications and Precautions

Propofol is contraindicated for patients with a hypersensitivity to propofol or any of the ingredients of its emulsion vehicle. It is also contraindicated during pregnancy and lactation. Propofol is relatively contraindicated in patients with a seizure disorder because they are at an increased risk of developing convulsions during the recovery phase. Propofol should be used with caution in patients with cardiac or peripheral vascular disease. The cardiovascular depressive and hypotensive effects of propofol can aggravate these conditions.

Propofol should be used cautiously in patients with cerebrovascular disease, impaired cerebral blood flow, or increased ICP because propofol can cause a significant reduction in mean arterial pressure and cerebral perfusion. Propofol is used with caution in patients who are hypotensive, hypovolemic, or hemodynamically unstable because of its hypotensive effects.

Disorders of lipid metabolism can be aggravated by the emulsion vehicle in which propofol is delivered. Patients with diabetic hyperlipidemia, pancreatitis, or primary hyperlipoproteinemia should be monitored closely.

Adverse Effects

The most common adverse effect to propofol is nausea and vomiting. Another frequent adverse effect is involuntary muscle movements. Propofol produces a dose-related degree of hypotension and decrease in systemic vascular resistance, which is not associated with a significant increase in heart rate or decrease in cardiac output. Apnea occurs in 50% to 84% of patients. Anaphylaxis may also occur. High-dose or long-term propofol use in the critical care setting is associated with inducing bright green urine.

Local adverse effects include pain on injection, transient muscle twitching, and tremor. The solution in which propofol is prepared can support bacterial growth because it contains soybean oil, glycerol, and egg phosphatide.

Drug Interactions

Propofol may interact with benzodiazepines, droperidol, CNS depressants, and theophylline (Table 16-4).

Assessment of Relevant Core Patient Variables

Health Status

The nurse should assess the patient for a history of hypersensitivity to propofol, soybean oil, glycerol, and egg phospholipids. The nurse should also assess the patient for diseases or disorders that would contraindicate the use of propofol.

Evaluate patients with a history of asthma or emphysema for use of theophylline. Evaluate patients with mental health issues for use of benzodiazepines or phenothiazines. Positive responses should be communicated to the anesthesiologist or nurse anesthetist prior to surgery.

When used in the setting of an intensive care unit (ICU), the nurse should obtain serum triglyceride levels prior to initiation of propofol and every 3 to 7 days of therapy.

Life Span and Gender

The nurse should document the age of the patient. Elderly, debilitated, and dehydrated patients are typically more sensitive to the effects of propofol than are younger patients. In addition, elderly patients typically have reduced total body clearance of propofol and should be given lower induction doses and slower infusion rates for anesthesia maintenance.

Environment

The nurse should be aware of the environment in which the drug will be administered. Propofol must be given in a controlled environment, such as an operating room, recovery room, or ICU. A cardiac monitor, blood pressure monitor, and ventilator are required.

Nursing Diagnoses and Outcomes

- Ineffective Breathing Pattern related to respiratory depression secondary to drugs used during anesthesia

  Desired outcome: The patient will maintain effective breathing despite respiratory depression by administration of oxygen as appropriate.
- Risk for Aspiration related to drug-induced nausea and vomiting, GI distention, hypoxia, and stimulation of the vomiting center

  Desired outcome: The patient's nausea and vomiting will be minimized by premedication with anticholinergic agents to reduce the risk of aspiration and nausea.
- Disturbed Sensory Perception, varied, related to CNS depression secondary to drugs used during anesthesia

  Desired outcome: The patient will remain free from sensory or perceptual alterations through careful reorientation, repeated as necessary.

Planning and Intervention

Maximizing Therapeutic Effects

For the surgical patient, preinduction and induction should be done in a low stimulus environment as with isoflurane. Preoperative patient teaching is imperative to minimize the patient's anxiety, thus maximize the therapeutic effects of propofol.

In the critical care setting, a low stimulus environment continues to be important. The nurse should interact with the patient only when necessary to avoid overstimulation. The nurse should evaluate the depth of analgesia and adjust the infusion of propofol according to the institute's standing orders.

TABLE 16-4 Agents That Interact With Propofol

Interactants	Effect and Significance	Nursing Management
benzodiazepines	The pharmacologic effects of propofol may be increased when coadministered with benzodiazepines.	Assess the clinical status of the patient and provide supportive therapy if needed.
central nervous system (CNS) depressants anesthetics opiates ethanol narcotics phenothiazines	Additive CNS and respiratory depression may occur with coadministration.	Monitor for respiratory depression. Adjust dosage as needed.
droperidol	Coadministration may increase frequency of postoperative nausea and vomiting.	Use propofol alone.
theophylline	Theophylline may antagonize the sedative effects of propofol.	Monitor sedation. Adjust dosage of propofol as needed.

Minimizing Adverse Effects

The nurse should visually inspect propofol for particulate matter and discoloration prior to administration. If the emulsion appears to be separated, do not use. Because propofol emulsions do not contain preservatives, it is important to time the duration of administration to avoid bacterial growth. If used for critical care sedation, propofol should be discarded after 12 hours if administered directly from the container provided from the pharmacy or within 6 hours if transferred to a syringe or other container.

Providing Patient and Family Education

- The nurse should provide preoperative teaching to explain the induction process to minimize fears of anesthesia.
- In the critical care unit, the nurse should explain the purpose of the light anesthesia state and reassure patients they are being constantly monitored.
- For outpatient surgery, the nurse should discharge the patient to the care of a responsible adult and instruct patient not to drive or engage in any activity that requires full alertness or coordination.

Ongoing Assessment and Evaluation

Patients receiving propofol as an induction agent for balanced anesthesia are monitored in the postanesthesia recovery room until they are awake and have stable vital signs.

In the critical care units, when propofol is used to maintain light anesthesia, the nurse should continuously monitor blood pressure, cardiac output, and pulmonary capillary wedge pressure. The patient's lung sounds should also be assessed frequently due to respiratory depression. Because the patient remains motionless, the nurse should turn the patient every 2 hours and assess for skin breakdown. The nurse should constantly monitor the level of sedation and titrate propofol to maximize sedation.

As previously mentioned, serum triglycerides should be monitored every 3 to 7 days. ■

MEMORY CHIP

P Propofol

- A parenteral anesthetic used in the management of general anesthesia, sedation induction or maintenance, and status epilepticus
- Significant contraindications: hypersensitivity to soybean oil, glycerol, or egg phosphatide
- Most common adverse effects: nausea, vomiting, involuntary movements
- Most serious adverse effects: apnea and anaphylaxis
- Maximizing therapeutic effects: low stimulus environment
- Minimizing adverse effects: time the administration to avoid potential bacterial growth
- Most significant patient education: reassure the patient that he or she is being constantly monitored

DRUGS CLOSELY RELATED TO P PROPOFOL

Thiopental

Thiopental (Pentothal) is a barbiturate anesthetic agent. Its rapid onset and short duration of action are ideal for an induction agent. Its onset of action after IV administration is less than 1 minute), and the hypnotic action lasts only a few minutes. Metabolism of thiopental takes place in the liver slowly, and it will accumulate in the tissues to a toxic level after repetitive administrations. Thus, thiopental differs from propofol because it is not used for the duration of anesthesia by continuous infusion. Thiopental does not provide any analgesia.

Etomidate

Etomidate (Amidate) is a nonbarbiturate, nonanalgesic anesthetic used primarily for induction, but it can be used for IV anesthesia when supplemented by a narcotic analgesic. Induction is rapid and recovery from a single dose takes only a few minutes because of rapid redistribution of drug to other tissues. Etomidate is metabolized by the liver and has a much shorter elimination than propofol. There appears to be less respiratory and cardiovascular depression than with barbiturates and propofol. Additionally, etomidate does not release histamine.

The popularity of etomidate has diminished because of its adverse effects, including involuntary movements during induction, a high incidence of nausea and vomiting during recovery, and adrenocortical suppression.

DRUGS SIGNIFICANTLY DIFFERENT FROM P PROPOFOL

Ketamine

Ketamine (Ketalar) closely resembles, both chemically and pharmacologically, phencyclidine, which is a street drug with a pronounced effect on sensory perception. Thus, ketamine produces pharmacologic actions distinctly different from other IV anesthetics. It produces dissociative anesthesia, resulting in catatonia, amnesia, and analgesia. The patient may appear awake and reactive but does not respond to sensory stimuli. Ketamine is used for short procedures not requiring muscle relaxation, including diagnostic tests and surgery. It can be used as a general anesthetic agent for children. Because of the high incidence of postoperative psychic phenomena (sensory and perceptual illusion and vivid dreams) associated with its use, ketamine is not commonly used in adult patients. It is considered useful for high-risk geriatric patients and patients in shock, because of its cardiostimulatory properties.

After IV administration, ketamine has an initial half-life of 10 to 15 minutes, which subsequently changes to a longer half-life of 2.5 hours corresponding with redistribution from the CNS and hepatic biotransformation. The metabolites of ketamine are excreted in the urine. Shortly after injection, there is cardiovascular and respiratory stimulation, which peaks within minutes and subsides within 15 minutes.

There is no muscle relaxation associated with ketamine use, and laryngeal and pharyngeal reflexes stay intact. The metabolites of ketamine are excreted in the urine.

Under ketamine anesthesia, the higher centers of the brain do not perceive auditory, visual, or painful stimuli. This effect is thought to occur through ketamine action at opioid and nonopioid receptors, including muscarinic receptors. It may be that different receptors are involved in analgesia and loss of consciousness.

Ketamine is contraindicated in patients for whom a significant increase in blood pressure would be hazardous. It is not used for patients with psychiatric disorders, because of the potential for an reaction during emergence, which may include hallucinations and agitation. It also should be avoided in cases of known hypersensitivity. Precautions should include patients with mild to moderate hypertension, pregnancy or lactation, alcohol abuse, acute intermittent porphyria, elevated intraocular pressure or ICP, and hyperthyroidism.

Hypertension and tachycardia are common cardiovascular effects and probably mediated through sympathetic stimulation. Nausea and vomiting also are common. In addition, ketamine may enhance the actions of the nondepolarizing neuromuscular blockers and prolong respiratory depression. Theophylline should not be coadministered with ketamine, because the two interact and may cause unpredictable seizures. In addition, patients on thyroid enhancement therapy may experience hypertension and tachycardia when administered ketamine.

Nursing care of the patient under ketamine anesthesia is largely protective because of the dissociative state that it causes and the likelihood of emergence reactions. Vital signs and a brief mental status examination are taken as pretreatment assessment.

The outcomes expected for ketamine anesthesia would be effective and safe anesthesia, adequate airway maintenance, and minimal emergence reaction. Emergence reactions may be avoided or diminished if the nurse is careful to reduce external stimuli during the recovery phase and allows the patient to wake up spontaneously. Frightening emergence symptoms may be stopped with diazepam. Because emergence reactions may occur up to 24 hours after anesthesia, the nurse should instruct the patient to avoid hazardous activities, including driving, for at least 24 hours. Ambulatory patients must be discharged into the care of a responsible adult. The nurse should instruct the patient to avoid alcohol and other CNS depressants for 24 hours. The nurse in the PACU and the nurse in charge of the patient on his or her return to the unit should evaluate outcomes achieved and compare them with what would be expected under conditions without complications.

Fentanyl

Fentanyl (Sublimaze) is a narcotic agent used in combination with a neuroleptic drug, such as droperidol, to produce a state of consciousness called neuroleptanesthesia. Fentanyl and droperidol are manufactured as the combination drug Innovar. To obtain neuroleptanesthesia, fentanyl and droperidol are administered IV in combination with nitrous oxide and oxygen. This type of anesthesia is useful for procedures, such as bronchoscopy, that require freedom from pain but the patient's ability to cooperate. The most significant adverse effect of neuroleptanesthesia is respiratory depression or arrest. Chapter 24 discusses narcotic agents in depth.

Benzodiazepines

Benzodiazepines (e.g., diazepam, lorazepam, midazolam) have been used as parenteral agents in balanced anesthesia. Midazolam is water-soluble at low pH and has been reported to cause less pain on injection and a lower incidence of venous thrombosis than diazepam. Additionally, midazolam can be administered IM. Chapter 17 discusses benzodiazepines in depth.

C LOCAL ANESTHETIC AGENTS

Local anesthetic agents are divided into esters and amides. There are important practical differences between these two groups. Esters are relatively unstable in solution and are rapidly hydrolyzed in the body by plasma cholinesterase and other esterases. One of the main breakdown products is paraamino benzoate (PABA), which is associated with allergic phenomena and hypersensitivity reactions. In contrast, amides are relatively stable in solution and are slowly metabolized by hepatic amidases; hypersensitivity reactions to amide local anesthetics are extremely rare. In current clinical practice, esters have largely been superseded by the amides.

Local anesthetics produce local or regional anesthesia by blocking nerve conduction and abolishing sensations in a limited and well-defined area of the body without loss of consciousness (Fig. 16-2). The blockade affects all nerve fibers sequentially: autonomic, sensory, then motor, with effects diminishing in reverse order. Clinically, the loss of nerve function affects temperature first, then pain, touch, proprioception, and finally, skeletal muscle tone.

Local anesthetics have the same mechanism of action, but they differ in their potency, onset of action, and duration (Table 16-5). Examples of local anesthetic agents include lidocaine (Xylocaine), bupivacaine (Marcaine), etidocaine (Duranest), and procaine (Novocain). The prototype discussed in this chapter is lidocaine (Xylocaine), an amide local anesthetic agent.

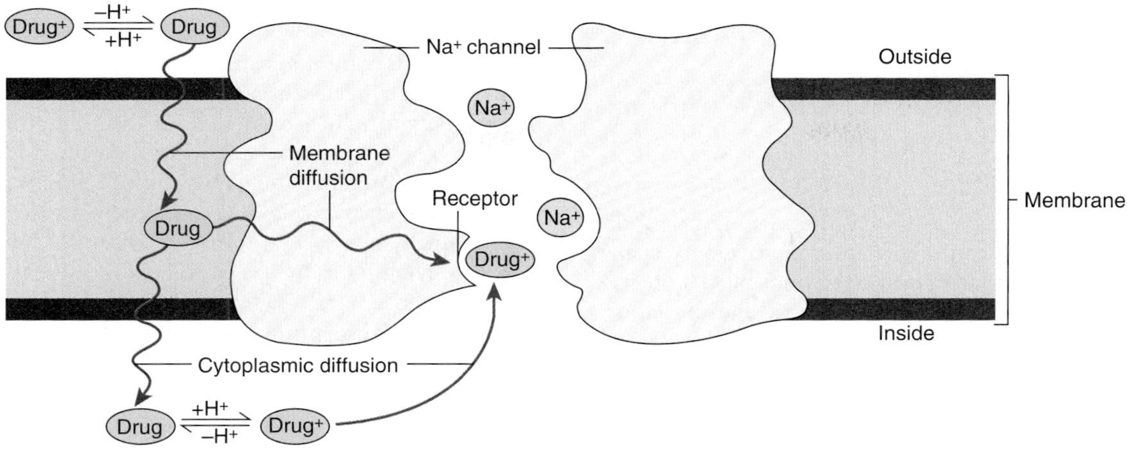

Figure 16-2. Local anesthetics' mechanism of action.

TABLE 16-5 Summary of Selected Local Anesthetic Agents

Drug (Trade) Name	Selected Indications	Route and Dosage Range	Pharmacokinetics
lidocaine (Xylocaine)	Infiltration anesthesia Topical anesthesia Peripheral nerve blocks IV regional nerve blocks Epidural and spinal blocks	*Adult and Child:* maximum, 3 mg/kg; with adrenalin: maximum: 7 mg/kg	*Onset:* Rapid *Duration:* 1–3 h $t_{1/2}$: 7–30 min
bupivacaine (Marcaine)	Infiltration anesthesia Peripheral nerve blocks Epidural and spinal blocks	*Adult and Child:* maximum: 2 mg/kg; with adrenalin, maximum: 2 mg/kg	*Onset:* 1–10 min *Duration:* 3–9 h $t_{1/2}$: neonates: 8.1 h $t_{1/2}$: adults: 3.5 h
etidocaine (Duranest)	Infiltration anesthesia Peripheral nerve block Extradural blocks	*Adult:* maximum: 4 mg/kg *Child:* maximum dose not established	*Onset:* 2–8 min *Duration:* 4.5–13 h $t_{1/2}$: neonates: 4–8 h $t_{1/2}$: adults: 2.7 h
mepivacaine (Carbocaine, Polocaine)	Infiltration anesthesia Peripheral nerve blocks	*Adults:* 400 mg as a single regional dose not to exceed 1000 mg/24 h *Child:* 5–6 mg/kg	*Onset:* 5–4 min *Duration:* 1–2 h $t_{1/2}$: neonates: 8.7–9 h $t_{1/2}$: adults: 1.9–3.2 h
prilocaine (Citanest)	Infiltration anesthesia Peripheral nerve blocks IV regional nerve blocks	*Adult and Child:* 6 mg/kg; with adrenalin, 9 mg/kg	*Onset:* <2 min *Duration:* 1–2 h $t_{1/2}$: 1.25 h
procaine (Novocain)	Dental anesthesia Infiltration Anesthesia Local anesthesia Peripheral nerve block Regional anesthesia Severe pain Spinal anesthesia Sympathetic nerve block	*Adult:* single dose of 350–600 mg *Child:* 15 mg/kg	*Onset:* 2–5 min *Duration:* 1 h $t_{1/2}$: 7.7 min

NURSING MANAGEMENT OF THE PATIENT RECEIVING LIDOCAINE

Core Drug Knowledge

Pharmacotherapeutics

Lidocaine is used as a local anesthetic in a variety of pathologies. They include infiltration anesthesia to repair full-thickness skin lacerations, regional blocks, nerve blocks, ophthalmic anesthesia, obstetric anesthesia, or dental anesthesia. It can be applied topically for dental pain, postherpetic neuralgia, neuropathic pain, or stomatitis. It has also been found effective for migraine headaches when administered intranasally.

In addition to its local anesthetic uses, lidocaine is also used intravenously for ventricular tachycardia or ventricular fibrillation. See Chapter 29 for a discussion of lidocaine as an antiarrhythmic.

Pharmacokinetics

Lidocaine may be administered topically, orally, subcutaneously, intradermally, submucosally, and IV. Only minimal amounts of lidocaine enter the circulation following subcutaneous injection. The duration of action of subcutaneously administered lidocaine is 1 to 3 hours, depending on the strength of the lidocaine preparation used. The addition of epinephrine 1:200,000 to 1:100,000 to lidocaine slows the vascular absorption of lidocaine and prolongs its effects.

Lidocaine is nearly completely absorbed following oral administration but undergoes extensive first-pass metabolism in the liver, resulting in a systemic bioavailability of only 35%. Some systemic absorption is possible when using oral viscous solutions.

Transdermal absorption of lidocaine is related to the duration of application and the surface area over which the patch is applied. When the lidocaine patch is used as directed there is very little systemic absorption. After topical administration of viscous solutions or jelly to mucous membranes, the duration of action is 30 to 60 minutes with peak effects occurring within 2 to 5 minutes.

Local anesthesia starts to occur within 2.5 minutes of application of the DentiPatch to intact mucous membranes and continues for approximately 30 to 40 minutes.

Pharmacodynamics

Lidocaine produces its analgesics effects through a reversible nerve conduction blockade by diminishing the nerve membrane's permeability to sodium. This action decreases the rate of membrane depolarization, thereby increasing the threshold for electrical excitability. Direct nerve membrane penetration is necessary for effective anesthesia, which is achieved by applying the anesthetic topically or injecting it subcutaneously, intradermally, or submucosally around the nerve trunks or ganglia supplying the area to be anesthetized.

Contraindications and Precautions

Lidocaine is contraindicated in patients with amide local anesthetic hypersensitivity and in patients with hypersensitivity to sulfites or methyl paraben. Epidural, local, nerve block, and spinal administration of lidocaine are contraindicated in patients with infection or inflammation at the injection site to avoid systemic absorption of lidocaine.

Applying lidocaine preparations to severely traumatized mucosa (large skin abrasions, eczema, burns) can increase its absorption, increasing the risk of systemic toxicity. Application to the oral mucosa can interfere with swallowing and increase the risk of aspiration. Lumbar and caudal epidural anesthesia should be used with extreme caution in patients with existing neurologic disease, spinal deformities, sepsis, and severe hypertension. Lidocaine should be used with caution during pregnancy and in patients who are breast-feeding.

Adverse Effects

Allergic reactions such as urticaria, angioedema, bronchospasm, and anaphylactic shock may occur with lidocaine administration. Some preparations contain sulfite and methyl paraben, which can cause severe allergic reactions, including status asthmaticus, in susceptible patients.

Local anesthetic agents are relatively free from adverse effects if they are administered in an appropriate dosage and in the correct anatomic location. However, systemic and localized toxic reactions may occur, usually from the accidental intravascular or intrathecal injection, or the administration of an excessive dose of the local anesthetic agent. Systemic reactions to local anesthetics involve primarily the CNS and the cardiovascular system.

Although lidocaine is a pregnancy category B drug, local anesthetics can cross the placenta rapidly when administered for epidural, paracervical, pudendal, or caudal block anesthesia, resulting in fetal bradycardia. The frequency and extent of toxicity are dependent on the procedure performed. Maternal hypotension can result from regional anesthesia, and elevating the feet and positioning the patient on her left side can alleviate this problem.

Transoral or transdermal application of lidocaine are unlikely to cause systemic adverse reactions due to the small amount of lidocaine absorbed. Potential local reactions include erythema, edema, and dysesthesia (abnormal sensations including numbness, tingling, prickling, or burning). These reactions are usually mild and transient resolving within a few minutes to hours.

Drug Interactions

Drug interactions occur most frequently with IV administration of lidocaine. Subcutaneous administration rarely causes drug interactions unless lidocaine is inadvertently administered into an artery or vein.

Local anesthetics can interact with antihypertensive agents, cholinesterase inhibitors, monoamine oxidase inhibitors, and opiate agonists (Table 16-6).

Assessment of Relevant Core Patient Variables

Health Status

The nurse should assess for hypersensitivity to lidocaine or any other drug with *-caine* in the name. Positive findings should be communicated to the provider prior to administration of lidocaine.

When using topical anesthesia, the nurse should inspect the area. Do not apply to abraded or denuded skin. For viscous lidocaine, the nurse should assess for the patient's ability to swallow prior to its use.

Life Span and Gender

When lidocaine is used as epidural anesthesia during labor and delivery, it may prolong the second stage of labor. The nurse should monitor for fetal or neonatal cardiovascular and CNS depression.

Lifestyle, Diet, and Habits

Viscous lidocaine may be provided for patients with stomatitis or chronic ulceration in the mouth. It is important that the patient assess the ability to swallow prior to eating or drinking to avoid biting the interior of the mouth or aspirating foods or fluids.

Environment

The nurse should be aware of the environment in which the drug will be administered. Lidocaine is used in a variety of settings including hospitals, outpatient surgical settings, clinics, private doctor's offices, and dental offices. Topical or viscous lidocaine may be administered in the home environment.

Nursing Diagnoses and Outcomes

- Fear related to traumatic injury and concern for pain during surgical procedure
  Desired outcome: *The patient will be assured pain will not occur during the procedure.*
- Risk for Peripheral Neurovascular Dysfunction related to action of drug
  Desired outcome: *The patient verbalizes the duration of action of the drug and refrains from activities that may induce injury while area is numb.*
- Impaired Swallowing related to administration of viscous lidocaine
  Desired outcome: *The patient will refrain from eating or drinking for 1 hour after swallowing viscous lidocaine.*

Planning and Intervention

Maximizing Therapeutic Effects

The nurse should assist with the administration of lidocaine after patient teaching is accomplished. The nurse should have a calm, reassuring approach and allow the patient to voice concerns prior to starting the procedure.

Minimizing Adverse Effects

The nurse should read the label carefully before assisting the provider with administration of lidocaine. Preparations containing preservatives should not be used for spinal or epidural anesthesia. Preparations with adrenaline should not be administered in areas such as fingers, toes, nose, or penis, because prolonged vasoconstriction

TABLE 16-6 Agents That Interact With Lidocaine

Interactants	Effect and Significance	Nursing Management
antihypertensive agents	Epidural administration of local anesthetics with antihypertensive agents may result in additive hypotensive effects due to loss of sympathetic tone.	Monitor vital signs.
cholinesterase inhibitors	Local anesthetics can antagonize the effects of cholinesterase inhibitors by inhibiting neuronal transmission in skeletal muscle.	Dosage adjustment of the cholinesterase inhibitor may be necessary to control the symptoms of myasthenia gravis.
monoamine oxidase inhibitors (MAOIS)	Concomitant administration of MAOIs and local anesthetics increases the risk of hypotension.	MAOIs should be discontinued 10 days before surgery requiring a regional block.
opiate agonists alfentanil fentanyl morphine sufentanil	Concomitant use of low-dose local anesthetics with opiate agonists may increase analgesia and decrease opiate dosage requirements.	Monitor for analgesic efficacy. Monitor CNS depression.

may result in a poor outcome. Food and fluids should be restricted for 1 hour after swallowing viscous lidocaine.

Providing Patient and Family Education

- The nurse should inform the patient and family of the action of local anesthetics such as lidocaine. The nurse should assure the patient the area will be without sensation prior to initiation of the procedure. The nurse should encourage the patient to verbalize any discomfort during the procedure.
- The nurse should advise patient receiving topical anesthesia at home to place the anesthetic on the dressing, then place the dressing on the site. The nurse should remind patients receiving viscous lidocaine that it causes numbness of the tongue, cheeks, and throat. The patient should not eat or drink for 1 hour to prevent biting cheeks or tongue and avoid aspiration.
- The nurse should advise the patient of the expected duration of lidocaine. The patient should contact the provider if sensation does not return.

Ongoing Assessment and Evaluation

The nurse should evaluate for the lack of sensation prior to starting a procedure. Remind the patient to assess for sensation before resuming food or fluid intake. ■

DRUGS CLOSELY RELATED TO LIDOCAINE

Bupivacaine

Bupivacaine (Marcaine) is a long-acting, local, amide anesthetic recommended for local or regional anesthesia. It has the ability to separate sensory and motor blockade, because its effect on motor function varies with concentration. With bupivacaine administration, analgesia persists longer than anesthesia, which postpones the need for postoperative narcotics. Bupivacaine is also used in epidural PCA in combination with narcotics.

Etidocaine

Etidocaine (Duranest) is a long-acting local anesthetic of the amide type. It is used for epidural, local, and retrobulbar anesthesia in surgical and dental procedures. Similar to lidocaine, etidocaine has a rapid onset of sensory and motor blockade, but duration of analgesia is 1.5 to 2 times longer than lidocaine. Its profound motor blockade may last up to 9 hours when given peridurally.

Mepivacaine

Mepivacaine (Carbocaine, Polocaine) is a local anesthetic of the amide type with an intermediate duration of action. Compared with lidocaine, it produces less vasodilation, and has a more rapid onset and longer duration of action. Mepivacaine is indicated for infiltration and transtracheal anesthesia, and peripheral, sympathetic, regional, and epidural nerve blocks in surgical or dental procedures.

Prilocaine

Prilocaine (Citanest) is another local anesthetic of the amide class used primarily for dental anesthesia. It has an intermediate duration of action and is longer acting than lidocaine. Prilocaine causes the least systemic toxicity of the amides but may cause methemoglobinemia at high doses.

Procaine

Procaine hydrochloride (Novocain) is a short-acting local anesthetic of the ester type used for local or regional anesthesia and dental applications. It has no topical anesthetic activity. Procaine is more likely to cause a hypersensitivity reaction and vasodilation than amide-type local anesthetics.

Topical Anesthetics

Local anesthetics may be applied to the skin, the eye, the ear, the nose, and the mouth, as well as other mucous membranes. In general, cocaine, lidocaine, and prilocaine are the most useful and effective local anesthetics for this purpose. When used to produce topical anesthesia, they usually have a rapid onset of action (5 to 10 minutes) and a moderate duration of action (30 to 60 minutes). Cocaine is a potent vasoconstrictor and is useful in the reduction of bleeding as well as topical anesthesia.

Absorption of local anesthetics through intact skin is usually slow and unreliable and high concentrations are re-

MEMORY CHIP

Lidocaine

- Used for infiltration anesthesia, regional blocks, nerve blocks, ophthalmic anesthesia, obstetric anesthesia, or dental anesthesia
- Significant contraindications: hypersensitivity to amide local anesthetics, sulfites, or methyl paraben; infection or inflammation at the site of administration
- Most common adverse effects: minimal adverse reactions unless accidental intravascular or intrathecal injection[a] occurs
- Most serious adverse effect: allergic reactions
- Maximizing therapeutic effects: calm reassurance by staff
- Minimizing adverse effects: read labels carefully. Be sure to use the right preparation for the right procedure
- Most significant patient education: safety due to lack of sensation

quired. EMLA cream is a mixture of local anesthetics (lidocaine and prilocaine in an emulsion) that may be used to provide surface anesthesia of the skin (particularly for children). Cutaneous contact (usually under an occlusive dressing) should be maintained for at least 60 minutes prior to venipuncture.

NEUROMUSCULAR BLOCKING AGENTS

Neuromuscular blocking agents are divided into two categories: **nondepolarizing drugs,** which prevent neural communication from depolarizing the muscle (i.e., the muscle remains in a relaxed state), and **depolarizing drugs,** which cause muscle depolarization and prevent repolarization (i.e., the muscle contracts and is unable to go into a relaxed state to receive further neurocommunication. Neuromuscular blockers are not mediated by the CNS. Rather, they work by directly interfering with transmission at the **end plate,** which is the site of communication between a nerve and a muscle (Fig. 16-3).

Physiology

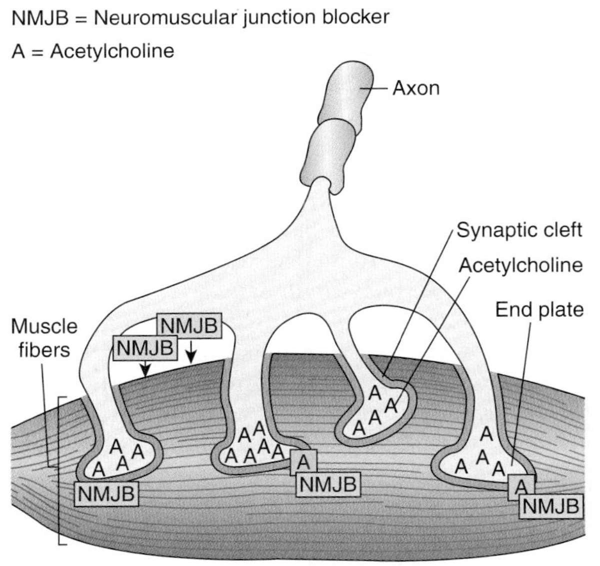

Figure 16-3. How neuromuscular blockers work. Motor end plates are the terminal branches of motor nerves. They are found within muscle fibers, but they are separated from the muscle itself by a synaptic cleft. Normally, the neurotransmitter acetylcholine is found in the axon of the motor nerve. However, when the nerve is stimulated, the acetylcholine is released and moves to receptor sites on surface of the muscle cell. Neuromuscular blockers inhibit the action of acetylcholine (muscle contraction) by competing for these receptor sites. (NMJB, neuromuscular junction blocker; A, acetylcholine.)

NONDEPOLARIZING NEUROMUSCULAR BLOCKING AGENTS

Nondepolarizing neuromuscular blocking agents include tubocurarine (Tubarine, Tubocuraine), pancuronium bromide (Pavulon), pipecuronium (Arduan), and vecuronium (Norcuron) (Table 16-7). The prototype drug of this class is tubocurarine.

NURSING MANAGEMENT OF THE PATIENT RECEIVING TUBOCURARINE

Core Drug Knowledge

Pharmacotherapeutics

Tubocurarine is a skeletal muscle relaxant used as an adjunct to general anesthetics to facilitate endotracheal intubation and to facilitate mechanical ventilation. In the ICU or cardiac intensive care setting, tubocurarine is used to minimize patients' movement to conserve energy or to reduce agitation that may increase ICP. It is also used to prevent trauma during electroconvulsive therapy and to diagnose myasthenia gravis.

Pharmacokinetics

Tubocurarine is only available for IV use. The onset of muscle paralysis occurs in 2 minutes after administration and peaks at 3 to 5 minutes. Muscle paralysis starts to subside within 20 to 30 minutes but may be prolonged to 90 minutes or more. Up to 75% of tubocurarine is excreted unchanged by the kidneys in the first 24 hours. Another 11% may undergo biliary excretion. Only a negligible amount of the drug is metabolized. Tubocurarine crosses the placenta; whether it enters breast milk is unknown.

Pharmacodynamics

Tubocurarine is found in certain plants in the Amazon rain forest. It is a component of curare, which is extracted from these plants. Tubocurarine and other NMJ blockers are antagonists of acetylcholine; they compete with the neurotransmitter for the cholinergic receptor sites at the motor end plate. This antagonism causes a decrease in the response of the muscle to acetylcholine, resulting in a flaccid or relaxed paralysis. Tubocurarine does not cross the blood–brain barrier and has no action on the CNS. For this reason, anesthesia is induced before neuromuscular blockade is started, otherwise the unanesthetized patient would have the frightening experience of paralysis and the inability to breathe. This is important to remember when NMJ blockers are used to facilitate mechanical ventilation in ICU or critical care unit patients.

It is also important to remember that NMJ blockers do not affect consciousness or alter sensation; therefore, benzodiazepines and analgesics are administered concurrently to manage fear, anxiety, or pain.

TABLE 16-7 Summary of Selected C Neuromuscular Blocking Agents

Drug (Trade) Name	Selected Indications	Route and Dosage Range	Pharmacokinetics
C Nondepolarizing Neuromuscular Junction Blockers			
P tubocurarine (Tubarine, Tubocuraine)	Moderate to long duration surgeries, adjunct to electroconvulsive therapy, diagnosis of multiple sclerosis	*Adult:* IV, 0.165 mg/kg for onset, then 0.04–0.1 mg/kg for maintenance; diagnosis, IV, 0.004–0.033 mg/kg *Child:* Same	*Onset:* 2 min *Duration:* 20–90 min $t_{1/2}$: 170–270 min
pancuronium bromide (Pavulon)	Endotracheal tube (ET) intubation Intensive care unit sedation	*Adult:* IV, 0.04–1 mg/kg *Child:* Same *Adult:* IV, 0.015 mg/kg every 25–60 min *Child:* Same	*Onset:* 2–3 min *Duration:* 45–60 min $t_{1/2}$: 90–140 min
pipecuronium (Arduan)	Long-acting (longer than 90 min) surgeries and ET intubation	*Adult:* IV, 70–85 μg/kg	*Onset:* 2–3 min *Duration:* 120–150 min $t_{1/2}$: 1.7 h
vecuronium (Norcuron)	Short to intermediate length surgeries	*Adult:* IV, 0.08–0.1 mg/kg, then 0.01–0.015 mg/kg for maintenance *Child:* > 10 y, same as adult; < 10 y, slightly higher initial dose and more frequent maintenance dosing; not for child <7 wk	*Onset:* 2–3 min *Duration:* 45–60 min $t_{1/2}$: 4 min
C Depolarizing Neuromuscular Junction Blockers			
P succinylcholine (Anectine)	Short inductions, ET intubation, endoscopy, electroconvulsive therapy (ECT), prolonged muscle relaxation	*Adult:* IV, short procedure, 0.3–1.1 mg/kg; long procedure, 2.5–4.3 mg/min; prolonged muscle relaxation by intermittent IV, 0.04–0.07 mg/kg *Child:* IV (infant and small child), 2 mg/kg; (older child and adolescent), 1 mg/kg; IM, 3–4 mg/kg	*Onset:* IV, 30–60 s; IM, 2–3 min *Duration:* IV, 4–6 min; IM, 10–20 min $t_{1/2}$: Unknown

The neuromuscular blocking actions of tubocurarine may be reversed with anticholinesterases, such as neostigmine, pyridostigmine, and edrophonium. These drugs block the normal breakdown of acetylcholine at the motor end plate, thereby leading to an accumulation of the neurotransmitter and return of muscle stimulation.

Contraindications and Precautions

Tubocurarine is contraindicated in patients who have ever shown hypersensitivity to the drug or to any other nondepolarizing blocker. Tubocurarine is classified as pregnancy category C. It is also contraindicated for use in early pregnancy because it can cause congenital fetal fractures.

Tubocurarine is used with caution in patients who have preexisting pulmonary disease or lung cancer. Neuromuscular blockade may be enhanced in these patients. Tubocurarine is also used with caution in patients with dehydration, electrolyte imbalance, or an acid-base imbalance because these disorders may alter its affects. In patients with hypothermia, the action or duration of tubocurarine may be decreased.

Patients with asthma, bronchospasm, hypotension, and cardiac disease may be affected by the histamine release and vasodilation effects of tubocurarine, which may exacerbate these conditions.

Tubocurarine should be used with extreme caution in patients with decreased renal function because the drug is excreted unchanged primarily by the kidneys. Tubocurarine should be used with caution in patients with myasthenia gravis, unless it is being used as a diagnostic aid.

Adverse Effects

The principal adverse effects of tubocurarine result from its blocking neuromuscular activity at all neuromuscular end plates. Prolonged paralysis can lead to pressure sores (decubitus ulcer formation) resulting from immobility. Prolonged apnea can result from the paralysis of the respiratory muscles. Therefore, assisted ventilation is needed until the drug's effects resolve or anticholinesterase administration is successful.

Neuromuscular blockade of the GI tract can result in decreased GI tone and mobility and may render the patient more prone to regurgitation, vomiting, and aspiration. Relaxation of arterial muscles results in vasodilation, which can promote flushing, hypotension, slow or rapid heart rate, or worsening of preexisting heart problems. Histamine release associated with the NMJ blockers may result in respiratory difficulty, including wheezing and bronchospasm. Occasionally, patients may respond to their first exposure to tubocurarine or other NMJ blockers with an extreme hypersensitivity reaction or even malignant hyperthermia, which is characterized by massive muscle contraction, sharply elevated body temperature, severe acidosis, and if uncontrolled, death.

Drug Interactions

Drugs that may decrease the effectiveness of tubocurarine include carbamazepine and the hydantoins and theophyllines. Drugs that potentiate the action of tubocurarine include antibiotics, inhalation anesthetics, ketamine, magnesium salts, quinine derivatives, thiopurines, trimethaphan, and verapamil. Table 16-8 discusses these potential drug interactions.

Assessment of Relevant Core Patient Variables

Health Status

The nurse should evaluate the patient for a history of hypersensitivity to any NMJ blocker or for any renal, hepatic, cardiovascular, or respiratory diseases. The nurse should place a note on the chart and the drug administration record (Kardex) identifying the need for close monitoring of patients with a history of any of these disorders.

Before administration, the nurse should perform a physical assessment. The physical examination should include body weight, temperature, state of hydration (skin turgor, pulses), reflexes and muscle tone, pulse,

TABLE 16-8 Agents That Interact With Tubocurarine

Interactants	Effect and Significance	Nursing Management
antibiotics aminoglycosides lincosamide polypeptides	Potentiate the action of tubocurarine, resulting in profound and severe respiratory depression	Avoid combination. Provide life support as needed. Provide anticholinesterases as indicated.
anticonvulsants carbamazepine hydantoins	In combination, may decrease the duration or efficacy of tubocurarine	Monitor for decreased muscle relaxant effectiveness. Titrate drug as necessary.
inhalation anesthetics	Potentiate the actions of tubocurarine	Monitor respiratory function. Titrate drug as necessary. Provide life support as needed.
ketamine	May enhance the actions of tubocurarine, resulting in profound and severe respiratory depression	Monitor respiratory function. Titrate drug as necessary. Provide life support as needed.
magnesium salts	May enhance the actions of tubocurarine, resulting in profound and severe respiratory depression	Monitor respiratory function. Titrate drug as necessary. Provide life support as needed.
quinine derivatives	Have a synergistic action with tubocurarine, resulting in profound and severe respiratory depression	Monitor neuromuscular function. Titrate drug as necessary. Provide life support as needed.
theophyllines	May antagonize the activity of tubocurarine	Monitor for efficacy of tubocurarine. Increase dose of tubocurarine if needed.
thiopurines	May inhibit phosphodiesterase, resulting in an anticurare action; may decrease the activity of tubocurarine	Monitor for efficacy of tubocurarine. Increase dose of tubocurarine if needed.
trimethaphan	Augments the neuromuscular blockade of tubocurarine, resulting in prolonged apnea	Avoid combination if possible. Monitor respiratory function. Titrate drug as necessary. Provide life support as needed.
verapamil	May enhance the action of tubocurarine because of its blockage of calcium channels in skeletal muscle	Avoid combination if possible. Monitor respiratory function. Titrate drug as necessary. Provide life support as needed.

blood pressure, respiratory rate, and adventitious breath sounds. The nurse should assess laboratory tests to establish baseline electrolyte values and renal and hepatic status.

Life Span and Gender

The nurse should assess women of child-bearing age for pregnancy. Tubocurarine is contraindicated in early pregnancy because of its potential for teratogenic effects. However, it can be used safely as an adjunct to anesthesia in cesarean deliveries. After birth, the nurse should closely observe the infant for any signs respiratory depression, because the drug crosses the placenta.

Environment

The nurse should be aware of the environment in which the drug will be administered. Like all neuromuscular blocking agents, tubocurarine causes respiratory impairment and paralysis. It should be administered only by a person skilled in administering NMJ blockers. Necessary equipment for intubation, controlled ventilation, and administration of oxygen must be immediately available.

Nursing Diagnoses and Outcomes

- Impaired Spontaneous Ventilation related to respiratory paralysis
  Desired outcome: *The patient will be maintained with artificial ventilation until the ability to sustain spontaneous respirations returns.*
- Impaired Skin Integrity related to paralysis
  Desired outcome: *The patient will remain free of skin breakdown.*
- Fear related to paralysis and helplessness
  Desired outcome: *The patient will be reassured and comforted to prevent fear and sympathetic effects of fear during paralysis.*

Planning and Intervention

Maximizing Therapeutic Effects

The nurse can maximize the therapeutic effects of tubocurarine by helping patients understand the reason for the therapy and by helping to decrease their fear and anxiety. The nurse should monitor the patient carefully for pain or distress; although not absolute, responses of the pupils, blood pressure, and heart rate are probably the most reliable guide to the patient's condition. The nurse should also reassure conscious patients frequently regarding personnel's awareness of their helplessness. Procedures and interventions should be explained to patients, because their hearing is not impaired.

Minimizing Adverse Effects

The nurse should have resuscitation equipment and drugs at the bedside throughout therapy. The nurse should evaluate the depth of paralysis by use of a stimulator and use cholinesterase inhibitors to overcome excessive or prolonged neuromuscular blockade.

If paralysis is prolonged, the nurse should change the patient's position frequently to prevent venous stasis or decubitus ulcer formation. The nurse should also provide frequent skin care to prevent skin breakdown.

Providing Patient and Family Education

- Before administration, the nurse should explain to the patient and family that this drug will paralyze muscles and the patient will be unable to speak, move, or breathe unassisted. It is important to explain that these effects should subside in a short period of time after the drug is discontinued.
- The nurse should advise the patient that adverse effects may occur after administration. These effects include sore muscles, constipation, difficulty voiding, and dizziness on arising. The nurse should explain to the patient the importance of reporting these symptoms to avoid potential injury.

Ongoing Assessment and Evaluation

The nurse should monitor the respiratory and cardiac status of the patient every 15 minutes during the administration of tubocurarine. For patients with prolonged paralysis, the nurse should monitor skin status frequently. Conscious patients should be monitored for any sign of distress. This is especially important because they are unable to talk or move. Keep in mind, however, that patients' hearing is intact. For patients with prolonged paralysis, the nurse should turn the patient every 2 hours and monitor for skin breakdown. The nurse should also provide protection to the corneas by taping eye pads in place and with use of artificial tears. The nurse needs to continue use of benzodiazepines and analgesic agents to provide a calm environment for this patient. ■

MEMORY CHIP

Tubocurarine

- A nondepolarizing neuromuscular junction blocking agent used to facilitate endotracheal intubation and mechanical ventilation
- Used in critical care patients to conserve energy and prevent agitation
- Significant contraindications: hypersensitivity, early pregnancy
- Most common adverse effects: flushing, hypotension
- Most serious adverse effects: prolonged paralysis, apnea, malignant hyperthermia
- Maximizing therapeutic effects: decrease anxiety and fear
- Minimizing adverse effects: have resuscitation equipment and cholinesterase inhibitor antidote at the bedside
- Most significant patient education: reassure the patient that he or she is being constantly monitored

DRUGS CLOSELY RELATED TO TUBOCURARINE

Pancuronium Bromide

Pancuronium bromide (Pavulon) is another IV nondepolarizing neuromuscular blocking agent. Although similar to tubocurarine, it is five times as potent. Pancuronium is used to induce relaxation of the skeletal muscles during surgery, to facilitate pulmonary compliance during mechanical ventilation, and to treat agitation in patients in intensive care.

Pancuronium is contraindicated for use in neonates. Some preparations of pancuronium contain benzyl alcohol as a preservative, which has been associated with a fatal toxic (gasping) syndrome.

One major difference between pancuronium and tubocurarine is that pancuronium produces little histamine release and no ganglion blockade. For this reason, hypotension and bronchospasm are not associated with its use.

Pipecuronium

Pipecuronium (Arduan) is a parenteral, long-acting, nondepolarizing neuromuscular blocker. Like other NMJ blockers, it is used as an adjunct to general anesthesia or for endotracheal intubation. Because of its long action, it should be used only for procedures expected to last more than 90 minutes.

Vecuronium

Vecuronium bromide (Norcuron) is a short-acting, IV, nondepolarizing neuromuscular blocking agent. Vecuronium is more potent than pancuronium in producing neuromuscular blockade. However, the blockade produced is short-lived in comparison with other NMJ blockers. The advantage of vecuronium is that it is the least active histamine releaser of the NMJ blockers and has minimal effect on cardiovascular function.

DEPOLARIZING NEUROMUSCULAR JUNCTION BLOCKERS

Depolarizing NMJ blockers work by causing the muscle cell membrane to depolarize or become excited, leading to muscle contraction. This leads to a paralysis of the muscle after repeated excitation. This differs from nondepolarizing NMJ blockers, which prevent excitation. Succinylcholine (Anectine) is the prototype depolarizing NMJ blocker.

NURSING MANAGEMENT OF THE PATIENT RECEIVING SUCCINYLCHOLINE

Core Drug Knowledge

Pharmacotherapeutics

Succinylcholine is used primarily for rapid endotracheal intubation and endoscopic procedures. It is also of value in modifying muscle contractions and preventing fractures during electroconvulsive therapy because it produces a rapid and complete neuromuscular blockade within 1 minute that lasts for a few minutes, allowing sufficient time to complete the therapy. The use of succinylcholine as an adjunct to anesthesia or to facilitate prolonged mechanical ventilation has been largely replaced by the use of more effective and less toxic NMJ blockers.

Pharmacokinetics

Succinylcholine is administered IV and IM. It has a rapid onset and a short duration of action. Following IV administration, complete muscle relaxation occurs in 30 seconds to 1 minute, lasts for 2 to 3 minutes, then dissipates within 10 minutes. After IM injection, muscle relaxation occurs in 2 to 3 minutes and lasts 10 to 30 minutes.

Succinylcholine is distributed in the extracellular fluid but does not readily cross the placental barrier. Succinylcholine has a complex excretion pattern. Approximately 10% of the dose is excreted unchanged in the urine. The majority of succinylcholine is hydrolyzed by plasma pseudocholinesterase to metabolites. One of the metabolites, succinylmonocholine, has nondepolarizing muscle relaxation properties. It, in turn, is excreted partly in urine, and the remainder is broken down into inactive metabolites. Succinylmonocholine is hydrolyzed slowly. If accumulation occurs, such as with hepatic dysfunction, prolonged muscle relaxation may cause apnea.

Pharmacodynamics

Succinylcholine acts as an agonist at the cholinergic nicotinic receptors of the motor end plate. Like the usual neurotransmitter acetylcholine, it depolarizes the postsynaptic membrane, producing repetitive excitation of the motor end plate. This causes muscular fasciculations (rapid contractions) followed by flaccid paralysis. Because of this effect, patients often experience postoperative muscle pain. The ensuing paralysis is short-lived because the succinylcholine is hydrolyzed by plasma pseudocholinesterase.

Contraindications and Precautions

Succinylcholine is contraindicated in any patient with a known hypersensitivity to the drug. Because it can induce malignant hyperthermia, it is also contraindicated in anyone with a personal or family history of malignant hyperthermia. Because it may interact with acetylcholine to produce prolonged apnea, it is contraindicated in patients with familial plasma pseudocholinesterase disorders. Succinylcholine is also contraindicated in patients with an open eye injury or acute narrow-angle glaucoma, because it causes a transient elevation in intraocular pressure immediately after injection.

Succinylcholine should be used with caution in patients prone to low pseudocholinesterase levels. Decreased concentrations of serum pseudocholinesterase, the major route for degradation of succinylcholine, can lead to very high levels of the drug and prolonged action.

It should also be used with caution in patients with hyperkalemia or in those at risk for hyperkalemia. Intense muscle contraction and potassium release from succinylcholine may induce hyperkalemia and provoke complications of hyperkalemia, such as cardiac arrhythmias. This is especially important in children and adults with compromised cardiac function, degenerative or dystrophic neuromuscular disease, or paraplegia. These patients tend to become severely hyperkalemic when succinylcholine is administered.

Adverse Effects

The principal adverse effects of succinylcholine result from muscle paralysis caused by the drug. Prolonged apnea can result from the paralysis of the respiratory muscles, and assisted ventilation is needed until the drug effects are known. Increased intraocular pressure can aggravate or precipitate glaucoma, and prolonged paralysis can result in decubitus ulcer formation due to immobility. A mild histamine release associated with succinylcholine may result in respiratory difficulty, including wheezing and bronchospasm, cardiac arrhythmias, hypotension, and even cardiac arrest in susceptible patients. Malignant hyperthermia has been reported infrequently. Other metabolic effects include hyperkalemia with its resultant muscular and cardiac effects and myoglobinemia and myoglobinuria associated with extreme muscle contraction. Patients may complain of intense muscle pain that may persist for several days after the drug is given.

Drug Interactions

Succinylcholine interacts with aminoglycosides, anticholinesterases, procaine, and trimethaphan (Table 16-9). It also interacts with drugs that decrease plasma cholinesterase, such as cyclophosphamide, echothiophate, lidocaine infusion, metoclopramide, and quinine derivatives.

Assessment of Relevant Core Patient Variables

Health Status

The nurse should assess the patient's personal or family history for low pseudocholinesterase levels. Patients at risk for low pseudocholinesterase levels include those with severe burns, malnutrition, dehydration, severe hepatic disease, cancer, severe anemia, or myxedema. The nurse should also assess for a history of slow recovery from anesthesia or difficulty during anesthesia.

Prior to administering succinylcholine, the nurse should perform a physical assessment. The physical examination should include body weight and temperature, state of hydration (skin turgor, pulses), reflexes

TABLE 16-9 Agents That Interact With Succinylcholine

Interactants	Effect and Significance	Nursing Management
aminoglycosides	Potentiate neuromuscular effects of succinylcholine	Use combination with caution. Delay administration of aminoglycosides as long as possible after recovery of spontaneous respirations. Monitor for respiratory depression. Have mechanical ventilation available.
anticholinesterases	Inhibition of plasma cholinesterase by anticholinesterases may delay hydrolysis of succinylcholine	Use this combination with caution. Monitor patients' spontaneous muscle activity, which must continue for 5 minutes before longer acting agents are administered.
plasma cholinesterase inhibitors cyclophosphamide echothiophate lidocaine infusion metoclopramide quinine derivatives oral contraceptives	Plasma cholinesterase (pseudocholinesterase) necessary to hydrolyze succinylcholine; decreased plasma cholinesterase interferes with the inactivation of succinylcholine, may prolong neuromuscular blockade	Measure serum cholinesterase levels for patients who have been receiving drugs that inhibit plasma cholinesterase. Reduce succinylcholine dosage if plasma cholinesterase levels are decreased. Monitor for respiratory depression. Have mechanical ventilation available.
procaine	Procaine and succinylcholine both hydrolyzed by plasma cholinesterase; competition for the enzyme possibly resulting in prolonged effects of succinylcholine	Monitor for respiratory depression. Have mechanical ventilation available.
trimethaphan	Potent noncompetitive inhibitor of plasma cholinesterase; directly decreases the sensitivity of the respiratory center, increasing risk for respiratory depression	Avoid this combination. Substitute nitroprusside for trimethaphan.

and muscle tone, pulse rate, blood pressure, respiratory rate, and adventitious breath sounds.

Life Span and Gender

The nurse should document the age and gender of the patient. The nurse should assess women of child-bearing age for pregnancy. Succinylcholine is used cautiously in children because it may cause severe bradycardia or cardiac arrest. The drug is in pregnancy category C. Although it is uncertain whether it causes fetal harm, it should be used cautiously during pregnancy because the drug places the patient at risk for increased drug effects, such as prolonged apnea. Succinylcholine is commonly used during cesarean section. If repeated dosing is required during delivery, the neonate should be monitored closely for apnea and flaccidity.

Environment

The nurse should be aware of the environment in which the drug will be administered. Like tubocurarine, succinylcholine causes respiratory impairment and paralysis. It should be administered only by a qualified clinician. Necessary equipment for intubation, controlled ventilation, and administration of oxygen must be immediately available.

Nursing Diagnoses and Outcomes

- Impaired Spontaneous Ventilation related to respiratory paralysis

  Desired outcome: The patient's breathing will be maintained with artificial ventilation until the ability to sustain spontaneous respiration returns.
- Impaired Physical Mobility related to drug-induced paralysis

  Desired outcome: The patient will remain free from disorders related to immobility, such as skin breakdown.
- Fear related to paralysis and helplessness

  Desired outcome: The patient will be reassured and comforted to prevent fear and sympathetic effects of fear during paralysis.

Planning and Intervention

Maximizing Therapeutic Effects

The nurse can maximize the therapeutic effects of succinylcholine by helping the patient understand the rationale for the therapy and by helping to decrease fear and anxiety.

Minimizing Adverse Effects

The patient should receive a small dose of a nondepolarizing NMJ blocker before succinylcholine is given to decrease muscle fasciculations. This is especially important when using succinylcholine for children.

MEMORY CHIP

Succinylcholine

- A depolarizing neuromuscular junction blocking agent used to facilitate endotracheal intubation and short procedures such as endoscopy or electroconvulsive therapy
- Significant contraindications: hypersensitivity, history of malignant hyperthermia, familial plasma pseudocholinesterase disorders, and narrow-angle glaucoma
- Most common adverse effects: increased ocular pressure, histamine release, muscle pain
- Most serious adverse effects: prolonged paralysis and apnea
- Maximizing therapeutic effects: decrease anxiety and fear
- Minimizing adverse effects: have resuscitation equipment at the bedside
- Most significant patient education: reassure the patient that he or she is being constantly monitored

Providing Patient and Family Education

- Before administration, the nurse should explain to the patient and family that this drug will paralyze muscles and the patient will be unable to speak, move, or breathe unassisted. It is important to explain that these effects should subside soon after the drug is discontinued.
- Because this drug may be used in an emergency situation, the nurse should explain the effects of the drug to the patient even if he or she appears to be unconscious.

Ongoing Assessment and Evaluation

The nurse should monitor for symptoms of malignant hyperthermia, such as muscle rigidity (especially the jaw), tachycardia, tachypnea, and elevated body temperature. Dantrolene should be on standby in case malignant hyperthermia occurs. The nurse should also monitor the cardiac and respiratory status of the patient while succinylcholine is being administered. ■

CHAPTER SUMMARY

- Anesthesia is a loss of feeling or sensation.
- Balanced anesthesia is a combination of anesthetic agents used to decrease the depth of anesthesia and keep the patient safe.
- Anesthetic agents are divided into inhaled or intravenous agents.
- Isoflurane (Forane) is a halogenated inhaled anesthetic. Nursing management of patients recovering from isoflurane anesthesia includes careful monitoring of residual CNS depression manifested as respiratory depression.
- Nitrous oxide is an inflammable gas used in combination with halogenated agents to increase their effectiveness without severely depressing the depth of coma.

DRUGS THAT ARE SEDATIVES, HYPNOTICS, AND ANXIOLYTICS

Sedative-hypnotic drugs

Barbiturates
- **phenobarbital**
- chloral hydrate
- mephobarbital
- pentobarbital
- secobarbital
- tuinal
- amobarbital
- butabarbital
- thiopental
- thiamylal
- methohexital

Benzodiazepines
- **lorazepam**
- alprazolam
- chlorazepate
- chlordiazepoxide
- clonazepam
- diazepam
- halazepam
- midazolam
- oxazepam
- prazepam
- buspirone
- flumazenil
- hydroxyzine
- meprobamate
- zaleplon
- zolpidem
- hypnotic benzodiazepines
  - estazolam, flurazepam, quazepam
  - temazepam, triazolam

The symbol C indicates the **drug class**.
Drugs in bold type marked with the symbol P are **prototypes**.
Drugs in blue type with no symbol are **closely related** to the prototype.
Drugs in red type with no symbol are **significantly different** from the prototype.
Drugs in black type with no symbol are **also used in drug therapy**; no prototype.

Anxiety disorders and insomnia are common problems. Anxiety disorders affect more than 23 million people in the United States each year at an estimated cost of more than $46 billion (Davis, 1999). **Anxiolytic** (antianxiety) drugs provide one of the mainstays of treatment. Some drugs are more **sedative** (causing relaxation); others are more **hypnotic** (producing sleep). Some are used for sedation only, whereas other are used for their hypnotic effects only. The class, however, is termed sedative-hypnotic. The drug classification of sedative-hypnotics is based on clinical uses rather than on similarities in chemical structures of mechanisms of action, because there is remarkable variation within this group.

Sedative-hypnotics are among the most widely prescribed drugs worldwide. This class of central nervous system (CNS) depressants is composed of several different subclasses that may be used as anxiolytics, hypnotics, or sedatives, depending on the dosage prescribed. In one sense, the uses and indications of these drugs form a continuum of CNS depression. At low doses, drugs classified as sedative-hypnotics will produce sedation, which is a decrease in responsiveness to a constant level of stimulation. The drug-induced sedation probably contributes to an anxiolytic effect but does not account for it entirely, because the amygdala contains many benzodiazepine receptors that presumably account for some control of emotional responses to stressful stimuli. At higher doses, these drugs will produce sleep. In fact, the continuum may progress to coma and death if excessively high doses are administered.

The two subclasses discussed in this chapter are the barbiturates and benzodiazepines. The barbiturates induce a state of generalized CNS depression. The benzodiazepines are thought to exert a potentiating effect on gamma-aminobutyric acid (GABA), an inhibitory CNS neurotransmitter. Thus, potentiation of GABA action results in CNS depression. The degree of CNS depression may be low, resulting in calming (anxiolysis) and sedation, or higher, resulting in hypnosis (a conscious state preceding sleep). In contrast to the benzodiazepines, the barbiturates in increasing doses will eventually result in anesthesia, coma, and death.

Historically, the barbiturates were extensively used as sedative-hypnotic and anxiolytic drugs. Except for a few specialized uses (occasionally as a preanesthetic, for emergency acute and chronic anticonvulsant effects, and for drug-induced coma for severe head trauma), the safer benzodiazepines and nonbenzodiazepines have now largely replaced the barbiturates. Although the chemical structure and pharmacologic properties of drugs described as nonbenzodiazepine nonbarbiturates (e.g., chloral hydrate, meprobamate) differ from the barbiturates, benzodiazepines, and each other, they are used for a similar pharmacotherapeutic effect—induction of sleep. Other unrelated nonbenzodiazepine nonbarbiturate hypnotic drugs (e.g., zaleplon and zolpidem) interact with a GABA-benzodiazepine receptor complex and share some of the pharmacologic properties of the benzodiazepines.

The prototype barbiturate for this chapter is phenobarbital. The prototype benzodiazepine for this chapter is lorazepam.

PHYSIOLOGY OF THE CENTRAL NERVOUS SYSTEM

The brain is responsible for processing incoming information and regulating affect, mood, and motor response. The brain stem, which connects the cerebrum to the spinal cord, includes the diencephalon, midbrain, pons, and medulla oblongata. The thalamus and hypothalamus are located in the diencephalon. The thalamus functions as a central relay station for ascending sensory impulses from other parts of the CNS to the cerebral cortex; all sensory pathways, except the olfactory, are connected to thalamic nuclei.

Located in the general area of the diencephalon is a complex of structures known as the limbic system. The limbic system works with the cerebral cortex, brain stem, and hypothalamus to normalize the expression of emotions, such as anxiety, anger, fear, pleasure, sorrow, and sexual feelings.

Scattered throughout the medulla oblongata, midbrain, and pons is a complex network of nerve fibers known as the reticular formation. This network has both motor and sensory functions. The motor function receives input from higher brain regions that control skeletal muscles. The sensory function of the reticular formation is known as the reticular activating system (RAS). The RAS alerts the cortex to incoming sensory signals. It also is responsible for maintaining consciousness and for awakening the person from sleep.

Neurons are the working components of the brain and transmit electrical impulses from one neuron to another across spaces called **synapses**. Such transmission is accomplished through the release and uptake of brain chemicals called **neurotransmitters**. After the impulse is transmitted, the neurotransmitter either remains in the synapse where enzymes break it down or is reabsorbed into the presynaptic neuron by the process of reuptake. Dysregulation of neurotransmitters appears to be the basis for most psychiatric disorders. Among the major neurotransmitters believed to be involved in mental illnesses are dopamine (DA), serotonin (5-HT), histamine, norepinephrine (NE), noradrenaline, acetylcholine, GABA, glutamate, and neuropeptides.

PATHOPHYSIOLOGY OF ANXIETY

The pathophysiology of anxiety disorders is complex and not well understood. Current hypotheses propose that anxiety disorders are biologic illnesses with an underlying genetic component. These disorders involve disruptions in several neurotransmitter systems, including NE, 5-HT, and GABA. It is believed that the disruption of these systems differs from one anxiety disorder to another. The benzodiazepines are thought to act by improving this function (Davis, 1999).

Although there has been evidence of structural brain abnormality in some psychiatric disorders (e.g., schizophrenia), evolving notions of the pathophysiologic processes underlying anxiety disorders are focused on functional abnormalities. New brain-imaging techniques for studying the metabolism and neurotransmitter activity in the living brain

Pharmacokinetics

Barbiturate absorption varies based on route of administration, with 70% to 90% of an oral dose absorbed. The rate of absorption increases if the sodium salt is in-

In sufficiently high therapeutic doses, it can induce anesthesia. Overdose can cause death from respiratory depression.

Phenobarbital decreases the excitability of both presynaptic and postsynaptic membranes in the cerebral

TABLE 17-1 Summary of Selected Barbiturates and Other Drugs

Drug (Trade) Name	Selected Indications	Route and Dosage Range	Pharmacokinetics
Barbiturates			
phenobarbital (*Canadian:* Barbita)	Sedation, alcohol withdrawal, grand and complex partial seizures, epilepsy	*Adult:* PO, 30–120 mg/d in two to three divided doses for sedation *Adult:* for anticonvulsant use, 60–200 mg/d	*Onset:* 30–60 min *Duration:* 10–16 h $t_{1/2}$: 79 h
butabarbital (Butisol; *Canadian:* Butalan)	Sedation, insomnia, preanesthetic sedation	*Adult:* PO, 15–30 mg/tid–qid (sedation), 50–100 mg/hs (hypnotic; effectiveness lost after 2 wk) *Reduced dosage in geriatric or debilitated patients* *Child:* PO, 7.5–30 mg (dosage calculated on age, weight, and degree of desired sedation)	*Onset:* 45–60 min *Duration:* 6–8 h $t_{1/2}$: 50–100 h
pentobarbital (Nembutal; *Canadian:* Novo-Pentobarb)	Sedation, insomnia, preanesthetic sedation, emergency anticonvulsant	*Adult:* PO, 20 mg/tid–qid (sedation), 50–100 mg/hs (hypnotic; effectiveness lost after 2 wk); IM, 150–200 mg; rectal, 120–200 mg; IV, 50–100 mg *Reduced dosage in geriatric or debilitated patients* *Child:* PO, 7.5–30 mg; IM/IV, 2–6 mg/kg; rectal, 30–120 mg (dosage calculated on age, weight, and degree of desired sedation)	*Onset:* PO: 10–15 min Rectal, IM/IV: Rapid *Duration:* 3–4 h $t_{1/2}$: 15–20 h

(*continued*)

fragmented sleep. Cycles of REM sleep occur approximately every 90 minutes throughout the night, and the time spent in REM increases toward the last 3 to 4 hours of sleep.

PATHOPHYSIOLOGY OF INSOMNIA

Insomnia affects as much as 10% of the U.S. population. It negatively affects quality of life, work production, and health. Studies have suggested that poor sleepers have a higher incidence of chronic illnesses (e.g., ischemic heart disease), absenteeism at work, and traffic accidents.

Insomnia occurs when an individual has measurable difficulty initiating or maintaining sleep. Primary insomnia is less common than secondary insomnia. The DSM-IV-TR classifies primary insomnia as difficulty falling asleep or maintaining sleep unrelated to any exogenous factors. It may result from individual variations in circadian rhythms, deviations from normal neurotransmitter activity, or both. Secondary insomnia has many possible causes: stress, environmental changes (e.g., noise, temperature, new surroundings), medications, medical or psychiatric illnesses, and substance use or abuse (Stimmel, et al., 2000). Either transient or chronic insomnia may be secondary to a preexisting medical condition (e.g., chronic obstruction pulmonary disease, sleep apnea) or to drug therapy. Many classes of drugs possess the ability to interfere with sleep, including over-the-counter (OTC) decongestants and caffeine. Some antidepressants (e.g., TCAs, SSRIs) may disturb normal sleep patterns. Many drugs that alter the sleep cycle by reducing REM and NREM stages 3 general effects of the sedative-hypnotic group of drugs used for hypnotic purposes is a decrease in stage 1 sleep, an increase in stage 2 NREM sleep, a decrease in REM sleep, and a decrease in slow wave sleep. Differing drugs have differing effects on sleep architecture, and some of the newer nonbenzodiazepine drugs (e.g., zapelon, zolpidem) are thought to be superior to the older drugs by virtue of producing minimal effects on normal sleep architecture. As a general rule, the effects of sedative-hypnotics on patterns of normal sleep are 1) decreased time to fall asleep, 2) increased duration of stage 2 NREM sleep, 3) decreased duration of REM sleep, and 4) decreased duration of slow-wave sleep (stages 3 and 4).

During slow-wave sleep, the secretion of adrenal steroids is at its lowest, whereas secretion of growth hormone is at its highest. Despite the sedative-hypnotic induced reductions in slow-wave sleep, there are no clinical reports of disturbances in the secretion of pituitary or adrenal hormones when either barbiturates or benzodiazepines are used as hypnotics. The use of sedative-hypnotics for more than 1 to 2 weeks, however, leads to some tolerance to their effects on sleep patterns.

Experimental studies have demonstrated that deliberate interruption of REM sleep causes anxiety and irritability followed by a rebound increase in REM sleep. A similar pattern of "REM rebound" is detected following discontinuation of drug treatment with most sedative-hypnotics.

SEDATIVE-HYPNOTIC DRUGS

Because of their narrow therapeutic index, numerous drug in-

TABLE 17-1 Summary of Selected Barbiturates and Other Drugs (Continued)

Drug (Trade) Name	Selected Indications	Route and Dosage Range	Pharmacokinetics
Nonbarbiturates/Nonbenzodiazepine			
buspirone (BuSpar; *Canadian:* Apo-Buspirone)	Anxiety	*Adult:* PO, 5 mg tid *Child:* Not established	*Onset:* Plasma levels, 1–6 mg/ml 40–90 min; therapeutic effect 7–10 d *Duration:* Unknown $t_{1/2}$: 2–11 h
chloral hydrate (Noctec; *Canadian:* PMS-Chloral Hydrate)	Nocturnal and preoperative sedation, adjunct to analgesics for postoperative pain control	*Adult:* PO/rectal, 250 mg/tid (sedation); 500–1000 mg/hs (hypnotic) *Child:* PO/rectal, 25 mg/kg (sedation—up to 500 mg); 50 mg/kg (hypnotic—up to 1000 mg)	*Onset:* PO/rectal—30–60 min *Duration:* 4–8 h $t_{1/2}$: 7–10 h
meprobamate (Equanil; *Canadian:* Novomepro)	Anxiety, sedation	*Adult:* PO, 1.2–1.6 g/d in divided doses *Child:* 6–12 y; 100–200 mg bid or tid; less than 6 y, dosage not established	*Onset:* 1 h *Duration:* 1–3 h $t_{1/2}$: 10–12 h
zaleplon (Sonata; *Canadian:* Starnoc)	Insomnia	*Adult:* PO, 5–10 mg for 7–10 d (2–3 wk maximum)	*Onset:* <15 minutes *Duration:* Not applicable $t_{1/2}$: 1 h
zolpidem (Ambien)	Insomnia	*Adult:* PO, 5–10 mg for 7–10 d (2–3 wk maximum)	*Onset:* 45 minutes *Duration:* Not applicable $t_{1/2}$: 2.6 h

cortex and reticular formation. Thus, it depresses the sensory cortex, decreases motor activity, and alters cerebellar function, which produces drowsiness and a sedative and hypnotic effect. This is thought to result from the GABA-like action and enhanced GABA effects by the barbiturates.

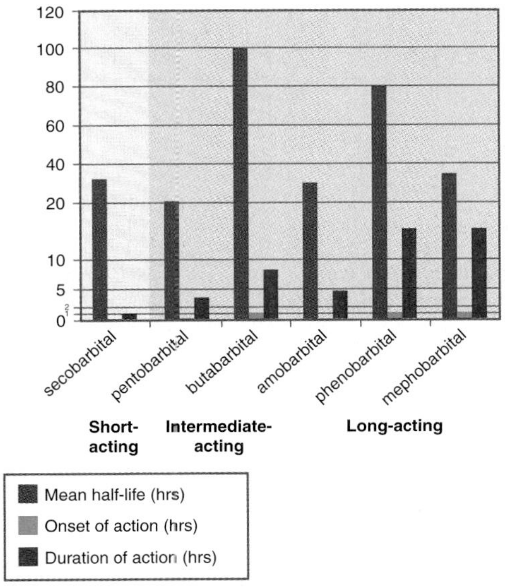

Figure 17-1. Comparison of the pharmacokinetic parameters of half-life, onset of action, and duration of action among the short-acting, intermediate-acting, and long-acting sedative-hypnotic barbiturates.

Phenobarbital and the other barbiturates are respiratory depressants; the degree of respiratory depression is dose dependent. With hypnotic doses, the respiratory depression is similar to that during physiologic sleep and is accompanied by slight decreases in blood pressure and heart rate.

Phenobarbital, like all other barbiturates, reduces REM sleep and decreases NREM sleep stages 3 and 4.

Contraindications and Precautions

Hypersensitivity is a contraindication to phenobarbital use. Tolerance or psychological and physical dependence may occur with continued use; phenobarbital should not be administered to individuals who are mentally depressed or have suicidal tendencies or a history of alcohol or drug abuse.

Phenobarbital should be used cautiously in patients with hepatic and renal function impairment, because metabolism is primarily by hepatic microsomal enzymes and urinary excretion is as either partially or completely unchanged drug. Marked hepatic or renal impairment contraindicates use of phenobarbital and the other barbiturates.

One specific precaution concerns IV administration. Too rapid IV administration may cause respiratory depression, apnea, laryngospasm, or hypotension from vasodilation. Solutions of barbiturates are highly alkaline; extravasation may cause local tissue damage with subsequent necrosis. Status epilepticus may result from abrupt discontinuation, even when administered in small daily doses in the treatment of epilepsy.

Adverse Effects

The major adverse effects of phenobarbital are CNS in nature and related to CNS depression. They include drowsiness, delirium, mental depression, and lethargy. Respiratory depression is a serious adverse effect of phenobarbital; the degree is dose dependent. Phenobarbital interferes with REM sleep and may cause chronic disruption of normal sleep patterns, which may make sleep less satisfying and restful. Phenobarbital may cause a "hangover" effect of residual daytime sedation and headache.

Other CNS effects include ataxia, confusion, dizziness, irritability, and sometimes stimulation. Occasionally, blood dyscrasias (e.g., agranulocytosis, thrombocytopenia, decreased serum folate levels) may develop. Non-CNS effects include hypersensitivity, nausea, vomiting, urticaria, and skin rash. Rarely a very serious exfoliative dermatitis (e.g., Stevens-Johnson syndrome) may occur. Like all barbiturates, phenobarbital can be habit-forming, and tolerance and dependence may occur with continued use.

Drug Interactions

Phenobarbital is a potent inducer of the CYP450 hepatic microsomal enzyme system and significantly alters the metabolism of many other drugs, such as digitalis compounds and phenytoin. Table 17-2 lists agents that interact with phenobarbital.

Assessment of Relevant Core Patient Variables

Health Status

The nurse assesses the patient for a history of pulmonary disorders, because such patients are extremely sensitive to the respiratory depressant effect of phenobarbital. The nurse also assesses for hepatic or renal dysfunction. Phenobarbital and the other barbiturates should be used with extreme caution in these patients, because the alterations in rate of metabolism and drug excretion increase the possibility of overdose.

The nurse performs a baseline and repeat electrocardiograms during phenobarbital therapy, because depression of cardiac contractility occurs with phenobarbital toxicity. Phenobarbital may increase vitamin D requirements, possibly by increasing the metabolism of

TABLE 17-2 Agents That Interact With Phenobarbital

Interactants	Effect and Significance	Nursing Management
alcohol, MAOIs, valproic acid	Increased sedative effects of phenobarbital, specifically CNS depression Increased risk of phenobarbital toxicity with valproic acid	Evaluate patient for potentially lethal additive CNS-depressant effects. Monitor serum levels (if appropriate) for therapeutic levels.
charcoal	Reduced absorption of phenobarbital	Assess patient for changes in seizure control or loss of sedative effect
chloramphenicol	Inhibition of phenobarbital metabolism or enhancement of chloramphenicol metabolism	Assess patient for signs of increased sedation or infection. Monitor serum levels (if appropriate) for therapeutic levels.
methoxyflurane	Increased risk of nephrotoxicity	Monitor patient's renal function status closely for changes.
rifampin	Increased hepatic microsomal enzyme system leading to decreased effectiveness of phenobarbital	Assess patient for changes in seizure control or loss of sedative effect. Monitor serum levels of phenobarbital as appropriate.
anticoagulants, beta blockers, carbamazepine, clonazepam, oral contraceptives, corticosteroids, digitoxin, doxorubicin, doxycycline, felodipine, griseofulvin, metronidazole, phenylbutazone, quinidine, theophylline, verapamil	Decreased effect of interactant drug	Assess the patient for effectiveness of therapy for concurrent disease states (e.g., cardiac or respiratory disease). Anticipate the need for dosage adjustment of interactant drug

vitamins D and K through hepatic microsomal enzyme induction. Supplemental vitamin therapy as prophylaxis may be necessary. Rarely, bone disease (e.g., osteomalacia) occurs following prolonged use of barbiturates.

Hypnotic drugs may cause sleep apnea, particularly in obese, middle-aged men. Thus, the nurse assesses the patient for this condition.

Life Span and Gender

The nurse assesses for age-related considerations during phenobarbital administration. Phenobarbital may produce a paradoxic excitement rather than depression in some individuals, especially children and occasionally the elderly. Barbiturates may produce irritability, excitability, inappropriate tearfulness, and aggression in children. Older adults may become confused and more wakeful. They may have difficulty falling asleep.

The nurse assesses the woman of child-bearing age for pregnancy or intention to become pregnant. Phenobarbital is FDA pregnancy category D. Barbiturates can cause fetal damage when administered to a pregnant woman, and studies suggest a connection between maternal use of barbiturates and increased incidence of fetal abnormalities. Barbiturates readily cross the placental barrier and are distributed throughout fetal tissues. Following parenteral use, fetal blood levels approach that of the maternal blood levels. Withdrawal symptoms (e.g., seizures, irritability) occur in infants born to mothers who receive barbiturates throughout the last trimester of pregnancy. Maternal ingestion of anticonvulsants, particularly barbiturates, may be associated with a neonatal coagulation defect (e.g., decreased levels of vitamin K-dependent clotting factors and prolongation of prothrombin time, partial thromboplastin time, or both) after birth, usually within 24 hours.

The nurse also assesses if the woman of child-bearing age is breast-feeding. Phenobarbital should be used cautiously during lactation, because small amounts are excreted in breast milk. Transfer of the drug through breast-feeding may cause drowsiness in the nursing infant.

Lifestyle, Diet, and Habits

The nurse determines whether the patient has a history of substance abuse, because use of phenobarbital can be habit-forming. Tolerance, psychological dependence, and physical dependence may occur, especially following prolonged use (90 days) of high doses.

The nurse specifically questions the patient about use of herbal medicines as well as prescription medications. Use of herbal or natural products is growing significantly, and many people fail to report such use. Thus, the risk for herb-drug interactions increases. Based on the mechanism of action, valerian and possibly ginger, goldenseal, and chamomile inhibit the enzyme responsible for catabolism of GABA. The interaction with phenobarbital will likely cause an additive sedative effect. The same type of additive interaction may occur with kava, because it has a synergistic GABA receptor site action. The nurse cautions the patient and family that the effect of these interactions with phenobarbital is increased sedation.

Nursing Diagnoses and Outcomes

- Risk for Ineffective Breathing Pattern related to barbiturate-induced respiratory depressant effect
  Desired outcome: *The patient will demonstrate satisfactory pulmonary function.*
- Disturbed Sleep Pattern related to barbiturate-induced alterations in normal sleep stages
  Desired outcome: *The patient will identify techniques to induce sleep and report an optimal balance of rest and activity.*
- Risk for Injury related to drug-induced CNS depressant effects
  Desired outcome: *The patient will identify factors that increase the risk for and relate intent to practice safety measures to prevent injury.*

Planning and Intervention

Maximizing Therapeutic Effects

When administering phenobarbital as a hypnotic, the nurse encourages good sleep practices. These include maintaining a regular bedtime, taking a soothing bath or shower close to bedtime, keeping a quiet sleep environment, and avoiding consumption of irritating foods near bedtime.

Minimizing Adverse Effects

Phenobarbital sodium may be administered IM or IV as an anticonvulsant for emergency use. IV phenobarbital should be administered no faster than 50 mg/minute. When administered IV, 15 minutes may need to elapse before phenobarbital reaches peak concentrations in the brain. Therefore, injecting phenobarbital sodium until the convulsions stop may cause brain levels to exceed those required to control the convulsions and may result in severe barbiturate-induced depression.

Immediately after the drug infusion, the nurse performs a thorough and careful assessment of the patient's neurologic, cardiovascular, and respiratory status. Resuscitation equipment should always be available.

The toxic dose of barbiturates varies considerably. In general, an oral dose of 1 g produces serious poisoning in an adult. Death commonly occurs after 2 to 10 g of ingested barbiturate.

Providing Patient and Family Education

- The nurse cautions the woman of child-bearing age to use an alternative, reliable, and consistent form of contraception during phenobarbital therapy. Phenobarbital decreases the effect of oral contraceptives because it induces hepatic microsomal enzymes. This inhibits the effectiveness of oral contraceptives, resulting in menstrual irregularities and unplanned pregnancy.

- The nurse advises the patient and family about behavioral interventions that may be effective for promoting a restful night's sleep. Insomnia may be resolved without the use of drugs by some simple behavioral changes: keeping a regular sleep schedule, creating a dark and comfortable bedroom environment, establishing a prebedtime ritual (e.g., soothing bath or shower), and avoiding known reasons for insomnia. The patient should eliminate alcohol for at least 3 to 4 hours before bedtime because it can interfere with the sleep cycle. Exercise, heavy meals, or caffeine can also interfere with the sleep cycle and should be avoided.
- The nurse advises the patient and family that drowsiness, light-headedness, or dizziness might occur with use of phenobarbital. He or she stresses the importance of avoiding activities requiring mental alertness or coordination until CNS effects are known.
- The nurse stresses that patients must limit the use of barbiturates for hypnotic effects to 2 weeks. If the patient is using phenobarbital or another barbiturate for insomnia, the nurse cautions that sleep disruption may occur following discontinuation of the drug, as rebound of REM sleep is common.
- Phenobarbital, along with the other sedative-hypnotic barbiturates, generally alters sleep stages; reduced REM sleep is a common effect. Pronounced REM deprivation from chronic use of hypnotics may produce personality changes. The disruption of the normal sleep pattern may make sleep less satisfying; therefore, dosages may be increased, possibly resulting in enhanced tolerance. A tolerance to the effects of the sedative-hypnotic effect of phenobarbital and the other barbiturates develops usually within 7 to 14 days; use for 1 month may lead to dependence. Barbiturates with long half-lives tend to have a cumulative effect, creating the feeling of a hangover upon awakening.
- The nurse emphasizes the importance of avoiding other CNS depressants (e.g., alcoholic beverages, narcotics, tranquilizers, antihistamines), because concomitant use may result in additional CNS depressant effects.
- The nurse explains to patients the importance of carrying identification (e.g., MedicAlert) to indicate the condition and drug treatment, including dosage. Advising patients to report any bothersome or persistent adverse effects is important. The nurse stresses the need to take the drug as directed and not to stop taking it abruptly. In addition, he or she emphasizes not to use OTC drugs and herbal preparations without approval from the health care professional.

Ongoing Assessment and Evaluation

The nurse assesses the patient for a positive clinical response. The patient should exhibit adequate sedative or hypnotic effects with minimal adverse effects.

The nurse notes any behaviors indicative of physical or psychological dependence and observes for signs of chronic intoxication (e.g., ataxia, slurred speech, vertigo). This medication may produce dependence.

Symptoms of dependence are similar to those of chronic alcoholism. They include a strong desire or need to continue taking the drug, a tendency to increase the dose, a subjective psychic dependence on the effects of the drug, and a physical dependence on the effects of the drug for maintenance of homeostasis that, when the drug is withdrawn, results in a definite, characteristic, and self-limiting abstinence syndrome. Minor withdrawal symptoms appear 8 to 12 hours after the last dose of a barbiturate and usually appear in the following order: anxiety, muscle twitching, tremor of the hands and fingers, progressive weakness, dizziness, distortion in visual perception, nausea, vomiting, insomnia, and orthostatic hypotension. Major withdrawal symptoms include convulsions and delirium, which may occur within 16 hours and last up to 5 days after abrupt cessation of these drugs. The intensity of withdrawal symptoms gradually decline in 15 days. Withdrawal symptoms can be severe and may cause death.

The treatment of dependence consists of cautious and gradual withdrawal of the drug, which takes an extended period. ■

MEMORY CHIP

Phenobarbital

- Used for seizure management and long-acting sedative-hypnotic effects
- Significant contraindications: marked hepatic or renal impairment, hypersensitivity
- Most common adverse effects: primarily CNS depression, such as drowsiness and delirium; chronic disruption in sleep patterns; hangover effect; possible tolerance and dependence with continued use
- Most serious adverse effect: respiratory depression (dose dependent)
- **Lifespan alert: possible paradoxic excitement instead of depression in children and the elderly; confusion, difficulty falling asleep when used in the elderly**
- Maximizing therapeutic effects: encourage use of good sleep practices
- Minimizing adverse effects: administer IV form no faster than 50 mg/min with close patient assessment immediately after infusion
- Most significant patient education: use of safety measures and avoidance of concomitant use of other CNS depressants, including alcohol

DRUGS CLOSELY RELATED TO PHENOBARBITAL

Chloral Hydrate

Chloral hydrate (Noctec) is effective as a hypnotic only for short-term use; it loses much of its effectiveness for inducing and maintaining sleep after 2 weeks of use. Hypnotic dosage produces mild cerebral depression and quiet, deep sleep. Although "hangover" is less common than with most barbiturates and some benzodiazepines, chloral hydrate has generally been replaced by safer and more effective agents. In therapeutic doses, chloral hydrate has little effect on respiration, blood pressure, and reflexes. It is metabolized in the liver and erythrocytes to its pharmacologically active metabolite, trichloroethanol, which has a half-life of 7 to 10 hours. Its toxic metabolite, trichloroacetic acid, is cleared very slowly and can accumulate with nightly administration. There are recurrent concerns regarding the possible carcinogenicity of chloral hydrate (or its metabolites) (Katzung, 1998).

Onset of action occurs within 30 minutes. Most frequent adverse effects are nausea, vomiting, and abdominal distress. Less frequent are ataxia, dizziness, and drowsiness. Hypnotic dosage produces mild cerebral depression and quiet, deep sleep. In therapeutic doses, chloral hydrate has little effect on respiration, blood pressure, and reflexes.

Mephobarbital

Mephobarbital (Mebaral) may be used as a sedative for the relief of anxiety, tension, and apprehension. It may also be used as an anticonvulsant for the treatment of grand mal and petit mal epilepsy; occasionally, it is combined with phenobarbital or phenytoin.

DRUGS SIGNIFICANTLY DIFFERENT FROM PHENOBARBITAL

Pentobarbital (Nembutal) and secobarbital (Seconal) are short-acting barbiturates primarily used for their hypnotic effects and occasionally for their sedative effects. They lose most of their effectiveness for inducing and maintaining sleep by the end of 2 weeks of continued drug administration, even with the use of multiple doses. Tuinal is a combination barbiturate drug that provides a more balanced sedative-hypnotic effect through the mixture of short-acting secobarbital and intermediate-acting amobarbital with differing rates of action and dissipation.

Amobarbital (Amytal) and butabarbital (Butisol) are intermediate-acting barbiturates used primarily for sedative purposes.

Thiopental, thiamylal, and methohexital are ultrashort-acting barbiturates that depress the CNS to produce hypnosis and anesthesia without analgesia. Methohexital does not possess muscle relaxant properties. These drugs are frequently used to provide hypnosis during balanced anesthesia with other agents for muscle relaxation and analgesia. The rapid onset and brief duration of action of these drugs are a function of their high lipid solubility. They quickly cross the blood-brain barrier but are rapidly redistributed from the brain to other body tissues, first to highly perfused visceral organs (e.g., liver, kidneys, heart) and muscle, and later to fatty tissues.

Administered IV as the sodium salts, these agents produce anesthesia within 1 minute. Recovery after a small dose is rapid, with somnolence and retrograde amnesia. Muscle relaxation occurs at the onset of anesthesia. The duration of anesthetic activity following a single IV dose is 20 to 30 minutes for thiopental and thiamylal, and somewhat shorter for methohexital.

Thiopental is readily absorbed by the rectal route when administered as a suspension; onset of action usually occurs within 8 to 10 minutes. Thiopental IV produces hypnosis within 30 to 40 seconds following administration. Repeated doses or continuous infusion of these agents causes accumulation. Slow release of the drug from lipid storage sites results in prolonged anesthesia, somnolence, and respiratory and circulatory depression. The plasma half-life is 3 to 8 hours.

BENZODIAZEPINES

Benzodiazepine receptors are linked with the GABA receptor, which has a major role in inhibitory mechanisms within brain functions. Their effects on the GABA receptor and chloride ion channels cause the antianxiety properties. At least two GABA receptors have been identified: GABA**A** and GABA**B**, with GABAA specific for the benzodiazepine receptors and having at least two subtypes itself. One of those subtypes is the BZ**1** (also known as the omega-1 receptor), believed to have a role in sleep onset and the sleep cycle. BZ**2** is thought to affect learning, memory, and sensory and motor function.

A distinctive feature of the benzodiazepines is their wide margin of safety between therapeutic and toxic doses. They generally have a relatively rapid onset of action and are classified according to their rate of effect and half-life. These factors influence their abuse potential, possibility for physiologic dependence, and rebound effects. Although safe overall, they are not without side effects, the most common of which is sedation.

Compared with the barbiturates or other nonbarbiturate nonbenzodiazepine anxiolytics (e.g., meprobamate), benzodiazepines are characterized by a relatively low abuse potential, produce less sedation with effective anxiolytic doses and less disruption of the normal sleep stages, do not affect the hepatic microsomal enzyme system, and produce less toxicity with acute overdosage. For these reasons, benzodiazepines are the most commonly used anxiolytics.

Lorazepam is the prototype benzodiazepine for this chapter. Drugs closely related to lorazepam include alprazolam (Xanax), clorazepate, chlordiazepoxide (Librium), clonazepam (Klonopin), diazepam (Valium), halazepam (Paxipam), midazolam (Versed), oxazepam (Serax), and prazepam (Centrax). Drugs significantly different from lorazepam are buspirone (BuSpar), flumazenil (Romazicon), hydroxyzine (Atarax, Vistaril), meprobamate (Equanil, Miltown), zaleplon (Sonata), and zolpidem (Ambien). In addition to their use as antianxiety agents, some benzodiazepines are also useful as hypnotics, anticonvulsants, and muscle relaxants. The hypnotic benzodiazepines include estazolam (ProSom), flurazepam (Dalmane), quazepam (Doral), temazepam (Restoril), and triazolam (Halcion) (Table 17-3).

NURSING MANAGEMENT OF THE PATIENT RECEIVING LORAZEPAM

Core Drug Knowledge

Pharmacotherapeutics

Lorazepam is one of a group of benzodiazepines used to manage anxiety disorders or for short-term relief of anxiety symptoms. Oral uses for lorazepam in adults include sedation and relief of anxiety. Parenteral uses include preanesthetic medication and a decreased ability to recall events related to diagnostic procedures or surgery.

Other therapeutic uses for the benzodiazepines include management of irritable bowel syndrome, depression, premenstrual syndrome, status epilepticus, chemotherapy-induced nausea and vomiting, acute alcohol withdrawal syndrome, and chronic insomnia. These "unlabeled" uses, however, are not FDA approved.

Pharmacokinetics

Lorazepam is readily absorbed following oral or IM administration, although at a slower rate than many of the other benzodiazepines. Sublingual lorazepam is absorbed more rapidly than following oral administration and is comparable to IM administration.

Lorazepam is highly lipid soluble, widely distributed in the body tissues, and highly bound to plasma proteins (70% to 99%). Its half-life (10 to 20 hours) and duration of action (12 to 24 hours) are related to its lipid solubility. Lorazepam half-life is not age dependent nor is it lengthened by hepatic disease. Lorazepam undergoes hepatic biotransformation to inactive compounds and

TABLE 17-3 Summary of Selected Benzodiazepines

Drug (Trade) Name	Selected Indications	Route and Dosage Range	Pharmacokinetics
lorazepam (Ativan; *Canadian:* Novo-Lorazepam)	Anxiety, anesthetic premedication, status epilepticus, alcohol withdrawal, chronic insomnia	*Adult:* PO, 2–6 mg/d; IM, 0.05 mg/kg; IV, 2 mg *Child:* Not recommended; IV/IM, oral dose not established	*Onset:* PO, 1–3 h; IM, 15–30 min; IV, 1–5 min *Duration:* 12–24 h $t_{1/2}$: 10–20 h
alprazolam (Xanax; *Canadian:* Nu-Alpraz)	Anxiety, panic disorder, agoraphobia	*Adult:* PO, 0.25–1.0 mg tid *Child:* Not established	*Onset:* 30 min *Duration:* 4–6 h $t_{1/2}$: 6.3–26.9 h
chlordiazepoxide (Librium; *Canadian:* Corax)	Anxiety, alcohol withdrawal, anesthetic premedication	*Adult:* PO, 5–10 mg tid–qid (50–100 mg for alcohol withdrawal); IM/IV, 50–100 mg *Child:* >6 y; PO, 5 mg bid–qid; IM/IV, 25–50 mg; not recommended under 6 y	*Onset:* PO, varies; IM, 10–15 min *Duration:* 48–72 h $t_{1/2}$: 5–30 h
diazepam (Valium; *Canadian:* Diazemuls)	Anxiety, status epilepticus, skeletal muscle relaxant	*Adult:* PO, IM, 2–10 mg/bid–qid; rectal, 0.2 mg/kg qd–bid; IV, 5–10 mg prn *Reduced dosage in geriatric or debilitated patients* *Child:* (2 y); PO, 1–2.5 mg tid–qid; IM and IV, up to 0.25 mg/kg; Rectal, 0.5 mg/kg	*Onset:* PO, 30–60 min; IM, 15–30 min; rectal, rapid; IV, 1–5 min *Duration:* 3 h (1 h IV) $t_{1/2}$: 20–50 h
flurazepam (Dalmane; *Canadian:* Somnal)	Insomnia	*Adult:* 15–30 mg at bedtime *Child:* Not for use < 15 y	*Onset:* 15–30 min *Duration:* 7–8 h $t_{1/2}$: 2–3 h; 47–100 h (active metabolite)
midazolam (Versed)	Preoperative sedation, anxiolysis, amnesia Sedation Anesthesia	*Adult:* IM, IV: 1–5 mg *Child:* 0.025–0.15 mg/kg *Dose individualized/reduced in patients >60 years of age, debilitated, or chronically ill.*	*Onset:* IM, *Adult:* 15 min; *Child:* 5 min; IV, 1–3 min *Duration:* 6 h $t_{1/2}$: 1.8–6.4 h
Benzodiazepine Antagonist			
flumazenil (Romazicon; *Canadian:* Anexate)	Benzodiazepine antagonist	*Adult:* IV, 0.2 mg q 60 seconds up to 1 mg (reversal of conscious sedation); 0.2 mg, then 0.3 mg q 30 seconds up to 3 mg (management of benzodiazepine overdose).	*Onset:* 20–30 sec *Duration:* 72 h $t_{1/2}$: 7–15 min; 41–79 min (repeated doses)

therefore has a relatively short half-life and duration of activity. Thus, it may be preferred in patients with liver disease and in older adults. Sustained clinical effects require multiple daily doses, and significant accumulation does not occur. The other agents with prolonged half-lives may be administered as a single daily dose at bedtime. Lorazepam is excreted almost entirely in the urine.

Little clinical evidence suggests that one benzodiazepine is more effective than another. The major differences are reflected in their pharmacokinetic profiles. Most other benzodiazepines are metabolized to active compounds (desmethyldiazepam is an active metabolite common to many benzodiazepines) with very long half-lives; cumulative effects occur with chronic administration. Figure 17-2 summarizes the major pharmacokinetic variables among these agents.

Pharmacodynamics

Lorazepam as well as the other benzodiazepines enhance the effects of GABA by increasing its affinity for its receptor. Three benzodiazepine receptors are recognized. They are benzodiazepine-1, located in the areas of the brain involved in sedation; benzodiazepine-2, highly concentrated in brain areas responsible for cognition, memory, and psychomotor functioning; and benzodiazepine-3, located in peripheral tissues and having no hypnotic efficacy. The benzodiazepine receptors are sometimes referred to as omega receptors.

Benzodiazepines can impair ability to store new memory (anterograde amnesia), whereas the ability to use and remember previously acquired knowledge remains intact. The impaired ability to consolidate new memory seems to be independent of sedation. There is some evidence that the patient will develop tolerance to the sedative and psychomotor effects of benzodiazepines, but not to the anxiolytic and amnesic effects.

Contraindications and Precautions

All benzodiazepines potentiate the effects of other CNS depressants (e.g., alcohol, antihistamines, barbiturates, narcotics); thus, lorazepam should not be combined with these agents. Safety and efficacy of lorazepam in patients younger than 12 years are not established.

Contraindications to benzodiazepine use are hypersensitivity, psychoses, acute narrow-angle glaucoma, clinical or biochemical evidence of significant liver disease, and age younger than 6 months. Benzodiazepines should not be administered to patients in shock or coma or with acute alcohol intoxication.

Lorazepam and the other benzodiazepines should not be injected intraarterially. Doing so may produce arteriospasm, resulting in gangrene.

Adverse Effects

Discontinuation of lorazepam and other benzodiazepine therapy because of undesirable effects is rare. Sedation and ataxia are the most common adverse effects. Older adults are especially sensitive to these effects, which increases their risk of injury from falls. Other adverse effects include anticholinergic effects, gastrointestinal (GI) disturbances, headache, incontinence, jaundice, and rash. Infrequently, a paradoxic reaction of excitation may occur. A disturbing effect of the benzodiazepines is anterograde amnesia, which is an inability to remember events for a period following drug administration. This effect may be used purposefully, however, when given prior to an unpleasant experience (e.g., chemotherapy, surgery). Overdose is rarely fatal, unless other CNS-depressant drugs (e.g., alcohol, barbiturates, opioids) are ingested concomitantly.

Adverse reactions of the hypnotic benzodiazepines include asthenia, hypokinesia, and hangover. The hangover effect is common—especially with the longer-acting

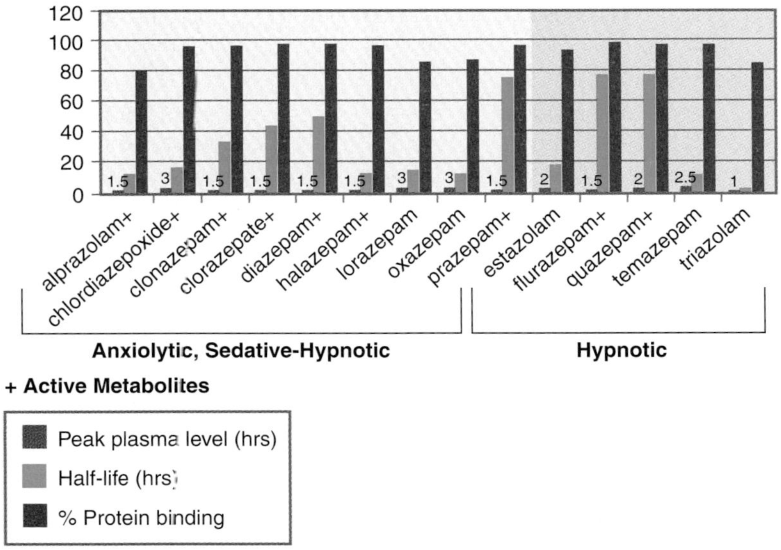

Figure 17-2. Comparison of the pharmacokinetic parameters of hours to reach peak plasma levels between the anxiolytic and sedative-hypnotic benzodiazepines, half-life, and percentage of drug that is bound to plasma proteins. Numbers shown are the average for peak plasma level.

hypnotic benzodiazepines. Patients may complain of headache, decreased mental alertness, and a feeling of slowness on awakening.

Adverse psychiatric effects from lorazepam and other benzodiazepines may include behavior problems, hysteria, psychosis, and suicidal tendencies. Mild paradoxic excitatory reactions during the first 2 weeks of treatment are possible.

Drug Interactions

Lorazepam and the other benzodiazepines produce fewer problematic interactions with other drugs than do the older sedative-hypnotics (e.g., barbiturates). Concomitant ingestion with antacids may alter the rate of absorption. Hypotension or muscular weakness is possible, particularly when lorazepam and other benzodiazepines are used with narcotics, barbiturates, or alcohol. Concomitant administration of the anticonvulsant drug, valproate, and benzodiazepines may produce psychotic episodes.

Drugs that inhibit CYP-450 oxidation (e.g., ketoconazole) have the potential to prolong the half-life and decrease plasma clearance of lorazepam and the other benzodiazepines. All benzodiazepines can decrease the elimination of digoxin, increasing the risk of toxicity (Table 17-4).

Assessment of Relevant Core Patient Variables

Health Status

A baseline assessment should include mental status, complete blood count, and renal and hepatic function. Renal function impairment may cause accumulation of lorazepam and other benzodiazepines. The benzodiazepines have little effect on respiratory and cardiovascular functions compared with other sedative-hypnotic drugs (e.g., barbiturates). The benzodiazepines, however, may compromise respiration for patients with chronic obstructive pulmonary disease or obstructive sleep apnea, so the nurse should check for these conditions. Some benzodiazepines (not lorazepam) may cause hepatic dysfunction, jaundice, and elevated levels of LDH, alkaline phosphatase, aspartate transaminase, and alanine aminotransferase. Liver function studies should be performed before and periodically throughout therapy.

Life Span and Gender

The nurse must consider the patient's age and related issues. Use in children and older adults begins with a small initial dose. Dosage increments are gradual to prevent ataxia or excessive sedation. Disinhibition and aggres-

TABLE 17-4 Agents That Interact With P Lorazepam

Interactants	Effect and Significance	Nursing Management
alcohol, CNS depressants (opioid narcotics, barbiturates)	Increased CNS effects of lorazepam	Evaluate patient for additive CNS-depressant effects. Monitor serum levels (if appropriate) for therapeutic levels. Avoid concomitant administration if possible.
antacids	Altered absorption of lorazepam	Administer antacid 1 hour before or 2 hours after lorazepam.
digoxin	Increased serum concentration of digoxin and possible toxicity	Assess serum digoxin levels closely. Monitor the patient's cardiac status frequently for changes.
levodopa	Decreased control of parkinsonian symptoms	Administer lorazepam cautiously to patients receiving levodopa for Parkinson disease. Assess patient for increasing muscle rigidity, tremors, and drooling.
oral contraceptives	Increased clearance of lorazepam	Anticipate change in lorazepam dosage.
phenytoin	Increased serum concentration of phenytoin leading to possible toxicity	Monitor serum phenytoin levels closely.
probenecid	Interference with hepatic conjugation leading to more rapid onset or prolonged effect of lorazepam	Assess patient for continued sedative effects. Anticipate need for dosage change as indicated.
rifampin	Increased hepatic microsomal enzyme metabolism of lorazepam leading to decreased effectiveness of lorazepam	Anticipate need for dosage change of lorazepam as indicated. Assess patient for changes in seizure control or decrease in sedative effect.
scopolamine	Increased sedation when administered with parenteral form of lorazepam	Institute safety measures. Assess patient for signs of increased drowsiness, dizziness, and ataxia.
theophylline	Possible antagonism of sedative effects of lorazepam	Anticipate need for lorazepam dosage adjustment.

sion may occur; children and adolescents with disruptive behavior disorders are especially prone to this effect. Although hypotension is rare, lorazepam use may cause cardiac complications resulting from a drop in blood pressure.

Lorazepam is frequently used in elderly patients, because it is metabolized to inactive compounds with a relatively short half-life and duration of action. Older individuals generally have diminished hepatic detoxifying capacity and often show cumulative effects to the usual adult dosage—especially for benzodiazepines that are metabolized to long half-lives (e.g., diazepam). Although dosage is generally reduced in older adults, it is reduced because of their greater sensitivity to the CNS depressant effects rather than because of the drug's metabolic accumulation. The elderly are particularly susceptible to the anterograde amnesia that occurs predominantly with the higher-potency benzodiazepines (i.e., alprazolam, clonazepam, lorazepam, midazolam, triazolam). Drowsiness, ataxia, and confusion have occurred, especially in the elderly and debilitated.

The nurse assesses the woman of child-bearing age for pregnancy or intent to become pregnant. Lorazepam is FDA pregnancy category D. The benzodiazepines and their metabolites freely cross the placenta and accumulate in the fetal circulation. Benzodiazepines have been found in maternal and cord blood, indicating placental transfer of drug. It is thought that the use of benzodiazepines during the first trimester of pregnancy may increase the risk of congenital malformations (e.g., cleft lip or palate); therefore, use of the benzodiazepines during this period should be avoided. The nurse advises patients that if they become pregnant or plan to become pregnant, they should consider discontinuing the drug.

Neonatal withdrawal consisting of severe tremulousness or flaccidity, respiratory problems, and irritability has been attributed to maternal ingestion of benzodiazepines. Prolonged CNS depression has been observed, apparently from an inability to biotransform benzodiazepines into inactive metabolites.

The nurse assesses the lactation status of the woman of child-bearing age. It is unknown whether lorazepam is excreted in the breast milk, although the other benzodiazepines are. Because neonates metabolize benzodiazepines more slowly than adults, accumulation of the drug and its metabolites to toxic levels is possible.

Lifestyle, Diet, and Habits

The nurse asks the patient whether he or she smokes. Sedative effects are decreased in heavy smokers.

Culture

The nurse should be aware of the patient's ethnic heritage. Pharmacokinetic studies suggest that Asians are more sensitive to effects of benzodiazepines. Clinical observations of lower dosage requirements for Asian patients correlate with higher plasma benzodiazepine concentrations and lower drug clearance compared with findings in whites (Rudorfer, 1993). Pharmacodynamic factors of altered dopamine-receptor-mediated responses are also thought to have a role in dosage differences.

Nursing Diagnoses and Outcomes

- Risk for Injury related to sensory-perceptual alterations secondary to benzodiazepine-induced cognitive alterations and anterograde amnesia

  Desired outcome: The patient will identify factors that increase the risk for and relate the intent to practice safety measures to prevent injury.
- Disturbed Sleep Pattern related to benzodiazepine-induced alterations in normal stages of sleep

  Desired outcome: The patient will identify techniques to induce sleep and report an optimal balance of rest and activity.

Planning and Intervention

Maximizing Therapeutic Effects

Injectable lorazepam (and diazepam) should not be mixed with other drugs or IV fluids. With IV administration, plastic containers, tubing, or both may absorb some of the drug. For anxiolytic or sedative purposes, the oral drug is usually given in divided doses, with the largest dose preferably taken before bedtime. For optimal effect, IM administration should occur at least 2 hours before an operative or diagnostic procedure with injection of undiluted drug deep into the muscle mass. For optimum effect, the nurse should give the drug 15 to 20 minutes before the procedure.

Light and temperature affect lorazepam stability. The nurse protects the solution from light and refrigeration. He or she does not use the solution if it is discolored or contains a precipitate. Tablets should be stored in light-resistant containers at 15 to 30°C. Sustained-release capsules should not be crushed or chewed.

Minimizing Adverse Effects

Lorazepam may be taken with food or water if stomach upset occurs. For anxiolytic effects, lorazepam (and other anxiolytic benzodiazepines) should be administered in the smallest possible dose over the shortest time possible.

Providing Patient and Family Education

- Anxiolytic and sedative-hypnotic compounds (e.g., barbiturates, benzodiazepines, and nonbarbiturate/non-benzodiazepines) are subject to restriction under the Federal Controlled Substances Act of 1970. Depending on the compound, they are classified as C-III or C-IV; the short-acting barbiturates classified C-II are an exception. The nurse stresses the importance of storing the drug in a safe place to avoid accidental ingestion by young, curious children. He or she cautions not to change (increase or decrease) the drug dosage without consulting the health care provider.

Patients must limit use of these drugs as sleeping aids to 2 weeks.

- Because of their related CNS depression, sedative-hypnotic and anxiolytic drugs may impair mental or physical abilities required for the performance of potentially hazardous tasks (e.g., driving, operating machinery). The nurse emphasizes the importance of avoiding potentially hazardous activities until effects of the drug are known.
- The nurse instructs the patient not to consume alcohol while taking benzodiazepines. Concurrent use of sedative-hypnotic or anxiolytic drugs with other CNS depressants (e.g., alcohol, narcotics, tranquilizers, antihistamines) may result in additional CNS depressant effects.
- The nurse explains to patients the importance of carrying identification (e.g., MedicAlert) to indicate the condition and drug treatment including dosage. He or she advises patients to report any bothersome or persistent adverse effects. The nurse stresses the importance of taking the drug exactly as directed and of not stopping therapy abruptly. In addition, he or she emphasizes not to use OTC drugs and herbal preparations without approval from the health care professional.
- The nurse counsels women of child-bearing potential to use effective contraceptive methods while taking benzodiazepines.
- Teaching patients to practice various relaxation techniques (e.g., guided imagery, meditation, yoga) may assist in lowering anxiety levels.
- The nurse informs the patient and family that if the patient misses or forgets a dose, he or she should take it as soon as possible. If several hours have passed or time for the next dose is approaching, however, the patient should not double the dose to "catch up," unless advised by the health care provider.
- The nurse alerts the patient and the family that benzodiazepine use may result in altered cognitive effects. Patients may experience anterograde amnesia.
- The nurse informs the patient and family that although lorazepam and the other benzodiazepines are relatively safe drugs, psychological and physiologic dependence are possible even with therapeutic use. Although withdrawal syndrome has occurred after as little as 4 to 6 weeks treatment, it is more likely if the drug is a short-acting benzodiazepine (e.g., alprazolam), has been taken regularly for more than 4 months, and is abruptly discontinued.
- The onset of the withdrawal syndrome occurs within 1 to 10 days, and its duration may be 5 to 30 days depending on the particular benzodiazepine, dose, and so forth. Symptoms generally begin with anxiety-like manifestations, sensory disturbances (e.g., paresthesias, photophobia, hypersomnia, metallic taste), concentration difficulties, fatigue, anorexia, dizziness, vomiting, insomnia, confusion, headache, muscle tension/cramps, tremor, dysphoria, muscle twitching, "psychosis" with paranoid delusions and hallucinations, memory impairment, and generalized tonic-clonic seizures.

Ongoing Assessment and Evaluation

The nurse assesses the patient for a positive clinical response, which is evident when the patient reports reduced feelings of anxiety and develops new coping strategies. The patient should exhibit adequate sedation with minimal adverse side effects and remain free from injury from orthostatic hypotension or sedation. The nurse notes any behaviors that indicate physical or psychological dependence and observes for signs of chronic intoxication (e.g., ataxia, slurred speech, vertigo). This medication may produce dependence if used in large doses or for longer than 4 months. Blood dyscrasias may occur during therapy. The nurse must determine any blood dyscrasias that could preclude administering the drug. If the patient complains of a sore throat, fever, or weakness, the nurse assesses for blood dyscrasias by obtaining a complete blood count with differential.

Because of isolated reports of neutropenia and jaundice, the nurse should perform periodic blood counts and liver function tests during therapy with lorazepam or other benzodiazepines. There have been reports of abnormal liver and kidney function test results following benzodiazepine use.

The nurse periodically reassesses the effectiveness of lorazepam as an anxiolytic or sedative-hypnotic. In some patients, depression or suicidal tendencies may accompany anxiety. The nurse must assess the patient for suicidal ideation and teach the family to recognize behaviors that might indicate the need for further treatment, hospitalization, or both. If suicide is a risk, giving the patient access to the smallest possible amount of drug is preferred. ■

DRUGS CLOSELY RELATED TO LORAZEPAM

Alprazolam

Alprazolam (Xanax) is an anxiolytic benzodiazepine metabolized into two metabolites with the same half-life as the parent drug. When alprazolam is discontinued, it is rapidly cleared from the system. Abrupt decrease of drug dosage or discontinuation of the drug may result in rebound CNS excitation; withdrawal seizures have occurred.

Chlorazepate

Chlorazepate is one of the most rapidly absorbed benzodiazepines and is metabolized to several active compounds. It has anxiolytic, sedative-hypnotic, and anticonvulsant actions. It is also used for relief of acute alcohol-withdrawal symptoms. Taking chlorazepate concurrently with CYP450-

MEMORY CHIP

Lorazepam

- Benzodiazepine used for management of anxiety disorders and short-term relief of anxiety symptoms
- Significant contraindications: hypersensitivity, psychosis, acute narrow-angle glaucoma, hepatic disease, and age patients younger than 6 months.
- Most common adverse effects: sedation and ataxia, hangover effect
- Most serious adverse effects: anterograde amnesia, psychosis, and suicidal tendencies
- **Lifespan alert: begin with smallest dose initially in children and the elderly with gradual increases in dosage as indicated; use reduced dosages in elderly patients.**
- Maximizing therapeutic effects: give oral form in divided doses with largest dose given at bedtime; give IM form 15 to 20 minutes before operative or diagnostic procedure; protect IM and IV preparations from light.
- Minimizing adverse effects: administer with food or water; use smallest dose possible for the shortest period of time.
- Most significant patient education: use of safety measures and avoidance of concomitant use of other CNS depressants.

inhibiting drugs (e.g., cimetidine, oral contraceptives, fluoxetine) may decrease elimination of chlorazepate and increase its pharmacologic effects (e.g., excessive sedation, impaired psychomotor function).

Chlordiazepoxide

Chlordiazepoxide (Librium) is a benzodiazepine used primarily for relief of acute alcohol withdrawal symptoms. Following drug administration, the patient should rest in bed and be monitored closely for several hours for decreases in respiratory rate, heart rate, and blood pressure. Chlordiazepoxide has several active intermediate metabolites. Taken concurrently with CYP450 inhibitors, its effects mimic those of chlorazepate.

Clonazepam

Clonazepam (Klonopin) suppresses the spike-and-wave discharge in petit mal seizures and decreases frequency, amplitude, duration, and spread of discharge in minor motor seizures. Five metabolites of clonazepam have been identified. The kidneys excrete clonazepam metabolites; the drug should be used cautiously in patients with impaired renal function or significant liver disease to avoid excess accumulation.

Abrupt withdrawal of clonazepam, particularly in those patients on long-term, high-dose therapy, may precipitate status epilepticus. Although clonazepam is being gradually withdrawn, another anticonvulsant should be substituted simultaneously. Other withdrawal symptoms include vomiting, diarrhea, and sweating.

Diazepam

Diazepam (Valium) is an anxiolytic and sedative-hypnotic benzodiazepine. Its plasma half-life increases with age, ranging from approximately 20 hours in young adults to several days for elderly patients. If diazepam is taken concurrently with CYP450 inhibitors, its effects mimic those that occur with chlorazepate.

Diazepam may cause hepatic dysfunction, jaundice, and elevations of low-density lipoprotein, alkaline phosphatase, ALT, and AST levels. Liver function studies should be performed before therapy and periodically throughout.

Chronic diazepam use in women who are breast-feeding reportedly caused infants to become lethargic and to lose weight. Thus, diazepam should not be given to nursing mothers. IM administration of diazepam results in slow erratic absorption and lower peak plasma levels than oral or IV administration, although IM administration into the deltoid muscle is more likely to be rapid and complete. When administered IV, the rate of infusion should not exceed 5 mg/min. Administered too rapidly, it may cause hypotension or respiratory depression.

Halezepam

Halezepam (Paxipam) is an anxiolytic benzodiazepine. It has a long half-life and active metabolites that may exert significant effects when multiple doses are administered. Elimination may take as long as several weeks. If halazepam is taken concurrently with CYP450 inhibitors, its effects mimic those that occur with chlorazepate.

Midazolam

Midazolam (Versed) is an injectable short-acting benzodiazepine used for induction or supplementation of general anesthesia, preoperative sedation, or conscious sedation for diagnostic procedures. Midazolam undergoes hepatic metabolism to pharmacologic active compounds by the CYP450 system. Multiple doses may lead to accumulation of metabolites. IV midazolam has been associated with respiratory depression and arrest in both adult and pediatric patients. The mean half-life of midazolam is increased (2.5 times) in patients with alcoholism. It is greater in patients with obesity (5.9 versus 2.3 hours).

Oxazepam

Oxazepam (Serax) is a benzodiazepine indicated for anxiety associated with depression and for treatment of acute alcohol withdrawal. Accumulation from multiple doses is minimal, and elimination is rapid. Its short half-life and duration of activity are of value in patients with liver disease and in the elderly.

Prazepam

Prazepam (Centrax) is used only as an anxiolytic. In comparison with the other benzodiazepines, it is one of the most slowly absorbed, and accumulation of active metabolites may be significant, with frequent reports of lethargy and increased fatigue.

DRUGS SIGNIFICANTLY DIFFERENT FROM LORAZEPAM

Buspirone

Buspirone (BuSpar) is an azaspirodecanedione anxiolytic that is neither chemically nor pharmacologically related to the benzodiazepines. It lacks anticonvulsant, hypnotic, muscle relaxant, ataxic, and dependence-producing properties. Its mechanism of anxiolytic action is unknown. Buspirone has anxiolytic effects similar to those of the benzodiazepines, which may take several weeks to be noticeable and up to 3 to 4 weeks to attain optimal response. Buspirone, however, does not produce the sedation or potentiate the CNS depressant effects of conventional sedative-hypnotic drugs, alcohol, or TCAs. Adverse effects include headache, nausea, lightheadedness, and excitement. Buspirone is in pregnancy risk category B. Its safety and efficacy in children younger than 18 years are unknown. No unusual adverse effects in the elderly have been identified. Buspirone undergoes hepatic metabolism and renal excretion; thus, it is contraindicated in patients with impairment of these systems. It may increase the risk of digitalis toxicity, because it displaces digoxin from its plasma protein-binding sites.

Flumazenil

Flumazenil (Romazicon) is an imidazobenzodiazepine with a high affinity for benzodiazepine receptors. It functions as a specific benzodiazepine antagonist that can rapidly reverse the sedative and CNS effects of benzodiazepines. It competitively inhibits benzodiazepine activity at the recognition site on the GABA-receptor complex (Cuthriell, 2000). Available only for IV administration, flumazenil has a half-life of 0.7 to 1.3 hours; its duration of clinical effect is brief (30 to 60 minutes). The primary indications for flumazenil are the reversal of sedative effects produced by benzodiazepines administered during general anesthesia or diagnostic or therapeutic procedures (1 mg over 1 to 3 minutes) or management of benzodiazepine overdoses (1 to 5 mg over 2 to 10 minutes). Flumazenil may precipitate seizures in patients who have developed benzodiazepine tolerance or dependence.

Hydroxyzine

Hydroxyzine (Atarax, Vistaril) is an antihistamine with an unknown mechanism of action; its anxiolytic effect may result from suppression of activity in selected subcortical areas of the CNS. Hydroxyzine has a rapid onset of action (15 to 30 minutes), a half-life of 2.5 to 3.4 hours, and duration of effect from 4 to 6 hours. Hydroxyzine undergoes hepatic metabolism and renal excretion. The most common adverse effect is sedation, which usually disappears after several days or with reduction of dosage.

Meprobamate

Meprobamate (Equanil, Miltown) is a nonbarbiturate/nonbenzodiazepine carbamate-derivative anxiolytic with mild tranquilizing, anticonvulsant, and skeletal muscle relaxant properties. Antianxiety effectiveness has not been established when used for longer than 4 months. Meprobamate is contraindicated for patients with acute intermittent porphyria. Caution should be used in patients with renal or hepatic impairment or in older adults. Meprobamate crosses the placenta and increases the risk of congenital malformations if used during the first trimester. It also crosses into breast milk. It is not recommended for children younger than age 6 years.

Physical and psychological dependence may occur, and abuse also is possible. Meprobamate should not be used in patients with alcoholism or other addictions. Adverse effects are neurologic (drowsiness, ataxia), GI (nausea, vomiting, diarrhea), and cardiovascular (palpitations, tachycardia) in nature.

Zaleplon

Zaleplon (Sonata), a rapidly absorbed non-benzodiazepine, has a rapid onset of effect, no active metabolites, and an elimination half-life of 1 hour. Its most frequent adverse effects are dizziness and headache. Zaleplon does not appear to cause rebound insomnia or have residual effects on performance and memory.

The characteristics that distinguish zaleplon from other hypnotics are its short duration of action and half-life. The short duration of action permits its unique use among the hypnotics in patients who have difficulty falling asleep. Like other hypnotics, it can be administered immediately before bedtime. But zaleplon can also be administered after the patient has gone to bed and experienced difficulty falling asleep. He or she must remain in bed for at least 4 hours, however, before becoming active again.

Studies have shown that drug concentrations of zaleplon are increased in Japanese patients. This finding is likely attributed to differences in body weight or, alternatively, may represent differences in enzyme activities resulting from differences in diet, environment, or other factors.

Zolpidem

Zolpidem (Ambien) is a non-benzodiazepine with a specific effect on the omega-1 receptor. Because of its specificity, zolpidem lacks anticonvulsant, muscle-relaxant, and anxiolytic effects. It also has fewer effects on sleep cycles and next-day performance when compared to the benzodiazepines, although its hypnotic efficacy is similar.

Hypnotic Benzodiazepines

Five drugs that belong to the benzodiazepine class are indicated for use as hypnotics (Fig. 17-3). They are listed next. In terms of mechanism of action, they are assumed to act similarly. The pharmacokinetics and pharmacodynamic effects produced by each, however, differ. Their neurochemical basis is not well understood. All hypnotic benzodiazepines decrease the time required to fall asleep (sleep latency), the amount of time spent in stage 2 sleep, and the number of awakenings. They shorten the length of stages 3 and 4 sleep, which are required for full rest. Additionally, they shorten the time spent in REM sleep.

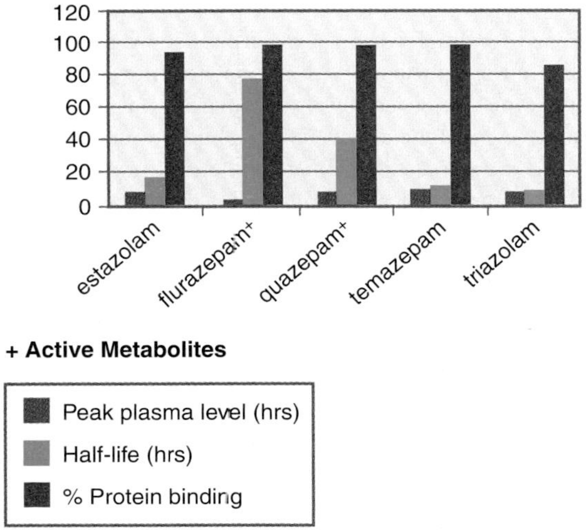

Figure 17-3. Comparison of the pharmacokinetic parameters of hours to reach peak plasma levels, half-life, and percentage of drug that is bound to plasma proteins between the hypnotic benzodiazepines.

Estazolam

Estazolam (ProSom) is characterized by a relatively long half-life (up to 24 hours). For this reason, it is less likely to cause rebound insomnia after drug withdrawal.

Flurazepam

Flurazepam (Dalmane) is a benzodiazepine hypnotic with an active metabolite that tends to accumulate with repeated doses and can prolong the half-life to as long as 5 days. Although the sleeping pattern will improve following the initial dose, 2 to 3 days may be required before flurazepam becomes fully effective. The long half-life minimizes the risk of rebound insomnia but makes morning hangover or daytime sedation more likely. Doses of 15 mg have been shown to impair coordination skills necessary for driving on the morning after use (Stimmel, et al., 2000). Flurazepam has been shown to be an effective treatment for insomnia for up to 28 days.

Quazepam

Quazepam is unique with specificity for the benzodiazepine-1 receptor. This effect is lost, however, from its metabolism into the same long-acting active metabolite as flurazepam.

Temazepam

Temazepam has a half-life of 6 to 20 hours. If temazepam is discontinued after 3 to 4 weeks of continued use, the patient may experience REM rebound.

Triazolam

Triazolam (Halcion) has a half-life of 2 to 6 hours. It differs from the other hypnotic benzodiazepines in that it does not suppress stage 4 sleep. Because it has no active metabolites, residual daytime sedation is less problematic than with longer-acting benzodiazepines.

CHAPTER SUMMARY

- Anxiety disorders may impair daily functioning. Anxiolytic drugs may be used to help an individual cope.
- Sedative and hypnotic drugs differ in their degree of CNS depression.
- Barbiturates cause a generalized CNS depression and are used primarily for anticonvulsant effects, although historically their use has been as sedative-hypnotics and anesthetics.
- Barbiturate-type sedatives, hypnotics, and anxiolytics depress the sensory cortex, decrease motor activity, and alter cerebral function to produce their effects.
- Phenobarbital therapy is complicated by many drug–drug interactions; it is used primarily to treat seizures.
- Benzodiazepines do not exert a general CNS-depressant effect and are among the most frequently prescribed drugs today; their wide range of selectivity of action allows them to be used for a variety of conditions (e.g., anticonvulsants, anxiolytics, hypnotics, muscle relaxants, pre-operative medications, and sedatives.
- Benzodiazepines have a broad spectrum of actions; actions may vary according to the actual chemical compound, dosage, and patient responsiveness. Benzodiazepine receptors are widely distributed in the CNS. Many of these receptors are associated with the GABA-receptor systems and chloride channels.
- Lorazepam given orally is indicated for the management of anxiety disorders, short-term relief of symptoms of anxiety, or anxiety associated with depressive symptoms. Parenteral use in adults includes preanesthetic medication producing sedation, relief of anxiety, and a decreased ability to recall events related to surgery. Unlabeled uses for parenteral lorazepam include control of status epilepticus, chemotherapy-induced nausea and vomiting, and acute alcohol withdrawal syndrome.
- Patient and family education should focus on safe self-administration. It is important for the nurse to emphasize that cognitive and physical performance may be impaired by many of these drugs and that their CNS-depressant effects will be enhanced when combined with alcohol or other CNS-depressant drugs.
- Individuals taking barbiturates or benzodiazepines are at risk for developing psychological and physiologic dependence.

QUESTIONS FOR STUDY AND REVIEW

1. Differentiate between a drug used for an anxiolytic effect, a sedative effect, and a hypnotic effect.
2. What problems may occur if an individual uses anxiolytic or sedative-hypnotic drugs to cope with the stresses of everyday life?
3. Name the clinical uses for the benzodiazepines. How do they exert their effects?
4. Discuss the reasons for a limited use of the barbiturates as anxiolytic and sedative-hypnotics.
5. In terms of nursing care, what difference does it make whether a benzodiazepine is metabolized to active or inactive metabolites?
6. What instructions must be emphasized for safe and effective use of an anxiolytic, sedative or hypnotic benzodiazepine?

NEED MORE HELP?

Chapter 17 of the study guide for *Drug Therapy in Nursing* contains exercises and activities to reinforce your understanding of the concepts presented in this chapter. For additional information see the text's accompanying website at *http://www.connection.lww.com*.

REFERENCES AND BIBLIOGRAPHY

American Psychiatric Association. (2000). *Diagnostic and statistical manual of mental disorders* (4th ed., text revision). Washington, DC: Author.

Bond, W. S. (1991). Ethnicity and psychotropic drugs. *Clinical Pharmacy, 10*(6), 467–470.

Brody, T. M., Larner, J., & Minneman, K. P., (Eds.). (1998). *Human pharmacology: Molecular to clinical.* St. Louis: Mosby—Year Book.

Burnham, T. H., & Short, R. M. (Eds.) (2000). *Drug facts and comparisons*. St. Louis: Facts and Comparisons.

Castellanos, D., & Hunter, T. (1999). Anxiety disorders in children and adolescents. *Southern Medical Journal, 92*(10), 946–954.

Cuthriell, A. M. (2000). Midazolam: Use in the pediatric intensive care population. *Pediatric Pharmacotherapy, 6*(1), 31–34.

Davis, W. M. (1999). Treating nonclassical psychiatric indications. *Drug Topics, 143*(22), 84–93.

Fauci, A., Braunwald, E., Wilson, J. D., Martin, J. B., Hauser, S. L., Longo, D. L., Kasper, D. L., & Isselbachter, K. J. (Eds.) (1999). *Harrison's Online.* New York: McGraw-Hill.

Hardman, J. G., Limbird, L. E., Molinof, P. B., Ruddon, R. W., & Gilman, A. G. (Eds.). (1997). *Goodman & Gilman's pharmacological basis of therapeutics.* (9th ed.). New York: McGraw-Hill.

Inder, T. (2000). *Advances and application of psychopharmacology in pediatrics.* Presented at the Joint Meeting of Pediatric Academic Societies and the American Academy of Pediatrics, Boston, Massachusetts.

Katzung, B. C. (Ed.) (2000). *Basic and clinical pharmacology.* (8th ed.). New York: McGraw-Hill.

Korn, M. L. (2000). *Perspectives in women's mental health.* Presented at the 153rd annual meeting of the American Psychiatric Association, Chicago, Illinois.

Long, S. F. (2000). Preventing and treating insomnia. *Drug Topics, 144*(13), 49–58.

Markowitz, J. S. (1998). Herbal medicines assuming larger role in psychiatric care. *Drug Topics, 142*(17), 50–53.

Nanko, S. (2000). *Psychiatric genetics: Clinical applications.* Presented at the 153rd annual meeting of the American Psychiatric Association, Chicago, Illinois.

Rainey, C. (2000). *New aspects of anxiety: Mental health and other sequelae of trauma.* Presented at the 153rd annual meeting of the American Psychiatric Association, Chicago, Illinois.

Rudorfer, M. V. (1993). Pharmacokinetics of psychotropic drugs in special populations. *Journal of Clinical Psychiatry, 54,* (Suppl. 9), 50–54.

Sanderson W. C., & Rego, S. (2000). *Empirically supported psychological treatment of panic disorder and agoraphobia.* Golden, CO: Accreditation Council for Continuing Medical Education.

Stimmel, G. L. & Dopheide, J. A. (2000). Sleep disorders: Focus on Insomnia. *U.S. Pharmacist, 25*(1), 69–80.

Chapter 18

DRUGS FOR TREATING MOOD DISORDERS

KEY TERMS

antidepressants
bipolar disorder
depression
mood
mood stabilizers
neurotransmitters

Learning Objectives

At the completion of this chapter the student will:

1. Identify risk factors for the development of depression.
2. Compare and contrast the symptoms of dysthymic disorder and major depression.
3. Name the types of drugs that are used in the treatment of bipolar disorder.
4. Identify the classes of antidepressant medications.
5. Identify core patient variables relevant to drugs that affect mood.
6. Describe nursing interventions to maximize therapeutic and minimize adverse effects for drugs that affect mood.
7. Determine key points for patient and family education for drugs that affect mood.

Antidepressants

Tricyclic antidepressants

- **desipramine**
- nortriptyline
- protriptyline
- amitriptyline
- amoxapine
- clomipramine
- doxepin
- imipramine
- trimipramine
- maprotilene
- mirtazapine

Monoamine oxidase inhibitors

- **phenelzine**
- isocarboxazid
- trancyclopromine
- selegiline

Selective serotonin reuptake inhibitors

- **fluoxetine**
- citalopram
- fluvoxamine
- nefazodone
- paroxetine
- sertraline
- trazodone
- venlafaxine

Mood stabilizers

- **lithium**
- carbamazepine
- gabapentin
- valproic acid

The symbol (C) indicates the **drug class**.

Drugs in bold type marked with the symbol (P) are **prototypes**.

Drugs in blue type with no symbol are **closely related** to the prototype.

Drugs in **red** type with no symbol are **significantly different** from the prototype.

Drugs in **black** type with no symbol are **also used in drug therapy**; no prototype.

Mood is defined as a conscious state of mind or predominant emotion. Mood normally fluctuates in response to the environment; however, this fluctuation may be abnormal or dysfunctional if it is pervasive, represents a change from previous functioning, or interferes with daily activities.

According to the fourth edition of the *Diagnostic and Statistical Manual of Mental Disorders* (DSM-IV-TR) (American Psychiatric Association, 2000), the mood disorders are depressive disorders (major depressive disorder and dysthymic disorder), bipolar disorders (bipolar I, bipolar II, and cyclothymic disorder), mood disorder arising from other medical conditions, and mood disorder that is substance-abuse related. This chapter discusses drug therapy to treat depressive disorders and bipolar disorder.

Depression, one of the most common mental health disorders, affects people of all ages, backgrounds, lifestyles, and nationalities. Risk factors for depression are poor physical health, female gender, chronic or malignant disease, old age, and drug or alcohol abuse. Chronic stress is also thought to precipitate depressive episodes, although its role is not clearly understood (Kubiak, 2000). Depression is often associated with decreased productivity, work absenteeism, unemployment, alcohol and drug abuse, and risk for suicide. Estimates are that depression costs more than $44 billion yearly. These costs include treatment and rehabilitation (28%), lost earnings from suicide (17%), and lost earnings from morbidity, absenteeism, lost productivity, and health care costs (78%).

Bipolar disorder, historically known as manic-depressive illness, is a serious, long-term mental illness with a variable course. It is characterized by recurrent episodes of depression, mania, or mixed states. Data strongly suggest that bipolar disorder is a genetic illness. It is thought to affect about 1% of the population.

Antidepressants are drugs used to treat depressive disorders. They may be thought of as belonging to different generations. The first-generation antidepressants include tricyclic antidepressants (TCAs) and monoamine oxidase inhibitors (MAOIs). These two drug subclasses significantly affect various neurotransmitter systems (especially cholinergic), causing many undesirable adverse effects. The "cyclic" antidepressants (i.e., tricyclic and heterocyclic) are so named because of their chemical structure. All the cyclic antidepressants, however, have similar pharmacologic and toxicologic properties. The prototype TCA discussed in this chapter is desipramine. The prototype MAOI is phenelzine.

The miscellaneous antidepressants (sometimes referred to as "second-generation" antidepressants) loosely refer to drugs that differ from these established antidepressants in terms of side effects, especially anticholinergic. They essentially lack anticholinergic action, and their adrenolytic and antihistaminic effects are weaker. Miscellaneous antidepressants (e.g., bupropion, venlafaxine) exert their actions by affecting one or more of the three main neurotransmitter systems associated with depression: serotonin (5-HT), norepinephrine (NE), and dopamine (DA).

The selective serotonin reuptake inhibitors (SSRIs) exert their therapeutic effects by selectively blocking the synaptic reuptake of 5-HT, making more 5-HT available to elevate mood. The prototype SSRI in this chapter is fluoxetine (Prozac).

Mood stabilizers are drugs that manage or prevent mood swings in patients with bipolar disorder. The prototype for the mood stabilizers is lithium carbonate (Eskalith).

PHYSIOLOGY

The brain processes incoming information and regulates affect, mood, and motor response. Although there has been evidence of structural brain abnormality in some psychiatric disorders (e.g., schizophrenia), evolving notions of the etiologic processes in mental health disorders focus on functional abnormalities. New techniques for studying the metabolism and neurotransmitter activity in the living brain have provided increased insight into brain pathophysiology and medication activity.

PATHOPHYSIOLOGY

MAJOR DEPRESSIVE DISORDER

Depression is a heterogeneous disorder. Its onset is usually gradual, unless a severe psychological stressor (e.g., grief, illness) precipitates the condition. This "reactive" type of depression is most common. Depression is chronic and recurrent in many individuals. Sometimes, major depressive disorder is referred to as endogenous depression. Following one major depressive episode, the likelihood of a second, third, and even fourth episode is significantly greater (St. Dennis, 1999). Major depression causes considerable impairment in social, occupational, and other areas of functioning. It can occur independently of bipolar disorder, bereavement, substance abuse, or an existing medical problem.

Approximately 15% of the general population experience a major depressive episode at some point; 10% to 15% of these cases are secondary to general medical illness or substance abuse (Fauci et al., 1999). Mild, chronic depression affects approximately 3.3% of the general population. The overall prevalence of late-life depression is approximately 15%, with much higher rates (30% to 40%) in some subpopulations (e.g., patients with Alzheimer disease) (St. Dennis, 1999). One in 10 children aged 6 to 12 years suffers from depression. Estimates are that 5% of those aged 12 to 19 years will experience at least one episode (prevalence is 10% for females in this age group); 50% will have a recurrent episode. Postpartum depression may affect as many as 30% of all new mothers. There are no differences in rates of depression among ethnic or racial groups (Quarles & Norton, 2000).

The DSM-IV-TR diagnostic criteria for major depression include a depressed mood for most of the day nearly every day; marked loss of interest or pleasure in activities; significant changes in sleep, appetite, and weight; feelings of worthless, guilt, malaise, and inertia nearly every day; diminished ability to think, concentrate, or make decisions; and thoughts of death or suicidal ideation (or both) with or without a suicide plan and suicide attempt. These signs must be present nearly daily for 2 or more weeks and represent a change from previous levels of functioning.

Suicide is the most devastating outcome of depression. Individuals with untreated severe depression have a suicide rate of 15%. Depressed men are especially at risk and account for most suicides. Substance abuse rates correlate positively with rates of depression; 32% of depressed people also suffer from drug or alcohol dependency.

Although depression is one of the most common mental health disorders, its cause is not clearly understood. Strong evidence supports a genetic component. Individuals who have a parent or sibling with major depressive disorder have a 1.5 to 3 times increased risk of also developing the disorder (Kubiak, 2000).

Historically, the etiology of depression has been linked with neurotransmitter deficiency. This theory evolved because patients with hypertension who were treated with reserpine developed depression. The mechanism of action of reserpine is to inhibit the storage of amine **neurotransmitters** (e.g., NE, 5-HT) in the vesicles of presynaptic nerve endings. The "biogenic amine" theory of depression proposes that depression results from alterations or deficiencies in neurotransmitters or neurotransmitter-receptor functions of endogenous monoamines in the brain, namely, NE, DA, and 5-HT. Reinforcement of this theory is seen in healthy individuals who develop depressive symptoms after dietary depletion of tryptophan, an essential amino acid that the body uses as a precursor to production of 5-HT.

Another theory is a "permissive" one, in that low levels of 5-HT cause the expression of an affective disorder. The level of NE determines the type of affective state. Low NE levels induce a depressive syndrome. Conversely, high NE levels cause a state of mania. To treat the affective disorder, a correction of the low 5-HT levels is necessary.

The "dysregulation" theory explains the origin of depression as a dysfunctional neurotransmitter system and an impairment of homeostatic mechanisms and receptor sensitivity. The result is erratic levels of neurotransmitters, especially 5-HT. Consequently, circadian rhythms are disrupted, and response to environmental stimuli is less selective. Although most hypotheses have focused on the neurotransmitters NE and 5-HT, some have suggested that DA may play a part in the etiology of depression and the mechanisms of antidepressant drug actions (Kubiak, 2000).

DYSTHYMIC DISORDER

Dysthymic disorder is a chronic condition with a lifetime prevalence estimated at 3% to 6%. Dysthymic disorder consists in a pattern of chronic (at least 2 years), ongoing, mild depressive symptoms that are less severe and disabling than those found in major depression. Onset is usually insidious in childhood, adolescence, or early adulthood. In adults, dysthymic disorder significantly affects psychosocial and occupational functioning. Incidence is significantly higher in women than in men. This disorder often occurs with other psychiatric disorders, particularly substance abuse and panic attacks and other anxiety disorders.

BIPOLAR DISORDER

Bipolar disorder is characterized by recurrent episodes of depression, mania, or mixed states. Although once thought rare in childhood, bipolar disorder is being more frequently diagnosed in prepubertal children. Bipolar disorder is difficult to recognize in youth because its symptoms can resemble or occur in combination with those of other common childhood-onset mental disorders, such as attention deficit hyperactivity disorder (ADHD) and conduct disorder (CD). The mean age of onset is 21 years, although symptoms may often first appear in adolescence. Data from the National Institute of Mental Health (NIMH) study suggest that bipolar disorder may be at least as common among youth as adults. In this study, 1% of adolescents (ages 14 to 18 years) were found to meet criteria for bipolar disorder.

Episodic depression and mania characterize bipolar disorder. The DSM-IV-TR subclassifies bipolar disorder as types I and II. The differentiation between bipolar disorder types I and II requires the occurrences of 1) a major depressive episode, 2) rapid cycling (four or more episodes per year), and 3) mixed states. These differences are important in regard to selection of pharmacotherapy (Benefield & Cohen, 2000).

The exact biologic disturbance in bipolar disorder is unclear; however, catecholamine-related activity and alterations in neurotransmitters (e.g., NE, 5-HT, DA) are thought to be dominant. Changes in the activity of gamma-aminobutyric acid (GABA) and acetylcholine (ACh) are also thought to be involved. Patients with cyclic attacks of mania have many symptoms characteristic of paranoid schizophrenia, including grandiosity, aggression, paranoid thoughts, and hyperactivity. There is a convincing genetic component to bipolar disorder, and suicide and substance abuse are common in patients with this mood disorder.

C ANTIDEPRESSANTS

The ideal antidepressant would have the following characteristics: rapid onset of action, convenient dosing schedule, minimal side effects, no drug interactions, and broad therapeutic activity to cover other possible coexisting psychiatric diagnoses. The antidepressants currently available fall short of meeting all these criteria (Table 18-1) (Fig. 18-1).

The antidepressant onset of effect is associated with downregulation of adrenergic or serotonergic postsynaptic receptors. This phenomenon, however, is not immediate. Downregulation is the development of a refractory or tolerant state as a result of repeated administration of a pharmacologically or physiologically active substance. It is often accompanied by an initial decrease in the affinity of receptors for the agent and a subsequent diminution in the number of receptors. For example, the initiation of treatment with an SSRI will result in increased concentrations of 5-HT at the somatodendritic sites. Continuous stimulation of the presynaptic serotonergic neurons ensues, leading to their downregulation. As a result, inhibition for cell firing decreases, release of 5-HT increases, and the synaptic cleft is flooded. Further transporter (reuptake) inhibition at the axonal level

TABLE 18-1 Summary of Selected Drugs for Treating Mood Disorders

Drug (Trade) Name	Selected Indications	Route and Dosage Range	Pharmacokinetics
Tricyclic Antidepressants			
desipramine (Norpramin; *Canadian:* Alti-Desipramine)	Major depression	*Adult:* PO, 100–200 mg/d *Child:* Not recommended for < 12 y	*Onset:* Varies *Duration:* 3–4 d $t_{1/2}$: 12–24 h
imipramine (Tofranil; *Canadian:* Apo-Imipramine)	Major depression	*Adult:* PO, 75–150 mg/d; IM, 100 mg/d *Child:* PO, 1.5 mg/kg/d	*Onset:* Varies *Duration:* Unknown $t_{1/2}$: 11–25 h
amitriptyline (Elavil; *Canadian:* Apo-Amitriptyline)	Major depression	*Adult:* 75–150 mg/d; IM, 20–30 mg qid *Child:* Not recommended for < 12 y	*Onset:* Varies *Duration:* > 20 h $t_{1/2}$: 31–46 h
clomipramine (Anafranil; *Canadian:* Gen-Clomipramine)	Obsessive-compulsive disorder	*Adult:* PO, 25–100 mg/d *Child:* PO, 25 mg/d with gradual increases to a maximum of 3 mg/kg/d or 100 mg/d	*Onset:* Slow *Duration:* 1–6 wk $t_{1/2}$: 19–37 h
doxepin (Sinequan; *Canadian:* Novo-Doxepin)	Major depression Depression, associated anxiety	*Adult:* PO, 75–150 mg/d *Child:* not recommended for < 12 y	*Onset:* Varies *Duration:* Unknown $t_{1/2}$: 8–24 h
trimipramine (Surmontil; *Canadian:* Nu-Trimipramine)	Major depression	*Adult:* PO, 75–150 mg/d *Child:* Use not recommended	*Onset:* Varies *Duration:* Unknown $t_{1/2}$: 7–30 h
amoxapine (Asendin)	Major depression	*Adult:* PO, 200–300 mg/d *Child:* Not recommended for < 16 y	*Onset:* Varies *Duration:* 2–4 wk $t_{1/2}$: 8–30 h
nortriptyline (Pamelor; *Canadian:* Norventyl)	Major depression	*Adult:* PO, 25 mg tid to qid *Child:* Use not recommended	*Onset:* Varies *Duration:* 2–4 wk $t_{1/2}$: 18–44 hr
protriptyline (Vivactil)	Major depression	*Adult:* PO, 15–40 mg/d divided into 3 or 4 doses *Child:* Use not recommended	*Onset:* Slow *Duration:* Unknown $t_{1/2}$: 67–89 h
maprotiline (Ludiomil)	Major depression, bipolar disorder	*Adult:* PO, 75–225 mg/d *Child:* Use not recommended; safety and efficacy have not been established	*Onset:* Slow *Duration:* 2–3 wk $t_{1/2}$: 61 h
mirtazapine (Remeron)	Major depression	*Adult:* PO, 15–45 mg/d single dose at bedtime *Child:* Safety and efficacy have not been established	*Onset:* Slow *Duration:* 2–4 wk $t_{1/2}$: 20–40 h
Selective Serotonin Reuptake Inhibitors (SSRIs)			
fluoxetine (Prozac; *Canadian:* Gen-Fluoxetine)	Major depression, obsessive-compulsive disorder, panic disorder, post-traumatic stress disorder, bulimia nervosa	*Adult:* PO, 20–60 mg/d not to exceed 80 mg/d *Child:* Safety and efficacy have not been established for < 18 y	*Onset:* Slow *Duration:* 10–12 h $t_{1/2}$: 1–3 d (7 to 9 d for S-norfluoxetine, active metabolite)
citalopram (Celexa)	Major depression	*Adult:* 20–40 mg/d *Child:* Safety and efficacy have not been established for < 18 y	*Onset:* Slow *Duration:* Unknown $t_{1/2}$: 35 h
fluvoxamine (Luvox)	Obsessive-compulsive disorder	*Adult:* PO, 50–300 mg/d *Child:* Safety and efficacy have not been established for < 18 y	*Onset:* Rapid *Duration:* 4–16 h $t_{1/2}$: 13.5–15.6 h

TABLE 18-1 Summary of Selected Drugs for Treating Mood Disorders (Continued)

Drug (Trade) Name	Selected Indications	Route and Dosage Range	Pharmacokinetics
paroxetine (Paxil)	Major depression, obsessive-compulsive disorder, panic disorder	*Adult:* PO, 20–50 mg/d *Child:* Safety and efficacy have not been established for < 18 y	*Onset:* 5.2 h *Duration:* 12–16 h $t_{1/2}$: 21 h
sertraline (Zoloft)	Major depression, obsessive-compulsive disorder	*Adult:* PO, 50 to 200 mg/d *Child:* Safety and efficacy have not been established for < 18 y	*Onset:* 4.5–8.4 h *Duration:* 12–20 h $t_{1/2}$: 26 h (104 h for active metabolite)
Monoamine Oxidase Inhibitors (MAOIs)			
phenelzine (Nardil)	Major depression	*Adult:* PO, 15 mg tid, increasing to 60 mg/d; maximum 90 mg/d	*Onset:* Approximately 4 wk *Duration:* 48–96 h $t_{1/2}$: Unknown
tranylcypromine (Parnate)	Major depression	*Adult:* PO, 30 mg/d maximum dose 60mg/d in divided doses	*Onset:* 7–10 d *Duration:* Unknown $t_{1/2}$: 2.5 h
Mood Stabilizers			
lithium (Eskalith; *Canadian:* Lithizine)	Mania of bipolar disorder	*Adult:* 1800 mg/d (slow release) for acute mania; 900–1200 g/d for maintenance *Child:* Safety and efficacy have not been established for < 12 y	*Onset:* 5–7 d *Duration:* Unknown $t_{1/2}$: 10–50 h
Other Antidepressants			
trazodone (Desyrel; *Canadian:* Trazorel)	Major depression	*Adult:* PO, 150–600 mg/d *Child:* Safety and efficacy have not been established	*Onset:* Varies *Duration:* Varies $t_{1/2}$: 4–9 h
nefazodone (Serzone)	Major depression	*Adult:* 200–600 mg/d *Child:* Safety and efficacy have not been established for < 18 y	*Onset:* Slow *Duration:* Unknown $t_{1/2}$: 11–24 h
venlafaxine (Effexor)	Major depression	*Adult:* PO, 75–225 mg/d in 2 to 3 divided doses *Child:* Safety and efficacy have not been established for < 18 y	*Onset:* Slow *Duration:* 48 h $t_{1/2}$: 5–13 h

eventually results in downregulation of postsynaptic 5-HT2 receptors. This sequence of events occurs over 1 to 4 weeks and explains the lag time between initiation of drug treatment and the appearance of any antidepressant effect (Ereshefsky, 1998).

According to dysregulation theory, treatment strategies that affect multiple transmitter systems may enhance antidepressant effects and cause receptor setpoints to change more quickly. This theory suggests that the ascending aminergic system of serotonergic, noradrenergic, and adrenergic arrangement in the brain is interconnected and disturbed in depression. Thus, therapies that alter multiple sites of action in this system may have a quicker onset of action or a more successful therapeutic outcome.

Although drug therapy can quickly correct neurotransmitter deficiencies, clinical antidepressant effects are seldom immediate. Currently, antidepressant effects are thought to result from chronic drug administration, which produces slow adaptive changes in the NE and 5-HT presynaptic and postsynaptic receptor systems. The emphasis of research has shifted from acute reuptake effects to the slower adaptive changes in NE and 5-HT receptor systems induced by chronic antidepressant therapy. Postsynaptic receptors participate in nerve impulse neurotransmission, whereas presynaptic receptors regulate neurotransmitter release and reuptake, an important mechanism of neurotransmitter inactivation. Long-term antidepressant treatment produces complex changes in the sensitivities of both presynaptic and postsynaptic receptor sites. Currently, antidepressant agents are thought to increase the sensitivity of postsynaptic alpha-1-adrenergic and 5-HT receptors and decrease the sensitivity of presynaptic receptor sites. The net effect is the correction (i.e., reregulation) of an abnormal receptor-neurotransmitter relationship, which hastens the patient's natural recovery process from the depressive episode by normalizing neurotransmission efficacy. In some cases, drugs themselves may have a depressive effect

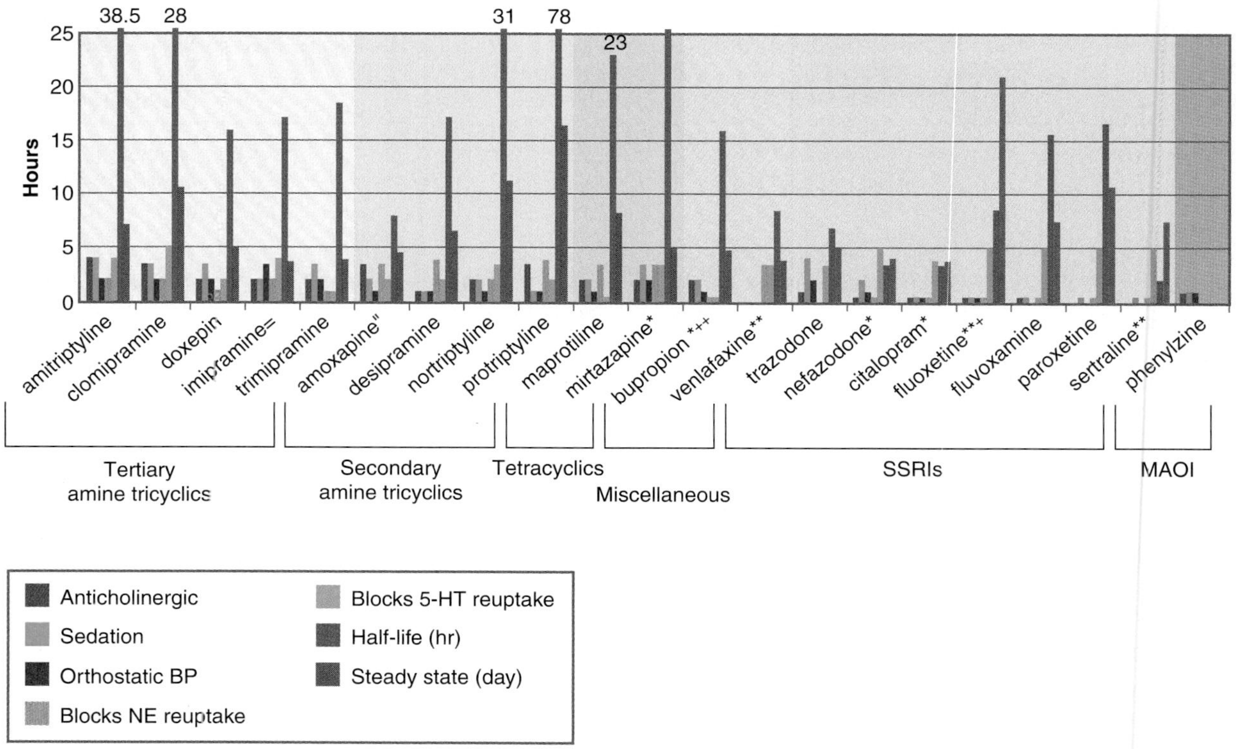

Figure 18-1. Comparison of antidepressant pharmacologic and pharmacokinetic parameters.

because of their pharmacodynamic influences on neurotransmitters (see the accompanying display, Drug Classes Associated With Depression).

A general rule in psychopharmacology is that the brain adapts to the presence of drugs. Reuptake inhibitors produce downregulation of the receptors for the specific neurotransmitter the uptake pump of which has been inhibited (for example, some 5-HT receptors [in the case of 5-HT uptake inhibitors] and beta-adrenergic receptors [in the case of NE uptake inhibitors]). In fact, such downregulation has been postulated to mediate the antidepressant efficacy of these drugs.

Such downregulation likely also mediates the withdrawal syndromes that can be seen when some antidepressants are abruptly stopped. Anticholinergic withdrawal syndrome can be seen when high-potency muscarinic cholinergic receptor blockers (e.g., tertiary-amine TCAs) are abruptly stopped. The symptoms of anticholinergic withdrawal syndromes (sometimes called "cholinergic rebound") are diarrhea, headache, excessive salivation, and urinary frequency.

Drug Classes Associated With Depression

Alcohol	H_2 antagonists
Anticonvulsants	Narcotic analgesics
Antihypertensive agents	Oral contraceptives
Antiparkinsonian agents	Psychotropic agents
Antituberculosis agents	Steroids

An SSRI withdrawal syndrome can be seen when SSRIs are abruptly discontinued. In comparison with the anticholinergic withdrawal syndrome, the SSRI withdrawal syndrome is more common, more severe, and easily mistaken for worsening of the underlying depression or even as the emergence of mania because it mimics those processes. A more gradual tapering of the drug to wean the patient from it can prevent the withdrawal syndrome.

Risk factors for antidepressant withdrawal syndromes are length of time on the drug, potency of the drug, and half-life of the drug. The SSRI withdrawal syndrome rarely occurs after nefazodone discontinuation. Withdrawal symptoms associated with discontinuation of antidepressant therapy may occur. These reactions usually start abruptly within a few days of stopping the antidepressant and are short lived, resolving in several days to several weeks. Tapering of antidepressant dosage is recommended for any individual who has been taking these drugs for longer than 8 weeks. Awareness of these reactions is important, because some may be severe or chronic and result in inappropriate therapy if not recognized (Haddad, 1998).

Serotonin reuptake inhibitor withdrawal syndrome can be remembered by using the mnemonic *FLUSH* (Preskorn, 1999):

*F*lu-like (e.g., fatigue, myalgia, loose stools, nausea)
*L*ight-headedness/dizziness
*U*neasiness/restlessness
*S*leep and sensory disturbances
*H*eadache

TRICYCLIC ANTIDEPRESSANTS

The tricyclics derive their name from their molecular structure: a three-ring nucleus. They are generally categorized as secondary or tertiary amines. In general, secondary amines (e.g., desipramine, nortriptyline, protriptyline) are better tolerated than tertiary amines (e.g., amitriptyline, chlomipramine, doxepin, imipramine, trimipramine). Comparatively, however, they are similar in clinical efficacy, although they differ in potency and selectivity. Tertiary amines are generally less well tolerated because of an increased incidence of anticholinergic effects, cardiotoxicity, and impairment of memory and cognition. The tertiary amines have a very narrow therapeutic index; even a moderate overdose (i.e., a dose greater than 1 g is toxic and can be fatal) can cause life-threatening cardiotoxicity, hypotension, and seizures.

All TCAs enhance the activity of NE and 5-HT by blocking their neuronal reuptake. Their lack of specificity affects other receptor systems and is associated with the anticholinergic, neurologic, and cardiovascular (CV) adverse effects.

The prototype TCA is desipramine (Norpramin), a secondary amine. Although secondary amines do not have many of the adverse effects of the tertiary amines, they unfortunately share the same cardiotoxic effect. Drugs closely related to desipramine include nortriptyline (Aventyl) and protriptyline (Vivactil). Drugs significantly different from desipramine are amitriptyline (Elavil), amoxapine (Asendin), clomipramine (Anafranil), doxepin (Sinequan), imipramine (Tofranil), trimipramine (Surmontil), maprotiline, and mirtazapine (Remeron). Because of their side effects, the TCAs are not considered a first-choice treatment for depression.

NURSING MANAGEMENT OF THE PATIENT RECEIVING DESIPRAMINE

Core Drug Knowledge

Pharmacotherapeutics

Desipramine (Norpramin) is used to relieve the symptoms of depression. Unlabeled uses in dosages of 75 to 300 mg/day include an analgesic adjunct for phantom limb pain and chronic pain (e.g., migraine, chronic tension headache, diabetic neuropathy, trigeminal neuralgia, cancer pain, painful peripheral neuropathy, postherpetic neuralgia, arthritic pain), cocaine withdrawal, panic disorder, bulimia nervosa, and premenstrual syndrome.

Pharmacokinetics

Desipramine and the other tricyclics are well absorbed from the gastrointestinal (GI) tract, with peak plasma concentrations in 2 to 4 hours. They undergo a significant first-pass effect. They are highly bound (more than 90%) to plasma proteins, lipid soluble, and widely distributed in tissues, including the central nervous system (CNS). There is wide individual variation in steady-state plasma levels at a given dosage, primarily because of differences in the rate of metabolism or first-pass effect. Effective dosage levels vary greatly and must be individualized. Hepatic metabolism of desipramine and the other TCAs occurs through the CYP450 enzyme system.

Pharmacodynamics

Desipramine specifically blocks reuptake of NE into nerve terminals, thereby allowing increased concentration at postsynaptic effector sites. The chemical structure and pharmacologic activity of the TCAs resemble those of the phenothiazine antipsychotics. The TCAs possess three major pharmacologic actions in varying degrees: blocking of the amine pump, sedation, and peripheral and central anticholinergic action. Other pharmacologic and clinical effects include inhibition of histamine, sedation, mild peripheral vasodilator effects, and possible quinidine-like actions.

Contraindications and Precautions

The TCAs should be used with extreme caution in patients with CV disorders because of the possibility of conduction defects, arrhythmias, congestive heart failure (CHF), sinus tachycardia, myocardial infarction (MI), stroke, and tachycardia. These patients require cardiac surveillance at all dosage levels of the drug. In high doses, TCAs may produce arrhythmias, sinus tachycardia conduction defects, and prolonged conduction time. Elderly patients and patients with a history of cardiac disease are at special risk of developing cardiac abnormalities with TCAs.

Patients with hyperthyroidism or those receiving thyroid medication require close supervision because of the possibility of CV toxicity, including arrhythmias.

At the upper limit of the therapeutic range, serious and potentially life-threatening cardiac and CNS effects may begin to develop. Overdosage produces symptoms that are primarily an extension of the common adverse reactions. Cardiac irregularities, especially tachycardia and conduction disturbances, are common and create the most serious hazards. Fatal arrhythmias may occur as late as 56 hours after overdose. Other problems include metabolic acidosis, respiratory depression, seizures, and hyperpyrexia (McEvoy, et al., 1997). See the accompanying display, Emergency Measures for TCA Overdose, for more information.

Emergency Measures for TCA Overdose

- Provide symptomatic and supportive care.
- Monitor cardiac changes continually.
- Administer phenytoin, lidocaine, or propranolol as prescribed for life-threatening cardiac arrhythmias.
- Avoid giving drugs such as quinidine, procainamide, and disopyramide. These agents depress myocardial conductivity and contractility.
- Reserve administration of the cholinergic agonist physostigmine for life-threatening, refractory anticholinergic symptoms.

Desipramine should be prescribed cautiously for patients with cardiac disease because, like the other TCAs, it has quinidine-like effects. Administration of desipramine can slow cardiac conduction and cause arrhythmias. Cross-sensitivity is also possible among the TCAs.

Because TCAs lower the seizure threshold, they should be used with caution in patients with a history of seizures or other predisposing factors (e.g., brain damage of varying etiology, alcoholism, concomitant drugs known to lower the seizure threshold). Seizures have also occurred following administration, however, in patients with no history of seizure disorders.

Adverse Effects

Adverse effects are related to the effects of TCAs on neurotransmitters. For example, tertiary amines cause sedation because of H-1 blockade; dry mouth, constipation, urinary retention, and memory impairment result from cholinergic-receptor blockade; and orthostatic hypotension or dizziness result from alpha-1 adrenergic-receptor blockade. Because of their anticholinergic effects, tertiary-amine TCAs should be used with caution in patients with a history of urinary retention, glaucoma, or increased intraocular pressure; even average doses may precipitate a recurrence. Occasionally, in susceptible patients or those receiving anticholinergics (e.g., antiparkinsonian agents), the atropine-like effects may become significantly more pronounced and cause major health problems (e.g., paralytic ileus).

In comparison, secondary-amine TCAs (e.g., desipramine) are less antihistaminergic, anticholinergic, and alpha-1 antiadrenergic. At usual therapeutic concentrations, they block NE reuptake. Patients report sedation and anticholinergic effects most frequently, although they usually develop tolerance to these effects. Other adverse effects include disturbed concentration and confusion (especially in older adults), headache, tremors, nausea, vomiting, bone marrow depression, urinary retention, sexual function disturbances, skin rash, nasal congestion, and weight gain.

Antidepressant drugs can cause skin rashes or "drug fever" in susceptible individuals. Rarely, these allergic reactions are severe. They are most likely during the first few days of treatment but may also occur later. The drug should be discontinued if the patient develops rash or fever. Table 18-2 lists strategies for managing other side effects of antidepressant drugs.

Drug Interactions

The TCAs, especially the tertiary amines, are associated with multiple pharmacokinetic and pharmacodynamic drug interactions because they are metabolized through the CYP-450 hepatic enzyme system. They interact pharmacodynamically with several other drugs, including sedative-hypnotics, alcohol, antihypertensives, antiarrhythmics, and anticholinergics. Because of their high degree of plasma-protein binding, competition for binding sites may exist between desipramine and other highly

TABLE 18-2 Management of Side Effects of Antidepressants

Symptoms	Strategies for Management
Gastrointestinal	
Nausea, anorexia	Administer with food (or antacids) if drug absorption is unaffected.
Diarrhea	Use antidiarrheal medication (if not contraindicated).
Constipation	Diet change (increase fiber and fluids), exercise, stool softener (avoid laxatives); wait for tolerance to drug effects.
Sexual dysfunction	Discuss methods available for satisfactory sexual expression.
Anorgasmia Erectile dysfunction Impaired ejaculation	Encourage talk with health care provider regarding dosage reduction or drug holiday.
Orthostatic hypotension	Use calf exercises, wear support hose, increase fluid intake.
Anticholinergic effects (dry eyes and mouth)	Use artificial tears, frequent dental hygiene, sugar-free chewing gum; wait to develop tolerance to drug effects.
Tremor/"jitteriness"	Slow gradual titration of increasing dosages; encourage discussion with health care provider regarding dosage reduction or drug holiday.
Insomnia	Take medication in the morning (exception is trazodone).
Sedation	Caffeine (if not contraindicated), take medication at bedtime (exception is bupropion in afternoon).
Headache	Evaluate diet, stress, other drugs used; suggest dosage reduction to health care provider.
Weight gain	Decrease carbohydrate intake; consume low-fat diet; exercise.

bound substances, such as aspirin, phenytoin, and phenothiazines. Other drugs, such as methylphenidate, oral contraceptives, and antipsychotics, may interfere with the metabolism of desipramine. Moreover, TCAs may prevent the antihypertensive action of some drugs by their primary and secondary effects at NE synapses. Concomitant administration of desipramine with MAOIs may result in severe CNS toxicity. Desipramine potentiates the sedative effects of alcohol. Table 18-3 provides more information.

Assessment of Relevant Core Patient Variables

Health Status

The nurse assesses patients for preexisting CV disease, because these patients are especially sensitive to the potential cardiotoxicity of desipramine. He or she routinely monitors patients with glaucoma during drug therapy because desipramine may precipitate an acute episode of angle-closure glaucoma. Patients with a history of seizure activity or organic brain disease require careful assessment; desipramine, like the other TCAs, lowers the seizure threshold. The nurse continually assesses depressed patients for suicidal tendencies during desipramine therapy.

Life Span and Gender

The nurse also considers age-related factors associated with desipramine therapy. Lower dosages are recommended for adolescents and older adults. Dosage increases should be gradual, depending on the clinical response and any evidence of intolerance.

Children are especially susceptible to the cardiotoxic and seizure-inducing effects of high doses of tricyclics. Since 1990, four cases of sudden death in children aged 8 to 12 years have been reported with desipramine (St. Dennis, 1999). Any overdose (in excess of 10 mg/kg) in children or infants should be considered serious and potentially lethal.

Elderly patients may be especially sensitive to the anticholinergic side effects of the TCAs and should receive initial doses that amount to one half to one third of the dose administered to younger adults, because confusion, disorientation, delusions, and hallucinations are common adverse effects in older adults. Furthermore, older adults may be at an increased risk for falls during drug therapy with desipramine.

The nurse assesses the woman of child-bearing age for pregnancy or intention to become pregnant. Desipramine is pregnancy category D; animal studies have demonstrated teratogenicity and embryotoxicity. Desipramine may cause neonatal withdrawal syndrome. With other

TABLE 18-3 Agents That Interact With Desipramine

Interactants	Effect and Significance	Nursing Management
alcohol	Increased sedative effects	Avoid coadministration
anticholinergic agents	Increased anticholinergic effects	Assess patient for increasing tachycardia, dry mouth, blurred vision, constipation, and urinary retention. Coadminister with caution.
barbiturates	Decreased serum concentration of desipramine Potential additive CNS depression	Anticipate need for increase in desipramine dosage. Institute safety measures. Monitor neurologic status closely.
cimetidine, haloperidol, SSRIs	Increased plasma concentration of desipramine	Monitor serum levels as appropriate. Assess for signs of desipramine toxicity.
clonidine	Increased risk for hypertension and hypertensive crisis	Monitor blood pressure closely. Avoid coadministration.
dicumarol	Increased anticoagulant effects	Assess for signs and symptoms of bleeding. Anticipate need for decreased dosage of dicumarol.
guanethidine	Antagonism of guanethidine action	Avoid coadministration. Monitor blood pressure closely.
disulfiram	Increased risk for organic brain syndrome Increased effect of desipramine	Avoid coadministration.
levodopa	Delayed levodopa absorption and decreased bioavailability	Assess for therapeutic effects of both drugs.
MAOIs	Hyperpyrexia, sweating, confusion, seizures, tachycardia, tachypnea, hypotension, coma, DIC, and death	Avoid coadministration. Discontinue MAOIs 7–10 days before starting desipramine.
oral contraceptives, phenothiazines	Inhibition of hepatic enzyme system metabolism of desipramine leading to increased plasma levels	Monitor for signs and symptoms of desipramine toxicity.

TCAs (e.g., amitriptyline, imipramine, nortriptyline), however, there have been clinical reports of congenital malformations and limb reduction anomalies. Safety for use during pregnancy has not been established; it should be used only when clearly needed and when potential benefits to the mother outweigh potential hazards to the fetus. The nurse also questions the female patient's lactation status. TCAs are excreted into breast milk in low concentrations.

Lifestyle, Diet, and Habits

The nurse asks the patient whether he or she performs activities that require mental alertness, manual dexterity, or motor coordination. Desipramine may impair concentration and coordination, so the patient receiving desipramine should perform such activities with caution until actual drug effects are known.

Culture

The nurse keeps in mind culture-related considerations that accompany desipramine therapy. Very little published information exists concerning differences in antidepressant pharmacology among African Americans, Hispanic Americans, and European Americans; however, some studies have suggested ethnicity influences the pharmacokinetics, pharmacotherapeutics, and pharmacodynamics of psychotropic drugs. For example, results of one study showed that plasma nortriptyline levels were 50% higher in African-American patients than whites. Another reported that Hispanic-American patients have an increased sensitivity to the anticholinergic effects of tricyclics and therefore require a lower dosage. Collected survey data from multiple Asian countries indicated that imipramine and amitriptyline dosages were much lower than those customary in the United States, suggesting that Asians achieve significantly higher plasma concentrations of tricyclics and had lower clearance rates than whites. These studies have been criticized for improper control of independent variables. For example, no controls were placed on dosage for body weight or environmental variables such as diet, smoking, and alcohol consumption (Wood & Zhon, 1991).

Nursing Diagnoses and Outcomes

Several nursing diagnoses may apply to the depressed patient on "cyclic" antidepressant therapy. Examples include *Risk for Self-Directed Violence*, *Ineffective Coping*, *Fatigue*, *Constipation* or *Diarrhea* related to medication, and *Disturbed Sleep Pattern* related to medication-induced somnolence or insomnia.

In addition to these, selected nursing diagnoses for treatment with the "cyclic" antidepressants include the following:

- Disturbed Sensory Perception related to exogenous chemical alterations secondary to TCA therapy
  Desired outcome: The patient will experience normal sensory perception.
- Risk for Poisoning related to TCA toxicity
  Desired outcome: The patient will identify factors that increase the risk for and verbalize practices to prevent poisoning.
- Risk for Injury related to adverse CNS effects (e.g., blurred vision, drowsiness, hypotension) secondary to TCAs
  Desired outcome: The patient will identify factors that increase the risk for and relate an intent to practice safety measures to prevent injury.
- Imbalanced Nutrition, More than Body Requirements related to adverse effect of TCAs
  Desired outcome: The patient will verbalize reasons why there is a risk for weight gain, identify normal nutritional needs, and discuss methods to control weight.

Planning and Intervention

Maximizing Therapeutic Effects

A single daily dose may be used for maintenance therapy. A single daily dose at bedtime, if convenient, will minimize the daytime side effect of sedation. The sedative effect at bedtime may be beneficial in patients with concomitant sleep disorders.

The nurse may use therapeutic drug monitoring (TDM) to monitor effective plasma drug levels for the greatest likelihood of antidepressant response and the smallest risk of adverse effects. Optimal serum concentrations for desipramine are 150 to 250 ng/mL.

Minimizing Adverse Effects

Although the half-lives of most TCAs are long enough to permit single daily dosing, adverse reactions often require divided dosing schedules. Because of their increased risk of CV and other complications, older adults may not tolerate single daily doses.

Regular electrocardiographic monitoring of cardiac rhythm is essential for any individual taking TCAs. Periodic monitoring of blood studies, including complete blood count (CBC) with differential, serum glucose levels, and renal and hepatic function, will help detect adverse effects so that intervention may occur before interrupted drug therapy or noncompliance compromises therapeutic effects.

Providing Patient and Family Education

- The nurse teaches the patient and family that the therapeutic response will not be immediate. Several weeks may pass before any measurable clinical effect is noted.
- The nurse stresses the importance of taking the drug exactly as prescribed and of not stopping the drug abruptly or without consulting with the health care provider. Abrupt discontinuation may cause nausea, headache, and malaise.
- The patient needs assistance to stay motivated to continue treatment. To promote compliance with the

therapeutic regimen, the nurse educates the patient and family about the medication effects—both therapeutic and adverse. He or she advises the patient about adverse effects that, if unidentified, may contribute to noncompliance. These include sweating, weight gain, and sexual dysfunction.
- The nurse makes the patient aware of the possibility of photosensitivity reactions. He or she cautions the patient to avoid prolonged exposure to sunlight or bright artificial light, to apply sunscreen before exposure, and to wear protective clothing.
- The patient needs to understand the importance of keeping the drug safely stored and away from curious children. Children are very susceptible to TCA-induced cardiotoxicity.
- Most antidepressants cause some degree of sedation and may impair mental alertness and physical coordination. Thus, the nurse cautions the patient to avoid operating machinery, driving a vehicle, or engaging in activities that require focus and concentration. Because certain drug combinations produce an additive CNS depressant effect, patients should not use antidepressants concurrently with alcohol or sleep-inducing drugs (e.g., sedative-hypnotics).
- The nurse cautions the patient about the consequences of abruptly discontinuing the medication, which include such withdrawal symptoms as anxiety, headaches, dizziness, and GI disturbances.
- The nurse advises the patient to wear or carry medical identification (e.g., MedicAlert) regarding antidepressant therapy, as interactions with many other drugs (as the result of hepatic CYP-450 isoenzymes) and foods (with MAOIs) are possible.

Ongoing Assessment and Evaluation

Because of the potential for drug-related cardiotoxicity, all patients, particularly those receiving higher than usual dosages of desipramine or other TCAs, should have periodic electrocardiograms (ECGs) regardless of normal cardiac functioning before treatment. TCAs may manifest a quinidine-like effect. Patients with preexisting CV disease should be closely monitored, with ECG tracings performed routinely. Patients on multiple drug therapies should be monitored for other effects as well, because other drugs, for example, antihypertensives, alcohol, and therapeutic hormones, may cause depression.

The nurse performs baseline and periodic leukocyte and differential counts and liver function studies. Fever or sore throat may signal serious neutrophil depression; therapy should be discontinued if there is evidence of pathologic neutropenia.

Most antidepressant drugs have a lag period of 10 days to 4 weeks before a therapeutic response is noted. Increasing the dose will not shorten this period but rather increase the incidence of adverse reactions. Signs of effectiveness include improved mood and sleep patterns and increased activity and socialization. Following remission, the patient may require maintenance medication for a longer time at the lowest dose that will maintain remission. Maintenance therapy should continue for at least 3 months to decrease the possibility of relapse. ■

DRUGS CLOSELY RELATED TO P DESIPRAMINE

Nortriptyline

Nortriptyline (Aventyl) is a secondary-amine TCA. It has an unlabeled use for panic disorder.

Protriptyline

Protriptyline (Vivactil) is a secondary amine and has an unlabeled use for obstructive sleep apnea. Tachycardia and postural hypotension may occur more frequently with protriptyline than other TCAs.

DRUGS SIGNIFICANTLY DIFFERENT FROM P DESIPRAMINE

Amitriptyline

Amitriptyline (Elavil) is biotransformed to the active metabolite nortriptyline. Amitriptyline causes significant anticholinergic side effects.

MEMORY CHIP

P Desipramine

- Tricyclic antidepressant used to treat symptoms of depression
- Significant contraindications: cautious use in patients with cardiovascular and seizure disorders
- Most common adverse effects: sedation and anticholinergic effects
- Most serious adverse effects: arrhythmias, conduction defects, congestive heart failure, MI, and stroke; severe CNS toxicity when used with MAOIs
- **Life span alert: lower dosages recommended for adolescents and elderly people with gradual dosage increases based on tolerance and clinical response; divided dosing possibly needed for older adults**
- Maximizing therapeutic effects: administer as a single daily dose at bedtime; maintain serum drug concentration at 150 to 250 ng/mL
- Minimizing adverse effects: regularly monitor ECG for prolongation of Q-T interval and arrhythmias; periodically review CBC with differential, serum glucose levels, and renal and hepatic function tests
- Most significant patient education: avoid alcohol and other CNS depressant drugs to prevent additive CNS depressant effects; use sunscreen or protective clothing to prevent photosensitivity reaction; adhere to drug therapy regimen and do not discontinue abruptly; may take several weeks for elevation of mood to occur

Amoxapine

Amoxapine (Asendin), a metabolite of the antipsychotic loxapine, retains some of the postsynaptic DA receptor-blocking action of the neuroleptics. Amoxapine is not an antipsychotic, but because it has substantial neuroleptic activity, it may cause similar serious adverse effects; namely, tardive dyskinesia, pseudoparkinsonism, dystonia, and neuroleptic malignant syndrome. Its onset of antidepressant action appears to be more rapid than that of desipramine. It is a less-sedating tricyclic, but it causes significant anticholinergic side effects.

Clomipramine

Clomipramine (Anafranil) is a tertiary amine and a TCA with a similar pharmacology and antidepressant effectiveness to that of desipramine. Unlike imipramine and the other TCAs that inhibit NE reuptake, clomipramine inhibits both serotonin and NE reuptake. Its approval by the Food and Drug Administration (FDA), however, is for obsessive-compulsive disorder (OCD) only. Anticholinergic and orthostatic hypotensive adverse effects are more pronounced for clomipramine than for the other TCAs. Clomipramine is the most specific of all TCAs with regard to its ability to inhibit 5-HT reuptake versus NE reuptake. An unlabeled use is major depression. Sexual dysfunction (e.g., ejaculatory failure, erectile dysfunction) is a frequent adverse effect.

Doxepin

Doxepin (Sinequan) is a TCA that also has antianxiety effects.

Imipramine

Imipramine (Tofranil) is biotransformed to the active metabolite desipramine. Imipramine is used to treat enuresis in children. The most common reactions are nervousness, sleep disorders, tiredness, and mild GI disturbances. These usually disappear with continued therapy or dosage reduction. Dosage should not exceed 2.5 mg/kg/day.

Trimipramine

Trimipramine (Surmontil) has been reported to increase bleeding times. If trimipramine and dicumarol are used concurrently, prothrombin time (PT) and international normalized ratio should be monitored frequently.

Maprotiline

Maprotiline (Ludiomil), although identified as a tetracyclic antidepressant, has a pharmacologic and therapeutic similarity to the TCAs. It is used for various types of depressive disorders, namely, unipolar depression, depressive neurosis, and the depressive phase of bipolar disorder. An unlabeled use is treating depression-associated anxiety. Maprotiline selectively inhibits the reuptake of NE at the neuronal membrane. Lower doses are generally recommended for adults older than 60 years. Dry mouth and drowsiness are common adverse effects. Between 2 or 3 weeks of therapy are usually required for therapeutic effects to be noticeable.

Mirtazapine

Mirtazapine (Remeron) has a very complex mechanism of action that involves increases in NE and antagonism of 5-HT-receptor sites. It is the first in the new class of antidepressants: the alpha-2 receptor antagonists. Unrelated to the tricyclics, it is a potent antagonist for central presynaptic and postsynaptic alpha-2 adrenergic, 5-HT, and histamine-1 receptors and a moderate antagonist of peripheral alpha-1 adrenergic receptors. These receptor effects help to explain prominent mirtazapine effects of sedation and orthostatic hypotension. Alcohol increases the sedative effects of mirtazapine. Mirtazapine augments noradrenergic and serotonergic activity by blocking 5-HT2,3, and alpha-2 receptors. Blockade of 5-HT2,3 minimizes the risk of GI side effects and sexual dysfunction; however, increased appetite and significant weight gain remain problems. Dizziness, somnolence, and other anticholinergic side effects may occur because of its antihistaminic and antimuscarinic activity, which is dose related. At low doses (15 mg/day), its antihistaminic effects predominate, and sedation occurs. At higher doses (30 mg/day), however, an increase in adrenergic activity counteracts the sedation.

Dosage is once daily (15 to 45 mg), preferably at bedtime. Other effects include neutropenia and increased levels of cholesterol, triglycerides, and liver enzymes. Mirtazapine is rapidly and completely absorbed orally, and peak plasma concentrations are achieved within 2 hours. It is extensively metabolized by the liver and excreted in the urine. Elimination half-life is characterized by a gender difference: mean half-life in women is 37 hours, compared with 26 hours in men. Drug clearance is reduced in patients with hepatic or renal function impairment and in older adults.

MONOAMINE OXIDASE INHIBITORS

Monoamine oxidase is a complex enzyme system widely distributed throughout the body. It is responsible for the metabolic degradation of biogenic amines, including NE, epinephrine, DA, and 5-HT. Drugs described as MAOIs inhibit MAO, increasing the concentration of the endogenous amines.

Specifically, there are two subtypes of MAO. MAO A, found primarily in the GI tract, liver, and peripheral adrenergic nerves, predominantly deaminates NE, 5-HT, and tyramine. MAO B, found in the brain, primarily breaks down DA. Consequently, inhibition of MAO results in increased concentrations of these amines throughout the body. Although the precise antidepressant mechanism of MAOIs is unclear, it is thought that the increases in 5-HT and NE or changes in other amine concentrations in the CNS are responsible.

Historically, MAOIs were used to manage tuberculosis. Patients taking these drugs often experienced CNS stimulation (mood elevation) and hypotension. Their very limited use as antidepressants and discontinued use as antihypertensives stem from their intense adverse effects and potentially fatal interactions (hypertensive crisis) rather than from ineffectiveness. Potentially fatal pharmacodynamic drug-drug interactions can occur with MAOIs when combined with a variety of drugs that are 5-HT or NE agonists or with foods rich in tyramine.

In general, nonselective MAOIs are indicated for patients with atypical (exogenous) depression and in some patients who are unresponsive to other antidepressant pharmacotherapy. They are rarely first-choice drugs. As irreversible inhibitors of MAO, they may require up to 2 weeks for normal amine metabolism to be restored following drug discontinuation. Studies have also indicated that chronic therapy with MAOIs causes downregulation in adrenergic and serotonergic receptors.

The prototype MAOI is phenelzine (Nardil). Drugs closely related to phenelzine are isocarboxazid (Marplan) and tranylcypromine (Parnate). A significantly different drug is selegiline (L-Deprenyl).

NURSING MANAGEMENT OF THE PATIENT RECEIVING P PHENELZINE

Core Drug Knowledge

Pharmacotherapeutics

Phenelzine is used mainly to treat atypical or neurotic depression that is refractory to other drug therapy or treatments. Patients may have mixed anxiety and depression and phobic or hypochondriacal features. In some cases, phenelzine is used to treat bulimia, cocaine addiction, and panic disorder associated with agoraphobia.

Pharmacokinetics

Monoamine oxidase inhibitors appear to be well absorbed following oral administration, and peak levels of phenelzine are reached in 2 to 4 hours. Maximal inhibition of MAO, however, does not occur for 5 to 10 days. Onset of antidepressant action can take from 7 days to 8 weeks. It is thought that the release of active metabolites metabolizes the hydrazine MAOIs (phenelzine, isocarboxazid). Inactivation is primarily by acetylation. The clinical effects of phenelzine may continue for up to 2 weeks after discontinuation of therapy. Phenelzine and isocarboxazid are excreted in the urine mostly as metabolites.

Half-life is fairly short and unrelated to the length of enzyme inhibition, which is prolonged. Slow acetylation of hydrazine MAOIs may yield exaggerated effects after standard dosing.

Pharmacodynamics

The MAOIs increase concentrations of 5-HT, NE, and DA within the neuronal synapse because they inhibit the MAO enzyme. Phenelzine, a hydrazine derivative, irreversibly inhibits both MAO A and MAO B.

Contraindications and Precautions

Hepatic dysfunction is a contraindication for using phenelzine because hydrazine compounds damage the hepatic parenchyma. Phenelzine is also contraindicated in patients with CHF and pheochromocytoma. Cautious use is advised in patients with ischemic heart disease, stroke, and MI, because phenelzine may produce depressant effects, such as orthostatic hypotension, bradycardia, and negative inotropic effects.

Adverse Effects

Hepatotoxicity that may accompany the use of phenelzine appears to be unrelated to dosage or treatment duration. Other adverse effects are anticholinergic, including blurred vision, constipation, and dry mouth. These effects are more pronounced at dosages above 45 mg/day. CNS-related adverse effects include akathisia, ataxia, dizziness, drowsiness, headache, insomnia, and nystagmus. Adverse effects related to other systems include agranulocytosis, anemia, leukopenia, thrombocytopenia, sexual function disturbances, and urinary retention.

The most serious adverse reactions involve changes in blood pressure and hypertensive crisis. Use of these drugs in elderly or debilitated patients or in patients with hypertension, CV problems, or cerebrovascular disease is inadvisable, as is coadministration with certain drugs or foods.

Drug Interactions

The mixed-acting sympathomimetics, such as pseudoephedrine and phenylpropanolamine (common ingredients in over-the-counter [OTC] decongestants, appetite suppressants, weight-loss products], release NE from adrenergic nerve endings. The indirect-acting sympathomimetics trigger NE release. Acute, severe, and potentially fatal hypertensive crises are possible when combining phenelzine with drugs from these classes, tyramine, or tryptophan (Table 18-4).

These drug-drug or drug-food interactions occur because phenelzine and the other agents act in peripheral adrenergic nerve endings to increase the build-up of NE, although they prevent the release of NE in response to normal nerve activity. Combined with the mixed-acting and indirect-acting sympathomimetics, however, NE release is not inhibited. The result is an intense adrenergic response because of the extra supply of NE. Ingestion of a tyramine-containing food (e.g., cured or fermented foods, aged cheeses, Chianti or other red wine, coffee, soy sauce) or a sympathomimetic drug may precipitate a hypertensive crisis. Normally hepatic MAO degrades these substances rapidly. When MAO is inhibited, tyramine remains underdegraded and triggers the release of accumulated NE, which in turn causes a hypertensive episode. The earliest symptom may be a severe headache. The necessity of avoiding these substances to prevent a life-threatening hypertensive crisis is the major limitation of MAOIs.

TABLE 18-4 Agents That Interact With Phenelzine

Interactants	Effect and Significance	Nursing Management
anesthetics	Adverse cardiovascular effects from sympathetic stimulation	Monitor heart rate, rhythm, and blood pressure for adverse effect from sympathetic stimulation.
antihypertensives (e.g., guanethidine, methyldopa)	Loss of antihypertensive effects	Monitor blood pressure for degree of control.
beta-adrenergic blockers	Bradycardia possible during concurrent use of MAOIs and beta adrenergic blockers	Monitor heart rate, rhythm, and cardiac output for adverse effect from bradycardia.
dextromethorphan	Hyperpyrexia, hypotension, and death associated with this combination*	Caution patients taking MAOIs to avoid OTC cold and cough preparations.
levodopa	Hypertensive reactions with combinations of levodopa and MAOIs	Avoid concurrent administration. Monitor cardiovascular status for adverse effect.
L-tryptophan	Coadministration resulting in hyperreflexia, confusion, disorientation, amnesia, ataxia, and Babinski signs	Caution the patient taking MAOIs to avoid food supplements, herbal/homeopathic, or home remedies without approval from the health care provider.
meperidine	Coadministration may result in agitation, seizures, fever, apnea, and death with possible adverse reactions weeks after MAOI withdrawal	Avoid concomitant administration of MAOIs and meperidine. For analgesia, administer other narcotic analgesics with caution.
SSRI, TCA, or venlafaxine antidepressants	Potential serious (occasionally fatal) reactions, including hyperthermia, rigidity, autonomic instability with labile blood pressure, myoclonus, and extreme agitation	Monitor neurologic and cardiovascular status for adverse effect.
sulfonamide compounds	Coadministration may cause either sulfonamide or MAOI toxicity	Avoid concurrent administration.
sulfonylurea antidiabetic agents	Possible potentiation of hypoglycemic response and delayed recovery from hypoglycemia	Monitor patients with diabetes for level of control and incidence of hypoglycemic episodes.
sumatriptan	Coadministration may cause sumatriptan toxicity	Avoid concurrent administration.
sympathomimetics (mixed acting or indirect acting, including anorexiants)	MAOI potentiation of sympathomimetic substances may cause severe headache, hypertension, hyperpyrexia possibly resulting in hypertensive crisis	Avoid concurrent administration.†
thiazide diuretics	Exaggerated hypotensive effects may result from concurrent use	Avoid concurrent administration. Monitor cardiovascular status and blood pressure for degree of control.

*Interaction inconclusive due to lack of adequate patient data.
†Direct-acting agents appear to interact minimally (if at all).

Assessment of Relevant Core Patient Variables

Health Status

Patients taking phenelzine should have a baseline CV assessment, CBC, and liver function tests. The nurse assesses the patient's orientation, mood, and affect as well, because phenelzine may cause memory and emotional changes, irritability, and nervousness.

Life Span and Gender

The nurse must consider the patient's age and its relation to phenelzine therapy. Phenelzine is not recommended for patients younger than 16 years. Because patients older than 60 years may be more prone to adverse drug effects, their dosages (less than 60 mg/day) should be increased gradually and adjusted accordingly.

The nurse asks the woman of child-bearing age if she is pregnant, intends to become pregnant, or is breastfeeding. Phenelzine is FDA pregnancy category C. It crosses the placenta and enters breast milk.

Lifestyle, Diet, and Habits

The nurse assesses the patient's lifestyle to determine whether he or she performs activities requiring alertness, physical coordination, or manual dexterity. Because of associated adverse effects (ataxia, drowsiness, blurred vision), patients need to exercise caution when driving or operating machinery. The nurse also must evaluate the patient's nutritional status. Because phenelzine is associated with pyridoxine deficiency (numbness, paresthesias, and edema), the patient may need a dietary pyridoxine (vitamin B6) supplement.

The nurse must ask the patient about his or her participation in outdoor activity. Phenelzine may cause photosensitivity. The patient should wear sunscreen and protective clothing in prolonged outdoor exposure, such as recreational or occupational pursuits.

Environment

The nurse must consider the environment in which phenelzine will be administered. The drug should be kept in a tightly closed container away from light and heat.

Culture

The nurse must consider the patient's ethnic background when beginning drug therapy with phenelzine. Acetylation inactivates phenelzine and its metabolites. About one half of the American and European populations (and more in Asia) are slow acetylators of hydrazine-type drugs, including phenelzine. This may contribute to the exaggerated effects observed in some patients who receive standard doses of phenelzine (Hardman, Limberd, Molinof, Ruddon, & Gilman, 1996).

Nursing Diagnoses and Outcomes

- Risk for Injury related to drug-nutrient, drug-drug, or drug-environment interactions or hypertensive crisis secondary to MAOI antidepressant therapy
  Desired outcome: The patient will remain safe and injury-free during drug therapy.
- Ineffective Therapeutic Regimen Management related to MAOI-required dietary restrictions
  Desired outcome: The patient will verbalize an understanding of the need to follow a low-tyramine diet and demonstrate appropriate dietary choices.
- Imbalanced Nutrition, More than Body Requirements related to adverse effect of MAOIs
  Desired outcome: The patient will verbalize reasons why there is a risk for weight gain, identify normal nutritional needs, and discuss methods to control weight.

Planning and Intervention

Maximizing Therapeutic Effects

Before MAOI therapy is initiated, platelet MAO activity (mostly B subtype) is usually measured. After therapy is under way, an inhibition of more than 85% is associated with therapeutic response (Hardman, et al., 1996). Platelet enzyme inhibition exceeding 95%, however, increases the risk of serious drug and food interactions.

Minimizing Adverse Effects

The difficulty with the MAOIs is found in the numerous dietary and medication restrictions that the patient must obey to avoid drug-food and drug-drug interactions. Taking an MAOI with foods high in tyramine or certain drugs (e.g., ephedrine, dextromethorphan, cocaine, decongestants, appetite suppressants) increases the potential for a hypertensive crisis. The symptoms of hypertensive crisis include severe occipital headache, stiff neck, nausea, vomiting, diaphoresis, and extremely elevated systolic and diastolic blood pressure.

The nurse advises the patient to avoid herbal preparations (e.g., St. John's wort, L-tryptophan, ginseng), alcohol, OTC products, or any stimulant or illicit drug. Use of these substances increases the likelihood of adverse effects or hypertensive crisis. Dosages exceeding 30 mg/day may result in postural hypotension, leading to syncope. If dosage increases are necessary, they should be made gradually. Other measures to minimize adverse effects include maintaining a tyramine/L-tryptophan-restricted diet during and for at least 2 weeks after phenelzine therapy and giving the drug with food or milk if GI discomfort is problematic. If the patient has been on fluoxetine therapy, at least 6 weeks should elapse before phenelzine therapy begins.

Providing Patient and Family Education

- The nurse warns all patients taking MAOIs against eating foods with high tyramine, DA, or tryptophan content and consuming alcohol during and for 2 weeks following phenelzine treatment. The patient taking MAOIs must understand and follow the special required dietary guidelines. Any high-protein food that is aged or undergoes breakdown by putrefaction process has the potential to produce a hypertensive crisis in patients taking MAOIs.
- The nurse cautions patients against self-medication with certain proprietary agents such as cold, hay fever, or weight-reduction preparations containing sympathomimetic amines while undergoing MAOI therapy.
- The nurse instructs patients not to consume excessive amounts of caffeine in any form.
- The nurse stresses the importance of not discontinuing the medication, adjusting dosage, or ingesting any other medication (including OTC items) except on the advice of the health care provider. He or she alerts the patient that phenelzine may cause drowsiness or blurred vision. The nurse warns the patient to exercise caution when driving or performing other tasks that require alertness, coordination, or physical dexterity until effects of the drug are known.
- The nurse alerts the patient to the possibility of orthostatic hypotension, dizziness, weakness, or fainting when arising from a sitting position.
- The nurse stresses to the patient and family that antidepressant effects may be delayed a few weeks. He or she cautions them to notify the health care provider if severe headache, palpitation, tachycardia, a sense of constriction in the throat or chest, sweating, dizziness, neck stiffness, nausea, vomiting, or other unusual symptoms occur.

Ongoing Assessment and Evaluation

Observation of the patient is necessary to identify the therapeutic effects of phenelzine. These may occur within 7 days after therapy begins, although in some, a therapeutic response may not occur for up to 6 to 8 weeks. Effectiveness of phenelzine is demonstrated by improved mood and sleep patterns, and increased socialization in depressed patients.

During therapy periodic hepatic function tests, such as aspartate transaminase, alanine transaminase, and bilirubin, should be performed. Phenelzine should be discontinued at the first sign of hepatic dysfunction or jaundice. Blood pressure should be monitored frequently to detect any abnormal pressor response. Therapy should be discontinued immediately if the patient reports palpitations or frequent headaches. These signs may signal a hypertensive crisis. ■

DRUGS CLOSELY RELATED TO P PHENELZINE

Isocarboxazid

Isocarboxazid (Marplan) is used to treat depression. It is characterized by a low incidence of altered liver function or jaundice. Cautious use in patients with hyperthyroidism is necessary because of increased sensitivity to pressor amines. Concomitant therapy of isocarboxazid with buspirone should be avoided because it may elevate blood pressure. At least 10 days should be elapse between discontinuation of isocarboxazid and institution of buspirone.

Trancyclopromine

Tranylcypromine (Parnate) resembles phenelzine in its pharmacotherapeutic and pharmacokinetic features. Pharmacodynamically, it reversibly binds to MAO. Tranylcypromine is contraindicated for patients older than 60 years, those with cardiac disease or hypertension, or those at risk for CV accident.

DRUG SIGNIFICANTLY DIFFERENT FROM P PHENELZINE

Selegiline (L-Deprenyl), an MAOB selective agent, is used therapeutically for the treatment of Parkinson disease.

MEMORY CHIP

P Phenelzine

- MAOI used to treat atypical or neurotic depression refractory to other drug therapy or treatment
- Significant contraindications: hepatic impairment, congestive heart failure, and pheochromocytoma
- Most common adverse effect: hepatotoxicity and anticholinergic effects
- Most serious adverse effect: hypertensive crisis, usually resulting from drug interaction with tyramine
- **Life span alert: dosage for elderly patients limited to less than 60 mg/day, increased gradually; not for use in patients less than 16 years of age**
- Maximizing therapeutic effects: Monitor platelet MAO activity with goal of inhibition more than 85% but less than 95%
- Minimizing adverse effects: avoidance of foods high in tyramine, OTC cold remedies, herbal preparations, alcohol, and any stimulants or illicit drugs; gradual increase in dosages; administration with food or milk
- Most significant patient education: avoid eating foods high in tyramine during and for at least 2 weeks after cessation of therapy; adhere to drug therapy regimen and do not discontinue abruptly; may take several weeks for antidepressant effects to occur

C SELECTIVE SEROTONIN REUPTAKE INHIBITORS

As a drug class, SSRIs are often the first choice for treating depression. Unlike the TCAs and MAOIs, they lack cardiotoxicity and have minimal anticholinergic and hypotensive effects. In comparison with the TCAs, SSRIs have similar efficacy but fewer side effects and significantly improved safety.

The prototype SSRI is fluoxetine (Prozac). Drugs closely related to fluoxetine include citalopram (Calexa), fluvoxamine (Luvox), nefazodone (Serzone), paroxetine (Paxil), sertraline (Zoloft), and trazodone (Desyrel). A drug significantly different from fluoxetine is venlafaxine (Effexor).

NURSING MANAGEMENT OF THE PATIENT RECEIVING P FLUOXETINE

Core Drug Knowledge

Pharmacotherapeutics

Fluoxetine, citalopram, fluvoxamine, paroxetine, and sertraline are similar in efficacy, and all have a wide therapeutic index. They are used to treat depression, obsessive-compulsive disorder, panic disorder, posttraumatic stress disorder, and bulimia nervosa. Unlabeled uses include ADHD, bipolar disorder, borderline personality disorder, schizophrenia, and migraine or tension-type headaches. Additional unlabeled uses for fluoxetine include alcoholism, anorexia nervosa, premenstrual syndrome, and social phobia.

Pharmacokinetics

Fluoxetine is well absorbed following oral administration, with peak plasma levels occurring within 4 to 8 hours. The onset of antidepressant activity is rather slow (1 to 3 weeks), with optimal therapeutic effects requiring 4 or more weeks of therapy.

Fluoxetine undergoes hepatic metabolism to its active metabolite, S-norfluoxetine. The elimination half-lives of both compounds (1 to 3 days for fluoxetine and 7 to 9 days for S-fluoxetine) appear prolonged in patients with impaired hepatic and renal function. They can be as long as 16 days.

SSRIs are extensively metabolized by the liver and should be used with caution in patients with severe liver impairment. The elimination half-life of fluoxetine was prolonged in a study of patients with cirrhosis, with a mean of 7.6 days. Norfluoxetine elimination was also delayed, with a mean duration of 12 days. Food does not appear to affect systemic bioavailability of fluoxetine, although it may delay absorption.

Pharmacodynamics

Fluoxetine is a potent and selective inhibitor of neuronal 5-HT reuptake and has a weak effect on NE and DA neuronal reuptake. The chronic administration of sertraline in animal studies was found to downregulate brain NE receptors.

The major pharmacologic difference between sertraline and TCAs is the incidence of adverse effects. Because the SSRIs do not have a high affinity for muscarinic, histaminergic, and alpha-adrenergic receptors, their capacity for causing anticholinergic, sedative, cardiac, and orthostatic hypotensive effects is considerably less than that of the TCAs.

Contraindications and Precautions

Fluoxetine should be administered with caution in patients with impaired renal or hepatic function. These patients may require a lower or less-frequent dosing schedule. Patients with a history of seizure disorder are at risk for seizures with the SSRIs.

Adverse Effects

Unlike the tricyclics, fluoxetine and the other SSRIs have fewer adverse anticholinergic and CV effects and usually do not cause weight gain. Adverse effects, which are mild and brief, include GI distress (anorexia, nausea, vomiting, diarrhea), headache, fatigue, insomnia, and sexual function disturbances (delayed ejaculation, anorgasmia). Some of these side effects are transient, subsiding within the first 1 to 2 weeks of therapy. Other adverse effects may include hematologic problems, such as blood dyscrasias, leukopenia, and altered platelet function. The most limiting adverse effects of the SSRIs are disturbances of sexual function.

Altered appetite and weight loss, especially in underweight depressed patients, has occurred with fluoxetine. Seizures have also occurred.

Drug Interactions

Fluoxetine inhibits hepatic drug-metabolizing CYP enzymes to a substantial degree and thus has the potential to cause clinically important pharmacokinetic drug-drug interactions. Drugs affected by this inhibition include antiarrhythmics, anticoagulants, antipsychotics, neuroleptics, and the TCAs (Table 18-5).

SSRIs are highly bound to plasma protein. Coadministration with another highly protein-bound drug may cause displacement of either drug and increased plasma concentrations of the free drug. Fluoxetine therapy may increase serum determinations of alkaline phosphatase, blood urea nitrogen, creatine phosphokinase, and uric acid. It may decrease levels of calcium.

Assessment of Relevant Core Patient Variables

Health Status

As with other SSRIs, the nurse reviews the drug history for current drugs used, the health history for any significant illnesses, and mental status, because SSRIs may precipitate mania or hypomania in susceptible patients. The nurse also investigates for a history of seizures, as SSRIs are used with care in patients with such a history. SSRIs should be discontinued if seizures occur.

Life Span and Gender

The nurse must consider the patient's age. Safety and efficacy have not been established for children. Elderly patients may not be able to tolerate once-daily dosing. Because of age-related changes, older adults are especially sensitive to the orthostatic hypotension that occasionally results from the SSRIs.

The nurse must ask a female patient of child-bearing age whether she is pregnant, intends to become pregnant, or is breast-feeding. The FDA classifies fluoxetine in pregnancy risk category C. The drug is excreted in breast milk.

Lifestyle, Diet, and Habits

The SSRIs can affect sexual functioning. Men most often report delayed ejaculation or ejaculatory failure, whereas women report the inability to achieve orgasm. The nurse inquires about any changes in sexual functioning, because they may lead to noncompliance.

During administration of fluoxetine, the nurse asks the patient about any changes in appetite and inquires about his or her eating habits. Fluoxetine may decrease appetite and stimulate the CNS; it has the greatest anorectic effect of the SSRIs. Patients who ingest caffeine-rich foods and beverages may report increased stimulation and even insomnia after SSRI therapy begins. Morning or early afternoon administration is advisable to prevent night-time sleep disturbances.

The nurse asks the patient about his or her consumption of alcohol. The combination of fluoxetine with alcohol or anxiolytics will increase CNS depression.

Culture

The nurse must consider the patient's cultural background. A polymorphism displayed by a CYP-450 isoenzyme means that some individuals may lack the enzyme, be poor drug metabolizers, and show SSRI tox-

TABLE 18-5 Agents That Interact With Fluoxetine

Interactants	Effect and Significance	Nursing Management
MAOIs	Potentiation of serotonin by fluoxetine and deamination of serotonin by MAOIs, leading to serotonin syndrome (confusion, seizures, severe hypertension)	Avoid concomitant use.
tryptophan, sumatriptan	Increased serotonin levels, leading potentially to serotonin syndrome	Avoid concurrent use.
cyclosporine	Increased cyclosporine concentrations	Monitor cyclosporine level carefully during administration and after discontinuance of fluoxetine.
TCAs	Increased serum TCA levels	Monitor for possible TCA toxicity.
haloperidol, pimozide	Increased risk for adverse effects of these drugs	Coadminister these drugs with fluoxetine with caution.
buspirone	Increased anxiety, resulting from opposite actions of these drugs (buspirone decreases serotonin; fluoxetine increases serotonin)	Avoid concomitant use.
carbamazepine, phenytoin	Impaired metabolism of carbamazepine and phenytoin, leading to possible toxicity	Monitor drug levels, and anticipate anticonvulsant dosage adjustments.
beta blockers: propranolol, metoprolol	Inhibited metabolism of beta blockers, leading to bradycardia and possibly heart block	Monitor cardiovascular status carefully.
lithium	Increased or decreased lithium level	Monitor lithium levels; intervene accordingly.
warfarin	Potentiation of hypoprothrombinemic effects, leading to bleeding/hemorrhage	Avoid concomitant use.
dextromethorphan	Possible hallucinations	Assess neurologic status, including cognition and thought processes. Avoid coadministration.
benzodiazepines	Decreased clearance of benzodiazepines cleared by the hepatic enzyme system	Monitor serum levels of benzodiazepine as appropriate. Assess for changes in psychomotor performance.
clozapine	Increased serum clozapine levels	Monitor for signs and symptoms of clozapine toxicity. Anticipate reduction in clozapine dosage.

icity even at low doses. Approximately 2% of African Americans lack this enzyme.

Nursing Diagnosis and Outcome

- Imbalanced Nutrition, Less than Body Requirements related to the adverse effect of anorexia secondary to fluoxetine

  Desired outcome: The patient will verbalize reasons why there is a risk for weight loss, identify normal nutritional needs, and discuss methods to maintain weight.

Planning and Intervention

Maximizing Therapeutic Effects

The patient needs encouragement to persevere with drug therapy, because he or she may not note improvement in mood and functioning for several weeks. Unfortunately, there is no delay in the appearance of adverse effects. For this reason, the patient may skip or double drug doses, which will impair therapeutic effects. Optimal serum concentrations for sertraline are 20 to 55 ng/mL.

Minimizing Adverse Effects

Patients with diabetes may lose glycemic control because fluoxetine alters glycemic control. Insulin or oral antidiabetic drug therapy may need adjustment. Hypoglycemia has occurred during fluoxetine therapy, and hyperglycemia has developed following discontinuation. Patients with diabetes may need to monitor blood glucose levels more frequently.

Photosensitivity is possible. Therefore, patients must take protective measures (e.g., sunscreens, protective clothing) against exposure to ultraviolet light or sunlight until tolerance is determined.

Providing Patient and Family Education

- The nurse informs patients about adverse effects (e.g., orthostatic hypotension) and advises against sudden position changes to prevent dizziness, accidental falls, or syncope.
- The nurse discusses the increased stimulant effect resulting from the combination of SSRIs and caffeine and advises the patient to modify the diet accordingly.
- Other instructions include cautioning the patient about driving and other activities requiring alertness,

because sertraline may cause drowsiness or dizziness and may adversely affect motor coordination.

Ongoing Assessment and Evaluation

Because fluoxetine is associated with GI upset, anorexia, and weight loss (or occasionally weight gain), the patient's weight should be monitored. Oral drugs may be given with food to minimize GI upset. Additionally, if the patient also has diabetes, the nurse should continue to assess glycemic control and inform the health care provider of any signs and symptoms of hypoglycemia reported by the patient. Evaluation of sexual functioning is important because changes in this area may have some impact on compliance with drug therapy. Effectiveness of fluoxetine therapy is demonstrated by the patient's report of fewer symptoms of depression and ability to manage adverse effects after sufficient time has elapsed for the therapeutic drug effects to occur. ■

DRUGS CLOSELY RELATED TO P FLUOXETINE

Citalopram

Citalopram (Calexa) is structurally unrelated to the other SSRIs, although it is highly selective. Citalopram has good oral bioavailability. Peak plasma levels are reached within 2 to 4 hours of administration, although there is a 2- to 3-week delay in the onset of the antidepressant activity.

MEMORY CHIP

P Fluoxetine

- SSRI used to treat depression, OCD, panic disorder, posttraumatic stress disorder, and bulimia nervosa
- Significant contraindications: cautious use in patients with impaired hepatic and renal function or seizure disorder
- Most common adverse effect: GI distress and sexual dysfunction
- Most serious adverse effect: hematologic problems, such as blood dyscrasias, leukopenia, and altered platelet function
- **Life span alert: possible inability to tolerate once-daily dosing and increased sensitivity for orthostatic hypotension in elderly people**
- Maximizing therapeutic effects: encourage to continue to adhere to drug therapy because improvement may take several weeks but adverse effects can occur at any time
- Minimizing adverse effects: monitor blood glucose levels frequently, especially in patients with diabetes, avoid exposure to ultraviolet light
- Most significant patient education: avoid alcohol and other CNS depressants to avoid possible additive depressive effects; avoid sudden position changes; may take several weeks for elevation of mood to occur

Half-life is 30 hours. Citalopram undergoes hepatic metabolism by CYP-450 enzymes to two active metabolites, although they do not contribute significantly to the antidepressant effects. Some clinical studies suggest that patients' aging may affect the area under the curve by 30% and half-life by 50%. Citalopram causes less sexual dysfunction than the other SSRIs, but can cause insomnia, dizziness, somnolence, and gastric side effects.

Fluvoxamine

Fluvoxamine (Luvox) has the shortest half-life of all the SSRIs and is the most likely to cause sedation. Anorexia and weight loss are less of a concern with fluvoxamine than with fluoxetine. Fluvoxamine is currently approved for use in obsessive-compulsive disorder. It is administered orally, and its absorption is rapid, nearly complete, and unaffected by food. Peak concentrations occur within 2 to 8 hours after oral administration. Steady-state serum concentrations are achieved after 10 days of therapy.

Fluvoxamine is less protein bound than other SSRIs (approximately 77%) and undergoes hepatic metabolism. Its inactive metabolites are renally excreted, and its excretion into breast milk is negligible. The elimination half-life is approximately 15 hours after administration of a single dose but increases with multiple dosing and hepatic function impairment. In older adults the clearance is reduced as well. Half-life does not change with renal impairment. A lower dosage or less frequent administration may be necessary in these situations. Fluvoxamine inhibits hepatic drug-metabolizing CYP enzymes to a substantial degree and thus has the potential for causing clinically important pharmacokinetic drug-drug interactions.

Nefazodone

Nefazodone (Serzone) is a new oral antidepressant with a distinct mechanism of action. Although nefazodone is structurally similar to trazodone, it causes less sedation and orthostatic hypotension. Similar in effectiveness to other antidepressants in treating major depression, nefazodone lacks the CV toxicity seen with the tricyclics and does not cause the restlessness, insomnia, or inhibition of REM sleep frequently associated with the SSRIs. The pharmacologic actions of nefazodone involve both the serotonergic and, to a lesser extent, the noradrenergic systems. Nefazodone antagonizes alpha-adrenergic receptors, and this blockade produces sedation, muscle relaxation, and CV effects (e.g., hypotension, reflex tachycardia, minor changes in ECG patterns). As with other antidepressants, nefazodone antidepressant effects may not be noticeable for several weeks.

Following oral administration, nefazodone is rapidly and completely absorbed, although food delays absorption and decreases bioavailability by about 20%. Peak plasma concentrations occur in about 1 hour, and steady-state concentrations are achieved in about 5 days. Nefazodone is distributed in most body tissues, including the CNS. Protein binding is approximately 99%. The half-life of nefazodone is 2 to 8 hours. Excretion of nefazodone and its metabolites (at least two are active) occurs through urine (55%) and feces (20% to 30%). Elimination is prolonged in patients with impaired hepatic or renal function.

Paroxetine

Paroxetine (Paxil) has the highest specificity for 5-HT of all the SSRIs. It is effective in depression that has proved resistant to other antidepressants or is complicated by anxiety. Paroxetine is administered orally and is completely absorbed. Individual patient response seems to vary, but steady-state concentrations are achieved in about 10 days. The therapeutic effects, however, may require 1 to 4 weeks. The drug is widely distributed and is 93% to 95% bound to plasma protein. It is extensively metabolized to several inactive metabolites. Excretion is primarily renal (about 62%) and fecal (about 36%). The elimination half-life is approximately 21 hours. Elderly patients or those with renal or hepatic impairment are prone to increased plasma concentrations. Paroxetine inhibits hepatic drug-metabolizing CYP enzymes to a substantial degree and thus has the potential to cause clinically important pharmacokinetic drug-drug interactions.

Sertraline

Sertraline (Zoloft) has been reported to increase bleeding times. If fluoxetine and Coumadin are used concurrently, PT and international normalized ratios should be monitored frequently.

Trazodone

Trazodone (Desyrel) is a weak 5-HT transporter inhibitor and blocks the 5-HT2 receptors. Blockade of these receptors diminishes some troubling adverse effects associated with 5-HT transporter inhibitors (e.g., insomnia, jitteriness, sexual dysfunction). Trazodone is also an alpha-receptor antagonist, so it can cause dizziness and orthostatic changes. Compared with the tricyclics, it is relatively free of antimuscarinic and adverse CV effects. It inhibits the reuptake of 5-HT, although this action is less potent than with fluoxetine. Administered orally, it is well absorbed, with food enhancing its absorption. Peak levels are achieved within 1 to 2 hours. Therapeutic response usually occurs within 2 weeks. Metabolism in the liver is extensive with none of its metabolites believed pharmacologically active. Elimination is mainly through the urine. Trazodone may cause priapism.

DRUG SIGNIFICANTLY DIFFERENT FROM P FLUOXETINE

Venlafaxine (Effexor) is a mixed noradrenergic-5-HT reuptake inhibitor. It has no significant affinity for alpha-adrenergic, histaminergic, or muscarinic receptors. Its pharmacologic effects are dose related, and it exhibits a triphasic pharmacologic effect over its useful dosage range. At the lowest effective dose, venlafaxine primarily affects 5-HT reuptake. Its noradrenergic and dopaminergic effects occur at higher concentrations (dosages of more than 300 mg/day). It may cause constipation, diaphoresis, disturbance in sexual function, dizziness, hypertension, nervousness, nausea, and somnolence. Thus, gradual titration of dosage increases is important to maximize venlafaxine's therapeutic effect. Minimizing side effects may be accomplished by an extended release formulation of venlafaxine, which provides a more stable plasma and CNS drug level than the rapidly absorbed and rapidly eliminated immediate-release drug formulation.

C MOOD STABILIZERS

Generally, manic episodes are initially treated with drugs that are described as mood stabilizers. Mood stabilizers control or prevent mood swings in patients with bipolar disorder. Lithium carbonate (Eskalith), usually simply called lithium, is the prototype antimanic drug. Other drugs used to treat bipolar disorder and stabilize mood include carbamazepine, gabapentin, and valproic acid. These drugs may be combined with lithium for a greater therapeutic effect.

NURSING MANAGEMENT OF THE PATIENT RECEIVING P LITHIUM

Core Drug Knowledge

Pharmacotherapeutics

Lithium is called a mood stabilizer because its primary action is to prevent mood swings. The drug has several unlabeled uses. It increases the neutrophil count in patients with cancer chemotherapy-induced neutropenia and in patients with acquired immune deficiency syndrome (AIDS) who receive zidovudine therapy. It also is useful in preventing cluster headache and in treating bulimia, alcoholism, and postpartum-affective and corticosteroid-induced psychoses. The therapeutic range for lithium is 0.5 to 1.2 mEq/L.

Pharmacokinetics

Nearly complete absorption from the GI tract occurs within 6 hours. Food does not significantly impair absorption. Peak plasma levels occur in 0.5 to 3 hours, and plasma half-life is about 20 hours. Onset of action is slow (5 to 7 days, with full therapeutic effects established in 10 to 21 days). Lithium is not protein bound or biotransformed into metabolites. Excretion occurs almost entirely in the urine (95%) and varies with pregnancy, age, and renal status. Lithium and sodium compete for resorption in the proximal renal tubule, so many factors (i.e., hypernatremia or hyponatremia, dehydration, or diuretic use) can affect lithium clearance. Dose-related adverse effects are not usually serious at serum levels maintained below 1.5 mEq/L.

Distribution approximates total body water and is complete within 6 to 10 hours. Higher concentrations occur in the bones, thyroid gland, and portions of the brain than in the serum. Lithium is not protein bound. Although distribution across the blood-brain barrier is slow, the cerebrospinal fluid level is 40% of the plasma concentration. Elimination half-life is 24 hours (range, 10 to 50 hours); steady state is reached in 5 to 7 days. In the kidneys, 80% of lithium is resorbed. Lithium and sodium compete for resorption in the proximal renal tubule.

During periods of sodium depletion (e.g., dehydration, diuretic use), the kidney will try to conserve sodium and lithium by resorbing more than 80% from the proximal tubule. The increased resorption causes the lithium serum level to rise, possibly leading to toxicity. Sodium loading will increase lithium excretion, and serum levels will decrease.

Pharmacodynamics

Lithium is a monovalent cation that competes with calcium, magnesium, potassium, and sodium in body tissues and at binding sites. It alters sodium transport in nerve and muscle cells and effects a shift toward intraneuronal catecholamine metabolism. The specific mechanism of action in mania is unknown, but it does affect the synthesis, storage, release, and reuptake of central monoamine neurotransmitters, including NE, 5-HT, DA, Ach, and GABA. Its antimanic effects may be the result of increases in NE reuptake and increased 5-HT receptor sensitivity. Lithium also affects distribution of sodium, calcium, and magnesium ions. The contribution of these effects to its antimanic qualities is uncertain, although its antimanic effects are thought to result from increases in NE uptake and 5-HT receptor sensitivity.

Contraindications and Precautions

Lithium is contraindicated in patients with CV or renal disease, brain damage, dehydration, hyponatremia, lactation, and diuretic therapy.

Adverse Effects

The adverse effects of lithium can be classified as acute, chronic, and toxic. Acute effects include polyuria, polydipsia, nausea, and a fine hand tremor (although patients commonly develop a tolerance to this effect). Chronic adverse effects include polyuria, weight gain, hair loss, acne, and cognitive impairment. Hypothyroidism and nephrogenic diabetes insipidus may also occur in patients receiving long-term lithium therapy, although discontinuing lithium reverses these effects. Long-term lithium therapy (exceeding 10 years) commonly impairs the ability of the kidneys to concentrate urine, although this is not associated with a reduced glomerular filtration rate or renal insufficiency (Benefield & Cohen, 2000). Toxic effects are dose related and most serious when serum concentrations exceed 2 mEq/L. Early symptoms include a coarse hand tremor, severe GI upset, blurred vision, and vertigo. Serious symptoms include seizures, coma, arrhythmias, and permanent neurologic impairment.

Hemodialysis is effective in removing lithium from the body. Chronic maintenance therapy is occasionally associated with hypothyroidism or acquired nephrogenic diabetes insipidus. Discontinuing lithium therapy usually will reverse these conditions.

Drug Interactions

Lithium interacts significantly with other drugs that deplete sodium. Examples of such drugs include thiazide diuretics and angiotensin-converting enzyme inhibitors, which may lead to toxicity secondary to decreased renal elimination of lithium (Table 18-6).

Assessment of Relevant Core Patient Variables

Health Status

In addition to taking a complete health history, the nurse performs a complete physical assessment and compiles a complete drug history, especially because lithium interacts with so many other drugs. Health conditions that increase sodium resorption, such as CHF, ascites, or cirrhosis, may increase resorption and lead to lithium toxicity. Signs of lithium toxicity include nausea, vomiting, drowsiness, mental dullness, slurred speech, confusion, dizziness, muscle twitching, irregular heartbeat, and blurred vision. A serious lithium overdose can be life threatening. Patients who are taking lithium should inform all health care providers, including dentists, of their use of this drug.

Life Span and Gender

The nurse considers the patient's age. Elderly patients should use lithium cautiously, because older adults experience more profound or toxic CNS effects. Older adults also are more likely to develop lithium-induced goiter, clinical hypothyroidism, and nephrogenic diabetes insipidus. The nurse asks the woman of childbearing age whether she is pregnant, intends to become pregnant, or is breast-feeding. Lithium is classified in pregnancy risk category D. It crosses the placenta, and serum concentration is equal in the mother and fetus. Lithium may cause fetal harm when given to a pregnant woman. Data from lithium birth registries suggest an increase in cardiac and other anomalies.

Lifestyle, Diet, and Habits

The nurse reviews the patient's diet and asks about use of alcohol and other drugs, including caffeine. Concurrent drug or alcohol abuse reduces responsiveness to drug therapy. Caffeine-containing foods and beverages, such as coffee and tea, have a diuretic effect and can lower the lithium level from loss of sodium.

The nurse considers the patient's daily activities. Lithium therapy causes drowsiness and may impair activities that require alertness or physical coordination.

TABLE 18-6 Agents That Interact With Lithium Carbonate

Interactants	Effect and Significance	Nursing Management
alkalinizing agents: potassium acetate, potassium citrate sodium bicarbonate, sodium citrate, sodium lactate, tromethamine	Increased renal clearance of lithium	Anticipate possible dosage adjustment.
caffeine	Reduced serum lithium concentrations	Counsel patients about possibly decreased effectiveness of therapy, and identify sources of caffeine (coffee, tea, chocolate, carbonated colas, and other beverages).
verapamil	Possible lithium toxicity	Avoid concurrent use.
diuretics	Increased or decreased lithium levels depending of diuretic: enhanced lithium reabsorption with diuretics that act in distal tubule (thiazides, spironolactone, triamterene) or enhanced renal clearance with diuretics that act at the proximal tubule (osmotic diuretics, carbonic anhydrase inhibitors)	Monitor lithium levels carefully; anticipate dosage adjustments accordingly.
methyldopa	Possible lithium toxicity	Coadminister cautiously.
NSAIDs	Elevated lithium serum concentration from reduced excretion	Monitor lithium levels carefully; observe for signs of toxicity.
phenothiazines, haloperidol, carbamazepine	Neurotoxicity (delirium, seizures, encephalopathy, hyperpyrexia, EPS)	Monitor lithium levels carefully; observe for signs of toxicity.
acetozelamide, theophylline	Increased excretion of lithium	Monitor lithium levels closely. Anticipate dosage adjustment.
TCAs	Increased pharmacologic effect of TCAs	Monitor patient carefully for signs and symptoms of TCA toxicity. Anticipate dosage adjustment for TCAs.
neuromuscular blocking agents	Increased neuromuscular blocking effect with severe respiratory depression	Assess respiratory and neurologic status closely. Anticipate dosage reduction of neuromuscular blocking agent. Coadminister with caution.
fluoxetine	Increased lithium levels	Monitor lithium levels closely. Assess for signs and symptoms of lithium toxicity.

Environment

The nurse must be aware of the environments in which lithium may be administered. Lithium can be administered safely in acute-care or chronic-care settings and in the home.

Culture

The nurse considers the patient's ethnic heritage. Japanese patients may be more sensitive to lithium's effects, because lower doses (with corresponding therapeutic plasma levels) are commonly used in Japan.

Nursing Diagnoses and Outcomes

- Ineffective Therapeutic Regimen Management related to side effects of therapy (e.g., narrow therapeutic index of lithium) or fear of drug-induced decrease in euphoria
  Desired outcome: The patient will comply with regularly scheduled blood tests to monitor serum lithium concentrations, which will remain within normal therapeutic margins.
- Excess Fluid Volume
  Desired outcome: The patient will verbalize an understanding of sodium and fluid intake requirements necessary with lithium therapy.
- Risk for Poisoning related to lithium toxicity
  Desired outcome: The patient will comply with regular monitoring of blood lithium levels to maintain a therapeutic serum level.

Planning and Intervention

Maximizing Therapeutic Effects

The nurse plays an important part in helping patients with bipolar disorder maintain their illness in remission. The patient should know about early warning signs of a relapse, how to manage psychosocial problems, and the importance of health-conscious behaviors, a restful night's sleep, regular diet, and exercise. If the patient cannot abstain from alcohol, the nurse advises moderate intake and management of work schedules to minimize stress.

Minimizing Adverse Effects

Consuming lithium with food or dividing the dose will minimize GI distress. Lithium is best taken with, or shortly after, meals. Administration should be accompanied by 10 to 12 glasses of water (8 oz) each day to prevent possible dehydration.

Providing Patient and Family Education

- The nurse cautions the patient against changing sodium intake, starting new drug therapy, or changing drug brands without first consulting the health care provider, because certain changes may foster toxic lithium levels. In addition, he or she explains the relationship between lithium activity and dietary sodium and teaches the patient how to maintain a constant level of sodium intake to avoid fluctuations in lithium action.
- The nurse teaches strategies to prevent dehydration during lithium therapy.
- The nurse cautions the patient to avoid OTC products containing nonsteroidal antiinflammatory drugs (NSAIDs), except for aspirin, because these products decrease renal clearance. Patients should not use NSAIDs without first consulting the health care provider.

Ongoing Assessment and Evaluation

The nurse monitors thyroid and CV function periodically during lithium therapy. To prevent toxic serum levels, blood specimens should be obtained 8 to 12 hours after drug administration and lithium concentrations measured. These studies should be performed once or twice weekly during initiation of therapy and monthly thereafter. The nurse stresses the importance of adhering to a schedule of follow-up laboratory and medical appointments.

The nurse observes the patient's neurologic and psychiatric functioning and routinely assesses neuromuscular, GI, CV, renal, and thyroid function. Serum drug levels should be monitored to determine whether dosage is within therapeutic ranges. To evaluate mood stability, the nurse can review pretreatment behaviors and the patient's adherence to the therapeutic regimen. ■

DRUGS SIGNIFICANTLY DIFFERENT FROM LITHIUM

Selective anticonvulsant agents, such as carbamazepine, valproic acid, and gabapentin, demonstrate antimanic effectiveness in patients who are refractory or intolerant to lithium (although these are unlabeled uses).

MEMORY CHIP

Lithium Carbonate

- Mood stabilizer used to prevent mood swings, especially mania, in bipolar disorder
- Significant contraindications: cardiovascular or renal disease, brain damage, hyponatremia, lactation, and diuretic therapy
- Most common adverse effects: polyuria, polydipsia, nausea, and fine hand tremor
- Most serious adverse effect: lithium toxicity (tremors, GI upset, arrhythmias, seizures)
- **Life span alert: profound or toxic CNS effects, drug-induced goiter, clinical hypothyroidism, and nephrogenic diabetes insipidus in older adults**
- Maximizing therapeutic effects: encourage health-conscious behaviors, restful sleep, and nutritious diet, including adequate fluid intake (at least 2 1/2 L/day) and dietary sodium intake
- Minimizing adverse effects: routinely monitor serum lithium concentrations; administer with food or in divided doses with consumption of 10 to 12 (8 oz) glasses of water daily
- Most significant patient education: do not change sodium intake, use OTC products containing NSAIDS, start new drug therapy or change brands without first consulting health care provider; maintain adequate hydration; continue follow-up monitoring of serum lithium levels

Carbamazepine

Carbamazepine (Tegretol) is an alternative to lithium for managing acute mania and for prophylactic therapy. It is thought to reduce the sensitization of the brain to repeated episodes of mood swing. Mood-stabilizing use of carbamazepine does not appear to cause the blood dyscrasias that complicate its use as an anticonvulsant.

Gabapentin

Gabapentin (Neurontin) appears effective in most patients who have bipolar disorder but have not responded to lithium or other mood stabilizers. Moreover, gabapentin may have significantly more anxiolytic and calming potency than either carbamazepine or valproic acid.

Valproic Acid

Valproic acid (Depakene) appears equally effective as lithium in treating mania but less effective in managing the depressive component of the disorder. Long-term therapy appears to reduce the frequency and severity of bipolar episodes.

CHAPTER SUMMARY

- Antidepressant therapy is used for the treatment of depressive disorders. The four major classes of antidepressants are the "cyclic" antidepressants, monoamine oxidase inhibitors (MAOIs), miscellaneous antidepressants, and selective serotonin-reuptake inhibitors (SSRIs).

- Lithium is considered the drug of choice for bipolar disorder.
- There is no ideal psychotherapeutic agent, because all produce adverse effects. An important function of the nurse is to teach the patient and family safe and accurate use of these agents.
- Hypertensive crisis is the most serious toxic effect of MAOIs. It may occur following the ingestion of certain foods containing high amounts of tyramine or concomitant use with several other drugs.

QUESTIONS FOR STUDY AND REVIEW

1. Identify three classifications of antidepressant drugs, describing how each exerts its effects.
2. What are common side effects produced by the TCAs?
3. What are some dietary restrictions of MAOIs?
4. What are the symptoms of an MAOI hypertensive crisis?
5. What disorders are amenable to treatment with the SSRIs?
6. How does lithium produce its therapeutic effect?
7. Identify the pharmacologic agents used to treat bipolar disorder?

NEED MORE HELP?

Chapter 18 of the study guide for *Drug Therapy in Nursing* contains exercises and activities to reinforce your understanding of the concepts presented in this chapter. For additional information see the text's accompanying website at *http://www.connection.lww.com*.

REFERENCES AND BIBLIOGRAPHY

American Psychiatric Association. (2000). *Diagnostic and Statistical manual of Mental Disorders* (4th ed., text revision). Washington, D.D.: Author.

Benefield, Jr., W. H. (1998). How to treat pediatric patients with psychiatric problems. *Drug Topics, 142*(17), 45–48.

Benefield, Jr., W. H., & Cohen, L. J. (2000). Understanding bipolar disorder: A treatment update. *U.S. Pharmacist, 25*(5), 99–109.

Bond, W. S. (1991). Ethnicity and psychotropic drugs. *Clinical Pharmacy, 10*(6), 467–470.

Burnham, T. H., & Short, R. M. (Eds.) (2000). *Drug facts and comparisons*. St. Louis: Facts and Comparisons.

Cada, D. J., Covington, T. R., Hebel, S. K., et al. (1998). New directions in treating depression. *Drug Topics, 142*(22), 85–94.

Carlson, G. A., Jensen, P. S., & Nottelmann, E. D. (Eds.) (1998). Special issue: Current issues in childhood bipolarity. *Journal of Affective Disorders, 51*(2), 77–80.

Davis, W. M. (1999). Treating nonclassical psychiatric conditions. *Drug Topics, 143*(22), 84–93.

Ereshefsky, L. (1998). Antidepressant pharmacodynamic, pharmacokinetic, and drug interaction issues. *U.S. Pharmacist, 23*, (Suppl. 12), 22–34.

Fauci, A., Braunwald, E., Wilson, J. D., Hauser, S. L., Longo, D. L., Kasper, D. L., Isselbachter, K. J. (Eds.) (1999). *Harrison's online*. New York: McGraw-Hill.

Fernandez, C. (1999). Antidepressant medication adherence in the geriatric patient. *Pharmacy Times, 65*(11), 58–67.

Hardman, J. G., Limbird, L. E., Molinof, P. B., Ruddon, R. W., & Gilman, A. G. (Eds.) (1997). *Goodman & Gilman's pharmacological basis of therapeutics* (9th ed.). New York: McGraw-Hill.

Haddad, P. M. (1998). Antidepressant discontinuation syndromes. Eccles, England: Cromwell House, Mental Health Services of Salford.

Kubiak, J. A. (2000). Major depressive disorder. *Pharmacy Times, 66*(10), 48–58.

Markowitz, J. S. (1998). Herbal medicines assuming a larger role in psychiatric care. *Drug Topics, 142*(17), 50–53.

McEvoy, G. K., Litvak, K., & Welsh Jr., O. H. (Eds.). (2000). *Drug information*. Bethesda, MD: American Hospital Formulary Service.

Preskorn, S. H. (1999). *Outpatient management of depression: A guide for the primary-care practitioner* (2nd ed.). Caddo, OK: Professional Communications.

Quarles, E., & Norton, J. (2000). Treatment guide to clinical depression. *U.S. Pharmacist, 25*(6), 28–37.

Rudorfer, M. V. (1993). Pharmacokinetics of psychotropic drugs in special populations. *Journal of Clinical Psychiatry, 549*, (Suppl.), 50–54.

Sax, B. W. (1999). Depression: Not uncommon and highly treatable. *Pharmacy Times, 65*(9), 73–74.

Scott, M. A., & McKenzie, C. A. (1999). Gloom and anger: Depression in the adolescent. *Pharmacy Times, 65*(5), 81–90.

St. Dennis, C. (1999). Therapeutic options in treating depression. *U.S. Pharmacist, 24*(10), 65–75.

Weller, E. (1999). *Pharmacologic treatment in childhood psychiatric disorders*. Presented at the 152nd Annual Meeting of the American Psychiatric Association, Washington, D.C.

Wood, A. J., & Zhon, H. H. (1991). Ethnic difference in drug disposition and responsiveness. *Clinical Pharmacokinetics, 20*, 350–373.

Zagaria, M. A. E. (2000). Depression: An undertreated illness. *U.S. Pharmacist, 25*(4), 111.

Chapter 19

DRUGS FOR TREATING THOUGHT DISORDERS

KEY TERMS

Alzheimer disease
antipsychotic agents
atypical antipsychotics
D2 receptor
dementia
extrapyramidal side effects
neuroleptics
neuroleptic malignant syndrome
psychosis
schizophrenia
tardive dyskinesia
typical antipsychotics

Learning Objectives

At the completion of this chapter the student will:

1. Explain the role of antipsychotic drugs in the management of schizophrenia.
2. Identify the classes of drugs used to manage schizophrenia.
3. Compare and contrast the typical and "atypical" antipsychotic drugs in terms of their therapeutic efficacy and side effects.
4. Identify key points for patient and family teaching for drugs that affect thought.
5. Describe the etiology, symptoms, and treatment of neuroleptic malignant syndrome.
6. Explain the progressive nature of dementia of the Alzheimer type.
7. Name the drugs and their mechanism of action that are used to manage Alzheimer disease.

Antipsychotics

Typical antipsychotics

Phenothiazines

Aliphatic compounds

- **chlorpromazine** (P)
- promazine
- triflupromazine

Piperidine compounds

- mesoridazine
- thioridazine

Piperizine compounds

- fluphenazine
- perphenazine
- prochlorperazine
- trifluoperazine

Thioxanthenes

- thiothixene

Phenylbutylpiperidines

- haloperidol
- pimozide

Dihydroindolones

- molindone

Dibenzoxazepines

- loxapine

Atypical antipsychotics

Dibenzapines

- **clozapine** (P)
- olanzapine
- quetiapine

Benzisoxazoles

- risperidone
- ziprasidone

Alzheimer's drugs

Acetylcholinesterase enzyme inhibitors

- **rivastigmine** (P)
- donepezil
- tacrine
- galantamine hydrobromide

The symbol (C) indicates the **drug class**.

Drugs in bold type marked with the symbol (P) are **prototypes**.

Drugs in blue type with no symbol are **closely related** to the prototype.

Drugs in **red** type with no symbol are **significantly different** from the prototype.

Drugs in **black** type with no symbol are **also used in drug therapy**; no prototype.

Thought disorders are characterized by disturbances of reality and perception, impaired cognitive functioning, and diminished or inappropriate mood (affect). Thought disorders include schizophrenia, dementia, and Alzheimer disease.

Antipsychotic agents are effective in the treatment of hallucinations, delusions, and thought disorders, regardless of etiology. They remain the cornerstones of acute and chronic treatment of schizophrenia. Prototypical antipsychotic agents discussed in this chapter include the typical antipsychotic, chlorpromazine, and the atypical antipsychotic, clozapine. Alzheimer drugs are used in the treatment of **Alzheimer disease** (AD), a common form of progressive dementia. The representative Alzheimer drug discussed in this chapter is rivastigmine.

PHYSIOLOGY

The cerebrum, the highest functional area of the brain concerned with activities such as creative thought, judgment, memory, and reason, is divided into two hemispheres by a deep groove—the corpus callosum. In most people, the left hemisphere appears to be dominant, controlling comprehension, logic, rational thinking, and speech. The largely nondominant right hemisphere, often referred to as the "creative" brain, is associated with affect, behavior, and spatial-perceptual functions. Each hemisphere further divided into four lobes with each lobe being named for the bones of the skull under which they lie. The frontal lobes control voluntary body movement, expression of feelings, perceptual interpretation of information, and thinking. The temporal lobes also play a role in the expression of emotions.

Other major central nervous system (CNS) functional systems include the extrapyramidal system responsible for muscle coordination; the limbic system responsible for the emotions of anger, anxiety, fear, pleasure, sorrow, learning, and memory; and the reticular activating system responsible for consciousness, filtering, and alerting to stimuli.

The CNS is made up of glial cells and neurons. Although not fully understood, glial cells are believed to be composed of many types of neurotransmitter receptors and ion channels. Neurons generate and transmit electrochemical impulses. They convey information through the body from one neuron to another by electrical and chemical transport of the message across a synapse—the junction point from one neuron to the next through neurotransmitters. Release of the neurotransmitter either stimulates or inhibits the activity of the postsynaptic neurons. Neurotransmitters play an important role in human emotion and behavior. Many neurotransmitters are the target for the mechanism of action of many psychotropic medications; for example, acetylcholine (ACh), dopamine (DA), norepinephrine (NE), and serotonin (5-HT). ACh, DA, NE, and 5-HT increase and decrease the rate of neuron stimulation, thus regulating changes in thought processes, mood states, and psychomotor responses.

Many areas of the brain secrete ACh; reduction in its amount causes cognitive changes. ACh has a number of functions including arousal, coordination of movement, memory acquisition, and memory retention. DA is secreted by neurons that originate in the midbrain that function in coordination, emotion, and voluntary decision making. It is believed that sensitivity of receptor sites to DA is an etiologic factor of psychotic behavior. Drugs that block DA transmission result in diminished disordered thinking and related behaviors. There are a variety of DA receptors in the brain but D1 and D2 are the primary ones involved with the antipsychotic agents.

DA pathways terminate in several areas including the frontal cortex and limbic system. Therapeutic cognitive and behavioral effects occur when DA receptors are blocked in these areas. Blockade of DA receptors in the brain stem produce an antiemetic effect. When DA receptors are blocked in the extrapyramidal system and hypothalamic-pituitary axis, respectively.

NE pathways in the CNS innervate a number of areas including the cerebral cortex and limbic system. NE is secreted by cell bodies in the reticular activating formation of the brain stem and hypothalamus. NE functions include arousal, cognition, perception, and regulation of mood. NE is associated with feelings of rage and aggression; it directs the release of chemicals that stimulate responses to emotional stimuli.

Alterations in 5-HT, which is secreted by areas of the nuclei of the brain, are associated with changes in behaviors and mood states.

SCHIZOPHRENIA

Schizophrenia refers to a complex and heterogeneous group of illnesses with uncertain etiology. It has afflicted people for centuries. Currently, schizophrenia afflicts approximately 1% to 2% of all populations worldwide, including 3 million Americans. In the United States, direct and indirect costs of schizophrenia are more than $30 billion annually, and this figure does not include the costs associated with homelessness (an estimated 33% to 50% of homeless Americans are schizophrenic) (Williamson & Wyandt, 2000). Schizophrenia is among the most chronic and debilitating mental illnesses. It interferes with a person's ability to think clearly, manage emotions, make decisions, and relate to others.

Schizophrenia usually begins during late adolescence and early adulthood. The onset is insidious. Peak incidence in men occurs between the ages of 15 and 24 years. In women, who are less frequently and severely affected, peak incidence occurs between the ages of 25 and 34 years (Beaumont, 2000). The syndrome generally has a poor outcome progressing from social withdrawal and perceptual distortions to a state of chronic delusions and hallucinations.

CHARACTERISTICS OF SCHIZOPHRENIA

The term psychosis denotes a variety of mental disorders. **Psychosis** is the inability to perceive and interpret reality accurately, think clearly, respond correctly, and function in a socially appropriate manner. **Schizophrenia** is a particular kind of psychosis that is characterized mainly by a clear sensorium but a marked disturbance in thinking.

Many people mistakenly believe that schizophrenia involves multiple personalities and that afflicted individuals are prone to violence. Schizophrenics do not suffer from multiple personalities and although their behavior may sometimes become violent, they are far more likely to withdraw from society.

Schizophrenia is characterized by symptoms described as positive, negative, and disorganized. The positive symptoms of schizophrenia, the most recognizable symptoms, include delusions, hallucinations, paranoia, and distorted perceptions. For example, individuals with schizophrenia may have ideas that are strange, false, and out of touch with reality, they may hear voices talking to them or about them and they may have difficulty making sense of everyday sights and sounds, so that ordinary events can appear strange and frightening. The negative symptoms of schizophrenia, the most common symptoms, include flat or blunted emotions, lack of pleasure or interest in things (anhedonia), and limited speech. For example, individuals with schizophrenia may have difficulty in understanding their feelings or in being able to clearly express their emotions. Furthermore, they view the world and society as very uninteresting and not worth participating in and very often may not say much or speak unless spoken to. Consequently, the individual may have trouble relating to others, which in turn can lead to periods of intense withdrawal and profound isolation. Disorganized symptoms of confused thinking and disorganized speech may cause schizophrenic individuals to have trouble thinking clearly and understanding what other people say, may make it difficult for them to carry on a conversation, plan ahead, or solve relatively small problems. The disorganized behavior may cause the individual to do things that do not make sense, such as repeat rhythmic gestures or make ritualistic movements.

Some symptoms of schizophrenia differ between men and women. For example, the negative symptoms are more often present in men; mood symptoms, especially depression, are more commonly seen in women. Additionally, delusions in women appear less bizarre, with more somatic and romantic preoccupation. Men are more concerned with political conspiracy and undercover activities and have more grandiose delusions of power, royalty, and divinity. Many individuals with schizophrenia have a combination of these symptoms.

PATHOPHYSIOLOGY OF SCHIZOPHRENIA

Although not fully understood, schizophrenia is believed to result from multiple causes rather than a single cause; for example, a genetic predisposition, environmental factors, and possible hormonal or neurotransmitter changes that alter the brain's chemistry. Family, twin, and adoption studies do indicate an important genetic contribution to the etiology of schizophrenia. Chromosomes 8, 13, and 22 are suspected to be the genetic locations of schizophrenia. The risk of developing schizophrenia is 1 in 10 if one parent suffers from the disease and increases to 1 in 4 with both parents diagnosed as schizophrenic. Otherwise, the risk is only 1 in 100 if there is no family history of the disease.

One hypothesis about the pathogenesis of schizophrenia is defective fetal development that leads to the structural abnormalities seen in the brains of schizophrenics, such as alterations in temporal lobes and limbic structures (including hippocampus and amygdala) and adjacent ventricles. Studies have reported an association between schizophrenia and problems surrounding birth, particularly those that cause oxygen deprivation.

Other hypotheses for the pathogenesis of schizophrenia exist, especially with regard to an alteration in the brain chemistry, because schizophrenia is associated with an unusual imbalance of neurotransmitters-for example, DA, 5-hydroxytryptamine, glutamate, and 5-HT. Of these, the DA hypothesis is the most fully developed. The DA hypothesis of schizophrenia is based on the unexpected discovery that agents that diminish dopaminergic activity have beneficial effects in reducing the acute symptoms and signs of psychosis, specifically agitation, anxiety, and hallucinations. Improvement of delusions and social withdrawal is less dramatic, however. Excessive DA activity is thought to be involved in schizophrenia as imaging studies have demonstrated this in parts of the brain—particularly the left side where positive symptoms occur. This imbalance does not appear to result from overproduction of DA, but rather from an increase in specific chemical receptors, particularly D1, which attract DA. Moreover, there appears to be low activity of D1 receptors in the prefrontal cortex of the brain where negative symptoms originate. Physiologic and anatomic factors supporting this hypothesis include:

1. Most antipsychotic drugs strongly block postsynaptic **D2 receptors** in the CNS, especially in the mesolimbic-frontal system.
2. Dopaminergic drugs (e.g., levodopa, amphetamines, and apomorphine) may either produce psychosis or exacerbate existing schizophrenia.
3. Increased DA receptor density in schizophrenic patients not treated with antipsychotics identified at postmortem examination.
4. Positron emission tomography has shown increased DA receptor density in both treated and untreated people with schizophrenia compared with scans of nonschizophrenic persons (Katzung, 2000).

The antipsychotic agents block D2 receptors stereoselectively; their binding affinity is very strongly correlated with clinical antipsychotic and extrapyramidal potency. Although five different DA receptors have been described, it is unknown whether antagonism of any receptor other than D2 plays any antipsychotic role (Katzung, 2000). Traditionally, schizophrenia has been treated with typical antipsychotic drugs (most commonly the phenothiazines) that block central D2 subtype DA receptors of the mesolimbic structures. Their ability to antagonize D2 receptors correlates with their antipsychotic efficacy.

It is likely that other neurotransmitters, including 5-HT, ACh, glutamate, and gamma-aminobutyric acid (GABA) also contribute to the pathophysiology schizophrenia. Another hypothesis suggests the involvement of excitatory amino acids. For example, concentrations of aspartate in the cerebrospinal fluid (CSF) have been found to be significantly higher in schizophrenic patients with tardive dyskinesia (slowed ability to execute voluntary movements). Additionally, there is evidence that "atypical" clozapine may differ from conventional antipsychotic agents in terms of its effect on glutamatergic receptors. Plus, differing effects on N-methyl-D-aspartate (NMDA) receptors may account in part for enhanced efficacy of atypical antipsychotics for negative symptoms and, possibly, decreased risk of tardive dyskinesia (Inada, 2000).

ANTIPSYCHOTIC DRUGS

Antipsychotic agents are used frequently in the treatment of acute and chronic management of schizophrenia. APs are used to manage the symptoms associated with psychosis. Regardless of the etiology, APs are effective in the treatment of hallucinations, delusions, and thought disorders. Their exact mechanism of action is not completely understood, but dopaminergic receptor blockade in the limbic system and basal ganglia appears to be an essential element.

Antipsychotic drugs (APs) are divided into two groups—**typical** and **atypical**. The term **neuroleptics** is used to refer to both typical and atypical agents, although typical APs are more commonly associated with the term, because they far more likely than atypical APs to produce neurologic adverse effects (e.g., extrapyramidal side effects) related to "neuroleptics." Table 19-1 summarizes selected antipsychotics.

TABLE 19-1 Summary of Selected Antipsychotics

Drug (Trade) Name	Selected Indications	Route and Dosage Range	Pharmacokinetics
Typical Antipsychotics			
Aliphatic Phenothiazines			
chlorpromazine (Thorazine; *Canadian:* Chlorprom)	Psychotic disorders, such as schizophrenia	*Adult:* PO, 10–25 mg, bid, tid, or qid to maximum of 2,000 mg/d; IM 25–50 mg repeated in 4 h if needed *Child:* 5–12 y, 23–46 kg, 75 mg/d; 6 mo–5 y (up to 23 kg), 40 mg/d; IM, 0.55 mg/kg q6–8h	*Onset:* PO, 30–60 min; IM, 10–15 min *Duration:* 4–6 h $t_{1/2}$: 23–37 h
Piperadine Phenothiazines			
thioridazine (Mellaril; *Canadian:* Apo-Thioridazine)	Psychotic disorders; agitation, depression, sleep disturbance, and fear in geriatric patients; hyperactivity and related symptoms in children	*Adult:* PO, 50–800 mg/d *Child:* 2–12 y, PO, 0.5–3.0 mg/kg/d	*Onset:* Varies *Duration:* 8–12 h $t_{1/2}$: 10–12 h
mesoridazine (Serentil)	Schizophrenia, alcohol withdrawal, acute/chronic alcoholism	*Adult:* PO, 50–400 mg/d (lower dosage for alcohol withdrawal)	*Onset:* Varies *Duration:* 4–8 h $t_{1/2}$: 24–48 h
acetophenazine (Tindal)	Psychotic disorders	*Adult:* PO, 20–80 mg/d in divided doses *Child:* Not recommended	*Onset:* 2–3 h *Duration:* 36–48 h $t_{1/2}$: 10–20 h
perphenazine (Trilafon; *Canadian:* Apo-Perphenazine)	Psychotic disorders	*Adult:* PO, 4–8 mg tid to qid; IM, 5–15 mg/d	*Onset:* Varies *Duration:* 6–12 h $t_{1/2}$: Unknown
fluphenazine enanthate (Prolixin; *Canadian:* Apo-Fluphenazine)	Psychotic disorders	*Adult:* IM/SC, 12.5–25 mg *Child:* Not recommended	*Onset:* 24–72 h *Duration:* 1–3 wk $t_{1/2}$: 3.7 d
Thioxanthenes			
thiothixene (Navane)	Psychotic disorders	*Adult:* PO, 2–30 mg/d; IM, 4–30 mg/d	*Onset:* 1–6 h *Duration:* 12–24 h $t_{1/2}$: 34 h
Phenylbutylpiperidines			
haloperidol (Haldol; *Canadian:* Peridol)	Psychotic disorders, hyperexcitability in children	*Adult:* PO, 0.5–2 mg bid to tid; IM, 5–30 mg/d *Child:* PO, 0.05–0.15 mg/d	*Onset:* PO, varies, IM, 15–30 min *Duration:* PO, 24–72 h; IM, 4–8 h $t_{1/2}$: 21–14 h

(*continued*)

TABLE 19-1 Summary of Selected Antipsychotics (Continued)

Drug (Trade) Name	Selected Indications	Route and Dosage Range	Pharmacokinetics
pimozide (Orap)	Tourette syndrome	*Adult:* PO, 1–10 mg/d in divided doses	*Onset:* Varies *Duration:* Unknown $t_{1/2}$: 55–154 h
Dihydroindolones			
molindone (Moban)	Psychotic disorders	*Adult:* PO, 50–225 mg/d in divided doses	*Onset:* Varies *Duration:* 24–36 h $t_{1/2}$: 1.5 h
Dibenzoxazepines			
loxapine (Loxitane; *Canadian:* Loxapac)	Psychotic disorders	*Adult:* PO, 10–100 mg/d; IM, 12.5–50 mg/d	*Onset:* PO, 30 min; IM, rapid *Duration:* 12 h $t_{1/2}$: 19 h
Atypical Antipsychotics			
Dibenzapines			
clozapine (Clozaril)	Schizophrenia unresponsive to other antipsychotic drugs	*Adult:* PO, 25–450 mg/d	*Onset:* Varies *Duration:* 4–12 h $t_{1/2}$: 8–12 h
olanzapine (Zyprexa)	Psychotic disorders	*Adult:* PO, 5–15 mg/d	*Onset:* Unknown *Duration:* Unknown $t_{1/2}$: 21–54 h, average 30 h
Benzisoxazoles			
risperidone (Risperdal)	Pyschotic disorders	*Adult:* PO, 1 mg bid to 16 mg/d	*Onset:* Varies *Duration:* Unknown $t_{1/2}$: 20 h

TYPICAL ANTIPSYCHOTIC DRUGS

The typical (also referred to as classical) APs have been used clinically for nearly 50 years and until recently have been the mainstay treatment for schizophrenia. The typical AP drugs block neuronal DA transmission. These drugs were developed on the premise that dopamine-receptor blockade was essential for antipsychotic effects. The typical APs are effective in controlling the symptoms of schizophrenia and other psychoses and allowing patients to function at a higher level. Because of adverse drug effects, however, therapeutic noncompliance is common and accounts for the high rate of relapse.

All of the typical APs are DA receptor antagonists with a greater affinity for D2 than D1 receptors. In general, these agents differ in their selectivity among the cortical DA systems and their binding affinities for nondopaminergic sites, such as cholinergic, alpha-1 adrenergic and histaminic receptors. The binding of the typical APs to these nondopaminergic sites helps to explain some of their side effects; for example, extrapyramidal syndrome (EPS), sedation, and orthostatic hypotension.

All of the typical APs are equally effective in the treatment of psychotic symptoms of schizophrenia, although they vary in potency and in their tendency to induce side effects.

Potency is one method of classifying the typical antipsychotics. Although the available typical APs differ in potency, they are essentially equivalent in their ability to relieve the symptoms of psychosis and schizophrenia. Potency refers to the size of the dose needed to elicit a certain response rather than to the drug's effectiveness. Even so, potency is important to consider in regard to undesired clinical responses—the greater the potency of the drug the more significant its adverse reactions (Table 19-2).

Another method of classifying typical APs is by chemical structure. They are grouped into one of five chemical classes:

1. Phenothiazines
2. Thioxanthenes
3. Phenylbutylpiperidines
4. Dihydroindolones
5. Dibenzoxazepines

This chapter organizes typical APs using that classification.

TABLE 19-2 Potency of Selected Antipsychotic Drugs

Low potency	mesoridazine (Serentil) thioridazine (Mellaril)
Moderate potency	chlorpromazine (Thorazine) loxapine (Loxitane) molindone (Moban)
High potency	fluphenazine (Prolixin) haloperidol (Haldol) thiothixene (Navane)

Phenothiazines stand out from other typical APs because they were the first modern example. Nine chemicals, classified as phenothiazines, belong to the largest group of APs currently in use. This group is subdivided into three subgroups: aliphatic, piperidine, and piperazine compounds—according to their chemical structure.

Chlorpromazine (Thorazine) is the prototypical AP. It belongs to the aliphatic subclass of phenothiazines. As the first AP, chlorpromazine has served as the basis for AP development for more than 40 years.

NURSING MANAGEMENT OF THE PATIENT RECEIVING CHLORPROMAZINE

Core Drug Knowledge

Pharmacotherapeutics

Schizophrenia is the primary therapeutic indication for chlorpromazine and other APs. Other uses include control of disturbed behavior in children and patients with Alzheimer disease. Nonpsychiatric indications include treatment of intractable hiccups. Unlabeled uses for chlorpromazine include psychosis induced by *Pneumocystis carinii* pneumonia and relief of migraine headaches.

Pharmacokinetics

Chlorpromazine is absorbed erratically and unpredictably from the gastrointestinal (GI) tract. Peak plasma levels occur 2 to 4 hours after administration. IM use provides 4 to 10 times more active drug than oral doses. Depot preparations for IM administration provide a long-acting effect (e.g., several weeks). Sustained release forms are unnecessary because of the long duration of action of these agents.

Once in the bloodstream, chlorpromazine is rapidly distributed throughout the body. Chlorpromazine is highly lipophilic and extensively bound to plasma proteins (91% to 99%). It accumulates in tissues with a high blood supply, such as the brain and lungs and traces of it may be found in the urine for up to 6 months following the last dose.

Chlorpromazine is slowly metabolized in the liver. Like other phenothiazines, chlorpromazine undergoes extensive hepatic biotransformation. Metabolites persist for prolonged periods; they themselves have important adverse effects and also contribute to the biologic activity of the parent drug. The persistence of these metabolites is thought to contribute to the slow rate of recurrence of psychotic episodes following cessation of drug therapy.

Elimination half-life is 20 to 40 hours and elimination occurs through renal excretion and enterohepatic circulation.

Pharmacodynamics

Therapeutic actions and adverse effects of chlorpromazine and related drugs stem from the blocking effects of various receptors, namely, D2, alpha1- adrenergic, muscarinic, H1, and 5-HT-2 receptors. The dopaminergic blockade occurs in the basal ganglia, hypothalamus, limbic system, brain stem, and medulla. The decrease in DA transmission correlates with the antipsychotic effects. The D2 blockade is also responsible for the moderate EPS observed with this drug. Blockade of alpha-1-adrenergic receptors produces sedation, muscle relaxation, and cardiovascular effects, such as hypotension, reflex tachycardia, and minor changes (e.g., prolonged QT interval, flattened T-wave) in electrocardiographic (ECG) patterns.

Chlorpromazine acts at D1 and D2 receptors. Its antiemetic action is the result of a central DA receptor blockade in the chemoreceptor trigger zone of the medulla and a peripheral blockade on the DA receptors in the stomach.

Contraindications and Precautions

Chlorpromazine is contraindicated in patients with hypersensitivity to a phenothiazine as cross-sensitivity may occur. Other contraindications include comatose or severely depressed states, bone marrow depression or blood dyscrasias, Parkinson disease, and severe hypotension or hypertension. Cholestatic jaundice may occur and this is regarded as a hypersensitivity reaction. Cautious use is required in patients receiving other CNS depressants and in patients with cardiovascular disease, history of glaucoma, compromised hepatic function or renal function impairment. Chlorpromazine and other APs should be used cautiously in patients with heart disease because they may precipitate hypotension. Increased pulse rates may exacerbate angina pectoris. Because the drug has a CNS depressant effect, it should be used cautiously in clients with chronic respiratory disorders such as asthma and emphysema. Hepatic and renal function should be monitored periodically in long-term therapy. Dosage reduction or cessation of drug therapy may be required in patients with abnormal blood urea nitrogen values.

Chlorpromazine is pregnancy category C. Safety for use during pregnancy has not been established. Chlorpromazine and other phenothiazines readily cross the placenta; however, most studies have found them safe for both mother and fetus if used occasionally in low doses. Use near term, however, may cause maternal hypotension and adverse neonatal effects (e.g., EPS, hyporeflexia, hyperreflexia, jaundice). Chlorpromazine and haloperidol have been detected in breast milk. Safety for use during lactation has not been established. Chlorpromazine is not recommended for children under 12 years of age.

Chlorpromazine, like all APs, is more difficult to use in the elderly because of pharmacokinetic factors. For example, lowered protein levels may produce toxicity from large amounts of circulating unbound drug, greater adipose tissue stores larger amounts of lipophilic drugs, and total body water decreases.

The nurse must use caution with IM and IV administration of chlorpromazine and other APs. These modes of administration are utilized when immediate effect of the drug is desired. Resuscitative equipment should be readily available in the event that severe hypotensive episodes or extrapyramidal responses occur.

Adverse Effects

Phenothiazine APs are notably safe drugs having a relatively flat dose-response curve that can be taken over a wide range of dose. The most disturbing and relatively common adverse effects of the typical APs are **extrapyramidal side effects**, which involve the nerves and muscles controlling movement and coordination. Patients generally develop EPS in the first few weeks of treatment; symptoms appear to be dose dependent. EPS effects include 1) acute dystonia, which comprises uncoordinated jerking or spastic movements of the eyes, tongue, face, neck limbs and worm-like movements of the tongue; 2) akathisia, which comprises agitation, compulsion to move or walk, facial tics, fine hand tremor, insomnia, and restlessness; 3) pseudoparkinsonism, which comprises akinesia, decreased or absent arm swing when walking, drooling, hypersalivation, mask-like face, pill-rolling hand tremor, shuffling gait, and stooped posture; and 4) **tardive dyskinesia** (TD, also known as lingual-facial-buccal dyskinesia), which comprises involuntary and often persistent movements of the facial muscles and tongue that develop as a late complication of some neuroleptic therapy, more likely with typical APs. See Figure 19-1 and the accompanying display, EPS Effects Associated with Chlorpromazine Therapy.

TD is considered to be an EPS effect; its pathophysiology remains poorly understood. Numerous theories have been proposed, including DA receptor supersensitivity, catecholamine hyperactivity, and GABA hypoactivity. Of these, the DA receptor supersensitivity theory has received the most attention. Although the "typical" APs affect many different neurotransmitters, it appears that their strong affinity for D2 receptors can be correlated with their high degree for producing TD. See the accompanying display, Risk Factors for Tardive Dyskinesia.

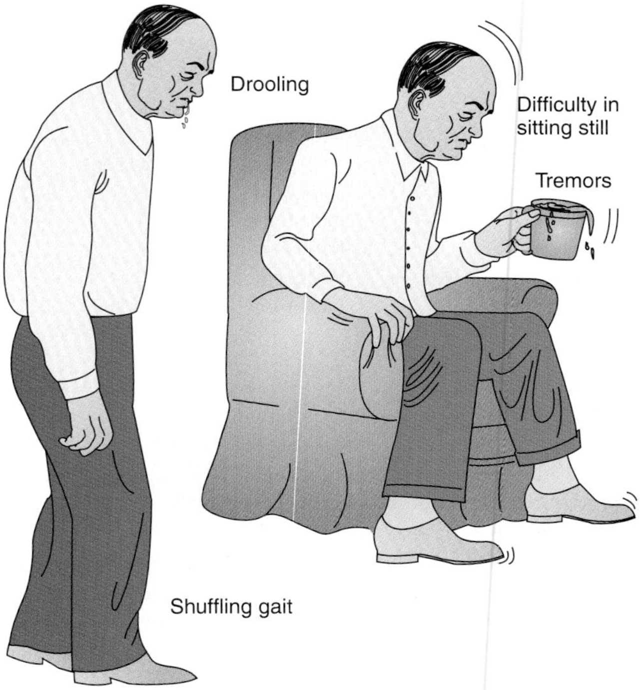

Figure 19-1. Extrapyramidal symptoms (EPS) refer to behaviors associated with functions of the cortex of the brain and the spinal cord. They include the following:

Dystonia—muscular jerkiness and uncoordination, facial grimacing, abnormal eye movements, wryneck

Akathisia—restlessness, inability to sit still, strong urge to move about

Pseudoparkinsonism—tremors and shakiness, masklike facial expression, depression, pillrolling, rigidity, drooling, shuffling gait

EPS are reversible, whereas tardive dyskinesia (protruding tongue, puffing cheeks, chewing movements, involuntary movement of trunk and extremities) is usually not.

Critical Thinking Scenario

EPS effects associated with chlorpromazine therapy

James Benjamin, a 26-year-old man, began taking chlorpromazine (Thorazine) 1 month ago after being diagnosed with schizophrenia. After 2 weeks in the hospital, he was discharged home to his family. Now he returns to the emergency department complaining of "agitation, compulsive walking, insomnia, and restlessness." The patient and his family are anxious that his schizophrenia is returning. His family wants him readmitted to the hospital.

1. What is a possible basis for this patient's symptoms?
2. What information should the nurse give to this patient and his family?
3. Is readmission to the hospital necessary for this patient? Explain your answer.

Risk Factors for Tardive Dyskinesia (TD)

If the patient is receiving treatment with "typical" antipsychotics, additional factors that place the patient at risk for TD include:

- 6 months of antipsychotic therapy
- Increased length of antipsychotic therapy
- Antipsychotic dosage change—either increased or decreased
- Diagnosis of organic mental disorder or mood disorder
- Increased age
- Diabetes
- Genetic predisposition
- Race (African Americans may be twice as likely to develop TD than whites)

Although some research supports the use of vitamin E in treating TD, there is no established treatment for TD. To minimize the risk of TD, APs are used in the lowest effective doses, and the patient is frequently assessed for early signs of TD.

Chlorpromazine (and other low potency aliphatic compounds, especially) lower the seizure threshold and induce discharge patterns in the electroencephalogram (EEG) that are associated with epileptic seizure disorders.

Muscarinic receptor blockade causes anticholinergic adverse effects of blurred vision, dry mouth, constipation, and urine retention. Moreover, the anticholinergic effects may precipitate angle closure and ocular changes (e.g., corneal deposits, pigmentary retinopathy, decreased night vision) may occur during prolonged therapy. Alpha-receptor blockade may cause cardiovascular effects of orthostatic hypotension and tachycardia. Priapism may occur with the typical and atypical APs. This may be due to their alpha-adrenergic blocking effects.

The antidopaminergic effects of chlorpromazine induce anterior pituitary secretion of prolactin that may stimulate the development of galactorrhea or breast engorgement in both genders. Hyperprolactinemia in men is associated with decreased libido, impotence, and sterility. Women may experience amenorrhea with long-term antipsychotic therapy.

Drug Interactions

Chlorpromazine can potentiate the CNS depressant action of other drugs (e.g., alcohol, barbiturates, benzodiazepines, general anesthetics, opiate agonists). Caution should be exercised during simultaneous use of these drugs because of the potential for excessive CNS effects (Table 19-3).

TABLE 19-3 Agents That Interact With Chlorpromazine

Interactants	Effect and Significance	Nursing Management
barbiturates, haloperidol, lithium, meperidine, methyldopa, metrizamide, pimozide, propranolol	Increased pharmacologic effects of chlorpromazine	Monitor cardiac rate and rhythm for evidence of first-degree AV block. Evaluate patient for additive CNS depressant effects. Assess patient for control of blood pressure. Assess patient for evidence of therapeutic effects of interacting drugs. Monitor patient for therapeutic serum levels (if appropriate) of interacting drugs.
aluminum salts, anticholinergics, barbiturates, carbamazepine, charcoal, phenytoin	Decreased pharmacologic effects of chlorpromazine	Evaluate patient for changes in seizure control. Assess patient for evidence of therapeutic effects of interacting drugs. Monitor patient for therapeutic serum levels (if applicable) of interacting drugs.
valproic acid, TCAs	Pharmacologic effects are increased by chlorpromazine	Appraise patient for changes in seizure control. Monitor patient for symptoms of depression and mental status. Assess patient for evidence of therapeutic effects of interacting drugs. Check for therapeutic serum levels (if applicable) of interacting drugs.
bromocriptine, epinephrine/norepinephrine, dopamine agonists, levodopa, guanethidine	Pharmacologic effects of interactants are decreased by chlorpromazine	Appraise the patient for therapeutic management of concurrent disease states (e.g., cardiac disease). Assess patient for evidence of therapeutic effects of interacting drugs. Check for therapeutic serum levels (if applicable) of interacting drugs. Monitor heart rate and blood pressure.

Assessment of Relevant Core Patient Variables

Health Status

It is important that the nurse gather baseline data from the client, family members, friends, other health team members, medical records, and community agencies. Additionally, the nurse should evaluate the client's general appearance; type and degree of behavioral dysfunction such as excitement, speech patterns, restlessness, tremors; and any psychological processes worthy of note such as affect, cognition, judgment, memory, mood, thought content and interpersonal patterns.

Past and present use of alcohol, nicotine, and medications including prescription, over-the-counter (OTC), herbal, illicit, or recreational should be identified. The nurse should note the length of time drug has been used and any undesired clinical responses.

It is important for the nurse to determine the client's mental and emotional status, insight, and comprehension of the problem and also assess the client's ability to communicate directly and accurately. This will help in identifying the patient's potential for compliance with the therapeutic regimen.

The nurse should obtain baseline measurements of blood pressure (standing and at rest), pulse rates, weight, complete blood count (CBC) with differential, liver function tests, urinalysis, ECGs, EEGs, and an ocular examination before administering any antipsychotic drug. Because long-term chlorpromazine therapy may affect vision, examination of the lens should be done as a baseline and evaluated at regular intervals. Blood glucose levels need to be monitored especially in patients with diabetes because long-term drug therapy may also cause changes in carbohydrate metabolism. Patients with diabetes may require a change in diet or drug therapy. Chlorpromazine may raise plasma cholesterol levels. Chlorpromazine may cause cholestatic jaundice—especially during the initiation of therapy. The nurse should observe for nausea, flu-like symptoms, rash, and yellowish skin. The offending drug should be immediately discontinued.

Life Span and Gender

The nurse should document the age of the patient. Studies have reported a strong negative correlation between age and chlorpromazine clearance in children between the ages of 4 months and 17 years (Rudorfer, 1993).

The elderly have slower hepatic metabolism and increased sensitivity of the brain to DA antagonism and anticholinergic effects. Elderly patients appear to be more susceptible to the cardiovascular and neuromuscular reactions of chlorpromazine and other antipsychotics. In general, lower doses should be used (about 25% of the dose for young adult), longer waiting periods before increasing doses and gradual increases in dosage (Gasbarro, 1999). Elderly patients receiving chlorpromazine are at particular risk for falls, cognitive dysfunction, cardiovascular effects, and TD associated with anticholinergic effects of the typical antipsychotic drugs. Chlorpromazine may cause thermoregulation problems—especially in the elderly. Hypothermia or hyperthermia may be induced by deviations in environmental temperature.

The nurse should assess the sexual patterns and reproductive goals of the patient, since reproductive effects (e.g., changes in libido, amenorrhea, irregular menses, breast engorgement, lactation, galactorrhea, gynecomastia, impotence, and ejaculatory failure) may occur. The nurse should also assess the woman for pregnancy and lactation. Female patients who think they may be pregnant should be advised to consult their health care providers without delay. The relative risks and benefits of psychotropic medication versus nonpharmacologic treatment must be individually considered for each pregnant patient (Rudorfer, 1993).

Lifestyle, Diet, and Habits

Photosensitivity occurs commonly in patients taking chlorpromazine. Therefore, the nurse should be aware of patients who regularly spend time out of doors (e.g., farmers, gardeners, construction workers, athletes).

It is important for the nurse to document the height and weight of the patient. Increased appetite is an adverse effect of chlorpromazine and other AP drugs. Significant weight gain may occur. Drug-nutrient interactions with chlorpromazine deplete riboflavin, vitamin B12, and ascorbic acid. Use of vitamin supplements may be necessary. High doses of vitamin C may reduce the effectiveness of chlorpromazine.

The nurse should document the patient's use of tobacco, because cigarette smoking decreases the antipsychotic effect of chlorpromazine by increasing its metabolism.

Environment

The nurse should document the climate in which the drug will be administered. From its actions within the hypothalamus, chlorpromazine interferes with temperature-regulating mechanisms. Body temperature changes, therefore, depend on the prevailing temperature. For example, hypothermia will occur in low environmental temperatures, hyperthermia in high temperatures. Additionally, a reduction in the body's tolerance to heat increases the patient's risk of heat stroke in hot weather or during exercise

Culture

It is necessary for the nurse to consider ethnic variations because they may affect drug therapy. Pharmacokinetics and pharmacodynamics may differ substantially among difference races; these differences can affect clinical outcome. Asians have a lower neuroleptic threshold and a more prominent antipsychotic-induced prolactin response; thus, they require lower doses of APs than whites (Bond, 1991).

Nursing Diagnoses and Outcomes

- Risk for Injury related to potential interactions and adverse effects associated with chlorpromazine

  Desired outcome: The patient will verbalize factors that contribute to potential injury from possible interactions and adverse effects.
- Ineffective Therapeutic Regimen Management related to lack of knowledge regarding the chronic nature of illness, need for life-long medication, and lifestyle adjustment.

  Desired outcome: The patient will describe the disease process and the regimen for disease control and will relate intent to practice needed health behavior.
- Sexual Dysfunction related to altered neurotransmitter function secondary to antipsychotic drug therapy

  Desired outcome: The patient will identify factual limitations on sexual activity caused by health problems, identify appropriate modifications in sexual practices in response to these limitations, and engage in alternative satisfying sexual activity.
- Ineffective Sexuality Patterns related to the need for reliable and consistent contraception secondary to potential teratogenic effects

  Desired outcome: The patient will identify appropriate modifications in sexual practices to facilitate contraception and experience no unplanned pregnancy.
- Noncompliance related to lack of insight and medication adverse effects

  Desired outcome: The patient will participate in the development of the treatment plan, describe reasons for the treatment regimen and measures to manage its adverse effects, and identify the barriers to adhering to the regimen.
- Impaired Physical Mobility related to antipsychotic adverse effects of sedation, EPS, and TD

  Desired outcome: The patient will use safety measures to minimize potential for injury and demonstrate measures to increase mobility.

Planning and Intervention

Maximizing Therapeutic Effects

Maintenance therapy can be administered as a single daily bedtime dose as a result of the long half-life of chlorpromazine. Oral liquid concentrates are light sensitive and are dispensed in amber or opaque containers for protection from light. The concentrates may be diluted in liquids, fruit juices, or semisoft foods to make it more palatable; mixtures using caffeine-containing fluids or foods (e.g., cola, tea) or pectinates (e.g., apple juice) should be avoided because a physical incompatibility may occur. The mixture should be administered immediately after dilution.

Minimizing Adverse Effects

Many patients stop taking these drugs because of the adverse effects. The adverse effects of sedation and orthostatic hypotension may be managed by giving small doses during the day and the major portion at bedtime. This facilitates sleep and decreases daytime drowsiness. Anticholinergic agents (e.g., benztropine, trihexyphenidyl) are sometimes administered prophylactically to decrease EPS symptoms by altering the balance of ACh and DA in the CNS. Chlorpromazine should be administered with food or a full glass or beverage to decrease gastric irritation.

To manage orthostatic hypotension and dizziness, the patient can use support stockings and learn to change positions slowly. For most patients, tolerance to this effect develops in 2 to 3 months. Increased fluid intake and using sugarless gum or hard candies may help manage xerostomia (a dry mouth). Xerostomia may affect the fitting of full or partial dentures; a dental referral may be necessary for this and other dental problems.

Parenteral administration of chlorpromazine greatly increases its effectiveness. Administered in this manner, however, it can cause pain. Thus, deep IM injection is necessary—preferably "Z" track; no more than 1 mL per injection site should be administered to lessen the risk of abscess formation, which is thought to result from large IV doses administered in a single area. Diluting the drug with 0.9% sodium chloride may reduce irritation of the tissue; occasionally the drug may be diluted with a local anesthetic to minimize the discomfort. Undiluted drug should not be administered IV; chlorpromazine and other APs should be diluted to at least 1 mg/mL and administered at a rate of 1 mg/minute for adults and 0.5 mg/minute for children. In both instances (IM or IV administration) the patient should be kept recumbent for at least 1 hour to minimize the hypotension and to be monitored closely.

Providing Patient and Family Education

- The nurse should help patients and families understand the danger of relapse associated with noncompliance as well as the benefit of remaining compliant with drug therapy. After experiencing improvement of psychotic symptoms for a period of time, many patients may choose to discontinue their medications; especially if they experience continued adverse effects with no obvious benefits. See the accompanying display, Improving Patient Compliance with Chlorpromazine.
- The nurse should stress to the patient and family that many of the antipsychotic drugs may impair mental or physical abilities and caution against activities requiring mental alertness and physical coordination (e.g., driving a car or operating machinery) until drug effects are known.
- Anticholinergic effects—although common, expected, and usually bothersome, can easily be managed. The

Critical Thinking Scenario

Improving patient compliance with chlorpromazine

Holly Hall walks into the clinic and asks to speak with the nurse about her 30-year-old son, Tom. She states that Tom has been taking chlorpromazine for 11 months and she has noticed some "strange" movements lately. The nurse asks her to describe the movements. It appears Tom cannot keep his feet still, blinks his eyes constantly, smacks his lips, and jerks his arms around. She is very concerned about his medication and is considering discontinuing the chlorpromazine. She also wants to know about a terrible side effect she has read about called tardive dyskinesia. How should the nurse respond?

nurse might provide comfort measures for dry mouth such as sucking on sugarless hard candies or ice chips or using a number of commercial products available for dry mouth. The nurse might suggest that blurry near vision can be relieved by use of magnifying glasses. The nurse might also recommend measures to alleviate constipation from slowed GI motility such as the use of stool softeners and increased fluid and fiber intake in the diet and exercise. The nurse should counsel patients to arise slowly from a chair or reclining position and to change positions slowly and carefully to prevent a fall caused by dizziness.

- The nurse should advise the patient that weight gain is a common side effect of all APs and it occurs because of an increase in appetite. This may be especially problematic if other health problems exist (e.g., diabetes, hypercholesteremia, hypertension, obesity) and can contribute to morbidity and mortality. The nurse should encourage the patient to follow a low-fat diet and engage in moderate exercise to help with weight control.
- Chlorpromazine promotes photosensitivity. The nurse should counsel the patient about using sunscreen, wearing protective cover-up clothing and hats, and avoiding prolonged exposure to sunlight.
- The nurse should encourage the patient on long-term therapy or moderate-to-high doses to have periodic ophthalmologic examinations. The incidence of ocular changes may be increased by exposure to light. The nurse should strongly encourage the use of sunglasses.
- The nurse should advise the patient that the use of alcohol and other CNS depressants increases such effects of chlorpromazine and other APs. Using these drugs concurrently increases the frequently and severity of EPS.
- Chlorpromazine may discolor urine from pink to red-brown; The nurse should advise the patient that this is a normal response and no cause for alarm.
- The nurse should alert the female patient of childbearing age that false-positive pregnancy test results have occurred but are less likely to occur when a serum test is used.
- The nurse should caution the patient and family about brand switching. There are bioavailability differences between dosage forms for various phenothiazines. The nurse should instruct them not to exceed prescribed dosage and not to discontinue the drug abruptly.

Ongoing Assessment and Evaluation

Ongoing assessment and evaluation is accomplished by measuring the patient's progress toward the identified goals. Is the patient using prescribed medications correctly? Can the patient perform activities of daily living (ADLs) independently? Does the patient spend time with others and interact appropriately? Whether the patient is adhering to the prescribed drug regimen is an ongoing concern that can be addressed by comparing baseline evaluations of behavior with present levels. Substance abuse and suicide are common in people with schizophrenia. It is essential for the nurse to routinely assess schizophrenic patients for these issues. The nurse needs to review the patient's level of orientation and therapeutic goals with the patient, family, and significant others to evaluate the degree to which the outcomes have been attained.

The pharmacologic effects of chlorpromazine may alter laboratory data. Laboratory assessment of blood, cardiac, renal and hepatic function should be done regularly. Alkaline phosphatase, bilirubin, transaminase, serum cholesterol, and urinary catecholamines may be elevated. Glucose tolerance, serum uric acid, follicle-stimulating hormone, growth hormone, and luteinizing hormone may be decreased. ■

DRUGS CLOSELY RELATED TO P CHLORPROMAZINE

Other Phenothiazines

As stated previously, phenothiazine APs are further classified according to their chemical structure, namely, aliphatic, piperidine, and piperazine compounds. Aliphatic compounds produce strong sedative and hypotensive effects and moderate-to-strong EPS. The most common aliphatic drug is chlorpromazine. Other aliphatic phenothiazines are promazine and triflupromazine. They are effective in treating psychotic symptoms of hallucinations and delusions.

Piperidine compounds have moderately strong anticholinergic effects and strong sedative affects but minimal EPS. Mesoridazine (Serentil) and thioridazine (Mellaril) belong to this group. These drugs are often used for short-term treatment of severe behavioral problems in children, sleep

MEMORY CHIP

Chlorpromazine

- Primarily used to treat schizophrenia
- Significant contraindications: hypersensitivity and severe depressed states
- Most common adverse effects: constipation, dry mouth, and orthostatic hypotension, sedation
- Most serious adverse effects: extrapyramidal side effects, tardive dyskinesia
- **Life span alert: not for use in children younger than 6 months of age; increased susceptibility to adverse effects—particularly anticholinergic effects in elderly; lower dosages are used initially and then gradually are increased**
- Maximizing therapeutic effects: take drug exactly as prescribed; avoid OTC drugs, herbal preparations and alcohol consumption
- Minimizing adverse effects: use sunscreen and protective clothing during sun exposure
- Most significant patient education: use caution in hot weather and avoid overheating and dehydration; this drug may increase susceptibility to heat stroke

disturbances, and dementia in the elderly. These compounds cause the greatest cardiovascular effects with the potential to cause serious arrhythmias. Thioridazine dosage above 1 g/day may cause pigmentary retinopathy characterized by diminution of visual acuity, brownish coloring of vision, impairment of night vision, and pigment deposits on the fundus. Ophthalmologic evaluation is recommended. Drug use should be discontinued if retinal changes occur.

Piperazine compounds cause the least sedation, fewer anticholinergic effects, but greater EPS. Fluphenazine (Prolixin), perphenazine (Trilafon), prochlorperazine (Compazine), and trifluoperazine (Stelazine) belong to this group. Piperazine compounds are particularly effective for withdrawn, apathetic individuals. One drug in this subgroup, prochlorperazine, is frequently used as an antiemetic. A cross sensitivity among the phenothiazines may occur.

Haloperidol

Haloperidol, an antipsychotic drug in the phenylbutylpiperidine subclass, is pharmacologically similar to the piperazine phenothiazines. Haloperidol is used to treat schizophrenia and the manic phase of bipolar affective disorder. Haloperidol comes in a depot drug formulation. This long-acting IM injection allows for maintenance therapy in patients who respond well to antipsychotics but are noncompliant. Long-acting depot formulations are available and may be useful in patients who cannot adhere to oral therapy; depot preparations require dosing every 2 to 4 weeks. Depot drugs have variable onset and duration; they are inappropriate for treating an acute psychotic episode. Small doses of haloperidol are effective in the control of acute agitation in the elderly. They may also be useful in treating some symptoms of dementia (e.g., hallucinations, hostility, hyperactivity, suspiciousness).

Anticholinergic activity and alpha-adrenergic blockade of haloperidol are less prominent than chlorpromazine, but its EPS are more prominent after long-term therapy. Haloperidol is contraindicated in patients whose medical conditions predispose them to developing EPS.

Neuroleptic malignant syndrome (NMS) is a rare idiosyncratic combination of EPS, hyperthermia, and autonomic disturbance manifested by catatonia, stupor, fever, unstable blood pressure, and myoglobinemia. All neuroleptic drugs have the potential to produce NMS, but it is most commonly associated with haloperidol and depot fluphenazines. It has occurred with thiothixene, thioridazine, and clozapine and may occur with other agents. The onset of NMS usually occurs within the first month of therapy but may occur long after drug initiation (months to years). Potentially fatal, NMS occurs in individuals who are extremely sensitive to the extrapyramidal effects of the APs, is believed to result from an excessively rapid blockade of postsynaptic DA receptors, and requires immediate discontinuation of the neuroleptic.

Haloperidol is pregnancy category C drug. It has been detected in breast milk. Safety for use during lactation has not been established. Haloperidol is not recommended for children less than 12 years of age.

Some evidence suggests that Asian patients have a greater sensitivity to haloperidol because metabolite levels are three times lower than in whites, suggesting a decreased capacity to reduce haloperidol to its primary metabolite. The difference may be accounted for either by better absorption or diminished hepatic first-pass effect in Asians (Wood & Zhon, 1991).

Thiothixene

Thiothixene, a thioxanthene agent, resembles the aliphatic and piperazine phenothiazine compounds in its antipsychotic efficacy, but generally produces fewer EPS.

Molindone

Molindone is the single typical AP in the dihydroindolone drug class. It is pharmacologically similar to chlorpromazine. Its most prominent adverse effects include EPS. Resumption of menses in previously amenorrheic women has been reported with molindone. Excessive weight gain has not occurred with molindone. It is not recommended for children less than 12 years of age.

Loxapine

Loxapine is structurally similar to chlorpromazine and causes few anticholinergic effects, yet produces a moderate degree of sedation and orthostatic hypotension and a high degree of EPS. Loxapine markedly lowers the convulsive threshold and most of its effects on the CNS resemble those produced by chlorpromazine. Seizures are likely when loxapine is added to existing treatment regimens, especially in patients with preexisting epilepsy. Loxapine may cause cardiac arrhythmias; an ECG should be performed as a baseline and then periodically. Loxapine is not recommended for children less than 16 years of age.

DRUG SIGNIFICANTLY DIFFERENT FROM CHLORPROMAZINE

Pimozide joins haloperidol in the phenylbutylpiperidine class. Pimozide blocks only at dopaminergic receptors. Its therapeutic use is restricted to suppression of motor and phonic tics in patients with Tourette disorder.

Pimozide may impair cardiac repolarization and lengthen the Q-T interval. A baseline ECG should be performed and periodically thereafter, especially during dosage adjustment. Information on the use and efficacy of pimozide in patients younger than 12 years of age is limited. Pimozide is not recommended for any childhood disorder other than Tourette syndrome.

ATYPICAL ANTIPSYCHOTIC DRUGS

Atypical APs were introduced with the development of clozapine. As a group, they have diverse pharmacodynamic profiles, but in general:

1. They have an increased affinity for 5-HT2 receptors compared with D2 receptors.
2. They act on several neurotransmitter systems including antagonism at one or more types of DA receptors (with a selectivity for limbic DA receptors); one or more 5-HT receptors; and alpha-1-adrenergic receptors.
3. They have activity at muscarinic, histamine (H1), or nicotinic receptors.

In contrast to typical APs, the atypical APs differ in their receptor profile. In addition to blocking D1, D3, and D4 receptors, atypical APs exert some degree of D2 receptor blockade. They also affect alpha-1- and alpha-2-adrenergic activity, influence the relationship between serotonergic (5-HT2) and D2 receptor activity, and bind to central 5-HT (5-HT2) receptors as well.

Studies indicate that atypical agents, unlike the typical APs, are effective in treating patients who are resistant to conventional antipsychotic therapy, may be more effective in relieving the negative as well as positive symptoms of schizophrenia, and exert minimal effects on serum prolactin levels.

Probably one of the most significant differences between typical and atypical agents is the type and severity of adverse effects. Figure 19-2 demonstrates a comparison of adverse effects between the typical and atypical APs. Primarily, atypical APs are considered for therapy because of their decreased ability or inability to induce EPS, a primary issue in maintaining patient compliance. Thus, the term atypical (also referred to as nonclassical) describes the lesser potential of these drugs to produce undesirable side effects including hyperprolactinemia and EPS, which are mediated by D2 receptor blockade. This may be accounted for by the fact that atypical antipsychotics tend to occupy a lower proportion of D2 receptors (40% to 60%) than typical drugs (70% to 80%) when used in clinically optimal doses. (Rakel, 2000).

Atypical antipsychotics are grouped into two chemical classes: dibenzapines and benzisoxazoles. Clozapine, a dibenzapine derivative with a greater potency in blocking 5-HT2 than the D2 receptor and a much higher affinity for the D4 than the D2 receptor, is considered the first and representative atypical AP. It was the first drug to demonstrate that antipsychotic activity could be separated from extrapyramidal activity. Unfortunately, the drug is associated with a high risk of agranulocytosis, requiring regular monitoring of the

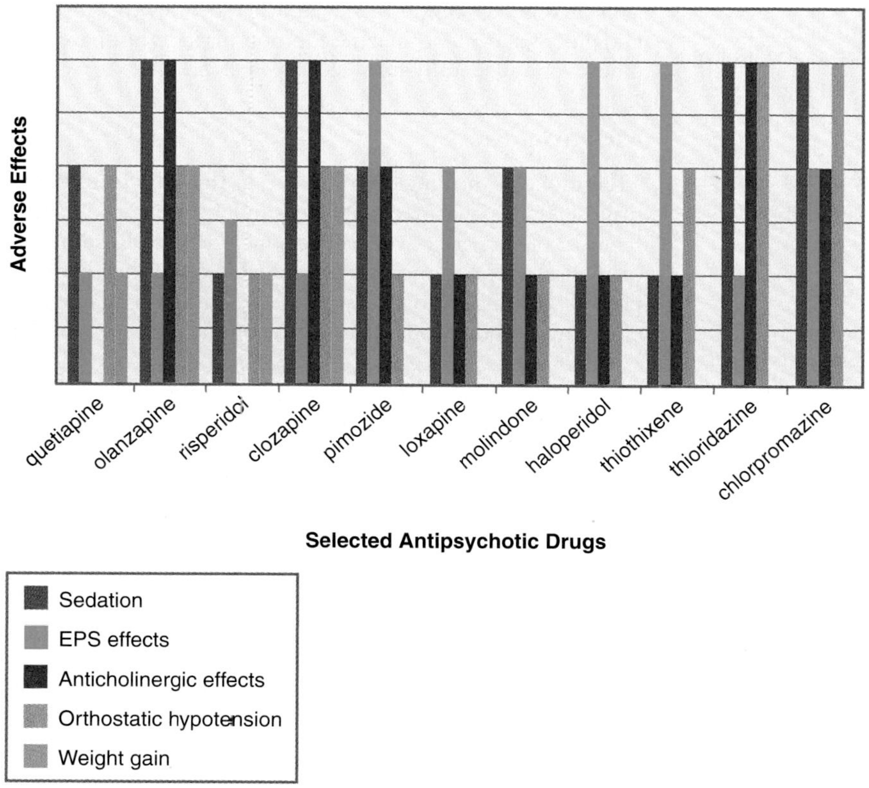

Figure 19-2. Comparison of typical and atypical antipsychotic agents.

patient's CBC. The higher efficacy of clozapine and risperidone, other atypical APs, in treating negative symptoms, along with the lower risk of TD, has stimulated the development of additional atypical antipsychotic agents that are likely to revolutionize the treatment of schizophrenia. Quetiapine, olanzapine, and two drugs now in phase III clinical trials (sertindole, ziprasidone) promise to have a therapeutic efficacy comparable with that of clozapine without the risk of agranulocytosis. Thus, the newer "atypical" APs are efficacious in treating the symptoms (both positive and negative symptoms) of schizophrenia, cause fewer EPS, block both DA and 5-HT receptors, and have a higher ratio of serotonergic (5-HT 2) to D2 antagonistic effects, leading to the suggestion that the neurotransmitter 5-HT also plays a role in schizophrenia. As a result, these agents have the potential to enhance patient compliance.

NURSING MANAGEMENT OF THE PATIENT RECEIVING CLOZAPINE

Core Drug Knowledge

Pharmacotherapeutics

Clozapine is an atypical AP drug with demonstrated efficacy for the management of severely ill schizophrenic patients. Due to its significant risk of causing agranulocytosis, the Food and Drug Administration (FDA) approves clozapine only for patients who fail to achieve adequate response with standard APs. Clozapine causes agranulocytosis (granulocyte count below 500/mm^3) in a small but significant number of patients, about 1% to 2%. The risk for clozapine-induced agranulocytosis appears to increase with age and affect more women than men. This is a serious—potentially fatal—effect that develops rapidly usually during the 6th to 18th weeks of therapy. Because of this risk, the drug is only available after registration in the "Clozaril Treatment/Patient Management System" (Cada, 2000). See the accompanying display, Clozaril Treatment/Patient Management System. It is unknown whether this adverse effect represents an immune reaction, but it appears to be reversible on discontinuation of the drug. Despite its demonstrated efficacy and minimal EPS potential, the FDA approves clozapine only for patients who fail to achieve adequate response with standard APs (Jessen, 1998).

Pharmacokinetics

Following oral administration, clozapine is rapidly absorbed and undergoes extensive hepatic first-pass metabolism, yielding at least one active metabolite. Clozapine is 95% protein bound and steady-state plasma concentrations are reached after 7 to 20 days of dosing. Smoking decreases concentrations by 60% to 80%. At equivalent doses, men who smoke have concentrations 20% to 30% lower than women who smoke. Widely distributed in tissues, concentrations in the central nervous system (CNS) exceed those in plasma. Because APs (both typical and atypical) are highly lipophilic, the drugs and their metabolites accumulate in the brain, lungs, and other tissues with high blood supply. They are stored in these tissues and may be found in urine for up to 6 months after the last dose. The onset of antipsychotic effect can take several weeks, but maximal effect may require several months.

Because clozapine is highly bound to serum proteins, competition for binding sites may occur with concurrent administration of other highly bound drugs. About 50% of clozapine excretion occurs through the kidneys; the remaining drug through enterohepatic circulation. Elimination half-lives range from 20 to 40 hours. Less than 1% is excreted as unchanged drug; it undergoes almost complete metabolism before excretion. Age-related decreases in hepatic elimination can occur; plasma concentrations may be increased in geriatric individuals. The bioavailability for clozapine tablets and solution is similar. There are pharmacokinetic differences between brand name and generic clozapine—patients should be monitored carefully when switching formulations.

Pharmacodynamics

Clozapine is a potent drug that exerts a greater activity at the limbic system than at the DA receptors by binding to 5HT-2, alpha-1 and H1 receptors, although there is some binding at DA receptors.

The pharmacology of clozapine differs from that of typical antipsychotic agents in that it blocks D2 recep-

COMMUNITY-BASED CONCERNS

Clozaril Treatment/Patient Management System

Results of early clinical studies with clozapine indicted that it was associated with 1% to 2% incidence of potentially lethal agranulocytosis. To minimize this risk, clozapine is available only through treatment systems that ensure a weekly or biweekly WBC testing prior to delivery of the next supply of medication. During the 5 years of WBC monitoring with the "Clozaril National Registry," the risk for agranulocytosis was reduced to approximately 0.38%. Guidelines for the Clozaril treatment/patient management system include:

- Treatment systems may include facilities with on-site pharmacies, facilities without on-site pharmacies, and individual treating physicians.
- Patients taking clozapine are enrolled in the "Clozaril National Registry."
- Clozaril is only available through weekly or biweekly distribution systems.
- WBC evaluation is required prior to initiation of therapy, weekly or biweekly during therapy, and for 4 weeks after discontinuation.
- All WBC evaluations (normal and abnormal results) must be promptly reported to the "Clozaril National Registry" within 7 days of collection.
- The "Clozaril National Registry" must be promptly notified of all patients who discontinue.

tors and has a high affinity for other DA receptors such as D1 and D4, serotonergic, alpha-adrenergic, histaminic, and muscarinic receptors. It does not disrupt dopaminergic function in the nigrostriatal pathway. These dopaminergic neurons are involved in the control of motor function. It is believed that clozapine selectively affects the dopaminergic neurons of the mesolimbic and mesocortical pathways. These pathways innervate the limbic and cortical areas and these neurons are involved in the control of behavior and emotion.

Clozapine reduces aggressive impulses and is thought to improve the negative symptoms, although this effect may not be evident for as long as 9 months (Bialek, 2000). Clozapine also exhibits a high affinity for several subtypes of serotonergic receptors.

Contraindications and Precautions

Clozapine should be used cautiously in patients receiving anticholinergic drugs, antihypertensive agents, and CNS-active drugs. It is contraindicated in patients receiving other bone marrow-suppressing drugs (e.g., carbamazepine).

The literature reports a few instances of sudden death from heart muscle injury associated with initial usage of clozapine, because the drug appears to increase triglyceride levels (Bialek, 2000).

Adverse Effects

Clozapine is associated with a high incidence of anticholinergic effects. Adverse effects include nasal congestion, constipation, drooling, fever, hypersalivation, hypotension, headache, insomnia, nausea, vomiting, and weight gain. Its potent anticholinergic effects may exacerbate glaucoma benign prostatic hypertrophy. Clozapine may cause new-onset diabetes.

The risk of agranulocytosis (white blood cell counts below $1{,}000^3$) is 1% to 2%, although it is not a predictable adverse effect and generally occurs during the first year of therapy. Older women are a higher risk for agranulocytosis although it can be reversed if the drug is withdrawn immediately (Bialek, 2000). A number of serious adverse effects may occur. The risk of seizures associated with clozapine use is related to dosage or plasma concentration. The occurrence of seizures is a concern even without a past history of seizures and may occur at higher doses (i.e., more than 600 mg/day) or with rapidly escalated doses.

Drug Interactions

Because of the risk for agranulocytosis, concurrent administration of clozapine with other drugs causing bone marrow suppression is contraindicated.

The concurrent administration of alcohol or CNS depressant drugs may enhance the CNS depressant effects of clozapine.

Clozapine is highly bound to plasma protein; it may increase the plasma concentration levels of other concurrently administered drugs that are also highly protein bound (e.g., digoxin, warfarin). Clozapine may potentiate the hypotensive effects of antihypertensive drugs and the anticholinergic effects of atropine-like drugs (Table 19-4).

TABLE 19-4 Agents That Interact With Clozapine

Interactants	Effect and Significance	Nursing Management
CNS depressants, alcohol	Increased CNS depression	Coadminister with caution.
bone marrow suppressants	Increased risk for agranulocytosis	Avoid coadministration. Monitor CBC with differential closely.
warfarin, digoxin	Increased plasma concentrations of interactant drugs	Monitor for increased effects of interactant, such as increased bruising, bleeding, or signs of digoxin toxicity.
cimetidine, erythromycin	Increased plasma concentration of clozapine	Monitor for evidence of increased adverse effects of clozapine. Anticipate reduced dosage of clozapine.
phenytoin	Decreased plasma clozapine levels	Assess for signs of ineffective control of schizophrenic symptoms. Anticipate need for possible increase in dosage of clozapine.
fluoxetine, fluvoxamine	Increased serum levels of clozapine	Coadminister with caution. Monitor for evidence of increased adverse effects. Anticipate reduced dosage of clozapine.
drugs metabolized by CYP-450 enzyme system (antidepressants, phenothiazines, carbamazepine, Type IC antiarrhythmics)	Increased plasma concentration of clozapine	Coadminister with caution. Monitor patient closely. Anticipate need for lower dosage of clozapine or other drug.

Assessment of Relevant Core Patient Variables

Health Status

The nurse should obtain the patient's baseline vital signs and other measurements, such as weight, serum glucose, and triglyceride levels and CBC, before clozapine therapy begins. The nurse should also assess for various individual patient factors that can alter drug response, for example, smoking, hepatic metabolism, gastric absorption, age, and possibly gender.

Life Span and Gender

The nurse should document the age and gender of the patient. The secondary elevation of prolactin secretion from AP use may diminish gonadal hormone levels, possibly leading to osteoporosis. The literature reports decreased bone mineral density in both male and female patients. The elderly patient on AP therapy should be considered at higher risk for fractures (Gasbarro, 1999). The nurse should also explore the sexual patterns and reproductive goals of the patient, because reproductive effects (e.g., changes in libido, amenorrhea, irregular menses, lactation, galactorrhea, gynecomastia, impotence, ejaculatory failure) may occur.

Lifestyle, Diet, and Habits

The nurse should evaluate the patient's caffeine intake and diet, because the potency of clozapine can be affected by fluctuations in caffeine intake.

The nurse should document the occupational and recreational activities of the patient, because drug-related dizziness and blurred vision may impair coordination and dexterity. Furthermore, orthostatic hypotension may occur in relation to increased activity.

Environment

The nurse should also document the climate in which the drug will be administered, because drug-related heatstroke may occur in hot weather and hypotension may occur with hot tubs, hot showers, or tub baths.

Nursing Diagnoses and Outcomes

- Imbalanced Nutrition: More Than Body Requirements related to increased appetite and polyphagia secondary to clozapine

  Desired outcome: The patient will describe reasons why there is a risk of weight gain and will identify the effects of a low-fat diet and exercise on weight control.
- Risk for injury related to drug-induced dizziness, blurred vision, orthostatic hypotension, drug-related heat stroke, blood dyscrasias (e.g., agranulocytosis)

  Desired outcome: The patient will identify factors that increase the risk for injury and will relate intent to use safety measures and practices to prevent injury.
- Disturbed Sleep Pattern related to clozapine adverse effect of insomnia

  Desired outcome: The patient will identify techniques to induce sleep and will report an optimal balance of rest and activity.

Planning and Intervention

Maximizing Therapeutic Effects

Clozapine's potency is affected the amount of caffeine consumed. Patients on clozapine therapy should limit the amount of caffeine in their diet. Patients who drink caffeinated beverages should be regularly monitored—particularly if their consumption or drinking habits change.

Minimizing Adverse Effects

Weight (5 to 20 kg) gain is common and frequently requires monitoring of food intake. Constipation from slowed GI motility can be relieved with stool softeners and increased fluid and fiber intake and exercise. Therapeutic effects of a single dose can last 24 hours, thus allowing for once-daily dosing to minimize undesirable reactions such as excessive sedation.

Providing Patient and Family Education

Much of the patient and family teaching done by the nurse for the typical APs also applies to the atypical APs. Selected patent and family education specific for atypical APs include the following:

- The nurse should advise the patient and family to report signs of lethargy, weakness, fever or sore throat. This may be an indication of developing agranulocytosis.
- Caution the patient and family to notify the health care provider before taking any prescription or OTC drug or herbal preparations.
- Some individuals may be unaware of how many foods, beverages, and OTC drugs contain caffeine. The nurse should teach the patient and family about such foods and OTC drugs and warn them to limit caffeine in the diet.
- To minimize the risks associated with drug-related dizziness and blurred vision, the nurse should advise the patient to avoid hazardous occupational or recreational activities until drug response is determined. Moreover, orthostatic hypotension occurs frequently, so the nurse should encourage the patient to modify activities for safety.
- The nurse should advise the patient that weight gain is a common adverse effect of all antipsychotic drugs, which occurs because of an increase in appetite. This may be especially problematic if other health problems exist (e.g., diabetes, hypercholesteremia, hypertension, obesity) and can contribute to morbidity and mortality. The nurse should encourage the patient to

follow a low-fat diet and engage in moderate exercise to help with weight control.

- The nurse should advise the patient receiving to take extra care to stay cool in hot weather to minimize the risk for heatstroke and hypotension.
- Due to the risk of agranulocytosis, the nurse should educate the patient and family about the importance of adhering to ongoing evaluations, particularly blood studies.
- The nurse should caution the patient and family about the adverse effects resulting from combined drug and alcohol use because of the hazards of enhanced sedation and decreased drug effectiveness.

Ongoing Assessment and Evaluation

The nurse should evaluate the patient for sedation during the first several weeks of therapy, because this adverse effect may be quite severe. Administering a single dose before bedtime may lessen this effect. ■

DRUGS CLOSELY RELATED TO P CLOZAPINE

Risperidone

Risperidone (Risperdal) is a structural relative of clozapine; it differs in that it is a more selective DA/5-HT antagonist. It is the first drug from a new class of atypical APs, the benzisoxazole derivatives. The most potent of atypical APs, it is indicated for the management of psychotic disorders. Unlabeled uses are management of childhood-onset schizophrenia, bipolar disorder, and dementia-related psychotic symptoms (Inada, 2000). It blocks both 5-HT and DA receptors and is effective for psychotic symptoms of apathy, delusions, depression, and hallucinations.

Dosages of 4 to 6 mg/day show optimal efficacy and lack of pseudoparkinsonism. Dosages higher than this have been associated with neurologic adverse effects like those of typical APs. Risperidone is metabolized by CYP-450-2D6 hepatic isoenzymes to an active metabolite, 9-hydroxy-risperidone, nearly as efficacious as risperidone itself. Risperidone's half-life is dependent on whether the individual is a "poor" or "fast" metabolizer. Between 5% and 10% of whites and 1% to 3% of Asians and African Americans have little or no activity at CYP2D6 and are considered "poor metabolizers." Poor metabolizers convert risperidone to its active metabolite at a slower rate, which can affect the half-life and time to steady state of the drug. No important differences in the incidence of adverse reactions have been noted among the poor metabolizers. The half-life ranges from 20 to 30 hours and from 3 to 21 hours, respectively. Risperidone and its metabolite are renally excreted.

When administered concurrently, drug interactions occur between risperidone and carbamazepine (increased risperidone elimination), clozapine (decreased risperidone elimination), and levodopa (decreased levodopa effects). Risperidone may adversely affect judgment, cognitive and motor skills, and activities requiring physical alertness (e.g., driving) and manual dexterity (operating dangerous machinery); consumption of alcohol should be avoided to minimize the risk for potentiating these effects. Common adverse effects include agitation, headache, insomnia, and weight gain. Orthostatic hypotension, tachycardia, and dizziness often occur during the dose-titration period. Other adverse effects include hyperprolactinemia, priapism, rhinitis, somnolence, and EPS. Relatively few EPS are seen at doses of less than 6 mg daily; doses above this result in significantly more EPS. The weight gain associated with risperidone is less than that associated with clozapine.

Nursing management of the patient receiving risperidone is similar to that of clozapine. One study demonstrated that the therapeutic benefit of risperidone may be optimized by monitoring serum concentrations of active drug (25 to 150 μg/L), although "this might be considered an enlarged therapeutic range" (Odou, et al., 2000). It is important that the nurse educate patients and their families about the importance of adhering to ongoing evaluations, particularly blood studies.

Olanzapine

Olanzapine is an atypical antipsychotic agent belonging to the dibenzapine class. The FDA has approved olanzapine as a short-term treatment of acute manic episodes associated with bipolar disorder. Olanzapine is slightly less potent than risperidone. Olanzapine is structurally and pharmacologically related to clozapine. Like clozapine, it is effective for positive and, at higher doses, the negative symptoms of schizophrenia. Also like clozapine, it binds to alpha-1, DA, H1, muscarinic, and 5-HT2 receptors. With olanzapine, EPS and the potential for interaction with other drugs are reduced. Unlike clozapine, olanzapine appears to have a low potential

MEMORY CHIP

P Clozapine

- Used in the treatment of schizophrenia
- Significant contraindications: myeloproliferative disorders, history of severe granulocytopenia, or clozapine-induced agranulocytosis
- Most common adverse effects: sedation, nausea, constipation, tachycardia, hypotension
- Most serious adverse effects: agranulocytosis, seizures
- **Life span alert: not for use in children; increased susceptibility to adverse effects in elderly; geriatric individuals are more susceptible to adverse effects; lower doses are given initially and then gradually are increased.**
- Maximizing therapeutic effects: limit caffeine consumption because this affects clozapine potency
- Minimizing adverse effects: closely monitor WBC count
- Most significant patient education: stress the importance of reporting signs of infection such as fever, sore throat, malaise, mouth ulcers and flu-like symptoms

for producing leukopenia or agranulocytosis. After oral administration, olanzapine is well absorbed, and peak serum levels occur in about 6 hours. The drug is metabolized in the liver.

Olanzapine is a substrate of CYP1A2, although it does not appear to inhibit or induce any of the P450 isoenzymes. Agents that induce or inhibit CYP1A2 may affect olanzapine metabolism. The clearance of olanzapine appears to be affected by patient age, gender, and smoking status, with clearance 50% lower in those older than 65 years, approximately 30% lower in women than in men, and 40% higher in smokers than in nonsmokers. Combinations of these factors can potentially lead to significant variations in olanzapine pharmacokinetics. Combination of olanzapine with any CNS depressant (e.g., benzodiazepines, alcohol) could result in additive effects with respect to sedation as well as psychomotor impairment.

High doses of olanzapine may cause greater EPS and akathisia. The nurse should provide patient teaching about adverse effects related to olanzapine such as sedation, mild anticholinergic effects, and weight gain.

Quetiapine

Quetiapine is an atypical antipsychotic agent belonging to the dibenzapine class. It is the least potent of the atypical APs and has fewer adverse effects, with sedation and weight gain the most prominent. Quetiapine acts as an antagonist at a number of receptors including 5-HT receptors (5-HT1A, 5-HT2) and DA (D1, D2) receptors. Its affinity for 5-HT2 is greater than that for D2. Quetiapine is also an antagonist at H1, and adrenergic (alpha-1, alpha-2) receptors. It has little effect on cholinergic receptors.

Oral clearance of quetiapine is induced by the prototype CYP3A4 inducer, phenytoin. Quetiapine should be used with caution with concomitant administration of potent enzyme inhibitors of CYP3A (e.g., erythromycin, fluconazole, ketoconazole). The efficacy of quetiapine may be diminished by concomitant administration of hepatic enzyme inducers (e.g., barbiturates, carbamazepine, glucocorticoids, rifampin). Thioridazine increases quetiapine clearance by 65%. Quetiapine reduces lorazepam clearance by 20%. Cimetidine reduces quetiapine clearance by 20%.

Quetiapine may cause hepatic enzyme elevation. Because the liver extensively metabolizes quetiapine, higher plasma levels will occur in hepatic function impairment and dosage adjustment may be needed.

Quetiapine also increases cholesterol and triglyceride levels. Quetiapine has demonstrated a dose-related decrease in total and free thyroxine (T_4) and TSH increases. Quetiapine adverse effects include agitation, anxiety, dizziness, headache, insomnia, nervousness, somnolence, and weight gain.

Ziprasidone

Ziprasidone, a 5-HT 5-HT1D antagonist, 5-HT1A agonist, and inhibitor of 5-HT and NE reuptake, is used to treat schizophrenia. The FDA has required a change in the brand name on approval from Zeldox to Geodon—to prevent medication errors due to look-alike or sound-alike confusion. Pharmacokinetics are not significantly affected by age, gender, smoking status, or renal impairment. Due to substantial hepatic clearance, a dosage adjustment with liver impairment is recommended. Ziprasidone is more likely than other atypical antipsychotic drugs to prolong the QT interval on ECGs. Significant prolongation of the QT interval can lead to a polymorphic form of ventricular tachycardia known as torsade de pointes; this can predispose patients to sudden death.

Use of ziprasidone in patients who have known cardiovascular disease, electrolyte abnormalities, congenital prolonged QT intervals, or who are taking medications that can have quinidine-like effects on ECG intervals (e.g., tricyclic antidepressants) may be at a greater risk.

DEMENTIA AND ALZHEIMER DISEASE

Dementia, a serious and common age-related health problem with many causes, affects more than 4 million Americans and costs society more than $50 billion annually. See the accompanying display, Risk Factors and Possible Causes of Dementia. It is a clinical syndrome of acquired impairments in memory and cognitive skills with memory the most common and most important cognitive ability lost. Other mental faculties such as attention, judgment, comprehension, orientation, learning, calculation, problem solving, mood, and behavior may also be affected. Agitation or withdrawal, hallucinations, delusions, insomnia, emotional apathy, and loss of inhibitions are also common.

The symptoms develop gradually and although the deterioration is not necessarily diffuse or "global," it often affects some areas of intellectual functioning while sparing others. Early in the disease, the patient may be aware of changes in

Risk Factors and Possible Causes of Dementia

Irreversible Risk Factors/Causes

- Age over 65 years
- Cerebral infarction or ischemia
- Diseases such as cardiovascular disorders, type 1 diabetes, degenerative (e.g., Parkinson disease), neoplasms
- Male gender
- Genetic factors such as apolipoprotein E gene on chromosome 19 and chromosome 10

Potentially Reversible Risk Factors/Causes

- Depression
- Diseases such as type 2 diabetes, hyperlipidemia, hypertension, infections
- Drugs with iatrogenic/idiosyncratic effect or polypharmacy
- Lifestyle habits such as excessive alcohol consumption, smoking, illicit drug use, among others
- Metabolic disorders
- Nutritional disorders
- Toxins
- Trauma

intellectual ability and become depressed or anxious and attempt to compensate by writing down information, attempting to structure routines, and simplifying responsibilities. Cognitive decline can severely diminish the possibility of independent living and is one of the main causes of disability and institutionalization among elderly individuals. There are considerable financial, social, and emotional costs associated with the burdens of caring for patients with dementia (Raker, 2000).

Alzheimer disease (AD), a form of progressive dementia, is one of the most common chronic conditions and causes of dementia in the elderly. Overall, it affects about 1 in 10 Americans older than the age of 65 with its incidence strikingly related to age. About 15% of the population between the ages of 75 and 84 and nearly 50% of those older than 85 are affected. Currently, AD is believed to affect 4 to 5 million persons. The number of people in the United States older than age 65, the most rapidly growing segment of the population, is expected to triple by the middle of the 21st century, making AD a public health problem of staggering proportions.

AD causes a gross, diffuse atrophy of the cerebral cortex with widening of sulci, narrow convolutions, lateral ventricular enlargement, reduction in white matter, extracellular plaques with beta-amyloid protein deposits, and neurofibrillary tangles in the cortical neurons with eventual loss of neurons. The earliest loss of neurons occurs in the nucleus basalis and the entorhinal cortex where cholinergic neurons are preferentially affected. As the illness progresses, up to 90% of cholinergic neurons in the nucleus basalis baseline may be lost. Cholinergic deficiency in AD is most prominent at the more advanced stages. Animal studies have demonstrated loss in these areas is associated with declines in learning capacity and memory (Farlow, 1999).

Typically, AD begins insidiously with memory loss, both short-term and long-term, and with the presence of other cognitive deficits that impair ADLs. Individuals with AD frequently repeat questions, forget phone messages and appointments, do not pay bills, or get lost driving. Individuals with AD may lose weight because they no longer shop for food, cook, or eat. Furthermore, the cognitive deficits are relentlessly progressive; affective, behavioral, and motor signs become more common as the disease advances.

In addition to the cognitive deficits, behavioral and psychiatric symptoms (e.g., abnormal sleep, delusions, depression, hallucinations, mania, pacing, paranoia, wandering) tend to occur at some point in most patients with dementia. The concept term "behavioral and psychological symptoms of dementia" (BPSD) has been proposed to explain these signs and symptoms. Although many psychotropics (e.g., anticonvulsants, antidepressants, atypical antipsychotics) are used to treat BPSD, none of these agents is currently labeled for such indications. As dementia progresses, patients inevitably lose function in the various ADLs (Doraiswamy, 2000).

The course of AD is prolonged. Generalized seizures may occur and death usually results from malnutrition, secondary infections, or heart disease. The typical duration of AD is 8 to 10 years, but the course can range from 1 to 25 years. Some AD patients show a steady downhill decline in function, whereas others have prolonged plateaus without major deterioration. The reasons for this are not known.

ALZHEIMER DRUGS

Acetylcholine is the neurotransmitter of several CNS neuronal circuits. One circuit projects from the basal forebrain to the hippocampus and parts of the cerebral cortex. Agents that augment this system have been under investigation for the treatment of AD for more than 20 years and numerous types of drugs that augment levels of ACh to compensate for losses of cholinergic function in the brain have been used in patients with AD. These drugs have included ACh precursors, muscarinic agonists, nicotinic agonists, and acetylcholinesterase inhibitors (AChEIs), which have been by far the most successful in terms of medications that have consistently verified cognitive and functional efficacy in AD and the only FDA-approved therapy to treat the symptoms of AD. AChEIs inhibit acetylcholinesterase (AChE) enzymes that break down ACh and prolong the activity of ACh on cortical cholinergic receptors and in the synapse, thus allowing for more effective transmission. The mechanism of action of the three AChEIs—tacrine, donepezil and rivastigmine—is essentially the same. These agents increase concentrations of the memory-regulating and cognition-regulating neurotransmitter ACh through reversible inhibition of the enzyme cholinesterase. Although these drugs have not been shown to alter the course of the dementing process, it is anticipated that disease effects will lessen as the disease process advances and fewer cholinergic neurons remain intact.

Drugs used in the treatment of dementia and AD include donepezil, rivastigmine, and tacrine. Rivastigmine (Exelon) is the prototypical Alzheimer drug. Table 19-5 summarizes selected Alzheimer drugs.

NURSING MANAGEMENT OF THE PATIENT RECEIVING RIVASTIGMINE

Core Drug Knowledge

Pharmacotherapeutics

Rivastigmine is indicated for the treatment of mild to moderate dementia of the Alzheimer type. In clinical studies it has shown enhanced cognition (memory, language, orientation) and improved function (in ADLs) in patients with mild to moderate AD.

Pharmacokinetics

Rivastigmine is rapidly and completely absorbed with peak plasma concentrations reached in 1 hour. Administration of rivastigmine with food delays its absorption (by about 1½ hours), although food does not impair absorption. Rivastigmine may be taken with food if GI adverse effects are problematic.

Rivastigmine is widely distributed throughout the body. It penetrates the blood–brain barrier, reaching CSF peak concentrations in 1.4 to 2.6 hours. Rivastigmine is 40% bound to plasma proteins.

Rivastigmine is rapidly and extensively metabolized by AChE; minimal metabolism occurs by the major

TABLE 19-5 Summary of Selected Drugs for Alzheimer Disease

Drug (Trade) Name	Selected Indications	Route and Dosage Range	Pharmacokinetics
rivastigmine (Exelon)	Mild to moderate Alzheimer type dementia	*Adult:* PO, 3 to 6 mg bid to a maximum of 12 mg/d *Child:* Not currently indicated	*Onset:* Intermediate *Duration:* 10 h $t_{1/2}$: 1.5 h
tacrine (Cognex)	Mild to moderate Alzheimer type dementia	*Adult:* 10 mg qid *Child:* Safety and efficacy not established	*Onset:* Unknown *Duration:* 6 h $t_{1/2}$: 2–4 h
donepezil (Aricept)	Mild to moderate Alzheimer type dementia	*Adult:* 5–10 mg/d *Child:* Safety and efficacy not established	*Onset:* Unknown *Duration:* Unknown $t_{1/2}$: 70 h

CYP450 isozymes. Thus, no CYP450 drug interactions have been observed. The elimination half-life is 1.5 hours, with most elimination as metabolites renally excreted. The oral solution and capsules may be interchanged at equal doses. It is about equally metabolized through the hepatic cytochrome P450 enzyme system and excreted as unchanged drug in the urine.

Pharmacodynamics

Rivastigmine is a carbamate derivative that is believed to exert its therapeutic effect by enhancing cholinergic function. This occurs by increasing the concentration of ACh through reversible inhibition of AChE. Rivastigmine does not alter the course of the underlying dementing process.

Contraindications and Precautions

Rivastigmine is contraindicated in hypersensitivity to carbamate derivatives. There are no adequate or well-controlled studies in children and pregnant or lactating women. Rivastigmine is placed in FDA pregnancy category B. It is not known whether rivastigmine is excreted in breast milk. Rivastigmine should be used cautiously in children and pregnant or lactating women.

Adverse Effects

Rivastigmine is associated with significant GI adverse reactions, including nausea and vomiting, anorexia, and weight loss. Other adverse effects include dizziness, headache, chest pain, peripheral edema, vertigo, arthralgia, agitation, nervousness, delusion, paranoid reaction, coughing, generalized rash, and urinary incontinence. Rivastigmine may have vagotonic effects on heart rates (e.g., bradycardia) because the drug increases cholinergic activity. These vagotonic effects may be particularly important in patients with "sick sinus syndrome" or other supraventricular cardiac conduction conditions. Again because of the increase in cholinergic activity, rivastigmine may cause urinary obstruction and may have some potential for causing seizures, although seizure activity also may be a manifestation of AD. Like other drugs that increase cholinergic activity, rivastigmine should be used with care in patients with a history of asthma or obstructive pulmonary disease.

Drug Interactions

Pharmacokinetic drug interactions are not believed to occur with rivastigmine, because only minimal metabolism of the drug occurs through the major CYP450 isozymes.

Synergistic effects may be expected when AChEIs are given concurrently with succinylcholine, similar neuromuscular blocking agents, or cholinergic agonists, such as bethanechol. Because of their mechanism of action, AChEIs have the potential to interfere with the activity of anticholinergic medications.

Assessment of Relevant Core Patient Variables

Health Status

The nurse should perform a thorough assessment of body systems. The patient's cardiac status may be adversely by AChEIs because these drugs increase cholinergic activity and may cause bradycardia from vagal effects on heart rate. The cholinergic activity of the AChEIs may cause urinary retention or obstruction; men with benign prostatic hypertrophy may be especially at risk.

The nurse should evaluate the patient's renal and hepatic function. Dosage adjustments may be necessary in patients with renal or hepatic function impairment. The nurse should review the patient's respiratory function because respiratory depression may occur. The nurse should carefully assess the patient's GI status as AChEIs such as rivastigmine may increase gastric acid secretion, cause gastritis, and exacerbate peptic ulcer disease. Individuals with a history of ulcer disease or those receiving nonsteroidal anti-inflammatory drugs should be assessed and closely monitored for symptoms of active or occult GI bleeding.

Life Span and Gender

The nurse should document the age of the patient. The mean oral clearance of rivastigmine is 30% lower in elderly individuals taking rivastigmine. The nurse should assess a woman of child-bearing age for pregnancy and lactation. If appropriate, the nurse should explore potential benefits of rivastigmine therapy against the potential risks to the fetus or child.

Lifestyle, Diet, and Habits

The nurse should assess the patient for tobacco use because nicotine use moderately increases the oral clearance of rivastigmine (23%).

Environment

The nurse should be aware of the environment in which the drug will be administered. If appropriate, the nurse should assess the patient's home or living environment. The patient's environment should be calm and predictable. A safe area in which the individual can move about should be provided, because wandering is common among patients with dementia.

Nursing Diagnoses and Outcomes

- Anxiety related to cognitive changes secondary to Alzheimer dementia
  Desired outcome: The patient will identify effective coping mechanisms.
- Risk for Injury related to adverse effect of sedation
  Desired outcome: The patient will establish appropriate sleep/rest patterns, participate in activities, and establish priorities for daily and weekly activities.
- Impaired Memory related to progressive Alzheimer dementia
  Desired outcome: The patient will identify at least two techniques to improve memory.
- Self-care Deficit related to the progressive dementia of AD
  Desired outcome: The patient will identify preferences in self-care activities, demonstrate optimal hygiene after assistance with care and participate physically and/or verbally in feeding, dressing, toileting, and bathing activities.
- Dysfunctional Family Processes related to impact of Alzheimer disease on family system
  Desired outcome: The family will participate in care of ill family member.
- Caregiver Role Strain related to emotional and physical stress secondary to managing the progressive deterioration associated with AD
  Desired outcome: The caregiver will share frustrations regarding caregiving responsibilities, identify one source of support and identify two changes that, if made, would improve daily life.
- The family will convey empathy to caregiver regarding daily responsibilities and establish a plan for regular and frequent support or help.
- Chronic Confusion related to progressive degeneration of the cerebral cortex secondary to AD
  Desired outcome: The patient will participate to a maximum level of independence in activities, experience decreased frustration when environmental stressors are reduced, have diminished or absent episodes of combative behavior, and increase hours of sleep at night.
- Risk for Injury related to lack of awareness of environmental hazards secondary to AD
  Desired outcome: The family will identify potentially hazardous factors in the environment and report safe practices in the home.
- Imbalanced Nutrition: Less Than Body Requirements related to decreased desire to eat secondary to nausea and vomiting from drug therapy
  Desired outcome: The patient will ingest daily nutritional requirements in relation to activity level and metabolic needs.

Planning and Intervention

Maximizing Therapeutic Effects

It is important to detect and correct any treatable factors causing or contributing to cognitive impairment. The nurse must be aware that any cognitive impairments may be exacerbated by hearing or visual deficits or medical conditions (e.g., heart failure, electrolyte imbalance, anemia). For example, impairment of the senses (e.g., auditory, visual) may affect the individual's performance on mental status tests that are used to evaluate for dementia. Additionally, it is necessary to rule out systemic diseases that can cause reversible dementia.

Minimizing Adverse Effects and Providing Patient and Family Education

The irreversible nature of AD and its progressive deteriorating course has devastating effects on affected individuals, their caregivers, and their families. Although drug therapy is directed toward enhancing cognitive and functional abilities, teaching considerations reflect more issues regarding the disease process and its progressive nature as well as the burdens facing the caregiver.

- The nurse should advise the patient and family of the high incidence of nausea and vomiting associated with the use of rivastigmine along with the possibility of anorexia and weight loss. The nurse should encourage them to monitor for these adverse events and inform the health care provider if they occur.
- The nurse should teach the patient and family to reduce disorientation by maintaining familiar physical surroundings with adequate night-time lighting and reducing excess auditory and visual stimulation.
- The family is often stressed because the demented individual is prone to wandering and unable to give his or her name or residence when found. The nurse should stress important safety measures such as providing a safe place to move about. The nurse should advise the family to have the affected person wear identification (necklace, bracelet) at all times.
- The nurse should advise the patient and family that a daily routine should be as simple and constant as possible, because variations and surprises may produce unnecessary anxiety and confusion.

- The nurse should offer helpful communication techniques such as using concrete language, maintaining social greetings and rituals, using a soft tone of voice, simplifying and repeating instructions frequently, and continuous reorientation (e.g., large clocks and calendars).

Ongoing Assessment and Evaluation

Correction of underlying issues (e.g., depression, drug toxicity, metabolic and endocrine disturbances, etc.) may result in cognitive improvement.

Rivastigmine, as with other AchEIs, produces modest improvement in some measures of cognitive functioning as well as in other areas of functioning in the patient with mild to moderate Alzheimer disease, apparently slowing the progression of the disease. However, the nurse must advise patients and their families to maintain realistic expectations regarding what the drug can do. ■

DRUGS CLOSELY RELATED TO RIVASTIGMINE

Tacrine

Tacrine (Cognex) is a centrally acting reversible AChEI. Tacrine was the first AChEI approved by the FDA for the treatment of AD. It has a short duration of action (about 6 hours) so the drug must be administered four times daily. Several studies have shown an improvement of cognitive symptoms in a minority of patients with mild to moderate AD by elevating ACh concentrations in the cerebral cortex and by slowing the degradation of ACh release by still-intact cholinergic neurons. Up to 50% of patients in these studies had to discontinue the drug due to adverse effects such as asymptomatic hepatotoxicity, nausea, vomiting, and diarrhea. Due to hepatotoxicity, the drug manufacturer recommends a slow increase of the dose of tacrine, checking serum transaminase levels weekly. Progression of the disease, however, lessens the effects of tacrine because there are fewer cholinergic neurons remaining intact.

Tacrine is primarily eliminated by the hepatic CYP450 enzyme system. Drug interactions may occur with drugs (e.g., phenytoin, theophylline) that undergo extensive metabolism by the same system.

Donepezil

Donepezil (Aricept) is a second-generation reversible AChEI that is indicated for the treatment of mild to moderate Alzheimer dementia. Donepezil has several advantages over tacrine, including a longer half-life. Its long half-life (about 70 hours) allows for once-daily dosing. Donepezil is usually well tolerated, causes limited and mild GI adverse effects of nausea, vomiting, and diarrhea, has no significant interactions with other drugs, and does not cause significant elevations of serum transaminase that requires monitoring of hepatic function.

Galanthamine Hydrobromide

Galanthamine hydrobromide (Reminyl), which was approved February 2001 by the FDA for treatment of AD, has a dual mechanism of action. It combines allosteric (influencing of an enzyme) modulation of nicotinic ACh receptors with reversible, competitive inhibition of ACh to potentiate the action of agonists at these receptors. In clinical trials, galanthamine was found to be effective at doses of 16, 24, and 32 mg/day, although the 32 mg/day dose was not associated with any additional cognitive benefit. In clinical trials, galanthamine improved ADLs in AD patients, which reduced the requirement for caregiver assistance with ADLs. Galanthamine is generally well tolerated with the majority of adverse effects—cholinergic and GI in nature—only mild to moderate in intensity and transient. Galanthamine has no clinically relevant effects on vital signs, hematologic or biochemical laboratory parameters and, importantly, no known hepatotoxicity.

MEMORY CHIP

Rivastigmine

- Used in the treatment of Alzheimer disease
- Significant contraindication: hypersensitivity to carbamates
- Most common adverse effects: high incidence of nausea, vomiting; possible anorexia and weight loss
- Most serious adverse effects: abnormal hepatic function, cholecystitis
- **Life span alert: increased susceptibility to adverse effects in the elderly; lower dosages are used initially then gradually are increased.**
- Maximizing therapeutic effects: administer on an empty stomach
- Minimizing adverse effects: administer with food only if severe GI upset occurs. Drug absorption is delayed by food
- Most significant patient education: avoid smoking; nicotine decreases therapeutic effects

CHAPTER SUMMARY

- Antipsychotic agents are commonly used in the treatment of psychotic disorders for the relief of psychotic symptoms such as hallucinations and delusions. Palliative rather than curative, they provide some symptomatic relief and may improve individual functioning and quality of life.
- Schizophrenia is a life-long illness and antipsychotic drugs must be used intermittently or continuously.
- Antipsychotic drug actions include an affinity to ACh, DA, histamine, and 5-HT receptors. Therapeutic and adverse effects relate to their specific receptor affinity as well as loci of action within the CNS.
- Typical antipsychotic drugs are described in terms of potency: high-potency drugs are generally associated with EPS, whereas low-potency drugs tend to cause greater anticholinergic effects.
- All typical APs share two major characteristics—they improve the positive and disorganized symptoms of schizophrenia and they produce a neurologic syndrome of extrapyramidal adverse effects (i.e., pseudoparkinsonism) by their action of ACh and DA neurotransmitters.
- EPS are the most significant undesired clinical responses associated with the typical neuroleptic drugs. These symptoms include acute

dystonia, akathisia, parkinsonism, and TD. The atypical drugs cause little to no pseudoparkinsonism.

- The largest class of the typical antipsychotics is the phenothiazines. They are divided into three distinct chemical categories. The aliphatic compounds (e.g., chlorpromazine, promazine) often produce strong sedative effects and moderate to strong EPS. They are particularly effective in controlling the psychotic symptoms of delusions and hallucinations. The piperidine compounds (e.g., thioridazine, mesoridazine) have moderate to strong anticholinergic effects, strong sedative effects, and minimal EPS. These drugs are often used for short-term treatment of severe behavioral problems in children and for sleep disturbances and dementia in the elderly. The piperazine compounds (e.g., trifluoperazine, fluphenazine, prochlorperazine) cause the least sedation and EPS. They are particularly effective for withdrawn, apathetic individuals.
- Atypical antipsychotic drugs are approximately equal in efficacy to the typical drugs for the positive and disorganized symptoms of schizophrenia. Their efficacy for the negative symptoms, however, is superior.
- Clozapine is an atypical antipsychotic that causes agranulocytosis and leukopenia. Patients taking clozapine must have their white blood cell counts carefully monitored during therapy.
- One of the major concerns for the nurse working with community-based chronically ill schizophrenic patients is to encourage compliance with the medical regime and treatment plan.
- Dementia typically evolves over many years; for much of this time the individual is not totally disabled and is more functional in a familiar and stable environment.
- Caregivers of AD patients experience profound emotional and physical stress in managing the progressive deterioration associated with AD.

QUESTIONS FOR STUDY AND REVIEW

1. Identify the etiology and pathophysiology of schizophrenia.
2. Differentiate between the positive, disorganized, and negative symptoms of schizophrenia.
3. Explain the difference in adverse effects between the typical and atypical antipsychotics.
4. Relate the important teaching points regarding antipsychotic drug therapy for the patient and family.
5. Discuss the occurrence of AD. Explain why it is considered to potentially be a major public health problem.
6. Identify the drugs used to treat AD and explain their mechanism of action.

NEED MORE HELP?

Chapter 19 of the study guide for *Drug Therapy in Nursing* contains exercises and activities to reinforce your understanding of the concepts presented in this chapter. For additional information see the text's accompanying website at *http://www.connection.lww.com.*

REFERENCES AND BIBLIOGRAPHY

Andreason, N. C. (1999). *Deconstructing schizophrenia.* Presented at the 51st Institute on Psychiatric Services, New Orleans, LA.

Andreason, N. C. (1999). *Schizophrenia: The fundamental questions.* Presented at the 51st Institute on Psychiatric Services, New Orleans, LA.

Beaumont, G. (2000). Antipsychotics—the future of schizophrenia treatment. *Current Medical Research and Opinion, 16*(1), 37–42.

Beyzarov, E. P. (2000). And then there were three. *Drug Topics, 144*(10), 19–20.

Bialek, D. (2000). Schizophrenia and its treatments. *Pharmacy Times, 66*(12), 10–71

Bond, W. S. (1991). Ethnicity and psychotropic drugs. *Clinical Pharmacy, 10*(6), 467–470.

Cada, D. J., Covington, T. R., Hebel, S. K., Hussar, D. A., Lasagna, L., Olin, B. R., Selevan, J. R., Sloan, R. W., Tatro, D. S., & Whitsett, T. L. (2001). *Drug facts and comparisons.* St. Louis: Facts and Comparisons.

Cummings, J. L. (1999). Cholinesterase inhibitors: A new class of psychotropic compounds. *American Journal of Psychiatry, 157,* 1–15.

Doraiswamy, P. M. (2000). Update on pharmacotherapy for Alzheimer's disease. Conference presented at the 13th annual meeting of the American Association for Geriatric Psychiatry, Miami, FL.

Farlow, M. R. (1999). *Therapeutic advances for Alzheimer's disease and other dementias.* Golden, CO: Accreditation Council for Continuing Medical Education (ACCME).

Fauci, A., Braunwald, E., Wilson, J. D., Martin, J. B., Hauser, S. L., Longo, D. L., Kasper, D. L., & Isselbachter, K. J. (Eds.). (1999). *Harrison's online.* New York: McGraw-Hill.

Gasbarro, R. (1999). The use of atypical antipsychotics in the elderly. *Pharmacy Times, 65*(8), 2HPT–6HPT

Gutierrez, M. A., Huang, L., & Wincor, M. Z. (1998). Olanzapine and its place in antipsychotic therapy. *U.S. Pharmacist, 23*(3), 78–87.

Hardman, J. G., Limbird, L. E., Molinof, P. B., Ruddon, R. W., & Gilman, A. G. (Eds.). (1997). *Goodman & Gilman's pharmacological basis of therapeutics* (9th ed.). New York: McGraw-Hill.

Hikal, A. H., & Hikal, E. M. (1998). Dementia in the elderly. *Drug Topics, 142*(19), 81–90.

Holcomb, H. (1999). *Functional neuroimaging applied to the syndrome of schizophrenia: Symptom, treatment, and etiologic observations.* Presented at the American Psychiatric Association's 152nd Annual Meeting, Washington, D.C.

Inada, T. (2000). *The treatment of schizophrenia: Practice and practicality.* Presented at the 153rd annual meeting of the American Psychiatric Association, Chicago, IL.

Jann, M. W. (2000). Rivastigmine, a new-generation cholinesterase inhibitor for the treatment of Alzheimer's disease. *Pharmacotherapy, 20,* 1–12.

Jessen, L. M. (1998). New treatment options for schizophrenia. *U.S. Pharmacist, 23*(5), 117–128.

Jeste, D. V., & Finkel, S. L. (2000). Psychosis of Alzheimer's disease and related dementias: Diagnostic criteria for a distinct syndrome. *American Journal of Geriatric Psychiatry, 54,* 257–263.

Katzung, B. C. (Ed.). (2000). *Basic and clinical pharmacology* (8th ed). New York: McGraw-Hill.

Nolan, S., & Scoggin, J. A. (1998). Serotonin syndrome: Recognition and treatment. *U.S. Pharmacist, 23*(2), 39–51.

Odou, P., Levron, J. C., Luyckx, M., Brunet, H. R. (2000). Risperidone drug monitoring: A useful clinical tool? *Clinical Drug Investigation, 19*(4), 283–292.

Rakel, R. E. (2000). *Conn's current therapy.* Philadelphia: W. B. Saunders.

Rauscher, M. (2000). Steady state dosing of antipsychotic may not be necessary. *Archives of General Psychiatry, 57,* 553–559.

Ross, B. S., & Ramsey, L. A. (2001). Novel antipsychotic drugs in the management of schizophrenia. *Drug Topics, 145*(9), 75–84.

Rudorfer, M. V. (1993). Pharmacokinetics of psychotropic drugs in special populations. *Journal of Clinical Psychiatry, 54,* (Suppl. 9), 50–54.

Saddock, B. J., & Saddock, V. A. (2000). *Kapla and Saddock's comprehensive textbook of psychiatry,* (9th ed.). Philadelphia: Lippincott Williams & Wilkins.

Sherman, C. (1999). Brief drug-free periods do no harm, may help. *Clinical Psychiatry News, 27*(8), 14.

Still, D. J. (1998). Schizophrenia patients learning to adjust to new treatment options. *Drug Topics, 142*(17), 36–45.

Tamminga, C. A. (1999). *Schizophrenia in the molecular age.* Presented at the American Psychiatric Association's 152nd annual meeting, Washington, D.C.

Thomas, S. H. L. (2000). Use of certain antipsychotic drugs may increase risk of arrhythmia. *Lancet, 355,* 1048–1052.

Tran, J. L., Stimmel, G. L., & Gutierrez, M. A. (2000). How to counsel patients on antipsychotic agents. *U. S. Pharmacist, 25*(2), 79–87.

Wickman, J. M., & Cold, J. (2000). Recognizing and treating tardive dyskinesia. *U.S. Pharmacist, 25*(5), 28–42.

Williamson, J. S., & Wyandt, C. M. (2000). Treating schizophrenia: New strategies. *Drug Topics, 144*(21), 64–73.

Wincor, M. Z., Wen, C. A., & Gutierrez, M. A. (1999). Donepezil in the treatment of Alzheimer's disease. *U.S. Pharmacist, 24*(2), 28–36.

Wood, A. J. & Zhon, H. H. (1991). Ethnic differences in drug disposition and responsiveness. *Clinical Pharmacokinetics, 20,* 350–373.

Chapter 20

DRUGS FOR TREATING SEIZURE DISORDERS

KEY TERMS

absence seizure
epilepsy
epileptogenesis
GABA
generalized seizure
glutamate
ictal
International Classification of Epileptic Seizures
partial seizure
postictal
seizure
status epilepticus
tonic-clonic seizure

Learning Objectives

At the completion of this chapter the student will:

1. Describe the purpose of the International Classification of Epileptic Seizures.
2. Identify common core drug knowledge about prototype drugs belonging to the major antiepileptic drug (AED) classifications.
3. Identify core patient variables of concern related to the major AEDs.
4. Generate a nursing plan of care based on the interactions between core drug knowledge and core patient variables for the major AEDs.
5. Describe nursing interventions to maximize therapeutic and minimize adverse effects for the major AEDs.
6. Relate key points for patient and family education for major AEDs.

Hydantoins

phenytoin
ethotoin
mephenytoin
fosphenytoin

Barbiturates

phenobarbital
primidone

Benzodiazepines

clonazepam
clorazepate
diazepam
midazolam
lorazepam

Succinimides

ethosuximide
methsuximide
phensuximide

Miscellaneous AEDs

carbamazepine
oxcarbazepine

Adjunct anticonvulsants

felbamate
gabapentin
lamotrigine
levetiracetam
tiagabine
topiramate
valproic acid
zonisamide
vigabatrin

Oxazolidinediones

trimethadione
paramethadione

The symbol C indicates the **drug class**.
Drugs in bold type marked with the symbol P are **prototypes**.
Drugs in blue type with no symbol are **closely related** to the prototype.
Drugs in **red** type with no symbol are **significantly different** from the prototype.
Drugs in **black** type with no symbol are **also used in drug therapy**; no prototype.

Seizures result from a disturbance in the electrochemical activity of the brain caused by excessive discharge of neurons. This abnormal electrical discharge in the brain produces paroxysmal involuntary alterations of behavior, movement, and sensation. Seizures, also referred to as convulsions, occur as a result of brain injury, developmental malformation, and genetic abnormalities. Seizures may also occur from known and reversible causes—most commonly, metabolic abnormalities (e.g., hypoglycemia, electrolyte imbalance), meningitis, uremia, preeclampsia and toxemia of pregnancy, hyperpyrexia, and drug and alcohol abuse. Seizures may also be related to nonreversible causes, such as cerebrovascular, neoplasm-related, and degenerative dementias. These are common causes of seizures in older adults. Refer to the accompanying displays, Causes of Seizures and Drugs and Other Substances That Can Cause Seizures.

Epilepsy is a chronic condition characterized by recurrent, unprovoked seizures that result from a related central nervous system (CNS) disorder. Epilepsy affects up to 3% of the American population. (Marks, et al., 1998) The prevalence is highest among older adults, primarily related to cerebrovascular accidents; the next highest prevalence is among children from birth to age 9 years, due to genetic syndromes and birth trauma. About half of all epilepsy cases are idiopathic (without known cause).

This chapter examines drugs that are used to control seizures. There are several drug classes that are used to prevent seizures. They include the hydantoins, (prototype phenytoin), the barbiturates (prototype phenobarbital), the benzodiazepines (prototype clonazepam), the succinimides (prototype ethosuximide), and carbamazepine, a drug that is a miscellaneous agent without a class. Many new anticonvulsants have been developed in the last few years. These drugs are unique to themselves. They are considered the adjuvant anticonvulsants and are each presented briefly. Magnesium sulfate is used to control seizures in severe preeclampsia or eclampsia in pregnancy without producing significant central nervous system (CNS) depression in the mother or infant, and in convulsions associated with very low levels of magnesium. Magnesium sulfate is discussed in more depth in Chapter 44.

Causes of Seizures

Neonates (younger than 1 month)
- Perinatal hypoxia and ischemia, intracranial hemorrhage, and trauma
- Acute CNS infection (bacterial and viral meningitis)
- Metabolic disturbances (hypoglycemia, hypocalcemia, hypomagnesemia, and pyridoxine deficiency)
- Drug withdrawal
- Developmental disorders (acquired and genetic)
- Genetic disorders

Infants and children (older than 1 month and younger than 12 years)
- Febrile seizures
- Genetic disorders (metabolic, degenerative, and primary epilepsy syndromes)
- CNS infection
- Developmental disorders (acquired and genetic)
- Trauma
- Idiopathic

Adolescents (12–18 years)
- Trauma
- Genetic disorders
- Infection
- Brain tumor
- Illicit drug use
- Idiopathic

Young adults (18–35 years)
- Trauma
- Alcohol withdrawal
- Illicit drug use
- Brain tumor
- Idiopathic

Middle and older adults (older than 35 years)
- Cerebrovascular disease
- Brain tumor
- Alcohol withdrawal
- Metabolic disorders (uremia, hepatic failure, electrolyte abnormalities, hypoglycemia)
- Alzheimer disease and other degenerative CNS diseases
- Complications of AIDS or other immune disorders
- Idiopathic

Drugs And Other Substances That Can Cause Seizures

Antimicrobials
- Lactams and related compounds
- Quinolones
- Isoniazid
- Ganciclovir

Anesthetics and antiarrhythmics
- Beta-adrenergic antagonists
- Local anesthetics (lidocaine)
- Class 1B agents

Immunosuppressants
- Cyclosporine

Psychotropics

Antidepressants
- Antipsychotics
- Lithium

Radiographic contrast agents

Theophylline

Sedative-hypnotic drug withdrawal
- Alcohol
- Barbiturates
- Benzodiazepines

Drugs of abuse
- Amphetamine
- Cocaine
- Phencyclidine
- Methylphenidate

PHYSIOLOGY

Within the CNS, information is transmitted through a series of neurons. The excitatory neurotransmitters acetylcholine and norepinephrine, and the amino acids aspartate and **glutamate** carry electrical impulses from one neuron to another.

*Diane Aschenbrenner reviewed and edited this chapter.

These neurotransmitters are released into the synaptic cleft when an action potential spreads across a presynaptic terminal. The neurotransmitter interacts with a specific receptor and depolarizes the nerve cell membrane.

The pH and levels of oxygen, glucose, amino acids, calcium, sodium, and potassium affect the cell membrane's stability and excitability. Transmission of electrical impulses, therefore, depends on homeostatic mechanisms that regulate the chemical environment inside and outside the cell and maintain an electrical gradient across the cell membrane.

Energy-dependent ion transport mechanisms and voltage-dependent sodium and calcium channels control electrolyte transport across the cell membrane. Uncontrolled generation of electrical impulses and excessive neuronal firing are prevented by the inhibitory neurotransmitter **gamma-aminobutyric acid (GABA)**, which counteracts the effect of excitatory neurotransmitters (glutamate and aspartate). GABA is present in 60% to 70% of all brain synapses (Davis, 1997). It is formed from glutamate by the enzyme glutamic acid decarboxylase. After synaptic release, GABA is taken up into nerve (or glial) cells. In the neuron, GABA is either re-released or degraded. In the glial cell, it is metabolized into the amino acid glutamine, which is then used by the neuron to synthesize more glutamate and GABA.

GABA inhibits neurologic firing; it acts on postsynaptic membranes to open chloride channels, thereby leading to membrane hyperpolarization. When released into the synapse, GABA can bind to two different receptor complexes, designated A and B.

GABA-A receptors can be stimulated by GABA, benzodiazepines, barbiturates, hydantoins, and neurosteroids. When GABA-A is activated, there is an increased inward flow of chloride ions through the special chloride channels in the nerve cell membrane. These negative charges hyperpolarize the nerve cell membranes and inhibit neuronal firing.

B-type receptors for the neurotransmitter GABA inhibit neuronal activity through G-protein-coupled second-messenger systems, which regulate the release of neurotransmitters and the activity of potassium and calcium ion channels. Physiologic and biochemical studies show variations in drug efficiencies at different GABA-B receptors, so it is postulated that GABA-B receptor subtypes exist. GABA is the main inhibitory neurotransmitter in the mammalian CNS, where it exerts through inotropic (GABA-A) receptors to produce fast synaptic inhibition and the metabotropic (GABA-B) receptors to produce slow, prolonged inhibitory signals.

PATHOPHYSIOLOGY

Seizures are a result of a shift in the normal balance of excitation and inhibition within the CNS, the sudden, excessive firing of a small number of neurons, and the spread of that electrical activity to adjacent neurons. There are numerous properties that control neuronal excitability and, therefore, many different ways to disturb this normal balance. Consequently, there are many different causes of both seizures and epilepsy; clinical understanding of the basic mechanisms involved, however, is limited. Although the pathophysiology of epilepsy is poorly understood, conceptually, three important clinical observations emphasize how a variety of factors determine why certain conditions may cause one seizure, several seizures, or epilepsy in a particular individual.

First, the normal brain is capable of having a seizure under the appropriate circumstances, and individuals differ in their susceptibility or threshold for seizures. For example, seizures may be induced by high fevers in children who are otherwise normal and who never develop other neurologic problems, including epilepsy. Other underlying, endogenous factors may influence the threshold for having a seizure; some of these factors are clearly genetic, because a family history of epilepsy has been shown to influence the likelihood of seizures occurring in otherwise normal individuals. Normal development also plays an important role, because the brain appears to have different seizure thresholds at different maturational stages.

Second, there are a variety of conditions that have an extremely high likelihood of resulting in a chronic seizure disorder. One of the best examples of this is severe, penetrating head trauma, which is associated with up to a 50% risk of leading to epilepsy. The high probability for severe traumatic brain injury to result in epilepsy suggests that the injury causes long-lasting, pathologic changes in the CNS that transform a presumably normal neural network into one that is abnormally hyperexcitable. This process is known as **epileptogenesis**, and the specific changes that result in a lowered seizure threshold can be considered epileptogenic factors. Other processes associated with epileptogenesis include stroke, infections, and genetic abnormalities of CNS development.

Finally, seizures are episodic. Patients with epilepsy have seizures intermittently and, depending on the underlying cause, many patients are completely normal for months, sometimes years, between seizures. Thus, there are important provocative or precipitating factors that induce seizures in patients with epilepsy or that are responsible for causing the single seizure in someone without epilepsy. These factors include those due to intrinsic physiologic processes (e.g., psychological or physical stress, sleep deprivation, or hormonal changes associated with the menstrual cycle) and exogenous factors (e.g., exposure to toxic substances, alcohol abuse, and certain medications).

These observations suggest that seizures and epilepsy have a number of causes and result from a dynamic interplay between endogenous factors, epileptogenic factors, and precipitating factors. Several experimental models have been developed to evaluate 1) how brain structure and function is affected by seizures, 2) if these effects relate to subsequent seizure activity or seizure susceptibility, and 3) the efficacy of antiepileptic drugs (AEDs). One model is an "acute seizure" model in which administration of a chemical convulsant induces **status epilepticus** (in which one seizure immediately follows another and consciousness is not regained). Another model is an intense course of electrical stimulation. A third model is an animal model of epilepsy known as the "kindling model" in which particular areas of the animal brain experience repeated low-intensity electrical stimulation to induce epileptogenic changes and ultimately achieve an epileptic state. In humans, kindling caused by traumatic brain injury may progress over a period of years, which explains the delay in development of epilepsy that may follow a traumatic brain injury.

INTERNATIONAL CLASSIFICATION OF SEIZURES

Seizures—whether from known (reversible) or idiopathic (nonreversible) etiologies—are classified according to the International League Against Epilepsy guidelines. This classification system is extremely important in determining diagnostic evaluation of the seizure, the AED selection, AED treatment, and duration of AED therapy. **The International Classification of Epileptic Seizures** divides seizures into two broad categories—partial onset and generalized onset (see the accompanying display).

International Classification of Epileptic Seizures

Partial seizures (generally involve one hemisphere of the brain at onset)

- Simple (consciousness not impaired)
  - With motor symptoms (aversive, Jacksonian)
  - With somatosensory or other special sensory symptoms
  - With autonomic symptoms
  - With psychic symptoms (disturbance of higher cerebral functions)
- Complex (consciousness impaired)
  - Simple partial onset followed by impaired consciousness
  - Impaired consciousness at onset
- Secondarily generalized
  - Simple partial seizures evolving to generalized tonic-clonic seizures
  - Complex partial seizures evolving to generalized tonic-clonic seizures
  - Simple partial seizures evolving to complex partial seizures, then to generalized tonic-clonic seizures

Generalized seizures (involve both hemispheres of the brain at onset; consciousness usually impaired)

- Absence
  - Typical
  - Atypical
- Myoclonic
- Clonic
- Tonic
- Tonic-clonic
- Atonic

Focal

- Idiopathic
- Symptomatic

Generalized epilepsy

- Idiopathic
- Symptomatic (e.g., infantile spasms, Lennox-Gastaut syndrome)

Special syndromes

- Febrile

Unclassified

PARTIAL SEIZURES

A **partial seizure** is a relatively common type of epileptic seizure caused by a neuronal dysfunction in the hemisphere of the brain where the electrical activity is localized. Partial seizures can occur at any age, although they are most common in older children and adults. Historically, partial-onset seizures have been referred to by a variety of names and occasionally to the area of brain involved; for example, "focal," "local," or Jacksonian-type seizures. Partial seizures are further subdivided into simple, complex, and secondarily generalized seizures.

Simple partial seizures may be associated with signs and symptoms of autonomic, motor, psychic, or sensory behaviors. Simple partial seizures do not impair consciousness, but generally cause confusion, jerking movements, tingling, or odd mental and emotional events, such as déjà vu, mild hallucinations, or extreme responses to smell and taste. After the seizure, the patient may have temporary weakness in some muscles. Simple partial seizures may develop into a complex partial seizure.

Complex partial seizures, also known as psychomotor or temporal lobe seizures, alter and impair consciousness. Other manifestations may include the onset of an aura (a warning sign characterized by an odd feeling, odor, or visual or auditory change); loss of judgment; involuntary or uncontrolled behavior; exaggerated emotions; appearance of intoxication; and repetitive movements such as chewing or lip smacking. Episodes usually last no more than 2 minutes and they may occur infrequently or as often as every day. A throbbing headache may follow this seizure. Complex partial seizures are more common in adults. The clinical manifestations of complex partial seizures in the elderly are not well defined because seizure-type behaviors may be subtle, prolonged, and mistakenly associated with dementia.

Both simple- and complex-partial seizures may become secondarily generalized. The progress may be so rapid the partial stage goes unnoticed.

GENERALIZED SEIZURES

Generalized seizures are caused by disturbances of nerve cells in more diffuse areas and both hemispheres of the brain. Thus, their effect on the individual is more serious than with partial seizures, unless the partial seizure is secondarily generalized. Types of generalized seizures are convulsive types also called "grand mal" (e.g., tonic-clonic), nonconvulsive types, also called "petit mal" (e.g., absence) and miscellaneous types (e.g., clonic, myoclonic, tonic).

Convulsive, Generalized Seizures

The first stage of a convulsive generalized seizure is the tonic phase in which the muscles suddenly contract, causing the patient to fall and momentarily lie rigidly (less than 30 seconds). Muscle spasms occur for about 30 seconds to 1 minute as the seizure enters the clonic phase, when the muscles begin to alternate between relaxation and rigidity. Loss of bowel or urinary control frequently occurs following this phase. Like the partial seizure, some people experience a premonition or aura before a convulsive, generalized seizure; however, most individuals lose consciousness without warning. If the throat or larynx is affected, a high-pitched musical sound called stridor may be heard when the patient inhales.

Nonconvulsive, Generalized Seizures

The most characteristic of the nonconvulsive, generalized disorders is the **absence seizure**; it was historically known as petit mal seizures. Absence seizures are further divided into typical and atypical. Absence seizures occur mainly in children, occasionally in adolescents and uncommonly in adults. Absence seizures may be so brief that they may go unnoticed by others. Absence seizures may consist of only a short cessation of physical movement and loss of attention or may impair consciousness. Small children may simply be observed staring or walking distractedly. Absence seizures may occur as often as 50 to 100 times a day—each lasting only few seconds. About 25% of patients with absence seizures (petit mal seizures) develop convulsive generalized seizures (grand mal seizures).

Miscellaneous Generalized Seizures

A tonic (also called akinetic, drop attack) seizure occurs when there is sudden loss of muscle tone. Sometimes only one part of the body may be affected (e.g., the jaw slackens and the head drops) In tonic seizures, the muscles contract and consciousness is altered for about 10 seconds, but the seizures do not progress to the clonic phase. Clonic seizures, which are uncommon, occur primarily in young children. Individuals experience spasms of the muscles but not the tonic rigidity. Myoclonic seizures are a series of brief, jerking muscle contractions of the face, extremities or trunk and occur in a series.

CLASSIFICATION OF EPILEPSY

Epilepsy is also classified by syndromes or grouped according to a set of common characteristics, such as age, type of seizure, or whether a cause is known or not known (idiopathic). Two of these include West syndrome (also called infantile spasms) and Lennox-Gastaut syndrome. West syndrome is a disorder that involves spasms and developmental delay in children within the first year of life—usually infants aged between 4 and 8 months. Lennox-Gastaut syndrome is a severe form of epilepsy in young children that causes developmental delay and retardation. This syndrome involves absence, tonic, and partial seizures.

NURSE'S ROLE IN SEIZURE ASSESSMENT

Nurses play a vital role in the assessment of the patient with seizures. It is important for the nurse to obtain information about patient activities prior to, during, and after the seizure (also known as the preictal, **ictal**, and **postictal** phases). Because alteration in consciousness often accompanies seizures, the patient may be unable to communicate this information. Family and friends who have witnessed the seizure at home may be able to supply this information. This information helps to identify a pattern or trend of seizure behavior and may be useful in determining the type of seizure and identifying the appropriate therapy. Nursing observation plays a critical role in seizure diagnosis. The nurse may have the opportunity to witness the seizure. Direct observation allows for exact description of data relevant to accurate diagnosis. When witnessing a seizure, the nurse should note and document if the following are present:

- Precipitating event or presence of a certain physical or psychic sensation that precedes a seizure (aura), if appropriate
- Area of the body where the seizure activity begins; progression and duration of the seizure
- Behavioral changes during the ictal and postictal periods; for example, alterations in consciousness, incontinence, evidence of tongue biting, periods of apnea and cyanosis, head deviations, falls, behavioral changes
- Motor weakness or paralysis, aphasia, and presence of headache

C ANTIEPILEPTIC DRUGS

The currently available AEDs are a heterogeneous group of drugs. Although there are some drug classes with several similarly structured drugs, many AEDs bear little resemblance to one another chemically and exhibit a broad array of biologic effects. In general, AEDs are believed to work either by blocking action potentials or by interfering with synaptic transmission (Fig. 20-1) (Table 20-1).

An AED possesses the pharmacologic ability to depress abnormal neuronal discharges within the CNS and in this way, inhibit seizure activity. The AEDs are discussed by groups because of differences in their pharmacology, their therapeutic use(s), and their potential for adverse reactions. The most frequently used AEDs are from the hydantoin, benzodiazepine, and succinimide drug classes and the newer miscellaneous adjuvant AEDs. Table 20-2 summarizes selected AEDs.

When selecting an AED, there are several factors for the prescriber to consider. These factors include the seizure type and the patient's medical history, age, gender, occupation, fatigue and stress levels, cost of therapy, personal habits (e.g., ingestion of large quantities of caffeine or alcohol), and acceptance of the treatment plan. The goal of pharmacotherapy is to reduce or eliminate seizure activity with minimal adverse effects. The ideal AED would suppress all seizure activity with minimal or no adverse effects. Unfortunately, no ideal AED exists, and the drugs used currently are not always effective and frequently cause adverse effects that vary in their degree of severity. One of the least serious adverse effects is mild CNS impairment; the most serious is death from hepatic failure or aplastic anemia. The trend is toward monotherapy, and the choice between drugs is debatable.

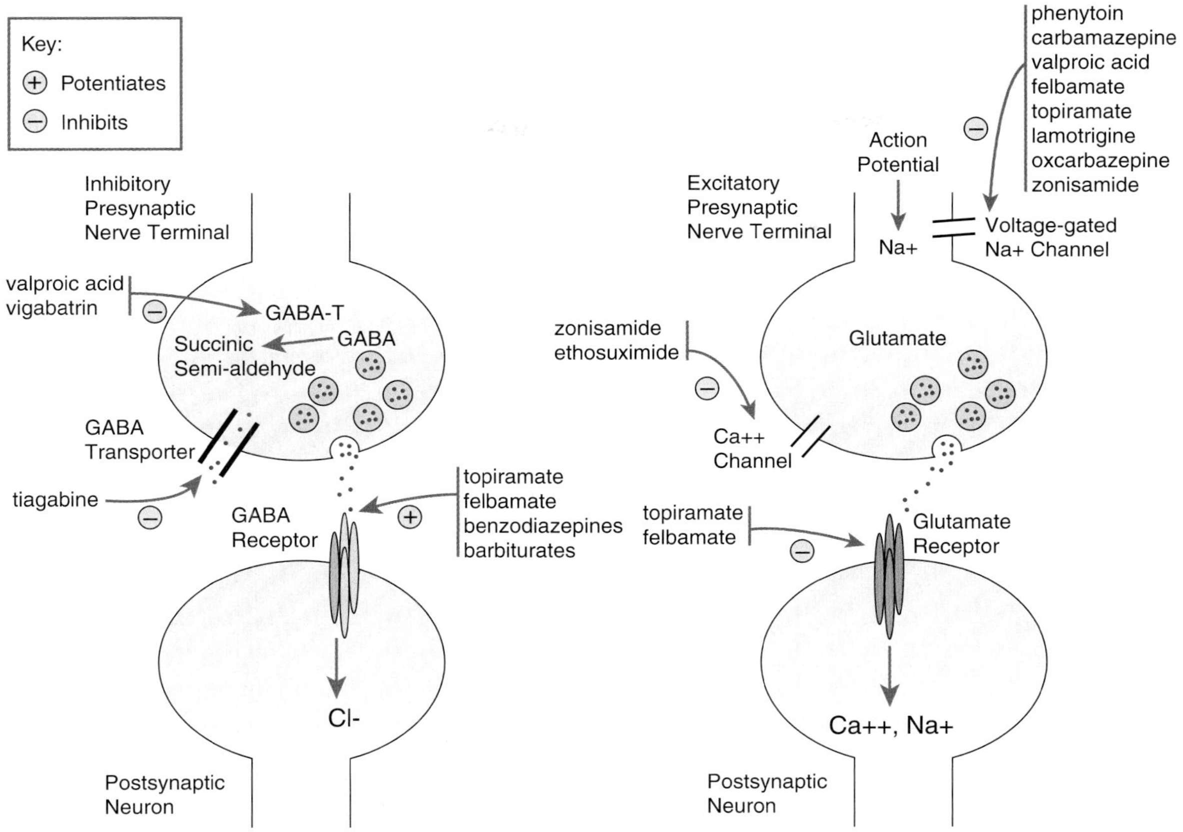

Figure 20-1. Mechanisms of antiepileptic drugs. Reprinted with permission from Drug Topics, Medical Economics Co., July 3, 2000.

TABLE 20-1 Mechanism of Action of AEDs

Mechanism of Action	Established AEDs	Newer AEDs	Antiepileptic Effects
Inhibition of Na^+ channels	Carbamazepine Phenytoin Valproate	Felbamate Gabapentin Lamotrigine Oxcarbazepine Topiramate	Stabilizes neuronal membrane Interferes with propagation of action potentials Decreases release of excitatory neurotransmitters
Interaction with voltage-sensitive Ca^{2+} channels	Ethosuximide Valproate Zonisamide	Felbamate Gabapentin Lamotrigine Topiramate	Decreased release of neurotransmitters Decreased release of glutamate
Reduced glutamate-mediated excitation	Phenobarbital	Felbamate Topiramate	Weak inhibitory effects on GABA receptor binding and benzodiazepine receptor binding
Enhanced GABA-mediated inhibition	Barbiturates Benzodiazepines	Felbamate Gabapentin Tiagabine Topiramate Vigabatrin Zonisamide	Enhanced GABA synthesis and decreased reuptake Re-establish balance between excitation and inhibition

The precise mechanism by which levetiracetam exerts its antiepileptic effect is unknown and levetiracetam is chemically unrelated to other AEDs.

TABLE 20-2 Summary of Selected Antiepileptic Drugs

Drug (Trade) Name	Selected Indications	Route and Dosage Range	Pharmacokinetics
Hydantoins			
phenytoin (Dilantin; *Canadian:* Diphenylan)	Tonic-clonic seizures, psychomotor seizures, status epilepticus	*Adult:* PO, use to serum levels of 5–20 μg/mL	*Onset:* Slow *Duration:* 6–12 h $t_{1/2}$: 6–24 h
fosphenytoin (Cerebyx)	Status epilepticus	*Adult:* IV, dilute in D_5W or 0.9% NaCl to a concentration of 1.5–25 mg phenytoin equivalent (PE)*/mL; administer at rate of ≤ 150 mg PE/mL	*Onset:* Rapid *Duration:* 1–2 h $t_{1/2}$: 6–24 h
Barbiturates			
phenobarbital (*Canadian:* Barbita)	Status epilepticus, cortical local, tonic-clonic seizures	*Adult:* PO, 60–100 mg/d to serum level of 10–40 μg/mL; IM/IV, 200–320 q6h *Child:* PO, 3–6 mg/kg/d; IM/IV, 10–15 mg/kg/d	*Onset:* PO, 30–60 min; IM, 10–30 min; IV, 5 min *Duration:* 8–15 h $t_{1/2}$: 53–140 h
Benzodiazepines			
clonazepam (Klonopin; *Canadian:* Rivotril)	Myoclonic seizures, absence seizures, akinetic seizures, variant absence seizures (Lennox-Gastaut)	*Adult:* PO, 1.5–20 mg/d *Child:* PO, 0.01–0.05 mg/kg/d	*Onset:* 20–60 min *Duration:* 6–12 h $t_{1/2}$: 18–60 h
clorazepate (Tranxene; *Canadian:* Apo-Clorazepate)	Partial seizures	*Adult:* PO, 7.5 mg tid *Child:* PO, 7.5 mg bid	*Onset:* 15–45 min *Duration:* 7–8 h $t_{1/2}$: 30–100 h
midazolam (Versed)	*Unlabeled use:* Treatment of refractory status epilepticus	*Adult:* IV, 10–15 mg	*Onset:* 3–5 m IV; 15 m IM *Duration:* 2–6 h $t_{1/2}$: 1.8–6.4 h
Succinimides			
ethosuximide (Zarontin)	Absence seizures	*Adult:* PO, 500 mg/d to serum level of 40–100 μg/mL *Child:* PO, 250 mg/d (3–6 y) or 500 mg/d (6 y or older)	*Onset:* Varies *Duration:* 3–7 h $t_{1/2}$: 40–60 h in adults; 30 h in children 7–9 y
Miscellaneous AEDs			
carbamazepine (Tegretol; *Canadian:* Carbamaz)	Tonic-clonic seizures, mixed seizures, psychomotor seizures	*Adult:* PO, 400–1,000 mg/d *Child:* 6–12 y, PO, 200–1,000 mg/d	*Onset:* Slow *Duration:* 4–5 h $t_{1/2}$: 25–65 h initially, 12–17 h with multiple dosing
oxcarbazepine (Trileptal)	Adjunctive treatment of partial seizures	*Adult:* PO, 1,200 mg/d as adjunctive therapy; 2,400 mg/d as monotherapy. *Child:* (4–16) y): PO, 30–46 mg/kg/d as adjunctive therapy	*Onset:* 1 h *Duration:* 3–13 h $t_{1/2}$: 2*–9**
Adjunct Anticonvulsants			
felbamate (Felbatol)	Adjunctive or monotherapy of partial seizures in adults; adjunctive therapy in children with Lennox-Gastaut syndrome	*Adult:* (less than 14 yo), 1,200–3,600 mg/d *Child:* (2–14) y): PO, 15 mg/kg/d	*Onset:* Rapid *Duration:* Dose proportional $t_{1/2}$: 20–23 h

TABLE 20-2 **Summary of Selected Antiepileptic Drugs** (Continued)

Drug (Trade) Name	Selected Indications	Route and Dosage Range	Pharmacokinetics
gabapentin (Neurontin)	Partial seizures in adults with and without secondary generalization	*Adult:* PO, 900–1,800 mg/d	*Onset:* Rapid *Duration:* 6–8 h $t_{1/2}$: 5–7 h
lamotrigine (Lamictal)	Adjunctive therapy for partial seizures (adults)	*Adult:* PO, 100–500 mg/d	*Onset:* Rapid *Duration:* 1.4–4.8 h (dose related) $t_{1/2}$: 33 h
valproic acid (Depakene; *Canadian:* Deproic)	Sole or adjunctive treatment for simple or complex absence seizures	*Adult:* PO, 10–60 mg/kg/d	*Onset:* Varies depending on dosage form *Duration:* 1–4 h $t_{1/2}$: 5–20 h (average, 10.6 h)
levetiracetam (Keppra)	Adjunctive treatment of partial seizures	*Adult:* PO, 1,000–3,000 mg/d	*Onset:* 1 h *Duration:* Unknown $t_{1/2}$: 7–8 h
vigabatrin (Sabril)	Adjunct to multidrug refractory complex partial seizures	*Adult:* PO, 1.5–3 g/d	*Onset:* Rapid *Duration:* 0.7–1.1 h $t_{1/2}$: 6–8 h
tiagabine (Gabitril)	Adjunctive treatment of partial seizures	Dosage ranges not established	*Onset:* Rapid *Duration:* 6–12 h $t_{1/2}$: Varies (4.5–13.4 h)
topiramate (Topamax)	Lennox-Gastaut syndrome, adjunct in adult partial-onset seizures	Dosage ranges not established	*Onset:* Rapid *Duration:* 2 h $t_{1/2}$: 21 h
zonisamide (zonegran)	Adjunctive treatment of partial seizures	*Adult:* PO, 100–400 mg/d	*Onset:* 2–6 h *Duration:* More than 105 h $t_{1/2}$: 63 h

* Parent drug
** Active metabolite

HYDANTOINS

The hydantoin AEDs are used primarily for their control of tonic-clonic seizures and partial seizures with complex or autonomic symptoms. Phenytoin is the prototype hydantoin. Other drugs represented by the prototype are ethotoin, mephenytoin, and fosphenytoin.

NURSING MANAGEMENT OF THE PATIENT RECEIVING PHENYTOIN

Core Drug Knowledge

Pharmacotherapeutics

Phenytoin is considered to be quite effective for the control of most types of seizures, particularly generalized-convulsive and complex-partial types. Other AEDs—especially the newer adjuvant drugs—are more effective than phenytoin in managing simple partial seizures. Phenytoin is not used for absence seizures, however, because it often worsens them. Phenytoin is also used for prophylaxis and treatment of seizures during or following neurosurgery or head trauma. Occasionally, phenytoin is used for status epilepticus.

Unlabeled uses for phenytoin include control of arrhythmias, particularly cardiac glycoside-induced arrhythmias; control of seizures associated with preeclampsia and toxemia of pregnancy; and treatment of trigeminal neuralgia.

Pharmacokinetics

Phenytoin is available in several oral forms—capsules, tablets, and suspensions; it is slowly absorbed from the small intestine. The rate and extent of absorption vary and are dependent on the product formulation. These dosage forms are relatively fast acting and cause peak blood levels to occur about 2 hours after administration.

Extended-release capsules are also available and peak plasma levels occur in approximately 12 hours. These produce a longer-lasting serum (blood) drug level because this dosage form is absorbed more slowly. Peak blood levels occur in about 6 hours. IM injection of phenytoin has a slow and unpredictable absorption that may continue for several days. Plasma (blood) levels vary following IM injection and are much lower than those achieved with the same oral dose. For these reasons it is not normally given by this route. Phenytoin is significantly bound (87% to 93%) to plasma proteins—primarily albumin.

Phenytoin metabolism is dose dependent; it is extensively metabolized by the liver and excreted in the urine. The plasma half-life is 6 to 24 hours with plasma levels that are less than 10 μg/mL. At higher plasma levels, drug elimination is dose dependent, and half-life increases. At therapeutic plasma levels of 10 to 20 μg/mL, half-life is 20 to 60 hours. Some individuals treated with hydantoins metabolize the drug slowly. Slow metabolism may be due to limited enzyme availability and lack of induction. It appears to be genetically determined. Phenytoin is excreted in breast milk.

Pharmacodynamics

The primary site of action of phenytoin appears to be the motor cortex where the spread of seizure activity is inhibited. Phenytoin promotes sodium efflux from the neurons. It is thought that this is how the cell membrane and seizure threshold are stabilized against hyperexcitability and seizure foci (points at which an electrochemical impulse originates) are prevented from spreading. This action causes little or no sedative or hypnotic effect.

Contraindications and Precautions

Some specific contraindications to phenytoin use include hypersensitivity to hydantoins.

Because of its effect on ventricular automaticity, phenytoin should not be used in sinus bradycardia, any type or degree of atrioventricular block, or in patients with Adams-Stokes syndrome. Phenytoin is a pregnancy class D drug. Some retrospective studies indicate that the risk of having a child with congenital defect is twofold to threefold higher in epileptic women who received AEDs, such as phenytoin, in the early stages of pregnancy. Other factors, such as genetics or the seizure disorder itself, may also contribute to this higher incidence of birth defects. Most women receiving phenytoin and other AEDs, however, deliver healthy infants.

Adverse Effects

Most of the common adverse effects with phenytoin are CNS related; for example, nystagmus, dysarthria, slurred speech, mental confusion, dizziness, insomnia, transient nervousness, diplopia, fatigue, irritability, drowsiness, depression, numbness, tremor, and headache. Other CNS effects include ataxia and motor twitching. There is a good correlation between plasma phenytoin concentration and CNS toxicity. With higher drug levels more serious effects will occur. Plasma levels exceeding 20 μg/mL may produce nystagmus, plasma levels exceeding 30 to 40 μg/mL will usually produce ataxia and gross mental changes, and levels exceeding 50 μg/mL oftentimes induce coma.

Adverse endocrine effects such as glycosuria and hyperglycemia may occur with phenytoin because of inhibition of insulin secretion. Osteomalacia with hypocalcemia and increased alkaline phosphatase activity may occur as a result of altered metabolism of vitamin D and the inhibition of intestinal absorption of calcium.

Phenytoin (and other AEDs) may cause skin rashes. Similar in appearance to measles, they usually occur within 3 to 8 weeks of the drug's initiation. These reactions are idiosyncratic in origin. Phenytoin induces hepatic CYP-450 drug-metabolizing enzymes; exposure to phenytoin (and other CYP-450-inducing AEDs) may cause an "AED hypersensitivity syndrome"; this is an uncommon, severe exanthematous rash with mucosal involvement that can progress into a purpuric or exfoliative dermatitis and may cause an accompanying carditis, eosinophilia, hepatitis, lymphadenopathy, and nephritis. Other serious integumentary syndromes, such as Stevens-Johnson syndrome and toxic epidermal necrolysis, may occur (Knowles, Shapiro, & Shear, 1999). On rare occasions, phenytoin and other AEDs have been associated with a "lupus-like" reaction.

Hematologic reactions from phenytoin include fever, agranulocytosis, megaloblastic anemia, aplastic anemia, hypoprothrombinemia due to phenytoin-induced vitamin K deficiency, leukopenia, and neutropenia. In vitro studies suggest that phenytoin-induced red blood cell aplasia is immunologic. Phenytoin alters folate absorption and metabolism; this is associated with megaloblastic anemia. Lymphadenopathy may occur secondarily as a result of deficiency in the production of immunoglobulins. Blood or bone marrow abnormalities that occur are not thought to be dose related or dose dependent. Marked depression of the blood count indicates the need for withdrawal of the drug.

Other miscellaneous adverse effects include gastrointestinal disturbances (e.g., nausea, vomiting, diarrhea, constipation, weight gain), harmless reddish-brown discoloration of the urine, immunoglobulin (Ig)A depression, pulmonary fibrosis, significant gingival hyperplasia (which may be disfiguring), and altered physical appearance due to an androgenic effect on the hair follicle (e.g., facial and body hair may increase, and acne may develop).

Additionally, IV phenytoin administered too rapidly (more than 50 mg/minute) may produce cardiovascular collapse, hypotension, severe cardiotoxic reactions, atrial and ventricular conduction depression, or ventricular fibrillation.

Teratogenic effects from phenytoin may include congenital malformations of cleft lip and palate; cardiac malformations; early neonatal coagulation defect; and a fetal phenytoin syndrome consisting of prenatal growth deficiency, microcephaly, mental retardation, craniofacial abnormalities, and nail and digital hypoplasia.

Drug Interactions

Phenytoin interacts with many other drugs. These interactions occur because of phenytoin inducing effects on hepatic microsomal enzyme (i.e., P450) systems. Pharmacologic induction of these enzymes enhances the metabolism of both endogenous and exogenous substances, including other AEDs (Table 20-3). Phenytoin may interfere with results of diagnostic endocrine tests that use dexamethasone.

Assessment of Relevant Core Patient Variables

Health Status

At normal therapeutic dosages, phenytoin causes few adverse effects; however, all body systems may be involved. Thus the nurse should obtain a thorough health history and baseline physical assessment from which to monitor the patient's health status during phenytoin therapy. Because phenytoin interacts with so many other drugs, the nurse needs to also complete a careful drug history. Phenytoin has significant depressant effects on cardiac electrical activity; the nurse should assess patients for sinus bradycardia, first-, second-, or third-degree heart block; or Stokes-Adams syndrome. Phenytoin may decrease serum thyroxine levels; the nurse should assess patients for hypothyroidism or goiter resulting from phenytoin use. Phenytoin undergoes hepatic metabolism. The nurse should assess the hepatic function of older adults, patients with impaired liver function, or patients with severe illness (e.g. systemic infections or chronic, debilitating diseases). These patients may show early signs of toxicity with phenytoin use.

Life Span and Gender

The nurse should assess the woman of child-bearing age for pregnancy and document her reproductive goals and contraceptive practices. Phenytoin is Food and Drug Administration (FDA) pregnancy category D. Evidence of the teratogenic effect of hydantoins in general—and phenytoin in particular—is well documented. The nurse should document the age and development level of the patient. There is some evidence that phenytoin therapy may have adverse effects on behavior and cognition in children. The pharmacokinetics of phenytoin and other AEDs may be affected by age-related changes. See the accompanying display, Age-Related Changes of Antiepileptic Drug Therapy.

Lifestyle, Diet, and Habits

The nurse should review the patient's dietary habits. Phenytoin therapy may result in folate deficiency, pos-

TABLE 20-3 Agents That Interact With P Phenytoin

Interactants	Effect and Significance	Nursing Management
allopurinol, amiodarone, benzodiazepines, cimetidine, clonazepam, disulfiram, ethanol, fluconazole, ibuprofen, isoniazid, metronidazole, miconazole, omeprazole, phenothiazines, salicylates, succinimides, sulfonamides, tricyclic antidepressants, trimethoprim, valproic acid	Increased pharmacologic effects of phenytoin from inhibition of its metabolism	Monitor patient for changes in seizure control. Monitor serum phenytoin levels. Assess for signs of phenytoin toxicity.
barbiturates, ethanol (chronic ingestion), rifampin, theophylline	Decreased pharmacologic effects of phenytoin due to its increased metabolism	Assess patient for increased seizure frequency and changed seizure control. Monitor serum phenytoin levels at regular intervals.
antacids, charcoal, sucralfate	Decreased phenytoin effects due to decreased absorption	Assess patient for increased seizure frequency and changed seizure control. Monitor serum phenytoin levels at regular intervals.
acetaminophen, carbamazepine, cardiac glycosides, corticosteroids, disopyramide, doxycycline, estrogens (and oral contraceptives), haloperidol, methadone, mexiletine, quinidine, theophylline	Decreased pharmacologic effects of interactants from increased metabolism by phenytoin Analgesic effects of acetaminophen may be reduced by concomitant phenytoin use; the potential hepatotoxicity of acetaminophen may be increased Corticosteroid use may mask systemic manifestations of phenytoin hypersensitivity reactions	Evaluate patient for changed seizure control. Assess patient for evidence of therapeutic effects of interacting drugs. Monitor patient for therapeutic serum levels (if applicable) of interacting drugs.

Age-Related Changes of Antiepileptic Drug Therapy

- Aging changes the pharmacokinetics of AEDs because altered physiologic processes affect absorption, distribution, metabolism, and excretion. The net result is reduced drug clearance. AED therapy, therefore, is usually initiated at lower doses and titrated upward more slowly.
- Gastric pH increases with aging; its effect on absorption is unknown.
- The ratio of body fat to lean body mass increases; therefore, fat-soluble drugs (e.g., benzodiazepines, barbiturates) have longer half-lives.
- Creatinine clearance is reduced; this affects the clearance for renally excreted AEDs (e.g., gabapentin, levetiracetam, oxcarbazepine).
- Albumin concentrations decline; unbound concentrations of highly protein bound AEDs (e.g., phenytoin) increase.
- Polypharmacy (e.g., three or more prescription medications for comorbid conditions) is common. Consequently, AED drug interactions are likely—particularly for AEDs that are highly protein bound or affect hepatic CYP450 enzymes by induction or inhibition.
- Over-the-counter medications, herbal preparations or dietary supplements may interfere with AEDs' pharmacokinetics.
- As a general rule, adverse effects of AEDs are exaggerated in the elderly because of preexisting comorbid conditions. Sedation, behavioral changes, ataxia, tremor, cognitive slowing, and hyponatremia may not be recognized as AED adverse effects and thus treated unnecessarily.

sibly progressing to megaloblastic anemia; vitamin D deficiency, possibly causing osteomalacia and serum hypocalcemia; and elevations in serum total cholesterol, high-density-lipoprotein (HDL) cholesterol, and triglyceride levels. The nurse should also assess the patient's alcohol intake. A drug-drug interaction exists between phenytoin and alcohol. A cross-tolerance develops in individuals who consume large quantities of alcohol. Furthermore, chronic alcohol use accelerates phenytoin metabolism by enzyme induction.

Environment

The nurse should be aware of the environment in which the drug will be administered and, if appropriate, assess the home or living environment of the patient. Oral phenytoin may be self-administered safely by the patient, parent, or caregiver in just about any health care, home, or other setting (school or office). Parenteral phenytoin is administered in a hospital where the patient may be observed throughout the period of peak serum phenytoin concentrations and electrocardiogram, blood pressure and respiratory function may be continuously monitored.

Culture

The nurse should document the ethnicity of the patient. A genetically determined limitation in the ability to metabolize phenytoin has been identified predominantly in Pacific Asians (Wood & Zhon, 1991).

Nursing Diagnoses and Outcomes

- Ineffective Management of Therapeutic Regimen related to lack of knowledge regarding potential chronic nature of illness, need for life-long medication and lifestyle adjustment.
  Desired outcome: The patient will describe the disease process, the regimen for disease control, and relate intent to practice needed health behaviors.
- Risk for Infection related to adverse drug effect of blood dyscrasias
  Desired outcome: The patient will experience no infections or injury related to abnormalities in blood components.
- Risk for Injury related to adverse drug effects of CNS-depression
  Desired outcome: The patient will identify types of drug-induced cognitive and/or motor deficits and take precautions to avoid harm.
- Disturbed Sensory Perception related to adverse drug effects of drowsiness and sedation
  Desired outcome: The patient will recognize and eliminate, if possible, potential risk factors and experience no injury.
- Ineffective Sexuality Patterns related to the need for reliable and consistent contraception secondary to potential teratogenic effects
  Desired outcome: The patient will identify appropriate modifications in sexual practices to facilitate contraception and experience no unplanned pregnancy.
- Ineffective Health Maintenance related to adverse drug effect of gingival hyperplasia
  Desired outcome: The patient will demonstrate knowledge of optimal oral hygiene and experience no deterioration in dental health.

Planning and Intervention

Maximizing Therapeutic Effects

It is important for the nurse to closely monitor the patient for therapeutic response to phenytoin. This is especially important when drug therapy is initiated, when dosages or drugs are changed, or when other illness occurs. As a general rule, phenytoin is usually begun at lower dosages and gradually titrated until a therapeutic dose is attained. The nurse should monitor blood levels of the drug for therapeutic ranges during initial use or dosage-adjustment periods. Some patients, however, will be therapeutically controlled when blood-drug levels are below the expected therapeutic range.

Phenytoin absorption is compromised when administered with enteral tube feedings. The nurse should therefore check gastric residuals and refrain from administering the drug for 1 to 2 hours if the residual is greater than 100 mL. Continuous tube feedings should be held for 1 hour before and after administering the phenytoin.

Minimizing Adverse Effects

Adverse effects from phenytoin are frequently related to excessively high blood drug levels. It is important to monitor the patient's blood levels of phenytoin as well as the patient's physical response to drug therapy. Drug levels should be monitored most closely at the initiation of therapy or after every increase in the dose. If the patient is demonstrating adverse effects the drug dosage may need to be decreased. It is important for the nurse to analyze the patient's mental and neurologic function and behavior regularly for changes from baseline behavior to determine whether CNS adverse effects are present. If the patient is having difficulty with dizziness, safety measures should be instituted to prevent falls and injury. The nurse should administer the drug with meals if the patient is experiencing nausea and GI distress; however, milk and antacids should be avoided because they may impair absorption. The diabetic patient may experience elevated glucose levels; their glucose levels should be measured more frequently until the effects of phenytoin on them are determined.

The nurse should report any signs and symptoms of skin rash. Although a rash is usually not serious, phenytoin may need to be discontinued to minimize the risk of severe reactions such as Stevens-Johnson syndrome.

It is important for the nurse to evaluate blood counts, bleeding tendencies, and white blood cell counts regularly to determine whether any hematologic adverse effects have occurred. Notify the prescriber if any abnormalities are detected to prevent serious adverse effects. Vitamin D and calcium supplements are recommended for patients showing symptoms of osteomalacia and also for those at high risk of developing osteomalacia.

The nurse should avoid administering IV push phenytoin faster than 50 mg/minute (or 25 mg/minute in older adults). Careful monitoring of the pulse and blood pressure is essential during IV administration. Follow the administration of phenytoin with sterile saline through the same IV catheter to avoid local venous irritation from the alkalinity of the phenytoin. Phenytoin is not given as a continuous IV infusion.

Providing Patient and Family Education

Patient education for phenytoin is similar to the teaching for any of the AEDs that may be prescribed. Please see the display, Patient and Family Education Common to AEDs, for more information. In addition, please consider the critical thinking scenario, What Happens When Antiepileptic Therapy Stops Abruptly? Patient and family education specific for phenytoin includes:

- The nurse should emphasize the necessity of not changing phenytoin products. Bioavailability may vary enough between products of different manu-

Patient and Family Education Common to AEDs

AEDs require that much of the same information be shared with patient and family. The nurse providing education for the epileptic patient should include the following information.

- AED therapy does not cure the seizure disorder; it suppresses seizure activity.
- The condition in which seizures recur so frequently that consciousness or normal function cannot be regained in the interval between seizures is known as status epilepticus; this is a medical emergency.
- Sudden withdrawal of the AED may cause epileptic control to be lost and the patient may experience seizures or status epilepticus.
- Double dosing of an AED should be avoided. If a dose is missed, instruct the patient to take the dose as soon as it is remembered unless it is close to the time for the next dose.
- Follow-up appointments with the health care provider and periodic laboratory testing are important because they provide an ongoing record of response (both positive and negative) to AED therapy.
- A "seizure record" should be kept. This record can provide information about changes in the type or frequency of seizures over time, the effect of different medications on seizure control, adverse effects of medications, and seizure-provoking factors. This record should include the date and time, as well as the type, of seizure. If a precipitating factor is suspected (e.g., lack of sleep, missed medication, stress, menstrual period), the patient should write it down. For women, it may be helpful to keep track of the relationship between seizures and the menstrual cycles. It is also helpful to record the medication, dosage, and blood drug levels (if known). Recommend that the patient and family (or caregiver) show this record to the health care provider during follow-up visits.
- A form of medical identification (e.g., MedicAlert) indicating the medical condition and the drugs prescribed for it, including dosage in case of an emergency, should be carried or worn by the patient.
- Use of OTC preparations, herbal preparations, and dietary supplements should be avoided unless approved by the physician or nurse practitioner.
- Transient mild drowsiness and dizziness are common in the first few days of therapy until the patient becomes accustomed to the drug therapy. Observe caution while driving, operating machinery or performing other tasks requiring mental alertness and motor coordination until effects of the drug are known.
- Alcohol consumption should be avoided because it may increase the CNS-depressant effect of the AED as well as precipitate incidence of seizures.
- Environmental factors (e.g., flashing lights, alcohol) and physiologic factors (e.g., hypoglycemia, fatigue, stress) may increase the frequency of seizures. If stress aggravates seizure activity, teach the patient to develop effective stress management techniques.
- AEDs can have significant effects on hormonal homeostasis, although epilepsy itself may play a role in causing these problems. Men may experience reduced libido and sexual potency; women may experience sexual arousal disorders. Seizure frequency may increase during menses because of the increase in sex hormones that alter the excitability of cortical neurons.
- The risk of having a child with a congenital defect may be 2–3 times greater in epileptic women who received AEDs in the early stages of pregnancy. Most AEDs are not recommended during pregnancy and lactation. Many women receiving AEDs, however, deliver healthy infants.

Critical Thinking Scenario

What happens when antiepileptic therapy stops abruptly?

Rudy Hernandez, 26 years old, is brought to the emergency department by his wife and brother. His brother states, "He's been having seizures off and on for an hour." In the emergency department, Mr. Hernandez cannot be aroused and is incontinent. His brother tells you that the patient has had epilepsy since childhood. His wife tells you he smokes two packs of cigarettes a day and stopped drug therapy a few weeks ago because "He didn't want to take it anymore."

1. Describe your impression of Mr. Hernandez's problem? Identify the potential causes and likely predisposing factors for what is happening.
2. Explain how you would counsel Mr. Hernandez in regard to his drug regimen.

facturers to cause toxicity or loss of seizure control from higher or lower plasma concentrations.

- The nurse should teach the importance of shaking suspension forms of phenytoin well, prior to pouring and measuring the dose.
- The nurse should teach the patient and family the importance of good dental hygiene to prevent gingival hyperplasia and gum softening. The nurse should encourage the patient to brush the teeth at least twice daily with a soft toothbrush and to floss daily.
- The nurse might suggest bleaching or electrolysis if hirsutism is a problem for female patients, because shaving or depilatories often leave a stubble.
- The nurse should suggest patients take with food to minimize GI distress.
- The nurse should teach the diabetic patient to frequently check capillary blood glucose.

Ongoing Assessment and Evaluation

Ongoing assessments include monitoring patients closely for therapeutic responses, seizure control, and adverse effects to drug therapy. This is particularly important when two or more AEDs are given in combination therapy. Regular monitoring of drug blood levels as well as the patient's clinical status is important until the effective dose is established and the patient's response to therapy is known. Patients may have seizure control even though blood levels show that the patient is not in the "normal therapeutic range." Conversely, adverse effects may also occur even if the patient is in "normal therapeutic range." Laboratory assessment is also needed periodically to assess for adverse effects on the hematologic system. The nurse should assess for drug interactions due to phenytoin's effect on hepatic enzyme metabolism every time total drug therapy is modified (i.e., any drug is discontinued or added, not just AEDs). Drug therapy is evaluated as being effective if the seizures are controlled and the patient is not exhibiting adverse effects. ■

BARBITURATES

The barbiturates produce a generalized CNS depression; they depress the sensory cortex, decrease motor activity, alter cerebellar function, and produce drowsiness and sedation. In addition to their use as sedatives and hypnotics, the barbiturates are used in the treatment of partial and generalized tonic-clonic seizures, and emergency control of certain acute convulsive episodes (e.g., status epilepticus, eclampsia, and meningitis.) Barbiturates include phenobarbital (the prototype) and mephobarbital. The full discussion of the prototype phenobarbital is in Chapter 17. This chapter will present some information about phenobarbital that is related to its use to treat seizures. Primidone is a drug that is significantly different than phenobarbital and will also be briefly discussed.

PHENOBARBITAL

Phenobarbital is a long-acting barbiturate AED that shares the same major indications as phenytoin does.

Phenobarbital may be used in conjunction with phenytoin to control generalized seizures. Phenobarbital is used to treat acute convulsive episodes that require emergency intervention (such as in status epilepticus, eclampsia, cholera, menin-

MEMORY CHIP

Phenytoin

- Used for most seizure types except absence seizures
- Significant contraindications: AV heart block, sinus bradycardia
- Most common adverse effects: sedation, nystagmus, ataxia, headache, nausea, gingival hyperplasia
- Most serious adverse effects: blood dyscrasias, lupus erythematosus, Stevens-Johnson syndrome
- **Life span alert: geriatric patients may have greater risk for toxicity from age-related decline in hepatic functions.**
- Maximizing therapeutic effects: take with food to enhance absorption and minimize GI upset; maintain therapeutic serum concentration (10–20 μg/mL)
- Minimizing adverse effects: maintain good oral hygiene and encourage frequent dental follow-up
- Most significant patient education: wear medical identification (e.g., MedicAlert) indicating condition and drug use/dosage; different brands of medication are not bioequivalent; abrupt withdrawal may cause status epilepticus

gitis, tetanus, and toxic reactions to strychnine or local anesthestics). An unlabeled use for phenobarbital is the treatment of febrile seizures in children. Phenobarbital's anticonvulsant activities are relatively nonselective. It stimulates GABA receptors, thereby elevating the seizure threshold and limiting the spread of seizure activity by affecting the CNS neuronal pathway neurotransmitters. Phenobarbital, at therapeutic concentrations, reduces the excitatory effects of glutamate and augments the inhibitory effects of GABA within the CNS. Tolerance does not occur to the anticonvulsant effects of phenobarbital.

Phenobarbital is classified as FDA pregnancy category D. Studies suggest a connection between maternal consumption of phenobarbital and a higher incidence of fetal abnormalities. Phenobarbital readily crosses the placental barrier and is distributed throughout fetal tissue. Reported effects on the infant include withdrawal symptoms including seizures and hyperirritability and a neonatal coagulation defect that may cause bleeding.

Adverse effects are related to CNS depression with respiratory depression the most serious. The degree of respiratory depression is dose dependent. The dosage used to control seizures is rarely involved with significant respiratory depression. Drowsiness occurs commonly with phenobarbital use in the treatment of seizures; tolerance to this effect, however, develops with chronic use. Other CNS effects may occur. In some instances, phenobarbital will produce CNS effects that are the opposite of what would normally be expected. Thus, agitation, hyperactivity, insomnia, irritability, and CNS stimulation may occur. Children and older adults are particularly prone to these paradoxic effects. Adverse cognitive effects in children may also include impaired short-term memory and deficits on neuropsychologic tests and memory concentration tasks. Fever may occur with chronic use. Status epilepticus may occur if phenobarbital is stopped suddenly after chronic use.

Phenobarbital induces the hepatic microsomal liver-enzyme system and significantly alters the biotransformation of a large number of other drugs. Phenobarbital is characterized by many drug-drug interactions. Because AED therapy often involves more than one drug, the nurse should carefully check to verify that a drug interaction is not likely to occur when phenobarbital is to be started.

When given for emergency use, phenobarbital is administered IV and may require at least 15 minutes before peak concentration is reached in the brain. Phenobarbital also has a long half-life. Therefore, administering phenobarbital continuously until the seizure activity ceases may lead to severe barbiturate-induced CNS depression, including respiratory depression and excessive hypotension. IV administration should not be faster than 50 mg/minute. Resuscitation equipment should always be available.

The nurse should assess the patient's alcohol intake before initiating long-term oral therapy with phenobarbital, because the combination of alcohol and phenobarbital may result in additional CNS depression and precipitate seizures. Additionally, alcohol abuse may cause the patient to be nonadherent with phenobarbital therapy. Finally, the nurse should take a careful drug history because the patient with a history of drug abuse may also be predisposed to abuse phenobarbital. Other nursing management is similar to that of phenytoin.

DRUG SIGNIFICANTLY DIFFERENT FROM P PHENOBARBITAL

Like phenobarbital, primidone (Mysoline) is used to control grand mal, psychomotor, or focal epileptic seizures, either alone or used in combination with other AED therapy. An unlabeled use of primidone is benign familial tremor. Although primidone is actually considered to be an adjuvant AED, one of the active metabolites of primidone is phenobarbital. The other active metabolite is phenylethylmalonamide (PEMA). Although primidone has anticonvulsant properties of its own, much of its effect comes from the anticonvulsant properties of phenobarbital and PEMA. Animal studies have shown that PEMA also potentiates the effects of phenobarbital. Phenobarbital accounts for between 15 and 25% of the metabolites formed by primidone.

Primidone has a half-life of 5 to 15 hours. PEMA and phenobarbital have longer half-lives (10 to 18 and 53 to 140 hours, respectively) and accumulate with chronic use. About 40% of primidone is excreted unchanged in the urine. The remainder of the drug is excreted as unconjugated PEMA and as phenobarbital and its metabolites.

The therapeutic effects and adverse effects of primidone are similar to those of phenobarbital and other AEDs. Nursing management of the patient is also similar.

C BENZODIAZEPINES

The benzodiazepines have multiple clinical uses, including treatment for anxiety, insomnia, muscle spasms, and seizures; benzodiazepines are also used to provide conscious sedation, and to prevent withdrawal symptoms from alcohol abuse. Their use in treating seizures will be discussed here. Benzodiazepines suppress the spread of seizure activity, they do not abolish the abnormal focal discharge. The current view of the anticonvulsant actions of the benzodiazepines is that they augment the inhibitory effects produced by stimulating various GABA-mediated pathways and enhance GABA-induced changes in membrane potential. Benzodiazepines appear to potentiate the effects of GABA and other inhibitory neurotransmitters by binding to specific benzodiazepine receptor sites. Recent evidence suggests there are two benzodiazepine receptors—BZ1 and BZ2. BZ1 is thought to be associated with sleep mechanisms; BZ2 with memory, motor, sensory, and cognitive functions. The antiepileptic activity of benzodiazepines (e.g., clonazepam) is thought to involve the brain stem.

Most benzodiazepines are FDA pregnancy category D. Use of benzodiazepines during the first trimester is believed to increase the risk of congenital malformations such as cleft lip and cleft palate. A neonatal withdrawal consisting of severe tremulousness and irritability or neonatal flaccidity and respiratory problems may occur as a result of maternal ingestion of benzodiazepines. Benzodiazepines are excreted in breast milk. Because neonates metabolize benzodiazepines more slowly than adults, accumulation of the drug and its metabolites to toxic levels is a distinct risk.

CNS adverse effects are common with benzodiazepines.

Many benzodiazepines have broad anticonvulsant characteristics, but only two (clonazepam and clorazepate) have been approved by the FDA for use in long-term treatment of certain types of seizures. Two other benzodiazepines—diazepam and midazolam—are used IV for status epilepticus. Lorazepam is the prototype benzodiazepine and is discussed thoroughly in Chapter 17. An unlabeled use of lorazepam is the treatment of status epilepticus. This chapter will briefly review the anticonvulsant use of the above mentioned benzodiazepines.

CLONAZEPAM

Clonazepam (Klonopin) may be used as monotherapy for seizure control. It may also be used as adjunctive treatment for various types of seizures, which include a variant form of absence seizures known as Lennox-Gastaut syndrome; akinetic and myoclonic seizures; and occasionally other types of seizures (e.g., absence seizures refractory to the succinimide AEDs, partial seizures with complex symptomatology, partial focal seizures, and some instances of infantile spasm.) Used in patients with multiple types of seizure disorders, clonazepam may sometimes increase the frequency of generalized convulsive seizures or precipitate them. Unlabeled uses for clonazepam include treatment of restless leg syndrome, dysarthria associated with parkinsonism, acute manic episodes of bipolar disorder, multifocal tic disorders, neuralgias, and as adjunctive therapy for schizophrenia.

Specifically, clonazepam appears to act at the limbic and subcortical levels of the CNS, producing anticonvulsant and sedative effects. It suppresses the spike-and-wave discharge in absence seizures and decreases the amplitude, duration, frequency, and spread of discharge in minor motor seizures.

Clonazepam is readily absorbed following oral administration. Peak plasma levels usually occur within 24 hours. Extremely lipid soluble, it is widely distributed in the body tissues including the brain and is highly bound to plasma proteins (97%). The long duration of action (half-life of 18 to 50 hours) is related to its lipid solubility and the fact that hepatic biotransformation oxidizes and reduces clonazepam to five identified metabolites. Because hepatic biotransformation is the predominant route for clonazepam metabolism, its disposition may be impaired by chronic liver disease.

Clonazepam is excreted almost entirely in the urine in the form of metabolites. The kidneys excrete clonazepam metabolites; use in patients with impaired renal function may result in excessive drug accumulation.

Clonazepam is an FDA pregnancy category C drug. Clonazepam freely crosses the placenta and accumulates in the fetal circulation.

Adverse effects related to the CNS are common with clonazepam as well as the other benzodiazepines. Transient mild drowsiness is common when therapy is first started. Drowsiness, ataxia, and confusion seem to occur most often in the older adult and in debilitated patients. Other CNS effects include problems with balance and movement, emotional changes, and speech difficulties. Paradoxic CNS stimulation may also occur. Constipation, diarrhea, dry mouth, and nausea are fairly common GI adverse effects from clonazepam. Potentially, serious adverse effects of cardiovascular and respiratory depression may occur after the IV administration of clonazepam. The most frequent drug interactions involving clonazepam and the other benzodiazepines occur with other CNS depressants. Alcohol will also potentiate the CNS adverse effects from clonazepam.

CLORAZEPATE

Clorazepate (Tranxene) is used as an adjunct in the treatment of partial seizures in adults and children older than 12 years of age. Peak plasma levels occur in 1 to 2 hours, elimination half-life is 40 to 50 hours, active metabolites prolong drug effects, and protein binding is about 98%. Pharmacodynamics, adverse effects and nursing management are similar to clonazepam.

DIAZEPAM

Anticonvulsant effects of diazepam (Valium) differ according to the mode of administration. Oral administration may be useful in adjunctive therapy. Some patients, stabilized on an AED, may require intermittent use of rectal diazepam to control episodes of increased seizure activity. Rectal dosing is based on age and weight. IV use is indicated for management of status epilepticus and severe recurrent convulsive seizures. IV diazepam has long been considered the drug of choice for status epilepticus, although drug selection may vary.

The IV route is preferred in the convulsing patient. IV administration of diazepam should avoid small veins or intra-arterial administration and the drug should be injected slowly so as to avoid reactions at the injection site. Seizures may return when given IV because of diazepam's short half-life by this route. Diazepam should not be infused nor mixed or diluted with other solutions because of the possibility of precipitation and instability. Additionally, diazepam interacts with plastic and introducing diazepam into plastic containers or administration sets will decrease availability of the drug. Emergency resuscitation equipment should be readily available when administering benzodiazepines IV for status epilepticus.

Injections of diazepam may be given IM if it is impossible to administer it IV. Absorption is unpredictable and erratic from IM injections. The deltoid muscle provides the best absorption, however, this site cannot accommodate more than 2 mL per injection (in adults) and is not suitable for multiple injections.

Safety and efficacy of diazepam have not been established in the neonate younger than 30 days of age. Prolonged CNS depression has been observed in neonates, apparently due to their inability to biotransform diazepam into inactive metabolites (Cada, Covington, Hebel, Hussar, Lasagna, Olin, et al., 2000)

Diazepam is also widely used for its many other benzodiazepine effects. See the discussion of benzodiazepines in Chapter 17.

MIDAZOLAM

Midazolam (Versed) is another benzodiazepine. Its primary use is as a general anesthetic (see Chapter 16). An unlabeled use of midazolam is an alternative treatment for status epilepticus. Despite the growing use of midazolam for the treatment of status epilepticus, little is known about its pharmacokinetics after prolonged use. Although midazolam is considered a "short-acting" benzodiazepine, its half-life is markedly increased after prolonged infusion.

LORAZEPAM

Lorazepam (Ativan), another benzodiazepine, is now often used to treat status epilepticus because of its longer duration of action in comparison with diazepam. This is, however, an unlabeled use for lorazepam. If given for status epilepticus, slow IV administration—similar to diazepam—is necessary to prevent respiratory and cardiovascular depression. The patient should be closely monitored while receiving IV lorazepam. Occasionally lorazepam may be given IM for status epilepticus. The antianxiety and other effects of lorazepam are discussed in Chapter 17.

SUCCINIMIDES

Succinimide-derivative AEDs are used mainly in managing absence seizures. The succinimide AEDs have replaced the oxazolidinedione AED drug class in the management and control of absence seizures. Succinimides include ethosuximide, methsuximide, and phensuximide. Ethosuximide is the prototype succinimide agent. The other drugs are represented by the prototype.

NURSING MANAGEMENT OF THE PATIENT RECEIVING ETHOSUXIMIDE

Core Drug Knowledge

Pharmacotherapeutics

Ethosuximide (Zarontin) is the drug of choice for treating absence seizures. There is some clinical evidence that ethosuximide is useful for managing and controlling myoclonic seizures or partial seizures with complex symptomatology.

Pharmacokinetics

Ethosuximide is readily absorbed from the GI tract. Absorption of ethosuximide appears to be complete; peak plasma concentrations occur within approximately 3 to 7 hours after a single oral dose and it is not significantly bound to plasma proteins. During long-term therapy the concentration in the cerebrospinal fluid is similar to the plasma concentrations. Therapeutic serum levels of ethosuximide range from 40 to 100 mL. Ethosuximide undergoes extensive hepatic metabolism and is excreted through the kidneys; approximately 20% is excreted unchanged. Ethosuximide plasma half-life in children is 30 hours and doubles to 60 hours in adults (Cada, et al., 2000). Therapeutic plasma-drug concentration is 40 to 100 μg/mL.

Pharmacodynamics

Ethosuximide elevates seizure threshold in the basal ganglia and the cortex; it also reduces the synaptic nerve response to low frequency repetitive stimulation. Typical and atypical absence seizures are characterized by a 3-cycle-per-second spike-and-wave pattern on the electroencephalograph. Thus, the ability of ethosuximide to reduce the synaptic response to repetitive stimulation explains its clinical efficacy for managing absence seizures.

Contraindications and Precautions

The clinical use of ethosuximide is contraindicated in hypersensitivity. Drug warnings emphasize that signs and symptoms of infection (fever, sore throat) should be thoroughly investigated because fatal blood dyscrasias have occurred, although they are not common. In addition, ethosuximide should be administered cautiously to patients with known liver or renal disease because liver and renal functional impairment have been reported as adverse effects of drug use. Ethosuximide is ranked in FDA pregnancy category C. Like other AEDs, an increased incidence of birth defects has been reported with use of ethosuximide during pregnancy. It should be administered cautiously to pregnant women. It should also be administered cautiously to breast-feeding women, children, and older adults.

Adverse Effects

Gastrointestinal adverse effects occur with the highest frequency in ethosuximide therapy. These include nausea, vomiting, vague GI upset, cramps, anorexia, diarrhea, weight loss, epigastric and abdominal pain, and constipation. Other common adverse effects include pruritus and urticaria.

Ethosuximide, like other succinimide AEDs, causes CNS-related adverse effects; the most common are drowsiness, dizziness, ataxia, irritability, nervousness, headache, and blurred vision. Other CNS effects are lethargy, euphoria, myopia, photosensitivity, hiccups, hyperactivity, insomnia, and fatigue. It is thought that some tolerance builds up to these effects. Emotional disturbances such as confusion, instability, mental slowness, depression, hypochondriacal behavior, sleep disturbances, night terrors, aggressiveness, and inability to concentrate have occurred in some patients, most commonly in patients who already have a reported psychiatric history.

Blood dyscrasias such as aplastic anemia and pancytopenia, both of which can be life threatening; various elevated white blood cell counts; and bone marrow depression are possible but uncommon adverse effects. Genitourinary adverse effects such as urinary frequency, renal damage, microscopic hematuria, and vaginal bleeding) are also possible but uncommon. Additional possible but uncommon adverse effects include dermatologic conditions (e.g., alopecia, erythematous skin rashes, hirsutism, pruritus, Stevens-Johnson syndrome, systemic lupus erythematosus); muscle weakness; periorbital edema; hyperemia; swelling of the tongue; and gingival hyperplasia.

Drug Interactions

Table 20-4 features drug interactions associated with ethosuximide. There are no significant drug-laboratory test or food-drug interactions with ethosuximide.

Assessment of Relevant Core Patient Variables

Health Status

The nurse should establish a baseline of hematologic, renal, and hepatic functions before starting ethosuximide therapy. It is also important for the nurse to monitor those functions at regular intervals to identify serious adverse drug reactions early. If dysfunction exists, succinimide AEDs must be used with caution. The drug should be discontinued if a skin rash develops or if the blood count (with differential) becomes depressed.

Life Span and Gender

As with all AEDs, the nurse should assess the woman of child-bearing age for pregnancy or lactation and explore her reproductive goals and contraceptive methods because of the potential risks to the fetus or breastfeeding infant.

Lifestyle, Diet, and Habits

The nurse should explore the patient's dietary and social habits to determine the patient's current use of alcohol, sedatives, and over-the-counter (OTC) drugs.

Environment

The nurse should be aware of the environment in which the drug will be administered. Ethosuximide may be administered by the health care provider or the patient in any setting.

Nursing Diagnoses and Outcomes

- Imbalanced Nutrition: Less than body requirements related to adverse GI drug effects of anorexia, abdominal complaints, nausea and vomiting

  Desired outcome: The patient will not experience significant nutritional imbalances while receiving ethosuximide.
- Risk for Injury from falls related to CNS adverse effects of ethosuximide

  Desired outcome: The patient will not sustain an injury while receiving ethosuximide.

Planning and Intervention

Maximizing Therapeutic Effect

As with all AEDs, one of the best ways to maximize therapeutic effect throughout therapy is to stress the importance of taking the drug as directed and not stopping it abruptly. The nurse should assess seizure control and drug-blood levels periodically.

Minimizing Adverse Effects

To minimize the CNS depressant effects of ethosuximide, the drug should not be mixed with other CNS depressants (e.g., alcohol, sleep-inducing medications) not approved by the health care provider. Additional strategies for minimizing adverse effects are similar to those for phenytoin.

Providing Patient and Family Education

Teaching about ethosuximide is much like teaching about the other AEDs. Please refer to the earlier display, Patient and Family Education Common to AEDs, for important patient education information. Specific teaching for ethosuximide is as follows:

- The nurse should instruct the patient to notify the health care provider if signs of infection (fever, sore throat) develop as blood work will likely need to be checked.

TABLE 20-4 Agents That Interact With P Ethosuximide

Interactants	Effect and Significance	Nursing Management
valproic acid	Increased pharmacologic effects of ethosuximide Both increases and decreases in ethosuximide levels have occurred	Monitor patient for changes in seizure control. Assess patient for evidence of therapeutic effects of interacting drugs.
phenytoin	Serum hydantoin levels may increase	Evaluate patient for changed seizure control. Assess patient for evidence of therapeutic effects of interacting drugs. Check for therapeutic serum levels of interacting drugs.
primidone	Lower primidone and phenobarbital levels may occur	Evaluate patient for changed seizure control. Assess patient for evidence of therapeutic effects of interacting drugs. Check for therapeutic serum levels of interacting drugs.

- The nurse should also instruct the patient to notify the physician if a severe rash develops.
- The nurse should teach the patient to take ethosuximide with food if GI distress develops.

Ongoing Assessment and Evaluation

Ongoing assessment and evaluation for ethosuximide are similar to that of phenytoin. ■

MISCELLANEOUS ANTIEPILEPTICS

Carbamazepine is a miscellaneous AED that is unique to itself. It is an iminostilbene derivative that is chemically related to the tricyclic antidepressants and unrelated to the other AEDs. It is an effective AED in the treatment of psychomotor and grand mal seizures and also an effective analgesic in the trigeminal neuralgia. Its mechanism of action is unknown. It appears to act by reducing polysynaptic responses and blocking posttetanic potentiation. Carbamazepine (Tegretol) is the prototype. A drug significantly different from carbamazepine is oxcarbazepine.

NURSING MANAGEMENT OF THE PATIENT RECEIVING CARBAMAZEPINE

Core Drug Knowledge

Pharmacotherapeutics

Carbamazepine is used in the prophylactic management of complex partial seizures, generalized tonic-clonic seizures, and mixed seizure types of these patterns. Its use is generally reserved for patients who have not responded satisfactorily to other AEDs, whose seizures are difficult to control, or who are experiencing marked adverse effects. Patients with complex partial seizures show the greatest improvement with carbamazepine. Unlabeled uses include several psychiatric disorders (e.g., bipolar disorder and unipolar depression, schizoaffective illness and resistant schizophrenia, posttraumatic stress disorder, and atypical psychosis).

Pharmacokinetics

Carbamazepine is slowly and adequately absorbed from the GI tract. It reaches peak serum levels in 4 to 5 hours. The suspension form of the drug is absorbed slightly faster than the tablet form, although both deliver the drug equally to the circulation. Peak and trough plasma levels are essentially equivalent between the suspension and tablet drug forms when the dosage regimen is three daily divided doses for the suspension and two for the tablets. Usual adult therapeutic levels are 4 to 12 μg/mL, although optimal levels have not been established.

Carbamazepine is 75% to 90% protein bound and is metabolized in the liver to an active metabolite. The drug has the ability to induce drug-metabolizing enzymes and this will increase its own metabolism. Initial half-life ranges from 25 to 65 hours, and with repeated doses, half-life decreases to a range of 12 to 17 hours. This change in half-life is explained by increased metabolism.

Following administration, carbamazepine's metabolites are primarily excreted in the urine (72%) with the remainder excreted in the feces. Approximately 3% of carbamazepine is excreted unchanged.

Pharmacodynamics

Some pharmacologic effects of carbamazepine resemble the pharmacologic effects of the hydantoin drug class; they have virtually identical actions on sodium channels, and they limit the spread of seizure activity by reducing polysynaptic responses.

Contraindications and Precautions

Carbamazepine is contraindicated in patients who are hypersensitive to it or to the tricyclic antidepressants. It is also contraindicated in patients with a history of bone marrow depression. Monoamine oxidase inhibitors should be discontinued at least 14 days before administering carbamazepine.

The drug should be used with caution in individuals with glaucoma. Carbamazepine has shown mild anticholinergic activity and should be used with caution in patients with increased intraocular pressure. Patients with a history of an adverse hematologic reaction to any other drug may be especially at risk for the hematologic effects of carbamazepine.

Teratogenic effects in animal studies have been demonstrated and a significant amount of carbamazepine is excreted in breast milk. Carbamazepine is FDA pregnancy category D. Epidemiologic data suggest that there

---

MEMORY CHIP

Ethosuximide

- Used to control absence seizures
- Significant contraindication: hypersensitivity
- Most common adverse effects: sedation, nausea, ataxia, headache, blurred vision, pruritus
- Most serious adverse effect: pancytopenia
- Maximizing therapeutic effects: maintain therapeutic serum concentration (40–100 μg/mL), store drug in a tight, light-resistant container at room temperature
- Minimizing adverse effects: establish baseline for CBC with differential; monitor periodically
- Most significant patient education: wear medical identification (e.g., MedicAlert) indicating condition and drug use/dosage; mental or physical abilities required for the performance of potentially hazardous tasks (e.g., driving, operating machinery) may be impaired; report unexplained fever, sore throat, unusual bleeding or bruising, and joint pain to health care provider; drug may harmlessly color urine pink, red, or reddish-brown; and abrupt withdrawal may cause status epilepticus

may be an association between the use of carbamazepine during pregnancy and congenital malformations, including spina bifida. A comparison of carbamazepine monotherapy or combination therapy with that of carbamazepine and another AED suggests that there may be a higher prevalence of teratogenic effects when carbamazepine is used in combination therapy. Therefore, carbamazepine monotherapy may be preferable for pregnant women. Carbamazepine and its epoxide metabolite are transferred to breast milk. Because of the potential for serious adverse reactions, breast-feeding should be avoided. Carbamazepine appears to be safe to use in children.

Adverse Effects

The most serious adverse effects of carbamazepine are fatal blood dyscrasias (e.g., aplastic anemia and agranulocytosis). Most adverse reactions produced by carbamazepine, however, are relatively minor and are minimized if drug therapy begins slowly at a lower dosage and advances gradually. The most common adverse effects are dizziness, drowsiness, unsteadiness, nausea, and vomiting.

Other adverse effects of carbamazepine are extremely varied and extensive. CNS effects may occur such as disturbed coordination, confusion, fatigue, headache, tinnitus, vertigo, visual hallucinations, speech disturbances, abnormal involuntary movements, peripheral neuritis and paresthesias, depression with agitation, talkativeness, tinnitus, abnormal sensitivity to sound, behavior changes in children, and paralysis and other symptoms of cerebral arterial insufficiency. Cardiovascular effects may also occur such as congestive heart failure, aggravation of hypertension, hypotension, syncope, edema, thrombophlebitis, thromboembolism, aggravation of coronary artery disease, arrhythmias, atrioventricular block, and adenopathy or lympadenopathy. GI effects may also occur, such as abdominal pain, gastric distress, constipation or diarrhea, anorexia, dryness of mouth or pharynx, glossitis, and stomatitis. Additionally, dermatologic effects may occur, such as photosensitivity, alterations in pigmentation, Stevens-Johnson syndrome, alopecia, diaphoresis, erythema multiforme and nodosum, purpura, aggravation of disseminated lupus erythematosus, and toxic epidermal necrolysis. Hepatitic effects may include abnormal liver function test results, cholestatic/hepatocellular jaundice, and hepatitis. Metabolic effects may include fever, chills, inappropriate antidiuretic hormone secretion syndrome, frank water intoxication, hyponatremia (may be serious) with confusion, and decreased plasma calcium levels). The following may also occur: musculoskeletal effects (aching joints and muscles, leg cramps); ophthalmic effects (transient diplopia and oculomotor disturbances, nystagmus, cortical lens opacities with pinpoint punctures on the surface, conjunctivitis, and blurred vision); pulmonary effects (pulmonary hypersensitivity); and miscellaneous effects (lupus erythematosus–like syndrome, aseptic meningitis [isolated reports]).

Drug Interactions

Numerous drug–drug interactions are possible with carbamazepine. For example, thiazide diuretics or furosemide used concomitantly with carbamazepine may produce a severe, symptomatic hyponatremia (Table 20-5).

Assessment of Relevant Core Patient Variables

Health Status

In addition to completing a health assessment, drug history, physical examination, and assessment of contraindicating conditions and allergies, the nurse needs to review results of baseline hematologic, hepatic, and renal function studies performed prior to carbamazepine therapy.

Life Span and Gender

The nurse should document the age and development of the patient. Safety and effectiveness for use in children younger than 6 years have not been determined and adverse effects on behavior and cognition have been noted.

The nurse should assess the woman of child-bearing for pregnancy and lactation because of potential effects on the fetus or nursing infant. The nurse should also explore the patient's reproductive goals and contraceptive practices because a nonhormonal method of birth control will be necessary.

Environment

The nurse should be aware of the environment in which the drug will be administered. Carbamazepine is easily administered in the acute care setting, or more often at home by the patient or family. The nurse should assess the patient for occupational environment that requires the operation of dangerous machinery, which may be problematic because of adverse effects of dizziness and drowsiness.

Nursing Diagnoses and Outcomes

- Imbalanced Nutrition related to adverse effect of nausea and vomiting
  Desired outcome: The patient will not have serious nutritional deficiencies while receiving carbamazepine.
- Risk for Injury related to falls from dizziness and unsteadiness
  Desired outcome: The patient will not become injured from a fall while receiving carbamazepine.

Planning and Intervention

Maximizing Therapeutic Effects

Extended release carbamazepine is for twice daily administration. The extended-release tablets must be swallowed whole and never crushed or chewed.

TABLE 20-5 Agents That Interact With Carbamazepine

Interactants	Effect and Significance	Nursing Management
antihistamines, barbiturates, cimetidine, danazol, diltiazem, isoniazid, lamotrigine, macrolide antibiotics, propoxyphene, selective serotonin reuptake inhibitors, tricyclic anti-depressants, verapamil	Increased pharmacologic effects of carbamazepine from alteration/inhibition in hepatic metabolism; risk of carbamazepine toxicity increased	Assess patient for control of concurrent disease Evaluate patient for changed seizure control Assess patient for evidence of therapeutic effects of interacting drugs Monitor patient for therapeutic serum levels (if applicable) of interacting drugs Check cardiac rhythm and function
charcoal, felbamate, phenytoin	Decreased pharmacologic effects of carbamazepine from alteration in hepatic metabolism Charcoal decreases carbamazepine effects by decreasing its absorption Serum levels of felbamate may also increase	Evaluate patient for changed seizure control Assess patient for evidence of therapeutic effects of interacting drugs Monitor patient for therapeutic serum levels (if applicable) of interacting drugs
acetaminophen, anticoagulants, barbiturates, bupropion, cyclosporine, doxycycline, felodipine, haloperidol, lithium, nondepolarizing neuromuscular blockers, oral contraceptives, succinimides, theophylline, valproic acid	Decreased therapeutic effects of interactants due to induction of hepatic CYP450 isozymes The analgesic effects of acetaminophen may be reduced by concomitant carbamazepine use; the potential hepatotoxicity of acetaminophen may increase The hypoprothrombinemic effect of the anticoagulants may decrease Concurrent administration of lithium and carbamazine may increase risk of CNS toxicity and lithium toxicity	Appraise the patient for management of concurrent disease states Monitor bleeding times/parameters Assess patient for evidence of therapeutic effects of interacting drugs Check for therapeutic serum levels (if applicable) of interacting drugs Evaluate patient for changed seizure activity and control.

Minimizing Adverse Effect

Carbamazepine should be added gradually to other AED therapy, and therapy should be started with the lowest doses of drug possible to minimize adverse reactions. Other AED dosages may need to be increased because of carbamazepine's enzyme-inducing properties.

The vast majority of minor hematologic changes that occur in patients on carbamazepine are unlikely to signal the occurrence of a serious abnormality. Complete pretreatment hematologic testing should be obtained as a baseline. If, in the course of treatment, a patient develops low or decreased white blood cell counts (i.e., less than 3/mm^3) or platelet cell counts, the nurse should monitor the patient closely. The nurse must monitor for signs of bone marrow suppression (e.g., infections, sore throat, bruising, unusual bleeding) and signs of hepatic dysfunction (e.g., jaundice, dark urine, light-colored stools). These changes should be reported to the health care provider immediately. Carbamazepine should be withdrawn if any evidence of significant bone marrow depression develops.

Providing Patient and Family Education

Most of the teaching for carbamazepine is similar to those of the AEDs in general. Please refer to the display Patient and Family Education Common to AEDs for more information. Patient and family education specific to carbamazepine follows:

- It is extremely important for the nurse to advise the patient or caregiver to immediately report symptoms such as sore throat, fever, easy bruising, petechiae, epistaxis, or other signs of infection or bleeding tendency, which may be indications of blood dyscrasias. Blood work will usually be required if these occur.
- The nurse should teach the patient to report any of the following symptoms immediately, if they occur: early signs of genitourinary dysfunction (e.g., urinary frequency, acute urinary retention, decrease urine output); and signs of cardiovascular adverse effects that require immediate attention (e.g., congestive heart failure, syncope, thrombophlebitis, cyanosis). Skin eruptions or changes in skin pigmentation may require drug withdrawal. In such cases, the nurse should instruct the patient to report these signs.
- The nurse should advise the patient to take carbamazepine with meals to minimize GI upset.
- The nurse should explain to the patient or caregiver that extended-release tablets should be taken twice daily and swallowed whole, never crushed or chewed. Alert the patient and family or caregiver that the extended-release tablet coating is not absorbed and is excreted in the feces; these coatings may be noticeable in the stool.

Ongoing Assessment and Evaluation

The ongoing assessment and evaluation of carbamazepine is similar to those for phenytoin. ■

MEMORY CHIP

Carbamazepine

- Used for refractory seizure disorders, partial seizures with complex symptomatology, generalized tonic-clonic seizures
- Significant contraindications: hypersensitivity to tricyclic antidepressants, history of bone marrow depression
- Most common adverse effects: sedation, dizziness, nausea, ataxia
- Most serious adverse effects: massive hepatic cellular necrosis, potentially lethal hematologic disturbances
- **Life span alert: Geriatric patients may experience agitation and confusion**
- Maximizing therapeutic effects: maintain therapeutic serum concentration (4–12 μg/mL)
- Minimizing adverse effects: establish baseline for CBC with differential and liver function; monitor regularly and discontinue if hepatic dysfunction occurs or evidence of bone marrow suppression
- Most significant patient education: wear medical identification (e.g., MedicAlert) indicating condition and drug use/dosage; mental or physical abilities required for the performance of potentially hazardous tasks (e.g., driving, operating machinery) may be impaired; report unexplained fever, sore throat, unusual bleeding, yellowing of the skin, and mouth ulcers; and abrupt withdrawal may cause status epilepticus

DRUG SIGNIFICANTLY DIFFERENT FROM CARBAMAZEPINE

Oxcarbazepine (Trileptal) is chemically similar to the metabolite of carbamazepine and was developed to mimic its efficacy while minimizing its adverse effects and potential for drug interactions. Oxcarbazepine is indicated for monotherapy or adjunctive treatment of partial seizures in adults and adjunctive therapy in children ages 4 to 16 years. An unlabeled use for oxcarbazepine is atypical panic disorder.

The AED activity of oxcarbazepine is primarily exerted through the 10-monohydroxy metabolite (MHD) of oxcarbazepine. The precise mechanism by which oxcarbazepine and MHD exert their AED effect is unknown; however, in vitro electrophysiologic studies indicate that they produce blockade of voltage-sensitive sodium channels, resulting in stabilization of hyperexcited neural membranes, inhibition of repetitive neuronal firing, and diminution of propagation of synaptic impulses. These actions are thought to be important in the prevention of seizure spread in the intact brain. In addition, increased potassium conductance and modulation of high-voltage activated calcium channels may contribute to the anticonvulsant effects of the drug. No significant interactions of oxcarbazepine or MHD with brain neurotransmitters or modulator receptor sites have been demonstrated.

Oxcarbazepine inhibits CYP-2C19 and induces CYP-3A4/5 with potentially important effects on plasma concentrations of other drugs that use this metabolic pathway. In addition, several AEDs that are cytochrome P450 inducers (e.g., carbamazepine, phenobarbital, phenytoin) can decrease plasma concentrations of oxcarbazepine and its metabolite, MHD, which is primarily responsible for the pharmacologic effect of oxcarbazepine. Oxcarbazepine induces the CYP-450 enzymes that are responsible for metabolizing sex hormones. Women of child-bearing age should be counseled that oral contraceptive failure may occur when taking oxcarbazepine and use of additional nonhormonal forms of contraception are recommended because of a reduction in hormonal contraceptive efficacy.

Oxcarbazepine is completely absorbed—food does not affect the rate or extent of oxcarbazepine absorption—and extensively metabolized to its pharmacologically active MHD metabolite. Approximately 40% of MHD is bound to serum proteins, predominantly to albumin. Clinically significant interactions with other drugs through competition for protein-binding sites are unlikely. The half-life of oxcarbazepine is 2 hours, whereas the half-life of MHD is 9 hours. Oxcarbazepine is renally excreted mostly in the form of metabolites; more than 95% of the dose appears in the urine. Fecal excretion accounts for less than 4% of the administered dose. Approximately 80% of the dose is excreted in the urine as metabolites.

With renal function impairment (creatinine clearance less than 30 mL/minute), dosage is usually begun at one half the usual starting dose (300 mg/day) and increased slowly to achieve the desired clinical response.

Oxcarbazepine is pregnancy category C. Oxcarbazepine and its metabolite are transferred through the placenta and excreted in human breast milk. There are no adequate and well-controlled clinical studies of oxcarbazepine in pregnant women; but as with other AEDs, oxcarbazepine may cause fetal effects and so should be used during pregnancy only if the potential benefit to the mother justifies the potential risk to the fetus.

Hyponatremia is common with oxcarbazepine therapy although the patients are often asymptomatic. The risk is greatest if the patient is receiving other drugs that deplete sodium levels.

The most common adverse effects from oxcarbazepine are dizziness, sleepiness, fatigue, diplopia, abnormal vision, nausea, vomiting, abdominal pain, dyspepsia, ataxia, tremor, and abnormal gait.

OXAZOLIDINEDIONES

Oxazolidinedione AEDs include trimethadione and paramethadione. These drugs, used therapeutically for refractory absence seizures, have limited use because of their relatively frequent and severe toxic effects (e.g., hepatic or renal damage, blood dyscrasias, systemic lupus erythematosus, and a myasthenia gravis-like syndrome). These agents are used only when other less toxic drugs have been found ineffective in controlling typical absence seizures. Newer drugs have essentially replaced them.

ADJUNCT ANTICONVULSANTS

Adjuvant anticonvulsants are newer agents that have been created to treat seizures. They are mostly used in combination with other AEDs, although some may be used in monotherapy. Nursing management for these drugs is similar to that for all AEDs.

FELBAMATE

Felbamate (Felbatol) is a dicarbamate AED structurally related to but pharmacologically distinct from the sedative meprobamate. The exact mechanism of felbamate action is unknown; it is thought to increase seizure threshold and reduce seizure spread. Peak plasma concentrations occur in 1 to 3 hours; half life is 14 to 22 hours. Felbamate is 24% to 35% protein bound, undergoes extensive hepatic metabolism, and a small amount (24%) is excreted unchanged by the kidneys. A therapeutic range has not been established.

Felbamate does interact with other AEDs—phenytoin concentrations are increased by approximately 20%, carbamazepine toxicity may be induced, and serum concentrations of valproate may be increased.

Common adverse effects include anorexia and GI disturbances, which may cause weight loss, insomnia, dizziness, blurred vision, headache, diplopia, and ataxia. Most patients have difficulty tolerating doses higher than 3,600 mg/day; the maximum recommended dose in children is 40 mg/kg. Felbamate has been associated with a significant risk for aplastic anemia and acute hepatic failure. Although an effective AED, felbamate poses substantial risks in several specific patient populations. Recognized risk factors, indicating a higher likelihood of aplastic anemia in certain patients, include

- Age: adults are at higher risk than children.
- Gender: aplastic anemia is more likely to occur in women.
- Concomitant autoimmune disorders (e.g., lupus).
- Previous significant hematologic adverse effects.

Specific patient management focuses on preventing toxic drug effects of aplastic anemia and hepatic failure. The nurse should carefully monitor the patient's complete blood count and liver function test results for such effects. Because of the serious potential toxicity of felbamate, it is generally used only for the treatment of refractory seizures.

GABAPENTIN

Gabapentin (Neurontin) is an AED that is structurally related to the inhibitory CNS neurotransmitter GABA, although it lacks direct GABA-mimetic action and its precise mechanism of action is unknown. It is thought to work at multiple sites by one or more of the following mechanisms:

- Competing with endogenous amino acids (e.g., leucine, phenylalanine) for transport carriers
- Inducing GABA synthesis in the brain
- Modulating calcium and/or sodium channels
- Inhibiting monoamine neurotransmitter release
- Inducing increased serotonin production

Therapeutic uses are as adjunct therapy for treatment of partial seizures with or without secondary generalization in adults and children over the age of 3 years. Gabapentin has also been demonstrated to be effective in treating neuropathic pain, migraine prophylaxis, bipolar depression, spasticity, postherpetic neuralgia, and diabetic neuropathy. The therapeutic range is 5 to 20 μg/mL.

Gabapentin does not bind to plasma proteins, is not appreciably metabolized, and does not induce hepatic enzyme activity. Peak plasma levels are related to creatinine clearance and occur in 2 to 3 hours with a half-life of 7 hours. Approximately 75% to 81% is renally excreted unchanged. Thus, excretion is decreased in patients with diminished renal function and in older adults. The pharmacokinetics of gabapentin are not substantially altered by concomitant administration of other AEDs. Conversely, gabapentin does not appear to alter the pharmacokinetics of commonly used AEDs (e.g., carbamazepine, phenytoin, valproate, phenobarbital, diazepam) or oral contraceptives. No drug interactions have been reported. When gabapentin is taken concurrently with antacids, its bioavailability is reduced by 20%. Two hours should elapse between administration of gabapentin and antacids. The only known contraindication to gabapentin is hypersensitivity to the drug.

The most common adverse effects of gabapentin are somnolence, dizziness, and ataxia. Patients often accommodate to these adverse effects. Starting with a low dose and gradually increasing the dose can minimize these adverse effects. Giving the first dose at bedtime is also helpful in minimizing the perception of adverse effects.

Cognitively impaired or developmentally delayed children may experience unacceptable behavioral effects—especially hyperactivity—from gabapentin (as well as other more-established and newer AEDs) may occur (Schachter, 2000). Gabapentin is FDA pregnancy category C as it has shown to be fetotoxic in laboratory animals.

LAMOTRIGINE

Lamotrigine (Lamictal) is a phenyltriazine AED that is used as adjunctive therapy in the treatment of partial seizures in adults with or without secondary generalization and as adjunctive therapy in the generalized seizures of Lennox-Gastaut syndrome in pediatric patients less than 16 years of age. An added benefit of lamotrigine therapy is improved attention and alertness—especially in patients with developmental or attention problems. Although the precise mechanism of action is unknown, it is thought to stabilize neuronal membranes by blocking voltage sensitive sodium channels, which inhibits the release of excitatory amino acid neurotransmitters (e.g., aspartate, glutamate) that play a role in the generation and spread of epileptic seizures.

Following oral administration, peak plasma concentrations occur from 1.4 to 4.8 hours and are dose related. The half-life is 24 hours. Plasma protein binding is 55% and there is no enzymatic induction. Extensively metabolized, approximately 10% of lamotrigine is renally excreted unchanged. Patients with renal and hepatic function impairment require cautious use of lamotrigine. Elimination of lamotrigine is markedly increased by the coadministration of hepatic-enzyme-inducing AEDs (e.g., carbamazepine, phenobarbital, phenytoin, primidone). When combined with valproic acid, however, lamotrigine elimination is decreased, and its half-life may be more than doubled. Because of this, if giving lamotrigine to a patient already receiving valproic acid, the dose of lamotrigine should be less than half of what would be used if the patient was not also receiving valproic acid.

Dosage of lamotrigine is based on the clinical response to drug therapy. Because of possible pharmacokinetic interactions when lamotrigine is given in combination therapy with other anticonvulsants, the monitoring of blood levels for lamotrigine and other anticonvulsants may be helpful, especially during times of dosage adjustment; but at the time of writing this chapter there is no established guideline or established therapeutic range of lamotrigine to do so. Monitoring blood levels is currently a clinical decision made by the physician or nurse practitioner.

Lamotrigine is FDA pregnancy category C. Many potential adverse effects from lamotrigine exist. The most frequently occurring adverse effects are ataxia, blurred vision, diplopia, dizziness, headache, somnolence, nausea, vomiting, and rash. Benign rashes may occur with lamotrigine. Severe, life-threatening rashes (e.g., Stevens-Johnson syndrome, toxic epidermal necrolysis) may also occur, although much less frequently. The incidence of life-threatening rashes is greater with increased dosage. Nearly all cases of life-threatening rashes associated with lamotrigine have occurred within 2 to 8 weeks of treatment initiation. The incidence of severe rashes appears to be higher in pediatric patients than in adults: 1% versus 0.3% (Yerby, 2001). The risk of serious rash is increased more than three times with co-administration of valproic acid. Because of the possible serious nature of some skin rashes, lamotrigine should be discontinued at once if a rash develops, although discontinuation of lamotrigine may not prevent a rash from becoming life-threatening, permanently disabling or disfiguring.

VALPROIC ACID

Valproic acid (Depakote, Depakene) is used as the sole therapy or as adjunctive therapy for patients with simple and complex absence seizures. It is also used as adjunctive therapy to treat complex partial seizures that occur either by themselves or with other types of seizures. Valproic acid is also approved for used in the treatment of mania from bipolar disorder, and for the prophylactic treatment of migraine headaches. Nonlabeled uses of valproic acid are numerous. They include as monotherapy or combination therapy in the treatment of atypical absence, myoclonic, and grad mal seizures; atonic, elementary partial, and infantile spasm seizures; intractable status epilepticus that has not responded to other treatments; prevention of recurrent febrile seizures in children; minor incontinence after ileoanal anastomosis; and in the management of anxiety disorders/panic attacks.

Valproic acid is chemically unrelated to other AEDs and its mechanism of action is not known. It may increase brain levels of GABA, potentiate postsynaptic GABA response, affect the potassium channel, or have a direct membrane stabilizing effect.

Valproic acid is rapidly absorbed when given orally and peaks within 1 to 4 hours. Absorption of the syrup form of the drug occurs more rapidly, in 15 minutes. Valproic acid is metabolized in the liver and its metabolites are excreted in the urine.

Valproic acid may cause fatal hepatic failure. Children younger than 2 years seem most at risk of this adverse effect. The incidence of fatal hepatotoxicity decreases significantly with age. Fatal liver disease usually occurs within the first 6 months of therapy. This may be preceded by nonspecific symptoms such as loss of seizure control, malaise, weakness, lethargy, facial edema, anorexia, jaundice, and vomiting. Patients should be closely monitored for these symptoms and liver function closely assessed during therapy with valproic acid.

Serious adverse effects of valproic acid include thrombocytopenia (increased risk with higher blood concentrations of valproic acid), and hyperammonemia (may occur with normal liver function test results).

Although there are many other possible adverse effects, the most common are sedation, nausea, vomiting, and minor elevations of liver enzymes (usually dose related). Valproic acid is a pregnancy category D drug. Drug interactions may occur with the use of many other drugs, especially phenytoin and other AEDs.

LEVETIRACETAM

Levetiracetam (Keppra) is used as adjunct therapy in the treatment of partial seizures in adults. A pyrrolidine derivative that is structurally unrelated to other currently available AEDs, its mechanism of action is unknown and it appears to inhibit hypersynchronization of epileptiform discharges rather than activity related to any known mechanisms involved in excitatory or inhibitory neurotransmission.

A potent AED, levetiracetam may be given without regard to food and is rapidly and almost entirely absorbed after oral ingestion. Peak plasma concentrations occur in 1 hour with a half-life of 6 to 8 hours and protein binding less than 10%. The half-life in adults is 6 to 8 hours. About 24% of an administered dose is metabolized to an inactive metabolite; its metabolism is independent of the hepatic CYP-450 isoenzyme system and no drug interactions have been reported. Approximately 67% of an administered dose is renally excreted unchanged. Patients with impaired renal function must have dosages modified according to the degree of impairment and based on creatinine clearance values. Dosage should be monitored carefully in older adults because of age-related decline in renal function. No dosage adjustment is needed in patients with hepatic impairment. Levetiracetam is FDA pregnancy category C. Compared with other AEDs, the incidence of adverse effects appears extremely low with somnolence, asthenia (loss of strength), and dizziness among the most frequently reported. Ataxia and other coordination problems may also arise. There are no potential fatal adverse effects.

TIAGABINE

Tiagabine (Gabatril) is a nipecotic acid derivative that is a potent inhibitor of GABA reuptake into neurons and glia. It is a "designer" drug the chemical composition of which allows passage across the blood–brain barrier. As monotherapy or when used in combination with other AEDs, it is effective against partial seizures in adults and children older than 12 years of age. It is usually administered orally with food.

Safety and efficacy have not been established for children younger than 12 years of age nor for adults older than

65 years of age. Peak concentrations of tiagabine occur within 30 minutes to 1 hour. Tiagabine undergoes extensive hepatic metabolism through the CYP-450 system and the plasma half-life (4.5 to 13 hours; mean, 7 hours) is decreased as much as 30% in patients concomitantly receiving an AED that induces hepatic microsomal enzymes. Tiagabine itself does not appear to induce or inhibit hepatic microsomal enzymes nor does it appear to have any clinically important interactions with other AEDs. Tiagabine is highly protein bound (96%).

Pharmacokinetics are similar among patients with normal and impaired renal function. Clearance is decreased in patients with hepatic impairment and these patients may require dosage adjustment. Tiagabine is well tolerated with few adverse effects. Most commonly experienced are dizziness, asthenia, somnolence, nervousness, and nausea.

TOPIRAMATE

Topiramate (Topamax) is structurally different from other currently available AEDs and possesses a spectrum of antiepileptic activity resembling those of carbamazepine and phenytoin. It is used in combination with other AEDs in the management of partial-onset seizures or primary generalized tonic-clonic seizures in adults and children younger than 2 years of age. Topiramate has a novel chemical structure derived from D-fructose that blocks voltage-sensitive sodium channels, enhances the activity of inhibitory GABA and blocks the action of excitatory glutamate. It is also a weak carbonic anhydrase inhibitor. Topiramate is administered orally without regard to food, is rapidly absorbed and time to peak plasma concentrations is 1.8 to 4.3 hours, half-life is 19 to 23 hours, and plasma protein binding is less than 20%. Topiramate is not extensively metabolized; some renal tubular reabsorption occurs and it is primarily eliminated unchanged in the urine (about 70% of an administered dose). Dosage adjustments should be made for renal and hepatic function impairment. In renally impaired patients (creatinine clearance less than 70 mL/min), 50% of the usual adult dose is recommended. Although topiramate does not cause enzyme induction, enzyme-inducing AEDs can increase topiramate clearance and reduce topiramate concentration. Topiramate does, however, increase valproate concentrations and reduces the concentrations of hormonal contraceptives.

Adverse effects that occur most often with topiramate are CNS related. Primarily they create psychomotor slowing or create somnolence or fatigue, although other CNS effects are possible. A tolerance to these adverse effects often develops. Additionally, topiramate is associated with adverse cognitive effects in children that may manifest as language dysfunction or behavioral changes (Schachter, 2000). Renal stones may occur from topiramate inhibition of carbonic anhydrase. The FDA pregnancy category is C.

ZONISAMIDE

Zonisamide (Zonegran) is a sulfonamide derivative AED that is indicated for use as adjunctive therapy for the treatment of partial seizures in adults (those older than 16 years of age). Zonisamide is also effective in generalized seizures as well as myoclonus, Lennox-Gastaut syndrome, and infantile spasms. The precise mechanism of zonisamide activity is unknown, although in vitro studies suggest that it exerts its antiepileptic effects through action within sodium and calcium channels, consequently stabilizing neuronal membranes and suppressing neuronal hypersynchronization. In vitro studies have demonstrated that zonisamide binds to the GABA/benzodiazepine receptor, suppresses synaptically driven electrical activity without affecting postsynaptic GABA or glutamate responses and facilitates dopaminergic and serotonergic neurotransmission. Peak plasma concentrations occur within 2 to 6 hours. Zonisamide is 40% bound to plasma proteins; half-life is 63 hours. Zonisamide's long half-life requires a slow titration of dosages with dose increases every 2 weeks. The therapeutic range is 20 to 30 µg/mL.

Zonisamide is metabolized through the hepatic CYP-450 enzyme system. Drug interactions occur between enzyme-inducing AEDs (e.g., phenytoin, carbamazepine, phenobarbital) and zonisamide; inducers increase zonisamide clearance and decrease the serum concentration. Zonisamide does not appear, however, to interfere with the metabolism of other drugs that are broken down by CYP-450 isozymes. Zonisamide is primarily renally excreted; thus drug clearance is decreased with impaired renal function.

Hypersensitivity reactions with zonisamide have occurred only rarely—usually as a result of severe reactions to sulfonamides. Hypersensitivity reactions include Stevens-Johnson syndrome, toxic epidermal necrolysis, fulminant hepatic necrosis, agranulocytosis, aplastic anemia, and other blood dyscrasias. Zonisamide should be immediately discontinued if hypersensitivity reactions occur. The most commonly observed adverse reactions are somnolence, anorexia, dizziness, headache, nausea, agitation, and irritability. Zonisamide is a FDA pregnancy category C drug.

VIGABATRIN

Vigabatrin (Sabril) is a structural analogue of GABA, the brain's primary inhibitory neurotransmitter. It binds selectively and irreversibly to GABA transaminase, the enzyme that breaks down GABA. This action is dose dependent and increases the brain and cerebrospinal fluid levels of GABA, thus increasing brain inhibition. Vigabatrin appears to be effective in the treatment of complex partial seizures, less effective for primary generalized seizures, and ineffective (i.e., it may even worsen) absence and myoclonic seizures. Vigabatrin currently is an investigational drug and has been deemed "approvable" for use in the United States; it is widely available now in Canada, Great Britain, and Europe.

A major advantage of vigabatrin is that it does not appear to be metabolized by the liver, nor does it influence hepatic metabolism so that the typical drug interactions frequently observed with the longer established AEDs (e.g., carbamazepine, phenobarbital, valproate) do not occur with vigabatrin. In clinical trials, vigabatrin decreased phenytoin levels by 20% to 30%; the reason for this was unclear. If used concomitantly, phenytoin levels should be monitored. Adverse effects are minimal and mild. Most commonly occurring in adults are somnolence, fatigue, irritability, dizziness, headache, depression, confusion, impaired concentration, abdominal pain, and anorexia; children frequently experience agitation and insomnia. There have been concerns of concentric visual field defects in human subjects in some studies (Yerby, 2001).

CHAPTER SUMMARY

- The goal of AED therapy is to control the seizures that the patient experiences. Most AEDs accomplish this goal primarily by altering sodium channels on the neuronal cell membrane (thereby limiting the spread of seizure activity) or by enhancing the activity (or concentrations) of the brain's inhibitory neurotransmitter, GABA.
- AED therapy is usually life long, although the drug choice and drug dose may change. Successful management of the seizures depends on the patient's cooperation with the treatment plan.
- Nurses play a vital role in the care of the patient with seizures. If the patient is hospitalized, the nurse's continuous interaction promotes recognition of abnormal behavior patterns, allows witnessing of the seizure, and provides an opportunity to assess and monitor the ictal and postictal behavior.
- Most AEDs try to restore a balance between excitatory and inhibitory neurotransmitters or block the spread of seizure activity. The choice of AED depends on various factors, including the type of seizures. Monotherapy for seizure control is preferred, although the use of more than one drug may be necessary to effectively control seizures.
- Sudden cessation of any AED therapy may initiate status epilepticus. Status epilepticus necessitates close monitoring. Resuscitative equipment should be on standby to treat possible cardiogenic or cardiovascular shock or cardiac arrest. Diazepam is most often the drug of choice to treat status epilepticus.
- Many of the AEDs share common adverse effects, especially on the CNS. Some AEDs have potentially fatal adverse effects. Monitoring serum drug levels, for many AEDs, is an important parameter in maximizing therapeutic effect and minimizing adverse effects of drug therapy.

QUESTIONS FOR STUDY AND REVIEW

1. What is status epilepticus?
2. Why are serum drug levels of phenytoin monitored when beginning drug therapy?
3. What risks exist if phenytoin is used by a pregnant woman?
4. Why should the nurse assess for use alcohol use if the patient is to be started on phenytoin therapy?
5. Which benzodiazepines are suitable as AEDs? For which seizure types are they effective?
6. Why is carbamazepine generally reserved for patients who have not responded satisfactorily to other AEDs, or whose seizures are difficult to control?

NEED MORE HELP?

Chapter 20 of the study guide for *Drug Therapy in Nursing* contains exercises and activities to reinforce your understanding of the concepts presented in this chapter. For additional information see the text's accompanying website at *http://www.connection.lww.com.*

REFERENCES AND BIBLIOGRAPHY

Cada, D. J., Covington, T. R., Hebel, S. K., Hussar, D. A., Lasagna, L., Olin, B. R., Selevan, J. R., Sloan, R. W., Tatro, D. S., & Whitsett, T. L. (2001). *Drug facts and comparisons.* St. Louis: Facts and Comparisons.

Davis, W. M. (1997). Advances in the pathophysiology and pharmacotherapy of epilepsy. *Drug Topics, 141,* 110–119.

Fauci, A., Braunwald, E., Wilson, J. D., Martin, J. B., Hauser, S. L., Longo, D. L., Kasper, D. L., Isselbachter, K. J. (Eds.). (1999). *Harrison's online.* New York: McGraw-Hill.

Feely, M. (1999). Drug treatment of epilepsy. *British Medical Journal, 318,* 106–109.

Hardman, J. G., Limbird, L. E., Milinoff, P. B., Ruddon, R. W., & Gilman, A. G. (Eds.). (1997). *Goodman and Gilman's pharmacological basis of therapeutics* (9th ed.). New York: McGraw-Hill.

Huffman, G. B. (2000). Newer medications for pediatric epilepsy. *American Academy of Family Physicians, 62,* 513–521.

Kirchner, J. T. (2000). Phenobarbital and phenytoin for seizures in newborns. *American Family Physicians, 62,* 17–24.

Knowles, S. R., Shapiro, L. E., & Shear, N. H. (1999). Anticonvulsant hypersensitivity syndrome-incidence, prevention and management. *Drug Safety, 21,* 489–501.

Karpa, K. D. (2000). Fits and starts. *Drug Topics, 144*(13), 28–30.

Ketter, T. A., Post, R. M., & Theodore, W. H. (1999). Positive and negative psychiatric effects of antiepileptic drugs in patients with seizure disorder. *Neurology, 53,* (Suppl. 2), S53–S67.

Kwan, P., & Brodie, M. (2000). Early identification of refractory epilepsy. *New England Journal of Medicine, 342*(5), 314–319.

McAbee, G. N., & Wark, J. E. (2000). A practical approach to uncomplicated seizures in children. *American Family Physician, 62,* 921–929.

McEvoy, G. K., Litvak, K., & Welsh Jr., O. H. (Eds.). (2000). *Drug information.* Bethesda: American Hospital Formulary Service.

McNamara, J. O. (1999). Emerging insights into the genesis of epilepsy. *Nature, 399,* (Suppl.), A15–A22.

Magill-Lewis, J. (2000). A promising antiepileptic drug gains approval for market.). *Drug Topics, 144*(3), 30.

Marks, W. J., Jr. & Garcia, P. A. (1998). Management of Seizures and epilepsy. *American Family Physician, 57*(7), 1589–1604.

Pellock, J. M. (1999). Managing pediatric epilepsy syndromes with new antiepileptic drugs. *Pediatrics, 104*(5), 1106–1116.

Privitera, M. D. (1999). Evidence-based medicine and antiepileptic drugs. *Epilepsia, 40*(Suppl. 5), S47–S56.

Rattya, J., Vainionpaa, L., Knip, M., Lanning, P., & Isojarvi, J. (2000). The effects of valproate, carbamazepine, and oxcarbazepine on growth and sexual maturation in girls with epilepsy. *Pediatrics, 103,* 588–593.

Rosser, E. M, & Wilson, L. C. (1999). Drugs for epilepsy have teratogenic risks. *British Medical Journal, 318,* 1289.

Schachter, S. C. (2000). *Critical issues in the use of antiepileptic drugs.* Symposium at the 27th annual meeting of the Southern Clinical Neurological Society, Ixtapa, Mexico.

Schachter, S. C. (1997). Seizures and epilepsy in the elderly. *Journal of Epilepsy, 10,* 151–153.

Semah, F., Picot, M-C., & Adam, C. (1998). Is the underlying cause of epilepsy a major prognostic factor for recurrence? *Neurology, 51,*1256–1262.

Sindrup, S. H., & Jensen, T. S. (1999). Efficacy of pharmacological treatments of neuropathic pain: An update and effect related to mechanism of drug action. *Pain, 83,* 389–400.

Timkin, N. R. (1999). Do antiepileptic drugs prevent epileptogenesis? Evidence from studies in humans. *Epilepsia, 40,* (Suppl. 7), 231.

Tomson, T., & Johannessen, S. (2000). Therapeutic monitoring of the new antiepileptic drugs. *European Journal of Clinical Pharmacology, 55* (10), 697–705.

Wood, A. J., & Zhon, H. H. (1991). Ethnic differences in drug disposition and responsiveness. *Clinical Pharmacokinetics, 20,* 350–373.

Yerby, M. S. (2001). *New antiepileptic drugs for the treatment of epilepsy.* Portland, OR: North Pacific Epilepsy Research Center.

Chapter 21

DRUGS AFFECTING MUSCLE SPASM AND SPASTICITY

Learning Objectives

At the completion of this chapter the student will:

1. Correlate the pathophysiology of muscle spasm and spasticity with appropriate pharmacotherapy.
2. Identify core drug knowledge about drugs that affect muscle spasm and spasticity.
3. Identify core patient variables related to drugs that affect muscle spasm and spasticity.
4. Relate the interaction of core drug knowledge with core patient variables for drugs that affect muscle spasm and spasticity.
5. Generate a nursing plan of care from the interactions between core drug knowledge and core patient variables for drugs that affect muscle spasm and spasticity.
6. Describe nursing interventions to maximize therapeutic effects and minimize adverse effects for drugs that affect muscle spasm and spasticity.
7. Determine key points for patient and family education about drugs that affect muscle spasm and spasticity.

KEY TERMS

centrally acting
clonic
peripherally acting
spasm
spasmolytics
spasticity
tonic

vironment of the myofilaments.

ness of the muscles and may interfere with gait, movement,

withdrawal may induce seizures. Treatment of overdose is supportive, following attempts to enhance drug elimination.

Chlorphenesin

Chlorphenesin (Maolate) is a drug used as an adjunctive treatment for discomfort in short-term, acute, painful musculoskeletal conditions. Like cyclobenzaprine, it works by CNS depression rather than by direct action on striated muscle. Chlorphenesin is given orally and is widely distributed throughout the body. It is given cautiously to patients with hepatic impairment. Chlorphenesin is not indicated for use in pregnant or breast-feeding women or in children. Therapy with chlorphenesin should be limited to fewer than 8 weeks.

Adverse effects are similar to those of cyclobenzaprine. In addition, chlorphenesin may induce hematologic effects such as leukopenia, thrombocytopenia, and agranulocytosis. Hypersensitivity reactions may occur in patients with a sensitivity to tartrazine, an ingredient in chlorphenesin.

Chlorzoxazone

Chlorzoxazone (Paraflex, Parafon Forte) is another centrally acting muscle relaxant. Although its exact mechanism of action is unknown, its effects are thought to be related to its CNS depression, resulting in reduced skeletal muscle spasms. Pain relief is thought to result from alterations in the perception of pain. Chlorzoxazone has been used for many years. It is widely distributed throughout the body, metabolized by the liver, and excreted by the kidneys.

Because chlorzoxazone is metabolized in the liver, it should be used with caution in patients with hepatic disease. A metabolite of chlorzoxazone is rapidly excreted in the urine; therefore, it should be used with caution in patients with renal impairment because it may alter excretion, possibly causing toxicity. Chlorzoxazone has not been evaluated for safe use during pregnancy, so its effects on the fetus are unknown. It should be used only when the benefits to the pregnant woman outweigh the risks to the fetus. It is not known whether chlorzoxazone is distributed into breast milk. Finally, chlorzoxazone is not recommended for use in older adults because of the potential for anticholinergic side effects, sedation, and weakness.

Adverse effects are sedation, dizziness, and hepatotoxicity. Hepatotoxicity ranges from a mild elevation in hepatic enzymes to hepatic necrosis.

Metaxalone

Metaxalone (Skelaxin), like other centrally acting muscle relaxants, has no direct effect on the contractile mechanism of striated muscle, the motor end plate, or the nerve fiber. Its mode of action may be related to its sedative properties. Administration is oral, metabolism is hepatic, and excretion is renal.

Metaxalone is contraindicated in patients with severe renal impairment. The drug is also contraindicated in patients with a history of drug-induced hemolytic anemia or other anemias. Because metaxalone is metabolized in the liver, it should be used with caution in patients with hepatic disease. Metaxalone is contraindicated in patients with severe hepatic impairment. Safety and effectiveness of metaxalone have not been established in children 12 years of age or younger. Metaxalone is not recommended for use in older adults because of the potential for anticholinergic side effects, sedation, and weakness. Metaxalone should be used during pregnancy only if the potential benefits to the pregnant woman outweigh the possible risks to the fetus. Distribution of metaxalone into breast milk is not known; therefore, it should be used with caution in breast-feeding women.

Adverse effects of metaxalone include elevated hepatic enzymes, such as increased serum concentrations of aspartate transaminase (AST), alanine transaminase (ALT), alkaline phosphatase, and bilirubin. Liver function tests should be performed periodically in patients receiving metaxalone. The most frequent reactions to metaxalone include nausea and vomiting, GI upset, drowsiness, dizziness, headache, anxiety, or irritability. Rare but serious adverse effects include leukopenia, hemolytic anemia, and jaundice.

Methocarbamol

Methocarbamol (Robaxin) is a centrally acting agent that may be administered by oral, intramuscular (IM), and intravenous (IV) routes. In addition to its use for muscle spasm, methocarbamol is used in the management of tetanus. As with other centrally acting agents, the exact mechanism of action is not understood but is thought to be its CNS depressant properties. Short duration of action limits methocarbamol therapy.

Methocarbamol is widely distributed throughout the body, crosses the placental barrier, and is concentrated in the liver and kidneys. It is extensively metabolized in the liver and renally excreted. Distribution into breast milk is unknown.

Contraindications for methocarbamol include hepatic or renal disorders, age younger than 12 years or older than 60 years, and pregnancy. It is used with caution in patients with seizure disorders, because it may exacerbate seizure activity.

When administering by the IV route, the rate should not exceed 3 mL/min. Because the solution is hypertonic, extravasation may occur, resulting in thrombophlebitis, sloughing, and pain at the injection site.

The most common adverse effects are related to its CNS depressant effects. Diplopia, dyspepsia, flushing, hypotension, metallic taste, mild muscular incoordination, nystagmus, sinus bradycardia, syncope, and vertigo have followed IM or IV administration of methocarbamol. IV injections occasionally have been associated with hemolysis, resulting in hematuria.

Orphenadrine

Orphenadrine (Norflex) is the last centrally acting muscle relaxant. Administration is by the oral or parenteral route. Orphenadrine is used as adjunct therapy for acute, painful musculoskeletal conditions and in the management of quinine-resistant leg cramps. It has also been used adjunctly in treating arteriosclerotic, idiopathic, or postencephalic parkinsonism. Like other centrally acting agents, it does not directly affect muscles but works by its depression of the CNS. Orphenadrine also possesses anticholinergic effects and some antihistaminic and local anesthetic action. Orphenadrine is distributed throughout the body and may cross the placenta. Distribution into breast milk is unknown.

Orphenadrine should be used with caution in diseases that are affected by its anticholinergic and antihistaminic effects. These include bladder obstruction, prostatic hypertrophy, GI obstruction, peptic ulcer disease, gastroesophageal reflux disease (GERD), asthma, glaucoma, and myasthenia gravis (MG). Orphenadrine should also be used with caution in older patients who do not tolerate anticholinergics well. Additionally, caution should be taken when administering to patients with cardiac insufficiency or thyrotoxicosis. The safety of orphenadrine in children or pregnant or breast-feeding women has not been established.

Orphenadrine interacts with haloperidol, worsening schizophrenic symptoms and possibly contributing to the development of tardive dyskinesia. It also interacts with amantadine, with resultant additive anticholinergic effects. When given concurrently with phenothiazines, orphenadrine decreases their actions. In addition to CNS effects similar to other centrally acting skeletal muscle relaxants, orphenadrine may induce aplastic anemia or anaphylactic reaction. The most common adverse effects to orphenadrine result from its anticholinergic and antihistaminic effects. They include dry mouth, agitation, blurred vision, constipation, dizziness, drowsiness, gastric irritation, hallucinations, and headache. Additionally, the peripheral anticholinergic effects of orphenadrine may decrease or inhibit salivary flow, thereby contributing to the development of caries, periodontal disease, oral candidiasis, or discomfort.

DRUG SIGNIFICANTLY DIFFERENT FROM P CYCLOBENZAPRINE

Diazepam (Valium) is a benzodiazepine. Diazepam can produce any level of CNS depression required, including sedation, hypnosis, skeletal muscle relaxation, anticonvulsant activity, or coma. Diazepam and baclofen are the only two centrally acting drugs that are used for spasticity as well as muscle spasm. Although diazepam is an extremely effective muscle relaxant, its use as a maintenance drug for spasms is limited because of its potential for physical and psychological dependence. Additionally, abrupt withdrawal of diazepam may induce seizure activity. For further information on benzodiazepines, see Chapter 17.

C CENTRALLY ACTING SPASMOLYTICS

The centrally acting spasmolytics work in the CNS to reduce excessive reflex activity and to allow muscle relaxation. This class includes baclofen and tizanadine. The prototype for the centrally acting spasmolytics is baclofen (Lioresal).

NURSING MANAGEMENT OF THE PATIENT RECEIVING P BACLOFEN

Core Drug Knowledge

Pharmacotherapeutics

Baclofen relieves some components of spinal spasticity–involuntary flexor and extensor spasms and resistance to passive movements. It is useful in multiple sclerosis and traumatic lesions of the spinal cord (paraplegia). Baclofen is not useful in treating spasms that follow a cerebrovascular accident (CVA) or those that occur in Parkinson disease or Huntington chorea (see Table 21-1).

Baclofen has been used in patients with focal dystonic movements, including torticollis (wry neck). It has been used with some success in Meige syndrome (blepharospasm-oromandibular dystonia) and stiff-man syndrome, aka Moersch-Woltmann syndrome. Stiff man syndrome occurs primarily in men. It is characterized by muscular rigidity accompanied by paroxysmal painful spasms precipitated by physical or emotional stimuli.

Baclofen has been effective in treating intractable hiccups. It may also be used in the management of trigeminal neuralgia and various types of neuropathic pain, including migraine headaches.

Surgically implanted pumps are used to deliver intrathecal baclofen to patients with long-term needs or with poor control with oral medications. This includes patients with MS or traumatic spinal cord lesions.

Pharmacokinetics

Baclofen is rapidly absorbed orally and peaks in 2 to 3 hours. It is distributed throughout the body and crosses the blood–brain barrier. Baclofen also crosses the placenta and passes into breast milk. The half-life ranges from 2½ to 4 hours. The kidneys excrete 70 to 85% of a dose as unchanged drug and metabolites. The liver metabolizes the remainder, which is excreted through the feces.

Pharmacodynamics

Baclofen is a derivative of the neurotransmitter gamma-aminobutyric acid (GABA) and acts specifically at the spinal end of the upper motor neurons at $GABA_B$ receptors to cause hyperpolarization. This reduces excessive reflex activity underlying muscle hypertonia, spasms, and spasticity and allows muscle relaxation. The mechanism of action explains why baclofen is not used for spasticity resulting from CVAs or Parkinson disease-these disorders involve lesional or functional impairment of basal ganglia coordination, an area of the CNS above the spinal motor neurons.

Contraindications and Precautions

Baclofen is contraindicated in anyone who has demonstrated previous hypersensitivity to it. It is contraindicated for spasticity of cerebral origin (cerebral palsy,

CVA), or for reducing the rigidity of parkinsonism or Huntington chorea because it is ineffective in these disorders.

Baclofen is classified as a pregnancy category C drug and should be used during pregnancy only when the benefits to the pregnant woman outweigh the risks to the fetus. Baclofen appears in small amounts in breast milk; therefore, caution should be used in breast-feeding women. Baclofen has not been approved for use in children younger than 12 years.

Baclofen should be used with caution in patients with any preexisting muscle weakness. Preexisting weakness may be exacerbated when decreased spasticity diminishes support for the legs. Extreme caution must be used when spasticity is necessary to maintain posture, balance in locomotion, or function.

Baclofen is used with caution in patients with seizure disorders. It has caused deterioration in seizure control and electroencephalographic changes in patients with epilepsy. When given to patients with CNS disorders, such as cerebral hemorrhage or a prior CVA (i.e., stroke), baclofen may increase the risk of developing CNS, respiratory, or cardiovascular depression and ataxia. Baclofen can increase blood glucose concentrations, so it should be used cautiously in patients with diabetes mellitus. Patients with preexisting psychiatric disorders are more likely to develop baclofen-induced psychiatric disturbances. Baclofen should also be used with caution in patients with renal impairment because most of the drug is excreted unchanged in the urine.

Adverse Effects

The most common adverse effects of baclofen therapy include drowsiness, weakness, dizziness and lightheadedness, headache, nausea and vomiting, hypotension, constipation, lethargy and fatigue, confusion, insomnia, and increased urinary frequency. Other effects in the CNS include euphoria, excitement, depression, and hallucinations. Baclofen may also cause paresthesias, myalgias, or tinnitus. The patient may experience difficulty with coordination, tremors, rigidity, or ataxia. The patient may also experience vision disturbances such as nystagmus, strabismus, miosis, mydriasis, or diplopia. Adverse effects in the GI system include xerostomia, anorexia, dysgeusia, abdominal pain, and diarrhea. Cardiovascular adverse effects, such as palpitations, angina, excessive diaphoresis, and syncope, are possible. Genitourinary (GU) effects may include urinary incontinence or retention, dysuria, erectile dysfunction, ejaculation dysfunction, and nocturia. Integumentary adverse effects may include rash and pruritus.

Drug Interactions

Baclofen has the potential to cause clinically important drug-drug interactions with other CNS depressants or TCAs. Baclofen has also been reported to cause positive results on tests for occult blood in the stool. Additionally, baclofen may induce elevations in levels of AST, alkaline phosphatase, or serum glucose (Table 21-3).

Assessment of Relevant Core Patient Variables

Health Status

The nurse should assess for a history of baclofen hypersensitivity or preexisting disorders that contradict the use of baclofen. The nurse should also assess for muscle spasms and their causes. Baclofen therapy will not affect skeletal muscle spasms resulting from CVA, cerebral palsy, or parkinsonism.

The nurse should perform a physical examination, including baseline assessments of neurologic function, cardiac function, kidney function, and muscle strength and spasticity. Laboratory assessments include baseline liver and kidney function values and blood glucose level.

Life Span and Gender

Older patients are more susceptible to baclofen-induced sedation and psychiatric disturbances, including hallucinations, excitation, and confusion. Thus, the nurse should continually assess older patients taking baclofen for such conditions. The nurse should evaluate the patient for pregnancy. Baclofen may be used during pregnancy when the benefits to the pregnant woman

TABLE 21-3 Agents That Interact With Baclofen

Interactants	Effect and Significance	Nursing Management
CNS depressants • sedatives • tranquilizers • alcohol • narcotics	In combination with baclofen, these drugs have additive effects, increasing CNS depression.	Avoid this combination. Monitor for sedation and dizziness. Provide ambulatory assistance. Ensure the patient's safety.
TCAs	Baclofen and TCAs have potentiation of muscle relaxation and enhancement of anticholinergic effects; this combination may result in severe weakness, memory loss, or loss of muscle tone.	Monitor for adverse effects. Provide ambulatory assistance. Increase fluids or consume sugarless candies for dry mouth.

outweigh the risks to the fetus. Baclofen should not be used in children younger than 12 years.

Lifestyle, Diet, and Habits

The nurse should caution the patient about the concomitant use of alcohol and baclofen. Alcohol may increase the risk of CNS depression and other CNS adverse effects. The nurse should also caution patients to assess their level of alertness (CNS depression) before attempting to drive, use machinery, or perform activities that require concentration.

Nursing Diagnoses and Outcomes

- Acute Pain related to headache, muscle pain, GI disturbances, or rash

  Desired outcome: The patient will be provided with comfort measures to decrease discomfort of drug therapy and possibility of noncompliance.
- Risk for Disturbed Sensory Perception related to visual changes, vestibular dysfunction, and somatosensory changes

  Desired outcome: The patient will be protected from injury if dizziness, weakness, visual changes, or perceptual changes occur.

Planning and Intervention

Maximizing Therapeutic Effects

The patient should take baclofen with a full glass of water at evenly spaced intervals.

Minimizing Adverse Effects

The nurse should ensure the patient's safety by keeping the bed in the lowest position and the side rails up. The nurse should assist ambulatory patients with locomotion because sedation and muscle weakness may increase. The nurse should advise the patient to change positions slowly to prevent dizziness.

Abrupt withdrawal of baclofen may result in agitation, auditory and visual hallucinations, seizures, psychotic symptoms, or, most commonly, acute exacerbations of spasticity. The nurse should ensure gradual reduction of the baclofen dosage over 1 to 2 weeks. For patients with GI distress, the nurse should coordinate small, frequent meals.

Providing Patient and Family Education

- Education for patients receiving baclofen is similar to that for patients receiving cyclobenzaprine. As with cyclobenzaprine, the nurse should caution patients to avoid sudden cessation of the drug; instead, patients should taper doses of the drug over 2 weeks.
- Another major point is to remind patients to refrain from alcohol or any other CNS depressant agents. The nurse should advise patients that full benefits from baclofen therapy may take up to 1 month.
- The nurse should advise patients of the importance of contacting the health care provider should they experience severe headaches, confusion, hallucinations, or sudden or increased weakness. The nurse should advise all female patients to contact the health care provider immediately if they become pregnant.
- Additionally, the nurse should instruct patients with diabetes to use capillary blood glucose monitoring, because baclofen may cause blood and urine glucose levels to rise. These patients should notify their providers if serum glucose level elevations are persistent.

Ongoing Assessment and Evaluation

Throughout therapy, the nurse should assess the patient for the CNS effects of baclofen to ensure safety. The nurse should also monitor for the emergence of hallucinations or psychotic episodes and consult with the prescriber immediately about the possibility of reducing the dose or discontinuing the drug. The nurse should also monitor the patient for integumentary, GI, or GU system complaints. The nurse should offer suggestions for minor symptoms such as analgesics for headache or small frequent meals for GI upset. The nurse should assist with establishing a bowel program if constipation occurs. He or she should refer the patient with complaints of GU problems, such as erectile dysfunction, to the provider and ensure that the patient does not abruptly stop the medication. See the accompanying display, Ensuring Successful Baclofen Therapy in the Home.

Therapeutic monitoring during baclofen therapy will show improvement in symptoms of spasticity and a decrease in resistance to passive movement of limb joints. ■

COMMUNITY-BASED CONCERNS

Ensuring Successful Baclofen Therapy in the Home

Surgically implanted drug delivery pumps are frequently used to deliver intrathecal infusions of baclofen in the long-term treatment of patients with spasms that are not adequately controlled by oral baclofen. These patients (particularly those with multiple sclerosis (MS) and traumatic spinal cord lesions) are being managed more frequently in the community setting, primarily because the cost of institutionalization for drug therapy is formidable. As a result, the community health system is facing an increasingly complex management issue.

Patients with neuromuscular diseases present a wide variety of management challenges—from feeding and providing for activities of daily living to promoting locomotion and the highest level of attainable function. Frequently, patients with painful, contracting muscle spasms related to MS or spinal cord injury

(*continued*)

COMMUNITY-BASED CONCERNS

Ensuring Successful Baclofen Therapy in the Home (Continued)

can benefit from continual intrathecal baclofen infusion. This therapy is accomplished with an indwelling catheter and a portable infusion pump.

Issues facing the community health nurse charged with supervising this therapy are the risk of infection introduced through the catheter and the need to maintain a continual infusion. The community health nurse needs to ensure that the infusion equipment remains patent and in good operating condition and that the patient receives effective nursing care.

When managing a patient receiving IV baclofen therapy at home, typical interventions include the following:

- Assess the home environment for designated "clean" areas needed for storing supplies, dressing, and so forth.
- Include at least one, and ideally more, significant others in all instructions about mixing drug solution, storage and care of the drug, and use and maintenance of the infusion pump and IV catheter insertion site.
- Identify community resources for ensuring that the patient does not run out of the drug and that the pump, whether battery operated or electrical, can be adequately and continually charged. Frequently, the power company in an area has provisions for these situations.
- Prepare and post a list of phone numbers of emergency and support systems in the patient's home, preferably near a telephone.
- Discuss the mechanics of baclofen therapy with other caregivers who may be working with this patient so that the entire health care team is aware of the associated needs and potential problems.
- Post a list of warning signs. Include signs of infection at the catheter insertion site, adverse drug effects, and increasing weakness. List telephone numbers of appropriate people to call for help.
- Consult the health resources in the area for support groups or respite services for family members or others involved in the patient's care and for the patient.

DRUG CLOSELY RELATED TO P BACLOFEN

Tizanidine (Zanaflex) is an oral agent used for the treatment of spasticity related to spinal cord pathology and MS. It is structurally and pharmacologically similar to clonidine, an alpha-2 adrenergic agonist. The efficacy of tizanidine in the treatment of spasticity has been found to be equivalent to that of baclofen.

Tizanidine is used cautiously in patients with hypotension, hepatic disease, psychosis, or renal impairment. An important drug-drug interaction with tizanidine occurs with oral contraceptives. When given concurrently, the clearance of tizanidine may be 50% lower, resulting in toxicity. Tizanidine also has additive effects when given with other antihypertensive agents, alpha-2 agonists, or ethanol. Adverse effects parallel those of other alpha-2 adrenergic agonists, including dry mouth, drowsiness, dizziness, GI disturbances, and liver function abnormalities. Because of the adrenergic action, hypotension and orthostatic hypotension may also occur. Tizanidine produces greater drowsiness and sedation than baclofen. Slow upward titration of the dose can minimize adverse effects.

MEMORY CHIP

P Baclofen

- Centrally acting spasmolytic is used for muscle spasms or spasticity
- Significant contraindication: patients who use spasticity to maintain posture or balance
- Most common adverse effect: sedation; safety is a nursing priority
- Most serious adverse effects: occur with abrupt withdrawal and include agitation, auditory or visual hallucinations, seizures, or psychotic symptoms
- **Lifespan alert: older patients are more prone to sedation and other effects on central nervous system**
- Maximizing therapeutic effects: administer at evenly spaced intervals
- Minimizing adverse effects: assist in changing positions slowly; withdraw medication over a 2-week period
- Most significant patient education: never abruptly stop medication

C PERIPHERALLY ACTING SPASMOLYTICS

Peripherally acting spasmolytics relax muscles through direct action within the skeletal muscle fibers. They do not interfere with neuromuscular communication, nor do they have CNS effects. Peripherally acting spasmolytics include dantrolene, botulinum toxin, 4-aminopyridine, ibuprofen, and glycine. Dantrolene (Dantrium) is the most frequently used peripheral agent and the prototype for the peripherally acting spasmolytics.

NURSING MANAGEMENT OF THE PATIENT RECEIVING P DANTROLENE

Core Drug Knowledge

Pharmacotherapeutics

IV dantrolene is the drug of choice, along with supportive measures, for acute treatment of malignant hyperthermia. Preoperatively, it can be used orally or intravenously to prevent malignant hyperthermia in patients considered at risk.

Dantrolene has several other pharmacotherapeutic uses. It has been effective in treating upper motor neuron disorders. It has also been used to treat heat stroke and to prevent and treat the rigors associated with amphotericin B. It is useful in the management of spasticity resulting from spinal cord and cerebral injuries, MS, cerebral palsy, and possibly CVA. Dantrolene is not effective in treating acute muscle weakness of local origin or muscle weakness resulting from rheumatoid spondylitis, arthritis, or bursitis.

Pharmacokinetics

Approximately 35% of an oral dose of dantrolene is absorbed; peak plasma concentrations are reached in approximately 5 hours. The liver metabolizes dantrolene to weakly active metabolites, which are excreted in the urine. The elimination half-life is reported to be about 9 hours in healthy adults and 7.3 hours in children. Therapeutic effects in patients being treated for upper motor neuron disorders may not appear for 1 week or more. Dantrolene crosses the placenta and enters breast milk.

Pharmacodynamics

Dantrolene reduces the force of contraction of skeletal muscle through a direct effect on muscle cells. It reduces the amount of Ca released from the sarcoplasmic reticulum, thereby uncoupling (relaxing) muscle contraction from excitation. Interference with the release of Ca from the sarcoplasmic reticulum may prevent the increase in intracellular Ca, which activates the acute catabolic events of malignant hyperthermia. Dantrolene has little or no effect on contraction of cardiac or intestinal smooth muscle. It may decrease hyperreflexia, muscle stiffness, and spasticity in patients with upper motor neuron disorders.

Contraindications and Precautions

Dantrolene is contraindicated in patients who rely on spasticity to maintain an upright posture and balance, such as patients with cerebral palsy. It is also contraindicated in patients with active liver disease because of dantrolene's associated liver toxicity. No contraindications apply to IV administration of dantrolene for prevention or acute treatment of malignant hyperthermia crisis.

Dantrolene should be used with caution in patients with preexisting myopathy or neuromuscular disease with respiratory depression. Risk of perioperative complications is increased in patients with these conditions receiving dantrolene for prevention of malignant hyperthermia.

Dantrolene should also be used with caution in patients with cardiac disease and pulmonary dysfunction, particularly chronic obstructive pulmonary disease (COPD). For patients with cardiac disease, dantrolene can precipitate pleural effusions or pericarditis. In patients with pulmonary dysfunction, dantrolene can precipitate respiratory depression.

Dantrolene is classified as a pregnancy category C drug; therefore, pregnant or lactating women should avoid its use.

Adverse Effects

The most common adverse effect of dantrolene therapy is muscle weakness. Manifestations of such muscle weakness may include drooling, slurred speech, drowsiness, dizziness, malaise, and fatigue. Serious adverse effects seen with dantrolene therapy include potentially fatal hepatitis, seizures, and pleural effusion with pericarditis.

In the GI system, symptoms include diarrhea, constipation, GI bleeding, anorexia, difficulty swallowing, abdominal cramps, and nausea and vomiting. Diarrhea is usually transient, but in some cases it can be severe, and the drug may have to be withheld. Hematologic adverse reactions with dantrolene therapy include aplastic anemia, leukopenia, and lymphocytic lymphoma.

Rash, acne, abnormal hair growth, and photosensitivity are possible integumentary effects. IV dantrolene may cause edema and thrombophlebitis. Rarely, IV administration may cause erythema and urticaria.

Drug Interactions

Drugs that interact with dantrolene include clofibrate, estrogens, verapamil, and warfarin. Table 21-4 discusses these potential interactions.

TABLE 21-4 Agents That Interact With Dantrolene

Interactants	Effect and Significance	Nursing Management
clofibrate	Clofibrate may decrease plasma protein binding of dantrolene, resulting in decreased effects of dantrolene.	Monitor for efficacy of therapy.
verapamil	In combination with dantrolene, verapamil may increase hyperkalemia and myocardial depression.	Monitor cardiac function. Monitor potassium levels. Avoid coadministration, if possible.
estrogens	Mechanism of action is unknown; women older than 35 years are at risk for hepatotoxicity when estrogens and dantrolene coadministered.	Monitor liver function.
warfarin	Warfarin may decrease plasma protein binding of dantrolene, resulting in decreased effects of dantrolene.	Monitor for efficacy of therapy.

Assessment of Relevant Core Patient Variables

Health Status

The nurse should elicit a comprehensive health history, including any history of active hepatitis, spasticity used to sustain upright posture and balance in locomotion or to obtain or maintain increased function, estrogen use in women older than 35 years, impaired cardiac or pulmonary function, or any liver disease. The nurse should communicate positive findings for any of these factors to the health care provider.

The nurse should perform a physical examination prior to initiation of therapy. Assessment of the musculoskeletal system should include the patient's posture, ability to walk, reflexes, and muscle tone. The nurse must document the amount and location of spasticity. Other assessments should include the CNS and GI systems. Laboratory tests should include complete blood count (CBC), AST, ALT, alkaline phosphatase, and total bilirubin levels.

Life Span and Gender

The nurse needs to consider the patient's age and its relationship to dantrolene therapy. Liver damage occurs most commonly in patients older than 30 years, especially women older than 35 years who are taking estrogens. Children younger than 5 years should not receive dantrolene. Older patients are more vulnerable to dantrolene's adverse effects. Prior to administration, the nurse must assess the patient for pregnancy and breastfeeding, because safety of dantrolene therapy has not been established for pregnant or lactating women.

Lifestyle, Diet, and Habits

Dantrolene capsules contain lactulose. Thus, the nurse should assess the patient for lactose intolerance before administration.

Environment

The nurse should caution the patient about the potential for photosensitivity. Patients should wear appropriate clothing and sunscreen whenever they are in direct sunlight. Because dantrolene causes muscle weakness, the nurse should also discuss with the patient environmental barriers in the home, such as stairs, that may affect dantrolene therapy. In addition, the nurse should caution the patient to assess the drug's effects before attempting to ambulate without assistance. See the accompanying display, Adjusting to Dantrolene Therapy.

Critical Thinking Scenario

Adjusting to Dantrolene Therapy

J. J. was born with cerebral palsy, which has been successfully managed medically for 18 years. He recently finished high school and enrolled in a junior college. During his second week at college, he began having uncontrollable muscle spasms that were painful and embarrassing to him. The college health service recommended treating the spasms with dantrolene.

1. Prioritize the assessment factors that the nurse must consider before and during therapy.
2. Suggest steps that may need to be taken at J. J.'s school as a result of the drug therapy.

Nursing Diagnoses and Outcomes

- Risk for Injury related to muscular weakness
  Desired outcome: The patient will be injury-free despite muscular weakness.
- Diarrhea or Constipation related to drug effects
  Desired outcome: The patient will maintain baseline bowel habits.
- Risk for Disturbed Sensory Perception: Kinesthetic related to dizziness, malaise, and fatigue
  Desired outcome: The patient will remain free of injury from adverse effects.
- Disturbed Body Image related to drug-related dermatologic effects
  Desired outcome: By the end of therapy, any adverse effects will be resolved.

Planning and Intervention

Maximizing Therapeutic Effects

The nurse should administer dantrolene with food or milk to avoid gastric distress. For patients with difficulty swallowing, the nurse should mix the contents of the capsule with fruit juice and administer immediately. If extended-release capsules or tablets are prescribed, they should not be opened or crushed.

Minimizing Adverse Effects

To avoid injury, the nurse should supervise the transfer or ambulation of patients taking dantrolene. The nurse should also provide frequent skin care and hygiene measures to prevent skin breakdown or request treatment for acne if appropriate. Protecting the patient from exposure to ultraviolet light is important, as is providing sunscreen if exposure is inevitable.

Therapy is initiated at low doses and gradually increased to minimize dose-related side effects. This also determines the minimum effective dose and allows a smooth induction of antispastic effects.

Providing Patient and Family Education

- Before administration, the nurse should explain to patients and family that this drug is being used to relieve spasticity and that muscle weakness may occur. Family members should assist patients with ambulation and ensure safety precautions.
- The nurse should inform patients that one of the most dangerous adverse effects of dantrolene ther-

apy is hepatitis. The nurse should write down a list of symptoms for patients to report to the health care provider immediately, including the following: loss of appetite, nausea, vomiting, yellowing of the skin or eyes, and changes in color of urine or stool. The nurse should also explain that regular follow-up medical care, including blood tests, is necessary to monitor the effects of this drug on the body.

- The nurse should advise patients that other adverse effects may occur, such as drowsiness, dizziness, GI upset, diarrhea or constipation, or rash. The nurse should discuss self-care measures to alleviate common symptoms and urge patients to contact the health care provider if the symptoms do not abate. To avoid photosensitivity, the nurse should advise patients to wear appropriate clothing and use sunscreen when in direct sunlight.

Ongoing Assessment and Evaluation

The nurse should monitor for improvement in symptoms of spasticity and decrease in resistance to passive movement of limb joint. Beneficial effects in spasticity may take 1 week or more to appear. The nurse should assist ambulatory patients with locomotion because muscle weakness may increase.

The nurse should monitor for signs of adverse effects, especially hepatitis and hematologic effects. The nurse should coordinate periodic laboratory tests to evaluate liver function and the CBC. The nurse should withhold dantrolene and contact the health care provider if clinical signs of hepatitis appear. ■

MEMORY CHIP

Dantrolene

- Peripherally acting spasmolytic is used for muscle spasms or spasticity
- Drug of choice for prevention or treatment of malignant hyperthermia
- Significant contraindications: patients who use spasticity to maintain posture or balance (e.g., patients with cerebral palsy) or have active hepatic disorders
- Most common adverse effect: muscle weakness; safety is a nursing priority
- Most serious adverse effect: fatal hepatitis, especially in women older than 35 years who are taking estrogens
- Maximizing therapeutic effects: give with food or milk to decrease gastrointestinal distress
- Minimizing adverse effects: assist with ambulation
- Most significant patient education: advise patients of symptoms of hepatitis and the importance of notifying the health care provider should any occur

CHAPTER SUMMARY

- Drugs used in the management of muscle spasm and spasticity are divided into muscle relaxants and spasmolytics.
- Muscle spasm is a sudden violent involuntary contraction of a muscle or group of muscles.
- Centrally acting muscle relaxants do not act on painful muscles; rather, they work by their CNS depressant activity.
- Most centrally acting muscle relaxants are not effective in the treatment of spasticity.
- In addition to their CNS depressant effects, centrally acting muscle relaxants have anticholinergic and antihistaminic effects.
- Safety is a primary concern for patients receiving centrally acting muscle relaxants and spasmolytics.
- Centrally acting muscle relaxants should be given with caution to older adults. They are not indicated for use in children.
- Spasticity is a prolonged increased tone in muscles that may lead to contraction.
- Baclofen (Lioresal) and diazepam (Valium) are centrally acting: drugs that are also used in the management of spasticity.
- Dantrolene (Dantrium) is a peripherally acting spasmolytic that affects spasticity within the muscle fibers.
- Spasmolytics should be used cautiously in patients who require spasticity to remain upright.

QUESTIONS FOR STUDY AND REVIEW

1. What is the difference between muscle spasm and muscle spasticity?
2. Your patient with a history of depression rammed his car into a light pole, sustaining multiple contusions and abrasions. The patient is taking amitriptyline (Elavil) four times a day and diazepam (Valium) as needed. The patient is placed on cyclobenzaprine for muscle spasms of the neck and back. What precautions would you take with this patient?
3. Which drugs are effective for the management of both muscle spasm and muscle spasticity?
4. Why is baclofen ineffective for spasms from CVAs or Parkinson disease?
5. What symptoms suggest hepatitis in the patient on long-term dantrolene therapy?

NEED MORE HELP?

Chapter 21 of the study guide for *Drug Therapy in Nursing* contains exercises and activities to reinforce your understanding of the concepts presented in this chapter. For additional information see the text's accompanying web site at *http://www.connection.lww.com*.

REFERENCES AND BIBLIOGRAPHY

CCIS System. (2001). *Computerized Clinical Information System.* Denver, CO: Microindex.
Clinical Drug Monographs. (2001). [CDRom]. Gold Standard Media.
Drug Facts and Comparisons. (2000). St. Louis: Facts and Comparisons.
Hardman, J. G., Limbird, L. E., Molinof, P. B., Ruddon, R. W., & Gilman, A. (eds.) (1997). *Goodman and Gilman's the pharmacological basis of therapeutics* (9th ed.). New York: McGraw-Hill.

Karch, A. (2001). *2001 Lippincott's nursing drug guide.* Philadelphia: Lippincott Williams & Wilkins.
Katzung, B. C. (2000). *Basic and clinical pharmacology* (8th ed.). New York: McGraw-Hill.
Lipetz, J. S., & Malanga, G. A. (1998). Oral medications in the treatment of acute low back pain. *Occupational Medicine, 13*(1), 151–166.
Melia, D. (1998). Spasticity. *Professional Nurse, 13*(12), 858–861.
Meythaler, J. M., Guin-Renfroe, S., & Hadley, M. N. (1999). Continuously infused intrathecal baclofen for spastic/dystonic hemiplegia: a preliminary report. *American Journal of Physical Medicine and Rehabilitation, 78*(3), 247–254.
Porth, C. (1998). *Pathophysiology: Concepts of altered health states* (5th ed.). Philadelphia: Lippincott Williams & Wilkins.
Reeves, R. R., et al. (1999). Carisoprodol (soma): Abuse potential and physician unawareness. *Journal of Addictive Diseases, 18*(2), 51–56.
Stolworthy, C., & Haas, R. E. (1998). Malignant hyperthermia: A potentially fatal complication of anesthesia. *Seminars in Perioperative Nursing, 7*(1), 58–66.
Tatro, D. (ed.) (2000). *Drug interaction facts* (6th ed.). St. Louis: Facts and Comparisons.
Tsutsumi, Y., et al. (1998). The treatment of neuroleptic malignant syndrome using dantrolene sodium. *Psychiatry and Clinical Neuroscience, 52*(4), 433–438.
Walker, P., Watanabe, S., & Bruera, E. (1998). Baclofen, a treatment for chronic hiccup. *Journal of Pain Symptom Management, 16*(2), 125–132.

Chapter 22

DRUGS FOR TREATING PARKINSON DISEASE AND OTHER MOVEMENT DISORDERS

KEY TERMS

akinesia
ballismus
basal ganglia
bradykinesia
bradykinetic episodes
bruxism
corpus striatum
dopaminergics
neuroleptic malignant syndrome (NMS)
paralysis agitans
parkinsonism
substantia nigra

Learning Objectives

At the completion of this chapter the student will:

1. Correlate the pathophysiology of movement disorders with appropriate pharmacotherapy.
2. Identify core drug knowledge about drugs that affect movement disorders.
3. Identify core patient variables related to drugs that affect movement disorders.
4. Relate the interaction of core drug knowledge to core patient variables for drugs that affect movement disorders.
5. Generate a nursing plan of care from the interactions between core drug knowledge and core patient variables for drugs that affect movement disorders.
6. Describe nursing interventions to maximize therapeutic and minimize adverse effects for drugs that affect movement disorders.
7. Determine key points for patient and family education for drugs that affect movement disorders.

Antiparkinson drugs

Dopaminergics

carbidopa-levodopa
levodopa
pramipexole
ropinirole
bromocriptine
selegiline
amantadine
pergolide
tolcapone
entacapone

Centrally acting anticholinergics

benztropine
diphenhydramine
trihexyphenidyl

Anti-ALS drugs

riluzole

DRUGS FOR OTHER MOVEMENT DISORDERS

Myasthenia gravis
neostigmine
pyridostigmine

Huntington disease
haloperidol
phenothiazines

Tourette syndrome
haloperidol
pimozide
clonidine
clonazepam
fluphenazine

Multiple sclerosis
dantrolene
baclofen
diazepam
glatiramer acetate

The symbol C indicates the **drug class**.
Drugs in bold type marked with the symbol P are **prototypes**.
Drugs in blue type with no symbol are **closely related** to the prototype.
Drugs in **red** type with no symbol are **significantly different** from the prototype.
Drugs in **black** type with no symbol are **also used in drug therapy**; no prototype.

Movement disorders can be chronic, severe, and debilitating. These disorders are incurable, and patients with them have various responses to treatment. As a result of the disorder's progression, patients may become socially isolated and depressed. As patients become increasingly disabled and the drugs are minimally effective, the primary role of the nurse changes from that of the medical model to psychosocial and functional care that assists the patient to maximize remaining capacities. This chapter limits the discussion to the nurse's pharmacologic role. Information on the nonpharmacologic role of the nurse can be found in a medical-surgical textbook or subject-specific website.

This chapter discusses two major movement disorders: Parkinson disease and amyotrophic lateral sclerosis (ALS), focusing on drugs used to inhibit the symptoms associated with these diseases. In addition, it discusses core drug knowledge, core patient variables, nursing management, potential nursing diagnoses, and patient education related to the use of these drugs.

PHYSIOLOGY

The extrapyramidal system is responsible for coarse control of voluntary muscles. This "system" is composed of basal ganglia, cortical areas of the brain that project to the basal ganglia, cerebellar areas of the brain that project to the basal ganglia, and parts of the reticular formation and thalamic nuclei that connect to the basal ganglia. Motor activity requires the integration of the actions of the cerebral cortex, basal ganglia, and cerebellum.

The **basal ganglia** are a group of functionally related nuclei located in each cerebral hemisphere in paired groups. Two primary nuclei are the **corpus striatum,** located deep within the cerebrum, and the **substantia nigra,** a group of darkly pigmented cells located in the midbrain. When the basal ganglia are stimulated, muscle tone in the body is inhibited, and voluntary movements are refined.

The inhibitory neurotransmitter dopamine is produced in the substantia nigra and adrenal glands. It is transmitted to the basal ganglia along a connecting neural pathway for secretion when needed. Recently, five dopamine receptors have been identified in the brain. Three of these receptors (dopamine-1, dopamine-2, and dopamine-3 - usually called D_1, D_2, and D_3, respectively) appear to play important roles in properly balancing the stimulation of the basal ganglia needed for normal motor function. Acetylcholine, the excitatory neurotransmitter, is produced by the basal ganglia and in the nerve endings in the periphery of the body. When the body wants to make a movement (anything from walking to picking up a cup of coffee), the striatum releases dopamine and acetylcholine through the nervous system to the appropriate muscles, which allows for the initiation, modulation, and completion of smooth, coordinated movement within a fraction of a second.

PATHOPHYSIOLOGY

PARKINSON DISEASE

Parkinson disease is also called idiopathic parkinsonism or **paralysis agitans.** This disease is naturally occurring in that an external stimulus, such as a virus or trauma, does not trigger it. Parkinson disease generally afflicts patients age 50 years and older and progresses slowly. In Parkinson disease, there is an unexplained loss of dopamine-containing neurons in the substantia nigra, resulting in reduced dopamine in the nerve terminals of the nigrostriatal tract. Consequently, an imbalance exists between inhibitory dopamine and excitatory acetylcholine (Fig. 22-1).

Additionally, unopposed acetylcholine stimulates the release of gamma-aminobutyric acid (GABA). The combina-

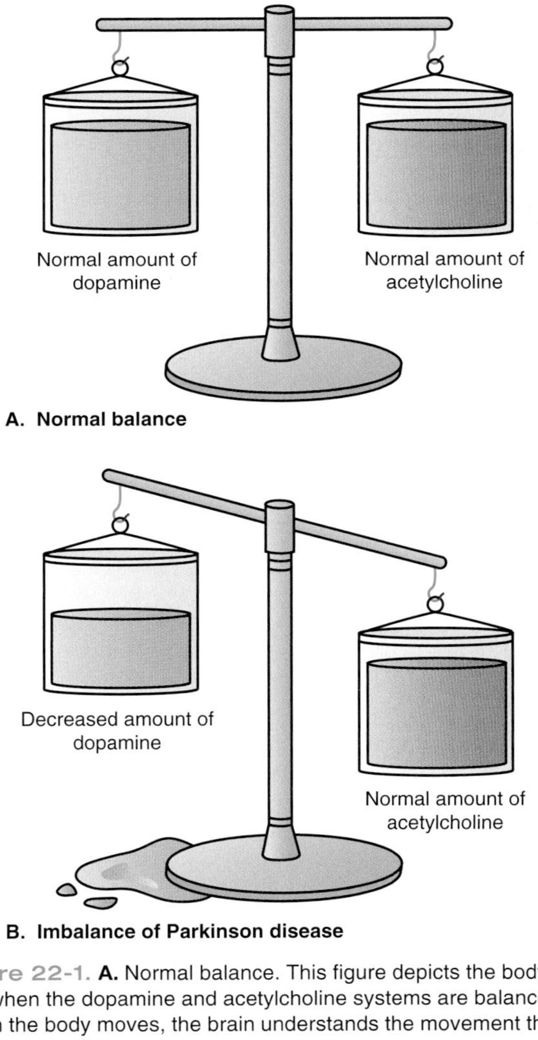

Figure 22-1. **A.** Normal balance. This figure depicts the body at rest when the dopamine and acetylcholine systems are balanced. When the body moves, the brain understands the movement the body wants to make, and it sends out a balance of dopamine and acetylcholine messages to keep that movement smooth. **B.** Imbalance of Parkinson disease. This represents Parkinson disease, in which the normal levels of acetylcholine and dopamine are imbalanced, and abnormal movement affects the body until chemical balance can be restored, to a degree.

tion of excessive acetylcholine and GABA is the basis for most symptoms of Parkinson disease, such as muscle rigidity, tremor at rest, **akinesia** (loss of voluntary movement) or **bradykinesia** (abnormal slowness of movement), and postural instability. As the disease progresses, patients may also experience depression, emotional changes, and sleep problems. Memory loss and slow thinking may develop, although the ability to reason remains intact. Whether people actually suffer intellectual loss (also known as dementia) from Parkinson disease is a controversial issue still being studied.

Parkinsonism is a syndrome with similar characteristics to Parkinson disease that are secondary to other conditions that structurally damage the dopaminergic pathway or interfere with dopamine's action within the basal ganglia. Well-known precipitants of parkinsonism are drugs such as the phenothiazines, metoclopramide, and reserpine. Drug-induced parkinsonism is usually reversible when the drugs are discontinued. Parkinsonism may also result from trauma, encephalitis, or heavy metal poisoning.

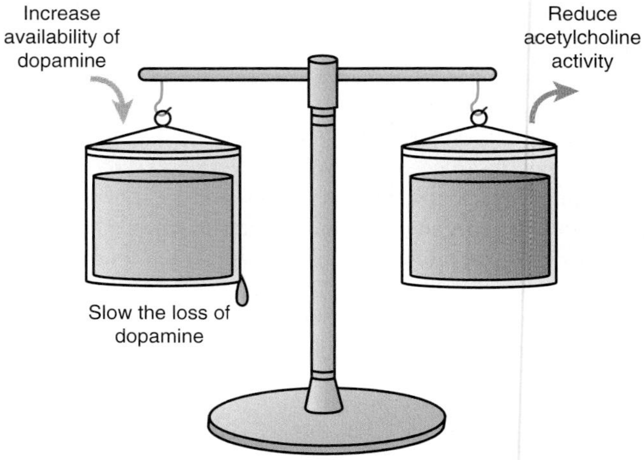

Figure 22-2. The goal of pharmacologic treatment for Parkinson disease is to restore the homeostatic balance between acetylcholine and dopamine. This can be accomplished by increasing the amount or availability of dopamine, slowing the loss of dopamine, or blocking the activity of acetylcholine.

AMYOTROPHIC LATERAL SCLEROSIS

Amyotrophic lateral sclerosis is a progressive neurologic disorder that affects motor function. It is also known as Lou Gehrig disease after the famous baseball player who succumbed to the disorder. The etiology of ALS is unknown. It presents in adulthood, usually between age 40 and 70 years, and affects men two to three times more often than women. ALS affects both the upper motor neurons in the cerebral cortex and the lower motor neurons in the brain stem and spinal cord. Although this disorder is neurologic, one of its classic features is that it spares the entire sensory system and the intellect. Additionally, it also spares the cranial nerves that innervate movement of the eye (i.e., cranial nerves III, IV, and VI).

The disease begins in the distal neurons and then progresses in a centripetal but asymmetrical direction. The loss of upper motor neurons results in spastic paralysis and hyperreflexia. The loss of lower motor neurons results in decreased muscle tone and reflexes and flaccid paralysis. Ultimately, neuronal cell death leads to muscular weakness, muscle atrophy and fasciculations, spasticity, dysarthria, dysphagia, and respiratory compromise. Although periods of remission may occur, ALS typically progresses rapidly, and death occurs within 5 years for 50% of patients diagnosed with the disease.

ANTIPARKINSON DRUGS

The relative lack of inhibitory dopamine combined with the relative excess of excitatory acetylcholine cause the symptoms of Parkinson disease. The goal of therapy is to restore the balance between dopamine and acetylcholine (Fig. 22-2). This can be accomplished by increasing the activity of dopamine or blocking the action of acetylcholine. Drugs that promote activation of dopamine receptors or slow the loss of dopamine are called **dopaminergics;** drugs that prevent the activation of cholinergic receptors are called anticholinergics. Both types of drugs are used to treat Parkinson disease at different stages. Dopaminergics are discussed fully in this chapter; however, anticholinergics are only briefly summarized here and discussed in depth in Chapter 15.

DOPAMINERGICS

The combination drug carbidopa-levodopa (Sinemet) is the prototype for the dopaminergics.

The logical solution to the imbalance in Parkinson disease is to administer dopamine to the patient; however, dopamine does not cross the blood–brain barrier. Levodopa, the precursor to dopamine, is occasionally used alone in treatment of Parkinson disease; however, it is largely deactivated in the periphery of the body. When levodopa is administered as a single drug, approximately 2% actually crosses the blood–brain barrier. To increase the amount of levodopa available to cross the blood–brain barrier, levodopa is combined with the drug carbidopa. Carbidopa does not cross the blood–brain barrier, but it decreases the peripheral destruction of levodopa.

In addition to carbidopa-levodopa and levodopa alone, other dopaminergics are used in the treatment of Parkinson disease. Dopamine agonists include pramipexole (Mirapex), ropinirole (Requip), bromocriptine (Parlodel), and pergolide (Permax). Amantadine (Symmetrel) is an oral antiviral dopaminergic. Selegiline (Eldepryl), another dopaminergic agent, inhibits monoamine oxidase type B (MAO-B). Tolcapone (Tasmar) and entacapone (Comtan) inhibit the enzyme catechol-O-methyltransferase (COMT), which degrades dopamine in the body's periphery.

NURSING MANAGEMENT OF THE PATIENT RECEIVING CARBIDOPA-LEVODOPA

Core Drug Knowledge

Pharmacotherapeutics

Carbidopa-levodopa (Sinemet) is a combination drug used in treating Parkinson disease. Carbidopa-levodopa is also used to treat restless-leg syndrome.

Pharmacokinetics

With oral administration, carbidopa-levodopa may begin acting after 2 to 3 weeks, although some patients require up to 6 months of therapy before noting effect. The plasma half-life of both carbidopa-levodopa and carbidopa alone is roughly 1 to 2 hours, and the duration of action of a dose is 5 hours. Most carbidopa-levodopa is metabolized into dopamine in the periphery of the body, whereas carbidopa itself is minimally metabolized. Carbidopa-levodopa is eliminated renally as dopamine metabolites and in small amounts as unchanged drug. In addition, carbidopa-levodopa crosses the placenta and is present in breast milk (Table 22-1).

Pharmacodynamics

Carbidopa-levodopa diffuses levodopa into the central nervous system (CNS), where it is converted to dopamine. The resulting change in dopamine-acetylcholine balance is believed to improve nerve impulse control and to be the basis of the drug's antiparkinsonian activity. Carbidopa does not cross the blood–brain barrier.

TABLE 22-1 Summary of Selected Drugs for the Management of Movement Disorders

Drug (Trade) Name	Selected Indications	Route and Dosage Range	Pharmacokinetics
Antiparkinson Agents			
Dopaminergics			
carbidopa-levodopa (Sinemet)	Parkinson disease	*Adult:* PO 25/100 bid–qid to a maximum of 200/2,000 mg/d *Child:* Not recommended	*Onset:* Rapid *Duration:* 6–12 h $t_{1/2}$: 1–2 h
levodopa (Dopar, Larodopa)	Parkinson disease	*Adult:* PO 500–1,000 mg/d in divided doses every 6–12 h maximum 8,000 mg/d *Child:* PO 0.5 g/m^2	*Onset:* Variable *Duration:* 6–12 h $t_{1/2}$: 1.2–2.3 h
amantadine (Symmetrel; *Canadian:* Endantadine)	Parkinson disease Antiviral agent	*Adult:* PO 100–400 mg/d as needed *Adult and child >9 y:* PO 100 mg bid *Child 1–9 y:* 2–4 mg/lb	*Onset:* 36–48 h *Duration:* Unknown $t_{1/2}$: 15–24 h
selegiline (Eldepryl)	Parkinson disease	*Adult:* PO 5 mg taken at breakfast and lunch *Child:* Not recommended	*Onset:* 1 h *Duration:* 24–72 h $t_{1/2}$: 9 min; 20.5 h for active metabolites
Dopamine Agonists			
pramipexole (Mirapex)	Parkinson disease	*Adult:* PO 1.5–4.5 mg/d *Child:* Not recommended	*Onset:* Rapid *Duration:* Unknown $t_{1/2}$: 8–12 h
ropinirole (Requip)	Parkinson disease	*Adult:* PO 1 mg tid *Child:* Not recommended	*Onset:* 30–40 min *Duration:* 16 h $t_{1/2}$: 6 h
bromocriptine (Parlodel; *Canadian:* Apo-Bromocriptine)	Parkinson disease Acromegaly Hyperprolactinemia	*Adult:* PO 5–50 mg bid *Adult:* PO 30–30 mg/d *Adult:* PO 5–7.5 mg/d *Child:* Not recommended	*Onset:* 1 h *Duration:* 14 h $t_{1/2}$: biphasic Initial 6–8 h Terminal 50 h
pergolide (Permax)	Parkinson disease	*Adult:* PO 1 mg tid *Child:* Not recommended	*Onset:* Varies *Duration:* Unknown $t_{1/2}$: 27 h

(*continued*)

TABLE 22-1 Summary of Selected Drugs for the Management of Movement Disorders (Continued)

Drug (Trade) Name	Selected Indications	Route and Dosage Range	Pharmacokinetics
COMT Inhibitors			
tolcapone (Tasmar)	Parkinson disease	*Adult:* PO 100–200 mg tid *Child:* Not recommended	*Onset:* 1 h *Duration:* Unknown $t_{1/2}$: 2–3 h
entacapone (Comtan)	Parkinson disease	*Adult:* PO 200 g with each dose of carbidopa-levodopa not to exceed 1,600 g qd *Child:* Not recommended	*Onset:* 1 h *Duration:* Unknown $t_{1/2}$: 1–2 h
Anticholinergics			
benztropine (Cogentin; *Canadian:* Apo-Benztropine)	Parkinson disease	*Adult:* PO/IM/IV, 0.5–6 mg/d *Child:* Not recommended	*Onset:* PO, 1 h; IM/IV, 15 min *Duration:* Unknown $t_{1/2}$: 6–10 h
diphenhydramine (Benadryl; *Canadian:* Allerdyl)	Parkinson disease	*Adult:* PO, 25–100 mg/d; IM/IV, 10–50 mg *Child:* PO > 10 kg 12.5–25 g 3–4 times daily, max 300 g qid; IV 5 mg/kg/d	*Onset:* PO, 15–30 min; IM 20–30 min; IV, rapid *Duration:* 4–8 h $t_{1/2}$: 2.5–7 h
trihexyphenidyl (Artane; *Canadian:* Apo-Trihex)	Parkinson disease	*Adult:* PO, 1–15 mg in divided doses *Child:* Safety and efficacy not established	*Onset:* Varies *Duration:* Unknown $t_{1/2}$: 5–10 h
C Anti-ALS Agent			
P riluzole (Rilutek)		*Adult:* PO 50 mg q 12 h *Child:* Not recommended	*Onset:* Rapid *Duration:* Unknown $t_{1/2}$: 2–3 h

The combination of carbidopa-levodopa is more effective than levodopa alone. When carbidopa is administered in combination with levodopa, it inhibits the conversion of levodopa to dopamine in the periphery of the body, thereby increasing the amount of levodopa available to diffuse into the CNS. Because the bioavailability of dopamine increases in the CNS, the dosing of levodopa can be reduced. This minimizes the potential for adverse reactions from levodopa. The carbidopa-levodopa combination also allows for a more rapid and even titration of effect.

Contraindications and Precautions

Patients with hypersensitivity to carbidopa-levodopa should not take this drug. Carbidopa-levodopa, marketed as Dopar, contains tartrazine. Thus, patients with tartrazine sensitivity should avoid carbidopa-levodopa if Dopar is the only formulation available. Carbidopa-levodopa can worsen malignant melanoma, so the drug is contraindicated in patients with undiagnosed pigmented lesions or a history of melanoma. Although carbidopa-levodopa may not be used in patients with closed-angle glaucoma, it may be used in patients with open-angle glaucoma if intraocular pressure is closely monitored and controlled. Simultaneous administration of carbidopa-levodopa with monoamine oxidase inhibitors (MAOIs) can result in hypertensive crisis. Thus, MAOIs should be discontinued 2 to 4 weeks before carbidopa-levodopa therapy begins.

Precautions to carbidopa-levodopa therapy include cardiac disease (especially myocardial infarction [MI] or arrhythmias), pulmonary disease, peptic ulcer disease, and diabetes mellitus. Carbidopa-levodopa may exacerbate symptoms in patients with these disorders.

Additionally, carbidopa-levodopa may cause mental status changes and should be used with caution in patients with a history of psychosis. All patients receiving carbidopa-levodopa should be monitored closely for signs of mental disturbances, including depression or suicidal thoughts.

Adverse Effects

Adverse gastrointestinal (GI) effects are common in patients receiving carbidopa-levodopa and include nausea and vomiting, anorexia, and weight loss. Another common adverse effect to carbidopa-levodopa therapy is orthostatic hypotension.

Of the more serious adverse effects of carbidopa-levodopa therapy, abnormal movements are the most common. These abnormal movements result from the increased dopamine in the brain. They include choreiform, dystonic reactions, and dyskinetic movements. Other involuntary movements that may develop include the following:

- **bruxism** (clenching the teeth, associated with forceful lateral or protrusive jaw movements, resulting in rubbing, gritting, or grinding the teeth)
- protrusion of the tongue
- opening and closing of the mouth
- bobbing of the head
- rhythmic movements of the feet or hands
- quick movements of the shoulder
- **ballismus** (jerking, flinging movements of an extremity)

Abnormal movements are usually dose related and may resolve with a reduction in dose. Unfortunately, with a dose reduction, the symptoms of Parkinson disease may recur.

Psychiatric disturbances may develop with the administration of carbidopa-levodopa. Symptoms include memory loss, anxiety, nervousness, agitation, restlessness, confusion, insomnia, nightmares, daytime somnolence, euphoria, malaise, and fatigue. Patients taking carbidopa-levodopa are also at risk for developing severe mental depression, suicidal tendencies, dementia, hallucinations, paranoid delusion, psychoses, and hypomania.

Cardiac arrhythmias can also occur during carbidopa-levodopa therapy but are relatively infrequent. Other cardiovascular symptoms include flushing and hypertension. For patients taking carbidopa-levodopa for a prolonged period, **bradykinetic episodes,** also known as the "on-off effect," may occur. Characteristics of this syndrome include akinesia, sudden return of effectiveness, and akinesia paradoxica (an abrupt hypotonic reaction in which the patient usually falls as he or she begins to walk). The akinetic episode can last from 1 minute to 1 hour. A sudden return of effectiveness may follow, and the cycle can recur many times each day.

Neuroleptic malignant syndrome (NMS) (parkinsonian crisis), which is characterized by an abrupt onset of marked rigidity, akinesia, tremor, and hyperpyrexia, can follow abrupt discontinuation of carbidopa-levodopa therapy. This occurs most frequently in patients who are also receiving antipsychotic drugs.

Other adverse effects associated with carbidopa-levodopa include episodic hyperventilation, bizarre breathing patterns, hoarseness, and increased nasal secretions. Urinary retention, polyuria, and urinary incontinence may also occur. Rarely, leukopenia may occur, necessitating temporary discontinuance.

Drug Interactions

Significant interactions may occur between carbidopa-levodopa and hydantoins, MAOIs, pyridoxine, phenothiazines, or tricyclic antidepressants (TCAs) (Table 22-2). Carbidopa-levodopa may also cause elevated serum and urinary pH levels, false-positive reactions for urinary glucose and ketones, and false elevations of urinary catecholamines.

Assessment of Relevant Core Patient Variables

Health Status

The nurse should assess the patient for tartrazine allergy, melanoma, and closed-angle glaucoma. The nurse should also assess for a history of psychiatric disorders necessitating the administration of MAOIs. The nurse must notify the health care provider before administration of carbidopa-levodopa if the patient has any of these disorders.

The nurse should assess for previous levodopa or carbidopa-levodopa therapy. After 2 to 5 years of continuous therapy, these drugs lose their overall effectiveness in controlling symptoms of Parkinson disease.

TABLE 22-2 Agents That Interact With Carbidopa-Levodopa

Interactants	Effect and Significance	Nursing Management
hydantoins	Mechanism of action unknown, but decrease effectiveness of carbidopa-levodopa	Monitor for decreased therapeutic effects. Consider alternative anticonvulsant therapy.
MAOIs	Inhibit peripheral metabolism of carbidopa-levodopa, resulting in increased levels of dopamine; may result in hypertensive crisis	Do not coadminister these drugs. If accidental administration occurs, phentolamine is the antidote.
pyridoxine	Increases the peripheral metabolism of carbidopa-levodopa, resulting in decreased dopamine levels	This effect is more pronounced in patients receiving levodopa as a single agent. Monitor for decreased therapeutic effects.
phenothiazines	May inhibit dopamine receptors in the CNS	Monitor for decreased therapeutic effects.
tricyclic antidepressants	Delay the absorption of carbidopa-levodopa and may decrease its bioavailability	Monitor for decreased therapeutic effects.

Administration of a higher dose may affect symptoms but will also increase the patient's risk for adverse effects.

The nurse should perform a complete physical examination, including mental status. Carbidopa-levodopa can exacerbate diseases or disorders in every body system; therefore, the nurse needs to evaluate baseline functioning. Appropriate laboratory or diagnostic tests are necessary, depending on the patient's preexisting conditions. Patients with cardiovascular disorders require a baseline electrocardiogram. Patients with pulmonary disorders should have baseline pulmonary function tests. Patients with glaucoma should have a baseline measurement of intraocular pressure. For patients with diabetes, a glycosated hemoglobin (Hb1AC) level should be obtained. Baseline hepatic function or renal function tests are included for patients with disorders in those body systems.

Throughout the physical examination, the nurse needs to document the signs and symptoms of Parkinson disease, such as abnormal posture and gait, muscle rigidity, and tremors. This baseline information will be used to assess the efficacy of carbidopa-levodopa therapy and progression of the disease.

Some patients receiving carbidopa-levodopa have experienced postoperative bleeding episodes; therefore, hematologic studies are recommended for all patients who undergo surgery while receiving carbidopa-levodopa.

Life Span and Gender

Carbidopa-levodopa is a pregnancy category C drug and therefore should be used with caution during pregnancy. It should not be given to breast-feeding women, because carbidopa-levodopa enters breast milk and may inhibit lactation. Thus, the nurse should assess all female patients for pregnancy or breast-feeding. In addition, carbidopa-levodopa should not be administered to children younger than 18 years, so the nurse needs to confirm that the patient is 18 years or older.

Lifestyle, Diet, and Habits

The nurse should coordinate a consultation with a nutritionist for patients taking carbidopa-levodopa. Patients should attempt weight control because increased body weight increases the work of the body, especially the muscles. A high-protein diet can slow or prevent absorption of carbidopa-levodopa. Therefore, moderate amounts of protein should be divided equally for consumption throughout the entire day. Pyridoxine (vitamin B_6) increases the action of decarboxylases that destroy levodopa in the periphery of the body, resulting in reduced effects of carbidopa-levodopa. Thus, patients should avoid foods containing large amounts of pyridoxine (e.g., avocados, bacon, beans, beef liver, dry skim milk, oatmeal, peas, pork, sweet potatoes, tuna). Patients should also increase dietary fiber and fluids to offset the potential for constipation.

Environment

Carbidopa-levodopa is usually administered in the home environment. The nurse must assess patients for their ability to understand the health care provider's directions and to physically self-administer drugs. Home care referrals are necessary for patients who cannot self-medicate. Because carbidopa-levodopa does not affect the progression of the disease, the nurse should coordinate counseling and physical and occupational therapies for the patient to optimize therapeutic outcome.

Culture

In decarboxylation, carbidopa-levodopa is metabolized by COMT, which antagonizes the therapeutic effects of carbidopa-levodopa. COMT activity destroys levodopa in the periphery of the body and is found in people of Chinese, Filipino, or Thai descent. Thus, the nurse should ask patients about their ethnic heritage.

Nursing Diagnoses and Outcomes

- Disturbed Thought Processes related to adverse CNS effects

  Desired outcome: The patient will remain oriented and communicate effectively.
- Disturbed Sleep Pattern related to drug therapy

  Desired outcome: The patient will report alterations in sleep patterns affecting activities of daily living.
- Impaired Physical Mobility related to on-off effect

  Desired outcome: The patient will immediately report incidents of the on-off effect to the health care provider.
- Risk for Injury related to drug-induced orthostatic hypotension

  Desired outcome: The patient will learn to change position slowly, carefully, and safely to minimize effects of orthostatic hypotension.

Planning and Intervention

Maximizing Therapeutic Effects

Carbidopa-levodopa should be taken on an empty stomach to facilitate absorption of the drug. The nurse should monitor the patient's diet to limit foods high in protein and pyridoxine. If the drug causes severe nausea, the nurse should give the patient a small amount of food 15 to 30 minutes after administering drug therapy.

Minimizing Adverse Effects

Carbidopa-levodopa should be administered at evenly spaced intervals; the dose should always be titrated. The dose is slowly increased to prevent nausea, vomiting, or orthostatic hypotension. The dose is slowly decreased to prevent NMS (parkinsonian crisis).

Providing Patient and Family Education

- The nurse should advise patients that carbidopa-levodopa therapy is palliative and will not cure the disease. Patients must understand that it takes weeks to months to notice benefits from therapy. The nurse should caution patients not to change the drug dosage in an attempt to hasten the therapeutic benefits, nor to discontinue the drug abruptly because they think treatment has failed.

- The nurse should advise patients to notify the health care provider about any of the following adverse reactions: uncontrollable movements of the face, eyelids, mouth, tongue, neck, arms, hands, or legs; mood or mental changes; irregular heartbeat or palpitations; difficult urination; severe or persistent nausea or vomiting; appetite loss; difficulty swallowing; or distorted taste.
- The nurse should demonstrate how to change positions slowly to avoid dizziness or fainting. He or she should advise patients to assess how the drug affects them before driving, using machinery, or performing tasks that require mental alertness.
- The nurse should discuss the potential for "on-off effect" described under the section on Adverse Reactions. He or she must ensure that patients understand that they are at risk for injury from falls during the off periods. The nurse should convey the importance of contacting the health care provider immediately if patients experience an akinetic episode.
- Patient education should also include necessary dietary changes. Patients should avoid vitamins or foods high in pyridoxine, high-protein foods when the drug is ingested, and alcohol.
- The nurse should caution patients with preexisting disorders, such as arrhythmias, pulmonary diseases, or peptic ulcer disease, that carbidopa-levodopa may exacerbate their condition. Patients must contact their health care provider if their symptoms increase in frequency or intensity. The nurse should caution patients with diabetes to monitor their glucose by capillary blood monitoring, because carbidopa-levodopa may induce false-positive urinary glucose results. Finally, carbidopa-levodopa sometimes darkens urine and sweat. The nurse should assure patients that this is no cause for concern.

Ongoing Assessment and Evaluation

The nurse should monitor for improvement in the patient's ability to perform activities of daily living and decreased muscle rigidity and tremors. During periods of dose adjustment, the nurse should monitor the blood pressure every 4 hours. When dose adjustment is done in the home, the nurse should teach a family member how to monitor the blood pressure.

The nurse should monitor for signs of adverse effects from carbidopa-levodopa therapy. Dosage changes may increase adverse effects, so notifying the health care provider if these signs occur is important. The nurse should remember to monitor for signs of personality, behavioral, or mental changes. Eliciting information regarding these potential changes from the family and patient is important. Patients should also receive a periodic eye examination because carbidopa-levodopa may affect intraocular pressure.

The nurse should monitor for signs or symptoms of NMS. If signs or symptoms of NMS develop, the nurse should assess for compliance of drug therapy to ensure proper dosing. The nurse, patient, or family should report any signs of NMS to the health care provider immediately.

With successful therapy, the nurse should observe decreased muscular rigidity and tremors and improved mobility. The patient should verbalize the importance of contacting the health care provider immediately if any adverse reactions occur. The patient should verbalize the importance of periodic reevaluation by the health care provider. ■

DRUGS CLOSELY RELATED TO CARBIDOPA-LEVODOPA

Levodopa

Levodopa (Larodopa, Dopar), a component of carbidopa-levodopa, may also be used as a single drug and works by promoting synthesis of dopamine in the striatum. When levodopa is administered as a single oral drug, less than 2% actually passes the blood–brain barrier for use in the CNS. Peripheral decarboxylation affects the remainder of the dose. Core drug knowledge and core patient variables are the same as for carbidopa-levodopa; however, abnormal movements

MEMORY CHIP

Carbidopa-Levodopa

- Dopaminergic drug used for the management of Parkinson disease
- Significant contraindications: known hypersensitivity, allergy to tartrazine, melanoma, closed-angle glaucoma, and breast-feeding
- Most common adverse effects: abnormal movements, orthostatic hypotension, and GI effects
- Most serious adverse effects: neuroleptic malignant syndrome, which may occur with abrupt cessation of the drug; precautions necessary with cardiac disease, pulmonary disease, peptic ulcer disease, diabetes mellitus, psychosis, and pregnancy
- Maximizing therapeutic effects: take drug on an empty stomach and reduce protein and pyridoxine in the diet
- Minimizing adverse effects: titrate the drug upward to avoid GI effects; titrate the drug downward to avoid neuroleptic malignant syndrome
- Most significant patient education: caution about hypotension and "on-off effect"

and psychiatric disturbances may be less intense and occur later in pharmacotherapy, when levodopa is administered as a single drug.

Dopamine Agonists

Pramipexole

Pramipexole (Mirapex) is one of four dopamine agonists used to treat Parkinson disease. The pharmacologic action of a dopamine agonist differs from that of carbidopa-levodopa. Carbidopa-levodopa is converted in the brain into dopamine. In contrast, dopamine agonists, such as pramipexole, act directly on dopamine receptors in the brain and thus can help alleviate the symptoms of Parkinson disease. Pramipexole is a selective agonist at D_2 and D_3 receptors in the brain. It is more selective for these receptors than either bromocriptine or pergolide.

Pramipexole has been approved for treating both early and late stages of Parkinson disease. With early stage monotherapy, pramipexole will delay the need for carbidopa-levodopa, thus extending the pharmacotherapeutic benefits of carbidopa-levodopa when it is used as treatment of more advanced stages of Parkinson disease. Additionally, in later stages of Parkinson disease, coadministration of pramipexole with carbidopa-levodopa can decrease the dosage of carbidopa-levodopa by 25%. This reduction decreases the potential for carbidopa-levodopa's adverse effects.

In the early stages of Parkinson disease, the most frequent adverse effects of pramipexole are nausea, dizziness, drowsiness, insomnia, and postural hypotension. In advanced stages of Parkinson disease, additional adverse effects include dyskinesias, extrapyramidal syndromes, and hallucinations. The nurse should inform all patients that postural hypotension may occur more frequently during initial treatment, and hallucinations can occur at any time during the course of treatment.

Ropinirole

Ropinirole (Requip), the second dopamine agonist, is similar to pramipexole. Like pramipexole, ropinirole may be used in early Parkinson disease or in later stages in conjunction with carbidopa-levodopa. With ropinirole, the dose of carbidopa-levodopa may be reduced, which may, in turn, help decrease the "on-off" fluctuations that affect some patients who have been on carbidopa-levodopa for some years.

Administration of ropinirole as monotherapy may induce adverse effects in every system of the body. In the autonomic nervous system, the most common adverse effects include diaphoresis, flushing, and xerostomia (dry mouth). In the overall body, the most common adverse effects include asthenia, chest pain, dependent edema, fatigue, malaise, pain, and peripheral edema. Cardiovascular adverse reactions include atrial fibrillation, extrasystoles, hypertension, hypotension, orthostatic hypotension, palpitations, sinus tachycardia, and syncope (sometimes with sinus bradycardia). Most syncope cases occurring with ropinirole therapy were reported more than 4 weeks after initiation and were usually associated with a recent increase in dosage. In the GI system, common adverse effects include abdominal pain, anorexia, dyspepsia, flatulence, and nausea and vomiting. The most common adverse reactions affecting the CNS and peripheral nervous system include dizziness, hyperesthesia, restlessness, and vertigo. The potential metabolic and nutritional adverse effect is weight loss, whereas potential respiratory adverse effects include bronchitis, dyspnea, pharyngitis, rhinitis, sinusitis, visual impairment, and xerophthalmia (conjunctival dryness).

Psychiatric adverse reactions include amnesia, impaired concentration, confusion, hallucinations, drowsiness, and yawning. There have been at least 60 postmarket reports of patients who have fallen asleep while driving or performing other normal daytime activities while taking ropinirole. The episodes occurred as late as 1 year after initiation of treatment. Some patients reported feeling completely alert prior to these events. It is not clear whether the medication, the sleep status of the patient, or Parkinson disease itself contributed to these episodes.

In addition to the above adverse effects, ropinirole in combination with carbidopa-levodopa may induce additional effects. These include dyskinesia, falls, headache, hypokinesia, paresis, paresthesias, tremor, constipation, diarrhea, dysphagia, flatulence, hypersalivation, anemia, upper respiratory infections, pyuria, urinary incontinence, and diplopia. Additionally, anxiety, abnormal dreaming, hallucinations, nervousness, and somnolence (drowsiness) may also occur. The potential advantage of ropinirole is a lower incidence of dyskinesia and lower propensity to induce adverse psychiatric effects compared with carbidopa-levodopa.

Bromocriptine

Bromocriptine (Parlodel), the third dopamine agonist, is an oral synthetic agent that has been used in the treatment of Parkinson disease for many years. Its other indications include acromegaly, amenorrhea, galactorrhea, infertility, and prolactin-secreting pituitary adenomas. It is being investigated for use as a treatment of insulin resistance in patients with type 2 diabetes mellitus.

Bromocriptine works by stimulating D_2 receptors and antagonizing D_1 receptors in the hypothalamus and striatum of the CNS. For treating Parkinson disease, the effect is to increase the availability of dopamine. Additionally, bromocriptine suppresses prolactin secretion from the anterior pituitary gland, enabling ovulation and ovarian function in amenorrheic patients and suppressing lactation in women with normal ovarian activity.

The adverse effects of bromocriptine therapy limit its use. Symptoms such as psychic disturbances, nausea, and orthostatic hypotension are very common. In patients with preexisting psychiatric illness, peripheral vascular disease, and peptic ulcer, bromocriptine exacerbates these conditions. Patients with a history of MI may experience serious cardiac problems.

Bromocriptine should not be administered with drugs that antagonize its actions. These include drugs that increase the concentration of prolactin, such as haloperidol (Haldol), loxapine (Loxatane), molindone (Moban), MAOIs, imipramine (Tofranil), amitriptyline (Elavil), methyldopa (Aldomet), phenothiazines, and reserpine (Serpalan). Estrogens or progestins can produce amenorrhea or galactorrhea and should not be given concurrently.

Pergolide

Pergolide (Permax), the last dopamine agonist, is an oral agent similar in action to bromocriptine, with ten times the potency of bromocriptine at the D_2 receptors. Unlike bromocriptine, pergolide stimulates the D_1 receptors as well. Pergolide causes direct activation of dopamine receptors in the striatum, inhibits the secretion of prolactin, and decreases luteinizing hormone. The effects on prolactin secretion persist much longer than the antiparkinsonian action.

Because pergolide is a potent dopamine-receptor agonist, it should not be administered concurrently with dopamine-receptor antagonists (e.g., neuroleptics such as phenothiazines, haloperidol, and thiothixene). Dopamine-receptor antagonists can antagonize the effects of pergolide.

Adverse effects of pergolide are similar to those of levodopa: nausea, vomiting, confusion, hallucinations, lightheadedness, and fainting. A rare side effect known as fibrosis (thickening or scarring of the membrane lining of body organs) has also been reported.

Dopaminergics

Amantadine

Amantadine (Symmetrel) is a dopaminergic agent that works differently than dopamine agonists. Amantadine is an oral antiviral drug that is also effective in treating Parkinson disease. Little is known about its precise mechanism of action in the brain. It has traditionally been considered a dopaminergic drug, but recent studies suggest that it may affect other neurochemical pathways containing the chemical messengers glutamate or acetylcholine. Like selegiline, amantadine's efficacy diminishes within a short time. Effects may decrease as soon as 3 to 6 months.

Amantadine tends to cause insomnia as well as daytime fatigue. Other side effects can include swelling of the feet, anxiety, dizziness, urinary retention, and hallucinations. The patient may also experience effects similar to those of anticholinergic drugs, such as blurred vision, constipation, urinary retention, and dry mouth. These effects may be enhanced when amantadine is given concurrently with other drugs with anticholinergic effects.

An adverse effect specific to amantadine is "livedo reticularis," a reddish-blue netlike mottling of the skin. Fortunately, this condition is benign and disappears with cessation of amantadine.

Selegiline

Selegiline (Eldepryl) is another dopaminergic agent that is not a dopamine agonist. It is an oral selective inhibitor of MAO-B, the chemical that breaks down dopamine. It should not be confused with the MAOIs used to treat depression. Selegiline decreases the destruction of dopamine, whether the dopamine is intrinsic or extrinsic, such as dopamine produced from carbidopa-levodopa. It is thought to slow the progression of Parkinson disease. Like pramipexole, selegiline delays the need for carbidopa-levodopa and effectively prolongs the efficacy of pharmacotherapy. Its action diminishes rapidly and is viable for only 12 to 24 months.

Selegiline is metabolized in the liver into two metabolites: amphetamine and methamphetamine. These metabolites may be responsible for the most common adverse effect of selegiline, which is insomnia. Concurrent administration of selegiline with carbidopa-levodopa may enhance adverse effects, such as orthostatic hypotension, dyskinesias, nausea, and psychologic disturbances.

DRUGS SIGNIFICANTLY DIFFERENT FROM CARBIDOPA-LEVODOPA

Tolcapone

Tolcapone (Tasmar) is a new adjunct to carbidopa-levodopa therapy. It inhibits the enzyme COMT, which degrades dopamine in the periphery of the body. The higher and more sustained plasma concentrations of levodopa result in more constant dopaminergic stimulation in the brain, leading to greater effects on the signs and symptoms of Parkinson disease. The decreased destruction of levodopa allows a decrease in the daily dosage of carbidopa-levodopa. Tolcapone is indicated for use in the treatment of Parkinson disease in patients who are experiencing fluctuations in symptoms and are not responding to or are not appropriate candidates for other adjunctive therapies.

In addition to levodopa, COMT metabolizes other medications, including dopamine, dobutamine, epinephrine, norepinephrine, isoproterenol, methyldopa, and bitolterol. It may be necessary to reduce the dosage of these agents in patients who are treated with tolcapone.

Because COMT and MAO are the two major enzyme systems involved in the metabolism of catecholamines, a possibility exists that the combined use of tolcapone and a nonselective MAO inhibitor, such as phenelzine or tranylcypromine, would inhibit most pathways involved in normal catecholamine metabolism. Therefore, the concurrent use of these agents should be avoided. Tolcapone can, however, be used concomitantly with the selective MAO-B inhibitor, selegiline, and these agents have been used together in antiparkinsonian regimens without difficulty.

The most frequent adverse effects of tolcapone are dyskinesia, nausea, sleep disorders, dystonia, orthostatic hypotension, diarrhea, dizziness, and hallucinations; also, there is a potential for elevation of liver transaminase concentrations in the blood. Because of reports of fatal liver injury, the manufacturers of tolcapone advise that its use should be reserved for patients who do not respond to or are not appropriate candidates for other available treatments. Extensive liver function testing is required of all patients before and during therapy.

Entacapone

Entacapone (Comtan) is the second COMT inhibitor to be approved and is indicated as an adjunct to levodopa/carbidopa to treat patients with idiopathic Parkinson disease who experience the signs and symptoms of end-of-dose "wearing-off." This agent has no antiparkinsonian effect of its own, and it must be administered in conjunction with levodopa/carbidopa. Like tolcapone, the addition of entacapone to a levodopa/carbidopa regimen increases the bioavailability of levodopa.

Entacapone has the same adverse effect profile as tolcapone, with the exception that entacapone is not associated with evidence of hepatotoxicity or significant elevation of liver enzymes. This represents an important advantage over tolcapone, because monitoring of liver function tests is not required. Potential drug-drug interactions with entacapone are similar to tolcapone.

Centrally Acting Anticholinergic Drugs

The centrally acting anticholinergic drugs work by blocking the access of acetylcholine to cholinergic receptors in the striatum. Centrally acting anticholinergic drugs are less effective than carbidopa-levodopa. They can be used as monotherapy in early Parkinson disease or in combination with dopaminergic drugs in later stages. They are used with caution in older patients because of the potential for severe CNS effects. The anticholinergics used most frequently in treating Parkinson disease are benztropine (Cogentin), diphenhydramine (Benadryl), and trihexyphenidyl (Artane). For additional information concerning anticholinergic drugs, see Chapter 15.

ANTI-AMYOTROPHIC LATERAL SCLEROSIS (ALS) DRUGS

Historically, there has not been specific pharmacotherapy for treating ALS. In December 1995, the Food and Drug Administration (FDA) approved the first drug for treatment of ALS, riluzole. Riluzole (Rilutek), the prototype anti-ALS drug, will not cure ALS. Rather, it is used to delay the need for tracheostomy or mechanical ventilation in patients with ALS. See the accompanying display, New Drugs for Amyotrophic Lateral Sclerosis, for information about ongoing research for additional ALS medications.

> **Focus on Research**
>
> **New drugs for amyotrophic lateral sclerosis (ALS)**
>
> **The Studies**
>
> Several clinical trials are ongoing for new drugs to combat ALS. Clinical trials of a new experimental ALS drug known as SR57746A are complete, and the data will be published at the end of 2000. This new drug is referred to as "the Sanofi drug," because of the company that makes it, Sanofi Pharmaceuticals (Montpellier, France). SR57746A seems to work by causing the body to produce more of various neurotrophic ("nerve-nourishing") factors, such as brain-derived neurotrophic factor, ciliary neurotrophic factor, and neurotrophic growth factor. Neurotrophic factors improve the survival of motor neurons, which are the cells affected in ALS, when tested in culture dishes and animal models of nerve damage.
>
> **Nursing Implications**
>
> The population of older adults is growing at an enormous rate. Unfortunately, as we grow older, we fall prey to a host of potential diseases, such as Alzheimer disease. As researchers find the causes of these diseases, and pharmaceutical companies use this information to develop drugs to combat neurologic diseases, the quality of life for older adults should vastly improve.

NURSING MANAGEMENT OF THE PATIENT RECEIVING RILUZOLE

Core Drug Knowledge

Pharmacotherapeutics

Riluzole is indicated for treating ALS because it slows down the disease's progression by delaying for several months the loss of muscle strength and limb function. The drug is given to extend survival time before tracheostomy is necessary, but it is not a cure.

Pharmacokinetics

Riluzole is administered orally in 50-mg doses every 12 hours. Its onset of action is slow, and its duration of action is 3 to 5 days. Well absorbed from the GI tract, riluzole has a half-life of 12 hours. Hepatic metabolism of riluzole is extensive, producing six major and several minor metabolites. The cytochrome P450 enzyme system is involved in hydroxylation and glucuronidation. The main isozyme involved in hydroxylation is CYP 1A2. Riluzole crosses the placenta and enters breast milk.

Excretion of riluzole is mainly renal and 5% fecal. Riluzole is largely excreted as metabolites with about 2% excreted as unchanged drug. Renal clearance of riluzole is individualized, possibly because of the variability of CYP 1A2.

Pharmacodynamics

The etiology of ALS is unknown. One of the leading theories of its pathogenesis is that glutamate injures motor neurons. Although the mode of action of riluzole in the treatment of ALS is also unknown, it may be related to riluzole's effects. Some of these effects include an inhibition of glutamate release, inactivation of voltage-dependent sodium channels, and interference with intracellular events that follow transmitter binding at excitatory amino acid receptors.

Contraindications and Precautions

The only contraindication to riluzole therapy is a hypersensitivity to any of its components. Many precautions, however, are issued.

Riluzole has affected fetal development and viability in animal studies; however, adequate studies on human pregnancy have not been completed. It is assigned to pregnancy category C and should be administered only when the benefits to the mother outweigh the risks to the fetus throughout pregnancy.

Hepatic disease, renal disease, or renal impairment can affect the clearance of riluzole, which is extensively metabolized in the liver and excreted in the urine. Patients with preexisting hepatic or renal disease should be given riluzole with caution.

Adverse Effects

The evaluation of adverse effects caused by riluzole presents some difficulty because ALS causes several manifestations that may be mistaken for adverse effects. In reviewing the adverse effects for patients taking riluzole, the nurse must also consider natural disease progression.

Potential side effects are fatigue, nausea, dizziness, diarrhea, anorexia, vertigo, and somnolence. When these symptoms become troublesome, treatment should be discontinued. Riluzole causes increased levels of hepatic enzymes in 50% of patients. This occurs in patients with no history of hepatic injury. Rarely, jaundice may also occur.

Many potentially adverse reactions have been reported with riluzole therapy, involving every system of the body. These adverse reactions, however, occurred in fewer than 1% of patients receiving riluzole. One of the most serious potential adverse effects is neutropenia. Although such reactions are rare, a complete blood count (CBC) should be monitored for the patient's safety.

Drug Interactions

As previously mentioned, riluzole may cause hepatic injury. There is a potential for increased risk of hepatic injury when riluzole is used concurrently with potentially hepatotoxic drugs, such as allopurinol (Zyloprim), methyldopa, sulfasalazine (Azulfidine), or aminoglycosides. Additionally, drugs that induce the hepatic enzyme system, such as barbiturates and carbamazepine, may also increase the risk for hepatic injury.

The principle isoenzyme involved in the metabolism of riluzole is CYP 1A2. Inhibitors of this enzyme may increase plasma concentrations, placing the patient at risk for toxicity. Conversely, inducers of CYP 1A2 may decrease plasma concentrations, resulting in a subtherapeutic dose of riluzole. Table 22-3 presents potential agents that may interact with riluzole.

Assessment of Relevant Core Patient Variables

Health Status

The nurse should elicit a careful history, including any preexisting hepatic or renal dysfunction. The nurse should also assess for a history of smoking cigarettes. He or she should communicate any positive findings to the health care provider.

Completing a physical examination of the patient prior to initiation of therapy is important. Riluzole can induce adverse effects in every body system. With the exception of hepatic injury, the chance of these adverse reactions is less than 1%. Baseline data are helpful should any of the reactions occur. All patients should have baseline CBC and renal and hepatic function tests documented.

Life Span and Gender

Older patients are more likely to have age-related changes in hepatic or renal function. No specific recommendations for dosage in older adults have been made,

TABLE 22-3 Agents That Interact With Riluzole

Interactants	Effect and Significance	Nursing Management
CYP 1A2 inhibitors caffeine theophylline amitriptyline quinolones	Potential for concurrent administration of riluzole with CYP 1A2 to decrease plasma concentrations of riluzole by increasing the rate of clearance	Monitor for efficacy of riluzole therapy. Monitor serum plasma levels.
CYP 1A2 inducers cigarette smoke charcoal-broiled foods rifampin omeprazole	Potential for concurrent administration of riluzole with CYP 1A2 to increase plasma concentrations of riluzole by inhibiting the rate of clearance	Monitor for toxicity of riluzole therapy. Monitor serum plasma levels.
hepatic enzyme inducers barbiturates carbamazepine	Potential for concurrent administration of riluzole with hepatic enzyme inducers to increase the risk for hepatotoxicity	Monitor liver function tests frequently. Monitor for signs of hepatic dysfunction.
hepatotoxic drugs allopurinol methyldopa sulfasalazine aminoglycosides	Potential for concurrent administration of riluzole with other drugs known for their hepatotoxic effects to increase the risk for hepatotoxicity	Monitor liver function tests frequently. Monitor for signs of hepatic dysfunction.

but the nurse should closely monitor older patients for adverse effects.

The metabolism of riluzole depends largely on the activity of a specific isozyme, CYP 1A2. This isozyme reportedly is more active in men than women. Higher blood concentrations of riluzole and its metabolites may be present in women. This may increase the risk of adverse effects in women, for which nurses should continually assess female patients.

Lifestyle, Diet, and Habits

The nurse needs to evaluate the patient's diet for high-fat content, use of caffeine products, and high intake of charcoal-broiled foods and to determine whether the patient is a smoker. The absorption of riluzole may be diminished by 20% in patients who consume a high-fat diet. Caffeine products can inhibit CPY 1A2, resulting in increased serum concentration of riluzole. Conversely, charcoal-broiled foods and tobacco smoking can induce CPY 1A2. Inducing the isozyme CYP 1A2 may increase the elimination of riluzole from the body.

Environment

Riluzole is usually administered in the home environment. The nurse must assess patients for their ability to understand the health care provider's directions and to physically self-administer drugs. Appropriate home care referrals are necessary for patients unable to self-medicate. Riluzole is extremely expensive. The nurse should evaluate patients' financial circumstances and refer patients and families for social services as appropriate.

Culture

The nurse should determine whether the patient is of Japanese descent. Riluzole clearance in native Japanese patients is 50% less efficient than in whites. It is uncertain whether this effect is related to a different metabolic function in native Japanese or to environmental factors, such as smoking, alcohol, coffee, or diet.

Nursing Diagnoses and Outcomes

- Risk for Injury related to hepatic dysfunction, anemia, and CNS and cardiovascular effects of riluzole therapy

  Desired outcome: The patient will immediately report any signs of hepatic dysfunction (fatigue, rash, jaundice), anemia (fatigue, sore throat, easy bruising), or CNS or cardiovascular events to the health care provider.
- Disturbed Thought Processes related to adverse CNS effects

  Desired outcome: The patient will remain oriented and able to communicate effectively.

Planning and Intervention

Maximizing Therapeutic Effects

The nurse should administer riluzole with a full glass of water. It is best for riluzole to be taken on an empty stomach, at least 1 hour before or 2 hours after meals. For patients who will be self-medicating, the nurse should explain the importance of correct administration.

Minimizing Adverse Effects

At the beginning of therapy, riluzole may cause dizziness or sedation. The nurse should caution the patient to refrain from driving, using machinery, or performing tasks that require mental alertness until the effects of riluzole have been established.

Providing Patient and Family Education

- The most important patient and family education is explaining that riluzole will not change the course of the disorder (see the accompanying display, Riluzole and Reality). At best, riluzole will delay the need for tracheostomy and mechanical ventilation. Patients must understand the eventual sequelae of ALS and have a legal document in place if they choose to refuse life-sustaining measures.
- The nurse should advise patients to take riluzole on an empty stomach at 12-hour intervals. He or she should present dietary concerns, such as a low-protein diet. The nurse should also advise patients to refrain from caffeine, alcohol, and charcoal-broiled foods.
- The nurse should advise patients of the potential adverse effects of riluzole. Because progression of the disease may mimic common adverse effects, patients should always contact the health care provider should any symptoms occur.
- The nurse should also advise patients about the importance of constant follow-up and the need for periodic blood testing. He or she should present symptoms of hepatic dysfunction and emphasize the importance of contacting the health care provider if any appear.

Critical Thinking Scenario

Riluzole and reality

Mrs. Baxter has been diagnosed with ALS. She has moderate weakness in her extremities and uses a walker to ambulate. During your home visit, Mr. Baxter tells you, "I'm so glad they have started my wife on riluzole. I was thinking of having our attorney come over and do all that paperwork about the will and stuff because I was so scared. Now I don't have to." How would you respond to Mr. Baxter? What specific topics would you cover with him?

Ongoing Assessment and Evaluation

The nurse should coordinate regular follow-up evaluations of the patient. At each visit, the nurse should evaluate the patient for the onset of adverse effects and complete a physical examination. CBC and alanine transaminase (ALT) levels should be drawn monthly during the first 3 months of treatment, then every 3 months for the remainder of the first year. After the first year, monitoring of ALT levels should continue periodically. Patients with elevated ALT levels require more frequent monitoring. Discontinuation of riluzole therapy should be considered when ALT levels become five times normal range. The nurse should reinforce dietary and smoking restrictions during each encounter with the patient.

Effective therapy should delay deterioration of the respiratory muscles. The patient should verbalize the importance of contacting the health care provider immediately if any adverse reactions occur. The patient should verbalize the importance of periodic reevaluation by the health care provider. ■

OTHER MOVEMENT DISORDERS AND RELATED DRUG THERAPY

The following disorders and the drugs used to treat them are important to include in any discussion of drugs used to treat movement disorders. The drugs commonly used to treat these disorders are covered in depth in other chapters in this textbook. Therefore, each disorder and the drugs commonly used to treat them are discussed briefly later in this chapter, and the reader is then referred to the appropriate chapter in the textbook for more detailed information about the specific drugs.

MEMORY CHIP

Riluzole

- Used in the management of ALS to delay need for mechanical ventilation
- Significant contraindication: hypersensitivity to any components of riluzole
- Most serious adverse effect: neutropenia; adverse effects possible in every body system but these may indicate progression of disease
- Maximizing therapeutic effects: recommend dietary decreases in protein and avoid caffeine, charcoal-broiled foods, tobacco, and alcohol
- Minimizing adverse effects: refrain from tasks that require concentration until the effects of riluzole are known
- Most significant patient education: have CBC and ALT monitored monthly for first 3 months, then every 3 months thereafter

MYASTHENIA GRAVIS

Myasthenia gravis (MG) is an autoimmune disorder that impairs the receptors for acetylcholine at the myoneural junction. In this disease, IgG antibodies to acetylcholine receptors form, block, and ultimately destroy the receptors; thus, the muscle cannot be stimulated. The patient experiences skeletal muscle weakness and rapid fatigue of the affected muscles.

The first symptoms of MG are usually weakness of the eye muscles and ptosis. The disease progresses from ocular weakness to generalized weakness. The proximal limbs are weaker than the distal limbs. Symptoms are generally worse in the afternoon or as environmental temperature rises.

Diagnosis of MG is based on the edrophonium (Tensilon) test. In this test, the patient is induced into weakness by being required to maintain a position. Edrophonium, a short-acting acetylcholinesterase inhibitor, is administered intravenously. Patients with MG will have a dramatic transitory improvement in muscle function.

As with other movement disorders, MG has no cure. The treatments of choice are neostigmine (Prostigmin) or pyridostigmine (Mestinon). Both are discussed in Chapter 15.

HUNTINGTON DISEASE

Huntington disease (chorea) is an inherited disorder that remains undiagnosed until midlife. Two main symptoms of the disease are progressive mental status changes, leading to dementia, and choreiform (rapid, jerky) movements. There is depletion of GABA, an inhibitory neurotransmitter in the basal nuclei and substantial nigra. Levels of acetylcholine in the brain also appear to be reduced. Dopamine, however, is unaffected.

The first symptoms of Huntington disease are restlessness and choreiform movements of the arms and face. Symptoms in early disease include intellectual impairment, such as loss of problem-solving skills, poor judgment, inability to concentrate, and memory lapses. As the disease progresses, personality changes, moodiness, and behavior disturbances occur. The dementia, which accompanies progressive disease, may be related to excessive amounts of dopamine. As atrophy of the brain continues, rigidity and akinesia develop.

There is no effective treatment for Huntington disease. Treatment of choreiform movements includes antipsychotic drugs, such as haloperidol (Haldol), or phenothiazines, which block dopamine receptors. These drugs are discussed in depth in Chapter 19.

GILLES DE LA TOURETTE DISEASE

Gilles de la Tourette disease (Tourette syndrome, TS) is an autosomal dominant inherited tic disorder appearing in childhood and characterized by multiple motor or vocal tics lasting more than 1 year. Patients may also have obsessive-compulsive behavior, attention-deficit/hyperactivity disorder, or other psychiatric disorders. Coprolalia (involuntary utterances of vulgar or obscene words) and echolalia (involuntary parrot-like repetition of a word or sentence just spoken by another person) can occur but are rare.

Motor and vocal tics from this disease may respond to haloperidol (Haldol) and similar D2 receptor blockers (see Chapter 19). Up to 80% of patients with TS initially benefit from haloperidol, sometimes dramatically; however, only approximately 20% of patients continue haloperidol for an extended period. Patients often discontinue the drug because of the emergence of side effects such as excessive fatigue, weight gain, dysphoria, parkinsonian symptoms, intellectual dulling, memory problems, personality changes, feeling "zombie-like," akathisia, school or social phobias, loss of libido, sexual dysfunction, and, especially after chronic use of high doses, tardive dyskinesia.

Pimozide (Orap) is another drug used for TS. It is chemically distinctive from haloperidol or phenothiazines, with potent dopamine-blocking properties. Its side effects are similar to haloperidol but may be less severe and appear in fewer patients. Routine electrocardiographic studies before and periodically during treatment are advised because of potential cardiotoxicity.

Other phenothiazines, particularly fluphenazine (Prolixin), may be effective alternatives to haloperidol and pimozide. Fluphenazine's side effects are potentially the same as those associated with haloperidol, but, as with pimozide, some patients tolerate them better. Other neuroleptics that have been reported to be effective in a few patients include thiothixene (Navane), chlorpromazine (Thorazine), and trifluoperazine (Stelazine). These drugs are also discussed in Chapter 19.

Another drug useful in the treatment of TS is clonidine (Catapres), an imidazoline compound with alpha-adrenergic agonist activity. In low doses, clonidine decreases the release of central norepinephrine, resulting in decreased motor tics. In addition to reducing the simple motor and phonic symptoms in TS, clonidine seems especially useful in improving attention problems and ameliorating complex motor and phonic symptoms. It has a low incidence of associated side effects. Perhaps of greatest importance is that it does not have the potential to cause tardive dyskinesia. Clonidine is covered in depth in Chapter 30.

MULTIPLE SCLEROSIS

Multiple sclerosis (MS) is a major cause of neurologic disability among young and middle-aged adults. It is characterized by demyelination in the white matter of the brain, brain stem, or spinal cord. Patients experience exacerbations and remissions over many years from several different sites in the CNS. Initially, functioning between exacerbations is normal to near-normal. As the disease progresses, however, less improvement and more neurologic dysfunction appear between exacerbations.

Pharmacotherapy for MS includes glucocorticoids to shorten the duration of an acute attack or delay the progression of optic neuritis. Abatement of symptoms includes the use of oxybutynin (Ditropan) for bladder incontinence; carbamazepine (Tegretol) or mexiletine (Mexitil) for shooting sensory pain; baclofen (Lioresal), carisoprodol (Soma), or benzodiazepines for muscle spasticity; and tizanidine (Zinaflex) for low back pain.

Interferon beta is also used in the treatment of MS. Interferon beta is available as interferon beta-1a (Avonex) and interferon beta-1b (Betaseron). There are many differences between these two drugs. A recombinant process produces both drugs, but the process differs greatly for each. In therapy, 1-mg interferon beta-1a represents 200 million units of activity, whereas 1 mg of interferon beta-1b represents 32 million units of activity. Interferon beta-1a shows relapse rate reduction and slows disease progression. Interferon beta-1b shows a very significant clinical benefit in decreasing relapse but has not been shown to slow disease progression. Interferon beta-1a is administered by intramuscular injection, whereas interferon beta-1b is administered by subcutaneous injection. Interferon beta-1a has not been associated with injection site necrosis, whereas roughly 85% of patients receiving interferon beta-1b experienced an injection site reaction.

Interferon beta should not be administered to patients with hypersensitivity to interferon beta or albumin. It is a pregnancy category C drug and should be avoided during pregnancy because of the risk of spontaneous abortion. It should also be avoided during breast-feeding because there is potential for serious adverse reactions in the infant. Interferon beta is also used with caution in patients with a history of cardiac arrhythmias, heart failure, or myocardial infarction. Suicidal ideation has occurred in patients on interferon beta therapy. It is unclear if this is related to the drug or to the disease process of MS.

A new drug approved for treating MS is glatiramer acetate (Copaxone). Glatiramer acetate is a synthetic chemical that is similar in structure to myelin basic protein. The action of glatiramer acetate is unclear; however, it is proposed that the drug serves as a decoy to locally generated autoantibodies. Glatiramer acetate is given daily as a subcutaneous injection. Adverse effects requiring immediate attention include chest pain, breathing difficulties, dizziness, flushing, hives, pounding heartbeat, uncontrolled eye movements, changes in vision, throat spasms, or swallowing problems.

Common adverse effects that should be reported to the health care provider are CNS symptoms such as anxiety, confusion, migraine, or mood changes; respiratory symptoms such as coughing or other bronchial irritation; and genitourinary (GU) symptoms such as vaginal discharge, frequent urination or blood in urine, impotence, and decreased libido. Other reportable symptoms include neck pain, tachycardia, skin rash, and swelling of the hands, lower extremities, or lymph glands. Other common adverse effects that are bothersome, but usually resolve with continued use, include irritation or swelling at the site of injection, runny nose, tremor, unusual tiredness or weakness, and weight gain.

Glatiramer acetate can alter the results of a Papanicolaou test (Pap smear); therefore, women should inform their obstetrician/gynecologist of its use.

CHAPTER SUMMARY

- Movement disorders are chronic, severe, and debilitating.
- Parkinson disease is a naturally occurring disorder characterized by rigidity, rest tremor, bradykinesia or akinesia, and postural instability.
- Parkinsonism is a syndrome of symptoms resembling Parkinson disease caused by trauma, drugs, or infection.
- Amyotrophic lateral sclerosis (ALS) is a muscle degenerative disease that progresses quickly until the patient experiences respiratory compromise and ultimately death.
- Drugs used to treat movement disorders are not curative.
- Dopaminergic drugs are used to treat Parkinson disease by increasing the action of dopamine in the CNS. The prototype dopaminergic drug is carbidopa-levodopa (Sinemet).
- Drugs that decrease the action of acetylcholine (e.g., anticholinergic drugs) are also used to treat Parkinson disease.
- The only FDA-approved anti-ALS drug is the prototype riluzole (Rilutek).
- Riluzole delays the need for tracheostomy and mechanical ventilation.
- Other movement disorders and the drugs used to treat them include myasthenia gravis (MG), neostigmine; Huntington disease (chorea), haloperidol or phenothiazines; Tourette syndrome, haloperidol, clonidine, fluphenazine, and clonazepam; and multiple sclerosis (MS), glucocorticoids, interferon beta, glatiramer acetate, and other medications to suppress specific symptoms.

QUESTIONS FOR STUDY AND REVIEW

1. How do the dopaminergic and anticholinergic drugs work to decrease the symptoms of Parkinson disease?
2. Why is carbidopa-levodopa considered more efficient than levodopa alone?
3. What is neuroleptic malignant syndrome? When is it most likely to occur?
4. What is a bradykinetic episode?
5. What diet restrictions should be discussed when a patient starts carbidopa-levodopa therapy?
6. What assessments should the nurse make throughout carbidopa-levodopa therapy?
7. What is the goal of riluzole therapy?
8. For patients taking riluzole, why is assessing adverse effects difficult?
9. What dietary restrictions should the nurse discuss with the patient starting riluzole therapy?

NEED MORE HELP?

Chapter 22 of the study guide for *Drug Therapy in Nursing* contains exercises and activities to reinforce your understanding of the concepts presented in this chapter. For additional information see the text's accompanying web site at *http://www.connection.lww.com*.

REFERENCES AND BIBLIOGRAPHY

Bryson, H. M., Fulton, B., & Benfield, P. (1996). Riluzole. A review of its pharmacodynamic and pharmacokinetic properties and therapeutic potential in amyotrophic lateral sclerosis. *Drugs, 52*(4), 549–563.

CCIS System: *Computerized Clinical Information System.* Denver, CO: Micromedex.

Clinical Drug Monographs, (2001). CDRom, Gold Standard Media.

Drug Facts and Comparisons. (2000). St. Louis: Facts and Comparisons.

Dooley M., & Markham, A. (1998). Pramipexole. A review of its use in the management of early and advanced Parkinson's disease. *Drugs Aging, 12*(6), 495–514

Freeman, R. D. (posted June 17, 1997). Diagnosis and management of Tourette syndrome: Practical aspects. *Medscape Mental Health (Online)* http://www.medscape.com/Medscape/MentalHealth/1997/v02.n07/ mh3053.freeman/mh3053.freeman.html.

Hardman, J. G., Limbird, L. E., Molinof, P. B., Ruddon, R. W., & Gilman, A. (Eds.). (1997). *Goodman and Gilman's the pharmacological basis of therapeutics* (9th ed.). New York: McGraw-Hill.

Hobson, D. E., Pourcher, E., & Martin, W. R. (1999). Ropinirole and pramipexole, the new agonists. *Canadian Journal of Neurological Science, 26*(Suppl 2), S27–33.

Hingtgen C. M., & Siemers, E. (1998). The treatment of Parkinson's disease: Current concepts and rationale. *Comprehensive Therapy, 24*(11–12), 560–566.

Kalra, S., Arnold D. L., & Cashman N. R. (1999). Biological markers in the diagnosis and treatment of ALS. *Journal of Neurological Science, 165*(Suppl 1), S27––32.

Korczyn, A. D., Brunt, E. R., Larsen, J. P., Nagy, Z., Poewe, W. H., & Ruggieri, S. (1999). A 3-year randomized trial of ropinirole and bromocriptine in early Parkinson's disease. *Neurology, 53*(5), 1162.

Kuzel, M. D. (1999). Ropinirole: A dopamine agonist for the treatment of Parkinson's disease. *American Journal of Health Systems Pharmacy, 56*(3), 217–224.

Lozano, A. M., Lang, A. E., Hutchison, W. D., & Dostrovsky, J. O. (1998). New developments in understanding the etiology of Parkinson's disease and in its treatment. *Current Opinions in Neurobiology, 8*(6), 783–790.

Micek, S. T., & Ernst, M. E. (1999). Tolcapone: a novel approach to Parkinson's disease. *American Journal of Health Systems Pharmacy, 56*(21), 2195–2205.

Miller, R. G., Anderson, F. A. Jr., Bradley, W. G., Brooks, B. R., Mitsumoto, H., Munsat, T. L., & Ringel, S. P. (2000). The ALS patient care database: goals, design, and early results. ALS C.A.R.E. Study Group. *Neurology, 54*(1), 53–57.

Piercey, M. F. (1998). Pharmacology of pramipexole, a dopamine D3-preferring agonist useful in treating Parkinson's disease. *Clinical Neuropharmacology, 21*(3), 141–151.

Porth, C. (1998). *Pathophysiology: Concepts of altered health states* (5th ed.). Philadelphia: Lippincott Williams & Wilkins.

Sethi, K. D., O'Brien, C. F., Hammerstad, J. P., Adler, C. H., Davis, T. L., Taylor, R. L., Sanchez-Ramos, J., Bertoni, J. M., & Hauser, R. A. (1998). Ropinirole for the treatment of early Parkinson disease: A 12-month experience. *Archives of Neurology, 55*(9), 1211–1216.

Tatro, D. (ed.). (2000). *Drug interaction facts* (6th ed.). St. Louis: Facts and Comparisons.

Ting, R. M., & Force, R. W. (1998). Pramipexole for Parkinson's disease. *Journal of Family Practice, 46*(1), 19–20.

Vickers, L. F., & O'Neill, C. M. (1998). An interdisciplinary home healthcare program for patients with Parkinson's disease. *Rehabilatative Nursing, 23*(6), 286–289, 299.

Chapter 23

DRUGS THAT STIMULATE THE CENTRAL NERVOUS SYSTEM

KEY TERMS

analeptics
anorectic
attention deficit-hyperactivity disorder
cataplexy
hypercapnia
hypnagogic hallucinations
narcolepsy
obesity
sleep paralysis

Learning Objectives

At the completion of this chapter the student will:

1. Describe the physiology of the central nervous system (CNS) as related to arousal and stimulation.
2. Describe the various therapeutic uses of CNS stimulants.
3. Identify core drug knowledge about drugs that stimulate the CNS.
4. Identify core patient variables relevant to drugs that stimulate the CNS.
5. Relate the interaction of core drug knowledge to core patient variables for drugs that stimulate the CNS.
6. Generate a nursing plan of care from the interactions between core drug knowledge and core patient variables for drugs that stimulate the CNS.
7. Describe nursing interventions to maximize therapeutic and minimize adverse effects for drugs that stimulate the CNS.
8. Determine key points for patient and family education for drugs that stimulate the CNS.

CNS STIMULANTS

Centrally acting stimulants

dextroamphetamine
methylphenidate
pemoline
cocaine
khat
betel

Anorectic agents

sibutramine

Adrenergic drugs
benzphetamine
diethylpropion HCl
mazindol
phendimetrazine
phentermine
phenylpropanolamine

Serotonergic drugs
fluoxetine
venlafaxine
sertraline

orlistat

Respiratory stimulants

caffeine
doxapram

The symbol indicates the **drug class**.
Drugs in bold type marked with the symbol are **prototypes**.
Drugs in blue type with no symbol are **closely related** to the prototype.
Drugs in **red** type with no symbol are **significantly different** from the prototype.
Drugs in **black** type with no symbol are **also used in drug therapy**; no prototype.

Many substances are used to stimulate the central nervous system (CNS). These substances, sometimes called **analeptics**, include drugs that are used for therapeutic effects and nontherapeutic effects, both legal and illegal. Substances with therapeutic effects are categorized as central, anorectic, or respiratory stimulants. Central and respiratory stimulants are generally used to stimulate the CNS, whereas **anorectic** agents depress the appetite. The central stimulants are used to treat narcolepsy and as adjuncts in the treatment of attention deficit-hyperactivity disorder (ADHD). The anorectic agents suppress appetite or the sensation of hunger, mainly through serotonergic activity or central sympathomimetic effects. They are used as adjuncts to diet and exercise in the short-term management of moderate to severe obesity. The respiratory stimulants are rarely used, but as analeptics they are representative of drugs that affect the brain stem and respiratory centers.

This chapter presents dextroamphetamine (Dexadrine), the prototype for centrally acting CNS stimulant drugs; sibutramine (Meridia), the prototype anorectic agent; and caffeine, the prototype respiratory stimulant. In addition, this chapter discusses core drug knowledge, core patient variables, nursing management, potential nursing diagnoses, and patient education related to the use of these drugs.

PHYSIOLOGY

The CNS is responsible for providing control systems and surveillance for many vegetative and conscious functions, including appetite, satiety, attention, arousal, activity, and respiration. The hypothalamus mediates appetite and satiety. Various sleep and arousal mechanisms are linked to the raphe nuclei and locus ceruleus in the pons and other parts of the reticular activating system (RAS).

The control of respiration occurs in the pons and medulla. Functional, structural, or lesional disorders may lead to disruptions in the usually smooth regulation of appetite, arousal, and activity. Figure 23-1 depicts a schema of the brain and shows the location of some regulatory centers involved in appetite, arousal, activity, and respiration.

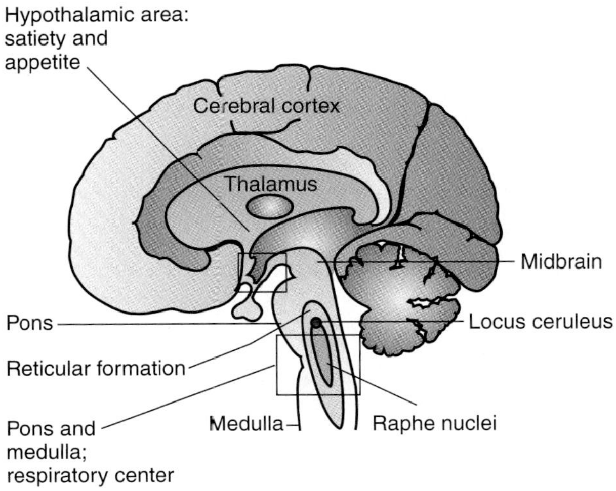

Figure 23-1. Regulatory centers of the brain.

At a synaptic level in the CNS, normal arousal mechanisms are effected through presynaptic release of neurotransmitters, such as norepinephrine, serotonin, and dopamine (Fig. 23-2). These transmitters diffuse across the synaptic cleft to the postsynaptic effector membrane, which is usually another neuron. The postsynaptic membrane contains receptors for the transmitters. In normal arousal, the transient combination of the transmitter with the receptor causes membrane changes and leads to propagation of the action potential. The transmitter can be metabolized by postsynaptic enzymes, such as monoamine oxidase (MAO), or removed from further activity through reuptake into the presynaptic storage vesicles. CNS stimulants may provoke an increased release of neurotransmitters, a decreased reuptake of neurotransmitters, or inhibition of postsynaptic enzymes. The result is a heightened postsynaptic response, leading to increased arousal. Similar mechanisms occur in the sympathetic nervous system, where drugs such as the amphetamines act as indirect adrenergic agonists.

PATHOPHYSIOLOGY

The CNS stimulants are indicated in various disorders and conditions, including narcolepsy, ADHD, obesity, and respiratory stimulation.

NARCOLEPSY

Narcolepsy, a neurologic condition that affects approximately one per 1,000 people, is characterized by irresistible bouts of rapid-eye-movement (REM) sleep during nonsleep cycles. Associated features include REM sleep disturbances, such as cataplexy, sleep paralysis, hypnagogic hallucinations, abnormal sleep-onset REM periods, and disturbed nocturnal sleep. **Cataplexy** is a brief, sudden loss of motor control. In the person with narcolepsy, cataplexy usually manifests itself as a postural collapse to the ground, even though the individual maintains full consciousness. **Sleep paralysis** usually precedes the onset of sleep and involves being unable to speak or move, even though awareness of external events remains intact. The elapsed time is usually brief but may seem inordinately long to the person who experiences it.

Hypnagogic hallucinations are the appearances of auditory, visual, or kinesthetic sensations without stimuli, occurring in the transition period between wakefulness and sleep. For example, the waking person may sense another person in the room but when fully awake recognizes that he or she is alone. Most people notice such hypnagogic hallucinations occasionally; however, they occur with greater intensity and frequency in patients with narcolepsy. Restoration of a more normal physiologic arousal leads to the return of more normal sleep-activity cycles, which forms the basis of CNS stimulant pharmacotherapy for narcolepsy.

ATTENTION DEFICIT-HYPERACTIVITY DISORDER

Attention deficit-hyperactivity disorder (ADHD) is characterized by a persistent pattern of inattention or hyperactivity-impulsivity that is more frequent and severe than typically

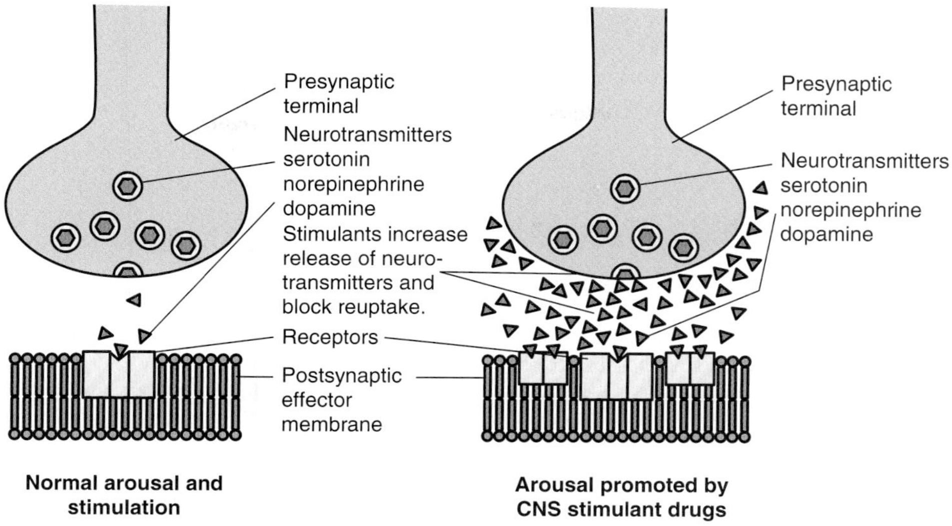

Figure 23-2. CNS arousal.

observed in individuals of a comparable developmental level. It afflicts between 3 and 5% of children and may persist into adult life at prevalence rates of 1 to 2%. Symptoms of ADHD include low frustration tolerance, short attention span, impulsivity, distractability, and usually hyperactivity. These symptoms may result in poor school performance and difficulty with peer or parental relationships. Some studies suggest that the etiology of ADHD involves a dopamine deficiency, because the three most effective stimulants for this disorder–dextroamphetamine, pemoline, and methylphenidate—all enhance dopamine concentrations. The management of the disorder may be complex but usually involves pharmacotherapy with one or more of the CNS stimulants. In people with ADHD, the stimulants act paradoxically and cause a quieting response. This allows for increased concentration and attention and decreased impulsivity and purposeless activity.

OBESITY

Obesity is an excessive accumulation of body fat. Generally, a person is considered obese if his or her body weight is 20% or more than his or her ideal body weight. Other parameters, however, such as triceps skinfold measurements (TSF), midarm circumference, midarm muscle circumference, and body mass index (BMI) are replacing crude weight measurements in the definition of obesity. For example, BMI is measured by taking the body weight in kilograms divided by the square of height in meters. About 32 million adults in the United States (25–74 years old) are obese (Table 23-1).

TABLE 23-1 Body Mass Index (BMI) Determination of Obesity

BMI	Description
25–30	Overweight
30–32	Mild obesity
32–35	Moderate obesity
>35	Severe (morbid) obesity

Children are typically diagnosed as obese when total body weight is more than 25% fat in boys and more than 32% fat in girls. The prevalence of obesity among children is uncertain, but it is estimated to be between 5 and 25%. Reports indicate that the prevalence of childhood obesity is increasing.

Weight regulation is multifactorial. Key endocrine systems involved in weight regulation include hypothalamic pituitary axis (HPA), the leptin system, insulin, neuropeptide Y, leptin-regulated hormones, and the autonomic nervous system. Although major endocrine dysfunction may cause obesity, by far the most common causes are overeating and a sedentary lifestyle.

Treatment of obesity is a combination of different modalities including modification of eating behavior, implementation and maintenance of an exercise program, and adjunctive pharmacologic therapy to reduce appetite. Drugs used to manage appetite include 5HT and norepinephrine reuptake inhibitors such as sibutramine, stimulants such as methylphenidate, lipase inhibitors such as orlistat, selective serotonin reuptake inhibitors (SSRIs) such as fluoxetine, and serotonin agonists such as phentermine. In morbidly obese patients, surgical intervention called "bariatric" surgery has been found to be most effective for long-term weight loss.

RESPIRATORY STIMULATION

In patients at risk for postoperative pulmonary complications, respiratory depression may be a complication arising from chronic obstructive lung disease and frequent hypercapnia. **Hypercapnia** is a buildup of carbon dioxide levels that may result from pulmonary compromise, frank lung disease, and changes in ventilatory efficacy. The increased levels of carbon dioxide depress the CNS, including the respiratory center, and further compound the problem.

Preterm infants may experience hypercapnia because of their immature respiratory systems. They are prone to postoperative respiratory depression and apnea severe enough to warrant pharmacologic respiratory stimulation. Pharmacologic management of respiratory depression includes administering CNS stimulants, such as caffeine and doxapram, that act directly on the respiratory center to stimulate effective ventilation and reverse hypercapnia.

CENTRALLY ACTING CNS STIMULANTS

The centrally acting CNS stimulants are drugs that stimulate the CNS directly or indirectly. This group of drugs includes the amphetamines, methylphenidate, pemoline, and cocaine (Table 23-2). Khat and betel are two naturally occurring CNS stimulants. The ideal and most widely used CNS stimulant is dextroamphetamine (Dexedrine), an amphetamine. This drug is the prototype for purposes of discussing the central CNS stimulants.

NURSING MANAGEMENT OF THE PATIENT RECEIVING DEXTROAMPHETAMINE

Core Drug Knowledge

Pharmacotherapeutics

The major therapeutic uses of dextroamphetamine include treatment of narcolepsy and ADHD and as an anorectic adjuvant in the treatment of obesity. Dextroamphetamine is occasionally used to treat refractory depression, although this is an unlabeled use.

Pharmacokinetics

Following oral ingestion, dextroamphetamine has an onset of 60 to 90 minutes and peaks in 2 to 3 hours. The sustained-release form of the drug peaks at 8 to 10 hours. The duration of action ranges from 4 to 24 hours, depending on the form of the drug used. The half-life ranges from 7 to 34 hours with an average of 10 hours.

Dextroamphetamine is metabolized by the liver and excreted, partly unchanged and partly in the form of inactive metabolites, in the urine. This process peaks at 12 to 24 hours.

Pharmacodynamics

The exact mechanism of action of dextroamphetamine is unknown, although it is likely that indirect alpha and beta adrenergic activity mediates both central and peripheral effects. Dextroamphetamine causes the release of norepinephrine and, in higher doses, dopamine in adrenergic nerve terminals. It also interferes with the reuptake of dopamine. The sites of action in the CNS are the cerebral cortex and the RAS. The drug's anorectic effects are likely secondary to CNS stimulation in the hypothalamic satiety-feeding center.

Contraindications and Precautions

Dextroamphetamine is contraindicated in patients with advanced arteriosclerosis, symptomatic cardiovascular disease, moderate to severe hypertension, hyperthyroidism, known hypersensitivity or idiosyncratic reactions

TABLE 23-2 Summary of Selected CNS Stimulants

Drug (Trade) Name	Selected Indications	Route and Dosage Range	Pharmacokinetics
dextroamphetamine (Dexedrine, Dexamin, Dexamyl, Delcobese, Obetrol)	Narcolepsy, attention deficit-hyperactivity disorder (ADHD) in children Exogenous obesity (short-term)	*Adult:* PO, 5–60 mg/d in divided doses q4–6 h *Child:* PO, 2.5–10 mg/d in single dose up to maximum of 40 mg/d *Adult:* PO, 5–30 mg/d in divided doses of 5–10 mg, 30–60 min before meals or 10–15 mg in the morning (long-acting form) *Child:* Not recommended for children younger than 12 y	*Onset:* 60–90 min *Duration:* 4–24 h $t_{1/2}$: 7–34 h
methylphenidate (Ritalin, Ritalin SR, *Riphenidate*)	ADHD, narcolepsy, postanesthetic shivering, narcoanalysis	*Adult:* PO, 10–60 mg/d in divided doses 30–45 min before meals *Child:* >6 y, PO, 5 mg bid to maximum of 60 mg/d	*Onset:* 1–2.5 h *Duration:* 4–6 h $t_{1/2}$: 2–7 h
pemoline (Cylert, Cylert chewable)	ADHD Narcolepsy and excessive daytime sleepiness	*Adult and child:* >6 y, PO, 37.5–112.5 mg/d *Adult:* PO, 50–200 mg/d in divided doses	*Onset:* 30–45 min *Duration:* 8–12 h $t_{1/2}$: 11–13 h (variable in children)
cocaine	Local anesthetic, hiccups, cluster headaches Ear, nose, and throat (ENT) surgery	*Adult:* SC, 1.5–2.5 mg/kg of 10% solution to total of 150–200 mg *Adult:* Topical gel, spray, or solution, 4% for ENT procedure or repair of dermal lacerations	*Onset:* 1 min *Duration:* 30 min $t_{1/2}$: 1 h

to other sympathomimetic drugs, glaucoma, or a history of drug abuse. Dextroamphetamine use in patients with these disorders places them at risk for hypertension, increased intraocular pressure, or abuse of the drug. Because of its pressor effects, dextroamphetamine is contraindicated during the first 14 days after the discontinuation of monoamine oxidase inhibitor (MAOI) therapy, because MAOI therapy itself may predispose the patient toward elevated blood pressure. Therefore, this 14-day washout period for MAOIs must be observed to prevent hypertensive crisis. Stimulant drugs should not be used in children with ADHD and concomitant Tourette syndrome or tics, because they will exacerbate the motor disorder.

Caution is warranted in older adult patients with even mild hypertension, because the adrenergic stimulation of the amphetamines increases blood pressure. When children take amphetamines, monitoring their growth and development is important, because amphetamines have been associated with increased growth hormone secretion. Moreover, growth suppression is common in children, although the two phenomena may be distinct. Dextroamphetamine is assigned to pregnancy category C, and women should not use it during the first trimester of pregnancy nor during lactation. If use is required during such periods, the provider should monitor treatment carefully to prevent fetal growth abnormalities or irritability in the breast-fed infant.

Some formulations of dextroamphetamine contain yellow dye No. 5 (tartrazine), which may cause allergic-type reactions (including bronchial asthma) in certain susceptible individuals. This sensitivity is rare, although it is frequently seen in patients who also have aspirin hypersensitivity.

Dextroamphetamine should be used with caution to avoid overdose and dependence. The least amount feasible should be prescribed or dispensed at any one time to minimize the possibility of overdosage. Patients should be advised not to discontinue therapy abruptly, because rebound symptoms may occur. As tolerance develops, particularly to the anorectic effects, the recommended dose should not be exceeded in an attempt to increase the effect. Instead, the drug should be discontinued. Patients who have recently ceased smoking cigarettes or using other products that contain nicotine may show a hypertensive sensitivity to dextroamphetamine, partly because of the absence of the vasoconstrictive toning effects of nicotine.

Adverse Effects

Dextroamphetamine produces the prototypical effects of all CNS stimulants: restlessness, dizziness, insomnia, and agitation. Other less common CNS adverse effects include overstimulation, euphoria, dyskinesia, dysphoria, tremor, headache, and exacerbation of motor tics and symptoms of Tourette syndrome. Anorexia and weight loss may occur as undesirable effects when amphetamines are used for ADHD or narcolepsy. Frequent cardiovascular adverse effects include palpitations, tachycardia, and elevation of blood pressure. Patients may experience gastrointestinal (GI) adverse effects, including dryness of the mouth, diarrhea, constipation, and an unpleasant taste.

Increased ocular irritation, resulting from decreased lacrimation, and mydriasis are two visual adverse effects that may interfere with activities such as driving. Occasionally, those with allergic tendencies may experience urticaria when taking dextroamphetamine. Finally, the pronounced sympathomimetic action of dextroamphetamine may lead to an inability to ejaculate and either increased or decreased libido.

Drug Interactions

Considerable care must be exercised when coadministering dextroamphetamine with many other classes of drugs. One noteworthy feature of anorectic drugs is their ability to cause rapid change in nutritional status, which may lead to cachexia and hypoproteinemia. This may alter the pharmacokinetics of other drugs. CNS depressants, if coadministered with CNS stimulants, will counteract each other and leave only residual adverse effects (see Table 23-2).

Dextroamphetamine may cause elevations in plasma corticosteroid levels beyond normal diurnal variations, which may interfere with serum or urinary steroid determinations. Dextroamphetamine use in children with ADHD has been associated with increased growth hormone levels and with hyperkalemia from rhabdomyolysis caused by the drug.

Maximal absorption of dextroamphetamine occurs in the alkaline environment of the small intestine. Therefore, acidic juices and fruits may impair GI absorption. In addition, foods that acidify urine increase the renal clearance of dextroamphetamine and may lower serum levels. This effect is seen with the anorectic influence of dextroamphetamine, because this prompts a form of fasting ketoacidosis and leads to enhanced excretion.

Assessment of Relevant Core Patient Variables

Health Status

During therapy, it is important to monitor for therapeutic effects, which will reveal the decrease in frequency or severity of target symptoms or the return of previously changed functioning. The nurse should evaluate the patient for advanced arteriosclerosis, symptomatic cardiovascular disease, moderate-to-severe hypertension, hyperthyroidism, known hypersensitivity or idiosyncrasy to the sympathomimetic amines, glaucoma, agitated states, a history of drug abuse, or a recent history of MAOI use. These are all contraindications for the use of dextroamphetamine. Dextroamphetamine must be used cautiously during pregnancy and lactation and by patients who have mild hypertension, are sensitive to tartrazine, or are undergoing smoking cessation.

Life Span and Gender

The nurse should ask if the patient is pregnant. If the patient is pregnant, dextroamphetamine should be used only if absolutely necessary, because it is not known if dextroamphetamine causes fetal abnormalities (pregnancy category C). If the patient is breast-feeding, monitoring the infant for CNS stimulation is important. If this occurs, the mother may need to discontinue the drug. Very young and very old patients may be at higher risk because of CNS adverse effects of agitation and restlessness. Monitoring children's growth is important, because dextroamphetamine may cause growth retardation. Children with ADHD and concomitant Tourette syndrome should not be treated with dextroamphetamine.

Lifestyle, Diet, and Habits

The nurse must support adherence to the drug regimen to enhance the patient's quality of life. People involved in shift work will need to adjust the timing of their doses to avoid sleep disturbances and to allow for normal appetite. Nurses must be aware of the high abuse potential for dextroamphetamine and should assess patients carefully for a history of drug or alcohol abuse.

Environment

Dextroamphetamine may be administered in any setting by health care providers, nurses, or patients themselves. Thus, the nurse must ensure safety of the patient's environment. When the patient is a child, it is advisable for parents to store and monitor the drugs.

Culture

In some immigrant populations, alternative therapies and drug use are a part of religious or cultural practice. Thus, it is important to determine the nature and type of alternative therapy or drug use to avoid drug–drug interactions and to maximize the therapeutic effects of dextroamphetamine.

Nursing Diagnoses and Outcomes

- Disturbed Sleep Pattern related to drug effects or caffeine use
  Desired outcome: The patient maintains normal sleep patterns through proper use of sleep hygiene measures and bedtime (hs) sedation.
- Delayed Growth and Development related to drug effects
  Desired outcome: The patient maintains normal growth and development profile.
- Disturbed Sensory Perception related to drug response
  Desired outcome: The patient remains free from sensory and perceptual disturbances.
- Imbalanced Nutrition: Less than body requirements, related to amphetamine abuse and anorexia
  Desired outcome: The patient maintains adequate nutrition.
- Noncompliance related to lack of motivation, poor self-image, or negative effects of prescribed drug
  Desired outcome: The patient adheres to the drug regimen.

Planning and Intervention

Maximizing Therapeutic Effects

It is important to administer dextroamphetamine with food in the morning and no fewer than 6 hours before bedtime, preferably longer for the sustained-release formulations. The nurse should inform patients and family members that improvements may not be seen until several weeks after the initiation of treatment. A great deal of emotional and psychological support is necessary during this interval, particularly because families often feel guilty about disorders. It is important to explain to the obese individual that anorectic agents are used only as adjuvants to supplement a combined program of calorie reduction, nutritional counseling and adjustment, and systematic exercise of large muscle blocks. The nurse can enhance support by encouraging the individual to attend self-support groups and psychotherapy. The nurse should explain that individuals suffering from narcolepsy, ADHD, or obesity will usually benefit from programs designed to foster and enhance self-esteem.

Minimizing Adverse Effects

In the event of toxicity or overdose, it is necessary to monitor vital signs and anticipate use of anticonvulsants and antipsychotics. Patients who are experiencing drug toxicity or overdose are vulnerable, and they must be placed in a nonstimulating yet supportive environment, where they are protected from self-harm or injury to others. The nurse should reassure the patient with drug toxicity or overdose, particularly because profound depression of systems initially stimulated by the drug may occur.

Providing Patient and Family Education

- An important component of health promotion is the encouragement and support of patients taking dextroamphetamine and of their families (see the accompanying display, Dextroamphetamine Therapy and ADHD). The nurse should ensure that patient and family education includes explaining the importance of adhering to dosing instructions, dosage scheduling, possible adverse effects, other drugs to avoid, drug storage, missed doses, abuse potential, and monitoring the effects of therapy.
- Cautioning all patients treated with dextroamphetamine therapy about adverse effects and the possibility of overdosing is important. The nurse should advise patients and their families about the management of adverse effects and when to consult with their caregivers if self-management is ineffective or if serious and persistent adverse effects continue. If toxicity or overdosing is suspected, it is important to decrease frequency of dosing.

Dextroamphetamine Therapy and Attention-Deficit/Hyperactivity Disorder (ADHD)

A family friend has a child who has been diagnosed with ADHD. The friend asks you what you think about treating this disorder with dextroamphetamine. Instead of giving an opinion, construct a patient-teaching plan to help this person understand the rationale for treating ADHD with dextroamphetamine. Present three topics for discussion with the family, and explain your prioritization of these topics.

- The nurse should encourage patients to avoid other stimulants during dextroamphetamine therapy, including caffeinated beverages, because these may lead to exaggerated CNS stimulation, irritability, and nervousness.
- The nurse must alert patients and parents or caregivers to keep dextroamphetamine in safe storage, out of children's reach.
- The nurse should advise patients to take dextroamphetamine early in the day, unless otherwise instructed, to avoid nighttime insomnia. If the tablets are sustained-release or long-acting, the nurse must advise patients not to crush or chew them. The nurse should tell patients to notify their health care provider if they experience nervousness, restlessness, insomnia, dizziness, dry mouth, diarrhea, constipation, or an unpleasant taste; a dosage adjustment may be necessary. It is also important to tell patients to avoid all other drugs (including over-the-counter [OTC] drugs) while taking dextroamphetamine unless they are prescribed or recommended by a health care provider.
- The nurse should teach patients and family members what to do if they miss a dose of dextroamphetamine. When the patient misses one dose, it is important for him or her to take that dose as soon as possible, but not later than 6 hours before bedtime for the short-acting form and not later than 10 to 14 hours before bedtime for the long-acting form to prevent trouble sleeping. If the patient does not remember the missed dose until the next day, he or she should skip the missed dose and return to the normal dosing schedule. The patient must never take double doses of the drug.
- The nurse should advise patients that dextroamphetamine may impair their ability to engage in potentially hazardous activities, such as operating machinery or driving vehicles, particularly if the effects of drug therapy are not yet known.

Ongoing Assessment and Evaluation

The nurse should obtain baseline patterns of growth and development data for children prior to starting CNS stimulant therapy to monitor and compare treatment effects. A full nursing history is essential to document any sleep disturbances, any evidence of seizure disorder, obesity, nervousness, depression, or any family history of endocrine problems. In addition, a complete diet history and normal patterns of activity and exercise are necessary to compare with treatment outcomes. The nurse should take baseline physical assessment data and should include height, weight, and vital signs. In addition, taking an ECG is important to rule out any cardiovascular abnormalities that CNS stimulants might exacerbate.

The nurse should ask the patient about his or her regular consumption of caffeine-containing drinks, such as tea, coffee, and cola, and whether he or she is taking any nonprescription drugs, particularly those with sympathomimetic effects. Checking the patient's history is important to rule out any contraindications to the therapy, including other drug therapies or drug and alcohol abuse. Patients often do not report the occasional use of OTC drugs unless questioned. It is important to monitor patients therapeutically, which involves the detection of improvements in mental and behavioral symptoms in children, decreased baseline rate of motor activity, weight loss, and decreased frequency of narcoleptic attacks. In addition, the nurse should monitor people receiving dextroamphetamine for the development of adverse and toxic adverse effects, such as hypertension, insomnia, irritability, hyperactivity, psychosis, hyperthyroxinemia (thyrotoxicosis), tolerance to dosage, and drug dependence.

The patient should show a reduction in symptoms or symptom severity. Patients receiving dextroamphetamines for ADHD should show improved attention span or decreased impulsivity. Patients receiving dextroamphetamines for obesity should have documented weight loss. Patients receiving dextroamphetamines for narcolepsy should have fewer or less severe episodes. The patient and family should show an increased understanding of how to recognize and manage adverse effects and explain how to store and administer drug therapy safely. ■

DRUGS CLOSELY RELATED TO DEXTROAMPHETAMINE

Methylphenidate

Methylphenidate (Ritalin) is an orally administered CNS stimulant that is chemically and pharmacologically similar to the amphetamines. It is clinically used in the treatment of narcolepsy and as adjunctive treatment in children with ADHD.

The CNS actions of methylphenidate are milder than those of the amphetamines and have more noticeable effects on mental activities than on motor activities. Methylphenidate shares the abuse potential of the amphetamines and is a Drug Enforcement Administration (DEA) schedule II controlled substance.

MEMORY CHIP

Dextroamphetamine

- Releases dopamine and norepinephrine in adrenergic nerve terminals and interferes with the reuptake of dopamine; sites of action in the CNS are the cerebral cortex and the reticular activating system
- Most common adverse effects: restlessness, insomnia, dizziness, overstimulation, palpitations, tachycardia, hypertension, dry mouth, unpleasant taste, and diarrhea
- Maximizing therapeutic effects: take with food in the morning and not less than 6 hours before bedtime
- Minimizing adverse effects: obtain a baseline nursing history and physical assessment to compare with treatment outcomes; important assessment items include sleep disturbances, nervousness, complete diet history (including use of caffeine), height, weight, ECG, and drug or alcohol abuse
- Most significant patient education: importance of adhering to dosing instructions, dosage scheduling, possible adverse effects, other drugs to avoid, drug storage, missed doses, abuse potential, and monitoring the effects of therapy

Pemoline

Pemoline (Cylert) is an oral CNS stimulant with pharmacologic actions similar to those of the amphetamines and methylphenidate; however, its sympathomimetic effects are minimal. Benefits to pemoline therapy include once a day dosing because of its long half-life and its classification as a DEA schedule IV controlled substance.

Pemoline is indicated for use in ADHD. Pemoline has been used off-label to fight fatigue in patients with multiple sclerosis (MS), as an alternative treatment for narcolepsy, and to fight fatigue associated with sustained military operations. Pemoline has caused hepatic dysfunction including autoimmune hepatitis, jaundice, and elevated hepatic enzymes and hepatic failure resulting in death. If no noticeable symptomatic improvement occurs within 3 weeks, pemoline should be discontinued because of its risk for hepatic failure.

Cocaine

Cocaine is used therapeutically as a local anesthetic. Its largest use, however, is as an illicit stimulant, which represents a significant abuse problem.

DRUGS SIGNIFICANTLY DIFFERENT FROM DEXTROAMPHETAMINE

Khat

Khat (pronounced "cot") is a natural CNS sympathomimetic stimulant from the *Catha edulis* plant, also known as qat, kat, chat, kus-es-salahin, mirra, tohai, tschat, catha, quat, Abyssinian tea, African tea, and African salad. This tall, flowering evergreen shrub grows in East Africa and southern Arabia, where it is widely used. In the United States, khat usage usually is seen among East African and Middle Eastern immigrants, particularly in large cities like New York, Washington, D.C., Los Angeles, Boston, Dallas, and Detroit, all of which have large representative subpopulations of these immigrants.

The active ingredients in khat are cathinone and cathine, both of which are structurally similar to dextroamphetamine. Fresh leaves contain both ingredients, whereas older leaves contain only cathine. The user typically chews a mouthful of fresh leaves, leaving the wad inside the mouth so that intermittent chewing will release further active components. Users report a mild euphoria similar to that experienced with amphetamine or cocaine but without the "rush" sensation. In addition to the euphoria, users report that khat sharpens and clarifies thinking and lifts the spirits; however, after the effects wear off, the user usually experiences a mild "let-down" or depressive mood.

Khat is used traditionally for religious and recreational purposes and is not considered a drug of abuse. Because khat is a sympathomimetic, users sometimes present with psychiatric symptoms from excessive use or with precipitated cardiovascular complaints. Under these circumstances, the nurse should complete a culturally sensitive assessment and ask about religious and recreational rituals.

Khat is freely available in shops and restaurants that cater to the ethnic and national groups of Yemen, Somalia, and Ethiopia, even though one of its ingredients, cathinone, is classified as a schedule I narcotic. Cathine, the ingredient that remains in khat after 48 hours, is classified as a schedule IV substance. Illegal drug trade laboratories have generated a synthetic variant of cathinone, known as methcathinone, or "cat," which has the same effects and uses.

Betel

Betel is the common name for the seeds of the *Areca catehu* palm, also known as betel nuts. Many people in the East Indies, southeast Asia, and the western Pacific use a masticatory mixture (betel quid or "pan") of Areca seeds, shell lime, and the leaves and flowers of *Piper betle* (a climbing pepper) as a euphoriant. The chief ingredient of Areca is arecoline, an alkaloid, which acts as a muscarinic agonist similar to pilocarpine. It has stimulant effects in the CNS, causing arousal and euphoria. Atropine can block its effects.

ANORECTIC AGENTS

Obesity is a complex problem that is very difficult to treat. Current views concerning the cause of obesity favor a disturbance in the hypothalamic set-point, which mediates caloric intake and use and energy expenditure. Although drug therapy is helpful, drugs alone cannot manage weight loss. Diet and exercise are equally important. Common agents used as anorectics include sibutramine, adrenergic drugs, serotonergic drugs, and orlistat (Table 23-3). This section focuses on sibutramine (Meridia), the prototype anorectic drug.

TABLE 23-3 Summary of Selected Anorectic and Respiratory CNS Stimulants

Drug (Trade) Name	Selected Indications	Route and Dosage Range	Pharmacokinetics
Anorectic Stimulants			
Sibutramine (Meridia)	Adjunct in obesity	*Adult:* 10 mg qd titrate to a maximum of 15 mg qd *Child* <16 y: not approved	*Onset:* Rapid *Duration:* Unknown $T_{1/2}$: 1.1 hr
benzphetamine (Didrex)	Adjunct in obesity	*Adult:* PO, 25–50 mg once daily *Child:* Not recommended for children younger than 12 y	*Onset:* NA *Duration:* NA $t_{1/2}$: NA
diethylpropion (Tenuate, Dospan, Tepanil)	Adjunct in obesity	*Adult:* PO, 25 mg tid 1 h before meals or 75 mg controlled release at midmorning	*Onset:* Within 1 wk *Duration:* 4–12 h $t_{1/2}$: 8 h
mazindol (Mazanor, Sanorex)	Adjunct in obesity Narcolepsy	*Adult:* PO, 1 mg tid 1 h before meals *Adult:* PO, 3–8 mg/d in single or divided doses	*Onset:* Within 2 wk *Duration:* NA $t_{1/2}$: 30–50 h
phendimetrazine (Adipost, Bontril)	Adjunct in obesity	*Adult:* PO, 35 mg tid; sustained release, 105 mg qid in AM	*Onset:* NA *Duration:* NA $t_{1/2}$: 2–4 h
phentermine (Adipex, Fastin, Minobese, Phentride, Obephen, Wilpowr)	Adjunct in obesity	*Adult:* PO, 24–30 mg/d 2 h after breakfast or 8 mg tid 30 min before meal *Child:* 12 y, PO, 5–15 mg/d	*Onset:* 1–2 wk *Duration:* Multiple dose, 12 wk $t_{1/2}$: 20 h
phenylpropanolamine (Dexatrim)	Adjunct in obesity	*Adult:* PO, 25 mg q4h or 50 mg q8h or 75 mg SR q12h, not to exceed 150 mg/d	*Onset:* rapid *Duration:* 24 hr $t_{1/2}$: 6 h
Orlistat (Xenical)	Adjunct in obesity	*Adult:* 120 mg TID with meals	*Onset:* 24–48 h *Duration:* Unknown $T_{1/2}$: 1–2 h
Respiratory Stimulants			
caffeine (OTC: Caffedrine, Tirend, NoDoz; prescription: caffeine and sodium benzoate)	Adjunct for analgesia (eg, headache), stimulant effects Postdural puncture headache Neonatal apnea	*Adult:* PO, 100–200 mg q3–4 h *Adult:* IV, 500 mg in 1 to 2 doses; PO, 300–400 as single dose (for postdural headache only) *Child:* IV/PO, 20 mg/kg as a loading dose, then 5–10 mg/kg maintenance dose	*Onset:* PO, 15–45 min *Duration:* NA $t_{1/2}$: 3–5 h
doxapram (Dopram)	Postanesthetic respiratory depression or postanesthetic shivering	*Adult:* IV, single injection of 0.5–1 mg/kg, not to exceed 1.5 mg/kg as single dose or 2 mg/kg as multiple doses at 5-min intervals	*Onset:* 20–40 s *Duration:* 5–12 min $t_{1/2}$: 3.4 h
	Drug-induced CNS depression	*Adult:* IV, inject priming dose of 2 mg/kg, repeat in 5 min and every 1–2 h until patient awakens	
	COLD	*Adult:* IV, mix 400 mg in 180 mL of IV infusion at 1–2 mg/min; do not use longer than 2 h *Child:* Do not give to children younger than 12 y	

NURSING MANAGEMENT OF THE PATIENT RECEIVING SIBUTRAMINE

Core Drug Knowledge

Pharmacotherapeutics

Sibutramine is used in the management of obesity, including weight loss and its maintenance. It is indicated for patients with an initial BMI greater than or equal to 30 kg/m^2 or greater than or equal to 27 kg/m^2 with other risk factors such as diabetes mellitus, dyslipidemia, or hypertension.

Pharmacokinetics

Following oral administration, sibutramine is rapidly absorbed from the GI tract and undergoes extensive first-pass metabolism into two pharmacologically active metabolites: M1 and M2. Sibutramine is rapidly and extensively distributed into tissues. It has a relatively low transfer to the fetus during pregnancy.

Sibutramine is metabolized primarily in the liver by the cytochrome P450 3A4 (CYP3A4) isoenzyme to the active metabolites M1 and M2. These active metabolites are further metabolized into pharmacologically inactive metabolites, M5 and M6. The primary route of excretion for M1 and M2 is hepatic metabolism; for M5 and M6, the primary route is renal excretion.

Pharmacodynamics

Sibutramine inhibits the central reuptake of dopamine, norepinephrine, and serotonin. Unlike other anorectic drugs, it does not release these neurotransmitters. Sibutramine's action on dopamine reuptake is less dramatic than its effects on norepinephrine and serotonin. It is thought that the serotonin mechanism enhances satiety, whereas the norepinephrine mechanism raises the metabolic rate. Sibutramine has no anticholinergic or antihistaminic activity.

Contraindications and Precautions

Sibutramine is contraindicated in patients taking other centrally acting appetite suppressant drugs or in patients who have anorexia nervosa because the drug is an appetite suppressant. Sibutramine is also contraindicated for use in patients with untreated or poorly controlled hypertension. Because sibutramine undergoes hepatic metabolism and renal excretion, it should not be used in patients with severe hepatic disease or severe renal impairment. Prior to prescribing sibutramine, the provider should exclude organic causes of obesity.

Sibutramine is a norepinephrine, serotonin, and dopamine reuptake inhibitor. The concomitant use of sibutramine with MAOIs is contraindicated. Because sibutramine substantially increases blood pressure and heart rate in some patients, it should be used cautiously in patients with a history of hypertension, coronary artery disease (CAD), congestive heart failure (CHF), cardiac dysrhythmias, or stroke.

Sibutramine can cause mydriasis and thus should be used cautiously in patients with closed-angle glaucoma. It should also be used cautiously in patients with a history of seizures. It should be discontinued in any patient who develops seizures while receiving the drug. Sibutramine should be used cautiously in patients with preexisting cholelithiasis because weight loss can precipitate or exacerbate gallstone formation.

Adverse Effects

Sibutramine is well-tolerated. The most common adverse reactions are anorexia, constipation, insomnia, headache, and xerostomia.

CNS adverse effects include dizziness, nervousness, emotional liability, and CNS stimulation. Cardiovascular adverse effects include tachycardia, vasodilation, hypertension, palpitations, and chest pain. In the GI tract, sibutramine may induce dyspepsia, dysgeusia, abdominal pain, and paradoxical increased appetite.

Because of its effects on serotonin uptake, sibutramine may have an effect on platelet function resulting in ecchymosis. Rarely, sibutramine may induce seizures.

Drug Interactions

Drug interactions with sibutramine may result in "serotonin syndrome" characterized by CNS irritability, motor weakness, shivering, myoclonus, and altered consciousness. This syndrome may occur when sibutramine is used in conjunction with dextromethorphan, ergot alkaloids, lithium, MAOIs, meperidine, 5-HT receptor agonists, and serotonin reuptake inhibitors. Drugs that are mediated by cytochrome P450 3A4 may also interact with sibutramine. Table 23-4 presents these drug interactions.

Assessment of Relevant Core Patient Variables

Health Status

The nurse should assess for disorders that contraindicate or require precautions with sibutramine therapy. The nurse should also assess for current or recent use of medications that may interact with sibutramine, especially MAOIs. The nurse should communicate positive findings to the health care provider prior to initiation of sibutramine therapy.

The nurse should perform a physical examination including calculation of BMI. Sibutramine is indicated for use only with morbidly obese patients. The nurse should obtain baseline blood pressure and heart rate parameters because sibutramine may increase both. Weight loss should occur slowly over time; therefore, the patient will receive this medication for a prolonged duration. Because of its prolonged duration of therapy, obtaining baseline laboratory tests is important, including complete blood count (CBC), liver function, and renal function tests.

TABLE 23-4 Agents that Interact with Sibutramine

Interactants	Effect and Significance	Nursing Management
dextromethorphan	Serotonergic effects of these agents may be additive.	Concurrent use is not recommended. If concurrent use is unavoidable, monitor patient for symptoms of serotonin syndrome.
ergot alkaloids dihydroergotamine ergotamine methysergide	Serotonergic effects of these agents may be additive.	Concurrent use is not recommended. If unavoidable, monitor patient for symptoms of serotonin syndrome.
lithium	Serotonergic effects of these agents may be additive.	Concurrent use is not recommended. If unavoidable, monitor patient for symptoms of serotonin syndrome.
MAOIs isocarboxazid phenelzine tranylcypromine	Serotonergic effects of these agents may be additive.	Concurrent use is contraindicated. Allow 2 weeks after stopping MAOIs before starting treatment with sibutramine. Allow 2 weeks after stopping sibutramine before starting treatment with MAOIs.
meperidine	Serotonergic effects of these agents may be additive.	Concurrent use is not recommended. If unavoidable, monitor patient for symptoms of serotonin syndrome.
SSRIs fluoxetine fluvoxamine nefazodone paroxetine sertraline venlafaxine	Serotonergic effects of these agents may be additive.	Concurrent use is not recommended. If unavoidable, monitor patient for symptoms of serotonin syndrome.
5-HT receptor agonists naratriptan risatriptan sumatriptan solmitriptan	Serotonergic effects of these agents may be additive.	Concurrent use is not recommended. If unavoidable, monitor patient for symptoms of serotonin syndrome.
cytochrome P450 3A4 drugs erythromycin clarithromycin danazol azole antifungal agents cimetidine quinidine diltiazem verapamil loratadine niacin propoxyphene	Concurrent use of drugs metabolized by cytochrome P450 3A4 may inhibit the metabolism of sibutramine, resulting in toxicity.	Monitor blood pressure and heart rate. Monitor for adverse effects.

Life Span and Gender

The nurse should assess female patients for current pregnancy or intention to become pregnant. Sibutramine is classified as pregnancy category C because adequate well-controlled studies with sibutramine have not been conducted in pregnant women. Women of child-bearing potential should use adequate contraception while taking sibutramine. The nurse should advise patients to notify their physician if they become or intend to become pregnant during sibutramine therapy. Additionally, it is unknown whether sibutramine or its metabolites are excreted in human milk; therefore, sibutramine is not recommended for breast-feeding mothers. Thus, the nurse must also assess female patients for lactation.

The nurse should assess for age-related considerations. In older adults, peak plasma concentrations are similar to those in young adults; however, dosing in older adults should be done cautiously, because of a greater frequency of decreased hepatic, renal, or cardiac function. Safety and effectiveness for patients younger than age 16 years has not been established.

Lifestyle, Diet, and Habits

The nurse should assess the patient's diet and make modifications to optimize therapy. Ingestion of sibutramine with food delays peak concentration but does not alter efficacy of therapy. Sibutramine is most effective when combined with a low calorie diet and behavior modification counseling.

Environment

Sibutramine may be administered in any setting by health care providers, nurses, or patients themselves. The nurse and patient should discuss the patient's environment to ensure safety.

Nursing Diagnoses and Outcomes

- Imbalanced Nutrition: Less than body requirements, related to anorexia
  Desired outcome: The patient maintains adequate nutrition.
- Noncompliance related to lack of motivation, poor self-image, or negative effects of prescribed drug
  Desired outcome: The patient adheres to drug regimen.

Planning and Intervention

Maximizing Therapeutic Effects

Patients should take sibutramine on an empty stomach to maximize peak concentration levels. They should take it only once a day. It is important to remember that sibutramine should be used in conjunction with a low-calorie diet and daily exercise routine for maximum results. Some patients benefit from writing a food journal to assess the amount of food intake and the types of foods consumed.

Minimizing Adverse Effects

Adverse effects are minimized when adhering to the contraindications and precautions for this medication. Refraining from using drugs that may induce "serotonin syndrome" or elevate the blood pressure and heart rate is especially important. At least 2 weeks should elapse between discontinuation of MAOI therapy and initiation of sibutramine therapy. Similarly, at least 2 weeks should elapse after stopping sibutramine therapy and starting MAOI therapy. It is also important to take precautions to avoid pregnancy and to contact the health care provider immediately should the patient become pregnant.

Providing Patient and Family Education

- An important component of health promotion is encouragement and support of the patient's commitment to weight loss. The nurse should remind the patient that sibutramine is only one component in the recipe for weight loss. Behavior modification and exercise are equally important to reach the patient's goal.
- The nurse should educate the patient and family regarding drugs that may interact with sibutramine and encourage the patient to contact the health care provider before adding any daily medications, even OTC drugs.
- The nurse should also instruct the patient regarding possible adverse effects to sibutramine therapy, especially the potential for hypertension. When possible the nurse should teach the patient and family how to take blood pressure and pulse.
- When working with women, the nurse must discuss contraception and the importance of notifying the health care provider should the patient become pregnant. The nurse should also discuss the need to refrain from sibutramine therapy if the patient is breastfeeding.

Ongoing Assessment and Evaluation

The nurse should calculate BMI at each follow-up visit in addition to obtaining gross weight measurement. Assessment of vital signs is equally important, with a focus on blood pressure and heart rate. When possible, the nurse should review the patient's food journal and assess the progress of the patient's behavior modification. The nurse should also reinforce the need for daily exercise to compliment sibutramine therapy. Finally, the nurse should arrange for serial laboratory tests including a CBC, liver function, and renal function tests.

Evaluating the patient routinely is important to assess progress. With sibutramine therapy, an adequate diet, and regular exercise, the patient should lose between 8 to 10 pounds per month. The patient should not remain on sibutramine therapy if weight loss does not occur. The time frame will depend on the individual's specific variables. ■

DRUGS CLOSELY RELATED TO SIBUTRAMINE

Adrenergic Drugs

The adrenergic drugs are primarily phenethylamines—drugs similar to amphetamine. These drugs were created by altering the side chain and ring structure of amphetamines to produce drugs with appetite-suppressing effects but markedly lower risks for CNS stimulation and abuse. Their mechanism of action is not fully known, but it is thought that they

MEMORY CHIP

Sibutramine

- Used only for patients with a body mass index diagnostic for morbid obesity
- Inhibits dopamine, norepinephrine, and serotonin
- Significant contraindications: uncontrolled hypertension
- Most significant adverse effects: "serotonin syndrome" and hypertension
- Most significant patient education: drug must be used in conjunction with a low-calorie diet and exercise plan

directly stimulate the satiety center in the hypothalamus. These drugs include benzphetamine (Didrex), diethylpropion (Tenuate), mazindol (Mazanor, Sanorex), phendimetrazine (Adipost, Bontril), phentermine (Adipex-P), and phenylpropanolamine (Dexatrim). With the exception of phenylpropanolamine, these drugs require a prescription. (See Chapter 35, Drugs Affecting the Upper Respiratory System, for more information on phenylpropanolamine.)

Serotonergic Drugs

Anorectic drugs that affect the serotonergic receptors in the brain include SSRIs, typically approved only as antidepressants. They do, however, induce weight loss in the short term. Fluoxetine (Prozac) is the SSRI known best for its ability to induce anorexia. Other SSRI drugs in this class that cause anorexia are venlafaxine (Effexor) and sertraline (Zoloft). These drugs are discussed in depth in Chapter 18.

DRUG SIGNIFICANTLY DIFFERENT FROM P SIBUTRAMINE

Orlistat is a GI lipase inhibitor indicated for weight loss and subsequent weight maintenance in morbidly obese patients. As with sibutramine, orlistat is used in conjunction with a reduced-calorie diet and physical activity. Orlistat works nonsystemically to block the absorption of dietary fat by approximately 30%. A thorough discussion of orlistat appears in Chapter 36.

C RESPIRATORY STIMULANTS

Respiratory stimulants are used for the management of postsurgical respiratory depression and apnea in preterm neonates. The primary respiratory stimulants are caffeine and doxapram (see Table 23-3). Caffeine is the prototype respiratory stimulant. It is used to manage postsurgical respiratory depression and apnea in preterm neonates. Because of its CNS stimulation, it is also used to maintain alertness and decrease fatigue. Caffeine is also used nontherapeutically in foods such as cocoa and chocolate and in beverages such as coffee, tea, and colas. It is chemically related to theophylline and possesses some bronchodilatory effects.

NURSING MANAGEMENT OF THE PATIENT RECEIVING P CAFFEINE

Core Drug Knowledge

Pharmacotherapeutics

Caffeine is used in the management of neonatal apnea, asthma, drowsiness, and fatigue. It is used in combination with many other drugs such as aspirin, acetaminophen, propoxyphene, and butalbital for treatment of migraine and other types of headache. Caffeine is also sold without a prescription in products marketed to treat drowsiness or mild water-weight gain.

Pharmacokinetics

Caffeine may be administered orally and intravenously. Orally administered caffeine in an adult is well absorbed from the GI tract, reaching peak plasma concentrations within 50 to 75 minutes. In neonates, oral administration results in peak concentrations in 30 to 120 minutes. Formula feedings do not affect the time to maximum concentrations after oral dosing. Caffeine is distributed rapidly to all body tissues and readily crosses the blood–brain and placental barriers. It is distributed into breast milk.

In adults, caffeine is partially metabolized in the liver. Caffeine metabolism in neonates is limited because of their immature hepatic enzyme systems. Unchanged caffeine and its metabolites are excreted in the urine.

Pharmacodynamics

Caffeine is a mild, direct stimulant at all levels of the CNS and also stimulates the cardiovascular system. Caffeine also stimulates the medullary respiratory center and relaxes bronchial smooth muscle. Caffeine stimulates voluntary muscle and gastric acid secretion, increases renal blood flow, and is a mild diuretic. Caffeine is preferred over theophylline in neonates because of the ease of once per day administration, reliable oral absorption, and a wide therapeutic window. The cellular mechanism of action is unclear.

Contraindications and Precautions

Caffeine should be used cautiously in patients with anxiety disorders, panic disorder, or both because, as a CNS stimulant, it can aggravate these conditions. Caffeine is contraindicated for patients suffering from insomnia because insomnia is one of its most frequent adverse effects. In overdoses, caffeine has been associated with seizures; therefore, it should be prescribed cautiously to patients with a seizure disorder.

Caffeine may stimulate the force of contraction and increase heart rate and blood pressure. It may also increase left ventricular output and stroke volume. Patients who have cardiac disease, angina, hypertension, or a history of cardiac dysrhythmias should be given caffeine cautiously. Patients should not take caffeine within 14 days of a myocardial infarction (MI).

Patients with chronic disorders such as diabetes mellitus, hyperthyroidism, and peptic ulcer disease should not receive or should minimize their intake of caffeine. In patients with diabetes, caffeine can either increase or decrease blood sugar. In neonates, both hypoglycemia and hyperglycemia have been observed with the use of caffeine. In patients with hyperthyroidism, the stimulatory effects of caffeine can be augmented. Because caffeine can stimulate gastric secretions, it may also aggravate stomach ulcerations.

Caffeine should be used cautiously in patients with hepatic disease or hepatic impairment. Caffeine clearance may be delayed, leading to toxicity. In neonates, who have underdeveloped hepatic metabolism, this is especially important. Additionally, renal impairment in premature neonates may delay caffeine clearance, as caffeine elimination depends more on renal clearance in neonates than in older infants or adults.

Adverse Effects

Many adverse reactions to caffeine are an extension of caffeine's pharmacologic actions. Caffeine can cause tremor, sinus tachycardia, and heightened attentiveness. Other adverse reactions include diarrhea, excitement, irritability, insomnia, headache, muscle twitches, and palpitations. Because caffeine is a mild diuretic, polyuria is a possibility.

Cardiac arrhythmias, seizures, and delirium are possible after deliberate overdoses. In neonates, intolerance or overdose of caffeine may manifest as tachypnea, hyperglycemia, azotemia, fever, or seizures.

High caffeine intake has been reported to cause spermatogenesis inhibition in male animals. Adverse effects may also occur when a patient abruptly discontinues use of caffeine. Caffeine withdrawal syndrome is characterized by lethargy, anxiety, dizziness, or headache.

Drug Interactions

Caffeine has many potential drug-drug interactions including oral contraceptives, psychostimulants, sympathomimetic agents, fluoroquinolone antibiotics, lithium, and MAOIs. Caffeine may also interact with grapefruit juice. Table 23-5 presents these potential drug interactions.

Assessment of Relevant Core Patient Variables

Health Status

The nurse should assess for disorders that contraindicate or require precautions with caffeine therapy. The nurse should also assess for current or recent use of medications that may interact with caffeine, especially MAOIs and sympathomimetic drugs. Assessing for the use of OTC drugs is important because many of these drugs have sympathomimetic ingredients. The nurse should communicate positive findings to the health care provider prior to initiation of caffeine therapy.

The nurse should obtain baseline vital signs. When caffeine is used for respiratory depression or neonatal apnea, appropriate monitoring equipment should be implemented.

TABLE 23-5 Agents that Interact with Caffeine

Interactants	Effect and Significance	Nursing Management
oral contraceptives	Serum concentrations of caffeine may be increased during concurrent administration with oral contraceptives.	Monitor for nausea or tremors. Limit caffeine intake with oral contraceptives.
fluoroquinolone antibiotics ciprofloxacin levofloxacin norfloxacin enoxacin	Fluoroquinolone antibiotics decrease the clearance of caffeine, resulting in the potential for caffeine toxicity.	Avoid concomitant use of caffeine with fluoroquinolone antibiotics if possible. Monitor for caffeine toxicity.
lithium	Caffeine reduces serum lithium concentration.	Monitor serum lithium levels. Counsel patients taking lithium regarding caffeine intake.
MAOIs	Dangerous cardiac arrhythmias or severe hypertension may occur because of potentiation of sympathomimetic effects.	Do not administer caffeine within 2 weeks of MAOI therapy. Counsel patient taking MAOIs of potential adverse effect with caffeine.
phenylpropanolamine	A combination of caffeine and phenylpropanolamine has resulted in cerebrovascular accident.	Do not combine these agents.
psychostimulants dextroamphetamine methylphenidate modafinil nicotine pemoline pseudoephedrine sympathomimetic agents	When combined with any of these medications, an additive effect may occur resulting in nervousness, irritability, insomnia, or cardiac arrhythmias.	Avoid these combinations when possible. Monitor blood pressure and heart rate. Monitor for adverse effects.

Life Span and Gender

The nurse should ask about the patient's desire to become pregnant or whether she is already pregnant. Couples who are pursuing pregnancy should probably limit excessive intake of caffeine. Caffeine drug products are generally classified in FDA pregnancy category B; however, injectable forms are classified in FDA pregnancy risk category C, because caffeine easily crosses the placenta. It is generally recommended that pregnant women avoid the intake of caffeine-containing beverages (e.g., coffee, teas, colas) or limit their use to no more than one or two caffeine-containing beverages per day. Likewise, pregnant women should limit use of caffeine-containing medications to only when absolutely necessary.

The American Academy of Pediatrics generally considers the usual use of caffeinated beverages to be compatible with lactation. Lactating women should use caffeine-containing drug products cautiously because of their high caffeine content. When breast-fed infants are prescribed caffeine for apnea, their mothers should avoid the use of caffeine.

In neonates, there is a possible association between the use of methylxanthines like caffeine and the development of necrotizing enterocolitis. All preterm neonates treated with caffeine should be monitored for the development of gastric adverse effects such as abdominal distension, vomiting, bloody stools, and lethargy. In addition, monitoring of serum caffeine levels is recommended. Neonates should receive caffeine without sodium benzoate.

The benzoate may displace bilirubin and induce kernicterus. In addition, elevated serum concentrations of benzoate have been associated with neurologic disturbances such as hypotension, gasping respiration, and metabolic acidosis.

Lifestyle, Diet, and Habits

Caffeine is found in many foods and beverages. To avoid toxicity, patients should limit their intake of these foods while taking drugs that contain caffeine. To avoid caffeine withdrawal syndrome, patients should decrease their intake of caffeine daily rather than stop caffeine ingestion abruptly. Patients should never take caffeine tablets with grapefruit juice, because it increases the effects of caffeine.

Environment

Oral preparations of caffeine may be administered in any setting by health care providers, nurses, or patients themselves. When used for respiratory depression or neonatal apnea, injectable caffeine must be administered in a monitored setting with appropriate life-sustaining equipment available.

Nursing Diagnoses and Outcomes

- Disturbed Sleep Pattern related to insomnia
  Desired outcome: The patient will maintain adequate sleep/rest cycles.
- Anxiety related to stimulatory effects of caffeine
  Desired outcome: The patient will remain calm throughout therapy.
- Deficient Fluid Volume related to diuretic effect of caffeine and potential diarrhea
  Desired outcome: The patient will remain well-hydrated.

Planning and Intervention

Maximizing Therapeutic Effects

The nurse should ensure that the patient takes the caffeine tablets or caplets as directed. It is very important that the patient does not take more than prescribed. If administering an extended-release form of caffeine, the nurse should advise the patient to swallow the tablet whole, not to crush or chew it. If administering chewable tablets, the nurse should advise the patient to chew well and then swallow. Consistent intake of caffeine results in tolerance to its effects. Patients obtain maximum therapeutic effects when they use caffeine intermittently.

Minimizing Adverse Effects

Adverse effects are minimized when patients adhere to the contraindications and precautions for caffeine therapy. Patients taking caffeine for its therapeutic effects should limit the ingestion of caffeine from food and beverage sources. The patient should also refrain from taking OTC products that contain caffeine, especially cold and cough medications that also have a sympathomimetic effect.

Providing Patient and Family Education

- The general public usually does not view caffeine as a drug. The nurse must convey to the patient that caffeine is a drug and as such may create serious adverse effects. The nurse should review the contraindications and precautions of caffeine therapy with the patient and family prior to initiation of therapy. The nurse should review potential drug-drug interactions and explain the importance of refraining from OTC drug use without the health care provider's knowledge.
- The nurse should instruct the patient regarding the potential adverse effects of caffeine and ways to minimize their potential. The nurse should inform the patient to contact the provider if symptoms such as anxiety or panic reactions, confusion, dizziness, lightheadedness, or fainting spells, fast or irregular breathing or heartbeat (palpitations), muscle

twitching, nausea and vomiting, seizures, or trembling occur.

- The nurse should alert women of childbearing age to the potential difficulty of becoming pregnant when they ingest large amounts (more than 500 mg/day) of caffeine daily. The nurse should inform men of the potential for spermatogenesis inhibition.
- The nurse should review dietary sources of caffeine and explain the importance of limiting caffeine from these sources while taking therapeutic caffeine. The nurse should also discuss the interaction between caffeine and grapefruit juice to avoid caffeine toxicity.

Ongoing Assessment and Evaluation

Caffeine is indicated for short-term or intermittent therapy. When used for respiratory depression or neonatal apnea, the nurse should monitor the patient's vital signs carefully. When administering for migraine or other types of headaches, the nurse should monitor for potential adverse effects, especially CNS and cardiovascular stimulation. Conversely, the nurse should also monitor for signs of caffeine withdrawal. ■

DRUG CLOSELY RELATED TO P CAFFEINE

Doxapram (Dopram), a parenteral analeptic agent, is used to stimulate postanesthesia respiratory depression or drug-induced CNS depression and for chronic pulmonary disease associated with acute hypercapnia. It has an unlabeled use for neonatal apnea. Doxapram works by activating the peripheral carotid chemoreceptors, thus increasing respiratory rate. It is not usually the drug of choice because of its narrow margin of safety. Adverse effects include hypertension, sinus tachycardia, arrhythmias, skeletal muscle hyperactivity, dyspnea, headache, dizziness, apprehension, disorientation, pupil dilation, convulsions, cough, tachypnea, laryngospasm, bronchospasm, nausea and vomiting, diarrhea, and urinary retention.

MEMORY CHIP

P Caffeine

- Used therapeutically for neonatal apnea, asthma, drowsiness, and fatigue
- Ingested nontherapeutically in cocoa, chocolate, coffee, tea, and cola
- Stimulates medullary respiratory center, CNS, and cardiovascular systems
- Most common adverse effects: usually an extension of its pharmacologic actions; caffeine withdrawal syndrome occurs with abrupt cessation after long-term or high intake of caffeine

CHAPTER SUMMARY

- The CNS acts as a control system and surveillance for many unconscious and conscious functions. Normal arousal mechanisms are effected through presynaptic release of neurotransmitters, such as norepinephrine, serotonin, and dopamine.
- The CNS stimulants are used therapeutically to treat several pathologic conditions, including narcolepsy, ADHD, obesity, and respiratory depression. CNS stimulants can be divided into three drug classes according to the specific effects they have on the body: central CNS stimulants, anorectic CNS stimulants, and respiratory CNS stimulants.
- The central CNS stimulants stimulate the CNS directly or indirectly, and drugs in this class include those that are used therapeutically and nontherapeutically. Those that are used therapeutically include dextroamphetamine, methylphenidate, pemoline, and cocaine. Those used nontherapeutically include amphetamines, cocaine, strychnine, nicotine, caffeine, khat, and betel.
- The prototype centrally acting CNS stimulant is dextroamphetamine. It is used to treat ADHD, narcolepsy, and obesity. Nursing management concerns regarding dextroamphetamine relate to prevention of abuse, adherence to the therapeutic regimen, and recognition and management of adverse effects.
- The anorectic CNS stimulants may directly stimulate the satiety center in the hypothalamus. These drugs include sibutramine, benzphetamine, diethylpropion, mazindol, phendimetrazine, phentermine, and phenylpropanolamine. Their mechanisms of action relate to adrenergic or serotonergic inhibition of the hypothalamic satiety center.
- Anorectic drug use is controversial and not effective as a monotherapy. These drugs should be used as part of an overall strategy to control obesity.
- All anorectic drugs, except phenylpropanolamine, are available by prescription only. They all exhibit a wide range of adverse effects.
- Nursing management for anorectic drugs should focus on careful pretreatment assessment, adequate therapeutic monitoring, and proper patient and family education.
- The respiratory CNS stimulants directly affect the brain stem and respiratory centers. Respiratory CNS stimulants include caffeine and doxapram.

QUESTIONS FOR STUDY AND REVIEW

1. When dealing with people from countries where use of khat or betel is endemic, what special knowledge must the nurse possess to manage care sensitively and effectively?
2. You have been telephoned by the daughter of your discharged patient, Mrs. Christo. Mrs. Christo was sent home last week with a diagnosis of narcolepsy and was taking dextroamphetamine 30 mg/d. Her daughter wants to know how effective this drug is. What questions would you ask her to answer her question properly?
3. You are talking with a colleague who tells you, "I must be allergic to my home. Every weekend I have a terrible headache. I feel tired, dizzy, and lethargic. I never feel this way at work. What could be wrong with me?"
4. Your patient has morbid obesity. She is prescribed sibutramine. What are the most important teaching points for this patient?
5. How do sibutramine and orlistat differ in their mechanisms of action?

Pain is a multidimensional, subjective experience encompassing the physiologic, sensory, affective, cognitive, behavioral, and sociocultural dimensions of a patient's life. By definition, pain is "an unpleasant sensory and emotional experience associated with actual or potential tissue damage, or described in terms of such damage" (International Association for the Study of Pain, Subcommittee on Taxonomy, 1979). Pain can truly be measured only by subjective data, because no objective finding is present in all painful experiences. Pain is "whatever the patient says it is, occurring whenever the patient says it occurs" (American Pain Society, 1992). Pain may accompany disease or treatment and may change over time. Pain may result from multiple simultaneous causes. If unrelieved, pain can affect the patient's psychological, social, physiologic, and spiritual health and prevent productive work and enjoyment of personal relationships. Despite the significant effects that pain has on health status, multiple studies over the years have shown repeatedly that health care providers undertreat pain, leading patients to suffer needlessly.

Pain may be a major indication for drug therapy, and the nurse will need knowledge of drug therapy based on core drug knowledge for prescribed drugs. Moreover, pain has a significant bearing on multiple core patient variables, which the nurse should consider during initial and ongoing assessments and evaluations of drug therapy.

PHYSIOLOGY

The peripheral nervous system and central nervous system (CNS) comprise an integrated system that provides a pathway for pain transmission. The physiologic mechanisms involved in the pain response are complex and are not yet completely understood. *Transduction* is the term used to describe the phenomena associated with the initiation of a pain signal. Pain receptors are found on the peripheral end plates of afferent neurons. Afferent neurons carry signals into the CNS, whereas efferent neurons carry signals from the CNS to the periphery. The sensation of peripheral pain begins in afferent neurons called **nociceptors**, which are found in the skin, muscle, connective tissue, circulatory system, and abdominal, pelvic, and thoracic viscera. Nociceptors may be stimulated by mechanical, thermal, hormonal (i.e., prostaglandins), or chemical (i.e., histamine, bradykinin, and serotonin, which are released during cellular destruction) stimuli. For example, with a stubbed toe, pressure in the surrounding tissue causes direct mechanical activation of pain receptors. Potassium, which leaks from the damaged cells into the tissues, then activates the inflammatory response, sending chemical mediators to the site of injury. These mediators are chemically caustic to the nociceptors. Stimulation of the receptors at the end plates then promotes cellular depolarization and the generation of an action potential.

There are two types of nociceptors: delta fibers and C fibers. Delta fibers are fast-traveling, myelinated, and responsive to mechanical stimuli. They sense sharp, stinging, cutting, or pinching pain. C fibers are slow-traveling, unmyelinated, and responsive to mechanical, chemical, hormonal, or thermal stimuli. They sense dull, burning, or aching pain. During inflammation, nociceptors become sensitized, discharge spontaneously, and produce ongoing pain. Prolonged firing of the C-fiber nociceptors allows cells to release glutamate, which has a role in the conduction of nerve impulses. Glutamate acts on specialized receptors in the spinal cord, known as N-methyl-D-aspartate (NMDA) receptors. Stimulation of the NMDA receptors causes the spinal cord neurons to become more responsive to all incoming stimuli, leading to a central sensitization to pain impulses (Bennett, 2000).

Once the nociceptor depolarizes, transmission of the pain signal has begun. Transmission is the process whereby the pain information is carried from the receptor end plate along the axon of the afferent neuron. Nociceptors enter the spinal cord and terminate in the dorsal horn, where they synapse in distinct regions. Substance P, a peptide in the unmyelinated fibers entering the dorsal horn, is released in response to painful stimuli. Substance P is a neurotransmitter and neuromodulator that activates special receptor sites. It appears to have a role in interpreting pain and regulating self-produced (endogenous) analgesic responses to nociceptor stimulation (Fig. 24-1).

From the dorsal horn, impulses are transferred, through the spinothalamic and spinoreticulothalamic tracts, to various higher brain areas for interpretation. Pain is mediated and modulated through forebrain mechanisms, which act at the spinal, brain-stem, and cerebral levels. The forebrain has the greatest control over nociceptor functioning. Indeed, pathology of the forebrain can cause pain, even if the nociceptors have not been activated peripherally (Casey, 1999). Multiple cerebral structures are now known to be involved in the perception of pain. During clinical studies of pain, brain imaging with positron emission tomography (PET) has identified some of the principal structures of this central network activated by pain. PET imaging has shown synaptically induced increases in regional cerebral blood flow in several regions of the brain when the person is exposed to painful stimuli. The intensity of the blood flow response in the brain correlates parametrically with perceived pain intensity (Casey, 1999). The areas of the brain involved in interpreting pain include the contralateral insula and anterior cingulate cortex, frontal inferior cortex, posterior cingulate cortex, bilateral thalamus and premotor cortex, and cerebellar vermis (Casey, 1999; Tolle et al., 1999). These brain regions are functionally diverse and involved with sensation, motor control, affect, and attention.

COMPONENTS THAT INFLUENCE PAIN

Pain is well known to have sensory-discriminative (physical) components and affective-motivational (emotional) components. The sensory dimension of pain encompasses pain's location, intensity, and quality. The quality of pain is the way it feels to the patient-for example, burning or gnawing. Affective aspects relate to the way that pain influences a patient's well-being, such as whether it is perceived as annoying, tortuous, or killing pain.

A study by Tolle et al. (1999) indicates that the different specific functions in pain processing appear to be attributable

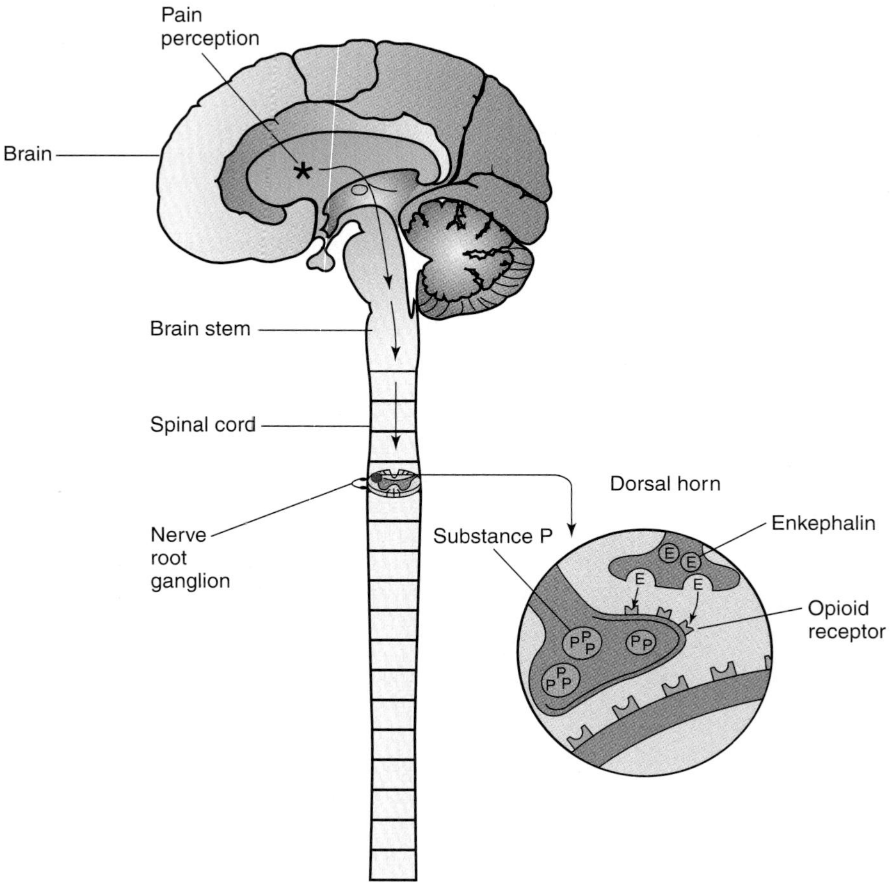

Figure 24-1. Inhibiting pain perceived over ascending pathways. Once the brain interprets a stimulus as pain, the nervous system responds along descending pathways. From the brain's perception of pain, an impulse is routed through the brain stem and into the spinal cord and travels through the dorsal horn to a dorsal root ganglion. Here, the impulses descending from the raphe nucleus system trigger the release of enkephalin (a peptide or endorphinlike substance). Enkephalin then stimulates the opioid receptors on the afferent neuron coming from the dorsal root ganglion. The release of enkephalin can excite or inhibit the release of the afferent neurotransmitters, which include substance P. If substance P is not released, the person will not sense pain. In some people, a sufficient release of endogenous enkephalin will change the membrane of the afferent neuron so that substance P cannot escape and cause pain. In others, exogenous opioids may be needed to achieve the same effect.

to specific brain regions. Pain threshold appears related to stimulation of the anterior cingulate cortex, frontal inferior cortex, and thalamus. Pain intensity is related to stimulation of the periventricular gray and posterior cingulate cortex. The feelings of unpleasantness or suffering associated with pain are from the posterior sector of the anterior cingulate cortex.

Other phenomena thought to influence the perception of pain are anxiety, fear, apprehension, attention, motivation, and other cognitive processes. For example, anxiety, fear, or apprehension appear to make the patient more sensitive to pain, allowing the patient to experience stimuli as painful when, under other circumstances, they might not. Conversely, the patient who is aware of his or her condition and wishes to control pain may deliberately use techniques (e.g., distraction by talking to others) to cope and decrease the pain experienced. Pain may delay healing and rehabilitation, prolong other symptoms, and leave the patient immunocompromised. Every effort should be mobilized to manage pain effectively, including stepped pharmacologic intervention (i.e., predetermined, progressive levels of intervention).

TYPES OF PAIN

Clinically, pain has been categorized as arising from somatic, visceral, or neuropathic processes or causes. Additionally, pain can be described according to its duration (e.g., acute or chronic) or underlying pathophysiologic cause (e.g., cancer). Differentiation of pain serves a critical role in diagnostic and therapeutic planning. Adequate pain management is based on accurate pain assessments.

Somatic pain results from ongoing activation of peripheral nociceptors found in structural tissues, such as bone, muscle, and soft tissue. It is characterized as well-localized, intermittent, or as constant, aching, gnawing, throbbing, or cramping. The bone and joint pain of arthritis is a common source of somatic pain. Muscle strains after intense physical exertion also result in somatic pain.

Visceral pain results from stimulation within the deep tissues or organs and surrounding structural tissues. Common visceral pain syndromes include pain associated with cholecystitis, pancreatitis, uterine and ovarian disease, and liver disease. Patients often describe visceral pain as deep, boring, diffuse abdominal pain. Visceral pain is less circumscribed than somatic pain and often has a referred component, such as pain from the liver, which can be referred to the right shoulder.

Neuropathic pain results from injury to the peripheral receptors, afferent fibers, or CNS. Neuropathic pain is unique in character and distribution. It can be described as shooting, burning, or stabbing and generally follows a radicular or radiating pattern. Several neuropathic pain syndromes may occur in patients with cancer. For example, direct tumor infiltration from adjacent soft tissues or lymph nodes or compression from metastases in the adjacent bony pelvis can damage the lumbosacral plexus. Postmastectomy syndrome is the result of nerve injury, with the development of a traumatic neuroma following surgery. It is characterized by a constricting, burning sensation in the posterior arm, axilla, and anterior chest and is aggravated by movement.

Acute pain, meaning the immediate phase of response to an insult or injury, results from tissue damage. It may be related to the treatment of an underlying disease process or to an injury that is expected to resolve. Medical procedures, operations, and trauma are examples of types of treatments resulting in pain. Postsurgical pain is the most common treatment-related pain.

Chronic pain is generally accepted to mean pain lasting longer than 6 months. In contrast to acute pain, chronic pain may persist well beyond actual tissue injury. Stress and other nonbiologic influences may exacerbate pain intensity, despite a reduction in the physiologic cause of the pain.

Cancer pain is one type of chronic pain. The pain is usually progressive as the disease advances to end stage and can be severe and debilitating. Additionally, acute episodes may occur, either in response to movement or activity or secondary to therapy or treatment of cancer, such as surgical removal of the tumor or skin irritation from radiation. Cancer pain may also be intermittent.

DRUG THERAPY TO MANAGE PAIN

When drug therapy is prescribed to treat pain, the pharmacotherapeutics and pharmacokinetics of the drug and relevant core patient variables help to govern which drug will be selected. Drug therapy may be used to correct the underlying pathophysiologic cause of the pain (e.g., nitroglycerin, a vasodilator, will be selected to treat angina pectoris from narrowed coronary vessels), or it may be used to decrease the pain response itself (e.g., morphine, codeine for postsurgical pain). The degree of pain that the patient is experiencing affects the pharmacodynamics of **analgesics** (drugs used to treat pain). Experts now know that preventing pain is easier than decreasing pain. It is also easier to treat pain at low levels than at severe levels. Pain that is allowed to escalate requires larger doses of drugs to obtain relief. These interrelationships between pain and core drug variables affect the therapeutic management of pain.

Drug classifications that are normally used for pain management are the **opioid** analgesics and the **nonsteroidal anti-inflammatory drugs** (NSAIDs). The opioids derive their name from opium, because they are natural alkaloids, semisynthetic analogues, or synthetic compounds of opium. Opioids, or **narcotics,** as they are more commonly called, act on the CNS to interfere with the pain experience. Morphine is the standard drug of choice in this category, and all other opioids are compared with it when evaluating their efficacy. NSAIDs act in the peripheral nervous system, interfering with prostaglandin synthesis and preventing the transmission of pain impulses. Some drugs are combinations of these drug classes, and they act on both the CNS and PNS simultaneously. (See Chapter 25 for more information on NSAIDs.)

Some other drug classes are used as secondary pain relievers, although their pharmacotherapeutics indicate that their primary uses are for other problems. When drugs are used secondarily for pain relief, they are known as **adjunct analgesics** or **co-analgesics.** Using multiple types of drugs to treat the exact symptoms of pain experienced is similar to using a combination of drugs (i.e., those that are cell cycle specific and those that are not cell cycle specific) to treat cancer. The outcome is more effective than that of any one drug alone. Adjuvant drugs can increase the efficacy of narcotics or provide independent analgesia for specific types of pain. Other CNS depressants that are primarily indicated for other diseases and disorders can be used as adjuncts. Included in this group are drugs that have antiemetic (i.e., against nausea) or mild tranquilizing effects. These are frequently used in acute pain (e.g., postsurgical pain). Classifications of other adjuvant drugs include antidepressants, corticosteroids, and anticonvulsants. Antidepressants are the treatment of choice for neuropathic pain described as burning or numbing. In clinical trials, tricyclic antidepressants are the only antidepressant drugs proven effective in managing neuropathic pain.

Steroids are useful for treating short-term, severe, episodic pain, such as that associated with nerve compression. They are also used in the management of cancer pain to relieve chronic pressure-related pain states, such as progressive visceral distention, severe lymphedema, increased intracranial pressure, soft-tissue infiltration unrelieved by NSAIDs and opioids, and continuing nerve compression.

Anticonvulsants are important adjuncts for neuropathic pain, particularly that described as stabbing or piercing. The anticonvulsants are used in nonmalignant states, such as trigeminal neuralgia, sciatica, migraine headache, and various neuropathic pain states in patients with cancer. These agents directly affect the peripheral nerve conduction of pain impulses, which is completely separate from their central effect.

Finally, in addition to pharmacologic interventions to treat pain, nonpharmacologic methods may be used. These are not substitutes for analgesics, especially in moderate to severe pain, but they are valuable adjuncts to therapy. The effective use of nonpharmacologic measures may decrease the required dose of a narcotic, thereby achieving pain control while minimizing adverse effects. Nonpharmacologic techniques include cognitive strategies for relaxation and physical strategies that interrupt pain transmission (Table 24-1).

NARCOTIC ANALGESICS

Narcotic analgesics are required for conditions, disorders, or treatments that are accompanied by moderate to severe pain. The narcotic analgesics are the most effective drugs for pain management.

The degree of pain relief that is achieved may be expressed in analgesic equivalents, which is the dose of an analgesic required to produce the same analgesic effect as a 10-mg dose of morphine (the standard measure of pain relief). Some equianalgesic dosages are presented in Table 24-2.

The narcotic analgesics include opiate agonists, mixed agonist-antagonists, and antagonists based on their activity

TABLE 24-1 Nonpharmacologic Techniques Used in Pain Control

Technique	Summary Description
Relaxation therapy	Uses progressive muscle relaxation techniques, controlled breathing, and simple hypnosis strategies to help patient achieve physical and emotional relaxation
Guided imagery	Uses visual and auditory imagery selected by the patient and specific to pain-relieving or stress-reducing feelings
Biofeedback	Teaches control of stress through patient's ability to monitor and manipulate some aspects of the autonomic nervous system
Music distraction	Uses music that is selected by the patient for the purpose of distracting the patient from pain and focusing instead on rhythm, tone, harmony, and other aspects of the music
Exercise	Promotes blood flow and tissue oxygenation, prevents muscle atrophy and stiffness, assists in building muscle to stabilize painful joints. An exercise plan defined by a physiatrist is extremely helpful in very debilitated patients. Heat promotes increased blood flow to the affected part, whereas cold reduces swelling associated with the inflammatory response. Take care not to use excessive heat, which can cause burns. Try alternating heat with cold.
Transcutaneous electrical nerve stimulation	Attempts to "confuse" the pain signal by activating other sensory circuits
Massage (various types)	Alleviates muscle stiffness and pain by breaking up fibrous tissue in muscle, increasing circulation, and promoting normal elongation of muscle fibers

at opioid receptors. Although there are five known types of opiate receptor sites (with the Greek names of mu, kappa, sigma, delta, and epsilon), activity at only three sites (mu, kappa, and delta) occurs with the narcotic analgesics available. From a nursing standpoint, comparing strong with mild to moderate analgesics within the opiate agonist classification may be beneficial. This will allow the examination of two important opiate agonist prototypes: morphine (opiate agonist and strong analgesic) and codeine (opiate agonist and mild to moderate analgesic). Some narcotic analgesics have mixed opioid effects, being an agonist at some receptors and an antagonist at others. Pentazocine (Talwin) is a mixed narcotic agonist-antagonist and the third prototype that is discussed in this chapter (Table 24-3).

Narcotics have an important role in pain management and control; however, they are typically underused. Research has repeatedly shown that major contributing factors to their underuse is lack of knowledge on the part of health care professionals regarding pain and pain control and misinformation regarding the pharmacokinetics and pharmacodynamics

TABLE 24-2 Equianalgesic Doses* (mg) of Selected Narcotic Analgesics

	Administration Route			
Drug	Oral	IM	Rectal	**Half-life (h)**
buprenorphine	—	0.3	—	2–3
butorphanol	—	2–3	—	2.5–4
codeine	200	120–130	—	3
fentanyl	—	0.1–0.2	—	1–6
hydromorphone	7.5	1.3–1.5	6	2–4
levorphanol	4	2	—	12–16
meperidine	300	75–100	—	3–5
methadone	10–20	10	—	15–30
nalbuphine	—	10	—	5
oxycodone	30	—	—	—
oxymorphone	(none)	1–1.5	5–10	—
pentazocine	180	60	—	2–3
propoxyphene	130	—	—	6–12

*In measuring pain relief, the analgesic equivalent compares the degree of pain relief achieved with that obtained by a 10-mg dose of morphine (the standard dose)

TABLE 24-3 Summary of Selected Narcotic Analgesics and Antagonists in Adults

Drug (Trade) Name	Selected Indications	Route and Dosage Range	Pharmacokinetics
morphine (Roxanol, RMS, *Canadian:* M-Eslon)	Moderate to severe acute and chronic pain, postoperative sedation, MI, pulmonary edema	*Adult:* q4h; 10–30 mg PO, IM, SC, 5–20 mg q4–6 h; IV, 2.5–15 mg diluted slow push; rectal, 10–20 mg q4h	*Onset:* PO, varies; IM, SC, rapid; IV, rapid *Duration:* 4–7 h $t_{1/2}$: 1.5 h
oxycodone (Roxicodone, Percodan, Percocet: *Canadian:* Supendol)	Moderate to moderately severe pain	*Adult:* PO, 5 mg q6h	*Onset:* 15–20 min *Duration:* 4–6 h $t_{1/2}$: Unknown
fentanyl (Sublimaze)	Analgesia during anesthesia, premedication, induction, maintenance and adjunct in anesthesia	*Adult:* IM/IV, 50–100 μg 30–60 min preoperative; adjunct or postoperative, 50–100 μg/kg; oral, 5–15 μg/kg as lollipop (oral transmucosal fentanyl citrate—OTFC)	*Onset:* IM/IV, 7–8 min; transdermal, gradual *Duration:* IM/IV, 1–2 h; transdermal, 72 h $t_{1/2}$: $1\frac{1}{2}$–6 h
hydrocodone (Hycodan, Lortab)	Cough, analgesia	*Adult:* PO, 5–10 mg tid or qid for cough; 5–10 mg q4–6h for pain	*Onset:* 10–20 min *Duration:* Varies $t_{1/2}$: 3.8 h
hydromorphone (Dilaudid; *Canadian:* Hydromorph Contin)	Mild to moderate pain	*Adult:* PO, 2–4 mg q4h; IM, IV, 1–2 mg q6h; rectal, 3–6 mg q6–8h	*Onset:* PO, varies; IM, 15–30 min *Duration:* 4–5 h $t_{1/2}$: 2–3 h
levorphanol (Levo-Dromoran)	Anesthesia adjunct, moderate to severe pain	*Adult:* IM, slow IV, PO, 1–2 mg; may repeat in 3–8 h	*Onset:* 30–90 min *Duration:* 6–8 h $t_{1/2}$: 12–16 h
meperidine (Demerol)	Analgesia, PCA analgesia	*Adult:* PO, IM, SC, 50–150 mg q3–4h; PCA, 15–35 mg/h	*Onset:* PO, 15 min; IM, SC, 10–15 min *Duration:* 2–4 h $t_{1/2}$: 3–8 h
methadone (Dolophine; *Canadian:* Methadose)	Analgesia, narcotic detoxification and withdrawal	*Adult:* PO, IM, SC, 2.5–10 mg q3–4h for analgesia; PO, 40–120 mg/d as liquid for methadone maintenance	*Onset:* PO, 30–60 min; IM, SC, 10–20 min *Duration:* PO, 4–12 h; IM, SC, 4–6 h $t_{1/2}$: 25 h
Moderate Narcotic Analgesics			
codeine	Cough, analgesia	*Adult:* PO, SC, IM, 15–60 mg q4h for pain, 10–20 mg q4h for cough	*Onset:* 15–20 min *Duration:* 4–6 h $t_{1/2}$: 3 h
Narcotic Agonist-Antagonist Analgesics			
pentazocine (Talwin, Talacen)	Moderate to severe pain, anesthesia adjunct	*Adult:* PO, 50–100 mg q3–4h; IV, IM, or SC, 30 mg q3–4h	*Onset:* PO, 15–30 min; IM, SC, 10–20 min; IV, 2–3 min *Duration:* PO, 3–4 h; IM, SC, 1–3 h; IV, 60 min $t_{1/2}$: 2–3 h
buprenorphine (Buprenex)	Pain	*Adult:* IM, IV, 0.3 mg q6h	*Onset:* IM, 15 min; IV, 10 min *Duration:* 6 h $t_{1/2}$: 2–3h
butorphanol (Stadol)	Pain, anesthesia adjunct	*Adult:* IV, 0.5–2 mg q3–4h for pain; 0.5–4 mg for anesthesia; IM, 2 mg q3–4h for pain	*Onset:* Rapid *Duration:* 3–4 h $t_{1/2}$: 2.1–9.2 h

(*continued*)

TABLE 24-3 Summary of Selected Narcotic Analgesics and Antagonists in Adults (Continued)

Drug (Trade) Name	Selected Indications	Route and Dosage Range	Pharmacokinetics
dezocine (Dalgan)	Pain	*Adult:* IM, 5–20 mg q3–6h, IV, 2.5–10 mg q2–4h	*Onset:* IM, 10–15 min; IV, 5 min *Duration:* Unknown $t_{1/2}$: 2.4 h
nalbuphine (Nubain)	Moderate to severe pain, anesthesia adjunct	*Adult:* IM, IV, SC 10 mg q3–6h for pain	*Onset:* IM, SC, <15 min; IV, 2–3 min *Duration:* 3–6 h $t_{1/2}$: 5 h

of narcotics. Because patients' pain may be incorrectly assessed and improperly treated, the nurse needs to be aware of current advances in the measurement, classification, and management of pain. See the accompanying display, Pain and Pain Treatment in AIDS Patients.

STRONG NARCOTIC AGONISTS

Strong narcotic agonists include morphine, hydromorphone, levorphanol, oxycodone, oxymorphone, meperidine, fentanyl, alfentanil, sufentanil, levomethadyl, methadone, and remifentanil. The prototype strong narcotic agonist is morphine. The narcotic antagonist naloxone is significantly different from morphine.

Focus on Research

Pain and pain treatment in AIDS patients

Pain and pain treatment in AIDS patients. A longitudinal study. Frich, L. M., & Borgberg, F. M. (2000). *Journal of Pain and Symptom Management, 19*(5), 339–347.

The Study

In all, 95 patients with AIDS were interviewed every 6 months for 2 years (or until they died) to determine the incidence and characteristics of pain associated with AIDS. Overall, most (88%) reported pain, and more than half (69%) had constant pain that interfered with daily living to either a moderate or severe degree. The most common sites of pain were the extremities, head, upper GI tract, and lower GI tract. Pain was related to opportunistic infections, Kaposi sarcoma, or lymphoma. Fewer than half these patients used morphine, either in a sustained-release form or as a continuous IV drip, or other short-acting opioids in pain management. Based on pain intensity assessment, the patients' pain was insufficiently treated. Although some patients felt that their pain was not taken seriously, few were dissatisfied with their pain management. This contradiction may have arisen from a belief that some pain was to be expected or that the optimal effect of therapy was being achieved. Patients stated that they feared addiction to narcotics and therefore did not like to take them for pain management.

Nursing Implications

Health care professionals need to assess and appropriately treat pain in patients with AIDS, because pain is a likely occurrence. Patients with AIDS need more education about pain management and realistic expectations of therapy. Health care professionals must address misconceptions about addiction so patients can take doses of narcotic adequate for pain management.

NURSING MANAGEMENT OF THE PATIENT RECEIVING MORPHINE

Core Drug Knowledge

Pharmacotherapeutics

The most significant clinical indication for morphine is moderate to severe acute or chronic pain, including postoperative pain and pain that is nonresponsive to nonnarcotic analgesics. Morphine is also used in dyspnea associated with acute left ventricular failure and pulmonary edema; it is the only narcotic agonist used to treat the pain of myocardial infarction (MI). Preoperatively, morphine can be used to sedate a patient, relieve anxiety, facilitate induction of anesthesia, or reduce the amount of anesthetic needed. The sustained-release form (MS Contin, Oramorph, or Kadian) is used only for patients who require an opioid analgesic for more than a few days and need around-the-clock pain control.

Pharmacokinetics

Onset of analgesic effect occurs within 15 to 30 minutes and lasts for about 3 to 7 hours. Morphine is metabolized in the liver and gut wall by conjugation to glucuronide, which is excreted along with unchanged morphine in urine and breast milk. It is also excreted in the feces through biliary and enterohepatic recycling. It has a half-life of 1½ to 2 hours.

Pharmacodynamics

Morphine is known to be an agonist at the mu, kappa, and possibly delta, opiate receptors. Its actions are related to the distribution of opioid receptors; high densities of opioid receptors are found in the brain stem, medial thalamus, hypothalamus, limbic system, and spinal cord. Many other areas with opioid receptors are excitatory nociceptive pathways, which morphine inhibits.

The general action of morphine in the spinal cord is to decrease the release of substance P, which modulates pain perception. Some specific effects can be attributed to agonist action at specific opioid receptors. Generally, it is thought that mu receptors are responsible for supraspinal analgesia, respiratory and physical depression, euphoria, miosis, and reduced gastrointestinal (GI) motility. Kappa receptors are linked to spinal analgesia, miosis, and sedation. The delta receptors have been linked with dysphoria and psychotomimetic effects that mimic psychotic effects (i.e., hallucinations). The secondary pharmacologic effects of morphine, like those of other narcotic agonists, are related to various effects of receptor stimulation. (See the accompanying display, Secondary Pharmacologic Actions of Morphine and Other Narcotics.)

Contraindications and Precautions

The main contraindications to the use of morphine are hypersensitivity, preexisting respiratory depression, acute or severe bronchial asthma, and upper airway obstruction. Morphine should also be avoided in premature infants or during labor when delivery of a premature infant is anticipated.

Other contraindications for morphine given by injection or immediate-release oral solutions include heart failure secondary to chronic lung disease, cardiac arrhythmias, increased intracranial or cerebrospinal pressure, head injury, brain tumor, acute alcoholism, or delirium tremens. Because of its stimulating effects on the spinal cord, morphine should not be used during convulsions.

Caution must be used when administering morphine to patients receiving other CNS depressants, because chances for respiratory depression increase. Morphine is generally considered contraindicated in cases of head injury and increased intracranial pressure; however, when its use is necessary, it must be given with extreme caution. Morphine, like all narcotics, may obscure clinical findings; the likelihood of respiratory depression and increased intracranial pressure is greater when morphine is given under these conditions. Caution should also be used when morphine is required for older or debilitated patients or those with renal or hepatic impairment. These patients may have altered pharmacokinetic processes and are more likely to exhibit adverse effects. Dose reduction may be necessary. Caution should also be used if morphine is given to patients who are sensitive to CNS effects because of concurrent alterations in their health status (e.g., respiratory compromise from chronic obstructive pulmonary disease).

Secondary Pharmacologic Actions of Morphine and Other Narcotics

Provision of analgesia is the primary action of morphine and other narcotics. In addition, these drugs have a wide variety of other effects on the body.

- **Respiration:** Tidal volume is first decreased, then decreased because of reduced sensitivity of the respiratory center to carbon dioxide. Depression is dose related. Deaths from overdose usually result from respiratory arrest.
- **Cough reflex:** Cough reflex is reduced because of direct effects on the cough center in the medulla. This may be useful, or it may promote a buildup of secretions, atelectasis, and airway obstruction.
- **Hypotension and orthostatic hypotension:** These result from peripheral vasodilation, reduced peripheral resistance, and inhibition of baroreceptors. Effect is exaggerated in the presence of hypovolemia.
- **Euphoria, dysphoria, alterations in mood, feelings of relaxation, drowsiness, apathy, mental confusion:** These result from stimulation of opioid receptors.
- **Nausea and vomiting:** These develop from direct stimulation of emetic chemoreceptor trigger zone (CTZ) in the medulla.
- **Itching, flushing, red eyes:** These are produced by release of histamine.
- **Miosis (pinpoint pupils):** This results from stimulation of oculomotor nuclei, which increases parasympathetic stimulation of the eye. No tolerance develops to this effect.
- **Abdominal pain, cramps:** These occur from decreased gastric motility; prolonged gastric emptying time; decreased biliary, pancreatic, and intestinal secretions; and delays in food digestion in small intestine. Resting tone of small intestine increases.
- **Constipation:** This happens because of diminished peristalsis, increased tone of large intestine before spasms occur, and inattention to the normal stimuli for defecation reflex.
- **Biliary colic and epigastric distress:** These are due to the constriction of the sphincter of Oddi.
- **Urinary retention, urinary urgency, and difficulty urinating:** These develop from increased tone of smooth muscles in urinary tract and spasms.

Adverse Effects

The most hazardous adverse effects relate to excessive CNS depression and include respiratory depression, hypoventilation, apnea, respiratory arrest, circulatory depression, cardiac arrest, shock, and coma. The most frequent adverse effects of morphine and other agonist narcotics are respiratory depression, apnea, bradycardia, light-headedness, dizziness, sedation, nausea and vomiting, and sweating.

In addition, patients may experience cardiovascular adverse effects (e.g., hypotension, orthostatic hypotension, flushing, peripheral circulatory collapse); CNS effects (e.g., euphoria, dysphoria, delirium, agitation, anxiety, drowsiness, miosis, blurred vision, increased intracranial pressure); GI effects (e.g., abdominal pain, biliary tract spasm, anorexia, constipation); genitourinary (GU) effects (e.g., urinary retention or hesitancy, dysuria, decreased libido, impotence); and decreased cough reflex. Overdoses of morphine may be life threatening and should be treated with naloxone (Narcan), a narcotic antagonist.

Drug Interactions

Generally, providers can anticipate that concurrent therapy of morphine and any other CNS depressant may produce additive CNS adverse effects and significant clinical effects. Increased respiratory and CNS depression effects are seen when morphine is given with barbiturate anesthetics, monoamine oxidase inhibitors (MAOIs), amitriptyline, cimetidine, clomipramine, and nortriptyline. Because morphine increases biliary tract pressure, levels of serum amylase or lipase may increase. One study showed that the bioavailability of oral morphine increased significantly following a high-fat meal (Table 24-4).

Assessment of Relevant Core Patient Variables

Health Status

The nurse must assess the patient for respiratory depression. Morphine should not be administered to any patient with respiratory depression, because it may precipitate respiratory arrest. It should not be given to anyone with a previous hypersensitivity to morphine.

The nurse should assess for current alterations in health status that place the patient at risk for increased sensitivity to CNS depressant effects. These include cardiac, renal, hepatic, or pulmonary disease; hypothyroidism; Addison disease; prostatic hypertrophy; or urethral stricture.

Prior to therapy, the nurse should perform a physical examination to establish a baseline to monitor the drug's effects. The nurse should evaluate orientation, affect, respiratory rate, adventitious sounds, and character of bowel sounds. If prolonged use is anticipated or the patient has a history of hepatic dysfunction, liver function tests should be done, because morphine is metabolized in the liver.

The nurse should assess the patient for the presence and severity of pain. The patient's self-report of pain will determine these conditions. Pain is extremely subjective and unique for each person. The current health status can indicate whether pain might be expected. Physiologic changes that may bring on a pain response and indicate the need for drug therapy with morphine include decreased oxygenation of cardiac cells during an MI, inflamed or infected organs, or inappropriate cell growth from tumors pressing on nerves, vessels, or adjacent organs. Some health states are the source of pain for the patient, whereas others bring pain from their diagnosis or treatment. An example would be postoperative pain.

Life Span and Gender

In using morphine, the nurse must assess for some special considerations that are characteristic of all narcotic analgesics. These include those related to age, pregnancy, labor and delivery, and lactation.

For many years, experts believed that pain perception was absent or diminished in the very young and very old, but this has been found untrue. Pain is an experience that all humans perceive regardless of age. Inability to verbalize that pain is occurring, however, may impair assessment of pain in both very young and very old patients. The patient's age also influences the treatment of pain. Age-related factors are important when using morphine, because it causes respiratory depression and hypotension.

The very young have impaired organ and system functioning because of immaturity. Dosages of pain-relieving drugs, therefore, need to be adjusted carefully to the child's body size and weight to prevent overdose and adverse effects.

Older adults are more likely to have age-related deterioration of organs, especially the liver and kidneys. Thus, they are more sensitive to adverse effects and can exhibit signs of overdosage unless dosage adjustments are made for them. Older adults should receive a reduced initial dose. Their response should be assessed before additional doses are determined.

Morphine is assigned to pregnancy category C. Like other narcotics, morphine crosses the placenta rapidly. Pregnant women who abuse narcotics can cause fetal dependency; infant withdrawal will occur after delivery. If given during labor, respiratory depression and psychophysiologic effects may appear in the neonate. Resuscitation equipment and the narcotic antidote, naloxone, should be available. The premature infant is at even greater risk of significant respiratory depression from exposure to morphine. For these reasons, morphine should not be given during labor if the delivery of a preterm infant is expected. Morphine has been shown to increase the length of labor. Morphine will cross into breast milk. Although this does not usually

TABLE 24-4 Agents That Interact With P Morphine

Interactants	Effect and Significance	Nursing Management
barbiturate anesthetics	Additive respiratory and CNS depression; apnea	Monitor respiratory function.
cimetidine	Additive CNS depression, respiratory depression	Monitor for excessive morphine response and toxicity.
esmolol	Esmolol toxicity—bradycardia, hypotension	Monitor cardiovascular function (may need to decrease esmolol dosage).
other CNS depressants (alcohol, other narcotic analgesics)	Additive CNC depression, respiratory depression	Avoid combinations if possible. Monitor respiratory function.

produce serious problems, withdrawal may be precipitated in breast-fed infants if morphine is discontinued rapidly after prolonged exposure. Waiting 4 to 6 hours after dosing with morphine will decrease the amount transferred to the infant.

Lifestyle, Diet, and Habits

Morphine acts by depressing the CNS. Patients who use morphine to control chronic pain, such as that caused by cancer, or who receive morphine for an extended period will eventually need higher doses to control their pain as they become tolerant to the drug's therapeutic effects. **Tolerance** means that the body has become accustomed to the effects of a substance and that the patient must use more of it to achieve the desired effect. With morphine, chronic usage may result in a degree of tolerance up to 35-fold. Clearly, as patients develop tolerance to morphine, they will require larger doses to achieve adequate pain control. In addition to developing tolerance to therapeutic effects, patients also develop tolerance to adverse effects-including lethal effects-of morphine. Patients in whom drug tolerance develops can thus take dosages that would be potentially lethal in patients who are opioid naive.

Patients who abuse alcohol, prescription drugs that suppress the CNS (such as opioid analgesics or benzodiazepines), or street or illicit drugs have special needs when they have pain. When a patient abuses such substances, he or she may develop a cross-tolerance to morphine's pain-relieving effects. Thus, these patients also require higher than normal doses to achieve the desired therapeutic effects of pain relief.

In long-term (i.e., longer than 3 months) use of morphine, physical **dependence** may also occur. Dependence is characterized by a withdrawal or abstinence syndrome on discontinuation of morphine and represents an exaggerated rebound from its acute effects. Dependence may occur in the treatment of cancer pain, and it is important in the clinical management of such pain to allow for proper agonist coverage during changes in drug dosages, schedules, or type of drug therapy. Otherwise, the patient may experience unnecessary pain and the discomfort of abstinence syndrome. Physical dependence is *not* the same as addiction. **Addiction** involves compulsive use of the drug for a secondary gain, not for pain control. Patients who receive morphine for pain management, even over a long period, will not normally seek morphine once the pain stimulus is gone. They will need, however, for their morphine dose to be decreased slowly before it is discontinued to prevent withdrawal. Patients who currently abuse or have a history of abusing opioids do have a risk of addiction from drug therapy in pain management. This is not a reason to withhold morphine or any other opioid if the patient is experiencing pain. Instead, health care providers in cooperation with the patient can accomplish careful drug selection and dosage adjustment. If addiction does occur after therapy concludes, it needs to be addressed separately. Patients should be helped to wean themselves away from drug use prior to discharge from the provider's care.

Environment

The nurse must closely monitor patients receiving morphine as part of monitored anesthesia care (MAC) or postoperatively for signs of serious adverse effects, particularly respiratory depression. Health care providers or patients themselves may administer narcotic analgesics, as in patient-controlled analgesia (PCA). Morphine, like all narcotics, is a controlled substance, and by law every dose must be properly accounted for and documented. This includes partial doses that may be wasted. Although oral doses may be administered in any setting, doses given by intravenous (IV) infusion, injection, and epidural and intrathecal catheters are normally given only in the hospital where the patient can be closely monitored. The exception is IV infusions, which may be used in the home during hospice care.

Culture

The experience of pain is personal and subjective; however, how individuals respond to painful stimuli reflects what they have learned about pain from their families, society, and cultures of origin. Learned messages about pain are indirect, and people react to them subconsciously. They include why people experience pain and what are appropriate responses to it. For example, some religions view pain as a punishment from God for sins. Others view pain as a test from God to develop inner strength and faith. Still others may believe that pain is merely an aspect of life like any other. Some cultures are very stoic and believe that people should tolerate pain without verbal complaints. British, German, and Asian groups are thought of as stoic cultures. Other cultural groups are very expressive about pain, see such expressiveness as acceptable, and may encourage it. Spanish, Italian, and Latin groups are thought to be expressive cultures. Although not everyone who shares a cultural background reacts identically to pain, nurses should consider these generalizations when patients have pain. The nurse may need to validate the expressive patient's pain, or encourage stoic patients to take needed pain medication. For both types of patient, the nurse needs to offer support as well as pain medication. See the accompanying display, Thinking Critically about Drug Therapy in Pain Management.

Nursing Diagnoses and Outcomes

- Ineffective Breathing Pattern, Hypoventilation, related to respiratory depression caused by the drug

  Desired outcome: The patient maintains effective breathing despite respiratory depression.
- Ineffective Airway Clearance secondary to cough suppression by the drug

  Desired outcome: The patient's airway remains patent and clear.

Critical Thinking Scenario

Thinking critically about drug therapy in pain management

Mr. Schneider is 60 years old. He is a second-generation German American. He has worked for 35 years in a local steel mill. He had surgery for a bowel obstruction yesterday. When you assess him, he states he does not have pain, yet he is restless in the bed and moaning. He says he will take something for pain when the pain is very severe.

1. Discuss factors that may be contributing to the inconsistencies between the patient's verbal report and nonverbal behavior.
2. Propose a teaching plan that you think would help this patient with effective pain management.

- Constipation secondary to activity of the drug
  Desired outcome: The patient remains free of constipation.
- Urinary Retention related to indirect anticholinergic effects of the drug on the urinary sphincters
  Desired outcome: The patient maintains normal urinary output.
- Risk for Injury related to orthostatic hypotension or sedation secondary to drug effects
  Desired outcome: The patient remains free of injury.
- Acute Pain related to trauma or disease process and insufficient analgesia
  Desired outcome: The patient remains free of pain.
- Deficient Knowledge related to morphine therapy
  Desired outcome: The patient has adequate knowledge of the drug and its adverse effects and their management.

Planning and Intervention

The key issue in morphine therapy is adequate control of pain balanced against the significant adverse effects of respiratory depression and excessive sedation. Goals of treatment include adequate pulmonary ventilation, a respiratory rate within 12 to 20 breaths per minute, minimal effects of constipation and urinary retention, freedom from injury, and adequate family and patient education for managing drug therapy. It is also important for the nurse to teach the patient possible adverse effects of morphine and how to manage them. Other goals relate to maintaining safety during potential episodes of orthostatic hypotension.

Maximizing Therapeutic Effects

Assessing Pain

The first step in maximizing the therapeutic effects of drug therapy with morphine or any other narcotic is to complete a full pain assessment. Recent position statements by the Joint Commission of Accreditation of Hospitals (JCAHO) state that patients have the right to appropriate assessment and management of pain. (See the accompanying display, JCAHO Standards on Pain Management for Hospital Accreditation.) The nurse must remember that pain is a subjective experience. It is whatever the patient says it is, occurring whenever the patient says it does. Objective data, such as elevated blood pressure or pulse rate, moaning, or grimacing, may accompany pain, but the absence of objective data does not indicate that pain does not exist. Many people actually cope with pain by using distraction techniques, such as smiling, talking, quiet rhythmic breathing, or watching television. Every patient has a different level of tolerance for what he or she feels is an acceptable level of pain. Careful assessment enables the nurse to assist the patient in identifying and achieving this level of control.

To begin the pain assessment, the nurse first determines the location of the pain. Location gives possible clues to the source of the pain and can help identify whether the pain is acute or of a more chronic or ma-

JCAHO Standards on Pain Management for Hospital Accreditation

The patient has a right to appropriate assessment and management of pain. To meet this goal the hospital will:

- Assess each patient initially, and then regularly reassess patients in pain or who are likely to develop pain.
- Educate relevant providers regarding the current knowledge of pain, how to assess pain and how to manage pain.
- Educate patients that pain management is an important part of their treatment.
- Educate the patient and their families regarding their roles in managing pain, and the potential limitations and adverse effects of pain treatments.
- Consider the personal, cultural, spiritual, and or ethnic beliefs of each patient and then communicate with patients and their families in an appropriate way that pain management is an important part of patient care.

Pain assessment of patients should include the following:

- Pain intensity, using an intensity rating scale
- Location of pain
- Quality and character of pain
- Onset, duration, variation, and patterns of pain
- Alleviating and aggravating factors for pain
- Present pain management regimen and its effectiveness
- Pain management history
- Effect of pain on patient (e.g., daily life, function, sleep, appetite, relationships, emotions)
- Patient's goal for pain control
- Physical exam and observation of the pain site
- A separate assessment for each site of pain
- Pain assessment incorporated in the clinical pathway (if this is used)

From http://www.jcaho.org

lignant nature. Many pain assessment tools incorporate a representation of the human body from a frontal and posterior view. The tools ask patients to shade or circle on the diagram to show the location of the pain. Such identification helps the patient define what he or she is experiencing and provides a starting point for further assessment. Each pain location should be recorded in the patient's chart along with its associated intensity and quality.

The next step is to determine the pain intensity. JCAHO stated in 2000 that all hospitals must use a tool to document pain assessment. Many assessment tools are available to rate pain intensity (Fig. 24-2). Each tool provides a continuum in some form to represent a range from "no pain" to the "worst pain imaginable." Asking the patient to rate pain using an imaginary scale in his or her head is *not* considered a tool. One of the most widely recognized pain assessment tools for reliability and ease of use is the visual analogue scale, which is numeric. It may be a scale from 0 to 5 or 0 to 10, but both ranges allow patients to rate their pain by assigning a number that demonstrates greater pain as they move up the scale.

Because research findings indicate that approximately 7 to 11% of adults cannot conceptualize well enough to use the visual analogue pain scale, other pain assessment tools may be helpful. One alternative is a descriptive pain-intensity tool in which words replace the numbers 0 to 5, again with the two extremes being no pain or the worst imaginable pain. The FACES scale, used frequently with children, shows a series of facial expressions ranging from very unhappy and crying to very happy and smiling. The patient is then asked to pick the face that most resembles how he or she feels. In the poker chip tool, four poker chips are placed in front of the patient. Each one is a "piece of hurt," with one piece being "just a little hurt" and four pieces being "the most hurt." Patients are asked to show how many pieces of hurt they have. This technique is also widely used for children.

Each patient may interpret the extremes of any of the scales differently based on his or her past experiences. With consistent use, however, the pain assessment tool gives the patient and the provider a common ground on which to plan treatment and understand the degree of relief from the treatments provided.

Intensity of pain is only one aspect of pain that should be assessed. JCAHO has also stated that pain quality and character (affective descriptions) should be measured. Not all pain assessment tools currently available assess for all these parameters. Some tools, such as the Pain-O-Meter (Gaston-Johansson, 1996), do measure severity, quality, and affective parameters. The Pain-O-Meter is a hand-held device with a sliding pointer that moves between the words "no pain" and "worst possible pain." On the back are two sections of words; one section describes the qualitative aspects of pain, whereas the other describes the affective aspects. Patients select at least one word from each section that describes current pain. The words have quality points assigned to them from 1 to 5. Patients who have no pain or do not select a word from a section receive no

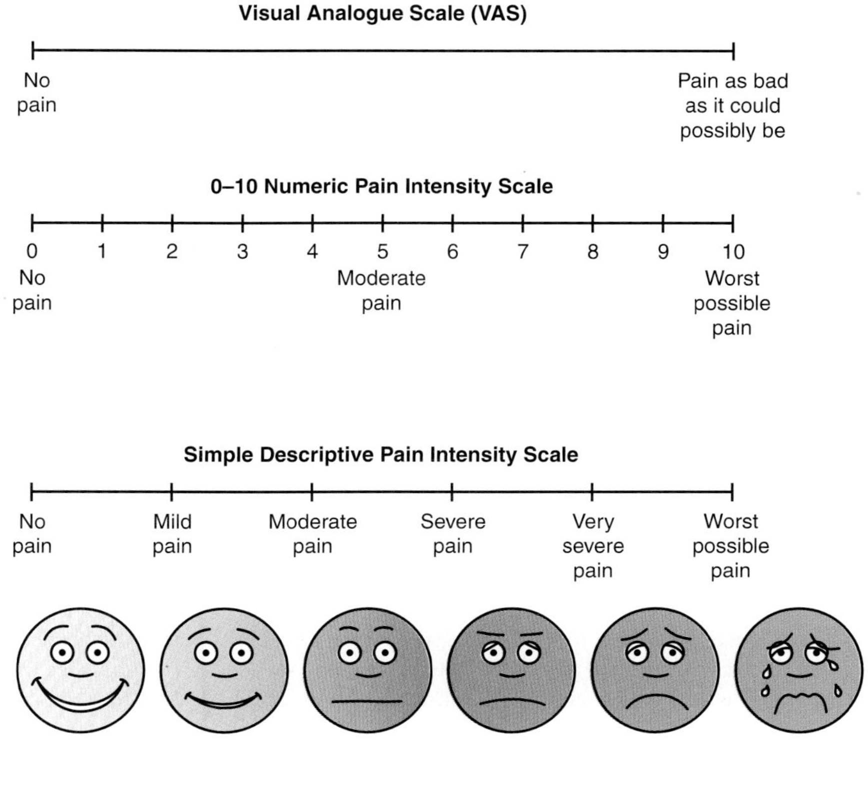

Figure 24-2. Pain assessment tools. Many pain intensity scales are available for ranking the pain of children and adults alike. Such scales as **(A)** the visual analogue, numeric pain intensity, and simple descriptive pain intensity rank pain from no pain to worst pain possible. Scales such as **(B)** the FACES pain rating scale are ideal for children and others who have difficulty with numeric concepts. To assist children with the FACES scale, the nurse explains that each face represents a person who feels happy because the person has no pain or a person who feels sad because the person has a lot of pain. Face 1 hurts a little bit, Face 2 hurts a little bit more, Face 3 hurts even more, Face 4 hurts a lot, and Face 5 has the biggest hurt you can have. Then, the nurse asks the child to choose the face that best describes his or her own pain and documents the selection. (Courtesy of Wong, D. L. [1995]. Whaley and Wong's *Nursing Care of Infants and Children* [5th ed.]. St. Louis: Mosby–Year Book.)

points for that section. The health care provider takes the word with the highest assigned quality points from each section and adds the scores to get a combined final score that will be between 0 and 10. This tool is useful not only because it measures both aspects of pain, but also because it can be used with patients who cannot speak or conceptualize a visual analogue scale.

Assessment of pain intensity and all aspects of pain is an important part of treating pain effectively. This may be especially true for patients who are stoic, who use coping mechanisms to deal with pain, or whose pain may be undertreated if the nurse offers drug therapy only to those who state that they are in pain.

Providing Analgesia

Morphine, like other drugs that relieve pain, is more effective when it is administered before the level of pain becomes severe. This is another reason why it is important to assess the patient's pain level frequently. When pain exists, analgesic dosages are best administered around the clock rather than as needed. Continual administration promotes a steady blood level of the drug, which prevents drug troughs that allow pain to escalate. In around-the-clock dosing, a baseline amount of the drug is administered over the 24-hour period when acute pain is expected or when severe, chronic pain occurs. Patients should be awakened for the analgesic; however, they may refuse the drug at any time.

The appropriate dose of morphine must be given to control the patient's pain. No one dose will be appropriate for every patient. Titration of dosage is usually required when therapy begins and continues for as long as the patient receives care. To titrate the morphine dose means to increase it incrementally. Aggressiveness of titration depends on pain intensity and response. Nurses need to remember that patients with a history of substance abuse or drug tolerance will need higher dosages of analgesics. Morphine is titrated until the desired therapeutic response, or efficacy, is achieved or until adverse effects occur. Efficacy is usually defined as a pain level below 4 out of 10 or a level determined by both the patient and health care provider. Nonopioids, such as NSAIDs, may be used in conjunction with morphine. Other adjunct drugs may be added to morphine if necessary for pain control. Finally, in addition to pharmacologic interventions, nonpharmacologic methods may be used in conjunction with morphine. These are not substitutes for morphine, but they are valuable adjuncts to therapy (Fig. 24-3).

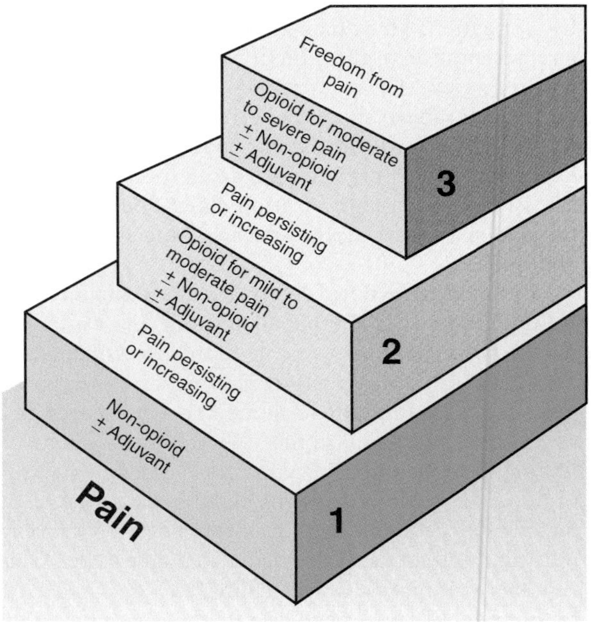

Figure 24-3. The World Health Organization's three-step analgesic ladder.

Minimizing Adverse Effects

Minimizing the adverse effects of morphine requires frequent and astute assessment and implementation of basic nursing care. (See the accompanying display, Minimizing Adverse Effects of Morphine.) Dosing the drug carefully to meet the needs posed by core patient variables can minimize adverse effects. In general, dosages will need to be lower for children, older adults, and patients with renal or hepatic impairment. Morphine should be administered before pain becomes severe. Because this dosing schedule is more effective, a smaller dose of the drug can be given, which helps to prevent or minimize adverse effects.

Breakthrough pain and incidental pain may occur during pain management with drug therapy. Clinicians use the term **breakthrough pain** to describe transitory flare-ups of pain over baseline in a patient receiving opioid therapy. Breakthrough pain is generally graded as moderate to severe in intensity. It may last from a few seconds to a few hours. It may or may not have a precipitating event. Spontaneous, or activity-related pain, is called **incidental pain.** An incident may be related to a specific movement or to all movements.

Factors to consider when assessing and treating breakthrough and incidental pain are those that relate to cause. When pain does occur, is it related to a specific time during the dosing schedule? If so, a change in the dosing interval or an increase in the drug dose may be beneficial. Does a certain movement cause pain, or is the pain unpredictable? Patients often have incidental or breakthrough pain associated with movement or activity. How long does the pain last? Although morphine has a fairly rapid onset, some severe pain may persist for less time than it takes for the analgesic to take effect.

All patients being treated for pain need access to **rescue doses** for breakthrough pain. The rescue dose should be equianalgesic to 10 to 30% of the dose the patient receives in 24 hours and is added to the established pain management. Patients who require more than three rescue doses in a day should have their analgesic dosage adjusted either by increasing the baseline dose or max-

Minimizing Adverse Effects of Morphine

For All

- Consult with the physician and pharmacist to individualize dosage and dosing intervals based on the patient's weight, age, pain intensity, diagnosis, concurrent medical status, and use of other CNS depressants.
- Because ambulation may increase occurrence of the frequent adverse effects, have patient lie down after the dose has been taken.
- Because low pain levels may increase occurrence of the frequent adverse effects, consider a nonnarcotic analgesic for patients with mild to moderate pain.

Respiratory Depression

- Assess vital signs, especially respiratory function, on a regular, frequent basis.
- Measure the oxygen concentration of the blood with a pulse oximeter on a regular and as- needed basis.
- Have the patient perform turning, coughing, and deep breathing, and reposition the patient to remove secretions and maintain adequate pulmonary ventilation.
- Place the patient on the side, not flat on the back, to maintain an open airway until condition stabilizes. If the patient must be placed on the back, remove pillow, and tilt the patient's head back slightly to prevent the tongue from occluding the airway. Use an oral airway if necessary.
- Withhold the next dose and notify the physician if the patient is bradypneic.
- Administer oxygen as needed.
- Have emergency respiratory equipment available.
- Keep naloxone, the narcotic antidote, on hand. Administer as needed.

Hypotension

- Monitor blood pressure carefully in postoperative patients, patients who have low circulating blood volume, or patients who are simultaneously receiving a CNS depressant (e.g., phenothiazine) or general anesthetics. These conditions make such patients more prone to hypotension.
- Monitor for orthostatic hypotension, especially during transport, for patients with decreased circulating blood levels or impaired cardiac function and for those receiving sympatholytic (blocking the action of the sympathetic nervous system) drugs.
- Monitor intake and output and replace fluids for patients who are hypovolemic.
- Assess ambulatory patients carefully for orthostatic hypotension.

Constipation

- Encourage dietary fiber when taking morphine orally.
- Encourage oral fluids when tolerated; keep patient well hydrated with IV fluids if NPO.
- Promote ambulation (assisted as necessary) as much as possible.
- Administer stool softeners or laxatives PRN.

Urinary Retention and Decreased Urinary Output

- Monitor intake and output at least every work shift.
- Question to determine whether the patient self-reports difficulty voiding, lack of voiding, frequent voiding of very small amounts, or feelings of bladder fullness or tenderness.
- Palpate the bladder to differentiate urinary retention from oliguria.
- Encourage oral fluids if allowed; provide adequate hydration with IV fluids if NPO.
- Use noninvasive means to promote voiding (ensure female patient sits upright, ensure male patient stands, run water in sink, pour water over perineum, use sitz baths).
- Obtain order and perform urethral catheterization if needed.

Light-headedness, Dizziness, and Sedation

- Assist the patient who is ambulating and getting out of bed.
- Ensure the use of side rails when the patient is in bed.

Nausea and Vomiting

- Keep the patient NPO during acute episodes; maintain the patient on IV fluids for hydration.
- Offer ice chips and clear liquids as symptoms diminish.
- Obtain order and administer antiemetics if indicated.

imizing the co-analgesics. A thorough assessment will assist the health care provider to decide whether the best option is to increase the dosage or to incorporate other therapies.

Providing Patient and Family Education

- Patients being treated for pain need to know what the treatment plan will be for managing their pain and that they are not expected to suffer. The nurse needs to assure patients that health care providers will listen to them and act when they report that they have pain.
- Patients need to know that they have an important role to play in managing their pain. The nurse should review the following with them:
  - Know how to use the pain assessment tools.
  - Report honestly how they feel during assessment.
  - Establish (with the health care team) what pain level will trigger automatic reevaluation of the pain management plan. Ideally, this should happen before pain develops or increases (e.g., in the preoperative period or early in the course of a disease) (see the accompanying display, Thinking Critically About Drug Therapy in Pain Management).
- The nurse should correct any fears or misconceptions, including the following:
  - Pain is inevitable.
  - Pain must be endured.
  - Patients will "lose control" of themselves if they take drugs for pain.
  - Patients will become addicted.
- The nurse should teach patients that drug therapy with morphine over a prolonged period (as in chronic or cancer pain) may produce physical dependence on the drug. The nurse should explain that physical dependence is not the same as addiction, nor is it a reason to withhold pain treatment. If the pain resolves, the patient can be weaned from the drug to prevent

withdrawal. Weaning is not appropriate with cancer pain because the pain will not resolve on its own.

- If the patient is discharged home on morphine, the nurse should teach the following:
  - How to administer
  - Adverse effects
  - To avoid driving and other hazardous activities during drug therapy
  - To avoid alcohol and concurrent CNS depressant therapy, unless a health care provider is managing the concurrent therapy
  - How to keep the drug secure from children and anyone likely to abuse it

Ongoing Assessment and Evaluation

Documentation of pain management should include the following:

- The pain scale used by the patient
- The rating given by the patient
- Sensory and affective components of pain
- Amount of morphine, route, and the time each dose is administered
- The degree of pain relief obtained from morphine therapy
- Nonpharmacologic interventions used and their effectiveness

Increasing pain in a patient previously stabilized on a certain dose of morphine should not be automatically attributed to tolerance without investigating for evidence of disease progression or complications. Cancer pain, for example, changes constantly. It may increase or decrease secondary to anticancer treatment, infectious processes, spreading tumors, or natural degenerative body changes (arthritis). Postoperative pain that morphine does not relieve may indicate postoperative complications, such as compartment syndrome.

The patient should have adequate pain control with minimal adverse side effects. Breakthrough pain should be minimal if the pain is adequately controlled. The patient should remain free from injury from orthostatic hypotension or sedation. The patient and family will show an understanding of adverse side effects if discharged on morphine and will be able to describe how to manage them if they occur. ■

MEMORY CHIP

Morphine

- Narcotic analgesic used in moderate to severe pain
- Standard against which all other narcotic analgesics are measured for effectiveness
- Significant contraindications: significant respiratory depression, increased intracranial pressure, and CNS depression
- Most common adverse effects: light-headedness, dizziness, sedation, nausea, and vomiting
- Most serious adverse effect: respiratory depression
- **Lifespan alert: avoid use in premature infants or during labor when delivery of premature infant is expected**
- Maximizing therapeutic effects: assess pain thoroughly before and during therapy and titrate the dose until the desired pain-relieving effect is achieved
- Minimizing adverse effects: individualize dose based on patient-related variables; monitor vital signs, especially respiratory rate, frequently; and have the antidote, naloxone, on hand
- Most significant patient education: for long-term use in cancer pain, physical dependency will develop. This is not the same as addiction and not an appropriate reason to withhold the drug.

DRUGS CLOSELY RELATED TO MORPHINE

Hydromorphone

Hydromorphone (Dilaudid) is a semisynthetic analogue of opium. Its effects on the body are almost identical to those of morphine. As an analgesic, hydromorphone is equally effective as morphine, although more potent. Between 1 and 1-1/2 (1 to 1.50) mg of subcutaneous (SC) or intramuscular (IM) hydromorphine is equal to 10 mg of morphine given through the same routes. Hydromorphone also has equal antitussive (cough suppression) effects; however, its ability to cause respiratory depression and physical dependency is less than that of morphine. Hydromorphone's ability to cause constipation, sedation, and emesis is unknown; thus, comparisons with morphine cannot be made. Unlike morphine, hydromorphone can cause transient hyperglycemia.

Levorphanol

Levorphanol (Levo-Dromoran), a synthetic compound, can be used to manage pain and as a preoperative agent. It has similar analgesic, constipating, respiratory depressive, sedating, and physical dependency qualities to those of morphine. It has fewer antitussive and emetic effects. Like hydromorphone, levorphanol is more potent than morphine with an SC dose of 2 mg equal to 10 mg of morphine.

Oxycodone

Oxycodone is a semisynthetic analogue of opium. Unlike morphine, it is only available as an oral preparation. It is available in regular-release (Roxicodone), timed-release (Oxycontin), and rapid-release formulas (OxyIR). Oxycodone has similar analgesic, antitussive, constipating, respiratory depressive, sedating, emetic, and physical dependency effects to those of morphine. It is often administered as a combination drug with either aspirin (Percodan, Roxiprin) or acetaminophen (Tylox, Percocet, Roxicet).

Oxymorphone

Oxymorphone (Numorphan) is a semisynthetic analogue of opium. It is used in pain control, as a preoperative medication, to support anesthesia, as an obstetric analgesic, and for the relief of anxiety in patients with dyspnea associated with pulmonary edema secondary to acute left ventricular dysfunction. Oxymorphone is available in injection and rectal forms. It has analgesic and constipating effects similar to morphine's; however, it causes more respiratory depression, emesis, and physical dependence. Oxymorphone has fewer antitussive effects than morphine; its sedating effects are unknown.

Meperidine

Meperidine (Demerol) is a synthetic compound used to treat pain as a preoperative medication, to support anesthesia, and during labor. Meperidine has similar analgesic and respiratory depressive effects and abilities to cause physical dependence as found with morphine. Meperidine has fewer sedative and constipating effects and significantly fewer antitussive effects than morphine. Meperidine has a longer half-life and is less potent than morphine, requiring 75 mg IM or SC to have an equianalgesic effect equal to that of 10 mg of morphine. A unique drug interaction occurs between meperidine and the hydantoins (anticonvulsants), which decreases the effectiveness of meperidine. This effect may result from an increased hepatic metabolism of meperidine.

The most significant difference between morphine and meperidine is related to the pharmacokinetics of meperidine. Meperidine is metabolized to an active metabolite, normeperidine. Normeperidine has a long half-life (15 to 30 hours) and will accumulate in the body with chronic dosing. Half-life is further extended in patients with renal impairment, which slows excretion of normeperidine. Normeperidine is a CNS toxin. Accumulated doses in the body can cause tremors, seizures, and changes in level of consciousness. Older adults are especially sensitive to the adverse effects of normeperidine, which may be the result of impaired renal function. For these reasons, the Clinical Guidelines for Acute Pain Management (U.S. Department of Health and Human Services, 1992) state that meperidine should normally be avoided in pain management when multiple doses will be given. The exception would be if the patient is allergic to morphine; however, the patient must have normal renal function.

Fentanyl

Fentanyl is a synthetic compound. Its major uses are as a preanesthetic, anesthetic, and analgesic. Fentanyl's analgesic properties are equal to those of morphine. It produces fewer respiratory and emetic effects. Its antitussive, constipating, sedating, and physical dependency effects are unknown in comparison with those of morphine. Fentanyl is much more potent than morphine, with 0.1 mg producing equianalgesia to that of 10 mg of morphine.

Fentanyl is available in various forms. Fentanyl as a liquid for injection (Sublimaze) is used as an anesthetic, an analgesic of short duration during anesthesia, and a supplement to general or regional anesthesia. An off-label use is pain control through epidural PCA, usually after surgery.

There are two types of fentanyl transmucosal systems. Fentanyl Oralet is used only as a premedication to anesthesia or to induce conscious sedation before a procedure such as cardiac catheterization. Use of this form carries a risk of hypoventilation; thus, it is administered only in hospital settings where anesthesia care can be monitored (e.g., operating rooms [ORs], emergency departments [EDs], and intensive care units [ICUs]). Trained personnel must monitor the patient throughout therapy with Oralet; emergency equipment and a narcotic antagonist must be available. Oralet is frequently used with children, although it may be used with adults. The lozenge is manufactured with a handle, similar in appearance to a lollipop. Administration should begin 20 to 40 minutes prior to the need for the desired therapeutic effect. The nurse should instruct the patient to suck on the lozenge. The nurse should remove the handle from the patient's mouth when effectiveness is adequate or if the patient develops complications.

The other transmucosal form of fentanyl (Actiq) is used only for the management of breakthrough pain in patients with cancer who are already receiving and tolerant to opioid therapy. Because of its potential for causing hypoventilation, fentanyl should never be used with opiate-naive patients. Only oncologists and pain specialists who are familiar with opioids should administer it to treat cancer pain. If used in the home, storage of the drug in a safe place is critical, because the dose found in this form may be fatal to children. Neither transmucosal form of fentanyl is used for acute or chronic pain (other than cancer pain).

Fentanyl is also available in a transdermal system (Duragesic). It is used in chronic pain, usually related to cancer, when the patient requires continuous opioid analgesia for pain that other methods cannot control. When first used, it takes approximately 24 hours for the full pain-relieving effect to occur. The patient should be treated with short-acting opioids during this period. Short-acting opioids are not needed when changing the patch after 72 hours, except for rescue doses for breakthrough pain. For more information, see the accompanying display, Teaching About Transdermal Fentanyl.

Alfentanil

Alfentanil (Alfenta) is used in the OR as an analgesic during anesthesia, to induce anesthesia when intubation and mechanical ventilation are required, and as the analgesic component of MAC. Its analgesic effects are similar to those of morphine. Its onset of action is immediate.

Sufentanil

Sufentanil (Sufenta) produces a greater analgesic effect than morphine. It is used as an anesthetic and analgesic adjunct to maintain balanced anesthesia when patients are intubated and on a ventilator. It is also used as an epidural analgesic during labor and vaginal delivery (when combined with low-dose bupivicaine).

Levomethadyl

Levomethadyl (Orlaam) is used in the treatment of narcotic addiction. Only approved treatment programs may dispense it. It is normally dosed three times a week. Patients should

COMMUNITY-BASED CONCERNS

Teaching About Transdermal Fentanyl

As more and more patients learn to manage their own health care and drug therapy at home, nurses may assume an even greater role in teaching patients and their caregivers about safe self-care and drug administration. For a patient who will be discharged while receiving transdermal fentanyl, some important drug administration teaching points for the patient or the caregiver follow.

1. Caregivers who administer a transdermal fentanyl patch should first put on gloves to avoid absorbing any of the drug themselves. They should also wear gloves when removing the patch.
2. Tear open a new patch packet carefully; never cut the patch with scissors.
3. Remove the liner on the sticky side of the patch.
4. Apply the fentanyl patch to nonirritated, smooth, hairless skin (clip hair; avoid shaving to avoid breaking the skin) on the chest, back, flank, or upper arm right after opening the patch package. If necessary, wash the skin with clear water and dry completely before applying the patch. Do not use soaps, creams, alcohol, oils, lotion or anything else that might irritate the skin or alter its characteristics.
5. Hold the patch in place for 30 seconds to ensure firm adherence.
6. Wear the system continually for 72 hours and then replace with a new patch, placed in a different location.
7. To discard a used patch, fold it in half with the sticky sides together (to prevent any residual drug from touching the skin) and flush the patch down the toilet. This is because active drug remains in the patch. (Patches discarded in the trash may be attractive to and accidentally come in contact with children or pets.)

be warned that the peak effect is not immediate. If they use other psychoactive drugs, including alcohol, while taking this drug, fatal overdose can occur. This is most problematic during the first few doses of levomethadyl. Levomethadyl has analgesic and constipating effects similar to those of morphine but fewer emetic and physical dependency effects.

Methadone

Methadone (Methadose, Dolophine) can be used for pain, to prevent withdrawal symptoms from heroin (detoxification), and as a maintenance treatment for narcotic abuse. Although its ability to produce analgesia and the duration of its analgesic effect (4 to 6 hours, compared with 3 to 7 hours) are similar to those of morphine, its half-life is much longer. The half-life of methadone is 15 to 30 hours compared with 1.5 to 2 hours for morphine. Adverse effects and signs of overdose may occur when methadone is used as pain management because of these pharmacokinetic properties. Methadone may be initiated in a hospital setting only for prevention of withdrawal. Only approved treatment programs for narcotic abuse may initiate treatment with methadone for maintenance treatment of addiction. If a patient is already in a maintenance treatment program with methadone and requires hospitalization, the hospital may provide the methadone, after personnel confirm the dose with the treatment center that normally observes the patient.

Remifentanil

Remifentanil (Ultiva), although classified as a narcotic agonist analgesic, is used as a general anesthetic and as part of monitored anesthesia care. Remifentanil has more analgesic effects than morphine but similar respiratory depressive and emetic effects. Physical dependence and constipation occur less often than with morphine.

DRUGS SIGNIFICANTLY DIFFERENT FROM P MORPHINE

Naloxone (Narcan) is a narcotic antagonist. It is believed to antagonize the effects of narcotics by competing for opioid receptor sites. It is used to reverse the effects of opiates (such as respiratory depression) and to treat opioid overdose. Although it can be given IM, SC, or IV, the most rapid onset is achieved with IV use, and this route is recommended in emergencies. IV onset is within 2 minutes; duration of action depends on the dose given and the route used. Careful monitoring of the patient beyond initial response is warranted, because the duration of action of the narcotic agonist may be longer than the duration of naloxone. Repeated doses may be necessary to maintain reversal of the opiate's effects. Abrupt reversal of narcotic depression may result in the adverse effects of nausea, vomiting, sweating, tachycardia, increased blood pressure, and tremors.

Naloxone's reversal of respiratory depression from buprenorphine (a mixed agonist and antagonist) may be incomplete, requiring mechanical assistance for respiration. Naloxone is not effective for respiratory depression caused by anything other than narcotic agonist analgesics. Administration of naloxone will precipitate withdrawal in persons physically dependent on narcotics. It will also reverse all the analgesic effects in those receiving morphine or other narcotic agonists for pain control if the dose is sufficient. Naloxone can be used in adults, children, and neonates.

C MILD NARCOTIC AGONISTS

The mild narcotic agonists include codeine, hydrocodone, and propoxyphene. Codeine is the prototype for the mild narcotic agonists.

NURSING MANAGEMENT OF THE PATIENT RECEIVING P CODEINE

Core Drug Knowledge

Pharmacotherapeutics

Codeine is used to control mild to moderate pain in adults and children. For this purpose, it is available in oral tablets and an injectable form for parenteral use. Orally, it may be combined with acetaminophen. Codeine is also used for cough suppression. The dose needed to achieve an antitussive effect is less than the dose required for analgesia. Although codeine has fewer antitussive effects than morphine (when comparing similar weights of the drugs), it is more widely used to suppress coughs, because it has low adverse effects at the antitussive doses. Codeine may be used alone, in the form of oral tablets, or in combination with other drugs that are expectorants (in a liquid or syrup form) to suppress coughs.

Pharmacokinetics

Codeine is well absorbed from the GI tract. Its peak effect occurs in 1 to 2 hours. (Other pharmacokinetic parameters are identified in Table 24-3). Codeine is metabolized in the liver and excreted in the urine. It crosses the placenta and enters breast milk.

Pharmacodynamics

Codeine has pharmacologic effects similar to those of morphine but its actions are milder. Codeine acts at specific opioid receptors in the CNS to produce analgesia, euphoria, and sedation. Codeine also acts directly on the medullary cough center to depress the cough reflex. It has a drying effect on mucous membranes and can increase the viscosity of respiratory tract secretions.

Contraindications and Precautions

Codeine should not be administered to patients receiving other narcotic analgesics for pain relief; such a combination can cause serious respiratory depression and sedation. Codeine should be used with caution in patients who need to cough to maintain the airways (i.e., postoperative patients and patients who have undergone major abdominal or thoracic surgery). Careful use is recommended for patients with asthma and emphysema, because cough suppression in these patients can lead to accumulation of secretions and a loss of respiratory reserve. Codeine is used with caution in patients with preexisting cardiac disease because of its potential to induce bradycardia and peripheral vasodilation.

Codeine is assigned to pregnancy category C. Like other opiate narcotics, it crosses the placenta, enters the breast milk, and can cause sedation and respiratory depression in the fetus or infant. Therefore, it should be used with caution during pregnancy and lactation. The closer it is given to delivery, the more likely it is for respiratory depression to occur in the newborn. Resuscitation equipment should be on hand if the mother has received codeine or other opiates during labor. Codeine should be avoided if the delivery of a premature infant is expected. Caution should also be used with patients who are hypersensitive to or have a history of addiction to narcotics; codeine is a narcotic and has a potential for addiction. Patients who need to drive or be alert should use codeine with extreme caution, because it can cause sedation and drowsiness. Caution is important when codeine is used for patients who have experienced a head injury or undergone a craniotomy. Codeine can increase intracranial pressure, which can be detrimental to these patients.

Adverse Effects

As already stated, codeine has a low incidence of adverse effects when dosed as an antitussive. The most frequent adverse effects observed with the use of codeine as a cough suppressant include drowsiness, sedation, dry mouth, nausea and vomiting, and constipation. When dosed as an analgesic, the adverse effects are similar to those of morphine, although they are less severe. Allergic reactions, including rashes and urticaria, have been noted in highly sensitive people. Respiratory depression and cardiovascular effects have occurred with higher doses.

Drug Interactions

An increased likelihood of respiratory depression, hypotension, or profound sedation exists when codeine is given with any other drugs that cause CNS depression, such as antihistamines, phenothiazines, barbiturates, sedative-hypnotics, tricyclic antidepressants, and alcohol. Codeine may also interact with histamine-2 antagonists, such as cimetidine (Table 24-5).

TABLE 24-5 Agents That Interact With P Codeine

Interactants	Effect and Significance	Nursing Management
antihistamines	Additive effects when given simultaneously, resulting in CNS depression	Monitor closely for CNS depression. Avoid coadministration if possible.
barbiturates	Additive effects when given simultaneously, resulting in CNS depression	Monitor closely for CNS depression. Avoid coadministration if possible.
histamine-2 receptor antagonists	Actions of narcotic analgesics enhanced, resulting in toxicity and increased risk for respiratory depression	Monitor for respiratory depression. Decrease dosage of narcotic analgesic as needed. Avoid coadministration if possible.
phenothiazines	Additive effects when given simultaneously, resulting in CNS depression	Monitor closely for CNS depression. Avoid coadministration if possible.

Assessment of Relevant Core Patient Variables

Health Status

The nurse should assess whether the patient needs to cough to maintain a patent airway. Such patients (e.g., postoperative patients) should not receive codeine. In this situation, the cough is a protective mechanism to rid the airways of potentially harmful substances that may lead to pneumonia. The same rationale is used when treating patients with asthma or emphysema. If they do not cough, they have the potential to retain secretions that may exacerbate their disease.

Prior to therapy, the nurse should perform a physical examination to establish a baseline to monitor the effects of the drug. Parameters to evaluate include orientation, affect, respiratory rate, adventitious sounds, and character of bowel sounds. If prolonged use is anticipated or the patient has a history of hepatic dysfunction, the nurse should ensure that liver function tests are done, because codeine is metabolized in the liver.

Life Span and Gender

The nurse should consider the patient's age before drug administration. Older adult patients are especially sensitive to respiratory depression with the use of narcotics. Therefore, a reduced dosage of codeine is advised. Codeine use is contraindicated in premature infants because of their sensitivity to respiratory depression. In addition, the nurse should carefully assess whether a female patient is pregnant before administering codeine. The drug should not be given to women in labor unless absolutely necessary.

Lifestyle, Diet, and Habits

Codeine has less potential for causing physical dependence than morphine. Withdrawal symptoms from codeine dependency are similar to those seen in withdrawal from morphine, although the symptoms are less severe. The nurse, however, should still assess patients for a history of drug abuse and administer codeine cautiously in such patients.

Environment

If the patient will be taking codeine as an outpatient, the nurse should assess his or her need to drive or operate potentially dangerous equipment. Patients must refrain from these activities until the nurse has assessed the drug's sedative effects.

Nursing Diagnoses and Outcomes

- Disturbed Sensory Perception related to drowsiness and sedation
  Desired outcome: The patient will be protected from injury related to sedation and drowsiness.
- Risk for Ineffective Airway Clearance related to suppression of cough reflex
  Desired outcome: The patient will maintain baseline respiratory function.
- Constipation secondary to activity of the drug
  Desired outcome: The patient remains free of constipation.

Planning and Intervention

Maximizing Therapeutic Effects

Actions are similar as for morphine.

Minimizing Adverse Effects

During therapy, the nurse should ensure the use of safety precautions, such as raising side rails and assisting with ambulation if the patient is having CNS adverse effects. The nurse should monitor movement of air and respiratory status periodically during drug use. The use of codeine should be avoided in patients who need a strong cough reflex. Other actions are similar to those of morphine.

Providing Patient and Family Education

- The nurse must remind patients that drowsiness and impaired orientation can occur. Thus, patients should not drive or perform other tasks requiring alertness until the effects of the drug are known.
- Teach the patient to avoid combining use of codeine with alcohol or other CNS depressants.
- Instruct patients and their families to report respiratory difficulty at once to the nurse or physician.
- The nurse should provide general pain control information, similar to that given for morphine.

Ongoing Assessment and Evaluation

The nurse should monitor the drug's effect on motor control and sedation. It is also important for the nurse to monitor the patient's respiratory status. By the end of therapy, the patient should be free from injury related to sedation and have open and functioning airways manifested by breathing without difficulty. Assessment and evaluation of pain control are the same as for morphine. ■

DRUGS CLOSELY RELATED TO CODEINE

Drugs similar to codeine include hydrocodone and propoxyphene. Hydrocodone, although classified as a narcotic agonist and possessing the ability to produce some analgesia, is used only for its antitussive effects. It is available only in combination with an expectorant in a syrup or elixir formula for coughs. Propoxyphene (Darvon) is used to treat mild to moderate pain. Compared with codeine, it has similar analgesic, respiratory depressive, sedative, emetic, and physical dependency effects. Whether they share codeine's antitussive and constipating effects remains unknown. Excessive doses

MEMORY CHIP

Codeine

- Used to treat mild to moderate pain and as a cough suppressant
- Significant contraindications: same as for all narcotics (e.g., respiratory depression, use of other CNS depressants)
- Most common adverse effects: as a cough suppressant—drowsiness, sedation, dry mouth, nausea and vomiting, and constipation (all incidence is low at this dose); as an analgesic—similar to those of morphine, although less severe
- Most serious adverse effect: respiratory depression (in overdoses)
- **Life-span alert: same as for morphine**
- Maximizing therapeutic effects: same as for morphine
- Minimizing adverse effects: avoid use if patient's health status requires a strong cough; other considerations are the same as for morphine
- Most significant patient education: provide general information on pain management as for all other narcotics

of propoxyphene, either alone or in combination with other CNS depressants (including alcohol), is a major cause of drug-related death. For this reason, propoxyphene and products that include it should not be prescribed to suicidal patients or those with addictive tendencies. The nurse should strongly warn patients not to exceed the dosage prescribed.

NARCOTIC AGONISTS-ANTAGONISTS

Some narcotic analgesics have mixed opioid effects, being an agonist at some receptors and an antagonist at others. Pentazocine (Talwin) is an example of a mixed narcotic agonist-antagonist and is also the prototype narcotic agonist-antagonist. Drugs similar to pentazocine include buprenorphine, butorphanol, dezocine, and nalbuphine.

NURSING MANAGEMENT OF THE PATIENT RECEIVING PENTAZOCINE

Core Drug Knowledge

Pharmacotherapeutics

In patients not previously exposed to opioids, pentazocine can be used as an agonist to control pain. In normal doses, pentazocine is effective for moderate to severe pain, such as postoperative pain or pain during labor. It is also used as premedication for anesthesia and a supplement to surgical anesthetics.

Pharmacokinetics

Pentazocine is well absorbed orally and from SC and IM sites. When given orally, it undergoes a significant first pass effect of hepatic metabolism, and bioavailability is less than 20% of the dose given. The peak serum levels from oral doses occur within 1 to 3 hours, with a duration of action of 3 hours (see Table 24-3). Pentazocine's metabolites and the small proportion of drug not metabolized are excreted in urine. Pentazocine crosses the placenta.

Pharmacodynamics

Pentazocine is a mixed agonist-antagonist. It stimulates kappa receptors much as morphine does but also exhibits weak antagonist effects at the mu receptors, the primary morphine receptors. In patients who abuse opioids or are receiving narcotic agonists, such as morphine, for pain control, this drug may precipitate a withdrawal syndrome because of its antagonistic effects. Pentazocine may increase intracranial pressure. When pentazocine is given intravenously, it elevates systemic and pulmonary arterial pressure, systemic vascular resistance, and left ventricular end diastolic pressure. These effects increase the workload of the heart.

Contraindications and Precautions

Pentazocine is contraindicated for patients with known hypersensitivity to it. Caution and low doses should be used if the drug is administered to patients with respiratory depression, severely limited respiratory reserves, severe bronchial asthma, obstructive respiratory conditions, and cyanosis. Pentazocine may cause allergic reactions in patients sensitive to sulfites. This is uncommon in the general population but more likely in patients with asthma.

Adverse Effects

The most common adverse effects of pentazocine are nausea, vomiting, dizziness or light-headedness, and euphoria. Pentazocine causes little respiratory depression because of its antagonist action at the mu receptors. Areas that may experience other possible adverse effects include cardiovascular (hypotension, hypertension, tachycardia, circulatory depression, and shock), CNS (sedation, headache, weakness, depression, disturbed dreams, insomnia, syncope, hallucinations, tremor, irritability, excitement, tinnitus, disorientation, and confusion), and dermatologic (soft tissue induration, nodules, cutaneous depression, ulceration with sloughing, sclerosis of the skin and subcutaneous tissues at site of injection, diaphoresis, stinging during injection, flushed skin, pruritus, and toxic epidermal necrolysis).

Drug Interactions

Pentazocine increases the action of alcohol and subsequently its accompanying CNS depressant effects. Barbiturate anesthetics increase the effect of respiratory and CNS depression from pentazocine because of additive pharmacologic activity (Table 24-6).

TABLE 24-6 Agents That Interact With Pentazocine

Interactants	Effect and Significance	Nursing Management
alcohol	Increased sedation	Avoid concurrent use. Caution against operating hazardous machinery or driving a motor vehicle.
thiopental	Increased CNS depression	Caution patient not to drive until effects subside completely. Avoid concurrent usage.
fluoxetine	Hypertension, diaphoresis, ataxia, flushing, nausea, dizziness, and anxiety	Monitor patient with caution if both drugs are used concurrently.
methohexital	Increased CNS depression	Consult prescriber about possible dosage adjustment.
zotepine	Increased risk of pentazocine-induced respiratory depression; enhanced sedation	Reduce dosage of pentazocine if necessary. Monitor for respiratory depression.
tobacco	Metabolism of pentazocine about 40% higher in smokers	Consult prescriber about increasing pentazocine dosage.

Assessment of Relevant Core Patient Variables

Health Status

The nurse should assess the patient for conditions that are contraindications or precautions to drug therapy as well as for hepatic disease, because decreased metabolism of the drug will occur, which predisposes the patient to greater adverse effects.

Because of the effect of increasing intracranial pressure, pentazocine may compound the clinical course of patients with head injuries. Its use in these patients should be avoided if at all possible; if pentazocine must be used, it should be done very cautiously, and the patient needs careful monitoring. Because of the cardiac effects, IV pentazocine should not be given to patients with an MI. If oral forms are given, they must be administered cautiously, with the patient monitored carefully.

Life Span and Gender

The nurse should assess female patients for pregnancy before administration. Pentazocine is a pregnancy category C drug. Infants born to mothers who abuse pentazocine will exhibit neonatal withdrawal and have lower birth weights than normal. The safety and efficacy of pentazocine in children younger than age 12 years have not been established; therefore, the nurse should clarify that the pediatric patient is age 12 years or older before administration.

Lifestyle, Diet, and Habits

A common form of pentazocine abuse is called "T's and Blues." The "T's" refers to oral doses of pentazocine (under its trade name Talwin), and the "Blues" refers to tripelennamine (trade name, PBZ), an H1 antihistamine. In this abused form, tablets are dissolved in tap water, filtered, and then injected IV as a substitute for heroin. The most frequent and serious complication of this form of addiction is pulmonary disease. Pulmonary disease results from blocking the pulmonary arteries and arterioles with unsterile particles of cellulose and talc from the tablets. Neurologic complications from "T's and Blues" may also occur, including seizures, strokes, and CNS infections. Pentazocine with naloxone (Talwin NX) has been produced in an effort to decrease the prevalence of this abuse. Giving pentazocine to patients who are dependent on opiates may induce withdrawal symptoms.

Environment

Pentazocine in parenteral form is administered in a hospital setting; oral forms may be administered in any setting by physicians, nurses, or patients themselves. The nurse and patient should discuss any possible risks in the home or living environment.

Nursing Diagnoses and Outcomes

- Disturbed Sensory Perception related to dizziness and lightheadedness
  Desired outcome: The patient will not be injured from falls while taking pentazocine.
- Imbalanced Nutrition secondary to nausea and vomiting
  Desired outcome: The patient's nutrition will not be compromised while on pentazocine.
- Ineffective Health Maintenance related to abuse of pentazocine
  Desired outcome: The patient will use drug therapy appropriately.
- Deficient Knowledge related to pentazocine therapy
  Desired outcome: The patient has adequate knowledge of the drug and its adverse effects and their management.

Planning and Intervention

Maximizing Therapeutic Effects

The nurse should be sure to provide environmental controls to reduce sensory stimuli and aid relaxation. For example, lights may be dimmed, noise reduced, and room temperature adjusted for greatest comfort. General actions for pain control are similar to those described for morphine.

Minimizing Adverse Effects

During therapy, the nurse should ensure that safety precautions are used, such as raising side rails and assisting with ambulation. In cases of overdosage, naloxone is indicated. General principles for pain control are the same as those followed for morphine.

Providing Patient and Family Education

- The nurse should teach patients that pentazocine may cause drowsiness. They must use it with caution while driving or performing tasks that require mental alertness, physical dexterity, or coordination.
- The nurse should emphasize that patients must avoid concurrent use of pentazocine with alcohol and other CNS depressants.
- The nurse should instruct patients to notify their physicians if skin rash, confusion, or disorientation develop.

Ongoing Assessment and Evaluation

The nurse should monitor the drug's effect on motor control, sedation, and pain. Adequate pain control should be achieved without adverse effects. Effectiveness of pain control is assessed similarly to morphine. ■

DRUGS CLOSELY RELATED TO PENTAZOCINE

Buprenorphine

Buprenorphine (Buprenex), used in the treatment of moderate to severe pain, has a high affinity at the mu receptors and disassociates from these sites slowly. This may explain its long duration of action (6 hours versus 3 hours for pentazocine) and its low ability to cause physical dependence. It also possesses very strong antagonist tendencies at opioid receptors, similar to the action of naloxone. How buprenorphine, a narcotic analgesic with strong receptor antagonist action, produces pain relief is not specifically known. Sedation is the most frequently occurring adverse effect, affecting more than half of the patients receiving buprenorphine. The next most common adverse effects, although their prevalence is much lower than sedation, are dizziness and vertigo, hypotension, headache, sweating, nausea and vomiting, miosis, and hypoventilation. Other adverse effects may also occur. There have been a few clinical reports of significant respiratory depression from buprenorphine; it should be used cautiously in patients with compromised respiratory status and those receiving additional drugs that cause respiratory depression. Like pentazocine, it is a pregnancy category C drug, and the safety of its use in children and during breast-feeding has not been established. Likewise, it should be used cautiously in those with hepatic disease. Like pentazocine, if buprenorphine is given to a patient who is opioid dependent, withdrawal will occur. The likelihood of this happening is greater than with pentazocine because of buprenorphine's strong antagonist action, whereas pentazocine has only weak antagonist properties.

MEMORY CHIP

Pentazocine

- Used for moderate to severe pain
- Is an agonist at some opioid receptors and a weak antagonist at others
- May precipitate withdrawal in patients physically dependent on narcotics
- Abused on the street (known as "T's and Blues")
- Most common adverse effects: nausea, vomiting, dizziness, lightheadedness, and euphoria
- Most serious adverse effects: respiratory depression and circulatory depression
- Maximizing therapeutic effects: same as for all narcotics
- Minimizing adverse effects: same as for all narcotics
- Most significant patient education: avoid alcohol and CNS depressants while taking drug

Butorphanol

Butorphanol (Stadol) is used as an analgesic, preoperative medication, supplement to balanced anesthesia, and pain reliever during labor. An intranasal form was shown effective in clinical trials in treating the pain of migraine headaches. The analgesic potency of butorphanol, compared by weight, is 20 times that of pentazocine and 3.5 to 7 times that of morphine. Like pentazocine, butorphanol has both narcotic agonist and antagonist effects. Its antagonist activity is approximately 30 times that of pentazocine but only 1/40 that of naloxone. Its mechanism for pain relief is not completely understood. Like pentazocine, it produces the same cardiovascular effects when given intravenously, increases intracranial pressure, is metabolized in the liver, is a pregnancy category C drug, and has no known safety data relevant to its use in children. It may induce withdrawal in patients who abuse opiates, although whether it is an antagonist at the mu receptors is not definitely known. Unlike pentazocine, its most common adverse effect is somnolence. Common adverse effects similar to pentazocine include nausea and vomiting and dizziness. Other adverse effects that occur with regularity include confusion, sweating, dry mouth, headache, vasodilation, insomnia, constipation, and an unpleasant taste.

Dezocine

Dezocine (Dalgan), a strong, narcotic analgesic with agonist and antagonist effects, is used IM or IV in acute pain. Its analgesic potency, onset, and duration of action in the relief of postoperative pain are comparable with those of morphine. Its use and effectiveness in chronic pain have not been adequately studied. Its antagonist effects are greater than those of pentazocine. Dezocine depresses respiratory function in a way similar to that of morphine, which is much greater than seen with pentazocine. In addition, unlike pentazocine, dezocine does not produce significant cardiovascular effects. Dezocine has adverse effects similar to all strong analgesics. The most common are nausea and vomiting, sedation, dizziness, and reactions at the injection site. Dezocine is not recommended for patients who are physically dependent on narcotics because of its antagonist effects.

Nalbuphine

Nalbuphine (Nubain) is a potent analgesic with agonist and antagonist effects. Its analgesic potency is essentially the same as that of morphine and about three times greater than that of pentazocine. Its antagonist activity is approximately 10 times that of pentazocine. Nalbuphine is used for moderate to severe pain, as a preoperative analgesic, as a supplement to balanced anesthesia, and as an obstetric analgesic during labor and delivery. Unlike pentazocine, nalbuphine does not increase pulmonary artery pressure, systemic vascular resistance, or cardiac work. Nalbuphine produces respiratory depression similar to morphine. Unlike morphine, the depressive effects seem to have a ceiling effect, with increases beyond 30 mg of nalbuphine producing no further respiratory depression. Like pentazocine, nalbuphine can produce an allergic response in patients with sulfite sensitivity and also trigger withdrawal in patients dependent on narcotics. The most common adverse effect is sedation, which occurs in about one third of the patients who use the drug. Other fairly common adverse effects are sweating, nausea and vomiting, dizziness and vertigo, dry mouth, and headache.

CHAPTER SUMMARY

- Pain is a subjective experience. Objective signs may or may not accompany pain. Lack of objective data does not mean that the pain is not present.
- Pain, a complex physiologic phenomenon, is not clearly or completely understood at this time.
- Pain is mediated through the CNS by nociceptors and perceived by the opiate receptors. When the opiate receptors are stimulated, perception of pain decreases.
- There are many types or classifications of pain. These are based on the physiologic origin of the pain (e.g., somatic, visceral, neuropathic), the length of time that the pain has been present (e.g., acute, chronic), or the pathologic source (e.g., cancer).
- To be treated appropriately, pain must be assessed with a pain assessment tool. Simply asking patients to rate their pain on a scale in their head is not the same as using an assessment tool.
- Pain is best controlled when patients take analgesics before pain becomes severe and doses are administered around the clock.
- Doses of analgesics should be titrated to obtain maximum efficacy with minimal adverse effects.
- Nonpharmacologic methods of pain management may be used to supplement drug therapy.
- Patients who have been receiving opioids for an extended period will develop tolerance to the pain relief from the analgesics and need increased doses. Patients who abuse substances will have cross-tolerance and need higher than expected doses to receive analgesia from drug therapy.
- Morphine is the standard narcotic analgesic. It is an agonist at the opioid receptors. All other narcotics are compared with morphine to measure their efficacy. Morphine is indicated in the treatment of moderate to severe pain.
- In addition to analgesia, morphine, like all narcotics, produces a wide variety of other effects on the body. The most serious of these is respiratory depression, which if severe, can be life-threatening.
- The antidote to morphine overdosage and respiratory depression caused by any narcotic is naloxone, a narcotic antagonist.
- Morphine, like all narcotics, is a controlled substance. By law every dose must be properly accounted for and documented. This includes partial doses that may be wasted.
- Patient-related variables are important to consider when providing morphine or other narcotics for pain control. The variables may alter the drug chosen, dose, frequency it is given, route it is given, patient's emotional response to pain, or frequency and depth of assessment made while the patient receives morphine or other narcotics.
- Codeine is another narcotic analgesic used for mild to moderate pain. It is also used to suppress coughs. It has similar effects to morphine but usually they are milder with codeine.
- Pentazocine, a different type of narcotic, is a combination of opioid agonists and opioid antagonists. Because of the antagonist effects at some receptors, it generally causes less respiratory depression than morphine and has less risk for inducing physical dependence. If given to a patient physically dependent on a narcotic, pentazocine may induce withdrawal.
- Patients and their families need education about the importance of pain control and what will be done when they report pain. Moreover, they need to know that they are not expected to suffer. Nurses should discuss with them any fears or misconceptions about analgesic use and dispel such mistakes with facts.
- Nurses should reassess patients for pain following changes in drug therapy, after every dose until a set dose controls pain, and periodically during the course of therapy.

QUESTIONS FOR STUDY AND REVIEW

1. Why should morphine not be administered to treat acute pain in a person with respiratory depression?
2. Can morphine be administered to treat chronic pain if the patient's respiratory rate is between 8 and 12 breaths per minute? Why?
3. Your patient has a history of opioid abuse, just came from surgery, and has a chest tube. Explain why he might need a larger dose of morphine to control his postoperative pain than other patients require?
4. What is a "rescue dose"?
5. Why might more than one dose of naloxone, a narcotic antagonist, be needed when a patient has severe respiratory depression from opiate overdose?
6. Why should codeine not be administered to anyone who needs to be able to cough to clear his or her airway?

NEED MORE HELP?

? Chapter 24 of the study guide for *Drug Therapy in Nursing* contains exercises and activities to reinforce your understanding of the concepts presented in this chapter. For additional information see the text's accompanying web site at *http://www.connection.lww.com*.

REFERENCES AND BIBLIOGRAPHY

American Pain Society. (1992). *Principles of analgesic use in the treatment of acute and cancer pain* (3rd ed.). Skokie, IL: American Pain Society.

Behrens, E. (1996). An ethical approach to pain management. *MEDSURG Nursing, 5*(6), 457–458.

Bennett, G. J. (2000). Update on the neurophysiology of pain transmission and modulation: focus on the NMDA-receptor. *Journal of Pain and Symptom Management, 19*(1 Suppl): S2–6.

Casey, K. L. (1999). Forebrain mechanisms of nociception and pain: analysis through imaging. *Procedures of the National Academy of Science USA, 96*(14), 7668–7674.

Coghil, R. C., Sang, C. N., Maisog, J. M., & Iadarola, M. J. (1999). Pain intensity processing within the human brain: A bilateral, distributed mechanism. *Journal of Neurophysiology, 82*(4), 1934–1943.

Fillingim, R. B., & Ness, T. J. (2000). Sex-related hormonal influences on pain and analgesic responses. *Neuroscience Biobehavior Review, 24*(4), 485–501.

Gaston-Johansson, F. (1996). Measurement of pain: The psychometric properties of the Pain-O-Meter, a simple, inexpensive pain assessment tool that could change health care practices. *Journal of Pain and Symptom Management, 12*(3).

International Association for the Study of Pain, Subcommittee on Taxonomy. (1979). Part II. Pain terms: A current list with definitions and notes on usage. *Pain 6,* 249–252 (updated 1982, 1986).

Joint Commission on Accreditation of Healthcare Organizations. (January 2001). http://www.jcaho.org.

McCaffrey, M., & Ferrell, B. R. (1997a). Influence of professional vs personal role on pain assessment and use of opioids. *Journal of Continuing Education in Nursing, 28*(2), 69–77.

McCaffrey, M., & Ferrell, B. R. (1997b). Nurses' knowledge of pain assessment and management: How much progress have we made? *Journal of Pain and Symptom Management, 14*(3), 175–188.

Sidebotham, D., Dijkhuizen, M. R. J., & Schug, S. A. (1997). The safety and utilization of patient-controlled analgesia. *The Journal of Pain and Symptom Management, 14*(4), 202–209.

Tolle, T. R., Kaufmann, T., Siessmeier, T., Lautenbacher, S., Berthele, A., Munz, F., Zieglgansberger, W., Willoch, F., Schwaiger, M., Conrad, B., & Bartenstein, P. (1999). Region-specific encoding of sensory and affective components of pain in the human brain: a positron emission tomography correlation analysis. *Annals of Neurology, 45*(1), 40–47.

U.S. Department of Health and Human Services. (1992). Acute pain management: Operative or medical procedures and trauma. Clinical practice guideline (AHCPR Pub. No 92-0032). Rockville, MD: Author.

U.S. Department of Health and Human Services. (1994). Management of cancer pain. Clinical practice guideline. (AHCPR Pub. No 94-0592). Rockville, MD: Author.

Chapter 25

DRUGS FOR TREATING FEVER AND INFLAMMATION

KEY TERMS

cyclooxygenase
nonsteroidal anti-inflammatory drug
para-aminophenol derivative
prostaglandin synthetase inhibitors
Reye syndrome
salicylates
salicylate poisoning
salicylism

Learning Objectives

At the completion of this chapter the student will:

1. Correlate the processes of inflammation, fever, and pain with salicylates, prostaglandin synthetase inhibitors, and para-aminophenol derivative drugs.
2. Identify core drug knowledge pertaining to salicylates, prostaglandin synthetase inhibitors, and para-aminophenol derivative drugs.
3. Identify core patient variables pertaining to salicylates, prostaglandin synthetase inhibitors, and para-aminophenol derivative drugs.
4. Relate the interaction of core drug knowledge to core patient variables for salicylates, prostaglandin synthetase inhibitors, and para-aminophenol derivative drugs.
5. Generate a nursing plan of care from the interactions between core drug knowledge and core patient variables for salicylates, prostaglandin synthetase inhibitors, and para-aminophenol derivative drugs.
6. Describe nursing interventions to maximize therapeutic and minimize adverse effects for salicylates, prostaglandin synthetase inhibitors, and para-aminophenol derivative drugs.
7. Determine key points for patient and family education for salicylates, prostaglandin synthetase inhibitors, and para-aminophenol derivative drugs.

Nonsteroidal anti-inflammatory drugs (NSAIDs)

Salicylates
- **aspirin**
- diflunisal
- salsalate

Prostaglandin synthetase inhibitors
- **ibuprofen**

Propionic acids
- fenoprofen
- flurbiprofen
- naproxen
- ketoprofen
- oxaprozin

Acetic acids
- diclofenac
- etodolac
- indomethacin
- ketorolac
- sulindac
- tolmetin

Pyrazolone derivative
- phenylbutazone

Fenamates
- mefenamic acid
- meclofenamate sodium

Oxicams
- piroxicam

Alkanones
- nabumetone

COX-2 inhibitors
- celecoxib
- rofecoxib

Para-aminophenol derivatives
- **acetaminophen**

The symbol C indicates the **drug class**.

Drugs in bold type marked with the symbol P are **prototypes**.

Drugs in blue type with no symbol are **closely related** to the prototype.

Drugs in **red** type with no symbol are **significantly different** from the prototype.

Drugs in black type with no symbol are **also used in drug therapy**; no prototype.

Fever, inflammation, and pain are symptoms of acute illness and frequently coexist. Inflammation and pain also can be symptoms of chronic diseases, such as arthritis and gout. Fever, inflammation, and pain are commonly treated with salicylates, prostaglandin synthetase inhibitors (PSIs) (also known as nonsteroidal anti-inflammatory agents or NSAIDS), or para-aminophenol derivative drugs.

This chapter discusses the therapeutic classes of drugs used for fever, inflammation, and associated pain and addresses the core drug knowledge, core patient variables, nursing management, potential nursing diagnoses, and patient education related to the use of these drugs.

PHYSIOLOGY AND PATHOPHYSIOLOGY

FEVER

Temperature regulation is a function of the hypothalamus. Normally, there is a homeostatic balance between body heat generated and body heat lost. In excessive heat, the regulatory mechanism is activated, and the body responds with integumentary vasodilation, resulting in perspiration and a net heat loss. When fever is present, the hypothalamus resets the regulating mechanism to tolerate a higher body temperature. Additionally, prostaglandin formation is stimulated when fever is present.

INFLAMMATION

The inflammatory response can be evoked by numerous types of stimuli, such as trauma, surgery, infection, and ischemia. The classic signs of local inflammation are swelling (tumor), heat (calor), redness (rubor), pain (dolor), and loss of function (functio laesa). Regardless of the etiology, the sequence of physiologic effects is similar.

Acute inflammation is divided into vascular and cellular responses. The vascular response occurs almost immediately after the injury. There is an initial vasoconstriction of the surrounding vessels, which is quickly followed by vasodilation of both the arterioles and venules in the area. The vasodilation allows an increased blood flow to the area, which accounts for the signs of redness and warmth. At the same time, there is an increase in capillary permeability, allowing fluid to accumulate in the surrounding tissues, causing swelling. With the swelling of the surrounding tissues and the release of chemical mediators from the injured tissues, pain and impaired function occur.

The cellular response is divided into four phases:

1. Margination of white blood cells (WBCs)—WBCs move to the periphery of the blood vessels to prepare for emigration.
2. Emigration of WBCs—The WBCs pass through the capillary walls and migrate into the tissue spaces.
3. Chemotaxis—Cellular debris or bacteria become more "attractive" to the WBCs.
4. Phagocytosis—Neutrophils and monocytes engulf and degrade the cellular debris.

Inflammation also is enhanced by the rupture of the mast cells, which release biochemical mediators, such as histamine, prostaglandins, and leukotrienes. Prostaglandins are thought to be pivotal in the inflammatory response by potentiating pain and edema caused by other chemical mediators.

PROSTAGLANDIN SYNTHESIS

Prostaglandins modulate some components of inflammation, body temperature, pain transmission, platelet aggregation, and many other body actions. They are derived from arachidonic acid, which is liberated from the cell membrane in response to physical, chemical, hormonal, bacterial, or other stimuli (Fig. 25-1). They are converted from arachidonic acid to prostaglandins by the enzyme **cyclooxygenase** (COX). There are two forms of the COX enzyme–COX-1 and COX-2. Compelling evidence suggests that COX-1 synthesizes prostaglandins that are involved in the regulation of normal cell activity, whereas COX-2 appears to produce prostaglandins mainly at sites of inflammation. For instance, in the gastrointestinal (GI) tract, COX-1 is responsible for secretion of cytoprotective mucus and bicarbonate, suppression of the output of gastric acid, and support for submucosal blood flow. In the renal system, COX-1 promotes vasodilation, resulting in increased blood flow to the kidneys. COX-2 is activated by arthritis and other stimuli and produces the prostaglandins that lead to inflammation, swelling, and joint pain. Most NSAIDs indiscriminately target both COX-1 and COX-2, thereby depleting the prostaglandins needed for normal cell function and protection. This explains the etiology of many of these drugs' adverse effects.

PAIN

The physiologic mechanisms involved in the pain response are complex (see Chapter 24). The sensation of peripheral pain begins in afferent neurons called nociceptors, which are found in skin, muscle, connective tissue, the circulatory system, and abdominal, pelvic, and thoracic viscera. Although these receptors may be activated by mechanical, chemical, or thermal stimuli, they also are activated by chemical mediators, such as prostaglandins, histamine, bradykinin, and serotonin, which are released during cellular destruction. It is theorized that the inhibition of prostaglandins may diminish the activation of peripheral pain sensors, resulting in decreased pain.

DRUGS TO TREAT INFLAMMATION AND FEVER

Salicylates, PSIs, and para-aminophenol derivative drugs are used to treat inflammation and fever in a variety of conditions. Salicylates are used in the management of conditions ranging from a simple headache to acute myocardia infarction. PSIs are used primarily for their anti-inflammatory effects but are also used extensively as an analgesic. The newest PSIs have been approved for other conditions such as familial adenomatous polyposis (FAP) and are undergoing exten-

Physiology

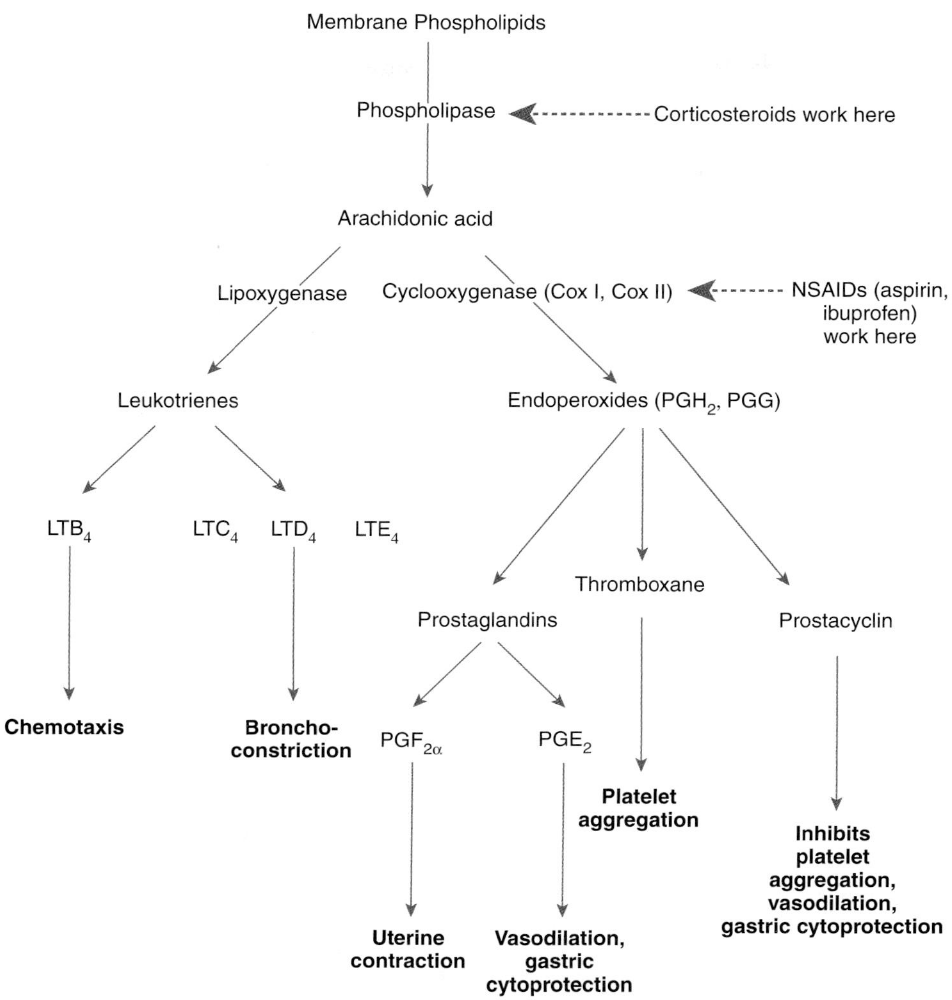

Figure 25-1. Synthesis of prostaglandins.

sive research into their viability to affect disorders such as Alzheimer and kidney disease.

NONSTEROIDAL ANTI-INFLAMMATORY AGENTS

By definition, a **nonsteroidal anti-inflammatory drug** is any drug that decreases inflammation but is not a steroid. NSAIDs are conventionally categorized as **salicylates** and **prostaglandin synthetase inhibitors**, although some of the literature refers to PSIs as NSAIDs. This is a subdivision of convenience because both salicylates and PSIs work by inhibiting COX and decreasing prostaglandins and thromboxane. A major difference is that salicylates irreversibly inhibit COX, whereas the action of the PSIs is reversible. The irreversible effects of aspirin, a salicylate, for example, account for the longer duration of its antiplatelet action. Salicylates are discussed first, followed by PSIs.

SALICYLATES

Since salicylates were isolated from the bark of the willow tree in 1829, they have become one of the mainstays of drug therapy in a variety of diseases and disorders. The therapeutic uses of salicylates continue to be researched in all areas of medicine. The prototype salicylate is acetylsalicylic acid, commonly known as aspirin.

NURSING MANAGEMENT OF THE PATIENT RECEIVING ASPIRIN

Core Drug Knowledge

Pharmacotherapeutics

Aspirin has a variety of therapeutic uses. It is indicated for mild to moderate pain, especially pain resulting from inflammation. It is used frequently to relieve headache, neuralgia, myalgia, arthralgia, postpartum pain, dental or oral surgery pain, and dysmenorrhea (painful menstruation).

Aspirin is the preferred agent for treating pain and inflammation associated with juvenile arthritis, rheumatoid arthritis, and osteoarthritis. It also is the preferred agent in treating fever, pleurisy, and arthritis. Other inflammatory conditions, such as tendonitis and bursitis, respond well to aspirin. In addition, it is used for treating pericarditis in patients with systemic lupus erythematosus (SLE).

Because of its antithrombotic and anti-inflammatory effects, aspirin is useful in preventing or reducing the risk of myocardial infarction (MI) and recurrent transient ischemic attacks. It is considered the drug of choice for treating Kawasaki syndrome (mucocutaneous lymph node syndrome).

Pharmacokinetics

Aspirin absorption usually occurs within 30 minutes depending on the dosage form, GI pH, and the presence of food or antacids in the stomach. Although a portion of aspirin is absorbed in the stomach, most is absorbed in the small intestine. Aspirin suppositories are slowly and variably absorbed. Buffered aspirin does not delay absorption; however, enteric-coated and extended-acting preparations do delay absorption.

Aspirin is 99% metabolized into salicylate and other metabolites by the liver. Aspirin and its metabolites are widely distributed throughout the body and body fluids, including breast milk. Additionally, they cross the placental barrier. Peak plasma levels occur within 2 hours. The half-life of aspirin is 15 minutes, whereas the half-life of salicylate is 2 hours. Aspirin and its metabolites are excreted by the kidneys (Table 25-1).

Pharmacodynamics

Aspirin is used for its analgesic, anti-inflammatory, antipyretic, and antithrombotic effects. It interferes with prostaglandin synthesis by irreversibly inhibiting COX. Antipyretic effects of aspirin are a result of inhibition of prostaglandin synthesis in the hypothalamus. Aspirin also may enhance peripheral vasodilation and sweating. Anti-inflammatory action is believed to be caused by peripheral inhibition of prostaglandin synthesis, but aspirin also may inhibit the action and synthesis of other mediators of inflammation. The antithrombotic effect of aspirin results from the inhibition of thromboxane A_2, a prostaglandin that induces platelet aggregation.

Contraindications and Precautions

Aspirin is contraindicated for patients with salicylate hypersensitivity. It also is contraindicated for patients with peptic ulcer disease, bleeding disorders, or patients on anticoagulation therapy because of its antiplatelet activity. Additionally, aspirin is contraindicated for patients with gout, *and* for those with renal or liver impairment. Aspirin is contraindicated in children with varicella or flulike illness because it is associated with the occurrence of **Reye syndrome**, a potentially fatal disease.

Aspirin is assigned to pregnancy category D and should be avoided by pregnant women because it can interfere with the prostaglandins that mediate uterine contraction, resulting in delayed or prolonged labor. In addition, aspirin's antiplatelet activity increases the risk of maternal or neonatal hemorrhage. Aspirin also should

TABLE 25-1 Summary of Selected Salicylates

Drug (Trade) Name	Selected Indications	Route and Dosage Range	Pharmacokinetics
Salicylates			
acetylsalicylic acid (aspirin, Bayer Aspirin; *Canadian:* Apo-ASA)	Minor aches, pains, or temperature Anti-inflammatory Acute rheumatic fever Prevention of transient ischemic attacks Prevention of myocardial infarction	*Adult:* PO, dependent on indication, in order of indications listed to the left: 325–1,000 mg q4h; 2.6–5.2 g/d in divided doses; 7.8 g/d in divided doses; 325 mg–1.3 g/d in two to four divided doses; 325 mg/d *Child:* PO, <25 kg; 60–90 mg/kg/d; >25 kg, 2.4–3.6 g/d in divided doses	*Onset:* 15–30 min *Duration:* 3–6 h $t_{1/2}$: 2–3 h
diflunisal (Dolobid; *Canadian:* Apo-Diflunisal)	Arthritis	*Adult:* PO, 250–500 mg bid not to exceed 1.5 g/d	*Onset:* 30–60 min *Duration:* 12 h $t_{1/2}$: 8–12 h
	Mild to moderate pain	*Adult:* PO, 1 g initially followed by 500 mg q12h (under 50 kg or elderly, 500 mg initially followed by 250 mg q12h)	
	Headache	*Adult:* PO, 500 mg q12h *Child:* Safe dosage not established	
salsalate (Disalcid)	Arthritis Musculoskeletal inflammation	*Adult:* PO, initially 500 mg–1 g bid or tid; maintenance, 2–4 g in divided doses *Child:* Safe dosage not established	*Onset:* 10–30 min *Duration:* 3–6 h $t_{1/2}$: 2–3 h

be avoided by lactating women because it crosses into breast milk and may exert its antiplatelet action in the infant.

Aspirin should be avoided by patients who smoke cigarettes and by patients with a history of alcohol abuse; both agents are known to be ulcerogenic. Aspirin should be given with caution to patients with asthma, nasal polyps, and hyperuricemia. Patients older than 60 years and those taking corticosteroids have a higher risk for aspirin's adverse effects.

Adverse Effects

Two adverse effects specific to aspirin therapy are salicylism and salicylate poisoning. **Salicylism** is mild aspirin toxicity, which may occur with long-term or high-dose aspirin therapy. Typical symptoms include headache, tinnitus, GI distress, paresthesias, and respiratory stimulation (i.e., increased respiratory rate secondary to stimulation in the central nervous system [CNS]). Patients may appear drowsy or confused. The only intervention needed for salicylism is a reduction of the dose of aspirin or cessation of the aspirin therapy.

Salicylate poisoning is a life-threatening event. The lethal dose of aspirin is 5 to 8 g for a child and 10 to 30 g for an adult. There is no antidote for salicylate poisoning. Treatment of salicylate poisoning includes gastric emptying, either with syrup of ipecac or gastric lavage; administration of activated charcoal; and life support, if indicated. Consequences of salicylate poisoning include respiratory alterations; fluid, electrolyte, and acid-base imbalances; seizures; high temperature; and shock leading to coma and death. Patients suspected of salicylate poisoning should be taken to an emergency department rather than a clinic or doctor's office for treatment. Children's aspirin has a pleasant flavor and may not be recognized as a drug by children. Therefore, it is important to keep aspirin in a safe place.

Common adverse effects related to aspirin are the result of the inhibition of prostaglandins. It is important to remember that prostaglandins are found in most body tissues and organs and frequently have opposing effects on the body. Adverse effects occur because of the inhibition of a particular prostaglandin necessary for normal cell function by inhibiting COX I.

The most common adverse effects of aspirin are related to the GI system. Aspirin may irritate the gastric mucosa, resulting in nausea, vomiting, abdominal pain, ulcerations, perforation, and bleeding. This occurs because of a direct irritating action to the mucosa of the GI tract and the inhibition of PGE_2, a prostaglandin that has a cytoprotective mechanism to the mucosa. Aspirin can be given with antacids to decrease its GI effects; however, antacids will also decrease the absorption of aspirin. Severe gastropathies occur most frequently with patients older than 60 years, those with a history of peptic ulcer disease, cigarette smokers, those who concomitantly use alcohol or corticosteroids, and those with dyspepsia during aspirin therapy.

Aspirin may cause hypersensitivity responses, such as rashes, hives, or bronchoconstriction, and possibly respiratory distress and anaphylaxis. Patients prone to these responses usually have severe corticosteroid-dependent asthma, nasal polyps, or chronic urticaria. High aspirin levels may induce ototoxicity manifested by tinnitus.

Another potentially serious adverse effect of aspirin is excessive or abnormal bleeding, especially in patients with hemophilia, anemias, or severe liver disease. Aspirin inhibits platelet aggregation by the inhibition of the prostaglandin thromboxane. Aspirin's antithrombotic action lasts for the life of the platelet (8 to 11 days). Other hematopoietic problems, such as agranulocytosis and aplastic anemia, have been reported infrequently.

Aspirin has been associated with hepatotoxicity in patients with juvenile arthritis, active SLE, rheumatic fever, or preexisting hepatic impairment. The hepatotoxicity is thought to be a direct toxicity to the liver and is associated with high-dose therapy.

In the renal system, acute renal failure may occur in susceptible patients. Patients with conditions associated with diminished renal blood flow, such as congestive heart failure (CHF), cirrhosis, renal insufficiency, and advanced age are at the highest risk. Prostaglandins play a role in opposing potent renal vasoconstrictors. Therefore, when the action of these prostaglandins is inhibited, vasoconstriction occurs and blood flow is diminished to the renal system, resulting in acute renal failure. Another problem inhibiting the renal prostaglandins is sodium and water retention. This is especially problematic for patients with conditions such as hypertension and CHF. Less common renal toxicities include interstitial nephritis and nephrotic syndrome. In addition to increased blood urea nitrogen (BUN) and creatinine levels, proteinuria occurs. Acute renal failure, water retention, interstitial nephritis, and nephrotic syndrome usually occur early in aspirin therapy and are reversible with the cessation of aspirin.

Additionally, aspirin decreases uric acid excretion by the kidneys; therefore, aspirin may potentiate gout.

Drug Interactions

Aspirin is a highly protein-bound drug and may interact with other drugs that are also highly protein bound. Because aspirin displaces the other active drugs into the serum, the pharmacologic effects of the displaced drug are enhanced. Drugs such as anticoagulants, oral hypoglycemics, insulin, methotrexate, and alcohol may be enhanced enough to cause toxicity. Conversely, drugs such as antacids, urinary alkalizers, probenecid, and corticosteroids may decrease the effectiveness of salicylates.

In addition, aspirin can cause false-negative results on the glucose oxidase test (Tes-Tape) and a false-positive result on the copper reduction test (Clinitest). These have become less important because of the widespread use of home blood glucose monitoring systems. A summary of drug-drug interactions for aspirin is provided in Table 25-2.

TABLE 25-2 **Agents That Interact With Aspirin**

Interactants	Effect and Significance	Nursing Management
antacids	Antacids increase urinary pH, thus reducing renal reabsorption of aspirin and increasing aspirin clearance. As more aspirin is cleared from the body, a potentially subtherapeutic aspirin level may result.	Monitor serum aspirin level when initiating or discontinuing antacid therapy.
anticoagulants	Aspirins inhibit platelet function, thus prolonging bleeding time. Aspirins displace anticoagulants from protein binding sites, thus increasing their effects. Both actions may result in hemorrhage.	Avoid administering aspirin or other salicylates if possible. If given, monitor prothrombin activity closely, and adjust the anticoagulant dose accordingly.
carbonic anhydrase inhibitors (CAI)	Aspirins displace CAI from protein binding sites and inhibit renal clearance. CAI accumulation and toxicity may result in central nervous system (CNS) depression and metabolic acidosis.	Coadministration should be avoided. When CAI is required, monitor plasma aspirin level and arterial blood gas (ABG) values. Monitor neurologic status.
corticosteroids	Corticosteroids stimulate metabolism of aspirins and increase renal elimination. Aspirin levels may become subtherapeutic.	Tailor aspirin dosage as needed. Monitor aspirin concentrations when adding or withdrawing corticosteroids.
ethanol (alcohol)	Both aspirin and alcohol damage the gastric mucosal barrier. The production of gastric acid stimulated by alcohol promotes the damage. Aspirin decreases the activity of gastric alcohol dehydrogenase, increasing bioavailability. Alcohol may potentiate aspirin-induced GI blood loss and prolong bleeding time.	Separate aspirin and alcohol intake by 12 h. Use buffered aqueous solutions or enteric-coated or extended-release aspirins.
insulin	Basal insulin concentrations are increased, and the acute insulin response to a glucose load is enhanced. This potentiates the serum glucose-lowering action of insulin and results in hypoglycemia.	Monitor blood glucose concentration, and tailor the insulin dosage regimen as needed.
methotrexate	Aspirins may decrease renal clearance and plasma protein binding of methotrexate, leading to methotrexate toxicity.	Decrease methotrexate dosage. Monitor methotrexate plasma level.
probenecid	Renal filtration of uric acid may be altered, leading to the inhibition of uricosuric action of either drug.	Avoid coadministration.
sulfonylureas	Hypoglycemic effect of sulfonylureas may be increased, but the mechanism of this action is not known.	Monitor blood glucose. If hypoglycemia occurs, consider decreasing the sulfonylurea dose.
urinary alkalizers	Aspirin excretion is enhanced in an increased pH environment, which results in decrease of therapeutic aspirin effect.	Anticipate need for possibly higher than expected aspirin doses.
valproic acid	Aspirin displaces valproic acid from protein binding sites. Coadministration may cause valproic acid toxicity.	Monitor serum valproic acid concentrations and liver enzyme levels.

Assessment of Relevant Core Patient Variables

Health Status

The nurse should assess the patient for potential medical conditions or drugs that contradict the use of aspirin or require close patient monitoring. It is important to assess for potential hypersensitivities to salicylates or other NSAIDs and for a history of asthma or nasal polyps, because patients with these conditions are prone to bronchospasm. The nurse should assess gross hearing as a baseline for possible ototoxicity.

For patients on long-term therapy, the nurse should obtain a baseline complete blood count (CBC), platelet count, and test results for renal and hepatic function. It is important to assess the patient's knowledge concerning the potential adverse effects and drug interactions associated with aspirin and to assess the patient for efficacy of the therapy.

Life Span and Gender

The nurse should determine whether the patient is pregnant. Aspirin should not be given to women in the last trimester of pregnancy because of an increased risk of maternal hemorrhage. In addition, taking aspirin during late pregnancy can result in adverse fetal effects, including low birth weight, increased intracranial hemorrhage, still births, and neonatal death. The nurse also should determine the patient's age before administering aspirin. Aspirin should never be given to children younger than 16 years with flulike symptoms because of its association with Reye syndrome. Aspirin should be given with caution to patients older than 60 years because of an increased risk for adverse effects, especially gastropathies. Recent studies indicate that men may metabolize aspirin faster than women, resulting in a decreased duration of action.

Lifestyle, Diet, and Habits

It is important to inquire about the patient's use of over-the-counter (OTC) drugs because many OTCs contain aspirin as an ingredient. Concomitant use will increase the risk for hepatic and renal toxicity. The nurse should assess for alcohol or drug abuse, because the patient may have undiagnosed preexisting hepatic dysfunction. Assessing for cigarette smoking also is important because smoking increases gastric acid production. With the loss of the cytoprotective mechanisms in the stomach from aspirin therapy, the risk for GI bleeding is increased.

Environment

The nurse should assess the patient's understanding of aspirin therapy. Aspirin has become the cheapest and most common of all household remedies. Because of its OTC availability and low cost, many people do not understand the potentially life-threatening effects it may cause. Interestingly, because of these two facts (availability and low cost), many people also do not believe aspirin is an important therapeutic intervention and are offended by receiving instructions to take aspirin. For these reasons, patient education is vital (see the accompanying display, Aspirin Therapy for Arthritis).

Critical Thinking Scenario

Aspirin Therapy for Arthritis

Mrs. Tyler, age 55, has been a patient at your clinic for the past 5 years. She has severe persistent asthma and takes oral prednisone as well as beta-adrenergic agonists as needed. She intermittently has an elevated glucose and follows a 2,400 calorie ADA diet. She was diagnosed with degenerative arthritis of her back today. The health care provider advised Mrs. Tyler to take two aspirin every 6 hours to relieve her discomfort and to increase the dose to three tablets every 6 hours if the pain continues. As Mrs. Tyler leaves she turns to you and states, "Aspirin—what a joke—I could have gotten that advice from a website on my computer." How would you respond to Mrs. Tyler? What patient education would you do? Does Mrs. Tyler's medical history predispose her to any problems with aspirin?

Nursing Diagnoses and Outcomes

- Acute or Chronic Pain related to ineffectiveness of aspirin

  Desired outcome: The patient will contact the health care provider if pain persists.
- Risk for Injury: GI bleeding, hepatic or renal toxicity related to aspirin therapy

  Desired outcome: The patient will avoid injury by contacting the health care provider if any signs of toxicity occur.
- Ineffective Protection related to blood dyscrasias or rash

  Desired outcome: The patient will contact the health care provider if any signs of blood dyscrasias or rash occur.
- Deficient Fluid Volume related to nausea and vomiting

  Desired outcome: The patient will avoid dehydration by contacting the health care provider if persistent nausea or vomiting occurs.
- Disturbed Sensory Perception (visual and auditory) related to blurred vision or tinnitus

  Desired outcome: The patient will contact the health care provider if blurred vision or tinnitus occurs.
- Risk for Injury related to self-medication

  Desired outcome: The patient will avoid injury by taking aspirin as prescribed.

Planning and Intervention

Maximizing Therapeutic Effects

The nurse may give aspirin with milk or food to decrease gastric distress, as needed.

Minimizing Adverse Effects

The nurse should not administer aspirin to a patient with a medical condition that contraindicates its use. It is important to monitor closely patients with preexisting medical conditions or those on drug therapy that may interact with aspirin. The nurse should arrange for periodic laboratory testing including a CBC, platelet count, and liver and renal function tests for patients on long-term therapy.

Providing Patient and Family Education

- The nurse should encourage the patient to take the drug exactly as prescribed by the health care provider to avoid adverse effects or overdose of aspirin.
- The nurse should caution patients not to take aspirin if they have problems with their kidneys or liver, are asthmatic and have nasal polyps (aspirin can cause an asthma attack), or are in their last trimester of pregnancy (aspirin may cause hemorrhage during delivery and adverse fetal effects).
- It is important to teach the patient about the potential side effects and adverse effects of aspirin and the

importance of contacting the health care provider if any occur. The nurse should advise the patient to contact the health care provider if any of the following serious adverse effects occur:
  - Confusion, dizziness, drowsiness
  - Seizures (convulsions)
  - Difficulty breathing, wheezing
  - Tinnitus (ringing in the ears)
  - Blurred vision
  - Black tarry stools, unusual bleeding or bruising, red or purple spots on the skin, dark urine, prolonged bleeding from a cut, vomiting blood or what looks like coffee grounds
- The nurse should caution patients that if aspirin is taken for a long time or in high doses, it can cause problems with the blood, kidneys, or liver.
- The nurse should advise patients to avoid drinking alcohol and smoking when taking aspirin, because these activities can increase the risk of gastric irritation and bleeding.
- The nurse should explain the importance of taking the drug exactly as prescribed to avoid the potential for GI distress or bleeding. For example, it is best to adhere to the following directions when taking different types of aspirin:
  - Chewable tablets can be chewed before swallowing, crushed and taken with food, or mixed in a drink.
  - Extended-release tablets should be swallowed whole, never crushed or chewed.
  - Tablets, caplets, or gel-caps should be swallowed with a full glass of water.
  - Suppositories should be removed from the foil, the tip moistened, and then placed in the rectum.
- It is important to caution the patient to contact the health care provider in the event of persistent nausea or vomiting to avoid fluid loss.
- The nurse should tell patients to take aspirin with food, milk, or antacid to prevent GI upset, and if they miss a dose, the dose should be taken as soon as possible. If it is time for the next dose, only that dose should be taken; double or extra doses should never be taken.
- It is important to encourage patients to read all OTC drug labels to avoid taking any drugs with aspirin or ibuprofen as an ingredient.
- The nurse should encourage patients with diabetes to use blood glucose monitoring rather than urine testing.
- The nurse must inform patients never to give aspirin to children younger than 16 years, unless directed by the health care provider, and to keep aspirin out of the reach of children.
- The nurse should tell the patient to keep aspirin in a cool, dry place to reserve its potency, and to discard any aspirin that smells like vinegar.
- The nurse should explain to the patient that, if the fever does not resolve in 3 days or pain does not go away in 10 days, he should see the health care provider.
- It is important for the nurse to instruct patients on long-term aspirin therapy to see their health care provider every 6 months for blood work to avoid serious adverse effects.

Ongoing Assessment and Evaluation

The nurse should monitor for signs and symptoms of GI distress or bleeding, anemia, hepatotoxicity, and renal failure. It is important to discontinue aspirin if the patient develops a rash, unexplained fever, or angioedema. The nurse should monitor for tinnitus and contact the health care provider immediately if this symptom occurs. The nurse should also monitor the patient for efficacy of aspirin therapy.

Therapy is considered effective if the patient is free of fever, pain, or inflammation, and does not develop serious adverse effects. In addition, the patient verbalizes the importance of contacting the health care provider immediately if any adverse reactions occur. ■

DRUGS CLOSELY RELATED TO P ASPIRIN

Diflunisal

Diflunisal (Dolobid) is similar to aspirin, but it does not metabolize into salicylic acid. It is used for acute or long-term relief of mild to moderate pain, acute and chronic rheumatoid arthritis, and osteoarthritis. It is not recommended for use as an antipyretic. Diflunisal has an onset of 1 hour, and peak action occurs in 2 to 3 hours. The half-life is 8 to 12 hours. Potential adverse effects are the same as for aspirin. The main advantage of diflunisal is its twice-a-day dosing schedule. The main disadvantage of diflunisal is its cost. Its efficacy for children has not been established.

MEMORY CHIP

P Aspirin

- Used for its analgesic, antipyretic, anti-inflammatory, and antiplatelet effects; irreversibly inhibits cyclooxygenase (COX)
- Significant contraindications: peptic ulcer disease, gout, renal or hepatic impairment, bleeding disorders, and patients on anticoagulation therapy
- Most common adverse effects: GI related
- Most serious adverse effects: hepatic and renal toxicity
- **Lifespan alerts: aspirin should not be given to children with varicella- or flu-like illness; it should not be given during pregnancy, especially during the third trimester; *monitor patients over the age of 60 carefully***

Salsalate

Salsalate (Disalcid) is the ester of salicylic acid. Salsalate is absorbed completely from the GI tract. However, this occurs in the small intestine because salsalate acid is practically insoluble in acidic gastric fluids. As an anti-inflammatory and analgesic drug, salsalate acid has the same efficacy as aspirin; however, it does not have antiplatelet or antipyretic effects. Salsalate is useful particularly for patients who cannot tolerate aspirin's GI effects or for patients at risk for anticoagulation. Peak action of salsalate occurs in 2 to 4 hours, and therapeutic levels may be maintained for up to 16 hours with twice-a-day dosing. Salsalate is not recommended for children.

PROSTAGLANDIN SYNTHETASE INHIBITORS

The PSIs are a subgroup of NSAIDs, although some health care providers use the term NSAIDs instead of PSIs. PSIs are grouped by chemical classes–propionic acid derivatives, acetic acids, alkanones, pyrazolones, fenamates, and oxicams. Despite the chemical differences of PSIs, they all inhibit COX and prostaglandin synthesis. Different PSIs may inhibit specific isoenzymes of the COX group, which may explain the differences in efficacy and adverse effects among the PSIs when used in specific disease states. Therapeutic efficacy of a PSI in a particular patient is based on clinical response and usually cannot be predicted before use. As previously mentioned, there are two distinct forms of COX. It is proposed that PSIs should be classified as either COX-1 specific, COX nonspecific, COX-2 preferential, or COX-2 specific.

Ibuprofen, a COX nonspecific agent, has had Food and Drug Administration (FDA) approval since the mid-1970s and currently is available in prescription and nonprescription dosages. Ibuprofen is the prototype for PSIs.

NURSING MANAGEMENT OF THE PATIENT RECEIVING IBUPROFEN

Core Drug Knowledge

Pharmacotherapeutics

Labeled uses for ibuprofen include rheumatoid arthritis, osteoarthritis, mild-to-moderate pain, primary dysmenorrhea, and fever. Unlabeled uses for ibuprofen include ankylosing spondylitis, juvenile rheumatoid arthritis, acute gout, and sunburn (Table 25-3). Table 25-4 presents labeled and unlabeled indications for selected PSIs.

TABLE 25-3 Summary of Selected Prostaglandin Synthetase Inhibitors

Drug (Trade) Name	Selected Indications	Route and Dosage Range	Pharmacokinetics
Prostaglandin Synthetase Inhibitors			
ibuprofen (Motrin, Advil; *Canadian:* Actiprofen)	Rheumatoid arthritis, osteoarthritis, dysmenorrhea, mild to moderate pain, fever	*Adult:* PO, 200–800 mg tid–qid not to exceed 3,200 mg/d *Child:* PO, 20–40 mg/kg/d in three to four divided doses	*Onset:* Rapid *Duration:* 24 h $t_{1/2}$: 2–4 h
diclofenac sodium (Voltaren; *Canadian:* Novo-Difenac)	Rheumatoid arthritis, osteoarthritis, ankylosing spondylitis	*Adult:* PO, 100–200 mg/d in two to four divided doses *Child:* Safety and efficacy not established	*Onset:* 1 h *Duration:* 4–6 h $t_{1/2}$: 1.2–1.8 h
etodolac (Lodine; *Canadian:* Ultradol)	Osteoarthritis, mild to moderate pain	*Adult:* PO, 600–1,200 mg/d in two to four divided doses, not to exceed 1,200 mg/d *Child:* Safety and efficacy not established	*Onset:* 30 min *Duration:* 4–8 h $t_{1/2}$: 6–8 h
fenoprofen (Nalfon)	Rheumatoid arthritis, osteoarthritis, mild to moderate pain	*Adult:* PO, 300–600 mg tid–qid not to exceed 3,200 mg/d *Child:* Safety and efficacy not established	*Onset:* 30 min *Duration:* 4–6 h $t_{1/2}$: 2–3 h
flurbiprofen (Ansaid)	Rheumatoid arthritis, osteoarthritis	*Adult:* PO, 50–100 mg bid–tid; maximum dose, 300 mg/d *Child:* Safety and efficacy not established	*Onset:* 1 h *Duration:* 4–8 h $t_{1/2}$: 2–4 h
indomethacin (Indocin; *Canadian:* Apo-Indomethacin)	Rheumatoid and osteoarthritis, ankylosing spondylitis, tendonitis, bursitis, acute painful shoulder, acute gout, closure of patent ductus arteriosus in premature infant	*Adult:* PO, 25 mg bid or tid up to total 150–200 mg/d *Child:* IV, 1.5–2.5 mg/kg/d in three to four divided doses	*Onset:* 30 min *Duration:* 4–6 h $t_{1/2}$: 2.6–11 h *Onset:* Immediate *Duration:* 15–30 min $t_{1/2}$: Same as above

(*continued*)

TABLE 25-3 Summary of Selected Prostaglandin Synthetase Inhibitors (Continued)

Drug (Trade) Name	Selected Indications	Route and Dosage Range	Pharmacokinetics
ketoprofen (Orudis; *Canadian:* Apo-Keto)	Rheumatoid and osteoarthritis, mild to moderate pain, primary dysmenorrhea	*Adult:* PO, 150–300 mg/d single or divided doses; maximum 300 mg/d *Child:* Safety and efficacy not established	*Onset:* 30 min *Duration:* 4–8 h $t_{1/2}$: 2–4 h
ketorolac (Toradol; *Canadian:* Acular)	Mild to moderate pain	*Adult:* PO, 10 mg q4–6h for maximum of 2 wk; IM/IV, 30–60 mg, followed by 15–30 mg q6h for a maximum of 5 d	*Onset:* PO, varies; IM/IV; 30 min *Duration:* PO, IM/IV; 6 h $t_{1/2}$: 2.4–8.6 h
meclofenamate sodium (Meclomen)	Rheumatoid and osteoarthritis, mild to moderate pain, dysmenorrhea	*Adult:* PO, 50–400 mg tid–qid *Child:* Not indicated for children <14 y	*Onset:* 30 min–1 h *Duration:* 6 h $t_{1/2}$: 1–4 h
mefenamic acid (Ponstel; *Canadian:* Apo-Fenamic)	Mild to moderate pain, primary dysmenorrhea	*Adult:* PO, initially 500 mg q6h, then decrease to 250 mg q6h; maximum dose, 1,000 mg/d, not to exceed 5–7 d *Child:* Not indicated for children <14 y	*Onset:* 1–2 h *Duration:* 6 h $t_{1/2}$: 2–4 h
meloxicam (Mobic)	Osteoarthritis	*Adult:* 7.5 mg once daily	*Onset:* Rapid *Duration:* Unknown $t_{1/2}$: 15–20 h
nabumetone (Relafen; *Canadian:* Apo-Nabumetone)	Rheumatoid and osteoarthritis	*Adult:* PO, 1,000 mg/d, not to exceed 2,000 mg/d *Child:* Safety and efficacy not established	*Onset:* 1–2 h *Duration:* 24–48 h $t_{1/2}$: 24 h
naproxen (Naprosyn; *Canadian:* Naxen)	Rheumatoid and osteoarthritis, ankylosing spondylitis, mild to moderate pain, primary dysmenorrhea, juvenile rheumatoid arthritis, tendonitis, bursitis, acute gout	*Adult:* PO, 250–750 mg bid, not to exceed 1,500 mg/d; acute gout, 750–825 mg initially, followed by 250–275 mg qid; moderate pain or dysmenorrhea, 500–550 mg, followed by 250–275 mg *Child:* PO, 10 mg/kg in two doses	*Onset:* 1–2 h *Duration:* 7–12 h $t_{1/2}$: 12–15 h
oxaprozin (Daypro)	Rheumatoid and osteoarthritis	*Adult:* PO, 600–1,200 mg once daily *Child:* Safety and efficacy not established	*Onset:* 1 h *Duration:* 24–48 h $t_{1/2}$: 26–92 h
piroxicam (Feldene; *Canadian:* Fexicam)	Rheumatoid and osteoarthritis	*Adult:* PO, 10–20 mg/d or in divided dose *Child:* Safety and efficacy not established	*Onset:* 15–30 min *Duration:* 24–48 h $t_{1/2}$: 30–86 h
sulindac (Clinoril; *Canadian:* Apo-Sulindac)	Rheumatoid and osteoarthritis, ankylosing spondylitis, bursitis, acute painful shoulder, acute gout	*Adult:* PO, 150–200 mg bid, not to exceed 400 mg/d *Child:* Safety and efficacy not established	*Onset:* 1 h *Duration:* 7–16 h $t_{1/2}$: 7–8 h
tolmetin (Tolectin; *Canadian:* Novo-Tolmetin)	Rheumatoid and osteoarthritis, juvenile rheumatoid arthritis, tendonitis	*Adult:* PO, initial 200–400 mg tid–qid; maintenance, 600–1,800 mg in divided doses, not to exceed 1,800 mg *Child:* PO, initial 20 mg/kg/d in three to four divided doses; maintenance, 15–30 mg/kg/d in three to four divided doses	*Onset:* Rapid *Duration:* 6–8 h $t_{1/2}$: 1–1.5 h
COX-2 inhibitors			
celecoxib (Celebrex)	Rheumatoid arthritis Osteoarthritis Bone pain FAP	*Adult:* PO, 100–200 mg bid 200 mg qd 400 mg qd 400 mg bid	*Onset:* <1 h *Duration:* Unknown $t_{1/2}$: 11 h
rofecoxib (Vioxx)	Dental pain, dysmenorrhea, mild-to-moderate pain Osteoarthritis	*Adult:* PO, 50 mg qd *Adult:* PO, 12.5–25 mg qd	*Onset:* 45 min *Duration:* 24 h $t_{1/2}$: 17 h

TABLE 25-4 **Indication for Selected Prostaglandin Synthetase Inhibitors**

Indications	Celecoxib	Diclofenac	Etodolac	Fenoprofen	Flurbiprofen	Ibuprofen	Indomethacin	Ketoprofen	Ketorolac	Meclofenamate	Mefenamic Acid	Nabumetone	Naproxen	Oxaprozin	Piroxicam	Rofecoxib	Sulindac	Tolmetin
Rheumatoid arthritis	•	•	X	•	•	•	•	•		•		•	•	•	•	•	•	•
Osteoarthritis	•	•	•	•	•	•	•	•		•		•	•	•	•	•	•	•
Ankylosing spondylitis		•	X		X	X	•						•				•	
Mild to moderate pain	•	X	•	•	X	•		•	•	•	•		•			•		
Primary dysmenorrhea	•				X	•	X	•			•		•		X	•		
Juvenile rheumatoid arthritis		X		X		X		X					•		X		X	•
Tendonitis			X		X		•						•		X		X	•
Bursitis			X		X		•						•				•	
Acute painful shoulder		X	X		X		•										•	
Acute gout			X		X	X	•						•				•	
Fever						•							X					
Sunburn		X		X	X	X	X	X		X	X		X		X		X	X
Migraine																		
Abortive					X					X	X		X					
Prophylactic				X			X	X					X					
Menstrual				X				X		X	X		X					
Cluster headache							X											
Polyhydramnios							X											

•, labeled use; X, unlabeled use.

Pharmacokinetics

Approximately 80% of ibuprofen is absorbed from the GI system after oral administration. Absorption is slower if the drug is taken with food; however, the extent of absorption is not affected. Peak serum concentrations occur in 1 to 2 hours. Analgesic and antipyretic effects occur in 2 to 4 hours, whereas a therapeutic inflammatory response takes a few days to 2 weeks. Ibuprofen is highly protein bound and is metabolized in the liver. Plasma half-life is 2 to 4 hours with urinary excretion within 24 hours (see Table 25-3).

Pharmacodynamics

Ibuprofen's effects are believed to be secondary to inhibition of synthesis or release of prostaglandins. Ibuprofen probably has a peripheral rather than a central action as an analgesic. Higher doses are required for an anti-inflammatory effect than for analgesia. Antipyretic activity may be the result of action on the hypothalamus, leading to an increased peripheral blood flow, vasodilation, and subsequent heat dissipation.

Contraindications and Precautions

Because chronic use of ibuprofen can result in gastritis, ulceration with or without perforation, or GI bleeding, ibuprofen is contraindicated in patients with a history of or active GI disease, including peptic ulcer disease, ulcerative colitis, or GI bleeding. Other patients at high risk for GI adverse effects are those who routinely consume alcohol or smoke tobacco products, because these behaviors are also conducive to ulcer development.

Ibuprofen should be used cautiously in patient with preexisting hepatic, renal, or hemopoietic dysfunction and patients older than 60 years. Liver dysfunction can occur during therapy with PSIs, resulting in jaundice and fatal hepatitis. Ibuprofen is metabolized in the liver, and accumulation can occur with liver dysfunction, increasing the risk of toxicity. Ibuprofen and its metabolites are excreted renally. Again, accumulation may occur in patients with renal impairment, increasing the risk of toxicity. Additionally, reduced renal blood flow caused by inhibition of prostaglandin synthesis can result in overt renal decompensation. Patients with the highest risk for renal decompensation are those with renal disease, hepatic disease, CHF, diabetes mellitus, SLE, edema, extracellular volume depletion; those taking diuretics or nephrotoxic drugs; and elderly patients.

Ibuprofen should be used cautiously in patients with preexisting coagulopathy or hemophilia, because of the effect of the drug on platelet function and vascular response to bleeding. Ibuprofen can prolong bleeding time. Anemia may be exacerbated with the use of ibuprofen.

Conditions associated with fluid retention, such as CHF, can be exacerbated with ibuprofen therapy.

Hypertension may be exacerbated by ibuprofen-induced fluid retention.

Ibuprofen is classified as a pregnancy category B drug until the third trimester, when ibuprofen enters pregnancy category D because of the potential for PSIs to cause premature closure of the ductus arteriosus in utero. Additionally, persistent pulmonary hypertension due to ductus arteriosus constriction is a potential complication. PSIs also have the potential to prolong pregnancy and inhibit labor if taken during the third trimester.

Adverse Effects

Ibuprofen, like salicylates, inhibits COX-1 and COX-2, resulting in adverse effects.

Gastropathies are commonly associated with ibuprofen. Nausea, vomiting, diarrhea, constipation, flatulence, and abdominal pain may be representative of minor adverse effects in some patients or serious GI toxicity in others. During long-term administration, the most serious effects are peptic ulcer disease or gastritis that leads to GI bleeding or even perforation. This can occur at any time, with or without warning.

Ibuprofen also can induce blurred vision, decreased visual acuity, and corneal deposits. The mechanism for visual disturbances is unclear. Vision generally improves after discontinuation of the drug. In addition, like aspirin, ibuprofen may induce tinnitus.

In the renal system, acute renal failure may occur in susceptible patients. Patients with conditions associated with diminished renal blood flow, such as CHF, cirrhosis, renal insufficiency, and advanced age, are at the highest risk. Vasodilatory renal prostaglandins and the potent vasoconstrictor angiotensin II work in concert to maintain renal blood flow. Inhibition of renal prostaglandins results in diminished renal blood flow, leading to acute renal failure. Less common renal toxicities include interstitial nephritis and nephrotic syndrome. In addition to increased BUN and creatinine levels, proteinuria occurs. Another problem resulting from the inhibition of the renal prostaglandins is sodium and water retention. This is especially problematic for patients with conditions such as hypertension and CHF. Acute renal failure, water retention, interstitial nephritis, and nephrotic syndrome usually occur early in ibuprofen therapy and are reversible with the cessation of the drug.

Ibuprofen may cause excessive or abnormal bleeding, especially in patients with hemophilia, anemias, or severe liver disease. Ibuprofen diminishes platelet aggregation by the inhibition of the prostaglandin thromboxane. This effect is transient and reversible. Other blood dyscrasias, such as agranulocytosis and aplastic anemia, have been infrequently reported.

Ibuprofen has been associated with hepatotoxicity, such as hepatitis or jaundice. This usually is infrequent, but patients should be monitored closely if on prolonged therapy.

Ibuprofen may have a cross-sensitivity to aspirin or other PSIs, including those in a different chemical class. However, cross-sensitivities are not always complete, and patients may be able to take other PSIs, even those in the same chemical class.

Drug Interactions

Ibuprofen is highly protein bound and has many interactions similar to those of salicylates. In addition to the drugs listed in Table 25-5, ibuprofen should not be given along with salicylates. There is no increased efficacy when these drugs are given together, but the risk for ad-

TABLE 25-5 Agents That Interact With Ibuprofen

Interactants	Effect and Significance	Nursing Management
anticoagulants	Ibuprofen inhibits platelet function and possibly produces gastric erosion. Anticoagulation effect is increased; hemorrhage may develop.	Avoid coadministering salicylates if possible. Monitor prothrombin activity closely if appropriate. Adjust the anticoagulant dose accordingly.
beta blockers	Ibuprofen inhibits renal prostaglandin synthesis, allowing unopposed pressor systems to produce hypertension. It also impairs antihypertensive effect of beta blockers.	Avoid coadministering if possible. Monitor blood pressure. Adjust beta blocker dosage as needed.
diuretics	Ibuprofen reduces natriuresis and antihypertensive response, resulting in decreased diuretic effect.	May need to administer a salicylate instead of ibuprofen. Anticipate possible need for higher dose of diuretic.
lithium	Ibuprofen is suspected to reduce renal elimination of lithium. Interaction may cause lithium toxicity.	Monitor lithium levels every 4–5 d until they stabilize after ibuprofen is added or withdrawn from treatment. Adjust lithium dosage as needed.
methotrexate	Ibuprofen is suspected to reduce renal elimination of methotrexate and may cause methotrexate toxicity.	Monitor methotrexate levels. Consider longer duration leucovorin rescue therapy in patients receiving ibuprofen.
sulfonylureas	Hypoglycemic effect of sulfonylureas may be increased, although the mechanism is not understood.	Monitor blood glucose levels. Anticipate an order to decrease the sulfonylurea dose if hypoglycemia occurs.

verse effects is maximized. Ibuprofen should be discontinued 72 hours before adrenal function tests are performed. Ibuprofen also may elevate sodium and chloride levels.

Assessment of Relevant Core Patient Variables

Health Status

The nurse should assess the patient for potential contraindications to ibuprofen therapy. It is important to obtain a drug history to identify potential drug-drug interactions and to assess for potential hypersensitivities to salicylates or other PSIs. The nurse should assess for a history of asthma or nasal polyps because patients with these conditions are prone to bronchospasm.

In addition, it is important to assess a patient's baseline gross hearing because of the potential for ototoxicity from ibuprofen use. For patients on long-term therapy, the nurse should obtain a baseline CBC, platelet count, and test results of renal and hepatic function. The nurse needs to assess the patient for efficacy of ibuprofen therapy; severe or visceral pain may not be affected by ibuprofen.

Life Span and Gender

The nurse should assess whether the patient is pregnant. Ibuprofen should not be given to women in the last trimester of pregnancy. The nurse also should determine the patient's age before administering ibuprofen. Although ibuprofen is considered safe for children, some of the other PSIs are contraindicated. Ibuprofen should be given with caution to patients older than 60 years because these patients have an increased risk of adverse effects. Ibuprofen, like aspirin, is thought to be metabolized faster in men, which may result in a shorter duration of action.

Lifestyle, Diet, and Habits

As with aspirin, it is important to inquire about the patient's use of OTC drugs because many OTCs contain ibuprofen or aspirin. Concomitant use of either or both will increase the risk for hepatic and renal toxicity.

The nurse needs to assess for alcohol or drug abuse because the patient may have undiagnosed preexisting hepatic dysfunction. In addition, the patient should be assessed for a history of cigarette smoking, because ibuprofen, like aspirin, decreases the cytoprotective mechanisms of the stomach.

Environment

The nurse should be aware of the setting in which ibuprofen may be administered. Ibuprofen may be self-administered at home or given in any health care setting. Because this drug first appeared on the market as a prescription drug, the lay public often believes that it is more effective than aspirin or acetaminophen. With its reasonable cost and high efficacy, some patients may take the drug at a higher dose than the labeling suggests or for a much longer duration without seeing a medical provider. This places the patient at a higher risk for adverse effects or other problems, because the etiology of their symptoms is not addressed.

Nursing Diagnoses and Outcomes

- Acute or Chronic Pain related to ineffectiveness of ibuprofen

  Desired outcome: The patient will contact the health care provider if pain persists.
- Risk for Injury related to incorrect self-administration or to drug-induced GI bleeding or hepatic and renal toxicity

  Desired outcome: The patient will remain free of injury by taking the drug only as directed.
- Risk for Deficient Fluid Volume related to nausea and vomiting

  Desired outcome: The patient will contact the health care provider immediately if intractable nausea or vomiting occurs.
- Ineffective Protection related to blood dyscrasias

  Desired outcome: The patient will contact the health care provider immediately if any signs and symptoms of blood dyscrasias occur.
- Disturbed Sensory Perception (visual) related to blurred vision

  Desired outcome: The patient will discontinue ibuprofen immediately and contact the health care provider if vision is affected.

Planning and Intervention

Maximizing Therapeutic Effects

The nurse should give ibuprofen with milk or food to decrease gastric distress, if needed.

Minimizing Adverse Effects

The nurse needs to monitor closely patients with preexisting medical conditions or drug therapy that may interact with ibuprofen. It is important to administer misoprostol to patients at high risk for developing gastropathies with ibuprofen (see the accompanying display, Misoprostol). Periodic CBC, platelet count, and liver and renal function tests should be obtained for patients on long-term therapy.

Providing Patient and Family Education

- The nurse should instruct patients to take the drug exactly as directed by the health care provider to avoid adverse effects or overdose with ibuprofen.
- It is important for the nurse to tell patients not to take ibuprofen if they have problems with their kidney or liver, to use ibuprofen cautiously during the first two trimesters of pregnancy, and not to take it at all during the third trimester of pregnancy. In addition, patients should not take ibuprofen if they are asthmatic and

Misoprostol

Misoprostol (Cytotec) increases bicarbonate and mucus production in the gastrointestinal tract. It may also inhibit gastric acid secretion. To minimize possible gastropathies in patients on long-term prostaglandin synthetase inhibitor (PSI) therapy, consider prophylactic therapy with misoprostol for patients with any of the following:

- Older than 60 years
- History of peptic ulcer disease
- Cigarette smoker
- Concomitant use of alcohol
- Concomitant use of corticosteroids
- Dyspepsia during salicylate or PSI use
- Poor surgical risk if ulcer complications occur

have nasal polyps, because ibuprofen could cause an asthma attack.

- The nurse should advise patients to take ibuprofen with food, milk, or possibly an antacid to prevent GI upset.
- The nurse should instruct the patient that if a dose is missed, it should be taken as soon as possible. If it is almost time for the next dose, only that dose should be taken; double or extra doses should never be taken.
- The nurse should caution patients that the drug can cause problems with the blood, kidneys, or liver if taken for a long time or in high doses.
- The nurse should caution patients that drinking alcohol and smoking while taking ibuprofen can increase the risk of GI irritation and bleeding.
- The nurse should advise patients to contact the health care provider if minor adverse effects such as diarrhea, dizziness, drowsiness, heartburn, nausea, and vomiting do not subside or if they are bothersome.
- It is important for the nurse to warn patients about serious adverse effects of ibuprofen and to advise them to seek medical attention immediately if they occur. Adverse effects include the following:
  - Black, tarry stools; blood in urine; dark yellow or brown urine
  - Difficulty breathing, wheezing; skin rash, redness, blistering, peeling, or itching; swelling of eyelids, throat, lips, or feet
  - Rapid heartbeat
  - Blurred vision
  - Fever, chills, muscle aches and pains
  - Weight change
  - Unusual bleeding or bruising, unusual tiredness or weakness, prolonged bleeding from a cut, vomiting blood or what looks like coffee grounds
- The nurse should instruct patients to change position slowly to avoid dizziness. If dizziness occurs, the patient should refrain from driving a car or operating machinery.
- It is important to tell patients to read the labels of all OTC drugs and to avoid any with aspirin or other NSAIDs as an ingredient.
- The nurse should warn patients to seek immediate medical assistance if they accidentally take too many tablets.
- The nurse should advise patients with diabetes to monitor their blood glucose levels rather than urine testing.
- The nurse should instruct patients to keep ibuprofen in a cool, dry place to preserve its potency.
- The nurse should tell patients to see their health care provider if their fever does not resolve in 3 days or their pain does not go away in 10 days.
- It is important to advise patients on long-term ibuprofen therapy to see their health care provider every 6 months for blood testing to make sure they are not having adverse effects from the drug.

Ongoing Assessment and Evaluation

The patient requires monitoring for signs and symptoms of GI distress or bleeding, anemia, tinnitus, hepatotoxicity, and renal failure. The nurse should monitor patients older than 60 years closely for these adverse effects. The nurse should arrange periodic laboratory tests for patients on long-term therapy or those at high risk for adverse effects. The nurse should monitor the patient for relief of pain and inflammation.

Therapy is considered effective if the patient is free of fever, pain, or inflammation, and does not develop adverse effects. In addition, the patient verbalizes the importance of contacting the health care provider immediately if any adverse effects occur. ■

DRUGS CLOSELY RELATED TO IBUPROFEN

Propionic Acids

In addition to ibuprofen, the following drugs are in the propionic class of PSIs: fenoprofen (Nalfon), flurbiprofen (Ansaid), ketoprofen (Orudis), naproxen (Naprosyn, Anaprox), and oxaprozin (Daypro). These drugs are similar to ibuprofen in action, indications, nursing management, and patient

MEMORY CHIP

Ibuprofen

- Used for its anti-inflammatory, analgesic, and antipyretic effects; reversibly inhibits cyclooxygenase (COX)
- Significant contraindications: active GI diseases; used with caution in patients with renal or hepatic impairment, hemopoietic dysfunction, preexisting coagulopathy, cardiac impairment, and those older than 60 years
- Most common adverse effects: GI related
- Most serious adverse effects: hepatic and renal toxicity
- **Lifespan alert: ibuprofen is in pregnancy category D in the third trimester; *monitor patients over the age of 60 carefully***

education. They differ only in their onset, peak, and duration of action. Although these drugs are chemically similar, patients may have relief of symptoms from one drug in this group but not another. Naproxen and ketoprofen, like ibuprofen, may be purchased OTC.

Acetic Acids

The acetic acids include diclofenac sodium (Voltaren), etodolac (Lodine), indomethacin (Indocin), ketorolac (Toradol), sulindac (Clinoril), and tolmetin (Tolectin). They are potent PSIs, highly protein bound, and may displace other protein-bound drugs, which may cause toxicities. They are associated with a high incidence of GI distress and should be given with meals or milk. They also may increase blood pressure or cause sodium and water retention. This group of PSIs also have an increased risk for causing liver dysfunction. Patients should have periodic liver function tests evaluated.

Patients taking indomethacin have an increased risk for adverse effects. It may aggravate depression, other psychiatric disturbances, epilepsy, and parkinsonism. Indomethacin is also associated with a high incidence of severe frontal headaches.

Ketorolac is the only PSI administered both orally and intramuscularly. It is administered for its analgesic effect alone. The efficacy of its intramuscular administration is similar to morphine and opioid analgesics. Despite its intramuscular (IM) administration, ketorolac also may induce GI distress including peptic ulcers and bleeding.

The advantage of acetic acids is their long-half life with resultant once or twice a day dosing. A major disadvantage is their high cost.

Pyrazolone Derivative

Phenylbutazone (Butazolidin) is a pyrazolone drug that has been used in the United States since 1949. It has a superior efficacy for rheumatoid arthritis; however, its anti-inflammatory and analgesic effects for other disorders are suboptimal. Even for rheumatoid arthritis, phenylbutazone is related to a high incidence of serious adverse effects. Therefore, it has limited uses compared with other PSIs. Phenylbutazone should be used for short-term therapy in acute exacerbations of rheumatoid arthritis or gout. It should be given with milk or antacids because of its effect on the GI system.

Fenamates

Mefenamic acid (Ponstel) and meclofenamate sodium (Meclomen) are the two fenamate drugs used in the United States. They have anti-inflammatory, analgesic, and antipyretic actions. They have no clear advantage over other PSIs and have an increased risk for adverse effects, especially diarrhea.

Oxicams

Piroxicam (Feldene) is the only oxicam currently available in the United States. It has anti-inflammatory, analgesic, and antipyretic effects. It is equivalent to aspirin, indomethacin, and naproxen in treating osteoarthritis and rheumatoid arthritis and is better tolerated. It may take up to 2 weeks for the effects of piroxicam to be noted. Its major advantage is its long half-life resulting in once-daily dosing. It major disadvantage is its high cost.

Alkanones

Nabumetone (Relafen) is a new type of PSI indicated for osteoarthritis and rheumatoid arthritis. Despite its high efficacy, it has a relatively low incidence of side effects. It appears to cause less gastric damage than other PSIs. It is assumed that its decreased GI effects are related to its decreased inhibition of COX-1. Like other drugs with a long half-life, nabumetone is administered once a day. The disadvantage of this drug is its high cost.

DRUGS SIGNIFICANTLY DIFFERENT FROM IBUPROFEN

COX-2 Inhibitors

There are currently two COX-2 inhibitors, celecoxib (Celebrex) and rofecoxib (Vioxx). These drugs exhibit anti-inflammatory, analgesic, and antipyretic activities by selectively inhibiting COX-2 prostaglandin synthesis, but not platelet aggregation. The discovery of COX-2 has made possible the design of drugs that reduce inflammation without removing the protective prostaglandins in the stomach and kidney made by COX-1. These highly selective COX-2 inhibitors may not only be useful in conditions such as rheumatic and osteoarthritis but also in colon cancer, Alzheimer disease, and kidney disease.

Current pharmacotherapeutics for both drugs include osteoarthritis (OA) and the treatment of dysmenorrhea or acute pain. Celecoxib is indicated for use in rheumatoid arthritis. In addition, celecoxib also is approved to reduce the number of adenomatous colorectal polyps in patients with FAP as an adjunct to usual care such as surgery and monitoring of the lower GI tract because COX-2 has been implicated in the development of these disorders.

COX-2 inhibitors should not be given to patients who have experienced salicylate hypersensitivity evidenced by asthma, urticaria, or allergic-type reactions after taking aspirin or other PSIs. Celecoxib is contraindicated absolutely in patients with known sulfonamide hypersensitivity because it contains a sulfonamide side chain. Precautions are similar to ibuprofen with the exception of hemophilia because COX-2 inhibitors do not inhibit platelet aggregation.

Potential adverse effects also are similar to ibuprofen. Theoretically, because of the specificity of these drugs for the COX-2 cyclooxygenase pathway, they have the potential to cause less gastropathy and risk of GI bleeding. However, serious GI bleeding or obstruction has been reported in patients receiving COX-2 inhibitors despite their cytoprotective properties.

PARA-AMINOPHENOL DERIVATIVES

Acetaminophen (Tylenol), a widely used analgesic and antipyretic, is the only **para-aminophenol derivative** available in the United States. Although similar to an NSAID and often grouped as such, it does not have an anti-inflammatory effect. It was first used in clinical medicine in 1893, but widespread use began after it received FDA approval in 1950. It is available without a prescription as an individual agent and in combination with a variety of other drugs.

NURSING MANAGEMENT OF THE PATIENT RECEIVING ACETAMINOPHEN

Core Drug Knowledge

Pharmacotherapeutics

Acetaminophen is indicated for treating fever or mild pain. It is used for patients with a hypersensitivity to aspirin or PSIs or intolerance to their GI effects and for patients who are receiving anticoagulant therapy (Table 25-6).

Pharmacokinetics

Acetaminophen is absorbed rapidly and completely from the GI tract or rectal mucosa. Peak concentrations occur within 60 minutes. The half-life is 1 to 3.5 hours, and the duration is 3 to 5 hours. Acetaminophen is metabolized in the liver and eliminated by the kidneys. Acetaminophen crosses the placenta and passes into breast milk.

Pharmacodynamics

Acetaminophen possesses both antipyretic and analgesic effects, but it has no peripheral anti-inflammatory effects. Thus, it may be less effective than other drugs for pain related to peripheral inflammation.

Acetaminophen's exact mechanism of action is unknown. It is centrally acting primarily, has no effects on platelet aggregation, and is a reversible weak inhibitor of COX. The antipyretic activity is thought to be produced by blocking the effects of endogenous pyrogen on the hypothalamic heat-regulating center, possibly by inhibiting prostaglandin synthesis. Heat is lost by vasodilation, increased peripheral blood flow, and sweating. The analgesic effect is believed to result from inhibited prostaglandin synthesis or from inhibited synthesis or actions of chemical mediators that sensitize the pain receptors to mechanical or chemical stimulation.

Contraindications and Precautions

Acetaminophen is contraindicated in patients with hepatic disease, viral hepatitis, or alcoholism. In these diseases, metabolism of the drug may be decreased, resulting in a risk for hepatotoxicity. Because acetaminophen is excreted primarily by the kidneys, serum concentrations may increase in patients with renal impairment, again resulting in an increased risk for toxicity.

Acetaminophen is also used with caution in patients with preexisting anemia because acetaminophen may exacerbate anemias. Patients who have phenylketonuria or who must restrict intake of phenylalanine should avoid acetaminophen products containing aspartame (Nutrasweet), such as Tempra chewable tablets, Alka-Seltzer Advanced Formula, Children's Anacin-3, Junior Strength Tylenol, Children's Tylenol, and Double-Strength Tempra.

Acetaminophen is assigned to pregnancy category B and therefore should be used cautiously in patients who are pregnant or lactating. However, it is the safest antipyretic analgesic drug to use, if necessary, during pregnancy or lactation.

Adverse Effects

Acetaminophen is generally well tolerated. Most adverse effects occur when the drug is taken in high doses or for prolonged periods. However, acetaminophen overdose is potentially fatal. Metabolites of acetaminophen can bind to tissue groups in either the kidney or liver, causing a loss of glutathione reserves and resulting in either nephrotoxicity or hepatotoxicity. Symptoms during the early stage of toxicity include anorexia, nausea, vomiting, pallor, and diaphoresis. During the intermediate stage (days 1 to 3), the patient may complain of right upper quadrant pain and experience decreased urine output. The late stage (days 3 to 5) is characterized by jaundice, elevated aspartate transaminase and alanine transaminase levels, and a dramatic rise in prothrombin time, indicating hepatic necrosis and symptoms of renal failure. During this stage, the patient also may experience CNS stimulation followed by CNS depression. Early administration of acetylcysteine, which replaces glutathione reserves, is the only antidote. Acetaminophen overdose is an emergency that must be treated in the hospital.

Acetaminophen may cause adverse effects in the hepatic, renal, hematologic, and GI systems. Hepatotoxicity and hepatic necrosis may occur in patients who are on high-dose or long-term therapy. Another potential adverse effect in patients with high-dose or long-term therapy is acute renal failure, renal papillary necrosis, or

TABLE 25-6 Summary of Para-Aminophenol Derivatives

Drug (Trade) Name	Selected Indications	Route and Dosage Range	Pharmacokinetics
Para-aminophenol Derivatives			
acetaminophen (Tylenol; *Canadian:* Atasol)	Fever, analgesia	*Adult:* PO, 325–650 mg q3–4h, not to exceed 4g/d *Child:* PO, 10 mg/kg q4–6h	*Onset:* 10–30 min *Duration:* 3–5 h $t_{1/2}$: 1–3.5 h

renal tubular necrosis. In the hematologic system, acetaminophen may cause anemia, leukopenia, thrombocytopenia, or pancytopenia. In the GI system, acetaminophen may cause GI bleeding. This occurs secondary to low prothrombin levels.

Drug Interactions

Acetaminophen may interact with activated charcoal, antacids, ethanol, hydantoins, and sulfinpyrazone. In rats, cimetidine decreases acetaminophen binding to hepatic microsomal proteins and has been shown to improve survival after acetaminophen overdose. The impact of these findings in the prevention of acetaminophen hepatotoxicity is uncertain; more studies are needed to evaluate the role of cimetidine in acetaminophen toxicity. Table 25-7 presents additional information about these interactions.

Assessment of Relevant Core Patient Variables

Health Status

The nurse should assess the patient for pain level and the potential for acetaminophen to be therapeutic because it is effective for mild to moderate pain. The nurse should assess for preexisting medical conditions or drug therapy that contraindicates using acetaminophen or necessitates close monitoring of the patient. For patients expected to be on long-term therapy, baseline CBC, platelet count, and renal and hepatic function values should be obtained and documented.

Life Span and Gender

The nurse should note the patient's age before administering acetaminophen. Acetaminophen is an excellent drug for treating fever and pain for children. Unlike aspirin, it is not associated with the occurrence of Reye syndrome. Elderly patients are more likely to develop hepatic and renal toxicity because of age-related decreases in hepatic and renal function. The nurse also should note whether the patient is pregnant. Acetaminophen is the drug of choice for pregnant women because it does not have any antiplatelet activity.

Lifestyle, Diet, and Habits

It is important to inquire about the patient's use of OTC drugs, because many of these products contain acetaminophen as an ingredient. Concomitant use will increase the risk for hepatotoxicity. The nurse should assess for alcohol or drug abuse, because the patient may have undiagnosed preexisting hepatic dysfunction.

Environment

The nurse should determine the patient's understanding of acetaminophen therapy. Acetaminophen is self-administered easily at home without medical supervision. Because of acetaminophen's low cost and availability, many people do not understand the potentially life-threatening adverse effects of acetaminophen. Patient education is important to avoid unintentional overdose or long-term complications.

TABLE 25-7 Agents That Interact With Acetaminophen

Interactants	Effect and Significance	Nursing Management
activated charcoal	Charcoal reduces gastrointestinal (GI) absorption of ingested drugs and adsorbs enterohepatically circulated drugs. Charcoal may actually remove drugs from the systemic circulation. Depending on the clinical situation, this will reduce the effectiveness or toxicity of a given agent.	Administer activated charcoal as soon as possible, in a situation involving toxicity of acetaminophen. Do not administer activated charcoal within 2–3 h of acetaminophen administration, in any situation using acetaminophen therapeutically.
antacids	Antacids can delay and decrease the oral absorption of acetaminophen.	Administer antacids and acetaminophen at least 2 h apart.
ethanol (alcohol)	Induction of hepatic microsomal enzymes by chronic ethanol consumption may be associated with acetaminophen-induced hepatotoxicity. Chronic consumption of ethanol may increase the risk of acetaminophen-induced liver damage.	Caution patient who consumes ethanol chronically and in excess about the potential interaction. Advise patients to avoid ethanol ingestion while taking acetaminophen. Monitor suspected ethanol abusers closely for hepatotoxicity.
drugs that increase the risk of hepatotoxicity hydantoins sulfinpyrazone	Hydantoins and sulfinpyrazone may induce hepatic microsomal enzymes, which accelerate the metabolism of acetaminophen. An unusually high rate of acetaminophen metabolism could lead to abnormally high levels of hepatotoxic metabolites. The potential hepatotoxicity of acetaminophen may be increased and the therapeutic effects of acetaminophen may be decreased when administered with chronic doses of hydantoins or sulfinpyrazone.	At usual therapeutic doses of acetaminophen and hydantoins or sulfinpyrazone, no special dosage adjustment is required. Risk is greatest when acetaminophen overdose accompanies chronic use of hydantoins or sulfinpyrazone. Monitor patients closely.

Nursing Diagnoses and Outcomes

- Acute or Chronic Pain related to ineffectiveness of acetaminophen
  Desired outcome: The patient will contact the health care provider if pain persists.
- Risk for Injury related to drug-induced hepatic and renal toxicity or to improper self-medication
  Desired outcome: The patient will take drug as directed and contact the health care provider if any signs of toxicity occur.
- Ineffective Protection related to potential blood dyscrasias
  Desired outcome: The patient will contact the health care provider if any signs of blood dyscrasias occur.

Planning and Intervention

Maximizing Therapeutic Effects

Acetaminophen can be administered without regard to meals. The nurse needs to monitor the patient for therapeutic effect of acetaminophen and relief of symptoms.

Minimizing Adverse Effects

It is important to assess patients for medical conditions that contradict the use of acetaminophen. The nurse needs to monitor patients carefully with preexisting medical conditions or drug therapy that may interact with acetaminophen. Periodic CBC, platelet count, and liver and renal function tests should be performed for patients on long-term therapy.

Providing Patient and Family Education

- It is important to tell patients to take the drug exactly as prescribed by the health care provider to avoid adverse effects or overdose.
- The nurse should warn patients not to take this drug if they have problems with their kidneys or liver.
- Because acetaminophen is manufactured in a variety of formulations, it is important to teach patients exact directions for correct administration.
- The nurse should teach patients with diabetes to monitor their blood glucose level for signs of hypoglycemia.
- The nurse should instruct the patient to read all OTC drug labels and to avoid any with acetaminophen as an ingredient.
- It is important to stress the potential for acetaminophen overdose and the importance of seeking medical attention should the patient accidentally take too many tablets.
- The nurse should advise patients to keep acetaminophen in a light-resistant container out of the reach of children.
- The nurse should encourage patients to contact the health care provider immediately if they have any adverse effects (e.g., signs of blood dyscrasias and signs of hepatic or renal toxicity), if fever does not subside within 3 days, or if pain is not relieved within 10 days.

Ongoing Assessment and Evaluation

The nurse needs to monitor the patient for sore throat, chills, easy bruising, and unusual bleeding, because these signs may indicate blood dyscrasias. It also is important to monitor the patient for any signs and symptoms of hepatotoxicity and renal failure. The nurse should not give acetaminophen if the patient develops a rash, unexplained fever, or angioedema. The patient needs to contact the health care provider immediately should any of these symptoms occur.

Therapy is considered effective if the patient is free of fever and pain. In addition, the patient should remain free of adverse effects and should verbalize the importance of contacting the health care provider immediately if any adverse effects occur. ■

MEMORY CHIP

Acetaminophen

- Used for mild to moderate pain and fever; usually well tolerated; and has no anti-inflammatory effect
- Significant contraindications: hepatic disease, viral hepatitis, and alcoholism
- Most common adverse effects: rash, urticaria, and nausea
- Most serious adverse effects: acetaminophen may cause hepatic or renal toxicity in susceptible patients
- **Lifespan alert: acetaminophen is the drug of choice for infants and children with flu or flu-like symptoms; analgesic of choice during pregnancy or lactation**

CHAPTER SUMMARY

- Prostaglandins are found in almost all body tissues and affect the body in a multitude of ways.
- Prostaglandins are subdivided into COX-1 and COX-2. COX-1 is involved in the maintenance of cells whereas COX-2 prostaglandins are generally found at the site of inflammation.
- Drugs for fever, inflammation, and pain include salicylates (aspirin), prostaglandin synthetase inhibitors (PSI) (ibuprofen), and para-aminophenol derivatives (acetaminophen). These drugs work by inhibiting the synthesis of prostaglandins.
- Aspirin and acetaminophen overdoses are common. Patients do not realize the potentially serious consequences of ingesting these drugs because they are easily obtained without a prescription.
- The most common adverse effects of aspirin and ibuprofen are GI in nature.
- The most serious adverse effects of aspirin and ibuprofen are hepatic dysfunction, renal dysfunction, and GI bleeding.

- COX-2 inhibitors decrease the potential for GI bleeding, although it may still occur in some patients.
- COX-2 inhibitors do not inhibit platelet aggregation.
- The most serious adverse effects of acetaminophen are hepatic and renal dysfunctions.

QUESTIONS FOR STUDY AND REVIEW

1. How do prostaglandins affect the processes of inflammation, pain, and fever?
2. How does prostaglandin inhibition induce adverse effects of salicylates, PSIs, and acetaminophen?
3. What are the most potentially serious adverse effects of salicylates, PSIs, and acetaminophen, and how might you decrease their occurrence?
4. Identify two major differences between PSIs that are nonselective and COX-2 inhibitors.

NEED MORE HELP?

Chapter 25 of the study guide for *Drug Therapy in Nursing* contains exercises and activities to reinforce your understanding of the concepts presented in this chapter. For additional information, see the text's accompanying web site at *http://www.connection.lww.com.*

REFERENCES AND BIBLIOGRAPHY

Andrade, S. E., et al. (1998). Comparative safety evaluation of non-narcotic analgesics. *Journal of Clinical Epidemiology, 51*(12), 1357–1365.

Bolten, W. W. (1998). Scientific rationale for specific inhibition of COX-2. *Journal of Rheumatology Supplement, 51,* 2–7.

CCIS System. (2001). *Computerized Clinical Information System.* Denver, CO: Micromedex.

Clinical Drug Monographs. (2001). [CD-ROM]. Gold Standard Media.

Drug Facts and Comparisons. (2000). St. Louis: Facts and Comparisons.

Hardman, J. G., Limbird, L. E., Molinof, P. B., Ruddon, R. W., & Gilman, A. (Eds.). (1997). *Goodman and Gilman's the pharmacological basis of therapeutics* (9th ed.). New York: McGraw-Hill.

Karch, A. (2001). *2001 Lippincott's nursing drug guide.* Philadelphia: Lippincott Williams & Wilkins.

Katzung, B. C. (2000). *Basic and clinical pharmacology* (8th ed.). New York: McGraw-Hill.

Levesque, H. & Lafont, O. (2000). Aspirin throughout the ages: A historical review. *Review of Internal Medicine, 21,* (Suppl. 1), 8s–17s.

Marnett, L. J. & Kalgutkar, A. S. (1999). Cyclooxygenase 2 inhibitors: Discovery, selectivity and the future. *Trends in Pharmacology Science, 20,* 465–469.

Mitchell, J. A. & Warner, T. D. (1999). Cyclooxygenase-2: Pharmacology, physiology, biochemistry and relevance to NSAID therapy. *British Journal of Pharmacology, 128*(6), 1121–1132.

Porth, C. (1998). *Pathophysiology: Concepts of altered health states* (5th ed.). Philadelphia: Lippincott Williams & Wilkins.

Tatro, D. (Ed.). (2000). *Drug interaction facts* (6th ed.). St. Louis: Facts and Comparisons.

Wolfe, M. M. (1998). Future trends in the development of safer nonsteroidal anti-inflammatory drugs, *American Journal of Medicine, 105*(5A), 44–52S.

Chapter 26

DRUGS FOR TREATING ARTHRITIS AND GOUT

KEY TERMS

antigout drugs
chrysotherapy
cytokine
disease-modifying antirheumatic drug
nitritoid crisis
pannus
tophi
tumor necrosis factor
uricosuric drugs

Learning Objectives

At the completion of this chapter the student will:

1. Correlate the processes of inflammation and pain with antirheumatic drugs, antigout drugs, and uricosuric drugs.
2. Identify core drug knowledge pertaining to antirheumatic drugs, antigout drugs, and uricosuric drugs.
3. Identify core patient variables pertaining to antirheumatic drugs, antigout drugs, and uricosuric drugs.
4. Relate the interaction of core drug knowledge to core patient variables for antirheumatic drugs, antigout drugs, and uricosuric drugs.
5. Generate a nursing plan of care from the interactions between core drug knowledge and core patient variables for antirheumatic drugs, antigout drugs, and uricosuric drugs.
6. Describe nursing interventions to maximize therapeutic and minimize adverse effects for antirheumatic drugs, antigout drugs, and uricosuric drugs.
7. Determine key points for patient and family education for antirheumatic drugs, antigout drugs, and uricosuric drugs.

DRUGS FOR ARTHRITIS AND GOUT

ARTHRITIS

Salicylates and prostaglandin synthetase inhibitors
(covered in Chapter 25)

- **auranofin** (P)
- aurothioglucose
- gold sodium thiomalate
- methotrexate
- hydroxychloroquine
- penicillamine
- leflunomide
- etanercept
- infliximab

GOUT

Acute

- **colchicine** (P)

Chronic

- **probenecid** (P)
- sulfinpyrazone
- allopurinol

The symbol (C) indicates the **drug class**.

Drugs in bold type marked with the symbol (P) are **prototypes**.

Drugs in blue type with no symbol are **closely related** to the prototype.

Drugs in **red** type with no symbol are **significantly different** from the prototype.

Drugs in **black** type with no symbol are **also used in drug therapy**; no prototype.

This chapter focuses on two inflammatory conditions, rheumatoid arthritis (RA) and gout. Rheumatoid arthritis is treated initially with a salicylate or prostaglandin-synthetase inhibitor (PSI), which are discussed in Chapter 25. More severe and chronic inflammation in patients with RA may require disease-modifying antirheumatic drugs (DMARDS). Drugs within the DMARD class include auranofin, aurothioglucose, gold sodium thiomalate, methotrexate (MTX), hydroxychloroquine sulfate, penicillamine, leflunomide, etanercept, and infliximab.

For inflammation caused by acute gout, antigout drugs are used. The only drug in this class is colchicine. Chronic gout is treated with uricosuric drugs, which decrease hyperuricemia associated with gout. Uricosuric drugs include probenecid, sulfinpyrazone (Anturane), and allopurinol (Zyloprim).

In addition to discussing the therapeutic classes of drugs used to treat RA and gout, this chapter also addresses the core drug knowledge, core patient variables, nursing management, potential nursing diagnoses, and patient education related to the use of DMARDS, antigout drugs, and uricosuric drugs.

PATHOPHYSIOLOGY

RHEUMATOID ARTHRITIS

Rheumatoid arthritis is a systemic inflammatory disease that affects all age groups, although it is more prevalent between the ages of 40 and 60. Women are more likely than men to have RA. In Yakima and Chippewa Native Americans, there is a fivefold greater risk for this disease.

It is thought to be an autoimmune disorder because 70% of patients have a substance found in their blood, synovial fluid, and synovial tissue called rheumatoid factor (RF), which is an antibody to their own immunoglobulin G (IgG). RF interacts with IgG or other antibodies to form immune complexes. These immune complexes activate the complement system, resulting in an inflammatory response. Leukocytes, monocytes, and lymphocytes are attracted to the area and phagocytize the immune complexes. During that process, lysosomal enzymes are released. These enzymes are capable of destroying joint cartilage, resulting in an inflammatory process that starts the cycle again. As the disease progresses, a destructive granular tissue called **pannus** extends through the synovial space, damaging the articular cartilage. Continued progression destroys the entire joint space, resulting in reduced joint motion and possible ankylosis (extreme stiffness or joint fusion) (Fig. 26-1).

The major characteristic of RA is symmetric polyarticular inflammatory arthritis. The clinical course is highly variable. Symptoms include morning stiffness that lasts more than 1 hour, symmetric involvement of joints, and rheumatoid nodules over bony prominences or extensor surfaces. Joints commonly affected include the proximal phalangeal (PIP), metacarpophalangeal (MCP), wrist, elbow, knee, ankle, and metatarsophalangeal joint (MTP).

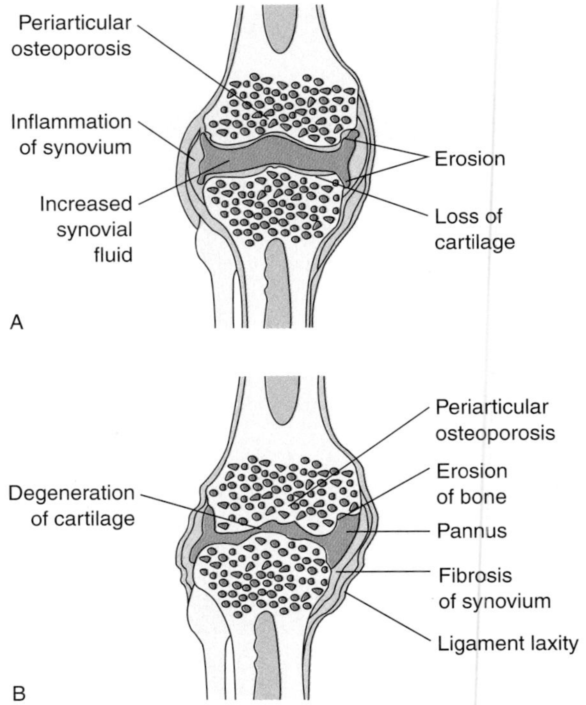

Figure 26-1. (**A**) Early rheumatoid arthritis with fluid accumulation and synovial swelling; (**B**) Late rheumatoid arthritis with pannus formation, eroded articular cartilage, and joint space narrowing.

GOUT

Gout is a disease of purine metabolism. Uric acid is a metabolite of the purines, adenine and guanine. Hyperuricemia may result from overproduction or underexcretion of uric acid. However, hyperuricemia does not always result in gout. Gout occurs when the hyperuricemia forms monosodium urate crystals, which precipitate into the synovial fluid and initiate an inflammatory response. As in RA, the inflammatory response attracts leukocytes to phagocytize the crystals. When the leukocytes die, they release lysosomal nodules called **tophi.** They can be found in bursas, synovium, tendons, and along the extensor surface of the forearm. Certain drugs, foods, or alcohol may precipitate an attack. Attacks are usually monoarticular and characterized by severe pain, erythema, and warmth of the affected joint (Fig. 26-2). Recurrent attacks damage the joint space, which results in gouty arthritis.

DISEASE-MODIFYING ANTIRHEUMATIC DRUGS

Disease-modifying antirheumatic drugs are used when salicylates and PSIs are ineffective or not tolerated. They are called DMARDs because they are capable of arresting the progression of RA and inducing remission in some patients. They also are known as slow-acting antirheumatic drugs (SAARDs) because of their delay in achieving a response. The most common DMARDs are gold salts, MTX, hydroxychloroquine, and penicillamine. The newest DMARDS are tumor necrosis factor (TNF) inhibitors and leflunomide

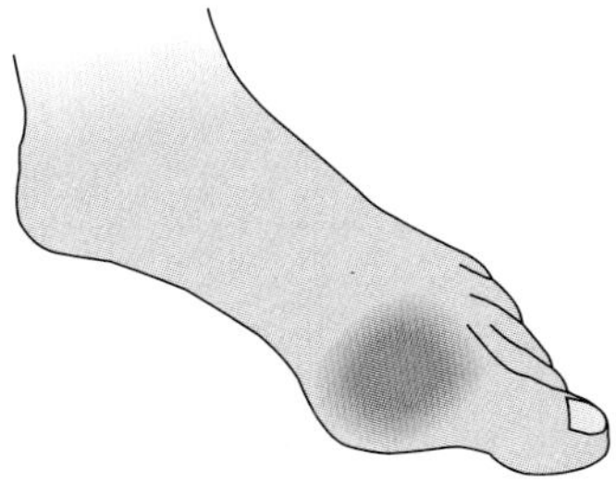

Figure 26-2. Gout in the first metatarsal phalangeal joint of the left foot.

(Arava). The major disadvantages of DMARDS are the slow onset of action, the delay in achieving a therapeutic response, and the potential for serious adverse and even fatal reactions. For these reasons, they are generally considered second-line drugs (drugs used when salicylates or PSIs fail). Auranofin (Ridaura), a type of gold salt, is the prototype DMARD.

NURSING MANAGEMENT OF THE PATIENT RECEIVING AURANOFIN

Core Drug Knowledge

Pharmacotherapeutics

Auranofin is used to treat early active cases of both adult and juvenile types of RA that have not responded to salicylates or PSIs. The drug is less effective against advanced, chronic cases of RA.

Pharmacokinetics

Auranofin is administered orally. About 25% of an orally administered dose of auranofin is absorbed from the gastrointestinal (GI) tract. Peak blood gold concentration usually is reached within 2 hours.

After multiple dosing, steady state is achieved in 8 to 12 weeks. Blood gold concentrations are generally higher than serum or plasma gold concentrations because the gold is bound within an erythrocyte. Gold concentration levels are significantly lower when given orally rather than parenterally. Auranofin is distributed widely throughout the body and is found in the lymph nodes, bone marrow, spleen, adrenals, liver, and kidneys. It crosses the placenta and is found in breast milk. Auranofin is metabolized in the liver, and approximately 60% is excreted by the kidneys; the remainder is excreted in feces (Table 26-1).

Pharmacodynamics

The administration of gold salts is called **chrysotherapy**. Auranofin contains about 29% gold and is the only gold compound available for oral administration. Auranofin exhibits antirheumatic, anti-inflammatory, and immunomodulating properties. The mechanism of action is unknown but may involve the inhibition of antigen processing by macrophages or the inhibition of lysosomal enzyme release, thus decreasing inflammation. Additionally, gold has a strong affinity for sulfur and may interfere with the cellular sulfhydryl system, which would inhibit the function of macrophages responsible for causing inflammation in rheumatic patients.

Contraindications and Precautions

Auranofin is contraindicated for use in patients with Sjögren syndrome, severe debilitation, systemic lupus erythematosus (SLE), uncontrolled congestive heart failure (CHF), marked hypertension, urticaria, eczema, colitis, or a history of sensitivity to gold compounds. Auranofin is contraindicated in patients with a history of disorders induced by the use of gold-based drugs, such as exfoliative dermatitis, pulmonary fibrosis, necrotizing enterocolitis, and anaphylactic reactions. It also is contraindicated in patients who have experienced severe toxicity from previously administered gold compounds or other heavy metal preparations.

Auranofin should be used with caution in patients with bone marrow aplasia, a history of blood dyscrasias, or bone marrow depression. Patients with recent radiation therapy are at high risk for blood dyscrasias because of radiation's depressant effect on the hematopoietic system. Patients receiving antimalarials, immunosuppressants, or phenylbutazone are at high risk for blood dyscrasias and should be monitored closely.

Auranofin also should be used with caution in patients with preexisting renal disease, inflammatory bowel disease, hepatic disease, or skin rash. These conditions indicate compromised organ systems, which could increase the risk of gold toxicity.

Auranofin is assigned to pregnancy category C. It crosses the placenta and is distributed in breast milk, and therefore should not be used in women who are pregnant or breast-feeding.

Adverse Effects

Chrysotherapy can produce severe toxic reactions. Therefore, patients receiving gold compounds must be monitored closely for early signs of adverse effects. The most serious adverse effect to auranofin is fatal bone marrow suppression. Other potential blood dyscrasias are leukopenia, thrombocytopenia, and anemia. The adverse effects of gold therapy may occur months after therapy discontinues.

The most common adverse effects to auranofin are GI in nature. Diarrhea is an expected response to the initiation of auranofin and, in some cases, may be severe. Other GI symptoms include nausea, vomiting, anorexia, abdominal cramps, and flatulence.

Chrysotherapy also can produce mucocutaneous reactions because of the deposits of gold in tissues. Pruritus, rash, skin pigment changes (gray to blue), conjunctivitis, glossitis, stomatitis, and alopecia may occur.

Additional adverse effects to auranofin involve the renal system. Transient and mild proteinuria may occur in about 50% of patients at some time during therapy. Less common effects include nephrotic syndrome and

TABLE 26-1 Summary of Selected Antirheumatic Drugs

Drug (Trade) Name	Selected Indications	Route and Dosage Range	Pharmacokinetics
auranofin (Ridaura)	Rheumatoid arthritis (RA)	*Adult:* PO, 6 mg/d, either as 3-mg bid or single dose; dosage may be increased to 9 mg/d in divided doses if response not adequate *Child:* PO, 0.1 mg/kg/d initially; titrate up to 0.15 mg/kg/d; do not exceed 0.2 mg/kg/d	*Onset:* Varies *Duration:* 6 mo $t_{1/2}$: 26 d
aurothioglucose (Solganal)	RA	*Adult:* IM, weekly IM injections: 1st injection, 10 mg; 2nd and 3rd injections, 25 mg; reassess after cumulative administration of 1 g; may continue 50-mg injections q3–4 wk if patient improves and has no symptoms of toxicity *Child:* IM, weekly IM injections: Administer ¼ of adult dose based on body weight; do not exceed 25-mg dose	*Onset:* Slow *Duration:* 6 mo $t_{1/2}$: 3–27 d
etanercept (Enbrel)	RA Juvenile RA	*Adult:* SC, 2 × wk *Child (4–17 y):* SC, 0.4 mg/kg 2 × wk, 2-mg/dose max	*Onset:* 2–4 wk *Duration:* unknown $t_{1/2}$: 2 wk
leflunomide (Arava)	RA	*Adult:* PO, 100 mg × 3 d, then PO, 20 mg qd	*Onset:* 1 mo *Duration:* wks–mos $t_{1/2}$: 2 wk
gold sodium thiomalate (Myochrysine)	RA	*Adult:* IM, weekly IM injections, 1st injection, 10 mg; 2nd and 3rd injections, 50 mg; maintenance, 25–50 mg every other week for 2–20 wk; if patient's condition remains stable, give 25–50 mg q3–4 wk indefinitely; do not exceed 100-mg dose *Child:* IM, initial dose of 10 mg, then give 1 mg/kg, not to exceed 5 mg/dose	*Onset:* Slow *Duration:* 6 mo $t_{1/2}$: 3–27 d
hydroxychloroquine (Plaquenil)	RA Discoid lupus erythematosus Malaria (suppression) Acute malaria	*Adult:* PO, (in order of indications at left) 400–600 mg/d with meals, 5–10 d later gradually increasing dosage to optimum effectiveness: maintenance: 200–400 mg/d; 400 mg qd–bid for several wk; prolonged use, 200– 400 mg d 310 mg base/wk on the same day each wk, beginning 2 wk before exposure and continuing for 6–8 wk after leaving the endemic area; if suppressive therapy is not begun before exposure, double the initial loading dose (620 mg base), and give in two doses, 6 h apart; day 1, 10 mg/kg; 6 h later, 5 mg/kg; day 2, 5 mg/kg; day 3, 5 mg/kg	*Onset:* Rapid *Duration:* Unknown $t_{1/2}$: 3–5 d
infliximab (Remicade)	RA Crohn's disease	*Adult:* IV, 3 mg/kg; additional, IV, 3 mg/kg in wk 2 and 6 p̄ 1st infusion *Adult:* IV, 5 mg/kg, followed by additional IV 5 mg/kg in wk 2 and 6 p̄ 1st infusion	*Onset:* 1–2 wk *Duration:* 12–48 wk $t_{1/2}$: 9.5 d
methotrexate (Rheumatrex)	RA Juvenile RA (JRA)	*Adult:* PO, 7.5 mg q/wk PO, 2.5 mg q 12 h for 3 doses, repeated at weekly intervals, max 20 mg q/wk *Child:* IM or PO, 5–15 mg m²/wk	*Onset:* 4–7 d *Duration:* 21 d $t_{1/2}$: 10–12 h
penicillamine (Cuprimine)	RA Wilson disease Cystinuria	*Adult:* PO (in order of indications listed at left), initial 125–250 mg/d; increase as tolerated; maintenance, 500–750 mg/d 250 mg qid 250 mg/d, increase gradually to 1–2 g in divided doses *Child:* PO (in order of indications at left), efficacy in JRA not established; 20 mg/kg/d in divided doses	*Onset:* 1–3 mo *Duration:* 1–3 mo $t_{1/2}$: Varies

glomerular nephritis. In rare instances, acute tubular necrosis and renal failure may occur. Gold therapy should be terminated if proteinuria does not resolve or hematuria occurs. Other rare but serious adverse effects include interstitial pneumonitis and fibrosis.

Drug Interactions

Auranofin should not be given to patients receiving penicillamine because of the possibility of causing potentially severe hematologic or renal effects. Although documentation of drug and auranofin interactions may not be available, drugs possessing toxic properties similar to those of auranofin should be avoided, if possible. Auranofin should be used cautiously in patients receiving drugs that can cause bone marrow toxicity or nephrotoxicity. Auranofin may enhance the response to a tuberculin skin test, resulting in a false-positive reaction. Nursing management of potential drug-drug interactions is presented in Table 26-2.

Assessment of Relevant Core Patient Variables

Health Status

The nurse should assess the patient for potential medical conditions or other drug therapy that contraindicates using auranofin or requires close patient monitoring. The nurse should assess for potential hypersensitivities to gold salts or previous reaction to heavy metal drug therapy. In addition, the nurse needs to assess joint involvement, deformities, and range of motion for use as baseline documentation. It is important to perform an examination of the skin and buccal mucosa before, and routinely throughout, therapy. A baseline complete blood count (CBC), platelet count, and tests for renal and hepatic function should be obtained (see the accompanying display, Auranofin Therapy).

Life Span and Gender

The nurse should determine whether the patient is pregnant or breast-feeding before administering auranofin. Because auranofin crosses the placental barrier and is excreted in breast milk, it should not be used in pregnant or lactating women.

Lifestyle, Diet, and Habits

Close monitoring of laboratory tests is mandatory when administering auranofin. Patients who cannot or will not undergo frequent blood monitoring should not take this drug.

Nursing Diagnoses and Outcomes

- Ineffective Therapeutic Regimen Management related to long-term use and adverse effects of auranofin
  Desired outcome: The patient will verbalize understanding of the risks and benefits of auranofin therapy, and will effectively manage the drug regimen.
- Diarrhea related to auranofin use
  Desired outcome: The patient will increase fluids to avoid dehydration and contact the prescriber if diarrhea persists.
- Risk for Impaired Skin Integrity related to pruritus and rash
  Desired outcome: The patient will contact the health care provider if integumentary reactions occur.
- Risk for Injury related to renal toxicity and to bone marrow depression, both induced by auranofin therapy
  Desired outcome: The patient will contact the prescriber if urinary changes, sore throat, easy bruising, or lethargy occurs.
- Risk for Deficient Fluid Volume related to nausea, vomiting, and diarrhea
  Desired outcome: The patient will contact the prescriber if GI symptoms occur.

TABLE 26-2 Agents That Interact With Auranofin

Interactants	Effect and Significance	Nursing Management
penicillamine	Concomitant administration of auranofin with penicillamine potentiates the action of both drugs, which may cause potentially severe hematologic or renal toxicity.	Do not administer these agents at the same time.
agents that cause bone marrow suppression: amphotericin B, antineoplastic agents, carbamazepine, chloramphenicol, clozapine, flucytosine, phenothiazines, zidovudine	Drugs possessing hematologic toxicities similar to those of auranofin may potentiate the action of both agents, resulting in bone marrow suppression.	Avoid coadministration if possible. Monitor complete blood count and platelet count frequently. Monitor patient for sore throat, chills, easy bruising, or bleeding tendencies.
agents that cause nephrotoxicity: amphotericin B, aminoglycosides, vancomycin, nonsteroidal anti-inflammatory drugs	Drugs possessing nephrotoxic potential similar to that of auranofin may potentiate the action of both agents, resulting in nephrotoxicity.	Avoid coadministration if possible. Monitor blood urea nitrogen and creatinine levels. Monitor for proteinuria. Monitor patient weight gain, fatigue, oliguria.

Critical Thinking Scenario

Auranofin therapy

Mrs. Spencer, a 68-year-old woman, has had rheumatoid arthritis for the past 6 years. Initially, Mrs. Spencer took up to 12 tablets per day until she complained of chronic tinnitus. Over the past year, Mrs. Spencer has been given four different types of prostaglandin synthetase inhibitors, producing only mild pain relief in both hips and her lower spine. Mrs. Spencer has been referred to a rheumatologist who has prescribed auranofin.

1. What assessments should the nurse document before administering auranofin?
2. Consider which laboratory tests you think should be done before administering auranofin.
3. Prepare patient teaching about auranofin for this patient.

Planning and Intervention

Maximizing Therapeutic Effects

The nurse can contribute to the best outcome by administering auranofin exactly as prescribed and by monitoring the patient for therapeutic effects regularly.

Minimizing Adverse Effects

The nurse needs to monitor closely patients with preexisting medical conditions or those undergoing drug therapy that may interact with auranofin. Monthly laboratory results also should be monitored. It is necessary to withhold the drug for patients who are experiencing adverse effects until the adverse effects resolve. The nurse should contact the prescriber immediately when adverse effects have occurred.

Providing Patient and Family Education

- It is important to teach patients to take auranofin as prescribed to avoid adverse effects or an overdose.
- The nurse should tell patients not to take gold salts if they have one of the following conditions: Sjögren syndrome, SLE, uncontrolled CHF, marked uncontrolled hypertension, urticaria, eczema, colitis, history of sensitivity to gold compounds, history of gold-induced complications or adverse effects from other heavy metal preparations, pregnancy, or breastfeeding.
- The nurse should caution patients not to take gold salts if they are taking penicillamine.
- The nurse should tell patients that if they miss a dose, they should take it as soon as possible. If it is almost time for the next dose, take only that dose; double or extra doses should never be taken.
- The nurse should tell patients to take auranofin with food or milk if GI upset occurs, and to drink plenty of fluids to avoid dehydration if experiencing nausea, vomiting, or diarrhea.
- It is important to tell patients that gold salts may cause minor adverse effects, such as a change in taste, diarrhea, pruritus, rash, discoloration of skin, indigestion, loss of appetite, nausea, vomiting, and stomach cramps. The nurse should tell patients to call their health care provider if minor adverse effects do not go away, if diarrhea lasts more than 3 days, or if the adverse effects are particularly annoying.
- The nurse should describe signs and symptoms of serious adverse effects, such as urinary changes, sore throat, easy bruising, bleeding, or lethargy, and emphasize the importance of notifying the health care prescriber if any occur.
- It is important to stress that patients must continue to take gold salts even if it seems that the drug is not working. Gold salt therapy may take weeks or months to become effective. The nurse should instruct patients to keep gold salts in the container in which they came because air and light can decrease their potency.
- If patients develop buccal ulcerations during therapy, the nurse should tell them to rinse their mouth with 1 teaspoon of salt in 8 oz of water and to notify the health care provider.
- The nurse should instruct patients to see their health care provider every month for blood and urine tests to be sure they are not having an adverse reaction to gold salts.

Ongoing Assessment and Evaluation

It is important to question the patient about sore throat, easy bruising, or unusual bleeding. Monthly CBC, platelet count, and urinalysis (to check for protein) for patients on long-term therapy should be obtained. The nurse needs to monitor for diarrhea or skin eruptions and should contact the health care provider immediately if these symptoms occur. The nurse should monitor for joint involvement, deformity, and range of motion and arrange for physical therapy to maximize the effects of auranofin. Finally, the patient needs to be monitored for efficacy of auranofin therapy.

Therapy is considered effective if the patient has a decrease in pain and inflammation within 6 months, and the patient remains free of side effects or adverse effects. The patient should verbalize the importance of contacting the health care provider immediately if any adverse effects occur. The patient should also verbalize the importance of monthly blood testing. ■

DRUGS CLOSELY RELATED TO AURANOFIN

Aurothioglucose

Aurothioglucose (Solganal) is an intramuscular dosage form of gold therapy. Its pharmacodynamics and pharmacotherapy are the same as auranofin. It is in a sesame oil suspen-

MEMORY CHIP

Auranofin

- Disease-modifying antirheumatic drug used for management of rheumatoid arthritis when aspirin or prostaglandin synthetase inhibitors are ineffective
- Significant contraindications: Sjögren's syndrome, severe debilitation, systemic lupus erythematosis, uncontrolled congestive heart failure, marked hypertension, urticaria, eczema, colitis, or a history of sensitivity to gold compounds
- Most common adverse effect: diarrhea
- Most serious adverse effect: fatal bone marrow suppression
- Maximizing therapeutic effects: administer exactly as prescribed
- Minimizing adverse effects: check complete blood count and urinalysis before administration
- Most significant patient education: explain that it takes a long time to see results from this drug; encourage the patient to continue taking the medication.

sion, which causes erratic and slow absorption. Aurothioglucose is about 50% gold.

The onset and duration of action are difficult to quantify because the therapeutic effects may not begin for several weeks and may last long after the drug has been discontinued. Between 1 and 2 months of weekly injections are required to achieve a steady-state serum level. Like auranofin, aurothioglucose is distributed throughout the body; however, it is not associated with circulating cells in most patients. The metabolic fate of aurothioglucose is unknown. About 40% is excreted each week during a standard weekly dosing schedule, and the remainder is excreted more gradually. About 70% is excreted in urine and 30% in feces. The half-life can be as long as 160 days.

When administering aurothioglucose, the nurse should be sure to have emergency life-support equipment available. Patients may experience anaphylactic shock, syncope, bradycardia, difficulty swallowing, and angioedema following an injection of aurothioglucose.

Another potential reaction of aurothioglucose is a **nitritoid crisis.** The symptoms of this *reaction* (e.g., flushing, feeling of warmth, light-headedness, or hypotension) resemble the response to a large dose of nitroglycerin, hence the term nitritoid. Patients are given a small test dose to assess for these responses. If there is no reaction to the test dose, a series of weekly or monthly injections may be given. Before each injection, a urinalysis and CBC are performed. Therapy must stop if the patient develops hematuria, proteinuria, or blood dyscrasias.

To administer the drug in uniform suspension, the nurse must immerse the vial in warm water, remove the drug with a dry needle and syringe, and inject the drug in the gluteal muscle, taking care to avoid IV administration. The patient should then remain in a recumbent position and be monitored for an allergic or nitroid reaction for at least 15 minutes after administration.

Patients should be reevaluated after receiving a cumulative dose of 1 g of aurothioglucose. Contraindications, precautions, and adverse effects are the same as for auranofin.

Gold Sodium Thiomalate

Gold sodium thiomalate (Myochrysine) is another aqueous solution of gold administered intramuscularly. Its pharmacodynamics and pharmacotherapeutics are similar to those of auranofin. Gold sodium thiomalate also may induce nitritoid or anaphylactic reactions. As with aurothioglucose, a urinalysis and CBC must be done before each injection. Contraindications, precautions, and adverse effects are similar to those of auranofin.

DRUGS SIGNIFICANTLY DIFFERENT FROM AURANOFIN

Methotrexate

Methotrexate (Rheumatrex) is an antineoplastic agent that is used for severe, disabling, rheumatic arthritis. Although not universally accepted, many rheumatologists consider MTX to be the first-choice DMARD after PSI therapy fails to manage symptoms of arthritis. It is the fastest acting of the DMARDs. Therapeutic effects may be seen in as little as 3 to 6 weeks.

The exact mechanism of action of MTX in RA is not well defined. It is used typically for intractable RA because many of its potential adverse effects may be fatal. MTX may induce bone marrow suppression, GI ulceration, hepatitic fibrosis, or pneumonitis. Because of its lower dosing in the management of RA, there is a decreased risk for severe adverse effects. However, this does not change the need for close monitoring for potential adverse effects.

Throughout MTX therapy the patient needs periodic laboratory testing. These tests should include liver and kidney function, CBC, and platelet count. Patients unwilling or unable to adhere to this close monitoring should not be placed on this drug.

Hydroxychloroquine Sulfate

Hydroxychloroquine (Plaquenil) is an antimalarial drug also used in the management of RA and discoid LE. In treating malaria, the mechanism of action is the same as for chloroquine. In the management of RA and discoid LE, the mechanism of action is unclear.

Hydroxychloroquine should be given with caution to infants or pregnant and lactating women because of the high potential to develop toxicity. In children, the dose must be calculated properly and the patient monitored closely, because toxicity has occurred with routine dosing. For patients on long-term therapy with hydroxychloroquine, the greatest concern is the development of irreversible retinal damage. Drug-drug interactions, adverse effects, nursing management, and patient education are the same as for patients taking chloroquine (see Chapter 55).

Penicillamine

Penicillamine (Cuprimine) is used in treating patients with early, mild, and nonerosive rheumatic arthritis. Its antirheumatic action may result from its ability to inhibit the formation of collagen. Penicillamine also appears to depress circulating levels of IgM RF but does not reduce the absolute levels of serum immunoglobulins. It also may decrease cell-mediated immune response by selectively inhibiting T-lymphocyte function.

In addition to its use as an antirheumatic drug, penicillamine is used as a chelating agent for removing excess copper from the blood of patients with Wilson disease and in reducing cystine excretion in patients with cystinuria.

Although penicillamine is a by-product of penicillin, it has no antibiotic activity. However, the possibility of cross-sensitization between penicillin and penicillamine exists; therefore, penacillamine should not be given to patients who are allergic to penicillin.

Penicillamine has potentially toxic adverse effects, including cutaneous lesions, blood dyscrasias, and a number of autoimmune disorders. Penicillamine is associated with a high incidence of potentially life-threatening adverse hematologic reactions because of bone marrow depression. Patients with a history of hematologic disorders or previous penicillamine-induced dyscrasias could experience these adverse reactions, which include leukopenia, thrombocytopenia, aplastic anemia, pancytopenia, sideroblastic anemia, agranulocytosis, and leukopenia. Penicillamine should be discontinued when the platelet count decreases to less than 100,000/mm^3, the leukocyte count to less than 3,000/mm^3, or if neutropenia occurs (see the accompanying display, Danger Signs: Adverse Reactions to Penicillamine).

Rare but serious adverse effects are myasthenia gravis (MG) syndrome and obliterative bronchiolitis. Penicillamine should be discontinued at the first sign of ptosis or diplopia (signifying MG syndrome) or exertional dyspnea, cough, or wheezing (signifying obliterative bronchiolitis). These symptoms should be reported immediately.

In the renal system, penicillamine may induce hematuria and proteinuria, which may indicate an impending immune complex membranous glomerulonephritis. This can degenerate into nephrotic syndrome. Penicillamine should be discontinued when proteinuria values exceed 1 g/24 hours.

The most common adverse effects involve the integumentary system. Rash and pruritus occurring in the first few months (early rash) are generally typical of drug hypersensitivity. Early rash usually disappears with discontinuation of the drug. Late rash during therapy may be accompanied with intense pruritus, fever, arthralgia, or lymphadenopathy. This rash may take weeks to disappear. Patients may also develop exfoliative dermatitis, increased skin friability, vesicular ecchymoses, and pemphigus.

Penicillamine also may cause GI upset, such as nausea, vomiting, anorexia, abdominal pain, and diarrhea. Patients with a history of peptic ulcer, hepatic dysfunction, and pancreatitis may experience reactivation of the disorder.

Because of the potential for adverse effects from penicillamine, patients should be taught carefully about this drug, including the signs and symptoms of potentially serious consequences. The nurse should inform female patients that this drug should not be taken if they are pregnant or breastfeeding. It also should not be taken by patients who have severe renal dysfunction or severe anemia; have taken penicillamine before and developed a high fever; or are taking gold salts by mouth or injection. Moreover, patients who are allergic to penicillin should inform their health care providers of this allergy.

The nurse should explain minor side effects, such as change in taste, diarrhea, loss of appetite, nausea, vomiting, and stomach pain, and advise patients to discuss these effects with the health care provider if the effects do not subside or are particularly annoying.

Patients should learn to take penicillamine at least 1 hour before or 2 hours after eating food. Patients taking penicillamine for Wilson disease must avoid foods that contain copper, such as chocolate, nuts, liver, and broccoli. In addition, patients should drink plenty of water to prevent kidney stones from forming. Patients should avoid taking antacids and iron preparations because they may prevent the drug from working properly.

A missed dose should be taken as soon as possible, but if it is almost time for the next dose, only that dose should be taken (double or extra doses should never be taken). The nurse should instruct patients to continue to take penicillamine even if it appears that it is not working. Penicillamine should be stored away from moisture (particularly away from a bathroom) and out of the reach of children. The nurse should urge patients to schedule monthly blood and urine tests to make sure they are not having any adverse effects to penicillamine.

Danger Signs: Adverse Reactions to Penicillamine

When educating patients about the potential adverse effects of penicillamine, the nurse should alert them especially to signs and symptoms of a potentially life-threatening adverse reaction. Patients should contact their health care providers should any of the following occur:

- Bloody, black, or tarry stools
- Bloody or cloudy urine
- Cough or hoarseness
- Fever, chills, or sore throat
- Wheezing or difficulty breathing
- Eye pain or vision problems
- Joint pain
- Lower back or side pain
- Mouth ulcers, sores, or white spots on the lips or in the mouth
- Ringing in the ears (tinnitus)
- Swelling of face, feet, or lower legs
- Unusual bleeding, bruising, pinpoint red spots on skin
- Unusual tiredness or weakness
- Swollen or painful glands

Leflunomide

Leflunomide (Arava) is a recently developed innovative DMARD. The pharmacologic activity of leflunomide is accomplished through its active primary metabolite A77 1726, also known as M1. M1 inhibits dihydroorotate dehydrogenase (DHODH), an enzyme located in cell mitochondria that inhibits a key step in de novo pyrimidine synthesis. Suppression of pyrimidine synthesis within T and B lymphocytes interferes with RNA and protein synthesis within the cells, and prevents further cell cycle progression. Reduction in the activity of lymphocytes leads to reduced cytokine and antibody mediated destruction of the synovial joints and decreases the inflammatory process. Because of its mechanism of action, the abatement of symptoms may occur in as little as 4 weeks. Additionally, because of its unique mechanism of action, it may be used in conjunction with other drugs such as PSIs and other DMARDS.

Leflunomide is contraindicated in patients with severe hepatic insufficiency and patients with diagnosed hepatitis B or hepatitis C. Leflunomide may increase liver function enzymes such as aspartate aminotransferase (AST) and alanine aminotransferase (ALT) and has been associated with inducing hepatoxicity, especially in these patients.

Leflunomide also is contraindicated for use during pregnancy or breast-feeding. Luflunomide is a category X drug because it has shown to induce fetal deformity. Women who have received leflunomide and wish to become pregnant must undergo a drug elimination process prior to conception. Cholestyramine (8 g) is administered three times a day for 11 days. The days do not have to be consecutive, but must total 11 days. Plasma drug levels are then evaluated twice, at least 14 days apart. The plasma drug level should be less than 0.02 μg/mL before conception is attempted. Without this procedure, blood levels greater than 0.02 μg/mL may remain for up to 2 years, depending on individual variations in clearance.

Precautions to leflunomide therapy include immunodeficiency, bone marrow dysplasia, and severe uncontrolled infections. Vaccinations with live vaccines are not recommended during therapy.

Common adverse effects include diarrhea, increased AST and ALT, alopecia, rash and respiratory infections. Less common adverse effects include dyspepsia, hypertension, and nausea.

Potential drug interactions include drugs that induce hepatotoxicity, cholestyramine, charcoal and rifampin. It does **NOT** appear to interact with triphasic oral contraceptives. This is important because women of child-bearing age need to be on a reliable contraceptive agent throughout leflunomide therapy.

Etanercept

Etanercept (Enbrel) is a TNF antagonist. It was produced by recombinant DNA technology. Etanercept is used in the management of RA to reduce signs and symptoms of the disease and delay structural damage in patients with moderately to severely active RA. It can be used in combination with MTX in patients who do not respond adequately to MTX alone. Etanercept also is indicated for reducing signs and symptoms of moderately to severely active polyarticular-course juvenile RA in patients who have had an inadequate response to one or more DMARDS.

Etanercept binds specifically to **tumor necrosis factor** and blocks its interaction with cell surface TNF receptors. TNF is a **cytokine** produced by macrophages and activated T-cells that plays an important role in RA by mediating cytokines that cause inflammation and joint destruction. TNF is elevated in rheumatoid synovial fluids in patients with severe disease or a high white blood cell count in the synovial fluid.

The only absolute contraindication to etanercept is hypersensitivity. However, there are several cautions to consider before using this drug. Etanercept has been associated with inducing sepsis and fatal infections in patients with predisposing diseases, such as advanced or poorly controlled diabetes. Therapy should be delayed until known infections have been resolved. In addition, etanercept may induce demyelinating disorders such as multiple sclerosis, myelitis, and optic neuritis, although such cases appear to be rare.

The possibility exists for anti-TNF drugs, including etanercept, to affect host defenses against infections and malignancies because TNF mediates inflammation and modulates cellular immune responses. The safety and efficacy of etanercept in patients with bone marrow suppression or other types of immunosuppression are not known. It also should be used cautiously in women who breast-feed because it is not known whether etanercept enters breast milk. Live vaccines should be avoided while on etanercept therapy because definitive clinical data on potential effects is not yet completed.

Common adverse reactions to etanercept include injection site reactions, upper respiratory infections, headache, nausea, and rhinitis. Less common symptoms include dizziness, cough, asthenia, abdominal pain, and rash.

Infliximab

Infliximab (Remicade) is another TNF. However, it specifically inhibits the activity of TNF-alpha. Initially, it was approved for the management of Crohn disease. It is now approved also for the management of RA when given in combination with methotrexate.

Infliximab reduces inflammation in patients with Crohn disease and RA by binding to and neutralizing TNF-alpha on the cell membrane and in the blood. TNF-alpha is a key inflammatory mediator, or **cytokine**, in RA, Crohn disease, and other autoimmune disorders. Overproduction of NF-alpha leads to inflammation in these chronic conditions.

Contraindications, precautions, and adverse effects are similar to those of etanercept. Unlike etanercept, infliximab is not approved for use in children.

C ANTIGOUT DRUGS

Antigout drugs are used to treat acute cases of gout and to prevent gout. As previously presented, gout is associated with hyperuricemia. Hyperuricemia occurs either because of an increased uric acid production, or by accumulation related to decreased renal excretion of uric acid. Antigout drug therapy focuses on either decreasing the inflammatory response caused by hyperuricemia or by reducing hyperuricema itself.

The prototypical antigout drug is colchicine, which has been used since 1763. It is an alkaloid of a plant called *Colchicum autumnale*. It was originally found in several gout mixtures sold by charlatans; however, its use was popularized in the United States by Benjamin Franklin.

NURSING MANAGEMENT OF THE PATIENT RECEIVING P COLCHICINE

Core Drug Knowledge

Pharmacotherapeutics

The most common use of colchicine is for treating acute gouty arthritis. It is occasionally effective for other types of arthritis. Non-FDA-approved uses of colchicine include amyloidosis, Behcet syndrome, biliary cirrhosis, hepatic cirrhosis, Mediterranean fever, Paget disease, pericarditis, and pseudogout.

Pharmacokinetics

Colchicine may be given either orally or IV. However, parenteral use is avoided because of potential toxicity. Colchicine should never be injected subcutaneously or intramuscularly, because this causes severe local irritation. Oral colchicine is rapidly absorbed, metabolized in the liver, and excreted primarily in the feces, with 10% to 20% eliminated unchanged in the urine (Table 26-3). Patients with hepatic disease may have an increased renal elimination. Enterohepatic recirculation occurs to a large extent and can lead to adverse GI effects with larger dosages. Colchicine distributes to the kidney, liver,

TABLE 26-3 Summary of Selected C Antigout and C Uricosuric Agents

Drug (Trade) Name	Selected Indications	Route and Dosage Range	Pharmacokinetics
C Antigout Agent			
P colchicine	Acute gouty arthritis Non-FDA approved uses: amyloidosis, Behcet syndrome, biliary cirrhosis, hepatic cirrhosis, mediterranean fever, Paget disease, pericarditis, pseudogout	*Adult:* PO, 1–1.2 mg initially, followed by 0.5–0.6 mg/h, or 1–1.2 mg q2h until pain is relieved or adverse effects occur; maintenance, 0.5–0.6 mg/d; IV, 2 mg infused over 12 h, followed by 0.5 mg q6h with a total 24 h dose not to exceed 4 mg *Child:* Safety and efficacy not established	*Onset:* PO, 0.5–2 h; IV, 30–50 min *Duration:* PO, unknown; IV, unknown $t_{1/2}$: PO, 20 min; IV, 20 min
C Uricosuric Agents			
P probenecid (Benemid; *Canadian*: Benuryl)	Chronic gout, serum urate levels above 9 mg/d, combination with antibiotic therapy	*Adult:* PO, 250 mg bid for 1 wk then 500 mg bid to a maximum dose of 2–3 g/d; combined w/antibiotic therapy, 1 g concurrent with oral antibiotics or 30 min before IM antibiotic *Child:* Not for child <2 y; other dosages based on weight	*Onset:* 30 min *Duration:* 4–6 h $t_{1/2}$: 4–7 h
sulfinpyrazone (Anturane; *Canadian*: Anturan)	Chronic gout Inhibition of platelet aggregation	*Adult:* PO (in order of indications listed to the left), 100–200 mg bid for 1 wk then increase to 200–400 mg bid, may reduce to 100 mg/d after serum urate levels are controlled; 200 mg bid–tid *Child:* Safety and efficacy not established	*Onset:* 30 min *Duration:* 4–6 h $t_{1/2}$: 3 h
allopurinol (Zyloprim; *Canadian*: Purinol)	Prevention of acute gouty attacks Uric acid nephropathy hyperuricemia Recurrent calcium oxalate renal calculus Prevention of acute gouty attacks during treatment of myeloproliferative neoplastic disease	*Adult:* PO (in order of indications listed at left), 100 mg qd increased by 100 mg weekly until serum urate concentration decreases below 6 mg/d or until maximum dose of 800 mg is achieved; same as above; 200–300 mg/d in divided doses; 600–800 mg/d in divided doses *Child:* PO (prevention of acute gouty attacks during treatment of myeloproliferative neoplastic disease), 6–10 y: 10 mg/kg in divided doses, <6 y: 150 mg/d in divided doses	*Onset:* 30 min–1 h *Duration:* 18–30 h $t_{1/2}$: 1–2 h metabolite, 18–30 h

spleen, and intestinal tissues and concentrates primarily in the leukocytes. It can be found in leukocytes for 10 days after administration.

Pharmacodynamics

Colchicine possesses anti-inflammatory properties. Although it is highly effective in treating acute gouty arthritis, it is not an effective analgesic for other types of pain, nor does it affect uric acid clearance. Colchicine inhibits the activity of leukocytes by decreasing their migration into the affected area, resulting in an interruption of the cyclic inflammatory response. Another action of colchicine is to prevent the release of an inflammatory glycoprotein from phagocytes, although it does not inhibit phagocytosis of uric acid crystals. Additional pharmacologic actions of colchicine include lowering body temperature, suppression of the respiratory center, and vasomotor stimulation, leading to hypertension. These actions can be extremely serious in cases of overdose.

Contraindications and Precautions

Colchicine is contraindicated in patients with severe cardiac disease, hepatic disease, and renal disease, because these patients are at risk for developing cumulative toxicity. Other patients at risk for cumulative toxicity are elderly or debilitated patients. These patients should be monitored closely.

Patients with renal impairment or elevated plasma levels of colchicine due to renal disease can develop a myoneuropathy characterized by proximal weakness and elevated serum creatine kinase levels. This reaction usually occurs with patients who have been taking colchicine for several years; however, it is prudent to monitor all patients with renal insufficiency for this reaction.

Colchicine is eliminated primarily through the biliary pathway. Patients with hepatic disease should be monitored closely during treatment with colchicine. Additionally, patients at risk for hepatic disease, such as those with alcoholism, also should be monitored closely.

Colchicine should be used cautiously in patients with preexisting GI disease or bone marrow depression. These patients are at a higher risk for adverse effects of colchicine.

Patients with myelosuppression are at risk for infections or bleeding. Dental work should be performed before initiating colchicine therapy or deferred until blood counts return to normal.

Oral colchicine is classified as pregnancy category C and therefore should be avoided by pregnant or lactating women. Parenteral colchicine is pregnancy category D and should never be taken by pregnant or breast-feeding women.

Adverse Effects

The most common adverse effects of colchicine are GI in nature. Up to 80% of patients may experience nausea, vomiting, diarrhea, abdominal pain, and paralytic ileus. These reactions may indicate toxicity, and the drug should be discontinued until the symptoms resolve.

Long-term therapy with colchicine may induce bone marrow depression, including aplastic anemia, pancytopenia, thrombocytopenia, leukopenia, or agranulocytosis. Patients receiving parenteral colchicine have a higher incidence of bone marrow depression. Signs and symptoms of serious adverse reactions that must be reported to the prescriber include fever, chills, or sore throat; wheezing or difficulty breathing; muscle weakness; numbness or tingling in hands and feet; skin rash, itching; stomach pain; swelling of face or mouth; unusual bleeding, bruising, and pinpoint red spots on skin; and unusual tiredness or weakness.

Other adverse effects include renal, integumentary, hematologic, and endocrinologic effects. In the renal system, potential adverse effects are bladder spasms, nephrotoxicity, proteinuria, hematuria, anuria, and acute renal failure. Integumentary effects include angioedema, urticaria, injection site reaction, skin necrosis, tissue necrosis, and median nerve neuritis. In the endocrine system, hypothyroidism may occur.

Drug Interactions

Colchicine can enhance the effects of radiation therapy or bone marrow depressants.

Colchicine also may interact with cyanocobalamin (vitamin B_{12}), cyclosporine, erythromycin, and nonsteroidal anti-inflammatory drugs (NSAIDs). Colchicine use may interfere with certain test results, yielding a false-positive finding when assessing for hemoglobin in urine. Table 26-4 presents potential drug interactions with colchicine.

Assessment of Relevant Core Patient Variables

Health Status

The nurse should assess the patient for potential medical conditions or drugs that contradict the use of colchicine or require close patient monitoring. The nurse should assess the joints for edema, erythema, or increased warmth. In addition, the nurse should assess for signs of hypothyroidism. A baseline CBC, platelet count, and tests for renal and hepatic function should be obtained.

Life Span and Gender

The nurse should determine whether the patient is pregnant or breast-feeding before administering colchicine. Pregnant or breast-feeding women should not receive parenteral colchicine. They may, however, receive oral colchicine if absolutely necessary.

Lifestyle, Diet, and Habits

The nurse should evaluate the patient's diet. Foods such as organ meats, oily fish, seafood, beans, peas, oatmeal, spinach, asparagus, cauliflower, and mushrooms should be avoided as these foods are high in purines. The nurse

TABLE 26-4 Agents That Interact With Colchicine

Interactants	Effect and Significance	Nursing Management
agents that cause bone marrow suppression: amphotericin B, antineoplastic agents, carbamazepine, chloramphenicol, clozapine, flucytosine, phenothiazines, zidovudine	Drugs possessing hematoxic properties similar to those of gold salts may potentiate the action of both agents, resulting in bone marrow suppression.	Avoid coadministration if possible. Monitor complete blood count (CBC) and platelet count frequently. Monitor patient for sore throat, chills, easy bruising, or bleeding tendencies.
cyanocobalamin	Administration of colchicine can result in a reversible decrease in the absorption of cyanocobalamin, resulting in anemia.	Monitor for signs and symptoms of anemia. Monitor CBC.
cyclosporine	Cyclosporine may cause hyperuricemia. Concomitant use of cyclosporine and colchicine may also increase cyclosporine concentrations, resulting in a high risk for nephrotoxicity.	Avoid coadministration, if possible. Monitor blood urea nitrogen, creatinine, and cyclosporine levels.
erythromycin	The addition of erythromycin to colchicine therapy may lead to colchicine toxicity.	Monitor for fever, gastrointestinal (GI) symptoms, myalgia, and leukopenia.
ethanol (alcohol)	Ethanol ingestion increases the risk of adverse GI effects and can increase serum urate concentration, thus decreasing the antigout effects of colchicine.	Avoid alcohol ingestion during therapy. Monitor for effectiveness of colchicine.
nonsteroidal anti-inflammatory drugs (NSAIDs)	Concomitant use of NSAIDs and colchicine increases the likelihood of developing adverse GI effects, especially ulceration or hemorrhage.	Avoid coadministration. Monitor for adverse GI effects. Monitor for easy bruising or bleeding.

also should evaluate the patient's intake of alcohol. Alcohol can cause both overproduction and underexcretion of uric acid. Because dehydration can trigger acute gout attacks, it is important that the nurse ensures that the patient consumes adequate amounts of fluids. Plasma uric acid levels rise during starvation. Therefore, the nurse should ensure the patient eats at regular intervals throughout the day.

Environment

The nurse should be aware of the setting in which colchicine may be administered. Colchicine is self-administered most frequently by patients in the home environment. Patients are advised to take the drug hourly until GI symptoms occur, then reduce the dosage. For severe attacks, colchicine can be given intravenously to avoid GI symptoms.

Nursing Diagnoses and Outcomes

- Acute Pain related to drug-induced abdominal cramps or paralytic ileus
  Desired outcome: The patient will contact the prescriber if abdominal pain occurs.
- Risk for Injury related to drug-induced renal toxicity or possible extravasation of IV colchicine
  Desired outcome: The patient administering colchicine at home will contact the prescriber if urinary changes occur. The hospitalized patient will remain free of extravasation of IV colchicine.
- Risk for Deficient Fluid Volume related to drug-induced nausea, vomiting, and diarrhea
  Desired outcome: The patient will contact the prescriber if GI symptoms occur.
- Ineffective Protection related to possible blood dyscrasias
  Desired outcome: The patient will contact the prescriber if sore throat, easy bruising, or lethargy occurs.

Planning and Intervention

Maximizing Therapeutic Effects

In an acute care setting, the nurse needs to administer colchicine with a full glass of water at evenly spaced intervals throughout the day. The patient who self-administers the drug should learn to do this as well. Adherence to diet and alcohol restrictions decreases hyperuricemia, thus allowing colchicine to achieve its maximum effect.

Minimizing Adverse Effects

The nurse should closely monitor patients with preexisting medical conditions or those on drug therapy that may interact with colchicine. The patient needs to be advised to take colchicine at the first sign of an acute gout attack.

It is important to question the patient about the possibility of pregnancy before the administration of IV colchicine. The nurse must administer IV colchicine cautiously and monitor frequently for signs of extravasation.

Providing Patient and Family Education

- The nurse should advise patients not to take colchicine if they have severe cardiac disease, hepatic disease, or renal disease.
- The nurse should make sure that pregnant or breast-feeding patients are not given IV colchicine.
- The nurse should advise patients to take colchicine at the first sign of a gout attack and to follow the directions on the drug container.
- The nurse should tell patients that if they miss a dose, they should take it as soon as they can. If it is almost time for the next dose, only that dose should be taken; double or extra doses should not be taken.
- It is important to tell patients that colchicine can cause minor side effects, such as loss of appetite and hair loss and that they should tell their health care provider if the adverse effects do not go away or if they are particularly annoying.
- The nurse should caution the patient to report GI adverse effects (e.g., nausea, vomiting, diarrhea, and abdominal pain) because these could indicate drug toxicity or lead to fluid loss over time.
- It is important to tell patients that colchicine can cause serious adverse effects and that they should call their prescriber immediately if any signs and symptoms occur, including sore throat, easy bruising, lethargy, or signs of renal toxicity (see preceding section, Adverse Effects).
- The nurse should advise patients to avoid alcohol because it can cause stomach problems and increase uric acid in the blood, which makes a gouty attack more likely. The nurse should review foods that are high in purines to decrease dietary intake of uric acid.
- It is important to inform patients that colchicine may produce severe adverse effects when coadministered with many prescription and over-the-counter (OTC) drugs and that they should never take any other drugs without consulting their health care provider.
- The nurse should tell patients to keep colchicine away from light and out of the reach of children.
- It is important to tell patients to see their health care provider every month for blood and urine tests to make sure they are not experiencing adverse effects from colchicine.

Ongoing Assessment and Evaluation

The nurse should monitor for hematopoietic and renal toxicity, joint involvement, deformity, and range of motion. The patient needs to be monitored for efficacy of colchicine therapy.

Therapy is considered effective if the patient reports a decrease in the frequency of acute gout attacks and remains free of adverse effects. The patient should understand and verbalize the importance of contacting the health care provider immediately if any adverse effects occur, scheduling periodic hematologic and renal testing, and contacting the health care provider before taking any other prescription or OTC drugs. ■

C URICOSURIC DRUGS

Uricosuric drugs increase urate excretion. Having no anti-inflammatory or analgesic activity, they are not useful in treating acute gout attacks. In fact, they can exacerbate an acute attack of gout when initiated. Uricosuric drugs include probenecid, sulfinpyrazone, and allopurinol. Probenecid (Benemid) is the prototype uricosuric drug.

NURSING MANAGEMENT OF THE PATIENT RECEIVING P PROBENECID

Core Drug Knowledge

Pharmacotherapeutics

Probenecid is used in treating chronic gout. It keeps the uric acid level below the saturation point, thereby preventing the formation and deposition of urate crystals. Probenecid should be discontinued at the time of an acute attack because its use can prolong the inflammatory response. Probenecid also is used in patients with visible tophi, those with serum urate levels above 9 mg/dL, and those with a family history of tophi or decreased uric acid excretion. It also is used in combination with antibiotic therapy to increase or prolong the serum concentration of antibiotics, such as penicillin, by delaying their renal clearance.

MEMORY CHIP

P Colchicine

- Decreases the inflammatory reaction of **acute** gout
- Significant contraindications: severe cardiac, hepatic, or renal diseases
- Most common adverse effects: related to gastrointestinal system
- Most serious adverse effects: blood dyscrasias, including bone marrow suppression
- Maximizing therapeutic effects: adherence to diet and alcohol restrictions to reduce hyperuricemia
- Minimizing adverse effects: take colchicine at the first sign of an attack, then only until the symptoms start to resolve
- Most significant patient education: related to diet and alcohol restrictions

Pharmacokinetics

Probenecid is administered orally and absorbed completely. The drug is distributed throughout the body tissues and is 75% to 95% bound to plasma protein, predominantly to albumin. Probenecid undergoes hepatic metabolism, resulting in active metabolites. Both parent drug and active metabolites have renal elimination. Small amounts of probenecid are excreted in the feces (see Table 26-3).

Pharmacodynamics

Probenecid interferes with tubular handling of organic acids within the nephron. It inhibits the active resorption of uric acid at the proximal convoluted tubules, resulting in an increased excretion of uric acid.

Contraindications and Precautions

Probenecid is contraindicated in patients with bone marrow depression or uric acid kidney stones because the drug can exacerbate these conditions. Probenecid should not be administered to patients with severe renal impairment (glomerular filtration rate under 50 mL/min) or patients with medical conditions in which uric acid production can increase acutely, such as cancer chemotherapy or radiation therapy.

Probenecid should be administered cautiously to patients with peptic ulcer disease because of a possible increase in GI adverse effects. Probenecid is assigned to pregnancy category C and therefore should be avoided, if possible, during pregnancy and while breast-feeding.

Adverse Effects

Therapeutic dosages of probenecid are generally well tolerated with few adverse effects. The most common adverse effects include headache, nausea, vomiting, and anorexia. Less frequent effects include dizziness, flushing, alopecia, polyuria, nephrotic syndrome, interstitial nephritis, leukopenia, and anemia. Reportable and very serious adverse effects signaling danger include blood in urine; fever, chills, or sore throat; wheezing or difficulty breathing; lower back or side pain; mouth sores; difficulty passing urine; rash and itching; swelling of feet, ankles, face, or lips; unusual bleeding, bruising, pinpoint red spots on the skin; or unusual tiredness or weakness.

Some patients with gout can experience an increased incidence of uric acid stones or the number of acute gouty attacks during the first 6 to 12 months of therapy. This occurs because of an increased uric acid renal clearance.

Drug Interactions

Uricosurics may interact with many drugs (Table 26-5). Probenecid reduces the renal tubular secretion of many drugs, which causes an increase in the serum concentration and increases the risk for adverse effects and toxicities. Conversely, it is the same action that allows probenecid to be used as adjunct therapy with antibiotics. Because the antibiotics are not excreted, the serum concentrations are elevated and prolonged.

Uricosuric actions of probenecid are inhibited by salicylates. When probenecid is used to treat hyperuricemia or gout, it is recommended that salicylates not be administered. Anticoagulant effects of heparin can be increased by concomitant administration of probenecid. Probenecid also can interfere with hepatic conjugation. This may result in prolonging the elimination half-life of lorazepam, thus risking toxicity. Probenecid interferes with laboratory tests for urinary 17-ketosteroids and may cause false-positive Clinitest results for patients with diabetes.

Assessment of Relevant Core Patient Variables

Health Status

The nurse must assess the patient for potential medical conditions or drugs that contraindicate the use of probenecid or require close patient monitoring. Baseline CBC, platelet count, and test values of renal function should be obtained. Neurologic functioning must be evaluated and pregnancy status ascertained. It is important to assess the patient's knowledge concerning the potential adverse effects and drug interactions associated with probenecid. Finally, the nurse needs to assess the efficacy of probenecid therapy.

Life Span and Gender

The nurse should determine if the patient is pregnant or breast-feeding before administering probenecid. Probenecid should not be given to pregnant or breast-feeding women. The nurse also should note the age of the patient before administering probenecid. Probenecid is not indicated for children younger than 2 years. Elderly patients taking probenecid must be monitored closely because they are at increased risk for developing uric acid stones related to decreased renal function.

Lifestyle, Diet, and Habits

The nurse should assess the patient's usual dietary patterns. Patients should be advised to limit their intake of vitamin C or cranberry juice. These tend to acidify the urine, which decreases the excretion of probenicid. There is an increased risk for toxicity when probenicid remains in the body.

Environment

The nurse should note whether the patient taking probenecid has diabetes and, if so, should advise him to monitor the blood glucose levels with capillary blood monitoring systems instead of Clinitest strips. This will help to ensure an accurate glucose level determination.

Nursing Diagnoses and Outcomes

- Risk for Injury related to probenicid-induced renal toxicity

TABLE 26-5 Agents That Interact With Probenecid

Interactants	Effect and Significance	Nursing Management
allopurinol	The antihyperuricemic effects of allopurinol and probenecid are additive when administered together.	Interaction may be therapeutic.
Antiviral Agents acyclovir famciclovir ganciclovir	Probenecid reduces the renal tubular secretion of antiviral agents, which increases the serum concentration and elimination regular half-life of antiviral agents. This results in an increased risk of adverse effects and toxicity.	Monitor serum concentration of antiviral agents. Assess patient for signs of antiviral toxicity.
Antibiotics penicillin cephalosporins aztreonam ciprofloxacin clofibrate imipenem cilastatin	Probenecid reduces the renal tubular secretion of antibiotic agents, which increases the serum concentration and elimination regular half-life of selected antibiotics. This results in an increased risk of adverse effects and toxicity.	Monitor serum concentration of antibiotic agents. Assess patient for signs of antibiotic toxicity.
Drugs That Cause Hyperuricemia ethacrynic acid diazoxide ethanol ethambutol thiazide diuretics triamterene pyrazinamide	Drugs that cause hyperuricemia decrease the effectiveness of probenecid.	Monitor for effectiveness of probenecid. Anticipate possible need for dosage adjustment.
Diuretics bumetanide furosemide indapamide	Probenecid can interfere with the natriuresis and plasma renin activity increases caused by certain diuretics. These diuretics can, in turn, increase the levels of serum uric acid, antagonizing the effects of probenecid.	Monitor for effectiveness of probenecid. Anticipate potential probenecid dosage adjustment.
dyphylline	Uricosurics directly affect the kidneys to decrease the active tubular secretion of dyphylline. May increase the half-life and decrease the total body clearance of dyphylline.	Consider use of theophylline in place of dyphylline. Monitor for signs of toxicity, such as nausea, tachycardia, and nervousness.
methotrexate	Probenecid is suspected to reduce renal elimination of methotrexate and may cause methotrexate toxicity.	Decrease methotrexate dosage. Monitor serum methotrexate concentration.
Prostaglandin Synthetase Inhibitors (PSIs) indomethacin ketoprofen ketorolac naproxen	Probenecid reduces the renal tubular secretion of selected nonsteroidal anti-inflammatory drugs (NSAIDs), which increases the serum concentration and elimination half-life of selected NSAIDs. This results in an increased risk of adverse effects and toxicity.	Do not coadminister ketoprofen and probenecid. Monitor for adverse reactions or toxicity to NSAIDs. Anticipate NSAID dose reduction.
salicylates	Salicylates inhibit actions of either drug alone.	Avoid coadministration. Advise patient to use acetaminophen for analgesic or antipyretic needs.
zidovudine	Probenecid may inhibit zidovudine glucuronidation. This may result in cutaneous eruption accompanied by systemic symptoms, including malaise, myalgia, or fever.	Coadminister with caution. Observe for possible rash and systemic symptoms.

Desired outcome: The patient will contact the prescriber if any urinary changes occur.

- Deficient Fluid Volume related to nausea and vomiting

  Desired outcome: The patient will contact the prescriber if nausea and vomiting persist.
- Ineffective Protection related to drug-induced blood abnormalities

  Desired outcome: The patient will contact the prescriber if sore throat, easy bruising, or lethargy occurs.

Planning and Intervention

Maximizing Therapeutic Effects

Do not administer probenecid with vitamin C or cranberry juice. Probenecid is excreted more easily in alkaline urine.

Minimizing Adverse Effects

The nurse should advise the patient to take probenecid with milk or food to decrease potential GI effects. Fluid intake should range between 2 and 3 L/d (unless contraindicated) to minimize potential for uric acid stone formation.

Providing Patient and Family Education

- The nurse should advise patients not to take probenecid if they have bone marrow depression, severe renal dysfunction, or uric acid kidney stones or if they are pregnant or breast-feeding.
- It is important to tell patients that if they miss a dose, they should take it as soon as they can. If it is almost time for the next dose, only that dose should be taken; double or extra doses should never be taken.
- The nurse should tell patients that probenecid can cause minor side effects, such as dizziness, flushing, hair loss, headache, loss of appetite, nausea, vomiting, and painful or swollen joints, and that they should let their doctor know about these side effects if they do not go away or if they are particularly annoying.
- It is important to tell patients that probenecid also can cause serious adverse effects and that they should call their health care provider immediately if they observe signs of renal toxicity (urinary changes), or signs of blood abnormalities (e.g., sore throat, easy bruising, or lethargy). (See the previous section, Adverse Effects.)
- The nurse should tell patients that it may take several months before the full effect of probenecid is seen.
- It is important to tell patients to avoid alcohol because it can cause stomach problems and increase uric acid in the blood, which makes a gouty attack more likely.
- The nurse should tell patients to avoid aspirin and drugs such as ibuprofen because they can make probenecid less effective.
- It is important to tell patients to drink at least 10 glasses of water a day to prevent kidney stones.
- Patients with diabetes should be instructed to use blood glucose monitoring.
- The nurse should warn patients to keep this drug out of the reach of children.
- It is important to tell patients to see their health care provider every month for blood and urine tests to make sure that they are not having any adverse reactions to probenecid.

Ongoing Assessment and Evaluation

It is important to obtain periodic CBC, platelet count, and renal function tests. The nurse should monitor for signs and symptoms of renal toxicity, headache, or dizziness and should contact the health care provider immediately if any of these symptoms occur. The patient needs to be monitored for efficacy of probenecid therapy.

Therapy is considered effective if the patient reports increased comfort or reduced pain and inflammation, and remains free of adverse effects. In addition, the patient should express an understanding of the need to contact the health care provider immediately if adverse effects occur, and of the advantages of increasing fluid intake and avoiding alcohol, aspirin, and PSIs. ■

DRUG CLOSELY RELATED TO PROBENECID

Sulfinpyrazone is an active metabolite of the PSI phenylbutazone, so it has some anti-inflammatory effects. Its action is the same as probenecid; however, it is longer acting and more potent. In addition to increasing uric acid excretion, sulfinpyrazone inhibits platelet aggregation, so it may be used in the prophylactic treatment of MI. Because of its antiplatelet action, the nurse should monitor the patient for signs of bleeding and should not administer sulfinpyrazone

MEMORY CHIP

Probenecid

- Used for the management of **chronic** gout
- Significant contraindications: bone marrow depression or uric acid kidney stones
- Most common adverse effects: headache, nausea, vomiting, and anorexia
- Most serious adverse effects: blood dyscrasias
- Maximizing therapeutic effects: do not administer with Vitamin C or cranberry juice
- Minimizing adverse effects: take with milk or food to decrease gastrointestinal distress
- Most significant patient education: taking the drug during an acute attack may worsen the symptoms

with other drugs, such as salicylates or anticoagulants (warfarin), that affect platelet aggregation. Sulfinpyrazone may induce GI distress, so it may be helpful to administer the drug with meals or milk.

DRUG SIGNIFICANTLY DIFFERENT FROM PROBENECID

Allopurinol is a uricosuric agent and a xanthine oxidase inhibitor. It differs from probenecid and sulfinpyrazone by its mechanism of action. Allopurinol works by inhibiting uric acid formation, whereas probenecid and sulfinpyrazone work by increasing uric acid excretion. Like the other agents, allopurinol is not recommended for use during an acute gouty attack because the decrease in plasma uric acid levels mobilizes urate deposits in the body, resulting in exacerbation of the acute attack. Allopurinol works best for patients who overproduce uric acid and for those with excessive tophi. In some critical care units, cardiothoracic surgeons use allopurinol with antioxidants preoperatively to prevent reperfusion-induced injury when blood flow is reestablished.

Potential adverse effects include skin rash, fever, GI distress, and liver toxicity. Drug interactions may occur with drugs that are metabolized by the hepatic microsomal enzymes, such as theophylline. Close monitoring is needed to avoid toxicity.

CHAPTER SUMMARY

- Arthritic inflammatory diseases are initially treated with salicylates and PSIs.
- For nonresolving symptoms, prescribers may initiate DMARDs, such as gold salts, hydroxychloroquine, penicillamine, methotrexate, leflunomide, and TNF antagonists.
- Because of their potentially fatal adverse effects, such as bone marrow depression, and the need for close monitoring, DMARDs are not used in the initial treatment of inflammatory diseases.
- Gout is a disease of altered purine metabolism resulting in hyperuricemia. However, hyperuricemia alone does not always result in gout.
- Antigout drugs resolve symptoms in two different ways: colchicine opposes leukocyte phagocytosis, which inhibits further urate deposits, whereas uricosuric agents reduce hyperuricemia.

QUESTIONS FOR STUDY AND REVIEW

1. What advantage do DMARDs have over salicylates, PSIs, and acetaminophen?
2. What is the major disadvantage to the use of DMARDs?
3. What is TNF?
4. When are TNF antagonists used in the management of RA?
5. Compare colchicine and probenecid.

NEED MORE HELP?

Chapter 26 of the study guide for *Drug Therapy in Nursing* contains exercises and activities to reinforce your understanding of the concepts presented in this chapter. For additional information, see the text's accompanying web site at *http://www.connection.lww.com.*

REFERENCES AND BIBLIOGRAPHY

Arava (leflunomide) package insert. (1998). Kansas City: Hoechst Marion Roussel.

CCIS System. (2001). *Computerized Clinical Information System.* Denver: Micromedex.

Clinical Drug Monographs. (2001). [CD-ROM]. Gold Standard Media.

Davis, J. C., Jr. (1999). A practical approach to gout. Current management of an 'old' disease. *Postgraduate Medicine, 106*(4), 115–116, 119–123.

Drug Facts and Comparisons. (2000). St. Louis: Facts and Comparisons.

Embrel (etanercept) package insert. (1999). Seattle: Immunex and Wyeth-Ayerst Laboratories.

Furst, D., Cannon, G. W., & Fox, R. (1998). Onset of effect and duration of response to leflunomide treatment of active rheumatoid arthritis compared to placebo or methotrexate. *Arthritis and Rheumatism, 41*, (Suppl. 9), 734.

Hardman, J. G., Limbird, L. E., Molinof, P. B., Ruddon, R. W., & Gilman, A. (Eds.). (1997). *Goodman and Gilman's the pharmacological basis of therapeutics* (9th ed.). New York: McGraw-Hill.

Karch, A. (2001). *2001 Lippincott's nursing drug guide.* Philadelphia: Lippincott Williams & Wilkins.

Katzung, B. C. (2000). *Basic and clinical pharmacology* (8th ed.). New York: McGraw-Hill.

Pascual, E. (2000). Gout update: From lab to the clinic and back. *Current Opinions in Rheumatology, 12*(3), 213–218.

Perkins, P., & Jones, A. C. (1999). Gout. *Annals of the Rheumatic Diseases, 58*(10), 611–617.

Pittman, J. R., & Bross, M. H. (1999). Diagnosis and management of gout. *American Family Physician, 59*(7), 1799–1806, 1810.

Porth, C. (1998). *Pathophysiology: Concepts of altered health states* (5th ed.). Philadelphia: Lippincott Williams & Wilkins.

Schuna, A., & Megeff, C. (2000). New drugs for the treatment of rheumatoid arthritis. *American Journal Health-System Pharmacy, 57*, 225–234.

Simko, L., & Walker, J. (1995). Allopurinol therapy for reducing reperfusion-induced injury in patients undergoing cardiothoracic surgery. *Critical Care Nurse, 16*, 69–73.

Tatro, D. (Ed.). (2000). *Drug interaction facts* (6th ed.). St. Louis: Facts and Comparisons

Walker, D. (1998). Early treatment of rheumatoid arthritis, *Practitioner, 242*(1592), 743–746, 748.

Weinblatt, M. E., et al. (1999). A trial of etanercept, a recombinant tumor necrosis factor receptor Fc fusion protein, in patients with rheumatoid arthritis receiving methotrexate, *New England Journal of Medicine, 340*, 253–259.

Angiotensin-converting enzyme inhibitors
see Chapter 30

Diuretics
see Chapter 31

Cardiac glycosides

- **digoxin**
- inamrinone
- milrinone
- carvedilol

Other drugs

beta blockers
carvedilol
see Chapters 14 and 30

angiotensin II receptor antagonists
see Chapter 30

The symbol (C) indicates the **drug class**.

Drugs in bold type marked with the symbol (P) are **prototypes**.

Drugs in blue type with no symbol are **closely related** to the prototype.

Drugs in **red** type with no symbol are **significantly different** from the prototype.

Drugs in **black** type with no symbol are **also used in drug therapy**; no prototype.

The heart is the muscle responsible for pumping blood through the circulatory system. When disease processes interfere with the ability of the heart to pump blood effectively, the organs and tissues are affected and damage may occur. One disease process that does this is congestive heart failure (CHF), sometimes now referred to as heart failure. In CHF, the heart does not pump effectively to meet the needs of the body.

The drugs classes primarily used to treat CHF are angiotensin-converting enzyme (ACE) inhibitors, diuretics, and cardiac glycosides. This chapter briefly discusses the various drug classes used in treatment of CHF and presents a thorough discussion of the cardiac glycosides, drugs used to increase the force of contractility of the heart. The prototype cardiac glycoside is digoxin (Lanoxin). Drugs significantly different from digoxin are inamrinone (Inocor), milrinone (Primacor), and carvedilol (Coreg).

PHYSIOLOGY

The heart is composed of four chambers–the left and right atria and the left and right ventricles. Blood is returned to the right atrium of the heart from the body. It progresses from the right atrium to the right ventricle to the lungs to be reoxygenated and have carbon dioxide removed. The reoxygenated blood returns to the left atrium, then to the left ventricle. The contraction of the left ventricle moves the blood back into systemic circulation (Fig. 27-1).

Blood is circulated throughout the body by a coordinated sequence of chamber contractions and valve openings and closings known as the **cardiac cycle**. The two phases of the cardiac cycle are systole and diastole. Together, it describes the timeframe from the beginning of one heartbeat to the beginning of another. During **systole**, the ventricles contract, and the aortic and pulmonic valves open, allowing ejection of blood into the aorta and pulmonary artery. During **diastole**, the ventricles relax and the mitral and tricuspid valves open, allowing blood to flow into the atria. This blood is sent to the ventricles by passive flow; atrial contraction contributes to the volume sent to the ventricle. Atrial contraction occurs at the end of diastole. As systole begins again, the increased pressure from ventricular contraction causes the mitral and tricuspid valves to shut.

The volume of blood that leaves the left ventricle in 1 minute is the **cardiac output**. Cardiac output consists of two elements, stroke volume and heart rate, and is the product of these two elements (cardiac output = stroke volume × heart rate). **Stroke volume** is the amount of blood that leaves the left ventricle with each contraction. Normally this is about 75 mL. **Heart rate** is how fast the heart is beating, or the number of contractions per minute. Normal adult range is 70 to 80 beats/minute. Cardiac output is affected by factors that alter either stroke volume or heart rate.

Stroke volume is dependent on three factors–preload, contractility, and afterload. **Preload** is the passive stretching force exerted on the ventricular muscle created by the amount of blood that has filled the heart by the end of diastole. Preload will be affected by the amount of blood that has returned to the heart (venous return), the ability of the atria to contract forcefully enough to move blood into the ventricles, and how much blood was left in the ventricle during the last contraction. **Contractility** is the force of the squeezing that the ventricle is able to achieve to eject the blood into the systemic circulation. **Afterload** is the amount of pressure the ventricular muscles must overcome to eject the blood into the systemic circulation. Contractility also is affected by the concentration of catecholamines in the heart muscle; the more catecholamines, the greater the contractility will be. Afterload is controlled by the diameter of the vessel and the pressure within the vessel, which is known as **peripheral resistance** (PR = pressure × diameter of vessel).

Contractions of the heart are dependent on the unique electrical conduction system of the cardiac muscle. The physiology of the conduction system of the heart is described within the physiology section of Chapter 29, Drugs Affecting Cardiac Output and Rhythm.

Physiology

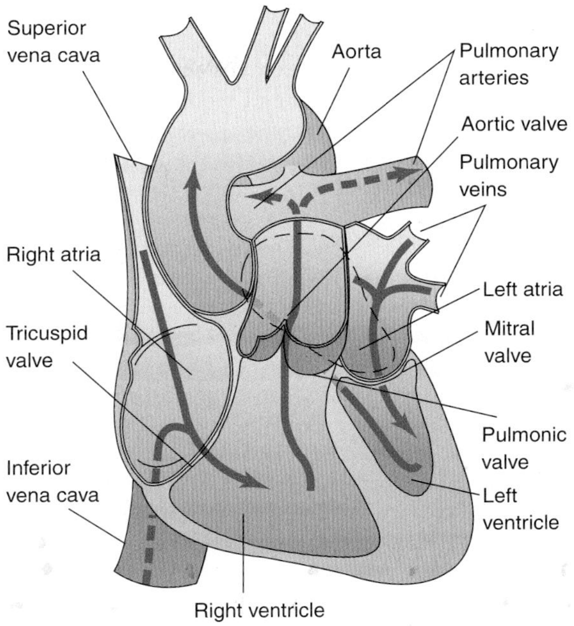

Figure 27-1. Cardiac circulation. The unoxygenated blood is returned via the superior and inferior vena cava to the right atrium, where it is moved to the right ventricle. Blood leaves the ventricle via the pulmonary artery to be reoxygenated in the lungs. The oxygenated blood returns to the left atrium via the pulmonary veins and then into the left ventricle. Blood is ejected from the ventricle to the body via the aorta.

PATHOPHYSIOLOGY

Congestive heart failure, a major pathologic problem in the United States, is associated with high morbidity and high mortality (Parra, Marshall, & Soisson, 1999; Parmley, 2000). Pathologic processes that may cause CHF occur either in the heart itself, such as an aortic stenosis or myocardial deficiency after an infarction; or systemically, such as from systemic hypertension, coronary artery disease, or renal failure. Coronary artery disease and hypertension are the primary causes of CHF.

Cardiac output will decrease when the left ventricle is unable to eject its normal volume of blood during systole; the **ejection fraction** (the amount leaving the ventricle with contraction compared with the total amount in the ventricle before contraction) is therefore decreased. For a while, the body attempts to compensate for the decreased cardiac output. The heart muscle enlarges (**cardiomyopathy**) to provide more force of contraction to try to improve cardiac output. Eventually, however, the heart becomes less and less effective in contracting. As output becomes diminished significantly, the kidneys retain sodium and water to increase circulating volume. Unfortunately, this mechanism places more of a burden on the already overworked heart, increasing preload and afterload. The ventricles then eject less and less. As blood accumulates in the ventricles, the pressure in the vessels coming to the heart increases. Build-up of blood in the left ventricle causes pulmonary congestion or left-sided heart failure. Symptoms include rales, rhonchi, and shortness of breath. Build-up of fluid in the right ventricle causes systemic congestion or right-sided heart failure. Symptoms include peripheral edema, positive jugular vein distention, and a third heart sound (S3).

Left-sided failure occurs first, then right-sided failure in CHF. This is sometimes referred to as backward failure. The compensatory hypertrophy of the heart muscle eventually, in most patients, will lead to some degree of "stiffness" or loss of elasticity of the ventricle. This "stiffness" alters ventricular diastolic function and does not allow the ventricle to fill completely, which further decreases cardiac output. Although most patients will develop systolic dysfunction first and then diastolic dysfunction, some patients do initially develop diastolic dysfunction. Diastolic dysfunction may also be from systemic hypertension and coronary artery disease. Additional causes of diastolic dysfunction are fibrosis from aging, infiltrative diseases (such as myocarditis), and constrictive pericarditis. Cardiac output will be decreased with diastolic dysfunction, although the ejection fraction may be normal. The compensatory mechanisms of the body will be identical in response to the diminished cardiac output. Initially with this type of failure, the body does not have a fluid overload, so the symptoms of fluid overload (such as S3, jugular venous distention, and peripheral edema) will not be present. For this reason, some practitioners believe the term heart failure is a more accurate description of the entire disease process than the term CHF, whereas other practitioners employ the term chronic heart disease. All of these terms may be used in practice.

DRUGS TO TREAT CONGESTIVE HEART FAILURE

When, for various reasons, the heart cannot achieve the normal cardiac output, a backlog of blood, or congestion, occurs, and heart failure develops. There are several drug classes used to treat CHF. These are ACE inhibitors, diuretics, and cardiac glycosides. These three drug groups together form what is considered the standard basis of care for CHF. The use of ACE inhibitors combined with diuretics has been found to decrease the mortality associated with congestive heart disease. Cardiac glycosides, of which digoxin is the prototype, have been found useful in the symptom management of CHF. Although digoxin does not decrease mortality, it has been shown to decrease the need for hospitalizations.

If these drug groups are unsuccessful in resolving symptoms, other drugs may be added to the regimen. If there is persistent dyspnea, hydralazine (a vasodilator) alone or combined therapy with nitrates is added. If there is persistent hypertension, a direct vasodilator or an alpha blocker is added. If the concomitant angina with the CHF, then nitrates and aspirin are added (Fig. 27-2).

Additionally, research is now examining the use of other drug classes, including beta blockers and angiotensin II receptor antagonists, and the diuretic drug, spironolactone, all of which may be used with the standard trio of ACE inhibitors, diuretics, and cardiac glycosides. It can be seen that polypharmacy is the standard treatment of choice for CHF.

ACE INHIBITORS

As circulating volume to the kidneys decrease in CHF, the renin-angiotensin-aldosterone systems are activated as the body attempts to "correct" for the low levels of circulating volume. Renin stimulates the production of Angiotensin I. Angiotensin I is converted by a special enzyme into an extremely potent vasoconstrictor, Angiotensin II. Angiotensin II also stimulates the production of aldosterone, which causes sodium and fluid to be retained, thus increasing circulating blood volume. This means that the already overworked heart must work harder. Vasoconstriction is designed to direct the diminished blood volume to vital organs. It also increases peripheral resistance, which decreases cardiac output and further increases the workload on the failing heart. ACE inhibitors prevent the conversion of angiotensin to the active vasoconstrictor form, thus preventing the deleterious effects from the renin-angiotensin-aldosterone systems. Certain ACE inhibitors have been approved for use in CHF. These are captopril (Capoten), fosinopril (Monopril), lisinopril (Prinivil), enalapril (Vasotec), and quinapril (Accupril). A recent, large clinical drug study of lisinopril (Assessment of Treatment with Lisinopril and Survival [ATLAS] study) found that the use of this drug with diuretics, digoxin, or both provided symptomatic relief of CHF. The study also showed that high doses of lisinopril reduced morbidity and mortality more than low doses of lisinopril (Simpson & Jarvis, 2000). Previously, low doses of ACE inhibitors have been used in CHF. Adverse effects of dizziness and renal insufficiency were more frequent in the high-dose group but there was no difference in the numbers of patients needing to stop taking the drug (Kulbertus, 1999). The ATLAS study also showed that lisinopril was at least as effective and as well tolerated by patients with CHF as other ACE inhibitors used in CHF treatment (Simpson & Jarvis, 2000). More information about ACE inhibitors is found in Chapter 30.

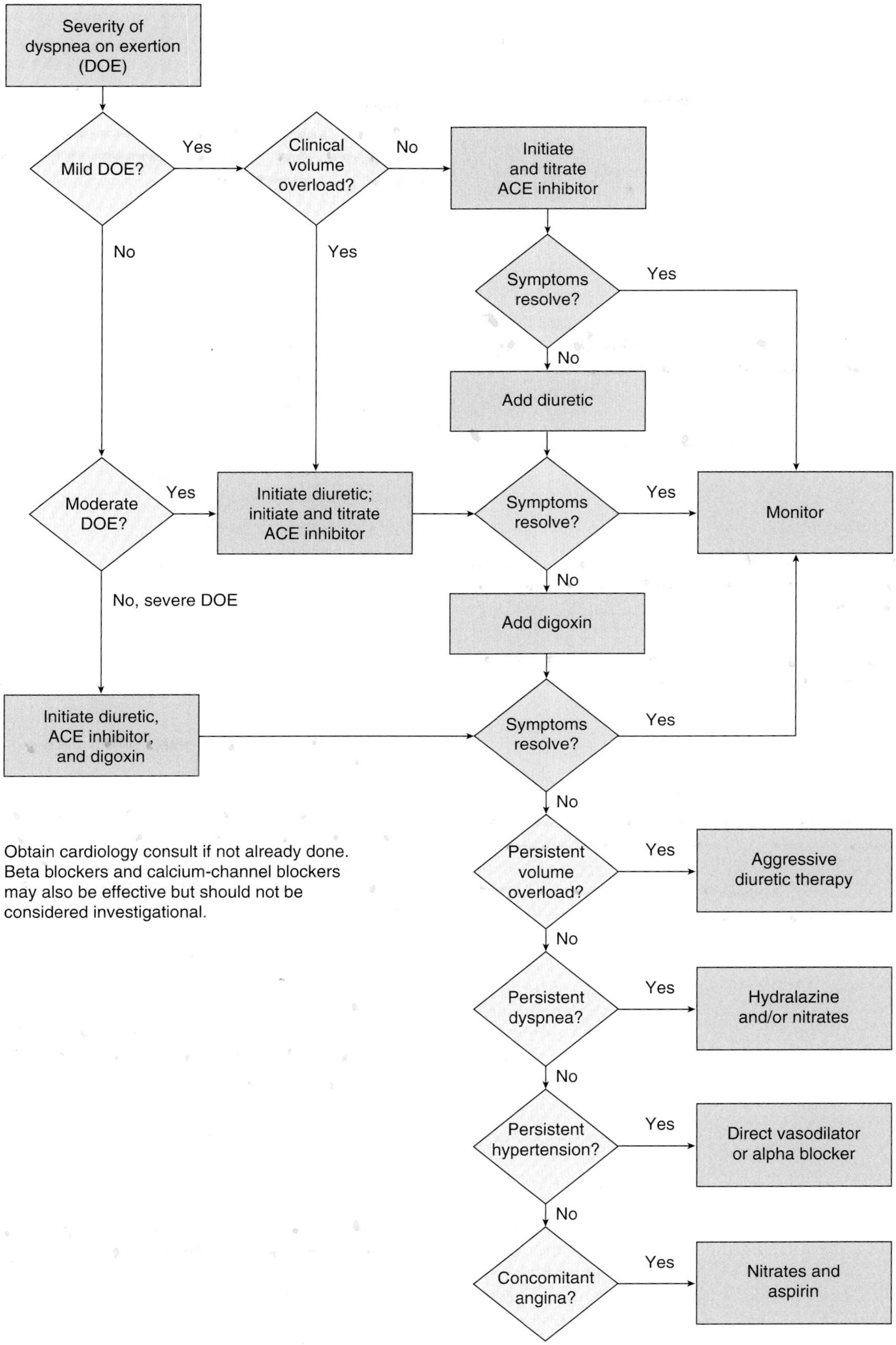

Figure 27-2. Pharmacological management of patients with heart failure. (From the Agency for Healthcare Research and Quality; http://hstat.nlm.nih.gov/tempfiles/is/tempBrPg38355.html?t=983547613.)

DIURETICS

Diuretics act in the nephrons of the kidney to increase urinary output. This decreases circulating volume and peripheral resistance, reducing the workload on the failing heart. Thiazide and loop diuretics are both used to treat the edema that occurs in CHF. Spironolactone is a potassium-sparing diuretic. Its potential use in CHF is currently being studied. See "Other Drugs" later in this chapter. Diuretics are discussed fully in Chapter 31.

CARDIAC GLYCOSIDES

The cardiac glycosides also are known as digitalis preparations or digitalis glycosides. These drugs increase the force of cardiac contraction, increasing cardiac output. This, in turn, increases perfusion to the kidneys. Higher renal perfusion causes increases in the production of urine. Thus, the drug reduces preload and afterload. Digoxin is the prototype cardiac glycoside discussed in this chapter.

OTHER DRUGS

Beta blockers, angiotensin II receptor antagonists, and spironolactone are additional drugs undergoing research and being used to treat CHF. In addition, new drug therapies for CHF are currently being researched.

Beta blockers inhibit the sympathetic nervous system, slowing the heart rate, and decreasing cardiac output. Historically, this was believed to be a contraindication for their use in CHF. In fact, beta blockers may worsen CHF before benefits are seen. However, beta blockers also cause vasodilation and reduce peripheral resistance, effects which are helpful in CHF. Clinical drug trials have shown that the nonselective beta-blocker carvedilol improves left ventricular function, improves quality of life, and reduces mortality in CHF (Cohn, Fowler, Bristow, Colucci, Gilgert, & Kinhal, 1997; Eichhorn, 1999). Carvedilol was the first beta blocker to be approved for use in CHF. It is discussed more fully at the end of this chapter. Recent studies have examined the use of other beta blockers in treating CHF. Controlled-release/extended-release metoprolol was found to improve survival, reduce the need for hospitalizations, improve the patient's functional class of CHF, and have positive effects on the patient's well-being (Hjalmarson, Goldstein, Fagerberg, Wedel, Waagstein, Kjekshus, et al., 2000). Further studies are ongoing in this area. Beta blockers are discussed in more depth in Chapters 14 and 29.

Angiotensin II receptor antagonists block the action of angiotensin II. It has been hypothesized that angiotensin II receptor antagonists may be more effective in controlling CHF than ACE inhibitors because of different pharmacodynamics. ACE inhibitors provide a cardiac protection by increasing bradykinin and nitric oxide. Although this is something that angiotensin II receptor antagonists do not do, it is believed that angiotensin II receptor antagonists provide cardiac protection through another, as yet unknown, mechanism (Kitakaze, Kuzuya, & Hori, 1999). Research is under way to learn whether angiotensin II receptor antagonists are effective in treating CHF, and whether they should be used instead of, or in addition to, ACE inhibitors. Angiotensin II receptor antagonists are discussed in Chapter 30.

Another drug that may be used with CHF is spironolactone, a potassium-sparing diuretic and aldosterone antagonist. Some studies have shown that spironolactone, when added to a drug regimen of an ACE inhibitor, diuretic, and digoxin, will reduce mortality. It is recommended for use in patients with severe CHF. Spironolactone is discussed further in Chapter 31.

C CARDIAC GLYCOSIDES

The prototype cardiac glycoside drug is digoxin (Lanoxin). Inamrinone (Inocor), milrinone (Primacor), and carvedilol (Coreg) are drugs significantly different from the cardiac glycosides.

NURSING MANAGEMENT OF THE PATIENT RECEIVING P DIGOXIN

Core Drug Knowledge

Pharmacotherapeutics

Digoxin (Lanoxin) is used in treating CHF and atrial flutter. Digoxin also is used in treating atrial fibrillation, especially if the ventricular rate is elevated (Table 27-1).

Pharmacokinetics

Absorption of digoxin varies with the type of preparation; tablet absorption is about 60% to 80%; elixirs, 70% to 85%; and solution-filled capsules, 90% to 100%. Taking digoxin with food slows down absorption, but total absorption usually is unchanged. The exception is when digoxin is taken with a meal that is very high in bran fiber, which may reduce absorption. Digoxin also may be administered IV. Digoxin is distributed widely in the tissues. High concentrations are found in the myocardium, skeletal muscle, liver, brain, and kidneys. Digoxin crosses the blood-brain barrier and the placenta. Serum drug levels are not affected significantly by changes in fat tissue weight, so dosing is best calculated on lean (ideal) body weight, rather than actual weight if the patient is obese. Metabolism takes place in the liver. However, much of the drug, 50% to 75%, is excreted unchanged by the kidneys. Digoxin is not removed by dialysis. Because of digoxin's long half-life, several days are required for steady state to be achieved and optimal clinical effects to be seen.

To increase the onset of therapeutic effects, a dose higher than normal, a **loading dose**, may be given to raise the blood level quickly to the desired range. This is known as **digitalization**. The total dose needed for digitalization is divided into several doses, with roughly half the loading dose given as the first dose. The remainder is divided and given at 6- to 8-hour intervals for oral dosage and 4- to 8-hour intervals for parenteral dosages.

TABLE 27-1 Summary of Selected Cardiac Glycosides

Drug (Trade) Name	Selected Indications	Route and Dosage Range	Pharmacokinetics
digoxin (Lanoxin; *Canadian:* Novo-Digoxin)	Congestive heart failure (CHF), atrial fibrillation, atrial flutter	*Adult:* PO, loading dose, 0.75–1.25 mg in divided doses; maintenance of 0.125–0.25 mg/d; IV, loading, 0.4–1.0 mg in divided doses; maintenance, 0.063–0.25 mg *Child:* Dosage individualized	*Onset:* PO, 30–120 min; IV, 5–30 min *Duration:* PO, 6–8d; IV, 4–5 d $t_{1/2}$: 30–40 h
inamrinone (Inocor)	CHF	*Adult:* IV, initially 0.75 mg/kg bolus slowly over 2–3 min with dose repeated in 30 min, if needed; maintenance infusion, 5–10 μg/kg/min; not to exceed 10 μg/kg daily *Child:* Safety and efficacy not established	*Onset:* Immediate *Duration:* 2h $t_{1/2}$: 3–6 h
milrinone (Primacor)	CHF	*Adult:* IV, loading dose, 50 μg/kg bolus over 10 min; maintenance, 0.375–0.75 μg/kg/min, not to exceed 1.13 mg/kg daily *Child:* Safety and efficacy not established	*Onset:* Immediate *Duration:* 8 h $t_{1/2}$: 2–3 h

The dose is lower if the loading dose is given IV instead of PO. Dosage adjustments must be made when there is renal failure or suspected age-related renal function deterioration to avoid cumulative and toxic effects.

Pharmacodynamics

The effect of digoxin on the heart is dose related. There is a direct action on both the cardiac muscle and the specialized electrical conduction system of the heart and an indirect effect on the heart from stimulation of the autonomic nervous system. The direct effect of digoxin is to strengthen the force of contraction of the heart. This is called a positive **inotropic** effect. This effect is believed to be due to digoxin increasing the movement of calcium ions across the myocardial cell membrane during depolarization discharge. As calcium is needed for contraction, a stronger contraction can occur with more calcium. Digoxin also directly increases the refractory period at the AV node. This is the period of time that the heart muscles cannot be stimulated into contracting again. Digoxin also is known to increase total peripheral resistance. The indirect effect of digoxin is to create a vagomimetic effect, one that mimics the action of stimulating the vagus nerve. This depresses the sinoatrial (SA) node and prolongs conduction to the atrioventricular (AV) node. This decrease in conduction is known as a negative **dromotropic** effect. Because of the prolonged conduction time, heart rate slows. This is termed a negative **chronotropic** effect. Cardiac output is increased as a result of these factors. The improved cardiac output results in an increase in renal perfusion, causing mild diuresis. In higher doses, digoxin increases sympathetic outflow from the central nervous system (CNS) to the cardiac and peripheral sympathetic nerves; this may increase atrial or ventricular rate. The additional sympathetic activity may be an important factor in digoxin toxicity.

Contraindications and Precautions

Digoxin is contraindicated in heart block, ventricular fibrillation, certain cases of ventricular tachycardia, some cases of sick sinus syndrome, presence of digitalis toxicity, beriberi-related heart disease, hypersensitivity to digoxin, and allergies, although allergies are rare. Caution must be used when administering digoxin over the long term to patients with CHF and who are difficult to regulate or who have a greater than normal risk for developing toxicity (such as those with unstable renal function or a tendency toward hypokalemia). For these patients, the physician may consider a cautious withdrawal of digoxin once the heart failure is controlled. The nurse must monitor these patients very carefully for signs of returning or recurrent heart failure.

Caution also should be used when giving digoxin to patients with severe carditis, acute myocardial infarction (MI), severe pulmonary disease, and severe heart failure because they may be more sensitive to digoxin-induced arrhythmias. Patients with renal insufficiency are more likely to have adverse effects and develop digoxin toxicity. Caution should be used in thyroid disorders because plasma levels of digoxin are proportional inversely to thyroid status. In untreated hypothyroidism, digoxin requirements are reduced; in thyrotoxic patients, larger doses of digoxin may be necessary. Patient response to digoxin is unchanged in compensated thyroid disease. The electrolyte imbalances of hypokalemia, hypomagnesemia, and hypercalcemia potentiate the effect of digoxin, and the patient may develop signs of toxicity even with normal serum levels. Hypocalcemia may nullify the effects of digoxin; serum calcium levels will need to be rectified to achieve therapeutic effects of digoxin.

Digoxin is a pregnancy category C drug and its safety for use in breast-feeding women has not been established. Children may receive digoxin; however, premature and immature infants are very sensitive to its effects.

Dosage must be titrated carefully in children, and they should be monitored closely for signs of toxicity.

Adverse Effects

Adverse effects are dose related and are signs of digoxin toxicity. Adverse effects occur in 5% to 20% of patients receiving digoxin, with between 1% and 4% experiencing serious reactions. The most common adverse effects are cardiac toxicity, followed by gastrointestinal (GI) disturbances and CNS toxicity. The cardiac toxicities include bradycardia, AV block, complete heart block, ventricular tachycardia, premature ventricular contractions, ventricular fibrillation, paroxysmal and nonparoxysmal nodal rhythms, AV dissociation, accelerated junctional nodal rhythm, paroxysmal atrial tachycardia, and atrial fibrillation. Almost any type of arrhythmia can be stimulated by digoxin toxicity. GI effects are anorexia, nausea, vomiting, diarrhea, and abdominal pain. CNS effects are headache, weakness, apathy, drowsiness, visual disturbances (e.g., blurred, yellow vision; halo effect in vision), confusion, restlessness, disorientation, seizures, electroencephalogram abnormalities, delirium, hallucinations, neuralgia, and psychosis.

When toxicity is suspected an electrocardiogram (ECG) may help identify whether digoxin toxicity has occurred. Digoxin causes a normal slowing of heart rate, a narrower QRS complex, and a depressed T wave. However, toxicity results in a prolonged P-R interval and a shortened Q-T interval. In the event of toxicity, the drug will be discontinued until all signs of toxicity are gone. Occasionally, if severe arrhythmias have occurred, additional treatment may be necessary. Potassium chloride may be given to help correct the arrhythmia, especially if hypokalemia is present. It may be given PO or IV if the need is urgent. Digibind (digoxin immune fab) is used as the antidote.

Drug Interactions

Digoxin interacts with many drugs. The interactions usually relate to decreased or increased serum levels of digoxin or increased incidence of adverse effects (Table 27-2).

Assessment of Relevant Core Patient Variables

Health Status

The nurse will determine whether the patient has ventricular fibrillation, ventricular tachycardia, heart block, sick sinus syndrome, beriberi-associated heart disease, or hypersensitivity to digoxin because these are contraindications to its use. A baseline ECG will be obtained by the nurse for comparison if digoxin toxicity is later suspected. The nurse also will determine if the patient is currently on drug therapy that promotes the loss of potassium, such as thiazide or loop diuretics, because hypokalemia increases the net effect of digoxin, placing the patient at increased risk of digoxin toxicity. The nurse should examine laboratory findings for indications of hypokalemia, hypomagnesemia, or hypercalcemia, which all predispose the patient to digoxin toxicity. The nurse will determine current thyroid function because this can alter the dosage requirement of digoxin. It also is important to determine whether the patient has renal impairment because poor renal excretion may allow digoxin levels to build up to toxic levels. Patients with renal impairment may require a lower dose of digoxin.

Life Span and Gender

The nurse should determine whether the patient is pregnant; digoxin is administered with caution during pregnancy because 50% to 83% of the maternal serum concentration of digoxin will affect the fetus. The nurse also needs to determine whether the patient is breast-feeding because safety in infants has not been established.

It is a good idea to note the patient's age before administering digoxin. Elderly patients must be administered digoxin carefully because they tend to have low body mass and decreased renal functioning, making them more prone to adverse effects of the drug. Lower drug dosage may be indicated. Accidental poisoning of children in their home is common with digoxin. Such digoxin normally had been prescribed for a parent or grandparent, not for a child.

Lifestyle, Diet, and Habits

The nurse should determine the patient's normal dietary intake of potassium, calcium, and magnesium because this may have a bearing on the serum levels of these electrolytes. St. John's wort, an herbal preparation, should not be started after digoxin therapy is begun because it has been known to reduce digoxin's therapeutic activity. Patients already using St John's Wort who stop using it after digoxin therapy has been regulated are at risk of having adverse effects from the higher serum levels of digoxin (Baede-van Dijk, van Galen, & Lekkerkerker, 2000).

Environment

The nurse should be aware of the environment in which digoxin will be administered. Digitalization of a patient most often occurs in the hospital where the patient can be monitored closely for adverse effects. In addition, IV doses of digoxin are administered in the hospital. Once the patient is stabilized and on an oral maintenance dose, administration of digoxin may be performed in any setting, including self-administration at home.

Nursing Diagnoses and Outcomes

- Decreased Cardiac Output related to altered cardiac function

TABLE 27-2 Agents That Interact With Digoxin

Interactants	Effect and Significance	Nursing Management
alprazolam, aminoglycosides (oral), amiodarone, anticholinergics, benzodiazepines, bepridil, captopril, cyclosporine, diltiazem, erythromycin, esmolol, felodipine, flecainide, hydroxychloroquine, ibuprofen, indomethacin, itraconazole, nifedipine, omeprazole, propafenone, propantheline, quinidine, quinine, tetracycline, tolbutamide, verapamil	Increased serum digoxin levels resulting from various mechanisms, such as altered GI flora, increased absorption, decreased clearance; may increase patient's risk for excessive levels and effects of digoxin	Monitor patient and blood tests for signs of digitalis toxicity.
aminoglutethimide, aminoglycosides (oral), aminosalicylic acid, antacids, antihistamines, antineoplastics, barbiturates, cholestyramine, colestipol, hydantoins, hypoglycemics (oral), kaolin/pectin, metoclopramide, neomycin, penicillamine, rifampin, sucralfate, sulfasalazine	Decreased serum digitalis level	Monitor patient to assess effects of drug therapy. Effect of digoxin may be reduced.
albuterol	Possibly enhanced skeletal muscle binding of digoxin	Monitor for therapeutic effect of digoxin.
beta blockers	Possibly complete heart block resulting from atrioventricular nodal conduction	Monitor ECG regularly.
disopyramide	Altered pharmacologic effect of digoxin	Monitor for therapeutic effect of digoxin.
nondepolarizing muscle relaxants and succinylcholine	Increased potential for toxic levels of either digoxin or interactant	Monitor patient and laboratory test values for signs of toxicities.
potassium-sparing diuretics	Unpredictable	Monitor patient, electrolyte levels, and laboratory values to detect signs of toxicities and decreasing therapeutic drug effects.
spironolactone	Increased or decreased serum digoxin level	Monitor patient, electrolyte levels, and laboratory values to detect signs of toxicities and decreasing therapeutic drug effects.
amiloride	Decreased inotropic effects of digoxin	Monitor for therapeutic effects of digoxin.
triamterene	Increased pharmacologic effects of digoxin	Monitor for adverse effects of digoxin.
sympathomimetics	Enhanced pacemaker activity, leading to increased risk for cardiac arrhythmias	Monitor pulse for arrhythmias, and evaluate ECG as indicated.
thiazide and loop diuretics and amphotericin B	Increased urinary potassium and magnesium loss, leading to increased effect and toxic levels of digoxin	Assess patient's electrolyte values. Replace electrolytes as needed.
thyroid hormones and thioamines	Decreased effect of digoxin with thyroid hormones; increased effect with thioamines	Report changes in laboratory and diagnostic test values to the prescriber in anticipation of need for dosage adjustment.

Desired outcome: The patient's CHF will be well controlled.

- Risk for Injury related to drowsiness, confusion, disorientation, seizures, delirium, hallucinations, and psychosis secondary to adverse effects of drug therapy

  Desired outcome: The patient will not sustain an injury related to adverse drug events while on drug therapy.

Planning and Intervention

Maximizing Therapeutic Effects

To achieve rapid onset of therapeutic effects, the patient is digitalized with an IV or PO loading dose. Roughly half the loading dose is given in the first increment, and the remainder is given in divided doses at appropriate intervals. The nurse should assess for therapeutic and adverse effects before each dose (see the accompanying display, Multiple Drug Therapy for Congestive Heart Failure).

Minimizing Adverse Effects

Digoxin has a narrow therapeutic index. This means that there is not much difference between the dosage needed to produce therapeutic effects and the dosage that will produce toxic effects. It is important to monitor the serum levels of digoxin to help prevent serious drug toxicity. The safe therapeutic serum level is 0.5 to 2.0 ng/mL. Unfortunately, some patients will exhibit signs of digoxin toxicity even when their serum levels are within "normal" range. Therefore, it is important to monitor also for signs of digoxin toxicity. For more information, see the accompanying display, Minimizing Adverse Effects From Digoxin Toxicity).

Providing Patient and Family Education

- The nurse should explain the reason for taking digoxin and the adverse effects of digoxin.
- The nurse teaches the patient how to check his own radial or carotid pulse. Instruct the patient to take the pulse for a full minute before taking digoxin. If the pulse is below 60 (or another parameter set by the health care provider for the patient), the patient should not take the drug without consulting with the health care provider.
- The nurse should caution the patient not to discontinue digoxin without approval from the health care provider. The accompanying display, Increasing Adherence to Drug Therapy, provides research and ideas on enhancing drug therapy compliance.
- It is important to tell the patient to avoid over-the-counter antacids and cough, cold, allergy, and diet drugs, except on the advice of the health care provider because these drugs frequently contain antihistamines that may interact with digoxin.
- The nurse should explain the importance of notifying the health care provider if any of the following occur while taking digoxin: loss of appetite, nausea, vomiting, diarrhea, stomach pain, unusual tiredness or weakness, drowsiness, headache, blurred or yellow vision, skin rash or hives, or mental depression.
- It is important to instruct the patient to return for requested laboratory work to check the serum digoxin level and electrolyte levels.
- The nurse should caution the patient to keep digoxin out of the reach of children (see the accompanying display, Digoxin).

Ongoing Assessment and Evaluation

The nurse should monitor the patient's pulse rate throughout therapy. It is important to assess serum digoxin levels after the drug is first started and has reached steady state, at each dosage change, and whenever signs of digoxin toxicity are present. Renal function will be monitored periodically throughout therapy by measuring blood urea nitrogen, creatinine, and electrolyte levels (potassium, calcium, and magnesium). Again, blood work will need to be monitored when digoxin is first started; recurrent blood work will be done based on the individual's response to therapy.

Symptoms of CHF should improve, and the patient should have increased urinary output, less edema, less shortness of breath, and fewer rales. When digoxin is given for atrial fibrillation or flutter, the arrhythmia should be corrected. The nurse will assess for development of arrhythmias. Development of arrhythmias may be a sign of digoxin toxicity. When the patient's CHF or arrhythmia is controlled without injury to the patient from adverse effects or toxicity, the drug therapy is considered effective. ■

Critical Thinking Scenario

Multiple drug therapy for congestive heart failure

Ms. Mahoney, a 65-year-old woman who lives alone in a two-story home, comes to the emergency department complaining of difficulty breathing. She reports increased shortness of breath, especially when climbing the stairs and walking; weakness; and ankle swelling. A diagnosis of congestive heart failure is made. She is hospitalized and stabilized on an oral regimen of digoxin 0.5 mg daily, the loop diuretic furosemide (Lasix) twice daily, the ACE inhibitor lisinopril, and an oral potassium supplement twice daily.

1. What is the desired therapeutic effect of this combination drug therapy?
2. Why should hypokalemia be prevented in Ms. Mahoney?
3. What blood work needs to be carefully monitored in Ms. Mahoney?

DRUGS SIGNIFICANTLY DIFFERENT FROM DIGOXIN

Inamrinone

Inamrinone (Inocor) was previously known as amrinone. The name was officially changed in the United States by the U.S. Pharmacopeia (USP) and the United States Adopted Names Council in July 2000 due to several drug errors that occurred when the drug was confused with a similar sounding drug, amiodarone, which is an antiarrhythmic. This name change has not yet been adopted internationally. The International Nonproprietary Name (INN) is still amrinone. If this drug is purchased from a source outside of the United States the label will list the ingredient as amrinone, not inamrinone. United

Minimizing Adverse Effects From Digoxin Toxicity

Monitor serum digoxin levels
- Measure levels at least 8 hours following the last oral dose and preferably 24 hours after the last dose if the patient is receiving maintenance therapy. Following this procedure will prevent reading falsely elevated digoxin blood levels.
- Monitor most closely when digoxin is first started, when the dose is changed, or when the patient has signs of toxicity.
- Periodic monitoring is needed when digoxin is used in long-term maintenance. The frequency of monitoring is based on patient response to drug therapy.

Assess for bradycardia
- Take the patient's apical pulse for 1 full minute to determine heart rate accurately before administering each dose of digoxin. If the pulse is below 60 beats/min, do not administer the dose without approval from the health care provider.

Correct electrolyte imbalances
- Monitor for low levels of potassium and magnesium and high levels of calcium because these altered levels place the patient at risk of developing digoxin toxicity.
- If potassium and magnesium levels are low, seek an order for replacement of the electrolyte.
- Electrolytes should not be administered rapidly. Calcium and potassium, especially, may bring on serious arrhythmias when administered by IV.
- Encourage the patient to follow a diet of potassium-rich foods while taking digoxin to prevent hypokalemia and digoxin toxicity. However, potassium intake should just be normal if the patient is on a potassium-sparing diuretic, ACE inhibitor, or a potassium chloride supplement.

Assess for other symptoms of digoxin toxicity
- Monitor for anorexia, nausea, vomiting, diarrhea, headache, blurred vision, confusion, *and* drowsiness
- Anorexia, nausea, vomiting, and diarrhea may also be evident when CHF is uncontrolled. This makes the assessment for digoxin toxicity more difficult.

Treatment of digoxin-induced arrhythmias
- Oral or slow IV potassium often is used as a treatment. IV doses are for more urgent problems.
  - Divided oral doses for adults should total 3 to 6 g (40 to 80 mEq), as long as normal renal function exists.
  - When given to adults by IV, 40 to 80 mEq are diluted in 5% dextrose and water (D_5W) to a concentration not greater than 40 mEq/100 mL. The drug should be administered at a rate not exceeding 20 mEq/h and more slowly if the patient reports pain at the catheter insertion site.
  - For children, oral doses totaling 1 to 1.5 mEq/kg or about 0.5 mEq/kg/h IV are given with careful ECG monitoring.
  - The ECG should be monitored for potassium toxicity (peaking of T waves). If the arrhythmia is corrected, the infusion should be stopped.
  - Potassium should not be used when renal failure exists or when complete heart block is secondary to digoxin toxicity and not related to tachycardia.
- Phenytoin, an anticonvulsant, may be used to treat atrial and ventricular arrhythmias.
  - Give 50 to 100 mg of phenytoin every 5 minutes. Total dose should not exceed 600 mg.
  - Phenytoin is used when potassium is *not* effective
- Lidocaine, an antiarrhythmic, is used to treat ventricular arrhythmias
  - Give IV for a dose of 1 mg/kg over 5 minutes, then 15 to 50 μg/kg per minute to maintain rhythm.
  - Lidocaine is used when potassium is not effective
- Atropine, an anticholinergic, may be used symptomatically to treat severe sinus bradycardia or slow ventricular rate due to secondary AV block.
  - Give 0.01 mg/kg IV
- Cholestyramine, colestipol (both are antilipids), or activated charcoal may be used to bind with digoxin in the intestine and prevent enterohepatic recirculation.

Use of the digoxin antidote
- The drug digoxin immune fab (Digibind) is considered the antidote to digoxin. This drug, used to treat potentially life-threatening toxicity, is given in approximately the same dosage as the digoxin in the patient's body. It combines with digoxin to make it unable to bind at its receptor site, therefore inactivating it.
- Improvement generally begins within 30 minutes of IV administration.
- Give digoxin immune fab over 15 to 30 minutes through a 0.22-mm filter, although it may be given as a bolus when cardiac arrest is imminent. This may be given to children or adults.
- Serum digoxin levels will remain high after administration of digoxin immune fab. Therefore, serum digoxin levels should not be used as a guideline of the antidote's effectiveness. Instead, the nurse should evaluate the patient's response to determine the antidote's effectiveness.

Miscellaneous
- Avoid administration of IM digoxin because it causes site pain.

States health care workers need to be very careful if faced with this situation to prevent making a drug error.

Like digoxin, inamrinone is used in treating CHF. However, it is only used for short-term management for those patients who have not responded positively to treatment with digoxin, diuretics, and vasodilators. Unlike digoxin, inamrinone is *not* a cardiac glycoside. Inamrinone has a positive inotropic effect and a vasodilatory effect similar to digoxin. However, inamrinone has a different structure and mode of action than digoxin. It also is different from catecholamines. Exactly how it works is unknown. The mechanism of action is believed to be related to its ability to inactivate cyclic adenosine monophosphate, which results in the contraction of myocardial muscle cells. Afterload and preload are reduced by inamrinone's direct relaxant effect on the vascular smooth muscle. These effects produce a prompt increase in cardiac output from the failing heart.

Inamrinone is administered by IV infusion. The peak of action of inamrinone is within 10 minutes; duration of action varies with the size of the dose. Duration of action is about 2 hours when larger doses are given. The main route of elimination is in urine.

Many of the adverse effects of inamrinone are common to those seen with digoxin. Inamrinone may cause supraventricular and ventricular arrhythmias, nausea, and less frequently, vomiting, abdominal pain, and anorexia. Unlike digoxin, inamrinone may cause two serious adverse effects—thrombocytopenia and hepatoxicity. Thrombocytopenia occurs in about 2.5% of patients receiving the drug, although it is more common in patients receiving prolonged

Focus on Research

Increasing Adherence to Drug Therapy

Fulmer, T. T., Feldman, P. H., Kim, T. S., Carty, B., Beers, M., Molina, M., & Putman, M. (1999). Enhancing adherence with drug therapy for CHF: An intervention study to enhance medication compliance in community-dwelling elderly individuals. *Journal of Gerontological Nursing, 25*(8), 6–14.

The Study

Community-dwelling adults, age 65 and older, who had had a primary or secondary diagnosis of congestive heart failure (CHF), were randomized into a study to test the effect of daily telephone or videotelephone calls on adherence to the prescribed drug therapy. Study subjects were either in a control group, receiving the usual care; in a group that received a daily telephone call reminder to take their medication; or in a group that received a daily videotelephone call reminder to take their medication. Over the course of the study, the groups that received a reminder call showed enhanced adherence over that of the control groups. There was no significant difference between the two treatment groups. During the study, the control group showed a decline in adherence to the treatment plan from 81% to 57%.

Nursing Implications

For drug therapy to be effective in the treatment and management of CHF, patients need to take medication regularly as prescribed. Telephone calls with or without video input are an effective means of increasing adherence with drug therapy than traditional methods, which include clinic visits, and preparation of prepoured pill boxes used at home. Telephone reminders may also be shown to be more cost effective, although this was not addressed in this study. Enhancing patient adherence is an important nursing action to maximize the therapeutic effect of the drug(s). Increased adherence to drug therapy should help minimize undesirable symptoms of CHF and prevent or decrease the need for hospitalization.

MEMORY CHIP

Digoxin

- Used in treating CHF, atrial fibrillation, and atrial flutter
- Direct effect is to strengthen force of cardiac contraction (positive inotropic effect)
- Indirect effect is to depress the SA node and slow conduction to the AV node (negative dromotropic effect), thus slowing heart rate (negative chronotropic effect)
- Can cause the same arrhythmias it is used to treat
- Antidote for digoxin overdose is digoxin immune fab
- Significant contraindications: heart block, ventricular fibrillation, certain cases of ventricular tachycardia, some cases of sick sinus syndrome, and presence of digitalis toxicity
- Most common adverse effects: cardiac toxicity; hypokalemia, hypomagnesemia, and hypercalcemia increase the risk of toxicity
- Most serious adverse effect: ventricular fibrillation
- **Lifespan alert: Older adults tend to have increased risk for adverse effects due to decreased renal function. Children are often poisoned accidentally by digoxin.**
- Maximizing therapeutic effects: achieve rapid onset of therapeutic effects with a loading dose ("digitalization")
- Minimizing adverse effects: monitor serum digoxin levels, assess for bradycardia (take apical pulse minute before giving drug), monitor and correct electrolyte imbalances, and assess for noncardiac signs of digoxin toxicity
- Most significant patient education: teach how to take pulse and to avoid taking the dose if pulse is below 60; keep digoxin out of the reach of children

therapy. Thrombocytopenia and hepatoxicity may be fatal; this is why the drug is not considered first-line therapy and is limited to short-term use.

Milrinone

Milrinone (Primacor) is also used to treat CHF. It is for short term, IV use in patients already receiving digoxin and diuretics. Unlike digoxin it is not a cardiac glycoside, but it increases the force of contraction similar to digoxin. Like inamrinone, milronone increases the force of contraction, is a vasodilator, and is different in structure and mode of action from digoxin and catecholamines. Milrinone inhibits cyclic adenosine monophosphate (cAMP) phosphodiesterase in cardiac and vascular muscle. In addition to improving cardiac contractility, milrinone improves left ventricular diastolic relaxation. Milrinone produces a prompt increase in cardiac output and decreases pulmonary capillary wedge pressure and vascular resistance. Milrinone is excreted primarily in the urine.

Adverse effects of milrinone are ventricular arrhythmias (most common adverse effect occurring in about 12% of patients), hypotension, angina, and ventricular tachycardia, which all occur in a small percentage of patients. Life-threatening arrhythmias are infrequent. Headache can occur from milrinone. Milrinone also can cause thrombocytopenia but much less frequently than inamrinone.

COMMUNITY-BASED CONCERNS

Digoxin

Digoxin can cause fatal effects if taken accidentally by children. Adults prescribed digoxin should be aware of these risks and take the following precautions in their homes:

- Store digoxin out of the reach of children.
- Have a child-safety cap placed on the medication container.
- Do not leave loose pills out where children can see them.
- Do not tell children that digoxin is "candy."

Carvedilol

Carvedilol is not a cardiac glycoside but is a nonselective beta blocker that also has alpha-blocking properties. It has been approved for treating mild-to-moderate CHF and is the first new drug approved for treating CHF in many years. Although beta blockers can decrease contractility of the heart, blocking the effect of the sympathetic nervous system can produce long-term clinical benefits to patients with CHF, even if coronary artery disease is the cause of heart failure. Carvedilol, although it decreases cardiac output (which is detrimental initially in CHF), also causes vasodilation and decreases peripheral vascular resistance (which is helpful to patients with CHF).

Carvedilol, when added to conventional therapy for CHF (digoxin, diuretics, and ACE inhibitors), may slow progression of heart failure and decrease the frequency of hospitalization. The patient should be started on a small dose and monitored carefully for signs of hypotension and worsening CHF. Dosage is increased gradually over several weeks until the therapeutic dosage range is reached. Full therapeutic effects may not occur for 1 to 3 months. At the initiation of each new dose, the patient should be observed for dizziness or lightheadedness for one hour. Transient worsening of CHF may occur when the drug is first started. This is usually well controlled by increasing the dose of the diuretic; sometimes the dose of carvedilol will need to be decreased or temporarily discontinued. Patients who have had initial difficulties with carvedilol are often successful on the drug when it is tried again.

Carvedilol, unlike digoxin, is highly protein protein bound (i.e., more than 98%). Additionally, unlike digoxin, carvedilol is metabolized by processes in the liver. Adverse effects of carvedilol that occur in a small percentage of patients with CHF include:

- Cardiovascular: bradycardia, hypotension and postural hypotension, syncope (these are the most common), cardiac failure, palpitations, extrasystoles, angina, dyspnea, and fluid overload
- CNS: depression, insomnia, hyperesthesia, and vertigo
- GI: flatulence, anorexia, dyspepsia, melena, and periodontitis
- Genitourinary: abnormal renal function and albuminuria
- Hematologic: anemia, decreased prothrombin time, and purpura
- Hepatic: increased alanine aminotransferase and aspartate transaminase levels
- Metabolic/Nutritional: hyperuricemia, hypoglycemia, hyponatremia, increased alkaline phosphatase, and glycosuria

For more information on beta blockers see Chapters 14 and 29.

CHAPTER SUMMARY

- CHF occurs when the heart is unable to effectively contract and pump out the volume of blood in the left ventricle.
- Digoxin is used in treating CHF; it also is used in treating atrial fibrillation and atrial flutter.
- Digoxin strengthens the force of contraction of the heart (positive inotropic effect), prolongs conduction to the AV node (negative dromotropic effect), and slows the heart rate (negative chronotropic effect).
- Digoxin does not increase the survival rate of patients with CHF but it does improve their symptoms and slows progression of the disease.
- ACE inhibitors, combined with diuretics, increase the survival rate of patients with CHF. Their use with digoxin are considered the standard treatment for CHF.
- Adverse effects of digoxin are dose related and are signs of digoxin toxicity. The most common adverse effects are cardiac toxicity, GI disturbances, and CNS toxicity.
- A low potassium level, low magnesium level, or a high calcium level potentiates the effect of digoxin, and digoxin toxicity may occur. This is true even if the serum level of digoxin is in "normal" range.
- Bradycardia is a clinical sign of excessive digoxin. Always check an apical pulse for 1 full minute to detect for bradycardia prior to administering digoxin. Notify the physician and do not give the drug if the pulse is less than 60 unless approved by the physician.
- Digoxin can be used to treat an arrhythmia, but it also may cause an arrhythmia.
- Inamrinone and milrinone also strengthen the force of contraction of the heart and are used in treating CHF. These drugs are only given IV and for short periods, never for chronic maintenance.
- Carvedilol is a beta blocker that is approved for use in the management of mild-to-moderate CHF. It is used in conjunction with digoxin, diuretics, and ACE inhibitors.

QUESTIONS FOR STUDY AND REVIEW

1. What are digoxin's primary effects on the heart?
2. What is the rationale for initially giving a larger than therapeutic dose (digitalization) for the first few doses of digoxin therapy?
3. What physical parameter should always be assessed before giving a dose of digoxin? What action should be taken if the finding is below normal range?
4. What effect may occur if digoxin is given to someone with decreased renal function? What actions could be taken to minimize this effect?

NEED MORE HELP?

Chapter 27 of the study guide for *Drug Therapy in Nursing* contains exercises and activities to reinforce your understanding of the concepts presented in this chapter. For additional information see the text's accompanying website at *http://www.connection.lww.com.*

REFERENCES AND BIBLIOGRAPHY

Anonymous. (2000). Heart failure drugs: what's new? *Drugs and Therapeutics Bulletin, 38*(4), 25–27.

Anonymous. (1999) Effect of metoprolol CR/XL in chronic heart failure: Metoprolol CR/XL Randomised Intervention Trial in Congestive Heart Failure (MERIT-HF). *Lancet, 353*(9169), 2001–2007.

Baede-van Dijk, P. A., van Galen, E., Lekkerkerker, J. F. (2000). Drug interaction of *Hypericum perforatum* (St. John's wort) are potentially hazardous [original in Dutch]. *Nederlands Tijdschrift voor Geneeskunde, 144*(17), 811–812.

Cohn, J. N., (2000). Heart failure: Future treatment approaches. *American Journal of Hypertension, 13*(5 Pt. 2), 74S–78S.

Cohn, J. N., Fowler, M. B., Bristow, M. R., Colucci, W. S., Gilbert, E. M., Kinhal, V., Krueger, S. K., Lejemtel, T., Narahara, K. A., Packer, M., Young, S. T., Holeslaw, T. L., & Lukas, M. A. (1997) Safety and efficacy of carvedilol in severe heart failure. The U.S. Carvedilol Heart Failure Study Group. *Journal of Cardiac Failure, 3*(3), 173–179.

Eichhorn, E. J. (1999). Experience with beta blockers in heart failure mortality trials. *Clinical Cardiology, 22,* (Suppl. 5), V21–V29.

Hjalmarson, A., Goldstein, S., Fagerberg, B., Wedel, H., Waagstein, F., Kjekshus, J., Wikstrand, J., El Allaf, D., Vitovec, J., Aldershvile, J., Halinen, M., Dietz, R., Neuhaus, K. L., Janosi, A., Thorgeirsson, G.,

Dunselman, P. H., Gullestad, L., Kuch, J., Herlitz, J., Rickenbacher, P., Ball, S., Gottlieb, S., & Deedwania, P. (2000). Effects of controlled-release metoprolol on total mortality, hospitalizations, and well-being in patients with heart failure: the Metoprolol CR/XL Randomized Intervention Trial in congestive heart failure (MERIT-HF). MERIT-HF Study Group. *Journal of the American Medical Association, 283*(10), 1295–1302.

Jelliffe, R. (2000). Goal-oriented, model-based drug regimens: Setting individualized goals for each patient. *Therapeutic Drug Monitor, 22*(3), 325–329.

Kitakaze, M., Kuzuya, T., & Hori, M. (1999). Efficacy of angiotensin II receptor antagonists as a novel drug: The treatment of chronic heart failure- in comparison with ACE inhibitors [original in Japanese]. *Nippon Rinsho. Japanese Journal of Clinical Medicine, 57*(5), 1148–1157.

Krum, H. (1999). Beta-blockers in heart failure. The "new wave" of clinical trials. *Drugs, 58*(2), 203–210.

Kulbertus, H. (1999). Clinical study of the month. The ATLAS study [original in French]. *Revue Medicale de Liege, 54*(12):952–4.

Parmley, W. W. (2000). Surviving heart failure: Robert L. Frye lecture. *Mayo Clinic Proceedings, 75*(1), 111–118.

Parra, D., Marshall, R., & Soisson, K. (1999). Clinical and pharmacologic management of chronic heart failure associated with left ventricular systolic dysfunction. *Lippincott's Primary Care Practice, 3*(3), 316–332.

Roberge, R. J., & Sorensen, T. (2000). Congestive heart failure and toxic digoxin levels: role of cholestyramine. *Veterinary and Human Toxicology, 42*(3), 172–173.

Simpson, K., & Jarvis, B. (2000). Lisinopril: A review of its use in congestive heart failure. *Drugs, 59*(5), 1149–1167.

Chapter 28

DRUGS USED TO TREAT ANGINA

KEY TERMS

angina
microvascular angina
myocardial infarction
Prinzmetal angina
stable angina
unstable angina
variant angina

Learning Objectives

At the completion of this chapter the student will:

1. Differentiate drug therapy for chronic stable angina from unstable angina.
2. Identify core drug knowledge about drugs used to treat angina.
3. Identify core patient variables relevant to drugs used to treat angina.
4. Relate the interaction of core drug knowledge to core patient variables for drugs used to treat angina.
5. Generate a nursing plan of care based on interactions between core drug knowledge and core patient variables for drugs used to treat angina.
6. Describe nursing interventions to maximize therapeutic and minimize adverse effects for drugs used to treat angina.
7. Determine key points for patient and family education for drugs used to treat angina.

Nitrates

nitroglycerin

isosorbide

The symbol indicates the **drug class**.

Drugs in bold type marked with the symbol are **prototypes**.

Drugs in blue type with no symbol are **closely related** to the prototype.

Drugs in red type with no symbol are **significantly different** from the prototype.

Drugs in **black** type with no symbol are **also used in drug therapy**; no prototype.

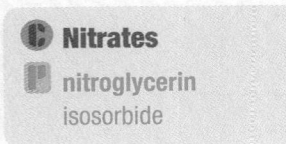

Angina is pain in the chest that occurs because the heart muscle is not receiving enough oxygen. Drug therapy to treat angina allows more oxygen to be delivered to the heart or decreases the oxygen needs of the heart, which stops the pain. This chapter discusses the three main drug therapies used in angina—beta blockers, calcium channel blockers, and nitrates. Because the prototypes for beta blockers and calcium channel blockers are presented in Chapters 14 and 29, respectively, only the nitrates are presented in this chapter.

PHYSIOLOGY

The heart is a muscle in the body that pumps oxygenated blood to the organs, muscles, tissues, and cells of the body. The heart itself requires oxygen delivered to its cells. The coronary arteries deliver oxygenated blood to the heart. Oxygen requirements of the heart increase as the heart pumps faster and works harder. Oxygen demands of the heart also increase if the heart has to overcome a greater peripheral resistance in the vessels to eject blood from the left ventricle.

PATHOPHYSIOLOGY

When the oxygen requirements of the heart are greater than the supply of oxygen it is getting, the heart muscle becomes ischemic. The oxygen imbalance may be from a reduced coronary blood flow or from a need for increased oxygen. Ischemia of the heart muscle will produce symptoms of chest pain in the patient. Chest pain that results from ischemia is termed **angina.** Angina is usually intermittent and substernal, although the pain may radiate, such as to the left arm or left shoulder. There are four types of angina:

- Stable angina
- Unstable angina
- Prinzmetal or variant angina
- Microvascular angina

In **stable angina,** oxygen need exceeds the ability of the body to supply oxygen. This may be due to a narrowing of the coronary arteries from atherosclerosis (deposits of fat in the vessel), or from an activity that increases the oxygen needs of the heart temporarily. Stable angina occurs during exercise, stress, or periods of increased physical exertion and is normally reversed with rest. No permanent damage to the heart usually occurs after an episode of stable angina. An episode of stable angina does not indicate that the patient is about to have a **myocardial infarction** (MI), and does not place the person at a greater risk of having a MI later.

Unstable angina is due to significantly decreased coronary blood flow. Pain in unstable angina occurs when the patient is resting; it can even occur during sleep and awaken the patient. Unstable angina may develop suddenly on exertion, which may the first time the patient has had anginal pain. It also can occur in patients who have previously had stable angina. For these patients, unstable angina is a marked increase in the frequency or the severity of their pain. Other presentations of unstable angina include non-Q wave MI, or post-MI onset of angina (more than 24 hours). Unstable angina results most frequently from plaque rupture in the vessel, followed by a local thrombus formation. Plaque rupture is caused by a complex sequence of events, including local inflammatory activity. Because of this, unstable angina is considered a critical phase of coronary heart disease and places the patient at high risk for having an MI. Special cardiac markers, not normally found in the blood, have been found in those with unstable angina. These regulatory contractile proteins are called cardiac tropin T and cardiac tropin I. Their presence has been shown to be a sensitive and specific marker for myocardial cell damage (Ottani, Galvani, Ferrini, Ladenson, Puggioni, Destro, et al., 1999). Tropins T and I, which can be measured by a special blood test, appear to be better indicators of damage and early risk from unstable angina than the traditionally used creatine kinase myocardial band (isoenzyme M). Death or nonfatal MI was more frequent in patients with unstable angina who had elevations of one or both of these markers (Ottani, et al. 1999). Patients who have had angina at rest within the last 48 hours and are tropin positive are considered to have a 20% risk of MI, death, or both within the next 30 days. Patients who have had angina at rest within the last 48 hours but who are tropin negative are believed to have only a less than 2% chance for MI, death, or both (Hamm, 2000). Many researchers are advocating testing of tropins T and I as standard treatment in emergency departments that treat patients with unstable angina.

Prinzmetal angina, also called **variant angina,** is due to sudden coronary artery spasms that induce ischemia in the heart muscle. These spasms, if lengthy, can lead to sudden death. However, this type of angina is rare. Prinzmetal angina may be precipitated by emotional stress, medications, street drugs (e.g., cocaine), or exposure to cold temperatures.

Microvascular angina is a newly discovered form of angina. Patients with this type of angina experience chest pain but have no apparent coronary blockages. The pain results from impaired function of the tiny blood vessels that perfuse the heart, arms, and legs. Microvascular angina can be treated with some of the same drugs as used to treat stable angina.

DRUGS TO TREAT ANGINA

Three main drug groups are used to treat angina—beta blockers, calcium channel blockers, and nitrates. Beta blockers prevent the beta-adrenergic receptors from being stimulated. These drugs have multiple effects on the heart and cardiovascular system, including slowing the heart rate, depressing atrioventricular (AV) conduction, decreasing cardiac output, and reducing systolic and diastolic blood pressure at rest and during exercise. These effects decrease the oxygen demands of the heart and thereby decrease angina. Beta blockers used commonly for treating angina are propranolol, atenolol, metoprolol, and nadolol. Other beta blockers that may be used in treating angina are bisoprolol (Zebeta), carteolol (Cartrol), and esmolol (Brevibloc), although this is an off-label use of these drugs. The beta blockers are discussed fully in Chapter 14.

Calcium is needed in the automatic and conducting cells of the heart to help create an action potential. In the cells of the heart that contract, calcium links excitation with contraction, and controls energy storage and use. Calcium travels to these cells through special channels. Calcium-channel blockers inhibit calcium from moving across cell membranes. The effects of this on the cardiovascular system are decreased contraction, depression of impulse formation (automaticity), and slowing of conduction velocity. These have the effect of decreasing the oxygen needs of the heart. Calcium-channel blockers are used in chronic stable angina when the patient cannot tolerate beta blockers or nitrates, or if the symptoms are not adequately controlled while on these therapies. The calcium-channel blockers used for chronic stable angina are verapamil (Calan), amlodipine (Norvasc), bepridil (Vascor), diltiazem (Cardizem), nicardipine (Cardene), and nifedipine (Procardia). The calcium-channel blocker used in unstable angina is verapamil. Amlodipine, nifedipine, verapamil, and diltiazem are used in treating Prinzmetal angina. The calcium-channel blockers are discussed more fully in Chapter 29.

Nitrates dilate vascular smooth muscle and both venous and arterial vessels (although there is more relaxation on the venous side). Venous dilation decreases the returning flow of blood to the heart (preload). Arterial dilation reduces systemic vascular resistance and arterial pressure (afterload). These effects decrease the workload on the heart and its oxygen needs. Nitrates also improve the circulation to the heart itself by redistributing blood flow to the collateral vessels.

Some other drug therapies are used as adjuncts to the main drug therapies for treating angina. These therapies are not designed to decrease oxygen demands on the heart. Rather, these therapies are used to slow down the progression of coronary artery disease or prevent complications that may arise with angina. Aspirin is one drug that is used in chronic stable angina and unstable angina. Aspirin has anticoagulant properties, which are helpful in preventing thrombus formation and a potentially resulting MI. Aspirin is discussed in more detail in Chapter 24. Heparin, an anticoagulant given IV or SC, is used in unstable angina to prevent thrombus formation. The use of low molecular weight heparin is being proposed instead of unfractionated heparin because it provides a more stable pharmacodynamic response and is easier to use. Low molecular weight heparin has been shown to be as effective as traditional, unfractionated heparin and appears to be most beneficial to patients who are at the highest risk for complications from unstable angina (Kaul, 2000). Heparin is discussed in Chapter 32. Lipid-lowering agents often are used in conjuncture with drugs to treat angina to slow the progression of coronary heart disease. Decreasing circulating fats in the blood will decrease the rate at which fatty deposits are deposited on the walls of the vessels. These fatty deposits narrow the vessel and block the blood flow, causing angina. This is especially problematic in the coronary arteries. Lipid-lowering agents are discussed in Chapter 34. If the pain of unstable acute angina is not controlled by nitrates or anti-ischemic therapy, morphine may be used. Morphine is discussed in Chapter 24.

New drug classes being examined in Europe for potential use in treating angina include potassium-channel openers and blockers, glycoprotein IIb/IIIa receptor antagonists, and direct thrombin inhibitors. There are no current clinical trials in the United States with these drugs, although some other research is being done. Potassium-channel openers are a novel class of vasodilators. By opening the potassium channel, the conductivity of potassium ions into the cells is increased, which results in hyperpolarization of smooth muscle membranes and produces vasodilation. Hyperpolarization of the cell membrane is a physiologic way of decreasing cell excitability (Lawson, 2000). Potassium blockers inhibit the cellular cardiac repolarization of potassium currents and multiple neuronal and vascular currents. This exerts an antiischemic and an antiarrhythmic effect on the body (Mitrovic, Oehm, Thormann, Pitschner, & Hamm, 2000). Glycoprotein IIb/IIIa receptor antagonists are a new class of platelet inhibitors that are more potent than aspirin because they target the final common pathway of platelet aggregation (Weitz & Bates, 2000). Finally, direct thrombin inhibitors are being studied because they appear to inhibit thrombin-mediated platelet aggregation and fibrin deposits (Weitz & Bates, 2000).

NITRATES

Nitrates include nitroglycerin (Nitrostat), which is the prototype, and isosorbide (Sorbitrate).

NURSING MANAGEMENT OF THE PATIENT RECEIVING P NITROGLYCERIN

Core Drug Knowledge

Pharmacotherapeutics

Therapeutic uses of nitroglycerin vary by the route of administration. Given sublingually or by transmucosal or translingual spray, nitroglycerin is used to treat acute angina. It also is used through topical, transdermal, translingual spray, and transmucosal or oral sustained-release methods to prevent chronic recurrent angina. When given IV, nitroglycerin is used to treat hypertension secondary to surgical procedures; to create controlled hypotension during anesthesia; to treat congestive heart failure (CHF) associated with acute MI; and to treat angina unresponsive to organic nitrates or beta blockers (Table 28-1).

Unlabeled uses for nitroglycerin include reducing cardiac workload in patients with acute MI and CHF (sublingual and topical), providing adjunctive treatment of Raynaud disease and other peripheral vascular diseases (topical), and managing hypertensive crisis (IV).

Pharmacokinetics

Nitroglycerin is absorbed rapidly sublingually; it also is absorbed through the skin. Metabolism occurs in the liver, and the drug has an extensive first-pass effect when given orally. It is excreted in the urine. Absorption of sublingual products depends on salivary secretion; dry mouth will decrease absorption. The drug is absorbed directly into the vascular system via this route; it is not swallowed and absorbed through the gastrointestinal

TABLE 28-1 Summary of Selected Antianginal Drugs

Drug (Trade) Name	Selected Indications	Route and Dosage Range	Pharmacokinetics
Nitrates			
nitroglycerin (Nitrostat, Nitrobid IV, Nitrol, Nitro-Dur, Nitrolingual)	Acute angina	*Adult:* SL, 1 tablet under tongue, every 5 min; total of 3 tablets	*Onset:* IV: 1–2 min; sublingual, 1–3 min; TL spray, 2 min; topical and transdermal, 30–60 min *Duration:* IV, 3–5 min; SL, 30–60 min; topical/transdermal, up to 24 h $t_{1/2}$: 1–4 min (IV)
	Prophylaxis	*Adult:* Topical (transdermal paste or patch), apply ½ inch q8h; increase by ½ inch to achieve desired results; translingual spray, 0.4 mg/metered dose into oral mucosa, not to exceed 3 doses/15 min	
	Hypertension	*Adult:* IV, 5 μg/min by infusion pump; increase by 5-μg increments every 3–5 min as needed *Child:* Safety and efficacy not established	
isosorbide dinitrate (Sorbitrate, Isordil; *Canadian:* Apo-ISDN)	Treatment and prevention of angina pectoris	*Adult:* SL, 2.5–5 mg; PO, 5–40 mg tablets or capsules *Child:* Safety and efficacy not established	*Onset:* PO, 20–40 min; SL, 2–5 min *Duration:* PO, 4–6 h; SL, 1–2 h $t_{1/2}$: Unknown
Beta Blocker			
atenolol (Tenormin; *Canadian:* Apo-Atenol)	Hypertension	*Adult:* PO, 50 mg/d; after 1–2 wk, dose may be increased to 100 mg *Child:* Dose has not been established	*Onset:* PO, varies; IV, immediate *Duration:* PO and IV, 24 h $t_{1/2}$: 6–9 h
	Angina pectoris	*Adult:* PO, 50 mg qd. If optimal response not achieved in 1 wk, increase to 100 mg/d, up to 200 mg/d	
	Acute myocardial infarction	*Adult:* IV, 5 mg over 5 min; follow with 5 mg, 10 min later; switch to 50 mg PO 10 min after last IV dose; follow with 50 mg PO 12 h later; administer 100 mg PO qd or 50 mg PO bid for 6–9 d *Child:* Safety and efficacy not established	
Calcium Channel Blocker			
nifedipine (Adalat, Procardia; *Canadian:* Apo-Nifed)	Angina pectoris Stable angina Hypertension	*Adult:* PO, 10 mg tid, titrate over 7–14 d; SR: PO, 30–60 mg/qd; titrate over 7–14 d *Child:* Safety and efficacy not established	*Onset:* PO and SR, 20 min *Duration:* 8–24 h $t_{1/2}$: 2–5 h

(GI) tract, thus bypassing the first-pass effect. Absorption of transdermal products is through the skin and into the vascular system. Ointments and transdermal systems provide a gradual release of drug into the circulatory system. The drug reaches its target organs before it is inactivated by the liver. Transdermal absorption will be increased with physical exercise, elevated external temperatures (e.g., saunas), and if the drug is applied to broken skin.

Pharmacodynamics

Nitroglycerin relaxes vascular smooth muscle and dilates both arterial and venous vessels. Dilation of veins is more predominant than dilation of arteries, resulting in peripheral pooling of blood and decreased preload. Blood pressure will decrease as a result of venous dilation. Reflex tachycardia may follow the drop in blood pressure. Arteriolar dilation reduces systemic vascular resistance and arterial pressure, thus reducing afterload. Myocardial oxygen consumption is decreased. Nitroglycerin redistributes blood flow in the heart, improving circulation to ischemic areas.

Tolerance to the vascular and antianginal effects may develop. This is minimized by starting with as small a dose as possible and removing the nitroglycerin (paste or transdermal patches) from the patient for 10 to 12 hours a day. The sublingual and translingual spray forms of the drug are the least likely to produce tolerance. The transmucosal form also appears to produce minimal tolerance.

Contraindications and Precautions

Nitroglycerin is contraindicated in hypersensitivity or idiosyncratic reactions to nitrates, severe anemia, closed angle glaucoma (intraocular pressure may increase), orthostatic hypotension, first hours to days of acute MI (sublingual), head trauma or cerebral hemorrhage (may increase intracranial pressure), and allergy to adhesives (transdermal). Caution also is advised when using nitroglycerin to treat patients with open-angle glaucoma. The IV route is contraindicated in hypotension, uncorrected hypovolemia, inadequate cerebral circulation, increased intracranial pressure, constrictive pericarditis, and pericardial tamponade. Caution also is advised when administering IV nitroglycerin to patients with hepatic disease and severe renal disease. Nitroglycerin is in pregnancy category C, and it is not known whether nitrates are excreted in breast milk, so cautious use is advised.

Adverse Effects

The most common adverse effect of nitroglycerin is headache, which may be persistent and severe. Cardiovascular effects may include hypotension, postural hypotension, tachycardia, palpitations, and syncope. Other effects on the central nervous system (CNS) include dizziness, vertigo, anxiety, and weakness. These adverse effects are related to the vasodilation and cardiovascular effects that occur with nitroglycerin use. Dermatitis can occur from topical application. Local burning under the tongue can occur with sublingual administration. Alcohol intoxication can develop in patients receiving high doses of IV nitroglycerin because many of the IV products contain alcohol as a dilutant.

Overdosage will result in hypotension, tachycardia, flushing, perspiring skin turning cold and cyanotic, headache, vertigo, palpitations, visual disturbances, diaphoresis, dizziness, syncope, nausea, vomiting, and anorexia. Other signs and symptoms of overdose include initial hyperpnea, dyspnea and slow breathing, heart block, and increased intracranial pressure exhibited by cerebral symptoms of confusion, moderate fever, and paralysis. These signs and symptoms are related to excessive cardiovascular action (see the accompanying display, Nitroglycerin).

Critical Thinking Scenario

Nitroglycerin

Peter Riley, 4 years old, is staying at his grandparents' house for the weekend. He finds his grandfather's nitroglycerin ointment in the bathroom. He squeezes some out and spreads it over his entire left arm. When his grandparents realize what he has done, they call the Advice Nurse hotline for their HMO.

1. If you were the Advice Nurse, what would you tell the grandparents to do?
2. What is the major risk to Peter?

Drug Interactions

A few drugs interact with nitroglycerin (Table 28-2). Nitroglycerin may interfere with the Zlatkis-Zak color reaction, causing a false report of decreased serum cholesterol levels.

Assessment of Relevant Core Patient Variables

Health Status

It is important for the nurse to ascertain whether the patient has acute angina or chronic recurrent angina. The nurse will assess the patient's pulse rate and blood pressure. The nurse also should determine whether the patient has any of the following conditions, which are contraindications to nitroglycerin use: closed angle glaucoma, orthostatic hypotension, severe anemia, head trauma or cerebral hemorrhage, first hours to days of acute confirmed MI, hypersensitivity to nitrates, and allergy to adhesives (if the patient is receiving a transdermal dosage form). If the patient is to receive IV nitroglycerin, the nurse must first be sure that the patient does not have hypotension or uncorrected hypovolemia, inadequate cerebral circulation, increased intracranial pressure, constrictive pericarditis, or pericardial tamponade because these are contraindications for this route. If hepatic or severe renal disease exist, caution must be used before IV administration.

Life Span and Gender

Nitroglycerin is in pregnancy category C, so the nurse needs to determine whether the patient is pregnant. The nurse also should assess whether the patient is breastfeeding because cautious use is advised. Safety and efficacy in children have not been established, so the nurse needs to note the age of the patient.

Lifestyle, Diet, and Habits

If the patient has chronic stable angina, it is important to determine how much or what type of activity precipitates an anginal attack, or if angina occurs at rest, which may indicate unstable angina. If the patient smokes cigarettes, this constricts the blood vessels and may cause angina. If the patient's diet is high in cholesterol or saturated fats, there is a risk for development of fatty deposits on the vessels, which contributes to narrowing of the vessels.

Environment

The nurse needs to be aware of the environment in which the drug will be administered. Nitroglycerin can be administered in any environment, with the exception of IV nitroglycerin, which is administered in the hospital while on continuous monitoring for blood pressure and heart rate. Sublingual tablets are likely to lose effectiveness if exposed to light, excessive heat, or moisture. Between 40% and 80% of the IV nitroglycerin dose will migrate

TABLE 28-2 Agents That Interact With Nitroglycerin

Interactants	Effect and Significance	Nursing Management
alcohol	Severe hypotension and cardiovascular collapse	Ensure patient does not consume alcohol. Educate patient about risks of interaction.
heparin	Decreased pharmacologic effects of heparin	Monitor for therapeutic effect of heparin.
fentanyl	Severe hypotension or increased fluid volume requirements that may cause decreased antimanic controls	Monitor hypotension and fluid levels.
lithium	Possible lithium toxicity and neurotoxic and psychotic symptoms	Give with caution and daily monitor serum lithium levels. Give drug with food or milk or after meals.
theophylline	Pharmacologic actions of theophylline potentially enhanced, particularly drug interactions	Have frequent blood tests to monitor drug effects, and ensure safe and effective dosage.

into many plastics. Therefore, the drug is diluted only into glass parenteral solution bottles and administered with IV tubing not made from polyvinyl chloride (PVC) that is provided by the manufacturer.

Nursing Diagnoses and Outcomes

- Acute Pain, chest, related to cardiac disease
  Desired outcome: Acute chest pain will be resolved with the use of drug therapy without injury to the heart occurring.
- Decreased Cardiac Output related to therapeutic effects of drug
  Desired outcome: Patient's blood pressure will decrease to therapeutic levels but will not decrease to the level of hypotension.
- Risk for Injury related to orthostatic hypotension and dizziness secondary to adverse effects of drug therapy
  Desired outcome: Patient will not sustain injury due to orthostatic hypotension and dizziness.
- Acute Pain, headache, related to adverse effects of drug therapy
  Desired outcome: Patient's headache, if it occurs, will be managed successfully by analgesics so that patient will adhere to drug therapy.

Planning and Intervention

Maximizing Therapeutic Effects

Sublingual Tablets

The nurse should place one tablet under the patient's tongue where it should be allowed to dissolve. It is important to administer a tablet every 5 minutes, up to three in 15 minutes if necessary, to achieve full therapeutic effect. The nurse should have the patient sit or lie down to allow for rest and decrease the oxygen needs of the heart.

It is a good idea to keep tablets in the original dark bottle and keep the lid on when not in use to prevent deterioration and loss of efficacy. Avoid exposure of tablets to high temperatures.

Topical Ointment and Transdermal Patches

The nurse should apply to areas that do not have excessive hair, to promote absorption. The nurse should apply to the chest, upper arm, or upper thigh to promote absorption and increase onset of systemic action. Do not apply to distal parts of extremities (i.e., near the hands or feet).

Translingual Spray

The nurse should spray nitroglycerin onto or under the tongue to promote absorption. Do not allow the patient to inhale the drug. If used to treat acute angina, the nurse should spray one or two metered doses. The dose may be repeated but not more than three times in 15 minutes. If used prophylactically, the nurse should administer one metered dose 5 to 10 minutes before onset of activity that may precipitate angina.

Transmucosal Tablets

The nurse should place one tablet between lip and gum above incisors or between cheek and gum to promote slow dissolving and extended absorption.

Intravenous

The nurse should use only the non-PVC IV administration tubing supplied by the manufacturer, and glass IV bottles for the diluted drug solution to prevent loss of active drug into the tubing or bag.

Minimizing Adverse Effects

All Routes

The nurse should assess the patient's pulse and blood pressure before administering drug therapy. It also is important to monitor for orthostatic hypotension and assist the patient to a standing position gradually when arising. The nurse should treat any headache that develops with aspirin or acetaminophen until tolerance to this adverse effect occurs. When withdrawing nitroglycerin as a treatment for angina, it is important to reduce the dosage gradually to prevent withdrawal reactions.

Sublingual

The nurse should not give more than three tablets—one every 5 minutes—to relieve acute angina. If three tablets do not alleviate angina, the patient is considered to be having an acute MI, and it is urgent to obtain emergency help immediately.

Transdermal

This route is not appropriate for acute angina. The nurse should not apply the drug to broken or irritated skin. It is important to remove the patch for 10 to 12 hours every 24 hours to prevent nitrate tolerance from developing. If anginal symptoms develop at night, the use of a beta blocker or calcium-channel blocker should be considered. Patients who normally have angina only during daytime hours are not at significant risk of developing nighttime angina with a nightly nitrate-free period.

The nurse should not discharge a cardioversion or defibrillation paddle through a transdermal system. Arcing may develop, which may concentrate local current, damaging the paddles and burning the patient.

Intravenous

The nurse should monitor the patient's blood pressure and heart rate while IV therapy continues. It is important to assess for alcohol intoxication if giving high doses for a prolonged period. The nurse also should use an IV pump to regulate the infusion rate.

Providing Patient and Family Education

All Routes

- The nurse should explain the purpose and adverse effects of nitroglycerin.
- The nurse should instruct the patient to sit or lie down when having angina.
- It is important to explain that postural hypotension may occur (especially if standing still after a dose). If feelings of dizziness, weakness, or fainting occur, the patient should lie down or place the head in a low position (if sitting), and take deep breaths.

Sublingual Tablets

- The nurse should teach the patient to place a sublingual tablet under the tongue at the first sign of an anginal attack, and not to wait for the pain to become severe (see the accompanying display, Sublingual Nitroglycerin).
- It is important to explain that if angina is not relieved, up to two more tablets may be taken; one 5 minutes after the first tablet and the other 5 minutes after the second tablet. The nurse should instruct the patient to go the nearest emergency department if angina is not relieved after the above measures are taken.
- The nurse should teach the patient to keep the sublingual tablets in their original bottle and to keep the cap on the bottle. It also is important to explain the importance of not storing the bottle in the sun.

Focus on Research

Sublingual nitroglycerin

Kimble, L. P., & Kunik, C. L. (2000). Knowledge and use of sublingual nitroglycerin and cardiac-related quality of life in patients with chronic stable angina. *Journal of Pain and Symptom Management. 19*(2), 109–117.

The Study

Knowledge of sublingual nitroglycerin and its use, general aspects of self care of angina, and quality of life were examined in this nursing research study. Older age, male gender, a recent diagnosis of coronary artery disease, and poor recall of instructions given about sublingual nitroglycerin were found to be predictors of poorer sublingual nitroglycerin knowledge. Having a bad experience (i.e., adverse effects) with sublingual nitroglycerin was associated with a poorer quality of life. Of the people in the study, 65% lacked knowledge about using sublingual nitroglycerin to prevent angina, and about one third took the drug for symptoms other than chest pain.

Nursing Implications

Nurses need to emphasize how to use nitroglycerin appropriately—both for acute angina and for prophylactic use. This teaching needs to be reinforced whether there is patient contact, such as at clinic or office visits, or during home visits. Additionally, if nurses help patients learn how to minimize or manage adverse effects of drug therapy, quality of life will be improved for patients.

Translingual Spray

- The nurse should instruct the patient on proper administration—spraying it onto or under the tongue, not inhaling it.
- It is important to explain that the drug may be used prophylactically or to treat the onset of angina.

Transmucosal Tablets

- The nurse should instruct the patient on the proper placement of the tablet—under the upper lip between the lip and gum above the incisor, or in the pouch between the cheek and gum. It is important to explain that it will dissolve slowly over a 3- to 5-hour period.
- The nurse must emphasize the importance of not chewing or swallowing the tablet.
- It is important to explain that the rate of dissolution may be increased by touching the tablet with the tongue, or by drinking hot fluids.

Sustained-Release Tablets

- The nurse should instruct the patient to swallow these tablets, not to chew them or place them sublingually because this alters onset of the drug effects.

Ointment

- The nurse should explain that ointments do not provide immediate relief of acute angina pain and should only be used prophylactically.
- It is important to instruct the patient to use an applicator or dose-measuring papers, not the hands, to measure and apply the prescribed amount of nitroglycerin ointment.

- The nurse should instruct the patient not to rub the drug into the skin.
- It is a good idea to teach the patient to choose a different area on the skin when applying a new dose. The nurse also should tell the patient to use a tissue to remove any old ointment left on the skin before applying a new dose.
- The nurse should instruct the patient to wipe off any ointment that gets on the outside of the tube to prevent it from getting on the hands, and to recap the tube securely.

Transdermal

- The nurse should teach the patient to apply the patch to as hairless a skin area as possible. The chest or upper arm are used typically; the patient should avoid placing the patch in the distal portion of the extremities.
- The nurse should instruct the patient to remove the patch for 10 to 12 hours as prescribed.
- The nurse should explain the importance of avoiding saunas and other environments that increase the external temperature.
- If the adhesive becomes loose during the "on" period, the nurse should instruct the patient to place additional tape over the patch to guarantee contact with the skin.
- There is still active nitroglycerin in the discarded patch, which can be a hazard for children and pets. Therefore, it is important to advise the patient to flush the used patch down the toilet (see the accompanying display, Chest Pain).

Ongoing Assessment and Evaluation

The patient's blood pressure and heart rate will be monitored throughout therapy. If given IV, this monitoring should be continuous. The nurse will assess for relief of angina or control of chronic angina. Therapy is effective when angina is controlled or prevented without the development of hypotension or damage to the heart. ■

DRUG CLOSELY RELATED TO NITROGLYCERIN

Isosorbide (Isordil) is a nitrate, like nitroglycerin, and is used for treating and preventing angina. It is not used to treat hypertension. Isosorbide is given sublingually or orally. Sublingual isosorbide has a slower onset and a longer duration of action compared to sublingual nitroglycerin. Because sublingual isosorbide does not relieve chest pain as rapidly as nitroglycerin, isosorbide is limited to treating acute angina in patients intolerant or unresponsive to sublingual nitroglycerin. Oral preparations include tablets, sustained-release tablets, and chewable tablets. Oral sustained-relief routes of isosorbide also have a slower onset and longer duration than comparable forms of nitroglycerin. Although nitroglycerin may be used occasionally with adequate monitoring during the early phases of an acute MI, isosorbide should never be used due to its greater sustained effects.

COMMUNITY-BASED CONCERNS

Chest Pain

Many community groups request health education topics for their members. Nurses are often the health care professionals who respond to these requests. If called on to discuss consumer response to chest pain be sure to include the following points when teaching families and the public how to respond appropriately when someone is experiencing an angina attack:

- Instruct them to have the person rest (sit or lie down).
- If the person is known to take nitroglycerin tablets, give one and have the person place it under the tongue.
- Repeat in 5 minutes and again in another 5 minutes if chest pain does not go away.

If after three tablets of nitroglycerin the pain does not go away, the person should be considered to be having a heart attack. Call the emergency medical number, and get the person to the nearest hospital.

OR

If the person with chest pain does not take nitroglycerin, have him or her sit or lie down If the pain does not go away within 5 minutes, assume that the person is having a heart attack. Call the medical emergency number and get the person to the nearest hospital.

MEMORY CHIP

Nitroglycerin

- Used in treating angina; IV route is used to decrease blood pressure (BP)
- Usually given sublingually topically, sometimes IV in acute care setting
- Relaxes smooth muscles and dilates vascular beds
- Most common adverse effect: headache followed by hypotension
- Most serious adverse effect: can be hypotension
- Maximizing therapeutic effects: keep tablets out of sunlight (keep in original dark bottle), moisture (keep cap sealed tightly when drug not in use), and excessive heat; give one tablet every 5 minutes, up to 3 in 15 minutes; and have patient rest or lie down during anginal attacks.
- Minimizing adverse effects: take BP before and during therapy; to prevent orthostatic hypotension, keep the patient lying down during therapy
- Most significant patient education: if three sublingual tablets do not alleviate pain, seek immediate emergency medical treatment; utilize prophylactic doses prior to activities that may precipitate angina; and remove patches or ointment for 10 or 12 hours out of every 24 to prevent tolerance.

CHAPTER SUMMARY

- Nitroglycerin is used to treat angina and to prevent angina. When given IV, it also is used to reduce hypertension.
- Nitroglycerin relaxes vascular smooth muscle and dilates both arterial and venous beds. Dilation of veins is more predominant than dilation of arteries, resulting in peripheral pooling of blood and decreased preload.
- Blood pressure will decrease as a result of venous dilation. Reflex tachycardia may follow the drop in blood pressure. Thus, the patient's blood pressure is assessed prior to each dose and during drug therapy with nitroglycerin and the pulse should be assessed during therapy.
- Arteriolar dilation reduces systemic vascular resistance and arterial pressure, thus reducing afterload. This decreases how hard the heart has to work to eject blood from the left ventricle, decreasing the oxygen needs of the heart.
- The most common adverse effect of nitroglycerin is headache.
- When nitroglycerin is given intravenously due to elevated blood pressure, the patient must be continually monitored in an intensive care setting. The drug should be administered via a pump for safety.

QUESTIONS FOR STUDY AND REVIEW

1. If the patient is taking nitroglycerin through a transdermal patch for prevention of recurrent angina, why should he or she only wear the patch 12 to 14 hours a day?
2. How often should a tablet of sublingual nitroglycerin be administered to treat an episode of angina? How many tablets can be administered?
3. Why should the nurse take the patient's blood pressure before administering a dose of nitroglycerin ointment topically?
4. When measuring the dose of nitroglycerin ointment, the nurse gets some on her hands. Later, she experiences a throbbing headache. What is the explanation for this?
5. How does nitroglycerin decrease anginal pain?

NEED MORE HELP?

Chapter 28 of the study guide for *Drug Therapy in Nursing* contains exercises and activities to reinforce your understanding of the concepts presented in this chapter. For additional information, see the text's accompanying web site at *http://www.connection.lww.com.*

REFERENCES AND BIBLIOGRAPHY

Agency for Health Care Research and Quality (AHRQ) (Formerly the Agency for Health Care Policy and Research (AHCPR). (1994) *Clinical practice guidelines: Unstable angina* [On-line]. Available: www.ahrq.gov.

Agrawal, B. (1999). The use of cardiac markers in acute coronary syndromes. *Scandinavian Journal of Clinical Laboratory Investigators Supplement, 230*, 50–59.

American College of Cardiology. (1999). Guidelines for the management of patients with chronic stable angina. *Journal of the American College of Cardiology, 33*(7), 2092–2197.

Godoy, I., Herrera, C., Zapata, C., Kunstmann, S., Abufhele, A., & Corbalan, R. (1998). Comparison of low-molecular-weight heparin and unfractionated heparin in the treatment of unstable angina. (in Spanish) *Revista Medica de Chile, 126*(3), 259–264.

Gokhan Cin, V., Gok, H., & Kaptanoglu, B. (1996). The prognostic value of serum toponin T in unstable angina. *International Journal of Cardiology, 53*(3), 237–244.

Hamm, C. W. (1996). New perspectives in therapy of unstable angina. (in German) *Herz, 21*(1), 37–43.

Hamm, C. W. (1998) Progress in the diagnosis of unstable angina and perspectives for treatment. *European Heart Journal, 19, (Suppl N), N48–50.*

Hamm, C. W., & Braunwald, E. (2000). A classification of unstable angina revisited. *Circulation*, 102(1), 118–122.

Hollenberg, N. K., Williams, G. H., & Anderson, R. (2000). Medical therapy, symptoms, and the distress they cause: Relation to quality of life in patients with angina pectoris and/or hypertension. *Archives of Internal Medicine,* 160(10), 1477–1483.

Iliadis, E. A., Klein, L. W., Vandenberg, B. J., Spokas, D., Hursey, T., Parrillo, J. E., & Calvin, J. E. (1999). Clinical practice guidelines in unstable angina improve clinical outcomes by assuring early intensive medical treatment. *Journal of the American College of Cardiology, 34*(6), 1689–1695.

Kaul, S., & Shah, P. K. (2000). Low molecular weight heparin in acute coronary syndrome: evidence for superior or equivalent efficacy compared with unfractionated heparin? *Journal of the American College of Cardiology, 35*(7), 1699–1712.

Lawson, K. (2000). Potassium channel openers as potential therapeutic weapons in ion channel disease. *Kidney International, 57*(3), 838–845.

Mitrovic, V., Oehm, E., Thormann, J., Pitschner, H, & Hamm, C. (2000). Potassium channel openers and blockers in coronary artery disease. Comparison to betablockers and calcium antagonists. *Herz, 25*(2), 130–142.

Mouallem, M., Schwartz, E., & Farfel, Z. (2000). Prolonged oral morphine therapy for severe angina pectoris. *Journal of Pain and Symptom Management, 19*(5), 393–397.

Ottani, F., Galvani, M., Ferrini, D., Ladenson, J. H., Puggioni, R., Destro, A., Baccos, D., Bosi, S., Ronchi, A., Rusticali, F., & Jaffe, A. F. (1999). Direct comparison of early elevations of cardiac troponin T and I in patients with clinical unstable angina. *American Heart Journal, 137*(2), 284–291.

Richards, S. B., Funck, M., & Milner, K. A. (2000). Differences between black and whites with coronary heart disease in initial symptoms and delay in seeking care. *American Journal of Critical Care, 9*(4), 237–244.

Weitz, J. I., & Bates, S. M. (2000). Beyond heparin and aspirin: New treatments for unstable angina and non-Q-wave myocardial infarction. *Archives of Internal Medicine, 160*(6), 749–758.

Chapter 29

DRUGS AFFECTING CARDIAC OUTPUT AND RHYTHM

KEY TERMS

action potential
arrhythmia
atrial flutter
atrial fibrillation
automaticity
cardiac cycle
depolarization
diastole
dysrhythmia
ectopic foci
proarrhythmia
re-entry phenomenon
resting membrane potential
repolarization
systole
transmembrane potential
ventricular fibrillation
ventricular tachycardia

Learning Objectives

At the completion of this chapter the student will:

1. Identify core drug knowledge about drugs that affect cardiac function.
2. Identify core patient variables relevant to drugs that affect cardiac function.
3. Relate the interaction of core drug knowledge to core patient variables for drugs that affect cardiac function.
4. Differentiate Class I, II, III, and IV antiarrhythmics.
5. Describe the varied therapeutic effects of beta blockers and calcium-channel blockers.
6. Generate a nursing plan of care from the interactions between core drug knowledge and core patient variables for drugs that affect cardiac function.
7. Describe nursing interventions to maximize therapeutic and minimize adverse effects for drugs that affect cardiac function.
8. Determine key points for patient and family education for drugs that affect cardiac function.

Class IA

quinidine
procainamide
dysopyramide

Class IB

lidocaine
tocainide
mexiletine
moricizine

Class IC

flecainide
propafenone

Class II

Beta blockers approved as antiarrhythmics

propanolol
acebutolol
esmolol

Beta blockers not approved as antiarrhythmics

atenolol
bisoprolol
metoprolol
nadolol
prindolol
timolol

Class III

amiodarone
sotalol
bretylium
ibutilide
dofetilide

Class IV

Calcium channel blockers approved as antiarrhythmics

verapamil
IV diltiazem

Non–calcium channel blocker

adenosine

Calcium channel blockers not approved as antiarrhythmics

amlodipine
bepridil
felodipine
isradipine
nicardipine
nifedipine
nimodipine
nisoldipine

Potassium removing resins

sodium polystyrene sulfonate

The symbol (C) indicates the **drug class**.
Drugs in bold type marked with the symbol (P) are **prototypes**.
Drugs in blue type with no symbol are **closely related** to the prototype.
Drugs in **red** type with no symbol are **significantly different** from the prototype.
Drugs in **black** type with no symbol are **also used in drug therapy**; no prototype.

The heart is the muscle responsible for pumping blood through the circulatory system. The contraction of the heart depends changes in electrical stimulation in cardiac muscle cells. These changes in electrical activity occur at regular, set intervals. This establishes a normal rhythm of the beating heart. When pathologic processes interfere with these normal changes in stimulation, the rhythm of the heart is altered. These alterations may be severe enough to be incompatible with supporting life. Arrhythmia is the term used to describe these alterations. **Arrhythmia,** literally meaning no rhythm, occurs any time there is an alteration in the normal rate or rhythm of the heart. The heart continues to beat but not in the expected pattern or manner. The term **dysrhythmia,** meaning abnormal rhythm, is used interchangeably with arrhythmia and is preferred by many health care providers. This chapter identifies drugs that are used to treat alterations in the rhythm of the heart.

Drugs to treat cardiac arrhythmias are grouped by class. There are three subclasses of Class I antiarrhythmics. The prototype for Class IA antiarrhythmics is quinidine (Quinaglute Dura-Tabs). Other drugs in this class are procainamide (Procan SR) and disopyramide (Norpace). Drugs similar to Class IA drugs are the Class IB antiarrhythmics, which include lidocaine (Xylocaine), tocainide (Tonocard), mexiletine (Mexitil), and moricizine (Ethmozine), and phenytoin (Dilantin), and the Class IC antiarrhythmics, which include flecainide (Tambocor) and propafenone (Rythmol).

Class II antiarrhythmics are the beta blockers. The prototype beta blocker is propranolol (Inderal). Of the other numerous drugs in this class, only acebutolol (Monitan) and esmolol (Brevibloc) are approved as Class II antiarrhythmics. Any of the other beta blockers may be used based on the clinical judgment of the physician.

Class III antiarrhythmics include the prototype amiodarone (Cordarone). Drugs similar to amiodarone are sotalol (Betapace) and bretylium.

Class IV antiarrhythmics are the calcium channel blockers; the prototype is verapamil (Calan). The other calcium channel blocker approved for treating arrhythmias is intravenous diltiazem (Cardizem). A drug significantly different from verapamil is adenosine (Adenocard). Calcium-channel blockers used to treat cardiac and circulatory pathologies other than arrhythmias are amlodipine (Norvasc), bepridil (Vascor), felodipine (Plendil), isradipine (DynaCirc), nicardipine (Cardene), nifedipine (Procardia), nimodipine (Nimotop), and nisoldipine (Sular).

Because hyperkalemia is an electrolyte imbalance that may cause potentially lethal arrhythmias, drugs to prevent arrhythmias are the potassium-removing resins. The prototype potassium-removing resin is sodium polystyrene sulfonate (Kayexalate).

PHYSIOLOGY

As stated in Chapter 27, the heart is composed of four chambers, the left and right atria and left and right ventricles. Blood is returned to the right atrium of the heart from the body. It progresses from the right atrium to the right ventricle to the lungs to be reoxygenated and have carbon dioxide removed. The reoxygenated blood returns to the left atrium, then to the left ventricle. The contraction of the left ventricle moves the blood back into systemic circulation.

Blood is circulated throughout the body by a coordinated sequence of chamber contractions and valve openings and closings known as the **cardiac cycle**. The two phases of the cardiac cycle are systole and diastole. Together they describe the timeframe from the beginning of one heartbeat to the beginning of another. During **systole,** the ventricles contract, and the aortic and pulmonic valves open, allowing ejection of blood into the aorta and pulmonary artery. During **diastole,** the ventricles relax and the mitral and tricuspid valves open, allowing blood to flow into the atria. This blood is sent to the ventricles by atrial contraction. Atrial contraction occurs at the end of diastole. As systole begins again, the increased pressure from ventricular contraction causes the mitral and tricuspid valves to shut.

Contractions of the heart are dependent on the unique electrical conduction system of the cardiac muscle. The conduction system connects to highly specialized cardiac cells that allow the heart to beat predictably and rhythmically. The system is composed of the sinoatrial (SA) node, the atrioventricular (AV) node, the bundle of His, the bundle branches, and the Purkinje fibers. The SA node is known as the pacemaker of the heart. It is influenced by both the sympathetic and the parasympathetic nervous systems. The progression of the electrical impulse that produces the heartbeat starts in the SA node. The action potential leaves the SA node traveling through the atria, causing them to contract. The impulse is slowed at the AV node so that the atria and the ventricles do not contract simultaneously. The impulse then travels through the bundle of His to the bundle branches and then through the Purkinje fibers. Depolarization and contraction of the ventricles then occur (Fig. 29-1).

To best comprehend how this unique conduction system works, it is important to understand how potassium, sodium, and calcium ions work to bring about electrical changes in the cardiac cells that stimulate contraction of the cardiac cells. The fibers of the heart muscle alternate between resting and contracting. Contraction of the muscle fibers is due to electrical and chemical changes within the cell. Potassium is predominantly an intracellular (i.e., within the cell) ion, and sodium and calcium are predominantly extracellular (i.e., outside the cell) ions (Fig. 29-2). Calcium also is stored in special places within the cell, but it is not active as long as it is stored.

These ions (potassium, sodium, and calcium) all flow following the normal concentration gradient (moving from areas of high concentration to areas of low concentration). Due to the intracellular and extracellular ions, there is an electrical gradient across the membrane of the cell. This is called the **transmembrane potential**. All changes that occur in the transmembrane potential during an entire cycle of contraction and relaxation are, as a unit, called the **action potential**. At rest, the electrical charge of the transmembrane potential, also known as the resting membrane potential, is –90 millivolts. This means that there is a 90-millivolt difference between the electrical charge inside and outside of the

Physiology

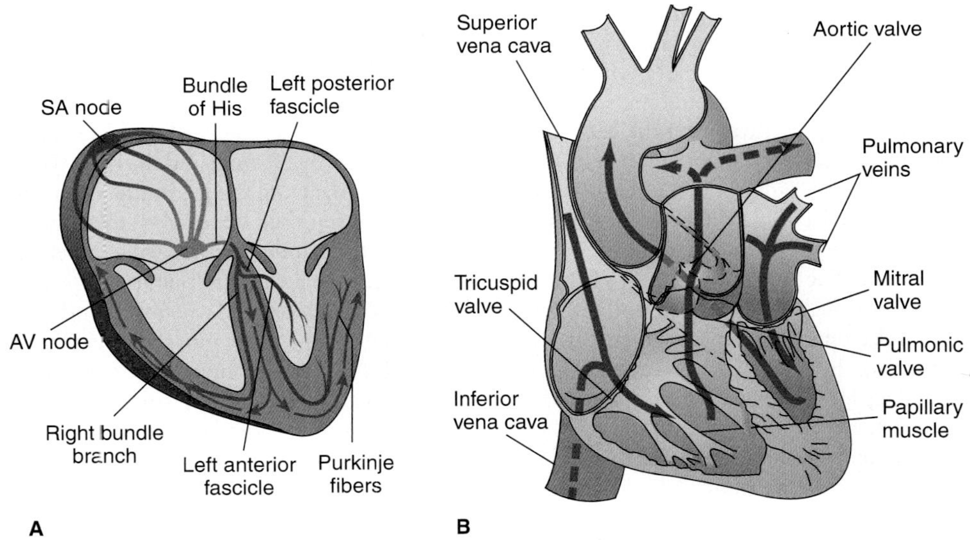

Figure 29-1. Cardiac conduction and circulation. The heart's electrical circuitry (**A**) has a profound effect on efficient blood flow to the tissues. An electrical impulse from the sinoatrial (SA) node travels over the atrial tracks to produce atrial contraction. The impulse slows slightly as it nears the ventricles at the atrioventricular (AV) node (the AV junction). After passing through the bundle of His, the impulse descends along the left and right bundle branches to the Purkinje fibers, stimulating ventricular contraction and proceeding on to the SA node to continue the cycle. The efficiency of the conduction system has a major influence on cardiac rhythm and output reflected by blood flow (**B**) and tissue perfusion. Drugs that affect cardiac output and rhythm work on the heart's electrical system or the mechanisms that promote efficient contraction and pumping.

cell, and that the charge is negative on the inside the cell, relative to the outside the cell. As sodium moves into the cell **depolarization** occurs. This means that there is a change in the transmembrane potential from a negative value toward 0 millivolts. Depolarization occurs rapidly and is called phase 0 of the action potential. During this rapid depolarization, the sodium channels open quickly for only a very short time. While these "fast channels" are open, sodium rushes into the cell. The influx of sodium ions into the cell increases the transmembrane potential to about +30 (meaning that the charge is now positive inside the cell relative to outside the cell). As soon as this positive charge is achieved, the voltage-regulated sodium channels close, and the cell begins to return to a negative state. This movement of the transmembrane potential away from a positive value and toward the negative resting potential is called **repolarization.** The initial downward movement toward zero is phase 1 of the action potential. As the charge reaches 0 millivolts, a plateau occurs. This plateau is what differentiates the action potential of cardiac muscle from the action potential of skeletal muscle. In this plateau phase, called phase 2, the calcium channels open slowly. These "slow channels" allow calcium ions to enter the cell. The positively charged calcium channels close, potassium channels open, and potassium again moves into the cell. The cell then begins a rapid acceleration of repolarization. This is phase 3 of the action potential. When full polarization is achieved once more, the cell is in phase 4 of the action potential and will remain there until stimulated again to depolarize. In other words, the cycle will start over again (Fig. 29-3).

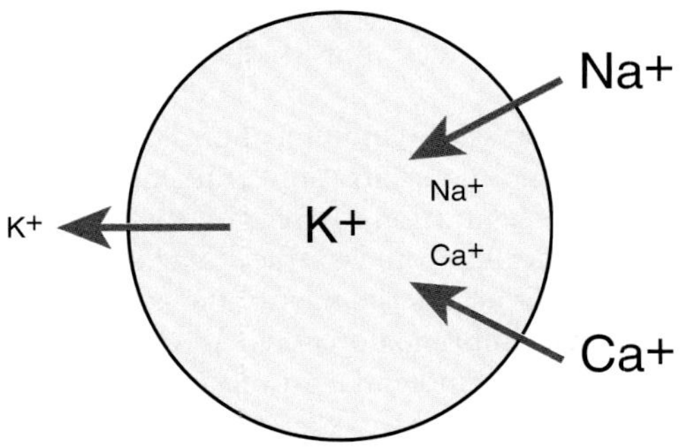

Figure 29-2. Intracellular and extracellular ions. Potassium is the predominant intracellular ion. It will move to the outside of the cell, following its concentration gradient. Sodium and calcium are predominantly extracellular ions; they will move into the cell.

After the cell depolarizes, and until it restores its normal electrical charge, it cannot be stimulated to fire again. This is termed the **refractory period.** Initially after depolarization, the cell cannot be stimulated to fire, no matter how great the stimulus. This is the absolute refractory period. As repolarization continues, the cell eventually becomes able to respond even though it is not at the resting state. However, the intensity of the stimulus needed to depolarize the cell is greater than when the cell is in the resting state. This ability to respond, but only to a larger than normal stimulus, is termed the relative refractory period.

Calcium is required for contraction of the heart. In contracting cells of the heart, calcium links excitation (from

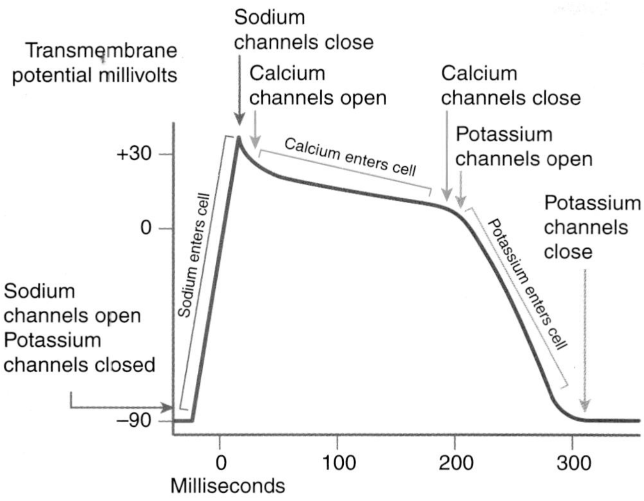

Figure 29-3. Movement of electrolytes during the action potential. As sodium enters the cell, rapid depolarization occurs. Once sodium channels close, the process of repolarization slowly begins. When calcium enters the cell, a plateau occurs. When the calcium channels close and potassium channels open, rapid repolarization occurs.

polarization) to contraction. The contraction of cardiac and vascular smooth muscle tissues is dependent on the movement of extracellular calcium into these cells. The influx of calcium, however, is approximately 20% of the calcium needed to initiate a contraction. The calcium that enters the cell stimulates the release of calcium that is stored inside the sarcoplasmic reticulum. This process is called calcium-induced calcium release. This process occurs during the plateau phase of the action potential. This additional release of calcium is what actually induces a contraction. Contraction will occur as long as calcium and energy are present.

The plateau phase is unique to the cardiac muscle. In contrast, repolarization of skeletal muscle occurs rapidly after depolarization. This allows the muscle to be stimulated to contract again almost immediately. Tetany, or constant contractions, may occur in skeletal muscles. This process would be life threatening if it occurred in the heart because no effective contractions would be present. Thus, this plateau phase can be considered a protective mechanism of the heart muscles to promote effective contractions (Fig. 29-4).

Imbalances of the electrolytes involved in the action potential, either greater than or less than normal serum levels, may produce changes in the action potential and cause various cardiac arrhythmias. Contractility of the heart is also affected by the concentration of catecholamines in the heart muscle—the more catecholamines, the greater the rate of contraction and the greater the force of contraction will be.

PATHOPHYSIOLOGY

Arrhythmias, also called dysrhythmias, are a disturbance in the electrical activity of the heart. Some arrhythmias are insignificant and do not create any problems for the patient. Others disrupt the function of the heart, increase the oxygen demand of the heart, and interfere with cardiac output. Some are considered life threatening and lethal.

Changes in the ionic currents through ion channels of the myocardial cell membrane are the main cause of cardiac arrhythmia (Borchard & Hafner, 2000). The ions are sodium, potassium, and calcium. These ionic changes allow arrhythmias to develop in one of three ways: through a disorder with impulse formation (the automaticity of the heart), through a disorder of the impulse conduction system, or through a combination of both. When there is a disorder of impulse formation the rate of SA nodal discharges is altered, allowing changes in the **automaticity** (ability to generate an impulse spontaneously) of the heart. Decreased automaticity results in sinus bradycardia; increased automaticity results in sinus tachycardia. These changes may be the result of drug toxicity, such as from digoxin, or from excessive sympathetic activity. Eliminating the contributing factor controls the arrhythmia. A different problem with automaticity occurs when the SA nodal rate decreases excessively and other excitable heart tissue reaches the threshold potential earlier than the SA node, thus generating an impulse. These abnormal sites of impulse formation are **ectopic foci**. These ectopic pacemakers may be due to hypokalemia, myocardial ischemia, emotional stress, or hypoxia. Ectopic foci may arise in atrial, nodal, Purkinje, or ventricular muscle.

Disorders of impulse conduction may be due to an alteration in the rate of impulse conduction or the pathway of conduction. When conduction of the impulses through the AV node is delayed, heart block occurs.

Reentry phenomenon is a more common source of alterations of impulse formation. Electrical impulses normally travel along a Purkinje fiber and divide at the small branch points in the fiber. When they meet each other in the connecting branch, they normally extinguish each other. However, where there is a temporary block in one of the branches because of an alteration in nerve impulse conduction, the impulse cannot continue to travel in its normal forward path, canceling itself out in the common branch. Instead, the impulse is carried through the unopposed side and reenters the branch from the opposite direction. **Reentry** or the **re-entry phenomenon** causes repetitive cardiac stimulation, firing, and arrhythmias (Fig. 29-5).

Arrhythmias can occur in the atria or in the ventricles. **Atrial flutter** is an arrhythmia originating in the atria; it has rapid atrial beating (approximately 300 times per minute) but a slower, usually regular, ventricular beating. **Atrial fibrillation** is an arrhythmia that is due to rapid, irregular discharges from multiple atrial ectopic foci. It results in a quivering of the atria without any true diastole occurring. Impulses are transmitted irregularly through the AV node, producing an irregular ventricular response, which is often rapid. Atrial fibrillation is the most commonly seen arrhythmia in clinical practice. Its incidence is increasing and it produces a great deal of morbidity and some mortality, although it is not directly life threatening. In the past, the goal of atrial fibrillation treatment was to slow the rate but not correct the rhythm. However, there are now compelling arguments that patients with atrial fibrillation should be converted and maintained in sinus rhythm. Animal studies have shown that an adverse electrical and structural remodeling of the atrium occurs with atrial fibrillation over time. These changes actually predispose the atria to perpetrate the arrhythmia—"atrial fibrillation begets atrial

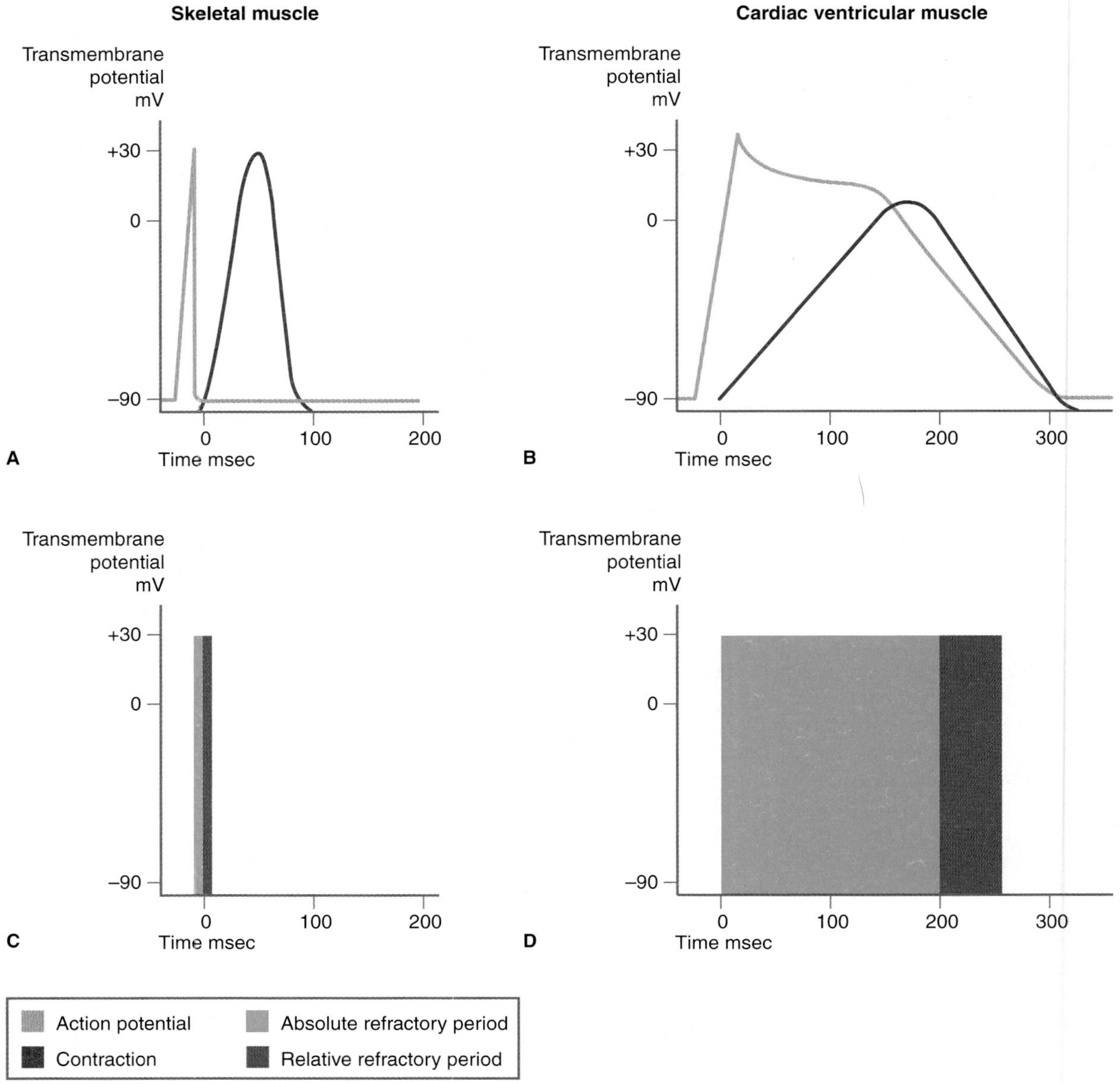

Figure 29-4. Comparisons of action potential, contraction, and refractory periods in skeletal and cardiac muscle.

fibrillation." Sustained sinus rhythm in a patient with atrial fibrillation leads to an increase in left ventricular ejection fraction, a decrease in left atrial size, an increase in maximal exercise capacity, and possibly an increase in the patient's quality of life (Singh, Mody, Lopez, & Sarma, 1999). Exactly which drug is best at maintaining sinus rhythm while causing the lowest adverse effects is not known at this time.

Ventricular tachycardia is rapid ventricular beating (greater than 100 beats per minute; usually 150–200 beats per minute) due to a ventricular ectopic foci. **Ventricular fibrillation** is a quivering of the ventricle without any systolic beat. If not terminated rapidly with defibrillation, brain damage will occur because the brain is not receiving oxygen. Ventricular tachycardia and ventricular fibrillation are serious and potentially life-threatening arrhythmias. They may occur after an acute myocardial infarction. These arrhythmias must be corrected within a relatively short timeframe or the patient is likely to die. This is because these contraction patterns do not allow the ventricle to fill appropriately, and when the contraction occurs, little blood is pushed out into the general circulation. Cardiac output therefore drops dramatically and blood pressure falls. After the patient has been converted to normal rhythm, there may be a tendency later to revert to ventricular tachycardia or ventricular fibrillation later. Patients who are deemed most at risk for this may be placed on long-term drug therapy.

DRUGS AND OTHER THERAPIES TO TREAT ARRHYTHMIAS

Drug therapy has been the mainstay for treating arrhythmias. As a more precise understanding of the reentrant and focal nature of many tachyarrhythmias has been achieved

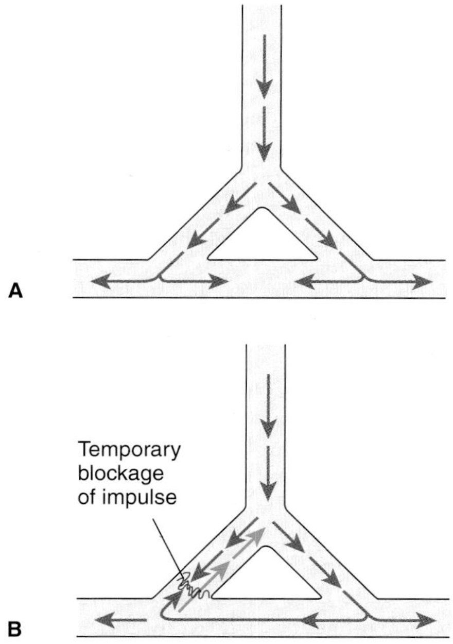

Figure 29-5. Reentry phenomenon. In normal cardiac conduction (**A**), electrical impulses cancel each other out. In reentry phenomenon, conduction is altered by a temporarily blocked impulse (**B**), allowing the impulse coming from the other direction to recycle and stimulate the Purkinje fibers to contract again. The result is a disturbance in cardiac rhythm. Antiarrhythmic drugs are used to treat these disturbances.

in recent years, it has become possible to prevent the recurrence of some arrhythmias with the use of implantable cardioverter defibrillators. Thus, technology has resulted in an extremely high rate of complete cure in many supraventricular arrhythmias and in some forms of ventricular arrhythmias, especially reentry arrhythmias. However, technology has not replaced the need for drug therapy. For example, atrial fibrillation is one type of arrhythmia that has not been responsive to correction from an implantable cardioverter defibrillator. Drug therapy remains the sole source of therapy for this arrhythmia. However, many clinicians and researchers believe that drug therapy and implantable cardioverter defibrillators should be viewed as complementary. (Singh, 1999a). Thus, concomitant use of drug therapy with implantable cardioverter defibrillators is often the rule. The question that is still being researched is which agent or agents are most effective when combined with implantable cardioverter defibrillators?

Antiarrhythmics are agents used to prevent, suppress, or treat a disturbance in cardiac rhythm. The primary outcome is decreased automaticity, decreased speed of conduction, and decreased reentry. Clinical trials are providing new information as to the effectiveness of different drugs in treating various arrhythmias. Selection of an antiarrhythmic drug is based on outcomes from these clinical trials, not solely on the electrophysiologic changes related to the drug class. One problem with all antiarrhythmics is that, due to their ability to modify the rhythm of the heart, they can cause a new arrhythmia or exacerbate the arrhythmia that they are treating. This adverse effect is termed **proarrhythmia.**

Many different drugs are used to treat arrhythmias. When antiarrhythmic drugs were developed, a system of classification was sought in an attempt to organize the complex information into a conceptually meaningful fashion. The classification system developed was fairly comprehensive, and was grouped by the drugs' actions (i.e., not the drugs, per se). Class I antiarrhythmic drugs block sodium channels. Several subtypes of sodium channels have been discovered, which depend on the kinetics of their sodium-channel properties (very fast, very slow, and intermediate.) Class IB antiarrhythmic agents are very fast; Class IC antiarrhythmic agents are very slow; and Class IA antiarrhythmic agents are intermediate. Class IA antiarrhythmic agents also are known to suppress sodium channel activity in all cardiac tissues, whereas Class IB antiarrhythmic agents suppress sodium channel action only in diseased or depolarized tissue.

Class II antiarrhythmic drugs block adrenergic receptors, producing antisympathetic properties. This slows the heart rate, lengthens the time needed for conduction, and increases the force of contraction. The effect seen in Class II antiarrhythmic drugs is depression of phase 4 of depolarization. Class III antiarrhythmic drugs lengthen the action potential duration. This prolongs phase 3 of repolarization. Class IV antiarrhythmic drugs block calcium channels. This depresses phase 4 of depolarization and lengthens phases 1 and 2 of repolarization (Fig. 29-6).

Although this classification system is widely used, it has significant limitations. Some drugs have characteristics of more than one class; other drugs, which are used in specific types of arrhythmias (such as digoxin and adenosine) do not fit within any of the classes within the system. Despite these limitations, the antiarrhythmics discussed in this

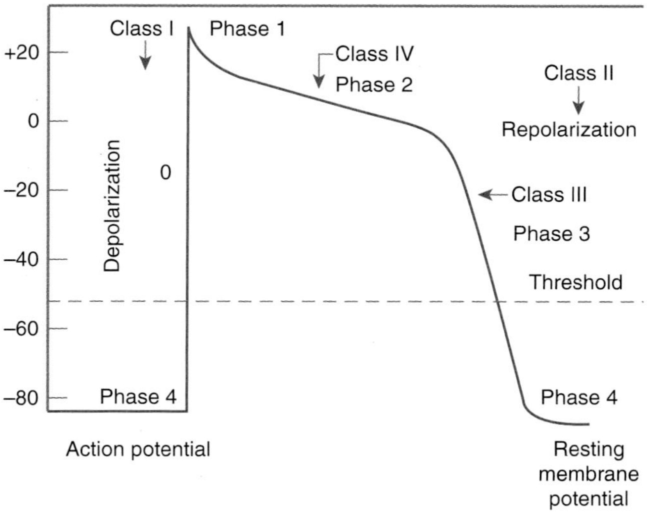

Figure 29-6. Action potential and antiarrhythmic drugs. The change in the charge of the myocardial cell that occurs when sodium (Na+) and calcium (Ca++) flow into the cell and potassium (K+) flows out is called the action potential. Different antiarrhythmic drugs act at different phases of polarization and repolarization. Class I drugs (quinidine) act during depolarization, class II drugs (propranolol) act during the resting period of repolarization, class III drugs (bretylium) act during rapid repolarization, and class IV drugs (verapamil) act during early repolarization.

chapter are presented in the traditional groupings of Class I, II, III, and IV.

The major goals of antiarrhythmic therapy are to alleviate symptoms (e.g., palpitations, presyncope, or syncope), improve quality of life, and prolong survival in patients with cardiac arrhythmias. The relief of symptoms in most patients can be achieved either by slowing the rate of the arrhythmia, or by preventing its recurrence. However, relief of the arrhythmia is not always associated with decreases in mortality. This was learned during the Cardiac Arrhythmia Suppression Trial (CAST) (1989), which was a study designed to evaluate the effects of individually titrated doses of encainide and flecainide (compared with placebo) on mortality in patients who had had myocardial infarction (MI) with frequent premature ventricular complexes. Although these drugs were found to markedly suppress the premature ventricular contractions, they were associated with increased mortality rates. Conversely, some drugs have a modest effect on suppressing arrhythmias (e.g., beta blockers) but have been shown to have a consistent and significant reduction in sudden death as well as in total mortality in many subsets of patients with heart disease. The reduction of mortality among patients with arrhythmias is evidently drug specific and is not mediated through suppression of the arrhythmia. Although it is important to suppress the arrhythmia to relieve symptoms, the selection of drug therapy should be such that mortality is not increased in the process (Singh, 1999b).

CLASS I ANTIARRHYTHMICS

Class I antiarrhythmics are local anesthetics or membrane-stabilizing agents that depress phase 0 in depolarization. The drugs in subgroups of A, B, and C are not interchangeable because they have different pharmacotherapeutics. Class IA antiarrhythmics include quinidine (Quinora, Quinidex Extentabs, Quinaglute Dura Tabs, Quinalan, quinidine sulfate, quinidine gluconate, Cardioquin), procainamide (Procan SR), disopyramide (Norpace), and moricizine (Ethmozine). Drugs similar to quinidine are the Class IB drugs lidocaine (Xylocaine), tocainide (Tonocard), mexiletine (Mexitil), and phenytoin (Dilantin) and the Class IC drugs flecainide (Tambocor) and propafenone (Rythmol). The prototype Class IA antiarrhythmic is quinidine.

NURSING MANAGEMENT OF THE PATIENT RECEIVING QUINIDINE

Core Drug Knowledge

Pharmacotherapeutics

Quinidine is used primarily to treat atrial arrhythmias, including premature atrial, AV junctional, paroxysmal atrial (supraventricular) tachycardia, paroxysmal AV junctional rhythm, atrial flutter, paroxysmal and chronic atrial fibrillation, and established atrial fibrillation when drug therapy is appropriate. It also is used as maintenance therapy after electrical conversion of atrial fibrillation or flutter. Other uses of quinidine include treating premature ventricular contractions, and paroxysmal ventricular tachycardia not associated with complete heart block. A noncardiac use of quinidine (quinidine gluconate only) is in treating life-threatening *Plasmodium falciparum* malaria. Normally given orally, quinidine may be given parenterally when oral therapy is not possible or when more rapid therapeutic effects are required (Table 29-1).

Pharmacokinetics

Quinidine is rapidly absorbed from the gastrointestinal (GI) tract. The concentration of quinidine varies among the different quinidine salts. Quinidine gluconate contains 62% active quinidine, whereas quinidine polygalacturonate contains 80% active quinidine and quinidine sulfate contains 83% active quinidine. Quinidine distributes to all body tissues except the brain. It is fairly highly protein bound at 80% to 90% and is metabolized by the liver and excreted unchanged by the kidneys. The influence of renal dysfunction on the disposition of quinidine is controversial; volume of distribution and renal clearance may be reduced. Acid urine promotes elimination of quinidine. Patients with cirrhosis may have a prolonged half-life and an increased volume of distribution. In congestive heart failure (CHF), total clearance and volume of distribution are decreased. In elderly patients, elimination half-life may be increased.

There appears to be some presystemic metabolism in the intestinal tract that occurs with quinidine. Normal subjects, in research studies, who were fed a high salt diet were shown to have a decreased bioavailability of quinidine. The locus of this effect appears to be at the intestinal level, not hepatic (Roden, 1999). The significance of these findings is still being explored.

Pharmacodynamics

Quinidine depresses myocardial excitability, conduction velocity, and contractility. The effective refractory period is prolonged, increasing conduction time. Reentry phenomenon is therefore prevented. Quinidine also exerts an indirect anticholinergic effect; it decreases vagal tone and may promote conduction in the AV junction.

It is important to examine the relationship of Class I antiarrhythmics to mortality. In patients without structural heart disease, the use of Class I drugs rarely causes proarrhythmia serious enough to be life threatening. However, in studies of patients with ventricular tachycardia and ventricular fibrillation, there is no decisive evidence from any controlled study demonstrating that Class I antiarrhythmics have the potential for prolonging survival for patients at high risk of dying suddenly. In fact, data from meta-analysis of several studies show that most, if not all, Class I antiarrhythmics are inclined to increase mortality (Singh, 1999b). Thus, drugs that prolong the action potential only (Class I) are not the answer for decreasing mortality in patients with arrhythmias and structural heart disease. Class I agents are still widely used to decrease the number of shocks that pa-

TABLE 29-1 Summary of Selected Class I Antiarrhythmics

Drug (Trade) Name	Selected Indications	Route and Dosage Range	Pharmacokinetics
quinidine (Quinaglute Dura-Tabs; *Canadian:* Quinate)	Premature atrial and ventricular contractions	*Adult:* PO, 200–300 mg three or four times daily *Child:* PO, 30 mg/kg/24 h or 900 mg/m^2/24 h in five divided doses	*Onset:* PO, 1–3 h; IM; 30–90 min; IV, rapid *Duration:* 6–8 h $t_{1/2}$: 6–7 h
	Paroxysmal supraventricular tachycardias	*Adult:* PO, 400–600 mg every 2 or 3 h until the paroxysm is terminated, administer after digitalization, dosage individualized *Child:* PO, 30 mg/kg/24 h or 900 mg/m^2/24 h in five divided doses	
	Atrial flutter	*Adult:* After digitalization dosage is individualized	
procainamide (Procan SR; *Canadian:* Apo-Procainamide)	Arrhythmia	*Adult:* PO, initially 50 mg/kg/d in divided doses every 3 h; PO maintenance 50 mg/kg/d in divided doses q6h; IV, loading (initial), 1 mL/min of 20 mg/mL solution or 100 mg every 5 min direct IV, up to 1 g total; maintenance 1–3 mL/min of 2 mg/mL solution *Child:* PO, 15–50 mg/kg/d divided every 3–6 h; max of 4 g/d; IV, initial 3–6 mg/kg/dose over 5 min; maintenance, 20–80 μg/kg/min continuous infusion; maximum, 100 mg/dose or 2 g/d	*Onset:* PO, 30 min; IM, 10–30 min; IV, immediate *Duration:* 3–4 h $t_{1/2}$: 2.5–4.7 h
lidocaine (Xylocaine HCl IV for cardiac arrhythmias)	Arrhythmia	*Adult:* Initial IV bolus 50–100 mg at rate of 25–50 mg/min; one-third to one-half the initial dose may be given after 5 min; do not exceed 200–300 mg in 1 h. Continuous infusion 20–50 mg/kg/min *Child:* AHA recommends bolus of 1 mg/kg IV, followed by 30 μg/kg per min w/caution	*Onset:* IM, 5–10 min; IV, immediate *Duration:* IM; 2 h; IV, 10–20 min $t_{1/2}$: 10 min, then 1.5–3 h
flecainide (Tambocor)	PSVT and PAF	*Adult:* Starting dose of 50 mg every 12 h; increase in 50-mg increments twice a day every fourth day until efficacy is achieved. Max dose is 300 mg per day. *Child:* Not recommended	*Onset:* 30–60 min *Duration:* 24 h $t_{1/2}$: 20 h
	Sustained ventricular tachycardia	*Adult:* 100 mg every 12 h; increase in 50-mg increments twice a day every fourth day until efficacy is achieved. Max dose is 400 mg per day. *Child:* Not recommended.	

PSVT = paroxysmal supraventricular tachycardia; PAF = paroxysmal atrial flutter.

tients with implantable cardioversion defibrillators receive. The efficacy for this use is unknown.

Contraindications and Precautions

Quinidine is contraindicated in the presence of hypersensitivity or a history of idiosyncratic reaction to quinidine or other cinchona derivatives. Hypersensitivity and idiosyncratic reaction are manifested by thrombocytopenia, skin eruption, or fever. Quinidine also is contraindicated in patients with the following conditions or findings:

- Myasthenia gravis
- A history of thrombocytopenic purpura associated with quinidine administration
- Digitalis intoxication manifested by arrhythmias or AV conduction disorders
- Complete heart block
- Left bundle branch block or other severe intraventricular conduction defects exhibiting marked QRS widening or bizarre electrocardiographic (ECG) complexes
- Complete AV block with an AV nodal or idioventricular pacemaker
- Aberrant ectopic impulses and abnormal rhythms due to escape mechanisms
- Drug-induced torsades de pointes (ventricular tachycardia associated with QT prolongation)
- Long QT syndrome

Quinidine should be used with extreme caution in patients with incomplete AV block because complete block may develop. Caution also must be used in digitalis toxicity because unpredictable arrhythmias may result.

Quinidine is used cautiously in patients with partial bundle branch block, severe CHF, and hypotension because quinidine will further depress myocardial contractility and arterial pressure. Caution must also be used when giving quinidine to patients with renal, hepatic, or cardiac insufficiency because toxicity is more likely to occur.

Quinidine crosses the placenta and achieves fetal serum levels similar to maternal levels. It is a pregnancy category C drug, indicating that safety has not been established. Quinidine also is excreted in breast milk. Milk:serum ratios have been found to be 0.71. Although safe use during breast-feeding has not been established clearly, the American Academy of Pediatrics considers the drug compatible with breast-feeding. Safety and efficacy in children have not been established.

Adverse Effects

The most common adverse effects involve the GI system and include nausea, vomiting, abdominal pain, diarrhea, and anorexia. These may occur after a fever. Arrhythmias also occur commonly, but most are not life threatening. Another common adverse effect is a syndrome of cinchonism, related to the tree bark source of quinidine, which may occur even after a single dose of quinidine. The symptoms of cinchonism include tinnitus, hearing loss, headache, nausea, dizziness, vertigo, light-headedness, and disturbed vision.

The most serious adverse effect is cardiotoxicity, which is manifested by increased PR and QT intervals, 50% widening of the QRS complex, ventricular tachyarrhythmias (including ventricular tachycardia, fibrillation, and torsades de pointes), frequent ventricular ectopic beats, or tachycardia. If signs of cardiotoxicity are present, quinidine should be discontinued at once, *and* the ECG of the patient should be monitored closely.

Other cardiovascular (CV) adverse effects include cardiac asystole, arterial embolism, ventricular extrasystole occurring at the rate of one or more for every six normal beats, complete AV block, ventricular flutter, and hypotension. Although large oral doses cause peripheral vasodilation that decreases blood pressure, the most serious hypotension is more likely to occur when quinidine is given IV.

Hepatic toxicity can occur, including granulomatous hepatitis. This reaction is believed to be the result of quinidine hypersensitivity. Fever occurs, and liver enzymes are elevated. Other hypersensitivity reactions, which are rare but may occur, are angioedema, acute asthma, vascular collapse, respiratory arrest, and purpura vasculitis. Other adverse effects that may occur include:

- Hematologic: acute hemolytic anemia, hypoprothrombinemia, thrombocytopenia, thrombocytopenic purpura, agranulocytosis, leukocytosis, neutropenia, and shift to left in white blood cell differentials
- Central nervous system (CNS): headache, fever, vertigo, apprehension, excitement, confusion, delirium, syncope, dementia, ataxia, and depression
- Ophthalmic: mydriasis and blurred vision, disturbed color perception, reduced vision field, photophobia, diplopia, night blindness, and optic neuritis
- Dermatologic: rash, urticaria, cutaneous flushing with intense pruritus, photosensitivity, exfoliative eruptions, psoriasis, and abnormalities of pigmentation
- Development of lupus erythematosus, which resolves after drug therapy stops

Quinidine overdosage may be associated with depressed mental function even if the patient is hemodynamically stable. In addition, CNS symptoms (e.g., lethargy, confusion, coma, respiratory depression or arrest, seizures, headache, paresthesia, and vertigo) may occur after the onset of CV toxicity. GI effects include vomiting, abdominal pain, diarrhea, and nausea. The CV effects are tachyarrhythmias, depressed automaticity and conduction, hypotension, syncope, and heart failure.

Some of the adverse effects of quinidine may be similar to reasons the drug is prescribed. For this reason, it is important to monitor blood levels to determine whether the drug is in therapeutic range or is elevated excessively.

Drug Interactions

Quinidine interacts with many other antiarrhythmic and cardiac drugs. It also interacts with anticoagulants and several drugs that affect the CNS (Table 29-2).

Assessment of Relevant Core Patient Variables

Health Status

Health care providers must determine if the patient has one of the types of atrial arrhythmias that are indications for therapy. It also is important to determine whether the patient has any of the following contraindications to quinidine therapy:

- Hypersensitivity to quinidine
- Myasthenia gravis
- A history of thrombocytopenic purpura from quinidine use
- Arrhythmias or AV conduction disorders from digitalis toxicity
- Complete heart block
- Left bundle branch block or other severe intraventricular conduction defects that exhibit marked widening of QRS complex
- Complete AV block with an AV nodal or idioventricular pacemaker
- Aberrant ectopic impulses and arrhythmias due to escape mechanisms
- A history of drug-induced torsades de pointes
- A history of long QT syndrome

The patient with renal, hepatic, or cardiac insufficiency is at greater risk of toxicity. If the patient has cirrhosis, the elimination half-life may be prolonged and the volume of distribution increased. This increases the

TABLE 29-2 Agents That Interact With Quinidine

Interactants	Effect and Significance	Nursing Management
antacids	Increases urinary pH affecting the rate of drug elimination	Stagger administration times of quinidine and antacids by at least 2 h.
barbiturates	May reduce serum level and half-life of quinidine	Monitor therapeutic effect of quinidine, and consult with prescriber about dosage adjustment.
cholinergic drugs	May result in failure to terminate paroxysmal supraventricular tachycardia (PSVT)	Use cautiously, if at all, in patients with myasthenia gravis.
cimetidine	Increased serum levels and risk of quinidine toxicity	Monitor serum levels of quinidine. Assess for signs of adverse effects.
hydantoins, nifedipine, rifampin, sucralfate, disopyramide	Decreased levels and effectiveness of quinidine	Monitor drug effectiveness.
verapamil	May cause hypotension, bradycardia, atrioventricular block, pulmonary edema	Monitor electrocardiogram. Check quinidine serum levels.
anticholinergics	Concurrent use may cause additive vagolytic effect	Consistently monitor and check quinidine serum levels.
anticoagulants	Potentiation of anticoagulation; hemorrhage possible	Assess coagulation times and patient for signs of bleeding.
beta blockers (metoprolol, propranolol)	Effects of metoprolol or propranolol may be increased in extensive metabolizers	Assess for adverse effects.
procainamide	Increased pharmacologic effects of procainamide and elevated NAPA (a major metabolite of procainamide) plasma levels	Watch for signs of toxicity.
succinylcholine	Prolonged neuromuscular blockade	Monitor drug levels, and attempt to stagger doses.
tricyclic antidepressants (TCA)	TCA clearance possibly reduced, thereby increasing effects	Same as above.

risk for adverse effects. If the patient has CHF, total clearance and volume of distribution will be decreased. This may result in increased risk for adverse effects or less significant therapeutic effects than expected.

The nurse needs to determine if the patient is on or has orders for cholinergic drugs. When these drugs are administered with quinidine, paroxysmal supraventricular tachycardia (SVT) may not be stopped. In addition, the nurse needs to assess which other drugs the patient is receiving to determine whether a drug interaction is likely to occur.

The patient's potassium level must be reviewed because potassium enhances the effect of quinidine, and hypokalemia will reduce the effectiveness. In addition, the risk for quinidine-induced torsades de pointes is increased with hypokalemia.

Life Span and Gender

The assessment should focus on whether the patient is pregnant or breast-feeding because safety and efficacy have not been established in these circumstances. Likewise, quinidine has not been proven safe or effective for children. If the patient is elderly, elimination half-life may be increased for quinidine.

Lifestyle, Diet, and Habits

The nurse assesses the patient's normal dietary patterns for adequate potassium intake, because hypokalemia decreases effectiveness and increases the risk of some adverse effects.

Environment

The nurse should be aware of the setting in which quinidine may be administered. Oral quinidine may be taken at home, in an acute care setting, or in a long-term care facility. Parenteral quinidine is given in a hospital where the patient can be closely observed and ECG and blood pressure can be monitored.

Nursing Diagnoses and Outcomes

- Imbalanced Nutrition, Less than Body Requirements related to nausea, vomiting, abdominal pain, anorexia, and diarrhea secondary to adverse effects of drug therapy
  Desired outcome: Patient will not develop adverse effects significant enough to alter nutrition.
- Decreased Cardiac Output related to cardiac changes secondary to adverse effects of drug therapy
  Desired outcome: Patient will not develop deleterious cardiac changes to alter cardiac output.
- Risk for Injury, such as hepatic toxicity, related to adverse effects of drug therapy
  Desired outcome: Patient will not incur hepatic toxicity while on drug therapy.

Planning and Intervention

Maximizing Therapeutic Effects

To maximize the therapeutic effects of quinidine, the nurse should adjust the dose to achieve a serum plasma drug concentration between 2 and 6 mg/mL. Additionally, the nurse needs to monitor the serum potassium level and maintain it in a normal range to promote action of quinidine.

Minimizing Adverse Effects

The nurse should administer oral quinidine with food to prevent GI upset and thus avoid altered nutrition. The nurse should give a test dose of a single 200-mg tablet or 200 mg IM to determine whether the patient has an idiosyncratic reaction to quinidine. It is important to connect the patient to a cardiac monitor and monitor rhythm continuously (when given IV) or obtain frequent ECGs (when quinidine is given orally).

The nurse should stop the quinidine and notify the health care provider if any of the following occurs:

- Increase exceeding 25% in duration of QRS complex
- Disappearance of P waves
- Restoration of sinus rhythm
- Decrease in heart rate to 120 beats/minute or less on the ECG

When using an IV infusion pump, it is important to dilute 800 mg of quinidine with 50 mL of D_5W and infuse slowly at 1 mL/min. The nurse should monitor serum quinidine levels to detect excessively high values and frequently monitor arterial blood pressure (when given IV). If blood pressure falls significantly, therapy should be discontinued and the health care provider notified.

The nurse should monitor blood counts and liver and kidney function tests. Discontinue if blood dyscrasias develop or if liver or renal function tests disclose elevated values.

Treatment of a drug overdose may include gastric lavage, emesis, or administration of activated charcoal. Other management includes symptomatic management of CNS and GI effects and checking ECG tracings, blood gases, serum electrolytes, and blood pressure. It also is important to institute measures to acidify the urine. Mechanical ventilation and other supportive measures may be needed. IV infusion of 1/6 molar sodium lactate may be used to reduce the cardiotoxic effects of quinidine.

Providing Patient and Family Education

- The nurse should explain the purpose of the drug and the potential adverse effects.
- It is important to explain the rationale for ECG monitoring and frequent blood testing, which is that these are methods used to detect early onset of adverse effects.
- The nurse should emphasize the importance of returning for follow-up tests.
- The nurse should teach patients not to chew oral, sustained-release tablets.
- It is a good idea to instruct patients to take oral doses with food to prevent GI upset.
- The nurse emphasizes the importance of notifying the health care provider or the nurse in the hospital if tinnitus, visual disturbances, dizziness, headache, nausea, skin rash, or breathing difficulty are experienced.

Ongoing Assessment and Evaluation

The patient's ECG will be monitored throughout therapy. Quinidine blood levels are checked to determine that they are therapeutic, not toxic. Periodically, liver enzymes, renal function, and complete blood counts also are monitored. Drug therapy is considered effective if the arrhythmia is converted and does not recur, and if the patient does not develop serious adverse effects from the drug. ■

DRUGS CLOSELY RELATED TO QUINIDINE: CLASS IB ANTIARRHYTHMICS

The Class IB drugs are similar to quinidine (Class IA) and Class IC drugs, because they depress phase 0 (although not as much). They also suppress automaticity. Like quinidine, these drugs also may cause arrhythmias in addition to treating them. Unlike quinidine, they are used primarily with ventricular arrhythmias, and they may shorten the action potential duration (see Table 29-1).

MEMORY CHIP

Quinidine

- Class I antiarrhythmic used in atrial arrhythmias, such as atrial flutter and fibrillation
- Decreases myocardial excitability, conduction velocity, and contractility
- Prevents re-entry phenomenon
- Exerts an indirect anticholinergic effect
- Significant contraindications: cardiac arrhythmias related to conduction abnormalities (complete heart block, left bundle branch block, complete atrioventricular block, long QT syndrome, and drug-induced torsades de points)
- Most common adverse effects: GI-related
- Most serious adverse effect: cardiotoxicity
- Maximizing therapeutic effects: adjust dose until reaching therapeutic range and maintain potassium at normal levels
- Minimizing adverse effects: monitor electrocardiogram and use an IV infusion pump if given IV
- Most significant patient education: take oral doses with food

Lidocaine

Lidocaine (Xylocaine) may be used with all acute ventricular arrhythmias that are related to cardiac surgery or acute myocardial infarction because these may be life threatening. In other strengths and routes, lidocaine also is used as a local and topical anesthetic. Lidocaine used to treat arrhythmias will, in therapeutic levels, weaken phase 4 diastolic depolarization, decrease the automaticity, and decrease or cause no change in the excitability and membrane responsiveness. Additionally, it decreases the action potential duration and the effective refractory period of Purkinje fibers and ventricular muscle. However, the ratio of the effective refractory period to the action potential duration is increased. The effective refractory period of the AV node may increase, decrease, or remain unchanged; atrial effective refractory period remains unchanged. Lidocaine raises the ventricular fibrillation threshold. This is why it is effective in treating ventricular fibrillation.

Clinical electrophysiological studies have demonstrated no change in sinus node recovery time, sinoatrial conduction time, and His- Purkinje fibers–conduction time. AV node conduction time is either unchanged or it may be shortened. Lidocaine does increase the electrical stimulation threshold of the ventricle during diastole. This allows for a longer diastole because the ventricle requires a longer period of time before it can be receptive to depolarization and contract again. This is helpful in treating ventricular arrhythmias. In therapeutic doses (serum levels of 1.5 to 6 μg/mL), lidocaine has no effect on the contractility of the heart, blood pressure, or the absolute refractory period.

Lidocaine is usually administered IV, because it is ineffective orally. Under certain circumstances it may be administered IM. Single IM doses are justified in the following exceptional circumstances: EGG equipment not available to verify diagnosis (but the potential benefits must outweigh the possible risk); and when the facilities for IV administration are not readily available. When given IM, higher and more rapid serum levels are achieved by injection into the deltoid muscle over the gluteus or vastus lateralis. Lidocaine is about 50% protein bound. Lidocaine is metabolized extensively in the liver into at least two active metabolites. These metabolites have both antiarrhythmic and convulsant (inducing convulsions) effects. Metabolism is impaired significantly by any condition that impairs liver function. Although renal elimination only processes about 10% of the dose given, it is highly involved in the excretion of the metabolites. Accumulation of one of the metabolites (known as GX) due to renal disease or impaired renal function contributes to lidocaine toxicity.

Lidocaine has a biphasic half-life. The half-life involved with the distribution phase is less than 10 minutes. This accounts for the short duration of action when an IV bolus is given. Due to the very short half-life, repeated boluses may be required to quickly achieve therapeutic level when a continuous IV infusion is required to maintain the therapeutic effects (see Table 29-1 for dosing). The elimination half-life is 1.5 to 2 hours. It may be 3 hours or more if the lidocaine infusion has lasted greater than 24 hours.

Lidocaine is a pregnancy category B drug. However, caution should be used because there are no adequate and well controlled studies in pregnant women. While safety and efficacy have not been established with children from clinical studies, the American Heart Association's Standards and Guidelines recommend using lidocaine when needed in children (see Table 29-1). Caution should be used, and lower doses are recommended, for patients who have CHF, reduced cardiac output, digitalis toxicity accompanied by AV block, hypovolemia and shock, in all forms of heart block, and when used in older adults.

Adverse effects of lidocaine are seen particularly in the CV and CNS systems. CV effects are related to serum levels, with the most severe cardiac depression coinciding with toxic levels of lidocaine. The most common CV effects are cardiac arrhythmias, and hypotension. Other effects include bradycardia, and CV collapse, which may lead to cardiac arrest. *CNS adverse* effects also are related to blood concentrations of lidocaine. The most common CNS effects are dizziness/light-headedness, fatigue, and drowsiness. These common, mild effects are seen with low blood levels of lidocaine and resolve rapidly. As blood levels of lidocaine rise, nervousness, confusion, mood changes, hallucinations, euphoria, tinnitus, blurred or double vision, and a sensation of heat, cold, or numbness may occur. In common health care jargon, these CNS effects are referred to as the "lidocaine crazies." With excessively high serum levels of lidocaine (greater than 6 μg/mL), toxicity is present and the patient develops seizures and loses consciousness.

It is very important to continually monitor the ECG of the patient receiving IV lidocaine. Emergency resuscitative equipment and drug therapy should be on hand in case the patient develops serious adverse effects. As soon as the patient is clinically stable, she or he should be switched to another antiarrhythmic that can be given orally.

Tocainimide

Tocainimide (Tonocard) is used to treat life-threatening ventricular arrhythmias. As a Class IB antiarrhythmic, it is similar to lidocaine, producing dose-dependent decreases in sodium and potassium conduction and thereby decreasing the excitability of the cardiac cells. Most patients who respond to lidocaine will respond to tocainimide. Failure to respond to lidocaine usually indicates that the patient will not respond to tocainimide either. The electrophysiologic effects of tocainimide are similar to those seen with lidocaine. Tocainimide does not prolong the QRS duration or QT intervals. Tocainimide slightly depresses the left ventricular function and left ventricular end diastolic pressure. Usually this produces no changes in the cardiac output. It does slightly, but significantly, increase the aortic and pulmonary arterial pressures. This is related most likely to increases in vascular resistance. Tocainimide has been used safely in patients with acute MI, post-MI, and with various degrees of CHF.

Tocainimide is given orally because it does not have the high metabolism of lidocaine. Bioavailability of tocainimide is nearly 100%; peak serum levels are reached in 0.5 to 2 hours after oral dosing. Protein binding is very low at 10% to 20%. It is inactivated by conjugation in the liver. About 40% of the drug is excreted in the urine unchanged.

It is important to use tocainimide cautiously in patients with known heart failure or minimal cardiac reserve, or when beginning or continuing antiarrhythmic therapy in the presence of signs of increasing depression of cardiac conductivity. Like all antiarrhythmics, tocainide can be proarrhythmic. The most common adverse effects are dizziness, vertigo, nausea, paresthesia, and tremor. These reactions are generally mild, transient, and dose related; they are reversible by reducing the dose, by taking the drug with food, or by discontinuing the therapy. The most serious adverse effect, although not common (less than 1% of patients) is the occurrence of blood dyscrasias (e.g., agranulocytosis, bone marrow depression, leukopenia, neutropenia, aplastic/hypoplastic anemia, and thrombocytopenia). These effects, which usually occur during the first 12 weeks of therapy, can be fatal in about one quarter of those patients who experience them. The nurse should monitor blood work weekly during this time period for signs of any of these effects. If any of these disorders are diagnosed, it is essential to discontinue the tocainide immediately. Blood work should return to normal within 1 month.

Fatalities also have occurred with patients who develop severe pulmonary disorders (e.g., pulmonary fibrosis, interstitial pneumonitis, fibrosing alveolitis, pulmonary edema, and pneumonia). The nurse should instruct patients to report immediately any pulmonary symptoms, such as shortness of breath on exertion, cough, or wheezing. Discontinue tocainimide if any of these disorders develop.

Other adverse effects that may occur include:

- CV: ventricular fibrillation, extension of acute MI, cardiogenic shock, angina, AV block, hypertension, increased QRS duration, pericarditis, prolonged QT interval, right bundle branch block, syncope, vasovagal episodes, cardiomegaly, sinus arrest, vasculitis, and orthostatic hypotension
- CNS: coma, convulsions/seizures, depression, psychosis, agitation, decreased mental acuity, dysarthria, impaired memory, increased stuttering, slurred speech, insomnia, sleep disturbances, local anesthesia, dream abnormalities, myasthenia gravis, and malaise
- Dermatologic: Stevens-Johnson syndrome, exfoliative dermatitis, erythema multiforme, urticaria, alopecia, pruritus, and pallor or flushed face
- GI: abdominal pain, constipation, stomatitis, dysphagia, dyspepsia, thirst, and dry mouth
- Hepatic: hepatitis and jaundice
- Respiratory: respiratory arrest and pulmonary edema/embolism

Mexiletine

Mexiletine (Mexitil) is another Class IB drug. It also is used in life-threatening ventricular arrhythmias and, like all antiarrhythmics, may produce arrhythmias. It only is administered orally. It has pharmacologic and electrophysiologic properties similar to those of lidocaine.

Phenytoin

Although treatment of arrhythmias is not a labeled use of phenytoin (Dilantin), it is used commonly in the treatment of digitalis-induced arrhythmias. It, like other Class IB drugs, depresses phase 0 slightly and may shorten the action potential. A full discussion of phenytoin and its use in treating seizures is in Chapter 20.

DRUGS CLOSELY RELATED TO P QUINIDINE: CLASS IC ANTIARRHYTHMICS

Class IC drugs are flecainide (Tombocor) and propafenone (Rythmol) (see Table 29-1). These drugs depress phase 0 considerably. In addition, they have a slight effect on repolarization and decrease conduction significantly. Flecainide is used in preventing paroxysmal atrial fibrillation or flutter and paroxysmal SVTs, including AV nodal reentry tachycardia and AV reentry tachycardia. It also can be used in preventing life-threatening ventricular arrhythmias. Propafenone is used in treating life-threatening ventricular arrhythmias. Unlabeled uses for propafenone include treatment of SVTs, including atrial fibrillation and flutter, and arrhythmias associated with Wolff-Parkinson-White syndrome. Both of these Class IC drugs are given orally; both, like quinidine and all antiarrhythmics, may induce arrhythmias.

In the National Heart, Lung, and Blood Institute's Cardiac Arrhythmia Suppression Trial, excessive mortality or nonfatal cardiac arrest rate was seen in patients treated with flecainide compared with those receiving placebo. These patients had non–life-threatening ventricular dysfunction and a history of MI more than 6 days but less than 2 years before the start of the study. The application of these findings to other patients, such as those without history of MI, or to other antiarrhythmics is unclear. However, based on this research it is recommended that the use of Class IC drugs be limited to patients with life-threatening arrhythmias, because the risks for patients with non-life-threatening arrhythmias are deemed too great (Epstein, Hallstrom, Rogers, Liebson, Seal, Anderson, et al., 1993). Even this limited recommendation for use has been recently called into question.

C CLASS II ANTIARRHYTHMICS

Antiarrhythmic class II drugs (beta blockers) depress phase 4 depolarization. The prototype class II drug is propranolol (Inderal). Other drugs in this class are acebutolol (Monitan) and esmolol (Brevibloc). It is important to keep in mind that only some of the beta blockers are approved for use as antiarrhythmics. What follows is a brief discussion of propranolol when it it is used solely as an antiarrhythmic. Propranolol is discussed in more depth in Chapter 14. Other uses of beta blockers relevant to CV function are found in Chapters 27, 28, and 30.

NURSING MANAGEMENT OF THE PATIENT RECEIVING P PROPRANOLOL

Propranolol is used for treating cardiac arrhythmias, specifically supraventricular, ventricular, and tachyarrhythmias secondary to digoxin toxicity. Propranolol also is used alone or in combination to treat hypertension. Other uses include treating angina, MI, and hypertrophic subaortic stenosis.

Propranolol blocks the beta-adrenergic receptor sites; thus, it is classified as a beta blocker. This blockage of the receptor sites occurs as the drug competes with beta-adrenergic agonists for available beta receptor sites. Propranolol blocks both the beta-1 sites, which are located chiefly in the cardiac muscle, and beta-2 receptors, which are located chiefly in the bronchial and vascular musculature.

Several mechanisms have been proposed by which propranolol achieves its effects on the CV system. One mechanism is that propranolol competitively blocks catecholamines at non-CNS adrenergic neuron sites, especially in the heart, thereby leading to decreased cardiac output. A second mechanism is a central effect that leads to reduced sympathetic outflow to the periphery. Third, because stimulation of beta receptors is responsible for the release of renin from the kidneys, beta blockade with propranolol prevents renin from being released. Total peripheral resistance initially increases slightly because of these mechanisms. However, it readjusts to the pretreatment level or lower with chronic use. Because the decrease in cardiac output is greater than the increase in peripheral resistance, blood pressure is lowered. Propranolol also has a membrane-stabilizing effect, like that of anesthetics, which depresses the cardiac action potential. This is what causes the antiarrhythmic response.

Propranolol is contraindicated in sinus bradycardia, greater than first-degree heart block, cardiogenic shock, CHF (unless secondary to a tachyarrhythmia treatable with beta blockers), overt cardiac failure, bronchial asthma or bronchospasm, severe chronic obstructive pulmonary disease, and hypersensitivity to beta blockers. For a full discussion of propranolol, refer to Chapter 14. ■

CLASS III ANTIARRHYTHMICS

Class III antiarrhythmics produce a prolongation of phase 3 (repolarization). The drugs in this class include amiodarone (Cordarone), sotalol, bretylium (bretylium tosylate, Bretylol), ibutilide (Corvert), and dofetilide (Tikosyn). The prototype Class III antiarrhythmic is amiodarone.

NURSING MANAGEMENT OF THE PATIENT RECEIVING P AMIODARONE

Core Drug Knowledge

Pharmacotherapeutics

Because of severe and potentially lethal adverse effects, amiodarone is only approved for use in life-threatening arrhythmias. Orally, amiodarone (Cordarone, Pacerone) is used in the treatment of only the following documented life-threatening recurrent ventricular arrhythmias that do not respond to documented adequate doses of other antiarrhythmics or when alternative agents are not tolerated:

- Recurrent ventricular fibrillation
- Recurrent, hemodynamically unstable ventricular tachycardia

If the patient is nonresponsive to other therapy, intravenous amiodarone is used in the initiation of treatment and as prophylaxis for frequently recurring ventricular fibrillation and hemodynamically unstable ventricular tachycardia. Intravenous amiodarone also can be used in patients who meet the requirements for oral amiodarone, but who cannot take oral medication.

As an unlabeled use, amiodarone may be helpful in the treatment of sustained or intermittent atrial fibrillation and intermittent supraventricular tachycardia. It also appears to be useful in treating symptomatic atrial flutter. Low doses (200 mg/day) may produce benefits in left ventricular ejection fraction, exercise tolerance, and ventricular arrhythmias in patients with CHF. Amiodarone is being studied currently as a drug that may have benefits in treating atrial fibrillation due to its multiple actions.

Pharmacokinetics

A modern view of the processes of pharmacokinetics is that they are established by the regulated activity of specific gene products (Roden, 1999). Thus, as genes vary among individuals, how the body processes the drug and the body's responses to drug therapy will also vary. This concept helps to explain the unusual pharmacokinetic and pharmacodynamic effects of amiodarone. At this time, very little is known about the molecular methods that produce these unusual effects, which include incomplete bioavailability, distribution to multiple tissue sites, extreme lipid solubility, biotransformation to an active metabolite, and extremely slow elimination of amiodarone and its metabolite.

With oral administration, amiodarone is absorbed slowly, and the absorption is highly variable. The bioavailability of a single dose of the drug (oral or IV) is about 50% of the dose given, although it can range from 35% to 65%. Some researchers suggest that the incomplete bioavailability is due to incomplete absorption related to amiodarone's high lipid solubility. This has ramifications for dosing when the patient is being switched from oral to IV (or vice versa). The patient may require a smaller IV dose than an oral dose.

Amiodarone is widely distributed throughout the body, with much variability. There is extensive distribution in some sites, such as adipose tissue and highly perfused organs (e.g., liver, lung, and spleen). Variability in distribution contributes to variability in response to drug therapy, which is exhibited by the patient. The drug is highly protein bound (96%). This high protein binding also complicates the distribution of amiodarone. Individual variability in protein levels may cause some of the variability of drug action. Free drug levels are difficult to measure in extensive protein binding. Because of its high lipid solubility, amiodarone and its metabolite are thought to concentrate in cell membranes especially of the liver, heart, and fat cells.

Research supports the idea that the slow distribution of amiodarone into tissue sites is an important component of the drug's unusual pharmacokinetic and pharmacodynamic activities.

Metabolism occurs in the liver, apparently by cytochrome P450 3A4, forming an active metabolite, diethanolamine (DEA). DEA accumulates in most tissues to an even greater extent than the parent, amiodarone. DEA has pharmacologic properties similar to amiodarone Like amiodarone, DEA is highly protein bound, although its distribution is concentrated in the heart.

The actual route of amiodarone elimination is not well understood. Amiodarone has a biphasic elimination with an initial one-half reduction of plasma levels after 2.5 to 107 days. A much slower terminal plasma elimination has a mean half-life of 53 days for amiodarone and 61 days for DEA. Thus, it takes almost a year for the drug to reach steady state with chronic oral administration. Because of this, a loading regimen of the drug is needed to achieve an initial pharmacologic effect. With prolonged administration, serum concentrations of amiodarone and DEA are similar. The main route of excretion is hepatic into the bile. Some enterohepatic recirculation may occur (Table 29-3).

Pharmacodynamics

Although amiodarone produces electrophysiologic changes characteristic of all four antiarrhythmic classes, it predominantly has Class III effects. There are two major properties of amiodarone: prolongation of the refractory period, and noncompetitive alpha- and beta-adrenergic inhibition. Amiodarone also modulates thyroid function (one molecule of amiodarone contains two iodine atoms, and amiodarone shares some structural similarities to thyroid hormones), phospholipid metabolism, and production of certain cytokine (extracellular factors that are important in controlling the inflammatory response). Which of these actions or combinations of actions is fundamental in creating its potent antiarrhythmic activity is not known (Kodama, Kamiya, & Toyama, 1999).

Like Class I antiarrhythmic drugs, amiodarone blocks the fast sodium channel. It may do this when the channel is in the inactivated state. Unlike Class I antiarrhythmic drugs, amiodarone also blocks potassium channels. These activities contribute to the slowing of conduction and increased refractory period. Amiodarone blocks multiple potassium channels, including inward and outward currents. Like Class II antiarrhythmic drugs, amiodarone has a noncompetitive antisympathetic action. Like Class IV antiarrhythmic drugs, it has a negative chronotropic effect (slowing heart rate) from blocking the slow calcium channel. All these actions (i.e., blocking sodium, potassium, and calcium channels, and inhibition of sympathetic action) have an effect on slowing conduction (negative dromotropic effect) at the SA node, and slowing conduction and increasing the refractory period at the AV node. Amiodarone does have some vasodilating effects, which decreases the oxygen needs of the heart.

The effect on sodium channels appears to be limited to acute dosing (by IV) and is not present in chronic dosing. The effect on calcium and potassium channels may be both acute and chronic. However, unlike oral dosing, IV dosing has little or no effect on the length of the sinus cycle, the refractoriness of the right atrium or

TABLE 29-3 Summary of Selected Class III Antiarrhythmics

Drug (Trade) Name	Selected Indications	Route and Dosage Range	Pharmacokinetics
amiodarone (Cordarone)	Ventricular fibrillation	*Adult:* PO, 800–1,600 mg/d in divided doses for 1–3 wk; reduce to 600–800 mg/d in divided doses for 1 mo *Child:* Not established	*Onset:* 2–3 q *Duration:* 6–8 h $t_{1/2}$: 2.5–10 d, then 40–55 d
sotalol (Betapace; *Canadian:* Sotacor)	Ventricular arrhythmias	*Adult:* PO, 80 mg bid; adjust gradually q2–3d; may require 240–320 mg/d	*Onset:* Varies *Duration and* $t_{1/2}$: 12 h
bretylium (Bretylol; *Canadian:* Bretylate)	Ventricular fibrillation	*Adult:* IV, 5 mg/kg by rapid bolus *Child:* IV, 5 mg/kg per dose followed by 10 mg/kg at 15–30 min intervals, maximum 30 mg/kg	*Onset:* IM, varies; IV, min *Duration:* IM, IV, 24 h $t_{1/2}$: 6.9–8.1 h
	Ventricular arrhythmias	*Adult:* IV, infuse diluted solution of 5–10 mg/kg > 8 min, and repeat q1–2h; IM, 5–10 mg/kg undiluted, repeated at 1–2 h intervals if arrhythmias persist *Child:* IV, 5–10 mg/kg per dose q6h	
ibutilide (Covert)	Atrial fibrillation Atrial flutter	*Adult* (≥ *60 kg*): IV, 1 mg infused over 10 min (< 60 kg): 0.01 mg/kg infused over 10 min; may repeat 1 ×	*Onset:* Within 10 min *Duration:* variable $t_{1/2}$: 2–12 h

right ventricle, repolarization, intraventricular conduction and infranodal (below or beneath the nodes) conduction. These differences suggest that the initial acute effects of amiodarone IV are focused predominantly on the AV node (because of sodium channel blockade).

Several electrophysiologic effects occur with the administration of amiodarone. An increased cardiac refractory period occurs, usually without influencing the resting membrane potential. Sinus rate decreases by 15% to 20%. The PR and QT intervals increase by about 10%. U waves appear and T waves are altered. These changes do not usually require discontinuation of amiodarone, although marked sinus bradycardia or sinus arrest and heart block can occur. QT prolongation can be associated with worsening of the arrhythmia, but this is rare.

After IV dosing, amiodarone relaxes the vascular smooth muscle, reduces peripheral vascular resistance (decreasing afterload) and slightly increases the cardiac index (ratio of cardiac output per minute to the body surface area). With oral dosing, amiodarone produces no significant change in left ventricular ejection fraction. After acute IV dosing, amiodarone may have a mild negative inotropic effect on left ventricular ejection fraction, decreasing the force of contractility. Oral dosing, however, produces no significant change in left ventricular ejection fraction.

Because of its ability to lengthen repolarization and refractoriness in atria and ventricles, while also blocking adrenergic stimulation, amiodarone is being considered as a potentially valuable drug in treating atrial fibrillation (see the accompanying display, Comparison of Drugs for the Treatment of New-Onset Atrial Fibrillation). One reason that amiodarone's use in atrial fibrillation is attractive to researchers is its ability to increase the action potential duration in atrial and ventricular tissues following chronic drug administration, while producing lesser effects in Purkinje fibers and M cells (special cardiac cells). Additionally, its effect on repolarization is not influenced by heart rate. Despite producing marked slowing of the heart rate and significant increases in the QT interval, the drug only seldom produces torsades de pointes (see Adverse Effects). Amiodarone is known to be effective in maintaining normal sinus rhythm, which is now considered crucial in treating atrial fibrillation. Low doses of amiodarone have been found to maintain sinus rhythm in patients with paroxysmal or chronic atrial fibrillation who were previously nonresponsive to other drug therapies. Furthermore, amiodarone has been found to effectively treat and prevent atrial fibrillation in patients who have CHF. Few other drugs have this benefit, yet almost 40% of patients with CHF develop atrial fibrillation.

Contraindications and Precautions

Contraindications for giving the drug orally include severe sinus-node dysfunction producing significant sinus bradycardia, second and third degree AV block, and in those instances when episodes of bradycardia have caused syncope (unless used with a pacemaker). Contraindications for giving the drug IV are similar and include marked sinus bradycardia, second and third degree AV block (unless the patient has a functioning pacemaker), and cardiogenic shock. Additionally, if patients have a known hypersensitivity response to the drug, it should be avoided.

Amiodarone inhibits peripheral conversion of thyroxine (T_4) to triiodothyronine (T_3), prompting increased T_4 levels, increased levels of inactive reverse T_3, and decreased levels of T_3. It also is a potential source of large amounts of inorganic iodine. Because it releases inorganic iodine, and perhaps for other unknown reasons, amiodarone can cause hypothyroidism or hyperthyroidism. Because of the slow elimination of amiodarone and its metabolite, high plasma iodide levels, altered thyroid function, and abnormal thyroid function tests may persist for several weeks or months following discontinuation of the drug.

Amiodarone is a pregnancy category D drug. It can cause congenital goiter/hypothyroidism or hyperthyroidism. Amiodarone is excreted into breast milk. In animal studies, nursing offspring are less viable and have reduced body weight gains.

Adverse Effects

Amiodarone has several adverse effects that are potentially fatal. Pulmonary toxicity is the most important of these serious adverse effects. The frequency of pulmonary

Focus on Research

Comparison of drugs for the treatment of new-onset atrial fibrillation

Joseph, A. P., & Ward, M. R. (2000). A prospective, randomized controlled trial comparing the efficacy and safety of sotalol, amiodarone, and digoxin for the reversion of new-onset atrial fibrillation. *Annals of Emergency Medicine*, *36*(1), 1–9.

The Study

In all, 120 patients with atrial fibrillation of less than 24-hours duration were randomly assigned to be treated with either sotalol, amiodarone, or digoxin. Patients received a single IV dose followed by 48 hours of oral treatment with their assigned drug. Conversion to normal sinus rhythm took significantly less time in the groups treated with sotalol and amiodarone than in the group treated with digoxin. Conversion to normal sinus rhythm also was more likely to occur if the patient received either sotalol or amiodarone. Fewer adverse effects also were noted in these groups compared with the group receiving digoxin.

Nursing Implications

Class III antiarrhythmic drugs (sotalol and amiodarone) appear to have a place in the treatment of atrial fibrillation. Although these drugs can have serious adverse effects in treating patients with atrial fibrillation, the findings of this study showed that these drugs actually caused fewer problems than the traditional therapy of digoxin. It is likely that these drugs will be used more often in clinical practice for treating atrial as well as ventricular arrhythmias.

toxicity with amiodarone is between 2% and 17%. About 10% of the patients who develop pulmonary toxicity will die. The syndrome, seen frequently with oral dosing, is cough, progressive dyspnea, and test findings (e.g., radiographic, gallium scan, or pulmonary function tests) consistent with pulmonary toxicity. Phospholipidosis (foamy cells, foamy macrophages) will be present in most cases of amiodarone-induced pulmonary toxicity. However, this is not a specific marker for amiodarone toxicity as these changes are also present in about 50% of patients on the drug.

Any new changes in the respiratory system warrant the patient being reexamined to determine if pulmonary toxicity is present. Amiodarone is prescribed to patients with life-threatening arrhythmias. Therefore, the drug must be discontinued cautiously if pulmonary toxicity is suspected because more patients die from sudden cardiac death (the most common cause of death for these patients) than from pulmonary toxicity. Before discontinuing amiodarone because of suspected pulmonary toxicity, other causes of respiratory impairment (e.g., infection) should be ruled out.

Another potentially fatal adverse effect of amiodarone is exacerbation of the arrhythmia it is treating. It also may make the arrhythmia more difficult to reverse. This occurs in about 2% to 5% of patients treated. The risk for exacerbation is increased if more than one type of arrhythmia is present. Exacerbation can include new ventricular fibrillation, incessant ventricular tachycardia, increased resistance to cardioversion, and polymorphic (more than one form) ventricular tachycardia associated with QT prolongation (torsades de pointes). Amiodarone also has caused symptomatic bradycardia, heart block, and sinus arrest with suppression of escape foci (ectopic foci picking up as pacemaker when SA is not functioning to maintain a heart beat) in 2% to 4% of patients. Drug-related bradycardia does not appear to be dose related.

A final potentially lethal adverse effect is liver disease. This is very rare, however. Some liver injury, evidenced only by elevated liver enzyme levels, is common with amiodarone, but this is normally mild and not serious.

Optic neuritis or optic neuropathy, although not a fatal adverse effect, can be a potentially serious adverse effect because visual impairment can occur and may result in permanent blindness. This adverse effect is rare however.

Other adverse effects include common CNS effects (e.g., malaise, dizziness, paresthesia, tremor, headache, and insomnia). These can occur in 20% to 40% of patients. The effects are not serious, rarely requiring discontinuing of the drug, and often are alleviated with dosage reduction or dividing the dose. GI complaints (e.g., nausea, vomiting, constipation, anorexia, and abdominal pain) also are common; about 25% of patients have these complaints. The drug rarely needs to be discontinued because of these effects. The GI effects are seen mostly with high doses, and usually are alleviated with dose reduction or divided doses.

Photosensitivity is a problem for about 10% of patients taking amiodarone. With long-term treatment, a blue-gray discoloration of the exposed skin may be seen. The risk, which may be increased in patients with fair complexions or excessive sun exposure, may be related to cumulative dose and the duration of therapy. It will reverse slowly after discontinuation of the drug, although sometimes it is irreversible. Hypothyroidism or hyperthyroidism may occur, as well as edema, coagulation abnormalities, flushing, epididymitis, vasculitis, pseudotumor cerebri, thrombocytopenia, and angioedema.

When amiodarone is given IV, hypotension is its most frequent adverse effect, although this is not normally serious. Clinically significant hypotension occurs in the first few hours of drug administration and appears to be related to the rate of infusion, not the drug concentration. Blood pressure should return to normal if the rate is slowed down (see the accompanying display, Amiodarone Therapy).

Drug Interactions

Amiodarone increases the plasma concentration of digoxin. This effect is believed to be due to amiodarone's inhibition of P-glycoprotein. P-glycoprotein pumps drugs entering the enerocyte back into the intestinal lumen. It also is active on the tubular side of the renal epithelium and the biliary side of hepatocytes, and serves to promote drug excretion at these sites. By inhibiting P-glycoprotein excretion, the elimination of digoxin is decreased, increasing blood levels of this drug.

Amiodarone also decreases the clearance of many other drugs, including flecainide and warfarin. There are most likely multiple mechanisms that underlie these

Critical Thinking Scenario

Amiodarone Therapy

Mr. Bowen is 74 years old. He was brought to the hospital emergency department by ambulance. He was diagnosed with myocardial infarction and was in ventricular fibrillation arrhythmia. He is cardioverted to sinus rhythm and started on amiodarone by IV infusion. When transferred to the intensive care unit, his blood pressure dropped to 88/50. The ICU nurse examines Mr. Bowen's laboratory results; the only unexpected finding is that he has a low serum albumin level.

1. What possible causes may account for the hypotension?
2. What action should the nurse take to manage Mr. Bowen's hypotension?
3. If the nurse in unable to correct the hypotension, what might the nurse do next?

effects. Amiodarone's impairment of flecainide elimination appears to be mostly renal. Its impairment of warfarin clearance is most likely related to amiodarone being an inhibitor of CYP 2C9 (another major isoenzyme of metabolism); warfarin relies solely on CYP 2C9 for metabolism. Research on amiodarone's effects on metabolism and elimination of other drugs is continuing. See Table 29-4 for additional information on drug interactions.

Amiodarone also interferes with laboratory tests. It alters thyroid function tests because of its effects on T_3 and T_4, and also may alter liver function tests (alanine aminotransferase [ALT], aspartate aminotransferase [AST]).

Assessment of Relevant Core Patient Variables

Health Status

The nurse determines the patient's cardiac status using an ECG. This will verify whether the patient has an arrhythmia that is responsive to amiodarone, and that none of the pathologic conditions that are contraindications to amiodarone's use is present. The nurse also obtains results of thyroid function tests and liver function tests as baseline data. It is important to assess respiratory status through chest x-ray, pulmonary function studies (including diffusion capacity), and auscultation of breath sounds before treatment.

Life Span and Gender

The nurse should determine the patient's age because safety and efficacy have not been established in children. The benzyl alcohol that is contained in some of these products as a preservative has been associated with a fatal "gasping syndrome" in premature infants. In older adults, amiodarone has a lower clearance rate and an increased half-life. It also is important to determine whether the patient is pregnant because amiodarone is a pregnancy category D drug. The drug should only be used if the potential benefits outweigh the significant risks to the fetus. If the patient is nursing, she should be advised to discontinue nursing while on amiodarone.

TABLE 29-4 Agents That Interact With Amiodarone

Interactants	Effect and Significance	Nursing Management
anticoagulants	Potentiation of anticoagulant response; protime may be increased	Dose decrease usually needed; monitor protime
beta blockers	May increase risk of bradycardia and hypotension from additive effect	Monitor pulse and blood pressure
calcium channel blockers	Increased risk of atrioventricular block or hypotension	Monitor for electrocardiographic (ECG) changes; monitor blood pressure
cyclosporine	Increased plasma levels of cyclosporine resulting in elevated creatinine	Reduce dose; monitor creatinine levels
dextromethorphan	Impairs metabolism of dextromethorphan	Assess for adverse effects
digoxin	Increased digoxin serum levels	Monitor digoxin levels; decrease dose of digoxin; consider stopping digoxin
disopyramide	Increases QT prolongation; may cause arrhythmias	Monitor for ECG changes
fentanyl	Increases effect of fentanyl and may cause hypotension and bradycardia	Monitor blood pressure and pulse
flecainide	Increases the effect of flecainide	Decrease the dose of flecainide, therapeutic levels will be maintained
hydantoins	Impairs metabolism of hydantoins; elevated serum levels of hydantoins may occur; amiodarone level also may be decreased	Monitor blood levels; assess for adverse effects
lidocaine	Increased levels of lidocaine	Monitor blood pressure (rare complications)
methotrexate	Impairs metabolism of methotrexate	Assess for adverse effects
procainamide	Increased procainimide serum levels may occur	Monitor for adverse effects
quinidine	Increased quinidine levels; potential for fatal arrhythmias	Assess ECG for changes
theophylline	Increased theophylline levels with toxicity	Monitor levels; assess for adverse effects
cholestyramine	Increased enterohepatic elimination of amiodarone, reduced serum levels and half-life may occur	Monitor for therapeutic effects
cimetidine	Increased serum levels of amiodarone may occur	Assess for adverse effects
ritonavir	Large increases in amiodarone blood levels may occur, increasing the risk of adverse effects	Assess for adverse effects; monitor ECG

Environment

The nurse should be aware of the setting in which amiodarone may be administered. IV amiodarone is given in an intensive care unit where the patient can receive continuous cardiac monitoring. Oral doses may be given in any environment, except when giving a loading dose; during this time the patient needs to be hospitalized. While on oral doses, the nurse should assess the patient's exposure to sunlight because photosensitivity may occur.

Culture

It is important to note that the variations in response to amiodarone may be genetically related. However, little is yet known about this.

Nursing Diagnoses and Outcomes

- Decreased Cardiac Output related to cardiac arrhythmia.
  Desired outcome: Cardiac rhythm will return to normal allowing for normal cardiac output.
- Risk for Injury related to adverse effects of drug therapy
  Desired outcome: The patient will not suffer permanent injury or death as a result of drug therapy.

Planning and Intervention

Maximizing Therapeutic Effects

To maximize the therapeutic effect of amiodarone, the nurse should administer the prescribed loading doses. When giving amiodarone IV, the nurse should mix the drug in glass bottles or polyolefin bags of 5% dextrose in water (D5W). Although some of the amiodarone dose is lost due to absorption from polyvinyl chloride administration tubing, this tubing should be used for administration, because the clinical trials that established dosage used this particular type of tubing. Thus, recommended doses account for this loss. Surface properties of solutions of amiodarone are altered so that drop size may be reduced. This size reduction can account for an underdosage of up to 30%. A volumetric infusion pump should be used to prevent an underdosage.

Minimizing Adverse Effects

Oral and IV Doses

It is important to correct electrolyte disturbances before beginning therapy. Hypokalemia and hypomagnesemia can exaggerate the degree of QT prolongation and increase the potential for torsades de pointes. The nurse should assess for proarrhythmia changes. In addition, the nurse should use pulse oximetry or arterial blood gases to assess for changes in respiratory function, including breath sounds, dyspnea, and oxygen delivery to the tissues. If changes occur, it is important to repeat the chest x-ray, physical examination, gallium scan, and pulmonary function tests to rule out pulmonary toxicity.

The nurse should assess for symptoms of visual impairment. Regular eye examinations are recommended throughout therapy. Ophthalmic examination should be sought immediately if impairment occurs. It also is important to assess T_3 and T_4 levels to determine thyroid function. Assess for signs of hyperthyroidism or hypothyroidism. Liver function studies also should be monitored.

Oral Doses

The nurse should monitor the patient closely during the loading phase until the risk of recurrent ventricular tachycardia or fibrillation has abated. It is important to attempt to discontinue prior antiarrhythmic drugs gradually. Reduce the dose of these other drugs by 30% to 50% several days after initiating amiodarone, when arrhythmia suppression should be present.

In patients who are not well controlled on amiodarone alone, the nurse should introduce other agents using half of the usual recommended dosage. It is a good idea to divide the dose or give amiodarone with food to minimize or prevent nausea, vomiting, and other GI effects.

IV Doses

The nurse should adjust the starting dose to suppress life-threatening arrhythmias based on varied individual response to therapy. The nurse must monitor the patient continuously using cardiac monitor during therapy. It is important to monitor blood pressure carefully as hypotension is most likely to occur in the early period, and to reduce the infusion rate if hypotension occurs.

The nurse should avoid administering amiodarone with aminophylline, cefamandole, cefazolin, mezlocillin, heparin, and sodium bicarbonate due to incompatibility and the formation of a precipitate. If possible, it is a good idea to administer amiodarone using a central venous catheter to prevent phlebitis.

The nurse should use an in-line filter. It is important to use IV therapy until the ventricular arrhythmia is stabilized. Transfer the patient to oral therapy either during or after IV treatment, and adjust the IV dose to a new lower, oral dose. If treated with IV infusion for less than 1 week, the nurse should give an oral dose of 800 to 1600 mg/day initially. If treated with IV for 1 to 3 weeks, the nurse should give an oral dose of 600 to 800 mg per day initially. If treated with IV for longer than 3 weeks, the nurse should give an oral dose of 400 mg/day initially.

Providing Patient and Family Education

- The nurse should explain the purpose of the drug and possible adverse effects of the drug.
- The nurse emphasizes the importance of returning for follow-up blood work and ECGs.
- It is important to teach the patient to use appropriate protection when out in the sun, and to limit sun exposure.
- The nurse must instruct the patient to notify the physician for new onset of cough, shortness of breath, and changes in visual acuity.

Ongoing Assessment and Evaluation

The patient's ECG should be monitored intermittently throughout therapy and after the initial stabilization and loading dose period for new arrhythmias or worsening of the current arrhythmia being treated. The nurse should make recurrent assessments of respiratory function, visual acuity, thyroid function, and liver function. Therapy is considered effective if the arrhythmia is corrected and the patient does not develop serious adverse effects. ■

DRUGS CLOSELY RELATED TO AMIODARONE

Sotalol

Sotalol also is categorized as a Class IC antiarrhythmic. Like amiodarone, it prolongs repolarization (phase 3). These Class III effects are seen in doses greater than 160 mg/day. Additionally, like amiodarone, sotalol decreases automaticity at the SA node and ectopic pacemakers. It also decreases conduction velocity at the AV node, although unlike amiodarone it does not decrease it at the atrium, bundle of His, or Purkinje fibers. ECG changes are similar except that sotalol does not lengthen the QT interval. Although sotalol and amiodarone both have antiadrenergic effects, they work by different mechanisms. Sotalol is actually a beta blocker, blocking both beta-1 and beta-2 sites. It is used in treating life-threatening ventricular arrhythmias. Because of its multiple sites of actions, it, like amiodarone, is being studied and recommended for use in treating atrial fibrillation (see Focus on Research). Sotalol has been shown to maintain sinus rhythm in about half the patients with atrial fibrillation after they were cardioverted to normal rhythm. Like all other antiarrhythmics, sotalol may induce arrhythmias as well as treat them. Torsades de pointes, although possible, is not likely to occur if the dose is controlled, if the patients have normal renal function, and if the patients do not have severe CHF. Sotalol is administered orally after the patient has been on IV antiarrhythmics for ventricular arrhythmias. It is considered safe to begin therapy in the outpatient setting if given for atrial fibrillation (see Table 29-3).

MEMORY CHIP

Amiodarone

- Class III antiarrhythmic used to treat life-threatening ventricular arrhythmias and prevent their recurrence
- Produces prolonged phase of repolarization (phase 3)
- Has properties of Classes I, II and IV also
- Has extremely long half-life and great variability in pharmacodynamics and pharmacokinetics
- Significant contraindications: severe sinus bradycardia and second- or third-degree atrioventricular heart block
- Most common adverse effects: central nervous system effects (e.g., malaise, dizziness, paresthesia, tremor, headache, and insomnia); gastrointestinal (GI) effects (e.g., nausea and vomiting); photosensitivity; and hypotension (IV use)
- Most serious adverse effects: pulmonary toxicity and cardiac arrhythmias
- **Lifespan alert: drug is in pregnancy category D; use only if benefit outweighs risk**
- Maximizing therapeutic effects: use a loading dose(s)
- Minimizing adverse effects: correct preexisting electrolyte imbalances before giving the drug; adjust IV dose to control ventricular arrhythmia; monitor blood pressure (IV dosing); monitor electrocardiogram for changes; and assess for respiratory changes
- Most significant patient education: take with food to minimize GI distress and notify the physician if cough or shortness of breath develops

Bretylium

Bretylium also is used in treating life-threatening ventricular arrhythmias when the patient has failed to respond to first-line drugs, such as lidocaine. Like amiodarone, bretylium prolongs phase 3 (repolarization) and the refractory period. Unlike amiodarone, bretylium increase the automaticity of the SA node and ectopic pacemakers and has no effect on the conduction velocity in the atrium and the AV node. Bretylium also does not produce the ECG changes that amiodarone does. Bretylium has a much shorter duration of action (6–8 hours) and half-life (5–10 days) than amiodarone. It is has a very low protein binding compared with that of amiodarone, which is very high. Bretylium is given only by IV infusion.

Transient tachycardia and elevated blood pressure may occur after administration of bretylium as a result of the initial release of norepinephrine. Subsequently, the release of norepinephrine is blocked, and orthostatic hypotension may occur.

The most frequent adverse effect is postural hypotension, occurring in about half the patients receiving the drug while they are supine. Other adverse effects include can be bradycardia, increased premature ventricular contractions, transient hypertension, initial increase in arrhythmias, and angina. Nausea and vomiting can occur, usually after rapid IV administration (see Table 29-3).

Ibutilide and Dofetilide

Ibutilide and dofetilide are both new drugs in what is termed the "pure" Class III antiarrhythmics. They are not as multifaceted as amiodarone. The goal of developing these new Class III drugs was to find a drug as effective as amiodarone but without its adverse effects.

Ibutilide was the first of the "pure" Class III drugs approved for use in the United States. It is approved only for IV use to convert atrial flutter and atrial fibrillation to normal sinus rhythm. It is about twice as effective in converting atrial flutter as atrial fibrillation. Ibutilide increases the atrial effective refractory period and causes a prolongation of the QT interval. The effect on the QT interval is dose dependent. There is also some blockade of potassium channels. As a result, there also is some prolonging of the action potential duration in the ventricles. Ibutilide is metabolized extensively in the liver; its high first-pass effect is the reason it must be given IV. Unlike amiodarone, ibutilide has a short half-life of 4 to 8 hours; its metabolites have a similar half-life. Ibutilide distributes rapidly to a large volume and its electrophysiologic effects decrease quickly after IV administration. Proarrhythmia effects are therefore greatest within the first hour of administration. There is an estimated 8% risk of torsades de pointes with ibutilide use. When it occurs, it often is transient. However, if ibutilide is given concurrently with beta blockers or calcium channel blockers, torsades de pointes is more likely to occur.

Dofetilide is used to convert patients in atrial fibrillation to normal sinus rhythm and maintain them in sinus rhythm. Dofetilide delays repolarization in the atria, ventricles, and Purkinje fibers by blocking some of the potassium channels. It has no effect on sodium or calcium channels and thus little effect on conduction velocity, force of contraction, and systemic hemodynamics. It increases repolarization and refractoriness in both atrial and ventricular tissue although the predominant effect is on the atrial tissue. It is well absorbed orally and has a bioavailability of moe than 90%. Most of the drug is excreted unchanged in the urine, and the rest is metabolized in the liver. Dofetilide has a reverse use-dependent effect, and at slow rates has the tendency to increase the QT interval. Dofetilide is not likely to cause torsades de pointes.

C CLASS IV ANTIARRHYTHMICS

Class IV antiarrhythmics depress phase 4 depolarization and lengthen phases 1 and 2 of repolarization (see Fig. 29-6). This class is composed of several calcium-channel blockers, but only two have been approved specifically as antiarrhythmics—verapamil (verapamil hydrochloride, Calan, Isoptin) and diltiazem (Alti-diltiazem [Canada]), Apo-Diltiaz [Canada]), Cardizem, Dilacor, gen-diltiazem [Canada], Novo-Diltazem [Canada], Tiamate, Tiazac). The prototype class IV antiarrhythmic calcium-channel blocker is verapamil.

Calcium-channel blockers, prescribed for other purposes, are amlodipine (Norvasc), bepridil (Vascor), felodipine (Plendil), isradapine (Dyna Circ), nicardipine (Cardene), and nifedipine (Procardia, Adalat). Other uses of calcium channel blockers are described in Chapters 28 and 30. Adenosine is a non–calcium-channel blocker drug that is significantly different from verapamil.

NURSING MANAGEMENT OF THE PATIENT RECEIVING P VERAPAMIL

Core Drug Knowledge

Pharmacotherapeutics

Verapamil, and another calcium-channel blocker, diltiazem, are used as antiarrhythmics. Verapamil used in conjunction with digoxin controls ventricular rate in chronic atrial flutter or fibrillation. It also can be used prophylactically for repetitive paroxysmal SVT. IV verapamil also is used to treat supraventricular tachyarrhythmias.

Verapamil also is used in treating angina (including Prinzmetal angina) and hypertension. Unlabeled uses include prevention of migraine headache, cluster headache, and exercise-induced asthma. Other unlabeled uses include treatment of hypertrophic cardiomyopathy, bipolar disorder (alternative therapy), and recumbent nocturnal leg cramps (Table 29-5).

The efficacy of sublingual verapamil in controlling acute rapid ventricular rate was assessed in a small group of patients with chronic atrial fibrillation. Mean heart rate was found to be significantly lower after 10 minutes, with the lowest rate achieved 60 minutes after administration. Thus, sublingual verapamil was shown an effective choice in acute control of rapid ventricular rate in atrial fibrillation. (Incze, Frigy, & Cotoi, 1998)

Pharmacokinetics

Well absorbed after oral administration, verapamil undergoes a significant first-pass effect, resulting in considerably less bioavailability. Verapamil is excreted by the kidneys. It crosses the placenta and appears in breast milk. When sustained-release verapamil is administered with food, it takes longer to reach maximum plasma levels. However, bioavailability is not affected significantly, so verapamil may be administered without regard to meals.

Pharmacodynamics

Verapamil acts by inhibiting the movement of calcium ions across the cardiac and arterial muscle cell membrane. This action results in slowing conduction through the AV node (conduction velocity), prolonging the effective refractory phase (automaticity), depressing myocardial contractility, and producing dilation of both coronary arteries and peripheral arterioles. Verapamil interrupts reentry at the AV node and thus can restore normal sinus rhythm in paroxysmal SVT. The other outcomes of verapamil therapy are decreased oxygen demand, decreased cardiac effort, and increased oxygen to the myocardium.

Contraindications and Precautions

The drug is contraindicated in sick sinus syndrome or second- or third-degree heart block (except with a functioning pacemaker), hypotension (with systolic pressure under 90 mm Hg), severe left ventricular dysfunction, cardiogenic shock, and severe CHF. Verapamil is a pregnancy category C drug. Verapamil in elderly patients may cause a greater hypotensive effect than in younger patients so that caution should be used. Caution should be used in patients with cirrhosis of the liver (the half-life is greatly increased) and with renal disease. Caution should be used if the patient has Duchenne muscular dystrophy

TABLE 29-5 Summary of Selected Class IV Antiarrhythmics and Selected Other Calcium Channel Blockers

Drug (Trade) Name	Selected Indications	Route and Dosage Range	Pharmacokinetics
verapamil (Calan, Isoptin)	Angina pectoris Supraventricular tachyarrhythmias	*Adult:* PO, 80–120 mg tid, increase q1–2d *Adult:* IV, 5–10 mg over 2 min; may repeat dose of 10 mg 30 min after first dose *Child:* IV, >1 y, 0.1–0.2 mg/kg over 2 min; 1–15 y, 0.1–0.3 mg/kg over 2 min; do not exceed 5 mg; repeat after 30 min, if necessary.	*Onset:* PO, 30 min; IV, rapid *Duration:* PO, 3–7 h; IV, 2 h $t_{1/2}$: 3–7 h
	Hypertension	*Adult:* PO, 240 mg qd; sustained-release form in morning; 80 mg tid	
diltiazem (Cardizem, Tiazac; *Canadian:* Apo-Diltiaz)	Angina pectoris Essential hypertension Atrial fibrillation or flutter (IV only)	*Adult:* PO, 30 mg qid before meals and hs, increase gradually at 1–2 d intervals to 180–360 mg in three to four divided doses; SR, cardizem CD, 180–240 mg/d PO for hypertension; 120–180 mg/d PO for angina IV, 0.25 mg/kg over 2 min; second bolus of 0.35 mg/kg given over 2 min IV infusion: 5–15 mg/h for up to 24 h *Child:* Safety and efficacy not established	*Onset:* PO and SR, 30–60 min; IV, immediate *Duration:* Unknown $t_{1/2}$: 3½–6 h; SR, 5–7 h
Non-antiarrhythmic Calcium Channel Blockers			
amlodipine (Norvasc)	Angina pectoris Essential hypertension	*Adult:* PO, 5 mg qd, may increase over 10–14 d to a max dose of 10 mg/d *Child:* Safety and efficacy not established	*Onset:* PO, unknown *Duration:* Unknown $t_{1/2}$: 30–50 h
nicardipine (Cardene)	Stable angina	*Adult:* PO, 20 mg tid; range, 20–40 mg tid; allow 3 d before increasing dosage *Child:* Safety and efficacy not established	*Onset:* 20 min *Duration:* Unknown $t_{1/2}$: 2–4 h
	Hypertension	*Adult:* PO, 20 mg tid; range 20–40 mg tid. Adjust dosage based on BP response; allow 3 d before increasing *Child:* Safety and efficacy not established	

because verapamil may decrease neuromuscular transmission. IV verapamil can induce respiratory muscle failure in these patients.

Adverse Effects

The most common adverse effect of verapamil is constipation. Other common adverse effects include dizziness/light-headedness, headache, nausea, hypotension, peripheral edema, bradycardia, AV block, pulmonary edema, rash, shortness of breath, and asthenia. Verapamil may produce potentially lethal ventricular arrhythmias.

Drug Interactions

Several drugs interact with verapamil. Verapamil may elevate serum transaminases with and without concomitant elevations in alkaline phosphatase and bilirubin. Usually, the elevations are transient, although several cases of hepatocellular injury have occurred. Verapamil will form a crystalline precipitate if administered into an infusion line containing 0.45% sodium chloride solution with sodium bicarbonate. A milky white precipitate forms when given IV push into the same line being used for nafcillin infusion (Table 29-6).

Assessment of Relevant Core Patient Variables

Health Status

The nurse should determine whether the patient has chronic atrial flutter or fibrillation, which is causing elevated ventricular rate, or chronic repetitive paroxysmal SVTs, both of which pose a need for therapy. The nurse also must identify whether the patient has any of the following conditions because they are contraindications to treatment with verapamil: sick sinus syndrome or second- or third-degree heart block (except with a functioning pacemaker), hypotension (with systolic pressure under 90 mmHg), severe left ventricular dysfunction, cardiogenic shock, or severe CHF. It also is important to determine whether the patient has renal or liver impairment or Duchenne muscular dystrophy, because verapamil must be used with caution in these patients.

Life Span and Gender

The nurse should determine whether the patient is pregnant because verapamil is in pregnancy category C and must be used cautiously. It also is important to note the patient's age before administering verapamil. Although

TABLE 29-6 Agents That Interact With Verapamil

Interactants	Effect and Significance	Nursing Management
barbiturates	Clearance of verapamil possibly increased and bioavailability decreased	Monitor pulse, blood pressure, and respiration carefully. Monitor patient responses and blood levels.
calcium salts	Antagonism of effects of verapamil with calcium	Administer 2 h apart.
hydantoins	Serum verapamil levels possibly decreased	Monitor for therapeutic effect.
quinidine	Hypotension bradycardia, ventricular tachycardia, atrioventricular (AV) block, and pulmonary edema possible	Use concomitantly only when no other alternatives exist.
rifampin	Possible loss of clinical effectiveness of oral verapamil	Use of IV verapamil may circumvent the interaction.
vitamin D	Therapeutic efficacy of verapamil possibly reduced	Stagger dosage and monitor vital signs.
beta blockers	Coadministration, potential increased adverse effects due to depressant effects on myocardial contractility of AV conduction	Concurrent use normally avoided.
cardiac glycosides (digoxin)	Possible increased digoxin levels	Monitor for adverse effects of cardiac glycoside.

the safety and efficacy of verapamil have not been established in children, experience has shown that treatment results are similar to those for adults. Intravenous verapamil is contraindicated in neonates and infants, but only when given to treat supraventricular tachycardia, because of a high risk of electromechanical dissociation. In children older than 5 years and in adolescents, IV verapamil may be administered with the same restrictions as in adult patients (i.e., a wide QRS complex tachycardia or significant hemodynamic compromise) (Paul, Bertram, Bokenkamp, & Hausdorf, 2000). Verapamil may have greater hypotensive effects on older adults.

Environment

The nurse should be aware of the setting in which verapamil may be administered. IV verapamil is administered only in the hospital where the patient is monitored constantly using ECG and blood pressure. IV verapamil solution must be protected from light. Oral verapamil may be administered in any setting.

Nursing Diagnoses and Outcomes

- Risk for Constipation related to adverse effects of the drug
  Desired outcome: Patient will prevent or minimize constipation by increasing fluid intake and adding fruit and fiber to the diet
- Decreased Cardiac Output related to decreased rate and force of contraction and return to normal rhythm related to therapeutic effects of drug
  Desired outcome: Patient's decreased cardiac output will decrease symptoms of cardiac alterations without development of adverse cardiac effects from drug therapy.

Planning and Intervention

Maximizing Therapeutic Effects

To maximize the therapeutic effects of verapamil, the nurse first verifies that the IV line is patent before IV administration. Once the infusion begins, the drug solution must be shielded from light. Digoxin may be given with verapamil to achieve the additive effect of slowing at the AV node.

Minimizing Adverse Effects

When administering verapamil in an IV route, the nurse should not dilute it with a sodium lactate injection in polyvinyl chloride (PVC) bags, which may not be stable. It is important to administer IV slowly (bolus 5–10 mg over 2 minutes, 5 mg/hour infusion), and to use an IV pump to regulate the drip rate.

The nurse should not administer IV verapamil simultaneously (or within a few hours) with IV beta blockers (both drugs suppress contractility and AV conduction). It is important to monitor the patient's ECG and blood pressure constantly during IV therapy. Throughout oral therapy, the nurse should monitor for ECG changes and hypotension. The nurse should encourage patients on oral verapamil therapy to increase fluid intake and include fresh fruit and fiber in their diet to help prevent constipation.

Providing Patient and Family Education

- The nurse should explain the purpose of the drug, and its adverse effects.
- It is important to stress the importance of adequate fluid intake and dietary fruit and fiber to help prevent constipation.
- The nurse should teach the patient how to take the pulse daily while on oral verapamil, instructing the patient to notify the health care provider if irregular beating (arrhythmias) occurs.

- The nurse should teach the patient how to take his own blood pressure, urging him to monitor the blood pressure on a regular basis. If the blood pressure falls below 90/60 or other parameter set by the health care provider, the nurse instructs the patient to contact the health care provider.
- It is important to emphasize the importance of scheduling follow-up visits and blood studies.

Ongoing Assessment and Evaluation

The nurse monitors the patient's ECG and blood pressure throughout therapy. It is important to monitor liver function periodically to detect elevated serum drug levels. Therapy is effective when normal rhythm is reestablished without onset of new arrhythmias, hypotension, or other significant adverse effects. ■

DRUG SIGNIFICANTLY DIFFERENT FROM VERAPAMIL

Adenosine, unlike verapamil, is not a calcium-channel blocker. Adenosine is not related chemically to verapamil or any other antiarrhythmic. It is an endogenous nucleoside occurring in all cells of the body. Adenosine, like verapamil, decreases automaticity, decreases conduction velocity at the AV node, and increases the refractory period at the AV node. It may produce first-, second-, or third-degree heart block of short duration. Unlike verapamil, it increases heart rate. It is used in the conversion of paroxysmal supraventricular tachycardia (PSVT) to normal sinus rhythm, and only is given as a rapid IV bolus (see Table 29-5). The IV boluses should be administered directly into the vein, or as proximally to the vein as possible, and followed by a rapid saline flush. The bolus may be repeated if necessary.

Adenosine is removed from the circulatory system very rapidly. It is taken up by erythrocytes and vascular endothelial cells. Its half-life is estimated to be less than 10 seconds. Adenosine is metabolized primarily to inosine and adenosine monophosphate (AMP). Conversion to normal sinus rhythm frequently occurs within 1 minute after dosing.

Adenosine is contraindicated in second- or third-degree AV block, sick sinus syndrome (unless a previously inserted pacemaker is functional), atrial flutter, atrial fibrillation, and ventricular tachycardia, because the drug does not convert these arrhythmias.

The most common adverse effects of adenosine are facial flushing and shortness of breath/dyspnea. Other adverse effects that may occur include:

- CV: sweating, palpitations, chest pain, hypotension (rare), prolonged systole, ventricular fibrillation, ventricular tachycardia, and transient increase in blood pressure
- CNS: headache, lightheadedness, dizziness, tingling in arms, numbness, apprehension, blurred vision, burning sensation, heaviness in arms, and pain in neck or back
- GI: nausea, metallic taste, tightness in throat, pressure in groin (rare)

MEMORY CHIP

Verapamil

- Class IV antiarrhythmic and a calcium channel blocker; may be given IV or PO
- Inhibits movement of calcium ions across the cardiac and arterial muscle cell membrane
- Slows conduction, depresses automaticity, depresses myocardial contractility, and dilates coronary arteries and peripheral arterioles
- Antiarrhythmic uses: controls ventricular rate in chronic atrial flutter or fibrillation; prophylactically with digoxin for repetitive paroxysmal supraventricular tachycardia; treat supraventricular tachyarrhythmias (IV administration)
- Also used in angina and hypertension
- Significant contraindications: significantly depressed cardiac function, including second- or third-degree heart block, severe hypotension, severe left ventricular dysfunction, severe congestive heart failure, or cardiogenic shock
- Most common adverse effect: constipation
- Most serious adverse effect: ventricular arrhythmias
- **Lifespan alerts: IV routes are contraindicated in neonates and infants; and older adults are more sensitive to hypotensive effects**
- Maximizing therapeutic effects: shield drug solution from light; give with digoxin for additive effect of slowing at the atrioventricular node
- Minimizing adverse effects: monitor electrocardiogram and blood pressure constantly while on IV; and monitor periodically throughout oral therapy
- Most significant patient education: techniques to prevent constipation

- Respiratory: chest pressure, hyperventilation, and head pressure (rare)

POTASSIUM-REMOVING RESINS TO PREVENT ARRHYTHMIAS

Because hyperkalemia may lead to cardiac arrhythmias, potassium-removing resins are drugs used to prevent arrhythmias from occurring. These resins bind with potassium and allow it to be excreted. The prototype and sole drug in this class is sodium polystyrene sulfonate (Kayexalate).

NURSING MANAGEMENT OF THE PATIENT RECEIVING SODIUM POLYSTYRENE SULFONATE

Core Drug Knowledge

Pharmacotherapeutics

Sodium polystyrene sulfonate is a potassium-removing resin used in treating hyperkalemia. It can be given orally or as an enema (Table 29-7).

TABLE 29-7 Potassium-Removing Resin

Drug (Trade) Name	Selected Indications	Route and Dosage Range	Pharmacokinetics
sodium polystyrene sulfonate (Kayexalate)	Treatment of hypokalemia	*Adult:* PO, 15 g 1–4 × day *Child:* PO 1 g/kg q6h *Adult:* Enema, 30–50 g q6h	*Onset:* PO, 2–12 h Enema, >12 h *Duration:* unknown $t_{1/2}$: unknown

Pharmacokinetics

The exchange of potassium ions after administration of sodium polystyrene sulfonate occurs in the large intestine. The drug is not absorbed systemically and is excreted through the GI tract. The onset of action after oral administration is 2 to 12 hours; after rectal administration, onset of action takes more time, although exact numbers are unknown (see Table 29-7).

Pharmacodynamics

As sodium polystyrene sulfonate moves through the intestine or is maintained in the intestine, it releases sodium ions that are replaced with potassium ions. The efficiency of this process is limited and unpredictable. The ion exchange capacity is approximately 1 mEq potassium/g of drug. Small amounts of calcium and magnesium also can be lost during the exchange process. Effective lowering of serum potassium may take several hours or days.

Contraindications and Precautions

Caution must be used when giving this drug to anyone who cannot tolerate a small increase in sodium intake, such as patients with severe CHF, hypertension, or marked edema. Because therapeutic effects are slow, this drug generally should not be used in patients with severe hyperkalemia in whom the hyperkalemia poses a medical emergency.

Adverse Effects

Hypokalemia may result from therapy and is the most serious adverse effect. Other electrolyte imbalances that may result include hypocalcemia and hypernatremia. Common adverse GI-related and include gastric irritation, anorexia, nausea, vomiting, and constipation. The constipation occasionally may be severe and cause fecal impaction. Diarrhea occurs occasionally.

Drug Interactions

When administered with nonabsorbable cation-donating antacids and laxatives, such as magnesium hydroxide and aluminum carbonate, systemic alkalosis can occur.

Assessment of Relevant Core Patient Variables

Health Status

The nurse should monitor the patient's serum potassium level, and if severely elevated, the patientNMs total physiologic condition and ECG should be reviewed. The nurse also needs to determine whether the patient has been receiving potassium supplements or replacements in IV fluids.

Life Span and Gender

The nurse should note the patient's age before administering sodium polystyrene sulfonate. Large doses of sodium polystyrene sulfonate can cause fecal impaction in elderly patients.

Lifestyle, Diet, and Habits

It is important to investigate the patient's dietary history and preferences, particularly if the patient normally consumes a potassium-rich diet.

Environment

The nurse should be aware that sodium polystyrene sulfonate is administered in the hospital.

Nursing Diagnoses and Outcomes

- Risk for Constipation related to adverse effects of drug therapy
  Desired outcome: Constipation will be prevented in the patient by administering sorbitol, orally or rectally, if warranted.
- Potential complication: hypokalemia.
  Desired outcome: Patient's potassium level will be lowered only to the normal range.

Planning and Intervention

Maximizing Therapeutic Effects

The nurse should clear the GI tract with a cleansing enema before administering the drug by enema. For adults, insert a soft large (28 French) rubber tube about

20 cm into the rectum. The nurse should mix the resin in an aqueous vehicle, such as 100-mL sorbitol or 20% dextrose to make a suspension; and infuse the drug by gravity. During infusion, it is important to stir the fluid to keep the particles in suspension.

After the fluid has run into the patient, the nurse should flush the tube with 50- to 100-mL fluid to make a total of 150- to 200-mL fluid as infused. It is important to clamp the tube and leave in place 30 minutes minimally but preferably several hours (keeping the solution in the colon allows the resin to work).

If back leakage develops, the nurse should elevate the patient's hips on pillows or have patient assume a knee-chest position temporarily. These positions will help keep the solution in the sigmoid colon.

The nurse should irrigate the colon using a Y tube connection with approximately 2 L of a nonsodium flushing solution at body temperature to remove resin. The Y tube allows the returns to drain as the colon is being irrigated.

When the drug is administered orally, the nurse should create a suspension of the powdered formula with water or syrup for greater palatability.

Minimizing Adverse Effects

If the potassium serum level is severely elevated, the nurse should use other methods to reduce potassium (sodium polystyrene sulfonate alone may be insufficient to correct an imbalance before a medical emergency occurs). Other methods include the use of IV calcium to antagonize the effect of hyperkalemia on the heart; IV sodium bicarbonate, glucose, insulin to cause an intracellular shift of potassium; and dialysis.

The nurse should monitor serum electrolytes for changes in potassium and other electrolytes. It also is important to monitor the ECG for changes indicative of hypokalemia (i.e., lengthened QT interval; widening, flattening, or inversion of T wave; prominent U waves; and arrhythmias).

The nurse should monitor the pulse rate for arrhythmias and irregularities. It is a good idea to administer sorbitol, orally or rectally, to prevent constipation if warranted.

Providing Patient and Family Education

- The nurse should explain the therapeutic and possible adverse effects of the drug.
- It is important to emphasize the importance of repeated blood work to monitor blood electrolyte concentrations.

Ongoing Assessment and Evaluation

The nurse should monitor serum electrolytes throughout therapy. The nurse will assess for signs of hypokalemia and monitor the patient's pulse and ECG periodically throughout therapy. Therapy is considered effective in patients whose serum potassium levels return to normal and who do not develop cardiac arrhythmias from hyperkalemia or hypokalemia, hypokalemia, or other electrolyte imbalances.

MEMORY CHIP

Sodium Polystyrene Sulfonate

- Used to lower serum potassium levels
- Given orally or as enema
- Significant contraindication: extremely high potassium levels
- Most common adverse effects: related to gastrointestinal system
- Most serious adverse effect: hypokalemia
- Maximizing therapeutic effects: give a cleansing enema first (if drug is given as enema); and leave resin in place at least 30 minutes after administering as enema
- Minimizing adverse effects: monitor serum electrolytes and electrocardiogram

CHAPTER SUMMARY

- Antiarrhythmics restore normal rhythm and rate by varied mechanisms.
- All drugs given to treat an arrhythmia also may cause an arrhythmia.
- Class I drugs block the influx of sodium in the myocardial membrane. They are local anesthetics or membrane stabilizing agents that depress phase 0 of the action potential.
- Quinidine, a Class I antiarrhythmic, is used for treating atrial fibrillation and flutter. Quinidine depresses myocardial excitability, conduction velocity, and contractility. The effective refractory period is prolonged, increasing conduction time. Reentry phenomenon is therefore prevented. Quinidine also exerts an indirect anticholinergic effect; it decreases vagal tone and may promote conduction in the AV junction.
- Potassium enhances the effect of quinidine, and hypokalemia will reduce the effectiveness.
- Class IB antiarrhythmics depress phase 0 of the action potential, but not as much as Class IA drugs do. They also suppress automaticity. Like quinidine, these drugs may also cause arrhythmias, in addition to treating them. Unlike quinidine, they are used primarily with ventricular arrhythmias, and . they may shorten the action potential duration. Lidocaine is a Class IB drug; it may be used with all acute ventricular arrhythmias that occur related to cardiac surgery or acute myocardial infarction.
- Class IC antiarrhythmics also depress phase 0 but markedly so. In addition, they have a slight effect on repolarization and decrease conduction significantly. They have been found to increase mortality significantly when used in patients who have had a myocardial infarction.
- All Class I antiarrhythmics have the potential to increase mortality; none have been proved to decrease mortality
- Class II antiarrhythmics block the beta-1 and beta-2 adrenergic receptors and stabilize the cardiac cell membranes. They depress phase 4 depolarization.

- Propranolol, a beta blocker and Class II antiarrhythmic, is used to treat supraventricular, ventricular, and tachyarrhythmias secondary to digoxin toxicity or due to excessive catecholamine action during anesthesia.
- Propranolol slows the sinus heart rate, depresses AV conduction, decreases cardiac output, reduces systolic and diastolic blood pressure at rest and on exercise, and reduces supine and standing blood pressure.
- Class II antiarrhythmics are the only antiarrhythmics that have been shown to decrease mortality.
- Class III drugs slow heart action by prolonging the action potential or myocardial repolarization (prolonged phase 3).
- Amiodarone, a Class III antiarrhythmic, is used to treat life-threatening ventricular arrhythmias. It also has actions from other classifications. These diverse actions of amiodarone are why the drug is being considered as potentially appropriate for treating atrial fibrillation as well.
- Amiodarone has unusual pharmacokinetic and pharmacodynamic properties. These unique effects include incomplete bioavailability, distribution to multiple tissue sites, extreme lipid solubility, biotransformation to an active metabolite, and extremely slow elimination of amiodarone and its metabolite. These effects may be attributable to genetic variations, although this is not known positively at this time. Because of these unique effects, the effect on patients is variable.
- Adverse effects of amiodarone can be serious and potentially fatal. The patient needs to be monitored closely while receiving it.
- Class IV drugs alter the action potential, decrease AV conduction, and prolong repolarization by inhibiting the influx of calcium in cardiac muscle cells. A few calcium-channel blocker drugs are in this class.
- Verapamil, a calcium-channel blocker and Class IV antiarrhythmic, controls ventricular rate in chronic atrial flutter or fibrillation (used in conjunction with digoxin). It is also used prophylactically for repetitive paroxysmal SVT. IV verapamil is used to treat SVT.
- Verapamil also is used in treating angina (including Prinzmetal angina) and hypertension.
- Sodium polystyrene sulfonate is a potassium-removing resin used in treating hyperkalemia. Because hyperkalemia may lead to cardiac arrhythmias, this drug prevents arrhythmias from occurring.
- Sodium polystyrene sulfonate is given orally or as an enema.
- Although sodium polystyrene sulfonate is in the GI tract, sodium ions are exchanged for potassium ions, which are then excreted in the stool. Onset is slow and unpredictable. Therefore, if the serum potassium level is quite elevated, other mechanisms of lowering the potassium level should be used.

QUESTIONS FOR STUDY AND REVIEW

1. Why are ventricular arrhythmias considered potentially life threatening?
2. What is meant by proarrhythmia?
3. Why do all antiarrhythmics have proarrhythmic qualities?
4. Describe the phase of the action potential affected by Class I, Class II, Class III, and Class IV antiarrhythmics.
5. Quinidine, a Class IA drug, is used to treat which type of arrhythmias?
6. Describe the clinical applications for beta blockers?
7. Why is a loading dose (or doses) necessary to administer when using the Class III drug amiodarone?
8. What suggestions can the nurse give to a patient taking verapamil, a Class IV antiarrhythmic, to prevent constipation?

NEED MORE HELP?

? Chapter 29 of the study guide for *Drug Therapy in Nursing* contains exercises and activities to reinforce your understanding of the concepts presented in this chapter. For additional information, see the text's accompanying web site at *http://www.connection.lww.com.*

REFERENCES AND BIBLIOGRAPHY

Borchard, U., & Hafner, D. (2000). Ion channels and arrhythmias [original in German]. *Zeitschrift für Kardiologie, 89,* (Suppl. 3), 6–12.

Cam, A. J., & Yap, Y. G. (1999). What should we expect from the next generation of antiarrhythmic drugs? *Journal of Cardiovascular Electrophysiology, 10*(2), 307–317.

Drug Facts and Comparisons. (2000). St. Louis: Facts and Comparisons.

Epstein, A. E., Hallstrom, A. P., Rogers, W. J., Liebson, P. R., Seals, A. A., Anderson, J. L., Cohen, J. D., Capon, R. J., & Wyse, D. G. (1993). Mortality following ventricular arrhythmic suppression by encainide, flecainide, and moricizine after myocardial infarction. The original design concept of the cardiac arrhythmia suppression Trial (CAST). *Journal of the American Medical Association, 270*(20), 2451–2455.

Goldschlager, N., Epstein, A. E., Naccarelli, G., Olshansky, B. & Singh, B. (2000) Practical guidelines for clinicians who treat patients with amiodarone. Practice Guidelines Subcommittee, North American society of Pacing and Electrophysiology. *Archives of Internal Medicine 160*(12), 1741–1748.

Incze, A., Frigy, A., & Cotoi, S. (1998). The efficacy of sublingual verapamil in controlling rapid ventricular rate in chronic atrial fibrillation. *Romanian Journal of Internal Medicine, 36*(3–4), 219–225.

Joseph, A. P., & Ward, M. R. (2000). A prospective, randomized controlled trial comparing the efficacy and safety of sotalol, amiodarone, and digoxin for the reversion of new- onset atrial fibrillation. *Annals of Emergency Medicine, 36*(1), 1–9.

Kodama, I., Kamiya, K., & Toyama, J. (1999). Amiodarone: Ionic and cellular mechanisms of action of the most promising Class III agent. *The American Journal of Cardiology, 84,* 20R–28R.

Koup, J. R., Abel, R. B., Smithers, J. A., Eldon, M. A., & deVries, T. M. (1998). Effect of age, gender, and race on steady state procainamide pharmacokinetics after administration of procanbid sustained release tablets. *Therapeutic Drug Monitoring, 20*(1), 73–77.

Kowey, P. R. (1998). Pharmacological effects of antiarrhythmic drugs. Review and update. *Archives of Internal Medicine, 158*(4), 325–332.

Nattel, S., & Singh, B. (1999). Evolution, mechanisms, and classification of antiarrhythmic drugs:focus on Class III actions. *The American Journal of Cardiology, 84,* 11R–19R.

Oudijk, M. A., Michon, N. M., Kleinmna, C. S., Kapusta, L., Stoutenbeek, P., Visser, G. H., & Meijboom, E. J. (2000). Sotalol in the treatment of fetal dysrhythmias. *Circulation, 101*(23), 2721–2726.

Paul, T., Bertram, H., Bokenkamp, R., & Hausdorf, G. (2000). Supraventricular tachycardia in infants, children, and adolescents [in German]. *Paediatric Drugs, 2*(3), 171–181.

Pollak, P. T., & Tan, M. H. (1999). Elevations of high-density lipoprotein cholesterol in humans during long term therapy with amiodarone. *The American Journal of Cardiology, 83,* 296–300.

Prystowsky, E. N. (2000). Management of atrial fibrillation: Therapeutic options and clinical decisions. *The American Journal of Cardiology, 85*(10A), 3D–11D.

Reiffel, J. A. (2000). Drug choices in the treatment of atrial fibrillation. *The American Journal of Cardiology, 85*(10A), 12D–19D.

Roden, D. M. (1999). Mechanisms underlying variability in response to drug therapy: implications for amiodarone use. *The American Journal of Cardiology, 84,* 29R–36R.

Singh, B. N. (1999a). Introduction to a supplement for The American Journal of Cardiology. *The American Journal of Cardiology, 84*(9A), 1R–2R.

Singh, B. N., (1999b). Overview of trends in the control of cardiac arrhythmia: Past and future. *The American Journal of Cardiology, 84*(9A), 3R–10R.

Singh, B. N., Mody, F. V., Lopez, B., & Sarma, J. S. M. (1999). Antiarrhythmic agents for atrial fibrillation: Focus on prolonging atrial repolarization. *The American Journal of Cardiology, 84,* 161R–173R.

The Cardiac Arrhythmia Suppression Trial (CAST) Investigators. (1989). Preliminary report: Effect of encainide and flecainide on mortality in a randomized trial of arrhythmia suppression after myocardial infarction. *The New England Journal of Medicine, 321,* 406–412.

Vardas, P. E., Kochiadakis, G. E., Igoumenidid, N. E., Tsatsakis, A. M., Simantirakis, E. N., & Chlouverakis, G. I. (2000). Amiodarone as a first-choice drug for restoring sinus rhythm in patients with atrial fibrillation: A randomized, controlled study. *Chest, 117*(6), 1538–1545.

Waldo, A. L., & Prystowsky, E. N. (1998). Drug treatment of atrial fibrillation in the managed care era. *American Journal of Cardiology, 81*(5A), 230–290.

Weirich, J., & Wenzel, Q. (2000). Current classification of anti-arrhythmia agents [in German]. *Zeitschrift für Kardiologie, 89*(Suppl. 3), 62–67.

Wooten, J. M., Earnest, J., & Reyes, J. (2000). Review of common adverse effects of selected antiarrhythmic drugs. *Critical Care Nursing Quarterly, 22*(4), 23–38.

Chapter 30

DRUGS AFFECTING BLOOD PRESSURE

KEY TERMS

diastolic blood pressure
essential hypertension
hypertension
hypertensive crisis
primary hypertension
renin-angiotensin-aldosterone system
secondary hypertension
shock
stepped-care approach
sympatholytic
sympathomimetic
systolic blood pressure

Learning Objectives

At the completion of this chapter the student will:

1. Describe stepped therapy as it is used in treating hypertension.
2. Identify the core drug knowledge for drugs that affect blood pressure.
3. Differentiate the antihypertensive drug classes.
4. Identify core patient variables relevant to drugs that affect blood pressure.
5. Relate the interaction of core drug knowledge to core patient variables for drugs that affect blood pressure.
6. Generate a nursing plan of care from the interaction between core drug knowledge and core patient variables for drugs that affect blood pressure.
7. Describe nursing interventions to maximize therapeutic effects and minimize adverse effects for drugs that affect blood pressure.
8. Determine key points for patient and family education for drugs that affect blood pressure.

Antihypertensives

Beta blockers
see Chapter 14

Diuretics
see Chapter 31

ACE inhibitors

- **captopril**
- benazepril
- enalapril
- enalaprilat
- fosinopril
- lisinopril
- moexipril
- quinapril
- ramipril
- trandolapril
- perinatopril

Angiotensin II receptor antagonists

- **losartan**

Alpha-beta blockers

- **labetalol**
- carvedilol

Centrally acting alpha-2 agonists

- **clonidine**
- guanabenz
- guanfacine

Peripherally acting alpha-1 blockers

- prazosin
- terazosin
- doxazosin

Peripherally acting antiadrenergics

- reserpine
- guanethidine
- guanadrel

Direct acting vasodilators

- **hydralazine**
- epoprostenol
- minoxidil

Drugs used in hypertensive crisis

- **nitroprusside**
- diazoxide
- fenoldopam mesylate
- trimethaphan
- phentolamine
- phenoxybenzamine
- metyrosine

Vasopressors

Drugs used in shock

- **dopamine**
- dobutamine
- epinephrine
- norepinephrine
- isoproterenol
- ephedrine
- mephentermine
- metaraminol
- methoxamine
- phenylephrine
- midodrine

The symbol (C) indicates the **drug class**.

Drugs in bold type marked with the symbol (P) are **prototypes**.

Drugs in blue type with no symbol are **closely related** to the prototype.

Drugs in **red** type with no symbol are **significantly different** from the prototype.

Drugs in **black** type with no symbol are **also used in drug therapy**; no prototype.

Hypertension occurs when systolic or diastolic blood pressure is elevated beyond normal ranges over time. If lifestyle changes are not enough to bring the blood pressure back into normal range, antihypertensive drugs are used to restore blood pressure to normal levels and to prevent the adverse effects of hypertension. The main drug classes used to treat hypertension are diuretics, beta blockers, calcium channel blockers, angiotensin-converting enzyme (ACE) inhibitors, angiotensin II receptor antagonists, alpha-2 stimulators, alpha-beta blockers, and direct vasodilators. Although many of these drug classes have multiple therapeutic indications, this chapter focuses on their capacity as antihypertensives. Diuretics, beta blockers, and calcium-channel blockers and their prototypes are discussed in greater depth elsewhere in the text. The prototype for ACE inhibitors is captopril (Capoten).

The prototype angiotensin II receptor antagonist is losartan (Cozaar). The prototype alpha-2 stimulator is clonidine. Two groups of drugs are considered significantly different from the alpha-2 stimulator prototype, clonidine. These are the peripherally acting alpha-1 blockers and the peripherally acting antiadrenergics. The category of peripherally acting alpha-1 blockers includes prazosin (Minipress), terazosin (Hytrin), and doxazosin (Cardura). The peripherally acting antiadrenergics are composed of reserpine (Serpalan), guanethidine (Ismelin) and guanadrel (Hylorel).

The prototype alpha-beta blocker is labetalol (Normodyne, Trandate). Another drug in the class, carvedilol (Coreg) also is used in the treatment of congestive heart failure (CHF) and is discussed further in Chapter 27. Hydralazine (Apresoline) is the prototypical direct-acting vasodilator. Drugs significantly different from the prototype are minoxidil (Loniten) and epoprostenol (Flolan).

This chapter also examines drugs used to treat hypertensive crises. The prototype drug used to treat hypertensive crises is nitroprusside. Drugs closely related to nitroprusside are diazoxide (Hyperstat), fenoldopam (Corlopam), and trimethaphan (Arfonad).

Finally, this chapter examines drugs used to raise blood pressure during shock, the vasopressors. The prototype vasopressor is dopamine (Intropin). Drugs similar to dopamine include: dobutamine (Dobutrex), norepinephrine (Levophed), isoproterenol (Isuprel), epinephrine, ephedrine, mephentermine (Wyamine), and metaraminol (Aramine). Drugs significantly different from dopamine include: phenylephrine (Neosynephrine), and midodrine (ProAmatine). Isoproterenol, epinephrine, ephedrine, and phenylephrine all are discussed in more depth in Chapter 14.

PHYSIOLOGY

Contractions of the heart propel blood through the vascular system. Each contraction increases outflow from the heart and pushes along the volume of blood already in the systemic circulation. As the blood moves through the circulatory system, the tightness or constriction (tension) of the vessels provides resistance. Arterial pressure, which results from these forces, is measured as blood pressure. The highest pressure is achieved during systole (when the heart contracts and ejects blood into the circulation). This is known as **systolic blood pressure.** The lowest pressure that can be measured is achieved during diastole (when the heart relaxes and fills with blood and the vessels propel the blood already in circulation). This is known as **diastolic blood pressure.**

Blood pressure is measured in millimeters of mercury (mmHg) and is calculated by measuring the amount of blood leaving the heart multiplied by the amount of resistance in the peripheral vessels. The formula for measuring blood pressure is blood pressure = cardiac output × peripheral resistance, or $BP = CO \times PR$ (Fig. 30-1).

When cardiac output or peripheral resistance increases, blood pressure increases. When cardiac output or peripheral resistance decreases, blood pressure decreases. Several innate mechanisms regulate blood pressure by affecting either cardiac output or peripheral resistance.

ROLE OF ADRENERGIC RECEPTORS

Adrenergic receptors in the nervous system have a role in blood pressure management. Adrenergic receptors are grouped into receptor sites–alpha-1, alpha-2, beta-1, and beta-2. When alpha-1 receptors are stimulated, they cause peripheral constriction, and blood pressure increases as a result. This effect, which is similar to stimulation of the sympathetic nerves, is called a **sympathomimetic** effect (mimicking the effect of the sympathetic system). Conversely, blockage of these receptor sites dilates resistance vessels (arterioles) and capacitance vessels (veins) and thus decreases pressure.

Alpha-2 receptor sites are located within the brain. Their stimulation inhibits the sympathetic system, causing a **sympatholytic** effect (stopping the effect of the sympathetic system). The resulting reduction in sympathetic outflow from the central nervous system (CNS) has two effects. It decreases the heart rate and, therefore, cardiac output. It also decreases vasoconstriction, which reduces peripheral resistance. The effect from both of these actions is a decrease in blood pressure.

Beta-1 receptor sites are located primarily in the heart. Stimulation of beta-1 receptor sites increases the heart rate, the speed of cardiac conduction, and the force of cardiac contraction. Cardiac output is increased, thus increasing blood pressure.

Beta-2 receptor sites are located primarily in the bronchial and vascular musculature. Stimulation of these sites induces bronchial and peripheral dilation. The peripheral dilation contributes to decreased blood pressure by decreasing peripheral resistance. If both beta-1 and beta-2 receptor sites are stimulated equally and simultaneously, the effect on blood pressure is negligible. (See Chapter 14 for more information about adrenergic receptors.)

ROLE OF VASOCONSTRICTORS

Another mechanism involved in blood pressure regulation is the renin-angiotensin-aldosterone system. Renin, which is synthesized by the kidneys, produces angiotensin I. Angiotensin I is a basically inactive substance until it is converted to the active angiotensin II by a special enzyme, ACE. Angiotensin II also is formed from various alternative pathways and also at the cellular level, thus there is an autocrine

Physiology

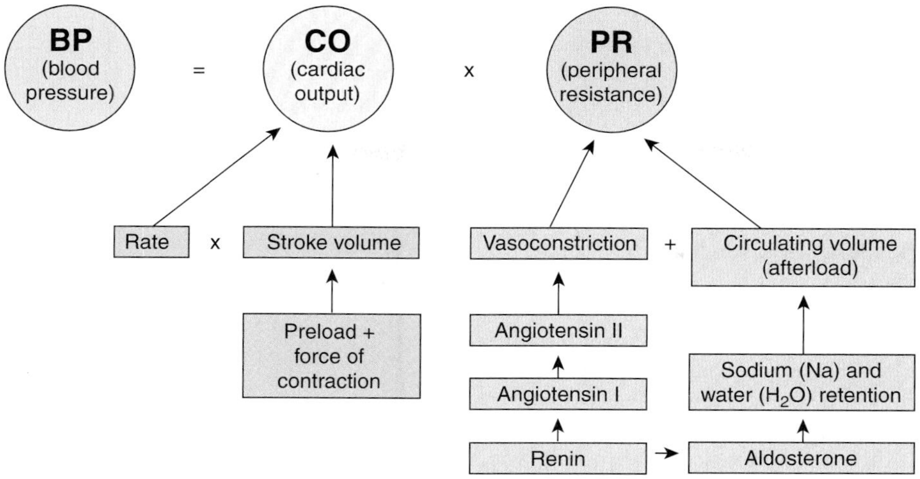

Figure 30-1. Mechanisms involved in regulating blood pressure. To alter blood pressure, either cardiac output or peripheral vascular resistance must change. The ideal is a balance between them. Some antihypertensive drugs alter cardiac output, and some change vascular resistance.

tissue renin-angiotensin system (RAS) (Meggs & Kodali, 1999). Angiotensin II is a potent vasoconstrictor. It also stimulates the secretion of aldosterone from the adrenal medulla. Aldosterone increases the retention of sodium and water in the body, which, in turn, increases circulating volume. The resulting vasoconstriction and increased circulating volume raise blood pressure by increasing peripheral resistance and cardiac output. When hypertension is present, angiotensin II also has been implicated in pathologic cell growth and cell death, and in the fundamental events that occur in the remodeling of the vascular wall and the myocardium (Meggs & Kodali, 1999).

PATHOPHYSIOLOGY

In the United States, hypertension is a chronic disorder that affects an estimated 40 million people, or 1 in 4 adults (Meggs & Kodali, 1999). One third of these people do not realize that they have high blood pressure (the American Heart Association www.americanheart.org). Hypertension is common to all racial groups, although some groups are more prone to hypertension than others. In the United States, American Indians have about the same, or somewhat higher, incidence of hypertension than the general population. Hispanics have generally the same, or a lower, rate than non-Hispanic whites, but African Americans have the highest rate. Compared with white Americans, African-Americans have an earlier onset, higher prevalence, and greater rate of stage 3 hypertension. These reasons explain why African Americans also have an 80% higher stroke mortality rate, a 50% higher heart disease mortality rate, and a 320% greater rate of hypertension-related end-stage renal disease compared with the general population (JNC-VI, 1997).

Women who take oral contraceptives have a small increase in both systolic and diastolic pressures, although the blood pressure usually continues to remain within the normal range. However, women who take oral contraceptives, smoke, and are over 35 years of age do experience hypertension. It is three times more common in this group than in women without these risk factors. High blood pressure is extremely common in older adults. Depending on their race, between almost two thirds and nearly three quarters of older adult Americans have hypertension. Older adults often are responsive to lifestyle changes, and this should be tried before drug therapy. Hypertension also is now a problem in children and adolescents due to high rates of childhood obesity, with accompanying lack of exercise and increasing prevalence of type I diabetes.

The American Heart Association defines hypertension as persistent elevation of systolic pressure equal to or greater than 140 mmHg or diastolic pressure equal to or greater than 90 mmHg. The diastolic pressure is based on the fifth Korotkov sound, which is the disappearance of sound. This criterion is now used for all age groups. Many factors, from exercise to stress to a variation in normal sodium intake, may increase blood pressure temporarily. Therefore, a definitive diagnosis of hypertension is not made until the average of two or more readings, each recorded at two or more visits, reveal persistent elevations (JCN-VI, 1997). There are two main categories of hypertension: primary hypertension and secondary hypertension. **Primary hypertension,** also known as essential hypertension, is responsible for 90% to 95% of all hypertension; secondary hypertension accounts for the remaining percentage. Primary hypertension has no identified cause. However, it can be managed successfully with drug therapy to prevent the adverse effects of hypertension. Risk factors associated with the development of primary hypertension include elevated blood lipid levels, smoking, diabetes, age older than 60 years, gender (male and postmenopausal women), and family history of cardiovascular disease (women younger than 65 years or men younger than 55 years).

Secondary hypertension occurs secondary to another condition, such as renal stenosis or renal tumor. Therapy aims to correct or remove the underlying cause. If this therapy is successful, the secondary hypertension will be eliminated. However, when the cause cannot be treated successfully, antihypertensive agents are used to control the blood pressure.

Hypertension, if untreated, can lead to stroke, myocardial infarction (MI), kidney disease, CHF, and even death. These diseases and disorders result from several physiologic changes. Persistently elevated pressure constricts the arterioles, which increases peripheral vascular resistance. This increases the workload of the left ventricle, which results in ventricular hypertrophy. The myocardium must work ever harder to overcome the increased resistance to outflow. Hence, the demand for oxygen increases. Eventually, the heart can compensate no longer and CHF results. At least 50% of people with untreated hypertension will develop CHF. Hypertension is the most common risk factor for CHF in the population (Himmelmann, 1999). Yet, as stated before, many people do not realize they have high blood pressure, and therefore do not seek any medical attention and their hypertension remains uncontrolled.

Another change resulting from persistent hypertension is a sclerosing (thickening and hardening) of the blood vessel wall, which narrows the blood vessel's lumen. The narrowed lumen inhibits blood flow, leading to decreased organ perfusion and, possibly, arterial thrombosis and tissue ischemia. Tissues at the greatest risk for damage include the brain, heart, eyes, and kidneys.

One study has shown recently that there is increased risk of late-age Alzheimer disease if hypertension is present and untreated in mid-life. Over 3,700 Japanese-American men were followed in the Honolulu Heart Program. Elevated, untreated blood pressure was found to be associated with dementia, although this was not true if the blood pressure was treated with antihypertensives (Launer, Ross, Petrovitch, Masaki, Foley, White, et al., 2000). Whether these results can be generalized to other races or to women is not known at this time.

People with primary hypertension are relatively symptom free for a long time. Hypertension often is detected initially at an incidental blood pressure screening or a during a routine physical examination. Because it is painless and symptom free, primary hypertension often remains undiagnosed until the symptoms of end-organ damage surface.

Hypertension is classified according to the degree of elevation. The treatment guidelines for hypertension from both the U.S. Sixth Joint National Committee on Prevention, Detection, Evaluation, and Treatment of High Blood Pressure (JNC-VI) and the joint report of the World Health Organization and the International Society of Hypertension (WHO/ISH) have similar classifications of hypertension. The major difference in the classifications is in the terminology. JNC-VI uses Stages 1, 2, and 3 whereas the WHO/ISH uses Grades 1 (mild), 2 (moderate), and 3 (severe) JNC-VI dropped the term mild, because it was believed that this led practitioners and patients not to treat the condition seriously. The WHO/ISH considered that the term "stages" indicates that blood pressure always progresses from one level to another and that this was misleading. Table 30-1 shows the classifications of blood pressure for individuals 18 years and older. If the systolic and diastolic blood pressure readings are in different categories, then the classification is based on the higher values.

HYPERTENSIVE CRISIS

When the patient's blood pressure is elevated acutely, the condition is termed a hypertensive crisis. This situation is defined as systolic blood pressure exceeding 210 mmHg and diastolic blood pressure exceeding 120 mmHg. When this occurs, and the patient is in danger of rapidly developing damage to one of the vital organs, such as the brain, heart, or kidneys, it is considered an emergency. The situation requires immediate assessment and intervention. The priority is to reduce the blood pressure as quickly as can be managed safely to prevent injury. Blood pressure does not need to be reduced to a normal level immediately. Although the pressure must be reduced, it must stay high enough to maintain perfusion of vital organs. The initial goal of treatment in hypertensive emergencies is to reduce the blood pressure by no more than 25% within minutes and up to 2 hours. Then it should be reduced toward 160/100 within 2 to 6 hours. The purpose of the gradual reduction is to avoid excessive falls in pressure that could induce renal, cerebral, or coronary ischemia (JNC-IV, 1997). The exact level of pressure reduction depends on patient-related variables.

TABLE 30-1 Blood Pressure and Hypertension Categories

Category	Systolic Pressure (mmHg)	Diastolic Pressure (mmHg)
Optimal	<120	<80
Normal blood pressure	<130	<85
High normal blood pressure	130–139	85–89
Stage 1 hypertension*/ grade 1 (mild) hypertension†	140–159	90–99
Stage 2 hypertension*/ grade 2 (moderate) hypertension†	160–179	100–109
Stage 3 hypertension*/ grade 3 (severe) hypertension†	≥180	≥110

*Joint National Committee on Detection, Evaluation, and Treatment of High Blood Pressure. (1997). Sixth report of the Joint National Committee on Detection, Evaluation, and Treatment of High Blood Pressure. *Archives of Internal Medicine, 157*, 2413–2446.

† World Health Organization: International Society of Hypertension (1999). Guidelines subcommittee of the World Health Organization: International Society of Hypertension (WHO-ISH) Mild Hypertension committee. 1999 World Health Organization: International Society of Hypertension Guidelines for the Management of Hypertension. Geneva: Author.

Hypertensive crisis may be caused by an ongoing condition, such as hypertensive encephalopathy, cerebral hemorrhage, eclampsia, pheochromocytoma (a tumor of the adrenal medulla), dissecting aortic aneurysm, unstable angina pectoris, acute MI, or acute left ventricular failure with pulmonary edema. It also could be induced from a drug-food interaction; for example, when monoamine oxidase inhibitors (MAOIs) are prescribed as drug therapy and tyramine-rich food is eaten. The symptoms manifest are acute and include decreased level of consciousness, neurologic deficits, decreased renal output, vomiting, and severe headache (cephalalgia). Emergencies initially are treated with IV administration of an appropriate agent for rapid onset.

A hypertensive crisis that is less serious is where it is desirable to reduce the blood pressure within a few hours, but in which there is no imminent risk for target organ damage. This is termed a hypertensive urgency. Examples of hypertensive urgencies are upper levels of stage 3 hypertension, hypertension with optic disc edema, and severe perioperative hypertension (JNC-IV, 1997). Urgent situations may be treated with oral doses of drugs with relatively fast onset of action, including loop diuretics, beta-blockers, ACE inhibitors, alpha-2 agonists, or calcium-channel blockers.

STEPPED-CARE APPROACH TO HYPERTENSION

The stepped-care approach to hypertension is based on the patient's response to therapy. A patient's therapy may be "stepped up" if she is nonresponsive or "stepped down" if the patient shows signs of good blood pressure control over time (Fig. 30-2). This approach reflects lifestyle modifications in addition to a progressive drug therapy approach. In step 1, hypertension is managed by lifestyle changes alone. These include reducing weight, restricting dietary intake of saturated fat, modifying alcohol intake, exercising regularly, reducing sodium intake, and stopping smoking (see the accompanying display, Lifestyle and Blood Pressure Control). Lifestyle changes also are believed to be essential in preventing hypertension, and patients should be encouraged to adopt them, especially if risk factors for cardiovascular disease are present.

A recent study examined the benefit of exercise alone versus exercise with weight control in decreasing hypertension. Both groups had reductions in their blood pressure, but the reduction was greater for the group that had aerobic exercise in combination with weight loss. Additionally, both groups showed decreased peripheral resistance, with the greatest decrease again being with the group that lost weight and exercised (Blumenthal, Sherwood, Gullette, Babyak, Waugh, Georgiades, et al., 2000).

All step 1 measures should be initiated before drug therapy is tried. This is true for patients with high normal blood pressure, or stage I as long as there is no target organ damage, clinical cardiovascular disease, and no more than one risk factor present. If these conditions are not met, or if the patient has stage 2 or 3 blood pressure, drug therapy is started at the same time as lifestyle modifications.

Based on the JNC-VI guidelines, if blood pressure remains at 140/90 or more after 6 to 12 months of lifestyle modification, the patient proceeds to step 2 and starts antihypertensive drug therapy. Lifestyle modification continues even when

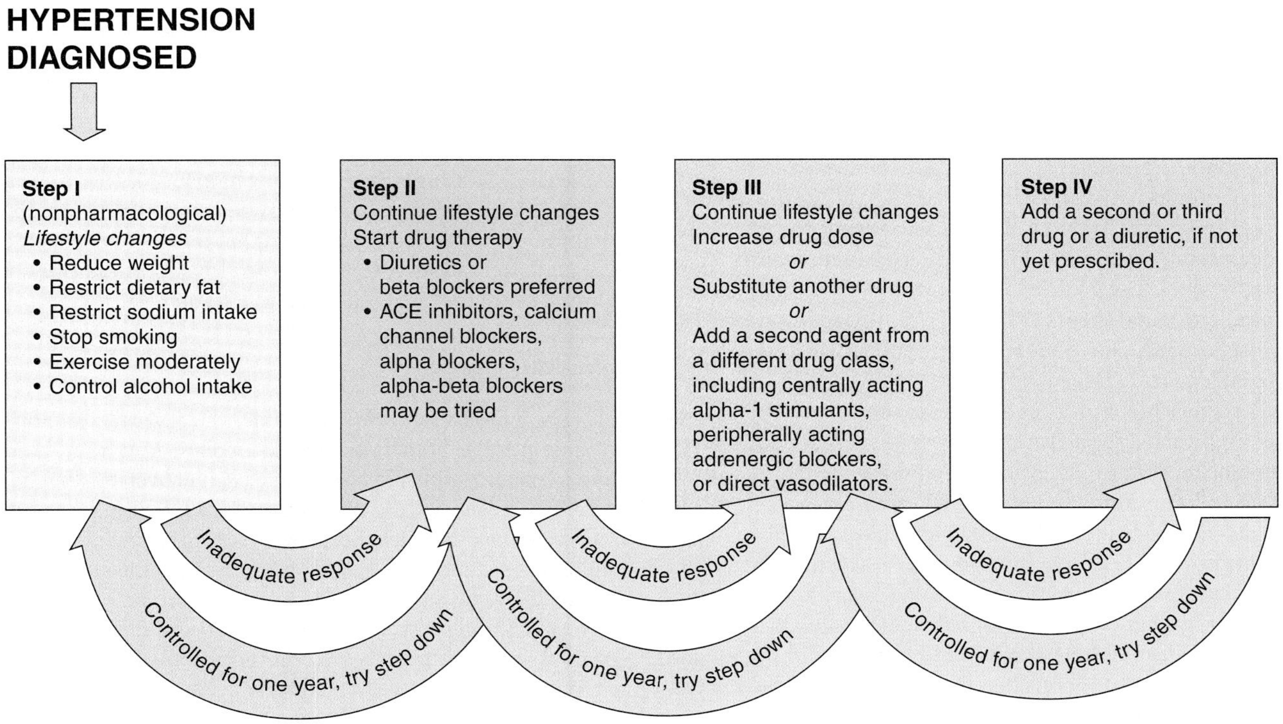

Figure 30-2. Steps in treating hypertension.

Focus on Research

Lifestyle and blood pressure control

Kim, M. T., Dennison, C. R., Hill, M. N., Bone, L. R. & Levine, D. M. (2000). Relationship of alcohol and illicit drug use with high blood pressure care and control among urban hypertensive black men. *Ethnicity and Disease, 10*(2), 175–183.

The Study

Baseline cross-sectional data from an ongoing study of the effectiveness of a high blood pressure care program was studied and described. Black urban men requiring treatment for their hypertension and who also consume alcohol and illicit drugs had different characteristics than hypertensive black urban men who did not abuse substances. Men who consumed alcohol and used illicit drugs were less likely to have medical insurance or a physician for their high blood pressure care, to engage in critical patient behaviors needed for blood pressure control, to receive antihypertensive drug therapy, or to comply with drug therapy if prescribed. Alcohol consumers and illicit drug users were more likely to have the lifestyle variations of eating a high fat/high salt diet and smoking cigarettes than nonusers. Men who abused alcohol or illicit drugs were significantly more likely to have uncontrolled blood pressure and higher systolic blood pressure.

Nursing Implications

Blood pressure was poorly controlled in black, urban hypertensive men who abuse alcohol or illicit drugs. It would be important for the nurse to assess for these lifestyle habits when beginning a patient on drug therapy for hypertension. Additional patient education or counseling may be necessary, as well as securing treatment for alcohol and drug use, as part of comprehensive high blood pressure care.

the patient "steps up" to drug therapy. Lifestyle modifications may decrease the dosage required in drug therapy (Fig. 30-3).

The decision to start drug therapy is based on consideration of several factors, including the degree of blood pressure elevation, the presence of target organ damage, and the presence of clinical cardiovascular disease or other risk factors. Drug therapy for treating hypertension has proven efficacy in decreasing cardiovascular morbidity and mortality. Additionally, their use has been found to be protective against stroke, coronary events, heart failure, progression of renal disease, progression to more severe hypertension, and deaths from all causes (JNC VI, 1997).

Drug therapy usually constitutes a single agent initially in uncomplicated hypertension. Preferred agents are diuretics or beta blockers because they have been shown to decrease morbidity and mortality. Sometimes hypertension occurs in conditions in which there is another complicating physiologic condition. These other conditions may respond best to other agents and are considered compelling reasons for starting with a drug class other than diuretics or beta blockers (Table 30-2). The drug dosage should be started at a low level and titrated up to what is considered the maximum dose for efficacy. Ideally the drug should have a therapeutic effect for 24 hours, requiring a dose to be taken only once daily.

If blood pressure remains uncontrolled, the patient advances another step, which involves adding an additional drug (particularly diuretics, if not already in use) or trying a different drug. If the patient tolerates the drug, the choice is to add another drug. If the patient is having adverse effects, a different drug should be tried.

If blood pressure still remains uncontrolled, step 4 is implemented. This involves adding a second or third drug to the therapy (see Figure 30-2). Patients who have achieved blood pressure control over a long time, usually at least 1 year, may be stepped down in therapy. This decreases the risk of adverse effects from drug therapy and may improve quality of life for the patient.

The advantage of the stepped approach is fairly clear. Through the use of drug combinations, the pharmacologic action of each drug increases. This reduces the required dose of each and consequently decreases the risk of adverse effects. This approach has been useful for all degrees of elevated blood pressure. Many antihypertensives are now available in combination with each other. This provides the patient with the benefits of both types of therapy, and the added advantage of needing to take only one pill, which improves adherence.

DRUGS TO TREAT HYPERTENSION

Drugs used to manage blood pressure primarily include those classified as diuretics, beta blockers, calcium-channel blockers, and ACE inhibitors. Additional therapy includes the angiotensin II receptors antagonists, alpha-2 stimulators, alpha-beta blockers, and direct vasodilators. Adjunct treatment includes the lipid lowering agents.

DIURETICS

Diuretics exert their effect in different areas of the renal tubules to promote the excretion of sodium and water from the body. Because water is not reabsorbed to as great an extent as usual from the kidneys, the volume of circulating fluid decreases. Although the exact mechanism of how diuretics reduce blood pressure is not known, it is generally accepted that the resulting decrease in peripheral resistance, from decreased circulating volume, is what lowers blood pressure. Diuretics are discussed in detail in Chapter 31.

BETA BLOCKERS

How beta blockers work is arguable, and several mechanisms of action have been proposed to explain how they reduce hypertension. Clinically, they have been proven to slow heart rate, decrease cardiac output, and lower blood pressure. Although beta blockers (at beta-2 receptor sites) increase peripheral resistance through vasoconstriction, this effect is outweighed by the significant decrease in cardiac output, thus lowering blood pressure. The peripheral vasoconstriction appears to be temporary, with resistance returning to baseline or lower levels with prolonged therapy. It also is believed that beta blockers have a central effect, which may decrease sympathetic outflow to the peripheral nervous system. Addition-

	Major Risk Factors	TOD/CCD (Target Organ Damage/ Clinical Cardiovascular Disease)
• Determine blood pressure stage. • Determine risk group by major risk factors and TOD/CCD. • Determine treatment recommendations (by using the table below). • Determine goal blood pressure. • Refer to specific treatment recommendations.	• Smoking • Dyslipidemia • Diabetes mellitus • Age > 60 years • Gender: –Men –Postmenopausal women • Family history: –Women < age 65 –Men < age 55	Heart diseases • LVH • Angina/prior MI • Prior CABG • Heart failure Stroke or TIA Nephropathy Peripheral arterial disease Hypertensive retinopathy

Blood pressure stages (mm Hg)	**Risk Group A** No major risk factors No TOD/CCD	**Risk Group B** At least one major risk factor not including diabetes No TOD/CCD	**Risk Group C** TOD/CCD and/or diabetes, with or without other risk factors
High-normal (130-139/85-89)	Lifestyle modification	Lifestyle modification	Drug therapy for those with heart failure, renal insufficiency or diabetes Lifestyle modification
Stage 1 (140-159/90-99)	Lifestyle modification (up to 12 months)	Lifestyle modification (up to 6 months) For patients with multiple risk factors, clinicians should consider drugs as initial therapy plus lifestyle modifications.	Drug therapy Lifestyle modification
Stages 2 and 3 (≥160/≥100)	Drug therapy Lifestyle modification	Drug therapy Lifestyle modification	Drug therapy Lifestyle modification

Example: A patient with diabetes and a blood pressure of 142/94 mm Hg plus left ventricular hypertrophy should be classified as having stage 1 hypertension with target organ disease (left ventricular hypertrophy) and with another major risk factor (diabetes). This patient would be categorized as Stage 1, Risk Group C, and recommended for immediate initiation of pharmacologic treatment.

Goal Blood Pressure	
<140/90 mm Hg	Uncomplicated hypertension, Risk Group A, Risk Group B, Risk Group C except for the following:
<130/85 mm Hg	Diabetes; renal failure; heart failure
<125/75 mm Hg	Renal failure with proteinuria > 1 gram/24 hours

Figure 30-3. JNC VI risk stratification and treatment recommendations. From the Sixth Report of the Joint National Committee on Prevention, Detection, Evaluation, and Treatment of High Blood Pressure (1997).

ally, beta-adrenergic receptors are responsible for the release of renin from the kidneys. This release is prevented by using beta blockers. For more information about beta blockers, see Chapter 14.

CALCIUM-CHANNEL BLOCKERS

Calcium-channel blockers inhibit the movement of calcium ions across cell membranes. This decreases the mechanical contraction of the heart, reduces impulse formation (automaticity), and lessens conduction velocity. Calcium-channel blockers also dilate coronary vessels and peripheral arteries, thus decreasing peripheral resistance and blood pressure. Cardiac output is not decreased, however, most likely because of reflex tachycardia secondary to vasodilation. Calcium-channel blockers also are discussed in Chapter 29.

ANGIOTENSIN-CONVERTING ENZYME INHIBITORS

In the renin-angiotensin-aldosterone sequence, a special enzyme is needed to convert the inactive angiotensin I to the active angiotensin II. Angiotensin II is a potent vasoconstrictor. Its presence increases the secretion of aldosterone. When aldosterone levels rise, the retention of sodium and water occur. The ACE inhibitors prevent the conversion of angiotensin I to angiotensin II. This in turn decreases peripheral arterial resistance and sodium and water retention.

ANGIOTENSIN II RECEPTOR ANTAGONISTS

Angiotensin II receptor antagonists, a fairly new class of drugs, block the action of angiotensin II from all the different pathways where it is formed, not just the single substrate

TABLE 30-2 Health Status Considerations for Selecting Drugs as First-Line Therapy for Hypertension

Health Status	Drug Class
Compelling Indications (unless contraindicated by comorbidity)	
Diabetes mellitus (type 1) with proteinuria	ACE inhibitors
Heart failure	ACE inhibitors, diuretics
Isolated systolic hypertension (older adults)	Diuretics (preferred), calcium channel blockers (long-acting dihydropyridine)
Myocardial infarction	Beta blockers (nonintrinsic sympathomimetic activity), ACE inhibitors (with systolic dysfunction)
Possible Indications	
Angina	Beta blockers, calcium channel blockers
Atrial tachycardia and fibrillation	Beta blockers, calcium channel blockers (nondihydropyridine)
Cyclosporine-induced hypertension (caution with the dose of cyclosporine)	Calcium channel blockers
Diabetes mellitus (types 1 and 2) with proteinuria	ACE inhibitors (preferred), calcium channel blockers
Diabetes mellitus (type 2)	Low-dose diuretics
Dyslipidemia	Alpha blockers
Essential tremor	Beta blockers (noncardioselective)
Heart failure	Carvedilol, losartan potassium
Hyperthyroidism	Beta blockers
Migraine	Beta blockers (noncardioselective), calcium channel blockers (nondihydropyridine)
Myocardial infarction	Diltiazem, verapamil
Osteoporosis	Thiazides
Preoperative hypertension	Beta blockers
Benign prostatic hypertrophy (BPH)	Alpha blockers
Renal insufficiency (caution in renovascular hypertension and creatinine level ≥265.2 micromol/L ≥3 mg/dL)	ACE inhibitors
Possible Precautions (Needs Special Monitoring) and Contraindications	
Bronchospastic disease	Beta blockers (contraindicated)
Depression	Beta blockers, central alpha stimulants, reserpine (contraindicated)
Diabetes mellitus (types 1 and 2)	Beta blockers, high-dose diuretics (precaution)
Dyslipidemia	Beta blockers (nonintrinsic sympathomimetic activity), diuretics (high dose) (precaution)
Gout	Diuretics (precaution)
2nd- or 3rd-degree heart block	Beta blockers (contraindicated), calcium channel blockers (nondihydropyridine) (contraindicated)
Heart failure	Beta blockers (except carvedilol), calcium channel blockers (except amlodipine, felodipine) (precaution)
Liver disease	Labetalol, methyldopa (contraindicated)
Peripheral vascular disease	Beta blockers (precaution)
Pregnancy	ACE inhibitors (contraindicated), angiotensin II receptor blockers (contraindicated)
Renal insufficiency	Potassium sparing diuretics (precaution)
Renovascular disease	ACE inhibitors, angiotensin II receptor blockers (precaution)

From the Sixth Report of the Joint National Committee on Prevention, Detection, Evaluation, and Treatment of High Blood Pressure. (1997). *Archives of Internal Medicine, 157*, 2413–2446.

altered by ACE inhibitors. These drugs are effective in lowering blood pressure. In addition they seem to block deleterious effects from angiotensin II at the end-organ stage, which is where serious complications of sustained hypertension occur. This effect seems to be independent of the antihypertension effect produced by the drugs (Meggs & Kodali, 1999). Continuing research is beginning to suggest that angiotensin II receptor antagonists eventually may be considered first-line agents for treating essential hypertension. The prototype for this class is losartan.

CENTRALLY ACTING ALPHA-2 STIMULATORS, PERIPHERALLY ACTING ALPHA-1 BLOCKERS, PERIPHERALLY ACTING ALPHA-BETA BLOCKERS, PERIPHERALLY ACTING ANTIADRENERGICS, AND DIRECT VASODILATORS

Centrally acting alpha-2 stimulators (also called agonists), peripherally acting alpha-1 blockers, peripherally acting alpha-beta blockers, peripherally acting antiadrenergic, and direct vasodilators are used in second-line treatment for hypertension and their use is restricted to step 3 or 4. These drug classes tend to cause significant adverse effects in patients.

Clonidine (Catapres), the prototype alpha-2 stimulator, stimulates the alpha-2 receptors centrally in the medulla oblongata, thereby inhibiting the sympathetic nervous system. Reduced sympathetic outflow from the CNS occurs, resulting in decreased heart rate, decreased blood pressure, decreased vasoconstriction, and decreased renal vascular resistance. The other second-line agents are significantly different from the alpha-2 stimulator prototype, clonidine. These are the peripherally acting alpha-1 blockers and the peripherally acting antiadrenergics. Peripherally acting alpha-1 blockers block postsynaptic alpha-1 adrenergic receptors, producing vasodilation of resistance vessels (arterioles) and capacitance vessels (veins), thereby decreasing blood pressure. Peripherally acting antiadrenergics either deplete the stores of norepinephrine or interfere with it release and distribution at the sympathetic neuroeffector junction. Therefore, less norepinephrine is available at the synaptic cleft. This causes depression of sympathetic nerve function, decreasing the heart rate and blood pressure.

Drugs that are combinations of alpha-1 adrenergic blockers and nonselective competitive beta-adrenergic blockers are known as alpha-beta blockers. The alpha-1 and beta-blocking properties decrease blood pressure.

The direct-acting vasodilators directly relax the arterioles, bringing about a decrease in peripheral resistance and lower blood pressure. These drugs are not suitable for monotherapy due to reflexive tachycardia and are used most frequently with two other drugs that each control blood pressure through different mechanisms.

ANTIHYPERLIPIDEMIC DRUGS

Antihyperlipidemic drugs reduce blood lipid levels. They are used as adjuncts to hypertensive drug therapy. Because hypertension can be caused or aggravated by the narrowed arterial passages when fat is deposited on the wall of the vessel, decreasing fat levels circulating in the blood is advantageous. Dietary modifications are a common first step for both hypertension and elevated cholesterol levels. Therefore, patient education should stress dietary modifications heavily for patients who are hypertensive and have elevated serum lipid levels. Antihyperlipidemic drugs are discussed in more detail in Chapter 34.

C ANGIOTENSIN-CONVERTING ENZYME (ACE) INHIBITORS

Captopril is the prototype ACE inhibitor.

NURSING MANAGEMENT OF THE PATIENT RECEIVING P CAPTOPRIL

Core Drug Knowledge

Pharmacotherapeutics

Captopril, like other ACE inhibitors, is used to lower blood pressure in hypertensive patients. Captopril also is used in treating CHF (usually in combination with diuretics and digitalis, although digitalis is not required for captopril to be effective). In addition, captopril is useful in treating diabetic nephropathy and left ventricular dysfunction after MI. Unlabeled uses include treating hypertensive crisis, neonatal and childhood hypertension, rheumatoid arthritis, hypertension related to scleroderma, renal crisis, idiopathic edema, Bartter syndrome (improves potassium metabolism and corrects hypokalemia), Raynaud syndrome (symptomatic relief), and hypertension of Takayasu disease. Captopril also is used to diagnose anatomic renal artery stenosis (captopril test) and primary aldosteronism (Table 30-3).

Pharmacokinetics

Captopril is absorbed rapidly after oral ingestion. Food decreases absorption. Captopril has a rapid onset of action. The drug is metabolized (50%) by the liver. It crosses the placenta and also appears in breast milk. It is ranked in pregnancy risk category C in the first trimester and category D in the second and third trimesters. Captopril does not cross the blood-brain barrier. It is eliminated unchanged (50%) by the kidneys. Half-life is less than 2 hours in normal renal function and 3.5 to 32 hours in renal impairment.

Pharmacodynamics

Captopril inhibits the ACE needed to change the inactive angiotensin I to the active form angiotensin II. This reduction of angiotensin II decreases the secretion of aldosterone, thus preventing sodium and water retention. Captopril, therefore, decreases peripheral vascular resistance and lowers blood pressure. Cardiac output is increased but there is no increase in the heart rate.

TABLE 30-3 Summary of Selected Antihypertensives

Drug (Trade) Name	Selected Indications	Route and Dosage Range	Pharmacokinetics
Angiotensin-Converting Enzyme (ACE) Inhibitors			
captopril (Capoten; *Canadian:* Apo-Capto)	Hypertension Heart failure LVD after MI Diabetic neuropathy	*Adult:* PO, 25–150 mg bid or tid *Adult:* PO, 25–100 mg tid *Adult:* PO, 50 mg tid *Adult:* PO, 25 mg tid	*Onset:* 15 min *Duration:* Dose related $t_{1/2}$: <2 h
benazepril (Lotensin)	Hypertension	*Adult:* PO, 20–40 mg/d	*Onset:* 1 h *Duration:* 24 h $t_{1/2}$: 10–11 h
enalapril (Vasotec)	Hypertension	*Adult:* PO, 10–40 mg/d *Adult:* IV, 1.25 mg over 5 min every 6 h	*Onset:* 1 h *Duration:* 24 h $t_{1/2}$: 1.3 h *Onset:* 15 min *Duration:* 6 h $t_{1/2}$: 1.3 h
fosinopril (Monopril)	Hypertension CHF	*Adult:* PO, maintenance: 20–40 mg/d *Adult:* PO, 20–40 mg/d	*Onset:* 1 h *Duration:* 24 h $t_{1/2}$: 12 h
lisinopril (Prinivil, Zestril; *Canadian:* Apo-Lisinopril)	Hypertension CHF Acute MI	*Adult:* PO, maintenance: 20–40 mg/d *Adult:* PO, 5 mg/d with diuretics and digitalis *Adult:* PO, maintenance: 10 mg/d	*Onset:* 1 h *Duration:* 24 h $t_{1/2}$: 12 h
moexipril (Univasc)	Hypertension	*Adult:* PO, maintenance: 7.5–30 mg/d	*Onset:* 1 h *Duration:* 24 h $t_{1/2}$: 2–9 h
ramipril (Altace)	Hypertension	*Adult:* PO, 2.5–20 mg/d	*Onset:* 1–2 h *Duration:* 24 h $t_{1/2}$: 13–17 h
quinapril (Accupril)	Hypertension CHF	*Adult:* PO, 20–80 mg/d *Adult:* PO, 20–40 mg/d with diuretics and digitalis	*Onset:* 1 h *Duration:* 24 h $t_{1/2}$: 2 h
Angiotensin II Receptor Antagonist			
losartan (Cozaar)	Hypertension	*Adult:* PO, 25–100 mg/d	*Onset:* 1 wk (therapeutic effect) *Duration:* Unknown $t_{1/2}$: 2 h
Alpha-Beta Adrenergic Blockers			
labetalol (Normodyne, Trandate)	Hypertension	*Adult:* PO, maintenance: 200–400 mg bid *Adult:* IV, 20 mg over 2 min up to 300 mg/d	*Onset:* Unknown *Duration:* 8–12 h $t_{1/2}$: 6–8 h *Onset:* Rapid *Duration:* Unknown $t_{1/2}$: 5.5 h
carvedilol (Coreg)	Hypertension	*Adult:* PO, 6.25–25 mg, bid	*Onset:* Rapid *Duration:* Unknown $t_{1/2}$: 7–10 h
Centrally Acting Alpha-2 Stimulators and Others			
clonidine (Catapres; *Canadian:* Apo-Clonidine)	Hypertension	*Adult:* PO, 0.2–0.6 mg/d in divided doses not to exceed 2.4 mg/d; transdermal, one, 0.1-mg–two 0.3-mg patches q7d	*Onset:* 30–60 min *Duration:* 12–24 h $t_{1/2}$: 12–16 h

TABLE 30-3 Summary of Selected Antihypertensives (Continued)

Drug (Trade) Name	Selected Indications	Route and Dosage Range	Pharmacokinetics
		Child: PO, 0.05–0.4 mg bid	*Onset (transdermal):* Slow *Duration:* 7 d $t_{1/2}$: Unknown
guanabenz (Wytensin; *Canadian:* Apo-Prazo)	Hypertension	*Adult:* PO, 4 mg bid, gradually increasing to maximum of 32 mg bid	*Onset:* 1 h *Duration:* Up to 12 h $t_{1/2}$: 6 h
prazosin (Minipress)	Hypertension	*Adult:* PO, maintenance, 6–15 mg/d in divided doses *Child:* PO, 0.5–7 mg tid	*Onset:* 2 h *Duration:* 6–12 h $t_{1/2}$: 2–3 h
terazosin (Hytrin)	Hypertension Benign prostatic hypertrophy	*Adult:* PO, maintenance, 1–5 mg/d up to 20 mg/d *Adult:* PO, 10 mg/d	*Onset:* Up to 15 min *Duration:* 12–24 h $t_{1/2}$: 9–12 h
doxazosin (Cardura)	Hypertension Benign prostatic hypertrophy	*Adult:* PO, initially 1 mg/d, increasing to maximum of 16 mg/d, if needed *Adult:* PO, 1–8 mg/d	*Onset:* Unknown *Duration:* Unknown $t_{1/2}$: 22 h
reserpine	Hypertension Psychiatric disorders	*Adult:* PO, 0.1–0.25 mg/d *Child:* not recommended; in exception, 0.02 mg/kg/d *Adult:* PO, 0.5 mg/d–1 mg/d	*Onset:* Slow *Duration:* 6–24 h $t_{1/2}$: 33 h
Direct-Acting Vasodilators			
hydralazine (Apresoline; *Canadian:* Apo-Hydralazine)	Hypertension	*Adult:* PO, 50 mg qid *Child:* PO, 7.5 mg/kg/d or 200 mg/d *Adult:* IV or IM, 20–40 mg, repeat as needed *Child:* IV or IM 0.1–0.2 mg/kg/dose every 4 to 6 h as needed	*Onset:* Unknown *Duration:* 6–8 h $t_{1/2}$: 3–7 h
	Hypertension in eclampsia	*Adult:* IV, 5–10 mg bolus every 20 min; after 20 mg, try another drug	*Onset:* 10–20 min *Duration:* 2–4 h

However, peripheral vascular resistance is lowered more than cardiac output is increased, resulting in a significant decrease in blood pressure. Captopril also increases renal blood flow but has no effect on the glomerular filtration rate. The serum potassium level may increase slightly as a result of decreased aldosterone levels.

ACE is similar to bradykinase (kinase II). Thus, ACE inhibitors increase the levels of bradykinin, and bradykinin stimulates the synthesis of prostaglandins. It has been hypothesized that the prostaglandins contribute to the antihypertensive effect of the ACE inhibitors.

Contraindications and Precautions

Captopril and all other ACE inhibitors can cause injury and death to a developing fetus during the second and third trimesters. It is contraindicated in patients with hypersensitivity to the drug, and there may be a cross-sensitivity to other ACE inhibitors. Captopril should be administered cautiously to patients with hypovolemia (from aggressive diuretic use or dialysis), aortic stenosis (theoretically, patients treated with vasodilators are at risk of decreased coronary perfusion because they do not develop the afterload reduction as other patients do), children (safety and efficacy not established), and breast-feeding women (concentrations of captopril in breast milk equal about 1% of maternal concentrations).

Adverse Effects

Chronic cough can occur with captopril and all ACE inhibitors, presumably because the drug inhibits the degradation of endogenous bradykinin. The cough is nonproductive and persistent. It resolves within 1 to 4 days after therapy stops but is a major reason for non-adherence to therapy. The next most common adverse effect is rash. Other adverse effects that may occur are first-dose hypotension (especially in severely salt or volume depleted patients [i.e., those treated aggressively with diuretics]), and hypotension, although this usually is limited to patients with CHF and is transient. Although uncommon, captopril, like other ACE inhibitors, carries the risk of two, serious, life-threatening effects–angioedema and neutropenia. Angioedema can occur after the first dose of captopril, or at any other time during therapy. Angioedema confined to face and lips may resolve untreated. Angioedema associated with laryngoedema can be fatal and needs immediate emergency care. The risk of neutropenia depends on the patient's clinical status. Most at risk are patients with collagen vascular diseases, such as systemic lupus erythematosus (SLE) and impaired renal function. Also at risk are patients with heart failure. Neutropenia generally resolves quickly after discontinuation of captopril. Fatalities have occurred, mostly in patients ill with the above-mentioned diseases.

Allergic reactions and anaphylaxis also are possible with captopril. Other adverse effects, which are not common, include:

- Proteinuria
- Cardiovascular (CV): chest pain, angina, MI, palpitations, orthostatic hypotension, tachycardia, and rhythm disturbances
- CNS: insomnia, paresthesia, dizziness, headache, fatigue, drowsiness, ataxia, confusion, depression, malaise, and nervousness
- Gastrointestinal/genitourinary (GI/GU): abdominal pain, nausea and vomiting, diarrhea, constipation, anorexia, oliguria, dry mouth, dyspepsia, pancreatitis, and hepatitis
- Respiratory: asthma, bronchospasm, and dyspnea
- Dermatologic: alopecia, pruritis, flushing, photosensitivity, erythema multiforme, and exfoliative dermatitis
- Miscellaneous: impotence, syncope, asthenia, anemia, blurred vision, fever, myalgia, arthralgia, eosinophilia, and vasculitis

Overdosage of captopril most frequently results in hypotension. Vascular reexpansion with IV normal saline solution is the treatment of choice.

Drug Interactions

Captopril interacts with several other drugs (Table 30-4). Captopril may cause a false-positive test result with urine acetone. Food significantly decreases the bioavailability of captopril by 30% to 40%, but it remains unknown whether the therapeutic effects of captopril are affected significantly.

Assessment of Relevant Core Patient Variables

Health Status

Blood pressure should be determined before captopril therapy begins. Patients receiving captopril for treatment of CHF are likely to be receiving concurrent diuretics. If the drug history reveals that the patient has received diuretics, especially high doses of diuretics, the patient should be assessed for signs of hypovolemia, because this places the patient at increased risk for hypotension. Other factors that may cause hypovolemia include excessive perspiration, vomiting, and diarrhea. The nurse should watch for signs of dehydration and determine whether the patient has renal impairment, because some patients have developed increases in blood urea nitrogen (BUN) and serum creatinine levels after blood pressure is reduced.

Patients with congestive heart disease may develop stable elevations of the BUN and serum creatinine with long-term captopril use, although discontinuation of treatment is not usually required. Electrolytes, especially potassium and sodium, should be in normal ranges to

TABLE 30-4 Agents That Interact With Captopril

Interactants	Effect and Significance	Nursing Management
antacids	Decreases bioavailability of captopril	Stagger drug administration by at least 2-h intervals.
capsaicin	Increases effect of captopril and may exacerbate coughing	Inform patient that coughing may attend coadministration, and suggest cough control measures. Assess for adherence to therapy.
indomethacin	Decreases effect of captopril, which may lead to an increase in blood pressure	Monitor blood pressure carefully to assess for therapeutic effect.
phenothiazines	Increases pharmacologic effects of captopril	Monitor blood pressure for hypotension.
probenecid	Increases effect of captopril, possibly raising serum levels and decreasing total clearance	Monitor blood pressure for hypotension.
allopurinol	Possibility for cross-sensitivity	Avoid concurrent administration. Monitor for signs of allergic reaction.
digoxin	Increases plasma digoxin levels	Monitor for possible bradycardia and other adverse effects.
lithium	Increases serum lithium levels	Monitor laboratory data for evidence of lithium level elevation and patient for symptoms of lithium toxicity.
potassium preparations or potassium-sparing diuretics	Increases serum potassium levels	Monitor electrolyte values. Observe patient for signs of hyperkalemia.

start therapy, because hyperkalemia and hyponatremia may result from therapy.

Life Span and Gender

The adverse effect of cough appears to affect women more than men. The nurse should determine whether the patient is pregnant. Patients who are pregnant should not receive captopril or other ACE inhibitors. If the patient becomes pregnant while taking captopril, therapy should be discontinued as soon as possible. The nurse also needs to determine whether the patient is breast-feeding, because captopril crosses into breast milk, and efficacy and safety have not been established in children.

Lifestyle, Diet, and Habits

The nurse should assess the patient's normal dietary habits before administering captopril. Poor oral intake and decreased sodium intake may predispose the patient to adverse effects of captopril. If the patient normally uses a salt substitute containing potassium or potassium supplements, these may need to be discontinued to avoid possible hyperkalemia. The nurse should also explore with the patient lifestyle changes intended to decrease blood pressure, such as weight loss, smoking cessation, increased exercise, and limited salt intake.

Environment

Although captopril may be given in any environment, it is important for the nurse to assess the safety of the patient's environment before taking the first dose because of the possibility of first-dose hypotension. One study found that patients living in the southeastern United States had significantly lower treatment success with captopril than patients living in other parts of the United States. Some unknown environmental factor has been hypothesized to cause this (Cushman, Reda, Perry, Willimas, Abdellatif, et al., 2000).

Culture

The nurse should note the patient's ethnic and cultural background before administering captopril. Captopril is effective even in hypertensive patients with low renin levels. In African Americans who are "low-renin hypertensive," there is a smaller antihypertensive response to captopril when it is used in monotherapy (Facts & Comparisons, 2000).

Nursing Diagnoses and Outcomes

- Risk for Injury from first-dose hypotension related to effect of drug therapy and from drug-induced neutropenia
  Desired outcome: The patient will not sustain injury from hypotensive event or neutropenia.
- Ineffective Therapeutic Regimen Management, noncompliance, related to persistent dry cough secondary to drug therapy
  Desired outcome: Adherence to drug therapy will be unaffected by chronic cough.
- Disturbed Sensory Perception related to possible electrolyte imbalance, hyperkalemia, and hyponatremia, related to effects of captopril
  Desired outcome: The patient's electrolyte levels will remain within normal ranges.
- Risk for Impaired Skin Integrity related to drug-induced rash and pruritus
  Desired outcome: Desired outcome: Skin integrity will not be impaired.

Planning and Intervention

Maximizing Therapeutic Effects

The nurse should administer captopril 1 hour before meals, because food decreases absorption.

Minimizing Adverse Effects

First-Dose Hypotension

The nurse should monitor the patient for at least 2 hours after the initial dose and until blood pressure stabilizes. Transient hypotension does not indicate that captopril should be discontinued; the dose can be restarted after blood pressure stabilizes. It is important to assist the patient to a supine position and give normal saline solution IV if severe hypotension occurs. The nurse should assess patients receiving diuretic therapy, especially when the diuretic dose increases, because salt deficiency or volume depletion increases risk.

Hypotension

The nurse should assess patients with CHF very carefully. It is important to start therapy with low doses or decrease the diuretic before starting captopril therapy, or increase salt intake about 1 week before starting captopril therapy.

Altered Laboratory Results

The nurse should assess blood reports for hyperkalemia, hyponatremia, and neutropenia, and urine for proteinuria.

Allergic Reactions

Extreme care is needed during dialysis of a patient on captopril, if a polyacrylonitrile dialyzer is used. Allergic reactions may occur suddenly with severe or fatal effects. The nurse should make sure that dialysis stops at the first sign of nausea, abdominal cramping, burning, angioedema, or shortness of breath leading to severe hypotension. The nurse must be prepared to intervene if the patient experiences anaphylactic reactions.

Providing Patient and Family Education

- The nurse should explain the purpose of the drug therapy and its possible adverse effects. If the patient is to start on captopril at home, the nurse should advise the patient to take the first dose at bedtime to minimize the possibilities of injury due to first-dose hypotension.

- The nurse should tell the patient to arise slowly from a lying or seated position in case of orthostatic hypotension and dizziness.
- The nurse should explain that the drug may produce a persistent dry cough, but that it is not serious. It is a good idea to encourage the patient to continue therapy and to provide ideas on minimizing the cough. However, the nurse should tell the patient to consult the prescriber if the cough becomes intolerable.
- The nurse should advise the patient to notify the prescriber promptly about the following adverse effects: sore throat, fever, swelling of hands or feet, irregular heartbeat, chest pain, swelling of face, eyes, lips, and tongue, difficulty breathing, or hoarseness. A rash may also appear and should be reported, although this is not as urgent as the other findings.
- The nurse should tell the patient not to use potassium supplements or salt substitutes containing potassium, because of the risk of hyperkalemia.
- It is important to explain the importance of adhering to schedules for follow-up blood tests.
- The nurse should counsel the patient to make lifestyle changes (e.g., diet, weight loss, and exercise) to reduce blood pressure. Positive reinforcement should be offered for changes made, and the patient should be encouraged to sustain these changes.
- The nurse should teach the patient how to self-monitor blood pressure to assess drug effectiveness.

Ongoing Assessment and Evaluation

Blood pressure should be monitored throughout captopril therapy. Blood pressure that decreases to a normal range is indicative of successful drug therapy. White blood cell counts, potassium and sodium levels, and urine protein values should be monitored throughout therapy as well. Levels that remain in the normal range demonstrate that adverse effects have not occurred. In patients with CHF, cardiac output will increase because of decreased peripheral resistance, and the patient's exercise tolerance time will increase. These findings also indicate effective drug therapy. The decreased peripheral resistance (afterload) will improve ejection fraction in patients who have left ventricular dysfunction resulting from MI. This reduces the incidence of overt heart failure that requires hospitalization.

Patients receiving captopril for diabetic nephropathy need to be monitored for renal insufficiency. Progressing renal insufficiency and serious clinical outcomes (need for dialysis, need for kidney transplant, and death) should be slowed. The nurse also should monitor these patients for proteinuria, even though captopril should decrease proteinuria. ■

MEMORY CHIP

Captopril

- Inhibits the angiotensin-converting enzyme (ACE) needed to change angiotensin I (inactive) to angiotensin II (active). Angiotensin II is a potent vasoconstrictor, so that less angiotensin II means less vasoconstriction.
- Decreased angiotensin II also decreases secretion of aldosterone, which thus prevents retention of sodium and water
- Lowers blood pressure by decreasing peripheral vascular resistance; smaller antihypertensive response (monotherapy) in African Americans than whites
- Most common adverse effect: chronic cough
- Most serious adverse effects: angioedema and neutropenia
- **Lifespan alert: captopril can cause injury and death to a developing fetus during the second and third trimesters**
- Minimizing adverse effects: monitor blood pressure for 2 hours after initial dose until stabilized; and monitor patient's blood pressure throughout therapy
- Most significant patient education: urge continuation of lifestyle changes while on drug therapy; and teach the signs and symptoms of hypotension

ANGIOTENSIN II RECEPTOR ANTAGONISTS

Losartan is the representative angiotensin II receptor antagonist.

NURSING MANAGEMENT OF THE PATIENT RECEIVING LOSARTAN

Core Drug Knowledge

Pharmacotherapeutics

Losartan is used to treat hypertension. It may be useful in treatment of heart failure, but this currently is an unlabeled use while additional research in being conducted.

Pharmacokinetics

Losartan undergoes a substantial first-pass metabolism and is converted to an active metabolite, which performs most of the antagonism at the angiotensin II receptors. Cytochrome P 450 2C9 and 3A4 isoenzymes are involved in losartan's metabolism. Both the drug and the active metabolite are highly protein bound. The peak concentration occurs in 1 hour for losartan, and in 3 to 4 hours for its metabolite. Half-life is about 2 hours for the drug and 6 to 9 hours for the metabolite. Excretion occurs in the urine and stool (see Table 30-3).

Pharmacodynamics

Angiotensin II receptor (type AT 1) antagonists (AIIRA) do not inhibit ACE. Instead, they block the vasoconstricting and aldosterone-secreting effects of angiotensin II by selectively blocking the binding of angiotensin II to the AT 1 receptors in many tissues, especially in the vascular smooth muscle and adrenal gland tissues. Although there is an AT 2 receptor, it does not seem to have an effect on the CV system. AIIRAs have a much greater affinity for AT 1 than AT 2 receptors. Losartan has about a 1000-fold increase in affinity for AT 1. Losartan is a reversible, competitive inhibitor of the AT 1 receptor. The active metabolite appears 10 to 40 times more potent by weight than losartan. It appears to be a reversible, but not competitive, inhibitor of the AT 1 receptor.

Losartan, like other AIIRAs, inhibits the pressor effect of angiotensin II, removing the negative feedback that occurs normally. This causes a two- to threefold increase in plasma renin activity and a rise in angiotensin II plasma levels. These increases are not enough to offset the positive effects that AIIRAs have on hypertension. Although there is a decrease in aldosterone secretion, potassium levels do not seem to be affected by losartan. There is a minimal decrease in serum uric acid when oral losartan is administered chronically.

Preliminary research indicates that losartan contributes to the regression of left ventricular hypertrophy that is associated with chronic hypertension. Additionally, losartan appears to increase exercise capacity in patients with either asymptomatic or symptomatic heart failure (Simpson & McLellan, 2000).

Contraindications and Precautions

The only contraindication to losartan is hypersensitivity to any component of the drug. Because of its anti-angiotensin II effect, and risk for fetal and neonatal morbidity and death, losartan is in the same pregnancy category as captopril (category C first trimester and category D second and third trimesters) and should not be used during pregnancy unless the benefit outweighs the risk.

Adverse Effects

A major advantage of losartan, and other AIIRAs, is that it does not cause the dry cough that occurs so frequently with ACE Inhibitors.

Overall, AIIRAs are well tolerated, with only about 2% of patients receiving losartan experiencing adverse effects bothersome enough to warrant discontinuing the drug. Of the adverse effects that do occur, the most frequent is upper respiratory infection; dizziness and diarrhea are the next two most frequent adverse effects. Other effects that may occur, but are not common, include anxiety and nervousness; musculoskeletal pain, cramps, and myalgia; nasal congestion, sinus disorder, and sinusitis; rash; tachycardia; and urinary tract infection.

Overdosage of losartan may produce hypotension, dizziness, and tachycardia. Bradycardia may be produced from parasympathetic (vagal) stimulation. Hypotension should be treated with supportive therapy. Valsartan cannot be removed by dialysis.

Drug Interactions

Losartan is known to interact with two drugs; whether these interactions are clinically significant is not known. Coadministration with cimetidine appears to increase the availability of losartan somewhat, but the active metabolite is not affected. Coadministration with phenobarbital reduces by about 20% the activity of losartan and its active metabolite. Food will slow the absorption of losartan but has minimal effects on the activity of the drug.

Assessment of Relevant Core Patient Variables

Health Status

Patients who have pathologies that are dependent on the renin- angiotensin-aldosterone system (such as patients with CHF), should not use AIIRAs because oliguria, progressive azotemia, or (rarely) acute renal failure or death may result. Patients receiving ACE inhibitors who have renal artery stenosis have shown elevated serum creatine or BUN and it is hypothesized that AIIRAs would have the same effect. The nurse should assess patients for these conditions and should monitor them for possible effects. Elevations in serum creatine or BUN also may occur in other patients on losartan. Of all patients who use losartan for hypertension, minor elevations in BUN and creatinine will occur in fewer than 1% of them. Although elevated serum levels of losartan have been found in patients with decreased creatinine clearance, the active metabolite is not affected. Therefore, no dose adjustment is required for these patients.

Patients who have impaired hepatic impairment do have increased bioavailability of losartan because metabolism is impaired. They should be given a lower starting dose of the drug and monitored for therapeutic and adverse effects. Small decreases in hemoglobin and hematocrit will occur in patients taking losartan. Although normally clinically insignificant, the nurse should monitor these patients.

Hypovolemia and salt depletion (usually from diuretic therapy) pose the same risk for hypotension to patients receiving losartan as to patients receiving captopril. It is important to correct these conditions before giving losartan.

Life Span and Gender

No dosage adjustments seem to be necessary for older adults because losartan is equally safe and effective in this group compared with in younger adults. The nurse should determine whether the patient is pregnant or breast-feeding before administering losartan. Due to adverse effects on the fetus and neonate, losartan should not be used during pregnancy. Animal studies indicate that losartan passes into breast milk; it is not known if this occurs with human milk as well. However, due to the serious effects that may occur, patients should not breastfeed while taking losartan. Additional concerns for women on losartan come from other animal studies showing that female rats receiving the drug have a slightly higher rate of pancreatic cancer and impaired fertility. Again, the effects in humans are not known. The safety and efficacy of losartan and other AIIRAs in children under 18 is not known.

Lifestyle, Diet, and Habits

The nurse should assess the patient's usual lifestyle. Lifestyle modifications that are general for all patients requiring hypertensive therapy should be followed for patients on losartan.

Environment

The nurse should be aware of the setting in which losartan may be administered. Losartan may be administered in any setting.

Culture

It is a good idea to note the patient's ethnic background before administering losartan. Like captopril, losartan is less effective when used as monotherapy in hypertensive African Americans than in other racial groups.

Nursing Diagnoses and Outcomes

- Risk for Infection (upper respiratory) related to adverse effects of drug therapy.
  Desired outcome: The patient will not develop an upper respiratory infection or if one develops it will be managed appropriately to minimize complications.
- Risk for Injury related to adverse effects on fetus and neonate.
  Desired outcome: The patient receiving losartan will report pregnancy to provider as soon as possible.
- Risk for Injury related to fall secondary to adverse effect of dizziness.
  Desired outcome: The patient will not fall.

Planning and Intervention

Maximizing Therapeutic Effects

Like all drug therapy for hypertension, the use of losartan should be accompanied by the recommended step-1 lifestyle changes. The nurse should determine whether the patient has made these changes and should provide encouragement to continue with them throughout drug therapy.

If losartan is ineffective alone, a diuretic should be added. Hydrochlorothiazide has been found to have an additive effect. The nurse should consult with the physician or nurse practitioner for additional drug orders if indicated.

Minimizing Adverse Effects

The nurse should help the patient out of bed when first started on losartan therapy in case dizziness is present. It is important to treat symptomatically for upper respiratory tract infections and diarrhea, if they occur. The nurse should monitor creatinine, BUN, hemoglobin, and hematocrit levels to verify that changes are not clinically significant.

Providing Patient and Family Education

- If the female patient is of childbearing age, the nurse should caution her about the adverse effects that losartan can have on the fetus and neonate. The nurse should urge the woman to notify the health care provider immediately if she becomes pregnant.
- The nurse should explain the importance of arising slowly until the effects of the drug are known or if dizziness is present.
- It is important to teach the patient to avoid hazardous activities until effects of the drug are known.
- The nurse should tell the patient to notify the health care provider if upper respiratory infection occurs.
- It is important to provide general teaching about hypertension, lifestyle changes, and losartan core drug knowledge.

Ongoing Assessment and Evaluation

The nurse should monitor blood pressure throughout therapy, and determine if desired blood pressure goal has been achieved. It is important to consider adding a diuretic if losartan not effective in monotherapy. The nurse should verify that the patient continues with life style changes. Treatment is effective if desired reduction in blood pressure occurs in either monotherapy or multidrug therapy without the patient having serious adverse effects. ■

ALPHA-BETA BLOCKERS

Labetalol is the prototype alpha-beta blocker.

NURSING MANAGEMENT OF THE PATIENT RECEIVING LABETALOL

Core Drug Knowledge

Pharmacotherapeutics

Labetalol is used for treating hypertension usually with other agents, especially thiazide and loop diuretics, although it may be used alone. The parenteral form is for managing severe hypertension and is given only in the hospital. Unlabeled uses include lowering of hypertension associated with pheochromocytoma, although higher IV doses may be needed, and paradoxic hypertensive responses have been reported. Labetalol also has been used in clonidine-withdrawal hypertension (see Table 30-3).

Pharmacokinetics

Labetalol is absorbed completely orally, and the peak action occurs in 2 to 4 hours. Maximum steady state blood pressure response occurs within 24 to 72 hours. The drug also can be administered parenterally with the onset occurring rapidly and peaking in 5 minutes. After discontinuation of IV therapy, blood pressure returns gradually to near-baseline levels in 16 to 18 hours. Labetalol has an extensive first-pass effect and is metabolized rapidly by the liver. It is excreted in the stool and urine. Labetalol penetrates the CNS, crosses the placenta, and appears in breast milk in minimal amounts (0.004% of maternal dose). It is a pregnancy category C drug.

Pharmacodynamics

Labetalol is an adrenergic blocking agent that has a nonspecific beta-blocking action at both the beta-1 and beta-2 receptor sites and a selective alpha-1 blocking action. The ratio of alpha:beta blocking action is 1:3 with oral use and 1:7 with IV use. The alpha blocking actions cause peripheral vasodilation. Because the alpha blocking action decreases standing blood pressure more than it decreases lying blood pressure, orthostatic hypotension may occur, although this is transient. The beta-blocking action prevents reflex tachycardia. It also prevents exercise-induced tachycardia and elevations in blood pressure, although there is no effect on respiratory rate. The beta-blocking effect also results in a decrease in the plasma renin level. Labetalol reduces blood pressure while maintaining glomerular filtration rate and renal blood flow.

Contraindications and Precautions

Labetalol is contraindicated with severe bradycardia, second- or third-degree heart block, bronchial asthma, overt, noncompensated heart failure, and cardiogenic shock due to stimulation of beta-1 and beta-2 receptor sites. Caution should be used in patients with a history of heart failure (who are well compensated). Heart failure has been known to occur, even in patients with no history of it. Caution is used with patients with nonallergic emphysema or bronchitis or diabetes mellitus due to beta blockade. Labetalol must be used cautiously in pregnancy, because there are no adequate controlled studies in pregnant women. Safety and efficacy in children have not been established. Administer with caution to patients with impaired hepatic function, because drug metabolism may be diminished.

Adverse Effects

Labetalol usually is well tolerated with the adverse effects being mild and transient. Orthostatic hypotension after oral dosage occurs in 2% of patients receiving labetalol. It usually is transient and unlikely to occur if the recommended starting dose and titration increments are followed closely. It is most likely to occur 2 to 4 hours after a dose, especially a large dose or dose change and if the patient was tilted or assumed an upright position within 3 hours of receiving the dose. Weakness, fatigue, and dizziness that can occur with administration are associated with postural hypotension. Other adverse effects include:

- GU: ejaculatory failure, impotence, priapism, difficulty in micturition, acute urinary bladder retention, and Peyronie disease
- GI: diarrhea, cholestasis with or without jaundice, and reversible increases in serum transaminase
- Respiratory: respiratory dyspnea and bronchospasm
- Miscellaneous: asthenia, muscle cramps, and toxic myopathy; rashes, reversible alopecia, bullous lichen planus, and facial reddening much like that of psoriasis; jaundice and hepatic dysfunction rarely are associated with labetalol but if they occur, they are reversible when the drug is stopped.

Signs of overdosage include excessive hypotension that is posture sensitive and excessive bradycardia.

Drug Interactions

The major drug interactions are shown in Table 30-5. Labetalol interacts with beta-adrenergic agonists, cimetidine, glutethimide, halothane, and nitroglycerin. There are no drug-food interactions. The metabolite of labetalol in the urine may cause a false increase in urinary catecholamine levels. Reversible increases in serum transaminase have been noted in 4% of patients taking labetalol; more rarely blood urea increases, which also is reversible.

Assessment of Relevant Core Patient Variables

Health Status

The nurse must determine whether the patient has CHF, second- or third-degree heart block, cardiogenic shock, severe bradycardia, bronchospastic disease, or diabetes mellitus because the beta-blocking action may be harmful to them. It is important to determine whether the patient has impaired hepatic function because metabolism may be decreased. The nurse also should determine if the patient is already receiving drug therapy with drugs that interact with labetalol.

Life Span and Gender

The nurse should determine the age of the patient because safety and efficacy has not been established in children. Because liver function may be deteriorated in the elderly, the first-pass effect may be diminished, increasing the absolute bioavailability of labetalol. It is important to determine whether the patient is pregnant or breast-feeding, because caution with administration is necessary.

pressure, urinary flow, cardiac output, and pulmonary wedge pressure closely throughout therapy.

The nurse should assess for a disproportionate rise in diastolic blood pressure (may be sign of predominant vasoconstriction). It is important to monitor patients with a history of occlusive vascular disease closely for changes in temperature or color of skin or extremities. If this is found, the nurse should consult with the physician to determine the benefits of dopamine versus possible necrosis.

It is important to infuse into a large vein (antecubital fossa preferred to those in hands or feet) to prevent extravasation (will cause necrosis and sloughing of tissue). The nurse should monitor the insertion site for patency and free flow. If extravasation does occur, it is important to treat immediately with phentolamine (causes sympathetic blockade), injecting into the SC space with a needle and syringe. The nurse should discontinue dopamine gradually to prevent hypotension.

Providing Patient and Family Education

- The administration of dopamine occurs during an acute medical crisis. Patient education will therefore be limited at this time.
- If the patient is awake and alert, the nurse should inform the patient that his or her blood pressure is low, and the medication will raise blood pressure to a normal level.
- It is important to reassure the patient that he will be monitored closely during drug administration. This also would be appropriate teaching for family members.

Ongoing Assessment and Evaluation

Dopamine therapy is effective if blood pressure stabilizes, urinary output returns to normal, cardiac output returns to normal, and the patient does not have serious adverse effects from the drug. ■

MEMORY CHIP

Dopamine

- Used to treat the hypotension resulting from shock as it stimulates alpha and beta receptors to increase cardiac output, blood pressure, and renal perfusion
- Correct hypovolemia prior to administering
- Significant contraindications: pheochromocytoma, uncorrected tachyarrhythmias, and ventricular fibrillation
- Most common adverse effects: ectopic beats, nausea and vomiting, tachycardia, angina, palpitations, dyspnea, headache, hypotension, and vasoconstriction
- Most serious adverse effect: ventricular arrhythmias
- Maximizing therapeutic effects: use an IV pump; titrate the dose upward until desired renal or hemodynamic response is achieved
- Minimizing adverse effects: monitor blood pressure, urinary output, cardiac output, and pulmonary wedge pressure throughout therapy

DRUGS CLOSELY RELATED TO DOPAMINE

Dobutamine

Dobutamine is chemically similar to dopamine. Like dopamine, its primary influence is on beta-1 receptors with similar effects on the force of contraction. Dobutamine is somewhat less effective than dopamine at increasing the rate at the sinoatrial (SA) node. Also like dopamine, dobutamine's beta-2 effects on vasodilation are minimal. Unlike dopamine, dobutamine has almost no effect on alpha receptors to cause vasoconstriction. Although cardiac output and blood pressure are similarly increased with both drugs, dobutamine does not produce the increased renal output that dopamine does. Furthermore, its effect on peripheral resistance is always to decrease it, whereas dopamine may increase or decrease peripheral resistance. Dobutamine does not cause the release of endogenous norepinephrine that dopamine causes.

The pharmacotherapeutic uses of dobutamine differ from dopamine. Dobutamine is indicated in the short-term treatment and support of patients experiencing cardiac decompression due to depressed contractility. The decreased contractility may be secondary to either organic heart disease or from cardiac surgery. Patients with atrial fibrillation and a rapid ventricular rate should be treated first with digoxin prior to dobutamine treatment to protect the ventricles.

Dobutamine is metabolized by two methods: methylation of the catechol and conjugation. Byproducts are excreted in the urine. Onset of action is 1 to 2 minutes but as long as 10 minutes may be needed to see the peak effect. A contraindication unique to dobutamine is the presence of idiopathic hypertrophic subaortic stenosis. Although elevated pulse usually does not occur when using dobutamine, tachycardia can occur with increases of 30 beats/minute or more. Accompanying the tachycardia is a rapid and substantial increase in blood pressure, with the systolic pressure rising 50% or greater. These adverse effects are usually dose related, and reducing the dose promptly corrects the problem. Interestingly, dobutamine also can cause significant hypotension if given in excessive amounts; again, decreasing the dose usually corrects the problem. Dobutamine may cause or exacerbate ventricular ectopic beats, although ventricular tachycardia is rare. Other rare adverse effects include nausea, headache, anginal pain, nonspecific chest pain, palpitations, and shortness of breath. Phlebitis and local inflammation at the IV site may occur; a large vein should be chosen to administer the drug to minimize this.

Patients receiving dobutamine, like dopamine, need to be monitored continuously on a cardiac monitor while receiving the drug. Blood pressures should be checked frequently. Pulmonary wedge pressure and cardiac output should be checked whenever possible.

Isoproterenol

Like dopamine, isoproterenol has a strong effect on beta-1 receptors, producing similar increases in contractility. However, isoproterenol's effect on the heart rate and vasodilation is much greater than dopamine's. Isoproterenol does not stimulate the alpha receptors for vasoconstriction. Isoproterenol increases cardiac output like dopamine. Renal perfusion also is effected, although unlike dopamine, it can increase or decrease it. Peripheral resistance always is decreased, but blood pressure may be increased or decreased by isoproterenol. Although isoproterenol may be used to treat shock, this is not a common practice due to the tachycardia that may occur. The other uses of isoproterenol and more complete information about it are found in Chapter 14.

Epinephrine

Epinephrine is also a vasopressor, as is dopamine. Epinephrine stimulates both alpha and beta receptors. Its effect on the contractility of the heart (beta-1) is similar to dopamine's effect, whereas its effects on SA node rate (beta-1), vasodilation (beta-2), and vasoconstriction (alpha-1) are stronger than dopamine's effects. Although epinephrine increases the cardiac output, its other pharmacodynamic effects differ from dopamine's. It decreases renal perfusion, decreases total peripheral resistance, and elevates systolic while lowering diastolic blood pressures. Epinephrine is indicated in the treatment and prophylaxis of cardiac arrest and attacks of transitory atrioventricular (AV) heart block with syncopal seizures (Stokes-Adams syndrome). Epinephrine is discussed completely in Chapter 14.

Norepinephrine

Norepinephrine is another vasopressor that stimulates the adrenergic system. Its beta-1 effects on contractility are less than dopamine's, whereas its effect on the SA node rate is similar. Similar to dopamine, norepinephrine has strong alpha receptor stimulation, producing vasoconstriction, but no effect on vasodilation from beta-2 receptors. Although peripheral resistance and blood pressure are raised, norepinephrine decreases renal perfusion, and either has no effect or decreases cardiac output. Norepinephrine is used to restore blood pressure when hypotension is due to one of the following conditions: pheochromocytomectomy, sympathectomy, poliomyelitis, spinal anesthesia, MI, blood transfusion, and drug reactions. It also is used as an adjunct in the treatment of cardiac arrest and severe hypotension. More information about norepinephrine is also found in Chapter 14.

Ephedrine

Ephedrine has less effect on contractility (beta-1 receptors) and less effect on vasoconstriction (alpha-1) than dopamine. Its effect on heart rate (beta-1) and vasodilation (beta-2) is similar to dopamine's effect. Ephedrine's pharmacodynamic effects of increasing blood pressure, increasing cardiac output, and increasing or decreasing peripheral resistance are similar to those of dopamine. Unlike dopamine, ephedrine decreases renal perfusion. Ephedrine is used clinically in acute hypotension, especially caused by spinal anesthesia, Stokes-Adams syndrome with complete heart block, use of a CNS stimulant in narcolepsy and depressive states, and acute bronchospasm (occasionally). It also is used as a vasopressor following sympathectomy or drug overdosage (from ganglionic blocking drugs, antiadrenergic drugs, *Veratrum* alkaloids, or other drugs used to lower blood pressure in the treatment of hypertension). Ephedrine also is used in enuresis and myasthenia gravis.

Mephentermine

Mephentermine has a weaker effect on the beta-1 receptors, causing less increase in contractility and heart rate than dopamine does. However, it has a stronger effect on the beta-2 receptors, producing moderate vasodilation. It only has a weak effect on alpha-1 receptors, causing a small increase in vasoconstriction. Its pharmacodynamics, when compared with those of dopamine, are in some ways similar. It increases cardiac output and blood pressure. It may have no effect on peripheral resistance or it may increase it, and renal perfusion may increase or decrease. Mephentermine is used to treat hypotension from ganglionic blockade or spinal anesthesia. It can be used on an emergency basis to maintain blood pressure during hypovolemic shock, but only until blood or blood substitutes become available.

Metaraminol

Metaraminol is similar to mephentermine in that it has only minor effects on beta-1 receptors, creating mild increases in contractility and heart rate. It has more effect on vasoconstriction from alpha-1 stimulation than mephentermine, but less than dopamine has. It has no effect on vasodilation from beta-2 stimulation. It primarily increases blood pressure by increasing peripheral resistance. Unlike dopamine, it lowers cardiac output and renal perfusion. Although the SA node is stimulated somewhat (which theoretically should increase the heart rate), the net effect on the heart is bradycardia, resulting from a strong reflexive response to the significant vasoconstriction. Metaraminol is used in the prevention and treatment of acute hypotensive states occurring with spinal anesthesia. It is an adjunct treatment for hypotension due to hypovolemia, reactions to drug therapy, surgical complications, and shock associated with brain damage due to trauma or tumor. Unlike dopamine, it can be given IM or SC in addition to IV infusion.

DRUGS SIGNIFICANTLY DIFFERENT FROM P DOPAMINE

Phenylephrine

Unlike dopamine, phenylephrine's effects are solely on alpha-1 receptors, producing strong vasoconstriction effects. Renal perfusion and cardiac output are decreased. Blood pressure is increased by the increase in peripheral resistance.

Phenylephrine is used in the treatment of vascular failure in shocklike states, drug-induced hypotension, or hypersensitivity. It also is used to overcome paroxysmal supraventricular tachycardia, to prolong spinal anesthesia, as a vasoconstrictor in regional analgesia, and to maintain an adequate blood pressure during spinal and inhalation anesthesia. Phenylephrine is discussed completely in Chapter 14.

Midodrine

Midodrine raises blood pressure, but it is not used as a vasopressor in shock. Instead, it is used in the symptomatic treatment of orthostatic hypotension in those patients whose lives are impaired significantly, despite standard clinical treatment. An unlabeled use is in the treatment of urine incontinence. It is administered orally. Midodrine is a prodrug that becomes active when it changes into the metabolite desglymidodrine. The metabolite is an alpha-1 agonist that increases the tone of the arteriolar and venous vasculature, increasing peripheral resistance. It results in increased standing, sitting, and lying blood pressures in orthostatic hypotension. Because it increases supine blood pressure it should not be given less than 4 hours prior to bedtime. Suggested dosing times are shortly before or just after arising in the morning, midday, and late afternoon. This should assist the patient to maintain his or her normal daytime activities and prevent supine hypertension during the night. If supine hypertension does occur, it may be controlled by preventing the patient from lying completely flat (i.e., lying with the head of the bed elevated).

CHAPTER SUMMARY

- Blood pressure is derived from the amount of blood leaving the heart times the resistance in the peripheries (blood pressure = cardiac output × peripheral resistance). When either cardiac output or peripheral resistance increases, the blood pressure will rise. Drug therapy to reduce hypertension is designed to decrease either cardiac output or peripheral resistance or both. Drug therapy to increase blood pressure increases either cardiac output, or peripheral resistance, or both.
- Hypertension is classified in four stages (from stage 1 to stage 4), according to the degree of blood pressure elevation.
- The stepped-care approach to hypertension is based on the patient's response to the therapy. Patients' therapy may be "stepped up" if they do not respond to therapy or "stepped down" if they show signs of good blood pressure control over time. This protocol reflects lifestyle modifications in addition to a progressive drug therapy approach.
- In step 1 hypertension, blood pressure is managed by lifestyle changes alone. These include weight reduction, dietary restriction of saturated fat, moderation of alcohol intake, regular physical activity, reduction of sodium intake, and smoking cessation. This step should be initiated before drug therapy is tried. Lifestyle modifications continue even if the patient steps up to drug therapy.
- Steps 2 though 4 include the addition of drug therapy with one or more drugs. Diuretics and beta blockers are generally recommended to be used as the drugs of first choice.
- Captopril, an ACE inhibitor, inhibits the ACE needed to change the inactive angiotensin I to the active form angiotensin II, thereby preventing sodium and water retention, decreasing peripheral vascular resistance, and lowering blood pressure. A significant adverse effect is a chronic cough, which may be so severe that the patient cannot tolerate or continue drug therapy. First-dose hypotension may occur.
- Losartan is an AIIRA; it does not inhibit ACE. Instead it blocks the vasoconstricting and aldosterone-secreting effects of angiotensin II by selectively blocking the binding of angiotensin II to the angiotensin receptors in many tissues, especially in the vascular smooth muscle and adrenal gland tissues.
- Labetalol is an adrenergic-blocking agent that has a nonspecific beta-blocking action at both the beta-1 and beta-2 receptor sites and a selective alpha-1 blocking action. The alpha-blocking actions cause peripheral vasodilation. Because the alpha-blocking action decreases standing blood pressure more than lying blood pressure, orthostatic hypotension may occur. The beta-blocking action prevents reflex tachycardia.
- Clonidine, an alpha-2 stimulator, stimulates the alpha-2 receptors centrally. This inhibits sympathetic nervous system responses. Reduced sympathetic outflow from the CNS occurs, resulting in decreased heart rate, decreased blood pressure, decreased vasoconstriction, and decreased renal vascular resistance. Initially, alpha receptors in the peripheries will be stimulated, producing vasoconstriction. However, the main effects are sympatholytic (reduced sympathetic outflow and vasodilation). Because of the sympatholytic effects, the drug may be used to control withdrawal symptoms from substances of abuse. Therefore, clonidine generally is not prescribed for hypertensive patients who are known substance abusers.
- Hydralazine, a direct-acting vasodilator, acts directly on the smooth muscles of the arterioles to produce relaxation and in turn, peripheral vasodilation. This promotes decreased arterial blood pressure and decreased peripheral resistance. As a reflex to peripheral vasodilation, the body increases heart rate, stroke volume, and cardiac output. The reflex mechanism is due to an increase in sympathetic stimulation.
- Nitroprusside, an agent used in hypertensive crisis, directly relaxes vascular smooth muscle. It is more active on veins than arteries, thereby promoting peripheral pooling of blood. This decreases venous return to the heart, reducing left ventricular end diastolic pressure and pulmonary capillary wedge pressure (preload). The resultant arteriolar dilation reduces systemic resistance and decreases mean arterial pressure (afterload). The result is markedly reduced blood pressure. The ability to decrease the blood pressure is seemingly unlimited. Nitroprusside is rapidly metabolized to cyanide through a reaction with hemoglobin. Cyanide poisoning may occur during its use. If after 10 minutes at the maximum infusion rate, blood pressure remains uncontrolled, the nurse should stop the infusion immediately. The nitroprusside infusion should be controlled by an administration pump, and the blood pressure must be monitored constantly.
- Dopamine, a vasopressor, is used to correct the hemodynamic imbalances present in shock. Dopamine is a naturally occurring catecholamine and a precursor to norepinephrine. It stimulates alpha-1 and beta-1 receptors through direct and indirect (releasing the stored epinephrine) methods. It has either no or only minimal effect on beta-2 receptors. It also has dopaminergic effects. The effects from dopamine are increased renal perfusion, increased cardiac output, increased or decreased peripheral resistance (depending on the dose), and increases in blood pressure. Dopamine is administered by IV continuous infusion. The patient must be monitored closely and continuously while on dopamine infusion.

QUESTIONS FOR STUDY AND REVIEW

1. What lifestyle changes constitute step 1 in antihypertensive therapy?
2. Which drug classes are generally recommended for step 2, initiating drug therapy?

3. How do ACE inhibitors like captopril lower the blood pressure?
4. Why is clonidine not recommended for antihypertensive patients who abuse narcotics?
5. Describe nursing actions that promote safety for the patient receiving nitroprusside.
6. Why is dopamine dosage determined by urinary output and CV response?

NEED MORE HELP?

Chapter 30 of the study guide for *Drug Therapy in Nursing* contains exercises and activities to reinforce your understanding of the concepts presented in this chapter. For additional information, see the text's accompanying web site at *http://www.connection.lww.com.*

REFERENCES AND BIBLIOGRAPHY

Adelman, R. D., Coppo, R., & Dillon, M. J. (2000). The emergency management of severe hypertension. *Pediatric Nephrology, 14*(5), 422–427.

Abramowicz, M. (Ed.). (1997). Safety of calcium channel blockers. *The Medical Letter, 39*(994), 13–15.

Abramowicz, M. (Ed.). (1997). Valsartan for hypertension. *The Medical Letter, 39*(999), 43–44.

American Heart Association. www americanheart.org

Blumenthal, J. A., Sherwood, A., Gullette, E. C. D., Babyak, M., Waugh, R., Georgiades, A., Craighead, L. W., Tweedy, D., Feinglos, M., Appelbaum, M., Hayano, J., & Hinderliter, A. (2000). Exercise and weight loss reduce blood pressure in men and women with mild hypertension. Effects on cardiovascular, metabolic, and hemodynamic. *Archives of Internal Medicine, 160,* 1947–1958.

Clinical Update. *1999 Guidelines for Hypertension Management* [Online]. Available:
http://pediatrics.medscape.com/CPG/ClinReviews/1999/v09.n06/c0906.02/pnt-c0906.02.html

Cushman, W. C., Reda, D. J., Perry, H. M., Willimas, D., Abdellatif, M., & Materson, B. J. (2000). Regional and racial differences in response to antihypertensive medication use in a randomized controlled trial of men with hypertension in the United States. Department of Veterans Affairs Cooperative Study on Antihypertensive Agents. *Archives of Internal Medicine, 160,* 825–831.

Deedwania, P. C. (2000). Hypertension and diabetes: New therapeutic options. *Archives of Internal Medicine, 160*(11), 1585–1594.

Fernandez-Gonzalez, R. Gomz-Pajuelo, C., Gabriel, R., de La Figuera, M., Moreno, E., of the Verapamil Frequency Research Group. (2000). Effect of verapamil on home self-measurement of blood pressure and heart rate by hypertensivepatients. Verapamil-Frequency Research Group. *Blood Pressure Monitor, 5*(1), 23–30.

Ford, E. S., Ahluwalia, I. B., & Galuska, D. A. (2000). Social relationships and cardiovascular disease risk factors: Finding from the Third National Health and Nutrition Examination Survey. *Preventive Medicine, 30*(2), 83–92.

Guidelines Subcommittee of the World Health Organization: International Society of Hypertension (WHO-ISH) Mild Hypertension Committee. (1999) World Health Organization: International Society of Hypertension Guidelines for the Management of Hypertension. *Journal of Hypertension, 17,* 151–183.

Hansson, L., Smith, D. H., Reeves, R., & Lapuerta, P. (2000). Headache in mild to moderate hypertension and its reduction by irbesartan therapy. *Archives of Internal Medicine, 160,* 1645–1658.

Himmelmann, A. (1999). Hypertension: An important precursor of heart failure. *Blood Pressure, 8*(5-6), 253–260.

Launer, L. J., Ross, G. W., Petrovistch, H., Masaki, K., Petrovitch, H., Masaki, K. Foley, D., White, L. R., & Havlik, R. J. (2000). Midlife blood pressure and dementia: The Honolulu-Asia aging study. *Neurobiological Aging, 21*(1), 49–55.

Meggs, L. G., & Kodali, P. (1999). Emerging concepts in antihypertensive therapy: The benefits of angiotensin II blockade. *Journal of the Association of Academic Minority Physicians, 10*(2), 34–43.

Moser, M. (1999). A critique of the World Health Organization: International Society of Hypertension Guidelines for the management of hypertension. *Cardiovascular Reviews and Reports, 4*(20), 1–4.

Mulrow, C., Lau, J., Cornell, J., & Brand, M. (2000). Pharmacotherapy for hypertension in the elderly. *Cochrane Database System Review,* (2):CD0000028.

Simpson, K. L., & McClellan, K. J. (2000). Losartan: A review of its use, with special focus on elderly patients. *Drugs and Aging, 16*(3), 227–250.

Skolnik, N. S., Beck, J. D., & Clark, M. (2000). Combination antihypertensive drugs: Recommendations for use. *American Family Physician, 61*(10), 3049–3056.

The Sixth Report of the Joint National Committee on Detection, Evaluation and Treatment of High Blood Pressure (JNC VI). (1997). *Archives of Internal Medicine, 157,* 2413–2446.

Volpe, M., Savoia, C., Panina, G., & Cangianiello, S. (2000). Therapeutic applications of angiotensin II receptor antagonists [in French]. *Annales d'Endocrinologie, Paris. 61*(1), 47–51.

Chapter 31

DRUGS AFFECTING DIURESIS

KEY TERMS

diuresis
diuretic
edema
glomerular filtration
hyperkalemia
hypertension
hypervolemia
hypokalemia
oliguria
osmolality
renal tubular reabsorption
renal tubular secretion

Learning Objectives

At the completion of this chapter the student will:

1. Describe normal kidney function and how diuretics work in the kidney.
2. Identify core drug knowledge about drugs that affect diuresis.
3. Identify core patient variables related to drugs that affect diuresis.
4. Relate the interaction of core drug knowledge to core patient variables for drugs that affect diuresis.
5. Generate a nursing plan of care from the interactions between core drug knowledge and core patient variables for drugs that affect diuresis.
6. Describe nursing interventions to maximize therapeutic and minimize adverse effects for drugs that affect diuresis
7. Determine key points for patient and family education for drugs that affect diuresis.

Thiazides

hydrochlorothiazide
chlorothiazide
benzthiazide
metolazone
chlorthalidone
bendroflumethiazide
hydroflumethiazide
trichlormethiazide
polythiazide
methychlothiazide
indapamide
quinethazone

Loop diuretics

furosemide
bumetanide
torsemide
ethacrynic acid

Potassium-sparing diuretics

triamterene
amiloride
spironolactone

Osmotic diuretics

mannitol
glycerin
urea
isosorbide

Carbonic anhydrase inhibitors

acetazolamide
dichlorphenamide
methazolamide

The symbol indicates the **drug class**.

Drugs in bold type marked with the symbol are **prototypes**.

Drugs in blue type with no symbol are **closely related** to the prototype.

Drugs in **red** type with no symbol are **significantly different** from the prototype.

Drugs in **black** type with no symbol are **also used in drug therapy**; no prototype.

Diuresis is the process of ridding the body of fluids through the increased production of urine and the excretion of water and electrolytes, such as sodium, by the kidneys. Diuresis occurs naturally if fluid intake has exceeded the body's normal requirements. This is a self-regulating or homeostatic mechanism to keep the body's fluid volume in balance.

A **diuretic** is a substance that causes diuresis. Drugs that are diuretics are used to decrease fluid volume in pathologic conditions in which the body cannot self-regulate fluid volume effectively. Diuretics decrease renal reabsorption of sodium and promote its excretion in water. The greater the sodium excretion, the greater the water excretion will be. During this process, reabsorption of other electrolytes (e.g., potassium) may also decrease, thereby promoting their excretion as well.

The various types of diuretics work differently in the body. Which diuretic is prescribed for a patient depends on the patient's underlying pathologies and the desired therapeutic effects. This chapter discusses five classes of diuretics–thiazide, loop, potassium-sparing, osmotic, and carbonic anhydrase inhibitors. The thiazide, loop, and potassium-sparing classes all are used to decrease circulating volume and complications related to excess volume. Thiazide diuretics work in the distal tubule of the kidney, whereas loop diuretics work in the loop of Henle. Potassium-sparing diuretics are used commonly in combination with other diuretics, and they work in the distal tubule.

Prototype drugs for thiazide, loop, and potassium-sparing classes are hydrochlorothiazide (HCTZ), furosemide, and triamterene, respectively. The osmotic diuretics, for which mannitol is the prototype, are used to decrease intraocular and intracranial pressure and to treat or prevent acute renal failure (ARF). The osmotic diuretics are filtered by the kidneys but poorly reabsorbed in the tubule. Acetazolamide, which is the prototype for the carbonic anhydrase inhibitors, induces diuresis by decreasing hydrogen ion secretion by the tubules and increasing excretion of sodium and water. Although the diuretic effect is limited, aqueous humor formation is reduced, thereby making these drugs useful for reducing intraocular pressure in glaucoma. This chapter also discusses nursing management strategies for patients on diuretic therapy.

PHYSIOLOGY

The renal system is a complex mechanism that has several important functions in maintaining health. It is the body's filtering and purifying center, ridding the body of impurities and waste by producing urine and excreting water, electrolytes, and other substances. Other functions of the renal system include regulating the body's acid-base balance, maintaining blood pressure, influencing circulating fluid volume, assisting in the production of red blood cells, and contributing to calcium metabolism (Fig. 31-1).

The renal system consists of the kidneys, ureters, and bladder. The kidneys are a pair of intricate, bean-shaped organs located behind the upper abdomen outside the peritoneal cavity. They are active in filtering, reabsorbing, and excreting fluid, electrolytes, and waste products. The ureters are tubes that transport waste products and excess fluid from the kidneys to the bladder, a balloon-like receptacle, for later excretion.

Urine formation, which occurs as a result of kidney function, involves three complex processes–glomerular filtration, renal tubular reabsorption, and renal tubular secretion. These mechanisms work together in a part of the kidney called the nephron, which processes blood plasma into urine.

The nephron has many parts, including the glomerulus, Bowman capsule, and various tubules and membranes. In the nephron, water and solutes move from the blood plasma across a glomerular capsular membrane into an area known as a Bowman capsule. This movement across the capsular membrane is called **glomerular filtration.**

As the blood flows through the kidney capillaries, pressure in the capillaries causes fluid to filter into the Bowman capsule. The glomerular capsular membrane (the basement membrane), which lies between the glomerulus and the Bowman capsule, allows fluid and electrolytes but not blood cells and plasma proteins to pass into the Bowman capsule. The average glomerular filtration rate is 125 mL/min (or about 180 L of plasma in 24 hours). More than 99% of the plasma filtered is reabsorbed in the tubules.

Usually, the kidneys produce less than 2 L of urine daily. However, changes in colloid osmotic pressure or capsular hydrostatic pressure can alter glomerular filtration. For example, a decrease in colloid osmotic pressure may increase filtration. Conversely, an increase in capsular hydrostatic pressure, which occurs in obstructive disease, may decrease filtration.

The conversion of the filtrate into urine occurs in the renal tubule by processes known as renal tubular reabsorption and renal tubular secretion. In **renal tubular reabsorption,** molecules move from the renal tubule across a semipermeable membrane into the peritubular blood (the blood surrounding the renal tubule).

In **renal tubular secretion,** molecules move from the blood surrounding the renal tubule into the tubule. In both reabsorption and secretion, diffusion and active transport are key mechanisms.

The strength, or concentration, of the urine produced is known as **osmolality,** which is the density of active particles in solution or the osmotic concentration determined by the ionic concentration of dissolved substances per unit of solution. Urine osmolality depends on the volume and composition of extracellular fluids. It also depends on a countercurrent mechanism in the renal medulla (a part of the kidney), which controls the flow of water and solute so that water is kept out of the area around the tubule and that sodium and urea are retained. An important contributor to this process is antidiuretic hormone (ADH), which is released when the osmolality of the extracellular fluid increases.

To enable water to move out of the tubule and into the surrounding capillaries, ADH increases the permeability of the collecting tubule to water; from the capillaries, it returns to the vascular system for circulation. As a result of increased water reabsorption, urine osmolality (concentration) increases. Without ADH, the renal tubules are impermeable to water, water is not reabsorbed, and dilute urine is produced.

The kidneys play a major role in regulating acid-base balance and maintaining a normal blood pH (7.35–7.45) by

Physiology

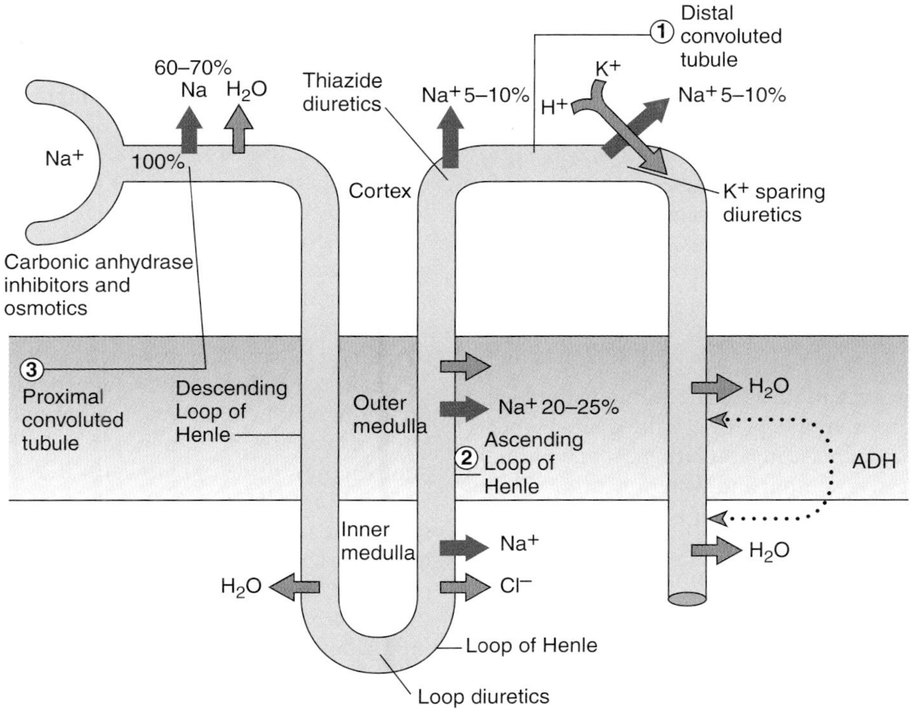

Figure 31-1. Diuretics work in the nephron. The main organ of the renal system is the kidney, which houses a tangled mass of nearly 1 million nephrons. The nephron is the structure known for its role in urine production. Different diuretic drugs work in different parts of the nephron: thiazide, thiazide-like, and potassium-sparing diuretics work in the distal convoluted tubule (**1**), loop diuretics in the ascending loop of Henle (**2**), and carbonic anhydrase inhibitors and osmotic diuretics in the proximal convoluted tubule (**3**). Fluid and electrolyte alterations depend on where the specific diuretic works in the kidney.

excreting hydrogen ions or reabsorbing bicarbonate. The kidneys regulate hydrogen ion secretion so that bicarbonate levels remain within normal limits. Most of the hydrogen ions excreted in the urine are secreted into the tubular fluid. Tubular fluid pH is acidic, and the kidney depends on buffers in the urine to combine with the hydrogen ion for excretion. The three buffers are bicarbonate (HCO_3), phosphate (HPO_4), and ammonia (NH_3).

The first step in bicarbonate reabsorption is the movement of carbon dioxide (CO_2) into a tubular cell where the CO_2 combines with water to form a hydrogen ion and a bicarbonate ion. The hydrogen ion is then secreted into the tubular fluid, and a sodium ion is reabsorbed. The sodium ion and bicarbonate ion pass into the extracellular fluid. The free hydrogen ion then combines with a filtered bicarbonate ion to form carbon dioxide and water. The water is eliminated in the urine, and the CO_2 diffuses into the tubular cell to combine with water, thereby forming a hydrogen ion and a bicarbonate ion to begin the process again.

Additional hydrogen ions are excreted in the urine in combination with a phosphate or ammonium buffer. The phosphate ion is filtered into the tubular fluid where it combines with a free hydrogen ion and is excreted. Ammonia is synthesized in the tubular cells and diffuses into the tubular fluid where it combines with a hydrogen ion to form an ammonium ion (NH_4), which is excreted.

Normally, the number of hydrogen ions secreted by the tubules is about equal to the bicarbonate ions filtered in the glomerulus. In metabolic acidosis, however, the number of hydrogen ions secreted exceeds bicarbonate filtration, and the urine becomes acidic. In metabolic alkalosis, bicarbonate filtration exceeds hydrogen ion secretion, and the urine becomes alkaline.

Additional work of the kidneys includes endocrine functions, whereby chemicals are produced to exert action elsewhere in the body. In this regard, the kidneys help maintain and regulate blood pressure and vascular resistance, red blood cell production, and calcium metabolism.

Blood pressure is affected by the kidneys' role in the renin-angiotensin-aldosterone mechanism. Renin, an enzyme, is synthesized and stored in the kidney and released in response to decreased blood flow or a change in the composition of fluid in the distal tubule. The release of renin plays a role in converting angiotensin I, a substance in the blood, into the powerful vasopressor angiotensin II. In response, the kidney decreases sodium and water excretion, causing blood pressure to increase. Angiotensin II also stimulates the adrenal cortex to secrete the hormone aldosterone, which promotes sodium and water reabsorption and increases blood pressure.

The kidney produces erythropoietin, which stimulates the bone marrow to produce and release red blood cells, particularly in response to hypoxia (oxygen deprivation). In kidney failure, loss of this ability contributes to anemia.

The kidneys play a vital role in the chemical transformation of compounds that are precursors to the active form of vitamin D, which is needed for the absorption of calcium from the gastrointestinal (GI) tract. Vitamin D also helps to regulate calcium deposition in the bones.

PATHOPHYSIOLOGY

When the body cannot maintain a balance of body fluid levels, fluid overload or volume depletion will occur. **Hypervolemia** (an abnormal increase in circulating blood volume) may result from excessive sodium and water retention. Fluid shifts into the interstitial spaces (**edema**) may occur with fluid volume excess. Peripheral edema increases the cardiac workload and decreases tissue perfusion. Moreover, other organ systems may be affected adversely by the congestion associated with edema. When systemic edema is severe, the congestion will back up into the lungs, affecting breathing and gas exchange.

Diuretic drugs are used in treating pathologic conditions in which fluid overload, and frequently edema, has occurred. These conditions include congestive heart failure (CHF), pulmonary edema, hypertension, and kidney disorders. Additionally, diuretics are used for treating adverse effects from long-term steroid or antiepileptic drug therapy, and such symptoms of fluid overload as increased intracranial and intraocular pressure and premenstrual syndrome.

Ineffective pumping of the heart can result in CHF because the heart does not empty well, and cardiac output is diminished. Approximately 5 million Americans have CHF, with 400,000 new cases diagnosed each year (Skrabal, Stading, Behmer-Miller, & Hilleman, 2000). Increased demands placed on the heart by other systemic problems can also cause the heart to fail. When the heart chambers do not empty well with each contraction, blood backs up into the body, and congestion occurs in the body tissues. Edema in CHF usually results from increased sodium and water retention and venous congestion, which increases capillary pressure in the peripheral and pulmonary circulation. As a result of the ineffective pumping ability of the heart, the kidneys receive a diminished blood supply. Impaired glomerular filtration and reduced blood flow to the renal tubules then occur. The kidney interprets these findings as signs of hypovolemia (insufficient circulating fluid or volume depletion) and activates mechanisms to retain sodium and water and increase circulating volume. Thus, volume is increased in an already congested system, and CHF actually worsens.

Drug therapy for CHF is now focused on improving survival. Drugs proven to reduce morbidity and mortality in CHF are angiotensin-converting enzyme inhibitors (ACE inhibitors), beta blockers, and the combination of hydralazine with a nitrate. The use of digoxin and diuretics, long considered standard treatment, has been found not to improve survival. However, these drugs are still an important aspect of drug therapy for CHF because they decrease symptoms and do help patients feel better. The increased urinary output resulting from diuretic therapy is useful in CHF because it reduces edema and circulating volume and prevents further fluid retention by the kidneys. These actions have a net effect of decreasing preload (volume returned to the heart) and afterload (resistance exerted by the vessels to blood pumped by the heart) and easing the heart's workload.

Other drug therapies that might be useful in treating CHF are calcium-channel blockers, phosphodiesterase inhibitors, catecholamine infusions, and amiodarone (Skrabal, et al., 2000). For more information on other drug therapies used to treat CHF, see Chapters 14, 27, 28, and 29.

Pulmonary edema, characterized by fluid-filled lungs, is a life-threatening condition. It commonly results from CHF, but it also can result from infections, exposure to toxic gases, and reactions to drugs. However, the pulmonary edema associated with CHF occurs because pulmonary capillary pressure is greater than capillary osmotic pressure (because of increased left ventricular end diastolic pressure). In addition, the capillary permeability of the pulmonary capillary membrane increases, thereby allowing fluid to leak into the lungs' interstitial spaces and the alveoli. This leakage impairs gas exchange, which stiffens the lungs and impairs expansion. Diuretics return fluid to the vascular space and increase fluid excretion, which eases breathing.

Hypertension (blood pressure that is chronically elevated above normal), one of the most common cardiovascular disorders in the United States, is closely associated with kidney function. Renin is released by the kidneys. The outflow of renin activates several mechanisms that lead to the activation of angiotensin II, a potent vasoconstrictor. Angiotensin II stimulates the secretion of aldosterone, which promotes sodium retention. Sodium retention promotes water retention. The resulting increased vascular resistance and the increased fluid volume elevate blood pressure.

Although hypervolemia is not necessarily present in the hypertensive patient, the action of diuretics effectively lowers the blood pressure. Blood pressure (BP) is cardiac output (CO) multiplied by peripheral resistance (PR) ($BP = CO \times PR$). By reducing circulating volume, diuretics decrease cardiac output and reduce blood pressure. In reducing circulating volume, fluid is pulled back into the vascular space, reducing edema and the symptoms associated with it. Peripheral vascular resistance is thus decreased, further promoting reduction in blood pressure and decreasing the workload on the heart.

The kind of diuretic drug prescribed depends on the patient's condition and the severity of the hypertension. Diuretics may be used alone or with antihypertensive drugs to lower blood pressure. For more information, refer to Chapter 30.

A kidney disorder characterized by generalized edema is nephrotic syndrome. This condition alters glomerular permeability to protein, allowing massive proteinuria as plasma proteins are lost by way of the kidney. This results in hypoalbuminemia (a lower-than-normal blood level of the protein albumin). Low albumin levels decrease colloid osmotic pressure, which allows fluid to move out of the vascular system.

This results in edema and decreased circulating volume. The kidneys attempt to compensate for the decreased blood volume by retaining sodium and water, which contributes to additional edema. Diuretics promote the excretion of sodium and water, and therefore decrease the circulating blood volume.

A potentially reversible condition, ARF results from an acute reduction of kidney function. Chronic renal failure, an irreversible and progressive reduction of kidney function, results from various conditions, including hypertension, diabetes mellitus, systemic lupus erythematosus, recurrent urinary tract infections, and obstruction. Renal failure is characterized by **oliguria** (abnormally reduced urine output, less than 400 mL/d); azotemia; sodium and water retention, leading to hypertension, CHF, and edema; metabolic acidosis; electrolyte imbalances; abnormalities of calcium, phosphorus, and vitamin D metabolism; and uremia in end-stage renal disease.

The effectiveness and safety of diuretics in treating ARF and chronic renal failure depend on kidney functioning. Osmotic diuretics are helpful in the early phases of ARF. Thiazide and loop diuretics may be used in the early stages of chronic renal failure. Once end-stage renal failure sets in, however, diuretics are of little value and may be harmful. Diuretics should be used cautiously in patients with renal impairment.

THIAZIDE DIURETICS

The thiazides comprise the largest group of diuretics. They are related structurally to the antibacterial sulfonamides, although a few drugs in the class differ slightly in chemical structure. These drugs are called thiazide-like diuretics and include indapamide (Lozol) and quinethazone (Aquamox). They exhibit the same diuretic mechanism of action, efficacy, and adverse reactions as the thiazides. Thiazide diuretics include hydrochlorothiazide (HydroDIURIL), benzthiazide (Exna), chlorothiazide (Diuril), chlorthalidone (Hygroton), and metolazone (Zaroxolyn). Additional thiazide diuretics include bendroflumethiazide (Naturetin), hydroflumethiazide (Diucardin), trichlormethiazide (Diurese), polythiazide (Renese), and methyclothiazide (Aquatensen, Enduron). The prototype thiazide diuretic is hydrochlorothiazide.

NURSING MANAGEMENT OF THE PATIENT RECEIVING HYDROCHLOROTHIAZIDE

Core Drug Knowledge

Pharmacotherapeutics

Hydrochlorothiazide is used widely in managing hypertension, either alone or with other drugs. Several days are required to see the antihypertensive effects, and full therapeutic effects may not occur for 2 to 4 weeks. Hydrochlorothiazide also is used in treating edema resulting from CHF, hepatic cirrhosis, renal disease, and long-term steroid or estrogen therapy (Table 31-1). Paradoxically, hydrochlorothiazide is used in diabetes insipidus as an antidiuretic, possibly because it enhances the action of ADH as a consequence of sodium depletion.

In investigational use, hydrochlorothiazide may be used alone or with amiloride or allopurinol to prevent the formation and recurrence of calcium stones in hypercalciuria by promoting the reabsorption of calcium.

TABLE 31-1 Summary of Selected Diuretic Drugs

Drug (Trade) Name	Selected Indications	Route and Dosage Range	Pharmacokinetics
Thiazide Diuretics			
hydrochlorothiazide (Esidrix, HydroDIURIL, Oretic; *Canadian:* Apo-Hydro)	Hypertension	*Adult:* PO, 25 mg/d; increase to 50 mg/d as a single or two divided doses *Child:* PO, infants up to 6 mo, 3.3 mg/kg/d in two doses; 6 mo–2 y, 12.5–37.5 mg/d in two doses, depending on body weight; 2–12 y, 37.5–100 mg/d in two doses depending on body weight	*Onset:* 2 h *Duration:* 6–12 h $t_{1/2}$: 5.6–14.8 h
	Edema	*Adult:* PO, 25–200 mg/d initially, then 25–100 mg/d *Child:* PO, 2.2 mg/kg/d in two doses	
Loop Diuretics			
furosemide (Lasix; *Canadian:* Apo-Furosemide)	Edema	*Adult:* PO, 20–80 mg/d in a single dose, may repeat 6 to 8 h later, titrate up to 600 mg/d in severe edema *Adult:* IM, IV, 20–40 mg, may repeat 2 h later	*Onset:* PO, within 1 h; IV, within 5 min *Duration:* PO, 6–8 h; IV, 2 h $t_{1/2}$: 2 h

(continued)

TABLE 31-1 Summary of Selected Diuretic Drugs (Continued)

Drug (Trade) Name	Selected Indications	Route and Dosage Range	Pharmacokinetics
	Hypertension	*Adult:* PO, 40 mg bid *Child:* PO, 2 mg/kg, may increase by 1–2 mg/kg, not to exceed 6 mg/kg	
	CHF, CRF	*Adult:* PO, IV, 2–2.5 g/d	
	Pulmonary edema	*Adult:* IV, 40 mg over 1–2 min, may increase to 80 mg *Child:* IV, 1 mg/kg, may increase by 1 mg/kg but not more than 6 mg/kg	
Potassium-sparing Diuretics			
triamterene (Dyrenium)	Hypertension	*Adult:* PO, 100 mg bid when used alone; decrease starting dose when given with other diuretics; decrease dose of each, adjust to need; not to exceed 300 mg/d	*Onset:* PO, 2–4 h *Duration:* 12–16 h $t_{1/2}$: 3 h
amiloride (Midamor)	Hypertension	*Adult:* PO, add 5 mg/d to usual antihypertensive or other diuretic therapy; increase up to 10 mg/d	*Onset:* 2 h *Duration:* 24 h $t_{1/2}$: 6–9 h
spironolactone (Aldactone; *Canadian:* Novo-Spiroton)	Hyperaldosteronism	*Adult:* PO, 100–400 mg/d	*Onset:* 24–48 h *Duration:* 48–72 h $t_{1/2}$: 20 h
	Edema	*Adult:* PO, 100 mg/d (range: 25–200 mg/d) *Child:* PO, 3.3 mg/kg/d in single or divided doses	
	Hypertension	*Adult:* PO, 50–100 mg/d, single or divided doses *Child:* PO, 1–2 mg/kg bid	
	Diuretic-induced hypokalemia	*Adult:* PO, 25–100 mg/d	
Osmotic Diuretics			
mannitol (Osmitrol)	Acute renal failure	*Adult:* IV, 50–100 g of 5%–25% solution (preventative) or 50–100 g of 15%–25% solution (treatment)	*Onset:* 0.5–1 h *Duration:* 6–8 h $t_{1/2}$: 15–100 min
	Intracranial pressure	*Adult:* IV, 1.5–2 g/kg as 15%–25% solution infused over 30–60 min	
	Intraocular pressure	*Adult:* IV, 1.5–2 g/kg as 15%–20% solution infused over 30 min	
	Diuresis in intoxications	*Adult:* IV, Up to 200 g	
	Urologic irrigation	*Adult:* Bladder catheter, 2.5% solution; add two 50-mL vials (25% mannitol) to 900-mL sterile water	
Carbonic Anhydrase Inhibitors			
acetazolamide (Diamox; *Canadian:* Apo-Acetazolamide)	Chronic open-angle glaucoma	*Adult:* PO, 250 mg–1 g daily in divided doses	*Onset:* PO, 1–1.5 h; IV, 2 min *Duration:* PO 8–12 h; IV, 4–5 h $t_{1/2}$: Unknown
	Secondary glaucoma/preoperative acute congestive closed-angle glaucoma	*Adult:* PO, IV, 250 mg q4h or 250 mg bid or 500 mg followed by 125 or 250 mg q4h *Child:* IM, IV 5–10 mg/kg/dose q6h; PO, 10–15 mg/kg/d in divided doses	
	CHF	*Adult:* PO, 250–375 mg (5 mg/kg)/d	
	Drug-induced edema	*Adult:* PO, 250–375 mg qd, give every other day or 2 d on then 1 d off *Child:* PO, IV 5 mg/kg/dose	
	Epilepsy	*Adult and child:* PO, IV, 8–30 mg/kg/d in divided doses	
	Mountain sickness	*Adult:* PO, 500–1,000 mg/d in divided doses; may use sustained-release preparation	

In addition, these drugs have been used to prevent osteoporosis in postmenopausal women.

Pharmacokinetics

Administered orally, hydrochlorothiazide is absorbed rapidly from the GI tract, and more than 50% of the circulating drug is bound to plasma proteins. Action begins within a few hours. The drug crosses the placental barrier and is secreted in breast milk. Hydrochlorothiazide is metabolized by the liver and excreted in the urine.

Pharmacodynamics

Hydrochlorothiazide acts in the distal tubule and possibly in the diluting segment of the ascending loop of Henle. It increases the excretion of sodium and chloride in the distal convoluted tubule by slightly inhibiting the ion pumps that work in sodium and chloride reabsorption. This also inhibits water reabsorption. Because most of the sodium is reabsorbed before the distal tubule, hydrochlorothiazide has a weak diuretic effect. It also increases excretion of potassium, bicarbonate, and magnesium and decreases the excretion of calcium. Water-soluble vitamins also are lost with the increased urine elimination from hydrochlorothiazide, as well as other diuretics (Suter, Haller, & Hany, 2000). Hydrochlorothiazide may decrease glomerular filtration rate and increase blood urea nitrogen (BUN).

Contraindications and Precautions

Important contraindications to hydrochlorothiazide therapy include severe renal impairment or anuria (urine output less than 250 mL daily), hepatic coma, and hypersensitivity to the drug or to sulfonamide antibiotics, which are similar chemically to hydrochlorothiazide and therefore increase the risk of cross-sensitivity. Thiazides should be used with caution in patients with renal disease, lupus erythematosus, liver disease, fluid and electrolyte imbalances, diabetes, gout, elevated cholesterol levels, elevated triglycerides, bronchial asthma, advanced arteriosclerosis, and heart disease. Hydrochlorothiazide is a pregnancy category B drug.

Adverse Effects

Adverse effects are due mostly to the effects of fluid loss or imbalance or from the effects of electrolyte imbalances, which may include hypokalemia, hyponatremia, hypochloremia, and hypercalcemia. The most common adverse effects affect various systems as follows: cardiovascular (hypotension), central nervous system (CNS; dizziness, lightheadedness, and vertigo), GI (anorexia, nausea, and vomiting), and genitourinary (GU; polyuria and nocturia).

Other adverse effects related to fluid and electrolyte imbalances include CNS effects, such as paresthesia (numbness and tingling), headache, and drowsiness. Cardiovascular effects include orthostatic hypotension, volume depletion, cardiac arrhythmias, and chest pain. GI disturbances include diarrhea, constipation, jaundice, and pancreatitis. Dermatologic effects include poor skin turgor and dry mucous membranes. Finally, the musculoskeletal system may be prone to weakness and muscle cramps or spasms resulting from potassium loss, and possibly gout resulting from increased uric acid levels.

Drug Interactions

Hydrochlorothiazide and other thiazide diuretics increase the effect of many drugs or drug classes, including allopurinol, anesthetics, antineoplastics, calcium salts, diazoxide, digitalis, lithium, loop diuretics, methyldopa, nondepolarizing muscle relaxants, and vitamin D. Thiazide diuretics decrease the effectiveness of anticoagulants and antigout agents. The effect of thiazides is increased by amphotericin B, corticosteroids, and anticholinergics. The effect of thiazides is decreased by cholestyramine, colestipol, methenamines, and nonsteroidal anti-inflammatory drugs (NSAIDs). Although no major drug-food interactions are associated with hydrochlorothiazide, some blood test findings may be altered. For example, decreased protein-bound iodine levels may occur without the patient's showing signs of thyroid disturbance (Table 31-2).

Assessment of Relevant Core Patient Variables

Health Status

The nurse must determine whether the patient is allergic to sulfa or to other thiazides because these are contraindications for use. Renal status must be assessed because severe renal impairment is a contraindication for hydrochlorothiazide use. Patients who have pre-existing renal disease, a creatinine clearance of 40 to 50 mL/min, a glomerular filtration rate of 25 mL/min, or a history of nonresponsiveness to thiazides most likely should be treated with loop diuretics instead of hydrochlorothiazide. If used, hydrochlorothiazide therapy in these patients must be monitored carefully.

The nurse should assess hepatic status because hepatic coma is a contraindication, and hepatic disease warrants cautious use. Other problems include a history of systemic lupus erythematosus, diabetes, gout, bronchial asthma, arteriosclerosis, heart disease, elevated triglyceride or cholesterol levels. In diabetic patients, blood glucose levels must be assessed; in patients with gout, uric acid levels must be assessed; and in patients with kidney disease or kidney failure, creatinine levels must be assessed because hydrochlorothiazide elevates blood glucose, lipid, and uric acid levels.

Before therapy begins, it is important to assess fluid and electrolyte status because hydrochlorothiazide will cause fluid and electrolyte losses. If the patient has fluid and electrolyte deficiencies before therapy, additional losses will increase the risk of significant adverse effects. Additional baseline measurements should include blood pressure and other vital signs; body weight; edema in the ankles, sacrum, and abdomen; and urinary elimination patterns and output volume.

Because many drugs interact with hydrochlorothiazide, the nurse should assess the patient's drug history,

TABLE 31-2 Agents That Interact With P Hydrochlorothiazide

Interactants	Effect and Significance	Nursing Management
allopurinol	May increase the incidence of hypersensitivity reactions to allopurinol	Monitor for allergic effects.
anesthetics	More anesthetic effect	Dosage may need to be decreased. Monitor/correct fluid imbalance prior to surgery if possible.
anticoagulants	Decreased anticoagulant effect	Monitor prothrombin time, partial thromboplastin time; dose may need adjustment.
antigout agents	Decreased effect with thiazides; increased uric acid levels	Monitor uric acid levels; dose may need to be adjusted.
antineoplastics	Induces leukopenia with prolonged use	Monitor white blood cell count.
calcium salts	Increased effect because thiazides promote calcium retention	Monitor calcium levels.
diazoxide	Hyperglycemia possible	Monitor blood glucose level.
digitalis glycosides	Hypokalemia from thiazides, which may induce digitalis toxicity	Monitor potassium level. Monitor for digitalis toxicity. Provide potassium in diet or supplements.
lithium	Sodium possibly lost instead of lithium ions, inducing lithium toxicity	Monitor blood lithium levels.
loop diuretics	Profound diuresis and serious electrolyte imbalance	Monitor electrolyte levels.
methyldopa	Rare occurrences of hemolytic anemia with concurrent use	Monitor complete blood chemistry.
nondepolarizing muscle relaxants	Possible prolonged neuromuscular blocking effects and respiratory depression	Assess respiratory status.
sulfonylureas, insulin	Increased blood glucose	Dose may need adjusting.
vitamin D	Biologic actions of vitamin D enhanced; hypercalcemia may have role	Monitor calcium levels.
amphotericin B, corticosteroids	Electrolyte depletion intensified	Monitor electrolyte levels, particularly potassium.
anticholinergics	Increased absorption of thiazides	Monitor blood pressure, electrolyte levels.
bile acid sequestrants (cholestyramine, colestipol)	Bind thiazides, reduce absorption	Give thiazides at least 2 h before resin.
methenamines	Possible decreased effect of thiazides due to alkalinization of urine	Monitor blood pressure, electrolyte levels; may need to adjust dosage.
nonsteroidal anti-inflammatory drugs	Reduced diuretic, natriuretic, and antihypertensive effect	Observe for therapeutic effect.

particularly the current drug regimen. Drug therapy that also causes electrolyte loss or that may be affected adversely by the electrolyte loss induced from hydrochlorothiazide therapy should be most closely assessed. For example, hydrochlorothiazide causes potassium loss (**hypokalemia**). Hypokalemia increases the effect of the drug digoxin. Therefore, patients receiving digoxin for CHF have an increased risk of digoxin toxicity if they become hypokalemic during hydrochlorothiazide therapy.

Life Span and Gender

It is important to determine whether the patient is pregnant or breast-feeding. Hydrochlorothiazide must be used with caution by pregnant or breast-feeding women. The nurse also should determine the patient's age before administering hydrochlorothiazide therapy. Efficacy and safety of hydrochlorothiazide have not been established in children. Some new research indicates that older adults with CHF who do not have left ventricular systolic dysfunction (i.e., their left ventricular function is normal) may have "diastolic heart failure" with impaired filling of the ventricles during diastole. By reducing intravascular volume, diuretics, such as hydrochlorothiazide may further impair ventricular diastolic filling in these patients. Long-term use of diuretics in these patients may provoke or aggravate hypotension on standing and after meals. The suggestion has been made that older adults with heart failure but intact left ventricular systolic function should not receive long-term diuretic therapy unless proven necessary to treat or prevent CHF. Thus, these patients should be evaluated to determine whether the dose may be tapered or the diuretic, hydrochlorothiazide or others, should be discontinued (van Kraaij et al 2000). Older adults also appear to be at increased risk for vitamin B1 deficiency while on hydrochlorothiazide or other diuretic therapy. This is due to vitamin loss with increased urination (Suter et al., 2000).

Lifestyle, Diet, and Habits

The nurse should assess the patient's normal fluid intake and dietary sources of electrolytes, particularly potassium, to evaluate whether the patient's nutritional intake can compensate adequately for electrolytes lost during drug therapy.

Environment

Some assessment factors related to hydrochlorothiazide therapy include whether the patient can get easily to a toilet, especially in the beginning of therapy when urine output increases. The patient's home must be set up for safety because falls may occur as a result of adverse effects of therapy. Hydrochlorothiazide can be self-administered at home or administered in acute-care, long-term care, or subacute-care settings.

Culture

The nurse should note the patient's ethnic background. In African-American patients, hydrochlorothiazide therapy is somewhat more effective than in patients who are of European descent. It is believed that hypertensive African Americans have features that are consistent with a theory of corrected volume status where the sodium and potassium pump is inhibited. Because hydrochlorothiazide stimulates the excretion of sodium and potassium, it exerts an additional effect in hypertensive African Americans.

From the findings of one small recent study of South African blacks, the recommendation was made that very low dose hydrochlorothiazide (12.5 mg daily) should not be used as monotherapy in blacks with mild to moderate hypertension because the ability to lower blood pressure is attenuated after 6 months of treatment, with most patients requiring an increase in the dose of hydrochlorothiazide and the addition of an ACE inhibitor to control blood pressure over 12 months (Radevski, Valtchenova, Candy, Hlatswayo, & Sareli, 2000).

Nursing Diagnoses and Outcomes

- Risk for Deficient Fluid Volume related to action and adverse effects of hydrochlorothiazide
  Desired outcome: The patient will not experience fluid imbalance while on hydrochlorothiazide therapy.
- Risk for Injury, falls, related to adverse effects of hydrochlorothiazide
  Desired outcome: The patient will not suffer injury from falls while on hydrochlorothiazide.
- Risk for Injury, drug interactions, related to multiple drug therapies
  Desired outcome: The patient will not have adverse effects from drug interactions while on hydrochlorothiazide.

Planning and Intervention

Maximizing Therapeutic Effects

The nurse should administer hydrochlorothiazide in the morning so that the maximum diuretic effect will not disturb sleep (assuming the patient is awake days and sleeps nights). It is important to provide ready access to a bathroom (or bedside urinal, bedpan, or commode) to ensure comfort during peak drug action.

The nurse should monitor fluid intake, urine output, and body weight for changes. It is important to encourage the patient to avoid foods high in sodium content and not to increase sodium intake greatly after hydrochlorothiazide dosage has been regulated (could counteract the effect of drug therapy). The nurse should encourage continued efforts at lifestyle changes that lower blood pressure (when used to treat hypertension).

Minimizing Adverse Effects

The nurse should monitor serum electrolyte levels for hypokalemia, hyponatremia, hypomagnesemia, hypercalcemia, hyperglycemia, and hyperuricemia, and also monitor serum triglyceride, cholesterol, and creatinine levels. Administer potassium supplements as indicated to maintain normal potassium levels.

It is important to assess the complete blood count (CBC) to detect blood abnormalities, and to inspect the skin for rashes or hives to detect sensitivity responses. The nurse should observe the patient for related signs and symptoms of fluid and electrolyte abnormalities. It also is important to weigh the patient regularly to determine extraordinary fluid loss (reflected in weight loss) and complications (reflected in weight gain). The patient might be weighed daily during the initial period of therapy and then weekly or biweekly once therapy is stabilized. A weight gain exceeding 3 lb in 1 day—a sign of fluid retention and complications—should be reported to the prescriber.

The nurse should caution the patient to avoid rapid position changes that may intensify orthostatic hypotension and precipitate falls. As needed, elderly or debilitated patients should be assisted with walking to the bathroom to prevent injury. Hydrochlorothiazide can be administered with meals or milk to prevent or minimize GI upset. It is important to assess for signs of drug interactions if the patient is currently receiving other drug therapies known to interact with hydrochlorothiazide.

Providing Patient and Family Education

- The nurse should explain the importance of follow-up blood work to monitor electrolyte levels.
- It is important to urge patients to report signs and symptoms of hypokalemia (irregular pulse rate, muscle weakness or cramps, constipation, or abdominal pain) to the physician or nurse practitioner.
- The nurse should tell the patient to take his pulse and compare the rate with former or normal rates. (The nurse may need to teach the patient how to take a pulse.)

- The nurse should encourage the patient to consume potassium-rich foods, such as bananas, apricots, and orange juice and other electrolyte-rich beverages and food to counter electrolyte losses, especially potassium.
- It is important to teach the patient to avoid injury from falls by rising slowly and balancing carefully to counter orthostatic hypotension.
- The nurse teaches the patient to take hydrochlorothiazide with food if he has problems with GI discomfort.
- The nurse explains the importance of wearing sunglasses, sunscreen, wide-brimmed hats, and cover-up clothing to avoid a possible photosensitivity reaction.
- It is important to store hydrochlorothiazide safely to prevent accidental poisoning of children, elderly or forgetful adults, or others.

Ongoing Assessment and Evaluation

The effects of therapy and the degree to which expected outcomes have been achieved should be evaluated. Most patients receiving hydrochlorothiazide can expect to have a reduction in fluid retention, edema, and blood pressure. To that end, edema and blood pressure may be compared with baseline values. Fluid balance may be evaluated by weighing the patient at the same time of day on the same scale, ideally with the patient wearing the same weight of clothing. Laboratory tests may be reviewed regularly to detect electrolyte imbalances and blood abnormalities. ■

LOOP DIURETICS

The loop diuretics work in the loop of Henle to inhibit the reabsorption of sodium and chloride. They exert a powerful effect on fluid and electrolyte balance. Loop diuretics are sometimes referred to as high-ceiling diuretics because the maximum diuretic effect that can be achieved is higher than with other diuretics. Loop diuretics include furosemide (Lasix), bumetanide (Bumex), ethacrynic acid (Edecrin), and torsemide (Demadex). The prototype drug in this class is furosemide.

MEMORY CHIP

Hydrochlorothiazide

- Widely used alone or with other agents to reduce blood pressure; also used to treat edema from CHF, hepatic or renal disease, or secondary to drug use
- Works in the distal tubule to promote excretion of sodium, chloride, potassium, and water
- Significant contraindication: severe renal disease
- Most common adverse effects: from fluid and electrolyte loss (dizziness, light-headedness, vertigo, nausea, and vomiting)
- Most serious adverse effects: aplastic anemia and thrombocytopenia (although not normally life-threatening)
- Minimizing adverse effects: monitor blood pressure, weight, intake and output, and serum electrolyte levels while on this drug
- Most significant patient education: explain the importance of periodic blood work to monitor electrolytes

NURSING MANAGEMENT OF THE PATIENT RECEIVING FUROSEMIDE

Core Drug Knowledge

Pharmacotherapeutics

Furosemide is a potent diuretic that is effective in reducing peripheral edema from CHF and hepatic and renal diseases, including nephrotic disease (see the accompanying display, Furosemide Infusion in Refractory Congestive Heart Failure). It is highly effective in

Focus on Research

Furosemide infusion in refractory congestive heart failure (CHF)

Paterna, S., Di Pasquale, P., Parrinello, G., Amato, P., Cardinale, A., Follone, G., Giubilato, A., & Licata, G. (2000). Effects of high-dose furosemide and small-volume hypertonic saline solution infusion in comparison with a high dose of furosemide as a bolus in refractory congestive heart failure. *European Journal of Heart Failure, 2*(3), 305–313.

The Study

A study of hospitalized patients with CHF who were unresponsive to high oral doses of furosemide, ACE inhibitors, digitalis, and nitrates was performed. The patients also all had an ejection fraction <35%, serum creatinine <2 mg/dL, BUN <60 mg/dL, a reduced urinary volume, and a low natriuresis. The patients either received an IV push bolus of furosemide (500 to 1,000 mg) bid or an IV infusion of furosemide (500 to 1,000 mg) in 150 mL of NaCl, bid over 30 minutes, over 6 to 12 days. Both groups also received KCL (20 to 40 mEq) IV to prevent hypokalemia. The group that received an IV push furosemide was hospitalized longer than the group that received an IV infusion of furosemide (11.67 ≤ 1.8 days versus 8.57 ± 2.3 days; $p < .001$). Both groups achieved a lower class rating of CHF (based on New York Heart Association [NYHA] classification) at discharge (this is an improvement). In a follow-up visit at 6 to 12 months, none of the patients who received the IV infusion of furosemide required readmission to the hospital and their NYHA classification remained as it was at discharge. This is contrasted with 40% of the patients who received IV push furosemide. These patients also reverted to a higher NYHA classification than they had achieved prior to discharge.

Nursing Implications

Patients with CHF who have been unresponsive to high doses of oral furosemide and other drugs may benefit from administration of furosemide as an IV infusion rather than an IV push, which is not diluted, when they are hospitalized for recurrent exacerbations of CHF. Nurses should consult with the other health care team members (nurse practitioners, physicians, and pharmacists) about this possibility of drug therapy for appropriate patients.

the treatment of pulmonary edema. It also is effective in the treatment of hypertension and is the first choice over thiazides in patients with pre-existing renal disease because, unlike thiazides, it does not decrease glomerular filtration rate (see Table 31-1). Some research indicates that inhaled furosemide reduces dyspnea. Further research is needed in this area, however, for this to become a common, accepted therapeutic use (Nishino, Ide, Sudo, & Sato, 2000).

Pharmacokinetics

After oral administration, furosemide is absorbed rapidly and well from the GI tract. However, after IV administration, furosemide acts even more rapidly—within 10 minutes. Duration of action is 2 hours. The drug is about 95% bound to plasma proteins. Furosemide is metabolized in the liver and excreted by the kidneys. It crosses the placenta and may enter breast milk.

Pharmacodynamics

Furosemide inhibits the reabsorption of sodium, chloride, and water in the ascending loop of Henle. It also has some effect in the proximal and distal tubules. As a result, the excretion of sodium, chloride, potassium, and water increases. Magnesium and calcium are excreted as well. Furosemide can increase blood glucose, low-density lipoprotein, total cholesterol, and triglyceride levels. In addition, furosemide decreases the excretion of uric acid, which may raise uric acid levels.

Furosemide influences the activity of vagally mediated mechanoreceptors in the airways. It is hypothesized that the vagal afferent fibers may play an important role in modulating the feeling of dyspnea. This would be the mechanism for inhaled furosemide alleviating dyspnea. One small study was able to alleviate the sensation of dyspnea that was induced experimentally by breath-holding and by a combination of inspiratory resistive loading and hypercapnia (Nishino et al., 2000).

Contraindications and Precautions

Furosemide should not be used in anuria or if hypersensitivity to the compounds or to sulfonylureas exists. Cautious use must be exercised in patients with poor renal function and lupus erythematosus. Furosemide is a pregnancy category C drug.

Adverse Effects

Most of furosemide's adverse effects relate to fluid or electrolyte imbalance. The most common adverse effects are CNS (dizziness, vertigo, paresthesias, xanthopsia, and weakness); GI (nausea, anorexia, vomiting, oral and gastric irritation, and constipation); CV (orthostatic hypotension); hematologic (leukopenia, anemia, and thrombocytopenia); GU (glycosuria and urinary bladder spasm); dermatologic (photosensitivity, rash, pruritus, and urticaria); and musculoskeletal (muscle cramps and muscle spasms).

Other adverse effects are CNS (headache, blurred vision, hearing loss [may be permanent], restlessness, and fever); GI (diarrhea, cramping, pancreatitis, jaundice, and ischemic hepatitis); CV (chronic aortitis); hematologic (purpura and aplastic anemia); dermatologic (necrotizing angiitis, interstitial nephritis, exfoliative dermatitis, erythema multiforme, rash, local irritation, and pain with parenteral use); and miscellaneous (hyperuricemia, hyperglycemia, and activation or exacerbation of systemic lupus erythematosus [SLE]).

Excessive diuresis from furosemide can result in dehydration, reduction in blood volume with circulatory collapse, and the possibility of vascular thrombosis and embolism, particularly in the elderly. Patients with hepatic cirrhosis and ascites must be monitored carefully because rapid electrolyte shifts resulting from furosemide therapy may induce hepatic encephalopathy and coma.

Ototoxicity can occur with rapid IV therapy, especially in patients with poor renal function and in those receiving high doses of furosemide. Although usually transient, ototoxicity may result in permanent damage. The Na- K- Cl cotransport system exists, not only in the kidney, but in the marginal and dark cells of the stria vascularis, which are responsible for endolymph secretion. Ototoxicity has been hypothesized to be an indirect effect on the body, related to changes in ionic composition and fluid volume within the endolymph (Humes, 1999).

Patients with SLE may have exacerbations of the illness when receiving furosemide. If increasing azotemia, oliguria, or BUN or creatinine levels occur in patients with renal impairment, furosemide therapy should be discontinued.

Drug Interactions

Furosemide increases the effect of aminoglycosides, anticoagulants, beta blockers, chloral hydrate, digitalis, and lithium. Furosemide decreases the effect of sulfonylureas and has an undetermined effect on nondepolarizing muscle relaxants and theophyllines. Thiazide diuretics, cisplatin, and clofibrate increase the effect of furosemide. Phenytoin, NSAIDS, probenecid, and salicylates all decrease the effect of furosemide. Bioavailability and degree of diuresis are reduced when furosemide is administered with food (Table 31-3).

Assessment of Relevant Core Patient Variables

Health Status

Initially, the nurse assesses for allergies to furosemide or other contraindications. A baseline assessment is then performed. This assessment is much like the one for a patient receiving HCTZ. It begins with taking blood pressure and vital signs and reviewing relevant blood test results and electrolyte levels. To assess fluid status and obtain baseline data for therapy, the nurse weighs the patient. Apparent edema is inspected and palpated. It is important to auscultate breath sounds, particularly

TABLE 31-3 Agents That Interact With Furosemide

Interactants	Effect and Significance	Nursing Management
aminoglycosides	Increased auditory toxicity; possible hearing loss	Monitor BUN and creatinine; adverse effects will increase if drugs are not excreted well. Assess for hearing problems. When giving furosemide IV, give very slowly.
anticoagulants	Enhanced anticoagulant action possible	Monitor PT, PTT.
beta blocker (propranolol)	Increased plasma levels of propranolol	Monitor therapeutic effect of propranolol.
chloral hydrate	Rare transient diaphoresis, hot flashes, hypertension, tachycardia, weakness, and nausea	Consider drug interaction if these effects occur.
digitalis glycosides	Furosemide-induced hypokalemia, possibly increasing digitalis toxicity	Monitor serum potassium level. Supply potassium in diet or as supplement. Monitor for signs of digitalis toxicity.
lithium	Possible increased plasma lithium levels and toxicity	Monitor lithium levels.
nondepolarizing muscle relaxants	Antagonized or potentiated action of muscle relaxants, perhaps depending on furosemide dose	Monitor for therapeutic effect.
sulfonylureas	Hyperglycemia	Sulfonylurea dosage may need adjustment.
theophylline	Theophylline effect enhanced or inhibited	Monitor for therapeutic effect of theophylline.
charcoal	Decreased absorption of furosemide	Monitor for therapeutic effect. May be antidote in case of furosemide overdose.
cisplatin	Additive ototoxicity	Monitor for hearing loss, tinnitus. Administer IV furosemide slowly.
clofibrate	Exaggerated diuretic response	Monitor intake and output, BP, edema, and fluid and electrolyte levels.
phenytoin	Decreased diuretic response	Monitor for therapeutic response.
NSAID	Decreased diuretic response	Monitor for therapeutic response.
probenecid	Decreased diuretic response	Monitor for therapeutic response.
salicylates	Diuretic response impaired in patients with cirrhosis and ascites	Monitor for therapeutic response.
thiazides	Profound diuresis and serious electrolyte levels	Monitor BP, edema, and fluid and electrolyte levels.

in patients with CHF or pulmonary edema. The nurse also should assess skin turgor and mucous membranes and measure fluid intake and urinary output.

During assessment, the nurse keeps the proposed route of administration in mind because IV furosemide may have a significantly more potent effect on blood pressure and vital signs (cardiac arrest has been reported) than oral furosemide. As with HCTZ, the nurse also assesses for gout, diabetes, and high serum cholesterol and triglyceride levels.

Life Span and Gender

The nurse should assess the patient for pregnancy. Furosemide is classified as a pregnancy category C drug and should not be used during pregnancy. It also is important to determine the patient's age before administering furosemide. Furosemide may increase the risk of developing patent ductus arteriosus when given during the first few weeks of life to premature infants with respiratory distress syndrome. Development of renal calcifications (kidney stones) also have been reported when furosemide is used in severely premature infants. Furosemide can be used safely in children, but doses should not exceed 6 mg/kg of body weight.

If severe diuresis occurs from use of the drug, acute hypotensive episodes may occur, especially in elderly people. Elderly patients are at increased risk for rapid changes in fluid volume, which can lead to circulatory collapse. Moreover, elderly adults also are less tolerant of the rapid changes in blood pressure, which may occur with furosemide therapy. In older adults, the rapid loss of plasma volume and the resulting hemoconcentration is likely to cause thromboembolic episodes, such as cerebral vascular thromboses and pulmonary embolism.

Lifestyle, Diet, and Habits

Furosemide may promote severe electrolyte imbalances, especially in patients who have high dosages and who are on sodium-restricted diets. Therefore, normal fluid intake and dietary preferences should be determined and evaluated for the adequacy of electrolyte content, especially potassium.

Environment

The nurse should assess whether the patient can get to a toilet easily when needed, especially in the beginning of therapy when urine output increases. The patient's home should be assessed for risk factors that may contribute to injuries (falls) resulting from adverse effects of drug therapy. Furosemide can be self-administered at home or administered by the nurse in acute-care, long-term-care, or subacute-care environments. Parenteral dosing is more common in an acute-care environment.

Nursing Diagnoses and Outcomes

- Risk for Deficient Fluid Volume related to action and adverse effects of furosemide
  Desired outcome: The patient will not experience fluid and electrolyte imbalance while on furosemide.
- Risk for Injury, falls, related to adverse effects of furosemide
  Desired outcome: The patient will not suffer injury while on furosemide.
- Risk for Injury, drug interactions, related to multiple drug therapies
  Desired outcome: The patient will not have adverse effects from drug interactions while on furosemide.

Planning and Intervention

Maximizing Therapeutic Effects

If therapy begins in the hospital, the patient will receive small doses that may increase gradually and incrementally. Otherwise, interventions are the same as for HCTZ.

Minimizing Adverse Effects

When giving furosemide, the nurse follows the same procedures as those for minimizing adverse effects of HCTZ therapy. The drug administration route must be considered carefully because furosemide may be given IV or orally. The nurse should administer 20 to 40 mg of IV furosemide over at least 1 to 2 minutes to decrease the risk of ototoxicity. It is a good idea to give oral furosemide with food or milk to minimize possible GI upset. The nurse should report the adverse effects of rapid onset or worsening of edema and deterioration in breath sounds. These signs indicate that dosage may need to be adjusted or that a complication is developing.

Providing Patient and Family Education

The patient's and family's educational needs are similar to the needs of patients taking HCTZ.

Ongoing Assessment and Evaluation

To judge an identified therapeutic outcome, such as a reduction in edema and blood pressure, ongoing assessments of the following parameters are performed: CBC, serum electrolyte and uric acid levels, and other test values are compared with baseline values to measure progress or complications. For example, in a patient with diabetes mellitus, it is important to monitor regularly serum glucose levels because furosemide therapy may alter the amount of insulin or oral antidiabetic needed. ■

POTASSIUM-SPARING DIURETICS

The potassium-sparing diuretics promote sodium and water excretion in the distal tubule. At the same time, potassium is not excreted; rather, it is reabsorbed. This group of drugs produces weak diuresis and antihypertensive effects when used alone. However, the drugs are used more frequently in combination with loop and thiazide diuretics to minimize potassium loss because they work synergistically with other diuretics. Patients on potassium-sparing diuretics are at risk for developing hyperkalemia. Potassium-sparing diuretics include triamterene (Dyrenium), amiloride (Midamor), and spironolactone (Aldactone). The prototype of the potassium-sparing diuretics is triamterene.

NURSING MANAGEMENT OF THE PATIENT RECEIVING TRIAMTERENE

Core Drug Knowledge

Pharmacotherapeutics

Like furosemide, triamterene is used to manage edema and hypertension. The edema may be associated with CHF, cirrhosis, nephrotic syndrome, steroid use, or sec-

MEMORY CHIP

Furosemide

- A potent diuretic used to treat edema from CHF, pulmonary edema, and in hepatic and renal disease; may be used as an antihypertensive
- First choice diuretic for treating hypertension with pre-existing renal disease
- Works in the loop of Henle to promote excretion of large amounts of sodium, chloride, potassium, and water
- Most significant contraindication: anuria in CRF
- Most common adverse effects: related to fluid and electrolyte loss, especially potassium loss
- Most serious adverse effects: permanent deafness and activation or exacerbation of SLE
- **Lifespan alert: teach that older adults are more sensitive to effects of rapid fluid loss**
- Minimizing adverse effects: administer IV push slowly; and monitor blood pressure, edema, breath sounds, weight, intake and output, and serum electrolyte levels while therapy continues

ondary hypoaldosteronism. It typically is used with other diuretics because it allows potassium to be reabsorbed and sodium to be excreted (see Table 31-1).

Pharmacokinetics

Triamterene is absorbed incompletely after oral administration. The drug is metabolized in the liver and excreted by the kidneys. Triamterene crosses the placenta and is excreted in small amounts in breast milk.

Pharmacodynamics

Triamterene achieves its diuretic effect by inhibiting transport of sodium in the distal tubules independent of aldosterone. This causes increased loss of sodium, chloride, water, bicarbonate, and calcium. The drug promotes the retention of potassium and magnesium. Triamterene does not inhibit uric acid excretion and thereby elevates serum uric acid levels as do the loop diuretics.

Contraindications and Precautions

Contraindications to triamterene include known hypersensitivity, use of other potassium-sparing diuretics, preexisting **hyperkalemia** (serum potassium level above 5.5 mEq/L), anuria, severe or progressive renal disease (except nephrosis), severe liver disease, and hepatic coma.

Precautions to its use include electrolyte imbalance, history of renal stone formation (it has been found in some renal calculi), diabetes (it can raise blood glucose), and when folic acid stores have been depleted (it is a weak folic acid antagonist). It is in pregnancy category B, and safety and efficacy have not been established in children.

Adverse Effects

Serious adverse effects include hyperkalemia (potentially fatal), electrolyte imbalance, and signs of fluid and electrolyte loss. Most common adverse effects are weakness, nausea, anorexia, vomiting, and dry mouth.

Other adverse effects include GI (diarrhea, jaundice, and liver enzyme abnormalities); renal (azotemia, elevated BUN and creatinine levels); hematologic (thrombocytopenia and megaloblastic anemia); CNS (fatigue, dizziness, and headache); and miscellaneous (anaphylaxis, photosensitivity, and rash).

Drug Interactions

Triamterene increases the effect of amantadine and potassium preparations. ACE inhibitors, cimetidine, and indomethacin all increase the effect of triamterene. Triamterene will interfere with the fluorescent measurement of serum quinidine levels (Table 31-4).

Assessment of Relevant Core Patient Variables

Health Status

Assessment activities include determining whether the patient has any known hypersensitivity to triamterene and carefully examining electrolyte values, especially potassium levels. As for other diuretic drugs, additional assessments include measuring blood pressure, edema, weight, and urine output; examining serum glucose and creatinine levels; and identifying preexisting conditions, such as diabetes mellitus, that may affect triamterene therapy.

Life Span and Gender

Triamterene must be used cautiously in pregnancy (risk category B). Triamterene crosses into breast milk, and because safety has not been established for children, the drug should not be used in breast-feeding women.

Glomerular filtration decreases with age; consequently, elderly patients do not excrete as much potassium as younger adults. Therefore, triamterene should be given cautiously to older adults because of the increased risk for hyperkalemia.

Lifestyle, Diet, and Habits

The nurse should determine if the patient normally eats a diet high in potassium, takes a potassium supplement, or uses a potassium chloride salt substitute.

Environment

Environmental concerns are the same as for thiazides.

Nursing Diagnoses and Outcomes

- Risk for Deficient Fluid Volume related to action and adverse effects of triamterene

TABLE 31-4 Agents That Interact With Triamterene

Interactants	Effect and Significance	Nursing Management
amantadine	Increased amantadine plasma levels and decreased urinary excretion; more risk for adverse effects	Monitor for adverse effects.
potassium preparations	Severe hyperkalemia; possible cardiac arrhythmias or cardiac arrest	Avoid concurrent use.
ACE inhibitors	Elevated serum potassium from ACE inhibitors; hyperkalemia	Monitor serum potassium level.
cimetidine	Increased bioavailability and decreased renal clearance of triamterene	Monitor for increased therapeutic effect.
indomethacin	Rapid progress into acute renal failure with concurrent use	Use together only if truly necessary.

Desired outcome: The patient will not experience fluid and electrolyte imbalance while on triamterene.

- Risk for Injury, related to adverse effects of triamterene, including risk for hyperkalemia

  Desired outcome: The patient will not suffer injury, and potassium levels will remain within normal limits while patient is on triamterene therapy.
- Risk for Injury, drug interactions, related to multiple drug therapies

  Desired outcome: The patient will not have adverse effects from drug interactions while on triamterene.

Planning and Intervention

Maximizing Therapeutic Effects

As with other diuretics, the drug dose should be administered in the morning so that increased diuretic effect occurs during waking hours.

Minimizing Adverse Effects

The nurse should monitor blood potassium levels, and assess for signs of hyperkalemia (nausea, diarrhea, muscle weakness or cramping, oliguria, weak pulse, and cardiac arrhythmias). It is important to limit the patient's intake of potassium-rich foods and avoid potassium supplements. The nurse should monitor for signs of fluid and electrolyte imbalance. Oral triamterene should be given with food or milk to prevent GI upset. It is a good idea to have the patient get out of bed slowly, and assist with ambulation to prevent falls from dizziness.

Providing Patient and Family Education

The main distinction between triamterene and other diuretics is the hyperkalemia that may develop with drug use. Because triamterene is usually added to therapy with other types of diuretics, patients may become accustomed to being at risk for hypokalemia. The patient needs to learn to cope with the different risks associated with triamterene (see the accompanying display, Adding Triamterene to Hypertension Therapy). Other patient and family education points are similar to those provided for the other diuretics.

- The nurse should teach the patient to avoid potassium-rich foods, supplements, and potassium chloride–salt substitutes
- It is important for the patient to learn the signs and symptoms of hyperkalemia.

Ongoing Assessment and Evaluation

The nurse needs to monitor the patient's potassium and other electrolyte levels, blood pressure, edema, weight, and urine output. Drug therapy with triamterene is effective when blood pressure is reduced to therapeutic levels or edema is reduced without the patient developing hyperkalemia. ■

DRUG CLOSELY RELATED TO P TRIAMTERENE

Amiloride, which has the same mechanism of action, efficacy, and adverse reactions as triamterene, has two additional uses. In inhalable form, amiloride may be used to treat cystic fibrosis. In patients taking lithium, amiloride can reduce lithium-induced polyuria without increasing lithium levels.

DRUGS SIGNIFICANTLY DIFFERENT FROM P TRIAMTERENE

Like triamterene, spironolactone works in the distal tubule to increase sodium and water loss and to retain potassium. Unlike triamterene, spironolactone is an aldosterone antagonist. It interferes with testosterone synthesis, which leads to altered estrogenic and androgenic activity. Like other potassium-sparing diuretics, spironolactone can be used as an adjunct therapy to treat hypertension and edema associated with CHF, nephrosis, and cirrhosis. In addition, it

Critical Thinking Scenario

Adding triamterene to hypertension therapy

Mr. Nixon is a 53-year-old white man being treated for hypertension with hydrochlorothiazide (Dyrenium). He also receives 20 mEq of potassium as a supplement daily. Mr. Nixon's drug therapy is not having the desired therapeutic effect, and Mr. Nixon's health care provider writes an order to add triamterene to his drug regimen.

1. Explain which major electrolyte imbalance may now be experienced by Mr. Nixon.
2. Suggest actions that a nurse can take to prevent an electrolyte imbalance.

MEMORY CHIP

P Triamterene

- Potassium-sparing diuretic used to manage edema and hypertension
- Significant contraindication: the patient already receiving a potassium-sparing diuretic
- Most common adverse effects: nausea, vomiting, anorexia, dry mouth, and headache
- Most serious adverse effect: hyperkalemia (electrolyte imbalance)
- **Lifespan alert: older adults are especially at risk for hyperkalemia**
- Most significant patient education: tell the patient to avoid eating potassium-rich food, taking potassium supplements, or using a salt substitute containing potassium chloride

also is used in preventing or treating hypokalemia in high-risk patients, particularly those also taking digitoxin for cardiac disease or those with cardiac arrhythmias. Because of its anti-aldosterone effects, a major use is in diagnosing and treating primary hyperaldosteronism. Spironolactone also has been used to treat hirsutism, familial male precocious puberty, symptoms of premenstrual syndrome, and acne vulgaris (short-term use).

The effect of spironolactone is delayed. Onset of action may not occur for 24 to 48 hours. This is because the drug blocks the effect of aldosterone, which then blocks the synthesis of the proteins required for sodium and potassium transport. The existing proteins continue to do their job, and diuretic effect does not occur until the existing proteins are inactive.

Nursing management unique to spironolactone therapy involves helping the patient understand and cope with such adverse effects as impotence, menstrual irregularities, and gynecomastia. Additionally, the nurse needs to teach the patient about the drug interaction between spironolactone and salicylates, such as aspirin, which decreases the diuretic effect of therapy.

OSMOTIC DIURETICS

Osmotic diuretics are filterable freely in the glomerulus and not reabsorbed by the tubules. They increase osmotic pressure and pull fluid into the vascular space. Because they are not reabsorbed by the tubules, they prevent water reabsorption as well. They also prevent the reabsorption of sodium and chloride. Osmotic diuretics include mannitol (Osmitrol), glycerin, isosorbide, and urea.

The prototype osmotic diuretic is mannitol. Structurally, it is a sugar. Mannitol is not used to treat hypertension or peripheral edema. Instead, it is used in more acute situations.

NURSING MANAGEMENT OF THE PATIENT RECEIVING MANNITOL

Core Drug Knowledge

Pharmacotherapeutics

Major uses of mannitol include preventing and treating ARF, reducing intracranial pressure in cerebral edema, reducing intraocular pressure when other drugs have not worked, and promoting excretion of toxic substances in urine.

In addition, mannitol is used diagnostically to measure glomerular filtration rate and postoperatively as an irrigant after transurethral procedures (see Table 31-1).

Pharmacokinetics

Mannitol usually is administered as an IV solution because it does not diffuse across the GI epithelium nor is it distributed like other sugars. It can be administered as a urinary irrigant but only in transurethral prostatic resections or other transurethral surgical procedures. It is metabolized poorly, and most of it is excreted in the urine. When used as an irrigant, mannitol has a rapid onset and a short duration of action. Mannitol crosses the placenta and may enter breast milk.

Pharmacodynamics

Mannitol increases the concentration of molecules in the glomerular filtrate. This increased osmolality causes the osmotic pressure to rise. The increased pressure inhibits water reabsorption, which leads to an increased and faster flow of water in the tubules and therefore water loss. Mannitol also decreases the reabsorption of sodium and chloride.

Contraindications and Precautions

Mannitol is contraindicated in severe renal disease, severe pulmonary congestion or frank pulmonary edema, active intracranial bleeding (except during craniotomy), severe dehydration, progressive renal damage or dysfunction after mannitol therapy, and progressive heart failure or pulmonary congestion after mannitol therapy.

Mannitol must be used very cautiously in CHF, hypovolemia, pseudoagglutination, and hemoconcentration. Mannitol is a pregnancy category C drug. Safety and efficacy for children 12 years and younger have not been established.

Adverse Effects

Several adverse effects result from mannitol use. They are related mostly to the fluid changes induced by its use. The most common adverse effects are CNS (dizziness) and GI (nausea, anorexia, dry mouth, and thirst). The most serious adverse effect is onset of acute CHF in susceptible patients resulting from to the sudden expansion of the extracellular fluid.

Other adverse effects related to fluid changes include CV (edema, thrombophlebitis, hypotension, hypertension, tachycardia, and angina-like chest pains); CNS (headache, blurred vision, and convulsions); GI (urinary retention and osmotic nephrosis); metabolic (fluid and electrolyte imbalance, acidosis, and dehydration); and miscellaneous (pulmonary congestion, rhinitis, local pain, skin necrosis, chills, urticaria, and fever).

Fluid and electrolyte alterations may occur suddenly with the rapid expansion of extracellular fluid. Therefore, the nurse needs to monitor for possible water intoxication and advise the patient to report chest pain or shortness of breath. These symptoms may occur when fluid or electrolyte losses induce hypotension or tachycardia.

Overdosage from larger than recommended doses may result in increased electrolyte loss, particularly sodium, chloride, and potassium. Electrolyte depletions may be severe enough to bring on hypotension and cardiac irregularities.

Drug Interactions

There are no major drug-drug interactions with mannitol. It does not interact with any foods nor interfere with any laboratory test results.

Assessment of Relevant Core Patient Variables

Health Status

The nurse initially determines any contraindications to mannitol therapy, including anuria resulting from severe renal disease, pulmonary congestion, impaired cardiac function or CHF, active intracranial bleeding, or severe dehydration. These conditions contraindicate therapy because they may worsen with mannitol, which increases extracellular fluid volume. If urine output does not range between 30 and 50 mL/hour after two test doses of mannitol, the drug should not be used.

The nurse should assess blood pressure, pulse rate and character, respiratory rate and character, and breath sounds. Other general assessments include checking skin color and edema, hydration status, level of consciousness, reflexes, and muscle strength before and during the mannitol infusion to detect adverse effects.

Life Span and Gender

The nurse should assess the patient for pregnancy and breast-feeding. Pregnant patients should only receive mannitol (pregnancy category C) if therapy is clearly warranted and the benefits outweigh potential fetal harm. The nurse should explain to breast-feeding patients that mannitol may or may not be secreted in breast milk. It also is important to note the patient's age before administering mannitol. Mannitol's effect on children younger than 12 years remains unknown. Elderly patients are at increased risk for developing dizziness, disorientation, and confusion due to rapid fluid loss when receiving mannitol.

Environment

The nurse should note that mannitol is administered only in an acute-care setting.

Nursing Diagnosis and Outcome

- Risk for Deficient Fluid Volume related to action of mannitol

  Desired outcome: The patient's fluid and electrolyte levels will remain in normal limits.

Planning and Intervention

Maximizing Therapeutic Effects

Concentrations of mannitol that exceed 15% have a tendency to crystallize. This is a characteristic of the drug, because it is a sugar; it is not a sign that the drug is old and should be discarded. Therefore, the drug vial should be warmed to no more than body temperature before administration to eliminate crystals. An in-line filter should be used for the infusion.

Minimizing Adverse Effects

The nurse should monitor the patient's hourly urine output. Accuracy is essential, so an indwelling catheter normally is required. It is important to adjust the drug infusion rate to maintain the patient's urine output between 30 and 50 mL/hour.

Adequacy of renal function is determined in patients with renal impairment by administering one or two test doses of 0.2 g/kg over 3 to 5 minutes before beginning an infusion. If urine output is less than 30 mL/hour after the test doses, mannitol is usually withheld.

The nurse should monitor blood pressure, pulse rate, electrocardiographic (ECG) tracings, intake-output ratios, renal function test results, and serum electrolyte levels to monitor for rapid fluid and electrolyte alterations. It is important to assess for water intoxication as evidenced by nausea, chest pain, and shortness of breath. Breath sounds and respiratory rate and character should be assessed regularly to detect complications, such as pulmonary congestion.

The nurse should provide mouth care and ice chips for dry mouth or thirst. It also is important to assess for hives, itching, or pain at the IV site, and to provide comfort and corrective measures as needed. It is a good idea to assist patients in rising slowly from bed and provide assistance when the patient ambulates, if the patient must get out of bed. Treatment of overdosage includes discontinuation of infusion therapy at once and institution of measures to normalize electrolyte levels. Hemodialysis may be needed to eliminate mannitol and reduce serum osmolarity.

Providing Patient and Family Education

- The nurse should explain the purpose of mannitol therapy.
- It is important to urge the patient to report any difficulty breathing, chest pain, or peripheral swelling (edema).
- The nurse should tell the patient that blurred vision or a runny nose (if these findings occur) should subside when therapy is discontinued.

Ongoing Assessment and Evaluation

Monitoring is ongoing throughout therapy and includes measuring urine output and checking for signs of fluid or electrolyte imbalance. Therapy is effective when urine output increases and intracranial or intraocular pressure is decreased without complications to the patient. ■

MEMORY CHIP

Mannitol

- Treats acute renal failure, increased intracranial pressure, and increased intraocular pressure
- A sugar that draws water into the vascular space through osmosis. Freely filtered but not reabsorbed; thereby causes diuresis
- Significant contraindications: anuria due to severe renal disease, pulmonary edema, and intracranial bleeding
- Most common adverse effects: dizziness and GI problems
- Most serious adverse effects: worsening of CHF; serious imbalances of fluid and electrolytes; and obscure or worsened hypovolemia
- Maximizing therapeutic effects: warm the drug vial in water before using if crystals are seen; and administer no warmer than body temperature using an in-line filter
- Minimizing adverse effects: give a test dose for patients with marked oliguria or inadequate renal function. If urine output does not increase after two test doses, discontinue use

DRUGS CLOSELY RELATED TO MANNITOL

Glycerin (Glycerol)

Glycerin is an osmotic agent given orally to reduce intraocular pressure before ophthalmic surgery and during acute glaucoma attacks. It is metabolized and eliminated by the kidneys. Peak reduction of intraocular pressure occurs 1 hour after administration. Duration of action is about 5 hours. Contraindications are similar to mannitol and include well-established anuria, severe dehydration, frank or impending acute pulmonary edema, severe cardiac decompensation, and hypersensitivity to any ingredient. Caution should be used if the patient has acute urinary retention, hypervolemia, congestive heart disease, diabetes, or cardiac, renal, or hepatic disease. It can cause adverse reactions similar to those caused by mannitol (e.g., nausea, vomiting, headache, confusion, and disorientation). Serious complications of severe dehydration, cardiac arrhythmias, and hyperosmolar nonketotic coma are possible and may be fatal. Glycerin is a pregnancy category C drug.

A suppository form (glycerin suppositories, Fleet Babylax, Sani-Sipp) also is available and used as a hyperosmolar laxative for temporary relief of constipation.

Isosorbide

Isosorbide (Ismotic) also is used to provide short-term reduction of intraocular pressure before and after intraocular surgery, and to interrupt acute attacks of glaucoma. Isosorbide causes less risk of nausea and vomiting, and it should be used in place of other osmotics when these adverse effects are undesirable for the patient. Like glycerin it is only given orally. It is a good idea to pour the drug over cracked iced and have the patient sip the drug to improve its taste and acceptance. Contraindications and adverse effects are similar to those of mannitol. Isosorbide is a pregnancy category B drug.

Urea

Urea (Ureaphil), like mannitol, is administered by IV infusion, and is used to decrease intracranial pressure (in the control of cerebral edema) and to reduce intraocular pressure. An unlabeled use has been to induce abortion. Contraindications are severely impaired renal function, active intracranial bleeding, marked dehydration, and frank liver failure. Urea is a pregnancy category C drug.

No serious adverse effects occur if urea is infused slowly, if there is adequate renal function, and if there is no intracranial bleeding. Adverse effects that occur are similar to those with mannitol and include headache, nausea, vomiting, syncope, and disorientation.

Urea should be mixed with 5% or 10% dextrose solution to prevent the hemolysis produced by pure solutions of urea. Infusions should be slow as rapid infusion may be associated with hemolysis and a direct effect on the cerebral vasomotor centers, causing increased capillary bleeding. It is important to avoid using veins in lower extremities of older adults as phlebitis and thrombosis of superficial and deep veins may occur. The nurse should monitor the infusion site carefully because extravasation may cause mild irritation to tissue necrosis.

CARBONIC ANHYDRASE INHIBITORS

Carbonic anhydrase is an enzyme that plays a role in renal excretion of acid urine and reabsorption of sodium and potassium in the proximal tubule. However, an agent that inhibits carbonic anhydrase promotes the excretion of sodium, potassium, bicarbonate, and water, resulting in an alkaline diuresis. Inhibition of carbonic anhydrase decreases aqueous humor formation and consequently decreases intraocular pressure. Carbonic anhydrase inhibitors include acetazolamide (Diamox), methazolamide (Neptazane), and dichlorphenamide (Daranide). The prototype carbonic anhydrase inhibitor is acetazolamide.

NURSING MANAGEMENT OF THE PATIENT RECEIVING ACETAZOLAMIDE

Core Drug Knowledge

Pharmacotherapeutics

Acetazolamide is used to treat chronic open-angle glaucoma. It also can be used in acute closed-angle glaucoma when delay of surgery is desired to reduce intraocular pressure; as an adjunct in treating edema resulting from CHF or use of drugs; as an adjunct in treating epilepsy; and in preventing and treating acute mountain sickness (see Table 31-1).

Pharmacokinetics

Acetazolamide is well absorbed from the GI tract and excreted unchanged by the kidneys.

Pharmacodynamics

Acetazolamide is a nonbacteriostatic sulfonamide that blocks the action of carbonic anhydrase, which is needed for active transport of ions across the proximal tubule. Inhibition of carbonic anhydrase results in decreased hydrogen ion secretion by the tubules and increased sodium, potassium, bicarbonate, and water excretion. The increased excretion of electrolytes reduces the pH of body fluids. Another effect of carbonic anhydrase inhibition is decreased formation of aqueous humor, which thereby lowers intraocular pressure.

Contraindications and Precautions

Contraindications to acetazolamide therapy are hypersensitivity, depressed sodium or potassium serum levels, marked kidney and liver disease or dysfunction, suprarenal gland failure, hyperchloremic acidosis, adrenocortical insufficiency, severe pulmonary obstruction, cirrhosis, and long-term use in chronic noncongestive closed-angle glaucoma.

Acetazolamide should be administered cautiously to patients with adrenocortical insufficiency because patients with this disorder are susceptible to electrolyte imbalances. Acetazolamide is a pregnancy category C drug. It is secreted in breast milk, although dosage received by the infant is minute. Safety and efficacy in children, however, have not been established.

Adverse Effects

Sulfonamide-type adverse reactions may occur due to cross sensitivity. Adverse effects are varied. The most common are GI related and include anorexia, nausea, vomiting, and constipation. Other adverse effects include:

- GI: melena, taste alteration, and diarrhea
- Renal: hematuria, glycosuria, urinary frequency, renal colic, renal calculi, crystalluria, polyuria, and phosphaturia
- CNS: convulsion, weakness, malaise, fatigue, nervousness, drowsiness, depression, dizziness, disorientation, confusion, ataxia, tremor, tinnitus, headache, lassitude, and flaccid paralysis
- Hematologic: bone-marrow depression, thrombocytopenia, thrombocytopenic purpura, hemolytic anemia, leukopenia, pancytopenia, and agranulocytosis
- Dermatologic: urticaria, pruritus, skin eruptions, rash, and photosensitivity
- Other: weight loss, fever, acidosis, absent libido, impotence, electrolyte imbalance, hepatic insufficiency, and transient myopia

Symptoms of overdose include drowsiness, anorexia, nausea, vomiting, dizziness, paresthesia, ataxia, tremor, and tinnitus. The electrolyte disturbance most likely to occur from overdosage is hyperchloremic acidosis. Treatment involves inducing vomiting or performing gastric lavage. Hyperchloremic acidosis may respond to bicarbonate administration. Potassium supplements may be required.

Drug Interactions

Acetazolamide increases the effect of cyclosporine but decreases the effect of primidone. Concurrent use of acetazolamide (or other carbonic anhydrase inhibitors) and salicylates increases the effect of both drugs. Diflunisal (Dolobid) will increase the effect of acetazolamide (or other carbonic anhydrase inhibitors). Because acetazolamide promotes excretion of bicarbonate ions, the patient's urine will be alkaline. This may cause some laboratory test results to be false-positive for urinary protein (Table 31-5).

Assessment of Relevant Core Patient Variables

Health Status

Assessment should focus on whether the patient is allergic to acetazolamide or to the chemically similar sulfonamide antibiotics and thiazide diuretics. The nurse also should investigate any history of chronic closed-angle glaucoma, renal or hepatic diseases, respiratory acidosis, and chronic obstructive pulmonary disease.

TABLE 31-5 Agents That Interact With Acetazolamide

Interactants	Effect and Significance	Nursing Management
cyclosporine	Increased trough levels of cyclosporine; possible nephrotoxicity and neurotoxicity	Monitor for signs of nephrotoxicity and neurotoxicity.
primidone	Decreased concentrations of primidone in blood and urine	Monitor for therapeutic effect.
salicylates	Accumulation and toxicity of acetazolamide, including CNS depression and metabolic acidosis; CAI-induced acidosis may allow increased CNS penetration by salicylates	Monitor for therapeutic effects.
diflunisal	Significant decrease in intraocular pressure; increased adverse effects possible	Monitor for therapeutic response. Monitor for adverse effects.

The nurse should review blood tests for electrolyte and fluid disturbances because the drug should be used cautiously in patients with fluid and electrolyte imbalances, especially hyponatremia, hypokalemia, and hyperchloremic acidosis; hepatic disease; adrenocortical insufficiency; respiratory acidosis; or chronic obstructive pulmonary disease.

Life Span and Gender

The nurse should determine the patient's breast-feeding status and age before administering acetazolamide. Safety has not been established for breast-feeding women because safety and efficacy have not been established in children. Elderly patients do not tolerate excessive diuresis and may experience hypotension and orthostatic changes. In these patients, dosage may need to be reduced.

Environment

The nurse should note the setting in which acetazolamide may be administered. Acetazolamide may be administered in any environmental setting. However, IV administration is performed only in the hospital.

Nursing Diagnoses and Outcomes

- Risk for Deficient Fluid Volume related to therapeutic action of acetazolamide

  Desired outcome: The patient will have desired fluid volume changes without experiencing complications from these changes.
- Risk for Injury related to adverse effects of acetazolamide (blood dyscrasias, metabolic acidosis, paresthesia)

  Desired outcome: The patient will not suffer injury while on acetazolamide.

Planning and Intervention

Maximizing Therapeutic Effects

The nurse should use acetazolamide with miotics or mydriatics for complementary effect when treating open-angle glaucoma. Best diuretic effects in CHF and drug-induced edema occur when the drug is given every other day or daily for 2 days, with the third day off. Palatability may be enhanced with honey or other sweet syrup for crushed oral tablets.

Minimizing Adverse Effects

It is important to allow the kidney to recover and prevent overdosage when used as diuretic to reduce edema. If reduction in edema ceases after first dose, the nurse should not increase the dose; instead a day of medication should be skipped. Overdosage can be treated by gastric lavage or by inducing vomiting.

The nurse should monitor CBC and platelet counts during therapy; bone-marrow suppression is rare but may occur. It also is important to monitor serum potassium levels (especially if severe cirrhosis is present or there is concurrent use of steroids or adrenocorticotropic hormones).

The nurse should administer orally or by IV injection; IM administration is painful. Do not add to syrups containing glycerin or alcohol if the drug must be crushed.

Providing Patient and Family Education

- The nurse should explain the importance of returning for follow-up blood work to check CBC and electrolyte levels.
- It is important to urge the patient to notify the health care provider if sore throat, easy bruising, petechiae, and mucosal ulcerations develop (signs of blood abnormalities).
- The nurse should tell the patient to notify the health care provider if nausea, fatigue, abdominal pain, tinnitus, hyperpnea, and numbness in extremities occur (signs of metabolic acidosis).
- The nurse should encourage the patient to take acetazolamide with food if GI upset occurs.
- It is important to caution the patient to avoid prolonged sunlight exposure.
- The nurse should tell the patient to use caution when performing activities requiring alertness until effects of the drug are known.

Ongoing Assessment and Evaluation

Throughout therapy, the patient should be alert for unusual vision problems and should maintain the follow-up schedule previously established. Drug therapy and nursing care are considered successful if ocular pressure remains controlled and the patient's fluid and electrolyte values stay within normal ranges. ■

MEMORY CHIP

Acetazolamide

- Used primarily in treating chronic, open-angle glaucoma because it prevents formation of aqueous humor and decreases intraocular pressure
- Inhibits hydrogen ion secretion in renal tubule, and therefore increases loss of sodium, potassium, bicarbonate, and water
- Significant contraindications: severe renal or hepatic disease
- Most common adverse effects: related to gastrointestinal system
- Most serious (although rare) adverse effect: bone marrow suppression
- **Lifespan alert: older adults may have hypotension and orthostatic changes; dosage may need to be reduced**
- Maximizing therapeutic effects (of CHF diuresis): give every other day or every 2 days, with the next day off
- Minimizing adverse effects: allow kidney to recover; and prevent overdosage when used to reduce edema
- Most significant patient education: explain the importance of follow-up blood work

CHAPTER SUMMARY

- Diuretics are used widely to treat conditions in which increased extracellular fluid and edema are problems. Examples include hypertension, CHF, cirrhosis, renal disorders, intracranial pressure, and intraocular pressure.
- Diuretics work along the renal tubule and inhibit sodium and water reabsorption to increase water loss. The degree of diuretic effect depends on the section of the tubule in which the drug works.
- Diuretic drugs affect the excretion and reabsorption of other electrolytes, especially potassium. This can lead to one of the major adverse effects of diuretic therapy, which is an electrolyte imbalance.
- Thiazide and loop diuretics are the two classes of diuretics most frequently used.
- To prevent hypokalemia, patients taking non-potassium-sparing diuretics may need to increase their dietary intake of potassium or take supplements. Conversely, patients taking potassium-sparing diuretics are at risk of hyperkalemia and need to avoid excess potassium intake.
- Osmotic diuretics work by increasing the osmotic pressure within the vascular space. They are used primarily in ARF, in increased intracranial pressure, in increased intraocular pressure, and to promote excretion in the urine of toxic substances.
- Carbonic anhydrase inhibitors work by a different mechanism to cause diuresis. They are used primarily in treating open-angle glaucoma.

QUESTIONS FOR STUDY AND REVIEW

1. Identify the physical assessments for health status that should be completed before a patient starts thiazide therapy for hypertension.
2. Identify at least three conditions treated by diuretic therapy.
3. Discuss at least three fluid and electrolyte problems likely to occur in patients receiving thiazide or loop diuretics.
4. Why is a patient more likely to develop hypokalemia when on loop diuretics than on thiazide diuretics?
5. How are osmotic diuretics different from thiazide or loop diuretics?
6. What is the primary therapeutic use of carbonic anhydrase inhibitors?

NEED MORE HELP?

Chapter 31 of the study guide for *Drug Therapy in Nursing* contains exercises and activities to reinforce your understanding of the concepts presented in this chapter. For additional information, see the text's accompanying web site at *http://www.connection.lww.com.*

REFERENCES AND BIBLIOGRAPHY

Brion, L. P., Primhak, R. A., & Ambrosio-Perez, I. (2000). Diuretics acting on the distal renal tubule for preterm infants with (or developing) chronic lung disease. *Cochrane Database System Review,* (3): CD001817.

Cifkova, R., Nakov, R., Novozamski, E., Hejl, Z., Petrzilkova, Z., Poledne, R., Stavek, P., & Compagnone, D. (2000). Evaluation of the effects of fixed combinations of sustained-release verapamil/trandolapril versus captopril/hydrochlorothiazide on metabolic and electrolyte parameters in patients with essential hypertension. *Journal of Human Hypertension, 14*(6), 347–354.

Frassetto, L. A., Nash, E., Morris, R. C., & Sebastian, A. (2000). Comparative effects of potassium chloride and bicarbonate on thiazide-induced reduction in urinary calcium excretion. *Kidney International, 58*(2), 748–752.

Freudenberger, R. S., Gottlieb, S. S., Robinson, S. W., & Fisher, M. L. (1999). A four-part regimen for clinical heart failure. *Hospital Practice (Office Edition), 34*(9), 51–56, 59–64.

Hoes, A. W., Grobbee, D. E., & Lubsen, J. (1997). Sudden cardiac death in patients with hypertension: An association with diuretics and beta blockers? *Drug Safety, 16*(4), 233–241.

Humes, H. D. (1999). Insights into ototoxicity. Analogies to nephrotoxicity. *Annals of New York Academy of Science, 884,* 15–18.

Naidoo, D. P., Sareli, P., Marin, F., Aroca-Martinez, G., Maritz, F. J., Jardim, P. C., Guerrero, A. A., Thompson, C. A., Bero, T., Drazka, J., Kosmalova, V., Dumortier, T., & Smith, R. D. (1999). Increased efficacy and tolerability with losartan plus hydrochlorothiazide in patients with uncontrolled hypertension and therapy-related symptoms receiving two monotherapies. *Advances in Therapy, 16*(5), 187–199.

Nishino, T., Ide, T., Sudo, T., & Sato, J. (2000) Inhaled furosemide greatly alleviates the sensation of experimentally induced dyspnea. *American Journal of Respiratory and Critical Care Medicine, 161*(6), 1963–1967.

Paterna, S., Parrinello, G., Amato, P., Dominguez, L., Pinto, A., Maniscalchi, T., Cardinale, A., Licata, A., Amato, V., Licata, G., & Di Pasquale, P. (1999). Tolerability and efficacy of high-dose furosemide and small-volume hypertonic saline solution in refractory congestive heart failure. *Advances in Therapy, 16*(5), 219–228.

Radevski, I. V., Valtchanova, Z. P., Candy, G. P., Hlatswayo, M. N. & Sareli, P. (2000). Antihypertensive effect of low-dose hydrochlorothiazide alone or in combination with quinapril in black patients with mild to moderate hypertension. *Journal of Clinical Pharmacology, 40*(7), 713–721.

Roy, B. D., Green, H. J., & Burnett, M. E. (2000). Prolonged exercise following diuretic-induced hypohydration: Effects on cardiovascular and thermal strain. *Canadian Journal of Physiology and Pharmacology, 78*(7), 541–547.

Skrabal, M. Z., Stading, J. A., Behmer-Miller, K. A., & Hilleman, D. E. (2000). Advances in the treatment of congestive heart failure: New approaches for an old disease. *Pharmacotherapy, 20*(7), 787–804.

Spence, J. D., Huff, M., & Barnett, P. A. (2000). Effects of indapamide versus hydrochlorothiazide on plasma lipids and pipiproteins in hypertensive patients: a direct comparison. *Canadian Journal of Clinical Pharmacology, 7*(1), 32–37.

Suter, P. M., Haller, J. & Hany, A. (2000). Diuretic use: a risk of subclinical thiamine deficiency in elderly patients. *Journal of Nutrition, Health, and Aging, 4*(2), 69–71.

van Kraaij, D. J., Jansen, R. W., Gribnau, F. W., & Hoefnagels, W. H. (2000). Diuretic therapy in elderly heart failure patients with and without left ventricular systolic dysfunction. *Drugs and Aging, 16*(4), 289–300.

van Kraaij, D. J., Jansen, R. W., Bouwels, L. H., Gribnau, F. W., & Hoefnagels, W. H. (2000). Furosemide withdrawal in elderly heart failure patients with preserved left ventricular systolic function. *American Journal of Cardiology, 85*(12), 1461–1466.

Unit VIII

Blood and Immune System Drugs

Chapter 32

DRUGS AFFECTING COAGULATION

KEY TERMS

anticoagulants
clotting cascade
clotting factors
coagulation
embolus
fibrin
fibrinolysis
hemophilia
hemostasis
International Normalized Ratio (INR)
plasmin
platelets
thrombin
thromboembolus
thrombus

Learning Objectives

At the completion of this chapter the student will:

1. Identify core drug knowledge about drugs affecting coagulation.
2. Differentiate between the anticoagulants heparin and warfarin.
3. Understand the differences between anticoagulants and thrombolytics.
4. Differentiate antiplatelet drugs from hemorrheologic drugs.
5. Differentiate clotting factors from hemostatic agents.
6. Identify core patient variables relevant to drugs affecting coagulation.
7. Relate the interaction of core drug knowledge to core patient variables for drugs affecting coagulation.
8. Generate a nursing plan of care from the interactions between core drug knowledge and core patient variables for drugs affecting coagulation.
9. Describe nursing interventions to maximize therapeutic and minimize adverse effects for drugs affecting coagulation.
10. Determine key points for patient and family education for drugs affecting coagulation.

HYPERCOAGULATION

Anticoagulants

Parenteral

- **heparin** (prototype)
- enoxaparin
- ardeparin
- dalteparin

Oral

- **warfarin** (prototype)

Antiplatelets

- **ticlopidine** (prototype)
- aspirin
- dipyridamole
- tirofiban
- eptifibatide
- abciximab
- anagrelide

Hemorrheologics

- **pentoxifylline** (prototype)

Thrombolytics

- **streptokinase** (prototype)
- alteplase, recombinant
- reteplase, recombinant

HYPOCOAGULATION

Clotting factors

- **antihemophilic factor** (prototype)
- Human factor IX complex
- coagulation factor VIIa, recombinant
- anti-inhibitor coagulant factor

Hemostatics

- **aminocaproic acid** (prototype)
- tranexamic acid

The symbol C indicates the **drug class**.

Drugs in bold type marked with the symbol P are **prototypes**.

Drugs in blue type with no symbol are **closely related** to the prototype.

Drugs in **red** type with no symbol are **significantly different** from the prototype.

Drugs in **black** type with no symbol are **also used in drug therapy**; no prototype.

This chapter examines drugs used to treat **coagulation** (blood aggregation, or clotting) disorders. Disturbances in the coagulation balance cause abnormalities in the body's ability to transport blood through the vessels to the cells or to form blood clots. Pathophysiologic effects may result from an excess of or a deficit in coagulation factors. When the body begins bleeding, a series of events occurs to slow blood flow, stop blood loss at the injury site, and prevent extensive blood loss. This process is known as **hemostasis.** Excessive coagulation, or hypercoagulation, will result in a **thrombus** (blood clot).

Several drug classes that are used to treat hypercoagulation disorders are discussed in this chapter. The first class is **anticoagulants** (substances that keep blood from clotting). Existing naturally and in drug form, anticoagulants prevent thrombus formation and the extension of existing thrombi. There are two types of anticoagulants—those that are given parenterally and those that are given orally. The prototype parenteral anticoagulant is heparin (Lipo-Hepin, Hep-Lock). Drugs similar to heparin are the low molecular–weight heparins (enoxaparin [Lovenox], ardeparin [Normiflo], dalteparin [Fragmin]). The prototype oral anticoagulant is warfarin (Coumadin). Other drugs in this class are dicumarol and anisindione (Miradone).

Other drug classes used to treat hypercoagulability include the antiplatelet agents, the hemorrheologics, and the thrombolytics. Antiplatelet agents interfere with platelet membrane function and platelet aggregation. The prototype for the antiplatelets is ticlopidine (Ticlid). Drugs in the same class are cilostazol (Pletal) and clopidogrel (Plavix); because clopidogrel produces fewer adverse effects, it is often more widely used than ticlopidine. A drug closely related to ticlopidine is aspirin. Drugs that are significantly different from ticlopidine are dipyridamole (Persantine), the glycoprotein II b/III a inhibitors (tirofiban [Aggrastat], eptifibatide [Integrilin], abciximab [Reo Pro]), and anagrelide (Agrylin).

Hemorrheologics reduce blood viscosity, increase the flexibility of red blood cells (RBCs), and decrease platelet aggregation. Pentoxifylline (Trental) is the prototype for the hemorrheologics.

Thrombolytics, unlike anticoagulants and other drugs that are used to treat hypercoagulation, actually dissolve existing clots. They are used to treat medical emergencies resulting from thrombus formations' blocking blood flow to the heart, lung, or deep veins of the legs. The prototype thrombolytic is streptokinase (Streptase, Kabikinase).

Other drugs in this class are anistreplase (Eminase) and urokinase (Abbokinase, Abbokinase Open-Cath). Drugs closely related to streptokinase are alteplase, recombinant (Activase) and reteplase, recombinant (Retavase).

This chapter also describes drug classes used when hypocoagulation, or subnormal coagulation, is a problem. These drug classes include clotting factors and hemostatic agents. Clotting factors are replacements for genetic deficiencies of normal clotting factors, which lead to **hemophilia** (uncontrollable bleeding). The prototype drug is antihemophilic factor (AHF, factor VIII). Other drugs in this class include coagulation factor VIIa (recombinant), anti-inhibitor coagulant complex, and factor IX concentrates.

Hemostatics inhibit **fibrinolysis,** the process of breaking down a formed clot. They are either systemic or topical. The prototype systemic hemostatic drug is aminocaproic acid (Amicar). Other drugs in this class include tranexamic acid (Cyklokapron) and aprotinin (Trasylol). Topical hemostatics are used to control minor bleeding, usually after surgery. The various agents work differently. No prototype is identifiable for topical hemostatics.

PHYSIOLOGY OF COAGULATION

Normal circulation requires blood to circulate freely through large and small blood vessels. However, blood must also be able to form clots to prevent excessive blood loss from injuries. To perform both of these functions requires the body's ability to balance coagulation and anticoagulation.

BLOOD COMPONENTS AND BALANCED BLOOD FLOW

Blood is composed of various cells and substances, each with a specific purpose that assists in maintaining a balance of coagulation and anticoagulation. Present in blood are **platelets** (also called thrombocytes), which are fragmented cells that assist in blood clotting and clot formation. In addition, the blood contains a number of other substances that promote coagulation but are inactive. These substances are the procoagulants (precursors to clotting factors) and **clotting factors,** which are plasma proteins that cause blood clotting. The clotting factors are inactive in the blood until an injury mobilizes them.

Circulating in an active form are the anticoagulants, which dominate the procoagulants, unless an injury to a blood vessel occurs that disrupts the dominance of the anticoagulants.

When a blood vessel is injured initially, the vessel goes into spasm (vasoconstriction), which decreases blood flow and limits blood loss. Because platelets have a surface composed of glycoprotein, they will then adhere to the endothelial surface of the damaged blood vessel. Next, with the help of enzymatic action, the platelets release a substance called adenosine diphosphate, which in turn is converted to thromboxane A_2. This activity attracts other platelets to the damage site. Together the platelets form a temporary plug that seals the injured vessel. Normally, this plug is effective because it is stabilized with **fibrin,** an insoluble protein.

CLOTTING CASCADE

Fibrin is a product of the **clotting cascade.** The cascade is initiated by the tissue damage and platelet activation, which mobilize the clotting factors circulating in the blood. Once active, these clotting factors work with calcium to form fibrin. At this point, blood coagulation is completed and blood loss stops.

The clotting cascade occurs over two pathways, intrinsic and extrinsic, to achieve hemostasis (Fig. 32-1). The intrinsic pathway—so named because all of the clotting factors are present in the blood—is activated by damage to the

Physiology

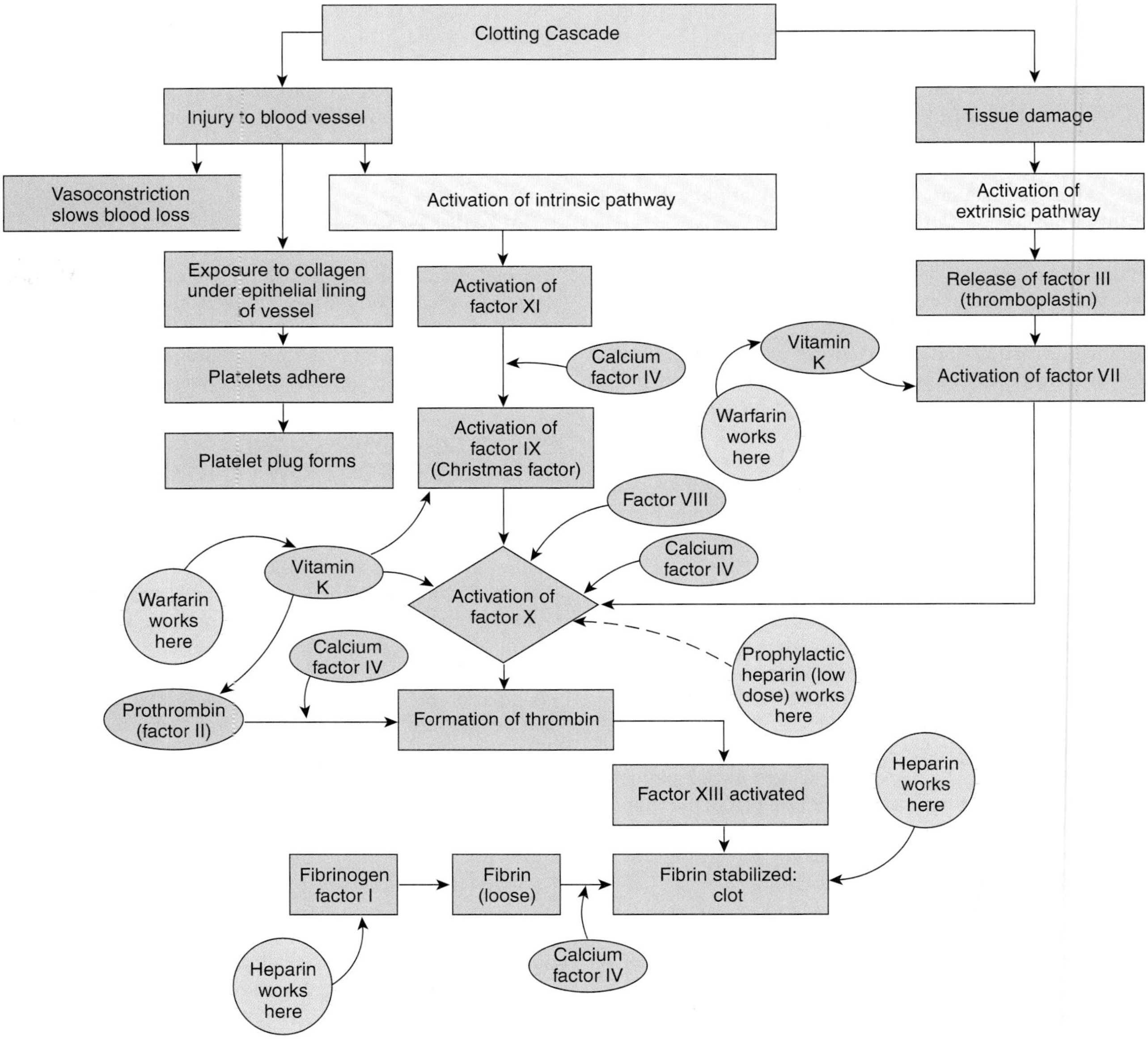

Figure 32-1. Events in the clotting cascade.

blood vessel. In the extrinsic pathway, the clotting factors are activated by the damaged tissue. One or both pathways may be activated in response to injury.

Intrinsic Pathway

Activity in the intrinsic pathway begins with an enzyme reaction that modifies factor XII from its inactive to active form. In turn, factor XII helps modify factor XI so that it can activate factor IX. Factor IX acts on factor VIII, and factor VIII activates factor X. Activated factor X affects factor V and promotes the conversion of prothrombin (factor II) to **thrombin.** Thrombin in turn converts factor I (fibrinogen) to fibrin. Thrombin also activates factor XIII, a fibrin-stabilizing factor. The fibrin threads that are produced trap the clotting factors that remain in the injured area, preventing the extension of the blood clot beyond the injury. The cascade thus ends in the formation of a stable blood clot.

Extrinsic Pathway

Activity in the extrinsic pathway begins with the activation of factor III followed by the activation of factor VII, then factor X. The remaining steps in this process follow those of the intrinsic pathway and are referred to as the final common pathway. The prevention of clot extension, which occurs at the end of the clotting cascade, is assisted by the release of heparin. Heparin, a naturally occurring anticoagulant normally found in small amounts in the blood, is released from mast cells at the time of the initial injury.

HEMOLYSIS

After a blood clot forms, the blood has a removal system that begins to lyse (decompose or break down) the clot about 1 to 2 days after bleeding stops. Plasma protein contains a substance known as plasminogen, which, along with other plasma proteins, is trapped in the blood clot. The damaged tissue releases tissue plasminogen activators, which change plasminogen to its active form, **plasmin.** Activated plasmin is the substance that lyses the blood clot.

PATHOPHYSIOLOGY

When blood flow is impeded and slowed in an area, coagulation occurs. This leads to a thrombus. Any excessive action from the coagulating factors may also produce a thrombus that obstructs blood flow. An **embolism** is any undissolved matter carried in a blood or lymph vessel to another location where it lodges and occludes the vessel. When a portion of a thrombus breaks off, the fragment may travel through the bloodstream and lodge in a vessel (**thromboembolus**), again occluding blood flow. When the thromboembolus is lodged in a coronary vessel, a myocardial infarction (MI) occurs. When it is lodged in the brain, a stroke, or cerebrovascular accident (CVA), occurs. When the thromboembolus is lodged in the pulmonary vessels it is called a pulmonary **embolus.** When a thromboembolus lodges in a blood vessel, blood flow through the vessel decreases or stops, depending on the size and position of the thromboembolus and the degree of obstruction. With decreased blood flow, tissues and cells do not receive necessary oxygen and nutrients, and necrosis (cell death) occurs.

Deep vein thrombosis (DVT) causes about 217,000 patients to be hospitalized every year in the United States (Merli, 2000). DVT may be secondary to surgery, trauma, malignancy, hereditary thrombotic disorders, stroke, spinal cord injury, or unexplained causes. The exact mechanism of the relationship between cancer and thrombosis is not known; however, it is known that cancer patients have an increased risk of developing thrombosis. Patients who present with thromboembolism of unknown causes are believed to have a higher risk for developing cancer, although there are no data to support thorough cancer screening with these patients (Valente & Ponte, 2000).

Acute coronary syndromes are also related to thrombus. Acute coronary syndromes include unstable angina, non–ST elevation MI, and ST-elevation MI (Reeder, 2000). All of these conditions have an underlying pathology of unstable coronary plaque on a coronary vessel, with an overlying intracoronary thrombus. Thrombus formation can also be a problem in atrial fibrillation. In this condition, the blood is not moving, which may lead to coagulation of the blood into clots.

Some conditions of hypercoagulability result from increased platelet activity. Constriction of, or fatty deposits in a blood vessel will narrow its lumen, leading to decreased or slowed blood flow through the vessel. The decreased flow causes stasis, which results in blood coagulation. Platelet activity is responsible for the formation of the blood clot. This is a particular problem for patients with chronic, obstructive vascular disease because blood clots will further impair or entirely block an already diminished blood flow, thereby posing a risk of tissue death from lack of oxygen and nutrients.

In peripheral vascular disease, the blood vessels in the extremities, particularly the legs, are narrowed. This prevents the flow of oxygenated blood to the tissues. Lack of oxygenation causes pain, especially with use of the extremity. This condition is known as intermittent claudication. Rest relieves the pain because it decreases the oxygen needed by the tissue. With the impaired circulation, venous stasis occurs, which in turn leads to platelet aggregation and thrombus formation. This thrombus further impairs circulation through the vessel to the tissue.

DRUG THERAPY FOR HYPERCOAGULATION

In general, disorders of hypercoagulability result from either an increase in platelets or an increase in the activity of the clotting system (Table 32-1). Treatment is aimed at interfering with the clotting cascade, with the effect desired to lengthen the time necessary for blood to clot. Anticoagulant drug therapy is used to prevent new clots from forming, to avoid extension of the thrombus, or to deter a thromboembolus. Cancer patients are considered eligible for primary prevention of thromboembolism if they are receiving chemotherapy, have a central venous catheter, are immobilized, or have undergone surgery (Valente & Ponte, 2000). Cancer patients have a significantly increased incidence of

TABLE 32-1 Risk Factors for Hypercoagulability

Core Patient Variable	Increased Platelet Activity	Increased Clotting Factor
Health Status		
Surgery	X	
Atherosclerosis		X
Congestive heart failure		X
Diabetes mellitus		X
Increased platelet count	X	
Malignant neoplasms	X	
Elevated blood lipid level		X
Life Span		
Pregnancy	X	
Oral contraceptives	X	
Lifestyle, Diet, and Habits		
Smoking	X	
Bed rest or other immobility	X	

recurrence of venous thrombosis compared to patients without cancer (Hutten, Prins, Gent, Ginsberg, Tijssen, Buller, et al., 2000).

When an existing clot may be fatal to the patient because of blocked blood flow to vital organs, thrombolytic agents are used to break it up. When the clot or obstruction blocks a coronary artery, the heart is affected; damage to the heart from a MI can be permanent or fatal. When the clot blocks the pulmonary artery, the blood supply to the lungs is altered; this in turn decreases the oxygenation of blood to be circulated. This is a life-threatening condition. When the thrombus is large and blocks the great veins in the legs, circulation is impaired in the limb. If the circulatory impairment is severe enough, the patient may be at risk of losing the limb as a result of tissue death. This also is considered a medical emergency. Thrombolytic agents are indicated in these emergency situations to prevent severe damage to the body or death.

When the patient has a less urgent need for therapy, antiplatelet drugs are used to decrease the clumping or aggregation of platelets. Platelet aggregation is also affected by hemorrheologic drugs. In addition, the hemorrheologics increase the flexibility of RBCs and decrease the blood viscosity.

Aspirin is also used for its effect on blood clotting. Aspirin in low doses is recommended to prevent MIs in high-risk patients, after MI to prevent future infarcts, and in patients with atrial fibrillation. Aspirin has been found to be an effective prophylactic treatment against stroke in patients with atrial fibrillation, unless strong risk factors are present (previous transient ischemic attack [TIA] or stroke, diabetes, advanced age–impaired left ventricular function, and a history of hypertension). If these risk factors are present in the patient with atrial fibrillation, the drug warfarin, adjusted to an international normalized ratio (INR) of 2.0–3.0, offers better protection against future stroke (Gornick, 2000). (See pharmacotherapeutics of warfarin, below, for more information on INR.) However, in diabetic patients, low-dose aspirin is a primary prevention therapy if the patient has cardiovascular risk factors (family history of coronary heart disease, cigarette smoking, hypertension, obesity, albuminuria, elevated lipid levels, and age older than 30 years). Aspirin is a secondary prevention strategy in patients with diabetes with large vessel disease; this would include history of MI, vascular bypass surgery, stroke or TIAs, peripheral vascular disease, claudication, and/or angina (Clinical guidelines, Aspirin Therapy in Diabetes, 1999). Aspirin is discussed more fully in Chapter 25.

ANTICOAGULANT DRUGS

Heparin, a naturally occurring anticoagulant, is produced by mast cells located in connective tissue throughout the body. The blood cells known as basophils produce a small amount as well. The areas that produce the largest amount of heparin are the lungs and to a lesser degree the liver. This is a natural protective mechanism of the body as these two areas receive the most small emboli.

All anticoagulants interfere with the clotting cascade and prolong blood clotting time. They vary by their route and their method of action. There are two types of anticoagulants, those that can only be administered parenterally and those that can only be administered orally. The parenteral anticoagulants work by preventing the conversion of fibrinogen to fibrin. The oral anticoagulants work by preventing the synthesis of factors dependent on vitamin K for synthesis, factors II (prothrombin), VII, VIII, IX, and X. Two different laboratory tests are therefore used to measure the therapeutic effects of these anticoagulants.

NURSING MANAGEMENT OF THE PATIENT RECEIVING HEPARIN

The prototype parenteral anticoagulant is heparin, which is unfractionated (containing both low molecular and high molecular weights) and stabilized with either sulfate (Lipo-Hepin, Liquaemin Sodium) or calcium (Calciparine).

Core Drug Knowledge

Pharmacotherapeutics

Heparin is the prototype parenteral anticoagulant. It interferes with the final steps of the clotting cascade. It is used to prevent the extension of a blood clot, particularly in patients with DVT or pulmonary embolism. It is also used prophylactically in patients with short-term increased risk of thrombus formation, such as in the postoperative period after a total hip replacement. When treating disseminated intravascular coagulation (DIC), heparin prevents further clotting in the microcirculation, leaving the procoagulants available to work at other sites in the body.

The heparin dosage is tailored to the patient and the severity of the condition. Continuous IV infusion of heparin is used to achieve full anticoagulation. In adults, a heparin IV drip is usually started by giving an IV bolus of the drug followed by continuous infusion. Selecting heparin dosage from a weight-based nomogram was found to achieve a therapeutic range more rapidly than methods of estimating the appropriate dose based on clinical experience alone or combined with general guidelines (Balcezak, Krumholz, Getnick, Vaccarino, Lin, & Cadman, 2000). Other ways to achieve full anticoagulating effects from heparin include using intermittent IV boluses or subcutaneous injections of heparin. In adults, subcutaneous administration of heparin may also prevent thromboembolic events (Table 32-2).

The duration of anticoagulation therapy for venous thromboembolism is based on the patient's level of risk for thrombosis if anticoagulation is stopped, as well as the patient's risk for bleeding if drug therapy is continued. Risk for recurrent thrombosis is considered low if it was precipitated by a reversible risk factor, such as

TABLE 32-2 Summary of Selected Drugs for Hypercoagulability

Drug (Trade) Name	Selected Indications	Route and Dosage Range	Pharmacokinetics
heparin (*Canadian:* Hepalean)	Anticoagulation	*Adult:* IV, 5,000 U bolus (or 35–70 U/kg) followed by 20,000–40,000 U/24 h or 15–25 U/kg/h *Child:* IV, 50 U/kg bolus, followed by 100 U/kg/4 h or 20,000 U/m²/24 h	*Onset:* immediate *Duration:* 2–6 h $t_{1/2}$: 60–120 min
	Prophylaxis	*Adult:* SC, 5,000 U q8–12h*	*Onset:* 20–60 min *Duration:* 8–12 h
enoxaparin (Lovenox)	Prophylaxis	*Adult:* SC, 30 mg, bid*	*Onset:* 20–60 min *Duration:* 12 h $t_{1/2}$: 4.5 h
warfarin (Coumadin; *Canadian:* Warfilone)	Prophylaxis and treatment	*Adult:* PO, 5–10 mg/day for 2–4 d, then adjust according to results of PT or INR values†	*Onset:* 24 h *Duration:* 2–5 d $t_{1/2}$: 1–2.5 d
ticlopidine (Ticlid)	Reduce risk of stroke	*Adult:* PO, 250 mg, bid†	*Onset:* 4 d *Duration:* up to 2 wk $t_{1/2}$: 12.6 h (single dose), 4–5 d (repeat dosing)
aspirin (Bayer; *Canadian:* APO-ASA)	Prophylaxis for MI Decrease risk of TIA in men	*Adult:* PO, 300–325 mg/d *Adult:* PO, 1,300 mg/d divided into two to four doses	*Onset:* 5–30 min *Duration:* varies $t_{1/2}$: 15–20 min
pentoxifylline (Trental)	Intermittent claudication	*Adult:* PO, 400 mg tid†	*Onset:* rapid *Duration:* unknown $t_{1/2}$: 0.4–0.8 h
streptokinase (Streptase)	Acute evolving MI	*Adult:* IV, 1.5 million IU over 1 h: intracoronary, 20,000 IU bolus, followed by 2,000 IU/min over 60 min†	*Onset:* immediate *Duration:* few hours (hyperfibrinolytic effect), up to 24 h (prolonged PT) $t_{1/2}$: 2 h (in vitro); 23 min (drug), 70–120 min fibrinolytic activity
	Pulmonary embolism (PE), deep vein thrombosis (DVT), arterial embolism, occluded arteriovenous cannulae	*Adult:* IV, 250,000 IU over 30 min initially, then 100,000 IU/h for 24–72 h for PE or arterial embolism; over 72 h for DVT; injected into cannula, 100,000–250,000 IU into each occluded port slowly, then clamp; cannula limb clamped for 2 h, then attempt to aspirate†	

*No dosage recommendation for children.
†Safety and efficacy not established in children.

surgery (i.e., surgery and postoperative period is past, so risk is no longer present). Risk for recurrence is high if the thromboembolism occurred with no apparent risk factors, or if the patient has persistent risk factors (such as cancer). Patients at low risk of recurrence should receive anticoagulation therapy for 3 months. Those at higher risk should receive anticoagulation therapy for 6 months to indefinitely, depending on the patient's variables (Couturaud, Grand' Maison, & Kearon, 2000).

Pharmacokinetics

Heparin is not absorbed from the gastrointestinal (GI) tract because it is destroyed by gastric acid, so it must be administered parenterally. When administered IV, heparin has an immediate onset of action. When administered subcutaneously, heparin's onset of action is 20 to 60 minutes. After administration, the drug is widely distributed in the body, although it does not cross the placenta, nor is it found in breast milk. Metabolism occurs in the liver where it is inactivated. It is eliminated from the body in the urine.

Pharmacodynamics

Heparin, along with antithrombin III, rapidly promotes the inactivation of factor X, which, in turn, prevents the conversion of prothrombin to thrombin. Heparin also has an effect on fibrin, limiting the formation of a stable clot. In blood tests measuring activated partial thromboplastin time (APTT), heparin prolongs the clotting time without affecting the bleeding time. Low-dose heparin therapy, which is prophylactic dosing, deactivates factor X but has minimal effect on already produced thrombin;

thus, it does not normally alter APTT levels. However, full anticoagulation effects can occur in some individuals. Heparin has no effect on blood clots that have already formed.

Contraindications and Precautions

Heparin is contraindicated in patients who are hypersensitive to beef or pork because some heparin products are derived from the intestinal mucosa of pigs and others from beef lung. Heparin is also contraindicated in patients with thrombocytopenia, bleeding disorders, and active bleeding other than DIC.

This drug should be used with caution in patients with the potential for hemorrhage, for example, in patients immediately after surgery or in those with peptic ulcer disease and liver disease.

Adverse Effects

The most common adverse effect of heparin is bleeding. Although heparin-induced thrombocytopenia (HIT) occurs rarely, it is potentially life threatening. Treatment for HIT includes discontinuing heparin, allowing the platelet count to return to normal, and treating any thrombosis. The only agent currently approved for treatment of HIT related thrombosis is lepirudin (Refludan) (Caiola, 2000). Other adverse effects of heparin, although uncommon, include hepatitis, rashes, urticaria, hypersensitivity, and fever.

If a patient receives an overdose of heparin or shows signs of bleeding, protamine sulfate, the antagonist for heparin, may be administered. Protamine sulfate, a strong base, will react with heparin, a strong acid, to form a stable salt, thereby neutralizing the anticoagulant effects of heparin. The protamine sulfate dose is based on the heparin dose: 1 mg of protamine sulfate/ 100 U of heparin or 0.5 mg of protamine sulfate/100 U of heparin if the heparin was administered more than 30 minutes before the protamine sulfate. No more than 100 mg of protamine sulfate should be given within a 2-hour period because this drug can cause anticoagulation in its own right. Administering protamine sulfate too rapidly may result in hypotension, bradycardia, dyspnea, and anaphylaxis. Hypersensitivity reactions may occur in some patients because of the fish base of protamine sulfate. Symptoms include flushing and feelings of warmth.

If the patient is not actively bleeding after heparin overdosage, the patient is usually monitored closely, and the protamine sulfate is not administered because heparin has a short half-life. The patient will recover from the overdosage without the added risk of complications from the protamine sulfate.

Drug Interactions

Several different drugs affect the action of heparin. Table 32-3 identifies these drugs and the significance of the reaction.

Assessment of Relevant Core Patient Variables

Health Status

Before administering the first dose of heparin, the nurse should review the patient's record for evidence of allergy or a preexisting prolonged bleeding time that would contraindicate administering heparin.

Life Span and Gender

The nurse should be aware that heparin is safe for pregnant women, although it places other patients at risk for injury, particularly those who are confused, cognitively impaired, unable to modify behavior to prevent injuries, or incapable of complying with requests to modify behavior.

Lifestyle, Diet, and Habits

Because heparin prolongs both internal and external bleeding, slight injuries may potentially cause serious adverse effects. The nurse should ask patients about their activity level. Patients who normally engage in active behaviors in which bumping or body injuries frequently occur are more at risk of injury when receiving SC heparin therapy at home.

TABLE 32-3 Agents That Interact With Heparin

Interactants	Effect and Significance	Nursing Management
cephalosporins	Additive effect with heparin is possible, which increases risk of bleeding.	Monitor for signs of bleeding. Monitor activated partial thromboplastin time carefully. Use drug cautiously when it is required.
nitroglycerin	Information is conflicting, but effect of heparin may be increased, increasing risk of bleeding.	Same as above.
penicillins	Parenteral administration can alter platelet aggregation and coagulation test findings. They may have additive effect with heparin to increase the risk of bleeding.	Same as above.
salicylate	Antiplatelet effect increases risk of bleeding.	Concurrent use is normally avoided.

Environment

The nurse should be aware of the environment in which the drug will be administered. Heparin is normally administered in an acute care setting.

Nursing Diagnosis and Outcome

- Risk for Injury, hemorrhage, related to heparin therapy

  Desired outcome: Hemorrhage will not occur.

Planning and Intervention

Maximizing Therapeutic Effects

The nurse should monitor laboratory values (e.g., APTT) to confirm that a therapeutic lengthening of the clotting time has been achieved. The therapeutic lengthening of the clotting time is generally measured as one and one half to two times the control APTT. Because control times vary from laboratory to laboratory depending on the test equipment used, the difference between the two times is used to measure effectiveness. For example, if the APTT control time is 30 seconds, a therapeutic level for the patient would be 45 to 60 seconds. Guidelines vary according to individual patients, who may require APTT values of less than one and one half times the control or more than two times the control to be therapeutic.

Heparin levels should be allowed to reach steady state before measuring APTT, usually 6 to 8 hours after the infusion starts. If the APTT is less than one and one half to two times the control, the nurse should contact the prescriber to seek new drug therapy orders. If the APTT is below the desired therapeutic range, the dosage needs to be increased. Repeated testing is needed after each dosage change has reached steady state (6–8 hours after the dosage change). In institutions with established protocols for adjusting heparin infusion rates to meet therapeutic levels, the rate may be changed by a registered nurse. If APTT values deviate from the protocol limits, the prescriber must be notified.

IV heparin therapy should not be interrupted because this will lower the blood levels of heparin and affect the therapeutic response. If occlusion or infiltration necessitates changing the IV site, the new IV line should be inserted as soon as possible to minimize the disruption of the infusion.

Doses of SC heparin should not be missed; they should be administered at the regularly prescribed times to maintain blood levels.

Minimizing Adverse Effects

Before initiating therapy, the nurse should review such laboratory values as APTT, hematocrit, and platelet count. These tests provide baseline information regarding clotting abilities and identify patients with conditions that contraindicate heparin therapy. However, these tests are not usually performed for prophylactic heparin use.

If the APTT during treatment exceeds the desired range, the dosage should be decreased. The nurse should contact the prescriber to seek new drug therapy orders, or act upon the standard protocol (if one is used).

An IV controller or pump should be used for continuous IV drip heparin to promote a steady rate of delivery and prevent rapid overdosage, which may occur when IV flow rates are regulated by gravity. Use of a pump is a standard safety precaution.

Administration of IV heparin should not be interrupted to give another drug. Doing so increases the risk of thrombus formation because therapeutic levels may not be maintained.

Other drugs should not be administered through the same tubing as heparin because heparin is incompatible with many other drugs and fluids. An additional peripheral IV line or a multilumen central venous catheter should be used instead.

The patient should be monitored for bleeding from the gums, nose, vagina, or wounds. Urine and stools should be examined to detect blood as well. The skin should be inspected for ecchymoses or hematomas that indicate bleeding into the tissues. If the patient develops active bleeding from an orifice or a wound, the prescriber needs to be notified immediately. Protamine sulfate is administered if active bleeding occurs.

IM injections should be avoided to prevent bleeding into the muscle. Pressure should be placed on IV sites when removing the line until bleeding stops.

For SC administration of heparin, a 25-gauge or finer needle should be used. Do not aspirate or massage the area after administration. See the accompanying display, Research-Based Subcutaneous Administration Techniques for Heparin.

To protect the patient from injury or falls, side rails should be raised or padded, particularly if the patient is

Research-Based Subcutaneous Administration Techniques for Heparin

Traditionally, the abdomen, 2 inches from the umbilicus, was the preferred site for injection because it was believed that this site carried less risk for developing hematoma. Research has shown, however, that site selection of the arm or thigh, as opposed to the abdomen, does not increase bruising or alter APTT (Fahs & Kinney, 1991). Research further indicates that technique affects hematoma formation. As early as 1988, Wooldridge found that changing the needle after drawing the drug into the syringe, having an air bubble in the syringe to follow the dose and lock the drug into the subcutaneous space, injecting at a 90-degree angle, and avoiding aspiration and massage after injection helped to prevent hematoma formation. The use of a 3-cc syringe rather than a 1-mL syringe has been found to cause smaller bruises when administering heparin (Hadley, Chang, & Rogers, 1996).

confused, disoriented, restless, or unable to comprehend or follow activity restrictions during therapy.

Providing Patient and Family Education

- Before heparin therapy begins, the nurse needs to inform the patient why the drug is needed and what it is expected to accomplish. Heparin should be described as an anticoagulant, not a blood thinner. Although this is a common description, it is not correct.
- The nurse should explain that frequent blood samples will need to be analyzed to measure the patient's clotting time and determine whether the patient is receiving a safe amount of heparin.
- The nurse should instruct the patient to report any blood in urine or stools and any bleeding from the gums, nose, vagina, or wounds.
- The nurse should educate the patient to use a soft toothbrush and an electric razor during therapy to prevent bleeding and to follow activity restrictions to prevent bruising and internal bleeding from injuries.

Ongoing Assessment and Evaluation

Throughout therapy, the nurse should monitor for signs of bleeding and review APTT values to maintain drug levels in the therapeutic range. Drug therapy is considered effective when a thrombus or extension of an existing thrombus is avoided. ■

DRUGS CLOSELY RELATED TO HEPARIN

Low-molecular-weight heparin is derived from standard heparin through either chemical or enzymatic depolymerization (breakdown of polymers into monomers, their basic building block). Whereas standard heparin has a molecular weight of 5,000 to 30,000 daltons, low-molecular-weight heparin ranges from 1,000 to 10,000 daltons, resulting in properties that are distinct from those of traditional heparin. Low-molecular-weight heparin binds to protein (although less strongly than traditional heparin), has enhanced bioavailability, interacts less with platelets, and yields a very predictable dose response, eliminating the need to monitor the aPPT. Low-molecular-weight heparin, like standard heparin, binds to antithrombin III; however, low-molecular-weight heparin also inhibits thrombin to a lesser degree (and actual factor X to a greater degree) than standard heparin.

Low-molecular-weight heparins also have prolonged half lives compared with unfractionated heparin (standard heparin that has not been depolymerized). This, in combination with the increased bioavailability, allows the drug to be dosed once daily SC. This means that treatment for stabilized patients can be done in their homes, while they are followed as outpatients.

Much research has been done on the effectiveness of low-molecular-weight heparins. In studies of heparin usage in patients with DVT of the legs, the anti-thrombotic effect of low-molecular-weight heparin was greater than the effect of calcium heparin. Low-molecular-weight heparin produced significantly higher maximum venous outflow than calcium heparin (Zanghi, Morici, Costanzo, Astuto, Salanitri, 1988). Low-molecular-weight heparins cause less bleeding when given in therapeutic doses, compared with unfractionated heparin. It appears that they also produce less heparin induced thrombocytopenia and osteoporosis as well (Pineo & Hull, 1998).

In multiple clinical trials and in meta analyses of trials, low-molecular-weight heparin treatment for DVT and pulmonary embolism resulted in decreased recurrent thromboembolism, major bleeding, and death when compared with standard, unfractionated heparin (Pineo & Hull, 1998). Other studies indicate that low-molecular-weight heparins are as safe and effective as unfractionated heparin in treating pulmonary embolism (Ageno & Turpie, 2000). Low-molecular-weight heparin appears to be safe to use within 2 hours prior to epidural anesthesia (Kassis, Fugere, & Dube, 2000). Low-molecular-weight heparin has also been found to be safe and effective for prophylaxis of venous thromboembolism in elective neurosurgery and does not cause an excessive risk for intracranial bleeding (Iorio & Agnelli, 2000). Low-molecular-weight heparin is safe to use during pregnancy and is effective in preventing venous thromboembolism in pregnant women (Ellison, Walker, & Greer, 2000; Sorensen, Johnsen, Larsen, Pedersen, Nielsen, & Moller, 2000). Based on the current research, the clinical guidelines from the Institute for Clinical Systems Improvement for managing DVT state that low-molecular-weight heparin is the preferred treatment for DVT (National Guideline Clearinghouse, 1999).

MEMORY CHIP

Heparin

- Anticoagulant that prevents formation or extensions of blood clots
- Has no effect on existing blood clots
- Parenteral administration (IV or SC)
- Significant contraindications: thrombocytopenia, bleeding disorders, and active bleeding other than DIC
- Most common adverse effect: bleeding (antidote for heparin overdose is protamine sulfate)
- Most serious adverse effect: thrombocytopenia
- **Lifespan alert: heparin is the anticoagulant that can be used during pregnancy**
- Maximizing therapeutic effects: monitor APTT for therapeutic range; adjust dose till therapeutic range achieved
- Minimizing adverse effects: use IV pump; assess for signs of bleeding
- Most significant patient education: instruct patients to report any blood in urine or stools or bleeding from gums, nose, vagina, or wounds

Enoxaparin

Enoxaparin (Lovenox), which is considered safer and equally effective as heparin, has an effect on activated factor X and has limited effect on thrombin. Thus, its effect on APTT is decreased. Enoxaparin also affects clotting factor C and antithrombin. Most enoxaparin is absorbed after SC administration and is widely distributed. Enoxaparin has been found to be superior to unfractionated heparin in reducing death, MI, and emergency revascularization in patients with Q wave MI. The beneficial effect of enoxaparin treatment lasted 43 days (Cohen, Antman, Gurfinkel, Turpie, Furst, Bigonzi, et al., 2000).

Patients who are to receive enoxaparin by SC injection after discharge should be taught how to administer the drug to themselves. It is important that they understand the reason for therapy, the necessity of taking the drug on time, and the importance of following a regular dosage schedule and having follow-up blood analyses done as recommended. They should also be advised about scheduling and keeping appointments with the prescriber.

Other important teaching points focus on safety, for example, clearing pathways, removing loose scatter rugs, wearing nonskid footwear, obtaining adequate lighting, and using handrails on stairways in bathtubs. Additional teaching and management concerns are similar to those for heparin therapy.

Ardeparin

Ardeparin (Normiflo) is a low molecular-weight heparin like enoxaparin. It is used to prevent DVT after knee replacement surgery. An unlabeled use is for secondary prophylaxis for recurrent thromboembolic events. Like enoxaparin, it should be administered only by deep SC injection. In contrast to enoxaparin, which is a pregnancy category B drug, ardeparin is a category C agent. One unique characteristic of ardeparin is its ability to increase lipoprotein lipase activity. However, it has been found to cause a paradoxic elevation of serum triglyceride levels in clinical trials. Another unique feature of ardeparin is that it contains metabisulfite, a sulfite that may cause allergic reactions, including anaphylaxis, in susceptible people. Adverse effects of ardeparin are similar to those of enoxaparin.

Dalteparin

Dalteparin (Fragmin), another low molecular-weight heparin, is used to prevent DVT. It is also used in the treatment of unstable angina and non-Q wave MI for the prevention of ischemic complication in patients on concurrent aspirin therapy. A unique feature of dalteparin is that the multiple dose vial contains benzyl alcohol as a preservative; benzyl alcohol has been associated with "fatal gasping" syndrome in premature infants. Because of this, dalteparin should not be used in infants or in pregnant women (because it crosses the placenta). Other characteristics of dalteparin are similar to those of enoxaparin.

NURSING MANAGEMENT OF THE PATIENT RECEIVING WARFARIN

Warfarin (Coumadin) is the prototype oral anticoagulant.

Core Drug Knowledge

Pharmacotherapeutics

Warfarin is an oral anticoagulant. It is administered after heparin therapy to complete treating a thrombus or embolism. Warfarin is also used prophylactically for patients with a long-term risk of thrombus formation, for example, when the mitral valve has been replaced or when hypercoagulability is a chronic concern related to venous stasis. It is also used prophylactically in patients with atrial fibrillation.

Dosage is based on achieving a therapeutic level as measured by changes in the prothrombin time (PT). The patient's PT is measured against a control PT. PT control times vary with laboratory test methods and equipment, so a standardized unit, known as the **International Normalized Ratio (INR)**, has been developed to measure therapeutic levels of warfarin. The INR is determined by a mathematic equation and reflects the patient's PT compared with the standardized PT value. Some institutions use one or the other laboratory test to measure warfarin effect. Others use both. For treatment or prophylaxis of a thrombus or embolus, the patient's PT should be 1.4 to 1.6 times the control time; the INR should be equal to 2 to 3. For prophylaxis in patients with mechanical heart valves, the PT should be 1.5 to 1.7 times the control or the INR should be 2.5 to 3.5. Patients with cancer who have been treated with warfarin for venous thrombosis have a lower incidence of recurrence when the INR is maintained at greater than 2.0, rather than less than 2.0 (Hutten et al., 2000).

Pharmacokinetics

After absorption, warfarin is bound to albumin in the plasma. The drug action peaks in 1 to 9 hours; however, the anticoagulant effects do not begin for 24 hours. Maximum effect occurs 3 to 4 days after dosing starts, which is the time required for the drug to reach a steady state in the blood. The time factor is related to previously activated factors that are still circulating in the blood. Each time the dose changes, another 3 to 4 days are needed for the drug to reach its full effect. The effects of warfarin will persist for 4 to 5 days after discontinuation. The drug crosses the placenta but is not present in breast milk. It is metabolized in the liver and excreted in the bile.

Patients receiving heparin therapy will begin taking warfarin before they discontinue heparin. This allows the warfarin to reach a therapeutic level before heparin is discontinued. The practice is safe because the two drugs affect different clotting factors (see Table 32-1).

Pharmacodynamics

Warfarin works by competitively blocking vitamin K at its sites of action. Thus, it prevents the activation of factors II (prothrombin), VII, IX, and X. It has no effect on factors that have already been activated. When warfarin is given immediately, the pharmacodynamic response to the drug is affected by the preoperative hemoglobin level. Lower preoperative hemoglobin is associated with an increased response to warfarin therapy (Messieh, 2000).

Contraindications and Precautions

Warfarin is contraindicated for patients with active bleeding, open wounds or ulcerations of the GI tract, or bleeding disorders, such as hemophilia or thrombocytopenia. It is not recommended for use in patients with subacute endocarditis, pericarditis, or pericardial effusions. Warfarin is also contraindicated for patients who are undergoing surgery in which hemorrhage is possible (spinal, eye, GI, cranial, and arterial bypass grafting). Usually, the drug is discontinued 7 days before elective surgery.

Cautious use is recommended in patients with renal and hepatic impairment. Warfarin use is primarily determined by comparing the risks of the drug versus the benefits to the patient.

Adverse Effects

The most frequent adverse effects of warfarin are bleeding and hemorrhage. Nausea, vomiting, diarrhea, and abdominal cramps can occur as well. Tissue necrosis is a rare adverse effect. A fetal warfarin syndrome has been identified when warfarin is given to pregnant women.

Drug Interactions

Several drug-drug and drug-food interactions need to be considered when a patient begins warfarin therapy (Table 32-4). Recent research suggests that high doses of acetaminophen (four or more 325-mg tablets daily for 7 days or longer) may increase the risk of bleeding in patients on warfarin (Hylek, Heiman, Skates, Sheehan, & Singer, 1998).

Assessment of Relevant Core Patient Variables

Health Status

Because deficiencies of vitamin K increase the bleeding risk for patients receiving warfarin, the availability of vitamin K should be assessed. Besides the body's production of vitamin K in the GI tract, one source of vitamin K is food. Vitamin K is a fat-soluble vitamin, and depends on the absorption of fat for its own absorption. Bile is necessary for fats to be digested and absorbed. A patient with decreased available bile, from obstructed bile ducts for example, will absorb less vitamin K. Patients with poor dietary intake of vitamin K will also be deficient in the vitamin.

Vitamin K deficiency may occur in adults whose normal GI flora have been affected by long-term antibiotic therapy or whose dietary intake consists of parenteral nutrition without vitamin K supplements.

Life Span and Gender

Patients with vitamin K deficiency experience decreased synthesis of normal clotting factors and are at greater risk of hemorrhage if they receive warfarin. Because vitamin K is continually produced in the GI tract, deficiencies are rare in healthy adults. Newborns, however, may have a vitamin K deficiency because intestinal flora is not active at birth. Warfarin should not be used during pregnancy because it is associated with a described syndrome of fetal defects, so it is important to determine the stage of the reproductive cycle for women.

The nurse should consider the patient's age before therapy begins. Bleeding complications with anticoagulant drugs appear to occur more frequently in older adults (those older than 75 years) than in younger adults. Older adults also have an increased sensitivity to the effects of warfarin, in both the early induction phase and maintenance phase of drug therapy. Congestive heart failure, malignancy, malnutrition, diarrhea, and unsuspected vitamin K deficiency, which are all more likely in older adults, enhance warfarin's effect on the PT (Sebastian & Tresch, 2000). Frail older adults who are in nursing homes may be more at risk of adverse effects from warfarin, according to one study, which found that anticoagulants were the most common medication associated with preventable adverse drug events (Gurwitz, Field, Avorn, McCormick, Jain, Eckler, et al., 2000). This may be related to multiple pathologies, deterioration of organ function from aging and disease states, or multiple drug therapies with potential for drug interactions.

Lifestyle, Diet, and Habits

The nurse should obtain information about the patient's dietary habits. Because vitamin K competes with warfarin, high vitamin K levels will decrease the effectiveness of warfarin. Diets rich in vitamin K, therefore, should be avoided. If the diet was normally rich in vitamin K when the warfarin dosage was adjusted, this is not as important. However, if the patient's diet does not normally include vitamin K–rich foods, these foods should be avoided. The nurse should consider lifestyle behaviors that place the patient taking heparin at increased risk of falls and injuries for the patient taking warfarin, as well.

Environment

The nurse should be aware that warfarin therapy may be started in the hospital, but most treatment is self-administered by the patient at home. The nurse and patient should explore potential risks in the home environment.

Nursing Diagnosis and Outcome

- Risk for Injury, bleeding, related to adverse effects of warfarin

  Desired outcome: The patient will not experience bleeding.

TABLE 32-4 Agents That Interact With Warfarin

Interactants	Effect and Significance	Nursing Management
acetaminophen, androgens, beta blockers, clofibrate, corticosteroids, cyclophosphamide, dextrothyroxine, disulfiram, erythromycin, fluconazole, gemfibrozil, glucagon, hydantoins, influenza virus vaccine, isoniazid, ketoconazole, miconazole, moricizine, propoxyphene, quinolones, sulfonamides, tamoxifen, thioamines, thyroid hormones, urokinase	They may increase the effect of warfarin by unknown or complicated mechanism, increasing risk of bleeding.	Monitor for bleeding carefully. Monitor PT or INR carefully. Anticipate dose adjustments of warfarin if these drugs are started after titrating the dose of warfarin.
amiodarone, chloramphenicol, cimetidine, ifosfamide, lovastatin, metronidazole, omeprazole, phenylbutazones, propafenone, quinidine, quinine, sulfamethoxazole-trimethoprim (SMZ-TMP), sulfinpyrazone	The effect of warfarin may be increased by inhibiting its metabolism, increasing the risk of bleeding.	Same as above.
chloral hydrate, loop diuretics, nalidixic acid	The effect of warfarin may be increased because of displacement from binding sites, increasing the risk of bleeding.	Same as above.
aminoglycosides, mineral oil, tetracyclines, vitamin E	The effect of warfarin may be increased because of interference with vitamin K, increasing the risk of bleeding.	Same as above.
cephalosporins, diflunisal, NSAIDs, penicillins, salicylate	The effect of warfarin may be increased because of effects on platelets and GI irritation (from NSAIDs), increasing the risk of bleeding.	Avoid administering NSAIDs and salicylates if possible. Other considerations are the same as above.
ascorbic acid, dicloxacillin, ethanol, ethchlorvynol, griseofulvin, nafcillin, sucralfate, trazodone	The effect of warfarin may be decreased by an unknown action.	Be aware that dose of warfarin may need to be adjusted to be in therapeutic range. Monitor PT or INR to assess drug effectiveness.
aminoglutethimide, barbiturates, etretinate, carbamazepine, glutethimide, rifampin	The effect of warfarin may be decreased by induction of the anticoagulant's hepatic microsomal enzymes.	Avoid variation in vitamin K–rich food after titrating warfarin dose. Vitamin K is considered antidote to warfarin. Otherwise nursing considerations are the same as above.
cholestyramine, contraceptives, oral estrogens, thiazide diuretics, thiopurines, spironolactone, vitamin K	The effect of warfarin may be decreased by various mechanisms.	Same as above.

Planning and Intervention

Maximizing Therapeutic Effects

Warfarin dosage should be individualized until PT or the INR is in therapeutic range. An initial loading dose is given to attain a rapid therapeutic level. This is then followed by a maintenance dose. Doses are usually given in the evening at 6 PM. This timing allows for early morning blood draws for PT or INR by hospital laboratory personnel.

Minimizing Adverse Effects

The patient's response to warfarin therapy is measured by using either the ratio of the patient's PT compared with the control PT, or the INR. The prescriber needs to be notified if the patient's clotting time is greater than the therapeutic level. Usually, drug dosage will be decreased if this occurs. Skipping one dose may be all that is required to lower the PT to the therapeutic level. In case of warfarin overdose, the antidote, vitamin K (phytonadione), is administered.

Falls may cause internal bleeding. The patient's home should be assessed for factors that may lead to falls. Encourage the use of proper lighting and handrails on stairways, which may help prevent falls.

Providing Patient and Family Education

- The nurse should teach the patient information regarding signs of bleeding and methods to prevent bleeding (which are the same as for heparin).
- The nurse should instruct the patient to take the drug at the same time each day because this helps prevent a drop in warfarin blood levels. After the drug level is stabilized and daily PT is not needed, the patient may switch to morning dosing. Doing so may increase absorption and improve adherence to drug therapy. The patient should be advised to return for follow-up blood work.
- The nurse should educate the patient that skipping a dose of warfarin could alter therapeutic levels. If patients forget a dose, they should take it as soon as they remember. However, they should not double up on the next dose to prevent bleeding.
- The nurse should instruct the patient that taking aspirin, large doses of acetaminophen, or other over-the-counter drugs with these ingredients can affect warfarin's action.
- The nurse should warm women to avoid becoming pregnant while on this drug.
- The nurse's dietary teaching should focus on the need to avoid increased intake of foods rich in vitamin K, primarily green vegetables.
- The nurse should emphasize to patients the importance of informing other health care providers (dentist, podiatrist, and so on) that they are on warfarin. Patients should also be instructed to wear or carry medical identification stating that they are receiving warfarin.

Ongoing Assessment and Evaluation

To determine the therapeutic effects of warfarin, the patient's PT or INR is monitored. Therapy is effective when a thrombus is prevented and bleeding does not occur. See the two accompanying displays, Solving Problems Related to Anticoagulant Therapy; and Impact of Chronic Conditions and Drug Therapies on Older Adults' Risk of Car Accidents. ■

ANTIPLATELET DRUGS

Drugs that prevent platelet aggregation are called antiplatelet drugs. They are used when overactive platelets pose long-term risks of hypercoagulability. The drugs differ in their modes of action and adverse effects. Although aspirin may be the most frequently prescribed antiplatelet drug, it is also used frequently for other clinical reasons. It is a prototype nonsteroidal anti-inflammatory drug (NSAID) and is discussed in Chapter 25.

Critical Thinking Scenario

Solving problems related to anticoagulant therapy

Melanie Graves is diagnosed with a left leg deep vein thrombosis (DVT). She is started on heparin 1,000 U/h by intravenous infusion. After 3 days, she will start taking warfarin in addition to the heparin.

1. Explain the rationale for starting warfarin while the patient is receiving heparin. Three days have passed. The first dose of warfarin (5 mg) is given at 6 PM. The following morning, blood is drawn to evaluate the PT. The control is 30 seconds, Ms. Graves' PT is 30 seconds, and the INR is 1.
2. Discuss the information about the dosage of the warfarin that can be obtained from this initial blood work. Explain how you arrived at this conclusion.

Ms. Graves complains that she doesn't like having her blood drawn so frequently. She says she cannot wait to go home so that she does not have to have any more blood work.

3. What elements will you develop in the initial teaching plan for her?

NURSING MANAGEMENT OF THE PATIENT RECEIVING TICLOPIDINE

The prototype of the antiplatelet drugs is ticlopidine (Ticlid).

Core Drug Knowledge

Pharmacotherapeutics

Ticlopidine inhibits platelet aggregation by altering the function of platelet membranes. It effectively prolongs the bleeding time. Ticlopidine is indicated for preventing thrombotic CVA (stroke) in patients who cannot tolerate aspirin (see Table 32-2). The drug has several unapproved uses: treatment of intermittent claudication (a demonstrated ability to decrease pain while walking), decreasing the incidence of occlusion in arteriovenous shunts or fistulas in patients with chronic renal failure, and preventing occlusions in patients after coronary bypass surgery. It has also been used to decrease the severity of the sickle cell crisis in patients with sickle cell disease.

Pharmacokinetics

Ticlopidine is well absorbed from the GI tract and is bound primarily to plasma proteins. Ticlopidine absorption is improved if the drug is administered with food. The drug is metabolized in the liver and eliminated by the kidneys and GI tract. After discontinuing the drug, it takes 4 to 10 days for the bleeding time to return to normal. For more information, see Table 32-2.

Focus on Research

Impact of chronic conditions and drug therapies on older adults' risk of car accidents

McGwin, G. Jr., Sims, R. V., Pulley, L., & Roseman, J. M. (2000). Relations among chronic medical conditions, medications, and automobile crashes in the elderly: a population-based case-control study. *American Journal of Epidemiology, 152*(5), 424–431.

The Study

Older drivers are known to have elevated crash rates and are more likely to be injured or die if they are involved in a crash. This study sought to identify medications and chronic conditions that are associated with a risk of at-fault crashes in older drivers. One study examined 901 drivers 65 years or older who were selected in a population-based case-controlled study in 1996 from Alabama Department of Public Safety driving records. More than half (497) had not been in car accidents. The rest had been involved in crashes; 244 were found at fault in the accident. Older drivers with heart disease or a history of stroke were more likely to be in car crashes and be the at-fault driver than older drivers without heart disease or stroke history. Women with arthritis were also more likely to be found at fault in car crashes. Drug therapies in older adults associated with an increased risk of being at fault in a car crash included nonsteroidal anti-inflammatory drugs, angiotensin-converting enzyme inhibitors, benzodiazepines, and anticoagulants. Calcium channel blockers and vasodilators were associated with a reduced risk of crash involvement.

Nursing Implications

Patient education about factors that increase the risk of car crashes has relevance for improving the health and safety of older adults. Nurses need to caution older patients that certain chronic conditions or drug therapies may increase their risk of having a car crash. It is not clear yet exactly how these factors are related to increasing the risk of car crashes. More research is needed in this area.

MEMORY CHIP

Warfarin

- Anticoagulant used to complete treatment with heparin after clot formation; is used prophylactically in patients at high risk of thrombus formation
- Administered orally
- May be given with heparin until therapeutic level of warfarin is obtained
- Significant contraindications: active bleeding, ulcerations of the GI tract, or bleeding disorders
- Most common adverse effect: bleeding (vitamin K is the antidote for warfarin toxicity)
- Most serious adverse effect: fetal warfarin syndrome
- **Lifespan alert: warfarin is not for use in pregnancy because it causes fetal defects**
- Maximizing therapeutic effects: monitor PT for therapeutic range; adjust dosage until therapeutic range is attained
- Minimizing adverse effects: monitor for signs of bleeding
- Most significant patient education: teach patients to monitor for bleeding, modify behavior to avoid injuries, and to avoid greatly increased vitamin K intake

Pharmacodynamics

Ticlopidine interferes with platelets binding with fibrinogen, thereby inhibiting aggregation. It also affects platelet interactions and prolongs the bleeding time (see Table 32-2).

Contraindications and Precautions

Ticlopidine is contraindicated in patients with hypersensitivity, active bleeding, bleeding disorders, and disorders that interfere with the formation of blood cells. Ticlopidine should not be used in patients with severe hepatic dysfunction. Assigned to pregnancy risk category B, it should be used only if absolutely necessary. The drug is not recommended for use in breast-feeding mothers; it is not known whether the drug enters breast milk. Cautious use of ticlopidine is recommended for patients with liver and renal impairment and those who are at an increased risk for bleeding.

Adverse Effects

Adverse reactions to ticlopidine may occur shortly after therapy begins or months after the patient has been on the drug. Adverse effects, which may affect several systems, may cease without stopping the drug.

The most common adverse effect is diarrhea. Serious, possibly life-threatening effects include neutropenia, although this is not common, and thrombocytopenia, although this is rare. Additional possible GI effects are nausea, vomiting, abdominal cramps, dyspepsia, flatulence, anorexia, abnormal liver function test results, and increased serum cholesterol levels (although lipid ratio is not affected). Other possible adverse effects include dizziness, ecchymoses, epistaxis, and skin rash.

Drug Interactions

Patients on digoxin who receive ticlopidine may have a decrease in digoxin plasma levels. Antacids decrease the effectiveness of ticlopidine.

Ticlopidine should not be administered with aspirin because it increases the risk of bleeding. Cimetidine interferes with the hepatic metabolism of ticlopidine, resulting in increased blood levels of ticlopidine. Ticlopidine interferes with the elimination of theophylline and thus increases risk of theophylline toxicity (Table 32-5).

Assessment of Relevant Core Patient Variables

Health Status

The nurse should review the patient's history and physical examination for any contraindications to the use of this drug. The patient should have a baseline complete blood count (CBC) with differential to determine platelet functioning. Liver function studies should also be done and serum lipid levels measured. Neurologic status should be assessed when ticlopidine is given to prevent stroke. Cardiovascular assessment is indicated when ticlopidine is used for other therapeutic effects.

TABLE 32-5 Agents That Interact With Ticlopidine

Interactants	Effect and Significance	Nursing Management
antacids	Decrease in ticlopidine plasma levels results in decreased effect of ticlopidine.	Do not give ticlopidine directly after antacids.
cimetidine	Chronic administration reduces the clearance of a single dose of ticlopidine by 50%, which increases the effect of ticlopidine.	Consult with prescriber; dose of ticlopidine may need to be decreased. Monitor for bleeding.
aspirin	Interaction results in potentiated effect of aspirin on collagen-induced platelet aggregation, which increases the risk of bleeding.	Do not coadminister ticlopidine and aspirin.
digoxin	Interaction decreases digoxin plasma level.	Monitor digoxin levels; dose may need to be adjusted.
theophylline	Theophylline half-life is increased; therefore, drug stays in blood longer, producing more effect from theophylline.	Monitor for signs of adverse effects from theophylline. Monitor theophylline levels.

Life Span and Gender

The nurse should consider the patient's age before therapy begins. Caution must be used in children younger than 18 years because safety has not been established and in patients who are pregnant or lactating. In older adults, adverse effects related to ticlopidine are more likely to develop.

Lifestyle, Diet, and Habits

Lifestyle behaviors that would place the patient at increased risk of bleeding while on this drug should be discussed with the patient.

Environment

The nurse should be aware of the environment in which the drug will be administered. Ticlopidine may be administered in the hospital. However, most of the time it is self-administered by the patient at home. The nurse should discuss with the patient potential risks in the home environment. Falls and activities that are likely to produce internal or external bleeding should be avoided while on ticlopidine.

Nursing Diagnoses and Outcomes

- Risk for Injury: intracerebral bleeding, neutropenia, and thrombocytopenia related to anticoagulant effects of ticlopidine

  Desired outcome: The patient will suffer no injury related to bleeding while on ticlopidine.
- Diarrhea, related to adverse effects of ticlopidine

  Desired outcome: Normal bowel elimination will be maintained.

Planning and Intervention

Maximizing Therapeutic Effects

Ticlopidine should be administered with food to increase absorption.

Minimizing Adverse Effects

Throughout therapy, CBC with differential needs to be assessed so that any decline in the neutrophil and platelet counts can be detected early. Laboratory tests should be performed every other week, starting in the second week of therapy until the end of the third month. If test results show normal ranges at this time, biweekly monitoring may stop. However, ticlopidine therapy should stop if neutropenia or thrombocytopenia occurs. More frequent monitoring is indicated when neutrophil counts begin to decline.

The nurse must also monitor for neurologic changes that may indicate intracranial bleeding. To minimize bleeding, pressure should be applied to all IV or injection sites.

Patients receiving both ticlopidine and digoxin need to have their digoxin levels assessed to ensure they are within the therapeutic range.

The drug should be taken with food to decrease GI problems. The home environment should be assessed for safety hazards that may contribute to falls or other accidents.

Providing Patient and Family Education

- The nurse needs to inform patients and families about laboratory tests that are needed on a regular basis and the reasons for their frequency.
- The nurse should also emphasize to patients and families the importance of informing all health care providers (such as dentists and other physicians) of the drug regimen. If surgery is needed, ticlopidine should be discontinued 10 to 14 days before the procedure to prevent excessive bleeding.
- The nurse should instruct patients and families to apply pressure on wounds until bleeding stops to avoid prolonging bleeding time.
- The nurse should emphasize to the patient that behaviors that may lead to injury should be avoided (e.g., roller-blading, ice skating, motorcycle riding, use

of nonmotorized scooters, walking on icy patches, and so on).

- The nurse should instruct patients and families to make the home environment more "fall proof" by removing scatter rugs, placing handrails on stairs, and fastening any loose carpet edges.

Ongoing Assessment and Evaluation

Laboratory tests are monitored as described in the section "Minimizing Adverse Effects." Therapy is evaluated as effective when the outcomes are achieved and a stroke has been prevented or other desired therapeutic effects have been obtained. ■

DRUG CLOSELY RELATED TO P TICLOPIDINE

Aspirin

Aspirin, a drug used for its antiplatelet properties, has a mechanism of action that differs from that of ticlopidine in that it irreversibly inhibits platelet cyclo-oxygenase and the subsequent synthesis of thromboxane A_2 for the life of the platelet. Thromboxane A_2 is a vasoconstrictor that facilitates platelet aggregation. Inhibiting its synthesis, therefore, inhibits platelet aggregation. Aspirin is used in prophylaxis against thromboembolic complications in cardiovascular disease, including MI and TIA. Aspirin does not pose the risk of neutropenia that ticlopidine does. For more information see Chapter 25.

DRUGS SIGNIFICANTLY DIFFERENT FROM P TICLOPIDINE

Dipyridamole

Unlike ticlopidine, dipyridamole is primarily a coronary vasodilator that increases functional levels of adenosine, which produces vasodilation. It also inhibits the enzyme phosphodiesterase, which increases cyclic adenosine monophosphate (cAMP). Although the substance cAMP is another coronary vasodilator, it also has an antiplatelet effect. Dipyridamole dilates coronary arteries, increasing flow in narrowed vessels. It does not usually produce significant systemic vasodilation. A mild positive inotropic effect has also been documented.

Dipyridamole is used with anticoagulants and other antiplatelets in patients after surgery, such as prosthetic heart valve placement and vascular grafting procedures, to prevent thrombus formation. Investigational uses include post-MI treatment and prevention of TIAs. It is used diagnostically during thallium myocardial perfusion imaging. In some parts of the United States, it is used more frequently than ticlopidine.

Dipyridamole is moderately absorbed after oral administration. Its distribution is widespread, crossing the placenta and entering breast milk. It is metabolized in the liver and excreted by the GI tract. It should be used cautiously in patients with hypotension because some vasodilation occurs.

The most frequent adverse effects are headache, dizziness, and nausea. After IV administration, MI, arrhythmias, and bronchospasm may occur, although they are uncommon.

Dipyridamole has additive effects on platelet aggregation when given with aspirin. There is increased risk of bleeding when used concurrently with anticoagulants, thrombolytics, NSAIDs, or sulfinpyrazone. Ingesting alcohol will increase the risk of hypotension. Theophylline may negate the effects of dipyridamole during diagnostic thallium imaging.

MEMORY CHIP

P Ticlopidine

- Antiplatelet that inhibits platelet aggregation; used to prevent thrombotic cerebral vascular accidents when aspirin is not tolerated
- Significant contraindications: active bleeding or bleeding disorders
- Most common adverse effect: diarrhea
- Most serious adverse effects: neutropenia or thrombocytopenia
- Minimizing adverse effects: monitor CBC with differentials and assess for bleeding
- Most significant patient education: teach patients about the importance of follow-up laboratory work and the need to inform their other health care providers that they are taking this drug

Glycoprotein IIb/IIIa Inhibitors

Tirofiban, eptifibatide, and abciximab (ReoPro) are all antagonists of the platelet glycoprotein IIb/IIIa receptor, the major platelet surface receptor involved in platelet aggregation. This receptor is found only on platelets and their progenitors. Activation of the glycoprotein IIb/IIIa receptors leads to the binding of fibrinogen and von Willebrand factor to platelets and thus, to platelet aggregation. Tirofiban and eptifibatide reversibly prevent fibrinogen and von Willebrand factor from binding to the glycoprotein IIb/IIIa receptor, thereby inhibiting platelet aggregation. Both tirofiban and eptifibatide are used in the treatment of acute coronary syndrome (unstable angina or non–Q wave MI). Tirofiban may also be used for patients who will be undergoing percutaneous transluminal coronary angioplasty; eptifibatide may also be used in the treatment of patients undergoing percutaneous coronary intervention. Both of these drugs are administered by IV infusion.

One difference between these two drugs is their rate of ability to bind with protein in the blood. Tirofiban is moderately protein bound (65%), whereas eptifibatide has low protein binding (25%).

Contraindications for the two drugs are the same and include: active internal bleeding or a history of bleeding within the last 30 days; a history of thrombocytopenia following a prior exposure to tirofiban; history of stroke within 30 days or any history of hemorrhagic stroke; a major surgical procedure or severe physical trauma within the last 30 days; severe hypertension; concomitant use of another parenteral glycoprotein IIb/IIIa inhibitor; any history of intracranial hemorrhage, intracranial, neoplasm, arteriovenous malformation or aneurysm; history, symptoms or findings suggestive of aortic dissection, acute pericarditis; platelet counts less than 1000,000/mm³; a serum creatinine level of 2 mg/dL or higher; or dependency on renal dialysis.

The most frequent adverse effect for both tirofiban and eptifibatide is bleeding, which can be a minor or major event. Nonbleeding adverse effects for tirofiban (when coadministered with heparin) include nausea, fever, and headache. The only nonbleeding adverse effect of eptifibatide is hypotension, which may be serious.

Abciximab is used as adjunct to percutaneous transluminal coronary angioplasty or atherectomy for the prevention of acute cardiac ischemic complications in patients at high risk of abrupt closure of the treated coronary vessel. It is used with aspirin and heparin. Like tirofiban and eptifibatide, bleeding is the major adverse effect of abciximab.

Anagrelide

Anagrelide is another antiplatelet agent that is significantly different from ticlopidine. It is used in the treatment of essential thrombocythemia (ET) to reduce the elevated platelet count and the risk of thrombosis and to reduce the associated symptoms of the disorder. Exactly how anagrelide reduces platelet counts is unknown at this time. It is hypothesized that dose-related reduction in platelet production results from a decrease in megakaryocyte hypermaturation. White blood cell counts and other coagulation factors are not affected. RBC counts may be altered, but these alterations are not clinically significant. The most common adverse effects of anagrelide are headache, diarrhea, edema, palpitations, and abdominal pain. Serious potential adverse effects include CHF, MI, cardiomyopathy, cardiomegaly, complete heart block, atrial fibrillation, CVA, pericarditis, pulmonary infiltrates, pulmonary fibrosis, pulmonary hypertension, pancreatitis, gastric/duodenal ulcers, and seizures. None of these serious adverse effects is common.

HEMORRHEOLOGIC DRUGS

The hemorrheologic drugs differ from the antiplatelet drugs in that they act on RBCs to reduce blood viscosity and increase the flexibility of RBCs. This aids in preventing thrombus formation and allows the RBCs to enter the microcirculation, thereby increasing oxygenation at the cellular level. These effects are helpful in treating peripheral vascular disease.

NURSING MANAGEMENT OF THE PATIENT RECEIVING PENTOXIFYLLINE

The prototype hemorrheologic drug is pentoxifylline.

Core Drug Knowledge

Pharmacotherapeutics

Pentoxifylline is used to manage the symptoms of intermittent claudication from peripheral vascular disease. Using this drug improves the patient's ability to walk for longer distances without pain. It has also been used to treat acute and chronic cerebral vascular disease because it improves the psychopathologic symptoms. Unlabeled uses include treating diabetic angiopathies, neuropathies, TIAs, chronic leg ulcers, Raynaud disease, and disorders of the circulation of the eye (see Table 32-2).

Pharmacokinetics

Pentoxifylline is absorbed readily from the GI tract. It undergoes first-pass effect in the liver with about 50% of the drug remaining. It is widely distributed. Onset of therapeutic effects takes 2 to 4 weeks. Full therapeutic effects are not evident, however, until 4 to 8 weeks after therapy starts. The drug is metabolized by RBCs and the liver and is excreted in urine.

Pharmacodynamics

Pentoxifylline increases the flexibility of RBCs by increasing cAMP levels. In turn, this decreases platelet aggregation and promotes vasodilation. Blood fibrinogen concentration is lowered. In addition, the drug increases cellular adenosine triphosphate levels, which stabilizes the cell membrane and reduces the RBC aggregation, thus lowering blood viscosity (see Table 32-2).

Contraindications and Precautions

Because pentoxifylline is derived from the methylxanthines (caffeine and theophylline), it is contraindicated in patients who have an intolerance to it or to the methylxanthines. Patients with impaired renal function may require a reduced dose to prevent toxicity. Pentoxifylline should be used cautiously in pregnant or nursing women. The drug is in pregnancy risk category C and is excreted in breast milk. Caution should also be used in children younger than 18 years because safety has not been established. Pentoxifylline should also be used with caution in patients with coronary artery or cardiovascular disease, such as angina, arrhythmias, or severe hypotension.

Adverse Effects

Pentoxifylline's adverse effects occur primarily in the central nervous, cardiovascular, and GI systems. The effects on these systems may be the result from this drug's similarity to caffeine and theophylline.

Headache, dizziness, tremor, dyspepsia, nausea, and vomiting are all common adverse effects. Other adverse effects can occur occasionally. These include agitation, nervousness, insomnia, angina, chest pain, arrhythmia, tachycardia, edema, hypotension, abdominal discomfort, bloating, belching, flatus, diarrhea, blurred vision, epistaxis, bad taste, rash, urticaria, pruritus, and brittle fingernails.

Drug Interactions

There may be an increased risk of bleeding when pentoxifylline is given with warfarin. Risk of theophylline toxicity may increase as well because pentoxifylline is a methylxanthine like theophylline. Smoking may decrease the effect of pentoxifylline. When caring for patients receiving pentoxifylline and warfarin, the nurse should monitor PT and INR values carefully.

Assessment of Relevant Core Patient Variables

Health Status

The nurse should determine whether the patient is hypersensitive to the drug or to methylxanthines prior to beginning therapy. Assess the patient's baseline walking tolerance, circulation, and pulses in the affected extremities. Ask the patient to describe any pain experienced with activity and the effect of rest on the pain.

Life Span and Gender

It is important for the nurse to determine whether the patient is pregnant or breast-feeding.

Lifestyle, Diet, and Habits

The nurse should find out whether the patient smokes tobacco. Usual patterns of exercise and activity should be compared with desired level of exercise and activity.

Environment

The nurse should be aware that pentoxifylline is generally self-administered in the home, although it may also be administered in the hospital. The nurse and patient should discuss potential risks in the home environment.

Nursing Diagnosis and Outcome

- Risk for Injury, related to adverse pentoxifylline effects (dizziness, drowsiness, blurred vision)
  Desired outcome: The patient will remain injury free while on pentoxifylline.

Planning and Intervention

Maximizing Therapeutic Effects

Pentoxifylline must be taken for several weeks before the full therapeutic effects are evident.

Minimizing Adverse Effects

Pentoxifylline may be given with food to minimize GI upset.

Providing Patient and Family Education

- The nurse should inform patients that there is not an immediate effect from pentoxifylline so that they should not stop taking the drug before it produces its therapeutic effects.
- The nurse should instruct patients to avoid driving or operating machinery until it is known whether dizziness or blurred vision will occur from the drug. If these problems continue after the initial phase of drug therapy, the prescriber should be contacted in case the dosage needs to be decreased.
- The nurse should advise patients not to smoke because this constricts the blood vessels.
- The nurse should instruct patients to keep all follow-up visits with the prescriber.

Ongoing Assessment and Evaluation

Peripheral circulation should be reassessed periodically to measure improvement. Throughout therapy, the patient's exercise tolerance should be assessed, with improvement being noted over time if therapy is effective. For patients also on antihypertensive drugs, blood pressure should be monitored throughout therapy. ■

C THROMBOLYTIC DRUGS

Thrombolytic drugs assist in breaking down formed blood clots. These drugs are used for patients who are diagnosed with an evolving, acute MI; a pulmonary embolism; acute, extensive DVT; or arterial thrombosis. They may also be given to unclog arterial catheters. These drugs may be given systemically or directly at the site of the blood clot. Although these drugs are given during emergency situations and can save lives, their adverse effects can be life threatening. Therefore, these drugs should be administered by clinicians who are familiar with them and skilled in using them. Patients receiving these drugs need to be monitored carefully for adverse effects. The prototype of the thrombolytic drugs is streptokinase.

Other drugs in this class are urokinase (Abbokinase) and anistreplase (Eminase). Drugs closely related to streptokinase are the tissue plasminogen activators (alteplase, recombinant [Activase] and reteplase, recombinant [Retavase]).

MEMORY CHIP

P Pentoxifylline

- Hemorrheologic agent that reduces blood viscosity and increases flexibility of red blood cells
- Used to manage symptoms of intermittent claudication
- Needs to be taken for several weeks before full therapeutic effect is seen
- Significant contraindication: sensitivity to methylxanthines
- Most common adverse effects: headache, dizziness, tremor, dyspepsia, nausea, and vomiting
- Most serious adverse effect: tachycardia

NURSING MANAGEMENT OF THE PATIENT RECEIVING STREPTOKINASE

Streptokinase (Streptase) is the prototype thrombolytic drug.

Core Drug Knowledge

Pharmacotherapeutics

Streptokinase is indicated in a number of thromboembolic conditions considered medical emergencies, for example, an evolving MI from an acute coronary artery thrombus. Therapy for this condition is most effective when it is initiated within 6 hours of onset of symptoms. Other conditions include massive pulmonary embolism; recent, massive DVT; and arterial thrombosis. Streptokinase can also be used in lower doses to open occluded arteriovenous catheters (see Table 32-2).

Pharmacokinetics

Streptokinase is infused intravenously or directly into the coronary arteries through a catheter. The onset of action is immediate, and peak effect is rapid. Streptokinase is metabolized by antistreptokinase antibodies. Plasma half-life of the streptokinase-plasmin complex is 23 minutes. After saturation of the antibodies, half-life is prolonged up to 90 minutes. The duration of action varies from 4 to 12 hours. Streptokinase is excreted in the urine and bile (see Table 32-2).

Pharmacodynamics

Streptokinase is produced by the hemolytic streptococci group C. It works by activating plasminogen, which causes its conversion to plasmin. Plasmin is the enzyme that dissolves fibrin, fibrinogen, and other clot-forming proteins.

Streptokinase effectively lyses a formed thrombus or embolism, with improved circulation resulting. The drug is nonselective and changes fibrin throughout the blood, not only at the site of the clot (see Table 32-2).

Contraindications and Precautions

Streptokinase should be used only in clinical settings where hematologic function and clinical response can be adequately monitored. It should be administered by a clinician with experience and knowledge in treating the thromboembolic disorders. The drug is contraindicated in patients with hypersensitivity, active internal bleeding, or severe uncontrolled hypertension. It is contraindicated in patients who have had a recent (within the last 2 months) cerebrovascular accident, intracranial surgery, intraspinal surgery, intracranial neoplasm, or thoracic surgery. The drug should be given with extreme caution to women in the early postpartum period (10 days) and to patients receiving oral anticoagulants.

Cautious use is recommended in patients with a history of recent (5 days to 6 months) streptococcal infection because they may have antibodies against the drug, resulting in increased resistance to its action. Caution should be used also when administering streptokinase in pregnancy, lactation, or childhood (safety not established) or in older adulthood (75 years or older, because there is increased risk of central nervous system [CNS] bleeding). Caution is recommended in patients who had minor surgery or trauma within the last 2 months, cerebrovascular disease, subacute bacterial endocarditis, diabetic hemorrhagic retinopathy, blood clotting defects associated with renal and hepatic disease, or in whom streptokinase was recently administered. In these patients, the risk of the therapy is considered against the need for treatment to maintain quality of life.

Adverse Effects

Because of the nonspecific action of streptokinase, severe bleeding occurs frequently. It may be external, from an orifice or invasive site, or it may be internal. Bleeding may be difficult to stop.

Fever is another frequent adverse effect, occurring in 30% of those who receive streptokinase. Urticaria is also a common adverse effect, and anaphylaxis, although not common, may be life threatening.

Other adverse effects include reperfusion arrhythmias, hypotension, periorbital edema, bronchospasm, and phlebitis near the injection site.

Drug Interactions

Anticoagulant therapy with heparin or warfarin increases the risk of bleeding. These drugs are used following streptokinase infusion, and patients who receive them need careful monitoring for bleeding. Other drugs that may increase the risk of bleeding with streptokinase administration include the antiplatelet drugs and NSAIDs (Table 32-6).

TABLE 32-6 Agents That Interact With Streptokinase

Interactants	Effect and Significance	Nursing Management
anticoagulants	Interaction prevents formation of new clots and increases risk of bleeding.	Monitor for bleeding closely. Monitor APTT, PT carefully.
antiplatelets	Interaction prevents platelet aggregation and increases risk of bleeding.	Monitor closely for bleeding.

Assessment of Relevant Core Patient Variables

Health Status

The nurse should assess the patient for conditions that contraindicate administering streptokinase. The nurse needs to investigate any recent streptococcal infections, because the drug may not be effective in these patients. Laboratory values, such as hematocrit, hemoglobin level, platelet count, PT, and APTT, can provide baseline clotting information.

The creatine phosphokinase and cardiac isoenzyme levels should be assessed in patients receiving streptokinase to treat MI.

Life Span and Gender

When considering life span and gender variables, the nurse needs to determine the patient's age, whether pregnancy is an issue, whether the patient has delivered a child within 10 days, or whether the woman is breastfeeding.

Nursing Diagnosis and Outcome

- Risk for Injury related to drug-induced bleeding and other adverse effects of streptokinase

  Desired outcome: The patient will not suffer injury from streptokinase.

Planning and Intervention

Maximizing Therapeutic Effects

The drug should be reconstituted in dextrose 5% in water (D_5W) or 0.9% sodium chloride (normal saline) solution. Dosage changes will be based on blood test findings and the patient's response to therapy.

Minimizing Adverse Effects

Throughout the time the drug is administered, the nurse should monitor vital signs (including temperature) and observe for signs of active bleeding. Frank bleeding may occur at access sites, such as IM injection or arterial puncture sites; from gums; or from orifices such as the vagina or rectum. Internal bleeding may be signaled by abdominal pain with coffee grounds–like emesis; black, tarry stools; joint pain; and changes in level of consciousness.

The nurse should assess vital signs and possible bleeding every 15 minutes for the first hour of therapy. For the next 8 hours, assess every 15 to 30 minutes depending on the patient's condition. After 8 hours, bleeding and vital signs should be monitored at least every 4 hours or more frequently if indicated by the patient's condition. If bleeding occurs, the infusion should be stopped and the physician notified.

Throughout therapy, hematocrit, hemoglobin level, platelet count, PT, thrombin time, and APTT need to be monitored. Notify the physician of any abnormal assessment findings or abnormal laboratory values.

Handle the patient gently and as little as possible to prevent internal injury. Avoid invasive procedures, such as IM injections, IV punctures, or arterial punctures. Multiple IV lines are usually indicated to allow for administration of the streptokinase and other drugs and to provide a route for obtaining blood samples during therapy. These lines should be started before initiating streptokinase therapy. Drugs that must be given parenterally should be given by the IV route instead of the IM route to prevent bleeding into the muscle. If invasive procedures must be performed, pressure should be applied to IV sites for at least 15 minutes and to arterial puncture sites for at least 30 minutes.

The patient's blood should be typed and cross matched. Blood should be available for transfusion should hemorrhage occur. Whole blood, packed RBCs, or fresh frozen plasma may be administered. Have aminocaproic acid available and give as needed as the antidote.

In case of anaphylactic reaction, have epinephrine, an antihistamine, and resuscitation equipment at hand.

In patients with drug-induced fever, acetaminophen may be administered to control fever.

Streptokinase is administered with an infusion pump to ensure accurate dosage. A 0.8-mm, pore-size filter is also used. Do not mix streptokinase with other drugs.

Systemic anticoagulation with heparin usually begins when thrombolytic therapy ends (after several hours).

The patient should be connected to a cardiac monitor, both during the treatment and afterward, if streptokinase is given as treatment for an MI. Arrhythmias may occur, especially after the clot has dissolved and the heart has been reperfused. Notify the physician if significant arrhythmias occur because IV lidocaine or procainamide may be needed prophylactically or to treat induced arrhythmias. Cardiac enzymes should also be monitored following the infusion. Any signs of reinfarction must be reported immediately.

When therapy is given to treat a pulmonary embolism, the nurse must monitor respiratory status carefully. Note respiratory rate, dyspnea, pulse oximetry, and arterial blood gas findings in addition to all the assessments described previously.

When streptokinase is given for DVT or acute arterial occlusion, the nurse should observe the extremities for color and perfusion and palpate peripheral pulses every hour. Notify the physician of circulatory impairment.

When streptokinase is used to clear occluded cannulas or catheters, the line should be aspirated carefully after the streptokinase has had at least 2 hours in the line to dissolve the clot. The cleared line can then be flushed with 0.9% sodium chloride solution. If the catheter cannot be aspirated, the physician should be notified.

Providing Patient and Family Education

- The nurse should emphasize to patients and families the need for frequent assessment, pressure dressings, and activity limitations.

- Patients should be instructed to notify the nurse if they experience signs of adverse reactions.
- At an appropriate time, the nurse should provide information about heparin and warfarin, because patients will usually be on heparin after the administration of a thrombolytic and could be discharged on warfarin for prophylaxis.

Ongoing Assessment and Evaluation

Vital signs, evidence of bleeding, and laboratory test results should be assessed throughout therapy as described previously. Therapy is judged effective if the patient sustains no injury or adverse effects of streptokinase, the clot dissolves and circulation is restored, and only minimal tissue damage occurs at the site of initial injury. ■

DRUGS CLOSELY RELATED TO STREPTOKINASE

Alteplase, Recombinant

Also a thrombolytic, recombinant alteplase (Activase) has been effective in the treatment of ischemic cerebrovascular accidents (CVAs). In a study conducted by the National Institute of Neurological Disorders and Stroke on the use of recombinant human tissue plasminogen activator (alteplase) in treating CVAs, researchers documented improvement in the patients' clinical condition 3 months after the stroke. The patients with demonstrated improvement were those treated with alteplase. Another group was treated with placebo and conventional methods. In the alteplase group, 6% of the patients experienced intracerebral bleeding. At the end of 3 months, minimal or no adverse effects from the CVA were demonstrated in 30% more study subjects in the experimental group than in the control group. The study findings indicate that recombinant alteplase is a treatment option for ischemic CVA. To be most effective, the drug should be given within 3 hours of the onset of symptoms of the CVA (Marler, 2000; NINDS t-PA Stroke Study Group, 1997). Based on these findings, recombinant alteplase is being used more frequently than streptokinase.

Unlike streptokinase, which works indirectly to activate plasminogen, alteplase attaches to the fibrin in a thrombus and converts the trapped plasminogen to plasmin. Unlike the other thrombolytic agents, it produces only limited conversion of plasminogen in the absence of fibrin and therefore produces fewer systemic effects (see Table 32-2). Bleeding is the most common adverse effect. Intracranial bleeding, a serious adverse effect, is possible, although not common. The risk for bleeding may be related to the concurrent use of heparin, which is not uncommon.

Reteplase, Recombinant

Recombinant reteplase (Retavase) is produced by recombinant DNA technology in *Escherichia coli*. It breaks the cleavage of endogenous plasminogen to generate plasmin. Plasmin degrades the fibrin matrix of the clot, thereby exerting its thrombolytic action. Recombinant reteplase is administered by IV infusion to treat acute MI. Treatment should be initiated as soon as possible after the onset of acute MI symptoms. Reteplase infusion has been found to produce a lower incidence of mortality, heart failure, and cardiogenic shock than streptokinase. Total incidence of stroke was similar between reteplase and streptokinase, but reteplase produced more hemorrhagic strokes than streptokinase. Reteplase, compared with alteplase, has been shown to produce a significantly more opened vessel, although reocclusion rates were similar for both drugs (Drug Facts and Comparisons, 2001). Like alteplase, bleeding is the most common adverse effect of recombinant reteplase and may be related to concurrent therapy with heparin.

MEMORY CHIP

Streptokinase

- Thrombolytic that breaks down formed blood clots; used in acute emergencies for evolving myocardial infarction, pulmonary embolism, arterial thrombosis, or acute, extensive, deep vein thrombosis
- Also used to clear occluded cannulas or catheters
- Significant contraindications: active internal bleeding and severe uncontrolled hypertension
- Most common adverse effects: bleeding and fever
- Most serious adverse effects: life-threatening bleeding and anaphylaxis
- Minimizing adverse effects: monitor vital signs, assess for bleeding, assess laboratory work showing clotting status/ability, keep patient on a cardiac monitor (post MI), and have emergency resuscitation equipment nearby
- Most significant patient education: teach patients about the need for safety precautions and limitations on activity

CLOTTING FACTORS

In addition to preventing blood coagulation, drug therapy may also be used to promote coagulation when the patient has a deficiency of normal blood clotting factors. These deficiencies, which are associated with prolonged bleeding and clot formation times, result from an inherited absence of the factor (hemophilia) or from a decreased synthesis of the factor or factors.

Replacement of these factors is the treatment of choice. The prototype drug for this class is antihemophilic factor (AHF). Other drugs in the class include anti-inhibitor coagulant complex and factor IX complex. AHF is from pooled human blood sources. It is screened for hepatitis antibodies and heated to prevent the transmission of hepatitis. Blood donors are screened for human immunodeficiency virus (HIV) as well, and positive sources are screened again. The chance of disease transmission, therefore, still exists but is quite small.

PATHOPHYSIOLOGY OF HEMOPHILIA

When clotting factors are deficient, blood clotting does not occur in a timely manner. A minor injury or trauma can cause prolonged bleeding, or hemorrhage, either internally or externally. Bleeding may occur into a joint, such as the elbow or knee, and cause serious damage.

Inherited deficiencies of specific clotting factors produce three major hemophilic conditions: hemophilia A (classic hemophilia), hemophilia B (Christmas disease), and von Willebrand disease. Hemophilia A results from lack of factor VIII. Hemophilia B results from lack of factor IX. Hemophilias A and B are transmitted on recessive, sex-linked genes. The genes are carried by women and transmitted to male children. Von Willebrand disease results from deficiency of factor VIII, factor VIII antigen, and von Willebrand factor. It is transmitted by an autosomal dominant gene and inherited by both sexes.

Decreased synthesis of clotting factors is characteristic of diseases that affect the liver, such as cirrhosis and hepatitis, because most clotting factors are produced in the liver. A second cause of decreased synthesis is an absence of vitamin K, which is necessary for the formation of four of the clotting factors: II (prothrombin), VII, IX, and X.

NURSING MANAGEMENT OF THE PATIENT RECEIVING P ANTIHEMOPHILIC FACTOR

Antihemophilic factor is the prototype clotting factor.

Core Drug Knowledge

Pharmacotherapeutics

In patients with a demonstrated deficiency of clotting factor VIII, hemophilia A, AHF is used to prevent and control excessive bleeding. The drug effect is short term because the factor is used up in the clotting process (Table 32-7).

Pharmacokinetics

Administered IV, AHF is totally absorbed. It is rapidly removed from the plasma because it is used in the clotting process. Its half-life is from 4 to 24 hours with a 12-hour average (see Table 32-7).

Pharmacodynamics

Factor VIII is an essential component of blood clotting. It is required for the conversion of prothrombin to thrombin. Patients with factor VIII deficiencies have markedly prolonged bleeding and clotting times.

Contraindications and Precautions

A contraindication to AHF is a hypersensitivity to mouse protein (this is limited to products that contain monoclonal antibodies). Considered a pregnancy risk category C drug, AHF should be used only if necessary. The pooled blood product may contain minute amounts of blood types A or B. If the patient receives a large quantity of the preparation, the risk of hemolysis from blood type incompatibility exists. In patients who have not previously received multiple infusions of blood or plasma products, signs or symptoms of some viral infections, especially hepatitis C, are likely to develop. These patients, particularly those with mild hemophilia, should receive single-donor products. There is also a risk of HIV transmission from AHF, although current viral-depleting processes and donor-screening practices have reduced the potential for transmission significantly.

Adverse Effects

Several adverse effects may result from AHF, although none is common. Allergic reactions include anaphylaxis, urticaria, nausea, and chills. Other adverse effects include

TABLE 32-7 Summary of Selected Drugs for Hypocoagulation

Drug (Trade) Name	Selected Indications	Route and Dosage Range	Pharmacokinetics
P antihemophilic factor (Alphanate, Bioclate, Helixate, Hemofil M, Humate-P, Koate-HP, Kogenate, Monoclate-P, Profilate HP, Recombinate)	Temporarily replaces clotting factors missing because of hemophilia Prevents or corrects bleeding episodes Prophylaxis	*Adult:* administered so that factor VIII level assay is 5% of normal or 30% of normal after trauma or surgery*	*Onset:* immediate *Duration:* unknown $t_{1/2}$: 12 h
	Mild to severe hemorrhage	*Adult:* IV, 10–50 IU/kg, single dose; followed by 10–25 IU/kg q8–12h if needed*	
anti-inhibitor coagulant complex (Autoplex T, Feiba VH)	Controls bleeding in patients with factor VIII inhibitors Joint hemorrhage	*Adult:* IV, 50–100 U/kg at 12-h intervals	*Onset:* immediate *Duration:* unknown $t_{1/2}$: unknown
P aminocaproic acid (Amicar)	Controls fibrinolysis and stops bleeding	*Adult:* PO or IV, 4–5 g over the first hour followed by 1–1.25 g/h for 8 h	*Onset:* PO, rapid; IV immediate *Duration:* IV, 2–3 h $t_{1/2}$: IV, 3 h

*Dosing is highly individualized to achieve desired results. See manufacturer's instructions.

tachycardia, hypotension, headache, drowsiness, lethargy, vision disturbances, loss of consciousness, vomiting, hepatitis, intravascular hemolysis, back pain, chest constriction, and wheezing.

Drug Interactions

No significant interactions are associated with AHF.

Assessment of Relevant Core Patient Variables

Health Status

Important assessments for patients with hypocoagulation problems include determining factor VIII level assays and reviewing test results, such as CBC, direct Coombs test, urinalysis, PTT, thromboplastin generation test, and prothrombin generation test. These test results provide data regarding current clotting times and serve as baseline information to determine whether reactions are occurring during therapy. In the physical examination, the nurse needs to be alert for signs of active bleeding and extent of the bleeding.

Life Span and Gender

Because the safety of AHF during pregnancy has not been established, the nurse needs to determine whether the patient is pregnant.

Lifestyle, Diet, and Habits

During assessment, any patient behaviors that are likely to result in injury, such as participation in contact sports, should be investigated.

Culture

Patients with religious views that forbid receiving blood products may be opposed to receiving AHF. The nurse and patient should discuss beliefs that may have an impact on drug therapy.

Nursing Diagnosis and Outcome

- Risk for Injury, hemorrhage, related to deficiency of clotting factor VIII
  Desired outcome: The patient will receive enough factor VIII to prevent injury.

Planning and Intervention

Maximizing Therapeutic Effects

Refrigeration is required for AHF until it is used. Before reconstitution, the nurse should warm the concentrate and the diluent provided by the manufacturer to room temperature. Only plastic syringes are used for the infusion because the AHF solution can stick to glass surfaces.

The diluent is added to the concentrate in the vial, and the vial is rotated carefully until the contents dissolve. To help prevent gel formation, the vial should not be shaken. If a gel forms during reconstitution of AHF, the pharmacy or blood bank is notified, and the AHF is withheld.

The nurse must monitor coagulation studies during therapy to assess the effectiveness of AHF.

Minimizing Adverse Effects

After dilution, AHF must be administered within 3 hours to prevent bacterial growth. Only the IV route can be used. The nurse should apply pressure to all venipuncture sites for at least 5 minutes. IM injections are avoided to prevent bleeding into the muscle. Other measures include monitoring intake and output ratios and inspecting urine for color. If there is discrepancy in ratios or if urine becomes red or orange, a sign of hemolytic reaction, the physician is notified.

The nurse should also monitor for decreased hematocrit and increased Coombs test, both of which are indications of hemolytic anemia, and assess for allergic reaction. If present, the infusion should be stopped and the physician notified.

Providing Patient and Family Education

- The nurse should instruct patients and families to observe for bleeding from gums, skin, urine, stools, or emesis.
- The nurse should caution patients to avoid products containing aspirin or ibuprofen because they may further impair clotting.
- The nurse needs to discuss strategies to prevent bleeding, such as using a soft toothbrush, avoiding IM and subcutaneous injections, and avoiding behaviors or activities that are likely to cause injury.
- The nurse should advise patients to wear medical identification that identifies their disease.
- The nurse should emphasize that improved screening factors have decreased the risk of transmission of hepatitis or HIV significantly, although there remains a slight risk of disease transmission.

Ongoing Assessment and Evaluation

Blood studies are monitored as previously described. Therapy is effective when prolonged bleeding is prevented or stopped. ■

DRUGS CLOSELY RELATED TO P ANTIHEMOPHILIC FACTOR

Human factor IX complex is used to treat hemophilia B (Christmas disease), although it is not a substitute for fresh-frozen plasma used in mild factor IX deficiency. The complex contains factors II (prothrombin), VII, IX, and X. Factors II (prothrombin), VII, and X are required for converting prothrombin to thrombin, and factor IX is necessary for prothrombin production. The complex prevents or controls bleeding in hemophilia B, controls bleeding episodes in

MEMORY CHIP

Antihemophilic Factor

- Provides factor VIII for those with hemophilia; made from pooled human sources
- Temporarily meets needs for clotting factor to prevent or stop bleeding
- Dosage is individualized to needs of patient
- No common adverse effects
- Most serious adverse effects: slight risk of hemolytic anemia and transmission of hepatitis or HIV
- Minimizing adverse effects: monitor hematocrit and Coombs test result (hemolytic anemia)
- Most significant patient education: teach patients to avoid injury to prevent bleeding, and to carry or wear identification of the disease

patients with factor VIII inhibitors, and reverses oral anticoagulant-induced hemorrhage. Human factor IX complex (Konyne 80, Profilnine SD, Proplex T, and AlphaNine SD) has one variant, mononine. Mononine contains factor IX, but after reconstitution has nondetectable levels of factors II (prothrombin), VII, and X. It also contains histidine, mannitol, and mouse protein.

Factor IX-human contains only factor IX. Human factor IX complex and factor IX are administered IV. Dosage depends on the condition of the patient and the manufacturer's instructions, which vary according to the manufacturer. For additional information, refer to Table 32-7.

Anti-Inhibitor Coagulant Factor

Made from pooled human plasma, anti-inhibitor coagulant factor is a concentrate of activated and precursor clotting factors. It differs from AHF in that it is useful in treating patients with hemophilia who have significant levels of factor VIII inhibitors. It therefore allows clotting to occur in patients with hemophilia who are not responsive to AHF (see Table 32-7).

HEMOSTATIC DRUGS

Hemostatics stop blood loss by enhancing blood coagulation. There are two types of hemostatic agents: systemic and topical. Systemic agents interfere with the breakdown of clots. Topical agents are used to control small amounts of bleeding or oozing, usually following surgery. The prototype systemic hemostatic drug is aminocaproic acid (Amicar). Tranexamic acid is also a hemostatic drug. Additional topical hemostatic drugs are presented in Table 32-8.

PATHOPHYSIOLOGY

Fibrinolysis normally occurs in balance with blood coagulation. A clot forms to prevent extensive blood loss. When the vessel heals, the clot is broken down (fibrinolysis) by activating plasminogen so that it becomes plasmin. Plasmin breaks down fibrin, fibrinogen, and other plasma proteins. When fibrinolysis is not in balance with the other phases of coagulation (i.e., there is an excess of plasmin), excessive bleeding occurs because the body cannot form a stable clot in response to injury.

NURSING MANAGEMENT OF THE PATIENT RECEIVING AMINOCAPROIC ACID

Aminocaproic acid is the prototype systemic hemostatic drug.

Core Drug Knowledge

Pharmacotherapeutics

Aminocaproic acid treats severe, life-threatening hemorrhage from systemic hyperfibrinolysis or urinary fibrinolysis. Systemic hyperfibrinolysis has occurred with heart surgery, abruptio placentae, cirrhosis of the liver, and neoplastic disorders. Urinary hyperfibrinolysis is associated with severe trauma, shock, prostatectomy, nephrectomy, and renal cancers.

An unapproved use of aminocaproic acid is in preventing recurrent subarachnoid hemorrhage. Aminocaproic acid is also used to treat overdoses of fibrinolytic drugs, such as streptokinase.

Pharmacokinetics

Aminocaproic acid is administered orally or by IV infusion. After oral administration, the drug is quickly absorbed; through both routes it is widely distributed. Most of the drug is excreted unchanged in the urine (see Table 32-7).

Pharmacodynamics

Aminocaproic acid prevents fibrinolysis in two ways. First, it blocks the action of plasminogen activators, thus interfering with the formation of active plasmin. Second, it interferes with the binding of active plasmin to fibrin, thus preventing breakdown of fibrin. The result is stabilization of the blood clot and control of bleeding.

Contraindications and Precautions

Aminocaproic acid should be used only in life-threatening situations and then only when the overactivity of the fibrinolytic system is verified by laboratory testing. The drug is not to be used in patients with active intravascular clotting, such as DIC.

This drug is used with caution in patients with uremia or hepatic disease. Cautious use is recommended in patients with upper renal tract bleeding and those with cardiac, liver, or renal disease. Cautious use is also recommended in pregnancy or lactation because safety has not been established.

TABLE 32-8 Topical Hemostatic Agents

Hemostatic Agent and Action	Indication	Dosage	Contraindications and Adverse Effects	Nursing Management
Topical thrombin (Thrombinar, Thrombogen, Thrombostat) When applied directly on the wound, thrombin converts fibrinogen to fibrin.	Used in oozing wounds after dental surgery, plastic surgery, neurosurgery, epistaxis, and graft procedures Also used with absorbable gelatin sponges for hemostasis during surgery	The amount of bleeding determines the strength of solution, 100 to 2000 U/mL.	This is included in pregnancy risk category C. The drug may cause a hypersensitivity reaction. If the drug enters the bloodstream, intravascular coagulation occurs and may result in death. Reported adverse effects include febrile episodes and allergic reaction when used to treat epistaxis.	Clean blood from affected area with gauze pads. Apply solution soon after it is reconstituted (within 3 h of reconstitution if it has to be refrigerated). Monitor the application site frequently to detect any recurrence of blood loss.
Microfibrillar collagen hemostat (Avitene, Hemostat, Hemotene, Hemoped) Attracts platelets when applied to a bleeding area. Platelet aggregation fills the space with a fibrin clot.	Adjunct in controlling bleeding when traditional methods are not effective or useful	The dose is impregnated into a web or sponge form. The amount used depends on the amount of bleeding.	The drug should not be resterilized after use; its use in infected wounds is not recommended. Its effect during pregnancy is not known. Excess drug should be removed after use to prevent complications. Adverse effects include increase in infection, formation of adhesions, and hypersensitivity.	Avoid handling the substance with wet gloves or instruments, because it will adhere to a wet surface. After application to the wound, apply pressure using a dry gauze sponge. Discard any unused material; this agent may not be resterilized.
Absorbable gelatin sponge (Gelfoam). Product absorbs and holds many times its weight in whole blood. Wound may be closed over sponge, which will dissolve slowly.	Used in dental and oral surgery, neurosurgery, and prostatectomy to control bleeding	It is supplied in several different sizes to match size of the wound and the amount of bleeding.	The preparation should not be resterilized using heat, because heat may alter the product's effectiveness. The sponge should not be used on incisions. It has no indication for use in postpartum bleeding. It should be used sparingly in areas where expansion may be detrimental to surrounding structures. Adverse effects include potential for infection or abscess formation.	Assess wound frequently for bleeding. Apply during surgery as recommended by the surgeon—either dry or saturated in saline solution. Squeeze sponge to remove any air bubbles when the sponge is to be moistened on application. After application, apply pressure with a gauze pad for 10 to 15 s.

Absorbable gelatin film (Gelfilm, Gelfilm Ophthalmic) Cellophane-like material that becomes rubbery when wet and may be implanted into body tissue will be slowly absorbed.	Used in neurosurgery, thoracic surgery, and ocular surgery	This is supplied in a standard size and cut to fit the area	Using this film in contaminated wounds is contraindicated.	Soak the film in a sterile saline solution until pliable. The surgeon will cut the film to the desired size.
Oxidized cellulose (Oxycel, Surgicel) Exact mechanism of action is unknown but provides hemostasis when applied directly on bleeding area. It does not affect normal blood clotting, but in contact with blood, this product forms an artificial clot.	Used to control bleeding when sutures or clipping are not possible Primarily for bleeding from capillaries, venioles, or arterioles Used for oral and dental surgery	This is supplied impregnated into pads, pledgets, and strips. Number used depends on amount of bleeding and size of wound.	This product is contraindicated for use as wound packing. Product should not be used in fractures or spinal surgery because it may interfere with bone regrowth or cause cyst formation. It is not recommended for use in bleeding from large arteries or with serous oozing. This drug product should not be used if it has been autoclaved because this method of sterilization causes it to break down. The product may be left in the wound, but its removal once hemostasis is achieved is recommended. If used during a laminectomy, it must be removed. Adverse effects include nasal burning, encapsulation of fluid, antibody reactions.	Use a surgical clamp to remove substance from its container. Do not wet the product; instead, apply it dry. Monitor wounds of patients using oxidized cellulose for signs of bleeding.

Adverse Effects

The most common adverse effect of aminocaproic acid is GI distress (anorexia, nausea). Life-threatening or serious adverse effects are rare; these include convulsions, rhabdomyolysis (acute, sometimes fatal disease with destruction of the skeletal muscle), and renal failure. Other adverse effects that may occur include headache, dizziness, seizures, malaise, thrombophlebitis, hypotension (after IV administration), arrhythmias, tinnitus, nasal congestion, vomiting, abdominal cramps, diarrhea, and diuresis. Symptoms of overdosage include nausea, diarrhea, delirium, hepatic necrosis, and thromboembolism.

Drug Interactions

An increase in clotting factors leading to hypercoagulation may occur if aminocaproic acid is administered concurrently with oral contraceptives or estrogen (Table 32-9).

Assessment of Relevant Core Patient Variables

Health Status

Initial assessments include identifying contraindications to the drug by determining clotting factor levels and platelet counts to assess the severity of the patient's condition.

Life Span and Gender

During assessment, the patient's possible pregnancy or breast-feeding status should be evaluated. If the patient is a child, his or her weight should be measured so that a correct dosage can be calculated.

Environment

The nurse should be aware of the environment in which the drug will be administered. Aminocaproic acid is administered in an acute care setting, such as a hospital.

Nursing Diagnosis and Outcome

- Risk for Altered Cardiovascular Perfusion, related to volume loss secondary to uncontrolled bleeding or thrombophlebitis secondary to adverse effects of aminocaproic acid

  Desired outcome: Adequate perfusion will be maintained as evidenced by presence of pulses, normal skin color and warmth, and capillary refill.

Planning and Intervention

Minimizing Adverse Effects

The nurse needs to monitor vital signs at start of therapy and throughout therapy at intervals appropriate to the patient's condition. Every 15 to 30 minutes, the patient should be assessed for bleeding, particularly at incision and old injection sites.

To administer aminocaproic acid, an IV infusion pump is used to regulate the flow rate. The IV site and line are assessed for patency. The nurse should verify that the line is secured to prevent thrombophlebitis. Aminocaproic acid is not to be mixed with other drugs.

The patient is connected to a cardiac monitor to detect arrhythmias and observed for signs of thromboembolic complications, such as chest pain, dyspnea, changes in skin color and temperature, pain in an extremity, or changes in peripheral pulses. The prescriber is notified if these changes occur.

Additional ways to guard against adverse drug effects include monitoring intake and output and monitoring neurologic status in patients with subarachnoid hemorrhage. The prescriber should be notified of significant discrepancies or changes.

To combat nausea, patients should be encouraged to eat small frequent meals.

Providing Patient and Family Education

- The nurse needs to teach patients and families about the role of aminocaproic acid in controlling bleeding. They also must understand the importance of reporting any bleeding or symptoms of thromboembolism immediately.
- The nurse should instruct patients to change positions slowly to prevent orthostatic hypotension.

Ongoing Assessment and Evaluation

The patient should be monitored throughout treatment and recovery for signs and symptoms of bleeding or embolism or any other untoward event. ■

DRUG CLOSELY RELATED TO P AMINOCAPROIC ACID

Tranexamic acid (Cyklokapron) is another systemic hemostatic agent. It competitively inhibits activation of plasminogen. It is used to reduce or prevent hemorrhage during and after tooth extraction in patients with hemophilia.

TABLE 32-9 Agents That Interact With P Aminocaproic Acid

Interactants	Effect and Significance	Nursing Management
oral contraceptives	Increase in clotting factors may lead to hypercoagulant state and may possibly increase risk of thrombus formation.	Monitor for signs of thrombus.
estrogens	Same as above.	Same as above.

MEMORY CHIP

Aminocaproic Acid

- Used to treat life-threatening bleeding from systemic hyperfibrinolysis or urinary fibrinolysis
- Prevents breakdown of the stable clot and controls bleeding
- Significant contraindications: use only in life-threatening situations and only when the overactivity of the fibrinolytic system is verified by laboratory testing; DIC
- Most common adverse effect: GI distress
- Most serious adverse effects: renal failure (rare), rhabdomyolysis (rare), thromboembolism, and arrhythmias
- Minimizing adverse effects: use IV pump, assess for bleeding or signs of thromboembolism, and place patient on cardiac monitor to detect arrhythmias
- Most significant patient education: teach patients to report symptoms of thromboembolism

After oral administration, between 30% and 50% of the drug is absorbed. The drug remains in serum for 7 to 8 hours and is excreted from the body in the urine.

The drug is contraindicated for patients with subarachnoid hemorrhage. It should be used cautiously in patients with acquired defective color vision because altered color vision is an early sign of visual toxicity. Caution should be used in pregnant or lactating women and in patients with renal insufficiency.

CHAPTER SUMMARY

- Anticoagulants do not break down existing clots; they prevent clots from forming.
- The parenteral anticoagulant heparin and the oral anticoagulant warfarin are used in treating thrombus or thromboembolic disorders to prevent extension of the clot or formation of an embolism. They are also used in high-risk patients to prevent formation of an initial clot. Patients may be on both drugs at the same time during dose regulation of the warfarin.
- Education for patients on anticoagulant therapy should include safety measures to prevent bleeding, instructions to be alert for signs of bleeding, and directions for what to do if bleeding occurs.
- Antiplatelet drugs prevent platelet aggregation and thereby prevent thrombus formation. They are used prophylactically to prevent CVAs (also called strokes) and MIs (also called heart attacks).
- Hemorrheologic agents promote the flexibility of the RBCs and decrease blood viscosity to prevent thrombus formation.
- Thrombolytic drugs break down existing clots. They are used in acute medical emergencies, such as evolving MI, pulmonary embolism, massive DVT, or arterial thrombosis. Although they can save lives, these drugs carry a great risk of inducing hemorrhage. The patient must be closely monitored during this drug therapy.
- Clotting factors are administered when the patient has a deficiency of clotting factors resulting from heredity or disease. These drugs allow natural clotting to occur and prevent massive blood loss.
- Hemostatics are drugs used to promote blood coagulation. There are systemic and topical forms of hemostatics. Systemic hemostatics also interfere with the breaking down of clots.

QUESTIONS FOR STUDY AND REVIEW

1. Describe how heparin and warfarin differ in their effects on the clotting cycle. What interventions would the nurse use to promote safety while the patient is receiving heparin by continuous IV infusion?
2. Describe which laboratory values need to be monitored if the patient is receiving heparin and warfarin. What criteria will the nurse use to determine whether these drugs are in a therapeutic range?
3. Why is it important to assess the usual vitamin K intake for a patient who will be receiving warfarin but not for the patient who will be receiving heparin?
4. Why is the antiplatelet drug ticlopidine reserved for patients who are unable to tolerate aspirin (when used for its antiplatelet function)?
5. What drug therapy would be used for a patient who has hemophilia and who requires an inguinal hernia repair?

NEED MORE HELP?

Chapter 32 of the study guide for *Drug Therapy in Nursing* contains exercises and activities to reinforce your understanding of the concepts presented in this chapter. For additional information, see the text's accompanying web site at *http://www.connection.lww.com*.

REFERENCES AND BIBLIOGRAPHY

Ageno, W., & Turpie, A. G. (2000). Low-molecular-weight heparin in the treatment of pulmonary embolism. *Seminars in Vascular Surgery, 13*(3), 189–193.

Balcezak, T. J., Krumholz, H. M., Getnick, G. S., Vaccarino, V., Lin, Z. Q., Cadman, E. C. (2000). Utilization and effectiveness of a weight-based heparin nomogram at a large academic medical center. *American Journal of Managed Care, 6*(3), 329–338.

Burke, M., & Rupprecht, H. J. (2000). Antithrombotic therapy in acute coronary syndromes. *EXS, 89*, 193–209.

Caiola, E. (2000). Heparin-induced thrombocytopenia: How to manage it, how to avoid it. *Cleveland Clinical Journal of Medicine, 67*(9), 621–624.

Cohen, M., Antman, E. M., Gurfinkel, E., Turpie, A. G., Furst, J., Bigonzi, F., & Radley D. (2000). Impact of enoxaparin low-molecular-weight heparin in patients with Q-wave myocardial infarction. *American Journal of Cardiology, 86*(5), 553–6, A9.

Couturaud, F., Grand' Maison, A., & Kearon, C. (2000). Optimal duration of anticoagulant treatment of venous thromboembolism. *Presse Medicale, 29*(24), 1379–1385.

DeLoughery, T. G. (2000). Anticoagulant therapy in special circumstances. *Current Cardiology Report, 2*(1), 74–79.

Drug Facts and Comparisons. (2000). St. Louis: Facts and Comparisons.

Ellison, J., Walker, I. D., & Greer, I. A. (2000). Antenatal use of enoxaparin for prevention and treatment of thromboembolism in pregnancy. *BJOG, 107*(9), 1116–1121.

Fahs, P. S. S., & Kinney, M. R. (1991). The abdomen, thigh, and arm as sites for subcutaneous sodium heparin injections. *Nursing Research, 40*(4), 204–207.

Gornick C. C. (2000). Anticoagulant use in nonvalvular atrial fibrillation. Determining risk and choosing the safest course. *Postgraduate Medicine, 108*(2), 113–116, 119–121, 125–126.

Gurwitz, J. H., Field, T. S., Avorn, J., McCormick, D., Jain, S., Eckler, M., Benser, M., Edmondson, A. C., & Bates D. W. (2000). Incidence and preventability of adverse drug events in nursing homes. *American Journal of Medicine, 109*(2), 87–94.

Hadley, S. A., Chang, M., & Rogers, K. (1996). Effect of syringe size on bruising following subcutaneous heparin injection. *American Journal of Critical Care, 5*(4), 271–276.

Hutten, B. A., Prins, M. H., Gent, M., Ginsberg J., Tijssen, J. G., & Buller H. R. (2000). Incidence of recurrent thromboembolic and bleeding complications among patients with venous thromboembolism in relation to both malignancy and achieved international normalized ration: A retrospective analysis. *Journal of Clinical Oncology, 18*(17), 3078–3083.

Hylek, E. M., Heiman, H., Skates, S. J., Sheehan, M. A., & Singer, D. E. (1998). Acetaminophen and other risk factors for excessive warfarin anti-coagulation. *Journal of the American Medical Association, 279*(9), 657–662.

Iorio, A., & Agnelli G. (2000). Low-molecular-weight and unfractionated heparin for prevention of venous thromboembolism in neurosurgery: A meta-analysis. *Archives of Internal Medicine, 160*(15), 2327–2332.

Kassis, J., Fugere, F., & Dube S. (2000). The safest use of epidural anesthesia after subcutaneous injection of low-dose heparin in general abdominal surgery. *Canadian Journal of Surgery, 43*(4), 289–294.

Kearon, C., Harrison, L., Crowther, M., & Ginsberg, J. S. (2000). Optimal dosing of subcutaneous unfractionated heparin for the treatment of deep vein thrombosis. *Thrombosis Research, 97*(6), 395–403.

Marler, J. R., Tilley, B. C., Lu, M., Brott, T. G., Lynden, P. C., Grotta, J. C., Broderick, J. P., Levine, S. R., Frankel, M., Horowitz, S. H., Haley, E. C. Jr, Lewandowski, C. A., & Kwiatkowski, T. P. (2000). Early stroke treatment associated with better outcome: the rt-PA stroke study. *Neurology, 55*(11):1649–1655.

McGwin, G., Jr., Sims, R. V., Pulley, L., & Roseman, J. M. (2000). Relations among chronic medical conditions, medications, and automobile crashes in the elderly: A population-based case-control study. *American Journal of Epidemiology, 152*(5), 424–431.

Merli, G. J. (2000). Low-molecular-weight heparins versus unfractionated heparin in the treatment of deep vein thrombosis and pulmonary embolism. *American Journal of Physical Medicine and Rehabilitation, 79,* (Suppl. 2), S9–16.

Messieh, M. (2000). Preoperative haemoglobin and warfarin response. *Journal of Bone and Joint Surgery British Volume, 82*(5), 728–730.

National Guideline Clearinghouse. (2000). Clinical guidelines: Aspirin therapy in diabetes. *Diabetes Care* [On-line], *23*(1), S61–S62. Available: www.summary.asp?guideline=001456&summary_type=brief_summary&view=brief_summary&sSe:9/29/00.

National Guideline Clearinghouse. (1999, June). *Clinical guidelines for deep vein thrombosis* [On-line]. Bloomington, MN: Institute for Clinical Systems Improvement. Available: www.summary.asp?guideline=001338&summary_type=brief_summary&view=brief_summary&sSe:9/29/00

NINDS t-PA Stroke Study Group. (1997). Intracerebral hemorrhage after intravenous t-PA therapy for ischemic stroke. *Stroke* (11): 2109–2118.

Pineo, G. F., & Hull, R. D. (1998). Heparin and low molecular weight heparin in the treatment of venous thromboembolism. *Baillieres Clinical Haematology, 11*(3), 621–637.

Reeder, G. S. (2000). Contemporary diagnosis and management of unstable angina. *Mayo Clinic Proceedings, 75*(9), 953–957.

Sebastian, J. L., & Tresch, D. D. (2000). Use of oral anticoagulants in older patients. *Drugs in Aging, 16*(6), 409–435.

Seo, P., & Locke, C. F. (2000). Current and potential uses of low molecular weight heparin: a review and an economic analysis. *American Journal of Managed Care, 6*(4), 498–506; quiz, 507–508.

Sorensen, H. T., Johnsen, S. P., Larsen, H., Pedersen, L., Nielsen, G. L., & Moller, M. (2000). Birth outcomes in pregnant women treated with low molecular weight heparin. *Acta Obstetrica et Gynecologica Scandinavica, 79*(8), 655–659.

Valente, M., & Ponte, E. (2000). Thrombosis and cancer. *Minerva Cardioangiologica, 48*(4-5), 117–127.

Zanghi, M., Morici, V., Costanzo, M., Astuto, L., & Salanitri, G. (1988). Deep vein thrombosis of the legs: New therapy by means of low molecular weight heparins. *Journal of Internal Medical Research, 16*(6), 474–484.

When anticoagulation goes too far. (1999). *Clinician Reviews, 9*(2), 130–131.

Chapter 33

DRUGS FOR MODIFYING BIOLOGIC RESPONSE

KEY TERMS

active immunity
anemia
antibodies
antigens
aplastic
B lymphocytes
basophils
biologic modifier
biologic modulator
cellular immune response
chemotaxis
complement
erythrocytes
erythropoiesis
erythropoietin
granulocytes
hematopoiesis
histocompatibility leukocyte antigens (HLAs)
immunoglobulins
interferon
interleukins
leukocytes
lymphocytes
lymphokines
macrophages
monocytes
myelopoiesis
neutropenia
neutrophils
phagocytosis
platelets
T lymphocytes
thrombocytopenia
thrombopoietin

Learning Objectives

At the completion of this chapter the student will:

1. Identify core drug knowledge about drugs that affect the biologic responses.
2. Identify core patient variables relevant to drugs that affect the hematologic-immune system.
3. Relate the interaction of core drug knowledge to core patient variables for drugs that affect hematologic and biologic responses.
4. Generate a nursing plan of care from the interactions between core drug knowledge and core patient variables for drugs that affect hematologic and biologic responses.
5. Describe nursing interventions to maximize therapeutic and minimize adverse effects for drugs that affect the hematologic-immune system.
6. Determine key points for patient and family education for drugs that affect the hematologic-immune system.

Hematopoietic growth factors

epoetin alfa
filgrastim
sargramostim
oprelvekin/interleukin-11

Cytokines

interferon alfa-2a
aldesleukin/interleukin-2
tumor necrosis factor

Polyclonal/monoclonal antibodies

rituximab
abciximab
palivizumab
muromonab-CD3
infliximab
daclizumab
basiliximab

Immune modulators

cyclosporine
the retinoids (ATRA, 9 cis-transretinoic acid, bexarotene)
levamisole
azathioprine
thalidomide
glatiramer
bacillus of Calmette and Guerin (BCG)

The symbol C indicates the **drug class**.
Drugs in bold type marked with the symbol P are **prototypes**.
Drugs in blue type with no symbol are **closely related** to the prototype.
Drugs in **red** type with no symbol are **significantly different** from the prototype.
Drugs in **black** type with no symbol are **also used in drug therapy**; no prototype.

Biologic modulators, or **biologic modifiers,** are a group of biopharmaceuticals that are naturally occurring proteins used to alter the body's hematologic or immunologic responses. This is sometimes called biologic therapy. The rapid growth of these therapies over the past decade is attributable to the refinement of recombinant DNA technology, which has enabled researchers to produce large quantities of these substances outside the body. Many agents are administered to enhance hematopoietic cell replacement. Others stimulate immunologic activity assistance to combat specific **antigens** (substances that induce the formation of antibodies). Similar drugs from this class may also be used to suppress the immune system to prevent rejection of foreign transplanted tissue, or when the body is inappropriately rejecting self, as in **autoimmune disease**. Moreover, some agents may both stimulate parts of the immune system and depress some parts of the immune system.

This chapter discusses four classifications of agents used to alter biologic responses: hematopoietic growth factors, cytokines, polyclonal/monoclonal antibodies, and immune modulators. Active and passive antibody-conferred vaccinations are addressed in Appendix G rather than in this chapter.

Hematopoietic growth factors are substances generated by the body to enhance production of blood cells. Some of these agents are actually classified as hormone substances (e.g., epoetin), whereas others are cytokine growth factors. For this text, epoetin alfa (Epogen, Procrit), a hematopoietic growth factor, is the prototype. Drugs significantly differently from the prototype are the colony-stimulating factors filgrastim (Neupogen) and sargramostim (Leukine), and oprelvekin (also known as interleukin-11) (Neumega).

Cytokines are immunologic toxins produced by white blood cells (WBCs, also called leukocytes) in response to foreign antigens such as microorganisms, transplanted tissue, or malignant cells. The prototype cytokine is interferon alfa-2a (Roferon-A). Drugs in the same class represented by the prototype are interferon alfa-2b (Intron-A), interferon alfa-n3 (Alferon N), interferon-n1 (Wellferon), interferon alfacon-1 (Infergen), interferon beta-1a (Avonex), interferon beta-1b (Betaseron), and gamma-1b (Actimmune). Drugs significantly different from the prototype interferon alfa-2a are aldesleukin (also known as interleukin-2) (Proleukin) and tumor necrosis factor (TNF).

Antibodies (complex proteins produced in response to the presence of antigens) are a heterogeneous class of agents that can contain multiple genetic clones (polyclonal) or a single genetic design (monoclonal). Polyclonal antibodies are now used less often since technology has permitted specific targeting of cells using the monoclonal agents. Using hybridoma technology, monoclonal antibodies can be engineered to attach to tumor cells for diagnosis or treatment of malignancies or target T-lymphocytes to prevent or suppress T-cell recognition of tissue from outside the receptor's body. Monoclonal antibodies are now used most frequently. The prototype monoclonal antibody is rituximab (Rituxan). Drugs in the same class and represented by the prototype are trastuzumab (Herceptin) and CMA-676 (Mylotarg). Monoclonal antibodies closely related to the prototype rituximab include abciximab (ReoPro) and palivizumab (Synagis). Drugs significantly different from rituximab are muromonab CD3 (Orthoclone), daclizumab (Zenapax), infliximab (Remicade), and basiliximab (Simulect).

The immune modulators are a group of several agents with distinctly different structures that alter T-cell or B-cell activity. The prototype is cyclosporine (Sandimmune, Neoral, SangCya). Drugs in the same class and represented by the prototype are tacrolimus (Prograf), sirolimus (Rapamune), and mycophenolate mofetil (CellCept). Drugs significantly different from cyclosporine are the retinoids (e.g., all transretinoic acid [ATRA]) (Tretinoin, Vesanoid), 9-cis transretinoic acid (Panretinide, isomer ATRA), and bexarotene (Targretin gel), levamisole (Ergamisol), azathioprine (Imuran), thalidomide (Thalomid), glatiramer (Copaxone), and bacillus of Calmette and Guerin (BCG) (ImmuCyst/TheraCys).

Research is now being conducted to determine whether other essential cell proteins, nutrients, and growth factors (such as dendritic cells, epidermal growth factor inhibitors, and tyrosine kinase inhibitors) can be manipulated to provide a clinical benefit (Lotze, Farhood, Cara, & Storkus, 1999). Some investigators are also attempting to combine cytokines and antibodies to create a group of agents called fusion proteins (Kinzler & Brown, 2001). The use of biopharmaceuticals bound to anti-neoplastic medications is also a growing field of study.

The body of knowledge about the components and actions of the hematologic and immune systems is growing and changing every day. As researchers make new discoveries and better understand biologic interactions, they will find more ways to modify the hematologic and immune systems and treat a variety of viral, autoimmune, hematologic, and neoplastic disorders.

PHYSIOLOGY

The immune system is composed of hematopoietic cells and multiple hematologic-immunologic production and storage sites. Hematopoietic tissue is found in the bone marrow, lymph nodes, and lymphatic channels of the body. Based on a negative feedback system, stem cells located in the red bone marrow, which is found in the long bones and vertebral skeleton, produce the three types of functional hematopoietic cells: **erythrocytes** (also called red blood cells [RBCs]), **platelets**, and **leukocytes** (also called WBCs). The reticuloendothelial system includes immunologically active tissue and cells found in the lymph system, spleen, liver, lungs, gastrointestinal tract, and brain. An integrated immune response involving hematopoietic cells and immune tissues provides the body's nonspecific and specific response to invasion by antigens identified as nonself. The essential components of the immune system are hematopoietic cells, barrier defenses, the nonspecific immune response, the specific immune response, and immunity.

HEMATOPOIETIC CELLS

Red blood cells (or erythrocytes) are mainly composed of hemoglobin, which allows the cells to carry oxygen to the cells in the body. The biconcave disc shape of the RBCs allows them to be flexible and maneuver through the small capillaries to deliver oxygen to the tissues.

The major peptide hormone, or glycoprotein, that stimulates the production of RBCs (called **erythropoiesis**) is **erythropoietin**. Erythropoietin is produced by the kidneys in response to tissue hypoxia and reduced oxygen carrying capacity. Chronic obstructive pulmonary disease (COPD) and anemia, which produce chronic hypoxic states, are examples of disorders that stimulate the production of erythropoietin, and consequently the production of RBCs. When hemoglobin levels fall (e.g., in anemia), erythropoietin production is stimulated. Erythropoietin in turn stimulates the progenitor stem cells to make RBCs that live about 120 days. Plasma erythropoietin levels vary from 0.01 to 0.03 U/mL and increase from 100- to 1000-fold during hypoxia or anemia. When hemoglobin levels are elevated, erythropoietin production is halted, ending the stimulation to produce new RBCs.

Iron is the primary ion reversibly bound to oxygen in the heme molecule and is necessary to support erythropoiesis. It is held stable in the ferrous form by the other atoms that are in heme. When there is iron deficiency, the final step in heme synthesis is interrupted.

Platelets are the formed element involved in blood coagulation. Platelets are small cells that arise from the bone marrow precursor cells called megakaryocytes. Platelet production, although stimulated by many cytokines, is mostly dependent on the action of interleukin-6 and a peptide called **thrombopoietin**. Thrombopoietin is produced in the liver. A low platelet count stimulates the production of thrombopoietin. Platelets are important in normal blood clotting. (For more information on blood clotting, see Chapter 32 Drugs Affecting Coagulation.)

Leukocytes (or WBCs) are key components of all immune system responses. During maturation in the bone marrow, WBCs differentiate into three main cell types—**granulocytes, monocytes**, and **lymphocytes**— that respond to cell injury or foreign invaders (Fig. 33-1). Granulocytes are the most common type of WBC. Production of granulocytes is regulated by colony-stimulating factors (CSFs), also known as growth factors. Granulocytes are further divided into neutrophils, eosinophils, and basophils. The formation of granulocytes (**myelopoiesis**) is stimulated by many cytokines. These cells are produced in response to infection, inflammation and tissue necrosis.

BARRIER DEFENSES

The human body has many physical barrier defense mechanisms to protect it from the outside environment. The skin is the first line of defense. Mucus is another barrier defense mechanism, providing protection for the respiratory and genitourinary tracts. A third barrier defense, the gastrointestinal (GI) tract, provides an acid protector that destroys many microorganisms.

NONSPECIFIC IMMUNE RESPONSES

If a pathogen gets past one of these barrier defense mechanisms and injures a cell, the body activates the nonspecific inflammatory reaction, initiating granulocyte and monocyte/macrophage activities to destroy the invader and repair the damage. **Neutrophils** are the most common granulocyte and are considered the "first line of defense" against pathogens that gain entry into the body. Neutrophils contain enzymes that kill bacteria in the blood stream when they are ingested by the neutrophil (endocytosis or **phagocytosis**). The life of the neutrophil is extremely short—only 6 to 8 hours. Normally, when an acute infection is present in the body, the number of both mature and immature neutrophils will rise and produce neutrophilia. The immature neutrophils are called bands. When large numbers of bands are present in the blood count it is termed a "shift to the left," and usually signals a bacterial infection. When the neutrophil level or count is low (neutropenia), infection is likely to occur. **Basophils** are granulocytes that are not capable of phagocytosis but contain chemical substances important for initiating and maintaining an immune response. These substances include histamine, heparin, and chemicals used in the inflammatory response. Monocytes differentiate into immunologically active cells called **macrophages**. Macrophages can be circulating phagocytes or can be fixed in specific tissues.

SPECIFIC IMMUNE RESPONSES

If an invader gets past the barrier and nonspecific immune systems and enters the tissues or blood stream, a specific immune response involving lymphocytes is initiated.

Bone marrow stem cells develop into two types of lymphocytes: **T lymphocytes**, or T cells, and **B lymphocytes**, or B cells. These T and B lymphocytes may also differentiate into specialized cells such as natural killer cells and lymphokine-activated killer (LAK) cells, which have been identified as the cells that aggressively attack and destroy neoplastic cells. Because research in the area of lymphocyte identification is relatively new and ongoing, other not-yet-identified lymphocytes may also take part in the immune response.

T cells are "programmed" in the thymus gland to develop into at least three different cell types. Effector or cytotoxic T cells are found in various areas of the body and aggressively attack nonself cells by releasing chemicals called **lymphokines**. These chemicals either directly destroy a foreign cell or mark it for destruction by phagocytes and elicit an inflammatory response. This is termed the **cellular immune response**. Foreign or nonself cells have different membrane-identifying antigens called **histocompatibility leukocyte antigens (HLA)**. Helper T cells respond to the chemical indicators of immune activity and stimulate other lymphocytes to be more aggressive and responsive. Suppressor T cells respond to rising levels of chemicals associated with an immune response and suppress or slow the reaction. The balance between these two systems permits a rapid response, which destroys invaders immediately, followed by a slowing reaction if the invasion continues. This slowing conserves energy and the components of the immune and inflammatory reaction.

B cells are found throughout the reticuloendothelial system in like groups called clones. These cells are "programmed" to identify specific antigens. When a B cell reacts with its specific antigen, it changes into a plasma cell. Plasma cells produce antibodies, or **immunoglobulins**, that circulate in the

Physiology

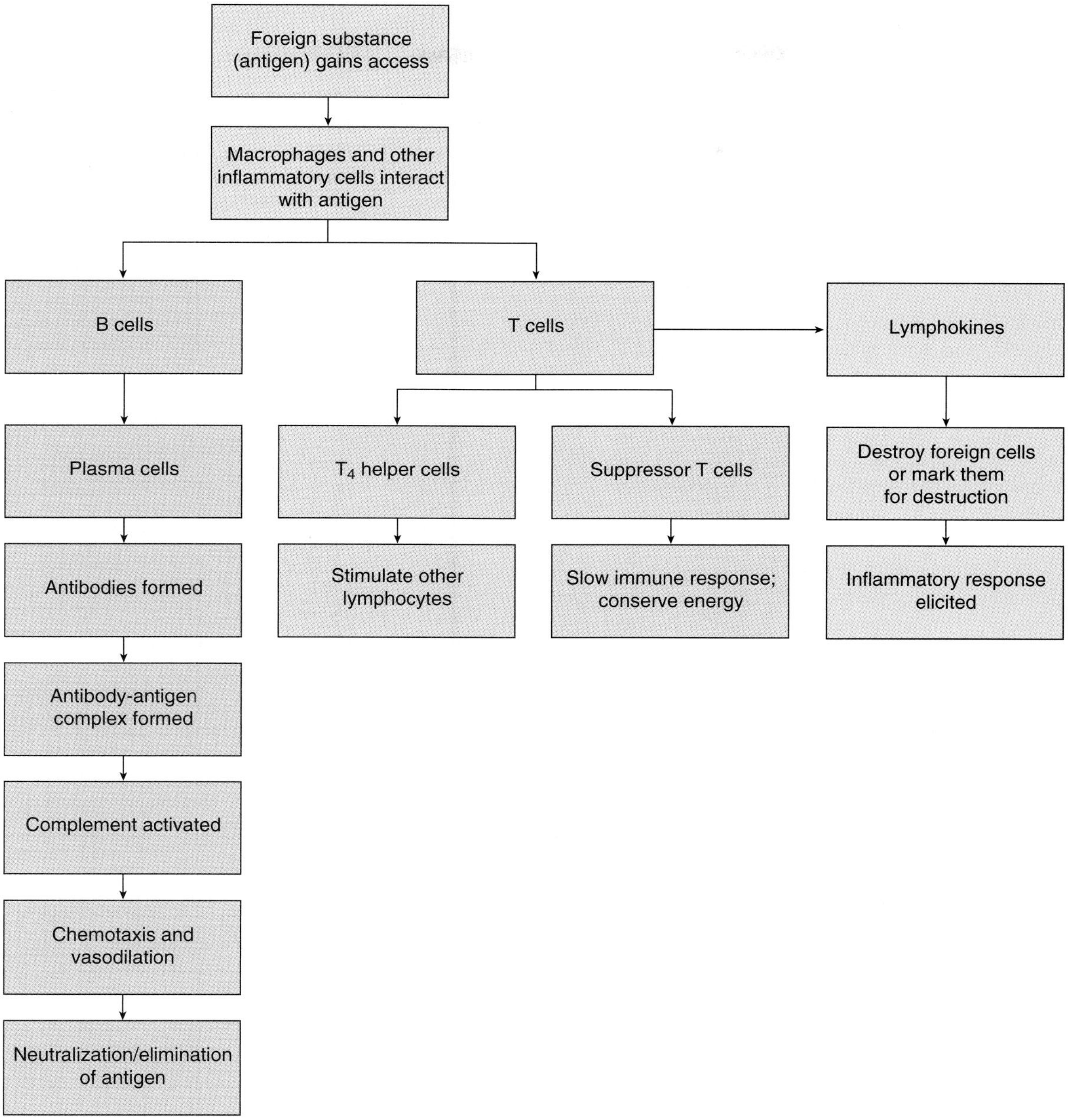

Figure 33-1. Response of T and B cells to invasion by foreign cells.

body and react with their specific "destiny" antigen when encountered. This is called a receptor-receptor site reaction and constitutes the humoral immune response. When the antigen and antibody react, they form an antigen-antibody complex, which reveals a new receptor site on the antibody that activates a series of plasma proteins in the body called **complement**. Complement proteins can destroy the antigen by altering the membrane and allowing osmotic inflow of fluid that bursts the cell. These proteins can also induce **chemotaxis** (attraction of phagocytic cells to the area) and increase the activity of phagocytes. In addition, they can release histamine, which causes vasodilation, increases blood flow to the area, and brings together all the components of the inflammatory reaction to destroy the antigen.

The initial formation of antibodies, called the primary response, takes several days. However, once the response is activated, the B cells form memory cells that, in turn, produce antibodies that are released immediately whenever the antigen is encountered. This process is a lifelong reaction called **active immunity**. B clones cluster in areas where they are most likely to encounter their specific antigen. For example, airborne antigens will meet B cells in the tonsils and upper respiratory tract. Experts believe that B cells are programmed genetically and are formed before birth. The introduction of a new antigen can result in widespread disease, because the body has no way of responding.

Chemical factors also play an important role in the specific immune reaction, acting as communication factors within the immune system to coordinate the immune response. For example, **interferons** are chemicals secreted by cells that have been invaded by viruses and possibly other stimuli. They prevent viral replication and suppress malignant cell replication and tumor growth. **Interleukins** are chemicals secreted by active WBCs to influence other WBCs. Interleukin-1 (lymphocyte-activating factor) stimulates T cells to initiate an immune response. Interleukin-2 (T-cell growth factor) is released from active T cells to stimulate the production of more T cells and to increase the activity of B cells, cytotoxic cells, and natural killer cells. Interleukin-2 also causes fever, arthralgia, myalgia, and slow-wave sleep-energy-conserving measures that help the body fight off invaders.

Several other factors released by lymphocytes and basophils have been identified. These include B-cell growth factor, macrophage-activating factor, macrophage-inhibiting factor, platelet-activating factor, eosinophil-chemotactic factor, and neutrophil-chemotactic factor. The presence or absence of these factors can influence the immune response.

The thymus gland, located in the mediastinal cavity, also releases a number of hormone types that circulate in the body to stimulate and communicate with T cells. Thymosin, a thymus hormone that has been replicated, is important in the maturation of T cells and cell-mediated immunity. Research is being done on using thymosin in certain leukemias and melanomas to stimulate the immune response (Wilkes, Ingwersen, & Burke, 1999). TNF is a chemical released by macrophages that inhibits tumor growth. It also interacts with other chemicals to make the inflammatory and immune responses more aggressive and efficient. Research is ongoing to determine the therapeutic effectiveness of this chemical as well (Oncology Nursing Society, 1995).

IMMUNITY

Immunity to a pathogen is achieved when the body has formed antibodies, which protect the body from developing an illness. Vaccines are used to stimulate an active immunity to commonly encountered antigens that could cause serious illness with first exposure. These vaccines are discussed in Appendix G. Sera are used to provide preformed antibodies, or passive immunity, in situations of acute exposure that could prove serious. In other words, by giving an antibody, rather than an antigen, which will then have to produce antibodies and which may cause illness, the immune response is started immediately, helping to prevent a serious, or potentially fatal, illness from occurring in the person exposed. Several drugs discussed in this chapter are used to affect immune system recognition or reaction to nonself proteins.

PATHOPHYSIOLOGY

Pathophysiologic conditions requiring drug therapy with immune modulators are varied and are related to either a hematologic failure or a dysfunction in any part of the immune response.

HEMATOLOGIC FAILURE

The pathophysiologic consequence of hematologic failure is inadequate cell production to meet the body's demands for transporting oxygen throughout the body, blood coagulation, or prevention of infection. Deficient cell production is named by the cell involved; when all cells are deficient, it is termed **aplastic**.

Anemia, a condition of reduced circulating RBCs, can be caused by deficient cell production (e.g., folic acid deficiency, iron deficiency, bone marrow failure) or abnormal hemolysis (e.g., sickle cell anemia, hemolytic anemia), or through loss of blood volume or cells, such as with overt bleeding. Anemia may also result from inadequate levels of the stimulating hormone erythropoietin. This most often occurs with chronic renal failure or bone marrow failure, conditions that cause insufficient production of erythropoietin. Anemias related to decreased erythropoietin levels can be treated with exogenous erythropoietin (epoetin alfa). In chronic renal failure, hemoglobin levels that are below 10 g/dL induce the heart to work harder to meet the tissue's needs for oxygen. This will eventually lead to left ventricular hypertrophy and left ventricular dilation, creating greater morbidity and severely altered quality of life. Normalization of the hemoglobin level can prevent the development of left ventricular dilation, as well as improve the quality of life. (Foley, Parfrey, Morgan, Barre, Campbell, Cartier, et al., 2000). To effectively manage early anemia in chronic renal failure, assume that there is an erythropoietin deficiency and rule out any iron deficiency that may be contributing to the problem. Therapy with replacement erythropoietin should begin whenever the hemoglobin levels fall below 10 g/dL. (Van Wyck, 2000).

A low platelet count is termed **thrombocytopenia**. Thrombocytopenia can result from decreased production, shortened survival, or loss of platelets. Decreased production is due to aplastic anemia, marrow infiltration, deficiencies of vitamin B12 and folate, radiation, and hereditary factors. Decreased survival of platelets is related to immune-mediated factors (idiopathic, systemic lupus erythematosus, drug induced, neonatal from maternal immunoglobulin G [IgG]); hypersplenism, disseminated intravascular coagulation, thrombotic thrombocytopenic purpura, hemolytic uremic syndrome; and prosthetic valves.

Abnormalities in WBC counts are fairly common, although abnormalities of WBC function are rare. Decreased numbers of neutrophils, called **neutropenia**, is related to two basic causes: decreased marrow activity and decreased neutrophil survival. When neutropenia is related to decreased marrow activity, it may be related to drug therapy (such as with antineoplastics, some antibiotics, gold, certain diuretics, antithyroid agents, antihistamines, and antipsychotics). Other causes include radiation exposure, megaloblastic anemia (anemia in which large nucleated abnormal RBCs are present in the blood), cyclic neutropenia (a benign disease), Kostmann (infantile) neutropenia, aplastic anemia (anemia from complete suppression, or loss of function, of the bone marrow), myelodysplastic syndrome, and marrow replacement by tumor.

IMMUNE DYSFUNCTION

Four abnormal conditions can weaken the immune system and stimulate the immune response: neoplasms, viral invasion, autoimmune disease, and transplant rejection. Neoplasms result from the growth of mutant cells that escape the normal surveillance of the immune system. Viral invasion of a cell changes the cell's membrane and antigenic presentation. In autoimmune disease, the body responds to specific self-antigens by producing antibodies against self-cells (autoantibodies). Organ transplantation weakens the immune system as the body reacts to the introduction of foreign cells.

HEMATOPOIETIC GROWTH FACTORS

Hematopoietic growth factors are exogenous replacements of endogenous growth factors. They are used when the internal mechanism of producing sufficient blood cells does not meet the body's needs. The prototype that will be presented is epoetin alfa, used to create RBCs.

Epoetin alfa is a 165 amino-acid glycoprotein manufactured by recombinant DNA technology. It is recombinant human erythropoietin. The product contains the identical amino acid sequence of natural erythropoietin. The human erythropoietin gene is introduced into mammalian cells, which then produce erythropoietin that has the same biologic effects as endogenous erythropoietin.

NURSING MANAGEMENT OF THE PATIENT RECEIVING EPOETIN ALFA

Core Drug Knowledge

Pharmacotherapeutics

Epoetin alfa (Epogen, Procrit), also referred to as erythropoietin or EPO, is used in the treatment of anemia associated with chronic renal failure to elevate or maintain the RBC level (assessed through the hematocrit or hemoglobin determinations) and to decrease the need for transfusion (Table 33-1). Epoetin alfa is also used to treat anemia related to zidovudine therapy in HIV-infected patients. It is used when the endogenous erythropoietin levels are below or equal to 500 mU/mL and the dose of zidovudine is less than or equal to 4,200 mg/week. It is also used to treat chemotherapy-induced anemia in cancer patients. It is intended to decrease the need for transfusions in patients who will receive chemotherapy for at least 2 months. Finally, epoetin alfa is used with anemic patients who will be undergoing elective,

TABLE 33-1 Summary of Selected Biotherapy Agents

Drug (Trade) Name	Selected Indications	Route and Dosage Range	Pharmacokinetics
Hematopoietic Growth Factors			
epoetin alfa or erythropoietin or EPO (Epogen, Procrit)	Anemia from chronic renal failure (CRF) Anemia related to ZDV therapy in HIV-associated illness Anemia related to chemotherapy in cancer patients	CRF: 50–100 U/kg 3 times/wk IV or SC injection to maintain Hct of 30%–36% HIV: 100 U/kg 3 times/wk for 8 wks IV or SC injection Cancer: 150 U/kg 3 times/wk SC injection (weekly injections under investigation)	*Onset:* IV, immediate SC within 5 to 24 h *Duration:* IV, ≥ 24 h SC levels fall slowly after 24 h $t_{1/2}$: 4–13 h
filgrastim, or granulocyte-colony stimulating factor (G-CSF) (Neupogen)	Neutropenia due to chemotherapy, after bone-marrow transplantation (BMT), or severe chronic neutropenia Prior to peripheral blood progenitor cell (PBPC) collection	Chemotherapy: 5 m/kg/d SC injection, or infusion, or IV BMT: 10 mck/kg/d IV or SC infusion Chronic: congenital 6 mg/kg bid SC injection Idiopathic or cyclic: 5 mg/kg once/d SC injection PBPC collection: 10 mg/kg/d SC (injection or infusion) starting at least 4 d prior to procedure	*Onset:* IV, immediate *Duration:* Unknown $t_{1/2}$: 3.5 h
oprelvekin or interleukin 11 (IL-11) (Neumega)	Thrombocytopenia from chemotherapy	*Adult:* 50 mg/kg/d SC injection *Child:* Safety and efficacy not established	*Onset:* Unknown *Duration:* Unknown $t_{1/2}$: 6.9 h

(continued)

Pharmacodynamics

Epoetin alfa has the same effects on the body as endogenous erythropoietin. It stimulates the production of RBCs. In patients with chronic renal failure, the first evidence that epoetin alfa is producing a positive response is an increase in the reticulocyte (immature RBC) count within 10 days. Next seen, within 2 to 6 weeks, is an increase in the counts of RBCs, hemoglobin, and hematocrit. Once the target hematocrit (30% to 36%) has been reached, it can be maintained by the use of epoetin alfa. The rate of hematocrit increases varies among patients and is dose dependent; however, doses over than 300 U/kg three times weekly produce no additional biologic response. Other factors affecting rate and extent of response include the availability of iron stores, baseline hematocrit, and concurrent illnesses.

Responsiveness of patients with HIV to epoetin alfa therapy is based on their endogenous erythropoietin levels. Those with levels above 500 mU/mL do not appear to respond to therapy (Wujcik, 2001). An increased hematocrit and a decreased need for transfusion are evidence of a response. Cancer patients who receive epoetin alfa are most likely to respond to therapy if they have lymphoid and solid cancers and do not have infiltration of the malignancy into the bone marrow.

Contraindications and Precautions

Avoid using epoetin alfa in uncontrolled hypertension and if there is hypersensitivity to mammalian cell-derived products or human albumin. Although there do not appear to be any direct vasopressor effects of epoetin therapy, blood pressure may rise during therapy. This is especially true during the early phase of treatment when the hematocrit is rising. An elevation in blood pressure is especially problematic for patients with chronic renal failure who are typically hypertensive already.

It is recommended that the hematocrit level not be increased more than four points in any 2-week period, because an excessive rate of increase may possibly be associated with an exacerbation of hypertension. Hypertension from increases in hematocrit has rarely been noted in patients with cancer receiving epoetin. Hypertensive encephalopathy and seizures have occurred in patients with chronic renal failure treated with epoetin.

The relationship of seizures to epoetin therapy in patients with chronic renal failure is unclear. Patients with chronic renal failure on dialysis seem to have a higher rate of seizures during the first 90 days of epoetin therapy than during the second 90-day period. It is hypothesized that there may be a relationship between rising hematocrit and seizures (Foley, et al., 2000). This possible relationship is another reason why the hematocrit level should not be allowed to rise more than four points in 2 weeks when treating patients with chronic renal failure. Thrombotic events, such as clotting of the artificial kidney during dialysis, myocardial infarction, transient ischemic attacks, or cerebral vascular accident can occur in chronic renal failure patients receiving epoetin. Patients receiving dialysis may need increased anticoagulation with heparin to prevent their artificial kidney from clotting. The risk of thrombotic events is greatly increased in patients with ischemic heart disease or congestive heart failure when the provider is trying to increase the hematocrit to normal levels (42%) with epoetin therapy.

In contrast, there does not seem to be any association between exacerbation of hypertension, seizures, and thrombotic events and epoetin therapy in patients with HIV. It is, however, still recommended that therapy should not be started until blood pressure is controlled.

Epoetin therapy is not to be used as a replacement for transfusion in patients with chronic renal failure who require correction for a severe anemia. In patients with HIV and cancer, epoetin should not be used for treatment of anemia caused by iron or folate deficiencies, hemolysis, or GI bleeding.

Adverse Effects

Adverse effects occurring during epoetin therapy appear to reflect the patients' underlying disease process or their postoperative state. It is difficult to determine then, exactly what the adverse effects of epoetin are. As discussed in the earlier precaution section, hypertension may occur in patients with chronic renal failure who are on dialysis. Headache, nausea and vomiting, and tachycardia are all frequently reported. Seizures have been reported less often, and more commonly in patients with renal disease. Porphyria (excretion of nitrogen containing compounds in the urine) may be exacerbated in patients with chronic renal failure, although this is rare.

Fever, headache, cough, rash, and nausea have been reported fairly frequently in patients with HIV. Patients with cancer report fever, diarrhea, vomiting, and edema often while on epoetin therapy. Patients who receive epoetin prior to surgery report fever, diarrhea, and vomiting. In clinical trials, all of these adverse effects were also reported by patients who received placebos instead of epoetin.

Drug Interactions

There are no known drug interactions with epoetin.

Assessment of Relevant Core Patient Variables

Health Status

Determine whether the patient has preexisting uncontrolled hypertension, because this is a contraindication for its use. If the patient does not have chronic renal failure, verify that the anemia is not caused by iron or folate deficiency, hemolysis, or GI bleeding, because these anemias should be treated differently. Determine whether the patient has preexisting vascular disease, because this may increase the patient's risk of developing thrombotic adverse effects. Prior to and during therapy, assess the patient's iron status, including transferrin saturation (serum iron divided by iron binding capacity) and serum ferritin (iron-phosphorous-protein complex that is the form in which iron is stored in the tissues). Transferrin saturation should be at least 20%, and ferritin should be at least 100 ng/mL. Iron is needed to support erythropoiesis. Absolute or functional iron deficiency may develop during therapy. Functional iron deficiency, in which the ferritin level is normal but the transferrin saturation is low, is believed to be caused by the body's inability to mobilize iron stores rapidly enough to support increased erythropoiesis.

Life Span and Gender

Determine whether the patient is pregnant, because epoetin is a pregnancy category C drug. Adverse effects have occurred in rats given epoetin in doses five times the comparable human dose; however, there are no adequate studies in humans. Caution should be used if administering to a woman who is breast-feeding because it is not known whether epoetin crosses into breast milk. Safety and efficacy in children is not established. If given to premature infants, use the form without the benzyl alcohol (i.e., preservative free) because benzyl alcohol has been associated with a fatal "gasping syndrome" in premature infants.

Lifestyle, Diet, and Habits

Verify that patients with chronic renal failure are continuing the dietary restrictions necessary in chronic renal failure. As patients begin to feel better when their hematocrit rises, they may feel that they no longer need a restrictive diet. Determine whether patients are at risk for iron deficiency; if so, they should be encouraged to consume foods high in iron.

Environment

Epoetin is administered in many ambulatory settings as well as the hospital or dialysis center. For patients who receive home dialysis or who intermittent ambulatory treatment (antiretroviral therapy, chemotherapy, or radiation therapy), therapy can be self-administered at home. The nurse should assess with the patient factors in the home environment that may affect adherence to drug therapy. The nurse should be careful to review reimbursement policies of the patient's health care insurance, because injectable medications are often not reimbursed as a home therapy.

Culture

There are no cultural barriers to the use of epoetin. If the nurse's assessment reveals that the patient has a religious affiliation (e.g., Jehovah's Witnesses) in which blood transfusions are forbidden, epoetin may still be administered. Epoetin is not considered a blood component by religious affiliations that object to transfusions and hence offers an excellent alternative to RBC transfusion for those individuals.

Nursing Diagnoses and Outcomes

- Impaired tissue oxygenation related to anemia
  Desired outcome: Tissues will be oxygenated satisfactorily, and hematocrit will reach desired level with epoetin alfa therapy.
- Risk for injury related to adverse effects of epoetin
  Desired outcome: Adverse effects will be prevented or minimized to prevent injury.

Planning and Intervention

Maximizing Therapeutic Effects

To maintain the biologic activity of epoetin, do not shake after reconstituting. Vigorous shaking may denature the glycoprotein, making it biologically inactive. Allow time for the hematocrit to rise before seeking an order to adjust the dose. When epoetin is given in chronic renal failure, the time required to elicit a clinically significant change in hematocrit is 2 to 6 weeks. The dose should not be adjusted more than once a month. After each dose adjustment, verify that the patient has an appointment to have his or her hematocrit measured twice a week for a least 2 to 6 weeks to verify that the hematocrit is in the correct range, showing that the drug is effective. If the hematocrit has not risen by five to six points in an 8-week period (and iron stores are adequate), the patient will require an increase in the dose. Seek orders and administer iron supplements IV, as needed, to help increase the effectiveness of the epoetin.

When epoetin is given to patients with HIV who are treated with zidovudine, the nurse should give an initial dose for 8 weeks. If the dose does not produce the desired response, seek an order to increase the dose. Evaluate the patient's response every 4 to 8 weeks thereafter and seek new orders to adjust the dose as needed. The nurse should monitor the hematocrit weekly during dose adjustment.

When epoetin is given to cancer patients on chemotherapy, the initial dose should be given for 8 weeks. After that period, seek orders to adjust the dose if needed. If patients still do not respond to therapy, it is unlikely that they will respond to higher doses.

When epoetin is given to presurgical patients with anemia, it should be given SC for 10 days before surgery, the day of surgery, and for 4 days postoperatively. Alternately, epoetin may be given in once-weekly doses at 21 days, 14 days, and 7 days before surgery, with a fourth dose on the day of surgery.

If a delayed or diminished response to epoetin occurs, the nurse should assess for other reasons that may be causing a low hematocrit (i.e., functional iron deficiency; underlying infectious, inflammatory, or malignant processes; occult blood loss; underlying hematologic diseases; folic acid or vitamin B12 deficiencies; hemolysis; aluminum intoxication; osteitis fibrosa cystica [overactivity of parathyroid gland resulting in disturbances in calcium and phosphorus metabolism]).

Minimizing Adverse Effects

The nurse should remember that the single-dose 1-mL vials have no preservative. To prevent contamination use only one dose per vial, do not reenter vial, and discard any unused portion. In contrast, the multidose 2-mL vial has preservative in it. Store at 2 to 8°C after initial entry and between doses. Discard 21 days after initial entry to prevent use of a possibly contaminated product.

Monitor the blood pressure of all patients receiving epoetin throughout therapy to assess for hypertension that may occur.

In patients who have chronic renal failure and are receiving epoetin, monitor the hematocrit to prevent adverse effects. Dosage adjustments to achieve the desired hematocrit are not uncommon. These adjustments, or titrations, may be stated in the original drug order, or in a unit or hospital protocol. If neither of these exists, the nurse needs to contact the prescriber for further orders. The nurse has a responsibility to verify that the dose being administered is safe, based on the patient's current physiologic status, and will not promote serious adverse effects If the hematocrit is approaching 36%, a dose reduction is indicated to maintain the suggested target hematocrit range. If the hematocrit rises above 36%, the nurse should notify the prescriber and withhold administering doses until the hematocrit begins to decrease. Epoetin should then be restarted with a lower, ordered dose. If the hematocrit increases by more than four points in a 2-week period, seek orders to immediately decrease the dose. After dose adjustment, monitor hematocrit twice a week for 2 to 6 weeks.

In patients who have HIV and are on zidovudine treatment while receiving epoetin, the hematocrit also needs to be closely monitored. If the hematocrit exceeds 40%, notify the prescriber and stop the dose until the hematocrit drops to 36%. When the prescriber resumes epoetin treatment, the dose should have been decreased by 25%; the nurse would then titrate the drug based on orders or protocol until the desired hematocrit is obtained.

Finally, when epoetin is being given to patients with cancer who are receiving chemotherapy, the hematocrit also needs to be monitored carefully. If the initial dose produces a rapid rise in hematocrit of more than 4% in 2 weeks, the nurse should seek an order to reduce the dose. If the hematocrit exceeds 40%, notify the prescriber and stop administering the dose until the hematocrit drops to 36%. When resuming epoetin therapy, the ordered dose should be 25% less than before. The dose may be titrated by the nurse, based on orders or protocols, until desired hematocrit is obtained.

Providing Patient and Family Education

- The nurse should teach the patient and family the purpose of the drug and the need for follow up blood work to check the hematocrit.
- The nurse should instruct patients to maintain adequate iron intake, which may aid in effectiveness of epoetin. Foods high in iron include green leafy vegetables, beans, and organ meats. High iron-content foods or supplements are best absorbed if taken with ascorbic acid, such as found with citrus drinks.
- The nurse should explain to patients with chronic renal failure the importance of continuing with diet restrictions and dialysis (if utilized) while on epoetin.
- For patients who will be self-administering epoetin at home, the nurse should teach proper SC injection technique and safe disposal of used needles and syringes.

Ongoing Assessment and Evaluation

Monitor patients' blood pressure and hematocrit throughout therapy. The hematocrit should be checked twice weekly until the target hematocrit has been achieved and the dose has been established. Monitor iron levels throughout therapy to verify enough iron is available to support erythropoiesis. Therapy is effective when the hematocrit rises to a desired treatment level, the need for transfusions is reduced, and the patient does not have significant adverse effects. ■

DRUGS SIGNIFICANTLY DIFFERENT FROM EPOETIN ALFA

Colony-Stimulating Factors

Colony-stimulating factors are glycoproteins that assist in the production of blood cells by binding to specific cell surface receptors and stimulating proliferation, differentiation com-

MEMORY CHIP

Epoetin Alfa

- Recombinant human erythropoietin works exactly as endogenous erythropoietin; it stimulates the production of RBCs (erythropoiesis)
- Used to treat anemia in chronic renal failure, HIV (when zidovudine is used), and cancer (when chemotherapy is used), and in preoperative anemic patients (when high blood loss and transfusion are anticipated)
- Significant contraindication: Uncontrolled hypertension
- Difficult to determine true adverse effects because those reported are also present in disease process or post procedure
- Most common adverse effects: hypertension (in chronic renal failure [CRF]); fever (all other uses)
- Most serious adverse effects: thrombotic effects (in CRF)
- Maximizing therapeutic effects: consult with prescriber about dose adjustment and verify iron availability
- Minimizing adverse effects: monitor hematocrit
- Most significant patient education: advise patients of the need for follow-up blood work and the importance of dietary iron

mitment, and some end-cell functional activation. Filgrastim is a granulocyte colony-stimulating factor (G-CSF), and sargramostim is a granulocyte-macrophage colony-stimulating factor (GM-CSF). Both have been produced by recombinant DNA technology. Interleukin-11, unlike other interleukins, primarily alters hematopoietic activity.

Filgrastim

Filgrastim (Neupogen) is produced by *Escherichia coli* bacteria, which have the human G-CSF gene inserted. G-CSF regulates the production of neutrophils within the bone marrow. Recombinant DNA G-CSF (filgrastim) acts the way that endogenous G-CSF does.

Filgrastim is licensed for use in patients with cancer to increase their neutrophil count. For cancer patients with nonmyeloid malignancies (cancers that are not related to blood cell components) who are receiving myelosuppressive chemotherapy (suppressing the production of blood cells in the bone marrow), it is used to decrease the incidence of infection, as manifested by febrile neutropenia. Primary administration of CSFs as prophylaxis should be reserved for patients expected to experience febrile neutropenia at an incidence equal or greater than 40%. Filgrastim is not recommended for routine use in neutropenic patients who are afebrile or who have uncomplicated fever and neutropenia (i.e., fever; less than 10 days duration of neutropenia; no evidence of pneumonia, cellulitis, abscess, sinusitis, hypotension, multiorgan dysfunction, or invasive fungal infection; and no uncontrolled malignancies) (Ozer, Armitage, Bennett, Crawford, Demetri, Pizzo, et al., 2000). It is also used for those patients with cancer who receive chemotherapy following bone marrow transplant to reduce the duration of neutropenia and neutropenia-related clinical sequelae (e.g., febrile neutropenia). Filgrastim is also used in patients with cancer prior to leukopheresis (removing WBCs from blood that are saved and then later transfused back into the patient). Filgrastim stimulates and mobilizes the cells that are the progenitor cells for neutrophils into the peripheral circulation. When this additional volume of progenitor cells is infused back into the patient, the neutrophil count will rise more rapidly.

Filgrastim is also used in patients with severe, chronic neutropenia that is congenital, cyclic, or idiopathic in origin. For these patients, the goal is to reduce the incidence and duration of sequelae of neutropenia (e.g., fever, infections, oropharyngeal ulcers).

Unlabeled uses of filgrastim include treatment of bone marrow suppression in patients with acquired immune deficiency syndrome (AIDS), aplastic anemia, hairy cell leukemia, myelodysplasia, drug-induced and congenital agranulocytosis, and alloimmune neonatal neutropenia.

Filgrastim is administered as a single daily SC injection bolus, by short IV infusion (15 to 30 minutes), or by continuous SC or IV infusion.

The only contraindication for administration of this agent is hypersensitivity to *E. coli*-derived proteins, filgrastim, or any of the product components. Caution should be used when a patient has a myeloid malignancy or requires concomitant cytotoxic (destructive to cells) chemotherapy or radiotherapy, because the rapidly dividing myeloid cells may be sensitive to these substances.

Do not use filgrastim from 24 hours before to 24 hours after chemotherapy with cytotoxic substances as extremely elevated WBC counts have occurred. Although no specific adverse effects have been noted with this, the WBC count should be monitored closely during therapy. Caution should be used to avoid discontinuing the treatment with filgrastim prematurely. Although there is a transient increase in neutrophil count 1 to 2 days after starting therapy, this should not be mistaken for the full therapeutic effect of drug therapy. Administer this agent throughout the time when the marrow-suppressing therapy's full nadir (lowest level) of neutrophils should have occurred before discontinuing therapy.

It is difficult to determine adverse effects to filgrastim in patients receiving chemotherapy, because all of the effects recorded during clinical trials with the drug are also consequences of the malignancy or the cytotoxic chemotherapy. In other words, adverse effects may mimic the disease being treated or other treatments for the disease. Medullary bone pain (within the marrow) is the only consistently observed adverse effect that can be attributed to drug therapy; it is mild to moderate in severity is reported in 24% of patients on filgrastim.

In patients receiving intensive chemotherapy or total body irradiation followed by bone marrow transplantation, few unique adverse effects have been attributable to the G-CSF therapy.

In patients in whom filgrastim is used in peripheral blood progenitor cell collection, adverse effects included decreased platelet count, anemia, mild to moderate musculoskeletal symptoms, medullary bone pain, headache, increases in alkaline phosphatase levels. Patients with severe chronic neutropenia have also experienced mild to moderate bone pain.

Drug interactions with filgrastim have not yet been fully evaluated. Drugs that may potentiate the release of neutrophils, such as lithium carbonate, should be used with caution as a synergistic effect may result.

Filgrastim is a pregnancy category C drug and should be used with caution. It is not known whether it is excreted in breast milk. Filgrastim has been used in pediatric patients ages 4 months to 17 years and no long-term risks have been identified. Safety and efficacy in neonatal autoimmune neutropenia have not been established. Long-term effects of this agent have also not been evaluated in neonates.

To achieve the maximum therapeutic effect from the filgrastim, the nurse should be sure to do the following:

- Dilute in 5% dextrose solution with albumin added to prevent absorption by plastic materials.
- Do not dilute in saline because it may precipitate.
- Avoid shaking because this may damage the protein.

To prevent adverse effects, the nurse should be careful not to decrease the dose prematurely (i.e., before the expected neutrophil nadir, or lowest point, is expected). Additionally, the nurse should discard any vial that has been at room temperature for more than 24 hours, use only one dose per vial, and never reenter a used vial. Because the filgrastim is preservative free, these actions will guard against bacterial growth.

Patients with neutropenia are at increased risk of contracting an infection. When providing patient education, the nurse should instruct the patient and those in contact with the patient to wash their hands frequently, avoid crowds, and avoid people with illnesses (see the accompanying displays, Neutropenia and Infection and Nosocomial Infections in Neutropenic ICU Patients).

Sargramostim

Sargramostim (Leukine) is produced by recombinant DNA technology in a yeast expression system. Sargramostim is a glycoprotein of 127 amino acids. The amino acid sequence differs from the natural human GM-CSF by substituting leucine at position 23; the carbohydrate portion may also be different than the native protein. Unlike G-CSF (filgrastim), which only induces the production of granulocytes, specifically neutrophils, GM-CSF induces partially committed progenitor cells to divide and differentiate into the granulocyte and the macrophage pathways. Sargramostim increases the cytotoxicity of monocytes toward certain neoplastic cell lines and activates neutrophils to inhibit the growth of pathogens or tumor cells.

Sargramostim is used in the treatment of patients with non-Hodgkin lymphoma, acute lymphoblastic leukemia, and Hodgkin disease undergoing autologous bone marrow transplantation (transplantation of their own bone marrow that was previously collected). It provides an acceleration of myeloid recovery in these patients. Sargramostim is also used in bone marrow transplant failure or where there are engraftment delays. It can be used after the induction of chemotherapy in older adults with acute myelogenous leukemia to shorten their neutrophil recovery time and reduce severe life-threatening infections. Sargramostim can also be used to mobilize the hematopoietic progenitor cells into the peripheral circulation where they can be collected by leukapheresis. The additional progenitor cells are then later returned after chemotherapy allowing for more rapid engraftment, decreasing the need for supportive care. The drug is also administered after peripheral blood progenitor collection transplantation to rapidly increase monocyte production. Sargramostim is also used after allogenic (from a matched donor) bone marrow transplant to accelerate the myeloid recovery.

Unlabeled uses of sargramostim include the following: to increase WBC counts in patients with myelodysplastic syndromes and in patients with AIDS who are receiving zidovudine; to limit the duration of leukopenia secondary to myelosuppressive chemotherapy and decrease myelosuppression in preleukemic patients; to correct neutropenia in aplastic anemia; and to decrease transplantation associated organ system damage, particularly liver and kidney disease (neutropenia correlates with organ system injury) (Wucjik, 2001).

Sargramostim is administered by IV infusion for most applications. It may be given SC when used after peripheral blood progenitor cell transplantation.

Contraindications to sargramostim use include excessive leukemic myeloid blasts in the bone marrow or peripheral blood, known hypersensitivity to the drug, and simultaneous administration of chemotherapy or radiotherapy or ad-

---

COMMUNITY-BASED CONCERNS

Neutropenia and Infection

Patients who are neutropenic are at increased risks if they contract an infection, because they cannot defend themselves against the infecting organism. The infection may become severe or even life threatening. This is true for even "common" infections, which most people can overcome fairly easily on their own. Patients who are immunocompromised by either disease or drug therapy should be taught how to minimize their risk of becoming sick with an infection, as follows:

- Wash hands frequently. Family members and others in the household should also wash their hands frequently.
- Avoid people with acute illnesses.
- Avoid going out in crowds, especially during cold and flu season. This would include such places as malls, movie theaters, and worship services.
- Handle food safely. Cook meats to an appropriately high temperature to kill bacteria. Clean thoroughly all surfaces that have come into contact with raw food products. Refrigerate leftover food as soon as possible.

Focus on Research

Nosocomial infections in neutropenic ICU patients

Gruson, D., Hilbert, G., Vargas, F., Valentino, R., Chene, G., Boiron, J.M., Reiffers, J., Gbikpi-Benissan, G., & Cardinaud, J. P. (2000). Impact of colony-stimulating factor therapy on clinical outcome and frequency rate of nosocomial infections in intensive care unit neutropenic patients. *Critical Care Medicine, 28*(9); 3155–3160.

The Study

Retrospective, consecutive case series analysis was performed in a medical intensive care unit (ICU) of a teaching hospital in France. The records of 28 patients with leukopenia who received filgrastim, the colony-stimulating factor, and 33 patients with leukopenia who did not receive drug therapy were reviewed. The purpose of the study was to determine whether filgrastim would reduce the mortality rate and the frequency rate of nosocomial infections of neutropenic patients in an ICU. Mortality and nosocomial infections occurred at the same percentage rate for both groups. More research is warranted.

Nursing Implications

Although this study may be flawed (small sample size, groups were not matched for characteristics, and no controlling was done for other possible variables that may have affected outcome), it may have interesting relevance to nursing. It is likely that patients who were already critically ill, requiring admittance to an ICU, were too ill to show benefits from filgrastim therapy. Because there was no difference between the groups, one might assume that what helped patients did not result from drug therapy. Help for these patients may be more closely related to basic nursing care than to drug therapy. Nursing actions that help to decrease the incidence of nosocomial infections include the following: frequent, thorough handwashing, especially between caring for different patients; strict use of medical asepsis when providing care and during procedures; use of protective equipment such as masks and gloves; close adherence to protective isolation as indicated; and limitation of traffic into the patient's room. The question for further study is this: If filgrastim does not decrease mortality and nosocomial rates in ICU restricted neutropenic patients, what other aspects of care do?

ministering sargramostim 24 hours preceding or following chemotherapy or radiotherapy.

Although the majority of the adverse effects that occur with sargramostim can also be attributed to the disease process or the chemotherapy used to treat it, there are some unique events that may occur with sargramostim for which the nurse should be alert. Occasional transient supraventricular arrhythmias occur during administration of sargramostim, especially if the patient has a history of cardiac arrhythmias. These arrhythmias are reversible when the drug is discontinued. Trapping of granulocytes in the pulmonary circulation has occurred following sargramostim infusion, sometimes producing dyspnea. The recommended treatment for patients who become dyspneic is to reduce the rate of infusion by half. In patients with preexisting pleural and pericardial effusions, sargramostim may aggravate fluid retention. This is usually reversible with dose interruption or reduction, although occasionally a diuretic is needed.

A first dose effect has occurred rarely following the first dose of sargramostim. In this syndrome, respiratory distress, hypoxia, flushing, hypotension, syncope, or tachycardia occurs. The syndrome should be treated by stopping the infusion and treating the patient according to symptoms. When symptoms have resolved, the infusion is resumed at half the rate. These effects do not usually happen again with future doses.

Excessively high WBCs have sometimes rapidly occurred with sargramostim therapy (absolute neutrophil count [ANC] above 20,000 cell/mm^3 or platelets above 500,000/mm^3). If this happens, the dose should be reduced or temporarily stopped.

In some patients with preexisting renal or hepatic dysfunction, sargramostim has induced elevation of serum creatinine or bilirubin and hepatic enzymes.

Like filgrastim, sargramostim is a pregnancy category C drug. It is not known whether it is excreted into breast milk. It does not appear to produce any greater toxicity in children than in adults.

Oprelvekin/Interleukin-11

Oprelvekin (Neumega) is produced in *E. coli* by recombinant DNA technology. The resultant polypeptide is 177 amino acids in length and differs from the 178 amino acid length of endogenous interleukin-11 by the missing amino-terminal proline residue. Bone-forming and bone-resorbing cells are potential targets of interleukin-11. Its primary hematopoietic activity is to stimulate the production of megakaryocyte cells and thrombopoietin.

Oprelvekin is used to prevent severe thrombocytopenia and to reduce the need for platelet transfusions following myelosuppressive chemotherapy in patients with nonmyeloid malignancies who are at high risk of severe thrombocytopenia. It is administered as a SC dose once daily.

Oprelvekin directly stimulates the formation of megakaryocyte progenitor cells and thrombopoietin. This stimulates production of platelets that are structurally and functionally the same as those platelets produced by endogenous interleukin-11. Platelet counts will begin to rise 5 to 9 days after starting drug therapy with oprelvekin. When treatment with oprelvekin is stopped, platelet levels will continue to rise for about 7 days, then will fall toward baseline in about 14 days.

Oprelvekin is contraindicated only if there is a hypersensitivity to the drug or any of its components. Caution should be used if oprelvekin is used in patients with preexisting cardiomyopathy or congestive heart failure, because fluid retention is a common effect of therapy. Do not use with, or immediately following, cytotoxic chemotherapy. Oprelvekin is a pregnancy category C drug and has caused increased fetal deaths in animal studies.

Fluid retention with weight gain is the most frequent adverse effect of oprelvekin. This may be evidenced by peripheral edema, dyspnea on exertion, an increase in pleural effusion (if it was present prior to therapy), and decreases of about 10% to 15% in hemoglobin concentration, hematocrit, and RBCs (dilutional anemia due to increase in plasma volume). The cardiovascular adverse effects of oprelvekin may also be related to fluid retention (tachycardia, vasodilation, palpitations, syncope, and atrial fibrillation and flutter). Transient, mild blurred vision and papilledema have occasionally been reported. Antibody production and transient rashes have occasionally been observed at the injection site after administration. This has not been associated with anaphylactic reactions or loss of clinical responsiveness to oprelvekin therapy.

The following adverse effects that are unique to oprelvekin (i.e., not likely to be associated with the cancer or its therapy) have been noted occasionally: dimmed vision, paresthesia, dehydration, skin discoloration, exfoliative dermatitis, and eye hemorrhage. There are no known drug interactions with oprelvekin.

Patient education should emphasize the importance of telling the physician and/or nurse if fluid retention occurs and the need to avoid activities that may cause bleeding until platelet counts are in normal range.

CYTOKINES

Cytokines are chemical mediators released by WBCs in response to antigenic invasion of the blood or tissues. Cytokines serve to enhance and accelerate the inflammatory and specific responses that will destroy the invading antigen. Cytokines are generally proinflammatory, but many also have anti-viral, anti-proliferative, and anti-neoplastic properties. Interferons and interleukins are cytokines produced by activated lymphocytes. The prototype is interferon alfa-2a (Roferon-A). Drugs in the same class as interferon alfa-2a include interferon alfa-2b, interferon alfa-n3, interferon-n1, interferon alfacon-1, interferon beta-1a, and interferon beta-1b. Drugs significantly different from interferon alfa-2a are aldesleukin (also known as interleukin-2) and TNF. One must recognize that these cytokines have considerable differences in action and adverse effects from the prototype.

The interferons available for pharmacologic use are produced by recombinant DNA technology from harvested human or animal WBCs. As stated, the prototype is interferon alfa-2a, produced by recombinant DNA technology using *E. coli* bacteria.

NURSING MANAGEMENT OF THE PATIENT RECEIVING INTERFERON ALFA-2A

Core Drug Knowledge

Pharmacotherapeutics

Interferon alfa-2a is licensed for treatment of hairy cell leukemia in selected patients 18 years and older, AIDS-related Kaposi sarcoma in selected patients 18 years and older, and chronic myelogenous leukemia in chronic phase Philadelphia chromosome-positive patients. Significant anti-neoplastic activity has been noted when this agent has been used to treat superficial bladder cancer, carcinoid tumors, cutaneous T-cell lymphoma, and low-grade non-Hodgkin lymphoma (see Table 33-1). It has also been widely used for treatment of select viral diseases such as hepatitis C, condylomata acuminata, cutaneous warts, and cytomegalovirus. It is normally administered SC or IM.

Pharmacokinetics

Interferon alfa-2a must be given by injection. If given IM, it is absorbed rapidly with peak effects in 3.8 hours; if given SC, absorption is slower with peak effects in 7.3 hours. The drug is metabolized in the liver and kidneys with a half-life of 3.7 to 8.5 hours. Direct lesional injection or instillation (as in the bladder) is indicated for some disorders. It crosses the placenta and may pass into breast milk. It is excreted in the urine.

Pharmacodynamics

Interferon alfa-2a inhibits the growth of tumor cells, prevents these cells from multiplying, and modulates the host immune response to help protect the body from tumor cells. It blocks specific viral infection by preventing viral replication in the body.

Contraindications and Precautions

Interferon alfa-2a is pregnancy category C, so its use during pregnancy may be risky to the fetus and is normally avoided. It should also be avoided during lactation and in patients with known allergies to interferon or its components. Caution should be used when administering the drug to patients with pancreatitis, hepatic or renal disease, bone marrow depression, cardiac disease, or a history of cardiac disease, or compromised central nervous system (CNS) function.

Adverse Effects

The most common adverse effects of interferon alfa-2a are dizziness, confusion, lethargy, flu-like symptoms, anorexia, nausea, and changes in taste. Depression, anxiety, and suicidal ideation have been reported in a significant number of cases. Disease processes that exacerbate these symptoms warrant careful monitoring. Hypothyroidism is problematic in as much as 10% of patients. Long-term therapy increases the risk of this complication. Other adverse effects include hypotension or hypertension, edema, arrhythmias, bone marrow depression, increased liver enzymes, rash, dry skin, and partial alopecia.

Drug Interactions

An increased risk of theophylline toxicity occurs when this drug is combined with interferon alfa-2a (Table 33-2). This is due to a decrease in theophylline clearance through the liver. Patients should be monitored to evaluate theophylline levels and have their theophylline dosages adjusted appropriately. Interferon alfa-2a can also cause increased effects and toxicity when combined with other neurotoxic, hematotoxic, and cardiotoxic drugs. Neurologic and hematologic toxicity has been particularly problematic for patients with HIV receiving concomitant anti-retroviral therapy. Renal toxicity is enhanced if given with interleukin-2. Anyone receiving drugs with overlapping toxicities must be carefully monitored.

Assessment of Relevant Core Patient Variables

Health Status

Before administering interferon alfa-2a, the nurse should review the patient's record to see whether the drug is contraindicated. Cardiovascular, pulmonary, and neurologic disorders may escalate the adverse effects of this agent. Glucose intolerance is a common effect of alfa-interferon therapies, and patients with diabetes mellitus are at particular risk for hyperglycemia crises. Patients with borderline thyroid function should also be carefully monitored for potential hypothyroidism. A complete

TABLE 33-2 Agents That Interact With Interferon Alfa-2a

Interactants	Effect and Significance	Nursing Management
theophylline/aminophylline	Decreased theophylline clearance in patients with hepatitis. This may raise theophylline levels	Monitor theophylline levels. If they increase significantly, dosage adjustments may be required.
cimetidine	May amplify the effects of interferon when used in treating melanoma; significance unknown	Monitor effects of interferon.
vinblastine	Enhances interferon toxicity in some patients	Monitor for adverse effects of interferon.

physical examination should be performed to establish a baseline for monitoring therapy. Next, the patient's weight, temperature, skin condition, orientation, reflexes, pulse, and blood pressure should be recorded. Because bone marrow depression and liver damage can be very serious, a complete blood count (CBC) and hepatic profile should be evaluated at least monthly during therapy.

Life Span and Gender

The nurse should determine whether the patient is younger than 18 years and is pregnant or lactating.

Lifestyle, Diet, and Habits

The nurse should assess whether patients consume alcohol or other unprescribed mood-altering drugs that may enhance the neurotoxicities of this agent.

Environment

The nurse should be aware of the environment in which the drug will be administered. Interferon alfa-2a may be given at home or in a clinic. If it is given at home, the patient needs a refrigerator so that reconstituted drug can be stored. It is important to explore with the patient any factors in the home setting that may affect compliance with drug therapy.

Nursing Diagnoses and Outcomes

- Risk for Infection related to possible bone marrow suppression, injections
  Desired outcome: The patient will be protected from exposure to infection and remain infection free.
- Altered Nutrition, Less Than Body Requirements related to GI effects and flu-like symptoms
  Desired outcome: The patient will maintain nutritional status.
- Risk for Injury related to CNS changes from drug therapy
  Desired outcome: The patient will not sustain injury while on drug therapy.

Planning and Intervention

Maximizing Therapeutic Effects

Following the manufacturer's guidelines for reconstitution and storage increases the therapeutic effectiveness of the drug. Obtaining baseline blood counts and chemistries before therapy and at least monthly during therapy helps direct therapy and ensures accurate dosage and treatment guidelines. Other nonpharmacologic immunologic boosting strategies, such as adequate sleep and proper nutrition, will assist patients in coping with therapy and may enhance their immunologic function.

Minimizing Adverse Effects

Most clinical experts recommend premedicating with drugs such as acetaminophen or diphenhydramine to reduce the flu-like adverse effects and administering interferon injections in the late evening to allow patients to sleep through most of the adverse effects. The nurse should observe how the patient and family members use sterile technique, perform the injection, and rotate injection sites. The patient should be advised to avoid crowds and people with known infections and to wash and treat injuries immediately to prevent infection. The nurse should warn the patient that interferon alfa-2a can cause confusion and dizziness, making falls and injury a risk. Consequently, the need for adequate lighting, bedside rails, assistance with walking, and avoidance of dangerous activities and driving should be stressed. Severe GI effects may warrant a nutritional consultation, and small, frequent meals or nutritional supplements may be prescribed.

Providing Patient and Family Education

- The nurse should explain that interferon alfa-2a inhibits the growth of tumor cells.
- The nurse should teach the patient or a family member how to reconstitute the powder into a solution and to date and refrigerate the reconstituted solution.
- The nurse should advise the patient to use reconstituted solution within 30 days and to mark drug days on the calendar so that the drug is taken when prescribed for maximum therapeutic effects.
- The nurse should teach the patient and family how to administer the drug, use sterile technique, and rotate injection sites. The nurse should also review injection technique periodically to ensure effectiveness and decrease adverse effects.
- When this drug is prescribed to a woman of childbearing age, the nurse should advise her to avoid pregnancy and to use barrier contraception.
- Because hypotension can occur for several days after drug administration, the nurse should advise patients to slowly move from a sitting to standing position and to avoid operating machinery or driving while adjusting to the therapy adverse effects.
- The nurse should also address the following teaching topics: avoiding infection and injury, maintaining good nutrition, getting regular blood tests and medical follow-up care, and watching for adverse effects.
- The nurse should emphasize the importance of calling the health care provider if fever, chills, sore throat, unusual bleeding or bruising, chest pain, palpitations, or changes in mental status occur. See the Critical Thinking Scenario, Interferon Alfa-2a in Hairy Cell Leukemia, for more information.

Ongoing Assessment and Evaluation

The nurse should monitor the patient's CBC and white cell differential, as well as liver and renal function before therapy and at least monthly during therapy to gauge the drug's effectiveness and to check for adverse effects (see the earlier display, Interferon Alfa-2a in Hairy Cell Leukemia). ■

Critical Thinking Scenario

Interferon Alfa-2a in hairy cell leukemia

Marla Barker, age 68, planned to spend her retirement years traveling, visiting her children and grandchildren, and playing golf. But 4 months ago, she was diagnosed with hairy cell leukemia. She was immediately started on interferon alfa-2a therapy. According to blood tests, the therapy is effective and her CBC is acceptable. When Mrs. Barker talks with you about treatment options, she reports that she feels depressed about her illness and fearful that she will never be able to travel or see her daughter get married next month. She also complains of stomatitis, exhaustion, anorexia, and continuing weight loss.

1. Consider the emotional and medical issues involved with this patient. Can she achieve emotional balance and a satisfactory quality of life within the limits set by her disease and drug therapy?
2. What restrictions on activity are imposed by interferon alfa-2a therapy? What special environmental needs will Mrs. Baker have when traveling?

DRUGS SIGNIFICANTLY DIFFERENT FROM INTERFERON ALFA-2A

Aldesleukin/Interleukin-2

Interleukins are cytokines produced by T cells to communicate between WBCs. Aldesleukin (Proleukin) is licensed for treatment of metastatic renal cell carcinoma and metastatic malignant melanoma, although many additional indications are emerging. The agent's immunostimulatory effects have been useful for stabilization of T-helper cell counts in HIV disease and for bone marrow engraftment protection post bone marrow transplantation, and its anti-viral effects have been promising for treatment of hepatitis.

This agent has been administered subcutaneously, intravenously and intralesionally. It is paradoxically more potent when given by continuous infusion than by bolus injections, and the adverse effect profile is widely variable due to dose ranges from 20,000 IU daily after bone marrow transplantation to 72,000,000 IU daily for treatment of metastatic renal cell carcinoma. The drug may be contraindicated in lactating patients, those with known allergies to aldesleukin, those with an abnormal thallium stress test or abnormal pulmonary function tests, and those with organ homografts. Aldesleukin should be used cautiously in patients with renal, liver, or CNS impairment. Its adverse effect profile is very similar to that of high dose interferon, but potentially more acute in onset and severe in intensity. Even severe adverse effects resolve with discontinuation of the agent, although hepatic, endocrine, and neurologic effects can persist for months after the conclusion of therapy. Concomitant administration of corticosteroids is not recommended based upon pre-clinical data suggesting that steroids may abrogate the immunostimulatory effects of this agent (Cuaron & Thompson, 2001).

MEMORY CHIP

Interferon Alfa-2a

- Inhibits growth of tumor cells, prevents their multiplication, and heightens the host immune response to help protect the body from tumor cells. Blocks specifically viral infection by preventing viral replication
- Used to treat some types of leukemia, AIDS-related Kaposi sarcoma, and various cancers
- Most common adverse effects: dizziness, confusion, lethargy, flu-like symptoms, anorexia, nausea, and altered taste
- Most serious adverse effects: depression and suicidal ideation
- **Life span alert: Usually avoided during pregnancy and breast feeding**
- Maximizing therapeutic effects: reconstitute and store following manufacturers' instructions
- Minimizing adverse effects: Premedicate patient with other drugs to reduce the flu-like adverse effects
- Most significant patient education: teach patients about the importance of avoiding infection

Tumor Necrosis Factor

Tumor necrosis factor (TNF), also known as cachectin, is a cytokine produced by activated macrophages. It apparently halts the cell cycle in the G2 phase, damaging the vascular endothelium of tumor capillaries and causing hemorrhage into the tumor. The agent can be administered intravenously, intramuscularly or subcutaneously. Severe inflammatory (high unremitting fever, rigors) and cardiopulmonary (arrhythmias, hypotension) adverse effects have been reported, limiting the drug's clinical utility. Currently, there are no licensed uses for this agent; it is only available as part of a research protocol. Research is still under way with this drug.

POLYCLONAL/MONOCLONAL ANTIBODIES

The earliest antibody preparations were general agents directed toward destruction of lymphoid cells (anti-lymphocyte globulins). They were derived after animals (horses and rabbits) were injected with human thymocytes (thymus gland is the source of T cells in humans) and RBCs, which stimulated the animal to produce nonspecific IgG antibodies. The most common of these were equine antithymocyte globulin (ATG, Atgam); antilymphocyte globulin (ALG); and antilymphocyte serum (ALS). These polyclonal antibodies are so named because they will react to more than one antigen. These agents have historically been administered to graft recipients, so that the foreign antibodies directly attack the host's T cells and reduce their circulating number. Since these agents are derived from nonhuman sources, they have caused the production of atypical antibodies and individuals easily become resistant to their beneficial effects. Because of production shortages, difficulty in purification, and scientific advances in specific antibody development, these agents are now rarely used. Instead, targeted antibody therapy called monoclonal antibodies are used which suppress one cell subtype or receptor site. Monoclonal antibodies can react with specific tumor receptor sites for diagnosis or treatment of malignancy. As our scientific body of knowledge regarding specific cellular defects with particular diseases grows, so does our ability to develop cell-targeted antibody therapy for abnormal cells, genes, or receptor sites. Several agents are in human clinical trials at the time of this publication.

Anti-tumor monoclonal antibodies include the prototype rituximab (Rituxan). Monoclonal antibodies available for use as immunosuppressants are considered significantly different from the prototype.

NURSING MANAGEMENT OF THE PATIENT RECEIVING P RITUXIMAB

Core Drug Knowledge

Pharmacotherapeutics

This agent is used to treat relapsed or refractory low-grade or follicular CD20 positive B-cell non-Hodgkin lymphoma.

Pharmacokinetics

Rituximab is given as a slow IV infusion at 375 mg/m^2 weekly for 4 weeks (days 1, 8, 15, 22). The serum half-life is 59.8 hours after the first infusion (375 mg/m^2) and 174 hours after the fourth infusion, although the drug is detectable for 3 to 6 months after completion of treatment. The actual drug infusion is calculated based upon the total dose the patient is to receive, not exceeding 50 mg/hour for the half hour of the first infusion. If no reactions are apparent after 30 minutes, the dose may be escalated every 30 minutes by 50 mg/hour until a maximum infusion rate of 400 mg/hour is reached. All subsequent infusions begin at 100 mg/hour and can be escalated by 100 mg/hour increments every 30 minutes until the maximum infusion rate of 400 mg/hour is reached.

Pharmacodynamics

Rituximab is a type of monoclonal antibody that binds specifically to CD20 antigen found on the surface of normal and malignant B lymphocytes and causes cell lysis. The CD20 antigen is expressed in more than 90% of B-cell non-Hodgkin lymphoma cells, but not on normal bone marrow cells, pre-B cells, or other normal tissues. One section of the drug binds to CD20 antigen and another section of the drug calls other immune activators to assist in cell lysis. Cell lysis is possibly due to complement dependent cytotoxicity or antibody-dependent cytotoxicity. Decreased IgG and IgM serum levels are evident for 5 to 11 months after the last infusion.

Contraindications and Precautions

The only contraindication to rituximab therapy is type 1 hypersensitivity or anaphylaxis to murine proteins or any components of the product. Safety in children or in pregnant or lactating women has not been tested. Experience with older adults is limited; its use needs to be carefully monitored.

Adverse Effects

Infusion-related effects occur in 80% of patients within 30 minutes to 2 hours after beginning the first infusion, although only 7% have severe reactions. Although less frequent with subsequent infusions (40%), the severity of the response is unchanged. Reactions may be related to dose because most of the reaction dissipates when slowing or interrupting the infusion rate. The most common infusional reactions include fever, flushing, chills, and rigors. Other reported symptoms include nausea, urticaria, fatigue, headache, pruritus, bronchospasm, dyspnea, hypotension, angioedema, dyspnea, rhinitis, vomiting, flushing, pain at disease sites, and throat swelling. Respiratory distress and hypotension are reportedly more common when tumors are larger than 10 cm (Wilkes, et al., 1999). As much as 16% of patients experience asthenia on retreatment. Other possible effects include tachycardia, arrhythmias, anorexia, peripheral edema, dizziness, and depression. Bone marrow effects such as leukopenia, thrombocytopenia, and anemia can be present for up to 30 days after the last dose.

About 1% of patients will develop antibodies to human anti-murine or chimeric antibodies producing severe allergic reactions, and limiting their future treatment with any antibody.

Drug Interactions

Concomitant vaccines of any type are not recommended due to theorized potential interactions; no research has been done on these potential interactions.

Assessment of Relevant Core Patient Variables

Health Status

Assess for preexisting cardiac and respiratory problems. This agent should be used cautiously in patients with pre-existing cardiac conditions such as arrhythmias or coronary artery disease because ventricular tachycardia, supraventricular tachycardia, angina, hypotension, and hypertension are not uncommon adverse effects. Patients with preexisting pulmonary conditions may also experience exacerbation of symptoms, particularly if the patient's tumor burden is larger than 10 cm.

The nurse should assess for other drug therapy used prior to giving rituximab. Rituximab has such potential for infusion reactions that concomitant administration of other agents that may cause severe allergic or anaphylactic reactions should be avoided during and within 2 hours before or after infusion. Agents to avoid include amphotericin, blood products, or first doses of antibiotics.

Life Span and Gender

The nurse should consider the patient's age. This agent is not recommended for use with children or in pregnant or lactating women. Experience with elderly patients is limited, so careful evaluation for contraindications is strongly recommended prior to starting therapy with this agent.

Environment

The nurse should be aware of the environment in which rituximab will be administered. Rituximab is usually given in the ambulatory care oncology clinic, although patients with specific risk factors for cardiac or pulmonary adverse effects may be admitted to the hospital for the first dose.

Nursing Diagnoses and Outcomes

- Altered Comfort related to fever, chills, or headache
  Desired outcome: Symptoms abrogated with premedications or relieved with mild analgesics/antipyretics.
- Potential Altered Cardiac Output related to drug infusion
  Desired outcome: Absence of cardiac symptoms.

Planning and Intervention

Maximizing Therapeutic Effects

Rituximab should be mixed in normal saline or dextrose solutions within a plastic bag, not in glass. The antibody will stick to glass, diminishing the amount of drug that will be administered.

Minimizing Adverse Effects

Because infusional adverse effects are common, many clinicians administer premedications to reduce their severity. Premedications often include antipyretics (e.g., acetaminophen) and anti-histamines (e.g., ranitidine). If patients experience infusional adverse effects, rituximab is stopped until symptoms resolve and is then restarted at half the dose that produced adverse effects. Subsequent infusions will begin slowly and can be escalated in the same manner, with temporary discontinuation if infusion effects reoccur.

For patients with hypertension, all anti-hypertensive agents are usually held for 12 hours prior to rituximab administration, and for 12 to 24 hours afterward.

Patients with cardiac or pulmonary risk factors should have continuous cardiac monitoring and frequent vital sign assessment. Infusion should be stopped at the first sign of adverse effects, because they may worsen before resolving. To reduce the risk of recurrence, medications such as nitrates or magnesium may be administered. After symptoms have resolved, the infusion may be resumed at a slower infusion rate with continuous monitoring.

Providing Patient and Family Education

- The nurse should instruct the patient and family about the purpose of the drug and common adverse effects. Patients should be instructed to notify the nurse if they begin to experience adverse effects.
- The nurse should assure patients that they will be closely monitored while receiving rituximab.
- Because immunologic effects persist for many weeks or months, the nurse should instruct patients to use birth control for 12 months after the completion of treatment and to avoid breast-feeding for the same amount of time.

Ongoing Assessment and Evaluation

Given the high rate of infusion reactions beyond the first dose, patients require premedications and close vital signs monitoring for all rituximab infusions unless no reactions have occurred. ■

DRUGS CLOSELY RELATED TO RITUXIMAB

Abciximab

Abciximab (ReoPro) is a monoclonal antibody and is actually a fragment called the Fab fragment. Unlike the prototype, rituximab, it does not have an anti-tumor function. It binds to a glycoprotein receptor on human platelets and inhibits their aggregation, leading to reduced hemostasis. The circulating half-life after IV bolus injection is 30 minutes, although

> **MEMORY CHIP**
>
> **Rituximab**
>
> - Binds specifically to CD20 antigen on the surface of malignant B lymphocytes and causes cell lysis.
> - Used in non-Hodgkin lymphoma
> - Most common adverse effects: infusion-related effects (fever, flushing, chills, and rigors)
> - Most serious adverse effects: respiratory distress and hypotension (more common when tumors are larger than 10 cm)
> - **Life span alert: Use birth control during therapy and for 1 year afterward and avoid breast-feeding during this time; use with caution in older adults**
> - Maximizing therapeutic effects: administer in saline or dextrose stored in plastic bags, not glass
> - Minimizing adverse effects: premedicate patient with other drug therapies
> - Most significant patient education: instruct patient to notify nurse of adverse effects.

clinical effects are evident for about 48 hours. In some patients, anti-platelet activity persists for up to 10 days. Many patients receive a 6 to 12 hour continuous intravenous infusion after the initial bolus to maintain optimal anti-platelet activity. This agent is used with a number of cardiovascular conditions, such as ischemic heart disease, or after percutaneous coronary interventions in which antiplatelet activity is desired. It is administered as an IV infusion prior to planned procedures, or at the onset of unstable angina. It may be contraindicated in patients with a recent history of stroke, major surgery or trauma, GI or genitourinary bleeding, vascular deformities, or uncontrolled hypertension. The primary adverse effect associated with abciximab is increased risk of bleeding.

Palivizumab

Palivizumab (Synagis) is a monoclonal antibody like rituximab; unlike rituximab, it has a unique function. This monoclonal antibody has been developed by deoxyribonucleic acid (DNA) recombinant technology to be directly cytotoxic to the respiratory syncytial virus (RSV), reducing the number of viral organisms in the lower respiratory tract. It is administered as prophylaxis in neonates at high risk for developing life-threatening pulmonary disease if infected with RSV (e.g., premature infants, children with cystic fibrosis). Its use in confirmed RSV infection has not been established. It is contraindicated in adults in whom serious illness with RSV infection has not been documented. It is administered as a monthly IM injection given fall through spring, having a half-life of 18 to 20 days. The reconstituted drug does not contain a preservative and should be administered within 6 hours of reconstitution. Common adverse effects include infection with other organisms, worsening respiratory symptoms, GI upset, hepatic dysfunction, injection site erythema, and flu-like syndrome. The serum blood levels of alanine aminotransferase and aspartate transaminase may be elevated as a consequence of this agent.

DRUGS SIGNIFICANTLY DIFFERENT FROM RITUXIMAB

Monoclonal antibodies used as immunosuppressants include the following drugs: muromonab-CD3, infliximab, basiliximab, and daclizumab.

Muromonab-CD3

Muromonab-CD3 (Orthoclone OKT3) is used to prevent allograft rejection in patients who have undergone renal transplantation and to treat steroid-resistant acute allograft rejection in heart and liver transplants. Muromonab-CD3 is a murine monoclonal antibody to the T3 complex of T cells. It acts on the T cell as an antigen and disables it. Muromonab-CD3 is available only for IV use.

Muromonab-CD3 is assigned to pregnancy category C. It is contraindicated in patients with known allergies to the drug or any murine product, and in cases of fluid overload. It should be used cautiously in patients with fever (give antipyretics before drug administration) and in those previously on muromonab-CD3, because serious reactions can occur.

The most common adverse effects of muromonab-CD3 are nausea, vomiting, diarrhea, tremor, fever, chills, dyspnea, and chest pain. Potentially serious adverse effects include acute pulmonary edema and cytokine-release syndrome (flu-like symptoms progressing to shock).

Muromonab-CD3 combined with other immunosuppressants poses a serious risk for infection and lymphoma. To decrease this risk, the dosage of other immune suppressants should be reduced and then returned to previous levels 3 days before muromonab-CD3 is finished. Encephalopathy and CNS effects are risks when muromonab-CD3 is combined with indomethacin (Indometh)—so this combination should be avoided.

Infliximab

Infliximab (Remicade) is a monoclonal antibody that is a chimeric human-murine IgG antibody that acts by blocking TNF. It is licensed for treatment of moderate to severe Crohn disease. Its safety and efficacy have not been established in children or in pregnant or lactating women, or beyond three doses. It has established efficacy but is not specifically licensed for use with methotrexate to treat rheumatoid arthritis. In studies with this disease, over 50% of patients achieved clinical remission, with a tolerable toxicity profile. It is administered once as a short IV infusion, and in severe Crohn disease, is readministered on a monthly basis for a total of three doses. Due to its low toxicity profile, many allogeneic bone marrow transplant protocols have been established to evaluate the efficacy of this agent in this population. The most common adverse effect is an infusion-related allergic-type reaction that includes fever, chills, pruritus, dyspnea, chest pain, and hypotension. Skin reactions such as rash, eczema, dry skin, acne, sweating, and flushing are also common. Autoimmune antibodies producing a lupus-like syndrome have been reported and warrant discontinuation of the drug. Infliximab is incompatible with polyvinyl chloride tubing and should be mixed in glass bottles and administered through polyethylene line infusion sets.

Basiliximab

Basiliximab (Simulect) is a monoclonal antibody that is an interleukin-2 receptor antagonist. It acts by binding to and blocking the CD25 antigen receptor site; this site is active in the cellular immune response involved in allograft rejection. Basiliximab is licensed as part of an immunosuppressive regimen that includes cyclosporine and corticosteroids for prevention of organ transplantation rejection in patients receiving renal transplantation. It is administered as an IV infusion over 20 to 30 minutes 2 hours prior to transplant surgery, and 4 days after surgery. The average duration of immunosuppressive interleukin-2 receptor blockade activity is 36 days. Readministration after initial therapy with basiliximab has not been studied, but excess immunosuppression or hypersensitivity reactions are projected. Pediatric patients in whom it has been used have demonstrated slower renal clearance, although no appreciable differences have been noted between adults and the elderly. This agent has not been tested with pregnant or lactating women because interleukin-2 is known to cross the placenta, and great risk to the fetus was suspected. The most common adverse effects relate to the infection risk associated with the immunosuppressive regimen; however, GI symptoms such as nausea, vomiting, and diarrhea were also common. Occasional reports of headache, tremors, insomnia, and electrolyte disorders warrant careful assessment within 48 hours of therapy.

Daclizumab

Daclizumab (Zenapax) saturates a subunit of the interleukin-2 receptor (Tac subunit), thus inhibiting interleukin-2 mediated cellular responses known to be important in allograft rejection. It is indicated as part of a three- or four-drug regimen for prophylaxis of acute organ rejection in adults receiving their first cadaveric kidney transplant. It is currently undergoing human trials for prevention and treatment of allograft rejection with other solid organ and bone marrow transplant. It is dosed at 1 mg/kg and administered within 24 hours prior to transplantation, then every 14 days for a total of five doses. It is known to effectively bind at the Tac subunit for as much as 120 days when the serum levels were 5 to 10 μg/mL. It has the same precautions and gender/age recommendations as basiliximab. Immunosuppression is the most important adverse effect; however, as with other immunosuppressive monoclonal antibodies, GI distress is common. Hypertension is agent specific and reported in both children and adults.

IMMUNE MODULATORS

Immune modulators appear to act directly on the function of T cells and B cells, stimulating or suppressing the immune response. Lymphocytic modulators are divided into subcategories according to their primary chemical structure and pharmacologic properties. Immune modulators may suppress or stimulate immune function. Some of these agents stimulate certain functions of the cell response and suppress others.

For this text, the immune suppressant cyclosporine (Sandimmune, Neoral) is used as the prototype. Cyclosporine is in the subclass of polypeptide antibiotics. Drugs that are also immune modulators and polypeptide antibiotics and are represented by the prototype include tacrolimus (Prograf), sirolimus (Rapamune), and mycophenolate mofetil (CellCept). Drugs that are also immune modulators but are significantly different from cyclosporine are the retinoids (all-trans retinoic acid [ATRA], 9-cis-transretinoic acid, and bexarotene); levamisole; azathioprine; thalidomide; glatiramer; and BCG. These drugs all cause some immune suppression and some stimulation.

The polypeptide antibiotics are a group of agents that were developed as antibiotics but were determined to be too toxic to hematopoietic cells for that use. What has evolved is a group of agents that destroys cells in the G_0 or G_1 phase of cell cycling, a long phase that is common for all lymphocytes. The first drug of this class to be licensed for use was cyclosporine, and it is the prototype agent. Immune modulators that act as immune suppressants block the normal effects of the immune system in the body. This action is beneficial in organ transplantation, in which the body destroys the foreign tissue, and in autoimmune diseases, in which the body destroys its own cells.

NURSING MANAGEMENT OF THE PATIENT RECEIVING CYCLOSPORINE

Core Drug Knowledge

Pharmacotherapeutics

Cyclosporine (Sandimmune, Neoral) is used as an adjunct treatment to prevent rejection in solid organ transplantation and to prevent graft versus host disease in allogeneic bone marrow or stem cell transplants. Other labeled uses include severe rheumatoid arthritis and extensive, refractory psoriasis. Unlabeled uses include alopecia areata, atopic dermatitis, biliary cirrhosis, Crohn disease, ulcerative colitis, dermatomyositis, Graves ophthalmopathy, lupus nephritis, multiple sclerosis, myasthenia gravis, nephrotic syndrome, pemphigus, polymyositis, and pulmonary sarcoidosis. It is used with corticosteroids to prevent rejection in kidney, liver, and heart transplantation and to treat chronic rejection in patients previously taking other immunosuppressants. The drug is being studied for use in pancreas, bone marrow, and heart and lung transplantation.

Pharmacokinetics

The absorption of cyclosporine from the GI tract is incomplete and variable; the lipid formulation has improved absorption characteristics. The absolute bioavailability of oral cyclosporine varies widely among patients. Factors that affect bioavailability include food, enterohepatic recirculation, and the type of assay used to measure levels. Ingestion of conventional cyclosporine with food high in fat may increase bioavailability. Cyclosporine is extensively metabolized by the cytochrome P450 enzyme system in the liver, and to a lesser degree in the GI tract and the kidneys. Many metabolites have been identified in the bile, feces, blood, and urine. Fortunately, these metabolites contribute little to drug toxicity. Excretion is primarily biliary, with less than 6% excreted in the urine. Neither dialysis nor renal failure significantly alters cyclosporine clearance. Children often need a larger oral dose, probably due to the limited absorptive area of their intestines. Patients with malabsorption may have difficulty achieving therapeutic levels with oral use.

The IV dose is not significantly related to age, body surface area, or bowel length.

Pharmacodynamics

Cyclosporine is a potent immunosuppressant that is produced as a metabolite by the fungus *Beauvaria nivea*. It suppresses some humoral immunity, but to a greater extent, cell-mediated immune reactions. The exact mechanism of action is not known but experimental evidence suggests it is caused by specific, reversible inhibition of immunocompetent T lymphocytes by targeting their cytotoxic effects to lymphocytes in the G_0 and G_1 phases of the cell cycle. The T-helper cell is the main target, but the T-suppressor cell may also be suppressed. It also inhibits lymphokine production and release, including interleukin-2 or T-cell growth factor. It does not cause bone marrow suppression.

Contraindications and Precautions

Cyclosporine that is injected (Sandimmune) is contraindicated in patients with hypersensitivity to polyoxyethylated castor oil. Oral cyclosporine (Neoral) should not be used concomitantly with psoralen ultraviolet A-range or ultraviolet B light therapy in patients with psoriasis. It is assigned to pregnancy category C and is used during pregnancy only if the potential benefit justifies the possible risk to the fetus. It readily crosses the placenta and is excreted in breast milk.

A significant risk of hepatotoxicity and nephrotoxicity exists with this drug. A form of chronic, progressive cyclosporine-associated nephrotoxicity is characterized by deterioration in renal function and morphologic changes in the kidney, which may persist despite discontinuation of the drug. Oversuppression of the immune system can increase susceptibility to infection. Liver and renal function tests should be monitored closely. If a severe reaction occurs, dosage should be decreased or the drug discontinued.

Adverse Effects

The most common adverse effects of cyclosporine are renal dysfunction, tremor, hirsutism, hypertension, and gum hyperplasia. Other less common adverse effects primarily involve the CNS and include confusion, lethargy, headache, ataxia, blurred vision, depression, encephalopathy, and convulsions. Studies have associated these symptoms with low cholesterol, low magnesium, aluminum overload, high-dose methylprednisolone, nephrotoxicity, and hypertension. The risk of malignancies in cyclosporine recipients is higher than in the healthy population but similar to that of patients receiving immunosuppressive therapies. Most commonly reported are lymphoproliferative and skin malignancies. Miscellaneous adverse effects include brittle nails, pruritus, anorexia, gastritis, hiccups, mouth sores, swallowing difficulty, pancreatitis, constipation, hypomagnesemia, anemia, conjunctivitis, hearing loss, edema, tinnitus, thrombocytopenia, joint pain, night sweats, hyperkalemia, and hyperuricemia.

Drug Interactions

Concomitant use of medications that affect the hepatic microsomal enzymes (P450 system) require monitoring and dose adjustment of cyclosporine. Drugs that may produce nephrotoxicity have an increased risk of producing renal dysfunction when used concomitantly with cyclosporine. Administration of oral cyclosporine (Neoral) within 30 minutes of food, particularly a high-fat meal, may decrease levels. Do not take cyclosporine with grapefruit juice unless instructed to do so; trough concentrations may be increased (Table 33-3).

TABLE 33-3 Agents That Interact With Cyclosporine

Interactants	Effect and Significance	Nursing Management
rifampin, phenytoin, phenobarbitol	Decrease plasma concentrations of cyclosporine. May decrease therapeutic effectiveness of cyclosporine	Monitor for effectiveness of cyclosporine.
azithromycin, clarithromycin, diltiazem, erythromycin, fluconazole, itraconazole, ketoconazole, nicardipine, verapamil, and grapefruit juice	Increases the concentrations of cyclosporine through altering metabolism. May increase risk of adverse effects	Monitor for adverse effects of cyclosporine.
aminoglycosides, amphotericin B acyclovir, SMZ-TMP, melphalan, ketoconazole, diclofenac, naproxen, sulindac, cimetidine, ranitidine, tacrolimus	These nephrotoxic drugs may increase cyclosporine nephrotoxicity.	Monitor for signs of nephrotoxicity; dosage adjustment may be required.
HMG-Co A reductase inhibitors (atorvastatin, cerivastatin, fluvastatin, lovastatin, simvastatin)	Increased risk of myositis, rhabdomyolysis, and acute renal failure from cyclosporine	Monitor for adverse effects carefully. The HMG-Co A reductase inhibitor may need to be stopped if serious adverse effects occur.
nifedipine	Increased risk of gingival hyperplasia.	Provide good oral hygiene to minimize risk of gingival hyperplasia.

Assessment of Relevant Core Patient Variables

Health Status

Before administering cyclosporine, the nurse should review the patient's record to see whether the drug is contraindicated. If it can be administered safely, a physical examination should be performed to establish a baseline for monitoring therapy. The nurse should assess the patient's skin color, temperature, and texture and note the appearance of any lesions to monitor for allergic reactions and signs of rejection. Hepatic function should be reviewed because the drug is metabolized primarily by the liver. Renal function should be evaluated because nephrotoxicity is a fairly common and irreversible adverse effect of the drug. A CBC and differential should be done as a baseline for potential hematologic changes that might occur during therapy. Vital signs should be assessed because hypertension is the most common adverse effect associated with cyclosporine administration.

Life Span and Gender

Assess whether female patients are of child-bearing age. Children may require higher doses of medications due to decreased drug absorption.

Lifestyle, Diet, and Habits

Determine whether the patient is frequently in crowds where he or she could be exposed to infection. Assess whether the patient has a lifestyle that allows frequent sun exposure. Determine whether the patient eats a high-fat diet because this will increase the bioavailability of one form of the drug (Sandimmune), but decrease the bioavailability of another form (Neoral).

Environment

The nurse should be aware of the environment in which cyclosporine will be given. Cyclosporine is usually started in the hospital after solid organ or bone marrow transplantation and then continued at home. The nurse should explore with the patient any factors in the home setting that might affect compliance with drug therapy.

Nursing Diagnoses and Outcomes

- Risk of Infection related to suppression of the immune system

  Desired outcome: The patient will be protected from exposure to infection, and infections will be prevented or decreased.
- Altered Renal Function related to nephrotoxic and hypertensive effects of medication

  Desired outcome: The patient will be monitored closely for deterioration in renal function and permanent renal damage will be prevented.
- Deficient Knowledge related to multiple drug interactions and adverse effects

  Desired outcome: The patient will be instructed in potential drug interactions, including both prescription and over-the-counter medications. The patient will be instructed in potential adverse effects of medications and the need for close monitoring after discharge.

Planning and Intervention

Maximizing Therapeutic Effects

The nurse should ensure that cyclosporine is started soon after transplantation. Medication should be administered as prescribed and according to recommendations to ensure therapeutic drug levels. Drug levels should be appropriately monitored to ensure adequate dosing. Although cyclosporine can be given IV, the oral form should be used as soon as possible. It can be mixed with juice (but not grapefruit juice) to increase palatability and should not be refrigerated. Cyclosporine should not be taken with foods, particularly those that are high in fat.

Minimizing Adverse Effects

The nurse should arrange for periodic blood tests to monitor for renal, hepatic, and hematologic effects of the medication. The drug should be held and the physician notified if signs of toxicity occur. The nurse should avoid mixing the drug with grapefruit juice. The patient should be protected from exposure to infection and immediate action taken at the first sign of infection. Patients should be assessed for adverse effects to the CNS and vital signs should be monitored for hypertension.

Providing Patient and Family Education

- The nurse should teach the patients how to take the oral form of this agent to maximize absorption.
- The nurse should caution patients not to discontinue this drug without consulting with their health care provider.
- Women of child-bearing age should be counseled of the potential adverse effects on the fetus, most commonly, premature birth.
- Patients on cyclosporine should be taught to avoid exposure to infection by avoiding crowds and to promptly report injuries or signs of infection.
- The nurse should advise patients to avoid sun exposure to decrease the risk of skin malignancies.

Ongoing Assessment and Evaluation

Cyclosporine is an agent with many drug interactions, issues of bioavailability, and significant adverse effects. It is important to follow cyclosporine serum drug levels and have the dose adjusted appropriately to achieve maximal immune suppression without excess adverse effects. ■

MEMORY CHIP

Cyclosporine

- Immunosuppressant that inhibits T-lymphocytes by causing cytotoxicity during the G_0 and G_1 phase.
- Used as an adjunct treatment to prevent rejection in solid organ transplantation and to prevent graft versus host disease in allogeneic bone marrow or stem cell transplants.
- Significant contraindication: hypersensitivity to polyoxyethylated castor oil
- Most common adverse effects: renal dysfunction, tremor, hirsutism, hypertension, and gum hyperplasia.
- Most serious adverse effects: renal toxicity and hepatic toxicity
- **Life span alert: Children may need higher doses; therapy usually avoided during pregnancy**
- Maximizing therapeutic effects: start as soon after transplantation as possible
- Minimizing adverse effects: monitor blood work
- Most significant patient education: teach patients about the importance of preventing infection

DRUGS SIGNIFICANTLY DIFFERENT FROM CYCLOSPORINE

Retinoids

The retinoids are a group of naturally occurring compounds that are derivatives of preformed (dietary) vitamin A or provitamin A carotenoid. Preformed vitamin A is primarily found in food substances, and the provitamin A group involves precursors to retinol. Retinol has long been recognized for its importance in vision, growth, reproduction, and epithelial cell differentiation. We now know that retinoids exert most of their effects through their influence on gene expression. It is essential for control of growth and differentiation of normal cells during embryonic development. Due to their ability to influence differentiation of some cells while arresting development of others, they have become an important part of chemoprevention protocols aimed at preventing cancer in high-risk individuals. Retinoids are known to enhance humoral-and cell-mediated immune responses as well. The agent that has been used the longest and most extensively is all-transretinoic acid (ATRA). Other similar retinoids include 9-cis-transretinoic acid (panretinide) and bexarotene.

All-Trans Retinoic Acid

This natural retinol metabolite is licensed for treatment of acute progranulocytic leukemia refractory to or relapsed from anthracycline chemotherapy; however, some unlabeled uses include treatment of myelodysplasia and chemoprevention in cervical dysplasia and precancerous skin lesions. The pharmacokinetics of ATRA (Tretinoin, Vesanoid) are poorly defined. ATRA for its licensed use is given IV as an infusion. Chemoprevention protocols use oral formulations, and some research protocols use a topical formulation.

Like all retinoids, ATRA is teratogenic and pregnancy category D; this precludes pregnancy during therapy and for an undefined period of time afterward. Egg or sperm donation prior to therapy is recommended for patients of childbearing age.

Acute hypervitaminosis A toxicity is a commonly described phenomenon with treatment doses of this agent. CNS symptoms prevail and include drowsiness, irritability, headache, and vomiting. More commonly are the dermatologic symptoms that include alopecia, dry desquamation, pruritus, and increased pigmentation. Constitutional symptoms are arthralgia, hepatosplenomegaly, and eye irritation. Symptoms are not usually life-threatening and resolve 1 to 4 weeks after the conclusion of therapy. Other significant toxicities of retinoids are hypercholesterolemia, teratogenesis, visual disturbances, and hyperleukocytosis.

Hyperleukocytosis with fever, respiratory distress, pulmonary infiltrates, and fluid retention are the characteristics of a syndrome called retinoic-acid syndrome, occurring in 20% to 30% of patients receiving therapy for progranulocytic leukemia. It so closely mimics infection and sepsis that it may be difficult to differentiate from the latter. High-dose steroids and leukopheresis have been used to supplement supportive care, usually help to resolve the symptoms without discontinuation of therapy.

ATRA has no known drug interactions.

9-Cis-Transretinoic Acid (Panretinide, isomer ATRA)

Like ATRA, this is a naturally occurring retinol derivative that acts on several sites and is licensed for topical treatment of Kaposi sarcoma lesions. Administration guidelines and adverse effects are similar to those of ATRA except for the absence of retinoic acid syndrome that is unique to ATRA.

Bexarotene (Targretin gel)

This naturally occurring retinol derivative is available in both a systemic and topical form for the treatment of cutaneous T-cell lymphoma (mycosis fungoides). This agent is also used for treatment of acne (Accutane).

Levamisole

Levamisole (Ergamisol) is used as an adjunctive therapy in patients being treated with fluorouracil (Adrucil) after surgical resection of Duke stage C colon cancer. The exact mechanism of synergy is unclear, but therapy responses are nearly doubled when administering the two agents concomitantly. Levamisole restores depressed immune function, stimulating antibody formation, enhancing T-cell response, and potentiating monocyte and macrophage activity. Levamisole is readily absorbed when given orally.

Levamisole is assigned to pregnancy category C, and should also be avoided with lactation.

Common adverse effects include dizziness, headache, depression, paresthesias, changes in taste, nausea, stomatitis, diarrhea, dermatitis, alopecia, fatigue, fever, arthralgia, myalgia, and infection. Bone marrow depression is a potentially serious, but infrequent, complication.

Increased phenytoin (Dilantin) levels and phenytoin toxicity can occur if this drug is combined with levamisole. Patients on this combination should be monitored closely and have phenytoin levels checked regularly, with changes in dosage made as appropriate. Because disulfiram (Antabuse)-like reactions can occur if levamisole is combined with alcohol, patients should be warned not to drink alcohol.

Azathioprine

Azathioprine (Imuran) is an intravenously infused anti-metabolite that splits into a precursor mercaptopurine. It is a unique anti-metabolite agent, as it is exclusively an immunosuppressant, not anti-neoplastic. Because of its action, it is highly mutagenic and has been associated with the development of secondary malignancies. It is indicated as part of a multidrug regimen to prevent rejection in renal transplantation and to treat rheumatoid arthritis not responsive to conventional management. Unlabeled uses include treatment of Crohn disease and myasthenia gravis, and prevention of rejection after cardiac transplantation. Notable drug interactions occur with allopurinol, angiotensin-converting enzyme (ACE) inhibitors, and anticoagulants. The most common and severe adverse event is infection, although GI distress may be significant enough to warrant limiting the dose. It is given cautiously with other immunosuppressants due to increased risk of infection, and dose reduction is necessary in hepatic dysfunction.

Thalidomide

Thalidomide (Thalomid) has been used for many years for various purposes. As a result of its early use in pregnant women and the resulting severe birth defects, it is classified as a pregnancy category X drug. There is the possibility that severe birth defects can occur with only one dose. In the United States, it is marketed under a special distribution program called "System for Thalidomide Education and Prescribing Safety." This means that it is a restricted drug that may only be prescribed by registered individuals. Male and female patients who are prescribed thalidomide must receive oral and written instruction about the need to use two methods of contraception; they must use the contraception for 1 month prior to starting thalidomide, during treatment, and for 1 month after stopping thalidomide. Periodic pregnancy testing is required while receiving thalidomide. Breast-feeding must also be avoided.

Thalidomide's licensed uses include treatment of cutaneous manifestations of erythema nodosum leprosum (a complication of the treatment for leprosy), rheumatoid arthritis, multiple myeloma, and after bone marrow transplant graft versus host disease refractory to standard therapy. It is an oral or IM injected agent given once daily.

Common adverse effects include thrombotic problems, drowsiness, photosensitivity, and peripheral neuropathies. Skin disorders, GI distress, secretory disorders (e.g., decreased lacrimation, dry mouth), and fluid retention have also been reported with some frequency. Patients taking thalidomide are advised to immediately report neurologic symptoms, because toxicity may not be reversible if the agent is not promptly stopped.

Glatiramer

Glatiramer acetate (Copaxone) is a synthetic copolymer of essential amino acids. It suppresses the specific immune processes involved in the pathogenesis of multiple sclerosis and reduces the frequency of relapses. Although the exact mechanism of action is unknown, it is thought to act by modulating T-cell autoimmune responses to myelin. The drug is given by daily SC injections and must be reconstituted and used immediately. A set of postinjection reactions—including chest pain, palpitations, anxiety, dyspnea, and urticaria—occurs in about 10% of patients with injection and is usually transient. Transient chest pain separate from the postinjection reaction has also been reported by about 20% of patients, but the symptom was self limiting and not associated with other life-threatening symptoms. This drug may interfere with normal immune function while blocking the mechanism that causes multiple sclerosis, so the patient should be protected from infection and injury. Photosensitivity is also common, necessitating use of sunscreen and protective clothing when outdoors.

Bacillus of Calmette and Guerin [BCG] (ImmuCyst/TheraCys)

Bacillus of Calmette and Guerin in the form of ImmuCyst is a suspension of an attenuated strain of *Mycobacterium bovis* that has been used as immunoadjuvant since the 1960s. TheraCys is live BCG. This agent in either of its forms is currently licensed for treatment of carcinoma in situ of the urinary bladder with or without papillary tumors, although its unlabeled uses also include hematologic malignancies. It has been given intradermally, although it is more frequently administered intravenously or instilled into the bladder. Acting as a nonspecific immunomodulatory agent, it stimulates both nonspecific and specific immune responses, although the precise mechanism of action is not known.

CHAPTER SUMMARY

- Blood cell components may be altered due to pathophysiology or drug therapy to treat a disease process.
- The mature blood cells differ in structure and function, but all develop from a common progenitor cell, or stem cell, from within the bone marrow.
- Recombinant human erythropoietin, also known as epoetin alfa, is used to treat anemias that result from a decrease in the production of RBCs (erythropoiesis). Tissue oxygenation cannot optimally occur if there is anemia.
- Iron is also needed to form RBCs. When epoetin therapy is not effective or has a diminished effect, it is likely due to iron deficiency, which may be absolute or functional. Most patients with chronic renal failure will need iron transfusions at some time in order for RBCs to be produced following epoetin administration.
- The CSFs are the granulocyte CSF and the GM-CSF factor. These stimulate WBC production. Low WBC counts, especially neutrophils, place the patient at increased risk of contracting an infection.
- Unlike other interleukins, interleukin-11 (oprelvekin) has hematopoietic properties and stimulates the production of platelets. Without an adequate number of platelets, proper blood clotting cannot take place.
- Drugs that promote production of blood cells should not be given at the same time as chemotherapy as the rapidly producing cells are likely to be killed by the drug therapy.

- The immune system is a complex system of cells and chemical mediators that prevents foreign pathogens or cells from invading the body.
- WBCs are active in the surveillance and initiation of inflammatory reactions to specific stimuli. WBCs include neutrophils, which digest foreign material; basophils, which release chemicals to initiate the immune response; mast cells, located in the skin and the respiratory and GI tracts; macrophages, which release chemicals to initiate the immune response; and eosinophils, which seem to be active in allergic reactions.
- Lymphocytes include T cells, which are important in modifying the immune response and in protecting the body from nonself cells, and B cells, which produce antibodies to specific antigens. The antibodies stimulate an immune and inflammatory reaction to the antigen and cause its destruction.
- Drugs that stimulate the immune system are hematopoietic growth factors, cytokines, and immune modulators. They are used to keep viral particles from replicating and to inhibit tumor growth.
- Interferons are produced by WBCs in response to viral invasion and other stimuli. They block viral replication and inhibit tumor cell growth. Interferons are used to treat various malignant and viral diseases.
- Interleukins are chemicals secreted by active WBCs to influence other WBCs.
- Antibodies may be used to target malignant cell clones, or to modify T or B lymphocytes. Antibodies may be polyclonal or monoclonal.
- Immune modulators may restore depressed immune function or stimulate immune function, stimulate antibody formation, or enhance T-cell response.
- Drugs that suppress the immune system are used to block T-cell activity in organ transplant patients, when the immune system tries to destroy the foreign cells, and to treat autoimmune diseases, when the immune system is mistakenly trying to destroy self cells.
- Patients taking drugs that modify the immune system need protection against infection, injury, and neoplasms because their susceptibility to these disorders is increased.
- These drugs often cause adverse GI effects, so efforts must be made to maintain nutritional status. A nutritional consultation; small, frequent meals; and supplemental feedings are often necessary.

QUESTIONS FOR STUDY AND REVIEW

1. What are the principle cytokines involved in hematopoiesis?
2. Why are people with chronic renal failure anemic?
3. What is the risk to people who are neutropenic after chemotherapy?
4. How are platelets produced?
5. What is the most common adverse effect from oprelvekin (interleukin-11)?
6. Which types of diseases are treated by interferon therapies?
7. What is the primary mechanism of action for monoclonal antibodies?
8. What is the most common adverse effect of rituximab?
9. What is the "retinoic acid syndrome" and why is it important for nurses to know about it?
10. Why is cyclosporine useful in preventing solid organ transplantation rejection?

NEED MORE HELP?

Chapter 33 of the study guide for *Drug Therapy in Nursing* contains exercises and activities to reinforce your understanding of the concepts presented in this chapter. For additional information see the text's accompanying website at *http://www.connection.lww.com*.

REFERENCES AND BIBLIOGRAPHY

Alafaci, C., Salpietro, F., Grasso, G., Sfacteria, A., Passalacqua, M., Morbito, A., Tripodo, E., Calapai, G., Buemi, M., & Tomasello, F. (2000). Effect of recombinant human erythropoietin on cerebral ischemia following experimental subarachnoid hemorrhage. *European Journal of Pharmacology, 406*(2), 219–225.

Brines, M. L., Ghezzi, P., Keenan, S., Agnello, D., de Lanerolle, N. C., Cerami, C., Itri, L. M., & Cerami, A. (2000). Erythropoietin crosses the blood-brain barrier to protect against experimental brain injury. *Proceedings of the National Academy of Science U.S.A., 97*(19), 10526–10531.

Caldwell, M. (1991). The immune challenge. *Discover, 12*(10), 56–61.

Cuaron, L., & Thompson, J. (2001). The interferons, In P. T. Rieger (Ed.), *Biotherapy. A comprehensive overview,* (2nd ed., pp. 125–194). Boston: Jones and Bartlett Publishers.

DiJulio, J. E. (2001). Monoclonal antibodies: Overview and use in hematologic malignancies. In P. T. Rieger (Ed.), *Biotherapy. A comprehensive overview,* (2nd ed., pp. 283–316). Boston: Jones and Bartlett Publishers.

Drug facts and comparisons. (2000). St. Louis: Facts and Comparisons. Physicians On-Line. Multimedia.

Du Bois, J. S., Udelson, J. E., & Atkins, M. B. (1995). Severe reversible global and regional ventricular dysfunction associated with high-dose interleukin-2 immunotherapy. *Journal of Immunotherapy with Emphasis on Tumor Immunology, 18*(2), 119–123.

Foley, R. N., Parfrey, P. S., Morgan, J., Barre, P. E., Campbell, P., Cartier, P., Coyle, D., Fine, A., Handa, P., Kingma, I., Lau, C. Y., Levin, A., Mendelssohn, D., Muirhead, N., Murphy, B., Plante, R. K., Possen, G., & Wells, G. A. (2000). Effect of hemoglobin levels in hemodialysis patients with asymptomatic cardiomyopathy. *Kidney International, 58*(3), 1325–1335.

Gale, D. M., & Sorokin, P. (2001). The interleukins. In P. T. Rieger (Ed.) *Biotherapy. A comprehensive overview,* (2nd ed., pp. 195–244). Boston: Jones and Bartlett Publishers.

Gong, J., Avigan, D., & Kufe, D. (1999). Dendritic-tumor cell fusions. In M. T. Lotze, & A. W. Thomson (Eds.), *Dendritic cells. Biology and clinical applications* (pp. 617–630). San Diego: Academic Press.

Gruson, D., Hilbert, G., Vargas, F., Valentino, R., Chene, G., Boiron, J. M., Reiffers, J., Gbikpi-Benissan, G., & Cardinaud, J-P. (2000). Impact of colony-stimulating factor therapy on clinical outcome and frequency rate of nosocomial infections in intensive care unit neutropenic patients. *Critical Care Medicine, 28*(9), 3155–3160.

Hoffman, R. L., & Reeder, S. J. (1998). Mycophenolate mofetil (CellCept): The newest immunosuppressant. *Critical Care Nurse 18*(3), 50–57.

Kinzler, D. M., & Brown, C. K. (2001). Cancer vaccines. In P. T. Rieger (Ed.) *Biotherapy. A comprehensive overview* (2nd ed., pp. 357–382). Boston: Jones and Bartlett Publishers.

Krouse, R. S., Royal, R. E., Heywood, G., Weintraub, B. D., White, D. E., Steinberg, S. M., Rosenberg, S. A., & Schwartzentruber, D. J. (1995). Thyroid dysfunction in 281 patients with metastatic melanoma or renal carcinoma treated with interleukin-2 alone. *Journal of Immunotherapy with Emphasis on Tumor Immunology, 18*(4), 272–278.

Kruit, W. H., Goey, S. H., Lamers, C. H., Gratama, J. W., Visser, B., Scmitz, P. I., Eggermont, A. M., Bolhuis, R. L., & Stoter, G. (1997). High-dose regimen of interleukin-2 and interferon-alpha in combination with lymphokine-activated killer cells in patients with combination with lymphokine-activated killer cells in patients with metastatic renal cell cancer. *Journal of Immunotherapy, 20*(4), 312–320.

Letizia, M, & Conway, A. M. (1996). Interleukin-2 therapy for renal cell cancer: Indications, effects, and nursing implications. *Critical Care Nurse, 16*(5), 20–26.

Lotze, M. T., Farhood, H., Cara, C. W., & Storkus, W. J. (1999). Dendritic cell therapy of cancer and HIV infection. In M. T. Lotze, & A. W. Thomson (Eds.). *Dendritic cells. Biology and clinical applications,* pp. 459–486). San Diego: Academic Press.

Mahon, P. M. (1991). Orthoclone and cardiac transplantation: An overview. *Critical Care Nurse, 11*(8), 42–50.

Medical letter on drugs and therapeutics. (1997). New Rochelle, NY: Medical Letter.

Meehan K. R., Verma, U. N., Cahill, R., Frankel, S., Areman, E. M., Sacher, R. A., Foelber, R., Rajagopal, C., Gehan, E. A., Lippman, M. E., & Mazumder, A. (1997). Interleukin-2 activated hematopoi-

Gemfibrozil

Gemfibrozil (Gemcor, Lopid) is used to treat hypertriglyceridemia and to reduce coronary heart disease risk in some patients who have not responded to other forms of treatment. It inhibits peripheral lipolysis and decreases the hepatic extraction of free fatty acids, thus reducing hepatic triglyceride production. It also leads to a decrease in VLDL production and an increase in HDL concentration for most patients. The exact mechanism of action for raising HDL levels is unknown. In addition, the drug may reduce the incorporation of long-chain fatty acids into new triglycerides. It may also increase the turnover and removal of cholesterol from the liver and increase excretion of cholesterol in the feces.

Gemfibrozil is well absorbed from the GI tract. Peak levels occur 1 to 2 hours after administration of the dose. Gemfibrozil is primarily oxidized to from hydroxymethyl and a carboxyl metabolite. Excretion is mostly renal.

Contraindications include hepatic or severe renal dysfunction, including primary biliary cirrhosis, preexisting gallbladder disease, or hypersensitivity. This drug is pregnancy category C and is recommended to be avoided in pregnancy and in breast-feeding.

Gemfibrozil may possibly increase the risk of hepatic malignancy and cholelithiasis. It also may occasionally be associated with muscle inflammation, which may be severe.

GI problems are the most common adverse effects for both gemfibrozil and clofibrate, with nausea and diarrhea most common with clofibrate, and dyspepsia very common with gemfibrozil. Abdominal pain and diarrhea are also fairly common for gemfibrozil, whereas nausea, vomiting, and constipation are possible. Like lovastatin, this drug may produce abnormal elevations of liver function enzyme levels. The effects are usually reversible when the drug is discontinued. A large variety of miscellaneous adverse effects is also possible with the fibric acid derivatives. Gemfibrozil produces a moderate hyperglycemic effect; special monitoring will be necessary for patients with diabetes who are receiving gemfibrozil.

Clofibrate

Clofibrate (Atromid-S) is used to treat hyperlipidemia with high triglyceride levels. Clofibrate primarily lowers serum triglyceride and VLDL levels. The exact mechanism of action is unknown, but it may increase the catabolism of VLDL to LDL and decrease hepatic synthesis of VLDL. Most of the effectiveness is seen in type III hyperlipidemia.

Clofibrate is hydrolyzed to chlorophenoxyisobutyric acid (CPIB), which is the active form of the drug. Peak action is seen within 3 to 6 hours after administration. Excretion occurs primarily through the kidneys.

Like gemfibrozil, contraindications for clofibrate include hepatic or severe renal dysfunction, including primary biliary cirrhosis, preexisting gallbladder disease, or hypersensitivity. This drug is also pregnancy category C and its use is suggested to be avoided in patients who are pregnant or breast-feeding.

Clofibrate has caused hepatic tumors (benign and malignant) in test animals and is associated with increased risk of cancer in humans. It has also been show to significantly increase the risk for cholelithiasis and to increase the mortality from cholecystectomy surgery (while on clofibrate therapy). Other serious adverse effects of clofibrate include cardiac arrhythmias and reactivation of peptic ulcers. Like gemfibrozil, this drug may occasionally be associated with severe muscle inflammation.

As already noted, adverse effects for clofibrate are similar to those for gemfibrozil. Clofibrate may also cause flu like symptoms.

Fenofibrate

Fenofibrate (Tricor) is used to treat hypertriglyceridemia. It is chemically similar to clofibrate and gemfibrozil. Exactly how fenofibrate works has not been clearly established. The metabolite of fenofibrate, fenofibric acid, lowers plasma triglycerides apparently by inhibiting the synthesis of triglycerides, which reduces the amount of VLDL that is released into the circulation. It also stimulates the catabolism of triglyceride-rich VLDL. Additionally, fenofibrate reduces the serum uric acid levels in patients with normal and elevated uric acid levels by increasing the urinary excretion of uric acid. Treatment of some patients with hyperlipoproteinemia may result in an increase of LDL cholesterol.

Fenofibrate is well absorbed from the GI tract; food increases absorption. Peak levels occur within 6 to 8 hours. Fenofibrate is highly protein bound (99%). It is rapidly hydrolyzed by esterases to the active metabolite, fenofibric acid. Fenofibric acid is primarily conjugated with glucuronic acid and then excreted in the urine. Fenofibrate has a half-life of 20 hours. It is excreted, in the form of its metabolites, in the urine.

Fenofibrate is contraindicated in hepatic or severe renal dysfunction (including primary biliary cirrhosis and patients with unexplained persistent liver function abnormality), preexisting gallbladder disease, and hypersensitivity.

Serious adverse effects of fenofibrate include pancreatitis, cholelithiasis, myopathy, myositis, and hepatic impairment. These adverse effects are similar to those for gemfibrozil and clofibrate, the fibric acid derivatives. Rash, the most common adverse effect, requires discontinuation of the drug. Other possibly adverse effects on the CNS vary. Effects include dizziness, increased appetite, insomnia, and paresthesia. Dermatologic reactions include pruritus. GI complaints such as dyspepsia, nausea and vomiting, diarrhea, abdominal pain, constipation, flatulence, and excessive burping may occur. Genitourinary effects include polyuria and vaginitis. Common respiratory symptoms include rhinitis, cough, and sinusitis. Eye irritation, blurred vision, conjunctivitis, earache, and eye floaters may be present. Miscellaneous effects include flu-like symptoms, pain, headache, asthenia and fatigue, arthralgia, and arrhythmia. Increases in blood urea and creatinine and decreases in hemoglobin and uric acid have occurred.

Nicotinic Acid

Nicotinic acid (niacin or vitamin B_3) is used to treat hyperlipidemia. Like lovastatin, nicotinic acid reduces levels of triglycerides LDL cholesterol and raises levels of HDL cholesterol. Triglycerides and VLDL levels are reduced by 20%

to 40% in 1 to 4 days. LDL level reductions may be seen in 5 to 7 days, with the maximal effect seen in 3 to 5 weeks. The effect on LDL is dose dependent. The decrease will be greater if the patient is also receiving bile acid sequestrants (40% to 60% decrease). HDLs are increased by 20%. Although the exact mode of action is unknown, nicotinic acid is known to inhibit lipolysis in adipose tissue, to decrease esterification of triglyceride in the liver, and to increase lipoprotein lipase activity.

Nicotinic acid is rapidly absorbed from the intestine with peak effects achieved 45 minutes after administration. It is excreted, mostly unchanged, in the urine. The newer sustained release forms have fewer adverse effects, making them more tolerable for patients and, therefore, excellent choices to elevate HDL levels (Chong & Bachenheimer, 2000).

Contraindications for this drug are hepatic dysfunction, active peptic ulcer, severe hypotension, and hemorrhaging.

Doses that are larger than those used to treat niacin deficiency (pellagra) are needed to achieve the lipid-lowering effects of nicotinic acid. These larger doses produce peripheral vasodilation, mostly in the cutaneous vessels of the face, neck, and chest. This results in flushing of the skin. The vasodilation and increased blood flow from niacin administration is due to histamine release. Flushing is usually transient. Other adverse effects of nicotinic acid include GI effects, such as activation of peptic ulcer, nausea, vomiting, abdominal pain, diarrhea, and dyspepsia. An increase in uric acid levels can also occur. The most serious adverse effect is hepatotoxicity, although this is uncommon. Liver enzyme levels should be closely monitored in patients who are receiving niacin.

Bile Acid Sequestrants

The bile acid sequestrants cholestyramine (LoCholest, Questran, Prevalite) and colestipol (Colestid) are now used as second- or third-line therapy for reducing elevated serum cholesterol levels in patients who have primary hypercholesterolemia. Cholestyramine and colestipol are also used to relieve pruritus associated with partial biliary obstruction.

Bile acid sequestrants are not absorbed orally but work in the GI tract. The reduction in LDLs is apparent in 4 to 7 days and may total 20%. A decline in serum cholesterol levels is usually apparent after 1 month of treatment. Once drug therapy is discontinued, cholesterol levels will return to baseline within 1 month.

A major difference between the bile acid sequestrants and lovastatin is how they achieve a decrease in the cholesterol levels. Unlike lovastatin, which works by decreasing the synthesis of cholesterol, the bile acid sequestrants promote the oxidation of cholesterol to bile acids. Cholesterol is the major, and perhaps the only, precursor to bile acids. Bile acids are secreted from the gallbladder and liver into the intestine during digestion. In the intestine, bile acids emulsify the fat and lipid particles from food, promoting absorption. Much of the bile acid that is secreted is reabsorbed and returned to the liver by hepatic circulation.

The bile acid sequestrants cholestyramine and colestipol bind with the bile acids in the intestine to make them nonresorbable. The bile acids are then eliminated in the stool. The decrease in available bile acid causes the body to increase the oxidation of cholesterol to bile acids, which in turn decreases the LDL and serum cholesterol levels. Although hepatic synthesis of cholesterol rises, serum cholesterol levels fall because there is an increased clearance of cholesterol-rich lipoproteins from the plasma. Serum triglyceride levels may increase somewhat initially but will then gradually fall below pretreatment levels within 4 weeks.

Patients with partial biliary obstruction have an increased bile acid concentration. Cholestyramine and colestipol, by decreasing circulating bile acid, reduce bile acid deposits in the skin tissues with a resultant decrease in pruritus.

The most common adverse effect of cholestyramine and colestipol is constipation, which can be severe and may lead to fecal impaction. Less frequently experienced are abdominal pain, distention, and cramping; GI bleeding; belching; bloating; flatulence; nausea and vomiting; diarrhea and loose stools; indigestion and heartburn; anorexia; and steatorrhea. Chronic use of cholestyramine can result in prolonged bleeding resulting from vitamin K deficiency. Headache can also occur with both cholestyramine and colestipol. In addition, dizziness, anxiety, vertigo, drowsiness, and fatigue have been noted with colestipol.

Absorption of fat-soluble vitamins, such as A, D, E, and K, may be impaired because cholestyramine interferes with the normal fat absorption and digestion. Because cholestyramine is a chloride anion exchange resin, prolonged use may cause hyperchloremic acidosis.

Because of their effect in the GI tract, the bile acid sequestrants interact with many different drugs and may impair the absorption of those drugs. The nurse should consult a drug guide to determine whether a drug interaction is likely before giving the bile acid sequestrants with any other drug therapy.

Before starting therapy with cholestyramine or colestipol, the nurse should determine whether both the patient's serum cholesterol and triglyceride levels are elevated. If so, elevated triglyceride levels should be treated first with other drug therapy, because these may rise initially from the treatment with cholestyramine.

Consideration should be given to the patient's life span prior to treatment with either of the bile acid sequestrants. Younger and smaller patients are more at risk of developing hyperchloremic acidosis. In adults more than 60 years old, constipation is more likely to develop with ongoing cholestyramine therapy. Cholestyramine and colestipol come in a powdered form, which needs to be diluted with fluid. Colestipol also comes in tablet form. Cholestyramine and colestipol should be administered before meals.

The bile acid sequestrants are no longer frequently used due to their GI adverse effects, cumbersome administration, and poor palatability.

Dextrothyroxine Sodium

A thyroid hormone, dextrothyroxine sodium (Choloxin) is also used to decrease serum cholesterol levels. It stimulates the liver to increase catabolism and excretion of cholesterol by way of the biliary route into the GI tract. Synthesis of cholesterol is unaffected. The predominant effect is the reduction of serum LDL cholesterol levels. Elevated beta lipoprotein levels and triglyceride fractions may also be reduced.

Dextrothyroxine sodium is contraindicated in patients who have normal thyroid function and any of the following conditions: organic heart disease, angina pectoris, history of MI, history of cardiac arrhythmia (including tachycardia), rheumatic heart disease, history of congestive heart failure, decompensated or borderline compensated cardiac status, hypertension (other than mild, labile systolic hypertension), advanced liver or kidney disease, and history of iodism (a condition induced by prolonged and excessive use of iodine or its compounds; iodine poisoning).

Increased serum thyroxine levels indicate absorption and distribution of the drug throughout the body and should not be interpreted as drug toxicity. If signs or symptoms of iodism develop, the drug should be discontinued. Some forms of this drug are prepared with tartrazine and should not be given to patients who are sensitive to this dye. This sensitivity is more frequently seen in patients who also have aspirin hypersensitivity.

Adverse effects of dextrothyroxine sodium are mainly due to the increase in body metabolism from elevated thyroid levels. Patients who have the least problems with adverse effects are those with normal thyroid function and who also have no signs or symptoms of organic heart disease. Adverse effects are varied. Cardiovascular effects include angina, arrhythmias, electrocardiographic evidence of ischemic myocardial changes, increase in heart size, and both fatal and nonfatal MI. CNS effects are insomnia, nervousness, tremors, headache, tinnitus, dizziness, psychic changes, and altered sensorium paresthesia. Dermatologic problems include hair loss, skin rash, and itching. GI effects such as dyspepsia, nausea, vomiting, constipation, diarrhea, decreased appetite, weight loss, gallstones, and cholestatic jaundice may occur. Ophthalmic problems include visual disturbances, exophthalmos, retinopathy, and lid lag. Other reported effects are sweating, flushing, hyperthermia, diuresis, menstrual irregularities, changes in libido, hoarseness, peripheral edema, malaise, tiredness, muscle pain, and worsening of peripheral vascular disease).

CHAPTER SUMMARY

- Hyperlipidemia is a known risk factor for atherosclerosis and the problems and complications associated with atherosclerosis. The blood lipids include the total cholesterol, HDL cholesterol, the LDL cholesterol, VLDL cholesterol, and triglycerides.
- Many patients being treated for elevated cholesterol levels do not achieve the recommended treatment goals of total cholesterol under 200 mg/dL, LDL under 130 mg/dL, and HDL above 35 mg/dL.
- Lovastatin, the prototype statin, lowers LDL, VLDL, triglyceride levels, and total cholesterol levels, and raises HDL levels. It has been shown to decrease mortality from cardiovascular complications associated with elevated cholesterol levels.
- Lovastatin is metabolized through the hepatic enzyme CYP3A4. All other drugs or agents that are inhibitors of this pathway may have a drug interaction with lovastatin, decreasing lovastatin's metabolism, and raising, sometimes dramatically, blood levels of lovastatin.
- All lipid-lowering drugs can elevate liver enzyme levels. This elevation is not normally serious although the patient's liver enzyme levels should be monitored closely for up to the first year of therapy. Liver enzyme levels usually return to normal with either a dose reduction or discontinuation of the drug.
- Dietary modifications to limit fat and cholesterol intake should be implemented prior to starting any drug to lower lipid levels. Diet modifications need to be continued once drug therapy has begun.
- The fibric acid derivatives of gemfibrozil, clofibrate, and fenofibrate lower triglycerides levels and increase HDL cholesterol. Their effect on LDL cholesterol can be either to lower it slightly or to increase it slightly. Gemfibrozil reduces hepatic triglyceride production. The mechanisms of clofibrate and fenofibrate are not clear.
- Nicotinic acid (niacin or vitamin B_3) reduces triglycerides, reduces LDL cholesterol, and increases HDL. Although the exact mode of action is unknown, nicotinic acid is known to inhibit lipolysis in adipose tissue, decrease esterification of triglyceride in the liver, and increase lipoprotein lipase activity.
- The bile acid sequestrants, cholestyramine and colestipol, decrease LDL. They work differently than other lipid-lowering drugs by binding with the bile acids in the intestine so that the bile acids are nonreabsorbable and are eliminated in the stool. The decrease in available bile acid causes the body to convert cholesterol to bile acids.
- Dextrothyroxine, a thyroid hormone, reduces LDL. It stimulates the liver to increase catabolism and excretion of cholesterol by way of the biliary route into the GI tract. Synthesis of cholesterol is unaffected.

QUESTIONS FOR STUDY AND REVIEW

1. Which of the forms of cholesterol is believed to provide some protective mechanism for the body and is termed "good" cholesterol?
2. How do elevated cholesterol levels contribute to hypertension?
3. Why is it important to determine if other drugs received by a patient taking lovastatin are metabolized by CYP3A4 or are inhibitors of CYP3A4?
4. Why is it important to monitor liver enzymes while a patient is receiving lovastatin or other lipid-lowering drugs?

NEED MORE HELP?

Chapter 34 of the study guide for *Drug Therapy in Nursing* contains exercises and activities to reinforce your understanding of the concepts presented in this chapter. For additional information see the text's accompanying website at *http://www.connection.lww.com.*

REFERENCES AND BIBLIOGRAPHY

American Heart Association. [On-line]. Available: http://www.americanheart.org/Heart_and_Stroke_A_Z_Guide/chols.html.

Beaird, S. L. (2000). HMG-CoA reductase inhibitors: assessing differences in drug interactions and safety profiles. *Journal of American Pharmaceutical Association 40*(5), 637–644.

Brown, W. V. (2000). Cholesterol lowering in atherosclerosis. *American Journal of Cardiology, 86,* (4 Suppl. 2), 29H–34H.

Chan, K. A., Andrade, S. E., Boles, M., Buist, D. S., Chase, G. A., Donahue, J. G., Goodman, M. J., Gurwitz, J. H., LaCroix, A. Z., & Platt, R. (2000). Inhibitors of hydroxymethylglutaryl-coenzyme A reductase and risk of fracture among older women. *Lancet, 355*(9222), 2185–2188.

Chong, P. H., & Bachenheimer, B. S. (2000). Current, new and future treatments in dyslipidaemia and atherosclerosis. *Drugs, 60*(1), 55–93.

Deedwania, P. C. (2000). Hypercholesterolemia. Is lipid-lowering worthwhile for older patients? *Geriatrics, 55*(5), 22–28.
Deslypere, J. P. (2000). Low density lipoprotein cholesterol lowering: are the treatment guidelines still appropriate? *International Journal of Clinical Practice, 54*(5), 307–313.
Farmer, J. A., & Torre-Amione, G. (2000). Comparative tolerability of the HMG-CoA reductase inhibitors. *Drug Safety, 23*(3), 197–213.
Gin, H., Rigalleau, V., & Aparicio, M. (2000). Lipids, protein intake, and diabetic nephropathy. *Diabetes Metabolism, 26,* (Suppl. 4), 45–53.
Eisenberg, D. (2000). Implications of the atorvastatin versus revascularization treatment (AVERT) study for the clinician. *Current Cardiology Report, 2*(5), 433–438.
Libby, P., Aikawa, M., Kinlay, S., Selwyn, A., & Ganz, P. (2000). Lipid lowering improves endothelial functions. *International Journal of Cardiology, 74,* (Suppl. 1), S3–S10.
Mack, W. J., Xiang, M., Shircore, A. M., Selzer, R. H., Hodis, H. N., & Azen, S. P. (2000). Efficacy of two lipid-lowering treatments on quantitative coronary angiographic endpoints. *Cardiovascular Drugs Theory, 14*(4), 411–418.
Meier, C. R., Schlienger, R. G., Kraenzlin, M. E., Schlegel, B., & Jick, H. (2000). HMG-CoA reductase inhibitors and the risk of fractures. *Journal of the American Medical Association, 283*(24), 3205–3210.
Miller, M. (2000). Current perspectives on the management of hypertriglyceridemia. *American Heart Journal, 140*(2), 232–240.
Packard, C., Caslake, M., & Shepherd, J. (2000). The role of small, dense low density lipoprotein (LDL): A new look. *International Journal of Cardiology, 74,* (Suppl. 1), S17–S22.
Pearson, T. A. (2000). The undertreatment of LDL-cholesterol: addressing the challenge. *International Journal of Cardiology, 74,* (Suppl. 1), S23–S28.
Pederson, T. R., Wilhelmsen, L., Faergeman, O., Strandberg, T. E., Thorgeirsson, G., Troedsson, L., Kristianson, J., Berg, K., Cool, T. J., Haghfelt, T., Kjekshus, J., Miettinen, T., Olsson, A. G., Pyorala, K., & Wedel, H. (2000). Follow-up study of patients randomized in the Scandinavian simvastatin survival study (4S) of cholesterol lowering. *American Journal of Cardiology, 86*(3), 257–262.
Rosenson, R. S. (1999). Non-lipid lowering effects of statins on atherosclerosis. *Current Cardiology Report, 1*(3), 255–232.
Safeer, R. S., & Lacivita, C. L. (2000). Choosing drug therapy for patients with hyperlipidemia. *American Family Physician, 61*(11), 3337–3382.
Su, S. F., Hsiao, C. L., Chu, C. W., Lee, B. C., & Lee, T. M. (2000). Effects of pravastatin on left ventricular mass in patients with hyperlipidemia and essential hypertension. *American Journal of Cardiology, 86*(5), 514–518.
Thuraisingham, S., Tan, K. H., Chong, K. S., Yap, S. F., & Pasamanikan, K. (2000). A randomized comparison of simvastatin versus simvastatin and low cholesterol diet in the treatment of hypercholesterolaemia. *International Journal of Clinical Practice, 54*(2), 78–84.
Tolman, K. G. (2000). Defining patient risks from expanded preventive therapies. *American Journal of Cardiology, 85*(12A), 15E–19E.
Vita, J. A., Yeung, A. C., Winniford, M., Hodgson, J. M., Treasure, C. B., Klein, J. L., Werns, S., Kern, M., Plotkin, D., Shih, W. J., Mitchel, Y., & Ganz P. (2000). Effect of cholesterol-lowering therapy on coronary endothelial vasomotor function in patients with coronary artery disease. *Circulation, 102*(8), 846–851.
Wang, P. S., Solomon, D. H., Mogun, H., & Avorn, J. (2000). HMG-CoA reductase inhibitors and the risk for hip fractures in elderly patients. *Journal of the American Medical Association, 283*(24), 3211–3216.

Unit **IX**

Respiratory System Drugs

Chapter **35**

DRUGS AFFECTING THE UPPER RESPIRATORY SYSTEM

KEY TERMS

antihistamines
antitussives
cilia
common cold
decongestants
expectorants
histamine
influenza
laryngitis
pharyngitis
rhinitis
sinuses
sinusitis

Learning Objectives

At the completion of this chapter the student will:

1. Describe the anatomy and physiology of the upper respiratory system.
2. Identify core drug knowledge pertaining to drugs that affect the upper respiratory system.
3. Identify core patient variables pertaining to drugs that affect the upper respiratory system.
4. Relate the interaction of core drug knowledge to core patient variables for drugs that affect the upper respiratory system.
5. Generate a nursing plan of care from the interactions between core drug knowledge and core patient variables for drugs that affect the upper respiratory system.
6. Describe nursing interventions to maximize therapeutic effects and minimize adverse effects for drugs that affect the upper respiratory system.
7. Determine key points for patient and family education for drugs that affect the upper respiratory system.

Antitussives
- **dextromethorphan**
- codeine
- hydrocodone bitartrate

Decongestants
- **pseudoephedrine**
- phenylpropanolamine
- oxymetazoline
- phenylephrine
- ephedrine
- dexamethasone

Antihistamines
- **fexofenadine**
- loratadine
- cetirizine
- oliphenhydramine
- brompheniramine
- chlorpheniramine

Expectorants
- **guaifenesin**
- terpin hydrate
- iodine preparations

The symbol (C) indicates the **drug class**.

Drugs in bold type marked with the symbol (P) are **prototypes**.

Drugs in blue type with no symbol are **closely related** to the prototype.

Drugs in **red** type with no symbol are **significantly different** from the prototype.

Drugs in **black** type with no symbol are **also used in drug therapy**; no prototype.

This chapter discusses drugs that affect the upper respiratory system. The upper respiratory system is essential for bringing oxygen into the body and body tissues. The classes of drugs that affect the upper respiratory system work to keep the airways open. The following drug classes are discussed in this chapter:

- **Antitussives**—drugs that block the cough reflex
- **Decongestants**—drugs that decrease the blood flow to an area and decrease the overproduction of secretions
- **Antihistamines**—drugs that block the release or action of **histamine,** a chemical released during inflammation, which increases secretions and narrows airways
- **Expectorants**–drugs that increase productive cough to clear the airways

PHYSIOLOGY

The respiratory system is composed of the upper and lower respiratory systems. The upper respiratory system, or conducting airway, is composed of the nose, mouth, pharynx, larynx, trachea, and the bronchial tree (Fig. 35-1). Air moves from the nasal cavity through the pharynx and into the larynx. The larynx contains the vocal chords and the epiglottis, the latter of which closes during swallowing to protect the lower respiratory tract from any foreign particles. From the larynx, air proceeds to the trachea, the main conducting airway into the lungs.

AIR FILTRATION

Air usually moves into the nasal cavity through the nose. Nasal hairs catch and filter foreign substances, and the air is warmed and humidified as it passes by blood vessels close to the surface of the epithelial lining in the nasal passage. This epithelial lining contains goblet cells that produce mucus, which traps dust, microorganisms, pollen, or other foreign substances. These actions help to purify the air and increase the efficiency of the gas for diffusion when it reaches the lower respiratory tract.

The cells of the epithelial lining also contain **cilia,** microscopic hair-like projections of the cell membrane. The cilia are in constant motion, moving the mucus and any trapped substance toward the throat where it will be swallowed and destroyed. There are three pairs of **sinuses** (air-filled passages through the skull) that open into the nasal passage. The epithelial lining of the nose is continuous with the lining of the sinuses, and the mucus produced in the sinuses drains into the nasal cavity. The mucus drains into the throat, is swallowed, and proceeds to the gastrointestinal (GI) tract where foreign materials are destroyed by the stomach acids.

OTHER AIR-PURIFYING MECHANISMS

The walls of the nasal cavity are sensitive to irritation. When receptors in the walls are stimulated, a central nervous system (CNS) reflex is initiated and a sneeze results. The sneeze causes air to push through the nasal cavity under tremendous pressure, cleaning out any foreign irritant and opening the passages for more efficient flow of gas. Throughout the airways, there are many macrophage scavengers that are free to move throughout the epithelium and destroy invaders. Mast cells are present in abundance and release histamine, serotonin, adenosine triphosphate, and other chemicals to ensure a rapid and intense inflammatory reaction to any cell injury.

PATHOPHYSIOLOGY

The most common conditions that affect the upper respiratory system can be classified as inflammatory responses. For example, the rhinovirus and adenovirus are two types of common cold viruses that invade the tissues of the upper respiratory tract, initiating the release of histamine and prostaglandins and causing an inflammatory response.

COMMON COLD

The **common cold** is a viral infection that starts in the upper respiratory tract, sometimes spreads to the lower structures, and may contribute to secondary infections in the eyes or middle ears. The main differences between the common cold

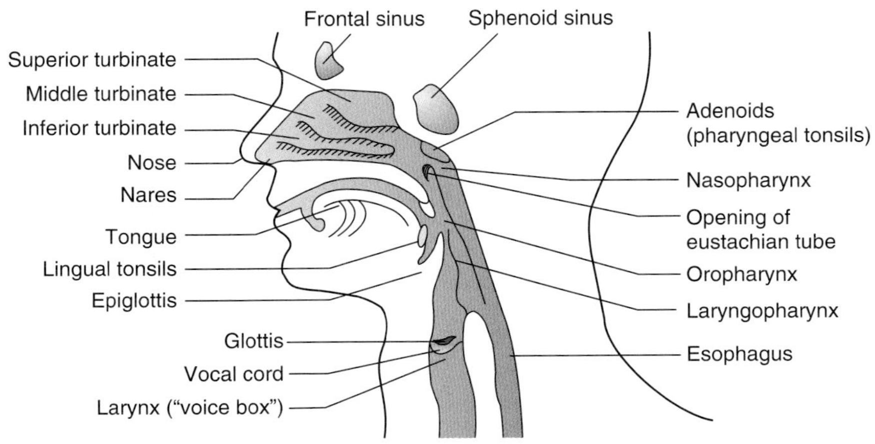

Figure 35-1. Structures of the upper airway.

and other respiratory infections are the absence of fever and the relative mildness of the symptoms. Cold symptoms vary from person to person. Manifestations may include sneezing, headaches, fatigue, chills, sore throat, inflammation of the nose (**rhinitis**), and nasal discharge. There is usually no fever. The secretions are generally watery and clear. Pathologic changes occurring in the mucous membrane that lines the nose, the nasal sinuses, the nasopharynx, and other upper respiratory passages may include tissue swelling, congestion of blood, and oozing of fluids.

ALLERGIC OR SEASONAL RHINITIS

A condition similar to the common cold that afflicts many people is called allergic or seasonal rhinitis. This inflammation of the nasal cavity also is commonly called hay fever. It occurs when the upper airways respond to a specific allergen (e.g., pollen, mold, or dust) with a vigorous inflammatory response, resulting in nasal congestion, sneezing, stuffiness, and watery eyes. Other areas of the upper respiratory tract can become irritated or infected, resulting in inflammation.

SINUSITIS

Sinusitis occurs when the epithelial lining of the sinus cavities becomes inflamed. It can be caused by bacteria or viruses. The resultant swelling that occurs often causes severe pain because the bony cavity cannot stretch and the swollen tissue pushes against the bone and blocks the sinus passages. The danger of a sinus infection is that if untreated, causative microorganisms can move up the sinus passages and into brain tissue.

PHARYNGITIS

Pharyngitis is an inflammation or infection of the pharynx (throat) caused by bacteria or viruses. The symptoms of pharyngitis caused by bacteria are generally redness and swelling of the throat, a pustulant fluid on the tonsils or discharged from the mouth, extreme soreness of the throat that is felt during swallowing, swelling of lymph nodes, and a slight fever. Viral pharyngitis infections produce raised whitish to yellow lesions in the pharynx that are surrounded by reddened tissue. They also cause fever, headache, and sore throat that lasts for 4 to 14 days. Lymphatic tissue in the pharynx also may become involved.

LARYNGITIS

Laryngitis is an inflammation of the larynx or voice box, caused by chemical or mechanical irritation, viral infections, or bacterial infections. Simple laryngitis usually is associated with the common cold or similar infections. Usually the mucous membrane lining the larynx is the primary site of infection; it becomes swollen and filled with blood, secretes a thick mucous substance, and contains many inflammatory cells.

When the epiglottis, which closes the larynx during swallowing, becomes swollen and infected by influenza viruses, the larynx can become obstructed, and suffocation may result. Excessive smoking, alcoholism, or overuse of the vocal cords may cause chronic laryngitis. The mucous membrane becomes dry and covered with polyps, small lumps of tissue that project from the surface. In addition, the wall of the larynx may thicken and become inflamed. Additional causes of laryngitis include diphtheria, tuberculosis, and syphilis, serious infections that require aggressive treatment.

INFLUENZA

Influenza is an infection caused by any of several strains of myxoviruses, categorized as types A, B, and C. Influenza is transmitted from person to person through the respiratory tract by inhalation of infected droplets resulting from coughing and sneezing. As the virus particles gain entrance to the body, they selectively attack and destroy the ciliated epithelial cells that line the upper respiratory tract, bronchial tubes, and trachea. The onset of symptoms is abrupt, with sudden and distinct chills, fatigue, muscular aches, and high temperature. A diffuse headache and severe muscular aches throughout the body are experienced and often are accompanied by irritation or a sense of rawness in the throat. Symptoms associated with respiratory tract infection, such as coughing and nasal discharge also may occur.

C ANTITUSSIVE DRUGS

Antitussives are drugs that suppress the cough reflex. Many disorders of the upper and lower respiratory tracts, including the common cold, sinusitis, pharyngitis, and pneumonia, are accompanied by an uncomfortable, nonproductive cough. Coughing normally is a protective mechanism that forces foreign irritants out of the respiratory system, opening it for more efficient flow of gas. However, persistent coughing can be exhausting, cause muscle strain, and further irritate the respiratory tract. A cough that occurs without an active disease process or that persists after treatment may be a symptom of another disease process and should be investigated before any drug is given to alleviate it. Antitussive drugs include dextromethorphan, codeine, and hydrocodone bitartrate. Dextromethorphan (Benylin) is selected as the prototype of the antitussives.

NURSING MANAGEMENT OF THE PATIENT RECEIVING P DEXTROMETHORPHAN

Core Drug Knowledge

Pharmacotherapeutics

Dextromethorphan is used in treating chronic, nonproductive cough. It is available widely in a variety of nonprescription forms, such as capsules, lozenges, syrups, extended-release oral suspension, and chewable tablets.

TABLE 35-1 Summary of Selected Antitussives

Drug (Trade) Name	Selected Indications	Route and Dosage Range	Pharmacokinetics
dextromethorphan hydrobromide (Benylin, Pedia Care, Pertussin; *Canadian:* Balminil DM)	Cough suppression	*Adult:* PO, 10–30 mg q4–8h *Child:* > 12 y: PO, 10–30 mg q4–8h 6–12 y: PO, 5–10 mg q4–6h	*Onset:* 15–30 min *Duration:* 5–6 h $t_{1/2}$: 11 h
codeine (*Canadian:* Omnituss)	Cough suppression	*Adult:* PO, 10–20 mg q4–6h *Child:* >12 y: PO, 10–20 mg q4–6h 6–12 y: PO, 5–10 mg q4–6h 2–6 y: PO, 2.5–5 mg q4–6h	*Onset:* 15–20 min *Duration:* 4–6 h $t_{1/2}$: 1.5–4 h
hydrocodone bitartrate (Hycodan; *Canadian:* Robidon)	Cough suppression	*Adult:* PO, 5–10 mg q4h *Child:* PO, 0.6 mg/kg in 3 to 4 divided doses	*Onset:* 10–20 min *Duration:* 3–6 h $t_{1/2}$: 3–8 h

Pharmacokinetics

Dextromethorphan is absorbed rapidly from the GI tract, with antitussive activity occurring within 15 to 30 minutes (Table 35-1). It undergoes extensive hepatic metabolism. Excretion is mainly renal with some drug being eliminated unchanged, but most eliminated as metabolites.

Pharmacodynamics

Dextromethorphan is related chemically to the opiate agonists and can suppress coughing as effectively as narcotics. Cough suppression occurs by several mechanisms, but mainly the drug directly affects the cough center in the medulla. Therapeutic doses do not affect ciliary activity.

Contraindications and Precautions

Dextromethorphan is contraindicated in treating chronic coughs resulting from emphysema and asthma. Because of its extensive hepatic metabolism, dextromethorphan is used with caution in patients with hepatic impairment. It also is used with caution during pregnancy. Although teratogenic effects have not been demonstrated by the drug, dextromethorphan is rated pregnancy category C.

Adverse Effects

Although adverse effects are generally rare, nausea and vomiting, drowsiness, dizziness, irritability, and restlessness can be indicative of dextromethorphan toxicity.

Drug Interactions

Dextromethorphan may potentiate sedation when used with other CNS depressants. It may interact with monoamine oxidase inhibitors (MAOIs), resulting in serotonin syndrome, which consists of nausea, hypotension, excitation, hyperpyrexia, and possible coma. It also may interact with amiodarone, quinidine, and selective serotonin reuptake inhibitor antidepressants (Table 35-2).

TABLE 35-2 Agents That Interact With Dextromethorphan

Interactants	Effect and Significance	Nursing Management
amiodarone	May inhibit the hepatic metabolism of dextromethorphan by inhibiting the hepatic cytochrome P450 2D6; may result in dextromethorphan toxicity	Avoid combination therapy if possible. Monitor for signs of dextromethorphan toxicity.
MAOIs	Dextromethorphan can block neuronal uptake of serotonin and may produce excessive concentration of serotonin in the CNS when used with MAOIs	Maintain an interval of at least 2 wk between administration of these two drugs. Monitor for serotonin syndrome.
quinidine	May inhibit the hepatic metabolism of dextromethorphan by inhibiting the hepatic cytochrome P450 2D6; may result in dextromethorphan toxicity	Avoid combination therapy if possible. Monitor for signs of dextromethorphan toxicity.
SSRI antidepressants fluoxetine paroxetine	Interfere with the metabolism of dextromethorphan, resulting in hallucinations or a serotonin syndrome-like reaction	Monitor for adverse effects. Decrease dose of SSRI antidepressant.

MAOI, monoamine oxidase inhibitor; SSRI, selected serotonin reuptake inhibitor.

Assessment of Relevant Core Patient Variables

Health Status

Before administering dextromethorphan, the nurse should review the patient's record to determine whether dextromethorphan may be administered safely. This drug is contraindicated for patients with emphysema or asthma. If coughing is suppressed in these patients, they may retain secretions that will exacerbate the disease.

The nurse also should review the patient's record for drugs that may interact with dextromethorphan, especially antidepressants. Finally, the nurse should evaluate the patient for a history of hepatic insufficiency because dextromethorphan is processed by the liver.

The nurse should perform a baseline evaluation of the head, eyes, ears, nose, and throat (HEENT) in addition to a complete lung assessment.

Life Span and Gender

The nurse should determine whether the patient is pregnant. Dextromethorphan, a pregnancy category C drug, should be used with caution during pregnancy. It also is important to be aware of the patient's age before administering dextromethorphan because it is not indicated for use in children younger than 6 years old.

Lifestyle, Diet, and Habits

The nurse should investigate the patient's need to drive or operate potentially dangerous equipment and advise the patient to refrain from these activities until the sedative effects of dextromethorphan use are known. It is important to assess the patient's typical intake of alcohol. The nurse should caution the patient about the potentially additive effects of dextromethorphan when used with alcohol because both are CNS depressants.

Environment

The nurse should be aware of the environment in which dextromethorphan will be administered. Dextromethorphan is used commonly in over-the-counter (OTC) cough and cold preparations, and prescribed dextromethorphan is just as commonly self-administered by patients at home. Therefore, the nurse should caution the patient to read labels of all drugs being taken to avoid a possible overdose.

Nursing Diagnoses and Outcomes

- Risk for Injury related to sensory-perceptual alteration from drug-induced drowsiness and sedation
  Desired outcome: The patient will remain free from injury related to sedation and drowsiness.
- Risk for Ineffective Airway Clearance related to suppression of cough reflex
  Desired outcome: The patient will maintain his or her baseline respiratory function.

Planning and Intervention

Maximizing Therapeutic Effects

In acute or long-term care settings, the nurse should administer dextromethorphan at evenly spaced intervals to maintain blood levels of the drug at steady state. The nurse also should provide environmental controls, including appropriate lighting, reduced noise, and comfortable temperature, to ease sensory-perceptual alteration and aid relaxation.

Minimizing Adverse Effects

During therapy, the nurse should ensure that safety precautions are used, such as side rails and ambulation assistance. It also is important to monitor movement of air and respiratory status periodically during drug use.

Providing Patient and Family Education

- The nurse should explain to patients and their families that taking dextromethorphan will help to quiet a cough.
- The nurse should emphasize that sedation, drowsiness, and impaired orientation can occur. Because it can be sedating, it is important to tell patients to take dextromethorphan only as directed and not to drive or perform other tasks that require alertness. Some patients may require assistance in walking if they react strongly to dextromethorphan.
- It is important to explain to patients that they should not take dextromethorphan if they are allergic to it, pregnant, breast-feeding, or have hepatic insufficiency.
- The nurse should alert patients not to take any OTC drugs or consume alcohol while taking dextromethorphan, because this could increase sedation.
- The nurse should caution patients to keep dextromethorphan out of the reach of children.
- It is important to tell patients to report immediately any chest tightness, difficulty breathing, noisy breathing, or shortness of breath.

Ongoing Assessment and Evaluation

The nurse should monitor the effect of dextromethorphan on the patient's motor control, sedation, and respiratory status. By the end of therapy, the patient should remain free of injury related to sedation and be relieved of his cough. ■

MEMORY CHIP

Dextromethorphan

- Used for the management of nonproductive cough
- Significant contraindication: cough resulting from emphysema or asthma
- Most common adverse effects: nausea, vomiting, and irritability
- Most serious adverse effects: drowsiness and dizziness
- Maximizing therapeutic effects: administer at evenly spaced intervals throughout the day
- Minimizing adverse effects: ensure safety precautions due to potential drowsiness or dizziness
- Most significant patient education: advise the patient to seek medical attention if cough does not resolve

DRUGS CLOSELY RELATED TO DEXTROMETHORPHAN

Codeine

Codeine is a controlled substance used in treating cough. Like dextromethorphan, it works directly on the medullary center to suppress the cough reflex. Codeine is more sedating than dextromethorphan and also may induce respiratory depression. Codeine is contraindicated for patients who must cough to maintain a patent airway (e.g., postoperative patients). Codeine is used with caution in patients who are pregnant or breast-feeding, and in patients with head injuries. It also is used cautiously in patients with chronic cough (e.g., from emphysema or asthma) or in patients with a history of drug addiction. Adverse effects include sedation, dry mouth, nausea or vomiting, and constipation. Codeine also is discussed in Chapter 24.

Hydrocodone Bitartrate

Hydrocodone bitartrate (Hycodan), also a controlled substance, is a derivative of codeine and acts directly on the cough reflex center in the medulla. It is somewhat more sedating than codeine and has the same properties, contraindications, and adverse effects.

DECONGESTANT DRUGS

Decongestants are drugs taken to decrease nasal congestion related to the common cold, sinusitis, and allergic rhinitis. These conditions are caused by an inflammatory response in the upper respiratory tract. They can be administered orally or topically. When decongestants are taken orally, they are absorbed in the body, thus increasing the chance of adverse effects. When used topically, the action of the drug is the same; however, the potential for adverse effects is diminished.

Drugs within the decongestant class include pseudoephedrine, phenylpropanolamine, ephedrine, oxymetazoline, and phenylephrine. The intranasal steroid dexamethasone sodium phosphate is not within the decongestant drug class but is used for its anti-inflammatory effect on nasal conditions. The prototype decongestant is pseudoephedrine (Sudafed), an orally administered decongestant.

NURSING MANAGEMENT OF THE PATIENT RECEIVING PSEUDOEPHEDRINE

Core Drug Knowledge

Pharmacotherapeutics

Pseudoephedrine may reduce the volume of nasal mucus and is recommended for the temporary relief of nasal congestion related to the common cold, allergic rhinitis, and sinusitis. It also is used to relieve the pressure of otitis media by promoting drainage of the Eustachian tubes.

Pharmacokinetics

Pseudoephedrine is absorbed readily from the GI tract with onset of activity occurring within 30 minutes. Duration of action ranges from 4 to 6 hours in regular formulations, to 8 to 12 hours in extended-release preparations (Table 35-3). Pseudoephedrine is metabolized by the liver and excreted in the urine. This drug also crosses the placenta and enters breast milk.

Pharmacodynamics

Pseudoephedrine mimics the actions of the sympathetic nervous system and achieves its nasal decongestant effects by causing vasoconstriction in the nasal mucous membranes. This shrinkage results in a decrease in membrane size and promotes sinus drainage and improved air flow. Stimulation of other sympathetic receptors while the patient is taking pseudoephedrine can result in cardiovascular stimulation, constriction of renal arterioles, and anxiety.

Contraindications and Precautions

Pseudoephedrine is categorized in pregnancy category C and should be used with caution during pregnancy or lactation because of its possible effects on the fetus and neonate. This drug should not be used in patients with severe hypertension and coronary artery disease because it produces sympathetic effects such as increased heart rate and blood pressure. Special caution should be used in patients with diabetes, thyrotoxicosis, coronary artery disease, benign prostatic hypertrophy, and increased intraocular pressure because of the risk of sympathomimetic adverse effects, which could aggravate these conditions.

Adverse Effects

Adverse effects related to pseudoephedrine are related primarily to the sympathetic effects on the CNS and cardiovascular system. They will occur almost immediately and include feelings of tension, anxiety, restlessness,

TABLE 35-3 Summary of Selected Decongestants

Drug (Trade) Name	Selected Indications	Route and Dosage Range	Pharmacokinetics
Oral Decongestants			
pseudoephedrine (Sudafed, Decofed, Dorcol Pediatric formula, Halofed, Novafed, Pediacare; *Canadian:* Eltor)	Relief of nasal congestion caused by common cold, hay fever, sinusitis Relief of Eustachian tube congestion	*Adult:* PO, 60 mg q4–6h not to exceed 240 mg in 24 h; topical spray, 2 sprays in each nostril bid *Child:* 6–12 y: PO, 30 mg q4–6h not to exceed 120 mg in 24 h 2–5 y: PO, 15 mg q4–6h not to exceed 60 mg in 24 h 1–2 y: PO (0.2 mL/kg), 7 drops q4–6h up to four doses per day 3–12 mo: PO, 3 drops/kg q4–6h up to four doses per day	*Onset:* 30 min *Duration:* 4–6 h $t_{1/2}$: 7 h
phenylpropanolamine (Propagest, Rhindecon)	Relief of nasal congestion caused by common cold, hay fever, sinusitis Relief of Eustachian tube congestion	*Adult:* PO, 25 mg q4h not to exceed 150 mg per day *Child:* 6–12 y: PO, 12.5 mg q4h not to exceed 75 mg per day 2–12 y: PO, 6.25 mg q4h	*Onset:* 30 min *Duration:* 4–6 h $t_{1/2}$: 6 h
Topical Decongestants			
ephedrine (Kondon's Nasal)	Relief of nasal congestion caused by common cold, allergic rhinitis, sinusitis	*Adult:* Topical, 0.1%, 0.25%, 0.5% solutions, apply locally as drops or spray or with a sterile swab, as required *Child:* >6 y: Topical, 0.1%, 0.25%, 0.5% solutions, apply locally as drops or spray or with a sterile swab, as required Do not use in children <6 y	*Onset:* 5–10 min *Duration:* 4–6 h $t_{1/2}$: 3–6 h
oxymetazoline (Afrin, Allerest, Dristan Long Lasting, Neo-Synephrine 12 hour, Sinex Long Lasting)	Relief of nasal congestion caused by common cold, allergic rhinitis, sinusitis	*Adult:* Topical, 2–3 sprays or 2–3 drops of 0.05% solution in each nostril bid *Child:* >6 y: Topical, 2–3 sprays or 2–3 drops of 0.05% solution in each nostril bid 2–5 y: Topical, 2–3 drops of 0.025% solution in each nostril bid	*Onset:* 5–10 min *Duration:* 6–10 h $t_{1/2}$: Unknown
xylometazoline (Otrivin)	Relief of nasal congestion caused by common cold, allergic rhinitis, sinusitis	*Adult:* Topical, 2–3 sprays or 2–3 drops of 0.1% solution in each nostril q3–4h *Child:* >6 y: Topical, adult dosage 2–12 y: Topical, 2–3 drops of 0.05% solution in each nostril q4–6h; do not use 0.1% solution in children <6 y	*Onset:* 5–10 min *Duration:* 5–6 h $t_{1/2}$: Unknown
phenylephrine (Neo-Synephrine, Sinex; *Canadian:* Dionephrin)	Relief of nasal congestion caused by common cold, allergic rhinitis, sinusitis	*Adult:* Topical, 2–3 sprays or 2–3 drops of 0.25% or 0.5% solution in each nostril q3–4h *Child:* >12 y: Topical, adult dosage 6–12 y: Topical, 2–3 sprays or drops of 0.25% solution in each nostril q3–4h *Infants:* Topical, 2–3 drops of 0.16% solution in each nostril q3h	*Onset:* 5–10 min *Duration:* 3–4 h $t_{1/2}$: Unknown
naphazoline HCl (Privine)	Relief of nasal congestion caused by common cold, allergic rhinitis, sinusitis	*Adult:* Topical, 1–2 gtt q3h or 0.05% spray solution q4–6h *Child:* >12 y same as adult	*Onset:* } Minimal systemic absorption *Duration:* $t_{1/2}$:

TABLE 35-3 Summary of Selected Decongestants (Continued)

Drug (Trade) Name	Selected Indications	Route and Dosage Range	Pharmacokinetics
tetrahydrozoline HCl (Tyzine)	Relief of nasal congestion caused by common cold, allergic rhinitis, sinusitis	*Adult:* Topical, 2–4 drops of 0.1% solution in each nostril q3–4h or 3–4 sprays in each nostril q4h *Child:* >6 y: Topical, adult dosage 2–6 y: Topical, 2–3 drops of 0.5% pediatric solution in each nostril q4–6h; do not use 0.1% solution in children <6 y	*Onset:* 5–10 min *Duration:* 6–10 h $t_{1/2}$: Unknown
Intranasal Steroid			
dexamethasone sodium phosphate (Turbinaire Decadron Phosphate; *Canadian:* Dexasone)	Allergic or inflammatory nasal conditions Nasal polyps (excluding polyps originating within the sinuses)	*Adult:* Topical, 2 sprays (168 μg) into each nostril two to three times a day, maximum 12 sprays per day *Child:* Topical, 1 or 2 sprays (84–158 μg) into each nostril two times a day, maximum 8 sprays per day	*Onset:*, *Duration:*, $t_{1/2}$: Minimal systemic absorption

tremor, insomnia, and weakness. Severe CNS reactions have included hallucinations, delusions, and convulsions. Adverse cardiovascular effects include palpitations, tachycardia, hypertension, and arrhythmias. Allergic reactions that have been reported with pseudoephedrine use include skin rashes and urticaria. Extreme dryness of the mucous membranes with resultant pain and irritation has been reported in some cases.

When sympathomimetic adverse effects occur, patients with concurrent diseases of diabetes, thyrotoxicosis, coronary artery disease, hypertension, benign prostatic hypertrophy, and increased intraocular pressure should discontinue using pseudoephedrine; patients without concurrent disease may continue taking the drug.

Drug Interactions

Increased hypertension may occur if pseudoephedrine is taken concurrently with MAOIs, guanethidine, methyldopa, or furazolidone. The nurse should instruct the patient to avoid such combinations. Increased duration of the effect of pseudoephedrine may occur if taken with any urinary alkalinizer (e.g., potassium citrate, sodium citrate, sodium lactate, tromethamine, sodium acetate, and sodium bicarbonate) because the drug cannot be excreted into an alkaline urine. An increased dose of pseudoephedrine may be necessary when given with urinary acidifiers, such as ammonium chloride, potassium phosphate, or sodium acid phosphate (Table 35-4).

TABLE 35-4 Agents That Interact With Pseudoephedrine

Interactants	Effect and Significance	Nursing Management
furazolidone	May increase the pressor sensitivity to mixed and indirect-acting sympathomimetics, such as pseudoephedrine, resulting in hypertension	Avoid coadministration. If used concurrently, monitor for hypertension. If hypertensive crisis results, consider the use of phentolamine.
guanethidine	Depletes norepinephrine stores, resulting in hypertension	Use an alternative antihypertensive therapy.
monoamine oxidase inhibitors	Increase the amount of norepinephrine available for release by pseudoephedrine, resulting in severe headache, hypertension, and hyperpyrexia; hypertensive crisis possible	Avoid coadministration. If these are used together and hypertension develops, administer phentolamine.
methyldopa	Coadministration of methyldopa and pseudoephedrine may result in an increased pressor response, resulting in hypertension	Monitor the blood pressure during coadministration. Discontinue pseudoephedrine if hypertension occurs.
urinary acidifiers	Tubular reabsorption of pseudoephedrine possibly decreased due to a decreased urinary pH by urinary acidifiers	Monitor possible need for an increased dose of pseudoephedrine to achieve desired results. Acidification of the urine may be useful in the treatment of sympathomimetic intoxication.
urinary alkalinizers	Tubular reabsorption of pseudoephedrine possibly increased due to an increased urinary pH by urinary alkalinizers	Decrease the dose of pseudoephedrine during coadministration of a urinary alkalinizer.

Assessment of Relevant Core Patient Variables

Health Status

The nurse should review the patient's health history and perform a physical examination to determine any contraindications to the use of this drug. Contraindications include hypersensitivity to the drug, thyrotoxicosis, diabetes, hypertension, benign prostatic hypertrophy, cardiovascular disorders, pregnancy, and lactation.

It is especially important for the nurse to assess patient orientation, affect, respiratory rate and auscultation, blood pressure, and pulse. In addition, the nurse should monitor cardiovascular effects carefully to prevent serious complications and arrange for dosage adjustment as appropriate.

Life Span and Gender

The nurse should be aware of the patient's age before administering pseudoephedrine. It is important to use caution when giving pseudoephedrine to elderly patients, because they may experience more serious adverse effects. It is recommended that sustained-release preparations be avoided and that shorter duration preparations be used. The nurse also should assess the patient for pregnancy. Pseudoephedrine is ranked in pregnancy category C and its use should be avoided by pregnant women unless the benefits are thought to outweigh the potential risks.

Nursing Diagnoses and Outcomes

- Risk for Injury caused by visual sensory-perceptual alterations (hallucinations) related to drug-induced CNS effects

  Desired outcome: The patient will be protected from injury related to drug use and will demonstrate safety procedures to use if these effects occur.
- Ineffective Tissue Perfusion: Cerebral or Cardiopulmonary related to sympathomimetic effects

  Desired outcome: The patient will be monitored and dosage adjusted to minimize potential perfusion deficits or CNS effects.

Planning and Intervention

Maximizing Therapeutic Effects

In conjunction with pseudoephedrine therapy, the patient should use a humidifier, drink plenty of fluids, and avoid smoke-filled rooms, because dry air, dry mucous membranes, and airborne irritants may render the drug less effective.

Minimizing Adverse Effects

The nurse should provide the patient with appropriate safety measures, such as side rails, adequate lighting, and assistance with movement to avoid injury if CNS effects are experienced.

Providing Patient and Family Education

- The nurse should explain to patients that the purpose of pseudoephedrine is to promote breathing and relieve congestion.
- The nurse should tell patients not to take pseudoephedrine if they are allergic to it, have high blood pressure, or are breast-feeding. In addition, the nurse should instruct patients to take the drug exactly as prescribed. Higher doses may cause nervousness, dizziness, chest pain, or sleeplessness.
- The nurse should tell patients not to take pseudoephedrine for more than 4 days. They should contact the health care provider and schedule an appointment if symptoms do not subside after 4 days.
- The nurse should caution patients to avoid the use of other OTC drugs, many of which also contain pseudoephedrine, because a serious overdose could occur.
- To avoid rebound congestion, the nurse should teach patients strategies for decreasing the discomfort of nasal congestion and how to decrease drug use (see the accompanying display, Prolonged Use of Nasal Decongestants).
- The nurse must outline safety measures that may be necessary if CNS effects occur, such as getting assistance with ambulation, using adequate lighting, and avoiding driving or tasks that require alertness.
- The nurse must urge patients to report excessive dizziness, weakness, palpitations, and sleeplessness, and to keep pseudoephedrine out of the reach of children.

Ongoing Assessment and Evaluation

The nurse should monitor for rebound congestion, sedation, dizziness, weakness, tremor, and urinary retention. By the end of therapy, the patient will be free from nasal congestion and free from potential CNS or cardiovascular adverse effects. ■

Critical Thinking Scenario

Prolonged use of nasal decongestants

Noah Rightman, age 16, comes to the clinic for a recheck of his allergic rhinitis. He uses a nasal decongestant daily. Lately, he has needed to use his nasal decongestant "10 times a day," and asks "what's wrong with this drug? I want something stronger." Understanding the sympathetic nervous system, how would you respond to Noah?

MEMORY CHIP

Pseudoephedrine

- Used for the relief of nasal congestion
- Significant contraindications: severe hypertension or severe cardiac disorders
- Most common adverse effects: tachycardia, palpitations, and nervousness
- Most serious adverse effects: dysrhythmias, hypertension, and coronary vasospasm
- Maximizing therapeutic effects: assist pseudoephedrine with use of humidifier and increase the fluid intake
- Minimizing adverse effects: adhere to safety precautions
- Most significant patient education: take pseudoephedrine exactly as prescribed to avoid rebound congestion

DRUGS CLOSELY RELATED TO PSEUDOEPHEDRINE

Phenylpropanolamine

Phenylpropanolamine (Rhindecon) is a drug used commonly in OTC decongestants. It is an indirect-acting sympathomimetic drug with decongestant properties from its peripheral adrenergic effects. Phenylpropanolamine has properties very similar to those of pseudoephedrine but produces somewhat fewer CNS effects.

The Food and Drug Administration has issued a public health advisory for consumers to stop using OTC or prescription drugs containing phenylpropanolamine because the drug has been associated with an increased risk for hemorrhagic stroke. The nurse should encourage patients to avoid any product containing the ingredient phenylpropanolamine, especially patients with a history of hypertension.

Oxymetazoline

Oxymetazoline (Afrin) stimulates alpha-adrenergic receptors in the nasal passages and thus causes a constriction in the nasal arterioles. As a result, the nasal membrane is reduced in size, swelling is limited, and the size of the nostril is increased, allowing for more efficient air flow. Although its action is similar to that of pseudoephedrine, its route of administration is topical. Oxymetazoline has the same adverse effects as pseudoephedrine. However, because it is not absorbed systemically, the potential for adverse effects is diminished. Oxymetazoline can be administered to children as young as 2 years old. However, the vascularity of the nasal membranes, developing nasal passages, and Eustachian tubes increases the risk of systemic absorption and adverse effects.

Use of oxymetazoline for longer than 5 continuous days can lead to rebound congestion. Rebound congestion occurs when the nasal passages become congested as the drug effect wears off. When this occurs, patients tend to use more of the drug to decrease the congestion, and a vicious cycle of congestion–drug use–congestion develops, leading to abuse of oxymetazoline. The nurse should instruct the patient to stop using the drug when this occurs.

Phenylephrine

Phenylephrine (Neo-Synephrine) is a powerful alpha-adrenergic stimulant that decreases nasal congestion when applied topically. Special caution must be taken to avoid use in abraded nasal membranes because systemic absorption of this drug can result in severe cardiac, CNS, and urinary effects. As with other decongestants, continuous use may induce rebound congestion.

Ephedrine

Ephedrine (Kondon's Nasal) is another powerful alpha-adrenergic stimulant found in many OTC topical preparations. Like phenylephrine, this drug can cause serious effects when absorbed systemically. In addition, this drug may cause rebound congestion if used continuously. Ephedrine is not recommended for use in children younger than 6 years old.

DRUGS SIGNIFICANTLY DIFFERENT FROM PSEUDOEPHEDRINE

Dexamethasone Sodium Phosphate

Although not within the decongestant drug class, topical steroidal preparations are used to treat seasonal allergic rhinitis for patients who do not respond to decongestant preparations. They are used frequently to relieve inflammation following the removal of nasal polyps. The exact mechanism of action of dexamethasone is unknown. It produces an anti-inflammatory effect by exerting a direct local effect, which blocks many of the complex reactions responsible for the inflammatory response. Its action is not immediate; up to 1 week may pass before the patient responds to therapy.

Because this drug blocks the inflammatory response, its use is contraindicated in patients with acute infections. Increased incidence of *Candida albicans* has been reported in patients using dexamethasone. This is probably related to its anti-inflammatory and anti-immune activities. Topical steroids do not have an effect on the adrenal glands; however, the patient should still be monitored for adverse effects. For more information about steroids, see Chapter 40.

ANTIHISTAMINES

Antihistamines are used to relieve symptoms of allergies. Because of their OTC availability, these drugs are often misused to treat colds and influenza. Their greatest effect is on allergic rhinitis, blocking the action of histamine as it is released as part of the inflammatory response to an antigen. Their action restores normal air flow through the upper respiratory system. Drugs within the antihistamine class can be separated into first generation and second generation. First-generation antihistamines include diphenhydramine, brompheniramine, and chlorpheniramine. Second-generation antihistamines include fexofenadine, loratadine, and cetirizine. Fexofenadine (Allegra) is the prototype for antihistamines.

NURSING MANAGEMENT OF THE PATIENT RECEIVING FEXOFENADINE

Core Drug Knowledge

Pharmacotherapeutics

Fexofenadine is used to relieve symptoms associated with seasonal and perennial allergic rhinitis, allergic conjunctivitis, uncomplicated urticaria, and angioedema. It is most effective if used before the onset of symptoms (Table 35-5).

Pharmacokinetics

Fexofenadine is taken orally and is absorbed rapidly. The peak drug effect is seen within 2 to 6 hours. Fexofenadine is only slightly (5%) metabolized in the liver and is excreted in the feces (80%) and urine (11%). This drug is assigned to pregnancy category C; it crosses the placenta and enters breast milk, so its use should be avoided or used with caution by pregnant and lactating women.

Pharmacodynamics

Fexofenadine selectively blocks the effects of histamine at the H_1-receptor sites, decreasing the allergic response. Fexofenadine also has anticholinergic (atropine-like) and antipruritic effects. However, fexofenadine, a second-generation antihistamine, has less of an anticholinergic effect than the first-generation antihistamines. This is because fexofenadine binds to lung receptors significantly more than it binds to cerebellar receptors, resulting in a reduced sedative potential.

TABLE 35-5 Summary of Selected Antihistamines

Drug (Trade) Name	Selected Indications	Route and Dosage Range	Pharmacokinetics
Second Generation			
fexofenadine (Allegra)	Relief of symptoms of allergic rhinitis, vasomotor rhinitis, conjunctivitis, urticaria	*Adult:* PO, 60 mg bid *Child:* 6–12 y: PO, 30–60 mg bid	*Onset:* 1–2 h *Duration:* 12 h $t_{1/2}$: 14 h
cetirizine (Zyrtec; *Canadian:* Reactine)	Allergic rhinitis, asthma, atopic dermatitis, urticaria	*Adult and child* >12: 10 mg qd *Child:* 6–11: 5–10 mg qd *Child:* 2–5 y 2.5–5 mg qd	*Onset:* 30 min *Duration:* 24 h $t_{1/2}$: 8–11 h
loratadine (Claritin)	Relief of symptoms of allergic rhinitis, vasomotor rhinitis, conjunctivitis, urticaria Amelioration of allergic reactions Relief of bronchospasm	*Adult:* PO, 10 mg qd *Child:* >12 y: PO, adult dosage *Note:* Patients with hepatic dysfunction should receive 10 mg QOD	*Onset:* 1–3 h *Duration:* 24 h $t_{1/2}$: 8.4 h
First Generation			
diphenhydramine (Benadryl; *Canadian:* Allerdryl)	Cough suppressant, allergic rhinitis, nighttime sleep aid, motion sickness	*Adult:* PO, 25–50 mg qid; IV/IM, 10–50 mg to maximum of 400 mg *Child:* PO, 5 mg/kg/d to maximum of 300 mg daily; IV/IM, same	*Onset:* PO, 15–30 min; IV, rapid; IM, 20–30 min *Duration:* 4–8 h $t_{1/2}$: 2.5–7 h
brompheniramine (Dimetane, Dimetapp)	Allergic rhinitis, allergic conjunctivitis, rhinorrhea, sneezing, vasomotor rhinitis, pruritis	*Adult and child* >12: 4–8 mg PO q6–8 h *Child* 6–11: 2–4 mg q6–8 h *Child* 2–5: 1 mg PO q4–6 h (in children 2–5 y, consult health care provider before administering)	*Onset:* 1 h *Duration:* 9–24 h $t_{1/2}$: 12–34 h
chlorpheniramine (Chlor-Trimeton; *Canadian:* Chlor-Tripolon)	Allergic rhinitis, allergic conjunctivitis, pruritis, urticaria, motion sickness, anaphylaxis	*Adult and child* >12: 4 mg PO q4–6 h max. 24/mg/d Exten release 8–12 mg q8–12h *Child* 6–11: 2 mg PO q4–6h max 12/mg/d *Child* 2–5: 1 mg PO q4–6 h max 4/mg/d *Adult:* SC, IM, IV; 5–40 mg single dose max. 40 mg/d *Child:* SC (only), 87.5 μg/kg q6h	*Onset:* PO, 15–30 min; Ex, unknown; SC, unknown; IM, unknown, IV, rapid *Duration:* PO, 4–12 h; Ex, 8–24 h; SC, 4–12 h; IM, 4–12 h; IV, 4–12 h $t_{1/2}$: 20–24 h

Contraindications and Precautions

Fexofenadine should not be used in the patient with a hypersensitivity to fexofenadine or terfenadine or any of its components, in children younger than 12 years old, or in pregnant or lactating women. Fexofenadine also should be used with caution in patients with renal impairment because the drug's half-life will be prolonged in these patients. In addition, the drug increases peak plasma levels in patients with renal impairment.

Adverse Effects

The most common adverse reactions associated with fexofenadine therapy include viral infection (e.g., cold and flu), nausea and vomiting, dysmenorrhea, drowsiness, dyspepsia, and fatigue. Fexofenadine is a metabolite of terfenadine. Terfenadine has been associated with QT prolongation and ventricular tachycardias and is no longer manufactured. Fexofenadine has not induced QT prolongation, but patients should still be monitored for this adverse effect.

Drug Interactions

No significant drug interactions have been reported for fexofenadine.

Assessment of Relevant Core Patient Variables

Health Status

The nurse should assess the patient's history for allergy to any antihistamine, pregnancy, lactation, or renal impairment. Before beginning therapy, the nurse should assess the patient's respiratory system, orientation and affect, and skin condition. For anticipated long-term therapy, renal function should be assessed as well.

Life Span and Gender

The nurse should note the age of the patient before administering fexofenadine. It is important to use special precautions in elderly patients who are more likely to experience dizziness, sedation, and syncope. The drug also should not be used by children younger than 12 years old. The nurse should determine if the patient is pregnant because fexofenadine should not be used during pregnancy.

Lifestyle, Diet, and Habits

Before driving a vehicle or performing tasks that require concentration, the nurse should assess patients for the level of sedation caused by fexofenadine.

Environment

The nurse should be aware of the environment in which fexofenadine will be administered. Fexofenadine usually is administered at home and in the community setting. The nurse should caution patients taking fexofenadine to read the labels of nonprescription products to be sure they are not taking another product that also contains an antihistamine, which could potentiate the effects of both drugs.

Nursing Diagnosis and Outcome

- Risk for Injury caused by drowsiness and fatigue related to drug-induced CNS effects

  Desired outcome: Safety precautions will prevent injury related to drug-induced CNS effects.

Planning and Intervention

Maximizing Therapeutic Effects

The nurse should institute measures to prevent dangers associated with thickening of respiratory secretions. Examples of appropriate measures include use of a humidifier, forcing fluids as appropriate, and encouraging the patient to avoid dry or smoke-filled areas.

Minimizing Adverse Effects

The nurse should administer the drug with food to decrease GI upset. The nurse should provide safety measures, such as side rails, controlled environment, and assistance with ambulation, if CNS effects occur.

Providing Patient and Family Education

- The nurse should explain that taking fexofenadine will relieve allergy symptoms.
- The nurse should caution patients not to take fexofenadine if they are allergic to it, pregnant, or breastfeeding. In addition, if patients miss a dose, they should take it as soon as they remember, unless it is almost time for the next dose; two doses should not be taken at the same time.
- It is important to tell patients to avoid the use of other OTC drugs, many of which contain similar antihistamines that could cause serious adverse effects. It is important to inform patients to avoid alcohol while taking fexofenadine and not to drive or perform tasks that require alertness until the drug's effect has been determined.
- The nurse should tell patients to take fexofenadine with food if GI upset occurs, and to suck on sugarless lozenges if dry mouth is a problem.
- The nurse must warn patients to report difficulty breathing, tremors, hallucinations, and palpitations and must teach patients and their families about safety measures that may be needed if these CNS effects occur. The nurse also should caution patients to keep fexofenadine out of the reach of children.
- The nurse should encourage patients to use a humidifier, drink fluids, and avoid overly dry spaces and smoke-filled areas to help decrease the problems associated with the drying effects of antihistamines.

Ongoing Assessment and Evaluation

After several days taking this drug, the patient should experience little discomfort associated with the drug's adverse effects. There will be no report of injury related to the CNS effects of this drug. The patient will not experience respiratory difficulty related to the anticholinergic effects of the drug. ■

DRUGS CLOSELY RELATED TO FEXOFENADINE

Loratadine

Loratadine (Claritin), like fexofenadine, is a second-generation antihistamine. It has fewer CNS effects than other H_1 receptor blockers and can be administered once a day. It is not indicated for children younger than 6 years old. Patients with hepatic dysfunction should take loratadine on an every-other-day regimen. Loratadine is most effective when taken on an empty stomach.

Cetirizine

Cetirizine (Zyrtec) is another of the H_1 receptor blockers. Like loratadine, it is given as a once-a-day medication. Cetirizine also is approved for use in children as young as 2 years of age.

DRUGS SIGNIFICANTLY DIFFERENT FROM FEXOFENADINE

Diphenhydramine

Diphenhydramine (Benadryl) is a first-generation antihistamine known as an ethanolamine. Other ethanolamine antihistamines are carbinoxamine, clemastine, dimenhydrinate, doxylamine, and phenyltoloxamine. Ethanolamine antihistamines have significant antimuscarinic activity and produce marked sedation in most patients. In general, GI effects are minimal. In addition to treating allergic symptoms, diphenhydramine is effective in relieving nausea, vomiting, and vertigo associated with motion sickness. It also is used commonly to treat drug-induced extrapyramidal symptoms and mild cases of Parkinson disease.

Brompheniramine and Chlorpheniramine

Brompheniramine (Dimetane) and chlorpheniramine (Chlor-Trimeton) are OTC antihistamines, which also may be used in conjunction with decongestants. They are nonselective H_1 blockers (first-generation antihistamines), and thus have sedative effects. Brompheniramine causes less sedation than other first-generation antihistamine agents. These drugs are given to treat allergies such as hay fever, allergic conjunctivitis, urticaria (hives), and angioedema (allergic swelling). They reduce sneezing, runny noses, and itching eyes in hay fever. In addition, they have a mild anticholinergic action that suppresses mucus secretion. Their advantage is that they are relatively inexpensive. The major detriment is that they must be taken every 4 to 6 hours.

MEMORY CHIP

Fexofenadine

- Used for allergic disorders
- Significant contraindication: use in children younger than 12 years old
- Most common adverse effects: flu-like symptoms, nausea and vomiting, dysmenorrhea, and drowsiness
- Most serious adverse effect: potential for QT prolongation
- Maximizing therapeutic effects: assist drug with use of humidifier and increase the fluid intake
- Minimizing adverse effects: adhere to safety precautions
- Most significant patient education: use for symptoms related to allergic disorders; do **not** use for symptoms related to common viral illness, such as colds

EXPECTORANT DRUGS

Expectorants are drugs that liquefy lower respiratory tract secretions. This results in a decrease in the viscosity of the secretions (which makes it easier for the patient to cough them up) and improves air flow. Expectorants are available in many OTC preparations, making them widely available to the patient without advice from a health care provider. Drugs within the expectorant class include guaifenesin and terpin hydrate. Although not within the expectorant class, iodine preparations have actions very similar to drugs within this class. Guaifenesin (Robitussin) is the prototype expectorant drug.

NURSING MANAGEMENT OF THE PATIENT RECEIVING GUAIFENESIN

Core Drug Knowledge

Pharmacotherapeutics

Guaifenesin is used for the symptomatic relief of respiratory conditions characterized by a dry, nonproductive cough. These disorders include the common cold, acute bronchitis, and influenza. Guaifenesin is often found in combination with antihistamines and decongestants (Table 35-6).

Pharmacokinetics

Guaifenesin is taken orally and is absorbed readily from the GI tract with an onset of action of 30 minutes. The duration of action is 4 to 6 hours. The half-life and metabolic rate of this drug are unknown. It is eliminated by the kidneys. Other pharmacokinetic parameters remain unknown.

TABLE 35-6 Summary of Selected Expectorants

Drug (Trade) Name	Selected Indications	Route and Dosage Range	Pharmacokinetics
guaifenesin (Robitussin, Scot-Tussin, Mytussin, Fenesin, and many more)	Relief of conditions characterized by dry, nonproductive cough Presence of mucus in the respiratory tract	*Adult:* PO, 100–400 mg q4h, not to exceed 2.4 g/d *Child:* >12 y: PO, adult dosage 6–12 y: PO, 100–200 mg q4h, not to exceed 1.2 g/d 2–6 y: PO, 50–100 mg q4h, not to exceed 600 mg/d	*Onset:* 30 min *Duration:* 4–6 h $t_{1/2}$: Unknown
terpin hydrate (various)	Symptomatic relief of dry, nonproductive cough	*Adult:* PO, 85–170 mg tid–qid *Child:* Do not give unless prescribed 10–12 y: 85 mg tid–qid 5–9 y: 40 mg tid–qid 1–4 y: 20 mg tid–qid	*Onset:* 30–60 min *Duration:* Unknown $t_{1/2}$: Unknown
iodine preparations (SSKI, Potassium Iodide)	Symptomatic treatment of COPD diseases in which tenacious mucus complicates the problem	*Adult:* PO, 300–1000 mg after meals bid–tid *Child:* PO, 150–500 mg after meals bid–tid	*Onset:* 30 min *Duration:* Unknown $t_{1/2}$: Unknown

Pharmacodynamics

Guaifenesin enhances the output of respiratory tract fluids by reducing the adhesiveness and surface tension of the respiratory fluids, allowing easier movement of the less viscous secretions. The result of this thinning of secretions is a more productive cough. With a more productive cough, the frequency of coughing should decrease.

Contraindications and Precautions

The only known contraindication to guaifenesin is a known allergy to the drug. The drug is assigned to pregnancy category C and therefore should be used with caution in patients who are pregnant or lactating. The most important consideration in the use of this drug is discovering the cause of the underlying cough. Prolonged use of the OTC preparation could result in the masking of important symptoms of a serious underlying disorder. The drug should not be used for more than a week, and if the cough persists, the nurse should encourage the patient to see a health care provider.

Adverse Effects

The most common adverse effects of guaifenesin use are GI symptoms, including nausea, vomiting, and anorexia. Some patients experience a headache or dizziness, and an occasional person will develop a mild rash.

Drug Interactions

Guaifenesin has no significant drug-drug interactions. However, it may interfere with colorimetric tests and give false results for 5-HIAA and vanillylmandelic acid urinary catecholamine determinations.

Assessment of Relevant Core Patient Variables

Health Status

The nurse should assess the patient for any past hypersensitivity to guaifenesin; history of persistent cough for more than 1 week; cough due to smoking, asthma, or emphysema; or a very productive cough. In addition, the nurse should perform a physical assessment, which should include an examination of the patient's skin condition (as a baseline if a rash develops), temperature (to monitor for underlying problems), respiratory status, and adventitious breath sounds.

Life Span and Gender

The nurse should determine whether the patient is pregnant. Guaifenesin is a pregnancy category C drug and so should be used very cautiously by pregnant patients.

Lifestyle, Diet, and Habits

It is important to assess the patient's smoking habits and typical alcohol intake. Smokers will not benefit from the action of guaifenesin because the etiology of their cough is irritation. When using guaifenesin, the patient should take care not to drink alcohol or use other drugs containing alcohol.

Nursing Diagnoses and Outcomes

- Imbalanced Nutrition: Less than Body Requirements related to GI symptoms of nausea and vomiting
  Desired outcome: The patient will maintain baseline weight and nutritional status.
- Ineffective Airway Clearance related to increased viscosity of secretions

Desired outcome: The patient will demonstrate effective coughing technique and make use of several methods to increase airway clearance.

Planning and Intervention

Maximizing Therapeutic Effects

The nurse should teach the patient about good pulmonary toilet, which includes coughing, deep breathing, drinking plenty of fluids, and using a humidifier. In addition, the nurse should show the patient how to perform effective coughing technique. Family members may assist with percussion and postural drainage as appropriate.

Minimizing Adverse Effects

The nurse should suggest that the patient eat small, frequent meals to alleviate GI upset. Additionally, the nurse can give the drug with meals if symptoms become intolerable.

Providing Patient and Family Education

- The nurse should explain to patients that guaifenesin will help make it easier to cough up secretions from the lungs.
- It is important that the nurse warn patients not to take guaifenesin if they are allergic to it, if their cough is due to smoking, or if their cough is chronic (unless approved by their provider).
- The nurse should tell patients not to use guaifenesin for longer than 1 week, and if the cough persists after that time, or if fever or rash develops, they should consult with their health care provider.
- It is important to caution patients not to take any other drugs while taking guaifenesin without their provider's approval and not to drink alcohol while taking this drug.
- The nurse should tell patients that if a dose is missed, it should be taken as soon as remembered unless it is time for the next dose. Two doses should never be taken at the same time.
- The nurse should teach patients ways to augment guaifenesin therapy, such as drinking a glass of water with each dose. Lots of water will help the body thin the secretions in the lungs and will help guaifenesin work better. Other ways to augment drug therapy include use of a humidifier, deep breathing, chest percussion, and positional drainage if needed. In addition, the nurse should teach patients good coughing technique and should encourage patients to use the technique regularly.

Ongoing Assessment and Evaluation

The nurse should monitor the patient's reaction to the drug carefully; fever, rash, or persistent cough may indicate a more serious underlying medical problem, and appropriate follow-up should be arranged. The patient will tolerate drug adverse effects through use of small, frequent meals and proper timing of dosage. Within 1 week, the patient will exhibit an increasingly productive cough and good movement of respiratory secretions as seen by productive cough and clearing breath sounds. ■

MEMORY CHIP

Guaifenesin

- Used for management of dry cough
- Significant contraindication: hypersensitivity
- Most common adverse effects: nausea, vomiting, and anorexia
- Maximizing therapeutic effects: good pulmonary toilet
- Minimizing adverse effects: small frequent meals to decrease GI distress
- Most significant patient education: seek medical attention if cough does not resolve

DRUGS CLOSELY RELATED TO GUAIFENESIN

Terpin Hydrate

Terpin hydrate stimulates the glands of the respiratory tract to increase the amount of fluid secreted. Actions and management related to this drug are very similar to those for guaifenesin. However, terpin hydrate contains about 42% alcohol, which crosses the placenta and may result in congenital abnormalities. The alcohol in terpin hydrate also is excreted in breast milk and can be harmful to infants.

Iodine Preparations

These drugs have been used for many years to stimulate an increase in the fluid produced by the lungs. They are used in treating chronic obstructive pulmonary disease and as adjunctive treatment in respiratory tract conditions, such as cystic fibrosis, and chronic sinusitis and after surgery to prevent atelectasis. These drugs tend to have a bitter flavor, limiting their popularity. They must be used with caution with many conditions because of the effect of iodine on the thyroid gland. Iodine preparations are assigned to pregnancy category X because of potential damage to the fetal thyroid.

CHAPTER SUMMARY

- The upper respiratory system is composed of upper or conducting airways, including the nares, nasal sinus, pharynx, larynx, and trachea.
- Disorders of the upper respiratory system include inflammation and irritation of the upper airways.
- Antitussives, such as dextromethorphan, are drugs used to suppress the cough reflex when dry, nonproductive coughing is tiring and irritating to the respiratory system.
- Decongestants, such as pseudoephedrine, are drugs used to decrease the swelling and blood flow to the mucosa of the respiratory tract. Oral decongestants are taken systemically and have the potential for more systemic adverse effects. Topical decongestants are applied directly to

the mucosa and have less potential for adverse effects. However, the topical decongestants have more potential for causing rebound congestion if used more than 5 days.

- Antihistamines, such as fexofenadine, are used to block the action of histamine as it is released in response to an inflammatory reaction. These drugs block the swelling and congestion that follow histamine release.
- Expectorants, such as guaifenesin, are drugs used to increase the viscosity and volume of the respiratory tract secretions, helping patients to clear the lower respiratory tract of tenacious secretions.

QUESTIONS FOR STUDY AND REVIEW

1. What is the difference between dextromethorphan and narcotic antitussive agents?
2. Why are antihistamines inappropriate for the treatment of the common viral cold?
3. What property of fexofenadine makes it an excellent antihistamine?
4. How does guaifenesin assist in the control of cough?

NEED MORE HELP?

Chapter 35 of the study guide for *Drug Therapy in Nursing* contains exercises and activities to reinforce your understanding of the concepts presented in this chapter. For additional information see the text's accompanying website at *http://www.connection.lww.com.*

REFERENCES AND BIBLIOGRAPHY

Bousquet, J. (1998). Antihistamines in severe/chronic rhinitis. *Clinical and Experimental Allergy, 28,* (Suppl. 6), 49–53.

CCIS System. (2001). *Computerized Clinical Information System.* Denver, CO: Micromedex.

Clinical Drug Monographs. (2001). [CD-ROM]. Gold Standard Media.

Drug Facts and Comparisons. (2000). St. Louis: Facts and Comparisons.

Ferguson, B. J. (1998). Cost-effective pharmacotherapy for allergic rhinitis. *Otolaryngology Clinics of North America, 31*(1), 91–110.

Hardman, J. G., Limbird, L. E., Molinof, P. B., Ruddon, R. W., & Gilman, A. (Eds.). (1997). *Goodman and Gilman's pharmacological basis of therapeutics* (9th ed.). New York: McGraw-Hill.

Howarth, P. H. (1999). Assessment of antihistamine efficacy and potency. *Clinical and Experimental Allergy, 29,* (Suppl. 3), 87–97.

Karch, A. (2001). *2001 Lippincott's nursing drug guide.* Philadelphia: Lippincott Williams & Wilkins.

Katzung, B. C. (2000). *Basic and clinical pharmacology* (8th ed.). New York: McGraw-Hill.

Mason, J., Reynolds, R., & Rao, N. (1999). The systemic safety of fexofenadine HCl. *Clinical and Experimental Allergy, 29,* (Suppl. 3), 163–170; discussion 171–173.

Mitchelson, F. (1998). Which cough mixture? *Australian Family Physician, 27*(11), 1041–1046.

Naclerio, R. M. (1998). Optimizing treatment options. *Clinical and Experimental Allergy, 28,* (Suppl. 6), 54–59.

Porth, C. (1998). *Pathophysiology: Concepts of altered health states* (5th ed.). Philadelphia: Lippincott Williams & Wilkins.

Pratt, C., et al. (1999). Cardiovascular safety of fexofenadine HCl. *Clinical and Experimental Allergy, 29,* (Suppl. 3), 212–216.

Tatro, D. (Ed.). (2000). *Drug interaction facts* (6th ed.). St. Louis: Facts and Comparisons.

Chapter 36

DRUGS AFFECTING THE LOWER RESPIRATORY SYSTEM

KEY TERMS

bronchodilators
bronchospasm
chemoreceptors
chronic airway limitation (CAL)
chronic obstructive pulmonary disease (COPD)
mucolytics
perfusion
respiration
ventilation

Learning Objectives

At the completion of this chapter the student will:

1. Describe the anatomy and physiology of the lower respiratory system.
2. Identify core drug knowledge pertaining to drugs that affect the lower respiratory system.
3. Identify core patient variables pertaining to drugs that affect the lower respiratory system.
4. Relate the interaction of core drug knowledge to core patient variables for drugs that affect the lower respiratory system.
5. Generate a nursing plan of care from the interactions between core drug knowledge and core patient variables for drugs that affect the lower respiratory system.
6. Describe nursing interventions to maximize therapeutic and minimize adverse effects for drugs that affect the lower respiratory system.
7. Determine key points for patient and family education for drugs that affect the lower respiratory system.
8. Compare and contract drugs used in the maintenance of lower airway disorders and drugs used in the management of acute exacerbations of lower airway disorders.

Mucolytics
- **acetylcysteine** (P)
- dornase alfa

Bronchodilators

Beta agonists
- **albuterol** (P)
- bitolterol
- epinephrine
- isoproterenol
- metaproterenol
- pirbuterol
- salmeterol
- terbutaline

Anticholinergics
- **ipratropium bromide** (P)

Xanthine derivatives
- **theophylline** (P)
- aminophylline
- diphylline
- caffeine

Anti-inflammatory agents

Inhaled glucocorticoid steroids
- beclomethasone
- dexamethasone
- flunisolide
- fluticasone
- triamcinolone

Mast cell stabilizers
- **cromolyn sodium** (P)
- nedocromil

Leukotriene receptor antagonists
- **zafirlukast** (P)
- montelukast
- zileuton

The symbol (C) indicates the **drug class**.

Drugs in bold type marked with the symbol (P) are **prototypes**.

Drugs in blue type with no symbol are **closely related** to the prototype.

Drugs in **red** type with no symbol are **significantly different** from the prototype.

Drugs in **black** type with no symbol are **also used in drug therapy**; no prototype.

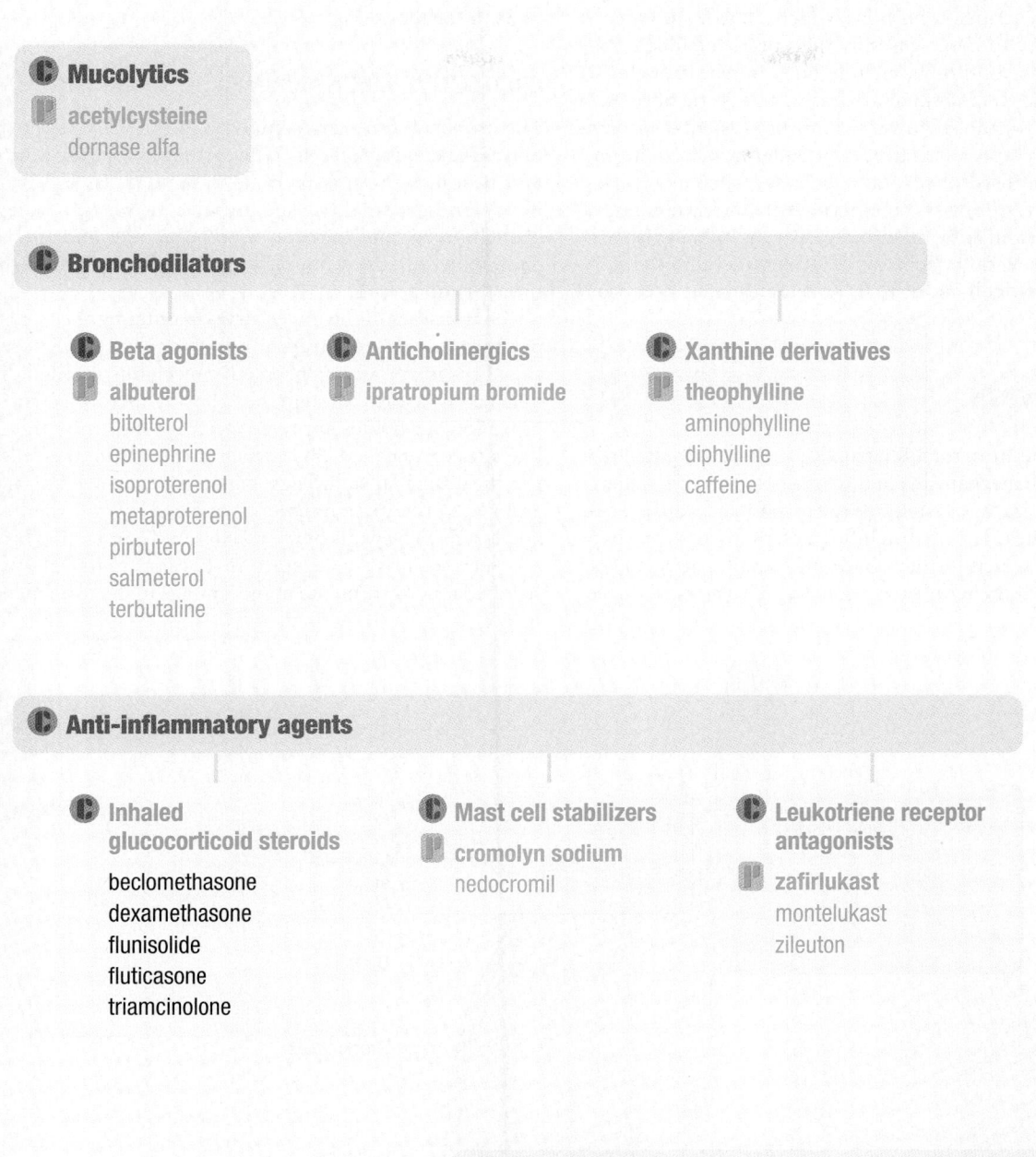

This chapter discusses drugs that affect the lower respiratory system. The lower respiratory system is affected by many serious conditions, which all, to some extent, affect the ability to move gases in and out of the lungs. Examples of these conditions include pneumonia, bronchitis, chronic obstructive pulmonary diseases, and cystic fibrosis.

Drugs used to manage lower respiratory system disorders include mucolytics such as acetylcysteine; bronchodilators, which are composed of several subclasses, such as sympathomimetics (respiratory beta-agonists), anticholinergics, and xanthines; and anti-inflammatory drugs, which also are composed of several subclasses of drugs, including glucocorticoids, mast cell stabilizers, and leukotriene receptor antagonists.

PHYSIOLOGY

The lower respiratory tract is virtually sterile as a result of the various defense mechanisms in the upper respiratory system. The lower respiratory system, or the respiratory airway, begins at the trachea. The trachea bifurcates, or divides, into two main bronchi, which further divide into smaller and smaller branches, hence the term *bronchial tree*. The bronchial tree flows into the paired lungs, which are composed of a network of blood vessels and small bronchi and alveoli: the functional units of the lungs (Fig. 36-1).

PROTECTIVE MECHANISMS

The bronchial tubes are composed of three layers: cartilage, muscle, and epithelial cells. The cartilage keeps the tube open and becomes progressively less abundant as the bronchi divide and get smaller. The muscles also help to keep the bronchi open, and they too become smaller and less abundant, with only a few muscle fibers remaining in the terminal bronchi and alveoli.

All the tubes in the lower airway contain goblet cells that produce mucus to entrap any particles that may have escaped the upper airway protective mechanisms. In addition, during the passage through the bronchi, microorganisms and other foreign bodies are removed from the air by tiny hair-like structures called cilia, which project from the cells that line the bronchial wall. These cilia exhibit a wave-like motion and sweep the foreign material upward toward the trachea and larynx. The walls of the trachea and conducting bronchi are very sensitive to irritation. Foreign material and the secreted mucus stimulate nerve endings in the bronchial wall

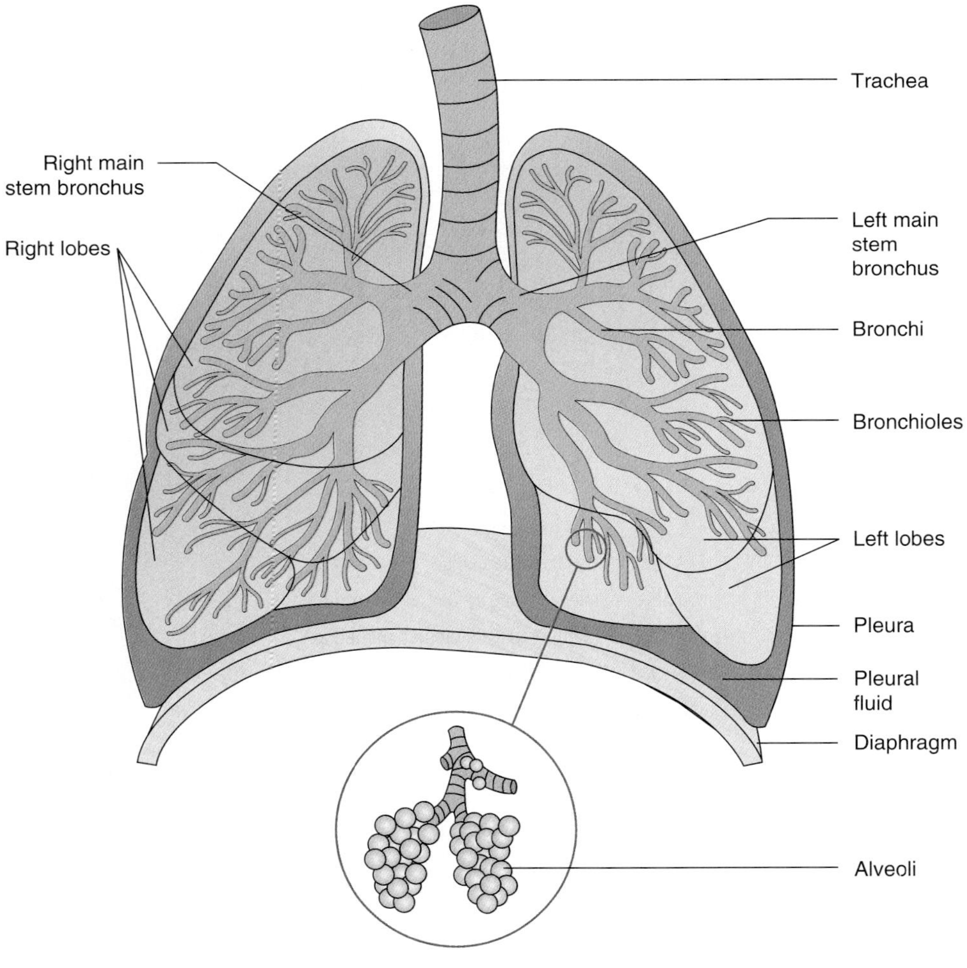

Figure 36-1. Lower respiratory system.

and initiate the cough reflex. Coughing then completes the expulsion of the foreign material and secreted mucus from the bronchial tree.

GAS EXCHANGE, PERFUSION, AND RESPIRATION

Lung tissue receives its blood supply from the bronchial artery, which branches directly off the thoracic aorta. The alveoli receive unoxygenated blood from the right ventricle by way of the pulmonary artery. The delivery of this blood to the alveoli is referred to as **perfusion.** In the alveoli, gas exchange occurs; carbon dioxide is removed from the blood while oxygen diffuses into the blood. This exchange of gases at the alveolar level is called **respiration.** The alveolar sac can stay open because the nitrogen and oxygen gases and the lipoprotein surfactant increase the tension of the cells, leading to alveolar collapse. Oxygenated blood is returned to the left atrium through the pulmonary veins. From there, it is pumped throughout the body to deliver oxygen and pick up waste products.

VENTILATION

Ventilation, or the act of breathing, is controlled by the central nervous system (CNS). The inspiratory muscles (i.e., diaphragm, external intercostal, and abdominal) are stimulated to contract by the respiratory center in the medulla. The medulla receives input from the **chemoreceptors** (neuroreceptors sensitive to carbon dioxide and acid levels) and increases the rate or depth of respiration to maintain homeostasis in the body. The vagus nerve, a predominant parasympathetic nerve, plays a key role in stimulating diaphragm contraction and inspiration. Vagal stimulation also leads to bronchoconstriction or tightening. The sympathetic system also innervates the respiratory system. Stimulation of the sympathetic system will lead to increased rate and depth of respiration and will dilate the bronchi to allow freer air flow through the system. It is interesting to note that during a physical examination the nurse documents vital signs as temperature, pulse, and respirations (TPR). To be accurate, the nurse is actually assessing the ventilatory rate, not the respiratory rate. However, the authors of this text do not recommend changing the long-standing method of charting vital signs.

PATHOPHYSIOLOGY

PNEUMONIA

Pneumonia is an inflammation of the lungs. It can be caused by bacterial or viral invasion of the tissue or by aspiration of foreign substances into the lower respiratory tract. The lung tissue progresses through an inflammatory reaction that will produce symptoms of difficulty breathing, fever, productive cough, shortness of breath, and sometimes chest pain. Pneumonia is more frequently seen when a person's immune system is compromised or when the person has an upper respiratory disorder that causes the normal protective mechanisms to be inefficient.

ACUTE BRONCHITIS

Acute bronchitis is most frequently caused by viruses. Therefore, it may be a sequela to the common cold, influenza, whooping cough, and measles. Bacterial organisms such as *Streptococci* and *Staphylococci* also may cause acute bronchitis. Furthermore, it can be precipitated by a variety of physical and chemical agents, such as fumes of strong acids, ammonia, or organic solvents. Symptoms of acute bronchitis include fever, a productive cough, and purulent mucus. Inflammation often narrows or obstructs a person's airway, making bronchitis a potentially serious condition. Treatment includes bronchodilators and expectorants as well as antibiotic therapy if indicated. The course of the disease is commonly short: 2 to 4 days. However, untreated acute bronchitis may develop into chronic bronchitis.

CHRONIC OBSTRUCTIVE PULMONARY DISEASES

Chronic obstructive pulmonary disease (COPD) also is known as **chronic airway limitation** (CAL). COPD is an umbrella term that describes gradually progressive, degenerative diseases, such as chronic bronchitis, emphysema, or repeated, severe asthma attacks. In COPD, the bronchioles become thick and edematous, the upper respiratory defense mechanisms are destroyed, and constant irritation and inflammation of the lower respiratory tract are present. With time, the fragile alveoli enlarge and collapse or fuse. Air is trapped in the lungs as the elastic fibers are lost, and increasing amounts of energy are required to try to move the air through the narrowed bronchial tubes. The lungs overinflate and the efficiency of gas exchange is lost. The person suffering from COPD complains of dyspnea and shortness of breath. A barrel chest develops as the lungs overinflate. The person is fatigued from the poor oxygenation of the blood and from the increased expenditure of energy with breathing.

Chronic Bronchitis

Chronic bronchitis is long-standing, largely irreversible, inflammation of the bronchial tree. The continuous injury to the lining of the bronchial tree has destroyed many of the cells, the cilia are absent, and the defense mechanism against invading foreign material is lost. The bronchial tubes are narrow, rigid, and distorted. There is hypersecretion of viscous mucous materials resulting in a chronic, deep, and productive cough. The cough is difficult to suppress and actually should not be because the abundant secretion has to be eliminated to avoid the danger of severe superimposed infection.

Excessive and prolonged tobacco smoking can be one of the causes of chronic bronchitis and is certainly one its most aggravating factors. Infections of the sinus cavities also provide a reservoir of available microorganisms, which can continually reinfect the lungs. Damaged bronchi are ideal sites for harboring infections and for accumulation of excess fluids and secreted mucus. Episodes of acute bronchitis and pneumonia are frequent because the respiratory tract is more susceptible to invasion by pathogenic microorganisms.

Emphysema

Emphysema is an abnormal distention of the lungs with air. The lungs show loss or degeneration of elastic tissue, disappearance of capillary walls, and breakdown of the alveolar walls. The alveoli first stretch and then tend to disintegrate. The lungs become filled with large pools of air, and loss of elastic support around small airways, or loss of small airways themselves, severely interferes with expiration. Like chronic bronchitis, smoking is the main cause of emphysema. Symptoms include severe breathlessness on exertion, weight loss, and swelling in the extremities. The skin takes on a bluish color from lack of sufficient gas exchange, there is tightness in the chest, and the affected person wheezes.

Bullous emphysema is a variety of emphysema in which the distended alveoli form large air cysts on one or both of the lungs and occasionally rupture, causing lung collapse.

Asthma

Asthma is a disorder characterized by recurrent episodes of **bronchospasm**, which is bronchial muscle spasm leading to narrowed or obstructed airways. Asthma has been classified as either intrinsic or extrinsic. Intrinsic asthma has no identifiable cause but has been associated with exercise and emotional stress. Extrinsic asthma occurs as a result of an allergic reaction to an environmental allergen. Exposure to the antigen causes a rapid and intense inflammatory reaction with the release of histamine, serotonin, and leukotrienes. These chemicals cause a severe bronchoconstriction and an increase in mucus production. In addition, with the increase in pressure in the system, movement of fluid into the tissues results in further obstruction. This reaction usually occurs within 5 to 30 minutes after exposure to the allergen. An extreme type of asthma is called status asthmaticus. This is a life-threatening bronchospasm, which occludes air flow into the lungs and requires emergency treatment (see the accompanying display, Classifications of Asthma).

CYSTIC FIBROSIS

Cystic fibrosis is a hereditary disease that affects the functioning of the body's exocrine glands: the mucus-secreting and sweat glands. In persons with this disease, a protein is produced that lacks the amino acid phenylalanine. This flawed protein distorts the movement of salt and water across the membranes that line the lungs and gut, resulting in dehydration of the mucus that normally coats these surfaces. Thus, the normal mucous secretions in the respiratory and digestive systems become abnormally thick, sticky, and concentrated. The thick, sticky mucus accumulates in the lungs, plugging the bronchi and making breathing difficult. This results in chronic respiratory infections, often bacterial. Chronic cough, recurrent pneumonia, and the progressive loss of lung function are the major manifestations of this disease. Treatment of these patients is aimed at keeping the secretions fluid and moving and maintaining airway patency as much as possible. Because the disease increases tenacious mucus secretions, acetylcysteine (Mucomyst), a mucolytic drug, is the drug of choice.

Classifications of Asthma

Mild Intermittent

- Symptoms occur two or fewer times per week
- Patient asymptomatic and normal peak flow between exacerbations
- Acute exacerbations tend to be brief but may range from moderate to severe
- Normal peak flow is greater than 80% of predicted value

Mild Persistent

- Symptoms occur more than twice per week but not daily
- Nocturnal symptoms occur more than twice per month
- Acute exacerbations interfere with daily activities
- Normal peak flow is greater than 80% of predicted value

Moderate Persistent

- Symptoms occur daily
- Rescue medication used daily
- Exacerbations affect activity
- Nocturnal symptoms occur more than once per week
- Acute exacerbations occur two or more times per week and may last for days
- Normal peak flow is 60% to 80% of predicted value

Severe Persistent

- Continued symptoms that limit physical activity
- Frequent acute exacerbations
- Frequent nocturnal symptoms
- Normal peak flow is less than 60% of predicted value

MUCOLYTIC DRUGS

Mucolytics break down mucus to help the high-risk respiratory patient cough up thick, tenacious secretions to improve breathing and air flow. The drugs may be administered by a nebulizer or by direct instillation into the trachea through an endotracheal tube or tracheostomy. Mucolytics usually are reserved for patients who have significant difficulty mobilizing and coughing up secretions. Mucolytic drugs include acetylcysteine and dornase alfa. Acetylcysteine is the prototypical mucolytic agent.

NURSING MANAGEMENT OF THE PATIENT RECEIVING ACETYLCYSTEINE

Core Drug Knowledge

Pharmacotherapeutics

Acetylcysteine is used to liquefy the thick, tenacious secretions of patients whose respiratory disorders make it difficult to mobilize and cough up these secretions.

These disorders include COPD, cystic fibrosis, pneumonia, and tuberculosis. It also is indicated for patients who develop atelectasis (a collapsing of alveoli) because of thick mucus secretions. It can be used during diagnostic bronchoscopy to clear the airway, to facilitate the removal of secretions postoperatively, and to facilitate airway clearance and suctioning in patients with tracheostomies. Acetylcysteine also is used orally to treat acetaminophen-induced hepatotoxicity.

Pharmacokinetics

Acetylcysteine is delivered directly to the respiratory system by nebulizer (inhalation) or direct instillation. Onset of effect occurs within 1 minute, with a peak effect occurring within 5 to 10 minutes. The drug is metabolized in the liver and is excreted in the urine (Table 36-1).

Pharmacodynamics

Acetylcysteine affects the mucoproteins in the respiratory secretions. It splits disulfide bonds that are responsible for holding the mucous material together. The result is a decrease in the tenacity and viscosity of the secretions. This drug also protects liver cells from being damaged during episodes of acetaminophen toxicity. It has this effect because it normalizes hepatic glutathione levels and binds with a reactive hepatotoxic metabolite of acetaminophen.

Contraindications and Precautions

Acetylcysteine is contraindicated in patients who are hypersensitive to the drug. It is assigned to pregnancy category C and therefore should be used with caution in pregnant or lactating women. The drug also should be used with caution in patients with a history of respiratory disease. For example, acetylcysteine should be used with caution in any condition that compromises the patient's ability to cough because the increased volume of secretions can compromise the airway if it is not cleared. It should also be used with caution with patients who have asthma because bronchospasm can occur.

Adverse Effects

This drug is administered directly into the respiratory tract. Therefore, the main adverse effects are bronchospasm, bronchoconstriction, chest tightness, a burning feeling in the upper airway, and rhinorrhea. Some patients report stomatitis and nausea as well. Less frequent adverse effects are fever, chills, drowsiness, and clammy skin.

Drug Interactions

No significant drug interactions have been reported for acetylcysteine.

Assessment of Relevant Core Patient Variables

Health Status

Before the nurse initiates therapy, a physical examination should be performed. This examination should include a baseline temperature, skin evaluation, and respiratory evaluation (including adventitious sounds and ability to cough).

TABLE 36-1 Summary of Selected Mucolytics

Drug (Trade) Name	Selected Indications	Route and Dosage Range	Pharmacokinetics
acetylcysteine (Mucomyst; *Canadian:* Parvolex)	Mucolytic adjuvant therapy for abnormal or viscous mucous secretions in acute and chronic bronchopulmonary disease Diagnostic bronchial studies Acetaminophen antidote	Nebulization with face mask, mouthpiece, tracheostomy 1–10 mL of 20% solution or 2–20 mL of 10% solution q2–6h Nebulization with tent, croupette: up to 300 mL per treatment Instillation: Direct or by tracheostomy 1–2 mL of a 10%–20% solution q1–4h Diagnostic bronchogram: Before the procedure, give two to three administrations of 1–2 mL of a 20% solution or 2–4 mL of a 10% solution by nebulization or intratracheal instillation Acetaminophen antidote: PO, 140 mg/kg loading dose followed by 17 maintenance doses of 70 mg/kg starting 4 h after the loading dose	*Onset:* Instillation and inhalation, 1 min *Duration:* 2–3 h $t_{1/2}$: 6–25 h
dornase alfa (Pulmozyme)	Management of respiratory symptoms associated with cystic fibrosis	*Adult:* Inhaled, 2.5 mg qid through nebulizer *Child:* >5 y, inhaled, adult dosage	*Onset:* Slow *Duration:* 1 wk $t_{1/2}$: Unknown

Life Span and Gender

The nurse should assess whether the patient is pregnant or breast-feeding because acetylcysteine should be avoided during pregnancy and lactation unless the benefit outweighs the potential risk to the fetus or child.

Environment

The nurse should note the environment in which acetylcysteine will be administered. Usually acetylcysteine is administered with the supervision of a respiratory therapist or specially trained nurse, although some patients or caregivers trained to administer it may give it at home.

Nursing Diagnoses and Outcomes

- Ineffective Airway Clearance related to drug effect and potential bronchospasm

  Desired outcome: The patient's airway will be maintained without increased difficulty breathing.
- Disturbed Sensory Perception: Olfactory, related to odor of drug and route of administration

  Desired outcome: The patient will remain comfortable and able to tolerate drug therapy.

Planning and Intervention

Maximizing Therapeutic Effects

The nurse should read the instructions regarding the inhalation mask before administering acetylcysteine. The nurse should monitor the nebulizer for any build-up in the drug from evaporation. Diluting the drug with sterile water for injection will prevent the concentrate from impeding drug delivery. The nurse should administer 20% solution if diluted with normal saline or sterile water and 10% solution if undiluted. The solution should be refrigerated and used within 96 hours to ensure effectiveness.

Minimizing Adverse Effects

The nurse should inform the patient that nebulization may produce an initially disagreeable odor, but that it is transient. It is best to use water to remove residual drug from the patient's face after administration by face mask; the drug may irritate the face and will make it feel sticky and uncomfortable. Finally, it is important for the nurse to establish a routine for pulmonary toilet to eliminate secretions as efficiently as possible; suction equipment should be kept available.

Providing Patient and Family Education

- The nurse should explain to patients that acetylcysteine will help to get rid of mucus in the lungs.
- The nurse should inform the patient that she or he must not take this drug without the assistance of a respiratory therapist or other health care provider unless he has been taught how to prepare the drug and how to use the nebulizer for administration.
- It is important for the nurse to warn patients not to take any other drugs without their provider's approval and not to drink alcohol while taking this drug.
- The nurse should teach patients and their family members all aspects of pulmonary toilet, including drainage, cupping, coughing, and deep breathing exercises. The nurse also can encourage other methods of keeping secretions loose: drinking plenty of fluids, using a humidifier, and avoiding dry or smoke-filled areas.
- The nurse should inform the patient that nebulization may produce a disagreeable odor, but that it is transient. In addition, it is helpful to explain to patients the need to wipe off their faces with water to remove the residual drug after administration by face mask because the drug may irritate the face and will make it feel uncomfortable. These patient education tips will help to increase compliance with drug therapy.
- The nurse should instruct patients to report all adverse effects, including difficulty breathing, severe nausea, and dizziness.

Ongoing Assessment and Evaluation

The nurse should assess the patient for proper techniques of pulmonary toilet. After a few days, the patient will have had no incidents of difficulty breathing. The patient will be tolerating and continuing with drug therapy. There will be evidence, by history and breath sounds, that secretions are loosening and the patient is having success coughing and moving secretions out. ■

DRUG CLOSELY RELATED TO ACETYLCYSTEINE

Dornase alfa (Pulmozyme) is a mucolytic prepared by techniques that use recombinant deoxyribonucleic acid (DNA). The drug selectively breaks down respiratory tract mucus by separating extracellular DNA from proteins. This drug is used to relieve the build-up of secretions in cystic fibrosis. It

MEMORY CHIP

Acetylcysteine

- Used to liquefy thick tenacious secretions
- Significant contraindication: hypersensitivity
- Most common adverse effects: nausea, vomiting, and rhinorrhea
- Most serious adverse effects: bronchospasm and bronchoconstriction
- Maximizing therapeutic effects: refrigerate the solution and use it within 96 hours
- Minimizing adverse effects: keep suction equipment close by
- Most significant patient education: correct use of special equipment

does not replace any other therapy for cystic fibrosis, but it does help to keep the airways open and functioning longer. Caution must be used in anyone with a history of hypersensitivity to hamster protein because the drug is manufactured using Chinese hamster ovary cells. It is not yet recommended in children younger than 5 years old. Adverse effects can include hoarseness and sore throat related to nebulizer use, skin rash, and conjunctivitis.

BRONCHODILATORS

Bronchodilators are drugs used to facilitate respiration by dilating the airways. Sympathomimetics (beta-2-adrenergic agonists), such as albuterol; anticholinergics, such as ipratropium bromide; and xanthine derivatives, such as theophylline, are commonly administered bronchodilators used in the treatment of respiratory diseases.

BETA-AGONISTS (SYMPATHOMIMETICS)

As discussed in Chapter 14, sympathomimetics are drugs that mimic the effects of the sympathetic nervous system. As a quick review, there are two subtypes of beta-receptors in the body: beta-1 and beta-2. Drugs that stimulate these receptors may be nonspecific or selective to either beta-1 or beta-2. Beta-2 receptors are more predominant in the lungs, whereas beta-1 receptors are more predominant in the heart. One of the actions of beta stimulation in the sympathetic nervous system is dilation of the bronchi and increased rate and depth of respiration. For respiratory disorders, the drugs of choice would be those that are beta-2 selective.

Included in the beta-agonist subclass of bronchodilators are albuterol, bitolterol mesylate, epinephrine, isoproterenol, metaproterenol, pirbuterol, salmeterol, and terbutaline. Albuterol (Proventil, Ventolin) is the prototypical beta-agonist agent.

NURSING MANAGEMENT OF THE PATIENT RECEIVING ALBUTEROL

Core Drug Knowledge

Pharmacotherapeutics

Albuterol is used as a bronchodilator in the management of COPD and asthma (Table 36-2).

TABLE 36-2 Summary of Selected Bronchodilators

Drug (Trade) Name	Selected Indications	Route and Dosage Range	Pharmacokinetics
Beta-Agonists			
albuterol (Proventil; *Canadian:* Asmavent)	Relief of bronchospasm in patients with reversible obstructive airway disease Prevention of exercise-induced bronchospasm Unlabeled use: Adjunct in treating serious hyperkalemia in dialysis patients; seems to lower potassium concentrations when inhaled by patients on hemodialysis	*Adult:* PO, 2–4 mg tid–qid; inhalation, 2 puffs q4–6h *Child:* >12 y: PO, adult dosage; inhalation, adult dosage 6–12 y: PO, 2 mg tid 2–6 y: PO, 0.1 mg/kg tid, not to exceed 2 mg tid Inhalation for <12 y: safety not established	*Onset:* PO, 30 min; inhalation, 5 min *Duration:* PO, 4–8 h; inhalation, 3–8h $t_{1/2}$: PO, 2–4 h; inhalation, 2–4 h
epinephrine, bitartrate (AsthmaHaler, Bronkaid Mist, Medihaler-Epi)	Respiratory distress	*Adult:* SC/IM, 0.3–0.5 mL of 1 : 1,000 solution q20min for 4 h; inhalation, 8–15 drops into nebulizer reservoir; repeat in 5 min *Child:* SC, 0.01 mg/kg or 0.3 mL/m² in 1 : 1,000 solution q20min for 4 h; topical nasal (>6 y), apply locally as drops or spray or with a sterile swab as indicated	*Onset:* SC, 5–10 min; IM, 5–10 min; inhalation, 3–5 min *Duration:* SC, 20–30 min; IM, 20–30 min; inhalation, 1–3 h $t_{1/2}$: SC, 5–6 h; IM, 5–6 h; inhalation, 5–6 h
isoproterenol sulfate (Medihaler)	Acute bronchial asthma COPD	*Adult:* Inhalation, 1:200 solution in 5–15 deep inhalations; IV, 0.01–0.02 mg of diluted solution; SL, 10 mg; do not repeat more than q3–4h or more than tid, do not exceed a total dose of 60 mg/d *Child:* Inhalation, 1 : 200 solution; do not use more than 0.25 mL of the 1 : 200 solution	*Onset:* Inhalation, rapid; IV, immediate; SL, rapid *Duration:* Inhalation, 50–60 min; IV, 1–2 min; SL, 2 h

(*continued*)

TABLE 36-2 Summary of Selected Bronchodilators (Continued)

Drug (Trade) Name	Selected Indications	Route and Dosage Range	Pharmacokinetics
		for each 10–15 min programmed treatment; SL, 5–10 mg; do not repeat more often than q3–4h or more often than tid; do not exceed a total dose of 30 mg/d	$t_{1/2}$: Inhalation, unknown; IV, unknown; SL, unknown
metaproterenol (Alupent)	Bronchodilation	*Adult:* PO, 20 mg q6–8h; inhalation, metered dose, 2–3 inhalations q3–4h; nebulizer, 5–10 inhalations of undiluted 5% solution q4–6h *Child:* >9 y: PO, 20 mg q6–8h 6–9 y; 10 mg q6–8h <6 y: 1.2–2.6 mg/kg/d in divided doses >12 y: Inhalation, same as adults <12 y: Inhalation, not recommended	*Onset:* PO, 15 min; inhalation, 1–4 min *Duration:* PO 4 h; inhalation, 3–4 h $t_{1/2}$: PO, unknown; inhalation, unknown
pirbuterol (Maxair)	COPD	MDI: 200 μg/puff *Adult and child:* 2 puffs q4–6h prn	*Onset:* Rapid *Duration:* 6 h $t_{1/2}$: 2–3 h
salmeterol (Serevent)	COPD	21 μg/puff *Adult and child:* 2 puffs q120h	*Onset:* 5–20 min *Duration:* 12 h $t_{1/2}$: 3–4 h
terbutaline (Brethine)	COPD Bronchospasm	*Adult:* PO, 2.5–5 mg tid at 6 h intervals; SC, 0.25 mg q15–30 min to a maximum of 0.5 mg q4h; inhalation, 2 inhalations separated by 60 s q4–6h *Child:* >12 y: Adult dosage for all routes <12 y: Safety and efficacy not established	*Onset:* PO, 30 min; SC, 30 min; inhalation, 5–30 min *Duration:* PO, 4–8 h; SC, 1.5–4 h; inhalation, 3–4 h $t_{1/2}$: PO, 3–4h; SC, 3–4 h; inhalation, 3–4 h
Combination Inhalers salmeterol and fluticasone DPI (Advair)	COPD Asthma	Diskus 100/50 (fluticasone 100 μg with salmeterol 50 μg Diskus 250/50 Diskus 500/50 *Adult and child > 12 years:* 1 inhalation bid	*Onset:* 30–60 min *Duration:* 12 h $t_{1/2}$: 5–7 h
Anticholinergic Agents			
ipratropium bromide (Atrovent)	COPD Rhinitis Common cold	*Adult:* Inhalation, metered dose inhaler, 2 inhalations qid no less than 4 h apart; intranasal (rhinitis), 2 sprays of 0.03% in each nostril bid–tid; intranasal (common cold), 2 sprays of 0.06% in each nostril tid–qid for up to 4 d	*Onset:* Inhalation, 15 min *Duration:* Inhalation, 3–4 h $t_{1/2}$: Inhalation, 2–3 h
Xanthine Derivatives			
theophylline (Slo-Phyllin; *Canadian:* Acet-Amp)	Acute asthma symptoms	*Adult:* (16–60 y): PO/IV, 300 mg/d in divided doses; titrate to maximum of 600 mg/d in divided doses; maintenance, up to 600 mg/d *Child:* (1–15 y): PO/IV, 12–14 mg/kg/d to maximum of 600 mg daily in divided doses; maintenance, up to 400 mg daily *Infant:* <53 wk: 0.2 mg × age in weeks; maintenance, 16 m	*Onset:* PO, varies; Peak: 2 h *Duration:* 2–3 d $t_{1/2}$: 3–5 h nonsmoker; 4–5 h smoker

TABLE 36-2 Summary of Selected Bronchodilators (Continued)

Drug (Trade) Name	Selected Indications	Route and Dosage Range	Pharmacokinetics
	Methotrexate toxicity Neonatal apnea Sleep apnea	*Adult and child:* >3 y: IV, 2.5 mg/kg Premature to 24 d: 1 mg/kg q12h 24 d+: 1.5 mg/kg q12h *Adults only:* 3.3 mg/kg bid	
aminophylline (Truphylline)	Acute asthma (child) Neonatal apnea Maintenance	*Adult and child:* >12: IV 0.7 mg/kg IV 0.5 mg/kg 0–24 d: 2 mg/kg/d divided dose q12h *Adult:* PO, 3 mg/kg q8h *Child:* 9–12 3 mg/kg q6h *Child:* 6–9 y 4 mg/kg q6h	*Onset:* PO 15–60/m IV rapid *Duration:* 6–8/h $t_{1/2}$: Variable
dyphylline (Dilor, Lufyllin)		*Adult:* 15/mg/kg qid PO 250–500 mg q6h IM *Child:* Safety not established	*Onset:* Unknown *Duration:* Unknown $t_{1/2}$: Unknown

Pharmacokinetics

Albuterol may be administered orally in tablet or liquid forms and by inhalation. Oral inhalation is by metered-dose inhaler (MDI) or by nebulizer (see the accompanying display, Types of Inhalation Devices). Following oral inhalation, bronchodilation occurs in 5 to 15 minutes, after which albuterol is absorbed over several hours from the respiratory tract. The kidneys excrete 80% to 100% of a dose within 72 hours whereas 10% may be eliminated in feces.

When albuterol is administered orally in tablet or liquid forms, bronchodilation occurs within 30 minutes. The kidneys excrete 75% of a dose within 72 hours as metabolites and 4% may be found in feces.

Pharmacodynamics

Albuterol is a moderately selective beta-2 agonist. It selectively stimulates receptors of the smooth muscle in the lungs, uterus, and vasculature supplying skeletal muscle. The main result of albuterol binding to beta-2 receptors in the lungs is relaxation of bronchial smooth muscles. This relaxation of bronchial smooth muscle relieves bronchospasm, reduces airway resistance, facilitates mucous drainage, and increases vital capacity.

Contraindications and Precautions

The only absolute contraindication to albuterol is hypersensitivity to the drug or any components of the delivery system, such as fluorocarbons.

Precautions include hypertension, cardiac disease, cardiac arrhythmias, ischemic heart disease, hyperthyroidism, diabetes mellitus, and seizures. It is important to remember that selectivity is relative. Therefore, potential beta-1 stimulation may exacerbate these conditions. Another precaution is pregnancy because beta-2 agonists may interfere with uterine contractility.

Adverse Effects

Adverse effects to albuterol are related to its sympathomimetic action. Adverse effects occur more frequently when albuterol is administered orally rather than by inhalation. The most common adverse effects to inhaled albuterol include throat irritation, palpitations, sinus tachycardia, anxiety, tremor, and increased blood pressure. Rarely, serious adverse effects such as bronchospasm, urticaria, or angioedema may occur.

Frequent adverse effects associated with oral albuterol include tachycardia or palpitations, anxiety, tremors, headache, insomnia, muscle cramps, and gastrointestinal (GI) symptoms such as dyspepsia, nausea, and vomiting.

Overuse of albuterol may induce rebound bronchoconstriction, regardless of the method of administration.

Drug Interactions

Albuterol may interact with other sympathomimetic agents, beta-adrenergic blocking agents, monoamine oxidase inhibitors (MAOIs) or tricyclic antidepressants, or thyroid agents. Table 36-3 presents these potential drug-drug interactions.

Assessment of Relevant Core Patient Variables

Health Status

The nurse should assess the patient for potential medical conditions or other drug therapy that contraindicates using albuterol or requires close patient monitoring. Any

Types of Inhalation Devices

Metered-dose inhaler (MDI)

- A small, hand-held device that delivers a set amount of drug with each activation
- Requires coordination to inhale medication correctly
- Optimally approximately 10% of drug reaches the lung
- Important to wait at least 1 minute between puffs
- May be used with a "spacer" to increase amount of drug delivered to the lungs
- Environmental hazard because it uses chlorofluorocarbon propellant that can damage the ozone layer

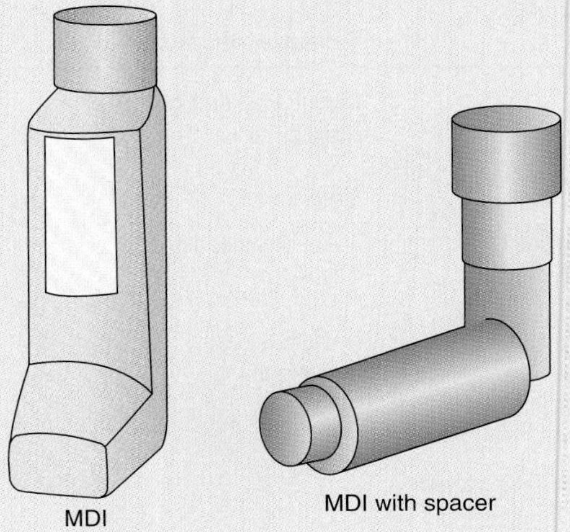

Dry-powder inhaler (DPI)

- A small, hand-held device that delivers a dry micronized powder with each inhalation
- Does not require coordination
- Optimally approximately 20% of drug reaches the lung
- Important to wait at least 1 minute between inhalations
- No environmental concerns because no propellant is used

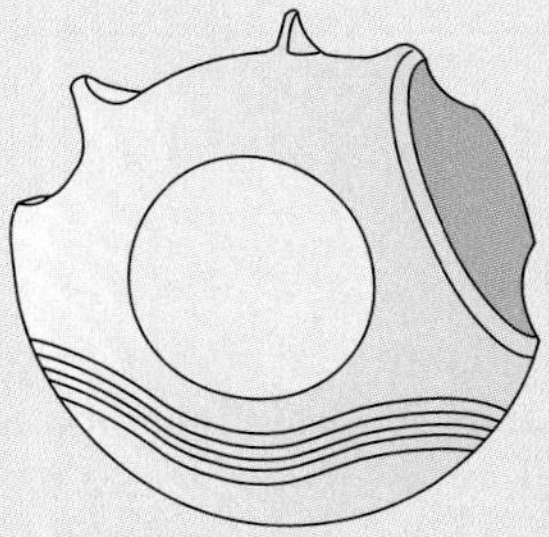

Nebulizer

- A small machine that delivers misted droplets of drug into the lungs
- Delivered through a mouthpiece or mask
- Takes longer time to deliver medication to the lungs than MDIs or DPIs
- More effective for some patients than MDIs or DPIs

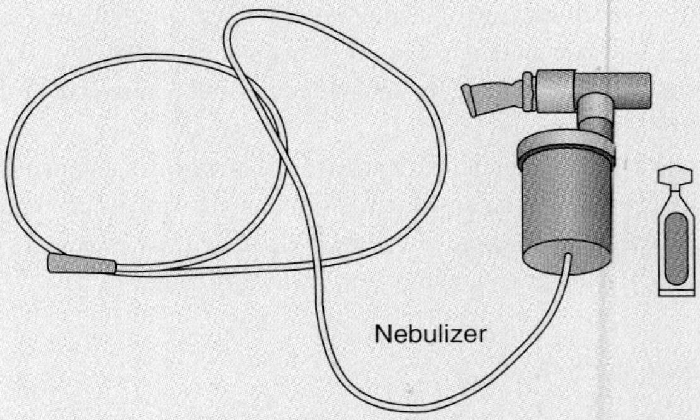

TABLE 36-3 Agents That Interact With P Albuterol

Interactants	Effect and Significance	Nursing Management
sympathomimetics	Additive effects may occur when albuterol is administered in combination with other sympathomimetic drugs. This increases the risk for cardiovascular adverse effects.	Monitor vital signs frequently. Avoid concurrent use if possible.
beta-adrenergic blocking agents	Albuterol has the exact opposite effect on the body as beta-adrenergic blocking agents. Coadministration will counteract each agent when given concomitantly.	Do not give concurrently.
MAOI or tricyclic antidepressants	MAOI and tricyclic antidepressants potentiate albuterol's effect on the peripheral vasculature. This may result in severe hypotension.	Monitor the patient's blood pressure. Avoid coadministration, if possible.
thyroid agents	Concomitant use of albuterol and thyroid hormones can enhance the effects of either drug on the cardiovascular system. Combined use of these agents may further increase this risk for coronary insufficiency.	Avoid coadministration, if possible. Monitor for signs of cardiac insufficiency.

positive findings should be communicated to the health care provider.

The nurse should perform a baseline physical examination concentrating on the cardiac and respiratory systems. The nurse should document the baseline findings to evaluate efficacy of treatment or potential adverse effects.

Life Span and Gender

The nurse should evaluate the pregnancy status of the patient, as needed. Albuterol is classified as a pregnancy class C because it can interfere with uterine contractility as a result of its beta-adrenergic-mediated relaxant effects on smooth muscle. This occurs more frequently when albuterol is administered orally rather than by inhalation.

It is important to be aware of the age of the patient before administering albuterol. Oral albuterol tablets and liquid have not been established as safe for children under the age of 6 years old. Extended-release tablets have not been approved for children under the age of 12 years old.

Lifestyle, Diet, and Habits

The nurse should assess the patient's intake of caffeine, including coffee, tea, soda, cocoa, candy, and chocolate. Caffeine has sympathomimetic effects that may increase the risk for adverse effects. The nurse also should assess for use of over-the-counter (OTC) medications such as pain relievers, appetite suppressants, and cold medicines because they frequently contain caffeine.

Environment

The nurse should note the environment in which the drug will be administered. Patients who self-administer albuterol may use their MDIs more frequently than recommended. This may result in rebound bronchoconstriction, then the patient increases the MDI use stimulating the cycle of rebound.

Nursing Diagnoses and Outcomes

- Anxiety related to sympathomimetic effects of albuterol administration

  Desired outcome: The patient will engage interventions that decrease anxiety.
- Ineffective Tissue Perfusion: Cardiopulmonary related to rebound bronchoconstriction due to overuse of albuterol

  Desired outcome: The patient will use albuterol as prescribed by the health care provider and contact that person if symptoms do not abate.

Planning and Intervention

Maximizing Therapeutic Effects

Because albuterol is most commonly administered by inhalation, it is important that the nurse supervise the patient's ability to use the MDI or nebulizer appropriately (see the accompanying display, How to Use a Metered-Dose Inhaler).

COMMUNITY-BASED CONCERNS

How to Use a Metered-Dose Inhaler

When a patient is first diagnosed with asthma and prescribed inhalation therapy, he or she may need to learn how to use the inhaler that will deliver drug therapy. The nurse may be the health care provider who supplies instructions such as these:

1. Hold the device upright and shake it.
2. Tilt the head back slightly.
3. Exhale and open mouth.
4. Position the inhaler in one of three ways:
   - Held 1–2 inches from the mouth (this is preferred)
   - Using a spacer
   - With the inhaler between the lips
   - When using dry powder inhalers, always place the mouthpiece between the lips.
5. Start to inhale slowly and press down on the inhaler to release the medication.
6. Breathe in for 3 to 5 seconds.
7. Hold your breath for 10 seconds to allow the drug to reach deep into the lungs.
8. Repeat for the ordered number of puffs, allowing 1 minute between each puff.

Spacers are recommended for children, older adults and anyone who has difficulty using a nebulizer alone. Spacers are indicated when using inhaled steroids.

Use the prescribed bronchodilator first to open air passages, and then use other prescribed medications.

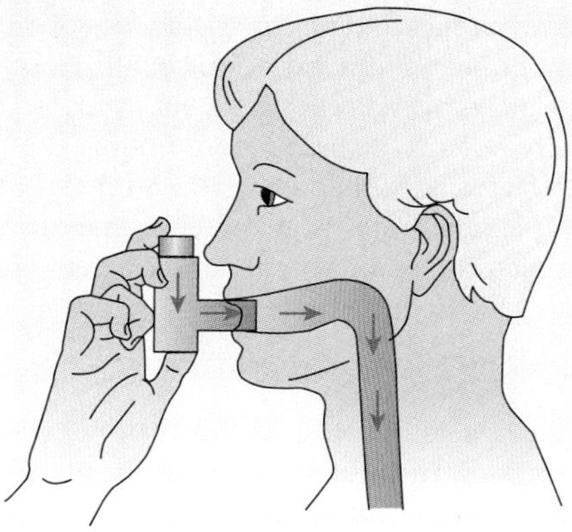

Minimizing Adverse Effects

The nurse should explain the need to adhere to the recommended frequency of administration. The patient should be encouraged to contact the health care provider if symptoms persist for adjunctive medications rather than increase the frequency of albuterol.

Providing Patient and Family Education

- The nurse should teach the patient that inhaled albuterol is referred to as a "rescue drug" and should be the *first drug* to use when symptoms of an acute attack occur.
- The nurse should teach the patient how to use an MDI. This includes the correct procedure for administration of medication, keeping the equipment clean, and how to assess when to change the canister (see the accompanying display, How to Care for Your Inhaler).
- The nurse should explain the importance of using the drug as prescribed and encourage contact with the health care provider if the symptoms do not abate with the recommended therapy.
- The nurse should explain the importance of limiting caffeine intake.
- The nurse should explain the importance of refraining from use of OTC drugs without the health care provider's knowledge.

Ongoing Assessment and Evaluation

The nurse should evaluate for abatement of the symptoms of asthma or COPD. The nurse should evaluate for symptoms of the central nervous system (CNS) such as anxiety, tremors, insomnia, or CNS disturbances. The nurse should evaluate the frequency of use and refer to the health care provider if albuterol is needed more frequently than prescribed. ■

COMMUNITY-BASED CONCERNS

How to Care for Your Inhaler

Keep the inhaler clean. Once a week, remove the medication canister from the plastic casing and wash the casing in warm, soapy water. When the casing is dry, replace the medication canister and place the cap on the mouthpiece. Ensure that the hole is clear. Check the expiration date. Keep a log of doses used to know when medication should be replaced. If in doubt about how much medication is left, estimate by placing the medication canister in a glass of water. If it floats on the top, it is time to replace your medication canister. This method is not always reliable.

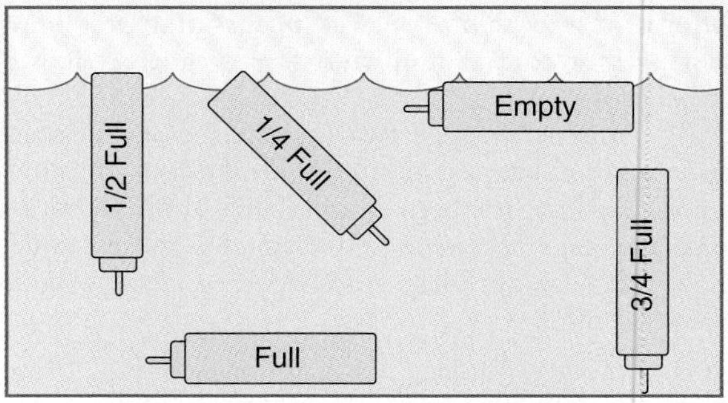

DRUGS CLOSELY RELATED TO ALBUTEROL

Several other beta-agonist agents are used as bronchodilators. The pharmacodynamics and pharmacokinetics of all of these drugs are very similar; slight variations or different vehicles make them the drugs of choice for different patients. A patient may need to try several of these before finding the one that works most effectively. Other sympathomimetics are bitolterol mesylate, epinephrine, isoproterenol, metaproterenol, pirbuterol, salmeterol, and terbutaline (see Table 36-2).

RESPIRATORY ANTICHOLINERGIC AGENTS

Anticholinergic agents diminish the effect of acetylcholine, the terminal neurotransmitter in the parasympathetic nervous system. In the respiratory system, use of inhaled anticholinergic drugs stops the bronchoconstriction that is caused by stimulation of the parasympathetic nervous system. Ipratropium bromide (Atrovent) is the prototypical respiratory anticholinergic agent.

NURSING MANAGEMENT OF THE PATIENT RECEIVING IPRATROPIUM

Core Drug Knowledge

Pharmacotherapeutics

Ipratropium is used for the maintenance treatment of bronchospasm associated with asthma, bronchitis, pulmonary emphysema, or COPD (see Table 36-2).

MEMORY CHIP

Albuterol

- Used for acute and chronic management of COPD and asthma
- Significant contraindication: hypersensitivity
- Most common adverse effects: throat irritation, palpitations, tachycardia, anxiety, tremors, and increased blood pressure
- Most serious adverse effects: bronchospasm, urticaria, and angioedema
- Maximizing therapeutic effects: correct use of inhalation device
- Minimizing adverse effects: do not use more than prescribed
- Most significant patient education: this rescue drug should be used first for all acute symptoms of shortness of breath or wheezing

Pharmacokinetics

Ipratropium bromide is administered through oral inhalation or intranasal spray. Following oral inhalation, onset occurs between 15 to 30 minutes, peaks in 1 to 2 hours, and lasts 4 to 5 hours. It is not readily absorbed into the systemic circulation after inhalation either from the surface of the lung or from the GI tract. Approximately 50% of the absorbed drug is excreted unchanged in the urine. After intranasal dosing, less than 20% of an ipratropium dose is absorbed from the nasal mucosa into the systemic circulation. The metabolism of intranasal ipratropium bromide is the same as the inhaled drug.

Pharmacodynamics

Ipratropium antagonizes the action of acetylcholine by blocking muscarinic cholinergic receptors. Blockade of these cholinergic receptors decreases the formation of cyclic guanosine monophosphate (cGMP) resulting in decreased contractility of smooth muscle.

Contraindications and Precautions

Ipratropium aerosol inhalation is contraindicated in patients who have soya lecithin hypersensitivity, including those patients with a history of peanut oil hypersensitivity or hypersensitivity to related foods and legumes such as soybeans and peanuts. Ipratropium should also not be used in patients with hypersensitivity to atropine or atropine derivatives, those with bromide hypersensitivity, or patients with hypersensitivity to propellant fluorocarbons.

Due to its anticholinergic effects, ipratropium should be used with caution in patients with bladder obstruction, prostatic hypertrophy, or closed-angle glaucoma. Ipratropium may precipitate urinary retention in patients with preexisting bladder obstruction or prostatic hypertrophy. It may increase intraocular pressure and aqueous outflow resistance in patients with closed-angle glaucoma, especially if the medication gets into the eyes.

Adverse Effects

Ipratropium aerosols can produce a paradoxic acute bronchospasm that can be life threatening in some patients. This rare problem, when it occurs, is usually seen with the first inhalation from a newly opened MDI. The patient should "test-spray" three times before using a new MDI for the first time. Another serious, but rare, adverse effect is anaphylactoid reactions. Symptoms include urticaria; angioedema of tongue, lips, and face; maculopapular rash; bronchospasm; laryngospasm; pruritus; and oropharyngeal edema. This may occur when a patient has an unknown allergy to soybeans, legumes, or soya lecithin.

More commonly, ipratropium may induce cough, hoarseness, throat irritation, or dysgeusia. The classic anticholinergic adverse effects dry mouth, constipation, urinary retention, and blurred vision may also occur, but not as frequently or intensely as with systemic anticholinergic drugs.

Nasal administration of ipratropium may induce epistaxis, headache, rhinitis, nasal congestion, rhinorrhea, and general nasal irritation.

Temporary ocular irritation, ocular pain, mydriasis, cycloplegia, blurred vision, conjunctivitis, or visual impairment may result from spraying ipratropium products inadvertently into the eyes.

Drug Interactions

No serious drug-drug interactions are associated with ipratropium. Ipratropium inhalation solution forms a precipitate with cromolyn sodium inhalation solution if mixed together in a nebulizer. Theoretically, there is a potential for ipratropium to have additive anticholinergic effects when administered with other antimuscarinics.

Assessment of Relevant Core Patient Variables

Health Status

The nurse should assess the patient for potential medical conditions or other drug therapy that contraindicates using ipratropium or requires close patient monitoring. The nurse should perform a baseline respiratory examination and document the findings. This baseline assessment will be used to evaluate the efficacy of treatment.

Life Span and Gender

The nurse should evaluate the pregnancy status of the patient, as needed. Ipratropium is classified as a pregnancy category B drug. However, human studies have not been done. Therefore, ipratropium should be used during pregnancy only when the benefits outweigh the risk to the fetus. Minimal amounts of Inhaled ipratropium reaches breast milk, therefore the potential risk to the fetus is negligible. Safety and effectiveness of ipratropium have not been established in infants or children younger than 5 years of age.

Lifestyle, Diet, and Habits

The nurse should assess the patient for the use of cigarettes. Smoking causes vasoconstriction, which is the opposite action of ipratropium.

Environment

The nurse should note the environment in which the drug will be administered. When ipratropium is self-administered, it is important that the nurse assist the patient identify the correct MDI that is used for acute symptoms. Beta-agonist drugs, such as albuterol, are the drugs of choice for acute symptoms, although ipratropium may still be delivered during exacerbations of asthma.

Nursing Diagnoses and Outcomes

- Risk for Injury (bronchospasm) related to use of new canister of ipratropium

Desired outcome: The patient will "test spray" a new canister three times before inhaling the medication.

- Risk for Injury (anaphylactoid reactions) related to allergies to soybeans, legumes, or soya lecithin.

  Desired outcome: The patient will review past allergic responses to assess whether any of the causative foods may have been implicated.

Planning and Intervention

Maximizing Therapeutic Effects

The nurse should explain the importance of taking ipratropium daily, despite the absence of symptoms. The nurse should watch the patient demonstrate the use of the MDI to assess correct use (see Community-Based Concerns: How to Use a Metered Dose Inhaler).

Minimizing Adverse Effects

The nurse should explain the importance of using the inhaler as prescribed to avoid systemic absorption that will lead to an increased risk for adverse effects.

Providing Patient and Family Education

- The nurse should advise the patient that ipratropium is used prophylactically to reduce the frequency and severity of future asthma attacks. It will not abort an asthma attack in progress.
- The nurse should advise patients to avoid the use of ipratropium if they have a history of allergy to soybeans, legumes, or soya lecithin.
- The nurse should remind the patient that ipratropium must be taken daily, despite the absence of symptoms of asthma.
- The nurse should remind the patient that overuse of ipratropium may induce adverse effects or increase their intensity.
- The nurse should teach the patient use of a MDI. This includes the correct procedure for administration of medication, keeping the equipment clean, and how to assess when to change the canister (see Community Based Concerns: How to Care for Your Inhaler).

Ongoing Assessment and Evaluation

The nurse should assess the patient for the need of beta-agonist drugs in addition to ipratropium. If the patient continues to need beta-agonists more that twice a week, refer the patient to the heath care provider for additional assessment. ■

XANTHINE DERIVATIVES

The xanthine derivatives, including theophylline, aminophylline, diphylline, and caffeine, come from a variety of naturally occurring sources. Theophylline is the prototype xanthine derivative bronchodilator.

MEMORY CHIP

Ipratropium

- Used for maintenance of COPD or asthma
- Significant contraindications: hypersensitivity to fluorocarbons or legumes, such as soybeans or peanuts
- Most common adverse effects: cough, hoarseness, throat irritation, dysgeusia, and anticholinergic effects
- Most serious adverse effects: bronchospasm and anaphylaxis
- Maximizing therapeutic effects: administer the medication daily, despite the absence of symptoms
- Minimizing adverse effects: use only as directed to decrease potential systemic absorption
- Most significant patient education: this drug will not abort an acute asthma attack

NURSING MANAGEMENT OF THE PATIENT RECEIVING THEOPHYLLINE

Core Drug Knowledge

Pharmacotherapeutics

Theophylline is indicated for the symptomatic relief or prevention of bronchial asthma and reversal of bronchospasm associated with COPD. An unlabeled use is to treat apnea and bradycardia in premature infants.

Pharmacokinetics

Theophylline is well absorbed when given orally. Its peak effects occur in 2 hours with a duration of effect from 4 to 8 hours. The drug is metabolized in the liver and excreted in the urine. It crosses the placenta and may enter breast milk (see Table 36-2).

Pharmacodynamics

Theophylline has a direct effect on the smooth muscle of the respiratory tract, both those in the bronchi and the blood vessels. The exact mechanism of action is not known. One theory suggests that theophylline works by affecting directly the mobilization of calcium within the cell. It acts through the stimulation of two prostaglandins and results in smooth muscle relaxation. This effect increases the vital capacity that has been impaired by bronchospasm or air-trapping. Theophylline also inhibits the release of slow-reacting substance of anaphylaxis and histamine, decreasing the bronchial swelling and narrowing that occur as a result of these two chemicals.

Contraindications and Precautions

Theophylline is contraindicated in patients with hypersensitivity to any xanthines, in association with status asthmaticus, or in patients with a peptic ulcer. It has been assigned to pregnancy category C and therefore is contraindicated or used with caution during pregnancy. The nurse should use caution with any patient with a cardiac problem, such as arrhythmia, coronary artery disease, congestive heart failure, or hypertension because of the drug's stimulatory effects. Caution also should be used in patients with renal or hepatic disease because the drug is metabolized in the liver and excreted through the kidneys. Also, it is not known whether theophylline enters into breast milk, but there is a possibility that the drug has a stimulatory effect on the infant. Therefore, the drug should be used with caution during lactation.

Adverse Effects

Adverse effects related to theophylline use are related directly to serum levels of the drug. If serum levels of theophylline are under 20 µg/mL, adverse effects are uncommon. At serum levels exceeding 20 to 25 µg/mL, the most common adverse effects are GI symptoms of nausea, vomiting, and diarrhea, and CNS effects of headache, insomnia, and irritability. When serum levels exceed 30 to 35 µg/mL, adverse effects, such as hyperglycemia, hypotension, arrhythmias, seizures, brain damage, and even death, may occur. Even at therapeutic doses, theophylline may cause CNS effects, such as irritability (especially in children), restlessness, and muscle twitching. It also may cause GI effects, such as loss of appetite, hematemesis, and gastroesophageal reflux. Potential cardiovascular effects include palpitations, tachycardia, and circulatory failure. In the respiratory system, theophylline may cause tachypnea. In the genitourinary system, urinary retention in men with prostate enlargement and diuresis may occur. Generalized effects, such as fever, flushing, rash, and elevated liver enzymes, also have occurred.

Drug Interactions

Theophylline levels and effects are influenced by a large number of other drugs. Increased effects and potential toxicity occur if the drug is taken concurrently with histamine-2 antagonists, such as cimetidine or ranitidine; macrolide antibiotics, such as erythromycin and troleandomycin; quinolone antibiotics, such as ciprofloxacin, norfloxacin, or ofloxacin; oral contraceptives; and rifampin.

Theophylline also may have significant interactions with halothane, barbiturates, charcoal, benzodiazepines, nondepolarizing neuromuscular blockers, and beta blockers. It also may interact with thyroid hormones, hydantoins, adenosine, disulfiram, mexiletine, and thiabendazole (Table 36-4).

TABLE 36-4 Agents that Interact With P Theophylline

Interactants	Effect and Significance	Nursing Management
activated charcoal	Can reduce absorption of theophylline and remove it from the systemic circulation, resulting in subtherapeutic levels of theophylline	Monitor for increased symptoms of respiratory distress if activated charcoal must be administered.
adenosine	Mechanism of action unclear; theophylline may decrease effectiveness of adenosine	Administer higher dose of adenosine.
barbiturates	May induce cytochrome P450, stimulating theophylline metabolism and increasing clearance, resulting in subtherapeutic levels of theophylline	Assess for need of increased theophylline dosage with coadministration of barbiturates.
benzodiazepines	Possible antagonistic action by competitive binding to intracerebral adenosine receptors, resulting in decreased sedative effects of benzodiazepines	Assess the clinical status of the patient, and tailor the dosage of benzodiazepines as needed.
beta blockers	May reduce the n-demethylation of theophylline, resulting in a decreased effect of one or both agents	Monitor patient for clinical changes. Monitor plasma theophylline levels when a beta blocker is added or deleted from a regimen. Beta-selective agents are preferred.
disulfiram	Inhibits the hydroxylation and demethylation pathways of theophylline metabolism, resulting in potential theophylline toxicity	Monitor theophylline levels closely when coadministered with disulfiram. Adjust theophylline dose as needed.
halothane	Catecholamine-induced arrhythmias possible when halothane is administered after theophylline	Do not administer halothane to patient taking theophylline.
histamine-2 antagonists	Inhibition of the hepatic metabolism of theophylline, resulting in potential toxicity	Monitor theophylline levels; 20%–40% reduction in dosage of theophylline may be necessary.
hydantoins	Phenytoin and theophylline metabolism increased, resulting in subtherapeutic levels of both drugs	Monitor plasma levels of both drugs and adjust as necessary.
macrolide antibiotics	Inhibit the metabolism of theophylline, and theophylline reduces the bioavailability and increases renal clearance of oral erythromycin, resulting in theophylline toxicity and macrolide ineffectivity	Monitor drug levels and adjust dosages as needed, with addition or deletion of macrolides.

(*continued*)

TABLE 36-4 Agents that Interact With Theophylline (Continued)

Interactants	Effect and Significance	Nursing Management
mexiletine	Inhibits the cytochrome P450 oxidase system, resulting in theophylline toxicity	Monitor theophylline levels and adjust dose as needed.
nondepolarizing muscle relaxants	Antagonistic activity between theophylline and nondepolarizing muscle relaxants—nontherapeutic effects of muscle relaxants	Assess the need for higher dosage of muscle relaxants.
oral contraceptives	Decrease the oxidative degradation of theophylline by cytochrome P448, resulting in theophylline toxicity	Monitor theophylline levels and adjust dose as needed.
quinolone antibiotics	Inhibition of the hepatic metabolism of theophylline resulting in potential theophylline toxicity	Monitor theophylline levels and adjust dose as needed.
rifampin	Appears to induce the hepatic metabolism of theophylline, resulting in subtherapeutic levels	Monitor theophylline levels and adjust dose as needed if rifampin is added or deleted.
thiabendazole	Possible metabolic inhibition of theophylline , resulting in theophylline toxicity	Monitor theophylline levels and adjust dose as needed
thyroid hormones and preparations	Direct correlation between plasma thyroid hormones/preparations and theophylline clearance; hypothyroid or hyperthyroid patients, alteration in theophylline clearance	Adjust dose according to plasma theophylline levels. Achieving a euthyroid state is critical in controlling theophylline clearance.

Assessment of Relevant Core Patient Variables

Health Status

When the nurse takes the patient history prior to theophylline therapy, the patient should be screened for any hypersensitivity to xanthines, peptic ulcer, active gastritis, status asthmaticus, coronary disease, hyperthyroidism, renal or hepatic disorders, pregnancy, and lactation.

Patients with cardiac disease should be monitored closely during theophylline therapy, because the drug may cause cardiovascular effects, such as palpitations, tachycardia, and elevated blood pressure.

The nurse should perform a physical examination, which should include a baseline for skin color, texture, and lesions; reflexes, orientation, and affect; and heart rate. It also is important to assess the respiratory system for rate, adventitious sounds, and the patient's forced expiratory volume in 1 second (FEV_1) (see the accompanying display, Using a Peak Flow Meter). For long-term therapy, the nurse must obtain baseline thyroid, liver, and kidney function test results.

Life Span and Gender

The nurse should assess the patient for pregnancy and lactation because theophylline is contraindicated during pregnancy; newborns of mothers who used theophylline exhibit tachycardia, jitteriness, and withdrawal apnea. The nurse also should assess older men carefully for possible enlarged prostate glands because special precautions should be taken when administering theophylline to these patients.

Lifestyle, Diet, and Habits

The nurse should assess whether the patient smokes. Smoking cigarettes may decrease serum theophylline levels. In fact, some patients who smoke require an increase in theophylline dosage of up to 50%. It is important to monitor patients who smoke for any change in smoking habits. It also is important for the nurse to assess the diet

COMMUNITY-BASED CONCERNS

Using a Peak Flow Meter

Patients receiving inhaled bronchodilators at home can monitor the effectiveness of drug therapy and lung function by using a peak flow meter to monitor peak expiratory flow rates (PEFR). These devices are inexpensive and may be available from the health care provider or by prescription from the pharmacist.

Peak flow values are a way to quantify and evaluate lung function. Daily monitoring helps to detect trends and subtle changes in lung function, sometimes even before the patient experiences symptoms. Daily monitoring also permits early and prompt intervention before the patient experiences a setback and needs to seek emergency care.

The peak flow meter consists of a mouthpiece connected to a sealed measuring device. The patient inhales as deeply as possible and then places the mouthpiece in the mouth, making a tight seal. Next, the patient blows out as hard and as fast as possible. The exhaled air propels an indicator up a scale to a number. This number, signifying liters of air per minute, represents the peak flow rate. After consulting with the provider, the patient can determine his or her normal PEFR. The patient can then keep a record of the readings and report any changes in PEFR to the health care provider.

of patients taking theophylline. Theophylline elimination is increased by a low-carbohydrate, high-protein diet and by charcoal-broiled beef. Theophylline elimination is decreased by a high-carbohydrate, low-protein diet. The effects of theophylline can be increased by foods containing xanthines, particularly caffeine. Caffeine is found in many beverages, such as coffee, tea, and cola, and in chocolate. OTC drug preparations also frequently contain caffeine.

Environment

The nurse should be aware of the environment in which the theophylline will be administered. Theophylline can be administered in the hospital or by the patient at home. If patients have frequent exacerbations of COPD, the nurse should determine the patient's ability to use peak flow meters in the home environment to assess the need for additional bronchodilation (see Community-Based Concerns: Using a Peak Flow Meter).

Nursing Diagnoses and Outcomes

- Disturbed Sensory Perception: Kinesthetic, related to CNS effects of irritability, insomnia, and dizziness
  Desired outcome: The patient will be protected from injury due to CNS effects, such as dizziness and loss of balance, occur.
- Ineffective Tissue Perfusion: Cardiopulmonary related to cardiac effects of drug
  Desired outcome: Adverse effects will be limited by proper administration and monitoring of drug serum levels.
- Risk for Injury related to headache, GI effects, and CNS effects
  Desired outcome: The patient will develop strategies to be able to tolerate the drug and remain injury free during drug therapy.

Planning and Intervention

Maximizing Therapeutic Effects

The nurse should screen the patient's diet, other drugs taken (including OTC drugs), smoking habits, and compliance with prescribed regimen if serum levels of theophylline have not been stabilized. In the hospital setting, the nurse should administer theophylline at a rate of 20 mg/minute.

Minimizing Adverse Effects

The nurse should monitor serum theophylline levels carefully and arrange for reduced or increased dosage to keep serum levels at 10 to 20 μg/mL, which is the optimal therapeutic level associated with few adverse effects. The nurse also should never infuse theophylline rapidly; rapid infusion may cause hypotension, arrhythmias, syncope, or even death.

The nurse should make sure the patient receives small meals and that immediate-release preparations are given with meals to alleviate GI distress. Sustained-release preparations must be given on an empty stomach, 1 hour before or 2 hours after meals. To prevent injuries, the nurse should be prepared to institute safety precautions if CNS effects occur. Additionally, the nurse should provide environmental control, including adjusting lighting, heat, and noise, if irritability, restlessness, or insomnia occur.

Providing Patient and Family Education

- The nurse must explain that theophylline will help make breathing easier.
- The nurse should caution patients not to take theophylline if they are allergic to it, if they have reactions to caffeine, or if they are breast-feeding.
- It is important to make sure that patients report the names of all drugs currently being taken to their health care providers.
- The nurse should explain the importance of taking theophylline exactly as prescribed and should instruct patients to make a list of things that can interfere with the drug concentrations (e.g., diet, OTC drugs, or smoking). The nurse should make sure that patients and their families are aware of precautions they should take and when to contact the health care provider if they change their diet, use OTC drugs, or change their smoking habits.
- It is important to teach patients never to chew or crush time-release capsules; they should be swallowed whole. In addition, the time-release capsules should always be taken on an empty stomach, 1 hour before or 2 hours after meals. If using a solution, it should be shaken well before use. Nurses should encourage the patient to take immediate-release and liquid preparations of the drug with food if GI upset occurs.
- The nurse should caution the patient not to change the drug dosage without consulting the health care provider, and to schedule regular check-ups or blood tests so that progress can be evaluated.
- It is important to instruct patients to take the drug around the clock; if a dose is missed, it should be taken as soon as it is remembered unless it is almost time for the next dose. However, two doses should never be taken at the same time.
- The nurse should instruct patients to avoid consuming large quantities of caffeine-containing foods (e.g., chocolates) or beverages (e.g., coffee, cola and tea) while taking theophylline, and to contact their health care providers if they change their consumption significantly. In addition, the nurse should alert patients to check the ingredients of any OTC drug for caffeine before using it.
- The nurse should advise the patient to take non-narcotic medications for headaches caused by theophylline therapy.

- The nurse should advise the patient to ingest small frequent meals if GI distress occurs.
- The nurse should advise a quiet environment or exercise to decrease agitation or insomnia from theophylline therapy.
- The nurse should caution against using theophylline for an acute asthma attack because its onset is not quick enough to subdue an acute attack.
- The nurse should urge the patient to report such adverse effects as headaches, insomnia, restlessness, muscle twitching, nausea, vomiting, severe GI pain, palpitation, and convulsions.
- For more patient education information on theophylline and other asthma therapies, see the accompanying display, Thinking About Theophylline and Other Asthma Therapies.

Ongoing Assessment and Evaluation

The nurse should monitor the patient for potential CNS and cardiovascular adverse effects. The patient's serum theophylline level should be maintained between 10 and 20 μg/mL for optimal therapeutic effects and minimal adverse effects. After 1 to 2 weeks on theophylline, the patient should report minimal discomfort from adverse effects and adhere to the therapy prescribed. ■

Critical Thinking Scenario

Thinking about theophylline and other asthma therapies

Martin Kell is a 12-year-old boy with a history of allergic asthma. Skin testing has revealed allergies to trees, molds, and dust. His mother, Mrs. Kell, is bringing him to the clinic for sensitization treatment. She reports that Martin has had a stuffy nose, dry cough, and occasional wheezing. On examination, scattered wheezes are noted throughout the lung fields. The physician orders the following:

Theophylline, 200 mg BID
Albuterol inhaler, 2 puffs BID
Beclomethasone inhaler, 2 puffs BID

The nurse reviews all of the medications with Martin's mother, who states, "All these medicines, how is he ever going to be able to take them all?"

1. Prioritize concerns to be discussed with Mrs. Kell.
2. Explain the rationale for using both inhalers.
3. Construct written instructions about using the inhalers for the nurse to give Mrs. Kell.
4. Consider what adaptations may be necessary to help ensure therapeutic adherence and effective drug therapy with Martin.
5. Propose some assessments that the nurse can anticipate making on the next visit to evaluate the effectiveness of therapy.

MEMORY CHIP

P Theophylline

- Used for symptomatic relief of bronchoconstriction and bronchospasm
- Significant contraindications: status asthmaticus and peptic ulcer
- Most common adverse effects: nausea, vomiting, headache, and insomnia
- Most serious adverse effects: seizures and arrhythmias
- Maximizing therapeutic effects: evaluate patient care variables if serum concentration not stable
- Minimizing adverse effects: monitor serum theophylline levels periodically
- Most significant patient education: take the drug exactly as prescribed to avoid adverse effects

DRUGS CLOSELY RELATED TO P THEOPHYLLINE

Aminophylline

Aminophylline (Truphylline) is pharmacologically identical to theophylline because it is a theophylline salt. It is more soluble than theophylline, thus it is preferred when IV administration is needed. It is important to administer IV aminophylline at a rate not to exceed 25 mg/minute. Aminophylline also may be administered orally by tablet or syrup and as a rectal suppository or solution.

Diphylline

Dyphylline (Dilor) is an oral and parenteral xanthine-derivative bronchodilator. It is used for the relief or prevention of bronchial asthma and for reversible bronchospasm. Dyphylline works by direct stimulation of the bronchial smooth muscles. It is approximately 1/10th as potent as theophylline, and therefore it induces fewer adverse effects.

Caffeine

Caffeine is a naturally occurring xanthine derivative used as a CNS and respiratory stimulant, or as a mild diuretic. Caffeine often is combined with analgesics or with ergot alkaloids for the treatment of migraine and other types of headache. Caffeine also is sold without a prescription in products marketed to treat drowsiness, or in products for mild water-weight gain.

Caffeine is administered both orally and parenterally as a respiratory stimulant in neonates with apnea of prematurity. It reduces the frequency of apneic episodes by 30% to 50% within 24 hours of administration. Some clinicians prefer using caffeine in neonates because of its once daily administration, reliable oral absorption, and wide therapeutic margin.

C ANTI-INFLAMMATORY AGENTS

In addition to bronchodilators, anti-inflammatory agents are used in the management of respiratory disorders, especially asthma. These agents include glucocorticoid steroids, mast cell stabilizers, and leukotriene receptor antagonists (Table 36-5). The most efficient anti-inflammatory agents are the glucocorticoid steroids (Table 36-6).

GLUCOCORTICOID STEROIDS

Glucocorticoid steroids are the most effective anti-inflammatory drugs available for the management of respiratory disorders. They may be given orally, parenterally, or by inhalation. When administered into the lungs by inhalation, steroids decrease the effectiveness of the inflammatory cells, which, in turn, decreases the swelling associated with inflammation and promotes the activity of the beta adrenergic receptors. This may promote smooth muscle relaxation and inhibit bronchoconstriction.

As with the anticholinergic ipratropium bromide, inhaled glucocorticoid steroids obtain their peak effect in 1 to 2 weeks of regular use. Therefore, inhaled glucocorticoid steroids are used as a maintenance drugs and not for acute respiratory symptoms. In an emergency, steroids such as

TABLE 36-5 Summary of Selected Anti-inflammatory Agents

Drug (Trade) Name	Selected Indications	Route and Dosage Range	Pharmacokinetics
Inhaled Glucocorticoid Steroids			
beclomethasone (Beclovent, Vanceril; *Canadian:* Alti-Beclomethasone)	Asthma COPD	Oral Inhalation (42 μg/spray): *Adult:* 2 puffs tid–qid; maximum: 20 puffs qd *Child:* > 6–12 y: 1–2 puffs tid–qid; maximum: 10 puffs/d	Onset: Rapid *Duration:* Week $t_{1/2}$: 3–15 h
(Vancenase AQ Nasal)	Rhinitis Nasal polyps prophylaxis	Nasal inhalation (42, 84 μg/spray): *Adult and child:* > 6 y: 1–2 sprays each nostril bid	
dexamethasone (Decadron Phosphate, Turbinaire; *Canadian:* Dexasone)	Asthma COPD	Oral inhalation (100 μg/spray) *Adult:* 3 sprays, tid–qid; maximum: 12 sprays d *Child:* 2 sprays, tid–qid; maximum: 8 sprays/d	*Onset:* 1–2 h *Duration:* 72 h $t_{1/2}$: 36–54 h
flunisolide (AeroBid; *Canadian:* Alti-Flunisolide)	Asthma COPD	Oral inhalation (250 μg/spray) *Adult:* 2 puffs bid; maximum: 8 puffs/d *Child:* > 6–15 y: 2 puffs bid; maximum: 4 puffs/d	*Onset:* 1 h *Duration:* Unknown $t_{1/2}$: 1.8 hr
(Nasalide)	Rhinitis	Nasal inhalation: *Adult:* 2 sprays each nostril bid–tid; maximum: 8 sprays/nostril/d *Child:* > 6–14 yr: 1 spray each nostril bid; maximum: 4 sprays/nostril/d	
fluticasone (Flovent)	Asthma prophylaxis COPD Rhinitis	Oral inhalation (44, 110, 220 μg/spray): *Adult:* 88–220 μg bid *Child:* > 4 yr: 88–220 μg bid	*Onset:* *Duration:* $t_{1/2}$:
(Flovent Rotadisk)	Asthma prophylaxis	Rotadisk inhalation (50, 100, 250 μg/spray) *Adult and child:* > 12 yr: 100–1000 μg bid Rotadisk *Child:* 4–11 yr: 50–100 μg bid	
(Flonase)	Rhinitis	Nasal inhalation (50 μg/spray): *Adult:* 1 inhalation each nostril bid *Child:* > 4 yr: 1 inhalation each nostril qd	
triamcinolone (Azmacort; *Canadian:* Oracort)	Asthma COPD	Oral inhalation (100 μg/spray): Adult: 2 puffs tid–qid; maximum: 16 puff/d *Child:* 6–12 yr: 1–2 puffs tid–qid; maximum: 12 puffs/d	*Onset:* 1 h *Duration:* 8–12 h $t_{1/2}$: 18–36 h
(Nasacort)	Rhinitis	Nasal inhalation (55 μg/spray): *Adult:* 2 sprays qd; maximum: 8/d *Child:* 6–11 yr: 1–2 sprays/d; maximum: 4/d	

(*continued*)

TABLE 36-5 Summary of Selected Anti-inflammatory Agents (Continued)

Drug (Trade) Name	Selected Indications	Route and Dosage Range	Pharmacokinetics
Mast Cell Stabilizers			
cromolyn sodium (Intal; *Canadian:* Nalcrom)	Asthma	Oral inhalation (800 μg/spray): *Adult and child:* > 5 yr: 2 puffs qid until stabilized then 2 puffs bid Exercise-induced asthma: 2 puffs 10–60 min before exercise *Child:* 2–4 yr: 20 mg Spinhaler qid until stabilized, then bid	*Onset:* 15 min *Duration:* Unknown $t_{1/2}$: 80–90 min
(Gastrocrom)	Mastocytosis	*Adult:* 200 mg PO qid *Child:* 2–12 y: 100 mg PO qid	
(Nasalcrom)	Allergic rhinitis	Nasal inhalation (40 mg/mL): *Adult and child:* > 6 yr: 1 spray each nostril 3–4/d	
(Crolom)	Allergic conjunctivitis	Ophthalmic (4% drops) *Adult and child:* >4 y, 1–2 drops each eye, 4–6/d	
nedocromil (Tilade)	Asthma Bronchospasm	Oral inhalation (1.75 mg/spray); *Adult and child:* >6 y: 2 sprays 4/d reduce to bid after being stabilized	*Onset:* Rapid *Duration:* 10–12 h $t_{1/2}$: 3.3 h
Leukotriene receptor antagonists			
zafirlukast (Accolate)	Prophylaxis and treatment of chronic asthma	*Adult and child:* >12: PO 20 mg bid *Child:* 7–11 yr: PO 10 mg bid	*Onset:* Rapid *Duration:* 12–24 h $t_{1/2}$: 10 h
montelukast (Singulair)	Prophylaxis and treatment of chronic asthma	*Adult and child:* >15: PO, 10 mg *Child:* 6–14: PO, 5 mg *Child:* 2–5: 4 mg	*Onset:* Rapid *Duration:* 12–24 h $t_{1/2}$: 5.5 h
zileuton (Zyflo)	Prophylaxis and treatment of chronic asthma	*Adult and child:* >12 y: 600 mg qid; maximum: 2400 mg/d *Child:* < 12 y not recommended	*Onset:* Rapid *Duration:* Unknown $t_{1/2}$: 2.5 h

prednisone may be administered intravenously in combination with bronchodilators such as theophylline or beta-adrenergic agonists.

Inhaled glucocorticoid steroids should be used with caution in any patient with an active infection of the respiratory system because the depression of the inflammatory response could result in serious illness. Adverse effects are limited with the use of inhaled glucocorticoid steroids because of the route of administration. Sore throat, hoarseness, coughing, dry mouth, and pharyngeal and laryngeal fungal infections are the most common adverse effects encountered.

The nurse should teach the patient to rinse the mouth after each administration to decrease the potential for fungal infections of the mouth. It also is important to teach the patient to use inhaled steroids daily, regardless of the absence of symptoms and to use a short-acting sympathomimetic inhaler for acute symptoms.

Commonly used inhaled glucocorticoid steroids include beclomethasone dipropionate, budesonide, dexamethasone, flunisolide, fluticasone propionate, and triamcinolone acetonide (see Table 36-5). For a more thorough discussion of glucocorticoid steroids, see Chapter 40.

MAST CELL STABILIZERS

Cromolyn sodium (Intal) is the prototype mast cell stabilizer.

NURSING MANAGEMENT OF THE PATIENT RECEIVING CROMOLYN SODIUM

Core Drug Knowledge

Pharmacotherapeutics

Cromolyn sodium is used as a prophylactic agent in the treatment of mild to moderate asthma. It also is used as a nasal inhaler to treat seasonal allergic rhinitis, as an ophthalmic solution to treat allergic conjunctivitis, and orally to treat systemic mastocytosis (a rare disease

TABLE 36-6 A Systematic Approach to Asthma: National Education and Prevention Program, Expert Panel Report II

Asthma Classification	Daily Medications	Rescue Drugs
Step 1: mild intermittent	No daily medications	Short-acting, inhaled beta-2 agonist*
Step 2: mild persistent	Inhaled anti-inflammatory: glucocorticoid (low dose) **or** cromolyn sodium **or** nedocromil **or** zafirlukast for patient > 12 years of age **or** Sustained release theophylline may be used but not preferred	Short-acting, inhaled beta-2 agonist*
Step 3: moderate persistent	Inhaled glucocorticoid (moderate dose) **or** Inhaled glucocorticoid (low-medium) dose **plus** long acting bronchodilator: • inhaled salmeterol • sustained-release theophylline • long-acting beta-2-agonist tablets	Short-acting, inhaled beta-2 agonist*
Step 4: severe persistent	Daily combined use of a high-dose inhaled corticosteroid **and** long-acting bronchodilator: • inhaled salmeterol • sustained-release theophylline • long-acting beta-2-agonist tablets **and** Systemic steroids (tablets or syrup) as needed (make every attempt to control with high dose inhaled steroids rather than systemic steroids)	Short-acting, inhaled beta-2 agonist*

* Use of short-acting inhaled beta-2 agonists on a daily basis, or increasing use, indicates the need for additional long-term control therapy

characterized by an abnormal increase in mast cells in various body organs and tissues) and ulcerative colitis (see Table 36-5).

Pharmacokinetics

Cromolyn sodium may be administered orally for a systemic effect to treat mastocytosis. There is no systemic absorption when used by either intranasal or ophthalmic administration. Approximately 10% of inhaled cromolyn reaches the lungs and may be decreased by the degree of bronchoconstriction present. About 98% of the drug is eliminated unchanged in feces. Minimal amounts of the drug cross the placenta or enter the breast milk. Improvement of symptoms requires several weeks of therapy.

Pharmacodynamics

Cromolyn sodium is an anti-inflammatory agent that works at the surface of the mast cell to inhibit degranulation after contact with an antigen. This, in turn, prevents the release of histamine and slow-reacting substance of anaphylaxis (SRS-A), mediators of type I allergic reactions. Cromolyn also may reduce the release of inflammatory leukotrienes. Although its exact mechanism of action is unclear, it is thought to produce these effects by inhibiting calcium influx.

Contraindications and Precautions

Cromolyn sodium is contraindicated absolutely in patients with a demonstrated hypersensitivity as anaphylaxis may occur. Cromolyn sodium is not a bronchodilator. Therefore, it is contraindicated in the treatment of acute bronchospasm or status asthmaticus. The aerosol preparation of cromolyn sodium is contraindicated in patients with coronary artery disease or cardiac dysrhythmias because the aerosol contains fluorocarbon as a propellant and fluorocarbons irritate cardiac cells.

Precautions include patients with lactose intolerance because oral preparations contain lactose. Patients with soft contacts should use ophthalmic cromolyn sodium cautiously because it contains benzalkonium chloride.

Adverse Effects

In general, cromolyn is well tolerated. When administered by oral inhalation, the most common adverse effects are bronchospasm, throat irritation, and cough.

Because oral inhalation preparations can contain lactose, patients with lactose intolerance may experience nausea and vomiting, bloating, abdominal cramps, and flatulence.

Intranasal cromolyn spray can produce sneezing and nasal irritation, but these are generally transient effects following application. Ocular cromolyn ophthalmic drops may produce ocular irritation, especially in patients with soft contact lenses. The most frequent adverse effects from cromolyn powder for oral solution are headache and diarrhea.

Drug Interactions

No clinically significant drug interactions are known with cromolyn sodium.

Assessment of Relevant Core Patient Variables

Health Status

The nurse should evaluate for previous adverse effects to cromolyn sodium before administration. The nurse should perform a baseline physical assessment including head, eyes, ears, nose, throat (HEENT), and lung sounds.

Life Span and Gender

Cromolyn sodium may be administered to both adults and children. The nurse should note whether the patient is pregnant or lactating. Cromolyn sodium is classified as a pregnancy category B drug because only a minimal amount of the drug passes the placenta or enters the breast milk.

Lifestyle, Diet, and Habits

The nurse should monitor patients with lactose intolerance for adverse effects to cromolyn sodium. The nurse should ask patients whether they experience exercise-induced bronchospasm because cromolyn sodium may be taken 15 to 20 minutes before exercise.

Environment

The nurse should be aware of the environment in which cromolyn sodium will be administered. Cromolyn sodium may be administered in any community or hospital setting. If administered at home, the nurse should remind the patient to administer it before engaging in a activity that causes bronchospasm.

Nursing Diagnoses and Outcomes

- Imbalanced Nutrition: Less than Body Requirements related to nausea and vomiting, bloating, abdominal cramps, and flatulence

  Desired outcome: The patient will maintain body weight throughout therapy.
- Ineffective Breathing Pattern related to bronchospasm and cough

  Desired outcome: The patient will have a patent airway throughout therapy.

Planning and Intervention

Maximizing Therapeutic Effects

Cromolyn sodium is available in a variety of administration vehicles such as a dry-powder inhaler (Spinhaler), a nebulizer, or an MDI. The nurse should evaluate the patient's ability to correctly use these devices (see the display, Community-Based Concerns: How to Use a Metered-Dose Inhaler). Cromolyn sodium is used for long-term management of respiratory disorders. With the exception of exercise-induced asthma, the patient should take the medication daily *regardless of the absence of symptoms.*

Minimizing Adverse Effects

The nurse should caution patients who have a known intolerance to lactose, or who experience symptoms of lactose intolerance (i.e., nausea and vomiting, bloating, abdominal cramps, and flatulence) while taking cromolyn sodium to contact the health care provider. Changing to a different drug may be necessary to avoid losing weight from GI effects.

Providing Patient and Family Education

- The nurse should stress that cromolyn sodium should not be taken by any patient who has a hypersensitivity to this drug.
- The nurse should emphasize that cromolyn sodium is not useful in the management of acute symptoms, and that it is used for prophylaxis only. The patient should use a short-term sympathomimetic drug for acute symptoms of respiratory distress.
- The nurse should demonstrate the correct use of administration devices and watch a return demonstration from the patient.
- The nurse should be sure that the patient understands that cromolyn sodium is taken on a daily basis *regardless of the absence of symptoms.*
- The nurse should instruct the patient to use cromolyn sodium 15 to 20 minutes prior to engaging in any activity that is a known precipitant to inducing bronchospasm in that patient (e.g., exercise).
- The nurse should teach the patient how to use a peak-flow meter to monitor his or her personal respiratory status.

Ongoing Assessment and Evaluation

The nurse should evaluate the effectiveness of cromolyn sodium demonstrated by a decrease in the frequency and severity of symptoms. For example, the patient should remain free from symptoms such as itchy, watery eyes, nasal congestion, or respiratory distress. The nurse should monitor for potential adverse effects in special populations, as previously mentioned. ■

DRUG CLOSELY RELATED TO CROMOLYN SODIUM

Nedocromil (Tilade) is an anti-inflammatory agent used in the maintenance treatment of mild to moderate asthma. Nedocromil is effective in the therapy of adult patients whose asthma is not controlled by beta agonists alone. It has actions similar to those of cromolyn and its safety and efficacy in the treatment of mild to moderate asthma is equivalent to cromolyn sodium. Although nedocromil is similar in some ways to cromolyn, distinct differences exist. Both cromolyn and nedocromil are similar in their ability to antagonize antigen-induced mast cell degranulation. Nedocromil differs from cromolyn by its ability to prevent bronchoconstriction secondary to non-antigenic stimuli at much lower doses.

LEUKOTRIENE RECEPTOR ANTAGONISTS

Within the last decade, leukotrienes have been identified as important mediators in the pathology and symptomatology of both acute and chronic asthma. Even patients with mild asthma show airway inflammation, including infiltration of the mucosa and epithelium with activated T cells, mast cells, and eosinophils. T cells and mast cells release the cytokines leukotriene, histamine, bradykinin, and serotonin that increase microvascular permeability, disrupt the epithelium, and stimulate neural reflexes and mucus-secreting glands. The result is airway hyperreactivity, bronchoconstriction, and hypersecretion, manifested by wheezing, coughing, and dyspnea. Leukotriene receptor antagonists include zafirlukast, montelukast, and zileuton. Zafirlukast (Accolate) is the prototypical leukotriene receptor antagonist.

MEMORY CHIP

Cromolyn Sodium

- Used for prophylaxis of allergic symptoms, including asthma
- Significant contraindications: hypersensitivity and acute symptoms
- Most common adverse effects: dry throat, cough, and wheezing
- Most serious adverse effects: bronchospasm and anaphylaxis
- Maximizing therapeutic effects: teach use of delivery systems
- Minimizing adverse effects: use only as directed
- Most significant patient education: take the medication daily, despite the absence of symptoms; the drug is to be used only for prophylaxis and not as a "rescue" drug.

NURSING MANAGEMENT OF THE PATIENT RECEIVING ZAFIRLUKAST

Core Drug Knowledge

Pharmacotherapeutics

Zafirlukast is used as prophylaxis or for treatment of chronic asthma. It is not indicated for symptoms of an acute attack. An unlabeled use of zafirlukast is chronic idiopathic urticaria and dermatographism (see Table 36-5).

Pharmacokinetics

Zafirlukast is administered orally. It is distributed to tissues to some degree, but it distributes minimally across the blood-brain barrier. In the treatment of asthma, the peak onset of action may be noted as early as day 1 of therapy, and usually within 2 weeks. For that reason, it is not useful in the management of an acute asthma attack.

Food reduces the bioavailability of zafirlukast by roughly 40%, and so it should be taken either 1 hour before or 2 hours after meals. Zafirlukast is metabolized extensively through the P450 (CYP 3A4 and CYP 2C9) system. Elimination is primarily in feces with approximately 10% excreted in urine.

Pharmacodynamics

Zafirlukast blocks receptors for the leukotrienes bound to the amino acid cysteine. The cysteinyl leukotrienes are potent bronchoconstrictors, approximately 100 to 1,000 times more potent than histamine. By blocking receptors that mediate bronchoconstriction, vascular permeability, and mucous secretion, zafirlukast significantly improves the wheezing, coughing, and dyspneic symptoms of asthma.

Contraindications and Precautions

Zafirlukast is contraindicated in any patient with a known hypersensitivity to zafirlukast or povidone, lactose, titanium dioxide, and cellulose derivatives, which are all inactive ingredients in the tablet. Zafirlukast is contraindicated for use in women who breastfeed since it is not approved for use in children younger than 6 years of age. Finally, it is contraindicated for use of acute symptoms of wheezing, shortness of breath, or bronchospasm.

Zafirlukast should be given cautiously to patients with hepatic disease due to the decreased clearance of zafirlukast. It also is used cautiously in patients taking warfarin because they use the same P450 metabolism pathway. Additionally, zafirlukast should be given cautiously to patients older than 60 years of age because of a decreased clearance.

Adverse Effects

The most common adverse reactions with zafirlukast are headache, gastritis, pharyngitis, and rhinitis. Other reported adverse effects include dizziness, nausea and vomiting, diarrhea, abdominal pain, arthralgia, myalgia, fever, and back pain.

Serious adverse effects include asymptomatic elevated hepatic enzymes, symptomatic hepatitis and hyperbilirubinemia or jaundice, and rarely, hepatic failure.

In patients taking zafirlukast at the same time that systemic steroids are being withdrawn, Churg-Strauss syndrome (CSS), a form of vasculitis with migratory lung infiltrates and eosinophilia, may occur. It is unclear whether this is caused by the use of zafirlukast or whether CSS was present previously but masked by the use of glucocorticosteroids.

Drug Interactions

Zafirlukast interacts with theophylline, warfarin, aspirin, erythromycin, and drugs metabolized through the P450 CYP2C9 or CYP3A4 isoenzymes. Table 36-7 presents these potential drug-drug interactions. Food decreases the bioavailability of zafirlukast by approximately 40%.

Assessment of Relevant Core Patient Variables

Health Status

The nurse should assess the patient for potential medical conditions, such as hepatic insufficiency or drug therapy that contraindicates using zafirlukast or requires close patient monitoring. It is especially important to assess the patient for use of theophylline, aspirin, warfarin, or other drugs that utilize the P450 metabolism pathway. The nurse also should assess for a hypersensitivity to

TABLE 36-7 Agents That Interact With Zafirlukast

Interactants	Effect and Significance	Nursing Management
aspirin	Co-administration of aspirin, acetylsalicylic acid 650 mg PO qid increases plasma concentrations of zafirlukast by approximately 45%.	Monitor for efficacy of zafirlukast therapy
erythromycin and clarithromycin	In asthmatic patients, erythromycin decreases the bioavailability of zafirlukast by approximately 40%.	Monitor for efficacy of antibiotic therapy
theophylline	Zafirlukast may increase the serum concentration of theophylline because it is thought to also inhibit CYP1A2, the hepatic isoenzyme that is responsible for the metabolism of theophylline.	Monitor serum theophylline levels Monitor for signs and symptoms of theophylline toxicity
warfarin	Zafirlukast increases the elimination half-life of S-warfarin by approximately 36% and prolongs the prothrombin time by 35%.	Prothrombin times and international normalized rates should be carefully monitored in patients on warfarin therapy The anticoagulant dosage should be adjusted as indicated
CYP3A4 metabolized drugs • alprazolam • carbamazepine • citalopram • some corticosteroids • cyclosporine • diazepam • calcium-channel blockers • irbesartan • lidocaine • lovastatin • midazolam • quinidine • sildenafil • simvastatin • tolterodine • triazolam • zonisamide	CYP3A4 metabolized drugs may be inhibited by zafirlukast because it is also metabolized through this pathway. Inhibition may result in increased serum concentrations of the inhibited drugs.	Monitor for toxicity of drugs Monitor for increased adverse effects
CYP2C9 metabolized drugs • amitriptyline • diclofenac • ibuprofen • imipramine • phenytoin • tolbutamide	CYP2C9 metabolized drugs may be inhibited by zafirlukast because it is also metabolized through this pathway. Inhibition may result in increased serum concentrations of the inhibited drugs.	Monitor for toxicity of drugs Monitor for increased adverse effects

povidone, lactose, titanium dioxide, and cellulose derivatives, all of which are ingredients in zafirlukast tablets. Finally, the nurse should evaluate the plan of care to see whether the patient is being withdrawn from glucocorticoid steroid therapy. Any positive findings should be communicated to the health care provider. The nurse should perform a baseline respiratory assessment and document the findings. This baseline will be used to evaluate the efficacy of zafirlukast therapy.

Life Span and Gender

The nurse should evaluate the pregnancy status of the patient, as needed. Zafirlukast is a pregnancy category B drug. However, human studies have not been performed. Zafirlukast should be administered during pregnancy only when the benefits outweigh the risk to the fetus. Zafirlukast enters breast milk. Therefore, it should not be administered to women who breast-feed because it is not approved for use in children younger than 5 years of age.

It is important to note the age of the patient taking zafirlukast. The nurse should arrange for frequent follow-up appointments for patients older than 60 years of age. Elderly patients may have a decreased renal clearance of zafirlukast, which increases the risk for adverse effects and toxicity.

Lifestyle, Diet, and Habits

The nurse should assess the patient's understanding that zafirlukast must be taken on an empty stomach. The nurse should remind the patient that food decreases the bioavailability of zafirlukast.

Environment

The nurse should note the environment in which the drug will be administered. Zafirlukast generally is administered in the home environment.

Nursing Diagnoses and Outcomes

- Risk for Injury (poisoning) related to interaction between drugs metabolized by the P450 enzyme system.
  Desired outcome: The patient will comply with dosage adjustment of medications, serial laboratory testing, and report adverse effects immediately to the health care provider.
- Diarrhea related to drug therapy
  Desired outcome: The patient will remain well hydrated throughout therapy.
- Acute Pain related to drug therapy
  Desired outcome: The patient will take non-narcotic analgesics should headache occur.

Planning and Intervention

Maximizing Therapeutic Effects

The nurse should assess that the patient takes zafirlukast twice daily, despite the absence of symptoms. The nurse should remind the patient to take zafirlukast on an empty stomach to increase the bioavailability of the drug.

Minimizing Adverse Effects

The nurse should ensure that the patient takes the medication only as prescribed. The nurse should assess for a change of COPD or asthma therapy when zafirlukast is added, especially if the patient is taking systemic glucocorticoid steroid medications. The nurse should carefully review the patient's medications to assess for other medications that utilize the P450 metabolism pathway.

Providing Patient and Family Education

- The nurse should explain that zafirlukast is used in the maintenance of COPD and asthma and should not be used if acute shortness of breath or wheezing occurs.
- The nurse should advise the patient to immediately report symptoms such as abdominal pain, jaundice, nausea, vomiting, and dark urine because these symptoms may indicate hepatic injury.
- The nurse can encourage the patient to take non-narcotic analgesics should headache occur, and to drink plenty of fluids if he or she experiences diarrhea while taking zafirlukast. The patient also should report these adverse effects to the health care provider.
- The nurse should caution the patient not to stop or decrease systemic glucocorticoid steroid therapy without speaking with the health care provider first.
- The nurse should emphasize the importance of contacting the health care provider if any new medications are prescribed by any other member of the health care team.

Ongoing Assessment and Evaluation

The nurse should assess the patient for the need of beta-agonist drugs in addition to zafirlukast. If the patient continues to need beta-agonist drugs more than twice weekly, refer the patient to the heath care provider for additional assessment.

The nurse should assess the patient for symptoms that may reflect hepatic injury. If the patient takes other medications that are metabolized by the P450 enzyme system, the nurse should evaluate the patient for potential adverse effects or toxicity of these drugs. ■

DRUGS CLOSELY RELATED TO P ZAFIRLUKAST

Montelukast

Montelukast (Singulair) is similar to zafirlukast in its mechanism of action. It has the advantage of once daily dosing as well as being approved for use in children 2 years of age and older. Unlike zafirlukast, montelukast does not inhibit specific hepatic cytochrome isozymes. Therefore, it is not

MEMORY CHIP

Zafirlukast

- Used for maintenance of COPD and asthma
- Significant contraindications: hypersensitivity to povidone, lactose, titanium dioxide, and cellulose; women who breast-feed
- Most common adverse effects: headache, gastritis, pharyngitis, and rhinitis
- Most serious adverse effects: hepatic failure and Churg-Strauss syndrome
- Maximizing therapeutic effects: administer the drug daily, despite the absence of symptoms
- Minimizing adverse effects: take the drug only as prescribed
- Most significant patient education: this drug will not abort an acute attack

expected to affect the hepatic clearance of drugs metabolized by these enzymes.

Zileuton

Zileuton (Zyflo) inhibits the first enzyme in the lipoxygenase pathway, thus preventing the formation of potent leukotrienes. Although this mechanism of action may be beneficial to disorders such as asthma, rheumatoid arthritis, and ulcerative colitis, it is only approved for the management of asthma at this time.

In animal studies, zileuton produced developmental defects. Therefore, it is assigned to pregnancy category C. During pregnancy, zileuton should be used only if the potential benefit to the mother outweighs the potential risks to the fetus. It is not known whether zileuton is excreted in human milk, and therefore, it should be avoided by women who breast-feed.

Most adverse effects attributed to zileuton administration have been mild and self-limited. Adverse effects include flu-like syndrome, headache, dizziness, dyspepsia, drowsiness, abdominal pain, and insomnia. In rare cases, hepatotoxicity and neutropenia have occurred.

CHAPTER SUMMARY

- Mucolytics, such as acetylcysteine, are drugs designed to break up the mucus produced in the respiratory tract, leading to a thinner secretion that is more easily moved.
- Drugs used in the management of COPD (CAL) are generally grouped into bronchodilators or anti-inflammatory agents.
- Bronchodilators are composed of several different subclasses, including sympathomimetics (albuterol), anticholinergics (ipratropium bromide), and xanthine derivatives (theophylline).
- Inhaled anticholinergics (ipratropium bromide) are used for maintenance treatment for asthma and COPD and are not used for acute symptoms. Short-acting sympathomimetic inhalers are the only type of inhaled drugs that help during acute episodes of asthma or exacerbations of COPD. They are known as "rescue drugs."
- Anti-inflammatory drugs are composed of several different subclasses, including inhaled glucocorticoids, such as beclomethasone, mast cell stabilizers (cromolyn sodium), and leukotriene receptor antagonists (zafirlukast).
- The mast cell stabilizer cromolyn sodium works by stabilizing mast cell rupture when exposed to an antigen. This stops the release of histamine, serotonin, bradykinin, and leukotriene; all of which induce bronchoconstriction.
- The glucocorticoids are the most effective anti-inflammatory drugs available for the management of respiratory disorders.
- The leukotriene antagonist receptor zafirlukast works by inhibiting the bronchoconstrictive properties of leukotrienes.
- Cromolyn sodium, inhaled glucocorticoid steroids, and leukotriene receptor antagonists are maintenance treatment for asthma and COPD, and are not used for acute symptoms.

QUESTIONS FOR STUDY AND REVIEW

1. In the management of lower respiratory tract disorders, which main classes of drugs are used?
2. Compare and contrast the pharmacodynamics of the different types of bronchodilators.
3. In a patient with acute respiratory distress, which of the bronchodilators would be most effective?
4. Which of the anti-inflammatory agents is the most effective?
5. What is the difference between glucocorticoid steroids given orally and by inhalation?
6. Compare and contrast the pharmacodynamics of the different types of anti-inflammatory agents?
7. In the patient taking inhaled steroids, an anticholinergic inhaler, and a beta-adrenergic agonist inhaler, which inhaler would you tell the patient to use first?

NEED MORE HELP?

Chapter 36 of the study guide for *Drug Therapy in Nursing* contains exercises and activities to reinforce your understanding of the concepts presented in this chapter. For additional information, see the text's accompanying website at *http://www.connection.lww.com.*

REFERENCES AND BIBLIOGRAPHY

CCIS System. (2001). *Computerized Clinical Information System.* Denver, CO: Micromedex.

Clinical Drug Monographs [CDRom]. (2001). Gold Standard Media.

Drug Facts and Comparisons. (2000). St. Louis: Facts and Comparisons Division.

D'Urzo, A. D., & Chapman, K. R. (2000). Leukotriene-receptor antagonists. Role in asthma management. *Canadian Family Physician, 46*(4), 872–879.

Hardman, J. G., Limbird, L. E., Molinof, P. B., Ruddon, R. W., & Gilman, A. (Eds.). (1997). *Goodman and Gilman's the pharmacological basis of therapeutics* (9th ed.). New York: McGraw-Hill.

Karch, A. (2001). *2001 Lippincott's nursing drug guide.* Philadelphia: Lippincott Williams & Wilkins.

Katzung, B. C. (2000). *Basic and clinical pharmacology* (8th ed.), New York: McGraw-Hill.

Konig, P. (2000). The effects of cromolyn sodium and nedocromil sodium in early asthma prevention. *Journal of Allergy and Clinical Immunology, 105*(2 Pt. 2), S575–S581.

Krawiec, M. E, & Wenzel, S. E. (1999). Use of leukotriene antagonists in childhood asthma. *Current Opinions in Pediatrics, 11*(6), 540–547.

Lim, S., Jatakanon, A., Gordon, D., et al. (2000). Comparison of high dose inhaled steroids, low dose inhaled steroids plus low dose theophylline, and low dose inhaled steroids alone in chronic asthma in general practice. *Thorax, 55*(10), 837–841.

National Education and Prevention Program, Expert Panel Report II. (1997). *Guidelines for the diagnosis and management of asthma.* Bethesda, MD: National Heart, Lung, and Blood Institute.

Pearlman, D. S., et al. (2000). Effectiveness and tolerability of zafirlukast for the treatment of asthma in children. *Clinical Therapy, 22*(6), 732–747.

Porth, C. (1998). *Pathophysiology: Concepts of altered health states* (5th ed.), Philadelphia: Lippincott Williams & Wilkins.

Silverman, R. (2000). Treatment of acute asthma. A new look at the old and at the new. *Clinical Chest Medicine, 21*(21), 361–379.

Simon, R. A. (1999). Update on inhaled corticosteroids: safety, compliance, and new delivery systems. *Allergy and Asthma Proceedings, 20*(3), 161–165.

Tatro, D. (Ed.). (2000). *Drug interaction facts* (6th ed.). St. Louis: Facts and Comparisons.

Warman, K. L. (2000). Management of asthma exacerbations: Home treatment. *Journal of Asthma, 37*(6), 461–468.

Zorc, J. J., & Pawlowski, N. A. (1999). Prevention of asthma morbidity: Recent advances. *Current Opinions in Pediatrics, 12*(5), 438–443.

Physiology

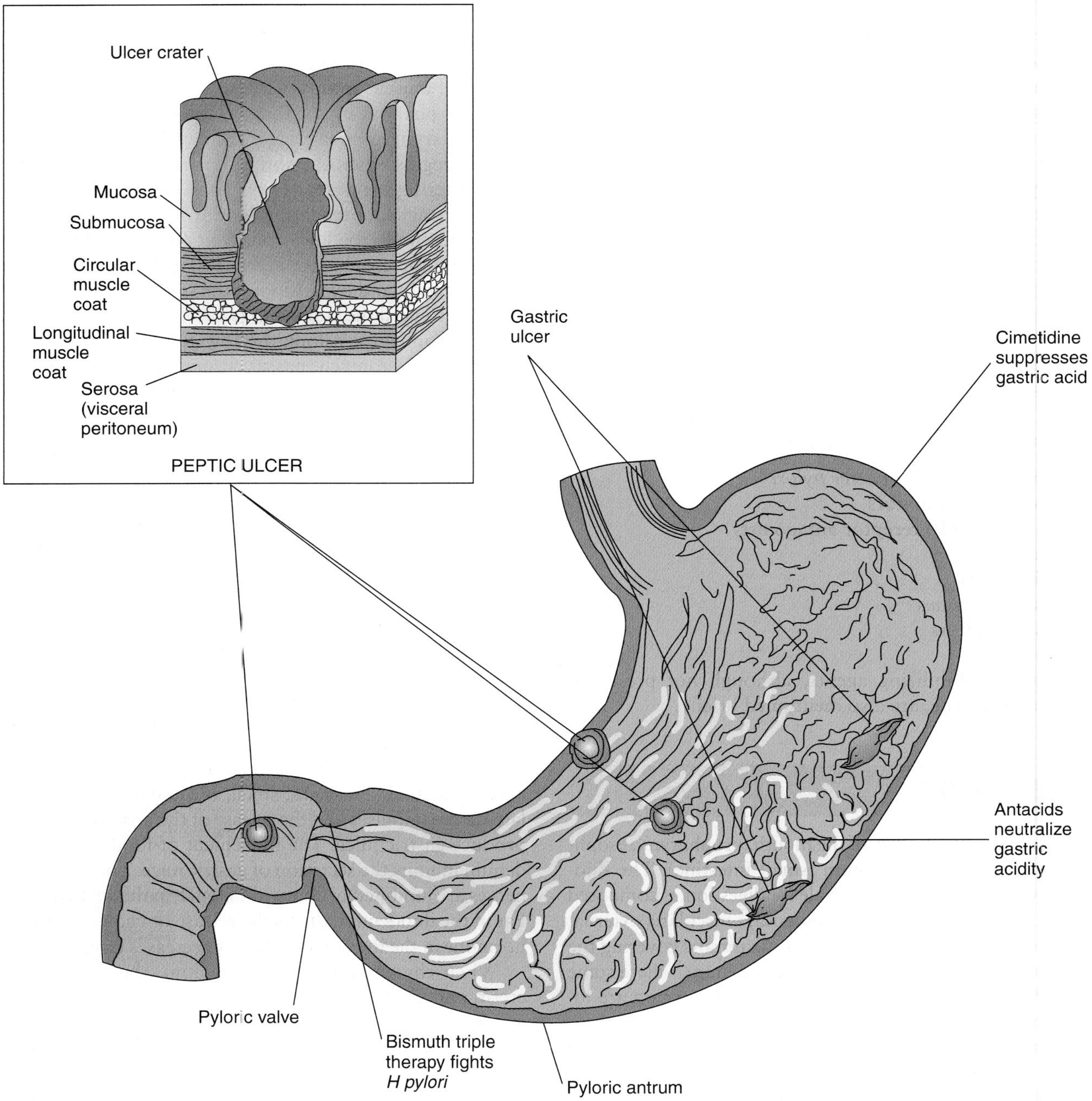

Figure 37-1. Drugs used in treating peptic ulcer disease need to retard further ulceration and promote healing. Lesions known as peptic ulcers are those that affect the mucosa of the stomach (gastric ulcer) or the duodenum (duodenal ulcer). With an advanced duodenal ulcer, gastric acid burrows through the gastric mucosa, submucosa, and muscle layers and perforates the peritoneum. As the illustration indicates, antacids neutralize excess acidity, H_2 receptor antagonists suppress gastric acid production; and bismuth triple therapy treats ulcers caused by *Helicobacter pylori.*

Additionally, the VC can be stimulated when the **chemoreceptor trigger zone** (CTZ) is stimulated. Located near the VC, the CTZ is stimulated by drugs, chemicals, toxins, radiation, hormonal changes, some disease states, and altered metabolic states. It also is stimulated by vestibular mechanisms. When the CTZ is stimulated, it acts on the VC, allowing it to maintain a state of excitability to other incoming vestibular impulses.

PATHOPHYSIOLOGY

GASTROESOPHAGEAL REFLUX DISEASE

When gastric acid abnormally moves into the esophagus, chronic symptoms of heartburn and dyspepsia and ulceration of the mucosal lining will occur. This is known as **gastroesophageal reflux disease** (GERD). Although GERD may sometimes occur alone, it often results from a hiatal hernia. A hiatal hernia exists when the cardiac portion of the stomach moves through a weakened opening in the diaphragm. The movement of the stomach into the diaphragm decreases the pressure of the lower esophageal sphincter so that the acid easily moves into the esophagus. Because cancer of the esophagus has the same symptoms as a hiatal hernia, cancer must be ruled out before drug therapy starts.

ULCERS

A **peptic ulcer** exists after erosion of all layers of the wall of the stomach or duodenum has occurred. Untreated, a peptic ulcer may erode through the serosa and result in perforation. Peptic ulcers may occur in any part of the upper GI tract that is in contact with gastric acid and pepsin. The symptoms depend on the location of the ulcer. Gastric ulcer pain usually occurs 1 to 2 hours after eating, whereas duodenal ulcer pain begins 2 to 4 hours after eating and often results in night pain. The complications of both types are perforation, hemorrhage, and obstruction. A **stress ulcer** is a peptic ulcer that is caused by acute or chronic stress. Stress ulcers occur frequently in critically ill patients. Clinically important complications of stress ulcers (i.e., bleeding that requires transfusion, bleeding associated with hemodynamic instability, and GI perforation) are believed to be relatively rare although the exact frequency has not been confirmed in clinical trials (Erstad, Barletta, Jacobs, Killan, Kramer, & Martin, 1999). The frequency of stress ulcers has not been studied in noncritically ill patients. Although several types of single system injuries (e.g., head, spinal cord, thermal, or hepatic) have been believed to be associated with higher incidence of clinically significant stress ulcers, and frequently receive prophylactic therapy in Intensive Care Units, only two risk factors have been found to be predictive of clinically important bleeding. These risk factors are respiratory failure requiring mechanical ventilation and coagulopathy (defects in the blood clotting mechanism).

HELICOBACTER PYLORI INFECTION

The bacterial organism *Helicobacter pylori* (***H. pylori***) is a gram-negative, spiral organism that colonizes the gastric mucosa. *H. pylori* is the most common chronic bacterial infection worldwide. It is found in over half of the human population. The natural history of *H. pylori* infection is still unknown. Person-to-person contact may possibly be responsible for transmission. Infection persists unless treated. Research has shown that there is an etiologic association between *H. pylori* infection and a number of important diseases, including chronic active gastritis, peptic ulcer disease, mucosa-associated lymphoid tissue lymphoma, gastric polyps, and gastric cancer. *H. pylori* has been identified in 90% to 95% of patients with duodenal ulcers, 50% to 80% of gastric ulcer patients, and in almost 100% of patients with chronic active gastritis. It is believed to be the causative agent for most incidences of ulcer disease. The link between gastric cancer and *H. pylori* is strong. Chronic *H. pylori* infection, particularly when acquired in early childhood, can predispose a person to an increased risk of developing gastric cancer. The world Health Organization has recently classified *H. pylori* as a type 1 human carcinogen because of this finding (Chelimsky and Czinn, 2000). The link between *H. pylori* and varied symptoms in children is considered controversial because it is frequently associated with nonulcerative gastritis in this age group (Tolia, 1999). A recent study, however, indicates that recurrent abdominal pain in children may be associated with gastritis induced by *H. pylori* (Frank, Stricker, Stallmach, & Braegger, 2000). There also have been suggestions in the literature that *H. pylori* may be involved in diseases outside the upper GI tract.

Historically, stress, caffeine intake, and smoking were considered contributors to excessive acid production, and the excess acid lead to ulcer formation. This theory has been abandoned because the link of *H. pylori* and peptic ulcers was found. Excess acid alone does not produce gastric ulcers. Still, 80% of people infected with *H. pylori* never develop an ulcer. Other factors in the person's internal environment play a role in creating peptic ulcers when *H. pylori* is present. These factors are not known yet. Diet may be one of these factors. In a review of the literature from 1966 to 1999, soluble fiber from fruit and vegetables seem to be a protection against developing duodenal ulcers. A diet with high amounts of refined sugars appears to be a risk factor for developing duodenal ulcers (Misciagna, Cisternino, & Freudenheim, 2000). Smokers do have a higher rate of peptic ulcer disease than nonsmokers; this most likely due to the detrimental effects on the gastric mucosa. Surface active phospholipids are believed to play a key role in protecting the gastric mucosa. Both *H. pylori* and smoking alter the concentrations of some of the phospholipid subclasses. This alteration makes the mucosa more vulnerable to damage from gastric acid that is present in the stomach (Wenner, Gunnarsson, Graffner, & Lindell, 2000). However, one study has shown that cigarette smoking did not increase the recurrence of peptic ulcers after eradication of *H. pylori* (Chan, Sung, Lee, Leung, Chan, Yung, et al., 1997). Persistent *H. pylori* infection, even after treatment, has been shown through a clinical study to be the only independent predictor of the recurrence of duodenal ulcer bleeding (Lai, Hui, Wong, Hu, Ching, & Lam, 2000).

PANCREATITIS

The pancreas contributes pancreatic juice and vital digestive enzymes to digestion. These enzymes are reduced or no longer produced in patients who have chronic pancreatitis or in those who have undergone a pancreatic resection or removal. In pancreatitis, digestive enzymes that are maintained normally in their inactive form in the pancreas become activated, destroying parts of the gland. With time, this destruction of the gland results in a decrease in the amount of enzymes that are produced due to cell loss. Chronic pancreatitis occurs following attacks of acute pancreatitis. The digestive enzyme pancrelipase is used to treat pancreatitis and other pancreatic deficiency states.

OBESITY

The incidence of overweight and obesity is increasing at an alarming rate both in the United States and worldwide. It has been estimated that a little more than half of American adults are now overweight or obese. This is an increase of over 25% over the past three decades. These increases have occurred among the three major racial groups in the United States and in both sexes (Flegal, Carroll, Kuczmarski, & Johnson, 1998). Obesity and overweight reflect how much a patient's body mass index (BMI) is larger than normal. The BMI is calculated as the weight in kilograms divided by the square of height in meters. Normal BMI is 18.5 to 24.9 kg/m^2. The term overweight is used if the patient's BMI is 25 to 29.9 kg/m^2, whereas the term obesity is used if the BMI exceeds 29.9 kg/m^2. Overweight and obesity are the result of a mismatch between energy consumed in calories and energy expended in activities. The lifestyle in industrialized countries is continuing to become more sedentary. The energy expenditure of the average American worker at the beginning of the 21st century is estimated to be about half of that of the American worker at the start of the 20th century. Additionally, a high-fat diet, common in these countries, also contributes to obesity.

Studies based on the data collected in the Third National Health and Nutrition Examination Survey showed that the prevalence of overweight and obesity were similar for white non-Hispanics, black non-Hispanics, and Mexican Americans (Must, Spandano, Coakley, Field, Coldity, & Diety, 1999). High blood pressure, type 2 diabetes, coronary heart disease, elevated blood cholesterol, gallbladder disease, and osteoarthritis are associated with overweight and obesity. High blood pressure is the most common overweight- and obesity-related health condition, and its incidence increases as weight increases (Must, et al., 1999). Type 2 diabetes, gallbladder disease, and osteoarthritis also are more prevalent as weight increases. Coronary heart disease did not have an elevated prevalence in overweight patients, but was significantly elevated if the patient was obese. Elevated blood cholesterol levels were found in all levels of overweight and obesity, but unlike the other morbidities, it did not increase progressively as weight increased (Must, et al., 1999). Prevention and treatment of obesity are important to control these lifelong morbidities, and the mortalities that accompany them.

NAUSEA AND VOMITING

Disorders of the upper GI tract are often accompanied by nausea and vomiting. Increased activity of neurotransmitters, for example, dopamine in the CTZ and acetylcholine in the VC, appears to have an important role in inducing vomiting. Serotonin also has a role in vomiting, and special serotonin receptors are located in the CTZ. The release of serotonin from the small intestine during chemotherapy stimulates these receptors and therefore stimulates vomiting.

Stimulation of the CTZ in the brain stimulates the VC. When the VC is stimulated, vomiting occurs. The VC also may be stimulated directly by conditions such as GI irritation, motion sickness, and vestibular neuritis. Inflammation, spasms, ischemia, and distention can also irritate nerve endings and activate the VC.

DRUGS USED TO TREAT *HELICOBACTER PYLORI* INFECTION

Elimination of *H. pylori* from the GI tract improves healing and decreases the recurrence of ulcers. Once the infection has been eradicated the reinfection rates are less than 0.5% per year; ulcer recurrence rates also are reduced dramatically. The cure rate from the various treatment options range from about 70% to 90% or higher. Eradication therapy is the standard of care for active or inactive peptic ulcer patients, including those using nonsteroidal antiinflammatory drugs (NSAIDS). No routine antimicrobial treatment is recommended if the patient has *H. pylori* infection but does not have an ulcer. In addition, the use of antibiotics to eradicate *H. pylori* in an attempt to prevent gastric cancer is not recommended due to lack of research (NIH Guidelines, 1998). Strong indications for treating *H. pylori* infections include mucosa-associated lymphoid tissue lymphoma, hyperplastic polyps, hyperplastic gastropathy, postendoscopic resection for gastric cancer, and acute *H. pylori* gastritis. Currently no single treatment is recognized as the standard, or best, treatment option. The Food and Drug Administration (FDA) has approved six different treatment options for treating *H. pylori* infections (Table 37-1). Other variations of combination drug therapy have been used in practice and in clinical trials.

Use of a single antibiotic is not recommended because of the potential for developing resistance to that antibiotic. Antibiotic resistance has been reported with metronidazole and clarithromycin but not with bismuth, amoxicillin, or tetracycline. Prior exposure to antibiotics increases the risk for drug resistance. Resistance to metronidazole often can be overcome if the dose and the duration of therapy are increased. Clarithromycin resistance can not be overcome by increasing the dose or the duration.

Use of a single antibiotic with a proton pump inhibitor has been shown to be effective in curing *H. pylori,* but only

TABLE 37-1 Therapies Approved by the Food and Drug Administration for *H. Pylori* Infection

Drug Therapy	Dose and Duration of Therapy
*lansoprazole +	30 mg bid for 10–14 d
clarithromycin +	500 mg bid for 10–14 d
amoxicillin	1 g bid for day to 14 d
omeprazole +	20 mg bid for 10 d
clarithromycin +	500 mg bid for 10 d
amoxicillin	1 g bid for 10 d
ranitidine bismuth citrate +	400 mg bid for 14 d
clarithromycin	500 mg tid for 14 d
followed by ranitidine bismuth citrate	400 mg bid for additional 14 d
bismuth subsalicylate +	525 mg qid for 14 d
metronidazole +	250 mg qid for 14 d
tetracycline +	500 mg qid for 14 d
H_2 receptor antagonist	per individual drug dosing for 28 d
†omeprazole +	40 mg qd for 10 d
clarithromycin	500 mg tid for 14 d
followed by additional omeprazole	20 mg once/daily for additional 14 d
†lansoprazole +	30 mg tid for 14 d
amoxicillin	1 g tid for 14 d

*This combination therapy has ≥90% or higher eradication rate of *H. pylori* infection.

† Practice guidelines from the American College of Gastroenterology do not recommend a single antibiotic combined with a proton pump inhibitor because cure rate is <70%.

30% to 70% of the time, so it is not recommended. Double antibiotic therapy with the addition of an antisecretory drug (one that prevents the secretion of gastric acid) is very effective and is the most preferred therapy. Triple and quadruple therapy regimens also are effective in curing *H. pylori* infection. They include bismuth subsalicylate (Pepto-Bismol), antibiotics, and an antisecretory agent. There is more risk of adverse effects from these therapies. Compliance also is a limiting factor for these therapies because of the number of drugs that must be taken every day.

Studies have concluded that the cure of *H. pylori* infection reduces significantly the risk of recurring ulcer disease. Thus, maintenance therapy with antisecretory agents is not needed for patients with a history of uncomplicated ulcer disease after eradication of *H. pylori*. For patients who have had complicated ulcer disease, the decision about whether they should continue on antisecretory drugs must be made on an individual basis. Factors that should be considered and may lead to a decision to continue with therapy are presence of comorbid disease; use of medications, such as NSAIDS and anticoagulants, which increase risk of recurrence or increase risk of complications; and the severity of the previous ulcer-related complications.

Ulcers that are refractory, or nonresponsive, to therapy for *H. pylori* infection often are related to the failure to eradicate the organism. Resistance to the therapy, patients' nonadherence with therapy, and concurrent NSAID use also may be involved in refractory ulcers. Retreatment regimens for treatment failure should not include antibiotics that might have acquired resistance. With antibiotic-resistant *H. pylori* infections, higher doses and longer durations of treatment usually result in better cure rates. When multiple treatment regimens fail, salvage therapy with quadruple therapy may be used. Furazolidone, another antibiotic for serious infections, may be substituted for the metronidazole (Graham & Qureishi, 2000).

In animal models, prophylactic and therapeutic vaccines have been described against *H. pylori*. Research for the development of vaccines for use in humans for *H. pylori* is now under way (Ernst & Pappo, 2000). Further discussion of the antimicrobials used to treat *H. pylori* is found in Chapter 49.

C PROTON PUMP INHIBITORS

The secretion of gastric acid can be suppressed by inhibiting the H+/K+ adenosine triphosphatase (ATPase) enzyme system at the secretory surface of the gastric parietal cell. Because this enzyme system is the "acid pump," also known as the "proton pump," within the gastric mucosa, drugs that work to inhibit this system are known as proton pump inhibitors. They work to block the final step of gastric acid production. The effect is dose related. These drugs inhibit acid secretion regardless of the stimulus producing the acid. The prototype drug is omeprazole. Another drug in this class is lansoprazole. A drug significantly different from omeprazole is sulcrafate.

NURSING MANAGEMENT OF THE PATIENT RECEIVING P OMEPRAZOLE

Core Drug Knowledge

Pharmacotherapeutics

Omeprazole is used in the symptomatic treatment of heartburn and other symptoms of GERD. It also is used in the treatment of duodenal ulcers associated with *H. pylori* infections. It is sometimes used in the short-term treatment (4 to 8 weeks) of active duodenal and gastric ulcer when *H. pylori* is not present. It also is used in the short-term treatment of erosive esophagitis, diagnosed by endoscopy, to maintain healing. It can be used long term in chronic hypersecretory conditions, such as **Zollinger-Ellison syndrome,** multiple endocrine adenomas, and systemic mastocytosis. Unlabeled uses are treatment of posterior laryngitis, and to enhance the efficacy of pancreatin in the treatment of steatorrhea in cystic fibrosis.

Pharmacokinetics

Omeprazole, and other proton pump inhibitors, are acid labile. Therefore, they are always formulated as enteric-coated granules. Absorption is rapid after leaving the stomach. Omeprazole is metabolized extensively by the liver and several metabolites are formed. These metabolites do not have an antisecretory function, expect perhaps minimally. Metabolism of omeprazole is via the cytochrome P450 system. The antisecretory effect of omeprazole is long acting and not related closely to elimination half-life from the plasma. The half-life is less than 2 hours in the plasma, whereas the antisecretory effect is longer than 24 hours. This extended effect is believed to be due to prolonged binding of the drug to the parietal H+/K+ ATPase enzyme. When the drug is discontinued, normal secretory activity returns within 3 to 5 days. Little of the drug is excreted unchanged. The metabolites are excreted mostly in the urine, although about a fourth of them are eliminated in the feces (Table 37-2). Duration of action is lengthened in Asians (compared with in whites). Therefore, dose adjustments may be necessary.

Pharmacodynamics

Omeprazole suppresses the last phase of gastric acid production by suppressing the H+/K+ ATPase enzyme system. Intragastric pH is therefore elevated. Because of this, blood flow in the antrum, pylorus, and duodenal bulb decreases. Omeprazole increases serum pepsinogen levels and decreases pepsin activity. The increases in gastric pH are associated with increases in nitrate-reducing bacteria and elevation of nitrate concentration in gastric juice in patients with gastric ulcers. Serum gastrin levels increase along with the inhibition of acid secretion. Continued treatment does not provoke serum gastrin levels to rise continually, but rather they reach a certain degree of elevation and remain there.

TABLE 37-2 Summary of Selected Antisecretory Drugs and Other Drugs Used in Peptic Ulcer Disease

Drug (Trade) Name	Selected Indications	Route and Dosage Range	Pharmacokinetics
Proton Pump Inhibitors			
omeprazole (Prilosec)	Active duodenal ulcer Gastric ulcer GERD Hypersecretory conditions *Helicobacter pylori*	20 mg/d PO × 4–8 wk 40 mg/day PO × 4–8 wk 20 mg/day × 4–8 wk 60 mg once daily PO initially 20 mg bid PO (in combination with other therapy)	*Onset:* Within 1 h *Duration:* 72 h $t_{1/2}$: 30–60 min
lansoprazole (Prevacid)	Active duodenal ulcer Erosive esophagitis, GERD Hypersecretory conditions *H. pylori*	15 mg/d PO × 4 wk 30 mg/day PO × 8 wk 60 mg/d 30 mg/d × 2 wk (in combination with other drug therapy)	*Onset:* Unknown *Duration:* 24 h $t_{1/2}$: 1.5 h
H_2 Receptor Antagonists			
cimetidine (Tagamet, Tagamet HB)	Alleviation of symptoms and prevention of complications due to peptic ulcer disease; heartburn and acid indigestion; part of multidrug program to eliminate causative *H. pylori* in peptic ulcer disease.	PO, 800 mg at bedtime, or 300 mg qid with meals and at bedtime for 4–6 wk (duodenal) or 8 wk (gastric); IV or IM, 300 mg q 6–8 h, not to exceed 2,400 mg/d	*Onset:* PO, varies; IV, rapid *Duration:* 4–13 h (depending on dose and regimen) $t_{1/2}$: 2 h
	Prevention of upper GI bleeding	IV, infusion at 50 mg/h	
	Erosive GERD	PO, 1,600 mg/d divided into 2 or 4 doses for 12 wk; IV or IM, dosing and regimen not established	
	Pathologic hypersecretory conditions	PO, 300 mg qid with meals and at bedtime not to exceed 240 mg/d, given as long as clinically needed.	
	Heartburn/acid indigestion	PO OTC, 200 mg twice daily; continuous IV infusion, 300 mg q 6–8 h	

(continued)

TABLE 37-2 Summary of Selected Antisecretory Drugs and Other Drugs Used in Peptic Ulcer Disease (Continued)

Drug (Trade) Name	Selected Indications	Route and Dosage Range	Pharmacokinetics
ranitidine (Zantac, Zantac 75, GELdose)	Same as cimetidine, for ulcers and related conditions	PO, 150 mg bid, or 300 mg at bedtime (duodenal) short-term use for active ulcers; maintenance dose, 150 mg at bedtime; parenteral (any use), IM, 50 mg (2 mL pre-mixed) q6–8h; IV push, 50 mg (2 mL) diluted with 0.09% NaCl solution (normal saline) to make 20 mL, over 5 min or more; intermittent IV, 50 mg diluted in 100 mL dextrose 5% in water (D_5W) or other compatible solution, run over 15–20 min, q6–8h, not to exceed 400 mg/d	*Onset:* PO, varies; IV, rapid *Duration:* 8–12 h $t_{1/2}$: 2–3 h
	GERD	PO, 150 mg bid	
	Pathologic hypersecretory conditions (i.e., Zollinger-Ellison syndrome)	PO, 150 mg bid, may give up to 6 g/d; continuous IV infusion (dilute in compatible solution to no more than 2.5 mg/mL); run at 1 mg/kg/h, after 4 h may be adjusted upward in 0.5 mg/kg/h increments up to 2.5 mg/kg/h	
	Erosive esophagitis	PO, 150 mg qid; maintenance 150 mg bid	
famotidine (Pepcid, Pepcid AC)	Same as cimetidine, for ulcers and related conditions	PO (acute duodenal ulcer), 40 mg/d at bedtime or 20 mg bid for 6–8 wk; maintenance, 20 mg/d at bedtime; (acute benign gastric ulcer), 40 mg/d at bedtime; IV (patient NPO), 20 mg q12h (dilute 2 mL, or 20 mg, in 5 or 10 mL normal saline or other) compatible solution, and inject over at least 2 min); intermittent IV, 20 mg (dilute in 100 mL D_5W or other compatible solution, infuse over 15–30 min)	*Onset:* PO, ≤1 h; IV, rapid *Duration:* 10–12 h $t_{1/2}$: 2.5–3.5 h
	Hypersecretory conditions	PO (individualize), 20 mg q6h to start, up to 160 mg q6h; continue as long as needed	
	GERD	PO, 20 mg bid up to 6 wk	
	Esophagitis due to GERD	PO, 20 or 40 mg bid for up to 12 wk	
	Heartburn, acid indigestion	PO (OTC), 10 mg (1 tablet); prevention 1 h before eating a meal expected to cause GI distress; up to 2 tablets in 24 h	
nizatidine (Axid AR)	Duodenal ulcer, benign active gastric ulcer	PO (active ulcer), 300 mg once daily at bedtime or 150 mg bid (less for patients with renal insufficiency); maintenance 150 mg once daily at bedtime	*Onset:* Varies *Duration:* 3–10 h $t_{1/2}$: 1–2 h
	GERD	Adult: PO, 150 mg bid	
C Miscellaneous			
misoprostol (Cytotec)	Prevention of NSAID-induced gastric ulcers	PO, 200 µg qid with food; if not well tolerated, may use 100 µg per dose	*Onset:* Rapid *Duration:* 3 h $t_{1/2}$: 20–40 min
sucralfate (Carafate)	Duodenal ulcer	1 g PO qid 1 h before meals and at bedtime for 4–8 wk	*Onset:* 30 min *Duration:* 5 h $t_{1/2}$: 6–20 h

Contraindications and Precautions

Omeprazole is contraindicated for patients who are hypersensitive to the drug or any of its components. Omeprazole is classified as a pregnancy category C drug.

Adverse Effects

Omeprazole is well tolerated generally. The most common adverse effects are headache and diarrhea. However, these effects also were found in patients receiving placebo during clinical trials. Other adverse effects reported in clinical trials include those present in the central nervous system (CNS) (dizziness and asthenia), GI (constipation, abdominal pain, nausea, and vomiting), and miscellaneous (upper respiratory infection, cough, rash, and back pain).

Rare adverse effects (occurring in fewer than 1% of patients in clinical studies) are numerous and diverse. They include confusion, drowsiness, blurred vision, tachycardia, diaphoresis, flushing, dry mouth, severe generalized skin reactions, elevated liver enzyme levels, and overt hepatic disease.

Overdosage with omeprazole has been reported rarely, and no serious outcomes have been reported from overdosage. When patients received 16 to 45 times the usual dose, the symptoms were transient and included confusion, drowsiness, blurred vision, tachycardia, nausea, diaphoresis, fusing, headache, and dry mouth.

Drug Interactions

Omeprazole may interact with other drugs that also are metabolized through the cytochrome P450 pathway. Examples of these drugs include cyclosporine, disulfiram, and the benzodiazepines. This may produce elevated levels of these other drug therapies as their metabolism is decreased. Because omeprazole causes prolonged and substantial decreases in gastric acidity, drugs that depend on an acid environment for absorption may not be absorbed as well (Table 37-3).

Assessment of Relevant Core Patient Variables

Health Status

The nurse should determine that the patient has a clinical indication for the use of omeprazole. Hepatic and renal disease do not require a decreased dosage.

Life Span and Gender

The nurse should assess female patients for pregnancy or breast-feeding. As stated previously, omeprazole is a pregnancy category C drug; there are no adequate or well controlled studies of the drug in pregnant women. Omeprazole should be used during pregnancy only if the potential benefit justifies the unknown risk to the fetus. It is not known whether omeprazole is secreted in breast milk. Animal studies showed decreased weight gain from nursing when the mother received large doses (35 to 345 times the human dose) of omeprazole. Therefore, use in breast-feeding is not recommended. The nurse also should note the patient's age. Its efficacy and use in children have not been established. Although bioavailability of the drug may be increased in older adults, no dosage adjustment is needed.

Lifestyle, Diet, and Habits

The nurse should assess the patient's diet and smoking habits. Highly acidic foods, such as tomato juice, and highly spiced foods may worsen the symptoms of GERD or peptic ulcer disease until healing of the ulcer occurs.

TABLE 37-3 Agents That Interact With Omeprazole

Interactants	Effect and Significance	Nursing Management
clarithromycin	Increases the plasma levels of both clarithromycin and omeprazole. This may be beneficial because the two are given as cotherapy to treat *Helicobacter pylori.*	Give as ordered. Assess for possible adverse effects.
sucralfate	Delayed absorption and reduced bioavailability of omeprazole by about 17% when the two are given at the same time. This decreases desired therapeutic effect.	Give omeprazole ≥30 min before sucralfate.
benzodiazepines (diazepam, flurazepam, triazolam)	Large increases (130%) in the half-life of the benzodiazepines, most likely due to decreased metabolism of the benzodiazepines. Plasma levels also increased and total clearance decreased.	Decreased dose of benzodiazepines may be indicated. Monitor for adverse effects.
phenytoin	Reduced plasma clearance of phenytoin and increased half-life, most likely caused by inhibition of its metabolism.	Decreased dose of phenytoin may be indicated. Monitor for adverse effects. Monitor blood levels of phenytoin.
warfarin	Prolong the elimination of warfarin due to inhibition of its metabolism.	Monitor for adverse effects. Assess protime carefully. Adjust dose if warranted.

Omeprazole should be taken before eating. Smoking also may aggravate the symptoms of peptic ulcer disease.

Environment

The nurse should be aware of the environment in which omeprazole will be administered. Omeprazole may be given in any environment.

Culture

The nurse should assess a patient's culture and genetic background before administering omeprazole. Asians may need a decreased dose because compared with whites who receive omeprazole, they may have elevated serum levels (up to fourfold higher).

Nursing Diagnoses and Outcomes

- Altered Comfort, related to symptoms of GERD, peptic ulcer disease, or chronic elevation of acid production.
  Desired outcome: Drug therapy will relieve the symptoms from the GI disorder.
- Imbalanced Nutrition: Less Than Body Requirements, related to symptoms of GERD, peptic ulcer disease, or chronic elevation of acid production.
  Desired outcome: Drug therapy will allow adequate dietary intake to be consumed.
- Collaborative Problem: *H. pylori* infection
  Desired outcome: Treatment regimen for H. pylori eradication will be effective with minimal adverse effects.

Planning and Intervention

Maximizing Therapeutic Effects and Minimizing Adverse Effects

The nurse should make sure that omeprazole is administered for the recommended time, based on the clinical indication for therapy, usually between 2 and 8 weeks. For chronic pathologic hypersecretory conditions, administer daily for as long as needed. Some patients are known to have received omeprazole for 5 years or longer. Daily dosages larger than 80 mg should be given in divided doses. Because the drug is enteric coated, it cannot be crushed before use.

Providing Patient and Family Education

- The nurse should teach the patient to take omeprazole before meals, and for the duration of prescribed therapy.
- The nurse should emphasize that the drug should not be crushed or chewed because this alters the absorption and effectiveness.
- The nurse can explain that antacids may be used while taking omeprazole for additional symptom management.

Ongoing Assessment and Evaluation

Therapy is effective when the symptoms of GERD, peptic ulcer disease, or hypersecretory conditions are controlled or the duodenal ulcer is healed. ■

DRUG SIGNIFICANTLY DIFFERENT FROM OMEPRAZOLE

Sucralfate (Carafate), like omeprazole, is used in treating duodenal ulcers (see Table 37-2). Unlabeled uses of sucralfate include accelerating the healing of gastric ulcers and long-term management of gastric ulcers. Other unlabeled uses include the treatment of reflux ulcers, reflux and peptic esophagitis, NSAID (and aspirin)-induced GI symptoms, and prevention of stress ulcers and GI bleeding in critically ill patients. Sucralfate suspension also has been used in treating oral and esophageal ulcers due to radiation, chemotherapy, and sclerotherapy.

Unlike omeprazole, sucralfate is not a proton pump inhibitor and does not prevent the secretion of gastric acid. Sucralfate is an aluminum salt of sulfated sucrose, a polysaccharide with antipeptic activity. In the acidic medium of gastric fluid, the aluminum ion splits off, leaving a highly polar anion. The basically nonabsorbent paste that forms adheres to the ulcer lesions and protects the lesion from acid, pepsin, and bile salts. This allows the ulcer to heal. There are minimal antacid effects of the drug, but these do not contribute to ulcer healing.

Sucralfate should be used cautiously in pregnancy (pregnancy category B) and in breast-feeding because it is not known whether the drug is secreted in breast milk. Safety and efficacy in children have not been established. In dialysis patients and others with chronic renal failure, sucralfate given concurrently with aluminum antacids increases the risk for aluminum toxicity because small amounts of aluminum, given off by sucralfate, are absorbed from the GI tract. This is not a problem for patients with normal renal function.

Adverse effects from sucralfate are usually mild. Rarely in clinical trials did the drug have to be discontinued. The most common adverse effect was constipation and this occurred in only 2% of patients. Sucralfate may decrease the effectiveness

MEMORY CHIP

Omeprazole

- Used to treat peptic ulcers resulting from *H. pylori*, GERD, erosive esophagitis, and chronic hypersecretory conditions (e.g., Zollinger-Ellison syndrome)
- May interact with other drugs metabolized by CYP 450
- Most common adverse effects: headache and diarrhea
- **Life span alert: use not recommended during breast feeding**
- Most significant patient education: take omeprazole before meals; do not crush or chew drug

of anticoagulants, digoxin, hydantoins, ketoconazole, quinidine, and the quinolones.

The nurse should teach the patient to take sucralfate at least 1 hour before meals and at bedtime to maximize the therapeutic effect. Antacids should be taken 30 minutes before or after sucralfate.

THE H_2 RECEPTOR ANTAGONISTS

Various terms are used to describe the H_2 receptor antagonists, including histamine-2 receptor antagonists, H_2 receptor blockers, H_2 antagonists, H_2 blockers, and histamine blockers. H_2 receptor antagonists block the effect of histamine at H_2 receptors, particularly those in the parietal cells of the stomach. Antihistamines that block histamine-1 (H_1) receptors, the most frequent site of action for antihistamines, do not have an effect on the H_2 receptor sites, and H_2 receptor antagonists do not block at H_1 sites; they also are not anticholinergic.

By blocking histamine at the parietal cells, gastric acid secretion is inhibited in all phases, and secretions caused by histamine, muscarinic agonists, and gastrin are inhibited. H_2 receptor antagonists also inhibit fasting, nocturnal secretions, and secretions stimulated by food, insulin, caffeine, pentagastrin, and betazole. These drugs also reduce the volume of, and the hydrogen ion concentration in, gastric secretions. H_2 receptor antagonists include cimetidine, which is the prototype. Other drugs in this class are ranitidine (Zantac), famotidine (Pepcid), and nizatidine (Axid AR). A drug significantly different from cimetidine is misoprostol.

NURSING MANAGEMENT OF THE PATIENT RECEIVING CIMETIDINE

Core Drug Knowledge

Pharmacotherapeutics

Cimetidine (Tagamet) is used to treat patients with active peptic and duodenal ulcers, maintenance therapy in duodenal ulcers, GERD (including erosive esophagitis), and pathologic hypersecretory conditions. It also is used in critically ill patients to prevent upper GI bleeding. In OTC strengths, it is used for treating heartburn, indigestion, and sour stomach (see Table 37-2).

Potential, unlabeled, uses include part of a therapy regimen to treat *H. pylori* infections; to prevent aspiration pneumonia; treating chronic idiopathic urticaria that does not respond to H_1 receptor drugs; preventing hepatotoxicity with acetaminophen overdosage (when given intravenously); preventing stress ulcers; preventing gastric damage from NSAID use; and treatment of primary and secondary (in chronic hemodialysis patients) hyperparathyroidism. It also may be used to treat tinea capitis, herpes virus infection, hirsutism in women, chronic viral warts in children, and improving the overall survival of patients with colorectal cancer.

Pharmacokinetics

Cimetidine is absorbed rapidly when taken after meals. Approximately 30% of the drug is metabolized during the first pass through the liver. The remaining 70% is absorbed from the GI tract. The drug is not highly protein bound (only 13% to 25%) and is distributed widely throughout the body. It crosses the blood-brain barrier and placenta readily. Cimetidine is metabolized by the liver to sulfoxide and 5-hydroxymethyl and is excreted in the urine.

Pharmacodynamics

Cimetidine reduces gastric acid production by blocking histamine at the H_2 receptor site of parietal cells, resulting in a reduction in the hydrogen ion concentration and volume of gastric acid. Cimetidine inhibits the basal secretion of acid and is effective when the parietal cells are stimulated by food, insulin, caffeine, and betazole. Another gastric secretion that is affected is pepsin. The effect of cimetidine on pepsin is related to the decrease in gastric acid production. When cimetidine is given at bedtime it reduces mean hourly H+ activity 85% to 100%, depending on the dose, over 8 hours in patients with duodenal ulcers. After a meal, the gastric acid secreted is reduced by 50% to 75% for about 4 hours. Another action of cimetidine is to inhibit the CYP450 enzyme system.

Contraindications and Precautions

Cimetidine is contraindicated in patients who are hypersensitive to the drug. It is a pregnancy category B drug, with no adequate, well-controlled studies of this drug in pregnant women. It also is not recommended for use by nursing mothers because it has been found in breast milk. The use of this drug in children is recommended if the benefits of use override the risks of the unknown. However, benzol alcohol, used as a preservative in many of the preparations for reconstitution has been associated with a fatal "gasping syndrome" in premature infants.

Cimetidine should be used cautiously in patients with hepatic or renal impairment because the drug is metabolized by the liver and excreted by the kidneys. Patients with gastric ulcers should be monitored closely when using cimetidine because the drug may mask symptoms of GI cancer temporarily. Such patients should be evaluated thoroughly to rule out cancer.

Adverse Effects

Cimetidine is well tolerated generally, and adverse effects that have been reported occur in 1% or fewer of patients receiving the drug. Many of them are rare. These adverse effects include:

- CNS: headaches, dizziness, fatigue, confusion, and hallucinations
- Dermatologic: alopecia and erythema multiforme

- GI: diarrhea, pancreatitis, and cholestatic/hepatocellular effects
- Hematologic: neutropenia, agranulocytosis, thrombocytopenia, and autoimmune hemolytic or aplastic anemia
- Miscellaneous: gynecomastia, cardiac arrhythmia, impotence, arthralgia, transient pain at site of IM injection, and hypersensitivity reactions.

In addition, cardiac arrhythmias and hypotension have been related to rapid IV administration in rare occasions. The CNS effects of confusion, agitation, psychosis, depression, anxiety, hallucinations, and disorientation occur mostly in severely ill patients, usually within 2 or 3 days of starting the therapy. The effects are reversible and will clear 3 to 4 days after stopping the drug.

There is no experience with deliberate overdosage. Ingestion of up to 20 g has been associated with transient adverse effects similar to those in normal dosing. Two deaths have occurred in adults who reportedly ingested more than 40 g in a single dose. In cases of overdosage, the stomach should be suctioned to remove unabsorbed cimetidine.

Drug Interactions

Cimetidine, because it inhibits the CYP450 enzyme system, decreases the hepatic metabolism of a long list of drugs and interacts with many other drugs in a variety of ways (Table 37-4). Because of the potential for multiple drug interactions, cimetidine use is decreasing and other drugs in this class (most commonly ranitidine) are being used as drugs of first choice. Ranitidine, famotidine, and nizatidine do not inhibit the cytochrome P450 system. Smoking decreases the effectiveness of cimetidine.

Assessment of Relevant Core Patient Variables

Health Status

Before administering cimetidine, the nurse assesses for epigastric, abdominal, and esophageal pain, commonly described as heartburn or a burning sensation that occurs after eating. The nurse also explores complaints of dyspepsia; nausea and vomiting; dark, tarry stools; hepatic dysfunction; and renal impairment. If the patient has a nasogastric tube in place, the nurse inspects for frank or occult bleeding.

The drug history should include the prescription and OTC drugs the patient is taking currently, because many drugs, including aspirin, other NSAIDs, and corticosteroids, can cause gastric irritation. Additional drug history involves determining whether the patient is taking any OTC H_2 receptor antagonists and asking how long and why the patient has been using these drugs.

TABLE 37-4 Agents That Interact With Cimetidine

Interactants	Effect and Significance	Nursing Management
ferrous salts	Decreased absorption of ferrous salts	Monitor for therapeutic effect.
indomethacin, ketoconazole, tetracyclines	Decreased effect of indomethacin, ketoconazole, and tetracyclines	Consult with prescriber about adjusting dosages if necessary.
carmustine	Possible enhanced bone marrow suppression due to additive effect or decreased metabolism of carmustine	Monitor for signs of bone marrow suppression, such as decreased hematocrit and low production of new red blood cells.
digoxin	Decreased serum digoxin levels; possible decreased effect of digoxin	Monitor serum levels and effect.
flecainide	Increased effect of flecainide	Monitor for adverse effects, such as dizziness, fatigue, cardiac arrhythmias.
fluconazole	Decreased plasma levels of fluconazole, possibly from decreased absorption	Monitor for therapeutic effect.
fluorouracil	Increased fluorouracil levels	Monitor for adverse effect of fluorouracil.
narcotic analgesics	Possible increased adverse effects of narcotic analgesic	Monitor for adverse effects (respiratory depression, constipation, urinary retention).
succinylocholine	Neuromuscular blocking effects may be prolonged; respiratory depression with extended periods of apnea	Monitor respiratory status carefully.
tocainide	Decreased effects of tocainide	Monitor for therapeutic effect.
antacids, anticholinergics, metoclopramide	Possible decreased absorption of cimetidine	Do not administer at the same time.
cigarette smoking	Reverses effect of cimetidine and hinders ulcer healing	Teach patient detrimental effects of smoking, and provide assistance with smoking cessation.

Life Span and Gender

The nurse should assess whether the patient is pregnant or breast-feeding because pregnant and breast-feeding patients should take cimetidine only if necessary. The nurse also should determine the patient's age. Elderly patients should be assessed carefully for decreased renal and hepatic function. The gynecomastia that may occur from cimetidine restricts its long-term use in children.

Lifestyle, Diet, and Habits

The nurse should assess the patient's diet and smoking habits. Caffeine, alcohol, and spicy foods may aggravate gastric symptoms from GERD, peptic ulcer disease, and hypersecretory conditions. Smoking reverses the drug-induced inhibition of nocturnal gastric acid production and hinders the ulcer in its healing. Cigarette smoking also is related closely to ulcer recurrence.

Environment

The nurse should note the setting in which cimetidine will be administered. Cimetidine can be administered in any setting. The oral form is self-administered easily. Administration through the IV or IM routes is done most commonly in an inpatient setting.

Culture

Cultural influences on dietary patterns need to be considered if the patient normally eats a diet consisting of highly spiced foods, such as jalapeño peppers, Thai curries, or Szechwan cuisine.

Nursing Diagnoses and Outcomes

- Chronic Pain, related to alteration in the gastric mucosa, ulceration, or irritation
  Desired outcome: The patient will report decreased pain while receiving drug therapy.
- Acute Pain, related to adverse drug effects, such as headache
  Desired outcome: The patient will not experience adverse while taking cimetidine.
- Risk for Injury related to drug-induced somnolence, dizziness, confusion, or hallucinations
  Desired outcome: The patient will not suffer injury from adverse effects of drug therapy.
- Diarrhea related to adverse effects of drug therapy
  Desired outcome: The patient's elimination pattern will remain normal while on drug therapy.
- Disturbed Body Image from gynecomastia related to cimetidine therapy
  Desired outcome: The patient's self-image will remain intact during drug therapy.

Planning and Intervention

Maximizing Therapeutic Effects

If both cimetidine and antacids are prescribed, the nurse should give them at least 2 hours apart to prevent decreased absorption of cimetidine.

Minimizing Adverse Effects

The nurse should monitor serum trough levels in patients with renal or hepatic impairment because CNS effects are more likely to occur when serum levels are elevated above the therapeutic level. Drug therapy may need to be discontinued if serious adverse effects occur.

The nurse should administer intravenous cimetidine therapy slowly to prevent hypotension and cardiac arrhythmias. It is important to administer single IV push doses, diluted in 20 mL of normal saline or other compatible solution over at least 2 minutes. Intermittent IV infusions of 300 mg in at least 50 mL of D_5W or other compatible solution should be administered over at least 15 or 20 minutes. The nurse should give a continuous IV infusion should be given at a rate of 37.5 mg/h.

Providing Patient and Family Education

- The nurse should instruct the patient to take the drug exactly as directed for the entire course of therapy, even if symptoms disappear (it usually takes 4 to 6 weeks for an ulcer to heal but less time for the symptoms to subside).
- The nurse should caution the patient not to take a double dose if a dose is missed.
- It is important to counsel the patient on smoking cessation. OTC or prescription smoking cessation aides may be recommended, if appropriate.
- The nurse should explain that alcohol, caffeine, spicy foods, products containing aspirin or ibuprofen, and smoking all contribute to gastric irritation and slow healing of the ulcer.
- The nurse should caution the patient not to drive until the effects of cimetidine on the patient are known.
- It is important to urge the patient to report immediately any tarry, black stools or coffee ground–like emesis, which are signs of gastric bleeding that must be treated.
- The nurse should caution the patient not to substitute OTC cimetidine for prescribed cimetidine (potency of the products varies) (see the accompanying display, Using Over-the-Counter Gastrointestinal Drugs Responsibly).
- It is important to teach the patient to stagger cimetidine and antacid dosing schedules to allow at least 2 hours between doses.

Ongoing Assessment and Evaluation

During therapy, the patient's blood counts should be monitored to detect signs of neutropenia with long-term use. Drug therapy is effective when epigastric pain decreases, peptic ulcers heal, hypersecretion of gastric acid declines, or GI bleeding is prevented without adverse effects. ■

COMMUNITY-BASED CONCERNS

Using Over-the-Counter (OTC) Gastrointestinal Drugs Responsibly

Various antacids, such as Maalox and Mylantin, and histamine-2 (H_2) receptor antagonists (also called H_2 blockers), such as cimetidine (Tagamet HB), ranitidine (Zantac HB), and famotidine (Pepcid AC), are available currently OTC. Nurses who provide home care or who treat patients on an outpatient basis need to be aware that many patients self-medicate with these preparations. They may use them alone, as an adjunct to prescribed therapy, or in place of their prescribed drug. The following guidelines may help nurses help such patients use these drugs responsibly:

- Assess specifically for OTC antacid and H_2-blocker use. The patient may not think of OTC products as "real drugs" and so fail to identify them during the drug history.
- Advise the patient taking a prescribed H_2 blocker to take only that drug and not to substitute any OTC preparation for it. Explain that the dosages and drug formulations may be different.
- Caution the patient not to take any OTC H_2-blocker in addition to the prescribed drug. In such cases, "more is not better."
- If a particular antacid has been prescribed for a patient, warn the patient not to switch brands or type of antacid without consulting the prescriber. Some forms of antacids are contraindicated in certain medical conditions (e.g., congestive heart failure and hypertension).
- Urge patient to consult own health care provider before taking antacids in conjunction with an H_2-blocker.

MEMORY CHIP

Cimetidine

- Blocks histamine competitively at histamine 2 (H_2) receptors in the gastric parietal cells; these receptors are not affected by H_1 antagonists
- Inhibits all phases of gastric acid secretion
- Used in GERD, duodenal ulcer, gastric ulcer, pathologic hypersecretory conditions, prevention of upper GI bleeding, and in heartburn/acid indigestion (OTC strength only)
- Interacts with numerous other drugs, many by decreasing their hepatic metabolism
- Most serious adverse effects: neutropenia, agranulocytosis, thrombocytopenia, autoimmune hemolytic, or aplastic anemia (all rare)
- **Life span alert: benzyl alcohol (a preservative present in some forms of the drug) causes fatal "gasping syndrome" in premature infants**
- Maximizing therapeutic effects: give cimetidine at least 2 h apart from antacids
- Most significant patient education: do not substitute OTC drug forms for prescription forms nor add them to prescribed drug therapy

DRUG SIGNIFICANTLY DIFFERENT FROM CIMETIDINE

Misoprostol (Cytotec), unlike cimetidine, is not an H_2 antagonist. It is a synthetic form of prostaglandin E and is used to prevent NSAID- (and aspirin)-induced gastric ulcers in high-risk patients (i.e., older adults, patients with other debilitating diseases, and patients with a history of gastric ulcers) (see Table 37-2). An unlabeled use is treating duodenal ulcers. Misoprostol may be useful in treating duodenal ulcers not receptive to treatment with H_2 receptor antagonists, but it does not prevent duodenal ulcers in patients on NSAIDs.

NSAIDs inhibit prostaglandin synthesis, causing diminished bicarbonate and mucus secretion in the gastric mucosa. Misoprostol binds at the prostaglandin receptors and can increase bicarbonate and mucus secretion, thereby protecting the stomach lining. This results in a decrease in peptic ulcer formation in patients taking NSAIDs. Misoprostol produces a moderate decrease in pepsin concentration during basal conditions but not during histamine stimulation. It has no significant effect on gastrin levels, either before or after meals. Misoprostol does decrease normal daytime and nocturnal gastric acid secretion. It also decreases the gastric acid that is produced in response to stimuli, including meals, histamine, pentagastrin, and coffee. Activity of the drug begins within 30 minutes of administration, and lasts for 3 hours or more.

Misoprostol is classified as a pregnancy category X drug because of its abortifacient properties. The drug causes uterine contractions and miscarriage. Women of child-bearing potential must receive written and oral warnings about the hazards of misoprostol, be able to comply with effective contraceptive measures, and have had a negative serum pregnancy test result in the previous 2 weeks before beginning therapy. Therapy should be started on the second or third day of the next normal menstrual cycle. It is not known whether the drug crosses into breast milk, so its use by nursing mothers is not recommended. Efficacy and safe use in children have not been established. Additionally, elderly patients may not be able to tolerate the usual dose. Cautious use is recommended for patients with renal failure. However, a dosage reduction is not normally necessary.

The most common adverse effect is diarrhea; the next most common is abdominal pain. Other adverse effects are nausea and vomiting, dyspepsia, flatulence, constipation, and headache. Possible gynecologic problems include spotting, cramps, and menstrual disorders.

When antacids are administered with misoprostol, the availability of misoprostol is reduced but this does not appear to be important clinically. Although food decreases the plasma concentrations of misoprostol, the specific receptors for misoprostol in the GI tract are still activated and a therapeutic response is evident. The effect of misoprostol is topical, rather than systemic. It is recommended that patients take misoprostol with food. If diarrhea is a problem, it can be diminished if the drug is taken after the meal.

ANTACIDS

Antacids are drugs that increase the gastric pH, thereby neutralizing gastric acidity. These preparations are used for various upper GI disorders, including symptoms of GERD (heartburn, indigestion, and upset stomach), esophagitis, hiatal hernia, gastritis, and peptic ulcer disease. Antacids are composed of inorganic salts of aluminum, magnesium, calcium, or sodium used alone or in various combinations. Antacids include aluminum hydroxide with magnesium hydroxide, aluminum, magnesium, calcium, and sodium bicarbonate. The prototype antacid is aluminum hydroxide with magnesium hydroxide (Maalox, Mylanta).

NURSING MANAGEMENT OF THE PATIENT RECEIVING ALUMINUM HYDROXIDE WITH MAGNESIUM HYDROXIDE

Core Drug Knowledge

Pharmacotherapeutics

The combination drug aluminum hydroxide with magnesium hydroxide is used in conditions of hypersensitivity to relieve the symptoms of upset stomach, heartburn, gastric reflux, and sour stomach associated with GERD, and the discomfort from peptic ulcers (Table 37-5). Unlabeled uses include treatment and maintenance therapy in duodenal ulcer.

Pharmacokinetics

A single dose of an aluminum- and magnesium-based antacid typically results in minimal absorption from the GI tract. Patients taking this type of drug for a prolonged period may absorb between 5% and 20% of the magnesium and very little of the aluminum. The small amounts of magnesium and aluminum that are absorbed are distributed widely throughout the body. Small amounts of the drugs are found in breast milk. Aluminum hydroxide with magnesium hydroxide is eliminated in the feces.

The onset of action is rapid. Duration of action varies according to when the drug was taken in relation to meals. If taken on an empty stomach, the duration is 20 to 60 minutes; if taken following a meal, the duration is 3 hours.

Pharmacodynamics

Antacids do not coat the lining of the stomach despite what is commonly believed. Aluminum hydroxide with magnesium hydroxide raises the gastric pH in the stomach and duodenal bulb above 4, resulting in inhibiting pepsin's proteolytic activity and increasing the tone of the lower esophageal sphincter. Antacids, in general, may have a local astringent effect. They also may increase the lower esophageal sphincter tone. Aluminum in this drug, and in other aluminum antacids, inhibits gastric emptying by inhibiting contraction of the smooth muscle of the stomach. The aluminum in the drug binds with phosphate in the GI tract and can lower phosphate levels effectively in patients with normal phosphate levels.

Antacids have different acid-neutralizing capacities (ANC). The ANC is expressed as mEq/mL. The definition is the mEq of HCl required to keep the antacid suspension at a pH of 3.5 for 10 minutes, in vitro (i.e., as measured in the laboratory). To be an antacid it must neutralize 5 mEq/dose or more. Antacids with high ANC are usually more effective in vivo (i.e., in the patient). Suspensions have the highest neutralizing capacity of the various forms in which antacids are available.

Contraindications and Precautions

Aluminum hydroxide with magnesium hydroxide may cause hypophosphatemia, especially if dietary intake of phosphorus is inadequate. Patients with renal insufficiency should use magnesium-containing antacids with caution because a small amount of magnesium is absorbed systematically and hypermagnesemia is possible, especially if the patient takes more than 50 mEq daily. Pregnant or breast-feeding patients should consult their health care provider before taking aluminum hydroxide with magnesium hydroxide.

Aluminum hydroxide with magnesium hydroxide should be used cautiously in patients who have recently had massive upper GI bleeding.

Adverse Effects

Antacids that contain aluminum alone can cause constipation, whereas antacids that contain magnesium alone can cause diarrhea. Aluminum and magnesium are combined to balance the constipating effects of aluminum with the diarrheal effects of magnesium. Other possible adverse effects include hypermagnesemia (in patients with renal failure) and hypophosphatemia. Less commonly, accumulation of aluminum in serum, bone, and the CNS (with large doses); osteomalacia; and encephalopathy may occur. Acid rebound may occur, although this may not be significant clinically because the buffers in the antacid may neutralize any elevation in acidity.

Drug Interactions

Magnesium and aluminum affect the action of many orally administered drugs (Table 37-6). This interaction may be from decreasing acidity of gastric juices, therefore affecting absorption; absorbing or binding to the surface of drugs, decreasing their bioavailability; or increasing urine alkalinity, changing the rate of drug elimination (slowing the excretion of basic drugs and speeding the elimination of acidic drugs).

TABLE 37-5 Summary of Selected Antacids

Drug (Trade) Name	Selected Indications	Route and Dosage Range	Pharmacokinetics
aluminum hydroxide with magnesium hydroxide (Maalox)	Hyperacidity; prevention of stress ulcer bleeding; treatment and maintenance of duodenal and gastric ulcers; initially for gastroesophageal reflux disease (GERD)	PO, 15–30 mL up to 4 × d	*Onset:* Immediate *Duration:* 20–40 min on empty stomach, 3 h if 1 h after meals $t_{1/2}$: Not systemically absorbed
magnesium hydroxide (Milk of Magnesia)	Hyperacidity; bleeding; treatment and maintenance of duodenal and gastric ulcers; initially for GERD	PO, liquid, 5–15 mL up to four times a day; liquid concentrate, 2.5–7.5 mL up to 4 × d; tablets, 622–1,244 mg up to 4 × d	*Onset:* Immediate *Duration:* 20–40 min on empty stomach, 3 h if 1 h after meals $t_{1/2}$: Not systemically absorbed
aluminum hydroxide (Amphojel)	Hyperacidity; prevention of stress ulcer bleeding; treatment and maintenance of duodenal and gastric ulcers; initially for GERD; reduction of phosphate absorption in hyperphosphatemia in chronic renal failure	PO, suspension, 5–30 mL as needed after meals and at bedtime; tablets/capsules, 500–1,500 mg three to six times a day between meals and at bedtime	*Onset:* Immediate *Duration:* 20–40 min on empty stomach, 3 h if 1 h after meals $t_{1/2}$: Not systemically absorbed
aluminum carbonate (Basaljel)	Hyperacidity; treatment, control, management of hyperphosphatemia; use with a low-phosphate diet to prevent formation of phosphate urinary stones	PO, suspension, 10 mL in water or juice up to every 2 h; tablets/capsules, 2 up to every 2 h	*Onset:* Immediate *Duration:* 20–40 min on empty stomach, 3 h if 1 h after meals $t_{1/2}$: Not systemically absorbed
calcium carbonate (Tums)	Hyperacidity (occasional use); calcium replacement	PO, tablets, 0.5–1.5 g as needed	*Onset:* Immediate *Duration:* 20–40 min on empty stomach, 3 h if 1 h after meals $t_{1/2}$: Unknown
magnesium oxide (Mag-ox)	Hyperacidity; magnesium replacement	PO, capsules, 140 mg tid–qid; tablets 400–800 mg/d	*Onset:* Immediate *Duration:* 20–40 min on empty stomach, 3 h if 1 h after meals $t_{1/2}$: Not systemically absorbed
magaldrate (Riopan)	Hyperacidity; treatment and maintenance of duodenal and gastric ulcers; initially for GERD	PO, suspension liquid, 5–10 mL between meals and at bedtime	*Onset:* Immediate *Duration:* 20–40 min on empty stomach, 3 h if 1 h after meals $t_{1/2}$: Not systemically absorbed
sodium bicarbonate (Bell/Ans)	Hyperacidity (occasional use)	PO, tablets, 0.3–2 g up to qid	*Onset:* Immediate *Duration:* 20–40 min on empty stomach, 3 h if 1 h after meals $t_{1/2}$: Unknown
sodium citrate (citra pH)	Hyperacidity (occasional use)	PO, liquid, 30 mL daily	*Onset:* Immediate *Duration:* 20–40 min on empty stomach, 3 h if 1 h after meals $t_{1/2}$: Unknown

No specific recommendations for a child's dose.

TABLE 37-6 Agents That Interact With C Antacids

Interactants	Effect and Significance	Nursing Management
allopurinol	Decreased effect with aluminum salts	Monitor for drug effectiveness. Alert prescriber to need for possible dosage adjustment. Do not administer both drugs at same time if significant interactions occur.
amphetamines	Increased effect with sodium bicarbonate	Same as above.
benzodiazepines	Increased effect with aluminum salts; decreased effect with magnesium salts, sodium bicarbonate, and magnesium/aluminum combination	Same as above.
captopril	Decreased effect with magnesium/aluminum combinations	Same as above.
chloroquine	Decreased effect with aluminum and magnesium salts	Same as above.
corticosteroids	Decreased effect with aluminum, magnesium, and magnesium/aluminum combinations	Same as above.
dicumarol	Increased effect with magnesium salts	Same as above.
diflunisal	Decreased effect with aluminum salts	Same as above.
digoxin	Decreased effect with aluminum and magnesium salts	Same as above.
ethambutol	Decreased effect with aluminum salts	Same as above.
flecainide	Increased absorption with sodium bicarbonate	Same as above.
fluoroquinolones	Decreased effect with calcium salts and magnesium/aluminum combinations	Same as above.
H_2 receptor antagonists	Decreased effect with aluminum salts, magnesium salts, and magnesium/aluminum combinations	Same as above.
hydantoins	Decreased effect with calcium salts, magnesium salts, and magnesium/aluminum combinations	Same as above.
iron salts	Decreased effect with all antacids	Same as above.
isoniazid	Decreased effect with aluminum salts	Same as above.
ketoconazole	Decreased effect with sodium bicarbonate and magnesium/aluminum combinations	Same as above.
levodopa	Increased effect with magnesium/aluminum combinations	Same as above.
lithium	Decreased effect with sodium bicarbonate	Same as above.
methenamine	Decreased effect with sodium bicarbonate	Same as above.
methotrexate	Decreased effect with sodium bicarbonate	Same as above.
nitrofurantoin	Decreased effect with magnesium salts	Same as above.
penicillamine	Decreased effect with aluminum salts and magnesium salts	Same as above.
phenothiazines	Decreased effect with aluminum salts, magnesium salts, and magnesium/aluminum combinations	Same as above.
quinidine	Increased effect with calcium salts, magnesium salts, sodium bicarbonate, and magnesium/aluminum combinations	Same as above.
salicylates	Decreased effect with calcium salts, sodium bicarbonate, and magnesium/aluminum combinations	Same as above.
sodium polystyrene sulfonate	Concurrent use, possible metabolic alkalosis in patients with renal impairment	Same as above.
sulfonylurease	Increased effect with magnesium salts and magnesium/aluminum combinations; decreased effect with sodium bicarbonate	Same as above.
sympathomimetics	Increased effect with sodium bicarbonate	Same as above.
tetracycline	Decreased effect with all antacids	Same as above.
thyroid hormones	Decreased effect with aluminum salts	Same as above.
ticlopidine	Decreased effect with aluminum salts, magnesium salts, and magnesium/aluminum combinations	Same as above.
valproic acid	Increased effect with magnesium/aluminum combinations	Same as above.

Assessment of Relevant Core Patient Variables

Health Status

The nurse should determine whether the patient has symptoms that warrant the use of aluminum hydroxide with magnesium hydroxide. The nurse should assess for GI bleeding; coffee-grounds–like emesis indicates GI bleeding, as do dark, tarry stools in a patient not on iron supplements. Patients who have had massive upper GI bleeding should use caution when taking products that contain aluminum. The nurse also should assess for renal insufficiency. Patients with a history of renal insufficiency should not receive aluminum hydroxide with magnesium hydroxide. Although antacids that are solely aluminum based are used to decrease elevated phosphate levels found in renal failure, aluminum in combination with magnesium hydroxide should be avoided because these patients do not excrete magnesium at the normal rate. The additional magnesium that can be absorbed from this product, and all magnesium-containing antacids, may be sufficient to cause hypermagnesemia in the renal failure patient. The nurse also should determine the patient's serum phosphate level (aluminum binds with phosphate).

Assessment issues to raise with the patient concern OTC drugs because the patient may not consider these important to mention during the drug history. The nurse should then assess which type of drugs these are, and why they are being used, to detect possible drug interactions.

Lifestyle, Diet, and Habits

The nurse should assess the patient's normal dietary, alcohol, and smoking habits. Caffeine, alcohol, spicy food, and smoking may contribute to the severity of symptoms experienced.

Environment

The nurse should be aware of the setting in which aluminum hydroxide with magnesium hydroxide will be administered. Aluminum hydroxide with magnesium hydroxide is easily self-administered. It may be used in any care setting, including the home.

Nursing Diagnoses and Outcomes

- Chronic Pain related to alteration in the gastric mucosa, ulceration, or irritation
  Desired outcome: The patient will report that pain has decreased while on drug therapy.
- Potential Complication: Electrolyte Imbalance related to hypophosphatemia, hypermagnesemia, hyperalbuminemia secondary to drug therapy
  Desired outcome: The patient's electrolyte levels will remain within normal limits.
- Diarrhea or Constipation secondary to drug therapy
  Desired outcome: The patient's elimination patterns will remain within normal parameters.

Planning and Intervention

Maximizing Therapeutic Effects

Liquid preparations are usually preferred because of their rapid action. The nurse should shake suspensions well before use to disperse the drug evenly. If tablets are used, they must be chewed thoroughly before swallowing and followed with a glass of water. These should be administered 1 to 3 hours after meals and at bedtime for the best therapeutic effects.

Minimizing Adverse Effects

The nurse should administer, or teach the patient to administer, aluminum hydroxide and magnesium hydroxide 2 hours after other drugs to prevent drug interactions. The nurse should assess for use of antacids and other OTC preparations during drug history; patients may not consider these to be drugs and fail to mention them unless asked.

It is important to monitor for signs of acid rebound, such as increased GI pain and complaints of acid reflux. It also is important to monitor serum phosphorus and magnesium levels in patients receiving high doses of aluminum hydroxide and magnesium hydroxide (i.e., the maximum dosage for more than 2 weeks), or in patients on long-term therapy or with renal impairment. The nurse should monitor for signs of aluminum deposits in serum, bone, and CNS and dialysis encephalopathy and osteomalacia syndromes when high doses are given to patients with renal failure.

Providing Patient and Family Education

- The nurse should teach the patient to take the antacid 2 hours after other drugs, and 1 hour after meals and at bedtime.
- The nurse should caution the patient not to take the maximum dose for longer than 2 weeks unless directed by the health care provider
- It is important to instruct the patient not to substitute this drug for prescription drugs to treat peptic ulcer disease
- The nurse should urge the patient to contact the health care provider if diarrhea or constipation occurs, if abdominal pain does not diminish, or if black, tarry stools or coffee grounds–like emesis is seen.
- The nurse should teach the patient to shake liquid forms well and measure the proper dose; the patient should not just drink some.
- It is important that the patient chews the tablet form thoroughly and then drinks water.

Ongoing Assessment and Evaluation

Drug therapy is considered effective if the patient's pain is decreased or eliminated, electrolytes remain in normal levels, and elimination patterns remain normal. ■

MEMORY CHIP

Aluminum Hydroxide With Magnesium Hydroxide

- Treats hyperacidity and its symptoms in GERD and peptic ulcers; prevents stress ulcer bleeding
- Interacts with many other drugs by increasing the pH (i.e., increasing alkalinity), which alters absorption, adsorption, or binding with drugs; or by increasing urinary pH (i.e., affecting drug elimination rate)
- Significant contraindication: avoid use in chronic renal failure (multiple doses)
- Most common adverse effects: constipation (aluminum antacids) and diarrhea (magnesium antacids); combination usually negates the adverse effect of each, although either may occur
- Most serious adverse effect: potential electrolyte imbalance
- Minimizing adverse effects: administer 2 h after other drugs to prevent drug interactions
- Most significant patient education: do not substitute this drug for prescription drugs to treat peptic ulcer disease

DRUGS CLOSELY RELATED TO ALUMINUM HYDROXIDE WITH MAGNESIUM HYDROXIDE

All antacid preparations are related closely and are used in various combinations to produce the desired results. In addition to the prototype aluminum hydroxide with magnesium hydroxide, aluminum preparations and magnesium preparations may be used individually. Additionally, sodium bicarbonate and calcium carbonate are used as antacids, either alone or in combination with other antacids. Various combinations of aluminum salts, magnesium salts, calcium carbonate, and sodium bicarbonate are useful. The aluminum salts used in antacids include aluminum carbonate, aluminum hydroxide, aluminum phosphate, and dihydroxyaluminum aminoacetate. The magnesium salts include magnesium carbonate, magnesium hydroxide, magnesium oxide, and magnesium trisilicate. The calcium salt calcium carbonate is often given with simethicone (an antiflatulent), magnesium carbonate, magnesium hydroxide, or aluminum hydroxide. However, it may be used alone.

The pharmacotherapeutics of the antacids vary. Unlike aluminum or magnesium preparations, neither calcium carbonate nor sodium bicarbonate is recommended for long-term use, such as treating peptic ulcer disease. Aluminum hydroxide is used to treat hyperphosphatemia associated with chronic renal failure. Aluminum carbonate may be used to treat, control, or manage hyperphosphatemia. It can also be used with low-phosphate diets to prevent phosphate-based renal calculi (i.e., kidney stones) from developing. Calcium carbonate is used in treating hypocalcemia. Magnesium sulfate is used to treat hypomagnesemia.

The pharmacokinetics of the antacids vary slightly because sodium bicarbonate and calcium carbonate undergo much more systemic absorption than the aluminum or magnesium preparations.

The main variation in pharmacodynamics is in the acid-neutralizing capacity of the antacids.

Sodium bicarbonate and calcium carbonate have the greatest acid-neutralizing capacity (see the accompanying display, Antacids' Acid-Neutralizing Capacity). Suspension forms of antacids have greater acid-neutralizing capacity than tablets.

Sodium bicarbonate and calcium carbonate can cause metabolic alkalosis and acid rebound because of their systemic absorption, especially with large doses and frequent use. When given together in large doses, they may cause milk alkali syndrome. Milk alkali syndrome can be acute (with symptoms of weakness, headache, nausea, and irritability) or chronic (with alkalosis, hypercalcemia, and possible renal impairment).

The major core patient variable that must be considered for the different forms of antacids is health status. Aluminum hydroxide may be used therapeutically in patients with renal failure, whereas multiple doses of magnesium oxide are avoided in renal failure because of the risk of magnesium toxicity. Because of the high sodium content, sodium bicarbonate should not be given to people on low-sodium diets or who have underlying pathologies that make sodium restrictions necessary, such as hypertension, congestive heart failure, or renal failure. Neither sodium bicarbonate nor calcium carbonate is recommended for peptic ulcer disease.

GASTROINTESTINAL STIMULANTS

The **gastrointestinal stimulants** increase the effect of acetylcholine on the GI system. Acetylcholine is responsible for normal GI function. GI stimulants increase peristalsis and gastric emptying. Drugs within the GI stimulant class include metoclopramide (Reglan) and dexpanthenol (Ilopan). The prototype GI stimulant is metoclopramide (Reglan).

Antacids' Acid-Neutralizing Capacity

The antacids listed below appear in descending order of their acid-neutralizing capacity (e.g., sodium bicarbonate most effective). Aluminum phosphate has the lowest acid-neutralizing effect.

- sodium bicarbonate
- calcium carbonate
- magnesium hydroxide
- magnesium and aluminum hydroxide mixtures
- magaldrate
- magnesium trisilate
- aluminum hydroxide
- aluminum phosphate

NURSING MANAGEMENT OF THE PATIENT RECEIVING METOCLOPRAMIDE

Core Drug Knowledge

Pharmacotherapeutics

Metoclopramide is used to relieve symptoms of diabetic gastroparesis, also known as diabetic gastric stasis. Symptoms of this disorder include nausea, vomiting, heartburn, persistent fullness after meals, and anorexia. Metoclopramide also is used short-term in the treatment of GERD in patients who fail to respond to usual therapy. It also can be used parenterally to prevent nausea and vomiting associated with postoperative states (if nasogastric suctioning is not desirable) or chemotherapy (Table 37-7). It may be administered as a single dose before small bowel intubation, especially in instances in which the tube does not pass through the pylorus easily. It may be used to promote the transit of barium through the GI tract after diagnostic procedure if the delayed passage of barium interferes with further radiographic diagnostic procedure of the stomach and small intestine.

Unlabeled uses include improving lactation (may increase milk production by elevating serum prolactin levels); minimizing nausea and vomiting in a variety of conditions, including during pregnancy and labor; treating gastric ulcers and anorexia nervosa; improving response to ergotamine, analgesics, and sedatives used in migraine headache; treating postoperative gastric bezoars (boluses of food that have hardened and remain in the stomach); treating diabetic atonic bladder; and treating esophageal variceal bleeding.

Pharmacokinetics

Metoclopramide is absorbed readily from the GI tract. The drug is distributed widely throughout the body; it crosses the blood-brain barrier and placenta and is found in breast milk. The drug is not highly protein bound (30%).

A small amount of the drug is metabolized by the liver, and most is excreted in the urine. Patients with renal insufficiency may require a dosage reduction.

Pharmacodynamics

Metoclopramide's mechanism of action is unclear. However, it appears to sensitize tissues to the effect of acetylcholine. It has the cholinergic-like effect on the upper GI tract of stimulating motility but does not stimulate gastric, pancreatic, or gallbladder secretions. Metoclopramide increases peristalsis of the duodenum and jejunum, thus shortening the transit time through the stomach and small intestine. It also increases the tone of the lower esophageal sphincter, increases gastric contractions, and relaxes the pyloric sphincter.

Dopamine produces nausea and vomiting by stimulation of the medullary CTZ. Metoclopramide is a dopamine-receptor antagonist with antiemetic effects that are exerted directly on the CTZ. It is believed to lessen the sensitivity of visceral nerves to stimuli that induce nausea and vomiting.

Contraindications and Precautions

Metoclopramide is contraindicated when stimulation of GI motility may be dangerous, as in GI hemorrhage, perforation, or mechanical obstruction. Other contraindications include hypersensitivity to the drug; pheochromocytoma (the drug may cause a hypertensive crisis that probably results from a release of catecholamines from the tumor); history of seizure disorders (seizure activity may increase with this drug); and patients who are receiving drugs that produce extrapyramidal effects (because these effects may increase).

Depression, from mild to severe, including suicidal ideation, has occurred in patients with and without a history of depression. Use caution in giving metoclopramide to patients with a history of depression; it should be given only if the benefits of the drug outweigh the potential risks from depression. Metoclopramide should be given very cautiously, if at all, to patients with Parkinson disease because they may experience an exacerbation of symptoms. Use caution if giving to patients with hypertension. Theoretically, metoclopramide may increase the pressure on a suture line following a gut anastomosis or closure. Although this has not been reported in the literature, use some caution when giving to post-

TABLE 37-7 Summary of Selected GI Stimulants

Drug (Trade) Name	Selected Indications	Route and Dosage Range	Pharmacokinetics
metoclopramide (Reglan, Octamide)	Diabetic gastroparesis, gastroesophageal reflux disease (GERD), prevention of postoperative nausea and vomiting, prevention of chemotherapy-induced vomiting	*Adult:* PO, 10 mg 30 min before each meal and at bedtime for 2–8 wk; IM, 10–20 mg near end of surgery; IV, infuse over at least 15 min, 30 min before chemotherapy, repeat every 2 h for two doses, then every 3 h for three doses; for highly emetogenic drugs, such as cisplatin and decarbazine, give 2 mg/kg for first two doses; for less emetogenic drugs, give 1 mg/kg	*Onset:* PO, 30–60 min; IM, 10–15 min; IV, 1–3 min *Duration:* PO, IM, IV 1–2 h $t_{1/2}$: PO, IM, IV, 5–6 h

operative patients. Elevated prolactin levels will persist during chronic administration of metoclopramide. One third of human breast cancers are prolactin-dependent in vitro. Therefore, use caution if the patient has previously detected breast cancer. Studies have not, however, shown a definite link between elevated prolactin levels and breast cancer in animals or in humans. Metoclopramide is classified as a pregnancy category B drug.

Adverse Effects

Approximately 20% to 30% of patients receiving metoclopramide experience adverse effects of the drug. The adverse effects are usually mild, transient, and reversible after discontinuing the drug. Incidence correlates with dose and duration of therapy. The possible adverse reactions are many. Effects on the CNS are common and include restlessness, drowsiness, fatigue, insomnia, headache, dizziness, confusion, anxiety, dystonia, mental depression (even in patients who had never experienced clinical depression before) with suicidal ideation and suicide, convulsive seizures, and hallucinations. Extrapyramidal symptoms, Parkinson-like reactions, tardive dyskinesia, and akathisia also may occur. Extrapyramidal symptoms are manifested primarily as acute dystonic reactions. They occur more commonly in children and young adults during the first 24 to 48 hours of treatment. They occur even more frequently when metoclopramide is used in high doses to control vomiting due to chemotherapy. Tardive dyskinesia is potentially irreversible, occurring most often in the elderly, particularly older women. Additional adverse effects are nausea, diarrhea, and transient hypertension.

Drug Interactions

Metoclopramide interacts with several drugs because it increases gastric motility, thereby altering absorption. The most significant drug interactions are with levodopa, anticholinergics, and narcotics. Levodopa and metoclopramide have opposite effects on dopamine receptors. The effects on GI motility from metoclopramide are antagonized by anticholinergics and narcotics (Table 37-8).

Assessment of Relevant Core Patient Variables

Health Status

Before beginning therapy with metoclopramide, the nurse should assess the patient for the presence of diabetic gastroparesis, GERD, cancer requiring chemotherapy, or postoperative status because these are indications for metoclopramide's use. The patient should also be assessed for depression, Parkinson disease, seizures, or hypertension, because these are precautions to its use. The nurse also should assess the patient's drug history; it should not include use of levodopa, anticholinergics, or narcotics. Any renal or hepatic impairment should be noted because the dosage may need to be adjusted.

TABLE 37-8 Agents That Interact With P Metoclopramide

Interactants	Effect and Significance	Nursing Management
alcohol	Increases the rate of absorption, raising blood levels more quickly	Teach patient to avoid alcohol while on drug therapy.
cimetidine	Decreases absorption so bioavailability may be reduced	Monitor for effectiveness of cimetidine.
cyclosporine	Faster gastric emptying, which may allow for increased absorption, possibly increasing immunosuppression and adverse effects from cyclosporine	Monitor white blood cell counts and watch for other adverse effects, such as tremor, hypertension, and renal dysfunction.
digoxin	Absorption, plasma levels, and therapeutic response may be decreased; capsule, elixir, and tablets with a high dissolution rate least affected	Monitor drug levels and therapeutic response. Consult with the prescriber regarding dosage or preparation change if therapeutic response declines significantly.
levodopa	Has the opposite effect on the dopamine receptors; bioavailability of levodopa may be increased; may decrease effect of metoclopramide on gastric emptying and lower esophageal pressure	Monitor for therapeutic and adverse effect of both. Administration of metoclopramide to patients with Parkinson's disease is relatively contraindicated.
monoamine oxidase inhibitors	Metoclopramide releases catecholamines in patients with essential hypertension; MAO inhibitors also have a sympathomimetic effect, blood pressure may be elevated	Use cautiously in hypertensive patients. Monitor blood pressure closely throughout therapy.
succinylcholine	Metoclopramide inhibits plasma cholinesterase, may increase the neuromuscular blocking effects of succinylcholine	Monitor respiratory function.
anticholinergics	Antagonize the effects of metoclopramide on GI motility	Monitor for therapeutic effects.

Life Span and Gender

The nurse should determine whether the patient is pregnant. Several case reports show no adverse effects on the fetus with the use of metoclopramide; however, no adequate and well-controlled studies exist. Although metoclopramide is excreted into breast milk, the levels are well below the maximum therapeutic infant dose. Therefore, there appears to be no contraindication to breastfeeding if the mother receives no more than 45 mg/day of metoclopramide. The nurse should note the patient's age and gender because older adults, especially older women, are more likely to develop the adverse effect of tardive dyskinesia.

Environment

The nurse should note the environment in which metoclopramide will be administered. Oral metoclopramide can be given in any setting and can be self-administered. IV administration of metoclopramide is administered in an acute care setting or an outpatient center.

Nursing Diagnoses and Outcomes

- Risk for Self-Directed Violence secondary to adverse effects of drug therapy
  Desired outcome: The patient will do no self-harm related to depression from drug therapy.
- Powerlessness related to extrapyramidal effects, Parkinson-like symptoms, or tardive dyskinesia secondary to adverse effect of drug therapy
  Desired outcome: The patient will make decisions regarding own care, treatment, and future (when possible) while on drug therapy.
- Risk for Injury related to drowsiness, fatigue, insomnia, confusion, and hallucination secondary to adverse effects of drug therapy.
  Desired outcome: The patient will not suffer injury while on drug therapy.

Planning and Intervention

Maximizing Therapeutic Effects

The nurse should give oral doses 30 minutes before each meal to allow for onset of action and should give an IM injection near the end of surgery to prevent postoperative nausea and vomiting. It is important to administer IV metoclopramide over at least 15 minutes, 30 minutes before the start of chemotherapy to prevent chemotherapy-induced vomiting. Repeat every 2 hours for two doses, then every 3 hours for three doses. The nurse should not administer metoclopramide concurrently with anticholinergic or narcotic drugs.

Minimizing Adverse Effects

The nurse should monitor for evidence of depression and report positive findings to the health care provider. Interventions should be instituted to protect the patient if he or she expresses suicidal ideas. It is important to withhold the dose, notify the prescriber, and seek orders for diphenhydramine (Benadryl) 50 mg IM or benztropine (Cogentin) 1 to 2 mg IM if extrapyramidal symptoms (i.e., involuntary movements of the limbs, facial grimacing, and rhythmic protrusion of the tongue) occur, especially during the first 48 hours of therapy. Either of these drugs usually reverses the symptoms.

The nurse should withhold the dose and notify the prescriber if Parkinson-like symptoms (i.e., bradykinesia, tremor, cog-wheel motions, and mask-like facies) occur, particularly in the first 6 months of therapy. Effects usually subside gradually within 2 to 3 months after drug discontinuation. The nurse should contact the provider regarding discontinuing the drug if signs of tardive dyskinesia (i.e., involuntary movements of face, tongue, mouth, or jaw and sometimes involuntary movements of trunk or extremities) occur because tardive dyskinesia may be irreversible.

Providing Patient and Family Education

- The nurse should tell the patient to take metoclopramide 30 minutes before meals.
- The nurse should caution the patient to prevent injury by avoiding activities that require mental alertness (e.g., operating motor vehicles or other heavy machinery), coordination, or physical dexterity until the effects of the drug are known.
- It is important to caution the patient to avoid alcoholic beverages, sedatives, and other CNS depressants during therapy because these substances may cause additive sedation.
- The nurse should explain to the patient how to recognize any involuntary movements of the eyes, face, or limbs, such as tremors or cog-wheel motion of the arms; depression; or serious diarrhea and report these to the provider at once. In such cases, the patient should not take any more of the drug without discussing these signs and symptoms with the prescriber.

Ongoing Assessment and Evaluation

With careful monitoring and follow-up assessments, nursing care and drug therapy may be considered successful if the patient's GI complaints diminish or subside and the patient does not experience depression or other adverse effects, such as nausea or Parkinson-like symptoms. ■

DRUG CLOSELY RELATED TO METOCLOPRAMIDE

Dexpanthenol

Dexpanthenol (Ilopan) is used prophylactically after major abdominal surgery to minimize the possibility of paralytic ileus. It also is used in treating paralytic ileus, intestinal atony

MEMORY CHIP

Metoclopramide

- Used as a GI stimulant in diabetic gastric stasis, and GERD; as an antiemetic postsurgery and with chemotherapy for cancer
- Most significant contraindication: when stimulation of GI motility might be dangerous
- Most common adverse effects: CNS complaints
- Most serious adverse effects: tardive dyskinesia and severe depression
- **Life span alert: older women are more likely to experience tardive dyskinesia as an adverse effect**
- Maximizing therapeutic effects: give metoclopramide 30 min before meals or chemotherapy
- Minimizing adverse effects: monitor for depression, Parkinson-like symptoms, extrapyramidal effects, and tardive dyskinesia; holding further drug administration and contact the prescriber if noted
- Most significant patient education: teach patient to recognize signs of serious adverse effects; to call prescriber at once when noted

causing abdominal distention, postoperative or postpartum retention of flatus, and postoperative delay in resumption of intestinal motility. Dexpanthenol contributes to the final step of acetylcholine production. Dexpanthenol is the alcohol analog of D-pantothenic acid. Pantothenic acid is a precursor of coenzyme A, which is a cofactor for enzyme-catalyzed reactions involving the transfer of acetyl groups. The final step in acetylcholine synthesis is the choline acetylase transfer of an acetyl group from acetylcoenzyme A to choline. Acetylcholine, the neurohumoral transmitter in the parasympathetic system, maintains normal intestinal function. Decreased acetylcholine results in decreased peristalsis. Thus, dexpanthenol contributes to the production of acetylcholine and promotes peristalsis.

Dexpanthenol is contraindicated in hemophilia and in an ileus if it is due to mechanical obstruction. It is a pregnancy category C drug. Dexpanthenol causes intestinal colic (30 minutes after administration), vomiting, and a slight drop in blood pressure. Other adverse effects include itching, tingling, difficulty breathing, red patches of skin, generalized dermatitis, and urticaria. Unlike metoclopramide, dexpanthenol does not cause extrapyramidal symptoms, parkinsonism, or tardive dyskinesia.

DIGESTIVE ENZYMES

Digestive enzymes are responsible for breaking down food into forms that can be absorbed easily in the GI tract. The digestive process normally begins in the mouth with salivary secretions, then continues in the stomach with the action of gastric acid and pepsin. It is completed in the duodenum with the release of the pancreatic enzymes that change protein, carbohydrate, and fat into absorbable forms.

Replacement of many of these enzymes is not necessary or truly useful, because rarely does a deficiency of endogenous enzymes actually cause GI problems. Many of the drug preparations of digestive enzymes are combinations of various enzymes, frequently paired with anticholinergics, barbiturates, or antacids. In those few situations in which an endogenous deficit does exist, it is nearly impossible to correct the deficit adequately with these combinations. In addition, combination therapy increases the risk of adverse effects from the other drug entities in the compound.

Pancreatic enzymes comprise one group of digestive enzymes that is an exception. Deficiencies of pancreatic enzymes do occur on a fairly frequent basis, usually in pancreatitis, duct obstruction, and following pancreatectomy. Replacement of these enzymes is indicated and therapeutic. Pancreatic digestive enzymes include pancrelipase (Pancrease, Cotazym, Ku-Zyme, Viokase, Ilozyme, Zymase, and Ultrase) and pancreatin (Dizymes, Entozyme, Donnazyme, Pancreazyme, Hi-Vegi-Lip, and Creon). The prototype for pancreatic digestive enzymes is pancrelipase.

NURSING MANAGEMENT OF THE PATIENT RECEIVING PANCRELIPASE

Core Drug Knowledge

Pharmacotherapeutics

Pancrelipase is enzymatic replacement therapy for patients with deficient exocrine pancreatic secretions; cystic fibrosis; chronic pancreatitis; postpancreatectomy; ductal obstructions caused by cancer of the pancreas or common bile duct; pancreatic insufficiency; steatorrhea from malabsorption syndrome and postgastrectomy; or post-GI surgery, such as Billroth II gastroenterostomy. Pancrelipase also can be used as a presumptive test to evaluate pancreatic function (Table 37-9).

Pharmacokinetics

Absorption, distribution, metabolism, and excretion are unknown. The onset, peak, and duration of this drug are also unknown. Because pancrelipase is affected by gastric acid, the drug is enteric coated. This may decrease absorption in the duodenum, however. The site of metabolism and how the drug is eliminated from the body are unknown.

Pharmacodynamics

Pancrelipase contains the enzymes lipase, protease, and amylase, which are responsible for the final phase of digestion. During this phase, fats are hydrolyzed to fatty acids, proteins to proteoses and derived substances, and starches to sugars and dextrins so that they can be absorbed in the small intestine. Pancreatic enzymes normally have an effect in the duodenum and in the first part of the jejunum.

Contraindications and Precautions

Pancrelipase is contraindicated in patients who are hypersensitive to pork protein or enzymes because the drug is derived from pork. It should not be used by patients with

TABLE 37-9 Summary of Selected Digestive Enzymes and Drugs Preventing Digestion

Drug (Trade) Name	Selected Indications	Route and Dosage Range	Pharmacokinetics
pancrelipase (Pancrease, Ku-Zyme, Viokase, Ilozyme, Zymase, Ultrase; *Canadian:* Creon)	Deficient exocrine pancreatic secretions	Adjust dosage until steatorrhea minimizes and good nutritional status is maintained	Unknown
	Pancreatic insufficiency, steatorrhea from malabsorption syndrome and postgastrectomy, or post-GI surgery, Billroth II gastroenterostomy	*Adult:* PO, 4,000 to 48,000 U with each meal and with snacks; severe deficiencies, increase to 64,000–88,000 units with each meal or increase hourly if tolerated *Child:* <6 mo, PO, dose not established; 6–12 mo, 2,000 U with each meal; 1–6 y, 4,000–8,000 U with each meal and 4,000 U with each snack; 7–12 y, 4,000–12,000 U with each meal and snack	
	Postpancreatectomy, ductal obstructions caused by cancer of the pancreas or common bile duct	*Adult:* PO, 8,000–16,000 U at 2 h intervals, or as prescribed	
	Cystic fibrosis	Use powder form: 0.7 g with meals	
pancreatin (Dizymes, Entozyme, Donnazyme, Hi-Vegi-Lip, Creon)	Same as above	*Adult:* PO, 1 or 2 tablets with meals and snacks; adjust according to individual meals *Child:* Dosage not established	Unknown
orlistat (Xenical)	Management of obesity	120 mg tid with meals that contain fat	*Onset:* Immediate *Duration:* Unknown $t_{1/2}$: Not absorbed
sibutramine (Meridia)	Management of obesity	10 mg/d PO; after 4 wk may titrate to 15 mg/d	*Onset:* Unknown *Duration:* To 24 h $t_{1/2}$: Unknown

acute pancreatitis or acute exacerbations of chronic pancreatitis. Pancrelipase is a pregnancy category C drug and should be used only if necessary. It is not known whether it crosses into breast milk, and so it should be administered with caution to nursing mothers.

Caution must be used not to spill the powder on one's hands because it may irritate the skin. Inhalation of the powder irritates the nasal mucosa and the respiratory tract, triggering an asthma attack in those susceptible.

Adverse Effects

Caution must be used with excessive dosing because it may cause nausea, abdominal cramps, and diarrhea. The adverse effects of hyperuricosuria and hyperuricemia have occurred with extremely high doses. Less often, allergic reactions may occur.

Drug Interactions

The antacids calcium carbonate and magnesium hydroxide can interfere with the beneficial effects of pancrelipase. Serum iron response to oral iron supplements may be decreased by concurrent dosing of pancrelipase (Table 37-10).

Assessment of Relevant Core Patient Variables

Health Status

The nurse must assess the patient's health history for chronic pancreatitis, cystic fibrosis, ductal obstructions from cancer, pancreatic insufficiency, pancreatectomy, gastrectomy, or other GI surgery. Results of laboratory studies to review include serum amylase and lipase

TABLE 37-10 Agents That Interact With Digestive Enzymes

Interactants	Effect and Significance	Nursing Management
calcium carbonate, magnesium hydroxide	May negate effect of enzymes	Administer 2 h apart. Monitor for therapeutic effect.
iron	Serum levels may not increase as expected with oral supplements	Monitor blood iron levels. Seek order to adjust dose if iron levels are significantly affected

levels to determine pancreatic functioning and findings of high quantities of fat in stool (steatorrhea). In addition, foul-smelling stools are a sign of steatorrhea. The nurse also needs to assess the patient's nutritional status because deficiency of pancreatic enzymes prevents the absorption of fats, proteins, and starches and may leave the patient malnourished. The nurse also should determine whether the patient is allergic to pork because pancrelipase is derived from pork.

Life Span and Gender

The nurse should determine whether the patient is pregnant or breast-feeding. Because pancrelipase is in pregnancy category C, it should be given only if clearly necessary. Caution should be used when administering pancrelipase to a breast-feeding woman. The nurse also should note the patient's age. The drug may be given to children, but the dosage for children younger than 6 months old has not been established.

Environment

The nurse should be aware of the settings in which pancrelipase may be administered. Pancrelipase can be administered in any setting, including the home.

Culture

The nurse should consider the religious affiliation of patients taking pancrelipase. Some religious groups, such as Moslems and Orthodox Jews, forbid the consumption of pork products in any form, and pancrelipase is pork based. Therefore, these patients may not accept the use of this drug therapy.

Nursing Diagnoses and Outcomes

- Imbalanced Nutrition: Less than Body Requirements related to impaired digestion secondary to insufficient pancreatic enzymes

  Desired outcome: The patient's nutrient absorption will be adequate to meet body needs while on drug therapy.
- Risk for Pain, acute abdominal, secondary to adverse effects of drug therapy

  Desired outcome: The patient will not develop pain as an adverse effect of drug therapy.

Planning and Intervention

Maximizing Therapeutic Effects

Brands of pancrelipase should not be changed without consulting the prescribing health care provider because the brands do not have equal bioavailability. If prescribed, the nurse may administer antacids or an H_2 receptor antagonist to maintain the patient's gastric pH within an alkaline range. This prevents pancrelipase tablets from dissolving in the stomach and becoming inactivated.

Minimizing Adverse Effects

The nurse must make sure to administer, or make sure the patient is administering, pancrelipase exactly as prescribed to prevent excessive dosing.

Providing Patient and Family Education

- The nurse should explain to the patient and family the need to learn about the role of the digestive enzyme in digestion and absorption of food. Insufficiency of the enzyme results in weight loss and steatorrhea (foul-smelling and frothy stools). Although it is not usually possible to dose pancrelipase to eradicate steatorrhea completely, pancrelipase should greatly decrease steatorrhea.
- The nurse should tell the patient to take the drug every time she or he eats, either before or with meals and snacks.
- It is important to caution the patient not to crush or chew pancrelipase because this will destroy the enzyme by exposing it to gastric acid.
- The nurse should urge the patient to notify the prescriber of any abdominal pain, diarrhea, nausea, or any return of steatorrhea.
- If the form of pancrelipase is a capsule that is to be opened and mixed with food, the nurse should caution the patient to avoid getting the powder on the hands or sniffing the powder contained in the capsules. Asthma attacks can occur in susceptible patients after sniffing pancrelipase powder.

Ongoing Assessment and Evaluation

The nurse should assess the patient for decreased steatorrhea, weight gain, and improved nutritional status. Drug therapy is successful if digestion and nutritional status improve without the occurrence of adverse effects. ■

DRUG CLOSELY RELATED TO PANCRELIPASE

Pancreatin is a digestive enzyme that has the same action and indication for use as pancrelipase (see Table 37-9). The difference between the two is that pancreatin is not as concentrated as pancrelipase and therefore may not control

MEMORY CHIP

Pancrelipase

- Used as enzyme replacement therapy for those deficient in this pancreatic enzyme
- Most common adverse effects: related to gastrointestinal system
- Most significant patient education: do not crush or chew tablets; take before or with meals

steatorrhea as well. Pancreatin may be from beef or pork sources.

C LIPASE INHIBITORS

There is one drug that inhibits the digestive enzyme lipase. This drug is orlistat (Xenical). It is used in the management of obesity. A drug significantly different from orlistat is the reuptake inhibitor, sibutramine (Meridia).

NURSING MANAGEMENT OF THE PATIENT RECEIVING P ORLISTAT

Core Drug Knowledge

Pharmacotherapeutics

Orlistat (Xenical) is used in the management of obesity, including weight loss and weight maintenance (see Table 37-9). It is to be used in addition to a weight-loss diet. Orlistat also is used to reduce the risk for regaining weight after weight loss, and for obese patients with an initial BMI of 30 kg/m^2 or more or BMI of 27 kg/m^2 of more if they have other cardiovascular risk factors (e.g., hypertension, diabetes, and dyslipidemia).

Pharmacokinetics

Very little orlistat is absorbed into the systemic circulation and most of its effect is from its local effect in the GI tract. In laboratory studies, orlistat is more than 99% protein bound. Metabolism appears to be predominantly within the GI wall. Two metabolites are formed but they do not seem to be pharmacologically significant. Fecal excretion is the main route of elimination.

Pharmacodynamics

Orlistat is a reversible lipase inhibitor. By inhibiting the action of lipase, the absorption of dietary fats is decreased. The therapeutic effect occurs in the lumen of the stomach and small intestine by preventing the formation of active gastric and pancreatic lipases. Thus, the inactivated enzymes are not available to hydrolyze dietary fat, in the form of triglycerides, into absorbable free fatty acids and monoglycerides. Undigested triglycerides are not absorbed, resulting in decreased calories being absorbed. This allows for weight loss. At the recommended therapeutic dose of 120 mg three times a day, orlistat inhibits dietary fat absorption by about 30%.

Weight loss was observed within the first 2 weeks of starting therapy with orlistat in clinical trials. For the first year of use the overall mean weight loss was between 12.4 and 13.4 pounds for people receiving orlistat, compared with 5.8 to 6.2 pounds for those receiving placebos. At the end of 1 year, 57% of the orlistat-treated patients (compared with 31% on placebo) had lost at least 5% of their baseline body weight. This comparison of the weight percentage lost was similar for the two groups after 2 years of therapy as well. In studies, patients on placebos regained between 52% and 63% of the weight lost, whereas orlistat patients regained only 26% to 35%.

Contraindications and Precautions

Orlistat is contraindicated if the patient has chronic malabsorption syndrome or cholestasis. It also is contraindicated if the patient is hypersensitive to the drug or any of its elements. Organic causes of obesity, such as hypothyroidism, should be ruled out before prescribing orlistat.

Some patients may develop increased levels of urinary oxalate following treatment. Caution should be used if the patient has a history of hyperoxaluria or calcium oxalate nephrolithiasis. The weight loss brought about by orlistat use may improve metabolic control in diabetic patients. They may require a reduced dose of oral hypoglycemic medication or insulin. Orlistat is a pregnancy category B drug.

Adverse Effects

The GI symptoms are the most common adverse effects and they are related to the pharmacodynamics of the drug. These adverse effects are generally mild and transient, although for some patients they may last for 6 months or longer and be severe enough to warrant discontinuing the drug. These GI symptoms are oily spotting, flatus with discharge of stool, fecal urgency, fatty or oily stool, oily evacuation, increased defecation, and fecal incontinence.

Other adverse effects that can occur, but are not common, include:

- CNS: anxiety, depression, dizziness, and headache
- Dermatologic: dry skin and rash
- GI: abdominal pain, gingival disorder, infectious diarrhea, nausea, rectal pain/discomfort, tooth disorder, and vomiting
- Musculoskeletal: arthritis, back pain, joint disorder, myalgia, tendonitis, and pain in lower extremities
- Reproductive, female: menstrual irregularity and vaginitis
- Respiratory: ear, nose, and throat symptoms, influenza, lower respiratory tract infection, and upper respiratory tract infection
- Miscellaneous: fatigue, otitis, pedal edema, sleep disorder, and urinary tract infection

No known adverse effects related to overdose are known. If necessary, stop the drug and observe the patient for 24 hours. The systemic effects attributable to lipase inhibition should be rapidly reversible.

Drug Interactions

Because of the impaired fat absorption from the use of orlistat the absorption of fat-soluble vitamins (A, D, E, beta-carotene) will decrease. A few other drug interactions are known (Table 37-11).

TABLE 37-11 Agents That Interact With Orlistat

Interactants	Effect and Significance	Nursing Management
cyclosporine	Exact clinical effect is unknown. Changes in cyclosporine absorption have been reported with variations in dietary intake.	Monitor for clinical effectiveness of cyclosporine.
fat-soluble vitamins	Decreased absorption rate of fat-soluble vitamins; 30% decrease in beta carotene and about 60% reduction in vitamin E absorption have been shown. Decrease in other vitamin levels not known exactly. Vitamin deficiency may result.	Teach patient to take a multivitamin that includes fat-soluble vitamins to prevent deficiencies.
pravastatin	Additive lipid lowering effect of pravastatin. Increases pravastatin serum levels about 30%. May possibly be a helpful adjunct therapy in hypercholesterolemia (not shown yet by research)	Monitor patient's HDL and LDL serum levels
warfarin	Possible decrease in Vitamin K absorption. No known effect on pharmacokinetics or pharmacodynamics of warfarin currently.	Monitor for changes in coagulation, increased effect of warfarin.

Assessment of Relevant Core Patient Variables

Health Status

The nurse should verify that the patient does not have a physiologic cause for obesity before starting orlistat.

Life Span and Gender

The nurse should determine whether the patient is pregnant or breast-feeding. As there are no adequate and well-controlled studies of orlistat in pregnant women, it is not recommended. It is not known whether orlistat is excreted in breast milk, and therefore, its use is not recommended. The nurse also should determine the patient's age because safety and efficacy in children have not been established yet.

Lifestyle, Diet, and Habits

A dietary history should be taken to determine how many current calories, and what percentage of the calories, come from fat. The patient should be on a nutritionally balanced, reduced calorie diet; no more than 30% of their caloric intake should come from fat while they receive orlistat.

Environment

The nurse should be aware of the setting in which orlistat will be administered. Orlistat is normally self-administered in the patient's home.

Nursing Diagnoses and Outcomes

- Imbalanced Nutrition: More Than Body Requirements
  Desired outcome: The patient will lose wait during drug therapy.
- Risk for Imbalanced Nutrition: Less Than Body Requirements related to impaired fat soluble vitamin absorption from drug therapy
  Desired outcome: The patient will not have serious vitamin deficiencies while on drug therapy.
- Risk for Bowel Incontinence related to adverse effects of drug therapy
  Desired outcome: Bowel incontinence will not occur or will be minimal and transient.
- Risk for Diarrhea related to adverse effects of drug therapy
  Desired outcome: Diarrhea will not occur or it will be minimal and transient

Planning and Intervention

Maximizing Therapeutic Effects and Minimizing Adverse Effects

Nursing actions are related to patient teaching.

Providing Patient and Family Education

- The nurse should teach the patient to limit dietary fat. Calories from fat should be no more than 30% of daily calories. This promotes weight loss and prevents and minimizes GI adverse effects.
- It is important for the patient to divide the daily fat intake equally between meals, and to take the drug with each meal containing fat (during or up to 1 hour after eating). The patient should skip a dose if the meal has no fat or if the meal is missed (see the accompanying display, Adverse Effects From Orlistat).
- The nurse should encourage the patient to take a vitamin supplement that includes fat-soluble vitamins.

Ongoing Assessment and Evaluation

Orlistat therapy is effective if weight loss occurs without significant GI adverse effects or vitamin deficiency occurring. ■

Critical Thinking Scenario

Adverse effects from orlistat

Ms. Benson has been taking orlistat, a lipase inhibitor, to promote weight loss for 1 month. She returns to the clinic for follow up. You, the nurse, ask her how she is tolerating the medication. She tells you that initially she only had some problems with "needing to go to the bathroom a couple of times a day." However, she says that in the last few days she has been bothered by "real oily poop." She tells you that she has to run to the bathroom "like mad, 'cause I can't hold it. Sometimes I can't get there fast enough and spot my panties with that stuff."

What questions should you ask Ms. Benson to assess her problem thoroughly?

MEMORY CHIP

Orlistat

- Used to promote weight loss in obesity; prevents absorption of dietary fat
- Most significant contraindication: chronic malabsorption syndrome or cholestasis
- Most common adverse effects: GI (oily spotting, flatus with stool, and fecal urgency)
- Most significant patient education: take with all meals containing fat; limit dietary fat to 30% of calories; take a multivitamin with fat-soluble vitamins

DRUG SIGNIFICANTLY DIFFERENT FROM ORLISTAT

Sibutramine (Meridia), like orlistat, is used in the management of obesity, including weight loss and maintenance of weight loss. Sibutramine works in a very different manner than orlistat, however. Sibutramine inhibits the reuptake of norepinephrine, serotonin, and dopamine. Norepinephrine levels are increased most, dopamine's least. The changes in neurotransmitter levels brings about appetite suppression, sibutramine is thus an anorexiant. It does not alter fat absorption or digestion as orlistat does. A full discussion of sibutramine is found in Chapter 14.

ANTIEMETICS

Antiemetics, which suppress the stimulation of the CTZ and the VC, are used to treat nausea and vomiting. Antiemetic drugs are primarily from three main drug classifications—selective serotonin receptor antagonists, antidopaminergics, and anticholinergics. A full prototype discussion of the selective serotonin receptor antagonists is presented next.

The antidopaminergic drugs (also referred to as phenothiazides) block the action of dopamine, which is found in both the GI tract and the CTZ; they also have sedative properties. These drugs also are considered antipsychotics. The prototype for phenothiazides, chlorpromazine (Thorazine), is discussed in Chapter 19. Other drugs in this class used as antiemetics include prochlorperazine (Compazine), triflupromazine (Stelazine), perphenazine (Trilafon), promethazine (Phenergan), thiethylperazine (Torecan), and metoclopramide (Reglan).

The anticholinergic antiemetics, such as meclizine, block the action of acetylcholine in the VC. Their effect on motion sickness is by reducing the sensitivity of the labyrinthine apparatus. This inhibits vestibular input to the CNS, reducing stimulation of the CTZ and the VC. The anticholinergics are used in treating nausea and vomiting, motion sickness, and some, such as meclizine (Antivert), are used in the treatment of vertigo. Anticholinergic drugs, such as the prototype atropine, are discussed in Chapter 15. Atropine is not used as an antiemetic. Other drugs in this class used as antiemetics include: scopalamine (Transderm-Scop), cyclizine (Marazine), buclizine (Buculadin-S Softabs), diphenhydramine (Benadryl), and trimethobenzamide (Tigan).

A different drug class altogether, the **emetics,** are drugs that induce vomiting. They are used when accidental ingestion of a noncorrosive agent has occurred. Ipecac is a product that is available OTC to inducing vomiting.

SELECTIVE SEROTONIN RECEPTOR ANTAGONISTS

The selective serotonin receptor antagonists, also known as the 5-HT3 receptor antagonists (to specify which of the serotonin receptors are blocked), prevent the stimulation of special serotonin receptors in the CTZ. Selective serotonin receptor antagonists include ondansetron (Zofran), dolastron (anzemet), and granisetron (Kytril). The prototype selective serotonin receptor antagonist is ondansetron.

NURSING MANAGEMENT OF THE PATIENT RECEIVING ONDANSETRON

Core Drug Knowledge

Pharmacotherapeutics

Ondansetron (Zofran) is used in the prevention of nausea and vomiting associated with cancer chemotherapy and radiotherapy, and in postoperative states when there is a high expectation that nausea or vomiting will occur or when nausea and vomiting must be avoided (see the accompanying display, Control of Postoperative Nausea and Vomiting).

Unlabeled uses of ondansetron include the treatment of nausea and vomiting associated with acetaminophen poisoning; treatment of acute levodopa-induced psychosis (visual hallucinations); nausea and vomiting due to prostacyclin therapy; reduction in bulimic episodes in patients with bulimia nervosa; and in the treatment of spinal or epidural morphine–induced pruritus. It also

Focus on Research

Control of postoperative nausea and vomiting

Loewen, P. S., Marra, C. A., & Zed, P. J. (2000). 5–HT_3 receptor antagonists versus traditional agents for the prophylaxis of postoperative nausea and vomiting. *Canadian Journal of Anaesthesia, 47*(10), 1008–1018.

The Study

A review of the literature that was published in English between 1966 and 1999 was conducted; it focused on studies that examined the control of postoperative nausea and vomiting. The effectiveness of "traditional" antiemetic therapy (i.e., metoclopramide, perphenazine, prochlorperazine, cyclizine, and droperidol [an off-label use of this anesthetic not approved by the Food and Drug Administration]) was compared to the effectiveness of 5–HT3 receptor antagonists (selective serotonin receptor antagonists), which include ondansetron, dolasetron, granisetron, and tropisetron. The review showed that the group of selective serotonin receptor antagonists was superior statistically to other drug treatments in the prevention of postoperative nausea and vomiting.

Nursing Implications

Nurses should be aware that the selective serotonin receptor antagonists are superior in their efficacy to other antiemetics for postoperative nausea and vomiting. This knowledge allows nurses to better meet the needs of patients who are at increased risk for postoperative nausea and vomiting, or who are having severe postoperative nausea and vomiting not controlled by other methods. Severe nausea and vomiting are also undesirable in certain postoperative patients because of strain on surgical incision and internal sutures. Nurses should seek orders for selective serotonin receptor antagonist antiemetics from physicians and other prescribers when the patient's situation warrants this drug therapy.

may have potential benefit in patients with social anxiety disorder.

New research is indicating that alcoholism that occurs earlier in life is associated with serotonergic abnormality and antisocial behaviors. Patients with early-onset alcoholism who received ondansetron in a clinical trial had fewer drinks per day, and more days without any drinking than patients who received placebos. Ondansetron appears to be effective treatment for these patients presumably by relieving an underlying abnormality from serotonin stimulation (Johnson, Roache, Javors, DiClemente, Cloninger, & Prihoda, 2000). More studies are needed in this area to confirm this finding.

Pharmacokinetics

Ondansetron is metabolized by the liver. It is moderately protein bound (about 75%). It crosses the placenta, may enter breast milk, and is excreted in the urine.

Pharmacodynamics

Serotonin receptors, of the 5-HT3 type, are located peripherally on vagal nerve terminal and centrally in the CTZ. During chemotherapy, special mucosal cells in the small intestine release serotonin, which stimulates these receptors. Ondansetron blocks these receptor sites preventing nausea and vomiting.

Contraindications and Precautions

Ondansetron is contraindicated if there is hypersensitivity to the drug or its components. Ondansetron is a pregnancy category B drug.

Adverse Effects

The most common adverse effects of ondansetron are headache, constipation, and malaise. Potentially serious adverse effects are arrhythmias, hypotension, extrapyramidal effects (e.g., Parkinson-like symptoms). Other adverse effects that can occur include:

- CV: hypertension
- CNS: anxiety, dizziness, drowsiness, and chills or shivering
- GI: abdominal pain, diarrhea, and xerostomia
- Miscellaneous: wound problems, musculoskeletal pain, cold sensation, fever, gynecological disorders, hypoxia, injection site reaction, paresthesia, pruritus, urinary retention, weakness, increases in aspartate transaminase and alanine aminotransferase, and pain.

Drug Interactions

As ondansetron is metabolized by the CYP450 enzymes, it is possible that there may be drug interactions with other drugs that are metabolized by CYP450 or that inhibit CYP450 metabolism. However, no dosage adjustment has been recommended based on available data regarding this finding.

Assessment of Relevant Core Patient Variables

Health Status

The nurse should verify that the patient has clinical indications for receiving the drug and is not known to have a hypersensitivity to it.

Life Span and Gender

The nurse should assess whether the patient is pregnant. Ondansetron is a pregnancy category B drug. Therefore, it should be used only if the potential benefit justifies potential unknown risks. The nurse also should determine the patient's age. Ondansetron is used to prevent nausea and vomiting associated with cancer chemotherapy in children. However, there is limited information about the correct dosage for children 3 years of age or younger. Dosage adjustment is not needed in older adults.

Environment

The nurse should note the setting in which ondansetron will be administered. Ondansetron normally is administered in the hospital.

Nursing Diagnoses and Outcomes

- Imbalanced Nutrition: Less Than Body Requirements related to severe nausea and vomiting
  Desired outcome: Nutritional needs will be met and ondansetron therapy will prevent severe nausea and vomiting.
- Risk for Altered Comfort related to severe nausea and vomiting
  Desired outcome: Comfort will be maintained and ondansetron therapy will prevent severe nausea and vomiting.
- Potential Complication: Altered Cardiac Output related to adverse effects of ondansetron
  Desired outcome: Cardiac output will not be affected adversely by possible hypotension and arrhythmias from ondansetron.

Planning and Intervention

Maximizing Therapeutic Effects

The nurse should administer ondansetron 30 minutes before the start of chemotherapy. Infusions should be over 15 minutes. Additional doses are used after treatment. When used for postoperative nausea and vomiting, it should be given immediately before induction into anesthesia. If used with radiation therapy the dose should be given orally, 1 to 2 hours before treatment. Oral disintegrating tablets should be removed from the pack by peeling back the foil, not by pushing the drug tablet through the foil. The nurse should place ondansetron on the patient's tongue and have the patient swallow it. Administration with a fluid is not needed.

Providing Patient and Family Education

- The nurse should explain the purpose of the drug.
- The nurse should teach the patient to report any tremor, gait problems, or other Parkinson-like symptoms.

Ongoing Assessment and Evaluation

Ondansetron therapy is considered effective if nausea and vomiting are controlled and adverse effects do not occur. ■

MEMORY CHIP

Ondansetron

- Used to prevent nausea and vomiting associated with cancer chemotherapy, radiation, and certain postoperative states
- Most common adverse effects: headache, constipation, and malaise
- Most serious adverse effects: arrhythmias, hypotension, and extrapyramidal effects
- Maximizing therapeutic effects: administer 30 mins before treatment
- Most significant patient education: notify the nurse if any adverse effects occur

TABLE 37-12 Summary of Selected Gallstone-Solubilizing Agents

Drug (Trade) Name	Selected Indications	Contraindications and Precautions	Adverse Effects	Route and Dosage Range
ursodiol (Actigall)	Dissolution of radiolucent, non-calcified, smaller than 20-mm gallstones in patients who are not candidates for surgery due to age, disease states, or idiosyncratic reactions to anesthesia	Will not dissolve calcified, radio-paque, or radiolucent bile pigment stones in patients with compelling needs for cholecystectomy	Nausea, vomiting, dyspepsia	*Adult:* PO, 8–20 mg/kg/d in two to three doses, for 1 y or more (if partial or full dissolution does not occur in 1 y, likelihood of success is reduced)
monoctanoin (Moctanin)	Dissolution of radiolucent gallstones retained in biliary tract after cholecystectomy when other means have failed or cannot be used	Impaired hepatic function, significant biliary tract infection, recent history of duodenal ulcer or duodenitis, portosystemic shunting, acute pancreatitis, or any life-threatening problem that would be complicated by biliary tract infusion	Abdominal pain, nausea, vomiting, diarrhea, anorexia, indigestion, fever	*Adult* (direct infusion into biliary tract only after a catheter has been placed endoscopically as close to the stones as possible): Dilute 120-mL vial with 13 mL of sterile water; perfuse stone 3–5 mL/h for 2–10 d

C GALLSTONE-SOLUBILIZING AGENTS

Gallstone-solubilizing agents, including ursodiol (Actigall) and monoctanoin (Moctanin), work to dissolve gallstones. They are used only under specific circumstances and are summarized in Table 37-12.

CHAPTER SUMMARY

- Drug therapy for the upper GI tract is related to problems from bacterial infection, acid production, digestion, and nausea and vomiting.
- Dietary factors may influence symptoms experienced from the disease process; may contribute to the effectiveness of the therapy; they may contribute to adverse effects from therapy. Current dietary habits should be explored, and additional dietary teaching provided as indicated, with all patients requiring drug therapy for upper GI problems.
- *Helicobacter pylori* causes a bacterial infection that has been shown to be a causative factor in peptic ulcers. When *H. pylori* is eradicated an ulcer rarely reoccurs. Treatment has various drug choices but includes the combination of usually two antibiotics and a proton pump inhibitor. A bismuth salicylate may be added as well. H_2 receptor antagonists are used sometimes instead of a proton pump inhibitor.
- Proton pump inhibitors, such as omeprazole, decrease gastric acid production. They are used to manage symptoms of, and to treat gastric disorders such as, GERD, peptic ulcers, and hypersecretory conditions.
- H_2 receptor antagonists, such as cimetidine, block histamine at the site of the parietal cells, resulting in a reduction in the hydrogen ion concentration and volume of gastric acid. Common uses of H_2 receptor antagonists include treatment of peptic ulcer disease, gastric esophageal reflux disease, hypersecretory conditions, and the prevention of stress ulcers. OTC cimetidine is used for heartburn and indigestion.
- Antacids are drugs that are base salts and increase the gastric pH, thereby neutralizing gastric acidity. These preparations are used for upper GI disorders, such as gastroesophageal reflux esophagitis, hiatal hernia, gastritis, and peptic ulcer disease. Antacids do not cure these conditions but help to manage the symptoms and discomfort associated with them. All antacids are closely related, and are used in various combinations to produce the desired effects and to minimize adverse effects.
- Two antacids are absorbed systemically, sodium bicarbonate and calcium carbonate. They can cause metabolic alkalosis in large doses. Sodium bicarbonate contains large quantities of sodium. It should not be given to patients who have pathologies who require salt restriction.
- Magnesium antacids should not be given to patients with chronic renal failure because they increase the risk of developing magnesium toxicity in such patients. Aluminum carbonate is used with patients with chronic renal failure because it binds with phosphorus, reducing serum phosphate levels.
- Sucralfate, although an aluminum salt, is not an antacid. With dissolution in the stomach, it forms a sticky paste that adheres to the ulceration, preventing gastric acids from touching the ulcer and allowing healing to occur.
- The GI stimulants, such as metoclopramide, are used in diabetic gastroparesis and with symptomatic gastroesophageal reflux. They increase GI motility, apparently by sensitizing the tissues to acetylcholine. Metoclopramide, because of its dopamine antagonist characteristics, also is used as an antiemetic postoperatively and during chemotherapy.
- Digestive enzymes are a replacement for the body's intrinsic enzymes when the body does not produce enough to meet the needs for digestion. The enzymes that are replaced most frequently with the greatest therapeutic effects are the pancreatic enzymes. They should be taken with meals and with snacks.
- Orlistat, a lipase inhibitor, prevents the absorption of dietary fat. It is used in obesity to promote weight loss and maintenance.
- Antiemetics prevent nausea and vomiting by preventing stimulation of the CTZ and the VC by interfering with neurotransmitter receptors. They are primarily either selective serotonin receptor antagonists, antidopaminergics, or anticholinergics.
- Selective serotonin receptor antagonists, such as ondansetron, are used to prevent the nausea and vomiting associated with cancer chemotherapy, radiation therapy, and after some types of surgery.

QUESTIONS FOR STUDY AND REVIEW

1. If a patient is treated for active peptic ulcer disease solely with an antisecretory drug, such as a proton pump inhibitor like omeprazole or an H_2 receptor antagonist like cimetidine, is it likely that the ulcer will recur?
2. Your patient is receiving the proton pump inhibitor omeprazole for GERD. Explain how dietary factors may interact with the therapeutic action of omeprazole.
3. Why is it important to assess the pharmacokinetics of other drugs that a patient is receiving when you are to start the patient on omeprazole therapy?
4. How do H_1 receptor antagonists differ from H_2 receptor antagonists?
5. What is the advantage of combining aluminum hydroxide with magnesium hydroxide as an antacid?
6. Why are aluminum antacids given to patients with chronic renal failure?
7. What are the main adverse effects from orlistat, a lipase inhibitor used in treating obesity?
8. Why is ondansetron especially helpful in preventing nausea and vomiting from cancer chemotherapy?

NEED MORE HELP?

Chapter 37 of the study guide for *Drug Therapy in Nursing* contains exercises and activities to reinforce your understanding of the concepts presented in this chapter. For additional information see the text's accompanying website at *http://www.connection.lww.com.*

REFERENCES AND BIBLIOGRAPHY

American College of Gastroenterology. (1999). *Treatment Guideline: Updated Guidelines for the Diagnosis and Treatment of Gastroesophageal Reflux Disease* [On-line]. Available: http://www.acg.go.org/acg-dev/staging/members/guides/gerdabs/html.

Axon, A. T. (2000). Treatment of *Helicobacter pylori:* An overview. *Alimentary Pharmacology and Therapeutics, 14,*(Suppl. 3), 1–6.

Ann Arbor/University of Michigan Health System. (1997). *Peptic ulcer disease. Guidelines* [On-line]. Available: http://www.summary.asp?guideline=001012&summary_type=brief_summary&view=brief_summary&sSe.

Bray, G. A. (2000). A concise review on the therapeutics of obesity. *Nutrition, 16*(10), 953–960.

Candelli, M., Carloni, E., Armuzzi, A., Cammarota, G., Ojetti, V., Pignataro, G., Santoliquido, A., Pola, R., Pola, E., Gasbarrini, G., & Gasbarrini, A. (2000). Role of sucralfate in gastrointestinal diseases. *Panminerva Medicine, 42*(1), 55–59.

Chan, F. K., Sung, J. J., Lee, Y. T., Leung, W. K., Chan, L. Y., Yung, M. Y., & Chung, S. C. (1997). Does smoking predispose to peptic ulcer relapse after eradication of *Helicobacter pylori? American Journal of Gastroenterology, 92*(3), 442–445.

Chelimsky, G., & Czinn, S. J. (2000). *Helicobacter pylori* infection in children: update. *Current Opinion in Pediatrics,12*(5), 460–462.

Cook, D. J., Fuller, H. D., & Guyatt, G. H. (1994). Risk factors for gastrointestinal bleeding in critically ill patients. *New England Journal of Medicine, 330,* 377–381.

Drug Facts and Comparisons. (2000). St. Louis: Facts and Comparisons.

Ernst, P. B., & Pappo, J. (2000). Preventive and therapeutic vaccines against *Helicobacter pylori:* Current status and future challenges. *Current Pharmaceutical Desig, 6*(15), 1557–1573.

Erstad, B. L., Barletta, J. F., Jacobi, J., Killan, A. D., Kramer, K. M., & Martin, S. J. (1999). *Survey of stress ulcer prophylaxis* [On-line]. Available: http://www.pubmedcentral.nih.gov/b.cgi?pubmedid=11056739.

Flegal, M. D., Carroll, R. J., Kuczmarski, R. J., & Johnson, C. C. (1998). Overweight and obesity in the United States: Prevalence and trends, 1960–1994. *International Journal of Obesity and Related Metabolic Disorders 22,* 39–47.

Frank, F., Stricker, T., Stallmach, T., & Braegger, C. P. (2000). *Helicobacter pylori* infection in recurrent abdominal pain. *Journal of Pediatric Gastroenterology and Nutrition, 31*(4), 424–427.

Gomollon, F., Sicilia, B., Ducons, J. A., Sierra, E., Revilla, M. J., & Ferrero, M. (2000). Third line treatment for *Helicobacter pylori:* A prospective, culture-guided study in peptic ulcer patients. *Alimentary Pharmacology and Therapeutics, 14*(10), 1335–1338.

Graham, D. Y., & Qureshi, W. A. (2000). Antibiotic- resistant *H. pylori* infection and its treatment. *Current Pharmaceutical Design, 6*(15), 1537–1544.

Hawkins, C., & Hanks, G. W. (2000). The gastroduodenal toxicity of nonsteroidal anti-inflammatory drugs: A review of the literature. *Journal of Pain and Symptom Management, 20*(2), 140–151.

Johnson, B. A., Roache, J. D., Javors, M. A., DiClemente, C. C., Cloninger, C. R., Prihoda, T. J., Bordnick, P. S., Ait-Daoud, N., & Hensler, J. (2000). Ondansetron for reduction of drinking among biologically predisposed alcoholic patients: A randomized controlled trial. *Journal of the American Medical Association, 284*(8), 963–971.

Kandel, G. (2000). Helicobacter and disease: Still more questions than answers. *Canadian Journal of Surgery, 43*(5), 339–346.

Lai, K. C., Hui, W. M., Wong, W. M., Wong, B. C., Hu, W. H., Ching, C. K., & Lam, S. K. (2000). Treatment of *Helicobacter pylori* in patients with duodenal ulcer hemorrhage—a long-term randomized, controlled study. *American Journal of Gastroenterology, 95*(9), 2225–2232.

Macleo, A. D. (2000). Ondansetron in multiple sclerosis. *Journal of Pain and Symptom Management, 20*(5), 388–391.

McManus, T. J. (2000). *Helicobacter pylori:* An emerging infectious disease. *Nurse Practitioner, 25*(8), 40, 43–44.

Misciagna, G., Cisternino, A. M., & Freudenheim, J. Diet and duodenal ulcer. *Digest for Liver Disease, 32*(6), 468–472.

Must, A., Spandano, J, Coakley, E. H., Field, A. E., Coldity, G., and Diety, W. H. (1999). The disease burden associated with overweight and obesity. *Journal of the American Medical Association* [On-line], *282*(16). Available: http://jama.ama-assn.org/issues/v282n16/rfull/joc81719.html.

Nakajima, S., Graham, D. Y., Hattori, T., & Bamba, T. (2000). Strategy for treatment of *Helicobacter pylori* infection in adults. Updated indications for test and eradication therapy suggested in 2000. *Current Pharmaceutical Design, 6*(15), 1503–1514.

National Institute of Health. (1998). *Helicobacter pylori* in peptic ulcer disease. *Guidelines* [On-line]. Available: http://www./summary.asp?guideline=000428&summary_type=brief_summary&view=brief_summary&sSe.

Powell, R. M., & Buggy, D. J. (2000). Ondansetron given before induction of anesthesia reduces shivering after general anesthesia. *Anesthesia and Analgesia, 90*(6), 1423–1427.

Therapeutic guidelines on stress ulcer prophylaxis. (1999). *American Journal of Health System Pharmacy, 56*(4), 347–379.

Tolia, V. (1999). *Helicobacter pylori* infection in pediatric patients. *Current Gastroenterology Report, 1*(4), 308–313.

Wadden, T. A., Berkowitz, R. I., Womble, L. G., Sarwer, D. B., Arnold, M. E., & Steinberg, C. M. (2000). Effects of sibutramine plus orlistat in obese women following 1 year of treatment by sibutramine alone: a placebo-controlled trial. *Obesity Research, 8*(6), 431–437.

Weiss, D. (2000). How to help your patients lose weight: Current therapy for obesity. *Cleveland Clinic Journal of Medicine, 67*(10), 739, 743–746.

Wenner, J., Gunnarsson, T., Graffner, H., & Lindell, G. (2000). Influence of smoking and *Helicobacter pylori* on gastric phospholipids. *Digestive Diseases and Science, 45*(8), 1648–1652..

Chapter 38

DRUGS FOR TREATING THE LOWER GASTROINTESTINAL TRACT

KEY TERMS

constipation
Crohn disease
diarrhea
fecal impaction
flatus
inflammatory bowel disease (IBD)
irritable bowel syndrome (IBS)
peristalsis

Learning Objectives

At the completion of this chapter the student will:

1. Identify core drug knowledge about drugs that affect the lower gastrointestinal (GI) tract.
2. Identify core patient variables related to drugs that affect the lower GI tract.
3. Relate the interaction of core drug knowledge to core patient variables for drugs that affect the lower GI tract.
4. Generate a nursing plan of care from the interactions between core drug knowledge and core patient variables for drugs that affect the lower GI tract.
5. Describe nursing interventions to maximize therapeutic and minimize adverse effects for drugs that affect the lower GI tract.
6. Determine key points for patient and family education for drugs that affect the lower GI tract.

Antiflatulants

- **simethicone**
- charcoal

Antidiarrheals

- **diphenoxylate HCL with atropine sulfate**
- difenoxin HCL with atropine sulfate
- loperamide
- bismuth subsalicylate
- kaolin and pectin

Laxatives

Saline laxatives

- **magnesium hydroxide**
- magnesium sulfate
- magnesium citrate
- sodium phosphate

Hyperosmotic laxatives

- polyethylene glycol electrolyte solution
- lactulose
- glycerin

Stimulant laxatives

- cascara sagrada
- calcium salts of sennosides A and B
- phenolphthalein
- senna
- castor oil
- bisacodyl

Bulk-forming laxatives

- polycarbophil
- psyllium

Stool softener

- docusate sodium

Lubricant laxative

- mineral oil

Drugs used to treat irritable bowel syndrome

- dicyclomine
- hyoscyamine

Drugs used to treat inflammatory bowel disease

- mesalamine
- sulfasalazine
- olsalazine
- balsalazide

The symbol C indicates the **drug class**.

Drugs in bold type marked with the symbol P are **prototypes**.

Drugs in blue type with no symbol are **closely related** to the prototype.

Drugs in **red** type with no symbol are **significantly different** from the prototype.

Drugs in **black** type with no symbol are **also used in drug therapy**; no prototype.

This chapter discusses drugs used to treat the most common alterations of the lower gastrointestinal (GI) tract, including flatus (gas), diarrhea, constipation, irritable bowel syndrome, and irritable bowel disease. All are digestive disorders. Their occurrence may be mild and episodic, or severe, debilitating and chronic. Patients may self treat these problems with over-the-counter (OTC) medications or they may seek medical attention. These problems may be related to other drug therapy, diet, emotions, or changes in activity. The drug classes used to treat flatus, diarrhea, and constipation are called antiflatulents, antidiarrheals, and laxatives, respectively. In addition, drugs used to treat irritable bowel syndrome and inflammatory bowel disease (including ulcerative colitis and Crohn disease) are presented briefly.

Some drugs begin acting in the lower GI tract. However, their therapeutic uses are for alterations of other systems. These drugs include potassium-removing resins, such as sodium polystyrene sulfonate (Kayexalate) and a lipid-lowering agent, such as cholestyramine (Questran). These drugs are discussed in Chapters 29 and 34, respectively.

PHYSIOLOGY

The large intestine is approximately 5 feet long (1.5 m) and 2-½ inches (6.5 cm) in diameter. The longitudinal muscle fibers on the outer surface of the large intestine are in three layers and do not cover the entire colon uniformly. The arrangement of the muscle in this way exerts a tension on the wall of the intestine, drawing it up and giving it a puckered appearance.

The large intestine is composed of the cecum, colon, rectum, and anal canal. The cecum, located on the right side of the abdomen, is a small pouch-like structure. The appendix is a blind tube of lymphoid tissue attached to the cecum. The colon has four sections—ascending, transverse, descending, and sigmoid. The area immediately after the sigmoid colon is the rectum, which is followed by the anal canal. The anal canal has two sphincters—the internal and the external.

The contents from the small intestine enter the cecum through the ileocecal valve. **Peristalsis,** wave-like muscular contractions and squeezing of the intestines, moves the contents through the small and large intestines. The movement of fecal material into the rectum triggers defecation. The distended rectum activates the defecation reflex, causing a relaxation of both the internal and external anal sphincters. As peristaltic action increases, the diaphragm lowers and the abdominal muscles contract, forcing the feces out of the body though the anus. Defecation is controlled in the healthy person by maintaining a contracted external anal sphincter. The normally brown color of fecal material is caused by the breakdown of bilirubin. The normal content of fecal matter includes dead bacteria, fat, inorganic matter, protein, dried digestive juices, and indigestible components of food.

Large amounts of mucus are secreted by goblet cells in the epithelial layer of the large intestine. This mucus protects the epithelial surface from abrasive fecal material and aids in holding the fecal material together. Certain bacteria normally present in the large intestine produce some vitamins needed in the body, including vitamin K, vitamin B_{12}, riboflavin, and thiamine. The bacteria produce gases that contribute to the formation of flatus.

During the movement of stomach contents through the large intestine, water and some electrolytes are reabsorbed. Absorption of fluid and electrolytes occurs primarily in the proximal colon. The longer the contents remain in the large intestine, the greater the amount of water that is reabsorbed (Fig. 38-1).

PATHOPHYSIOLOGY

FLATUS

Flatus is a normal byproduct of digestion. Flatus becomes problematic, causing discomfort or pain from excessive production (ingestion of gas-producing foods) or from an inability to pass it through the large intestine (disruption of peristalsis, such as occurs temporarily after surgery).

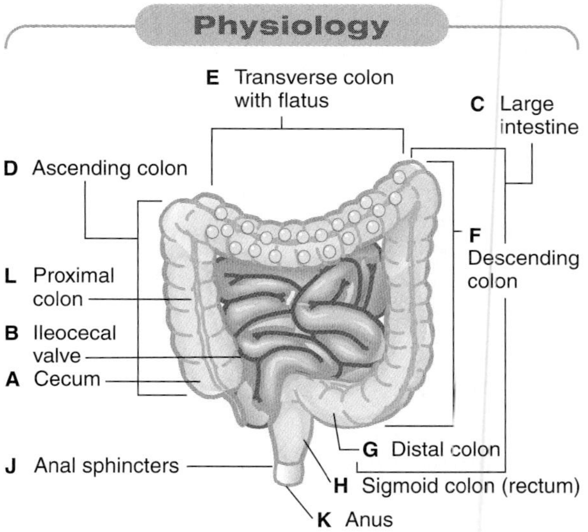

Figure 38-1. Moving through the lower gastrointestinal tract. Once the contents of the small intestine enter the cecum (**A**) through the ileocecal valve (**B**), they are transported through the large intestine (**C**) by peristalsis (wave-like propulsion of gastric contents). The three segments of the large intestine are termed the ascending colon (**D**), the transverse colon (**E**), and the descending colon (**F**). When the contents leave the distal colon (**G**) and enter the sigmoid colon (**H**) (rectum), the distended rectum activates the defecation reflex, which causes the internal and external anal sphincters (**J**) to relax. As peristaltic activity increases, the diaphragm lowers and the abdominal muscles contract, forcing the feces out of the body through the anus (**K**). Certain bacteria normally present in the intestine produce gases that are commonly known as flatus. Absorption of fluid and electrolytes occurs primarily in the proximal colon (**L**), although some absorption occurs throughout the length of the large intestine. The longer the contents remain in the large intestine, the more water is absorbed.

DIARRHEA

When peristalsis occurs too rapidly and stomach contents move more quickly than normal through the large intestine, diarrhea results. **Diarrhea** occurs when frequency of stools increases and the content of the stools is loose and watery. Normal absorption of nutrients cannot occur with diarrhea.

The causes of diarrhea may include malabsorption syndrome, bacterial or viral infections, irritable bowel syndrome, ulcerative colitis, lactose intolerance, cancer, and laxative abuse. The cause of the diarrhea should be determined before instituting treatment. If the cause is an infection, drug therapy may not be recommended.

Diarrhea may be acute or chronic. Acute diarrhea is most often the result of bacterial infection, food poisoning, viral infection, or drug toxicity. It is usually self-limiting and responds to treatment within 48 hours. Chronic diarrhea is most often secondary to a disease process, such as irritable colon, ulcerative colitis, diverticulitis, or cancer, or secondary to removal of some of the bowel through surgery. Treatment of the disease usually eliminates the diarrhea. When diarrhea becomes chronic, antidiarrheal drug therapy may be needed for an extended time.

CONSTIPATION AND FECAL IMPACTION

Constipation is infrequent or incomplete passage of hard stools that results from a decrease in peristaltic activity and slow movement of fecal material through the colon. This slow movement through the colon allows more water to be absorbed from the feces, resulting in hard, dry stools. The hard, dry fecal material is more difficult to pass and can cause painful defecation. Prolonged constipation may lead to **fecal impaction,** in which the patient is unable to pass the hardened mass of feces. The many causes of constipation include:

- Inadequate fiber in the diet
- Not defecating when the urge is felt
- Inactivity
- Decreased fluid intake
- Irritable bowel syndrome
- Weakened abdominal muscles due to aging or disease
- Inability to perform the Valsalva maneuver effectively
- Hemorrhoids
- Cancer
- Hypothyroidism
- Adverse effects from drug therapy

Patients' definitions of constipation reflect what their normal patterns are. This may or may not reflect the actual slowed movement through the colon with resultant dry, hard stools.

IRRITABLE BOWEL SYNDROME

Irritable bowel syndrome (IBS) is a common disorder of the intestines. It affects an estimated one in five adult Americans and three times as many women as men. IBS is the most common GI diagnosis among gastroenterology practices in the United States. IBS is a problem with colonic motility with no known cause. It is called a functional disorder because when the colon is examined there is no evidence of disease. IBS does not lead to any serious, organic diseases. IBS has not been linked to inflammatory bowel diseases such as Crohn disease or ulcerative colitis. Neither does IBS cause cancer of the bowel.

In IBS, the bowel is hypersensitive and overreacts to mild stimulation by going into spasms. The normal distention of the bowel that can occur with food intake, gas, or a high-fiber diet can be enough to trigger IBS. Thus, IBS patients exhibit pain and discomfort at lower volumes of gastric distention than occurs in patients who do not have IBS. The symptoms of IBS are painful diarrhea or constipation, or diarrhea that alternates with constipation. Other symptoms are crampy abdominal pain, bloating, gas pain, excessive flatulence, increased belching, mucus in the stool, small stools ("rabbit-like pellets"), or flat, "ribbon" stools. Bleeding, fever, weight loss, and persistent severe pain are NOT symptoms of IBS and may indicate other problems.

The symptoms of spastic contractions may be triggered by stress because the bowel is controlled partly by the nervous system. IBS, however, is *not* related to a personality disorder; it is a disorder of digestion. Stress management or stress-reduction instruction may help relieve some of the symptoms or make them less severe. Diet also can trigger flares of IBS. An increase in peristalsis is normal after eating. For people with IBS, strong contractions of the colon may come sooner after eating than usual, accompanied with cramps and diarrhea. Because fat is a strong stimulus for colonic contractions, eating a high-fat meal will bring on contractions that may be stronger or more violent. Large meals also can cause cramping and diarrhea in people with IBS. Finally, women with IBS have more symptoms when they have their menstrual period. It is hypothesized that female sex hormones increase the susceptibility of the colon to spasm. To some patients, IBS may be a mild annoyance; to others it may be disabling, affecting their ability to work, socialize, or travel (see the accompanying display, Irritable Bowel Syndrome and Quality of Life).

INFLAMMATORY BOWEL DISEASE

Inflammatory bowel disease (IBD) is a general term that includes both ulcerative colitis and Crohn disease. IBD has no known cause but inflammation of the large or small intestine is present. **Ulcerative colitis** is an inflammatory disease of the large intestine. Ulcers form in the mucosa of the colon or rectum. Diarrhea, blood, and pus may result. **Crohn disease** is an inflammation extending into the deeper layers of the intestinal wall. It is most often found in the ileum and the first part of the large intestine (cecum). Crohn disease can develop, however, anywhere along the entire GI tract. It may cause ulcers along the entire colon, form a string of ulcers in one part of the colon, or cause multiple scattered clusters of ulcers in the colon. The main symptom of IBD is diarrhea, which may, especially in ulcerative colitis, contain blood. Constipation also may develop during active flare-ups. Cramps and intestinal pain may occur. Fever, fatigue, loss of appetite, and weight loss also may occur.

Focus on Research

Irritable bowel syndrome (IBS) and quality of life

Luscombe, F. A. (2000). Health-related quality of life and associated psychosocial factors in irritable bowel syndrome: a review. *Quality of Life Research, 9*(2), 161–176.

The Study

A review of the literature on characteristics of IBS and associated health-related quality of life was performed. The literature shows significantly lower scores on both the physical and mental health scales for those with IBS symptoms compared with both asymptomatic controls and the established United States norms. IBS symptoms were found to affect general health, vitality, social functioning, bodily pain, diet, sexual function, and sleep negatively. IBS symptoms also were related to time lost from work. Impairment of health-related quality of life and concomitant psychosocial problems appear to correlate with the decision to seek medical care for IBS.

Nursing Implications

The symptoms of IBS have a negative impact on a person's life. People often do not seek help for symptoms of IBS until this negative impact is significant. Because this is a common disorder, nurses should be aware of the impact that IBS has on patients. When interviewing and assessing patients initially, nurses should ask whether the patient has any IBS symptoms. If these symptoms are present, the patient should be encouraged to seek medical help for these problems. Hope should be offered; explain that drug therapy may be helpful. Additionally, when working with patients diagnosed with IBS, the nurse should assess the impact of the disease on the individual patient. The nurse needs to offer appropriate emotional support. Teaching may be very helpful in providing the patient with some strategies to minimize and deal with the symptoms of IBS.

Approximately 1 to 2 million Americans suffer from IBD (the wide variation is due to the difficulty of diagnosing IBD, and because people may have long remissions and not be identified). Male and female sufferers seem to be affected equally. IBD most often is diagnosed between 15 and 40 years of age. Jewish Americans of European descent have a risk of IBD that is five times that of the general population. IBD is more common among city dwellers than country dwellers and is more prevalent in developed countries.

Although the exact cause is not known, it is known that genetic factors have a role. Up to 25% of people with IBD have family members with the disease. Genetic abnormalities for the two disorders may share locations on chromosomes 1, 3, 4, 7, 12, and 16. Some researchers believe that the disease develops in people who have a genetic susceptibility that allows an agent, such as a virus or bacterium, to trigger an abnormal immune response. In a normal, healthy person, when an organism injures the lining of the intestine, the immune system reduces the inflammation and injury by producing suppressor T cells. In people with IBD, however, when an organism injures the lining of the intestine, the immune system produces helper T cells. Helper T cells produce a protein called a cytokine. Cytokines cause intestinal inflammation and damage, which attract even more helper T cells to the area. Because IBD is more prevalent in industrialized countries, it has been hypothesized that environmental factors, such as diet, also play a role in producing IBD. No clear insight into this is yet available from research.

ANTIFLATULENTS

Antiflatulents decrease gas production, coalesce gas bubbles, and facilitate the passage of gas through belching and expelling flatus. Antiflatulents include simethicone and charcoal. The prototype antiflatulent is simethicone (Mylicon). It is available alone or in combination with antacids and digestants (see Chapter 37).

NURSING MANAGEMENT OF THE PATIENT RECEIVING SIMETHICONE

Core Drug Knowledge

Pharmacotherapeutics

Antiflatulents are drugs used to relieve the discomfort of excess gas in the GI tract caused by swallowing air, postoperative gas distention, peptic ulcer, spastic or irritable colon, or diverticulitis. These drugs relieve pain and discomfort by promoting belching and the passing of flatus (Table 38-1).

Pharmacokinetics

Simethicone is inert and is not absorbed from the GI tract. Because the drug is inactive, it is excreted unchanged in feces and does not interfere with absorption of water or nutrients or secretion of mucus in the GI tract. Simethicone is not distributed systemically in the body and is excreted unchanged in the feces. Simethicone begins to act immediately in the GI tract and has a duration of approximately 3 hours. Its peak and half-life are unknown.

Pharmacodynamics

Simethicone has a defoaming action that alters the surface tension of gas bubbles. As the surface tension is changed, gas bubbles unite, forming larger gas bubbles that are eliminated more easily by belching or expelled as flatus. It also is used in combination with antacids to decrease flatulence but has no antacid properties. An unlabeled use is treating the symptoms of infant colic.

Contraindications and Precautions

Simethicone has no contraindications or precautions.

Adverse Effects

No significant adverse reactions have been reported with the use of simethicone.

Drug Interactions

No drug interactions with simethicone are known.

TABLE 38-1 Summary of Selected Antiflatulent and Antidiarrheal Drugs

Drug (Trade) Name	Selected Indications	Route and Dosage Range	Pharmacokinetics
Antiflatulents			
simethicone (Mylanta Gas, Gas Relief, Gas-X, Major-Con, Phazyme, Flatulex, Mylicon)	Relief of symptoms and pressure from excess gas in the intestinal tract	*Adult:* PO, 125-mg capsules qid with meals; 40–125-mg tablets qid with meals; 40–80-mg drops qid up to 500 mg/d *Child:* PO, <2 y, 20 mg qid up to 240 mg/d; 2–12 y, 40 mg qid	*Onset:* Not absorbed systemically *Duration:* None $t_{1/2}$: None
Antidiarrheals			
diphenoxylate HCl with atropine sulfate (Lomotil, Logen, Lonox, Lomanate)	Diarrhea	*Adult:* PO, 5 mg qid *Child:* 0.3–0.4 mg/kg/d in 4 doses	*Onset:* Unknown *Duration:* Unknown $t_{1/2}$: 12–14 h
loperamide (Imodium, Kaopectate II Caplets, Pepto Diarrhea Control)	By prescription: control of acute nonspecific diarrhea or chronic diarrhea associated with inflammatory bowel disease	*Adult:* acute: PO, 4 mg initially, then 2 mg after each loose stool, not to exceed 16 mg/d; chronic, 4 mg initially, then 2 mg after each loose stool until diarrhea controlled *Child* (acute): PO, first day, 13–20 kg weight, 1 mg tid; 20–30 kg weight, 2 mg bid; >30 kg weight, 2 mg tid; after first day, 1 mg/10 kg after loose stools (not to exceed first day recommended doses); chronic, not established	*Onset:* Unknown *Duration:* Unknown $t_{1/2}$: 9.1–14.4 h
	OTC: traveler's diarrhea (acute diarrhea)	*Adult:* PO, 4 mg initially, then 2 mg after each loose stool, no more than 8 mg/d for no more than 2 d *Child* (9–11 y): PO, 2 mg initially then 1 mg after each loose stool up to 6 mg/d for no more than 2 d; (6–8 y): 1 mg initially and after each loose stool up to 4 mg/d for up to 2 d	
bismuth subsalicylate (Pepto-Bismol, Bismatrol, Pink Bismuth)	Indigestion, nausea, diarrhea (including traveler's diarrhea), abdominal cramps	*Adult:* PO, 2 tablets or 30 mL every 30 min to 1 h as needed, up to 8 doses in 24 h *Child* 9–12 y: PO, 1 tablet or 15 mL; 6–9 y: 2/3 tablet or 10 mL; 3–6 y: 1/3 tablet or 5 mL, same dosing schedule as adults	*Onset:* Bismuth, unknown; salicylate, rapid *Duration:* Bismuth, unknown; salicylate, 3–6 h $t_{1/2}$: Bismuth, unknown; salicylate, 2–3 h

Assessment of Relevant Core Patient Variables

Health Status

Before administering simethicone, the nurse will assess for abdominal pain, distention, and bowel sounds.

Lifestyle, Diet, and Habits

The nurse will assess the patient's dietary choices for gas-producing foods such as cucumbers, cabbage, onions, beans, and radishes.

Environment

The nurse should note the setting in which simethicone will be administered. Simethicone is easily self-administered and can be given in any setting. Some preparations are available OTC.

Nursing Diagnosis and Outcome

- Acute Pain related to the presence of flatus

  Desired outcome: Within 2 to 3 hours of using simethicone, the patient will experience a decrease in abdominal pain and distention.

Planning and Intervention

Maximizing Therapeutic Effects

It is important to administer simethicone after meals and at bedtime to increase its effectiveness. The nurse also should have the patient chew tablets thoroughly or allow them to dissolve in the mouth to promote dispersion. It is important to shake the suspension form of the drug to ensure active ingredients are dispersed throughout.

The nurse should use, or teach the patient to use, a calibrated dropper to administer liquid forms. This will ensure accuracy of the dosage. It is important to mix simethicone with 30 mL of a suitable liquid, preferably formula or cool water, when administering to infants.

Providing Patient and Family Education

- The nurse teaches the patient to take simethicone after each meal and at bedtime; to chew tablets thoroughly before swallowing; or to shake the liquid suspension form well before measuring a dose.
- The nurse should tell the patient to expect to pass gas and have increased belching after taking this drug.
- It is important to caution the patient not to increase the dosage unless instructed to do so by a health care provider.
- The nurse instructs the patient to avoid gas-producing foods. A high-fiber diet will increase peristalsis, and a low-fat diet will decrease production of carbon dioxide gas.

Ongoing Assessment and Evaluation

The nurse will assess abdominal pain and distention periodically throughout therapy to monitor the effectiveness of the drug. Simethicone is effective if abdominal distention is decreased and the patient reports feeling more comfortable. If effectiveness is not observed, the dose may need to be increased. Verify that the patient does not have any increase in abdominal pain, nausea, vomiting, or fever, because these findings are not symptoms of excessive flatus and may indicate that the patient requires medical attention. ■

DRUG CLOSELY RELATED TO P SIMETHICONE

Charcoal is an absorbing, detoxicating, and soothing agent. The drug relieves gas and cramping by absorbing toxins and gas on the surface of carbon particles. Like simethicone, it is useful for the relief of gas, diarrhea, and GI distress associated with indigestion and cramping.

Unlike simethicone, it is used as an antidote in poisonings from drug overdose because it reduces the absorption of certain drugs and chemicals and can actually remove them from the systemic circulation. Charcoal also is used for preventing nonspecific pruritus associated with kidney dialysis. Charcoal should not be given to children younger than 3 years of age. Charcoal can be combined with simethicone to treat gas pains; the charcoal decreases the amount of gas produced, and the simethicone promotes the elimination of gas.

> **MEMORY CHIP**
>
> **P Simethicone**
>
> - Relieves the pain of excess gas in the GI tract; antifoaming action changes surface tension of gas bubbles, causing them to coalesce and pass more easily
> - Most significant patient education: chew tablets to promote effectiveness; take after meals and at bedtime

C ANTIDIARRHEALS

Antidiarrheals slow intestinal motility, allowing time for fluid reabsorption and formation of a more formed stool. The most effective antidiarrheal drugs include opiate derivatives, the opiates themselves, and loperamide, a drug related to the antipsychotic haloperidol. These drugs act systemically to reduce intestinal motility and slow peristalsis. Several locally acting drugs are available OTC and are effective in mild cases of diarrhea.

The drugs discussed in the following sections include diphenoxylate HCl, difenoxin, loperamide, and locally acting agents, bismuth subsalicylate, kaolin, and pectin. The prototype antidiarrheal drug is diphenoxylate HCl with atropine sulfate.

NURSING MANAGEMENT OF THE PATIENT RECEIVING P DIPHENOXYLATE HCL WITH ATROPINE SULFATE

Core Drug Knowledge

Pharmacotherapeutics

Diphenoxylate HCl with atropine sulfate (Lomotil, Lomanate, Lonox, Logen) is used as an adjunct in treating diarrhea (see Table 38-1).

Pharmacokinetics

Diphenoxylate HCl with atropine sulfate is absorbed readily in the GI tract. When the tablet form is used instead of solution, the bioavailability is decreased by approximately 10%. Diphenoxylate HCl with atropine sulfate is found in breast milk; however, the distribution is unknown. The drug is metabolized in the liver to difenoxin, which is an active metabolite that produces the desired therapeutic effects. It leaves the liver as bile and is excreted in feces. A tiny amount is excreted unchanged in the urine.

Pharmacodynamics

This drug is a synthetic narcotic similar in structure to meperidine. The dosage used in treating diarrhea is not high enough to provide pain relief. The drug acts on the smooth muscle of the intestine to slow intestinal motility and prolong intestinal transit time, allowing for the reabsorption of fluid. A small amount of atropine sulfate is combined with diphenoxylate to discourage deliberate abuse. When excessive dosages are taken, the adverse reactions of atropine sulfate are particularly unpleasant. This preparation is very effective in treating diarrhea.

Contraindications and Precautions

Hypersensitivity to the drug or to atropine sulfate is a contraindication. Treatment with diphenoxylate HCl with atropine sulfate is contraindicated for diarrhea caused by GI organisms that penetrate the gastric mucosa (e.g., *Shigella, Salmonella,* and some toxic strains of *Escherichia coli*) because the drug slows peristalsis and may aggravate and prolong the diarrhea. The drug is contraindicated in patients with pseudomembranous colitis that occurs with broad-spectrum antibiotic therapy because it may worsen and prolong diarrhea. It also is contraindicated in patients with obstructed jaundice due to hepatic impairment. Diphenoxylate HCl with atropine sulfate is contraindicated in children younger than 2 years of age. The drug is a pregnancy category C drug.

Caution is used when administering the drug to patients with advanced hepatic and renal disease due to risk of hepatic coma; ulcerative colitis due to risk of inducing toxic megacolon; and severe dehydration, because it may cause variability of drug response and may predispose the patient to delayed diphenoxylate intoxication. Caution should be used in lactating women and in children because adverse effects from the atropine sulfate are more likely. Children with Down syndrome are at special risk for atropine sulfate toxicity when taking diphenoxylate, even when the drug is taken in recommended doses. Although diphenoxylate HCl with atropine sulfate in recommended dosages does not produce morphine-like effects or addiction, in high doses, addiction can occur.

Adverse Effects

The most common adverse effects of diphenoxylate HCl with atropine sulfate are drowsiness and dizziness related to the drug's having a chemical structure similar to meperidine, an opioid. Dry mouth and other anticholinergic effects (e.g., flushing, tachycardia, hyperthermia, and urinary retention) from the atropine in the drug are not common in adults receiving normal, therapeutic doses of diphenoxylate HCl. There is greater risk that children will experience these adverse effects. Diphenoxylate HCl with atropine sulfate also may have the following adverse effects:

- GI: nausea, vomiting, abdominal discomfort, paralytic ileus, toxic megacolon, and pancreatitis
- Central nervous system (CNS): sedation, headache, malaise, lethargy, restlessness, euphoria, depression, and numbness of extremities
- Allergic: pruritus, swelling of gums, angioneurotic edema, urticaria, and anaphylaxis

Drug Interactions

When diphenoxylate HCl with atropine sulfate is given to patients taking monoamine oxidase inhibitors (MAOIs), the combination of the two drugs could precipitate a hypertensive crisis because diphenoxylate is similar chemically to meperidine. Diphenoxylate HCl with atropine sulfate may potentiate the depressive effects of alcohol, barbiturates, and tranquilizers (Table 38-2).

Assessment of Relevant Core Patient Variables

Health Status

Before administering diphenoxylate HCl with atropine sulfate, the nurse will assess the patient for abdominal pain and distention to have a baseline for monitoring therapy. The nurse will auscultate bowel sounds. Patients with diarrhea will usually have frequent high-pitched bowel sounds. The nurse will then determine whether the patient has a diagnosis of hepatic impairment, obstructive jaundice, pseudomembranous colitis, or ulcerative colitis. Pertinent information about stools includes frequency, color, consistency, and odor; these will be assessed and documented by the nurse. The nurse will examine laboratory reports of stool specimens and will not administer diphenoxylate HCl with atropine sulfate if stool cultures are positive for *E. coli, Salmonella, Shigella,* or *Clostridium difficile.* During drug history, the nurse will determine whether the patient is receiving MAOIs and check the condition of

TABLE 38-2 Agents That Interact With Diphenoxylate HCl With Atropine Sulfate

Interactants	Effect and Significance	Nursing Management
monoamine oxidase inhibitors	Chemical structure of diphenoxylate similar to meperidine—hypertensive crisis possible	Administer together cautiously. Monitor BP while on both drugs.
barbiturates, tranquilizers, and alcohol	Depressant effect on central nervous system may be potentiated, leading to respiratory depression or sedation	Closely observe patient when patient is receiving both drugs. Monitor level of consciousness and respirations.

mucous membranes and the skin for signs of dehydration. If the patient is a child, the nurse will observe for Down syndrome.

Life Span and Gender

The nurse will determine whether the patient is pregnant or breast-feeding, and if the patient is a child, the nurse will verify that he or she is older than 2 years of age.

Lifestyle, Diet, and Habits

The nurse will determine whether the patient has a history of substance abuse because this may make the patient more likely to use diphenoxylate HCl with atropine sulfate inappropriately.

Environment

The nurse should be aware of the setting in which diphenoxylate HCl with atropine sulfate will be administered. Although diphenoxylate HCl with atropine sulfate requires a prescription, oral doses are easily self-administered and can be given in any setting.

Culture

Cultural and social variations exist as to how frequently bowel movements should occur to be considered regular and when diarrhea has occurred. The nurse should determine the patient's perception of normal elimination and diarrhea.

Nursing Diagnoses and Outcomes

- Diarrhea related to the causative factor (if identified)
  Desired outcome: Diarrhea will be controlled through use of diphenoxylate HCl with atropine sulfate.
- Risk for Injury related to drowsiness and dizziness secondary to drug therapy
  Desired outcome: The patient will not sustain injury from drug therapy.

Planning and Intervention

Maximizing Therapeutic Effects

To maximize the therapeutic effect, the nurse should administer diphenoxylate HCl with atropine sulfate as ordered, four times daily to obtain therapeutic results. The nurse also should use the dropper provided when administering liquid preparations to administer the correct dose.

Minimizing Adverse Effects

The nurse should decrease the dosage of diphenoxylate HCl with atropine sulfate when the number of stools decreases. The recommended dosage should not be exceeded. If the patient's condition does not improve with the maximum daily dose for 10 days, diarrhea symptoms are unlikely to be controlled by further use of this drug. In such cases, the nurse should assess for adverse effects. The nurse should assess for toxic megacolon (abdominal distention and pain are possible indications). The massive dilation and atony of the colon from toxic megacolon can result in serious complications. It is important to report signs of abdominal distention immediately.

The nurse also should assess for and report signs of atropine sulfate toxicity (i.e., dry mouth, flushing, hypothermia, tachycardia, and urinary retention) because this condition requires immediate treatment. It is important to assess children very carefully because they are especially susceptible.

Providing Patient and Family Education

- The nurse teaches the patient not to exceed the prescribed dosage, and to lower the dosage as instructed as soon as symptoms of diarrhea are controlled. Furthermore, if a dose is missed, the patient should not take two doses.
- The nurse should instruct the patient to notify the primary care provider if diarrhea persists longer than 10 days.
- The nurse should encourage the patient to avoid alcohol and other CNS depressants, and not to drive or perform tasks that require mental alertness until the effects of diphenoxylate HCl with atropine sulfate are known.
- It is important to caution the patient to maintain adequate fluid intake during periods of diarrhea to prevent dehydration and electrolyte imbalance.
- The nurse should caution the patient to store diphenoxylate HCl with atropine sulfate out of the reach of children.
- For liquid forms of diphenoxylate HCl with atropine sulfate, it is important to tell the patient not to use a household teaspoon to measure doses but rather a specially marked dropper or measuring spoon.
- If dry mouth occurs, the nurse recommends that the patient suck on hard candy or sip water.

Ongoing Assessment and Evaluation

It is important to assess skin turgor and mucous membranes for loss of moisture because these signs indicate dehydration. Monitoring electrolyte laboratory reports for electrolyte imbalance that may occur with the loss of fluid through diarrhea is a priority. Weakness, muscular cramping, or dizziness should be reported because these are subjective symptoms of electrolyte imbalance. Any change in amount, color, consistency, or odor of stools should be noted. Drug therapy is effective when diarrhea is controlled without any adverse effects occurring (see the accompanying display, Diphenoxylate in Antidiarrheal Therapy). ■

DRUGS CLOSELY RELATED TO P DIPHENOXYLATE HCL WITH ATROPINE SULFATE

Difenoxin (Motofen) is the principal active metabolite of diphenoxylate and is effective at one fifth the dose of diphenoxylate. It is metabolized to an inactive form. Loperamide (Imodium) is chemically similar to haloperidol, an antipsychotic drug. Unlike diphenoxylate, loperamide may be used for chronic and acute diarrhea. Loperamide comes in prescription and OTC strengths. Because loperamide does not contain the anticholinergic drug atropine sulfate, the contraindications and adverse reactions related to atropine sulfate are not applicable. It may be better tolerated for this reason.

DRUGS SIGNIFICANTLY DIFFERENT FROM P DIPHENOXYLATE HCL WITH ATROPINE SULFATE

Bismuth Subsalicylate

Bismuth subsalicylate (Pepto-Bismol, Bismatrol, Pink Bismuth), a locally acting antidiarrheal, is available without a prescription and is used widely as an antidiarrheal agent. The subsalicylate component of this drug seems to have an antisecretory effect, whereas the bismuth component has a direct antimicrobial effect against bacteria and viral pathogens in the GI tract. Bismuth subsalicylate is used to treat diarrhea, indigestion, nausea, and abdominal cramps. Unlabeled uses include treatment of chronic infantile diarrhea and symptoms of Norwalk virus–induced gastroenteritis and prevention of traveler's diarrhea. Bismuth subsalicylate is not given to children or adolescents with viral diseases because of the possibility of Reye syndrome's developing from its salicylate component.

Critical Thinking Scenario

Diphenoxylate in antidiarrheal therapy

Mr. Rothberg is 46 years old. He enters the emergency clinic with complaints of acute diarrhea for the last 36 hours. He also complains of abdominal pain and cramping. "Every time I eat," he says, "I have to run to the bathroom. I can't seem to keep anything in."

1. What questions you would ask when assessing Mr. Rothberg's condition?
2. After assessment is completed, Mr. Rothberg is diagnosed as having diarrhea secondary to an acute viral illness of the GI tract. He is given a prescription for diphenoxylate HCl with atropine sulfate. What additional core patient variables need to be assessed to provide patient education geared to Mr. Rothberg's personal learning needs?

MEMORY CHIP

P Diphenoxylate HCL With Atropine Sulfate

- Used to treat diarrhea not responsive to symptomatic and supportive treatment
- This drug is related chemically to meperidine, an opioid, but lacks any analgesic effect. Atropine is added to discourage abuse.
- Significant contraindications: diarrhea associated with organisms that penetrate intestinal mucosa; pseudomembranous enterocolitis
- Most common adverse effects: drowsiness, dizziness, and dry mouth
- Most serious adverse effects: atropine overdose and toxic megacolon
- **Life span alert: children are more likely to have adverse effects from atropine, especially if they have Down syndrome; variable response in children; avoid use if patient is <2 years old**
- Minimizing adverse effects: decrease the dose when diarrhea becomes less frequent; monitor for signs of atropine overdose (in children) and toxic megacolon
- Most significant patient education: do not exceed the prescribed dose

Kaolin and Pectin

Kaolin and pectin (Kaopectate) are locally acting antidiarrheals frequently used in combination. These drugs are used widely to treat mild diarrhea, even though clinical studies have not firmly established their effectiveness. Kaolin and pectin are different from the prototype, diphenoxylate. These drugs act as adsorbents; that is toxins, bacteria, and other irritants in the GI tract bind to their surfaces. Commercial products usually contain two or more adsorbents. For example, Kaopectate is a combination of kaolin and pectin. The adsorptive action is not selective and therefore can interfere with normal GI absorption, particularly absorption of other drugs.

C LAXATIVES

Drugs used to treat constipation are referred to as laxatives. Laxatives are drugs that act directly on the intestine to promote peristalsis and evacuation of the bowel. Laxatives are classified as saline, hyperosmotics, stimulants, bulk forming, stool softeners (surfactants), and lubricants.

C SALINE LAXATIVES

Saline laxatives include magnesium hydroxide, magnesium sulfate, magnesium citrate, and sodium phosphate. The prototype saline laxative is magnesium hydroxide.

NURSING MANAGEMENT OF THE PATIENT RECEIVING MAGNESIUM HYDROXIDE

Core Drug Knowledge

Pharmacotherapeutics

Magnesium hydroxide is used for acute or chronic constipation, preoperatively to prepare the bowel for surgery, and before or after radiologic and other diagnostic studies to clear the lower bowel tract (Table 38-3). Magnesium hydroxide also is used as an antacid (see Chapter 37).

Pharmacokinetics

Magnesium hydroxide has a local effect in the lower GI tract and is absorbed poorly. Approximately 15% to 30% of the magnesium in magnesium hydroxide is absorbed in the small intestine. Onset of action is 30 minutes to 3 hours after administration. A bowel movement usually occurs within 6 hours of administration. Excretion occurs in the kidneys and GI tract.

TABLE 38-3 Summary of Selected Laxatives

Drug (Trade) Name	Selected Indications	Route and Dosage Range	Pharmacokinetics
Saline Laxatives			
magnesium hydroxide (Milk of Magnesia)	Constipation, preparation for diagnostic tests of lower GI tract, post-GI diagnostic tests	*Adult:* PO, 30–60 mL/d; 15–30 mL/d (if concentrated) *Child:* 2–5 y, PO, up to 30 mL depending on age	*Onset:* 0.5–3 h *Duration:* Unknown $t_{1/2}$: None
magnesium sulfate (epsom salts)	Same as above	*Adult:* PO, 10–15 g in glass of water *Child:* PO, 5–10 g in glass of water	*Onset:* 0.5–3 h *Duration:* Unknown $t_{1/2}$: None
magnesium citrate (Citrate of Magnesia, Citro-Nesia)	Same as above	*Adult:* PO, 240 mL *Child:* PO, 120 mL	*Onset:* 0.5–3 h *Duration:* Unknown $t_{1/2}$: None
sodium phosphate (Phospho-Soda, sodium phosphates)	Same as above	*Adult:* PO, 20–30 mL mixed in half glass cool water *Child:* PO, 5–15 mL mixed in half glass cool water	*Onset:* 0.5–3 h *Duration:* Unknown $t_{1/2}$: None
Hyperosmotic Laxatives			
polyethylene glycol-electrolyte solution (PEG-ES) (Colovage, CoLyte, Golytely, OCL)	Induce diarrhea to cleanse bowel tract before GI examination	*Adult:* PO, 240 mL every 10 min until 4 L consumed or effluent is clear; may be given through nasogastric tube 20–30 mL/min *Child:* 25–40 mL/kg/h for 4–10 h	*Onset:* 30–60 min *Duration:* About 4 h $t_{1/2}$: None
lactulose (Cephulac, Cholac, Chronulac, Constilac, Constulose, Duphalac, Enulose)	Constipation	*Adult:* PO, 15–30 mL/d up to 60 mL/d if needed *Child (infants):* PO, 2.5–10 mL in divided doses; older children and adolescents, 40–90 mL	*Onset:* 24–48 h *Duration:* Unknown $t_{1/2}$: None
	Prevention and treatment of portal-systemic encephalopathy, including hepatic precoma and coma	*Adult:* PO, 30–45 mL tid or qid; adjust dose every day or two to produce two or three soft but formed stools; may give hourly doses to induce rapid effect initially *Adult:* rectal, 300 mL in 700 mL water or normal saline solution, retain for 30–60 min; repeat every 4–6 h until patient is awake enough to take oral form	
glycerin (Sani-Supp, Fleet Babylex)	Constipation	*Adult and child:* Rectal, 1 suppository, retain 15 min (sized for adults and children)	*Onset:* 0.25–0.5 h *Duration:* Unknown $t_{1/2}$: None

TABLE 38-3 Summary of Selected Laxatives (Continued)

Drug (Trade) Name	Selected Indications	Route and Dosage Range	Pharmacokinetics
Stimulant Laxatives			
cascara sagrada (cascara sagrada fluid extract aromatic)	Constipation	*Adult:* PO, 325 mg tablet at bedtime or 5 mL *Child:* No recommended dosage	*Onset:* 6–10 h *Duration:* Unknown $t_{1/2}$: None
calcium salts of sennosides A and B (Ex-Lax Gentle Nature)	Same as above	*Adult:* PO, 20–40 mg with water at bedtime *Child:* PO, 6 y or older, 20 mg/d	*Onset:* 6–10 h *Duration:* Unknown $t_{1/2}$: None
senna (Senokot, Senexon, Senolax, Senna-Gen, Senokotxtra, Black Draught, Gentlax, Dr. Caldwell Senna Laxative, Fletcher's Castoria)	Same as above	*Adult:* PO, 187-mg tablets, 2 tablets up to eight times daily; 374-mg tablets, 1 tablet up to qid; 600-mg tablets, 2 tablets up to tid *Child:* PO, 6–12 y, 187-mg tablets, 1 tablet up to qid	*Onset:* 6–10 h *Duration:* Unknown $t_{1/2}$: None
castor oil (Fleet flavored Castor Oil, Purge, Emulsoil)	Same as above	*Adult:* PO, 15–60 mL, depending on the product *Child:* PO, 2–12 y, 5–15 mL, depending on product	*Onset:* 2–6 h *Duration:* Unknown $t_{1/2}$: None
bisacodyl (Dulcagen, Dulcolax, Fleet laxative, Bisco-Lax)	Same as above, pre- and postdiagnostic studies of lower GI tract	*Adult:* PO, 10–15 mg/d up to 30 mg/d prediagnostic study *Child:* PO, 6–12 y, 0.3 mg/kg/d *Adult:* Rectal, suppository form of 10 mg/d *Child:* 6–12 y, rectal, suppository form of 5 mg/d	*Onset:* 0.25–1 h *Duration:* Unknown $t_{1/2}$: None
Bulk-Forming Laxatives			
polycarbophil (Fibercon, Equalactin, Mitrolan, Fiber-Lax, Fiberall)	Constipation or diarrhea associated with conditions such as irritable bowel syndrome and diverticulitis; acute nonspecific diarrhea	*Adult:* PO, 1 g/d to qid not to exceed 6 g/d; severe diarrhea, repeat every 30 min not to exceed maximum dose *Child:* PO, 3–6 y, 500 mg/d to bid not to exceed 1.5 g/d	*Onset:* 12–24 h *Duration:* Unknown $t_{1/2}$: None
psyllium (Fiberall, Hydrocil Instant, Konsyl, Metamucil, natural vegetable powder, Reguloid, Serutan, Syllact, Konsyl-D, Modane Bulk, V-Lax)	Constipation, promotion of regularity	*Adult:* PO, 1 rounded teaspoon in 8 oz water one to three times daily	*Onset:* 12–24 h *Duration:* Unknown $t_{1/2}$: None
Stool Softener			
docusate sodium (Colace, Regutol, Disonate, DOK, DOS Softgel, D-S-S, Modane Soft, Pro=Sof, Regular SS, Dioeze, Surfak Liquigels, DC Softgels, Pro-Cal-Sof, Sulfalax Calcium, Diolose, Diocto-K, Kasof)	Softens stool to prevent constipation and straining in defecation	*Adult:* PO, 50–500 mg/d *Child:* PO, 6–12 y, 40–120 mg/d; 3–6 y, 20–60 mg/d; <3 y, 10–40 mg/d	*Onset:* 24–72 h *Duration:* Unknown $t_{1/2}$: None
Lubricant Laxative			
mineral oil (Neo-Cultol, Milkinol, Agoral Plain, Kondremul Plain)	Constipation	*Adult:* PO, 5–45 mL/d *Child:* PO, 5–20 mL/d	*Onset:* 6–8 h *Duration:* Unknown $t_{1/2}$: None

Pharmacodynamics

Magnesium hydroxide is a salt. It works in the small and large intestine by attracting and retaining water in the intestinal lumen, thereby increasing pressure within the intestine. The retention of fluid in the intestine results in stimulation of the stretch receptors and an increase in peristalsis, which promotes prompt evacuation of the bowel.

Contraindications and Precautions

Magnesium hydroxide should not be used if the patient has abdominal pain or any symptoms that are indicative of an acute abdomen (e.g., nausea, vomiting, or diarrhea). Magnesium salts must be used with caution in patients with renal failure because retention of magnesium could result in magnesium toxicity. Safe use in children younger than 2 years old has not been established. Large doses in pregnancy may lead to serious fluid and electrolyte imbalances.

Adverse Effects

Adverse effects can occur with large doses. Overactive bowel activity (i.e., cramps, diarrhea, or nausea) is the primary adverse effect. Fluid and electrolyte imbalance can occur with large doses given frequently.

Drug Interactions

Magnesium hydroxide decreases the effect of benzodiazepines, chloroquine, corticosteroids, digoxin, histamine-2 antagonists, hydantoins, iron salts, nitrofurantoin, penicillamine, phenothiazines, tetracyclines, and ticlopidine. Magnesium hydroxide increases the effect of dicumarol, quinidine, and sulfonylureas (Table 38-4).

Assessment of Relevant Core Patient Variables

Health Status

Assessment of the patient receiving magnesium salts involves obtaining a history to determine whether there is a history of renal insufficiency. Assessment before administration includes listening for bowel sounds, palpating for abdominal distention, and asking questions about the patient's usual pattern of bowel function. Be sure to determine whether the patient is receiving drug therapy that may interact with magnesium hydroxide.

Life Span and Gender

The nurse should determine the patient's age before administering magnesium hydroxide. The patient must be 2 years old or older to receive magnesium hydroxide. Older adults may have weakened abdominal muscles and decreased peristalsis due to aging. They also may engage in less regular activity and eat fewer foods containing roughage. All of these factors may contribute to constipation.

Lifestyle, Diet, and Habits

It is necessary to determine whether the patient's normal fluid intake is adequate (at least between 1,000 and 1,500 mL daily); whether the normal diet includes an adequate amount of fruits, vegetables, and roughage; and whether the patient engages in any regular physical

TABLE 38-4 Agents That Interact With P Magnesium Hydroxide

Interactants	Effect and Significance	Nursing Management
benzodiazepines	Decreased effect of benzodiazepines	Monitor for effect. When possible, give drugs 2 h apart.
chloroquine	Decreased effect of chloroquine	Same as above
corticosteroids	Decreased effect of corticosteroids	Same as above
dicumarol	Increased effect of dicumarol	Same as above
digoxin	Change in gastric pH, decreasing rate of absorption of digoxin, possibly resulting in decreased effect	Same as above
H_2 antagonists	Decreased effect of H_2 antagonists	Same as above
hydantoins	Decreased effect of hydantoins	Same as above
iron salts	Decreased effect of iron salts	Same as above
nitrofurantoin	Decreased effect of nitrofurantoin	Same as above
penicillamine	Decreased effect of penicillamine	Same as above
phenothiazines	Decreased effect of phenothiazines	Same as above
quinidine	Inhibition of excretion of quinidine, possibly leading to increased effect	Same as above
sulfonylureas	Increased effect of sulfonylurea	Same as above
tetracyclines	Binds to the surface of tetracycline, preventing absorption, decreasing effect	Same as above
ticlopidine	Decreases effect of ticlopidine	Same as above

activity. The nurse also will assess whether the patient must frequently ignore the urge to defecate because of lifestyle patterns. These variables can contribute to constipation. Whether the patient uses laxatives regularly also is important because chronic use of laxatives may lead to dependency on the laxative to expel a bowel movement.

Environment

The nurse should note the setting in which magnesium will be administered. Magnesium hydroxide is sold OTC and patients frequently self-medicate for constipation. The drug also is used in acute care settings before rectal and colonic examinations or diagnostic tests and preoperatively. Patients in an inpatient facility frequently are less active than when they are at home, which can contribute to constipation. Thus, magnesium hydroxide also may be used in a hospital setting to treat constipation.

Culture

Cultural and social variations exist as to how frequently bowel movements should occur for the individual to be considered regular or constipated. The nurse needs to ascertain what the patient means by normal elimination and constipation.

Nursing Diagnosis and Outcome

- Constipation related to dietary factors, fluid restrictions, decreased peristalsis, lack of activity, changes in activity, postoperative state, GI disease or malfunction, or adverse effects from other drug therapy.
  Desired outcome: The patient will have a bowel movement after taking magnesium hydroxide.

Planning and Intervention

Maximizing Therapeutic Effects

It is important to follow administration of magnesium hydroxide with a full glass of water to prevent dehydration and to promote a speedier effect.

Minimizing Adverse Effects

Use of magnesium hydroxide should be limited to short-term treatment of constipation to prevent fluid and electrolyte imbalance. The nurse should administer magnesium hydroxide with caution, if at all, in patients with renal disease. It is important to allow at least 2 hours between administration of drugs that are known to interact with magnesium hydroxide.

Providing Patient and Family Education

- The nurse should educate the patient that magnesium hydroxide should be used for short-term use only, and that long-term use may cause electrolyte imbalance and dependency on laxatives.
- The nurse should caution the patient not to take magnesium hydroxide within 2 hours of other interacting drugs.

Ongoing Assessment and Evaluation

The nurse should assess color, consistency, and amount of stool produced to monitor effectiveness of the drug (see the accompanying display, Educating Patients in the Community About Laxative Use). ■

DRUGS CLOSELY RELATED TO MAGNESIUM HYDROXIDE

Magnesium sulfate (Epsom salts), magnesium citrate (Citrate of Magnesia), sodium phosphate (Phospho-Soda) are all saline laxatives like magnesium hydroxide. Pharmacological actions are similar to magnesium hydroxide.

COMMUNITY-BASED CONCERNS

Educating Patients in the Community About Laxative Use

Individual misuse of OTC and prescription laxatives is encountered commonly by nurses practicing in the community. Nurses have a vital educational role to play in this area by providing teaching programs for individuals or groups. These programs may focus on general principles of elimination and bowel health so that patients learn to use laxatives responsibly and to avoid laxative abuse. A general teaching program may include the following features:

- Assessing elimination patterns. Teach patients how to assess their own usual habits and daily elimination routines to identify what is a "normal bowel movement" pattern for them.
- Defining normality. Show patients how to analyze their assessment findings and recognize patterns that are normal for the individual. Emphasize that what is normal for one person may not be normal for another.
- Eating to promote regularity. Identify dietary measures that promote peristalsis and regular bowel movement. Emphasize adequate fluid intake of 1,000 to 2,000 mL/d and fiber-rich foods, such as whole-grain breads, cereals, and vegetables, and fluids, such as pulpy fruit juices.
- Exercising to promote regularity. Assist patients to incorporate regular exercise into their daily activities. Explain how exercise promotes peristalsis and regular bowel movements.
- Dealing with altered elimination patterns. Teach patients to observe for changes in the normal pattern, form, and color of stools. Help them to decide when occasional use of laxatives, preferably bulk or stimulant types, may be appropriate and when medical attention may be advisable. Also point out the potential for dependence on laxatives and the disadvantages of dependence.

MEMORY CHIP

Magnesium Hydroxide

- Laxative for short-term use. Works by pulling water into the bowel by distending it and promoting peristalsis.
- Significant contraindications: signs of an acute abdomen and renal failure
- Most common adverse effect: overactive GI activity
- Most serious adverse effect: Fluid and electrolyte imbalance (large, frequent doses only)
- Maximizing therapeutic effects: follow administration with a glass of water
- Most significant patient education: magnesium hydroxide is not for long-term use

HYPEROSMOTIC LAXATIVES

The hyperosmotics act similarly to the saline laxative magnesium hydroxide. Drugs in this laxative subclass include lactulose (Cephulac, Cholac, Chronulac, Constilac, Constulose, Duphalac, Enulose), glycerin suppository (Sani-supp, Colace, Fleet Babylax), and polyethylene glycol-electrolyte solution (PEG-ES; GoLYTELY, CoLyte, NuLytely, OCL).

Like the saline laxative magnesium hydroxide, lactulose pulls water into the colon. Unlike magnesium hydroxide, lactulose is a synthetic disaccharide of lactose. In the colon, lactulose is metabolized by bacteria into acids and carbon dioxide. These products increase the oncotic pressure in the colon and draw water into the stool. The acids formed also draw ammonia into the stool. Lactulose is used, therefore, to treat constipation and decrease blood ammonia levels in hepatic coma and hepatic encephalopathy. Lactulose also can be given by enema.

Glycerin suppositories are inserted into the rectum. They pull moisture into the bowel and provide local irritation to stimulate a bowel movement. Glycerin suppositories are considered a rather gentle laxative.

Another drug that stimulates bowel evacuation by drawing water into the bowel is PEG-ES, a nonabsorbable solution with sodium sulfate and electrolytes. This combination prevents reabsorption of sodium and ion absorption or loss. PEG-ES induces diarrhea, usually within 4 hours. Unlike the saline laxative magnesium hydroxide, PEG-ES is not used to treat constipation but is used for bowel cleansing in preparation for GI examinations. PEG-ES is available by prescription.

STIMULANT AND IRRITANT LAXATIVES

The stimulant and irritant laxatives are similar to the saline laxative magnesium hydroxide. Stimulant laxatives include bisacodyl (Dulcolax, Fleet Laxative, Modane, Women's Gentle Laxative, Bisac- Evac, Caroid, Correctol, Feen-a-mint, and Reliable Gentle Laxative), cascara sagrada (Cascara Aromatic, Aromatic Cascara Fluidextract), sennosides (Senexon, Ex-lax, Senokot, Senna-Gen, SenokotXTRA), and castor oil (Purge, Emulsoil, and Neoloid). These drugs have a direct effect on the intestinal mucosa and stimulate peristalsis. They all alter water and electrolyte secretion. In addition, they all work in the colon, with the exception of castor oil, which works in the small intestine. Therapeutic uses are similar to the saline laxative magnesium hydroxide.

BULK-FORMING LAXATIVES

Polycarbophil (Fibercon, Equalactin, Mitrolan, Fiber-Norm, Konsyl Fiber, and Fiberall) and psyllium (Fiberall, Genfiber, Metamucil, Hydrocil Instant, Konsyl, Natural Fiber Laxative, Reguloid, Serutan, Syllact, Modane Bulk, and Perdiem Fiber Therapy) are bulk-forming agents. They work by keeping water in the stool, thus distending the colon mechanically and promoting a bowel movement. They work in the small and large intestines. Their onset of action, 12 to 24 hours normally but rarely up to 72 hours, is more prolonged than that of the saline laxative magnesium hydroxide. Some of these preparations contain sodium, and therefore, they must be used cautiously in patients for whom excess sodium can cause problems (e.g., patients with congestive heart failure or hypertension). Despite this, these agents are considered the safest and most physiologic of the laxatives. Psyllium also appears to be useful in reducing cholesterol levels as an adjunct therapy to dietary control. This is an unlabeled therapeutic use. Polycarbophil, in addition to its laxative use, also can be used for diarrhea because it absorbs free fecal water and produces formed stools.

STOOL SOFTENERS

Docusate is a stool softener (surfactant). It has detergent activity and facilitates the addition of fat and water into the stool to soften it. It does not stimulate peristalsis. It is used prophylactically to prevent constipation in patients who are at risk of developing constipation, such as elderly patients after orthopedic surgery or patients for whom straining at stool is contraindicated (e.g., after myocardial infarction, eye surgery, or anorectal surgery).

Docusate is available in two formulations, either as docusate sodium (Colace, D-S-S, Modane Soft, Regulax SS, Diocto, Ex-lax Stool Softener, Non Habit Forming Stool Softener, Stool Softener, Genasoft, Phillips Liqui-Gels, Docu, and Silace) or as docusate calcium (Surfak, DC Softgels).

LUBRICANT LAXATIVES

Mineral oil (Kondremul, Milkinol, NeoCultol) is an emollient or a lubricant. It coats the stool and thus retards the colonic absorption of fecal water. The stool is thus softened because it has more water in it. Mineral oil when given orally may decrease the absorption of fat-soluble vitamins. Mineral oil also is used as an enema in fecal impaction.

DRUGS USED TO TREAT IRRITABLE BOWEL SYNDROME

At this time, there are no drugs with the sole use of treating IBS approved by the FDA. However, antispasmodics may be used to help manage the symptoms of IBS. Dicyclomine

(Bentyl, Byclomine, Di-Spaz, Antispas, Or-Tyl) and hyoscyamine (Levsin, Anaspaz, ED-SPAZ, Donnamar, Gastrosed, Cytospaz-M, and Levsinez Timecaps) are two antispasmodics prescribed commonly for IBS (Table 38-5). Both of these drugs have a nonspecific direct relaxant effect on smooth muscle. Dicyclomine can be given orally or by IM injection. IM administration may cause local irritation and temporary lightheadedness. There have been reports of children 3 months old and younger experiencing respiratory distress, seizures, syncope, asphyxia, pulse rate fluctuation, muscular hypotonia, and coma within minutes of ingesting dicyclomine. These effects appear to be a result of local irritation or aspiration rather than a pharmacologic drug effect. Because of these possible problems, however, dicyclomine should not be used in infants younger than 6 months old. Hyoscyamine also has been used in infant colic. Hyoscyamine is available in oral forms and by SC, IM, or IV injection.

DRUGS USED TO TREAT INFLAMMATORY BOWEL DISEASE

Drug therapy cannot cure IBD but it is effective in reducing inflammation and IBD symptoms in up to 80% of patients. The drug groups used to treat IBD include the 5-aminosalicylic acid (5-ASA) preparations, corticosteroids, and drugs that suppress the immune system. Corticosteroids are discussed in Chapter 40, and drugs that suppress the immune system are discussed in Chapter 33.

5-ASA PREPARATIONS

The 5-ASA preparations include mesalamine, sulfasalazine, olsalazine, and balsalazide (see Table 38-5). Mesalamine is a 5-ASA; the other drugs are converted to 5-ASA (mesalamine) when they reach the colon. 5-ASA has a chemical structure similar to that of aspirin. Therefore, the 5-ASA preparations should not be used in people who have an allergy to aspirin.

Mesalamine (Asacol, Pentasa, Rowasa) is used in mild-to-moderate ulcerative colitis and Crohn disease and for preventing relapse of ulcerative colitis. The exact mechanism of action is not known but it is believed that mesalamine diminishes inflammation by blocking cyclooxygenase and inhibiting prostaglandin production in the colon. It appears to have a local effect rather than a systemic effect. About 28% of the drug is absorbed after oral dosing. Only what is not absorbed provides therapeutic action in the colon. Mesalamine is generally well tolerated and the adverse effects are mild and transient. The most common adverse effect was headache. Mesalamine is available in tablet, capsule, suppository, and rectal suspension formulations.

Sulfasalazine (Azulfidine) is used in treating ulcerative colitis; it also is used in treating rheumatoid arthritis. It is a combination of mesalamine (5-ASA) with sulfapyridine, a sulfa antibiotic that prevents mesalamine from being absorbed until it reaches the colon. In the colon, the intestinal bacteria break sulfasalazine into the two main components. The sulfapyridine plays no active role in the treatment of IBD. All of the therapeutic effects come from the mesalamine. Because of the sulfa component of sulfasalazine, it should not be used in people allergic to sulfa. The sulfa component accounts for most of the adverse and allergic reactions in up to 33% of the people who take the drug. These common adverse effects are heartburn, headache, loss of appetite, nausea, vomiting, and temporarily lower sperm count in men. Sulfasalazine also may turn the urine bright orange-yellow. Rare but serious adverse effects include a lupus-like disorder, pancreatitis, liver damage, and blood disorders (including aplastic anemia, leukopenia, and neutropenia), which may be life threatening.

TABLE 38-5 Summary of Selected Drugs to Treat Irritable Bowel Syndrome and Drugs to Treat Inflammatory Bowel Disease

Drug (Trade) Name	Selected Indications	Route and Dosage Range	Pharmacokinetics
dicyclomine (Bentyl, Byclomine, Di-Spray, Antispas, Or-Tyl)	IBS	80 mg/d PO or IM divided into 4 doses; may increase to 160 mg/d; give 30 min before a meal	*Onset:* 1–2 h *Duration:* up to 4 h $t_{1/2}$: Initial: 1.8 h Terminal: 9–10 h
mesalamine (Asacol, Pentason, Rowasa)	Ulcerative colitis	*Oral tablets:* 800 mg tid 6 wk *Oral capsules:* 1 g qid up to 8 wk *Suppository:* suppository (500 mg) bid for 3–6 wk *Enema:* 4 gm rectally qd for 3–6 wk	*Onset:* Unknown (oral); 3–21 d (rectal) *Duration:* Unknown $t_{1/2}$: Oral: 2–15 h Rectal: 5–10 h
balsalazide (Colazal)	Ulcerative colitis	2.25 g PO tid for 12 wk	*Onset:* Within 1 h *Duration:* Unknown $t_{1/2}$: Unknown
sulfasalazine (Azulfidine, Azulfidine Entabs)	Ulcerative colitis Rheumatoid arthritis	*Ulcerative colitis:* 1 g tid-qid PO *Rheumatoid arthritis:* 500 mg–2g/d in two to four divided doses	*Onset:* Unknown *Duration:* Unknown $t_{1/2}$: 5.7–10 h

Olsalazine (Dipentum) is used in the maintenance of remission of ulcerative colitis when the patient is intolerant of sulfasalazine. It is a sodium salt of a salicylate compound that is bioconverted to 5-ASA, mesalamine, in the colon by bacteria. The very slow absorption rate from the colon results in very high local concentrations in the colon. Olsalazine produces diarrhea in about 17% of patients taking the drug. This finding may be difficult to distinguish from that caused by IBD.

A recently approved drug, and the first new drug for IBD in 10 years, is balsalazide (Colazal). Balsalazide is delivered intact into the colon where it is cleaved to release mesalamine. More free and active mesalamine is delivered by balsalazide than other preparations. Balsalazide is used in the treatment of mildly to moderately active ulcerative colitis. It should not be used in patients with sensitivity to aspirin. The most common adverse effect is headache, followed by abdominal pain, nausea, and diarrhea. Balsalazide is a safe and effective first-line drug for treating ulcerative colitis.

CHAPTER SUMMARY

- Drugs used to treat digestive disorders of the lower GI tract include antiflatulents, antidiarrheals, laxatives, and drugs used to treat IBS and IBD.
- Antiflatulents are drugs used to decrease the production of gas and to cause gas bubbles to coalesce, facilitating the passage of gas through belching and expelling flatus. These drugs are used to provide relief from postoperative gastric distention, dyspepsia, peptic ulcer, spastic colon, and diverticulosis. Simethicone is the prototype antiflatulent.
- Charcoal is another antiflatulent. Unlike simethicone, it interferes with the absorption of many drugs and is therefore useful in the treatment of drug overdosage and poisonings.
- Diarrhea occurs when motility through the GI tract is too rapid, which prevents water from being reabsorbed from the stool. Infections of the GI tract may cause this. Changes in diet and emotional stress also may contribute to diarrhea.
- Antidiarrheals are used to slow motility through the GI tract. OTC antidiarrheals are used widely, although there are no specific data on their efficacy. The prototype antidiarrheal is diphenoxylate HCl with atropine sulfate. This drug is similar structurally to meperidine. A small amount of atropine sulfate is combined with diphenoxylate to discourage deliberate abuse. It acts systemically to reduce intestinal motility and slow peristalsis.
- Constipation occurs when excessive water is reabsorbed from the stool while it is in the colon, drying the stool and preventing passage. A lack, or deficiency, of effective peristalsis, dietary factors, and changes in activity also may contribute to this. Laxatives are used to treat constipation. Types of laxatives include saline, hyperosmotics, stimulants and irritants, stool softeners, and lubricants.
- Laxatives are contraindicated in patients who have severe abdominal pain that has not been diagnosed, are nauseated and vomiting, or have a bowel obstruction.
- Magnesium hydroxide, the prototype saline laxative, works by attracting water into the colon, increasing intracolonic pressure, and increasing peristalsis. It should not be used if the patient has renal failure because the additional magnesium will not be excreted renally and may cause hypermagnesemia.
- Lactulose, a hyperosmotic laxative, also attracts water into the colon. A unique feature of this laxative is that additionally it produces acid in the colon, which attracts ammonia from the blood. Lactulose also is used therapeutically to decrease serum ammonia levels in those patients with hepatic coma.
- Antispasmodics may be used to treat the symptoms of IBS. They have a nonspecific direct effect on the muscle in the GI tract.
- The inflammation of IBD is treated with 5-ASA preparations (like mesalamine), corticosteroids, and immunosuppressant agents.

QUESTIONS FOR STUDY AND REVIEW

1. What instructions should be given to the patient taking simethicone tablets?
2. Why is atropine sulfate added to diphenoxylate HCl?
3. What classification of laxative would be used prophylactically for a patient recovering from a cataract extraction?
4. Should a patient with severe constipation and renal failure receive magnesium hydroxide?
5. What nonlaxative effect of lactulose is desired for patients with severe hepatic disease?

NEED MORE HELP?

Chapter 38 of the study guide for *Drug Therapy in Nursing* contains exercises and activities to reinforce your understanding of the concepts presented in this chapter. For additional information see the text's accompanying website at *http://www.connection.lww.com.*

REFERENCES AND BIBLIOGRAPHY

Colazal (balsalazide disodium) [On-line]. Available: http://www.fda.gov/cder/foi/label/2000/206101bpl.pdf.

FDA approves Colazal (balsalazide disodium) for ulcerative colitis [On-line]. Available: http://www.docguide.com/dgc.nsf/NewsPrint/86B08264D3613F24852569260048FE05.

Irritable bowel syndrome [On-line]. Available: http://www.discoveryhealth.com/DH/ihtIH?t=9735&p=~br,DSC|st,20809|~r,WSDSCooo|~b,*|11/12/00

Irritable bowel syndrome [On-line]. Available: http://thedailyapple.com/level3/ds3/kiddig/ibhmkd3.htm

Ulcerative colitis [On-line]. Available: http://www.helioshealth.com/digestive/ulcerative_colitis/index.html

What is inflammatory bowel disease? [On-line]. Available: http://my.webmd.com/content/dmk/dmk_article_40052

Unit **XI**

Endocrine System Drugs

Chapter **39**

DRUGS AFFECTING PITUITARY, THYROID, PARATHYROID, AND HYPOTHALAMIC FUNCTION

KEY TERMS

acromegaly
bone resorption
cretinism
diabetes insipidus
gigantism
Graves disease
hyperthyroidism
hypopituitarism
hypothyroidism
myxedema coma
osmolarity
Paget disease
thyrotoxicosis
thyrotoxic crisis

Learning Objectives

At the completion of this chapter the student will:

1. Identify drugs commonly used for pituitary hypofunction and hyperfunction, thyroid hypofunction and hyperfunction, and parathyroid hypofunction and hyperfunction.
2. Identify core drug knowledge about drugs affecting the pituitary gland and its hormones, the thyroid gland and its hormones, and the parathyroid glands and their hormones.
3. Identify core patient variables relevant to drugs affecting the pituitary gland and its hormones, the thyroid gland and its hormones, and the parathyroid glands and their hormones.
4. Generate a nursing plan of care from the interactions between core drug knowledge and core patient variables for drugs affecting the pituitary gland and its hormones, the thyroid gland and its hormones, and the parathyroid glands and their hormones.
5. Describe nursing interventions to maximize therapeutic and minimize adverse effects for drugs affecting the pituitary gland and its hormones, the thyroid gland and its hormones, and the parathyroid glands and their hormones.
6. Determine key points for patient and family education for drugs affecting the pituitary gland and its hormones, the thyroid gland and its hormones, and the parathyroid glands and their hormones.

PITUITARY

Pituitary drugs

Growth hormones
- **somatropin** (P)
- somatrem

GH antagonists
- octreotide acetate
- bromocriptine mesylate

Posterior pituitary hormone regulators
- **desmopressin** (P)
- vasopressin
- lypressin
- terlipressin

THYROID

Thyroid hormone drugs
- **levothyroxine** (P)
- desiccated thyroid
- liothyronine
- liotrix

Antithyroid drugs
- **propylthiouracil** (P)
- methimazole
- iodide or iodine solutions
- radioactive sodium iodine (I-131)
- propranolol

PARATHYROID

Antihypercalcemic drugs
- **calcitonin, salmon** (P)
- alendronate
- etidronate
- residronate
- tiludronate
- plicamycin
- furosemide
- gallium

Antihypocalcemic drugs
- **calcitriol** (P)
- dihydrotachysterol
- doxercalciferol
- paricalcitol

The symbol (C) indicates the **drug class**.
Drugs in bold type marked with the symbol (P) are **prototypes**.
Drugs in blue type with no symbol are **closely related** to the prototype.
Drugs in **red** type with no symbol are **significantly different** from the prototype.
Drugs in **black** type with no symbol are **also used in drug therapy**; no prototype.

The functional goal of the endocrine system is promotion of homeostasis. This goal is accomplished through an intricate coordination of glandular activities involving the stimulation and suppression of glands and hormones. Hyperactivity and hypoactivity of these glands upset the homeostasis of the body, producing specific disorders. The drugs presented in this chapter are used to manage these disorders by correcting the imbalances caused by hyperactivity or hypoactivity of the pituitary, thyroid, and parathyroid glands.

Agents that affect pituitary function are used mainly to mimic or antagonize the effect of pituitary hormones and have several purposes, including replacement therapy for conditions resulting from an underactive pituitary gland, diagnosis, and inhibition of pituitary function for conditions resulting from an overactive pituitary gland.

Agents that affect thyroid function may be used to replace deficient or to antagonize excessive thyroid hormone.

Serum calcium and phosphate are regulated by vitamin D, calcitonin, and parathyroid hormone (PTH). PTH is the single most important hormone regulating ionic serum calcium levels; pharmacologic agents used routinely to regulate serum calcium primarily increase or decrease serum calcium levels, rather than replacing or inhibiting PTH activity.

PHYSIOLOGY

A combination of neural and endocrine systems, originating in the hypothalamus, regulates the central nervous system (CNS), autonomic nervous system, and endocrine functions. The hypothalamus, known as the master gland of the body, has great direct regulatory effects over the neurologic and endocrine systems of the body (Fig. 39-1). Major hypothalamic regulatory functions consist of somatic and visceral reactions including the following:

- Temperature regulation
- Perspiration
- Gastrointestinal (GI) activity
- Appetite and thirst regulation
- Blood pressure
- Respiration
- Regulation of basic body rhythms (e.g., sleep and menstrual cycles)
- Complex behavioral and emotional reactions (e.g., sexual behavior and defensive reactions of fear and rage)

To promote homeostasis, the hypothalamus transmits stimuli to the pituitary gland, causing hormonal release or hormonal inhibition. The pituitary gland rests in the bony sella turcica under a layer of dura mater and consists of three lobes—an anterior lobe, a posterior lobe, and an intermediate lobe. A stalk of neurosecretory fibers connects it to the hypothalamus. Several hypothalamic hormones have characteristic controlling effects on the anterior lobe of the pituitary. This control comes from a group of releasing hormones (sometimes referred to as releasing factors). These releasing hormones and their actions include the following:

- Growth hormone-releasing hormone (GHRH), also known as sermorelin, stimulates anterior pituitary release of growth hormone (GH). It is used as a single IV injection for evaluating the ability of the somatotroph of the pituitary gland to secrete GH. Sermorelin (Geref) has orphan drug status for idiopathic or organic GH deficiency in children with growth failure; *and* as an adjunct to gonadotropin in ovulation induction, and catabolism associated with the acquired immunodeficiency syndrome (AIDS), weight loss, and cachexia.
- Thyroid-releasing hormone (TRH), also known as protirelin, stimulates the anterior pituitary to produce thyrotropin (thyroid-stimulating hormone), which in turn stimulates the thyroid to produce thyroxine. A TRH infusion test is the most sensitive method for diagnosing mild hypothyroidism and hyperthyroidism. TRH has orphan-drug status for the prevention of infant respiratory distress syndrome associated with prematurity. Timely high-dose TRH is under investigation for improving the outcome of spinal cord injuries (Katzung, 1998). Other clinical indications include as an adjunct to other diagnostic procedures in patients with pituitary or hypothalamic dysfunction, and as replacement or supplemental therapy in hypothyroidism. Unlabeled uses include treatment of obesity; they are ineffective, however, and should not be used for this condition.
- Gonadotropin-releasing factor (GnRH) controls the release of the gonadotropins: follicle-stimulating hormone (FSH) and luteinizing hormone (LH). Analogues of GnRH include goserelin, histrelin, leuprolide, and nafarelin. Goserelin is used in the palliative treatment of advanced breast and prostate cancer and endometriosis. Histrelin is used for the treatment of central precocious puberty (i.e., gonadotropin dependent) in children of both sexes. The uses of leuprolide are similar to goserelin and histrelin. Nafarelin is used in the management of endometriosis and central precocious puberty.
- Corticotropin-releasing factor (Xerecept) stimulates release of adrenocorticotropic hormone (ACTH). It is stimulated by serotonin, dopamine and other neurotransmitters in response to stress (emotional, physical, or chemical). It may be used for diagnostic purposes of adrenocortical hyperfunction (e.g., Cushing disease) and endogenous depression. An unlabeled use is in peritumoral brain edema.

PITUITARY GLAND FUNCTION

Anterior Lobe of the Pituitary Gland

The pituitary, once described as the "master" gland of the body—a role now assumed by the hypothalamus, has many important functions. Through various feedback mechanisms, the pituitary regulates the function of many other endocrine glands. Six major hormones of the anterior pituitary lobe participate in the control of reproductive function, body growth, and cellular metabolism. These hormones are:

- GH
- TSH
- ACTH

Physiology

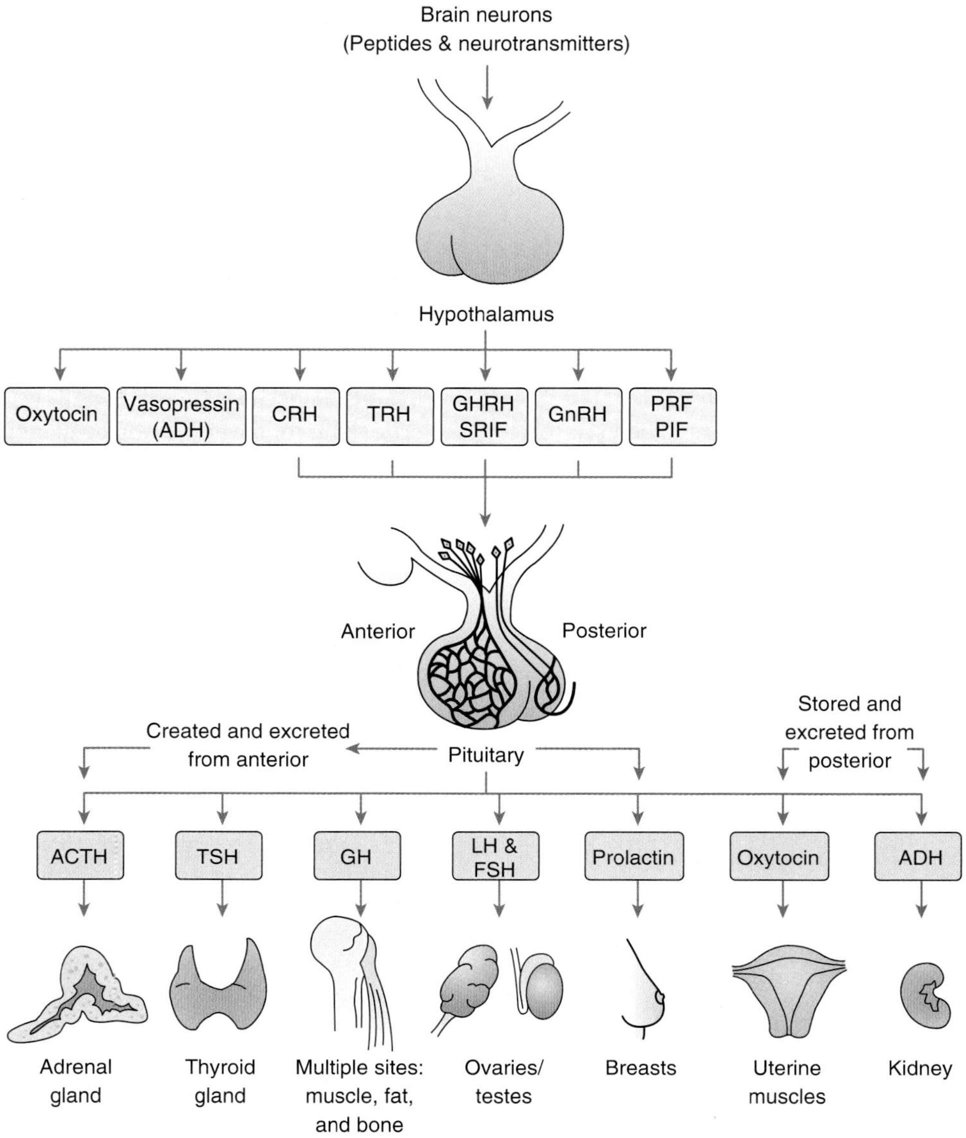

Neurohormones excreted by hypothalamus	Hormones released by pituitary
Corticotropin-releasing hormone (CRH)	Adrenocorticotropic hormone (ACTH)
Thyrotropin-releasing hormone (TRH)	Thyroid-stimulating hormone (TSH)
Growth hormone-releasing hormone (GHRH)	Growth hormone (GH)
Somatotropin release-inhibiting factor (SRIF)	Luteinizing hormone (LH)
Gonadotropin-releasing hormone (GnRH)	Follicle-stimulating hormone (FSH)
Prolactin-releasing factor (PRF)	Prolactin
Prolactin-inhibiting factor (PIF)	Oxytocin
	Antidiuretic Hormone (ADH)

Figure 39-1. Governed by the brain, the pituitary gland has many effects on peripheral target tissues and glands. Some hypothalamic hormones influence the functions of the anterior pituitary gland. Anterior gland tropic hormones, in turn, affect the production and secretion of various responsive glands. The secretions of these glands influence metabolism of various peripheral tissues and exert feedback effects on the adenohypophysis and the hypothalamus. The neurohypophysis stores and releases other hypothalamic hormones that also affect the functioning of peripheral target tissues. Adapted from Boyd, M. A., Nihart M. A. (1998). *Psychiatric nursing; Contemporary practice.* Philadelphia: Lippincott-Raven.

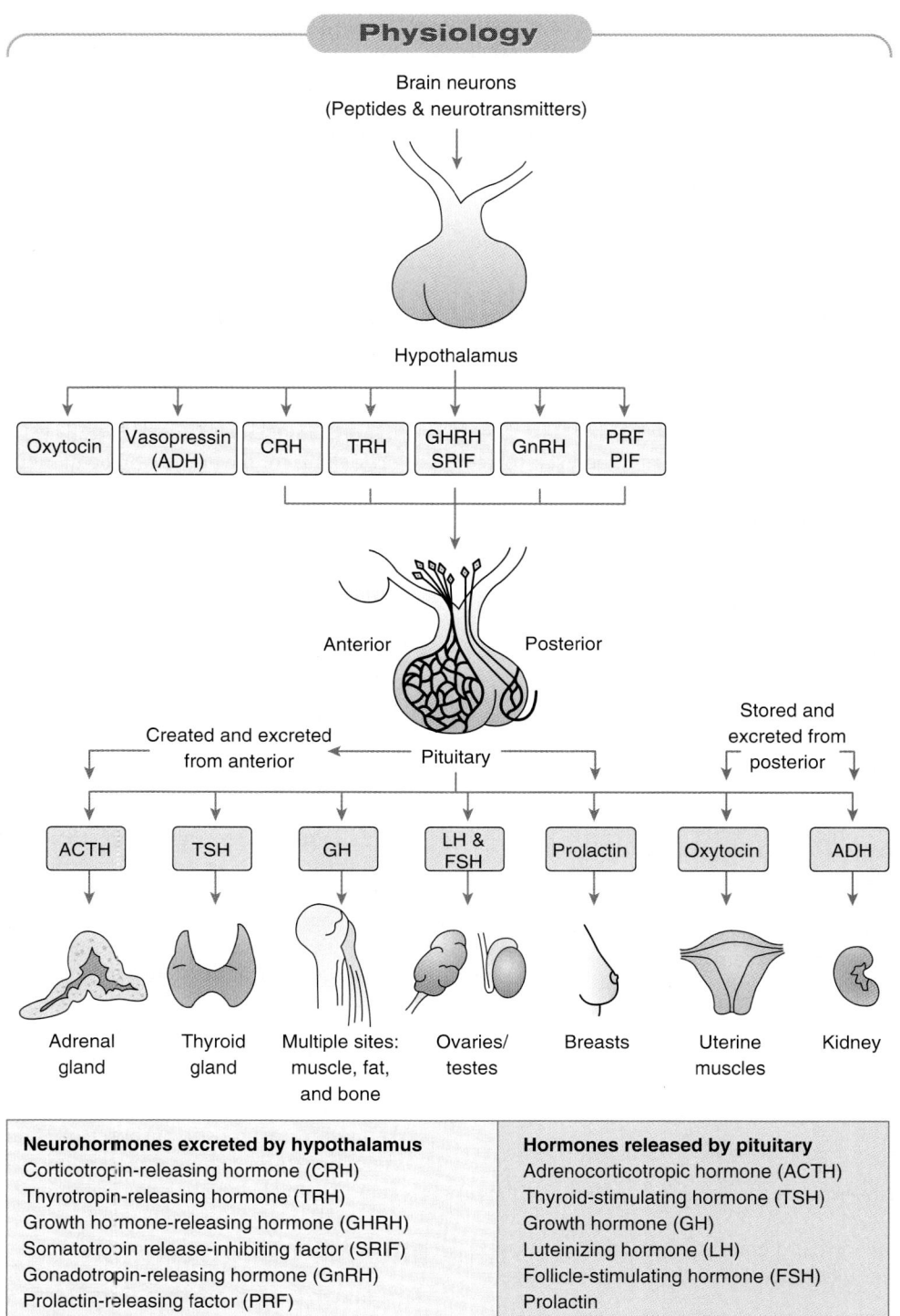

- FSH
- LH
- Prolactin

Deficiency or overproduction of these tropic hormones disrupts this control. All anterior pituitary hormones are released in a pulsatile manner into the bloodstream, and their secretion varies with time of day or physiologic activities, such as exercise or sleep. Their synthesis or release is affected by a number of variables, for example, the CNS, hypothalamic hormones, hormones of the peripheral endocrine glands, some diseases, and a variety of drugs.

GH has no specific target gland. Instead, GH stimulates linear body growth in children and regulates cellular metabolism in a variety of tissues in both children and adults. It facilitates the transport of amino acids across cell membranes, thereby stimulating an anabolic effect. GH causes stimulation of lipolysis, enhanced production of free fatty acids, elevated blood glucose, and a positive nitrogen balance. Many of its anabolic actions are mediated by enhanced production of an insulin-like growth factor (IGF-1), a protein produced in the liver and peripheral target tissue in response to GH.

GH is released in a pulsatile, episodic manner and it is the most pronounced of the pituitary hormones. GH serum levels are the result of strong controls by hypothalamic hormones—GHRH and somatostatin. GH is released during sleep, with maximum release occurring about 1 hour after the onset of sleep. GH also is released after exercise, by hypoglycemia, stress, emotional excitement, and in response to arginine and levodopa.

Posterior Lobe of the Pituitary Gland

The posterior pituitary stores two hormones that are produced in the hypothalamus. These hormones are vasopressin (also known as antidiuretic hormone [ADH], which possesses antidiuretic, hemostatic and vasopressor properties) and oxytocin. Vasopressin and oxytocin are synthesized in the hypothalamus and transported through the neurosecretory fibers within the stalk to the posterior pituitary lobe, from which they are released into the circulation. ADH is released in response to increases in plasma **osmolarity** (the concentration of osmotically active particles in solution) or decreases in blood volume. Oxytocin stimulates uterine smooth muscle contraction in late phases of pregnancy, and can be used to induce or improve uterine contractions in labor. It also causes milk release in lactating women (see Chapter 8 for a thorough discussion of oxytocin).

Intermediate Lobe of the Pituitary Gland

The hormones of the intermediate pituitary lobe have melanocyte-stimulating properties, which are important in animals that use skin color changes as an adaptive mechanism. These hormones are not yet identified as discrete hormones in humans, and they have no present role in clinical pharmacology. However, they are being investigated as neurostimulators.

THYROID GLAND FUNCTION

The thyroid gland is a vascular, bilobar gland that is located in the neck where it surrounds the trachea. The gland is made up of cells arranged in circular follicles. The center of each follicle is composed of colloid tissue made of thyroglobulin synthesized in the thyroid cells and extruded into the follicle where the thyroid hormone is stored. The thyroid gland uses iodine from food, water, or medication to produce two slightly different thyroid hormones:

- Thyroxine (T_4) contains four iodine atoms and triiodothyronine
- Liothyronine (T_3) contains three iodine atoms

An adequate dietary intake of iodine is necessary for optimal production of thyroid hormones. The thyroid cells remove iodine from the blood, concentrate it, and oxidize the iodine for attachment to the amino acid tyrosine. This molecule is then oxidized further to form a molecule that attaches to thyroglobulin. It is stored in the thyroid colloid. When thyroid hormone is needed, the molecule is taken up into the cells where T_3 and T_4 are broken off and released into circulation. Once released into the bloodstream, these hormones are more than 99% bound to plasma proteins and are measured as protein-bound iodine. The thyroid gland produces more T_4 than T_3, but T_3 is approximately four times more active than T_4. At the tissue level, T_4 is converted to T_3, and the half-life of T_4 is approximately 1 week, compared with 12 hours for T_3. Because of these factors, T_4 is thought to be the more important thyroid hormone.

TSH regulates the release of thyroid hormone (Fig. 39-2). TSH causes the thyroid to grow and increases the glandular production of thyroid hormone. The secretion of TSH is regulated by a hypothalamic-regulating factor, TRH. A delicate balance exists among the thyroid, pituitary, and hypothalamus in regulating the levels of thyroid hormone. If the thyroid produces increased thyroid hormone in response to increased levels of TSH, the increased thyroid hormone levels will send a negative message to the pituitary to decrease TSH release and to the hypothalamus to decrease TRH release. A drop in TRH levels will result in a drop of TSH levels, which will in turn lead to a drop in thyroid hormone levels when the thyroid gland is no longer stimulated. The drop in thyroid hormone level will be sensed by the hypothalamus and the pituitary and will result in an increase in TRH and TSH levels. This results in stimulation of the thyroid to produce more hormones. Through this intricate feedback loop, the body can maintain the thyroid hormone level within a narrow, effective range.

Thyroid hormone regulates the rate of metabolism in almost all body cells (Table 39-1). Specifically, the thyroid hormone controls the rate at which body cells consume energy. The hormones synthesized and released by the thyroid gland affect such fundamental processes as heat production and body temperature, oxygen consumption and cardiac output, blood volume, enzyme system activity, and metabolism of carbohydrates, fats, and proteins. The mechanisms by which thyroid hormones exert these physiologic effects

Physiology

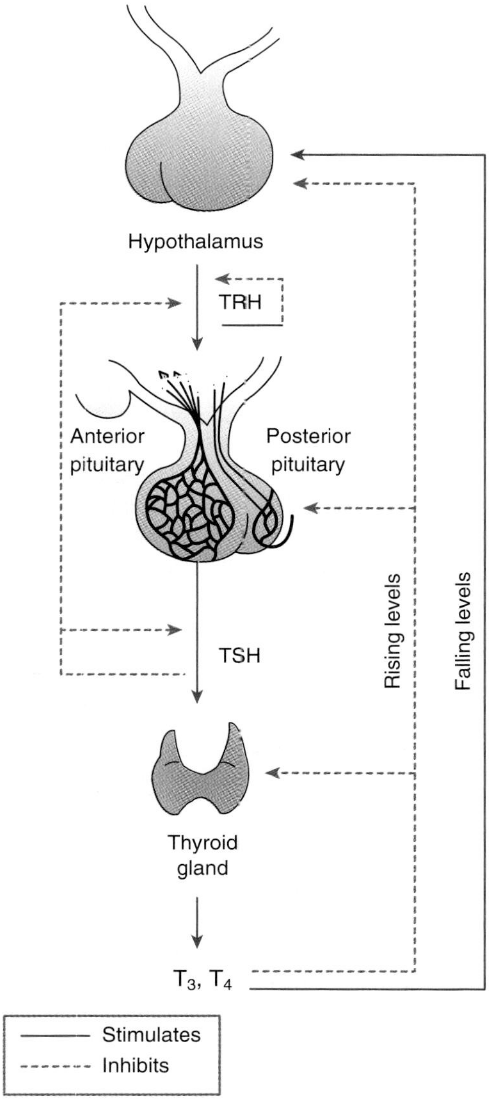

Figure 39-2. Thyroid-releasing hormone (TRH) from the hypothalamus stimulates the anterior pituitary to release thyroid-stimulating hormone (TSH). It also inhibits the hypothalamus from releasing TRH. TSH stimulates the thyroid gland to release T_3 and T_4, it also inhibits the hypothalamus from releasing TRH and the anterior pituitary from releasing more TSH. The release of T_3 and T_4 from the thyroid gland inhibits TRH release from the hypothalamus, TSH release from the pituitary, and further T_3 and T_4 release from the thyroid gland. Falling T_3 and T_4 levels will stimulate the hypothalamus to release TRH, and the process repeatedly continues to maintain effective hormone levels.

are not well understood. Thyroid gland hormones affect nearly all body tissues and orchestrate the regulation and maintenance of normal body homeostasis, metabolism, and growth and development. Any disorder of the thyroid gland will have systemic effects throughout the body.

The thyroid hormones have important, but not necessarily identical, effects on most body tissues. They appear to be required for the optimal functioning of other hormones (e.g., catecholamines, corticosteroids, and ADH).

TABLE 39-1 Effects of Thyroid Hormone

Target Physiologic Process or Body System	Primary Effects
Carbohydrate metabolism	Increases cellular glucose uptake Increases gluconeogenesis and glycolysis Increases GI carbohydrate absorption Increases insulin secretion
Cardiovascular system	Increases heart rate, cardiac output, arterial pressure
Central nervous system	Increases mental processes Increases activity in spinal cord areas controlling muscle tone
Fat metabolism	Increases fat metabolism, including lipid mobilization from fat tissues and free fatty acid oxidation
GI function	Increases appetite, food absorption, digestive enzyme secretions, GI motility
Growth metabolism	Accelerates growth (in children) Accelerates food use for energy, speeds protein synthesis and catabolism, excites mental processes Increases other endocrine gland functions

PARATHYROID GLAND FUNCTION

The parathyroid glands are four pea-sized, highly vascular glands of the endocrine system, which are located behind the thyroid. Their sole purpose is the regulation and maintenance of calcium and phosphate homeostasis through the interaction of three substances—PTH, calcitonin, and vitamin D. Plasma calcium concentration usually is maintained within narrow limits—approximately 4.5 to 5.7 mEq/L—and exists in three forms: namely, ionized (50%), protein bound (46%), and complexed to organic ions (4%) (Craig & Stitzel, 1998). When the concentration falls outside this range, the functions of many tissues are affected. Neuromuscular excitability and tetany may occur from hypocalcemia, whereas hypercalcemia can result in life-threatening cardiac dysrhythmias, renal damage, soft-tissue calcification, and CNS abnormalities.

Plasma calcium concentration is the most powerful factor that regulates parathyroid gland secretory activity. The primary function of PTH is to elicit the adaptive changes that maintain a constant concentration of serum calcium. PTH achieves this through promoting calcium conservation by the kidneys, stimulating calcium release by the bone, working with vitamin D to enhance calcium absorption from the GI tract, and reducing serum phosphate levels. PTH secretion increases, and hyperplasia and hypertrophy of the parathyroid glands result, if the hypocalcemia is sustained.

There is a negative feedback mechanism that controls PTH secretion. When serum calcium concentration is low, PTH release is stimulated. An increased serum calcium level suppresses PTH release. Magnesium also affects PTH secretion by mobilizing calcium and by inhibiting its release when concentrations rise above or fall below normal. An increased serum phosphate level stimulates parathyroid activity indirectly. Renal tubular phosphate reabsorption triggers calcium secretion into the urine with the resulting serum calcium decrease stimulating PTH secretion.

PATHOPHYSIOLOGY

PITUITARY GLAND DYSFUNCTION

Pituitary dysfunction may occur as a result of developmental abnormalities or congenital defects, circulatory disturbances (e.g., hemorrhage or infarction), acute or chronic inflammation, and neoplasms. A single or multiple hormone(s) may be affected.

Anterior Pituitary Gland

Growth hormone deficiency and excess are characteristic conditions of anterior pituitary dysfunction.

Growth Hormone Deficiency

Growth hormone deficiency may be congenital or acquired. Idiopathic GH deficiency is the most common type in children. GH deficiency in children results in short stature (dwarfism).

Although there are no obvious problems in GH-deficient adults, some studies suggest that adults with GH deficiency may manifest metabolic disorders that affect their physical mobility, socialization, and energy levels. It also may affect their life expectancy; GH-deficient adults may also be at greater risk of cardiovascular disease. Adults with GH deficiency may have **hypopituitarism** (diminution or cessation of anterior pituitary function) as a result of pituitary tumors or trauma, or they may have been treated for GH deficiency as children.

Growth Hormone Excess

Two different syndromes may occur as a result of GH excess, depending on the patient's age. GH hypersecretion before the epiphyseal plates of the long bones fuse causes an acceleration in linear skeletal growth to produce **gigantism** of 7 to 8 feet in height with fairly normal body proportions.

In adults after epiphyseal closure, linear growth is impossible. Instead, enlargement takes place in the peripheral parts of the body such as the hands and feet and in internal organs, especially the heart. **Acromegaly** is the term used to describe the onset of excessive GH secretion occurring after puberty and epiphyseal plate closure. Acromegaly is an uncommon disorder and is characterized by enlargement and thickening of bony surfaces still responsive to GH effects. For example, hands and feet will increase in size, while enlargement of facial bones and thickening of cartilage and soft tissues will result in coarsened facial features. Other adverse effects associated with acromegaly include cardiovascular disease, diabetes mellitus, hypertension, muscle weakness, and peripheral neuropathy.

Posterior Pituitary Gland

Posterior pituitary gland disorders—secondary to metastatic cancer, lymphomas, disseminated intravascular coagulation, and septicemia—affect ADH and may be acute or chronic in nature. Two major disorders of the posterior pituitary are diabetes insipidus resulting from deficient ADH secretion and syndrome of inappropriate antidiuretic hormone (SIADH) from excessive secretion.

Diabetes Insipidus

Antidiuretic hormone is released in response to increases in plasma osmolarity or decreases in blood volume. It produces its antidiuretic activity in the kidney, causing the cortical and medullary parts of the collecting duct to become permeable to water, thereby increasing water reabsorption, reducing plasma osmolarity, and increasing blood volume.

Diabetes insipidus (DI) is a disease of impaired renal conservation of water due to either an inadequate secretion of vasopressin from the neurohypophysis (may be referred to as central or cranial DI) or to an insufficient renal response to vasopressin (may be referred to as nephrogenic DI). DI is characterized by the excretion of very large amounts (more than 30 mL/kg per day) of dilute urine containing no glucose and of low specific gravity (less than 1.005) causing dehydration and extreme thirst. DI, characterized by polyuria, polydipsia, and dehydration, is an infrequent metabolic disorder in which patients produce large quantities of dilute urine and are constantly thirsty. DI may occur as a result of glandular disease or glandular injury (e.g., head trauma, surgery, or tumors) and can be acute in nature and of short duration or a chronic, life-long problem.

Syndrome of Inappropriate Antidiuretic Hormone

Syndrome of inappropriate antidiuretic hormone (SIADH) is a disease of impaired water excretion accompanied by hyponatremia and hypoosmolality caused by the excessive and inappropriate secretion of vasopressin. The clinical manifestations of plasma hypotonicity secondary to SIADH may include lethargy, anorexia, muscle cramps, nausea, vomiting, seizures, coma, and death. A number of disorders can induce SIADH including pulmonary diseases, CNS injuries or diseases (e.g., head trauma, infections, or tumors), and a variety of drugs (see the accompanying display, Drugs that May Cause Syndrome of Inappropriate Antidiuretic Hormone Secretion).

THYROID GLAND DYSFUNCTION

Thyroid dysfunction can produce dramatic changes in the pattern of growth and development, and in the functioning of the cardiovascular, GI, skeletal, neuromuscular, and

Drugs That May Cause Syndrome of Inappropriate Antidiuretic Hormone Secretion (SIADH)

carbamazepine (Tegretol)
chlorpropamide (Diabinese)
clofibrate (Atromid S)
cyclophosphamide (Cytoxan)
isoproterenol (Isuprel)
morphine
oxytocin (Pitocin)
phenothiazines
prostaglandins
thiazide diuretics
tricyclic antidepressants
vasopressin
vincristine (Oncovin)

reproductive systems. Two thyroid gland disorders include hypothyroidism and hyperthyroidism (Table 39-2).

Hypothyroidism

Hypothyroidism (HOT) results from inadequate secretion of the thyroid hormones. It is a common finding in the elderly. The symptoms of HOT are varied, vague, and frequently overlooked, or may be mistaken for signs of normal aging. HOT occurs when there is a lack of effect of thyroid hormone—T_4 or T_3—on body tissues. Primary HOT refers to a defect within the thyroid gland itself causing decreased production of thyroid hormone. Hypothalamic or pituitary failure may cause a secondary form of HOT and this is due to a lack of TRH or TSH. In the United States, the primary form of HOT is the most common, usually occurring because of autoimmunity.

Adult HOT is called **myxedema.** This usually develops gradually as the thyroid slowly stops functioning adequately. However, it also can develop as a result of autoimmune thyroid disease (Hashimoto thyroiditis), viral infection, drug-induced by antithyroid drugs (e.g., I-131, PTU) or drugs which inhibit thyroid activity (e.g., amiodarone, lithium), iron deficiency, surgical removal of thyroid tissue (subtotal or total thyroidectomy), and thyroid cancer.

The clinical manifestations of HOT involve virtually every body system and, generally there is a slowing of physical and mental activity and a functional slowing of the cardiovascular, GI, and neuromuscular systems. These affected individuals may exhibit many symptoms of decreased cellular metabolism—anxiety, constipation, increased diastolic blood pressure, lethargy, hypoactive reflexes, hypotension, bradycardia, pale and coarse skin, loss of hair, intolerance to the cold, decreased appetite, decreased body temperature, puffiness of the hands, feet, and face, thickening of the tongue and vocal chords, decreased sexual function, menstrual irregularities, and infertility.

Failure to diagnose and treat HOT can have serious consequences. For example, poorly controlled HOT can result in bradycardia and respiratory depression. In addition, elderly individuals with severe HOT are at risk for **myxedema coma**—a life-threatening condition manifested by coma, hypothermia, bradycardia, hypoglycemia, and hypoventilation. Myxedema coma often is precipitated by an intercurrent illness (e.g., infection, stroke, or congestive heart failure [CHF]) or by sedative-hypnotic drugs.

In children, HOT can have devastating effects, including impairment of physical growth and mental development. Children born without a thyroid gland or with a nonfunctional or dysfunctional gland develop a hypothyroid condition called **cretinism,** which results from HOT during development and infancy. If untreated, cretinism is marked by retardation of both physical and mental development. Cretinism is not apparent at birth but becomes manifest over the ensuing weeks to months and by the time the clinical picture is obvious the changes are largely irreversible. Early manifestations of cretinism include constipation, failure to thrive, feeding problems, hoarse cry, and somnolence. Development of newborn screening programs for early detection of HOT in neonates can prevent these complications by providing early treatment.

Hyperthyroidism

The term **hyperthyroidism** (HRT), also referred to as **thyrotoxicosis,** refers to a heterogenous group of disorders in which the body tissues are exposed to excessive amounts of T_3, T_4, or both. Excessive amounts of thyroid hormone may occur from overproduction of thyroid hormone (e.g., Graves disease), "leaking" hormone from thyroid destruction (e.g., subacute thyroiditis), drugs, and tumors. Approximately 2% of females and 0.2% of males are affected. The two most common forms of HRT are toxic multinodular goiter and Graves disease.

Patients with HRT may exhibit many signs and symptoms of overactive cellular metabolism; for example, increased body temperature, tachycardia, palpitations, hypertension, flushed and thin skin, intolerance to heat, amenorrhea, weight loss, and diffuse, vascular goiter. Often, mild HRT produces no apparent effects. As the condition progresses, however, the manifestations are related to increased metabolic function of all body systems and thyrotoxicosis is said to occur when the HRT causes noticeable signs and symptoms. When assessing an individual for HRT, the nurse should be alert for the following signs and symptoms: dyspnea, diaphoresis, goiter, exophthalmos, fatigue, heat intolerance, increased appetite, irritability and nervousness, muscle weakness, tremor and wasting, and weight loss.

Graves disease is a poorly understood autoimmune condition caused from circulating immunoglobulins that bind to and stimulate the TSH receptor, which results in sustained overactivity of the thyroid gland, stimulation of thyroid hormone production and growth of the entire thyroid gland (goiter). Infiltrative ophthalmopathy (exophthalmos) and skin lesions (dermopathy) are additional manifestations of Graves disease. Exophthalmos occurs more than 50% of the time and is characterized by increased retroorbital tissue and lympho-

TABLE 39-2 Clinical Comparison of Hypothyroidism and Hyperthyroidism

Body System	Clinical Picture of Hypothyroidism	Clinical Picture of Hyperthyroidism
Central nervous system	General slowing of mental processes Lethargy Neuropathies	Emotional lability Hyperkinesia Nervousness
Cardiovascular system	Decreased peripheral vascular resistance, heart rate, stroke volume, cardiac output, pulse pressure ECG changes: bradycardia, increased PR interval, flat T wave, low voltage Low-output congestive heart failure Pericardial effusion	Increased peripheral vascular resistance, heart rate, stroke volume, cardiac output, pulse pressure High-output congestive heart failure Increased inotropic and chronotropic effects Angina Arrhythmias
EENT	Enlarged tongue Eyelid drooping Periorbital edema Puffy, nonpitting face	Diplopia (Graves disease) Exophthalmos (Graves disease) Periorbital edema Retraction of upper lid with wide stare
Gastrointestinal system	Decreased appetite Decreased frequency of bowel movements Ascites	Increased appetite Increased frequency of bowel movements Hypoproteinemia
Hematopoietic system	Decreased erythropoiesis Anemia	Increased erythropoiesis Anemia
Metabolic system	Decreased basal metabolic rate with slight positive nitrogen balance Delayed degradation of insulin with increased insulin sensitivity Increased cholesterol and triglycerides Decreased hormone degradation Decreased requirements for fat- and water-soluble vitamins Decreased drug detoxification	Increased basal metabolic rate with negative nitrogen balance Hyperglycemia Increased free fatty acids Decreased cholesterol and triglycerides Increased hormone degradation Increased requirements for fat- and water-soluble vitamins Increased drug detoxification
Musculoskeletal system	Stiffness and muscle fatigue Decreased deep tendon reflexes Increased alkaline phosphatase, LDH, AST	Weakness and muscle fatigue Increased deep tendon reflexes Hypercalcemia Osteoporosis
Renal system	Impaired water excretion Decreased renal blood flow Decreased glomerular filtration rate	Mild polyuria Increased renal blood flow Increased glomerular filtration rate
Reproductive system	Hypermenorrhea infertility* decreased libido* Men: impotency, oligospermia decreased gonadal steroid metabolism*	Women: menstrual irregularities decreased fertility, decreased gonadal steroid metabolism*
Respiratory	Pleural effusions Hypoventilation Hypercarbia	Dyspnea Decreased vital capacity
Skin	Pale, cool, puffy skin (myxedema) Dry, brittle hair Brittle nails Cold intolerance	Warm, moist, diaphoretic skin Fine, thin hair Heat intolerance

*Both men and women

cytic infiltration of the extraocular muscles, which gives the eyes of these affected patients their characteristic protruding appearance. Exophthalmos associated with Graves disease is usually independent of the thyrotoxic aspect and is essentially unchanged by drug treatment.

A rare, yet life threatening and potentially fatal **thyrotoxic crisis** (thyroid storm) may occur spontaneously, as HRT progresses without treatment, or it may be precipitated by a number of factors including infection, radioactive iodine, trauma, or surgery. Manifestations of thyroid storm include extreme tachycardia with arrhythmias, dehydration, extreme hyperthermia, profound weakness, high-output heart failure, delirium, or coma. Treatment includes administration of propylthiouracil (PTU) as the antithyroid drug of choice, corticosteroids, beta-adrenergic blockers, fluids and electrolytes, sedation, oxygen, and measures to control hyperthermia.

Treatment of HRT is directed at reducing the excessive secretion of thyroid hormones. The usual therapeutic regimens to treat HRT include thyroid-hormone-antagonist drugs to inhibit thyroid secretion, and surgery or radioactive iodine to reduce the amount of functional thyroid tissue and achieve a state where the thyroid is functioning normally (i.e., euthyroid state).

PARATHYROID GLAND DYSFUNCTION

Hyperparathyroidism

Hyperparathyroidism (HRPT) is a disorder caused by overactivity of one or more of the parathyroid glands. Primary HRPT develops when the normal regulatory relationship between serum calcium levels and PTH is interrupted by an adenoma or hyperplasia of the gland. It occurs twice as often in women and most frequently during the 6th to 7th decades of life. It causes excessive serum and urinary levels of calcium (hypercalcemia) (Table 39-3). Although the urine phosphate level is high, the serum level is normal to low. Potential complications that occur from these imbalances can be remembered by the rhyme, "moans, groans, stones, and bones." Complications include severe osteoporosis and osteopenia, pathologic bone fractures, kidney stones, peptic ulcers, pancreatitis, and nervous system complaints. Secondary HRPT usually occurs in patients with chronic renal failure (CRF) but may occur in Paget disease, multiple myeloma, and bone metastases. Tertiary HRPT occurs when PTH production is autonomous in individuals with normal or low serum calcium levels. Regardless of cause, HRPT is characterized by bone decalcification and the deposition of calcium salts in body tissues. The severity of the hypercalcemia in primary HRPT is reflective directly of the quantity of hyperfunctioning tissue. The excessive quantities of PTH stimulate the transport of calcium into the blood from the intestine, kidney, and bone. Nephrolithiasis develops secondary to calcium deposits in the soft tissues of the kidney.

PTH has a very powerful influence on the cells of the bones, which causes them to release their calcium into the bloodstream. Under its presence, the bones will give up their calcium in an attempt to increase the blood level of calcium. Under normal conditions, this process is very highly regulated and the amount of calcium in bones remains at a normal level. Under the presence of too much PTH, however, the bones will continue to release their calcium into the blood at too high of a rate, which results in bones which have too little calcium—the conditions of osteopenia and osteoporosis (Fig. 39-3). Another way in which PTH acts to increase blood levels of calcium is through its influence on the intestines. Under the presence of PTH, the lining of the intestine becomes more efficient at absorbing dietary calcium (Table 39-4).

CRF and hyperphosphatemia cause secondary HRPT. As the glomerular filtration rate decreases in CRF, serum phosphorous levels increase, which in turn decreases serum calcium levels, which stimulates PTH secretion.

Serum calcium acts as a sedative on the body. As serum calcium rises above 11 mg/dL, neuromuscular irritability is depressed. Hypercalcemia is most often associated with HRPT but can occur secondary to immobilization or neoplastic disease in which there is increased movement of calcium out of the bones and decreased renal excretion of calcium in renal failure.

Hypoparathyroidism

Hypoparathyroidism (HOPT), whether hereditary or acquired, is characterized by hypocalcemia and frequently hypophosphatemia. Tetany, convulsions, muscle spasm, and cardiac dysrhythmias may develop as a result of hypocalcemia. Historically, "acquired" HOPT—secondary to surgery in the neck—was more common, although the fre-

TABLE 39-3 Disorders of Bone and Calcium Metabolism

Disorder	Examples	Management
Hypocalcemia	• Inadequate dietary intake of Ca++ and/or vitamin D • Malabsorption caused by vitamin D lack or end-organ resistance • Hypoparathyroidism, pseudohypoparathyroidism • Renal failure	• Treatment with calcium and vitamin D compounds
Hypercalcemia	• Hyperparathyroidism • Hypervitaminosis D • Neoplasia • Hyperthyroidism • Immobilization	• Treatment with fluids, low calcium diet, calcitonin, bisphosphonates, glucocorticoids, loop diuretics
Impaired bone remodeling	• Osteoporosis	• Treatment with bisphosphonates, calcitonin, calcium, estrogen (female)

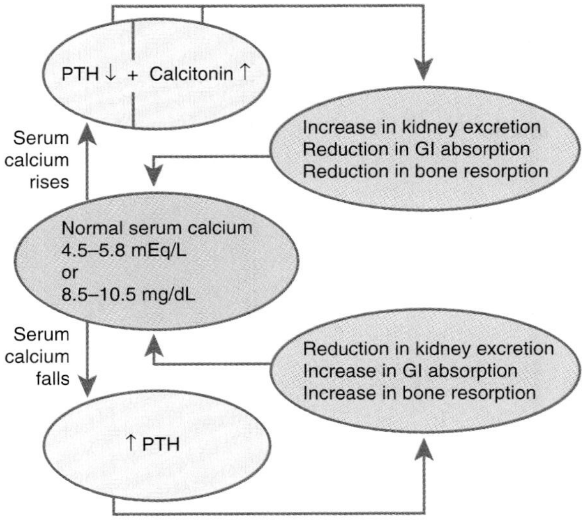

Figure 39-3. Regulation of serum calcium. Parathyroid hormone (PTH) and calcitonin regulate normal serum calcium. As serum calcium rises, PTH is inhibited by calcitonin. The kidney then excretes more calcium, the GI system absorbs less, and a reduction in bone resorption occurs. As serum calcium falls, PTH is secreted and raises the calcium level by decreasing the amount of calcium lost in the kidney, increasing the amount absorbed in the GI tract, and increasing bone resorption.

quency of surgically-induced HOPT has diminished as a result of improved surgical techniques and the increased use of nonsurgical therapy for HRT (e.g., I-131). Vitamin D deficiency leads to rickets in children and osteomalacia in adults.

PITUITARY DRUGS

Drugs used to affect pituitary function are designed mainly to mimic or antagonize the effects of pituitary hormones. The drugs most frequently used include GH, somatostatin, ADH, and oxytocin.

GROWTH HORMONES

Historically, GH deficiency was treated with GH injections extracted from cadavers' pituitary glands; thus, the supply of GH was limited. However, this practice was suspended due to several reported cases of Creutzfeldt-Jakob disease (encephalopathy caused by an obscure infectious agent in the GH resulting in neurologic disturbances and progressing rapidly to coma and death). Synthetic human GH (rhGH) is now readily available from recombinant DNA sources. Although expensive, it is used increasingly to treat GH deficiencies. Somatropin (Humatrope) is the prototype rGH discussed in this chapter.

NURSING MANAGEMENT OF THE PATIENT RECEIVING SOMATROPIN

Core Drug Knowledge

Pharmacotherapeutics

Somatropin is a recombinant-DNA formulation of GH (rGH) that has the same amino acid sequence as pituitary-derived GH and is used as long-term replacement therapy for children who have a growth failure due to inadequate endogenous GH secretion (Table 39-5).

Currently, GH is suggested to have antiaging effects. There are serious consequences, however, because the high dosage needed is possibly carcinogenic and will cause some serious adverse effects such as gynecomastia, acromegalic facial changes, and carpal tunnel syndrome.

Pharmacokinetics

Somatropin is well absorbed and distributed. The absolute bioavailability of somatropin is 75% and 63% after SC and intramuscular IM administration, respectively. GH localizes to highly perfused organs, most notably the liver and kidney. In the kidney, GH is filtered

TABLE 39-4 Actions of Parathyroid Hormone (PTH) and Vitamin D

	PTH	Vitamin D (and metabolites)
Bone	• High doses—calcium and phosphate resorption increased • Low doses—may increase bone formation	• Increased calcium and phosphate resorption by calcitriol • Increased bone formation
Kidney	• Decreased calcium excretion • Increased phosphate excretion	• Calcium and phosphate excretion may be decreased by calciferol and calcitriol
Intestine	• Increased calcium and phosphate absorption by increased calcitriol production	• Increased calcium and phosphate absorption by calcitriol
Effect on serum levels	Serum calcium is increased and serum phosphate is decreased	Serum calcium and serum phosphate are both increased

TABLE 39-5 Summary of Selected Pituitary Drugs

Drug (Trade) Name	Selected Indications	Route and Dosage Range
Growth Hormones		
somatropin (Genotropin, Humatrope, Norditropin, Saizen, Serostim)	Growth hormone replacement therapy Treatment (long-term) of growth failure in children from: growth-hormone deficiency chronic renal failure† (prior to transplant) AIDS wasting syndrome	*Child:* SC: up to 0.0125 mg/kg/d *Child:* IM, SC; mg/kg/d or 3qwk Dosage is based on individual response *Child:* SC; 0.35 mg/kg weekly *Adult:* 4–6 mg hs
somatrem (Protropin)	Treatment (long-term) of growth failure in children Short stature of Turner's syndrome (orphan use)	*Child:* IM; up to 0.1 mg/kg 3qwk Dosage is based on individual response *Child:* IM; <0.1 mg/kg 3qwk
Growth Hormone Antagonists		
octreotide acetate (Sandostatin)	Acromegaly (reduce growth hormone levels) Severe diarrhea	*Adult:* SC; 50–600 µg bid–qid *Child:* safety and efficacy not established
bromocriptine mesylate (Parlodel)	Acromegaly Parkinson disease (idiopathic) Suppression of physiologic lactation following parturition Hyperprolactinemia	*Adult:* PO; 1.25–30 mg/d *Adult:* PO; 2.5–100 mg/d; efficacy for >2 yr not established *Adult:* PO; 2.5 mg bid × 14–21 d *Adult:* PO; 5–10 mg/d
Posterior Pituitary Hormone Regulators		
desmopressin (DDAVP, Stimate⊕)	Neurogenic diabetes insipidus	*Adult:* Intranasal, 0.1–0.4 mL/d qd or bid; 1 spray (300 mg)/nostril; SC, IM—0.5–1.0 mL/d bid PO—0.05 mg bid *Child* (3 mo-12 y): Intranasal—0.05–0.3 mL/d qd or bid; 1 spray (300 mg)/nostril; SC, IM—0.5–1.0 ml/d bid; PO—0.05 mg bid (*Dosage adjusted according to water turnover pattern*)
	Primary nocturnal enuresis Hemophilia A (with factor VIII >5%) Von Willebrand's disease	*Adult/Child* (>6 y): Intranasal 20–40 µg hs: *Adult/child:* IV, 0.3µ/kg (*Repeated administration based on patient response*)
	Neurogenic diabetes insipidus	*Adult:* IM, SC, intranasal; 5–10 U repeated q3–4 h as needed
vasopressin (Pitressin)	Abdominal distention Antiflatulent effect for abdominal roentgenography	*Adult:* IM; 5–10 U repeated q3–4 H intervals *Adult:* IM, SC; 10 U at 2 h and 10 U at ½ hr before procedure *Child:* decrease dosage proportionately
lypressin (Diapid)	Neurogenic diabetes insipidus	*Adult:* Intranasal; 1–2 sprays qid in one or both nostrils (*Dosage dependent on urination or significant thirst*)

†Nutropin only
⊕Used for hematological effects only
ϕSpecific use for patient sensitive to animal products

by the glomerulus, reabsorbed in the proximal tubule, and is broken down within renal cells into amino acids that return to the circulation. The mean half-life of IV somatropin is 0.36 hours, in comparison with SC and IM administered somatropin doses that have mean half-lives of 3.8 and 4.9 hours, respectively. The liver and kidney are major elimination organs for exogenously administered CH; severe hepatic and renal function impairment will reduce its clearance.

Pharmacodynamics

Treatment with GH has powerful effects on growth and metabolism. It stimulates cell growth and cellular mitosis, facilitates cellular uptake of amino acids for protein synthesis, and promotes fatty acid utilization for energy. These effects are not caused directly by GH, however, but rather through an intermediary peptide known as IGF-1. In vitro and clinical testing has demonstrated that somatropin is equivalent therapeutically to GH of pituitary origin in adults. Treatment of GH-deficient children produces increased growth rate and IGF-1 concentrations similar to those seen after therapy with GH of pituitary origin.

Contraindications and Precautions

Somatropin is pregnancy category C. It should be given only when clearly needed. It is unknown whether somatropin is excreted in breast milk. Somatropin therapy is contraindicated in patients with closed epiphyses. It also is contraindicated in patients who have evidence of intracranial tumor activity because tumor growth rate may increase. Cautious use also is advised in diabetic patients because a state of insulin resistance resulting in hyperglycemia may develop. Some product formulations contain diluent preservatives that may cause hypersensitivity.

Adverse Effects

Adverse effects include headache, hypertension, joint and back pain, peripheral edema, muscle aches, and rhinitis. Many of these adverse effects occur initially and then either resolve spontaneously or in response to dosage adjustments. Others include HOT, hyperglycemia, glycosuria, and pain at the injection site. Recurrent growth of intracranial tumor also may occur. Leukemia has occurred in a small number of children receiving somatropin or somatrem. The relationship, however, is uncertain.

A small percentage of patients (approximately 2%) may develop antibodies to the rGH protein molecule. However, GH antibody binding capacities (2 mg/L) have not been associated with any growth reduction.

Drug Interactions

GH reduces the activity of hepatic mixed-function oxidases. This reduction may alter drug metabolism. Glucocorticoid or other corticosteroid therapy may inhibit the growth-promoting effect of rGH. Patients with coexisting ACTH deficiency may need their glucocorticoid replacement dosage adjusted carefully to avoid an inhibitory effect on growth. Therefore, patients should be monitored closely if this combination must be used. Use of somatropin with anabolic steroids, androgens, estrogens, or thyroid hormones may accelerate epiphyseal maturation.

Assessment of Relevant Core Patient Variables

Health Status

Before administering somatropin, the nurse should review the patient's record to determine whether somatropin can be administered safely. Before beginning therapy, the nurse should perform a physical assessment to establish a baseline from which to monitor the effects of the drug. This assessment should include height and weight measurements, thyroid function tests, glucose tolerance tests, and levels of GH. Radiographs of the hip should be obtained before initiating therapy. Funduscopic examination of patients is recommended at the initiation and periodically during the course of GH therapy.

HOT may develop during GH therapy and, if untreated, may prevent an optimal response. Periodic thyroid function tests should be performed and thyroid hormone used if indicated.

Serum levels of inorganic phosphorus, alkaline phosphatase, and PTH may increase with somatropin therapy. Changes in thyroid hormone laboratory measurements may develop during treatment in children who lack adequate endogenous GH secretion.

Untreated HOT prevents optimal response to therapy. Therefore, it is important to periodically test thyroid function and include treatment with thyroid hormone if indicated. Insulin resistance may be induced by GH. Patients with diabetes or glucose intolerance should be observed closely during somatropin therapy. Individuals with GH deficiency secondary to an intracranial lesion should be evaluated regularly for progression or recurrence of the underlying disease process. Individuals should be assessed routinely for any malignant transformation of skin lesions. Individuals with growth failure secondary to chronic renal insufficiency should be monitored regularly for progression of renal osteodystrophy progression because slipped capital femoral epiphysis or avascular necrosis of the femoral head may be seen in children with advanced renal osteodystrophy. It is uncertain whether these problems are affected by GH therapy.

Life Span and Gender

The nurse should assess whether the patient is pregnant or breast-feeding. Somatropin is classified as pregnancy category C by the Food and Drug Administration. It should be given to a pregnant or lactating woman with caution and only if clearly needed. It is not known whether somatropin is excreted in breast milk. Available literature data suggest that rGH clearances are similar in adults and children. The treatment with GH is a long-term regimen. Children receiving this drug will need continual monitoring and once therapy has begun, the patient's height and weight should be measured and recorded at regular intervals.

Lifestyle, Diet, and Habits

The nurse should assess the patient's ability and willingness to comply with the drug regimen. Somatropin dosage is individualized. SC injections each evening are most effective; nightly injections mimic the natural hormone surge that occurs after sleep. Stimulation of growth is most effective when treatment begins early, and injections are continued until the epiphyses close.

Environment

The nurse must be aware of the setting in which somatropin will be administered, the ability of the patient or caregiver to administer the drug properly, and the patient's and family's financial situation. Somatropin may be administered in the home, clinic, or office setting. The nurse, parent, or caregiver must reconstitute the drug using the manufacturer's instructions and then refrigerate the drug following reconstitution. If unable to perform self-care, the patient will need access to someone capable of proper reconstitution and to refrigeration. The drug is very expensive, and sources of financial support may need to be solicited. Parents or caregivers often learn to perform the injections to decrease health care visits. If home use is desired, the nurse should give instructions on appropriate use, including a review of the contents of the patient information insert. Thoroughly instruct patients and parents or caregivers in the importance of proper disposal and caution against any reuse of needles and syringes. Regular follow-up health care is necessary.

Nursing Diagnoses and Outcomes

- Delayed Growth and Development related to deficiency of GH
  Desired outcome: The patient will demonstrate an increase in linear growth.
- Imbalanced Nutrition: More (or Less) than Body Requirements related to endocrine changes and rapid changes in height and weight
  Desired outcome: The patient will receive adequate nutrition for growth appropriate to age and need.
- Altered Comfort related to headache, joint, and muscle discomfort secondary to somatropin effects
  Desired outcome: The patient will describe measures to improve comfort.

Planning and Intervention

Maximizing Therapeutic Effects

Hypothyroidism may develop during somatropin therapy and, if untreated, may prevent an optimal response. Periodic thyroid function tests should be performed, and thyroid hormone replacement therapy should be used if indicated. Patients with coexisting ACTH deficiency need their glucocorticoid replacement dosage adjusted carefully to avoid an inhibitory effect on growth. Guidelines for optimizing somatropin therapy in patients requiring dialysis suggest that hemodialysis and chronic ambulatory peritoneal dialysis patients take their dose before bedtime. The nurse should make certain that patients using chronic cycling peritoneal dialysis receive their dose in the morning after the dialysis is completed.

Minimizing Adverse Effects

Insulin resistance may be induced by GH therapy. The nurse should observe the patient closely for glucose intolerance. Children being treated with rGH for growth failure secondary to chronic renal insufficiency may develop problems of renal osteodystrophy (generalized bone changes resembling osteomalacia and rickets). Slipped capital femoral epiphyses or avascular necrosis of the femoral head may occur in these patients. Radiographs of the hip should be obtained before initiating therapy with GH, although it is uncertain whether these problems are a direct result of GH therapy. Health care providers and parents should be alert to the development of a limp or complaints of hip or knee pain. Slipped capital femoral epiphysis may occur more frequently in patients with endocrine disorders or in patients undergoing rapid growth. Pain and discomfort related to headache, bone, and muscle discomfort may be treated with appropriate analgesics and environmental controls.

Sudden growth spurts and changes in growth and development coupled with potential thyroid changes and insulin resistance may cause nutritional imbalance that can complicate the desired effect of the GH. The nurse should consider nutritional assessment and appropriate replacement of necessary nutrients.

Providing Patient and Family Education

- The nurse should explain that this drug is replacing an important hormone (GH) that is necessary for normal growth and development.
- It is important to explain to patients and their families that the drug can only be given by injection. The nurse should teach patients, family members, or care givers how to reconstitute and administer the drug. A review of site rotation is important to maximize therapeutic effect and avoid problems of lipodystrophy. Periodic review of technique is important in ensuring effectiveness and decreasing adverse effects.
- The nurse should instruct patients to refrigerate reconstituted solution.
- It is important to alert diabetic patients to the insulin resistance that may develop. The nurse should instruct these patients to monitor blood sugar closely and to report variations to their health care provider.
- The nurse should instruct patients or their families to report any adverse drug effects and should emphasize the importance of reporting a limp or any hip or knee pain as soon as possible. Slipped capital femoral epiphysis may occur more frequently in patients with endocrine disorders or in patients undergoing rapid growth.

Ongoing Assessment and Evaluation

The nurse should evaluate thyroid function at regular intervals because HOT will compromise rGH drug effects. The nurse should be alert for signs of glucose intolerance because insulin resistance may develop and disrupt control of diabetes. As with all protein pharmaceuticals, a small percentage of patients may develop antibodies to the protein. An evaluation of compliance with the prescribed treatment program, thyroid status, and testing for GH antibodies should be done in any patient who fails to respond to therapy. The nurse should stress the importance of follow-up appointments and periodic analysis of thyroid function, glucose tolerance, and GH levels to evaluate the effectiveness of the drug and possible development of adverse effects. Therapy is considered effective when anticipated growth occurs. The patient and family should demonstrate appropriate drug administration and the important of monitoring for adverse effects and reporting significant ones to the health care provider. ■

DRUGS CLOSELY RELATED TO SOMATROPIN

There are a large number of commercially available preparations of somatropin. They include Genotropin, Norditropin, Nutropin, Saizen, and Serostim. With one exception (Nutropin AQ), all are powders that need reconstitution. They differ in the amounts of rGH IU (international units) contained in the vial, single- or multiple-dose vials, and diluents (some diluents are preservative free).

Nutropin is indicated for the chromosomal disorder, Turner syndrome, which affects females exclusively and is characterized partly by short stature and incomplete sexual development.

Serostim is indicated for HIV-associated cachexia (wasting syndrome) with treated patients showing increased lean muscle mass and body weight. Serostim is FDA pregnancy category B.

Somatrem (Protropin) is an artificial human GH with therapeutic effects very similar to somatropin. Its chemical structure differs from somatropin in the addition of one amino acid. Approximately 30% to 40% of all somatrem-treated individuals develop persistent antibodies to GH. Other adverse effects include a decrease in thyroid function and insulin resistance.

MEMORY CHIP

Somatropin

- Genetically engineered (recombinant DNA) human growth hormone used for long-term treatment of children with deficient endogenous growth hormone
- Significant contraindications: closed epiphyses and cranial lesions
- Most common adverse effects: joint and muscle pain
- Most serious adverse effects: development of antibodies to growth hormone, hypothyroidism, and insulin resistance
- Maximizing therapeutic effects: reconstitute drug according to manufacturer's directions
- Minimizing adverse effects: periodic testing of glucose tolerance, thyroid function, and presence of growth hormone antibodies
- Most significant patient education: proper preparation and storage of medication; proper SC or IM injection technique

Sermorelin (Geref) is an analogue of GHRH that may be used for treatment of idiopathic GH deficiency by stimulating its release from the anterior pituitary. Once-daily dosage of 30 μg/kg is effective in promoting growth in some prepubertal children. Common adverse effects include transient facial flushing and pain at the injection site. Less common adverse effects include headache, dizziness, and hyperactivity.

DRUGS SIGNIFICANTLY DIFFERENT FROM SOMATROPIN

Growth hormone antagonists decrease GH secretion. Almost all conditions of GH hypersecretion are caused by pituitary tumors and are usually treated by radiation therapy or surgery. Pharmacotherapy for GH excess includes two groups of drugs; the somatostatin analogues (octreotide acetate) and the dopamine agonists (bromocriptine) (see Table 39-5). Although an effective GH inhibitor, hypothalamic somatostatin from the hypothalamus is used rarely because of its short initial half-life (1 to 3 minutes) and its multiple effects on many secretory systems (e.g., inhibits release of gastrin, glucagon, insulin).

Octreotide Acetate

Octreotide acetate (Sandostatin) is a more potent GH-inhibiting analogue of somatostatin with less of an inhibitory effect on insulin release. The therapeutic indications for octreotide acetate include pituitary disorders causing excessive secretion of GH (e.g., acromegaly), hyperinsulinemia from insulinomas and secretions from GI endocrine tumors, and carcinoid tumors that cause severe diarrhea (see the accompanying display, Sandostatin LAR Depot Versus Surgery for Treating Acromegaly). Octreotide also may be used to control the severe diarrhea associated with AIDS unresponsive to other treatments.

Unlabeled uses include reduction of output from GI and pancreatic fistulas, control of bleeding varices, irritable bowel syndrome, and dumping syndrome.

The half-life is 1.7 hours with about 32% of the dose excreted unchanged in the urine. In elderly patients, dosage adjustments of octreotide may be necessary due to a 46% increase in the half-life and a 26% decrease in the clearance. In patients with severe renal failure requiring dialysis, octreotide half-life may be increased, also necessitating adjustment of the maintenance dose.

Octreotide mimics the actions of the natural hormone somatostatin. It suppresses GH, serotonin, and several of the gastroenteropancreatic peptides (e.g., gastrin, glucagon, insulin, and secretin).

Mild hypoglycemia or hyperglycemia may occur during therapy. Individuals with acromegaly are especially prone and this may result in overt diabetes mellitus or require dosage changes in insulin or other hypoglycemic agents.

Transient side effects of GI discomfort (e.g., changes in bowel habits—constipation or diarrhea, flatulence, and nausea), headache, sinus bradycardia or other cardiac arrhythmias, and decreased glucose tolerance may occur. Octreotide therapy may cause acute cholecystitis, cholestatic jaundice,

Focus on Research

Sandostatin LAR depot versus surgery for treating acromegaly

National Institute of Diabetes and Digestive and Kidney Diseases (NIDDK). Sandostatin LAR Depot vs. Surgery for Treating Acromegaly.

The Study

The purpose of this study is to compare the efficacy of Sandostatin LAR Depot to transsphenoidal surgery in previously untreated acromegalic patients with macroadenomas. The primary goal is to normalize insulin-like growth factor-1 (IGF-1) levels. Secondary goals are to compare Sandostatin LAR Depot treatment and transsphenoidal surgery to achieve the following goals: suppress growth hormone GH levels to less than or equal to 2.5 ng/mL, relieve the clinical signs and symptoms of acromegaly, reduce the size of the macroadenomas, produce few side effects, assess the prognostic value of baseline pituitary adenoma size, extension and baseline growth hormone level on posttreatment growth hormone and IGF-1 levels, and assess the resource use of each treatment type.

More information about the study can be obtained at *http://clinicalstudies.info.nih.gov.*

Nursing Implications

1. The goal of treatment in acromegaly is to reduce GH and IGF-I levels to normal.
2. Sandostatin LAR Depot can be used in patients for whom surgical resection is not an option.
3. In patients with acromegaly, octreotide reduces GH to within normal ranges in 50% of patients and reduces IGF-I to within normal ranges in 50% to 60% of patients. Because the effects of pituitary irradiation may not become maximal for several years, adjunctive therapy with octreotide to reduce blood levels of growth hormone and IGF-I offers potential benefit before the effects of irradiation are manifested.
4. Octreotide suppresses secretion of thyroid stimulating hormone; patients may develop a hypothyroid state. Baseline and periodic assessment of thyroid function (TSH total or free T_4) is recommended during chronic therapy.
5. Octreotide inhibits gallbladder contractility and decreases bile secretion; the incidence of gallstone or biliary sludge formation is markedly increased.

biliary tract obstruction, or pancreatitis. It frequently causes cholelithiasis unrelated to age, gender, or drug dosage. Dietary fat absorption may be altered in some patients. Periodic fecal fat and serum carotene determinations should be performed to aid in the assessment of possible drug-induced fat malabsorption. It is important to stress the importance of reporting icterus, jaundice, dark urine, or clay-colored stools to the health care provider immediately. The nurse should advise the patient to notify the health care provider of any abdominal pain, edema, chest pain, shortness of breath, or fainting.

Octreotide interacts with cyclosporine and may cause rejection of transplanted organs. Drug and food interactions include alteration of dietary fat absorption of dietary fats, decreased vitamin B12 levels, and abnormal Schilling test results.

Unused drug should be stored in the refrigerator. At room temperature, octreotide is stable for 14 days if protected from light. If refrigerated, the solution should be allowed to warm to room temperature before administration. Octreotide must be administered SC. Therefore, the nurse should teach the patient and family details on sterile technique, injection site rotation, and signs of infection for which to watch. The patient receiving octreotide therapy will require long-term follow-up and regular evaluation for signs of acromegaly and other endocrine dysfunction (e.g., thyroid or insulin resistance), which may require dosage adjustment. The nurse should emphasize the importance of regular follow-up visits with the health care provider. Responsiveness to octreotide therapy may be evaluated by assessment of GH and IGF-1 serum levels.

Bromocriptine Mesylate

Bromocriptine mesylate (Parlodel), a semisynthetic ergot alkaloid, inhibits prolactin secretion with no effect on other pituitary hormones, except in acromegaly, in which it lowers elevated blood levels of GH. It may be used alone or as an adjunct to irradiation. Bromocriptine produces a prompt and sustained reduction in circulating levels of serum GH. It also is used to treat Parkinson disease (see Chapter 22 for a complete drug discussion). Dopamine agonists inhibit GH secretion in some patients with acromegaly; paradoxically, the opposite effect occurs in normal individuals. The GH-inhibiting effect of bromocriptine may be explained by the fact that dopamine increases somatostatin release from the hypothalamus. Unlabeled uses for bromocriptine include the treatment of hyperprolactinemia associated with pituitary adenomas, neuroleptic malignant syndrome, cocaine addiction, and cyclical mastalgia. Bromocriptine is administered orally and it has a substantial hepatic first-pass effect; 28% of an oral dose is absorbed from the GI tract. Bromocriptine undergoes first-pass metabolism and only a small percentage (6%) of the absorbed dose reaches the systemic circulation unchanged. Plasma half-life is 6 to 8 hours. Bromocriptine is highly bound (90% to 96%) to serum albumin. Bromocriptine is metabolized completely before excretion. About 85% of the dose is excreted in the feces and less than 5.5% is excreted in the urine. The major route of excretion of absorbed drug is biliary. Sensitivity to ergot alkaloids, severe ischemic heart disease, or peripheral vascular disease are contraindications to use of bromocriptine. Safe use of bromocriptine has not been demonstrated in pregnancy and use in pregnancy is contraindicated. If pregnancy occurs, treatment should be discontinued immediately and these patients should be observed carefully throughout the pregnancy.

C POSTERIOR PITUITARY HORMONE REGULATORS

The posterior pituitary stores two hormones that are produced in the hypothalamus. These hormones are vasopressin (also known as ADH, which possesses antidiuretic, hemostatic, and vasopressor properties) and oxytocin.

Synthetic analogues of the naturally occurring posterior pituitary hormone, vasopressin, including desmopressin, lypressin, and vasopressin, predominantly are used to treat DI. Oxytocin elicits milk ejection in lactating women and, in pharmacologic doses, can be used to induce or improve uterine contractions in labor (see Chapter 8 for a complete drug discussion). The prototype posterior pituitary hormone is desmopressin acetate. It is the preferred treatment for most individuals with chronic DI because it has a longer duration of action, a more specific antidiuretic action, and an antidiuretic-to-pressor ratio significantly greater than that of vasopressin.

NURSING MANAGEMENT OF THE PATIENT RECEIVING P DESMOPRESSIN

Core Drug Knowledge

Pharmacotherapeutics

For the management of central DI, desmopressin (DDAVP, Stimate) may be administered intranasally, orally, or parenterally (IV or SC). It is ineffective for the treatment of nephrogenic DI, however. Intranasal desmopressin also is effective in managing primary nocturnal enuresis and episodes of spontaneous or trauma-induced bleeding. Administered 2 hours before the procedure, parenteral desmopressin will maintain homeostasis in association with hemophilia A and von Willebrand disease (Type I) during the intraoperative and postoperative periods (see Table 39-5).

An unlabeled use for intranasal desmopressin is treatment of chronic autonomic failure characterized by nocturnal polyuria, overnight weight loss, and morning postural hypotension. There is considerable variability in the intranasal dose of desmopressin required to maintain normal urine volume so that dosage must be tailored individually.

Pharmacokinetics

Administered parenterally, desmopressin has a biphasic half-life—7.8 and 75.5 minutes for the fast and slow phases, respectively. When administered by injection, desmopressin has an antidiuretic effect 10 times that of an equivalent dose administered intranasally. The half-life of the nasal spray is approximately 3.5 hours. Plasma concentrations of the nasal spray are maximal 40 to 45 minutes after dosing. It is metabolized rapidly by the liver and excreted by the kidneys.

Pharmacodynamics

The naturally occurring posterior pituitary hormone, vasopressin (ADH), and its synthetic analogues (desmopressin, lypressin) interact with two types of receptors—V1 receptors and V2 receptors. V1 receptors have a pressor response and V2 receptors have an antidiuretic and hemostatic response. Binding with V1 receptors causes a general vasoconstriction by smooth muscle contraction of most blood vessels. At higher concentrations, ADH interacts with these receptors and this vasoconstriction is marked in the portal and splanchnic vessels, somewhat less in cerebral, coronary, peripheral and pulmonary vessels, and slightly in intrahepatic vessels. GI motility and tone are also enhanced. V2 receptors are found on renal tubule cells and mediate antidiuresis through increased water permeability and water resorption in the renal collecting tubules. Binding with V2 receptors mediates a release and increase in circulating levels of two proteins that are involved in blood coagulation—factor VIII and von Willebrand factor.

Adverse Effects

Most adverse effects are mediated through the V1 receptor acting on vascular and GI smooth muscle. Adverse reactions are less common and severe with desmopressin and frequently disappear with dosage reduction; these include mild abdominal pain, transient headache, nasal congestion, nausea, and rhinitis. The most serious effects, however, are on the coronary circulation. The use of posterior pituitary agonists should be used with extreme caution in individuals with vascular disease, especially coronary artery disease. Other cardiac complications include arrhythmias and decreased cardiac output.

The major V2 receptor-mediated adverse effect is water intoxication. Rare severe allergic reactions have been reported with desmopressin. Allergic reactions, ranging from urticaria to anaphylaxis, may occur. Intranasal administration may cause local adverse effects in the nasal passages such as edema, scarring, rhinorrhea, congestion, irritation, pruritus, and ulceration.

Drug Interactions

Although desmopressin pressor activity is very low, large intranasal or parenteral doses (more than 0.3 µg/kg) should be used cautiously with other pressor agents because of the potential for additive or synergistic effects. Carbamazepine, chlorpropamide, and nonsteroidal anti-inflammatory drugs (NSAIDs) enhance the antidiuretic response to vasopressin; thus, these drugs may potentiate the effects of desmopressin.

Assessment of Relevant Core Patient Variables

Health Status

The nurse should assess for preexisting health conditions that require cautious use of desmopressin. It is important for the nurse to establish a baseline from which to evaluate drug effects. This baseline should include measurements of weight, serum and urine osmolality, and serum sodium. The nurse also should monitor patients carefully for cardiac reactions while taking desmopressin. Posterior pituitary agonists should be used extremely cautiously in patients with vascular disease, especially coronary artery disease, as small doses may precipitate anginal pain and myocardial infarction with larger doses. Desmopressin should be used cautiously in patients with asthma, epilepsy, heart failure, and migraine because these conditions may be further compromised by a rapid rise in extracellular water. Water intoxication may occur; early signs include confusion, drowsiness, listlessness, and headache.

Life Span and Gender

The nurse should assess if the patient is pregnant or breast-feeding. There are no adequate and well-controlled studies in pregnant women and safety and efficacy for use during pregnancy and lactation have not been established. Thus, use in pregnancy and lactation should only occur when the potential benefits outweigh the potential hazards to the fetus.

It is important to note the age of the patient before administering desmopressin. Clinical trials have demonstrated that desmopressin is an effective agent in both adults and children and has few side effects. For the treatment of DI, safety and efficacy of parenteral desmopressin in children (younger than 12 years of age) or intranasal desmopressin in infants (younger than 3 months of age) have not been established. Infants and children, especially, require careful fluid intake restriction to prevent possible hyponatremia and water intoxication. This is likely to cause seizures in children.

Lifestyle, Diet, and Habits and Environment

It is important for the nurse to assess the individual's lifestyle in terms of work, leisure activities, rest patterns, and use of social or recreational drugs. Factors that stimulate ADH secretion include decreased plasma volume, pain, stress, sleep, exercise, and certain drugs (e.g., barbiturates, nicotine, morphine, and vincristine).

Nursing Diagnoses and Outcomes

- Risk for Excessive Fluid Volume related to administration of desmopressin secondary to diabetes insipidus

  Desired outcome: The patient will maintain a urine specific gravity within a normal range and demonstrate no signs and symptoms of water intoxication.
- Risk for Ineffective Therapeutic Regimen Management related to lack of knowledge of diabetes insipidus, management, and signs and symptoms of complications.

  Desired outcome: The patient will describe the disease process, causes, and factors contributing to symptoms, and the regimen for disease or symptom control, relate intent to practice health behaviors needed or desired for disease control and prevention of complications, and relate less anxiety from fear of the unknown and loss of control.

Planning and Intervention

Maximizing Therapeutic Effects

The nurse should establish baseline values for weight, blood pressure, electrolytes, and urine specific gravity. The dosage should be individualized according to the diurnal pattern of water elimination, control of nocturia, and adequate duration of sleep. The nurse should assess periodically the condition of nasal passages during long-term therapy. Inappropriate administration may lead to nasal ulceration and subsequent administered doses may be inadequate as a consequence.

As with all protein preparations, ADH solutions must be protected from temperature extremes (e.g., heat, freezing) and agitation. It is important to refrigerate nasal and parenteral solutions of desmopressin to maintain potency.

Minimizing Adverse Effects

The nurse should assess the patient for preexisting cardiovascular disorders and monitor patients carefully for cardiac reactions from desmopressin. Infants and children, especially, require careful fluid intake restriction to prevent possible hyponatremia and water intoxication. It is important to teach patients that drinking one to two glasses of water with each dose of desmopressin may help to reduce some of the GI effects of the drug.

Severe vasoconstriction and local tissue necrosis may result if desmopressin extravasates during IV infusion. When administering the drug via IV infusion, the nurse should insure patency of venous access, preferably in a larger vein and use an infusion control device.

Providing Patient and Family Education

- The nurse should provide information about antidiuretic drugs, including action, use, adverse effects and drug interactions that may occur. It is important to emphasize to the patient and family that sudden changes in weight, pulse rate, and blood pressure may indicate serious fluid imbalance.
- It is important to caution the patient against consuming alcohol during therapy because alcohol may alter the therapeutic response. Discuss the necessity of reading over-the-counter (OTC) drug labels because alcohol may be found in OTC products. Advise the patient to carry appropriate medical identification to alert medical personnel in case of an emergency.
- The nurse should review with the patient and family or caregiver the proper administration technique for nasally administered dosage forms. Intranasal preparations should not be inhaled. Proper technique may help to lessen the nasal irritation that may occur. Nasal congestion may impair absorption when desmopressin is administered intranasally.
- The nurse should stress the importance of taking the drug as directed and of not stopping it abruptly without first consulting the health care provider.

Ongoing Assessment and Evaluation

The nurse should encourage the patient to monitor urine specific gravity, keep track of intake and output, and weigh daily to observe efficacy of drug therapy. Therapeutic drug response will be observed by decreased urine output and decreased thirst. It is important to assess bowel sounds and presence or absence of flatus if desmopressin is being used for abdominal distention. During prolonged therapy, electrocardiographic (ECG), fluid, and electrolyte status should be monitored at frequent intervals. ■

DRUGS CLOSELY RELATED TO DESMOPRESSIN

Lypressin

Lypressin (Diapid) is a synthetic derivative of vasopressin and acts principally as an ADH. It is used to treat DI. Lypressin possesses little pressor or oxytocic activity. It is a short-acting nasal spray that has a prompt onset of action, a duration of activity of 3 to 8 hours, and minimal cardiovascular pressor effects when administered in therapeutic doses. Large doses may cause coronary artery constriction. Safety of lypressin use during pregnancy and lactation has not been established.

Nasal congestion, allergic rhinitis, or upper respiratory tract infections may decrease lypressin effectiveness because of decreased absorption by the nasal mucosa and larger doses may be required. Infrequent and mild adverse effects include localized ones of rhinorrhea, nasal congestion, irritation, and pruritus, and systemic ones of headache, conjunctivitis, and heartburn secondary to excessive intranasal use.

MEMORY CHIP

Desmopressin

- Synthetic analogue of human ADH; for treatment of neurogenic diabetes insipidus
- Significant contraindications: presence of hemophilia A with factor VIII levels 5% or less
- Most common adverse effects: localized erythema with intranasal administration; burning pain with parenteral injection
- **Life span alert: infants, children, and the elderly require careful fluid intake restriction to prevent possible hyponatremia and water intoxication**
- Maximizing therapeutic effects: keep solutions (nasal, parenteral) refrigerated
- Minimizing adverse effects: monitor urine volume/osmolality, plasma osmolality; patients with conditions associated with fluid/electrolyte imbalances are prone to hyponatremia
- Most significant patient education: inform patients that medication bottle accurately delivers 25 to 50 doses and any solution remaining after 25 to 50 doses should be discarded because the amount delivered thereafter may be substantially less than prescribed. The remaining solution should not be transferred to another bottle.

Terlipressin

Terlipressin (Glypressin) has orphan-drug status for the treatment of bleeding esophageal varices.

Vasopressin

Diabetes insipidus resulting from a partial or complete deficiency in the production and secretion of posterior pituitary ADH may be effectively treated with synthetic vasopressin (Pitressin). Vasopressin also may be used to prevent or treat postoperative abdominal distention, and to facilitate abdominal radiography (see Table 39-5).

An unlabeled use of vasopressin is the management of bleeding esophageal varices. Synthetic vasopressin aqueous solution has a plasma half-life of 10 to 20 minutes following SC, IM, or IV injection and the duration of antidiuretic activity is 2 to 8 hours. It is metabolized rapidly by the liver and is excreted by the kidneys.

Use of vasopressin is contraindicated in hypersensitivity or chronic nephritis with increased levels of blood urea nitrogen (BUN). Vasopressin is pregnancy category C and its effect on lactation is unknown. The literature reports that vasopressin, used during pregnancy in doses sufficient for an antidiuretic effect, is not likely to produce tonic uterine contractions that could be harmful to the fetus or threaten the continuation of the pregnancy.

THYROID DRUGS

Thyroid hormones influence essentially every organ system in the body with numerous biologic effects, including stimulation of the basal metabolic rate, which affects protein, carbohydrate, and lipid metabolism. Thyroid hormones are essential for normal growth and development for the entire life cycle. The thyroid gland, like most endocrine glands, can secrete too much hormone (HRT) or too little hormone (HOT).

Thyroid disorders generally involve an alteration in the quantity of thyroid hormone secretion and/or enlargement of the thyroid gland (goiter) and are classified as either HRT or HOT.

The prevalence of HRT (also known as thyrotoxicosis) and HOT are similar—approximately 2% of women and 0.2% of men are affected. The incidence of HOT increases with age; over the age of 60, 6% of women and 2.5% of men have TSH levels greater than twice the upper limit of normal. In some cases HOT may be mistaken for the normal aging process (Haupt, 2000).

THYROID HORMONES

Thyroid hormones are the only treatment for HOT, and treatment usually involves life-long replacement of thyroid hormone adequate to meet the individual's metabolic needs. HOT can be corrected completely by a number of pharmacologic preparations of endogenous thyroid hormone, including levothyroxine, thyroid dessicated, liothyronine, and liotrix. Levothyroxine (T_4; Levothroid, Synthroid) is the preferred treatment for HOT and is used almost universally.

NURSING MANAGEMENT OF THE PATIENT RECEIVING LEVOTHYROXINE

Core Drug Knowledge

Pharmacotherapeutics

Levothyroxine (T_4) is used as replacement therapy in HOT. It also may be used for pituitary suppression of TSH in the treatment and prevention of euthyroid goiter, in the management of HOT secondary to thyroid cancer, and as a treatment for myxedema coma. T_4 also may used in conjunction with antithyroid drugs to prevent goiter formation, HOT, and thyrotoxicosis during pregnancy (Table 39-6).

Pharmacokinetics

Levothyroxine is well absorbed from the GI tract and absorption is increased in an empty stomach. It must be converted to triiodothyronine (T_3) for its clinical effects, however. When given orally, the onset of effect occurs very slowly with the peak effect occurring in 1 to 3 weeks. When given IV to treat myxedema coma, the onset of effect is 6 to 8 hours with a peak effect in 24 to 48 hours. The half-life of T_4 is 6 to 7 days. Levothyroxine is metabolized in the liver and excreted in the bile. It crosses the placenta and enters breast milk.

Pharmacodynamics

Levothyroxine acts as replacement for natural thyroid hormone. It increases the basal metabolic rate of body tissues, thereby increasing oxygen consumption, respiration, heart rate, rate of fat, protein and carbohydrate metabolism, and growth and maturation.

Contraindications and Precautions

Levothyroxine is FDA pregnancy category A and is safe for maintaining and regulating thyroid function during pregnancy. It should be used with caution in lactating women because it crosses into breast milk and can affect the infant's thyroid-pituitary balance. It also should be used with caution in patients with CAD or coronary insufficiency because the resulting increase in basal metabolic rate may aggravate angina pectoris because of the increased myocardial oxygen demand. Use of T_4 in cardiovascular disease should be initiated at a low dosage and titrated upward gradually.

Levothyroxine is contraindicated in hypersensitivity; in thyrotoxicosis, in which T_4 would further aggravate the signs and symptoms of thyroid overactivity, and in acute myocardial infarction (MI) complicated by HOT in which the metabolic stimulating effects of T_4 could extend the MI, cause arrhythmias, and lead to further complications. Patients with adrenocortical insufficiency (e.g., Addison disease) should first be stabilized on corticosteroid therapy before adding T_4 to the therapeutic regimen.

Adverse Effects

Adverse effects observed with the use of thyroxine include the signs and symptoms of HRT (e.g., hypertension, tachycardia, hyperreflexia, anxiety, and increased sweating). Allergic reactions, including rash and dermatologic lesions, also may occur. Alopecia may occur in the first few months of treatment.

Drug Interactions

There is an increased risk of bleeding if T_4 is given with anticoagulants; bleeding times (e.g., international normalized ratio, prothrombin time [PT], partial thrombo-

TABLE 39-6 Summary of Selected Thyroid Hormones

Drug (Trade) Name	Selected Indications	Route and Dosage Range	Pharmacokinetics
levothyroxine (L-thyroxine; Synthroid, Levothroid)	Replacement therapy for hypothyroidism, including cretinism	*Adult:* PO, 50–200 μg/d *Child:* PO, 0–6 mo, 8–10 μg/kg/d; 6–12 mo, 6–8 μg/kg/d; 1–5 y, 5–6 μg/kg/d; 6–12 y, 4–5 μg/kg/d; over 12 y, 2–3 μg/kg/d	*Onset:* Slow *Duration:* 3 wk $t_{1/2}$: 2–7 d
	Emergency treatment of myxedema coma	*Adult:* IV, 0.2–0.5 mg in solution of 0.1 mg/mL	
thyroid dessicated (T_3 and T_4; Armour Thyroid)	Same as above	*Adult:* PO, 16 mg/d for 2 wk, increasing to 32 mg/d for 2 wk, then 65 mg/d to a maximum of 195 mg/d *Child:* PO, 4 mg/kg/d up to 65 mg/kg/d for cretinism	*Onset:* Slow *Duration:* 3 wk $t_{1/2}$: 2–7 d
liothyronine (T_3; Cytomel, Triostat)	Same as above	*Adult:* PO, 25 μg/d increase every 1–2 wk by 12.5–25 μg; maintenance, 25–75 μg/d *Child (and elderly adult:)* PO, 5–50 μg/d	*Onset:* Varies *Duration:* 3–4 d $t_{1/2}$: 1–2 d
liotrix (T_4 and T_3; Thyrolar)	Same as above	*Adult:* PO, 15–30 mg/d increase every 2 wk to a maximum of 60–120 mg/d	*Onset:* Slow *Duration:* 3 wk $t_{1/2}$: 2–7 d

plastin time [PTT]) should be monitored closely, and the anticoagulant dosage may need adjustment. Digitalis levels may be reduced when given with T_4. If this combination of drugs is used, the serum digoxin levels should be monitored closely and appropriate dosage adjustments made. Beta-adrenergic blockers and theophylline effects may be altered as the individual returns to a euthyroid state. If these drugs are given in combination with T_4, the patient should be monitored closely, and dosage of the theophylline or beta-blockers should be adjusted as needed (Table 39-7). Medicinal or dietary iodine interferes with all in vivo tests of radioactive iodine uptake thus reflecting a false decrease in hormone synthesis.

Certain drugs may interfere with thyroid hormone absorption or metabolism. Antilipemic agents (e.g., cholestyramine, lovastatin), aluminum-containing antacids, ferrous sulfate, and sucralfate may inhibit absorption. Administration of these drugs should be separated by a four or five hour interval from the administration of T_4. Some anti-epileptic drugs (phenytoin, carbamazepine), amiodarone, or rifampin may require an adjustment in T_4 dosage because these agents may affect drug metabolism. Dosages of oral anticoagulants, insulin, oral hypoglycemic agents, cardiac glycosides, tricyclic antidepressants, catecholamines, and sympathomimetic agents may require adjustment when a client is started on thyroid replacement or when the dosage is changed to avoid serious adverse consequences.

Assessment of Relevant Core Patient Variables

Health Status

Before administering T_4, the nurse should review the patient's record to determine whether the drug can be administered safely. It is important that the nurse perform a physical examination to establish a baseline from which to monitor the effects of the drug. The nurse should note skin color, temperature, texture, and presence of any lesions to monitor for allergic reactions and to assess thyroid hormone effectiveness. It also is important to note muscle tone, weight, temperature, blood pressure, pulse, and respirations to assess for the desired therapeutic effects of T_4 and to monitor for toxic or adverse effects. The nurse should make sure that thyroid function tests, ECGs, and serum laboratory analyses are done as a baseline for dosage and response to the drug.

Individuals with a known cardiac problem should begin drug therapy with a smaller dose of thyroid hormone replacement due to the cardiac stimulant effect of T_4. The nurse should carefully monitor the individual for angina and cardiac arrhythmias.

Life Span and Gender

It is important to determine the patient's age before administering T_4. The nurse should begin geriatric patients on low dosages of thyroid hormone replacement with gradual dosage increases to prevent serious cardiovascular and neurologic adverse effects. The T_4 dose should be held if the pulse rate is over 100. It is important to monitor closely elderly patients who are receiving beta-blockers or digitalis glycosides because of the potential for increased toxic effects. Long-term T_4 therapy has been associated with decreased bone density in the hip and spine in premenopausal and postmenopausal women. It may be beneficial to obtain a basal bone density measurement and then monitor closely for development of osteoporosis.

It is important to monitor children for growth and development when maintained on T_4. It also is important to monitor for toxic effects of the drug because children are more susceptible to them. The nurse should be aware that the dosage will need to be adjusted as the child grows.

The nurse should assess the patient for pregnancy. Pregnant patients who are receiving thyroid hormone replacement may require a dosage increase during pregnancy; thyroid hormone deficiency may have an adverse

TABLE 39-7 Agents That Interact With P Levothyroxine

Interactants	Effect and Significance	Nursing Management
cholestyramine and colestipol	Loss of efficacy of thyroid hormone; potential for hypothyroidism	Monitor thyroid hormone levels closely; administer drugs 4–6 h apart.
anticoagulants	Increased effect of anticoagulant; bleeding problems possible	Monitor INR, PT, PTT tests closely; assess patient for signs of overt or occult bleeding Anticoagulant dose may need adjustment.
beta-adrenergic blockers	Actions of beta blockers possibly blocked as patient returns to euthyroid state	Assess for decreased beta blocking action; consider alternative therapy or increased beta blocker dose.
digitalis glycosides	Reduced serum levels of digitalis and decreased therapeutic effects	Evaluate serum digoxin levels; adjust dose as needed for therapeutic effects.
theophylline	Increased theophylline levels as patient reaches euthyroid state and normal theophylline clearance	Monitor serum theophylline levels closely; increase dose as needed to maintain therapeutic levels.

effect on fetal nervous system development and on the outcome of the pregnancy.

Lifestyle, Diet, and Habits and Environment

The nurse should assess the patient's ability to adapt to a long-term drug regimen. Patients maintained on T_4 will most likely be taking the drug for life. They will need to establish a routine to take the drug daily; it is best taken as a single daily dose, preferably before breakfast.

T_4 is usually given in the home. Caution the individual to avoid changing from one brand of this drug to another without consulting the pharmacist or health care provider. Products manufactured by different companies may not be equally effective and bioavailability differences have occurred with different preparations of T_4. IV T_4 is reserved for cases of myxedema coma and is only used for a short time until the patient is able to switch to the oral drug.

Nursing Diagnoses and Outcomes

- Imbalanced Nutrition: More Than Body Requirements related to dietary intake in excess of metabolic demands secondary to hypothyroidism

  Desired outcome: *The patient will describe reasons why weight gain may occur, discuss nutritional needs related to age, lifestyle and diagnosis, and discuss the effects of exercise and diet on weight control.*
- Risk For Injury related to adverse drug reactions

  Desired outcome: *The patient will not demonstrate adverse reactions to thyroid hormone replacement.*
- Risk For Injury related to pre-existing health status that requires cautious use of a thyroid agent

  Desired outcome: *The patient exhibits no complications of pre-existing health conditions linked to the prescribed thyroid hormone replacement therapy; for example, coronary artery disease, angina, myocardial infarction, and hypertension because of increased metabolic demands on the heart and acute adrenal crisis because thyroid agents increase tissue demand for adrenal hormones.*
- Deficient Knowledge related to thyroid dysfunction and the necessity for thyroid hormone replacement

  Desired outcome: *The patient and family express an accurate understanding of the teaching regarding the disease process and the prescribed thyroid hormone replacement therapy; for example, avoidance of myxedema coma from interrupted drug therapy.*

Planning and Intervention

Maximizing Therapeutic Effects

Replacement therapy is to be taken for life. Taken as a single daily dose on an empty stomach, preferably before breakfast, T_4 absorption is increased. During drug therapy, the nurse should monitor cardiovascular response and serum thyroid function tests to determine the appropriate dosage and response to T_4. The nurse should regularly monitor children to assess the need to change dosage to allow for appropriate growth and development. If the patient is on other drugs, the response to these drugs and to T_4 should be monitored periodically, especially as the patient achieves a euthyroid state. The nurse should offer support and encouragement to deal with the need for lifelong therapy.

Minimizing Adverse Effects

Young adults who have no evidence of coronary artery disease can usually begin a full replacement dose of T_4. Older individuals and those with or at risk for coronary artery disease and/or atrial arrhythmias should begin low doses (e.g., 25 to 50 μg/day) with a slow upward titration of the dosage.

It is important to check adrenal function in hypothyroid clients because some of these individuals also will have adrenal insufficiency. Without appropriate glucocorticoid replacement in these individuals, institution of thyroid replacement can precipitate an acute adrenal crisis because thyroid agents increase tissue demand for adrenal hormones.

Thyroid agents may potentiate the hypoprothrombinemic effect of oral anticoagulants by increasing the catabolism of vitamin K. Administration of thyroid agents to diabetic patients may cause an increase in the required dosage of insulin or oral agent.

Providing Patient and Family Education

- The nurse should explain to patients and their families that this drug is a hormone that is being used to replace the thyroid hormone that their body is not able to produce (see the accompanying display, Levothyroxine and Weight Control). This hormone is responsible for regulating the body's metabolism or

Critical Thinking Scenario

Levothyroxine and weight control

A woman comes to the clinic and asks for a prescription for thyroid hormone. She has tried multiple diets without success and is convinced that she must have a "glandular" problem. She tells you that she read that thyroid hormone is an effective way to lose weight because it increases your metabolism, and she wants to try it. After obtaining thyroid function tests, it is determined that this patient has normal thyroid function.

1. Think about the problems that could occur if thyroid replacement hormone is given to a euthyroid patient. Outline the normal controls of thyroid activity, and predict what could happen.
2. Develop a patient education tool to explain this situation to the patient, and propose other ways of dealing with her weight problem.

the speed with which the body's cells burn energy. The nurse should explain that this drug will most likely need to be taken for life and that it should be taken every day, preferably at the same time each day.
- The nurse should explain that there are few adverse effects to this drug but that the patient should report any skin rash or lesions and any increase in the symptoms of thyroid dysfunction, such as weight changes, nervousness, skin changes, lethargy, and sleeplessness.
- The nurse should advise patients to avoid over-the-counter (OTC) drugs and to check with the health care provider if they feel they are needed.
- Because many of these drugs contain ingredients that interfere with thyroid function, patients may want to obtain a medical identification tag or card so that people taking care of them in an emergency are aware of the need for this drug.
- The nurse should tell patients to keep this drug out of the reach of children.
- It is a good idea to stress the importance of notifying the health care provider if manifestations of HRT (e.g., headache, nervousness, chest pain, palpitations, increased pulse rate, diarrhea, diaphoresis, heat intolerance) occur.

Ongoing Assessment and Evaluation

The nurse should monitor serum thyroid hormone levels periodically. As a patient reaches a euthyroid state, the nurse should reassess the potential for drug interactions and the need to adjust the dosage of other drugs appropriately. It is important to monitor pulse rate and rhythm and respiratory rate to assess the effect of the thyroid hormone on these systems and possible need for dosage adjustment. Medications are administered to the patient with HOT very cautiously because of altered metabolism and excretion and depressed metabolic rate and respiratory status.

Long-term use of T_4 may cause decreases in hip and spine bone density in women. Bone density should be measured before beginning T_4 therapy to establish a baseline and then should be monitored routinely.

Thyroid hormones may increase blood glucose levels, which may necessitate adjustment in doses of insulin or oral hypoglycemic agents for diabetic patients. HOT patients are characterized by an increased susceptibility to all hypnotic and sedative agents, analgesics, and anesthetics. These drugs, even in small doses, may induce profound somnolence lasting far longer than anticipated. Respiratory depression is likely as a result of the decreased respiratory reserve and alveolar hypoventilation that occur with HOT.

As the patient moves from a hypothyroid to a euthyroid state, the body's response to many drugs may be changed. Patients on multiple drugs should be monitored closely as they return to a euthyroid state and dosages of the other drugs may require adjustment. For example, the actions of some beta-adrenergic blockers may be impaired, serum digitalis levels may be reduced with a reduced therapeutic effectiveness of digitalis glycosides, and theophylline clearance will be altered. Nursing management of drug therapy is considered effective if the patient adheres successfully to drug therapy, can recognize various signs and symptoms of HOT, and seeks appropriate attention from the health care provider. ■

DRUGS CLOSELY RELATED TO LEVOTHYROXINE

Desiccated Thyroid

Desiccated thyroid (Armour Thyroid) is composed of desiccated bovine and porcine thyroid glands and is much less pure, stable, and predictable than synthetic preparations of thyroid hormone. The active thyroid hormones (T_4 and T_3) are available in their natural state and at their natural ratio. Although these preparations are cheapest, their standardization by iodine content or bioassay is inexact. Optimal dosage is determined by the patient's clinical response and laboratory findings. Therapy is instituted using low doses, with increments that depend on cardiovascular status. The usual starting dose is 30 mg, with increments of 15 mg every 2 to 3 weeks. However, a lower dose (15 mg/day) is used in patients with long-standing myxedema, particularly if cardiovascular impairment is suspected. The drug dosage should be reduced if angina occurs. These natural products, desiccated thyroid and thyroglobulin, are derived from beef or pork. Although these preparations are most economical, standardization by iodine content or bioassay is inexact.

Liothyronine Sodium

Liothyronine sodium (Cytomel [PO form]; Triostat [parenteral form]) is a synthetic form of the natural thyroid hormone T_3, has pharmacologic activities of the natural

MEMORY CHIP

Levothyroxine

- Synthetic thyroid hormone replacement
- Significant contraindications: acute myocardial infarction, thyrotoxicosis; use cautiously in hypoadrenalism
- Most common adverse effects: symptoms of hyperthyroidism, alopecia with initial therapy (particularly in children)
- Maximizing therapeutic effects: monitor drug response carefully at the start of therapy; administer oral drug as a single daily dose before breakfast
- Minimizing adverse effects: monitor cardiac response as increased basal metabolic rate may exacerbate angina pectoris
- Most significant patient education: have patient wear medical ID (tag or bracelet) to alert emergency medical personnel of drug therapy

hormone, and has a short duration of activity that permits quick dosage adjustment and facilitates control of overdosage. It can be used in patients allergic to thyroid extract derived from pork or beef. Liothyronine injection is for IV use only—not IM or SC—and should be stored between 2 and 8°C (36 to 46°F).

Liotrix

Liotrix (Thyrolar) is a uniform mixture of synthetic T_4 and T_3 in a 4:1 ratio by weight. Optimal dosage is determined by patient's clinical response and laboratory findings.

ANTITHYROID COMPOUNDS

The pharmacotherapeutic antithyroid compounds used clinically to manage HRT include the thioamide drug class, radioactive iodine (I-131), and iodides (Lugol solution). PTU, a thioamide drug, is the prototype antithyroid compound.

NURSING MANAGEMENT OF THE PATIENT RECEIVING PROPYLTHIOURACIL

Core Drug Knowledge

Pharmacotherapeutics

The usual therapeutic regimens to treat HRT are thyroid-hormone-antagonist drugs to inhibit thyroid secretion, surgery, or radioactive iodine to reduce the amount of functional thyroid tissue. Drugs in the thioamide class are used in the palliative treatment of HRT, as adjunct therapy in preparation for surgery (thyroidectomy) or radioactive iodine therapy, and to control thyrotoxic crises that may complicate thyroidectomy. PTU also is used when thyroidectomy is contraindicated or not advisable. An unlabeled use for PTU is in the management of alcoholism-associated liver disease; 300 mg/day appears helpful in reducing the hypermetabolic state induced by alcohol (Table 39-8).

Pharmacokinetics

Propylthiouracil is well absorbed from the GI tract. The onset of action varies between 10 and 21 days, and the effect lasts for weeks. The half-life of PTU is 1 to 2 hours. PTU is metabolized in the liver and excreted in the urine. PTU is highly protein bound (80%) and must be administered twice or three times daily around the clock. PTU is metabolized in the liver and excreted in the urine.

Pharmacodynamics

Propylthiouracil inhibits thyroid synthesis by interfering with the incorporation of iodine within thyroglobulin, inhibiting the formation of iodothyronine, and inhibiting the peripheral tissue conversion of T_4 to T_3. PTU does not, however, deactivate the existing T_4 to T_3 stored in the thyroid or circulating in the blood and it has no effect on exogenous thyroid hormones. Because the synthesis rather than the release of hormones is affected, the onset of action is rather slow—often requiring 3 to 4 weeks before stores of T_4 are depleted.

There is some clinical evidence suggesting the thioamide drugs have immunosuppressant effects. Thus, they are beneficial for suppressing the immune-mediated HRT of Graves disease.

Contraindications and Precautions

Propylthiouracil is contraindicated with any known allergies to antithyroid drugs.

TABLE 39-8 Summary of Selected Antithyroid Drugs

Drug (Trade) Name	Selected Indications	Route and Dosage Range	Pharmacokinetics
propylthiouracil (PTU)	Treatment of hyperthyroidism Attain euthyroid state before thyroidectomy, radioactive iodine therapy	*Adult:* Initial dose, PO, 300–900 mg/d maintenance; PO, 100–130 mg/d *Child:* PO, 6–10 y, 50–150 mg/d; ≥ 10 y, 150–300 mg/d; maintenance, based on response	*Onset:* 10–21 d *Duration:* Weeks $t_{1/2}$:1–2 h
methimazole (Tapazole)	Treatment of hyperthyroidism Amelioration of hyperthyroidism before thyroidectomy, radioactive iodine	*Adult:* PO, 15 mg/d for mild hyperthyroidism; 30–40 mg/d for moderate hyperthyroidism; 60 mg/d for severe hypothyroidism *Child:* PO, 0.4 mg/kg/d; maintenance, ½ initial dose	*Onset:* 1 wk *Duration:* Weeks $t_{1/2}$: 5–13 h
sodium iodide I-131 (Iodotope, Sodium iodide I-131 [therapeutic])	Treatment of hyperthyroidism, thyroid cancer	*Adult:* PO, hyperthyroidism, 4–10 mCi; thyroid cancer, 50 mCi; then 100–150 mCi as needed	*Onset:* Rapid *Duration:* Unknown $t_{1/2}$: 7.61 d
strong iodine solution (Lugol solution, Thyro-Block)	Treatment of hyperthyroidism Expectorant	*Adult:* PO, 2–6 drops tid	*Onset:* 24–48 h *Duration:* 6 wk $t_{1/2}$: Unknown

Adverse Effects

Adverse effects occur in fewer than 1% of treated patients. The most common adverse effects include paresthesias, vertigo, drowsiness, pruritic skin rash, hypoprothrombinemia, bleeding, nausea, and epigastric distress. PTU may cause a transient increase in liver transaminase levels; these elevations require close monitoring but are not indications to discontinue use of the drug. Jaundice may occur and may persist for several weeks after discontinuing the drug. The most serious adverse reactions associated with PTU are hepatitis and an idiosyncratic agranulocytosis. Not considered to be dose related, agranulocytosis usually develops suddenly within the first 3 months of therapy. The incidence of agranulocytosis varies from 0.3% to 0.6% and the risk appears to be higher in individuals over 40 years of age and in doses of 900 to 1200 mg/day (Haupt, 2000).

Drug Interactions

Propylthiouracil exerts an anti-vitamin K effect. Thus, increased anticoagulant effect may be seen if PTU and oral anticoagulants are taken concomitantly. Patients receiving this combination need to be monitored closely for signs of bleeding, and the anticoagulant dosage may need to be adjusted accordingly.

Assessment of Relevant Core Patient Variables

Health Status

Before administering PTU, the nurse should review the patient's record to determine whether the drug can be administered safely. PTU is contraindicated during pregnancy and in patients with a known allergy to antithyroid drugs. The nurse should use caution when administering the drug to a woman who is lactating.

Before beginning drug therapy, the nurse should perform a physical examination to establish a baseline to monitor the drug's effects. The nurse should note skin color, temperature, texture, and presence of any lesions to monitor for allergic reactions and to assess thyroid hormone effectiveness. It also is important to review liver and renal function tests because the drug is metabolized in the liver and excreted in the urine. A complete blood count (CBC) with differential should be done as a baseline for potential hematologic changes that can occur during therapy. In addition, thyroid function tests should be performed to monitor the effect of the drug on thyroid function.

Life Span and Gender

The nurse should determine whether the patient is pregnant or breast-feeding. The nurse should counsel women of childbearing age to avoid pregnancy while using this drug because serious fetal effects can occur. PTU is FDA pregnancy category D. An effective drug in HRT complicated by pregnancy, it crosses the placenta and can induce goiter (approximately 10% of patients will develop neonatal goiter) and even cretinism in the developing fetus. In many pregnant women, the thyroid dysfunction diminishes as the pregnancy proceeds, thus making a reduction of dose possible. In some instances, these products can be withdrawn 2 or 3 weeks before delivery. Postpartum patients receiving antithyroid preparations should not nurse their babies. However, if necessary, the preferred drug is PTU.

The nurse also should note the patient's age before administering PTU. Hepatotoxicity has occurred in some pediatric patients. The nurse should monitor children closely to ensure that thyroid function is maintained and that growth and development proceed normally. Dosage adjustment may be needed with prolonged use.

Lifestyle, Diet, and Habits and Environment

The nurse should assess the patient's ability to adapt to a long-term drug regimen. Patients on PTU may require prolonged therapy to achieve full effectiveness. The drug needs to be taken every 8 hours around the clock. The nurse should help the patient establish a schedule that will cause the least interference with the patient's sleep pattern. Weakness, drowsiness, and vertigo are frequent effects of this drug. Therefore, the nurse should caution the patient to avoid driving or performing tasks that require precision and alertness if these effects occur.

This drug is usually given in the home. The nurse should teach patients the importance of taking the drug around the clock and the necessity of making special arrangements in their schedule and routine to facilitate this need.

Nursing Diagnoses and Outcomes

- Imbalanced Nutrition: Less Than Body Requirements related to increased metabolic demands secondary to hypothyroidism

  Desired outcome: The patient will describe reasons why weight loss may occur and discuss nutritional needs related to age, lifestyle, and diagnosis.
- Risk For Injury related to blood dyscrasias (e.g., agranulocytosis) or related to drowsiness, dizziness, vertigo secondary to adverse reactions of PTU

  Desired outcome: The patient will demonstrate no adverse hematologic reactions to thyroid therapy (e.g., hypoprothrombinemia, bleeding), identify factors that increase the risk from injury (e.g., from CNS side effects), relate intentions to practice and use safety measures to prevent injury.
- Noncompliance related to long-term use of the antithyroid agent.

  Desired outcome: The patient will describe the reasons for the therapeutic regimen, identify barriers to adhering to the regimen and identify the behaviors desired to change to facilitate compliance.

Planning and Intervention

Maximizing Therapeutic Effects

The nurse should ensure around-the-clock administration of the drug with administration of three equal doses at 8-hour intervals to maintain serum concentration. Fluid intake of 3 to 4 L/day should be encouraged unless contraindicated. PTU may be given with meals to minimize GI irritation.

Minimizing Adverse Effects

During drug therapy, the nurse should arrange for periodic blood tests to monitor for hematologic and thyroid functions. The nurse also should arrange for frequent, small meals to alleviate GI symptoms and to help maintain nutrition while the patient is taking PTU. The nurse should provide side rails and adequate lighting to prevent falls and injury. It also is important to encourage the patient to avoid driving or performing hazardous tasks if drowsiness, dizziness, vertigo, and paresthesias occur. Monitor the patient's bone marrow function. It is important to obtain a baseline assessment of the CBC with a differential. The nurse should emphasize the importance of regular follow-up care and the monitoring of bone marrow, CBC, and thyroid functions at regular intervals.

Providing Patient and Family Education

- The nurse should explain to patients and their families that this drug is an antithyroid drug that blocks the production and activity of the thyroid hormone. This hormone is responsible for regulating the body's metabolism, that is, the speed with which the body's cells burn energy. The nurse should explain that this drug will most likely need to be taken for a prolonged time to achieve the desired effect.
- The drug must be taken every 8 hours around the clock. The nurse should work with patients and the family to establish a schedule that will cause the least interference with sleep.
- The nurse should explain that because adverse effects of this drug include dizziness, drowsiness, numbness, and tingling, the patient should avoid driving or performing hazardous tasks while on this drug and should take extra precautions to prevent falls and injuries.
- Other adverse effects include nausea, vomiting, and epigastric distress. The nurse should suggest small, frequent meals to maintain nutrition and alleviate some of the discomfort associated with these adverse effects.
- The nurse should tell patients that they will need to have periodic blood tests while on this drug to monitor its effectiveness and possible adverse effects. The nurse should stress the importance of reporting fever, sore throat, unusual bleeding or bruising, and headache to the health care provider.
- It is important to tell patients to keep this drug out of the reach of children.

Ongoing Assessment and Evaluation

The nurse should monitor serum thyroid hormone levels periodically to evaluate the effectiveness of the drug and to assess for the need for replacement thyroid hormone as the thyroid gland is suppressed. With continued antithyroid therapy, an insidious goitrogenic HOT may appear. The nurse should alert the patient to watch for signs of this, such as decreased cardiac rate, intolerance to cold, and weight gain. Thyroid function tests are used to evaluate drug therapy and these should be measured routinely (every 4 to 6 weeks). It is important to review periodically the signs of HOT and HRT with the patient and significant others. As the patient reaches euthyroid state, the nurse should assess the need for dosage adjustment with drugs affected by metabolic rate and activity. Therapy is evaluated as successful when normal thyroid status is maintained, and the patient can verbalize and demonstrate self-monitoring techniques. ■

DRUG CLOSELY RELATED TO P PROPYLTHIOURACIL

Methimazole (Tapazole) is a thioamide with similar characteristics to PTU. Hematologic effects are more common with this drug, and the patient needs to have CBC and differentials monitored regularly. GI effects are somewhat less pronounced with this drug, and it may be a drug of choice in patients unable to tolerate PTU. It has a longer half-life so that once-daily dosing is possible. In contrast to PTU, methimazole 0% protein bound and has high transfer across the

MEMORY CHIP

P Prophylthiouracil (PTU)

- Inhibits the synthesis of thyroid hormones; antithyroid agent
- Significant contraindications: pregnancy or lactation; may induce hypothyroidism or cretinism in fetus
- Most common adverse effects: paresthesias, GI (nausea, vomiting, epigastric pain), and urticaria
- Most serious adverse effects: hepatitis, exfoliative dermatitis, agranulocytosis, hypoprothrombinemia
- Maximizing therapeutic effects: administer drug around the clock at 8-hour intervals
- Minimizing adverse effects: periodic blood tests to assess bone marrow depression and bleeding tendencies
- Most significant patient education: drug must be taken for a prolonged period to achieve the desired effects (months); report fever, sore throat, unusual bleeding or bruising, and malaise

placental membrane and secretion into breast milk. Cholestatic jaundice is an infrequent, but serious adverse reaction. Agranulocytosis may occur and the drug should be discontinued; it is considered to be a dose-related effect.

DRUGS SIGNIFICANTLY DIFFERENT FROM P PROPYLTHIOURACIL

Iodine-131

Iodine-131 (radioactive iodine) is the most common and preferred treatment for HRT. It also is effective in treating thyroid cancer. While destroying thyroid tissue, it exposes only the thyroid tissue to the altering radiation, eliminates the problems of surgery, and allows outpatient treatment. The goal of therapy with radioactive iodine is to affect enough thyroid tissue to achieve euthyroidism; however, HOT and the requirement for temporary or lifelong thyroid hormone replacement therapy may result.

The total amount needed to achieve a clinical remission of HRT without destruction of the entire gland varies widely. The average single dose administered is 10 to 15 mCi, but doses of 25 to 29 mCi are not unusual and dosage for thyroid carcinoma may range from 50 to 200 mCi.

The exposure level around a patient treated with I-131 depends on the dose given, the time elapsed following treatment, and the amount absorbed by thyroid tissue. Hospital radiation-safety protocols (based on the U.S. Nuclear Regulatory Commission regulations for radiopharmaceutical therapy) must be followed strictly during the hospitalization. Radioactive iodine therapy is considered safe. Some individuals, particularly the elderly, may be treated with antithyroid drugs prior to I-131 therapy to minimize the risk of exacerbating the HRT.

I-131 has orphan-drug status for detection of hepatocellular carcinoma, hepatoblastoma, and alpha-fetoprotein-producing germ-cell tumors; detection of tumors that produce human chorionic gonadotropin; adrenal cortical imaging; B-cell lymphomas and leukemias; and as a diagnostic adjunct in pheochromocytoma.

I-131 is absorbed readily from the GI tract and distributed primarily within the extracellular fluid of the body. It is trapped and rapidly converted to protein-bound iodine by the thyroid, concentrated by the stomach and salivary glands and excreted within several days principally through the urine. The physical half-life of I-131 is 8.5 days. Biotransformed I-131 becomes nonradioactive xenon-131.

I-131 is FDA pregnancy category X and is contraindicated for pregnant or lactating women because it crosses the placenta, is distributed into breast milk, and destroys the fetal thyroid gland. It also is contraindicated in pre-existing vomiting because if the patient vomits during the first few hours after therapy, the vomitus will be highly radioactive.

The immediate adverse reactions following treatment I-131 treatment for HRT are usually mild but may be more severe following larger doses such as those used in thyroid carcinoma. Depression of the hematopoietic system and signs of radiation sickness may occur. Manifestations may include bone marrow depression, acute leukemia, anemia, thrombocytopenia, nausea, and vomiting. Itching of the skin, rash, and hives also may occur. Tenderness and swelling around the neck area, pain on swallowing, sore throat, and cough may occur 72 hours after treatment. These manifestations usually respond to treatment with analgesics.

The uptake of I-131 will be affected by recent intake of iodine in any form, and thyroid and antithyroid agents. Antithyroid therapy (e.g., propylthiouracil) of a severely hyperthyroid patient is usually discontinued 3 to 4 days before administration of I-131.

I-131 is not usually used for the treatment of HRT in patients younger than 30 years of age unless circumstances prevent other forms of treatment. Historically, fears of radiation-induced genetic damage, leukemia, and neoplasia have shaped this practice, although these fears have not been realized over several decades of clinical experience. Studies indicate that the risk of infertility and birth defects following I-131 treatment is not increased when pregnancy is avoided for at least 1 year following treatment.

Patients with Graves disease may be given an antithyroid drug, such as PTU, for several months preceding radiotherapy to establish chemical euthyroidism. I-131 dosing is then based on the ability of the abnormal thyroid tissue to absorb and eliminate I-131.

The nurse should question the patient regarding previous medication and procedures involving radiographic contrast media, because the uptake of I-131 will be affected by recent intake of these agents. It is a good idea to reassure patients that they need not be isolated from other household members. Instead, caution them to avoid prolonged, close contact with others, particularly children and pregnant women, for about 1 week following therapy with I-131.

Household contamination is not a great risk, but saliva and urine may be contaminated for a several days following treatment. The nurse should advise the patient to avoid oral contact with others. It is helpful to give the patient and family verbal and written instructions specific to their living situations. Eating utensils should be washed thoroughly with soap and water after every meal. It is important to emphasize the importance of handwashing. Typically, the toilet is the most contaminated item because most of the iodine-131 dosage is excreted in the urine. The NRC recommends an annual radiation dose limit of 100 mrem for the general public; this excludes exposure to family members of outpatients receiving radiation, however. Hyperthyroid patients treated with I-131 typically emit only low levels of radiation beyond a 1-m distance. The nurse should make certain household members understand that they can minimize their exposure by staying 1 m away from the patient for a few days. It is important to reassure any anxious household member that exposure from diagnostic X-rays (typically 10 to 2,000 mrem) is considerably greater than exposure results from minimal contact with the patient.

The nurse should advise the patient that temporary thinning of the hair may occur 2 to 3 months after treatment. It is important to teach the patient and family to recognize the signs and symptoms of HOT that may occur following I-131 therapy.

Iodine (Lugol solution, Thyro-Block [tablets])

Iodine is the oldest of the antithyroid drugs. Low doses of iodine are needed in the body for the formation of thyroid hormone. High doses, however, tend to inhibit thyroid function. A hyperfunctioning thyroid gland responds to iodine by promptly inhibiting the release of hormone. Iodine helps to firm the thyroid gland by reducing its size and vascularity; this helps prevent postoperative hemorrhage and the surgical complication called thyroid storm.

Potassium iodide or occasionally strong iodine solution is used preoperatively to reduce the vascularity of the gland prior to thyroidectomy and in the management of thyrotoxic crisis (thyroid storm), usually in conjunction with other antithyroid agents (e.g., PTU) alone or combined with propranolol. When used preoperatively, potassium iodide is administered 10 to 14 days before surgery.

Manifestations of iodism (chronic toxicity, which is dose dependent) may occur when potassium iodide is given in large doses or over a long duration. Iodism is usually manifested as a metallic taste, burning in the mouth and throat, soreness of the teeth and gums, increased salivation, and eye irritation with swelling of the eyelids. Gastric irritation is common and diarrhea may occur. When the drug is discontinued, the clinical manifestations of iodism generally subside spontaneously within a few days.

Hypersensitivity reactions to iodides may result in angioedema, cutaneous and mucosal hemorrhage, and clinical signs resembling serum sickness (e.g., fever, arthralgia, lymphadenopathy, and eosinophilia).

Prolonged use or excessive doses of iodides may result in thyroid gland hyperplasia, thyroid adenoma, goiter, and severe HOT.

Concomitant use of lithium salts, other iodides or antithyroid agents and potassium iodide may result in an additive or synergistic hypothyroid effect. If these drugs are used together, the patient should be monitored closely for signs and symptoms of HOT. Simultaneous use of potassium iodide and potassium-containing drugs or potassium-sparing diuretics may result in hyperkalemia.

Initial administration of potassium iodide should be done cautiously because some individuals are markedly sensitive to iodides. Persons at highest risk are those with goiter or autoimmune thyroid disease (i.e., Hashimoto thyroiditis). Some commercially available formulations of potassium iodide contain sodium bisulfite, a sulfite that may cause allergic-type reactions, including anaphylaxis and life-threatening asthmatic episodes, in certain susceptible individuals. The nurse should question the patient carefully in regards to the presence of goiter, autoimmune thyroid disease, or asthma because this sensitivity occurs more frequently in asthmatic individuals.

Propranolol

Propranolol (Inderal), a beta-adrenergic blocker, is used commonly IV in the treatment of thyroid storm to minimize the excessive cardiac stimulation that results from the catecholamine activity.

PARATHYROID DRUGS: C ANTI-HYPERCALCEMIC, CALCIUM-REGULATOR DRUGS

Calcium-regulator drugs used to treat PTH excess or high levels of serum calcium include the calcitonins (human and salmon) and the bisphosphonates-alendronate, etidronate, gallium, pamidronate, risedronate, and tiludronate. These drugs act on the serum levels of calcium and not directly on the parathyroid gland or PTH.

Calcitonin is a polypeptide hormone secreted by the thyroid gland. Commercially available calcitonin drugs are calcitonin, salmon and calcitonin, human. Both derivatives are derived synthetically and are used when the hypercalcemia is related to HRPT. The prototype calcium-regulator drug is calcitonin, salmon.

NURSING MANAGEMENT OF THE PATIENT RECEIVING P CALCITONIN, SALMON

Core Drug Knowledge

Pharmacotherapeutics

Calcitonin, salmon (Calcimar) is used to treat Paget disease. Paget disease of bone (osteitis deformans) is an idiopathic disease characterized by chronic, focal areas of bone destruction complicated by concurrent excessive bone repair, affecting one or more bones. These changes result in thickened but weakened bones that may fracture or bend under stress. Signs and symptoms may be bone pain, deformity, fractures, neurologic disorders resulting from cranial and spinal nerve entrapment and from spinal cord and brain-stem compression, increased cardiac output to the involved bone, increased serum alkaline phosphatase levels (reflecting increased bone formation), or urine hydroxyproline excretion (reflecting increased bone resorption). Calcitonin, salmon is also used to treat postmenopausal osteoporosis and as an emergency treatment for severe hypercalcemia. This drug is given SC, IM, or intranasally. Because of the risk of allergic reaction to the salmon antigens in this calcitonin, a skin test should be given before the drug is used. The skin test consists of 0.1 mL of a 10-IU/mL solution given SC. If no reaction is noted within 15 minutes, the drug can be given safely (Table 39-9).

Calcitonin, human (Cibacalcin) is a synthetic form of the hormone produced by the human thyroid gland. Calcitonin, human is used for the treatment of Paget disease. It must be given SC up to three times weekly and should be discontinued as soon as symptoms are relieved.

Calcitonin, salmon is structurally the same as calcitonin produced by the human thyroid gland, but it has a significantly greater potency (about fifty-fold) and duration of action. It works to inhibit **bone resorption** (pathologic or physiologic loss or destruction of bone tissue, which may occur as a result of neoplasms, HRPT, osteoporosis, or prolonged immobility) and increase the ex-

TABLE 39-9 Summary of Selected Antihypercalcemic Drugs

Drug (Trade) Name	Selected Indications	Route and Dosage Range	Pharmacokinetics
calcitonin, salmon (Calcimar, *Miacalcin; *Canadian:* Caltine)	Treatment of Paget disease Postmenopausal osteoporosis with calcium and vitamin D Emergency treatment of hypercalcemia	*Adult:* Paget disease, initial dose, SC or IM, 100 IU/d; maintenance, 50 IU/d or qod; postmenopausal osteoporosis, SC or IM, 100 IU/d; hypercalcemia, SC or IM, 4 IU/kg q12h, may increase to 8 IU/dg q6h *Child:* Safety and efficacy not established	*Onset:* 15 min *Duration:* 8–24 h $t_{1/2}$: 1.2 h
calcitonin, human (Cibacalcin)	Treatment of Paget disease	*Adult:* Initially, SC, 0.5 mg/d may use up to 1 mg/d SC for 6 mo *Child:* Safety and efficacy not established	*Onset:* 15 min *Duration:* 8–24 h $t_{1/2}$: 1 h
alendronate (Fosamax)	Treatment of Paget disease in patients at risk for complications	*Adult:* Osteoporosis, PO, 10 mg/d; Paget disease, PO, 40 mg/d for 6 mo *Child:* Safety and efficacy not established	*Onset:* Slow *Duration:* Days $t_{1/2}$: Unknown
etidronate (Didronel)	Treatment of Paget disease Heterotopic ossification Hypercalcemia resulting from malignancy	*Adult:* Paget disease, PO, 5–10 mg/dg/d for up to 6 mo; heterotopic ossification, PO, 20 mg/dg/d, total treatment should not exceed 4 mo; hypercalcemia, IV, 7.5 mg/kg/d	*Onset:* Slow *Duration:* 6 h; 6 h (serum) $t_{1/2}$: 90 d
furosemide (Lasix; *Canadian:* Apo-Furosemide)	Promotes renal excretion of calcium	Up to 100 mg IV	*Onset:* 5 min *Duration:* 2 h $t_{1/2}$: 2 h
gallium nitrate (Ganite)	Treatment of malignancy-related hypercalcemia	*Adult:* IV, 200 mg/m²/d for 5 consecutive d *Child:* Safety and efficacy not established	*Onset:* Slow *Duration:* 3–4 d $t_{1/2}$: Unknown
pamidronate (Aredia)	Treatment of hypercalcemia resulting from malignancy Paget disease Osteolytic bone lesions Postmenopausal osteoporosis	*Adult:* Hypercalcemia, IV, 60–90 mg over 24h; Paget disease, IV 30 mg/d over 4 h for 3 d; osteolytic bone lesions, IV, 90 mg over 4 h each month *Child:* Safety and efficacy not established	*Onset:* Rapid *Duration:* 72 h $t_{1/2}$: 1.6 h, then 27.3 h
plicamycin (Mithracin)	Hypercalcemia and hypercalciuria in symptomatic patients associated with advanced neoplasms	Base dose on body weight. Use ideal weight if patient has abnormal fluid retention. 25 μg/kg/d for 3 or 4 d; may repeat at intervals of ≥1 wk to maintain serum and urinary calcium excretion at normal levels.	*Onset:* Rapid *Duration:* Unknown $t_{1/2}$: Unknown
risedronate (Actonel)	Treatment of Paget disease Prevention of bone loss in postmenopausal women	*Adult:* PO, 30 mg/d for 2 mo *Child:* Safety and efficacy not established	*Onset:* Rapid *Duration:* Unknown $t_{1/2}$: 220 h
tiludronate (Skelid)	Treatment of Paget disease	*Adult:* PO, 400 mg/d for 3 mo *Child:* Safety and efficacy not established	*Onset:* 2 h *Duration:* Days $t_{1/2}$: Unknown

*Nasal spray.

cretion of calcium, sodium, and phosphorus by the kidney, thereby lowering serum calcium levels. Calcitonin, given intranasally, increases spinal bone mass in postmenopausal women with established osteoporosis, but not in early postmenopausal women.

Pharmacokinetics

Calcitonin is inactivated in the GI tract. Parenterally administered, it is metabolized rapidly, primarily in the kidneys, but also in the blood and peripheral tissues. A small amount of unchanged hormone and its inactive metabolites are excreted in the urine. Half-life is 1.2 hours for salmon and 1 hour for human calcitonin.

Pharmacodynamics

Calcitonins are polypeptide hormones secreted by parafollicular cells of the thyroid. Calcitonin has a role in the regulation of calcium and bone metabolism and it has direct renal effects and actions on the GI tract. Single injections of calcitonin transiently inhibit bone resorption. With prolonged use, there is a persistent, smaller decrease in the rate of bone resorption associated with decreased resorptive activity and number of osteoclasts. Osteocytic resorption also may be decreased. Endogenous calcitonin, in conjunction with PTH, regulates blood calcium. High blood calcium levels increase secretion of calcitonin, which inhibits bone resorption.

Contraindications and Precautions

The most important contraindication to use of calcitonin, salmon is allergy. Allergy to fish products also limits its use. The possibility of a systemic allergic reaction exists. Patients with multiple allergies should consider skin testing prior to calcitonin treatment, particularly patients with suspected sensitivity.

Adverse Effects

Adverse effects are generally infrequent and mild. GI disturbances such as nausea and vomiting are most evident when treatment is initiated and tend to decrease with continued use. Other adverse effects include dermatologic effects of skin rash and flushing of the face and hands, nasal irritation, and localized inflammatory reactions at the injection site.

Drug Interactions

There is a risk of hypercalcemia with decreased therapeutic effects if calcitonin, salmon is taken with calcium supplements, antacids, or vitamin D. The nurse should advise patients against the use of OTC vitamin and mineral preparations and antacids since many of these contain calcium. Concurrent administration of theophylline may increase bone resorption.

Assessment of Relevant Core Patient Variables

Health Status

Before administering calcitonin, the nurse should review the patient's record to determine whether calcitonin can be administered safely. In addition, the nurse should perform a physical examination to establish a baseline from which to monitor the drug's effects. It is important to evaluate muscle tone, bone pain, bowel sounds, serum calcium levels, and renal function test results. It is important for the nurse to collect a thorough health history, specifically asking about bone disease, endocrine disorders, kidney stones, or ulcer diseases. The nurse also should collect a complete drug history, including use of prescription and OTC drugs. Thiazide diuretics and excessive ingestion of vitamin D can produce hypercalcemia.

The family history should be included because primary HRPT occurs in a number of familial syndromes. The nurse should use caution when administering calcitriol to patients with renal dysfunction or upper GI disease. A nasal examination should precede calcitonin administered intranasally and repeated at any time nasal complaints occur.

Life Span and Gender

It is important to assess for pregnancy and lactation. Calcitonin is FDA pregnancy category C because it may decrease fetal birth weight. Although calcitonin does not cross the placenta, it does inhibit lactation. It is not known whether it is excreted in breast milk, and therefore, safety for use during nursing has not been established. The nurse should determine the patient's age because geriatric individuals should have their dosages monitored closely.

Lifestyle, Diet, and Habits and Environment

Long-term treatment with calcitonin occurs in the home or community. The patient's responses should be monitored closely to detect adverse effects or previously unrecognized effects of the drug. Significant responses include dehydration due to diuresis and loss of sodium and water, abnormal serum calcium levels, and signs of allergy, which diminishes the therapeutic response.

It is important to obtain a thorough health history to identify any factors that relate to the cause of HRPT, such as vitamin D intoxication, osteolytic bone metastases, and hyperphosphatemia. The nurse should obtain a broad database about the patient for comparison during therapy; for example, dietary practices, allergic tendencies, visible bone deformities, deformities interfering with activities, emotional lability, and lethargy.

Nursing Diagnoses and Outcomes

- Imbalanced Nutrition: Less Than Body Requirements related to GI effects of drug therapy

  Desired outcome: The patient will relate the importance of good nutrition and ingest daily nutritional requirements in accordance with activity level and metabolic needs.
- Pain, Acute or Chronic related to complications of calcium and/or phosphate imbalances (e.g., renal stones, pathologic fractures, osteoporosis)

  Desired outcome: The patient will practice pain relief measures to avoid or manage the pain.

Planning and Intervention

Maximizing Therapeutic Effects

The nurse should monitor serum calcium levels before drug therapy begins and periodically thereafter. Reconstituted solution should be used within 6 hours. The nasal spray should be taken with adequate calcium (at least 1,000 mg elemental calcium per day) and vitamin D (400 IU/day).

Minimizing Adverse Effects

The drug should be administered at bedtime to minimize nausea and vomiting. During drug therapy, it is important to measure serum calcium levels at least weekly. It may be necessary to arrange for small, frequent meals to alleviate GI discomfort and to provide adequate nutrition. The nurse can divide the dose if GI effects are severe. The nurse should monitor bone pain and the progression or status of the disease.

Providing Patient and Family Education

- The nurse should teach the patient or family members correct techniques for administering the parenteral and nasal forms of the drug. It also is important to teach patients how to evaluate regularly the mucous membranes if using the nasal spray.
- The nurse should explain to the patient and family that this drug is designed to decrease the level of calcium in the blood. Calcium is needed for many of the body's activities, and it is important to keep the blood calcium levels in an effective range.
- The nurse should explain that some of the adverse effects of the drug include GI upset with nausea, vomiting, and epigastric distress. It is important to explain to patients that the drug should be taken once a day and at the same time each day. The nurse can suggest small, frequent meals to maintain nutrition and decrease the unpleasant effects of the drug.
- The nurse should explain that there might be an exacerbation in Paget disease bone pain when the drug is started. It is important to assure patients that this usually passes with time. The nurse teaches the patient the following ways to manage bone pain associated with Paget disease. In Paget disease, bone resorption and formation are both increased, leading to thickening and softening of bones and bending of weight-bearing bones.
  - Nonnarcotic analgesics (e.g., NSAIDs, cytochrome-C-oxidase-2 (COX-2) inhibitors)
  - Applications of heat
  - Massage
  - Bracing
  - Guided imagery
  - Relaxation techniques
  - Biofeedback
  - Meditation
- The nurse should ask patients to report twitching, muscle pain, severe diarrhea, or dark urine.
- It is important to tell patients to keep this drug out of the reach of children.
- The nurse should alert the patient and family that skeletal deformities (e.g., bowing of tibia or femur, kyphosis, and barrel-shaped chest) are not corrected by treatment. The nurse can teach the patient to camouflage deformities using clothing (e.g, slacks for women, tunic-style tops, and loosely fitted apparel).

Ongoing Assessment and Evaluation

Calcitonin can cause a drop in the serum calcium level, with tetany and cardiac arrhythmias. In addition, antibodies may form after several months of therapy, causing resistance to the drug and decreased therapeutic effects. Those in long-term therapy should be monitored for their hormone status and clinical response.

Nursing management of drug therapy is judged effective when calcium levels are maintained within a normal range. The patient should verbalize the importance of self-monitoring for adverse effects and of reporting significant effects to the prescriber. ■

DRUGS CLOSELY RELATED TO CALCITONIN, SALMON

Bisphosphonates

The bisphosphonates are calcium-regulator drugs closely related to calcitonin. The major pharmacologic action of the bisphosphonate drugs is primarily on bone; namely, the inhibition of normal and abnormal bone resorption. Reduction of abnormal bone resorption is responsible for therapeutic benefit in hypercalcemia. Bisphosphonate drugs are used in the long-term management of hypercalcemia to increase bone resorption of calcium, in the treatment and prevention of osteoporosis in postmenopausal women (see Chapter 43), and management of Paget disease.

Unlabeled uses for the bisphosphonates include:

- Etidronate: treatment of postmenopausal osteoporosis, prevention of bone loss in early postmenopausal women, and glucocorticoid-induced bone loss in postmenopausal women
- Pamidronate: postmenopausal osteoporosis, HRPT and prevention of glucocorticoid-induced osteoporosis, control of bone pain in prostatic carcinoma, and immobilization-related hypercalcemia
- Risedronate: prevention of bone loss in postmenopausal women

MEMORY CHIP

Calcitonin, Salmon

- Calcium regulator used to treat postmenopausal osteoporosis, Paget disease, hypercalcemia
- Significant contraindications: hypersensitivity to fish products
- Most common adverse effects: nausea, vomiting, and diarrhea
- **Life span alert: *children*—safety and efficacy not established**
- Maximizing therapeutic effects: store unopened bottle (nasal drug formulation) in the refrigerator between 36° and 43°F; once the pump has been activated, store at room temperature
- Minimizing adverse effects: periodically examine urine sediments of patients on chronic therapy; coarse granular casts and renal tubular epithelial cell casts result from therapy and may cause renal calculi
- Most significant patient education: with intranasal dosing, alternate nostrils daily; notify health care provider if significant nasal irritation occurs

The nurse should caution patients taking bisphosphonates that the expected drug benefits may only be obtained when each tablet is taken with a full glass of plain water (6 to 8 oz) first thing in the morning and then waiting in an upright position 30 minutes before the first food, beverage, or medication of the day improves drug absorption. Even dosing with juice or coffee markedly reduces the absorption (especially alendronate). Supplemental calcium and vitamin D should be consumed along with the bisphosphonates if dietary intake is inadequate. Weight-bearing exercise along with the modification of certain behavioral factors (e.g., cigarette smoking, alcohol consumption) may help to diminish the bone resorption. Bisphosphonates may cause significant GI upset (e.g., nausea, diarrhea).

Alendronate

Alendronate (Fosamax) is a bisphosphonate and calcium regulator drug that slows normal and abnormal bone resorption without inhibiting bone formation and mineralization. It is indicated for the treatment of postmenopausal osteoporosis and for Paget disease. If not contraindicated, it is usually recommended that the patient take concomitant hormone replacement therapy when being treated for osteoporosis.

Etidronate

Etidronate (Didronel) has a similar therapeutic action to that of alendronate and by blocking the calcium removal from bone, it promotes a lowering of serum calcium levels. It is used for managing Paget disease and treating hypercalcemia related to malignancy. Etidronate is excreted unchanged in the urine, has a serum half-life of 6 hours, and a bone half-life of 90 days. Etidronate crosses the placenta and may enter breast milk.

Etidronate should be used cautiously with renal dysfunction or upper GI tract disease. The most common adverse effects of etidronate are GI complaints, such as metallic taste sensation, nausea, and diarrhea. Exacerbation of Paget disease with bone pain can occur when drug therapy first starts, but this usually resolves as therapeutic levels are reached. Hypersensitivity reactions are rare but have included angioedema, urticaria, rash, and pruritus.

Residronate

Residronate (Actonel) is a bisphosphonate that affects osteoclast activity by reducing the enzymatic and transport processes that lead to resorption of the bone and by inhibiting the osteoclast protein pump, leading to a rate of bone turnover near normal in patients with Paget disease. Supplemental calcium and vitamin D should be ingested concurrently if dietary intake is inadequate. Agents containing calcium, aluminum, and magnesium should be taken at a different time of the day to prevent interference with risedronate absorption. Risedronate is not recommended for use in patients with severe renal impairment (i.e., creatinine clearance less than 30 mL/min).

Tiludronate

Tiludronate (Skelid), a bisphosphonate drug similar in action to risedronate, is used for the treatment of Paget disease. Patients with Paget disease should receive supplemental calcium and vitamin D if dietary intake is inadequate. Administer a single 400-mg daily oral dose of tiludronate with 6- to 8-oz plain water only for a period of 3 months. Beverages other than plain water (including mineral water), food, and some medications (e.g., indomethacin) are likely to reduce the absorption of tiludronate and should not be taken within 2 hours. Calcium or mineral supplements should be taken 2 hours before or after tiludronate; antacids containing aluminum or magnesium should be consumed 2 hours after taking tiludronate. Following therapy, an interval of 3 months should be allowed to assess response. The effectiveness of this drug beyond 3 months is not known. The tablets should not be removed from the foil strip packaging until they are to be used.

Plicamycin

Plicamycin (Mithracin) is a cancer chemotherapeutic agent that is very effective at lowering serum calcium levels. The dose is about 10% of that used for cancer treatment, so the adverse effects are significantly lower. The dosage is based on body weight; ideal weight should be used if the individual has abnormal fluid retention. Administered only IV, extravasation may cause local irritation and cellulitis at injection sites. Plicamycin demonstrates a consistent calcium-lowering effect not related to its tumoricidal activity. It blocks the hypercalcemic action of pharmacologic doses of vitamin D, acts on osteoclasts, and blocks the action of PTH. Plicamycin inhibition of DNA-dependent RNA synthesis renders osteoclasts unable to fully respond to PTH with the biosynthesis necessary for osteolysis. Decreases in serum phosphate levels and urinary calcium excretion accompany the lowering of serum calcium concentrations. It is cleared rapidly from blood within the first 2 hours; excretion also is rapid (90% in the first 24 hours after injection). Contraindications to use are thrombocytopenia, thrombocytopathy, coagulation disorders, impairment of bone marrow function, and pregnancy (FDA pregnancy category X). Most common adverse effects include GI symptoms (anorexia, nausea, vomiting, diarrhea, and stomatitis). Electrolyte disturbances and depression of serum calcium, phosphorus, and potassium may occur. Calcium supplements are sometimes needed during plicamycin therapy.

DRUGS SIGNIFICANTLY DIFFERENT FROM CALCITONIN, SALMON

Furosemide

Furosemide (Lasix) is a loop diuretic that promotes renal excretion of calcium. Dosage is up to 100 mg IV and adverse effects include dehydration, hypokalemia, hypochloremic alkalosis, hyperuricemia, and hypomagnesemia. It is important for the nurse to carefully monitor fluid balance, pulse and blood pressure, and serum electrolytes.

Gallium

Gallium (Ganite) inhibits calcium resorption from bone and reduces bone turnover; these actions result in a lowered serum calcium level. Gallium is administered IV over 5 days to treat cancer-related hypercalcemia that is symptomatic and does not respond to conventional treatment. There is a risk of acute renal failure with this drug and renal function tests must be monitored very closely for any sign of renal failure. It is crucial to maintain adequate hydration in patients receiving gallium and to monitor serum electrolytes closely.

ANTIHYPOCALCEMIC DRUGS

Replacement therapy with vitamin D compounds combined with calcium salts and a high dietary intake is usually enough to regulate blood calcium and phosphate levels satisfactorily. Calcitriol (1,25-dihydroxy-vitamin D3) (Rocaltrol [capsules]; Calcijex [parenteral]) is the active form of vitamin D and the prototype anti-hypocalcemic.

NURSING MANAGEMENT OF THE PATIENT RECEIVING P CALCITRIOL

Core Drug Knowledge

Vitamin D compounds regulate absorption of calcium and phosphate from the small intestine, mineral resorption in bone, and reabsorption of phosphate from the renal tubules. Considered a hormone, although not a natural human hormone, the commonly used term "vitamin D" refers to both ergocalciferol (D2) and cholecalciferol (D3). Vitamin D2, essentially a plant vitamin, is used predominantly to fortify milk and cereals; it can, however, substitute for D3 in every metabolic step.

Biologically active vitamin D metabolites control the intestinal absorption of dietary calcium, the tubular reabsorption of calcium by the kidney, and, in conjunction with PTH, the mobilization of calcium from the skeleton. They act directly on bone cells (osteoblasts) to stimulate skeletal growth and on the parathyroid glands to suppress PTH synthesis and secretion. Vitamin D also is involved in magnesium metabolism.

Working along with PTH and calcitonin to regulate calcium homeostasis, vitamin D actually functions as a hormone. HOPT is treated primarily with vitamin D and, if necessary, dietary supplements of calcium. Vitamin D products are used to treat patients with HOPT because deficient levels of PTH result in hypocalcemia. Vitamin D stimulates calcium absorption from the intestine and restores the serum calcium to a normal level. Vitamin D is a fat-soluble vitamin derived from natural sources (fish liver oils) or from conversion of provitamins. In humans, natural supplies of vitamin D depend on ultraviolet (UV) light for conversion to vitamin D3 or vitamin D2. Following exposure to UV light, vitamin D3 must then be converted to its active forms by the liver and kidneys. Vitamin D is hydroxylated by the hepatic microsomal enzymes to calcifediol and then further hydroxylated primarily in the kidney to calcitriol and doxercalciferol. Calcitriol (Rocaltrol [capsules, solution]; Calcijex [parenteral]) is believed to be the most active form of vitamin D in stimulating intestinal calcium and phosphate transport.

Pharmacotherapeutics

There are several clinical indications for calcitriol. They are the management of hypocalcemia and resulting bone disease in patients on chronic renal dialysis; reduction of elevated PTH levels; management of secondary HRPT and metabolic bone disease in predialysis patients with moderate to severe chronic renal failure (creatinine clearance 15 to 55 mL/min); and management of hypocalcemia and its clinical manifestations in patients with HOPT (e.g., postsurgical or idiopathic HOPT, pseudohypoparathyroidism). An unlabeled use (oral, topical) is decreased severity of psoriatic lesions (Table 39-10).

Pharmacokinetics

Calcitriol can be given orally or IV. It is absorbed readily from the small intestine and bile is essential for adequate absorption. Absorption is reduced in liver or biliary disease. In either administration form, the onset of action is 2 to 6 hours with a peak effect occurring in 10 to 12 hours. Stored chiefly in the liver, vitamin D also is found in fat, muscle, skin, and bones. In plasma, it is bound to globulins and albumin. Vitamin D undergoes hydroxylation by the hepatic microsomal enzyme system to calcifediol; then calcifediol undergoes hydroxylation by the kidney to doxercalciferol. Calcitriol half-life is 5 to 8 hours and its pharmacologic activity persists for 3 to 5 days. Calcitriol half-life increases at least twofold in chronic renal failure and hemodialysis patients. The primary route of vitamin D excretion is in the bile; only a small percentage is found in the urine.

Pharmacodynamics

Vitamin D is a fat-soluble vitamin derived from natural sources (fish liver oils) or from conversion of pro-vitamins, 7-dehydrocholesterol, and ergosterol. In humans, natural supplies of vitamin D depend on UV light for conversion of 7-dehydrocholesterol to vitamin D3 or ergosterol to vitamin D2. Following exposure to UV light, vitamin D3 must then be converted to the active form of vitamin D, calcitriol, by the liver and kidneys. Calcitriol is believed to be the most active form of vitamin D3 in stimulating intestinal calcium and phosphate transport. Calcitriol is a fat-soluble vitamin that helps to regulate calcium homeostasis, bone growth, and maintenance. Calcitriol increases calcium absorption from the intestine, increasing serum calcium levels; it decreases alkaline phosphatase and possible PTH levels.

Biologically active vitamin D metabolites control the intestinal absorption of dietary calcium, the tubular reabsorption of calcium by the kidney, and, in conjunction with PTH, the mobilization of calcium from the skeleton. They act directly on bone cells (osteoblasts) to stimulate skeletal growth and on the parathyroid glands to suppress PTH synthesis and secretion. Vitamin D also is involved in magnesium metabolism.

TABLE 39-10 Summary of Selected Antihypocalcemic Drugs

Drug (Trade) Name	Selected Indications	Route and Dosage Range	Pharmacokinetics
calcitriol (Calcijex, Rocaltrol)	Management of hypocalcemia in chronic renal dialysis Reduction of elevated PTH levels	*Adult:* PO, 0.25 μg/d may be increased to a maximum of 0.5–1 μg/d; 0.5 μg IV three times a week at end of dialysis *Child:* >6 y, PO, 0.5–2 μg/d; 1–5 y, PO, 0.25–0.75 μg/d	*Onset:* 2–6 h *Duration:* 3–5 d $t_{1/2}$: 3–6 h
dihydrotachysterol (DHT, Hytakerol)	Treatment of hypoparathyroidism Postoperative or idiopathic tetany	*Adult:* PO, 0.8–2.4 mg/d initially; maintenance, PO, 0.2–1 mg/d to maintain serum calcium levels	*Onset:* 10–24 h *Duration:* 3–5 d $t_{1/2}$: 16 d
doxercalciferol (Hectorol)	Reduction of elevated parathyroid hormone levels in the management of secondary hyperparathyroidism in patients undergoing chronic renal dialysis	10 μg administered three times a week; initial dose adjusted as needed to lower blood PTH into 15- to 300-pg/mL range. Increase dosage at 8-week intervals by 2.5 μg. The maximum recommended dose is 20 μg administered three times a week at dialysis for a total of 60 μg/week.	*Onset:* 10–24 h *Duration:* 4 d $t_{1/2}$: 3.2–3.7 h
paricalcitol (Zemplar)	Prevention and treatment of secondary hyperparathyroidism associated with chronic renal failure	Initial dose is 0.04 to 0.1 μg/kg (2.8 to 7 μg); dose may be increased by 2–4 μg at 2–4 wk intervals to maximum of 0.24 μg/kg (16.8 μg) administered as a bolus dose every other day during dialysis.	*Onset:* 10–24 h *Duration:* 16 d $t_{1/2}$: 15 h

Contraindications and Precautions

Hypercalcemia may develop and calcium phosphate may precipitate if the product of serum calcium multiplied by phosphate (i.e., Ca × P) exceeds 70. If hypercalcemia develops, it is necessary to discontinue the drug immediately. However, once normal calcium levels are achieved, calcium may be readministered at a lower dosage. Chronic hypercalcemia can lead to generalized vascular calcification, nephrocalcinosis, and other soft tissue calcification. In patients with normal renal function, chronic hypercalcemia may be associated with an increase in serum creatinine levels. Although this is usually reversible, it is important for the nurse to pay careful attention to factors that may lead to hypercalcemia. The kidneys of end-stage renal disease (ESRD) patients cannot adequately synthesize calcitriol, the active hormone formed from the precursor vitamin D. Resultant hypocalcemia and secondary HRPT are a major cause of the metabolic bone disease of renal failure.

Dynamic bone lesions may develop if PTH levels are suppressed to abnormal levels. The kidneys of uremic patients cannot adequately synthesize calcitriol, the active hormone formed from precursor vitamin D.

Some vitamin D products contain tartrazine, which may cause allergic-type reactions (including bronchial asthma) in susceptible individuals. Although the incidence of sensitivity is low, it is frequently seen in patients with aspirin hypersensitivity. Products containing tartrazine are identified in product listings on the label.

Adverse Effects

The most common adverse effects seen with calcitriol are associated with the GI system, and include nausea, vomiting, metallic taste, dry mouth, and constipation. Common too are CNS effects of weakness, headache, somnolence, and irritability. Other effects that can occur include polyuria, nocturia, decreased libido, muscle and bone pain, and cold symptoms. Potentially dangerous adverse effects include cardiac arrhythmias and hypertension, which can occur as serum calcium levels increase.

Drug Interactions

There is a risk of hypermagnesemia if calcitriol is taken with magnesium-containing antacids. These drugs should be spaced 2 to 4 hours apart if the combination cannot be avoided. Reduced absorption of calcitriol occurs if taken with cholestyramine or mineral oil. This combination also should be avoided or spaced 2 to 4 hours apart. A possible risk of hypercalcemia occurs in some patients when thiazide diuretics and calcitriol are combined (Table 39-11).

Assessment of Relevant Core Patient Variables

Health Status

It is important to obtain a thorough health history to identify any factors that relate to the cause of HOPT such as a history of previous neck surgery (e.g., thyroidec-

TABLE 39-11 Agents That Interact With Calcitriol

Interactants	Effect and Significance	Nursing Management
Cholestyramine, ketoconazole, mineral oil, phenytoin, phenobarbital, thiazide diuretics	Decreased pharmacologic effects of vitamin D Intestinal absorption of vitamin D may be reduced Ketoconazole may inhibit both synthetic and catabolic enzymes of calcitriol Absorption of vitamin D is reduced with prolonged use of mineral oil Hypoparathyroid patients on vitamin D may develop hypercalcemia due to thiazide diuretics Endogenous synthesis of calcitriol will be inhibited; higher doses of calcitriol may be necessary with concurrent administration of phenytoin and phenobarbital	Appraise the patient for management of concurrent disease states. Assess the patient for evidence of therapeutic effects of interacting drugs. Check for therapeutic serum levels (if applicable) of interacting drugs.
Mg^{++}-containing antacids, digitalis glycosides, verapamil	Increased pharmacologic effects from interaction with vitamin D Hypermagnesemia may develop in patients on chronic renal dialysis Hypercalcemia in patients on digitalis may precipitate cardiac arrhythmias.	Assess the patient for control of concurrent disease states. Evaluate patient for evidence of therapeutic effects of interacting drugs. Measure therapeutic serum levels (if applicable) of interacting drugs. Monitor cardiac rhythm and function.

tomy) that may have resulted in inadvertent removal of the parathyroid glands.

Calcitriol should be used with caution in elderly patients, especially those with coronary disease, renal function impairment, and arteriosclerosis. Before administering calcitriol, the nurse should review the patient's record to determine if calcitriol can be safely administered. The nurse should use caution when administering the drug to patients with renal stones.

Before beginning drug therapy, the nurse should perform a physical examination to establish a baseline from which to monitor the effects of the drug. It is important to monitor skin color, temperature, orientation, and status of mucous membranes. The nurse also should determine serum blood levels of calcium, phosphorus, magnesium, alkaline phosphatase, and renal and liver function to establish a baseline to measure drug activity and adverse effects.

Life Span and Gender

The nurse should assess the patient for pregnancy or breast-feeding. Calcitriol is FDA pregnancy category A, but this changes to category C when used in doses that exceed the RDA. Safety of vitamin D in amounts over 400 IU/day is not established, and doses greater than the RDA during a normal pregnancy should be avoided because animal studies have shown fetal abnormalities associated with hypervitaminosis D. There are no adequate and well-controlled studies in pregnant women; it should be used during pregnancy only if the potential benefits outweigh the potential hazards to the fetus. Therefore, the nurse should use caution when administering calcitriol to women of child-bearing age and these women should be advised to avoid conception while on this drug and to use barrier contraceptives.

Vitamin D is excreted in breast milk in limited amounts, and lactation should be avoided when taking calcitriol. However, if drug therapy is necessary, monitoring of the infant's serum calcium concentration is essential because large doses of vitamin D may cause hypercalcemia.

The nurse should note the age of the patient. Safety and efficacy of vitamin D and its metabolites in children in doses exceeding the RDA and in children undergoing dialysis have not been established. Long-term calcitriol therapy is well tolerated by pediatric patients not undergoing dialysis. Pediatric doses should be individualized and monitored closely.

Lifestyle, Diet, and Habits

Calcitriol is generally given in the home setting. IV doses can be given following dialysis to increase calcium levels. The nurse should evaluate vitamin D ingested in fortified foods, dietary supplements, and other concomitantly administered drugs. It may be necessary to limit dietary vitamin D and its derivatives during treatment.

Patients receiving calcitriol are likely to experience multiple GI effects. It is important to explain that small, frequent meals may help alleviate some of these symptoms. A bowel-training program may be needed for severe constipation. The nurse should closely monitor nutritional status.

Nursing Diagnoses and Outcomes

- Imbalanced Nutrition: Less Than Body Requirements related to reduced absorption of fat-soluble vitamins (hypovitaminosis), including calcitriol, in presence of very low-fat diet

Desired outcome: The patient will ingest a nutritionally balanced diet to allow for normal absorption of fat-soluble vitamins.

- Imbalanced Nutrition: More Than Body Requirements (hypervitaminosis) related to drug-vitamin interaction of vitamin D and calcium supplements

  Desired outcome: The patient will identify sources of dietary vitamin D and calcium and consume these foods in moderation and refrain from consuming vitamin/dietary supplements containing vitamin D and calcium.
- Acute Pain related to headache and general discomfort secondary to drug effects

  Desired outcome: The patient will not experience undue pain and discomfort as a result of drug therapy.

Planning and Intervention

Maximizing Therapeutic Effects

Calcitriol capsules should be swallowed whole rather than crushed or chewed. Eating a balanced diet and periodic exposure to sunlight usually satisfies normal vitamin D requirements. The nurse should caution the patient and family to avoid using vitamin supplements as a substitute for a balanced diet. The nurse should monitor serum calcium levels before the patient begins drug therapy and during treatment as adequate dietary calcium is necessary for a clinical response to vitamin D therapy. Therapy should begin at the lowest possible dose, with dosage increases made after careful analysis of the serum calcium and dosage adjustment made as soon as there is clinical improvement. It is essential to estimate the daily dietary calcium intake and adjust that intake when indicated. Patients with normal renal function taking calcitriol should maintain an adequate fluid intake to avoid dehydration, because the range between therapeutic and toxic doses is narrow. When high therapeutic doses are used, frequent serum and urinary calcium, phosphate, and BUN determinations are necessary.

HOPT and dialysis patients should have their serum calcium, phosphate, magnesium, and alkaline phosphatase levels monitored routinely. Serum calcium levels should be maintained between 9 and 10 mg/dL.

Minimizing Adverse Effects

During drug therapy, the nurse should monitor serum calcium levels at least weekly. Use of mineral oil should be avoided. Chronic dialysis patients should avoid magnesium-containing antacids while taking these drugs. It is important to arrange for small, frequent meals to alleviate GI discomfort and to provide adequate nutrition. The nurse should monitor bowel function and begin a bowel-training program as appropriate. The nurse should monitor environment—light, noise, and temperature—and provide analgesics as appropriate to decrease discomfort and pain related to drug effects.

Providing Patient and Family Education

- The nurse should explain to patients and their families that this drug is a form of vitamin D and that it is being used to increase their calcium levels, which are low. Calcium is needed for many of the body's activities, and it is important to keep calcium levels in the blood in an effective range.
- The nurse should explain that some of the adverse effects of the drug include GI upset with nausea, vomiting, and epigastric distress. The nurse can advise patients to eat small, frequent meals to maintain nutrition and decrease some of the unpleasant side effects of the drug.
- It is important to explain that headache, muscle ache, and irritability also are common adverse effects of the drug. The nurse can advise patients to monitor noise, temperature, and light and to take prescribed analgesics as needed to decrease discomfort.
- The nurse should ask patients to report lethargy, weight loss, severe bone pain, excessive urine output, or constipation.
- It is important to tell patients to keep this drug out of the reach of children.

Ongoing Assessment and Evaluation

Dosage adjustment is required as soon as there is clinical improvement. Therapy should be started at the lowest possible dose, with increases made after careful monitoring of the serum calcium. It is important for the nurse to estimate daily dietary calcium intake and adjust the intake when indicated. Patients with normal renal function taking calcitriol should avoid dehydration by maintaining adequate fluid intake. In some conditions (e.g., vitamin D-resistant rickets), the range between therapeutic and toxic doses is narrow. When high therapeutic doses are used, it is especially important to chart the progress with frequent determinations of serum and urinary calcium, phosphate, and BUN and to periodically monitor serum calcium, phosphate, magnesium, and alkaline phosphatase levels; and also to monitor 24-hour urinary calcium and phosphate levels. These laboratory determinations are especially important in hypoparathyroid and dialysis patients. Serum calcium levels should be maintained between approximately 9 and 10 mg/dL.

Nursing management in drug therapy is considered effective when calcium levels are maintained within a normal range, the patient recognizes and verbalizes the importance of self-monitoring for adverse effects, and the patient takes responsibility for reporting significant adverse effects to the health care provider.

MEMORY CHIP

Calcitriol

- Vitamin D; management of hypocalcemia and resultant bone disease in patients undergoing chronic renal dialysis
- Significant contraindications: hypercalcemia, hypervitaminosis D, malabsorption syndrome, and decreased renal function
- Most common adverse effects: weakness, headache, somnolence, nausea, vomiting, dry mouth, constipation, muscle or bone pain, and metallic taste
- Most serious adverse effect: chronic hypercalcemia can lead to generalized vascular calcification, nephrocalcinosis, and other soft tissue calcification
- **Life span alert: use caution in elderly patients, especially those with coronary disease, renal function impairment, and arteriosclerosis**
- Maximizing therapeutic effects: patients with normal renal function taking calcitriol should maintain adequate fluid intake and avoid dehydration; periodically monitor serum calcium, phosphate, magnesium, alkaline phosphatase, and 24-hour urinary calcium and phosphate, especially in hypoparathyroid and dialysis patients
- Minimizing adverse effects: maintain serum calcium levels between 9 and 10 mg/dL
- Most significant patient education: adequate dietary calcium is necessary for a clinical response to vitamin D therapy; compliance with dosage instructions, diet, phosphate-binder use, and calcium supplementation is essential; avoid use of nonprescription drugs, including magnesium-containing antacids

DRUGS CLOSELY RELATED TO CALCITRIOL

Dihydrotachysterol

Dihydrotachysterol (DHT; Roxane) is another vitamin D derivative used in the treatment of postoperative tetany and idiopathic tetany. DHT has a rapid onset of effect and is normally used in high doses until the serum calcium level is within normal range. Then maintenance doses and a calcium supplement are used. DHT may be toxic in doses as low as 25 mg/day; toxicity is manifested by symptoms of hypercalcemia. It is important that the nurse carefully monitor standard hypercalcemia-related metabolic parameters (e.g., serum levels of calcium, phosphate, magnesium, potassium).

Doxercalciferol

Doxercalciferol (Hectorol), a vitamin D analogue, is indicated for the treatment of secondary HRPT in ESRD and hemodialysis patients. It has a mean half-life of 32 to 37 hours. Doxercalciferol is a pro-hormone of vitamin D that undergoes hepatic conversion to active vitamin D. Hyperphosphatemia lessens its effectiveness. A drug interaction of decreased absorption may occur when combined with agents known to interfere with the absorption of fat-soluble vitamins (e.g., cholestyramine, mineral oil). Frequent adverse effects include edema, headache, dizziness, malaise, nausea, and vomiting.

Paricalcitol

Paricalcitol (Zemplar) is a parenterally administered synthetic vitamin D analogue that reduces PTH levels. Mean half-life is 15 hours. Paricalcitol suppresses PTH levels in patients with CRF and is not likely to cause hypercalcemia and hyperphosphatemia. Paricalcitol must be administered IV. Paricalcitol may also reduce serum total alkaline phosphatase levels. It is important to inform the patient that effective therapy with paricalcitol requires a dietary regimen of calcium supplementation and phosphorus restriction. Phosphate-binding compounds may be needed; excessive use of aluminum-containing compounds should be avoided.

CHAPTER SUMMARY

- A combination of neural and endocrine systems, originating in the hypothalamus, regulates CNS, autonomic nervous system, and endocrine functions.
- The hypothalamus produces two hormones—oxytocin and vasopressin—that are stored in and released from the posterior lobe of the pituitary gland. The hypothalamus releases a series of stimulating and inhibiting factors to promote the release of stimulating hormones from the anterior pituitary gland. These stimulating hormones affect several other endocrine glands.
- The anterior lobe of the pituitary gland produces GH, a hormone important for the regulation of growth and development. Release of GH is determined by inhibiting and releasing factors and by chemical signals for growing tissue.
- The thyroid gland is a bilobar gland located in the neck around the trachea. This vascular gland uses dietary iodine to produce two thyroid hormones (T_3 and T_4). These hormones affect the way many body cells burn energy and maintain metabolism. A fine balance among TRH, TSH, and the thyroid hormone levels regulates these hormones.
- The parathyroid glands are four very small groups of tissue located on the back of the thyroid gland. These cells produce PTH (parathormone), the most important regulator of serum calcium levels in the body. Parathormone stimulates osteoclasts to release calcium from the bone, increases intestinal absorption of calcium, and increases calcium resorption from the kidneys. It also stimulates cells in the kidney to produce calcitriol, the active form of vitamin D, which stimulates intestinal transport of calcium into the blood. Calcium is a vital anion that is used in many of the body's metabolic processes, including membrane transport processes, conduction of nerve impulses, muscle contraction, and blood clotting. To be effective, the serum levels of calcium must be maintained between 9 and 11 mg/dL.
- The GH, somatropin, is an example of a drug used to replace a pituitary hormone. It is given by injection to children with GH deficiency, to some adults with GH deficiency, and to girls with Turner syndrome.
- Release of GH is blocked by octreotide, bromocriptine, and GH-inhibiting factor (somatostatin). These drugs can be used to treat acromegaly and must be given by injection.
- Vasopressin (or ADH) is administered by injection or intranasally to regulate water loss when levels of ADH are low or absent. Vasopressin blocks the release of water in the nephron and increases vascular volume while decreasing osmolarity. The dosage of this drug is determined by patient response and water balance.

Glucocorticoids

prednisone
hydrocortisone
methylprednisolone
dexamethasone
betamethasone

Inhaled glucocorticoids
beclomethasone
budesonide
flunisolide
fluticasone
triamcinolone

Topical glucocorticoids
hydrocortisone
methylprednisolone
betamethasone
dexamethasone
triamcinolone

Mineralocorticoids

fludrocortisone

Steroid hormone antagonists

aminoglutethimide
corticosterone and desoxycorticosterone
cyproheptadine
ketoconazole
mifepristone
mitotane

The symbol C indicates the **drug class**.

Drugs in bold type marked with the symbol P are **prototypes**.

Drugs in blue type with no symbol are **closely related** to the prototype.

Drugs in **red** type with no symbol are **significantly different** from the prototype.

Drugs in **black** type with no symbol are **also used in drug therapy**; no prototype.

Corticosteroids are used for replacement therapy to maintain adequate levels of hormones in patients with inadequate adrenal function. Corticosteroids also are used for their physiologic stress management, and for their anti-inflammatory, antiallergenic, and immunosuppressive effects on many inflammatory diseases (see the accompanying display, Therapeutic Uses for the Corticosteroids).

There is a definite risk: benefit ratio with pharmacotherapeutic use of the corticosteroids. Unfortunately, the benefits derived from chronic use of corticosteroids are often accompanied by a number of undesirable effects. Corticosteroid complications vary from mild to life threatening and are a function of the dosage, route of administration, and duration of therapy.

PHYSIOLOGY

The hormones of the endocrine system are important negotiators in the communication between cells. In addition, the nervous system, adrenal glands, and other endocrine glands contribute to homeostasis, thus allowing physical and emotional adaptation to internal and external changes.

Two adrenal glands, one located at the top of each kidney, are composed of two distinct parts—the medulla and the cortex. The medulla and cortex are crucial to metabolism, the body's stress response, and fluid and electrolyte balances. The adrenal medulla synthesizes and secretes catecholamines—epinephrine and norepinephrine. These hormones are important in counteracting short-term stress.

The adrenal cortex is involved primarily in the synthesis and secretion of **glucocorticoids** and **mineralocorticoids** (collectively referred to as the corticosteroids) from plasma-derived, low-density lipoproteins and high-density lipoproteins (cholesterol). Corticosteroids are characterized by mineralocorticoid and glucocorticoid effects, depending on the predominant pharmacologic action of the agent. Adrenal corticosteroids exert effects on almost every organ in the body; their pharmacologic actions are generally an extension of their physiologic effects. Their primary actions include carbohydrate, protein and fat metabolism; electrolyte and water metabolism; cardiovascular functions; and immune effects. The zona reticularis region of the adrenal cortex also is capable of producing and secreting other steroid hormones, including adrenal androgens, progesterone, and the estrogens.

Therapeutic Uses for the Corticosteroids

Physiologic Doses
- Adrenocortical insufficiency*†
- Adrenogenital syndrome (salt-losing)*†

Pharmacologic (Supraphysiologic) Doses
- Acute allergic conditions (e.g., bronchial asthma, serum sickness)*
- Acute spinal injury (e.g., 30 mg/kg methylprednisolone rapid IV injection within 8 hours of injury)*
- Cerebral edema*
- Collagen diseases, rheumatic disorders (e.g., systemic lupus erythematosus, and acute rheumatic carditis)*
- Dermatologic diseases (e.g., seborrheic dermatitis, severe psoriasis)*
- Gastrointestinal diseases (e.g., Crohn disease, intractable sprue, ulcerative colitis)*
- Hematologic disorders (e.g., autoimmune hemolytic anemia, thrombocytopenia)*
- Hepatic diseases (e.g., liver cirrhosis with ascites)*
- Joint inflammation (e.g., bursitis)*
- Meningitis*
- Neoplastic diseases (e.g., leukemias, lymphomas)*
- Nephrotic syndrome*
- Ocular disorders (e.g., allergic conjunctivitis, chorioretinitis, iritis, keratitis)*
- Organ transplants*
- Respiratory diseases (e.g., interstitial pulmonary fibrosis, pulmonary emphysema with bronchial edema)*
- Thyroiditis*

*Glucocorticoid.
†Mineralocorticoid.

GLUCOCORTICOIDS

The glucocorticoids acquired their name from their role in glucose metabolism; they increase blood glucose concentrations by:

- Stimulating gluconeogenesis and glucose secretion by the liver
- Increasing the hepatic sensitivity to the gluconeogenic actions of glucagon and catecholamines
- Decreasing glucose uptake and utilization by peripheral tissue
- Increasing proteolysis and decreasing protein synthesis in muscles to support the gluconeogenesis activities

The glucocorticoid **cortisol** is necessary for the maintenance of life. Synthesized in the zona fasciculata of the adrenal cortex, it exerts a wide range of physiologic effects.

Glucocorticoids exert potent and diverse actions on glucose, protein, and bone metabolism and possess anti-inflammatory, antiallergenic, and immunosuppressant actions. Metabolic effects of glucocorticoids include gluconeogenesis, the primary metabolic effect that occurs by actions on the liver and peripheral tissues, mobilization of amino acids from protein in striated muscle, protein catabolism, fat synthesis and lipolysis, and hepatic enzymatic activities that convert amino acids to glucose with most of the excess glucose stored in the liver as glycogen. The metabolic effects of the glucocorticoids result in the following:

- An increase in circulating amino acid levels
- An overall depletion of muscle protein
- A negative nitrogen balance
- Mobilization of fatty acids, converting cell metabolism from using glucose for energy to using fatty acids for energy

In addition to the glucocorticoids' diverse and varied effects on metabolism, other physiologic effects include antagonistic effects on antidiuretic hormone to maintain water balance, lowering of the threshold for electrical excitation in the brain, and reduction in the amount of new bone synthesis. Glucocorticoids also have actions that allow the body to cope effectively with physiologic or psychological stress (e.g., overwhelming illness or trauma). For example, cortisol sensitizes the arterioles to norepinephrine for vasopressor effects and allows epinephrine and glucagon to activate gluconeogenesis and glycogenolysis.

Hypothalamic corticotropin-releasing factor (CRF) stimulates the release of pituitary adrenocorticotropic hormone (ACTH). This hypothalamic-pituitary-adrenal (HPA) axis regulates and stimulates cortisol synthesis release by the adrenal cortex. Each of these substances is regulated by a complex feedback loop as the production of one substance is regulated by the plasma concentrations of the other two. Glucocorticoid, androgen, and estrogen secretion depend on adrenocortical stimulation by ACTH from the anterior pituitary. CRF, produced by the hypothalamus, controls ACTH release into the bloodstream (Fig. 40-1). Three factors are significant in regulating ACTH secretion:

- Circulating cortisol levels
- Stress
- Circadian (diurnal) rhythms

Pituitary production of ACTH is very sensitive to suppression by exogenous glucocorticoids. Long-term or chronic administration may result in adrenocortical atrophy and subsequent impaired endogenous glucocorticoid biosynthesis.

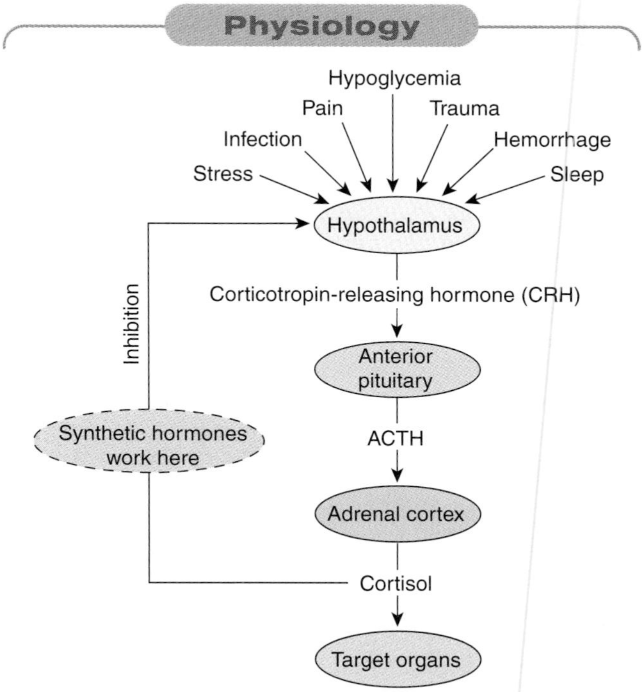

Figure 40-1. The hypothalamic-pituitary-adrenal (HPA) feedback system regulates and stimulates cortisol synthesis and release by the adrenal cortex. Each hormone in the HPA axis is influenced by a complex feedback loop because synthesis of one substance is regulated by plasma concentrations of the others. For instance, secretion of glucocorticoid, androgen, and estrogen depends on adrenocortical stimulation by adrenocorticotropic hormone (ACTH) from the anterior pituitary. Corticotropin-releasing factor, produced by the hypothalamus, controls ACTH release into the bloodstream. Circulating cortisol levels, stress, and circadian rhythms are also significant in regulating ACTH secretion. ACTH in turn regulates cortisol release. The objectives of replacement and pharmacologic drug therapy involve maintaining balance in the HPA feedback system.

MINERALOCORTICOIDS

The mineralocorticoids (**aldosterone** is the most prevalent naturally occurring mineralocorticoid) exert a major influence on regulating potassium, sodium, and water balance. Mineralocorticoids are produced in the outer layer of cells of the adrenal cortex (zona glomerulosa). Numerous systemic factors, including angiotensin II, plasma potassium levels, ACTH, and circadian rhythms affect the synthesis and secretion of aldosterone; angiotensin II is the most potent of these factors. In the distal renal tubules, aldosterone promotes the reabsorption of sodium into the blood in exchange for potassium secreted into the tubular distillate for urinary excretion.

Several mechanisms control aldosterone levels. They include 1) extracellular sodium and potassium levels—when serum sodium levels are low or potassium levels are high, aldosterone levels rise; 2) renal renin release—a reduction in renal blood flow increases aldosterone levels by the renin-angiotensin-aldosterone system; and 3) ACTH—the glucocorticoid hormones produced in the adrenal cortex have mineralocorticoid effects.

SEX STEROIDS

As stated previously, the adrenal cortex produces small amounts of sex steroids (e.g., testosterone and estrogens) and some weak anabolic androgens (e.g., dehydroepiandrosterone and androstenedione). These hormones are produced by the adrenal glands in males and females. The amounts, however, are usually insignificant, in normal circumstances, compared with the hormone amounts secreted by the gonads. However, under certain conditions (e.g., tumors, cushingoid effects) their excess may cause a significant endocrine imbalance. These gonadal hormones are discussed in depth in Chapters 42 and 43.

PATHOPHYSIOLOGY

ADRENAL INSUFFICIENCY

There are two forms of adrenal insufficiency—primary and secondary. Primary adrenal insufficiency (**Addison disease**) results from the destruction of the adrenal cortex due to infection or hemorrhage, resulting in hyposecretion of all adrenocortical hormones-most significantly the glucocorticoid, cortisol and the mineralocorticoid, aldosterone. Characteristics of Addison disease include those related to glucocorticoid deficiency, such as hypoglycemia, anorexia, nausea, vomiting, flatulence, diarrhea, hyperpigmentation of skin, anxiety, depression, and loss of mental acuity; and those related to mineralocorticoid deficiency, such as fluid and electrolyte imbalance, orthostatic hypotension, hyponatremia, hyperkalemia, general malaise, muscle weakness, muscle pain, and cardiac arrhythmias.

The major complication of Addison disease is a sudden, life-threatening exacerbation called **addisonian crisis** (adrenal crisis). The patient experiences the extremes of hypotension, hyponatremia, dehydration, hyperkalemia, and hyperthermia in the absence of disease. A stressor usually triggers addisonian crisis. Characterized by shock and hypotension unresponsive to standard therapy (e.g., vasopressors, plasma expanders), the initial treatment of adrenal crisis involves immediate replacement of adrenocortical hormone (e.g., intravenous [IV] hydrocortisone [Solu-Cortef]), salt, and fluids to restore normal blood volume and blood pressure.

In secondary adrenal insufficiency, the deficiency of cortisol secretion is secondary to insufficient secretion of ACTH by the anterior pituitary. There is little or no alteration in aldosterone secretion. Thus, there is glucocorticoid insufficiency, but mineralocorticoid levels are not affected. The most common cause is long-term treatment of nonendocrine disorders (e.g., certain malignancies, asthma, severe obstructive lung disease, and immunosuppression for transplanted organs) with pharmacologic doses of glucocorticoid drugs. Because it bypasses the negative feedback loop, this treatment results in gradual loss of adrenal and pituitary hormonal reserves and some degree of atrophy of both the ACTH-secreting cells of the pituitary and the adrenal cortex. Sudden withdrawal of the glucocorticoid drug will then result in secondary adrenal insufficiency, manifested clinically by acute adrenal insufficiency. HPA axis suppression resulting from glucocorticoid therapy may last for as long as 1 year after drug therapy has been discontinued.

A patient receiving pharmacologic doses of glucocorticoids for more than 2 weeks may have some degree of HPA axis suppression. Prevention of secondary adrenal insufficiency following prolonged administration of glucocorticoid drugs can be avoided by "weaning" the patient from the drug over weeks or months, depending on the patient's dosage and the duration of therapy. A common guideline is a 5% to 10% reduction per week.

CUSHING SYNDROME

Cushing disease is a rare disorder resulting from increased adrenocortical secretion of cortisol, resulting in chronic elevation in glucocorticoid and adrenal androgen hormones; mineralocorticoid hormone levels are usually not affected because increased ACTH production is usually the causative agent. Cushing syndrome may be caused by any one of the following sources:

- ACTH-dependent adrenocortical hyperplasia
- Tumor
- Ectopic ACTH-secreting tumor
- Chronic administration of large doses of any steroid that is a potent glucocorticoid (Cushing syndrome medicamentosus or iatrogenic Cushing syndrome)

The term *cushingoid* refers to the variable number of the physiologic changes associated with Cushing syndrome (see the accompanying display, Cushingoid Characteristics).

SALT-LOSING ADRENOGENITAL SYNDROME

Salt-losing adrenogenital syndrome, a congenital condition, is characterized by an inherited enzymatic interference with the normal biosynthesis of glucocorticoids and mineralocorticoids. The resulting low levels of these corticosteroids stimulate the body's feedback mechanism to produce large amounts of corticotropin (i.e., ACTH). The adrenal glands are only able to respond to the increased ACTH by increasing their production of adrenal androgens. Consequently, testosterone levels are abnormally high, which results in masculinization.

HYPERALDOSTERONISM

Hyperaldosteronism is another abnormality of adrenal hormone production. Certain tumors of the adrenal cortex produce excessive amounts of aldosterone (or occasionally another mineralocorticoid). Two problems occur as a result of hyperaldosteronism: hypertension secondary to sodium and water retention and hypokalemia-induced muscle weakness. Both problems represent excessive aldosterone actions on the distal renal tubule. Treatment ultimately involves surgical removal of the tumor.

STEROID HORMONE AGONISTS

GLUCOCORTICOIDS

The primary endogenous glucocorticoids produced by the adrenal gland are cortisol (hydrocortisone) and cortisone. Although cortisone is slightly less active than cortisol, hepatic conversion renders them virtually identical. Cortisol and cortisone are used only for replacement therapy in patients with adrenal insufficiency (i.e., deficiency of endogenous glucocorticoids); they have no role in any anti-inflammatory therapeutic regimen because of their high mineralocorticoid activity relative to their anti-inflammatory activity. Synthetic glucocorticoids include prednisone, methylprednisolone, dexamethasone, and betamethasone (Fig. 40-2).

All natural and synthetic glucocorticoids act by binding to a specific cytoplasmic glucocorticoid receptor. Currently, glucocorticoids are available in numerous formulations, including oral, topical, ophthalmic solutions and ointments, oral inhalers, nasal formulations, parenteral, and rectal preparations. The main therapeutic uses of glucocorticoids include replacement therapy for individuals with adrenal insufficiency, as an anti-inflammatory-immunosuppressive agent, and adjunctive treatment in selected malignant disorders.

A common adverse effect of synthetic glucocorticoids administered in supraphysiologic doses for anti-inflammatory and immunosuppressant effects (combined or separately) is suppression of the HPA axis. This effect appears within days

Cushingoid Characteristics

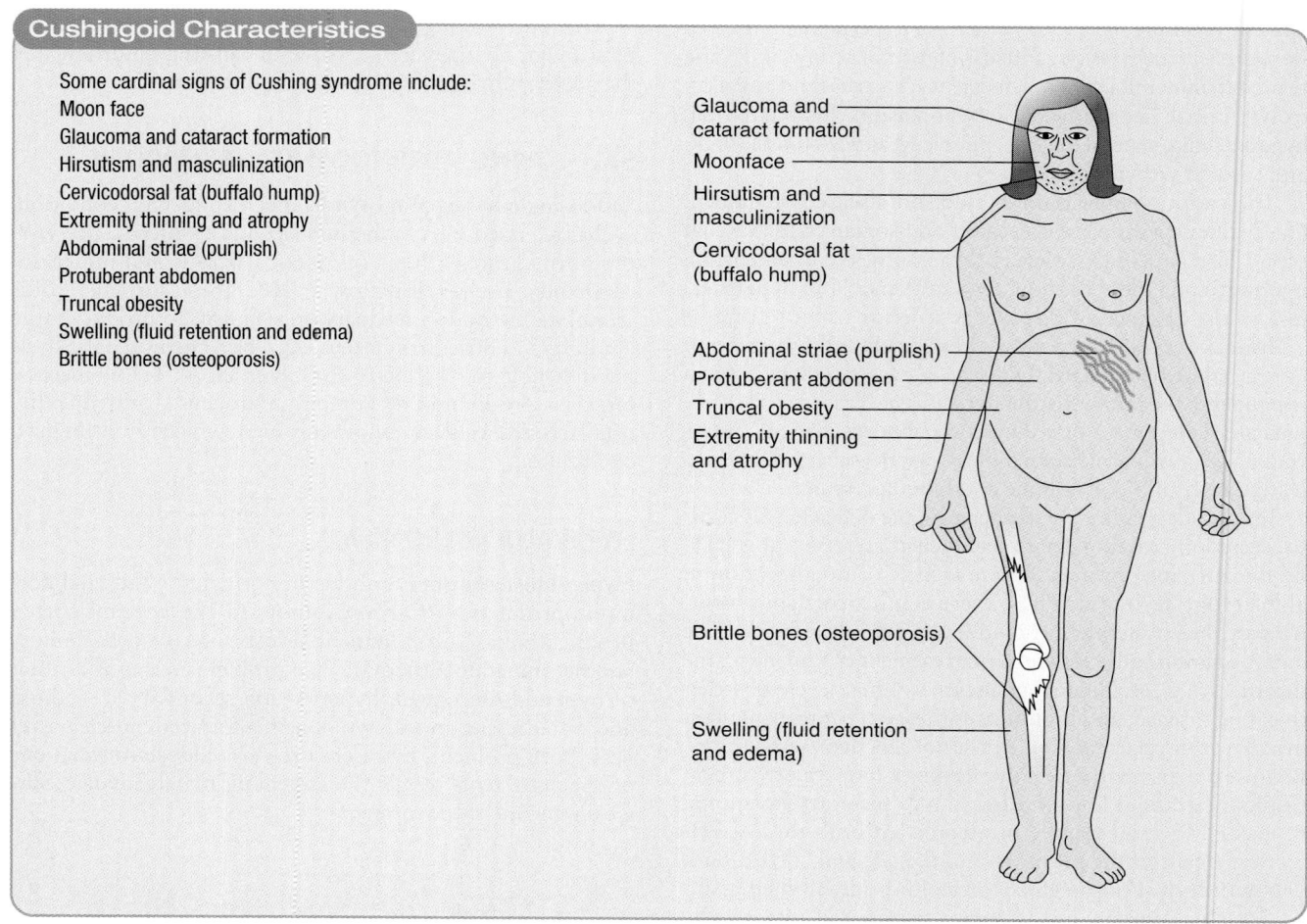

Some cardinal signs of Cushing syndrome include:
Moon face
Glaucoma and cataract formation
Hirsutism and masculinization
Cervicodorsal fat (buffalo hump)
Extremity thinning and atrophy
Abdominal striae (purplish)
Protuberant abdomen
Truncal obesity
Swelling (fluid retention and edema)
Brittle bones (osteoporosis)

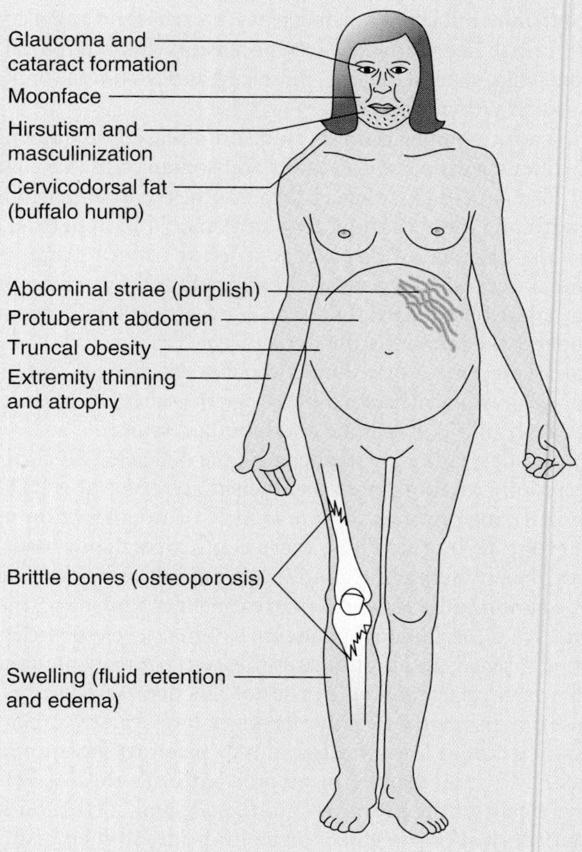

after glucocorticoid therapy is begun. It is thought that patients who receive glucocorticoids in doses equivalent to 5 mg or more of prednisone daily for more than 2 weeks should be considered as having some degree of HPA axis suppression. The time needed for the HPA axis to recover depends on the type of glucocorticoid given, the dose and frequency of administration (e.g., daily dosing versus alternate-day dosing), and the duration of treatment. Recovery may take 1 year or longer. Occasionally, the patient's HPA axis remains permanently suppressed by glucocorticoid anti-inflammatory therapy. Consequently, the corticosteroid therapy reverts to replacement therapy.

Abrupt discontinuation of a glucocorticoid following a prolonged administration time may result in acute adrenal insufficiency from a lack of both exogenous and endogenous glucocorticoids. Also known as addisonian crisis, acute adrenal insufficiency is characterized by serious morbidity and sometimes mortality. To prevent acute adrenal insufficiency, exogenously administered glucocorticoids must be withdrawn gradually so that the HPA axis can resume secretion of cortisol at a normal level and rate.

Prednisone is considered the prototype synthetic glucocorticoid. Although prednisone is a synthetic analogue of cortisone, its results are longer acting with a more potent anti-inflammatory activity and less mineralocorticoid effect. Prednisone and its derivatives are the most commonly used glucocorticoids for the treatment of inflammatory conditions and a variety of autoimmune diseases.

NURSING MANAGEMENT OF THE PATIENT RECEIVING PREDNISONE

Core Drug Knowledge

Pharmacotherapeutics

Prednisone is significantly more potent (four times) than naturally occurring cortisol. It has primarily glucocorticoid activity, although some mineralocorticoid activity is present and more apparent when the drug is administered in high doses (see Figure 40-2). This may cause salt and water retention, resulting in edema and hypertension. Therapeutic uses of prednisone include replacement therapy for adrenal deficiency states and as anti-inflammatory and immunosuppressive treatment for a variety of chronic conditions such as rheumatoid arthritis, asthma, chronic obstructive pulmonary disease, ulcerative colitis, or Crohn disease. It may be used in a variety of ways. For example, at the beginning of treatment for a chronic condition to manage symptoms until other drugs become effective; during periods of

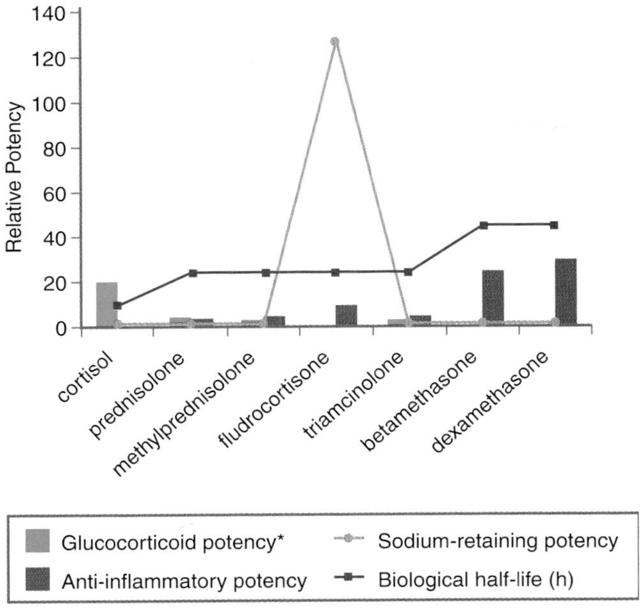

*Glucocorticoid activity signifies the stimulation of glucose formation, a reduction in its utilization, and the promotion of its storage as glycogen.

Figure 40-2. Comparison of glucocorticoids.

acute exacerbation; or long-term high-dose or low-dose therapy depending on the underlying condition (e.g., transplant) or disease (e.g., rheumatoid arthritis) being treated (Table 40-1).

Pharmacokinetics

Prednisone, like other glucocorticoids, is absorbed readily from the gastrointestinal (GI) tract due to its lipophilic nature. Glucocorticoids also are absorbed from the synovial and the conjunctival spaces and very slowly through the skin. Consequently, topical administration is used only briefly for a localized action. Long-term use of nasal spray may lead to nasal and pulmonary epithelial atrophy. Excessive and prolonged local application may result in enough absorption to cause systemic effects. In contrast to oral dosage forms, injectable preparations (e.g., esters, suspensions) have greatly altered onsets and durations of action; they are, however, absorbed slowly and completely. Prednisone—inactive on its own—must be metabolized in the liver into pharmacologically active prednisolone. Prednisolone is excreted in the urine, crosses the placenta, and enters the breast milk.

The liver and kidney are the major sites of glucocorticoid inactivation. Drugs that are cyproheptadine (CYP) inducers (e.g., phenobarbital, phenytoin, rifampin) may accelerate the hepatic biotransformation of

TABLE 40-1 Summary of Selected Glucocorticoids

Drug (Trade) Name	Selected Indications	Route and Dosage Range	Pharmacokinetics
prednisone (Deltasone, Prednisone; *Canadian:* Apo-Prednisone) or prednisolone (Delta-Cortef; *Canadian:* Novo-Prednisolone)	Rheumatic disorders Collagen disorders Dermatologic disorders Allergic states Ophthalmic disorders Respiratory diseases Hematologic disorders Neoplastic diseases GI diseases	*Adult:* PO, 5–60 mg/d	*Onset and duration:* Vary with administration and dosage preparation Plasma $t_{1/2}$ (for prototype glucocorticoid prednisone): 60 min Biologic $t_{1/2}$: 18–36 h
betamethasone (Celestone)	Anti-inflammatory and immunosuppressant effects (similar to those of prednisone)	*Adult:* PO, 4–60 mg/d	*Onset and duration:* Vary with administration and dosage preparation
betamethasone dipropionate† (Alphatrex; *Canadian:* Taro-Sone)	Localized anti-inflammatory effects	Topical	
betamethasone sodium phosphate* (Cel-U-Jec, Selestoject; *Canadian:* Betnesol)	Anti-inflammatory and immunosuppressant effects (similar to prednisone)	*Adult:* IM, IV, up to 9 mg/d	Plasma $t_{1/2}$ (for betamethasone): 300+ min
betamethasone sodium phosphate† betamethasone acetate* (Celestone Soluspan)	Localized anti-inflammatory effects	*IL, 0.5–2 mL (1 mL = 3 mg each compound)	Biologic $t_{1/2}$: 36–54 h
betamethasone valerate+ (Valisone)	Localized anti-inflammatory effects	Topical	
cortisone acetate (Cortone Acetate)	Glucocorticoid replacement therapy for adrenocortical insufficiency	*Adult:* PO, 25–300 mg/d	

(continued)

TABLE 40-1 Summary of Selected Glucocorticoids (Continued)

Drug (Trade) Name	Selected Indications	Route and Dosage Range	Pharmacokinetics
dexamethasone*† (Decadron; *Canadian:* Dexasone)	Anti-inflammatory and immunosuppressant effects (similar to prednisone) Cerebral edema Chemotherapeutic antiemetic Diagnostic aid for Cushing syndrome and major (endogenous) depression	*Adult:* PO, 0.75–9 mg/d	*Onset and duration:* Vary with administration and dosage preparation Plasma $t_{1/2}$ (for dexamethasone): 110–210 min
dexamethasone acetate (Decadron-LA) or	Anti-inflammatory and immunosuppressant effects (similar to those of prednisone)	*Adult:* IM, 8–16 mg; *IL, 00.8–16 mg	Biologic $t_{1/2}$: 36–54 h
dexamethasone sodium phosphate† (Decadron Phosphate, Hexadrol)	Localized anti-inflammatory effects	*Adult:* IV, 0.5–9 mg/d *IL, 0.4–4 mg	*Duration:* 2–3 d (PO, IM, or IV)
flunisolide (AeroBid; *Canadian:* Bronalide)	Localized anti-inflammatory effects Bronchial asthma	Aerosol	*Onset:* Slow *Duration:* 4–6 h
fluocinolone acetonide	Localized anti-inflammatory effects	Topical	Plasma $t_{1/2}$: 1–2 h
fluticasone propionate (aerosol, Flonase; topical, Cutivate)	Localized anti-inflammatory effects	Aerosol, topical	Biologic $t_{1/2}$: wk
cortisone/hydrocortisone† (Cortef)	Primary or secondary adrenal cortical insufficiency (hydrocortisone or cortisone is drug of choice; synthetic analogues, however, may be used in conjunction with mineralocorticoids)	*Adult:* PO, 20–240 mg/d	*Onset and duration:* Vary with administration and dosage preparation Plasma $t_{1/2}$ (for hydrocortisone): 80–120 min Biologic $t_{1/2}$: 8–12 h
hydrocortisone sodium phosphate (Hydrocortisone Phosphate) or	Localized anti-inflammatory effects	*Adult:* IM, IV, SC, 15–240 mg/d	
hydrocortisone sodium succinate (Solu-Cortef)		*Adult:* IM, IV, 100–500 mg at 2-, 4-, or 6-h intervals; *IL; 12.5–75 mg	
hydrocortisone acetate*†	Localized anti-inflammatory effects		
methylprednisolone (Medrol; *Canadian:* Meprolone)	Anti-inflammatory and immunosuppressant effects (similar to those of prednisone)	*Adult:* PO, 4–48 mg/d	*Onset and duration:* Vary with administration and dosage preparation Plasma $t_{1/2}$ (for methylprednisolone): 78–188 min Biologic $t_{1/2}$: 18–36 h
methylprednisolone acetate*† (Depo-Medrol; *Canadian:* Medrol Veriderm)		*Adult:* IM, 40–120 mg/wk	
Methylprednisolone sodium succinate (Solu-Medrol)		*Adult:* IM, IV, 10–40 mg; *high-dose therapy,* 30 mg/kg	
prednisolone acetate (Prednisolone Acetate, Predcor) or	Anti-inflammatory and immunosuppressant effects (similar to those of prednisone)	*Adult:* IM, IV, 4–60 mg/d *IL, 4–100 mg	*Onset and duration:* Vary with administration and dosage preparation
prednisolone sodium phosphate (IV-Predate, IM-Hydeltrasol)	Localized anti-inflammatory effects	*Adult:* IM, IV, 4–60 mg/d *IL, 5–20 mg/d	
prednisolone tebutate (Prednisolone Tebutate, Hydeltra-T.B.A.)	Localized anti-inflammatory effects	*Adult:* *IL, 4–30 mg *Child:* Individualize dosage depending on severity of condition and patient's response	
triamcinolone (Aristocort, Kenacort; *Canadian:* Oracort)	Anti-inflammatory and immunosuppressant effects (similar to those of prednisone)	*Adult:* PO, 4–48 mg (in divided doses depending on the disease)g	*Onset:* Varies with administration and dosage preparation

TABLE 40-1 **Summary of Selected Glucocorticoids** (Continued)

Drug (Trade) Name	Selected Indications	Route and Dosage Range	Pharmacokinetics
triamcinolone diacetate (Aristocort)	Localized anti-inflammatory effects	*Adult:* IM, Up to 40 mg/wk *IL, 5–48 mg	Plasma $t_{1/2}$: 200† min Biologic $t_{1/2}$: 18–36 h
triamcinolone hexacetonide (Aristospan Intralesional, Aristospan Intraarticular)	Localized anti-inflammatory effects	*IL, 2–20 mg	

*May be administered for localized effects (e.g., intraarticular, intrabursal, intradermal, intralesional, intrasynovial, or soft tissue [IL]). Dosage varies according to size of treatment area and desired local effects.

†May be administered topically (e.g., dermatologic, inhalation, or ophthalmic).

glucocorticoids. Hypothyroidism, conversely, may cause the hepatic metabolism to be decreased.

Pharmacodynamics

Prednisone affects virtually all body cells but not in the same way. Anti-inflammatory effects include retardation of the migratory polymorphonuclear leukocytes, suppression of tissue repair and granulation, reduction in the erythrocyte sedimentation rate, decrease in fibrinogenesis, and diminished C-reactive protein. Prednisone does not, however, affect antigen-antibody or immediate hypersensitivity reactions.

Its immunosuppressant effects are due to suppression of phagocytosis, decrease in the number of circulating eosinophils and lymphocytes, suppression of delayed hypersensitivity reactions, decrease in antigen-antibody tissue reactions, and a decrease in plasma immunoglobulins.

Glucocorticoid effects on carbohydrate, fat, and protein metabolism are responsible for both the beneficial and adverse effects. The normal physiologic role of prednisone (other systemic glucocorticoids are included) is increased gluconeogenesis and decreased glucose use; these actions provide for glucose production (and energy) during periods of stress or decreased carbohydrate intake (see the accompanying display, Pharmacodynamic Effects of Glucocorticoids).

Pharmacodynamic Effects of Glucocorticoids

Metabolic
- Increased glycogenolysis and gluconeogenesis
- Increased protein catabolism and decreased protein synthesis
- Decreased gastrointestinal absorption of calcium
- Decreased secretion of thyroid-stimulating hormone
- Decreased activity and formation of osteoblasts

Anti-inflammatory (systemic and local effects)
- Decreased production of prostaglandins, cytokines, and interleukins
- Decreased proliferation and migration of lymphocytes and macrophages

Contraindications and Precautions

Contraindications to prednisone use are a hypersensitivity to the drug, systemic fungal infections, IM use in clotting disorders, and after administration of live virus vaccines (e.g., smallpox) in immunosuppressed patients.

Some glucocorticoid drug preparations contain tartrazine or sulfites. Individuals with sensitivity to these additives may develop severe allergic or anaphylactic reactions.

Abrupt withdrawal of systemic prednisone for replacement with an inhaled glucocorticoid preparation should be avoided. A corticosteroid-withdrawal syndrome (e.g., malaise, myalgia, nausea, headache, and low-grade fever) and asthma relapse are problems encountered when systemic glucocorticoids are withdrawn too quickly after beginning inhalation therapy.

Adverse Effects

Initial treatment with prednisone may produce mild adverse effects. These include central nervous system (CNS) complaints of euphoria, headache, and vertigo. GI complaints include nausea, vomiting, increased appetite, weight gain, and dyspepsia. Endocrine changes of menstrual irregularities, hyperglycemia, and suppression of pituitary ACTH release (after 2 to 3 days) are common with continued prednisone use. In addition, dermatologic and integumentary adverse effects include acne, suppression of skin test reactions, and delayed healing of wounds. Other effects of continued prednisone use include muscle weakness, increased susceptibility to infections (especially herpesvirus, varicella virus, *Candida* spp., and *Mycobacterium* spp.), masked signs of infection, sodium and fluid retention, fatigue, insomnia, and malaise.

Administration of prednisone produces a negative feedback effect on the HPA axis; this results in the suppression of endogenous cortisol production. Significant suppression of ACTH release and cortisol secretion has been shown to occur with 50 mg/day of oral prednisone for as few as 5 days. Although long believed to be important, high doses and long-term use of glucocorticoids are no longer thought to be reliable predictors of a probable HPA axis deficiency. There appears to be considerable patient variability in responses to dosages and duration of therapy. Acute adrenal insufficiency due to HPA axis suppression following drug withdrawal is one of the most serious complications of prednisone therapy (see the accompanying display, Complications of Prednisone (and Other Glucocorticoid Therapy).

Definite adverse reactions occur with long-term administration of supraphysiologic (pharmacologic) doses of prednisone. Cushingoid characteristics, such as redistribution of fat deposits (e.g., buffalo hump [also known as dowager hump], moon facies, and truncal obesity), and signs of protein catabolism, such as loss of muscle mass and thinning of the extremities, muscle aches, and weakness develop with long-term, supraphysiologic doses of prednisone (and other glucocorticoids). Visual acuity may be affected by the development of cataracts and glaucoma. Hyperlipidemia and thrombus formation also may occur. Other adverse effects from long-term therapy (doses above 5 mg/day) include undesired dermatologic responses of acne, hirsutism, delayed wound healing, skin tearing, and striae; women and the elderly of both genders are more prone to these effects.

A clinically significant adverse effect of long-term prednisone therapy is osteoporosis, which is often considered to be a major limitation of long-term prednisone therapy. Long-term prednisone therapy (doses over 7.5 mg/day) enhances calcium loss, which in turn increases bone resorption from increased parathyroid hormone levels. Bone resorption increases and decreases bone mineral density thereby promoting an osteoporotic condition that increases the risk of hip, pelvic, rib, or vertebral fractures.

Both men and women (premenopausal and postmenopausal) are at high risk for developing glucocorticoid-induced osteoporosis, but postmenopausal women, individuals who are old, debilitated, or immobile, and children are most susceptible to this adverse effect. Significant bone effects (e.g., suppression of bone growth) may occur when these drugs are used in the long-term and intermittent treatment of a variety of childhood in-

Complications of Prednisone (and Other Glucocorticoid Therapy)

Central Nervous System Problems
- Emotional lability
- Paresthesias
- Seizures
- Increased intracranial pressure with papilledema
- Insomnia
- Nervousness
- Psychosis
- Paradoxical suicidal depression
- Aggravation of preexisting psychiatric disorders

Endocrine/Metabolic Problems
- Antagonistic effects on insulin, parathyroid, and thyroid hormones
- Glucose intolerance
- Hirsutism
- Suppression of HPA axis
- Hyperglycemia
- Hyperlipidemia
- Iatrogenic diabetes
- Obesity
- Increased serum lipids
- Increased serum triglycerides (in transplant and asthmatic patients and those with organ transplantation treated with >5 mg/d of prednisone)
- Protein wasting
- Amenorrhea
- Postmenopausal bleeding

Cardiovascular Problems
- Thromboembolism (fat embolism)
- Arrhythmias secondary to K+ alterations
- Hypertension
- CHF

Gastrointestinal Problems
- Fatty liver infiltrates
- Pancreatitis
- Increased appetite (which leads to weight gain)
- Ulcerative esophagitis
- Nausea and vomiting
- Peptic ulceration with perforation or hemorrhage

Fluid and Electrolyte Problems
- Fluid retention
- K+ loss (hypokalemia)
- Na+ loss (hyponatremia)
- Negative Ca++ balance

Hematologic and Immunologic Problems
- Altered inflammatory response
- Eosinopenia
- Leukocytosis
- Direct correlation between opportunistic infections and higher doses and prolonged duration of glucocorticoids
- Leukopenia

Musculoskeletal Problems
- Aseptic necrosis (femur, humerus head)
- Growth failure
- Myopathy
- Osteopenia
- Osteoporosis

Ophthalmic Problems
- Increased intraocular pressure
- Cataracts
- Glaucoma
- Exophthalmos

Integumentary Problems
- Acne
- Ecchymoses
- Petechiae
- Thinning of skin (increased friability and fragility)
- Striae purpura
- Subcutaneous fat atrophy

General Problems
- Cushingoid characteristics
- Withdrawal syndrome

flammatory diseases (e.g., asthma). The bones most often affected are the vertebrae, ribs, and long bones, although all bones are at risk. There is a high incidence of vertebral compression fractures in patients who receive extended prednisone treatment.

Several mechanisms mediate adverse bone effects of prednisone and other glucocorticoids. Osteoblastic collagen synthesis, osteoid formation, and bone formation are reduced; bone resorption is enhanced; and intestinal malabsorption of calcium occurs. Increased urinary excretion of calcium suggests that bone calcium is mobilized to maintain plasma calcium concentration to balance renal losses. There appears to be a direct correlation between the extent of bone loss and the duration of prednisone therapy; research suggests that the majority of bone loss occurs within the first 3 to 12 months with a slowing of bone loss thereafter. Although alternate-day therapy has been shown to decrease some of the adverse effects of long-term prednisone therapy, it does not appear to decrease the risk for development of osteoporosis. The prevalence of osteoporosis is difficult to assess when corticosteroids are used in diseases in which the risk of osteoporosis is already great (e.g., rheumatoid arthritis and renal disease).

Finally, glucose tolerance is affected by prednisone (and other glucocorticoids). This occurs in as many as 15% of individuals on long-term therapy. The risk of iatrogenic diabetes mellitus increases with age, obesity, a previous history of glucose intolerance, and a family history of diabetes. Even low-dose therapy can impair glucose tolerance in patients with types 1 and 2 diabetes. Patients with diabetes may need changes in diet or hypoglycemic therapy (e.g., insulin, oral drugs) to maintain control of blood sugar.

Drug Interactions

Significant interactions may occur between prednisone and a variety of drugs. Prednisone also causes some interactions with laboratory measurements. Urine glucose and serum cholesterol levels may be increased. Serum levels of K+ may be decreased. Triiodothyronine (T_3), thyroxine (T_4), thyroid I-131 uptake, and protein-bound iodine concentrations may be decreased, making it difficult to monitor the therapeutic response of patients receiving the drugs for thyroiditis or assessing patients for thyroid dysfunction. Prednisone also may produce a false-positive result in some tests for systemic bacterial infections. In addition, reactions to skin tests may be suppressed. Prednisone alters glucose tolerance tests. Diabetics should be monitored closely and adjustments in dosage of insulin or oral antidiabetic drugs made accordingly (Table 40-2).

TABLE 40-2 Agents That Interact With Prednisone

Interactants	Effect and Significance	Nursing Management
troleandomycin	May increase therapeutic and toxic effects of troleandomycin	Monitor patient for these effects.
ketoconazole	Prednisone clearance possibly decreased	Observe for excess effects of prednisone.
oral contraceptives	Possible increased prednisone half-life and concentration and decreased clearance	Evaluate for excess effects of prednisone. Dosage may require adjustment.
ambenonium, edrophonium, neostigmine, pyridostigmine	May cause severe deterioration of muscle strength in patients with myasthenia gravis	Monitor muscle strength in patient.
barbiturates, phenytoin, rifampin	Decreased pharmacologic effects of prednisone	Observe for subtherapeutic effects of prednisone. Dosage may require adjustment.
salicylates	Prednisone will reduce serum salicylate levels and may decrease their effectiveness	Evaluate for subtherapeutic effects of salicylate. Dosage may require adjustment.
hydantoins	Possible increased prednisone clearance, resulting in reduced therapeutic levels	Observe for subtherapeutic effects of prednisone. Dosage may require adjustment.
oral anticoagulants	Anticoagulant dose requirements possibly reduced; conversely prednisone may oppose the anti-coagulant action.	Monitor prothrombin time and coagulation tests.
isoniazid	Isoniazid serum concentrations possibly decreased	Monitor for subtherapeutic effects of isoniazid. Dosage may require adjustment.
potassium-depleting agents (diuretics)	May increase the depletion of potassium	Observe patients for muscular and systemic effects of hypokalemia.
somatrem	Growth-promoting effect of somatrem possibly inhibited	Increased dosage of somatrem may be necessary. Monitor closely for pharmacologic side effects.
theophylline	Alterations in the pharmacologic activity of either agent possible	Observe for subtherapeutic effects of either drug. Dosage adjustments may be necessary.

Assessment of Relevant Core Patient Variables

Health Status

Before administering prednisone, the nurse should assess the patient's drug history for use of prescription, over-the-counter (OTC), recreational, or illicit drugs. In addition, it is important to review the patient's medical history for GI problems of frequent upset, reflux disease, presence or history of stomach ulcers, or epigastric pain. The patient's nutritional status, weight control, and disease or trauma history should be compiled. The nurse should perform a complete physical examination and review current laboratory data (e.g., electrocardiogram, x-ray films of spine and chest, glucose tolerance test results, tuberculin skin test results, complete blood count with differential, ocular pressure, HPA axis function, and blood pressure). In addition, muscle strength and body proportions should be observed, as should patterns of hair growth and distribution. Depending on the findings, the nurse may coordinate further testing (e.g., hepatic and renal function studies). Throughout therapy, the nurse should continue to assess for signs of adrenal insufficiency.

Life Span and Gender

The nurse should determine whether the patient is pregnant or breast-feeding. Prednisone is Food and Drug Administration (FDA) pregnancy category C. It is excreted in breast milk and may suppress growth or cause other adverse effects in nursing infants. It also is important to note the patient's age before administering prednisone. Growth failure can occur in children receiving prolonged prednisone therapy. Irreversible loss of height may occur if prednisone is administered during periods of greatest growth (i.e., before 2 years of age or during puberty when the epiphyses of the long bones close). Growth suppression is proportional to the dose and frequency of prednisone administered; divided daily doses are more growth inhibiting than a single daily dose.

Elderly patients are more prone to adrenal suppression from prolonged prednisone administration because of the prevalence of ongoing prednisone therapy for chronic diseases (e.g., rheumatoid arthritis and bronchial disease). Elderly patients may require lower doses because of physiologic changes resulting from aging, such as decreased muscle mass and plasma volume or impairment of hepatic or renal functions. Blood pressure and blood glucose and electrolyte levels should be monitored regularly. Sudden withdrawal of prednisone can lead to acute adrenal insufficiency.

Lifestyle, Diet, and Habits

The nurse should assess the patient's typical diet and blood pressure. Foods high in sodium will help compensate for the resulting mineralocorticoid deficiency. It also is important for the patient to maintain an adequate blood pressure and to avoid drugs or foods high in potassium because of the tendency to retain this electrolyte. Increased salt and fluid intake during periods of diaphoresis (e.g., hot weather or strenuous exercise) to avoid imbalances is necessary.

A diet that controls carbohydrate and calorie intake is important (unless contraindicated) due to the increased gluconeogenesis, decreased glucose use, increased appetite, and weight gain effects of pharmacologic glucocorticoid therapy.

It also is important to assess the patient's typical daily activities. The weak muscles and fatigability characteristic of glucocorticoid excess predispose the patient to accidents. The osteoporosis and vertebral-compression effects of excessive glucocorticoid therapy may make bone fractures more likely. Passive and active range-of-motion exercises to offset the tendency toward muscle weakness and atrophy are important. Physical or occupational therapy referrals may be necessary.

Nursing Diagnoses and Outcomes

- Disturbed Body Image related to cushingoid characteristics or physical changes secondary to glucocorticoid therapy

  Desired outcome: The patient will verbalize and demonstrate acceptance of appearance (grooming, dress, posture, presentation of self), verbalize and demonstrate increased positive feelings, and demonstrate healthy adaptation and coping skills.
- Excess Fluid Volume related to sodium and water retention secondary to corticosteroid therapy

  Desired outcome: The patient will relate causative factors and methods of preventing edema and exhibit decreased peripheral and sacral edema.
- Risk for Infection or Risk for Injury related to anti-inflammatory, immunosuppressive and metabolic effects of chronic corticosteroid therapy

  Desired outcome: The patient will demonstrate knowledge of risk factors associated with potential for infection or injury and will practice appropriate precautions for prevention.
- Imbalanced Nutrition: More Than Body Requirements related to altered satiety patterns secondary to corticosteroid medications

  Desired outcome: The patient will describe reasons why weight gain is a risk, discuss current nutritional needs, and discuss the effects of exercise on weight control.

Planning and Intervention

Maximizing Therapeutic Effects

Hormone production by the adrenal gland is influenced by many factors. Normal cortisol production follows a diurnal cycle. Levels peak in the early morning hours (6 AM to 8 AM) and decline throughout the day with a second, lower peak in the late afternoon (4 PM to 6 PM). Cortisol secretion from the adrenal gland also is increased in response to stress (physical or emotional) and low endogenous glucocorticoid levels. Thus, the most opportune time for administration of daily doses of glucocorticoids is early in the morning.

When prednisone is prescribed for replacement therapy, the nurse should advise the patient regarding glucocorticoid imbalances and should teach the patient how to monitor the response to therapy. It is important to advise the patient that timing of the dose is important; the preferred drug schedule follows the normal diurnal pattern of cortisol secretion (i.e., two thirds of the dose before 9 AM and the remaining third late in the afternoon).

The nurse also should teach the patient to determine what constitutes stress (e.g., physical illness, injury, trauma, or emotional upset) and how to manage stress. It is important to explain that the prednisone dosage needs to be increased during periods of stress or illness. The nurse should emphasize the importance of making a special effort to avoid injury and infection.

When prednisone is prescribed for its anti-inflammatory effects, the nurse should obtain a thorough drug history, including previous corticosteroid therapy and indication(s) for drug therapy, duration of drug therapy, and dosage and method of administration.

The nurse should alert the patient that following intra-articular injection, the injected joint should not be overused. Weight-bearing joints (e.g., knee) should be rested 24 to 48 hours post injection.

Minimizing Adverse Effects

The nurse should emphasize the importance of adherence to the drug regimen and should warn patients that they must not abruptly stop either short-term or long-term prednisone therapy because of the danger of acute adrenal insufficiency associated with abrupt discontinuation.

Prednisone administration (especially at high doses and during prolonged therapy) can lead to the formation of a peptic ulcer complicated by hemorrhage and perforation or a previously healed ulcer may be reactivated. Therefore, the nurse should teach the patient that gastric irritation may be reduced if prednisone is consumed with milk (unless contraindicated), food, nonsystemic antacids (e.g., Al+, Ca++, or Mg+ salts), or, preferably, with concomitant antiulcer drug therapy (e.g., antiulcer agents—H_2-receptor antagonists, proton-pump inhibitors). It also is important to recommend limiting intake of caffeine and alcohol and products containing aspirin. These factors increase the secretion of gastric acid, which irritates the gastric mucosa and increases the risk of GI bleeding.

The nurse should assess children for growth periodically during therapy, since there is risk of altered growth and development with glucocorticoid. Inhaled glucocorticoids may cause coughing, dry mouth, fungal infections, hoarseness, and throat irritation. The nurse should advise the patient to rinse the mouth with water following use of the inhalant to minimize the risk of oral, laryngeal, or pharyngeal fungal infections.

Alternate-day administration (i.e., glucocorticoids given every other day instead of daily) of long-term, systemic glucocorticoids has been used to lessen the suppression of the hypothalamus, the anterior pituitary and the rate of bone growth. This mode of administration may pose some problems, however. In some individuals, this dosing regimen may not be enough to control the inflammatory process. Alternate-day dosing minimizes HPA-axis suppression and reduces the incidence of most glucocorticoid adverse effects. By dosing glucocorticoids every other morning, the HPA-axis recovers in the last 12 hours of the off day of therapy. Intermediate-acting glucocorticoids, such as prednisone, are most appropriate for alternate-day therapy. Long-acting agents, such as dexamethasone, do not allow the HPA-axis to recover on the off day. Short-acting agents, such as hydrocortisone, may not provide sufficient glucocorticoid effects to manage symptoms on the off day. Alternate-day dosing does not minimize the risk of osteoporosis or cataract formation. In addition, a too-abrupt switch from daily doses to alternate-day dosing may cause signs and symptoms of adrenal insufficiency (e.g., fatigue, nausea, vomiting, and hypotension) on the days between doses.

Patients taking corticosteroids who require surgery should receive a preoperative dose of a rapid-acting corticosteroid. This should be continued postoperatively in decreasing doses for several days. This will help the patient cope with the stress of surgery.

Providing Patient and Family Education

- The nurse should instruct patients to take the drug exactly as prescribed. It is important to caution individuals and their families or caregivers of the dangers associated with abrupt discontinuation of drug therapy (e.g., acute adrenal insufficiency). The nurse should instruct patients on how to take the drug correctly and what to do if a dose is missed. This will depend on the type of dosing strategy that has been prescribed for the patient (see the accompanying display, Home Dosing Strategies).
- Prednisone replacement therapy is used to treat the chronic, lifelong conditions of adrenal cortical insufficiency. Therefore, the patient may need emotional support and assistance in the grieving process over loss of health and loss of control. The nurse should stress the importance of maintaining the drug regimen to regain and maintain health and control.
- It is important to advise the patient to wear a medical identification device with the diagnosis and drug therapy clearly indicated. The nurse also must emphasize the importance of the patient's notifying any health care professional about glucocorticoid therapy before undergoing treatment for another medical problem.
- The nurse should discuss the adverse effects of drug therapy with the patient and family and should

Home Dosing Strategies*

One Dose Every Other Day

If a dose is missed, it is important to take the missed dose as soon as possible if it is remembered the same morning, then go back to the regular schedule.

If the dose is not remembered until later, wait and take it the following morning, and then skip a day and start the regular dosing schedule.

One Dose Every Day

If a dose is missed, it is important to take the missed dose as soon as possible, then go back to the regular schedule.

If the missed dose is not remembered until the next day, skip it and do not double the next dose.

Several Doses Every Day

If a dose is missed, it is important to take the missed dose as soon as possible, then go back to the regular schedule.

If the missed dose is not remembered until the next dose is due, double the next dose.

*The nurse should make sure that the directions for dosage adjustment (for example, doubled with minor stress, such as common cold or dental visit, tripled with severe stress, such as serious illness or surgery) are clearly indicated on the drug label.

clearly identify those that should be reported to the health care provider immediately.
- The nurse should warn the patient and family that long-term glucocorticoid therapy will cause alterations in appearance and this may cause disturbances in self-concept. The nurse should assist the patient and family in dealing with the changes that occur. Many changes (e.g., truncal obesity, thinning of extremities, "buffalo hump") may be camouflaged with loosely fitted clothing. Make-up may be used to cover the acne and hyperpigmentation that may occur.
- Supplemental daily intake of 1500 mg of oral calcium and 400 IU of vitamin D is usually recommended to minimize the loss of bone density that occurs with chronic glucocorticoid therapy.
- Any individual who has received a significant amount of glucocorticoid is at risk for some degree of adrenal cortical atrophy. What dosage is responsible and how long it will persist is unknown. What is known, however, is that too abrupt a withdrawal of glucocorticoid therapy will cause acute adrenal insufficiency. The nurse should instruct the patient to be alert for the symptoms of anorexia, hypoglycemia, lethargy, malaise, nausea, psychologic despondency, restlessness, and weakness; the patient should report them immediately to the health care provider if any occur.
- The patient and family or other caregivers need to be informed about the importance of rest, sleep, and health-maintenance behaviors. The nurse should teach patients ways to avoid infection and how to recognize signs of infection, including elevated temperature, feelings of malaise, or localized swelling; these signs should receive prompt medical attention. Patients treated with alternate-day corticosteroid therapy seldom develop infectious complications. The nurse should discuss self-medication for minor illnesses with the patient. It is important to identify probable situations previously handled at home alone (e.g., flu with vomiting and diarrhea), which will now require dosage adjustments, medical intervention, or hospitalization. The nurse should provide patients and their families with written instructions on what to do in these situations.
- Safety issues are important to discuss with patients. Prevention of falls is of vital importance because of the occurrence of osteoporosis with long-term or high-dose use of prednisone and other systemic glucocorticoids. The nurse should evaluate the safety of the home environment. The nurse also should stress the importance of reporting bone pain, because aseptic necrosis or pathologic fractures may occur spontaneously.

Ongoing Assessment and Evaluation

Pharmacologic prednisone therapy represents a drug regimen in which the patient must be monitored for therapeutic drug response, adverse drug reactions, and indications of drug toxicity. Patients who are to undergo dental, medical, or surgical procedures will usually require an increase in corticoid dosage, because their "normal" adrenocortical response to stress has been inhibited as a result of the supraphysiologic dosages of corticoids. It is important to assess for infection during and after hospitalizations or minor surgery. Used for its anti-inflammatory effect, prednisone will delay wound healing; the nurse should assess for any abrasions or incisions that are not healing well. In addition, common indicators of infection (e.g., temperature elevation, erythema, and leukocytosis) will not occur, because corticosteroids block these inflammatory responses. Instead, the patient may report changes in energy level, activity level, and appetite as indicators of infection.

The glucocorticoid effect of increased gluconeogenesis and decreased glucose use may cause hyperglycemia to occur; the nurse should monitor patients for the development of iatrogenic diabetes mellitus. Patients with existing diabetes may need to reestablish control. Prophylactic antitubercular-drug therapy may be required because high glucocorticoid levels are likely to reactivate encapsulated tuberculosis.

The nurse should be particularly vigilant about assessing patients receiving long-term prednisone (and other glucocorticoids) therapy. Adrenal suppression may occur; alternately, usual effects of endogenous glucocorticoid hormones on the body may be exaggerated. Indications of adrenal suppression may be anorexia, diarrhea, fluid and electrolyte imbalances (especially decreased Na^+, decreased glucose and increased K^+), fatigue, nausea, vomiting, and weight loss. If fluid volume deficit occurs, it is important for the nurse to assess for hypotension, pyrexia, tachycardia and tachypnea, dry skin, and dry mucous membranes. The nurse also should assess for exaggerated, undesired effects from prednisone (and other glucocorticoids), including changes in mood or affect (e.g., agitation, depression, euphoria, and insomnia), edema, muscle weakness, nausea, vomiting, and weight gain.

The metabolic end products of adrenocortical and androgenic hormones are 17-ketosteroids. Actual serum levels of cortisol and ACTH may be determined by a 24-hour urine collection with subsequent measurement of 17-ketosteroids. Either a dexamethasone suppression test or an ACTH stimulation test may disclose the function of the HPA axis feedback system. Finally, the nurse should monitor patients receiving digoxin or other digitalis-based drugs for toxicity.

It is essential for the nurse to evaluate for relief of the signs and symptoms that precipitated the use of glucocorticoid drugs. Used as replacement therapy, the patient should report an increased state of health (e.g., absence of fatigue, hypoglycemia, hypovolemia, and weakness) and a feeling of well being. Used for chronic inflammatory conditions (e.g., rheumatoid arthritis), the patient should experience less pain and discomfort and increased joint mobility. Lymphocyte levels (primarily T_4) should decrease when used for immunosuppressive effects. ■

MEMORY CHIP

Prednisone

- Anti-inflammatory or immuno-suppressive therapy
- Hepatic dysfunction may impair prednisone conversion into active prednisolone
- Prednisone use may cause HPA axis suppression if given for more than 2 weeks and is then withdrawn too abruptly, placing the patient at risk for acute adrenal insufficiency
- Significant contraindications: hypersensitivity to prednisone; systemic fungal infections
- Most common adverse effects: CNS complaints of euphoria, headache, and vertigo; GI complaints of nausea, vomiting, increased appetite, weight gain, and dyspepsia
- Most serious adverse effect: acute adrenal insufficiency due to HPA axis suppression following prednisone withdrawal
- Maximizing therapeutic effects: administer prednisone according to established schedule (preferably one that follows the normal diurnal pattern of cortisol secretion); increase the dosage in times of stress to prevent drug-induced adrenal insufficiency
- Minimizing adverse effects: give prednisone with meals and/or antacids
- Most significant patient education: advise the patient to wear medical identification so that any emergency medical personnel will know about this drug therapy

DRUGS CLOSELY RELATED TO PREDNISONE

Among the glucocorticoids closely related to prednisone are hydrocortisone, methylprednisolone, betamethasone, dexamethasone, inhaled glucocorticoids, and topical glucocorticoids.

Hydrocortisone

Hydrocortisone is bound reversibly to corticosteroid-binding albumin and globulin; the endogenous hormone is bound to a greater degree than the exogenous hormone. Hydrocortisone is metabolized by the liver and excreted in the urine; the synthetic corticosteroids undergo a similar biotransformation and excretion. Hydrocortisone is absorbed partially following rectal administration. Rectal preparations of hydrocortisone (e.g., retention enema, intrarectal foam) are absorbed as much as 50% and used as adjunctive therapy in patients with ulcerative colitis. Contraindications to rectal hydrocortisone use are systemic fungal infections, recent ileocolostomy or intestinal anastomoses, abscess, obstruction, peritonitis, and perforation.

Methylprednisolone

Methylprednisolone (Medrol) and its derivatives, methylprednisolone sodium succinate (Solu-Medrol), such as betamethasone, dexamethasone, and triamcinolone, are synthetic glucocorticoids characterized by potent anti-inflammatory and immunosuppressive effects. These drugs have little mineralocorticoid activity and usually are not used to manage adrenal insufficiency unless a more potent mineralocorticoid is administered concomitantly. Pharmacokinetics, pharmacodynamics, contraindications, and adverse effects are similar to those associated with prednisone.

Methylprednisolone is useful for the following:

- Short-term management of inflammatory and allergic disorders, such as rheumatoid arthritis
- Collagen diseases, such as systemic lupus erythematosus, and skin diseases, such as pemphigus
- Status asthmaticus and autoimmune disorders
- Cancer-related hypercalcemia
- Ulcerative colitis, acute exacerbations of multiple sclerosis, and palliative therapy in some leukemias and lymphomas
- Blood disorders, such as thrombocytopenia purpura

Unlabeled uses for methylprednisolone are severe alcoholic hepatitis (to reduce mortality), adult respiratory distress syndrome and septic shock (these uses are controversial), and acute spinal cord injury (to improve neurologic function).

Methylprednisolone is metabolized by the liver, crosses the placenta, and enters breast milk. It is excreted in the urine. Dosages are individualized according to patient and dosage form. Methylprednisolone is administered orally, whereas methylprednisolone sodium succinate may be given by IM or IV injection. Methylprednisolone acetate may be administered by IM, intra-articular, intralesional, or soft-tissue injection. As in prednisone therapy, systemic methylprednisolone must be discontinued gradually to prevent acute adrenal insufficiency.

Adverse effects of methylprednisolone therapy are many. Common ones include vertigo, headache, weight gain and increased appetite, sodium and fluid retention, immunosuppression, and impaired wound healing. The nurse should teach patients to avoid people with known infections; to avoid receiving live virus vaccines while taking methylprednisolone; and to report adverse effects, such as unusual weight gain, edema, muscle weakness, black or tarry stools, and prolonged cold-like infections (see the accompanying display, Concerns Raised by Methylprednisolone and Other Glucocorticoids).

Dexamethasone

Dexamethasone exhibits essentially no mineralocorticoid activity and maximal anti-inflammatory activity with a prolonged plasma half-life (see Figure 40-2) and pronounced growth-suppressing and bone demineralizing properties. Thus, it is used almost exclusively in short-term situations requiring maximum anti-inflammatory activity (e.g., cerebral edema and septic shock). Dexamethasone, given for cerebral edema, may alter the results on a brain scan because of a decreased uptake of radioactive contrast medium. It also may be used to diagnose Cushing disease (idiopathic adrenocortical hyperfunction). Following drug administration, urine is collected for 24 hours to determine the amount of 17-hydroxycorticosteroid excretion. Unlabeled uses for dexamethasone include acute mountain (altitude) sickness, chemotherapy hyperemesis, bronchopulmonary dysplasia in preterm infants, bacterial meningitis (to decrease incidence of auditory impairment), diagnosis of major (endogenous) depression, and hirsutism.

Critical Thinking Scenario

Concerns raised by methylprednisolone and other glucocorticoids

Mr. Vito, 62 years old, is admitted to the emergency department with acute respiratory distress related to chronic obstructive pulmonary disease. Emergency treatment consists of respiratory inhalation therapy and IV methylprednisolone sodium succinate (Solu-Medrol), after which Mr. Vito is transferred to the telemetry unit. The nursing history that accompanies him discloses that he has type 2 diabetes that is controlled by diet and oral antidiabetic drugs.

1. Discuss assessment data needed to ensure safe administration of methylprednisolone to Mr. Vito, identifying any condition that represents a need for particularly cautious drug administration.
2. Define any concerns the nurse may have related to respiratory therapy and diabetes control. As Mr. Vito recovers, plans are made for him to begin long-term, anti-inflammatory corticosteroid therapy. At discharge, he will be on oral prednisone 5 mg qid and a beclomethasone (Vanceril) inhaler as needed.
3. Identify any important screening tests that should be done to ensure safe administration of prednisone. In addition, propose important points to include in a patient education program.

Betamethasone

Betamethasone binds to intracellular corticosteroid receptors to produce anti-inflammatory and immunosuppressive effects. Clinical uses and adverse effects for betamethasone are similar to those for dexamethasone and methylprednisolone. In an unlabeled use, betamethasone is given to prevent respiratory distress syndrome in premature neonates.

Inhaled Glucocorticoids

Beclomethasone dipropionate, budesonide, flunisolide, fluticasone, and triamcinolone acetonide constitute a new family of synthetic inhalant/intranasal steroids, possessing enhanced topical anti-inflammatory activity and low systemic potency. Inhaled glucocorticoids are metabolized in the lung before they are absorbed, thereby reducing their systemic effects. These drugs are relatively equal in potency and clinical effectiveness and thought to have negligible systemic activity and complications. One published study has demonstrated that a dose-related systemic effect occurred in a substantial proportion of patients using high-dose inhaled corticosteroids. Dosages in excess of 1.5 mg/day (0.75 mg/day) for fluticasone were associated with a significant reduction in bone density (Lipworth, 1999).

Dysphonia and oropharyngeal *Candida albicans* infection are the most frequently encountered adverse effects associated with inhaled corticosteroids; these effects are related to daily use of the active drug. Because the inhaled corticosteroids are supplied in metered-dose inhalers (MDIs), the nurse should teach correct use of the unit. The newer MDIs have spacers, which help to alleviate dysphonia by filtering larger aerosol particles that ordinarily deposit in the oropharynx and extrathoracic airways (thereby reducing the risk of oropharyngeal candidiasis) and by increasing the intrapulmonary delivery of the drug if the patient's inhalation technique is poor.

These drugs are inhaled through the mouth to treat asthma and sprayed into the nose to treat rhinitis. Nursing management concerns with these drugs should focus on teaching about the importance of good oral hygiene, teaching the proper use of metered-dose inhalers, and teaching the patient to report signs and symptoms of oropharyngeal candidiasis (e.g., mouth ulcers, white spots on oral mucous membranes, and painful swallowing).

Topical Glucocorticoids

Topical glucocorticoids include hydrocortisone, methylprednisolone, betamethasone, dexamethasone, and triamcinolone. These are applied topically rather than ingested. For the most part, topical application of corticosteroids does not produce systemic effects. Applied to the conjunctiva or external ear, these drugs are not absorbed systemically. However, they may be absorbed systemically if applied to the nasal mucosa or large areas of abraded skin, inhaled excessively for prolonged periods, or large doses are used.

Another topical application form is intra-articular injection, which produces localized effects for symptomatic relief (e.g., analgesia, increased joint mobility). Patients receiving this form of the drug need to be cautioned to allow time for the treated area to heal; the pain-induced limitation may be eliminated, but overusing the joint may still aggravate the active inflammatory process. Frequent intra-articular injections may damage joint tissues.

Topical preparations are effective therapy for a variety of inflammatory skin conditions. Topical glucocorticoids are available in various formulations (e.g., creams, gels, lotions, ointments, and solutions). This formulation has a major impact on percutaneous absorption and penetration. Ointment-based formulations are preferred generally for most regions of the body. Ointments facilitate steroid absorption and penetration by trapping the moisture in the epidermis.

Adverse effects with topical application are usually milder and more transient than those seen after systemically administered steroids. However, adrenal function may be suppressed when potent topical agents are used in large amounts for long periods, especially when the skin surface is denuded or when occlusive dressings are used. Occlusive dressings significantly increase percutaneous absorption and efficacy and increase the risk of local adverse effects (e.g., skin atrophy) and systemic adverse effects. Increased skin temperature, hydration, and application to skin with a thin surface layer also enhance absorption. The primary therapeutic effects of the topical corticosteroids are their anti-inflammatory activity, which is nonspecific in that they act on most causes of inflammation, including chemical, immunologic, mechanical, and microbiologic. When the glucocorticoids are applied to inflamed skin, they inhibit the migration of macrophages and leukocytes into the area by reversing the vascular dilation and permeability. The clinical result is a decrease in edema, erythema, and pruritus.

MINERALOCORTICOIDS

Aldosterone, the naturally occurring mineralocorticoid, is expensive and requires parenteral administration. Therefore, fludrocortisone (Florinef Acetate) is the prototype exogenous mineralocorticoid. This adrenal corticosteroid has both high mineralocorticoid and glucocorticoid activity (its glucocorticoid potency is 15 times greater than that of hydrocortisone). However, it is used only for its mineralocorticoid activity as replacement therapy in adrenocortical deficiency.

NURSING MANAGEMENT OF THE PATIENT RECEIVING FLUDROCORTISONE

Core Drug Knowledge

Pharmacotherapeutics

Fludrocortisone is used for partial replacement therapy for primary adrenocortical insufficiency and for treating salt-losing adrenogenital syndrome. An unlabeled use for fludrocortisone is management of severe orthostatic hypotension.

Pharmacokinetics

Orally administered, fludrocortisone is absorbed readily from the GI tract with peak concentration in 1.7 hours. It is metabolized in the liver and excreted by the kidney. Plasma half-life is approximately 3.5 hours, but biologic half-life ranges from 18 to 36 hours. Fludrocortisone crosses the placenta and enters the breast milk. The usual adult dosage is 0.1 mg/day (range, 0.1 mg three times a week up to 0.2 mg/day).

Pharmacodynamics

Fludrocortisone acts on the distal renal tubule to enhance the reabsorption of sodium and to increase the urinary excretion of both potassium and hydrogen ions. In small oral doses, the mineralocorticoid effects of fludrocortisone predominate—urinary excretion of potassium, marked sodium retention, and a rise in blood pressure as a result of the physiologic effects of these electrolyte levels. Larger doses of fludrocortisone result in predominance of glucocorticoid effects.

Contraindications and Precautions

Hypersensitivity to fludrocortisone and conditions not requiring intense mineralocorticoid activity are contraindications to use. Fludrocortisone's glucocorticoid activity places patients at risk for infection; its use is contraindicated in systemic fungal infections. Patients should be monitored for evidence of intercurrent infection. The drug should be used cautiously during lactation because it is secreted into breast milk, and safety and efficacy are not established in children. It should also be used cautiously in patients with cardiovascular disease, because it can elevate sodium and fluid levels.

Adverse Effects

In small oral doses, fludrocortisone produces marked sodium retention and increased urinary potassium excretion. It also causes a rise in blood pressure, apparently because of these effects on electrolyte levels. In larger doses, fludrocortisone inhibits endogenous adrenal cortical secretion, thymic activity, and pituitary corticotropin excretion. It promotes the deposition of liver glycogen, and, unless protein intake is adequate, it induces negative nitrogen balance.

Adverse effects usually occur if the dosage is too high or if the drug is withdrawn too rapidly. Cardiovascular adverse effects may include edema, hypertension, congestive heart failure, and cardiomegaly. Dermatologic adverse effects may include bruising, diaphoresis, urticaria, or allergic skin rash. Hypokalemic alkalosis may occur. Additionally, because fludrocortisone possesses potent glucocorticoid activity, fludrocortisone may cause adverse effects similar to those seen with the glucocorticoids.

Drug Interactions

Fludrocortisone interacts with many of the same drugs as prednisone due to its high glucocorticoid activity. The drugs with which fludrocortisone interacts include barbiturates, hydantoins, rifampin, anticholinesterases, and salicylates (Table 40-3).

Assessment of Relevant Core Patient Variables

Health Status

Before administering fludrocortisone, the nurse should assess the patient's fluid and electrolyte balance, nutritional status, and weight control history. Fludrocortisone acts on the distal renal tubule to enhance the reabsorption of sodium. It increases urinary excretion of both potassium and hydrogen ions. In small doses, it produces marked sodium retention, increased urinary excretion of potassium, and elevated blood pressure. In larger doses, the glucocorticoid effects of fludrocortisone promote the deposition of liver glycogen, and unless protein intake is adequate, may induce a negative nitrogen balance. Depending on the patient's condition before drug administration, the nurse should coordinate appropriate laboratory or diagnostic tests, such as hepatic or renal function studies, because of fludrocortisone's pharmacokinetics.

Fludrocortisone therapy in patients with cardiovascular disease (e.g., hypertension), congestive heart failure, or impaired renal function may increase sodium and water retention and worsen these conditions.

Life Span and Gender

The nurse should determine whether the patient is pregnant or breast-feeding. Fludrocortisone is FDA pregnancy category C, which means that safety for use during pregnancy has not been established. If given during pregnancy, the newborn should be observed for signs of adrenocortical insufficiency because of adrenal suppression. Fludrocortisone enters breast milk. Therefore, it should be given cautiously to lactating women. It is important to note the patient's age before administering fludrocortisone. Growth and development of infants and children on long-term therapy should be monitored routinely.

Lifestyle, Diet, and Habits

The nurse should assess the patient's diet because sodium retention and potassium loss are accelerated by a sodium-rich diet while taking fludrocortisone.

Culture

It is prudent for the nurse to determine the cultural background of a patient before administering fludrocortisone. Traditional foods and herbal and home remedies consumed by patients of various ethnic or cultural groups may be high in sodium. For example, Chinese foods are traditionally prepared with soy sauce and monosodium glutamate (MSG). Preserved and fermented foods are also high in sodium. A complete dietary history, including usual dietary intake, food preferences and intolerances, and use of home remedies should be gathered. This information will allow the nurse to assess the patient's risk of developing weight gain or edema while taking fludrocortisone. It will also provide the nurse with knowledge to aid in patient teaching. For example, discussing ways to reduce sodium intake by gradually reducing dietary sodium from food sources and food preparation (e.g., the use of soy sauce, MSG, or salt-cured or salt-processed foods).

Nursing Diagnoses and Outcomes

- Excess Fluid Volume related to mineralocorticoid-induced sodium and water retention

TABLE 40-3 Agents That Interact With Fludrocortisone

Interactants	Effect and Significance	Nursing Management
barbiturates, hydantoins, rifampin	Decrease the effects of fludrocortisone	Observe for signs of adrenal insufficiency. Increased dosage of fludrocortisone may be necessary.
anticholinesterases	Decrease the effects of the anticholinesterase in myasthenia gravis (MG)	Observe for signs of exacerbation of MG. Increased dosage of the anticholinesterase may be required.
salicylates	Decrease serum levels and effectiveness of salicylates	Evaluate for ineffectiveness of salicylate therapy. Increased dosage of the salicylates may be necessary. Measure serum salicylate levels.

Desired outcome: The patient will relate causative factors and methods of preventing fluid retention and exhibit decreased peripheral and sacral edema.

- Risk for Injury related to adrenocortical insufficiency

  Desired outcome: The patient will demonstrate knowledge of risk factors associated with potential for injury and will practice appropriate precautions for prevention.

Planning and Intervention

Maximizing Therapeutic Effects

The nurse should explain to the patient that the dosage should be increased during times of stress to prevent drug-induced adrenal insufficiency. It also is important for the nurse to assess the patient's drug history for potential drug interactions with fludrocortisone; drugs that may interact include barbiturates, cholestyramine, oral contraceptives, and salicylates.

Minimizing Adverse Effects

The nurse should review the patient's history for preexisting conditions that require cautious use of fludrocortisone (e.g., diabetes mellitus, hypertension, osteoporosis, or impaired renal function).

Monitoring of fluid balance is vital; it is important to measure blood pressure and electrolyte status. Patients with a history of renal or cardiovascular dysfunction may be more likely to develop adverse effects from fludrocortisone. The nurse should encourage the patient to select potassium-rich foods. This will help to prevent potassium loss and secondary hypokalemia associated with the sodium-retaining activity of the mineralocorticoids. It also is important to teach patients to moderate their sodium intake to prevent weight gain and edema. Sodium restriction may be necessary if edema or hypertension develops.

Providing Patient and Family Education

- The nurse should instruct patients to adhere to drug therapy as prescribed. It is important to stress the importance of regular follow-up visits with the health care provider.
- It is important to encourage the patient to wear a medical identification bracelet that states the patient's medical condition and the specific drug therapy.
- The nurse should teach patients to report unusual weight gain, lower extremity edema, muscle weakness, and severe or continuing headache. It also is important to monitor blood pressure and serum electrolytes (including calcium) regularly to prevent fludrocortisone overdosage.
- The nurse should discourage the consumption of high-sodium foods and encourage the consumption of high-potassium foods.
- The nurse should instruct the patient to weigh herself or himself daily; any sudden increase indicates fluid retention.

Ongoing Assessment and Evaluation

Fludrocortisone exerts major effects on sodium and potassium. The nurse should monitor closely for edema, weight gain, hypertension, cardiac arrhythmias, or muscular weakness, which may develop because of the drug's sodium-retaining and kaliuretic effects. Potassium supplementation may be necessary. Periods of stress (e.g., trauma, surgery, or severe illness) may require supportive mineralocorticoid and glucocorticoid dosage to avoid drug-induced adrenal insufficiency.

The nurse should assess the patient for adverse reactions to fludrocortisone, which include fluid retention (e.g., increased blood pressure, sudden weight gain, such as more than 2 lb in 24 hours), ankle edema, or respiratory crackles. The nurse also should monitor for acute adrenal insufficiency or characteristic adverse glucocorticoid reactions. Fludrocortisone replacement therapy is effective when the patient exhibits a normal blood pressure, and fluid and electrolyte balance is within normal limits. The patient should verbalize the importance of self-monitoring for adverse effects and of reporting to the health care provider any significant ones, such as sudden weight gain, weakness, undue fatigue, change in sleep patterns, tarry or black stools, infections, or injuries. ■

C STEROID HORMONE ANTAGONISTS

Adrenal steroid inhibitors act to inhibit or suppress the adrenal cortex, thus controlling the symptoms of Cushing syndrome. Drugs within this class include aminoglutethimide,

MEMORY CHIP

Fludrocortisone

- Fludrocortisone is given for adrenal insufficiency (Addison disease)
- Fludrocortisone may cause HRA axis suppression if given for more than 2 weeks and withdrawn too abruptly; this places the patient at risk for acute adrenal insufficiency
- Significant contraindications: hypersensitivity to fludrocortisone; conditions not requiring intense mineralocorticoid activity
- Most common adverse effects: sodium retention and increased urinary potassium excretion
- Most serious adverse effects: congestive heart failure, cardiomegaly, and hypokalemic alkalosis
- Maximizing therapeutic effects: increase the dosage in times of stress to prevent drug-induced adrenal insufficiency
- Minimizing adverse effects: monitor fluid balance
- Most significant patient education: eat potassium-rich foods and moderate sodium intake

cyproheptadine, ketoconazole, mifepristone, and mitotane. Aminoglutethimide (Cytadren) suppresses adrenal cortical function and is the prototype steroid hormone antagonist.

NURSING MANAGEMENT OF THE PATIENT RECEIVING AMINOGLUTETHIMIDE

Core Drug Knowledge

Pharmacotherapeutics

Aminoglutethimide is used to treat hypercortisolism (Cushing syndrome). However, it does not affect the underlying pathology of the hypercortisolism and is usually used only for a short period (less than 3 months) until more definitive therapy (e.g., surgery or pituitary radiation) can be done. Unlabeled uses for aminoglutethimide include metastatic prostate carcinoma and advanced breast carcinoma in postmenopausal women.

Pharmacokinetics

Aminoglutethimide is well absorbed orally and is bound minimally to plasma proteins. Its plasma half-life of 5 to 9 hours (initially 11 to 16 hours) decreases following 1 to 2 weeks of therapy because of its action as a hepatic enzyme inducer. Aminoglutethimide crosses the placenta and passes into breast milk. It is excreted in the urine. The usual adult dosage for Cushing syndrome is 250 mg every 6 hours up to a maximum of 2 g/day.

Pharmacodynamics

Aminoglutethimide blocks the conversion of cholesterol to $\Delta5$-pregnenolone and reduces the synthesis of all hormonally active steroids.

Contraindications and Precautions

Hypersensitivity to glutethimide (a nonbarbiturate sedative-hypnotic) or aminoglutethimide is a contraindication to use. Under conditions of stress, aminoglutethimide may cause cortical hypofunction. Patients should be monitored carefully, and glucocorticoid (hydrocortisone) and mineralocorticoid supplements may be needed.

Adverse Effects

The most frequently occurring adverse reactions include drowsiness, skin rash, nausea, headache, myalgia, and anorexia. These effects usually disappear spontaneously within 1 to 2 weeks of therapy. Because hypothyroidism may occur, baseline thyroid function should be established, and supplemental thyroid hormone may be necessary. Hematologic abnormalities have been reported. Elevations in levels of aspartate aminotransferase (AST), alkaline phosphatase, and bilirubin have been reported.

Cardiovascular adverse effects of orthostatic hypotension and tachycardia may occur. Adverse effects of the CNS are headache and dizziness, possibly caused by decreased vascular resistance and orthostasis. Rash and cholestatic jaundice are considered to be allergic or hypersensitivity reactions. Masculinization and hirsutism in females and precocious sex development in males have occurred occasionally.

Drug Interactions

Drug interactions with aminoglutethimide occur because of its action as an enzyme inducer. Aminoglutethimide interacts with coumarin, warfarin, oral anticoagulants, theophylline, digoxin, medroxyprogesterone, and dexamethasone (Table 40-4).

Assessment of Relevant Core Patient Variables

Health Status

Hypothyroidism and hematologic abnormalities (e.g., agranulocytosis, anemia, leukopenia, neutropenia, and thrombocytopenia) have occurred with aminoglutethimide. Therefore, the nurse should establish thyroid function studies and baseline complete blood count with differential.

Before administering aminoglutethimide, the nurse should assess the patient for indications of excessive

TABLE 40-4 Agents That Interact With Aminoglutethimide

Interactants	Effect and Significance	Nursing Management
dexamethasone	Dexamethasone metabolism accelerated by aminoglutethimide	Observe for subtherapeutic glucocorticoid effects.
coumarin, warfarin, theophylline, digoxin, medroxyprogesterone	Therapeutic effects of interacting drugs diminished by aminoglutethimide	Monitor PT and PTT profiles; anticoagulant effects may be subtherapeutic. Assess for subtherapeutic serum levels of theophylline. Evaluate patient for exacerbation of respiratory disease. Evaluate serum digoxin levels. Monitor patient for worsening of cardiac disease. Advise women to use alternate form of contraception.

steroid levels (e.g., cushingoid effects). Important also is the history of prescription, OTC, recreational, or illicit drug use; GI upset; ulcers; or epigastric pain. Other assessments should focus on nutritional status, weight control, and medical, disease, or trauma history.

The nurse should perform a complete physical examination, including orthostatic vital signs. It also is important to review current laboratory data, including serum electrolyte levels, electrocardiogram, x-ray films of spine and chest, glucose tolerance test results, tuberculin skin test results, complete blood count with differential, ocular pressure, HPA axis function, and blood pressure. In addition, muscle strength and body proportions should be observed as should hair growth and distribution patterns. Depending on the findings, the nurse may coordinate further testing, for example, hepatic and renal function studies. Throughout therapy, the nurse continues to assess for signs of adrenal insufficiency.

Life Span and Gender

The nurse should determine whether the patient is pregnant or breast-feeding. Aminoglutethimide is assigned to pregnancy category D, and so it should be avoided during pregnancy. It is unknown whether it enters breast milk, but safety in lactation and safety and efficacy in children remain unestablished. It is important to note the patient's age before administering aminoglutethimide. Geriatric patients may have increased sensitivity to CNS effects and may become lethargic.

Lifestyle, Diet, and Habits

The nurse should assess the patient's typical daily activities. Dizziness and drowsiness may occur with aminoglutethimide use, and caution performing activities requiring alertness and concentration is necessary until drug effects are known. It also is important to determine the patient's alcohol intake because alcohol potentiates aminoglutethimide's effect.

Nursing Diagnoses and Outcomes

- Disturbed Body Image related to hirsutism and masculinization (in females)
  Desired outcome: The patient will identify and incorporate methods for camouflaging the adverse hormonal effects of aminoglutethimide therapy.
- Risk For Injury related to CNS effects of hypotension and sedation, endocrine effects of hypothyroidism, or hematologic effects of agranulocytosis, leukopenia, and thrombocytopenia
  Desired outcome: The patient will remain injury free during aminoglutethimide therapy.
- Imbalanced Nutrition: Less Than Body Requirements related to adverse effects of anorexia and nausea
  Desired outcome: There will be no change in nutritional status, and, ideally, it will improve.

Planning and Intervention

Maximizing Therapeutic Effects

The nurse should advise the patient to carry some type of medical identification and to inform other health care professionals that aminoglutethimide is being taken. An intercurrent injury, infection, or illness may cause adrenocortical insufficiency, and the patient may require supplemental doses of steroids.

Minimizing Adverse Effects

Suppression of aldosterone production may cause orthostatic or persistent hypotension. Therefore, the nurse should help the patient to change positions slowly and to avoid situations or environments that enhance hypotension (e.g., consumption of alcohol, overheated areas) to decrease the risk of accidental injury from postural hypotension.

Providing Patient and Family Education

- Aminoglutethimide may cause dizziness or drowsiness; it may also cause fainting, weakness, or headache. The nurse should caution patients about driving or performing other tasks that require alertness, coordination, or physical dexterity until the effects of the drug are known.
- The nurse should inform patients and their family or caregiver that this drug may cause nausea and anorexia in the first weeks of treatment. Small, frequent meals of bland foods may help to lessen these problems.
- The nurse should tell patients to report skin rash, severe drowsiness or dizziness, headache, or severe nausea immediately to their health care provider.
- It also is important to discuss with female patients the necessity of avoiding pregnancy while taking this drug, which is in pregnancy category D, because fetal harm is well documented.

Ongoing Assessment and Evaluation

During aminoglutethimide therapy, adrenal insufficiency may occur, especially under stressful conditions (e.g., surgery, trauma, or acute illness). Mineralocorticoid or glucocorticoid replacement therapy (e.g., fludrocortisone, hydrocortisone) may be necessary. The nurse should monitor blood pressure and assess for hematologic abnormalities and physical and mental changes associated with hypothyroidism during therapy. Thyroid hormone replacement may be necessary.

Nursing management of aminoglutethimide therapy is considered successful when the patient sustains a reduced plasma cortisol level. When subjected to stress, the patient will understand the need for increasing mineralocorticoid and glucocorticoid dosages. The patient should also be able to state the importance of self-monitoring for adverse effects and of reporting significant ones to the health care provider. ■

DRUGS SIGNIFICANTLY DIFFERENT FROM AMINOGLUTETHIMIDE

Corticosterone and Desoxycorticosterone

Corticosterone and desoxycorticosterone (Metyrapone) are potent inhibitors of endogenous adrenal corticosteroid synthesis and are used as diagnostic drugs for testing hypothalamic-pituitary ACTH function. The pharmacologic effect is to reduce cortisol and corticosterone production by inhibiting a hydroxylation reaction in the adrenal cortex. The response to metyrapone does not occur immediately; peak steroid excretion occurs during the subsequent 24-hour period. Adverse effects include headache, dizziness, and sedation from actions in the CNS; allergic rash; GI complaints of nausea, vomiting, and abdominal pain or discomfort; and, rarely, decreased white blood cell count or bone marrow depression.

Cyproheptadine

Cyproheptadine (Periactin) is a potent serotonin and cholinergic antagonist that inhibits secretion of ACTH from pituitary microadenoma cells. It is used for treatment of ACTH hypersecretion and Cushing syndrome secondary to pituitary disorders. Remission of Cushing syndrome usually occurs 1 to 3 months after beginning therapy.

Ketoconazole

Ketoconazole (Nizoral) is an antifungal, which also strongly inhibits all gonadal and adrenal steroid hormone synthesis.

> **MEMORY CHIP**
>
> **Aminoglutethimide**
>
> - Used to treat adrenocortical hormone excess (Cushing syndrome); it suppresses adrenal cortical function
> - Significant contraindication: hypersensitivity to glutethimide
> - Most common adverse effects: drowsiness, skin rash, nausea, headache, myalgia, and anorexia
> - Most serious adverse effects: orthostatic hypotension and tachycardia
> - Maximizing therapeutic effects: provide supplemental doses of steroids during times of injury, infection, or illness
> - Minimizing adverse effects: help the patient change positions slowly to decrease the risk of injury related to orthostatic hypotension
> - Most significant patient education: take the drug with small, frequent meals to lessen GI effects; do not drive or perform other tasks that require alertness, coordination, or physical dexterity until the effects of the drug are known

In an unlabeled use (dosages of 800 to 1,200 mg/day), ketoconazole effectively treats Cushing syndrome because of its ability to inhibit adrenal steroidogenesis.

Mifepristone

Mifepristone (RU-486) is a synthetic progesterone and glucocorticosteroid receptor antagonist. It also weakly binds to the androgen receptor. Its antagonistic activity at the glucocorticoid receptor disrupts the negative pituitary feedback resulting from the normal morning rise in cortisol levels. Mifepristone is absorbed rapidly following oral administration with peak plasma levels occurring 1 to 3 hours after administration. The anti-glucocorticoid action of mifepristone (dosages of 20 mg/kg per day) is useful in some patients for the treatment of Cushing syndrome. Common adverse effects include abdominal pain, mild to moderate nausea and vomiting, headache, and diarrhea. These adverse effects can usually be controlled with mild analgesic and antiemetic agents.

RU-486 has been used to treat endometriosis and breast cancer. It can be used as a contraceptive drug that acts by inhibiting follicle maturation, ovulation, and egg implantation. It also is used to interrupt pregnancy through the release of prostaglandins and increased uterine contractions.

Mitotane

Mitotane (Lysodren) is an adrenal cytotoxic agent, although it can cause adrenal inhibition without cellular destruction. It is used for palliative treatment of inoperable functional or nonfunctional adrenal cortical carcinoma. Its biochemical action is unknown, but it reduces production of adrenal steroids and is thought to modify the peripheral metabolism of steroids and directly suppress the adrenal cortex. Approximately 40% of oral mitotane is absorbed; it is primarily stored in fat and undergoes hepatic metabolism. It is excreted in the urine (10% to 25%) and feces (up to 60%). Its blood levels, detectable for up to 10 weeks after discontinuation of therapy due to the drug's lipophilic nature, do not appear to be related to therapeutic or toxic effects.

Mitotane is assigned to FDA pregnancy category C. Therefore, reliable contraceptive measures are recommended during therapy. Precautions include concomitant drug therapy, hepatic enzyme induction, and the possibility that adrenal insufficiency may develop.

Protein-bound iodine levels and urinary 17-hydroxycorticosteroids may be decreased by mitotane (high values are seen in Cushing syndrome and extreme stress). Adverse reactions include GI distress, lethargy and somnolence, and transient skin rashes.

CHAPTER SUMMARY

- Corticosteroids affect nearly every body system and have the potential to cause severe adverse effects. Prolonged corticosteroid therapy with supraphysiologic doses increases the incidence of potentially disabling or lethal effects.
- Glucocorticoids occupy a chief role in the pharmacologic management of various inflammatory diseases despite the numerous complications

that may occur from therapy. Therapeutic uses for the corticosteroids include replacement therapy and anti-inflammatory or immunosuppressive effects. Glucocorticoids are used as replacement therapy in Addison disease, as pharmacologic anti-inflammatory drugs for serious inflammatory disorders and autoimmune diseases, and for a chemotherapeutic effect in certain malignant neoplasms.

- Glucocorticoids are potentially useful in many situations, although subsequent complications can be serious. A clear understanding by the nurse, patient, and family about the drugs' actions and uses is essential in preventing or managing complications.
- Glucocorticoids used therapeutically are usually synthetic analogues of the naturally occurring adrenal corticosteroid cortisol, also known as cortisone. The prototype glucocorticoid is prednisone.
- Some patients are at high risk for the serious adverse or toxic effects of the glucocorticoids. For example, patients with systemic viral infections and those receiving live virus vaccines. Glucocorticoids require cautious use in children, pregnant or lactating women, and patients with diseases and disorders, such as cardiovascular disease, renal impairment, peptic ulcer disease, diabetes mellitus, osteoporosis, and treatment-resistant infections.
- Adverse effects, also known as cushingoid effects or characteristics (similar to the signs and symptoms of idiopathic Cushing disease) may be debilitating and life threatening. Cushingoid effects occur with long-term supraphysiologic dosages of systemic glucocorticoids.
- Acute adrenal insufficiency may occur after abrupt withdrawal of pharmacologic dosages of glucocorticoids. A patient experiencing acute adrenal insufficiency is in a potentially life-threatening situation because of the multiple body systems involved.
- Whether treatment is for replacement therapy or for achieving anti-inflammatory or immunosuppressant effects, the patient receiving glucocorticoid therapy and the family have a variety of needs. The underlying disease or condition and its extent will suggest the therapeutic goal that in turn will influence the nursing care. Patient and family education is fundamental to nursing management.
- Mineralocorticoids are essential for fluid, sodium, and potassium homeostasis.
- Fludrocortisone is the prototype mineralocorticoid. It is used therapeutically with a glucocorticoid for treating patients with adrenocortical insufficiency (Addison disease).
- Episodes of acute stress (e.g., surgery, trauma) may require an adjustment of the mineralocorticoid dosage to prevent acute adrenal insufficiency.
- Aminoglutethimide, an adrenal steroid inhibitor, suppresses adrenal cortical function. It is used for disorders chiefly characterized by adrenocortical hormone excess (Cushing syndrome).

QUESTIONS FOR STUDY AND REVIEW

1. What are the main effects of glucocorticoids on metabolism?
2. What is the result of untreated acute and chronic adrenal insufficiency (Addison disease)?
3. What is Cushing syndrome? What is the effect of chronic pharmacologic dosage of glucocorticoids? How is Cushing syndrome different from "cushingoid" characteristics?
4. What are the three major actions of the adrenal steroids?
5. Why should glucocorticoid therapy not be stopped suddenly in a patient who has been receiving long-term therapy?
6. What are the advantages and disadvantages of glucocorticoid alternate-day therapy?
7. What are the two major clinical uses of adrenal steroids?
8. When are water-soluble glucocorticoid preparations preferred over suspension preparations?
9. What drug interactions commonly occur with glucocorticoids?
10. What is the major clinical use of fludrocortisone? What steroid characteristics does it possess?
11. What patient teaching should be done with fludrocortisone?
12. What is the major clinical indication for use of the adrenal steroid inhibitors? Name the prototype adrenal steroid inhibitor. Explain its function.

NEED MORE HELP?

Chapter 40 of the study guide for *Drug Therapy in Nursing* contains exercises and activities to reinforce your understanding of the concepts presented in this chapter. For additional information, see the text's accompanying website at *http://www.connection.lww.com*.

REFERENCES AND BIBLIOGRAPHY

Brody, T. M., Larner, J., Minneman, K. P., & Neu, H. C. (1998). *Human pharmacology: Molecular to clinical* (3rd ed.). St. Louis: C. V. Mosby.

Bello, C. E., & Garrett, S. D. (1999). Therapeutic and adverse effects of glucocorticoids. *U. S. Pharmacist, 24*(10), 100–110.

Dipiro, J. T., et al. (1999). Pharmacotherapy: A pathophysiologic approach (4th ed.). New York: McGraw-Hill.

Fauci, A., Braunwald, E., Wilson, J. D., Martin, J. B., Hauser, S. L., Longo, D. L., Kasper, D. L., Isselbachter, K. J. (Eds.). (1999). *Harrison's Online*. New York: McGraw-Hill.

Gennaro, A. (Ed.). (2000). *Remington: The Science and Practice of Pharmacy* (20th ed.). Philadelphia: Lippincott Williams & Wilkins.

Hardman, J. G., Limbird, L. E., Molinoff, P. B., Ruddon, R. W., & Gilman, A. G. (Eds.). (1996). *Goodman and Gilman's pharmacological basis of therapeutics* (9th ed.). New York: McGraw-Hill.

Katzung, B. C. (Ed.). (2000). *Basic and clinical pharmacology* (8th ed.). New York: McGraw-Hill.

Lipworth, B. J. (1999). Systemic adverse effects of inhaled corticosteroid therapy: A systematic review and meta-analysis. *Archives of Internal Medicine, 159*, 941–955.

McEvoy, G. K., Litvak, K., & Welsh, O. H., Jr. (Eds.). (2000). *Drug information*. Bethesda: American Hospital Formulary Service.

Stockley, I. H., & Stockley, I. H. (1999). Drug interactions: *A source book of adverse interactions, their mechanisms, clinical importance and management*. Nottingham, UK: Pharmaceutical Press.

Stone, T., et al. (2000). *Pills, potions and poisons: How medicines and other drugs work*. Oxford, U.K.: Oxford University Press.

Chapter 41

DRUGS AFFECTING BLOOD GLUCOSE LEVELS

KEY WORDS

dawn phenomenon
diabetic ketoacidosis
diabetes mellitus
gluconeogenesis
glycogenolysis
glycosylated hemoglobin
hyperglycemia
hyperosmolar hyperglycemic state
hyperosmolar
hypoglycemia
insulin
insulinopenia
islets of Langerhans
lactic acidosis
lipodystrophy
Somogyi effect
sulfonylureas

Learning Objectives

At the completion of this chapter the student will:

1. Discuss the significance of diabetes in terms of prevalence and costs.
2. Compare the characteristics of type 1, type 2, gestational, and secondary diabetes; describe their pathophysiologic processes.
3. Explain the principles and practices of insulin therapy, including measures to prevent and treat hypoglycemia.
4. Identify core drug knowledge and core patient variables about the oral hypoglycemic drugs.
5. Generate a nursing plan of care from the interactions between core drug knowledge and core patient variables for drugs that affect blood glucose.
6. Describe nursing interventions to maximize therapeutic and minimize adverse effects for the drugs that lower blood glucose.
7. Identify the peak action time for the four types of insulin and determine when a hypoglycemic episode is most likely to occur.
8. Determine key points for patient and family education for insulin and the oral hypoglycemic drugs that affect blood glucose levels.

Protein hormone injectable hypoglycemics

- **regular insulin**
- aspart
- lispro
- regular concentrated iletin II
- NPH insulin
- lente insulin
- ultralente insulin
- glargine insulin

Oral hypoglycemics

Sulfonylureas

- **glyburide**

First-generation sulfonylureas

- acetohexamide
- chlorpropamide
- tolazamide
- tolbutamide

Second-generation sulfonylureas

- glimepiride
- glipizide

Meglitinides

- repaglinide
- nateglinide

Alpha glucosidase inhibitors

- **acarbose**
- miglitol

Biguanides

- **metformin**
- phenformin (investigational)

Thiazolidinediones

- **rosiglitazone**
- pioglitazone

Glucose elevating agents

- **glucagon**
- diazoxide
- glucose

The symbol (C) indicates the **drug class**.

Drugs in bold type marked with the symbol ■ are **prototypes**.

Drugs in blue type with no symbol are **closely related** to the prototype.

Drugs in **red** type with no symbol are **significantly different** from the prototype.

Drugs in **black** type with no symbol are **also used in drug therapy**; no prototype.

"It is time for all health professionals to treat diabetes aggressively." Almost 16 million Americans (about 6% of the U.S. population) have diabetes mellitus (DM), and its overall incidence is increasing each year (ADA website, October 2001). Furthermore, one out of every three people with diabetes—5.4 million of the 16 million Americans with diabetes—have not been diagnosed according to the Centers for Disease Control and Prevention (Campbell, 2000). Between 90% and 95% of individuals who have diabetes have type 2 and most of the remainder have type 1. Although the exact incidence of each type of diabetes varies widely throughout the world, DM and its complications are a major cause of morbidity and mortality. DM is the sixth leading cause of death by disease and the leading cause of kidney failure, adult blindness, and lower-extremity amputation (ADA website, October 2001). The annual economic impact of DM in the United States is estimated to be nearly $100 billion (ADA website, October 2001).

PHYSIOLOGY

Glucose is made available to the body from food that is ingested and production of glucose by the liver. Unable to store or synthesize glucose, the brain depends on a steady supply of glucose from the circulation and extracts its energy on nearly a continuous basis.

Three body systems are involved in the regulation and utilization of glucose—the liver, pancreas, and skeletal muscle tissue. The liver synthesizes its own glucose supply (**gluconeogenesis**) in addition to storage and release of glucose that has been ingested from the diet. Normally, the liver releases some of its stored or synthesized glucose when blood levels are low and stops producing and releasing glucose when blood levels are high.

The pancreas is both an exocrine and endocrine gland. Exocrine pancreatic functions are the production of digestive enzymes. Endocrine functions are the synthesis and secretion of peptide hormones—insulin, glucagon, and somatostatin by the islets of Langerhans. The **islets of Langerhans** are cellular structures that lie in the interstitial tissue of the pancreas and are innervated richly by adrenergic and cholinergic nerves. Insulin, glucagon, and somatostatin play an important role in regulating the metabolic activities of the body as well as in regulating and maintaining the homeostasis of blood glucose. The islets of Langerhans contain the following:

- Beta cells, which secrete the hypoglycemic hormone insulin
- Alpha cells, which secrete the hyperglycemic hormone glucagon
- Delta cells, which release somatostatin, a hormone that inhibits both glucagon and insulin secretion
- F cells, which synthesize and secrete pancreatic polypeptides used in digestion

The muscle tissue is the target organ for the action of insulin; it contains the majority of insulin receptor sites. When insulin binds with receptor sites on the skeletal muscle, glucose is able to cross over the membrane and enter the cell. When muscle tissue has fewer available receptor sites than are needed by the cells for glucose entry, a condition called insulin resistance occurs. Insulin resistance plays a major role in the development of type 2 diabetes (Semb, 2000).

INSULIN

Insulin is a small protein, consisting of two polypeptide chains, which is synthesized as a precursor protein (proinsulin) and undergoes enzymatic splitting to form insulin and peptide C—both of which are secreted by the pancreatic beta cells. Measurement of circulating C peptide provides an index of insulin levels.

Insulin secretion is regulated tightly by a coordinated interaction of blood glucose levels, gastrointestinal (GI) and pancreatic hormones, and autonomic neurotransmitters. Insulin secretion is most commonly triggered by high blood glucose. Glucose is one of the body's most important energy sources and some tissues—especially those in the brain—are highly dependent on glucose for energy, particularly the glucose extracted from the blood. Therefore, careful regulation of blood glucose levels and cellular uptake is essential (Fig. 41-1).

Numerous hormones are involved with regulating blood glucose levels. Two hormones—insulin and glucagon secreted by the pancreas—exert the most direct influence, however.

Functions of Insulin

Insulin has a number of important actions. Primarily, it regulates carbohydrate metabolism but it also plays an important role in metabolizing fats and proteins. Insulin and its analogues lower blood glucose levels by stimulating peripheral glucose uptake–especially by skeletal muscle and fat. In the muscle cells, insulin promotes the uptake and metabolism of glucose. Insulin resistance leads to an inappropriately elevated hepatic glucose output and impaired glucose uptake by the muscle tissue. In the liver, insulin has several functions; insulin promotes the uptake and storage of glucose in the form of glycogen, promotes the conversion of excess glucose into fat, and suppresses hepatic gluconeogenesis (production of glucose) and glycogenesis (breakdown of glycogen to glucose). Most cells in the body need insulin so that glucose can enter the cell (Fig. 41-2). Exceptions to this are tissues of the brain, nerves, intestine, liver, retina, erythrocytes, and renal tubules.

Insulin Synthesis and Release

The plasma glucose level is the single most important factor in controlling the rate of insulin synthesis and release. Other factors that directly or indirectly influence insulin release or its action include sugars (fructose, sucrose, and other types), oral-hypoglycemic drugs from the sulfonylurea class, rising levels of free fatty acids, growth hormone, thyroid-stimulating hormone, glucagon, sympathetic and parasympathetic stimulation, adrenocorticotropic hormone, and cortisol.

Stimulated by plasma glucose levels, insulin secretion occurs in two phases. During the first phase, insulin secretion peaks after 1 to 2 minutes and is short lived. Delayed onset and a longer duration of action characterize the sec-

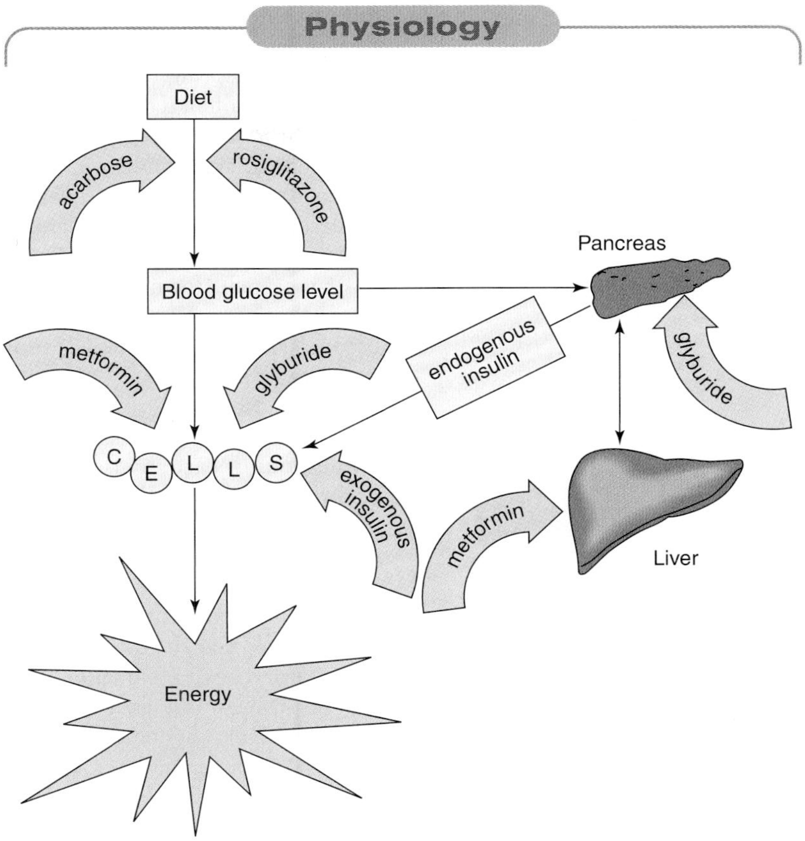

Figure 41-1. Glucose balance. When the body's delicate glucose balance is disrupted because processes involving insulin secretion are impaired, diabetes mellitus results. The figure above represents the glucose balance, which is integral to cellular functions. External dietary factors and internal insulin secretion and release must work together to transport the glucose needed by the body's cells for energy. When diet and insulin fail to perform properly, drug and diet therapy may help to restore the balance. This figure identifies the antidiabetic drugs commonly used to restore balance and their sites of action.

ond phase. The exact mechanism by which glucose stimulates insulin release is not fully understood.

Blood glucose levels may be influenced by several factors other than insulin. Any of the following can cause changes in blood glucose levels:

- Stress or illness
- Secretion of insulin-antagonistic hormones (counter-regulatory hormones) that affect glucose metabolism (e.g., cortisol, epinephrine, growth hormone, glucagon, and somatostatin)
- Rates of hepatic synthesis of glucose (gluconeogenesis) or its conversion of glycogen to yield glucose (**glycogenolysis**)
- Presence and levels of insulin antibodies
- Use of glucose by peripheral cells or tissues
- Number of cellular insulin receptors

Typically, in response to postprandial elevations of blood glucose levels, insulin is released into the bloodstream by the beta cells. A prompt rise in insulin release occurs so that absorbed carbohydrates are transported rapidly to the liver and other tissues where carbohydrates are stored or used, preventing the serum glucose level from rising too much. As a result, the blood glucose levels decline, and the stimulus for insulin secretion is suppressed. When the level of serum glucose decreases, the alpha cells release glucagon into the bloodstream. This raises the blood glucose level by stimulating the release of glycogen from hepatic storage sites to prevent the serum glucose level from falling too low.

Between periods of food intake, insulin levels remain low, and sources of stored glucose and amino acids are mobilized to meet the energy needs of glucose-dependent tissues. Hepatic glycogen stores are depleted within 6 hours after a meal. If additional food is not ingested by this time, muscles begin to release amino acids that are converted to glucose. Lipolysis occurs in adipose tissue, and serum levels of free fatty acids rise. Free fatty acids are used for energy by muscle and liver cells, thus conserving glucose for use by the brain.

GLUCAGON

Glucagon also plays a role in regulating the blood glucose level. Glucagon is a small protein hormone, and declining blood glucose levels stimulate its release from pancreatic islet alpha cells. Sympathetic nerve impulses, exercise, infection,

Physiology

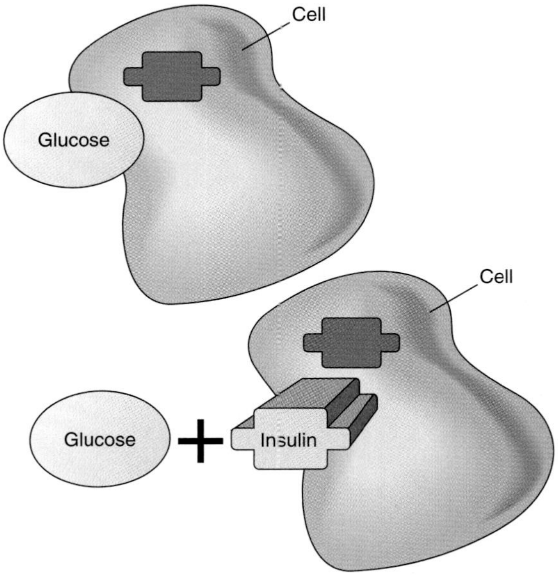

Figure 41-2. Insulin functions to transport glucose into the cell, providing the key that unlocks the cellular membrane to allow entry.

and trauma also stimulate its release. In the liver, glucagon stimulates glycogenolysis and gluconeogenesis, resulting in a release of glucose into the blood.

PATHOPHYSIOLOGY

Diabetes mellitus is a serious chronic disease, affecting people of all ages and ethnic groups. Type 2 diabetes appears in a disproportionately higher prevalence in some minority groups in the United States, including African Americans, Hispanic Americans, and Native Americans.

TYPES OF DIABETES

Most cases of DM fall into two broad categories—type 1 (formerly called juvenile-onset or insulin-dependent diabetes mellitus [IDDM]), and type 2 (formerly called adult-onset or non–insulin-dependent diabetes mellitus [NIDDM]) (Table 41-1). Other types include gestational, disease-induced (e.g., carcinoma, pancreatitis, and infections), hormonal (e.g., acromegaly and Cushing syndrome), drug- or chemical-induced (e.g., corticosteroids), and genetic defects of the beta cell.

Gestational diabetes mellitus (GDM) is a condition characterized by glucose intolerance with its onset during pregnancy. Approximately 4% of all pregnancies in the United States are complicated by GDM. This rate may be much higher in certain populations, such as Asians, Hispanics, Native Americans, and Pacific Islanders (Caffrey & Flaherty, 2000; Zagaria, 2000). Treatment may include diet, exercise, and insulin. Generally, glucose regulation returns to normal following delivery, although women with a history of GDM carry a high risk of developing type 2 diabetes later in life as do their offspring. Type 1 diabetes is the result of a lack of sufficient insulin or a total absence of insulin. This type of diabetes is most commonly a result of cellular-mediated autoimmune destruction of the beta cells of the pancreas.

Formerly described as "juvenile-onset" because its onset occurred commonly during childhood or puberty, type 1 DM can develop at any age. In fact, another small peak of onset is seen during midlife. Type 1 DM was previously referred to as insulin-dependent diabetes mellitus (IDDM) because it required administration of insulin by injection to maintain health.

Type 2 diabetes is the result of insulin resistance by the tissues and usually a decrease in insulin production. Abnormalities of carbohydrate, fat, and protein metabolism occur in Type 2 diabetes. Type 2 DM—previously described as "adult-onset," "maturity-onset," or "non-insulin-dependent diabetes mellitus (NIDDM)" is developing at younger ages. Type 2 DM is linked closely to obesity, sedentary lifestyle, and lack of physical activity; scientific experts declare that the dramatic rise in the population of patients with diabetes is due, in significant part, to America's weight problem (see later discussion). Type 2 DM may be treated with oral hypoglycemics or injections of insulin.

The American Diabetes Association (ADA) recommends eliminating the categories of IDDM and NIDDM because they are based on treatment rather than etiology, they vary considerably, and they do not indicate the underlying problem (ADA, 2000a). The current classifications of diabetes are based on clinical presentation.

Type 1 Diabetes Mellitus

Type 1 DM is characterized by an abrupt failure of the pancreas, which depletes the reserve of insulin and results in hyperglycemia and ketoacidosis. By the time signs and symptoms of type 1 DM appear, most pancreatic beta cells have been destroyed. Although the pathogenesis is unclear, considerable evidence (e.g., islet cell and insulin autoantibodies) suggests that the destructive process is autoimmune with genetic and environmental components as well. The autoimmune destruction of the pancreatic beta cells may occur over a period of months to several years before the onset of clinical disease is observed. The final result of type 1 DM is an extensive and selective loss of pancreatic beta cells and a state of absolute insulin deficiency (**insulinopenia**). Therefore, insulin therapy is indicated in all cases of type 1 DM (hence, the former name "insulin-dependent diabetes mellitus"). Insulin is used as replacement therapy in managing insulinopenia by supplementing the deficient endogenous levels and temporarily restoring the ability of the body to use carbohydrates, fats, and proteins properly.

Type 2 Diabetes Mellitus

Insulin resistance and type 2 DM are correlated closely with obesity. Over 60% of the U.S. adult population is either over-

TABLE 41-1 Comparison of Type 1 and Type 2 Diabetes Mellitus

Patient Characteristics	Type 1 (Absolute Insulin Deficiency)	Type 2 (Relative Insulin Deficiency)
Age at onset	Usually before 20 y; onset sudden	Usually after 40 y with incidence increasing as age and weight increase; gradual onset; may occur in youth
Incidence	5%–10%	90%–95%
Body weight	Usually thin/underweight or normal weight	Usually overweight/obese
Endogenous insulin production/activity	Significantly decreased/absent	Slightly decreased; normal or may be increased; insulin effects reduced by inadequate tissue (receptor) response.
Insulin receptors/resistance	Normal receptors/no resistance	Decreased or defective receptors/definite insulin resistance
Dietary modifications	Necessary	Beneficial for blood glucose and weight control
Exogenous insulin requirement	Required for all patients with type 1 diabetes	May be necessary for patients with type 2 diabetes
Clinical signs/symptoms	Hyperglycemia, significant polyphagia/polydipsia/polyuria, weight loss	Hyperglycemia, fatigue, weakness, mild polyphagia/polydipsia/polyuria, fungal infections (especially skin, vaginal), blurred vision
Complications		
Acute - ketoacidosis	Likely	Unlikely; may occur in the presence of severe illness/stress
Chronic - microvascular and macrovascular disorders	Frequent	Frequent
Etiology/genetic susceptibility	Not fully known; related to human leukocyte antigen (HLA-DR3, HLA-DR4), proposed beta-cell destruction by viral infection or autoimmune process	Not fully known; strong familial component
Clinical management	Insulin injections, dietary controls, exercise regimen	Weight reduction, dietary controls, exercise regimen, oral drug therapy (hypoglycemics: sulfonylureas, meglitinides; antihyperglycemics: biguanides, alpha glucosidase inhibitors, thiazolidenediones), insulin

weight or obese. Body mass index (BMI = weight in kg/height in m^2) is based on an individual's height and weight and is a reliable indicator of over- and underweight in adults. Although BMI compares well to body fat, it cannot be interpreted as a certain percentage of body fat. The relationship between degree of fatness and BMI is influenced by age and gender. For the same BMI, women are more likely to have a higher percentage of body fat than men. Furthermore, at the same BMI, older people have more body fat than younger adults. A healthy BMI for adults is between 18.5 and 24.9 kg/m^2 (see the accompanying display, Body Mass Index). BMI ranges are based on the effect body weight has on morbidity and mortality; obesity itself is a strong risk factor for morbidity (e.g., diabetes, coronary heart disease, cancer, and high blood pressure) and premature mortality. On a cultural note, however, the World Health Organization (WHO) criteria that define overweight and obesity in morbidity and mortality terms are not necessarily appropriate for Asian populations. In Asians a BMI range of 23 to 24.9 kg/m^2 has a risk equivalent for type 2 that a BMI of 25 to 29.9 kg/m^2 does in those of European ancestry (Zimmet, 2000).

Type 2 DM historically has been believed to be rare in children, adolescents, and young adults. This is no longer the case, however, as type 2 DM is increasing in these younger age groups as the childhood population becomes increasingly overweight. Type 2 DM is now seen as an emerging epidemic in the pediatric population (Beyzarov, 2000). This increased incidence is occurring worldwide; research has shown increases

Body Mass Index (BMI)

BMI values for adults (regardless of age or gender):
Underweight: BMI < 18.5
Normal weight: BMI 18.6–24.9
Overweight: BMI 25.0–29.9
Obese: BMI 30.0–34.9
Clinically severe obesity (i.e., morbid obesity): BMI >35.0

in Japan, Libya, Bangladesh, Australia, and Canada (ADA 2000a).

Insulin resistance can be considered the primary defect in type 2 DM. An insulin-resistance syndrome known as "metabolic syndrome" (also known as "Syndrome X") is a precursor to the development of type 2 DM. This syndrome is a combination of conditions, namely: insulin resistance with a compensatory hyperinsulinemia to maintain glucose homeostasis; obesity (especially abdominal or visceral obesity); dyslipidemia of the high-triglyceride and/or low-high density lipoprotein type; and hypertension. The locus of these signs and symptoms is an increasing inability to use insulin.

There is no significant loss of pancreatic beta cells or cellular activity from the islets in type 2 DM. The plasma concentrations of insulin are essentially normal or may even be increased because the pancreas tries to overcome the resistance by producing more insulin and the peripheral tissue resistance to the hormone's actions. Individuals with type 2 DM are described as being relatively insulin deficient, meaning that there is a decrease in the responsiveness of the peripheral tissues to effects of insulin.

Undiagnosed type 2 DM is common in the United States with estimates that about 8 million individuals are undiagnosed (see the accompanying display, Criteria for Testing for Diabetes in Asymptomatic, Undiagnosed Individuals). Hyperlipidemia linked to insulin leads to atherosclerotic plaques in the vessels. Thus, patients with undiagnosed type 2 DM are at significantly increased risk for coronary heart disease, stroke, and peripheral vascular disease.

In many cases, type 2 DM can be controlled with weight reduction, age-appropriate physical activity, dietary modifications, and oral drug therapy (e.g., sulfonylureas, biguanides, alpha-glucosidase inhibitors, meglitinides, or thiazolidinediones).

COMPLICATIONS OF DIABETES

The consequences of uncontrolled diabetes are serious and can result in acute or chronic complications.

Criteria for Testing for Diabetes in Asymptomatic, Undiagnosed Individuals

- All patients at age 45 years and older; if normal result, repeat at 3–year intervals
- Testing at younger age or more frequent intervals if individual:
  Is obese (>120% ideal body weight or a BMI >27)
  Has a first-degree relative with diabetes
  Is a member of a high-risk ethnic group (e.g., African American, Asian American, Hispanic American, Native American, or Pacific Islander)
  Has delivered a baby weighing >9 lb or has been diagnosed with gestational diabetes
  Is hypertensive (i.e., *BP*>140/90)
  Has an HDL cholesterol level >35 mg/dL and/or a triglyceride level >250 mg/dL
  Has had impaired glucose tolerance or impaired fasting glucose on previous testing

Acute Complications

Hypoglycemia is a significant drop in blood glucose level (less than 60 mg/dL) that may result from excessive insulin's entering the bloodstream or from a failure of the glucose release rate to meet tissue demands. The earliest signs of hypoglycemia are neurologic in nature because the brain uses only glucose for fuel. They include fatigue and malaise, nervousness, trembling, irritability, headache, cold sweats, and rapid heart beat.

Hyperglycemia is an abnormally high concentration of glucose in the circulating blood. According to the 2000 ADA guidelines, this is a non-fasting plasma glucose value of more than 200 mg/dL. The classic signs of hyperglycemia include excessive urination (polyuria) and excessive thirst (polydipsia) because of the osmotic pull of glucose. Other symptoms include fatigue, dry or itchy skin, poor wound healing, and vision changes (often blurred vision).

Diabetic ketoacidosis (DKA) and **hyperosmolar hyperglycemic state (HHS)** are two serious acute complications of diabetes that significantly contribute to the morbidity and mortality among patients with diabetes. These disorders are extreme manifestations of impaired carbohydrate regulation that can occur in diabetes.

Severe hyperglycemia in type 1 DM results in DKA, which is associated with blood glucose levels exceeding 200 mg/dL and usually 400 to 800 mg/dL or higher. Severe hyperglycemia in type 2 DM results in HHS, which is associated with blood glucose levels exceeding 600 mg/dL and frequently exceeding 1,000 mg/dL. Patients with type 2 DM typically produce enough insulin to prevent ketosis. HHS has a mortality rate of approximately 15%, which increases substantially with aging and the presence of concomitant life-threatening illnesses. Historically known as "hyperglycemic hyperosmolar nonketotic coma" or hyperglycemic hyperosmolar nonketotic state," these terms have been replaced with the term HHS to reflect that alterations in sensorium often may be present without coma, and the hyperosmolar, hyperglycemic state may consist of variable degrees of clinical ketosis (Kitabchai, Umpierrez, Murphy, Barrett, Kreisberg, Malone, et al., 2001).

The basic underlying pathogenesis of HHS is a reduction in the net effective concentration of circulating insulin, which minimizes ketosis but does not control the hyperglycemia, combined with a concomitant elevation of counterregulatory stress hormones such as glucagons, epinephrine, cortisol, and growth hormone. This leads to severe dehydration and impaired renal function leading to decreased renal excretion of glucose. Furthermore, inadequate fluid intake contributes to the hyperosmolarity usually without ketosis, which is the hallmark of HHS.

Chronic Complications

The chronic complications of diabetes are usually classified as microvascular or macrovascular, according to the type of blood vessel damage that underlies the problem. Among the macrovascular chronic complications are atherosclerotic vascular disease, myocardial infarction, and cerebral vascular accident. Among the microvascular complications are cataracts, glaucoma and blindness from retinopathy, lower-extremity infections and gangrene, foot ulcers and Charcot joints resulting in amputation from peripheral neuropathy, renal failure from nephropathy and gastroparesis, and sexual dysfunction as a result of autonomic neuropathy.

DIABETES CONTROL AND COMPLICATIONS TRIAL (DCCT)

The DCCT is a landmark study that was conducted from 1983 to 1993 by the National Institute of Diabetes and Digestive and Kidney Diseases. This study demonstrated conclusively that the onset and progression of chronic complications of diabetes (e.g., retinopathy, nephropathy, and neuropathy) are slowed by keeping blood sugar levels as close to normal (about 70 to 100 mg/dL) as possible. The study also showed that any sustained lowering of the blood glucose level helps, even in patients with a history of poor control. Although the DCCT studied patients with type 1 diabetes exclusively, the findings have been clinically extrapolated to patients with type 2 DM. A fasting blood glucose level of 126 mg/dL is considered diagnostic for diabetes. A fasting blood glucose level of 110 to 125 mg/dL indicates impaired fasting glucose (ADA, 2000d).

Insulin therapy is indicated for type 2 DM when weight reduction, dietary modifications, and oral hypoglycemics fail to maintain satisfactory serum blood glucose levels. This does not make the individual insulin dependent, however. Tight glycemic control and decreased hyperlipidemia can be readily achieved in patients with type 2 DM who do not succeed with oral therapy by an intensive regimen of conventional split-dose insulin therapy combined with frequent monitoring of capillary blood glucose levels, for example. Because of the associated insulin resistance with type 2 DM, large doses of exogenous insulin may be required. This may result in peripheral hyperinsulinemia and weight gain. Patients with type 2 DM will require insulin in the presence of major surgery, severe trauma, infections (including gangrene), fever, hepatic or renal dysfunction, hyperthyroidism or other endocrine dysfunction, and pregnancy.

Other studies have replicated the DCCT's rationale for intensive glycemic control. The Japanese Kumamoto Study evaluated the effect of intensive glycemic control on microvascular complications of type 2 DM. This study demonstrated a more than 2% reduction in A_{1C} levels and a decrease in the progression of retinopathy and nephropathy by 69% and 70%, respectively. The Veterans Affairs Cooperative Study on Glycemic Control and Complications in type 2 DM evaluated the risks and benefits of intensive treatment compared with standard insulin treatment. In this study, approximately 42% of patients attained normal A_{1C} levels compared with approximately 4% of patients who received standard therapy. The United Kingdom Prospective Diabetes Study is the largest study performed to date in patients with type 2 DM and provides substantial evidence of the link between glycemic control and diabetic complications. Results of this study demonstrated A_{1C} levels, risk of microvascular complications, progression of retinopathy, and incidence of microalbuminuria significantly lower with intensive treatment (Campbell, 2000).

PROTEIN HORMONE INJECTABLE HYPOGLYCEMICS: INSULIN

Insulin is a normal body protein produced by the pancreas. It is necessary for normal carbohydrate, protein, and fat metabolism. Insulin for human use was historically obtained from bovine or pork pancreas; it can now be synthesized by recombinant DNA technology or genetic engineering to create human-like insulin. Modifying the amino acid sequence of the human insulin molecule has resulted in new, rapid acting insulin analogs, such as aspart or lispro (rDNA). Human-sourced insulin is considered the standard therapy, although beef- or pork-based insulins may be used with some patients. Beef-based insulins are no longer available in the United States. In comparison, animal-based insulins are slower acting than human insulin and are more antigenic than human insulin.

Insulin is available in rapid-, short- (also known as "regular"), intermediate- and long-acting types. Type usually refers to the action time of a particular produce; this includes the onset, peak, and duration of effects. Some insulins are injected separately whereas others may be mixed together in a syringe. Some are available premixed in standard concentrations in one vial.

The potency of insulin is expressed as United States Pharmacopeia (USP) units. Most types of insulin currently used clinically are prepared in solutions of 100 units per milliliter. The numbers after the "U" indicate the number of units per milliliter (e.g., U-100). Insulin is available commercially in concentrations of 100 or 500 U/mL, (U-100 or U-500). In the U.S., U-100 is the standard insulin preparation; U-500 is used only in rare cases of insulin resistance when the patient requires extremely large doses. The syringe that is used to administer the insulin should be calibrated to provide the same concentration per unit as the insulin (i.e., a U-100 syringe should be used with a U-100 insulin). U-500 and rapid-acting rDNA insulins (aspart, lispro) require a prescription, whereas the other insulins do not. Different types and species sources (e.g., porcine, rDNA) of insulin have different pharmacologic properties. Consequently, the properties of insulin-concentration, type, and species source—as well as injection technique, presence of insulin antibodies, site of injection, and individual patient response differences can all affect the onset, peak, degree, and duration of insulin activity.

Short-acting regular insulin is the prototype insulin.

NURSING MANAGEMENT OF THE PATIENT RECEIVING REGULAR INSULIN

Core Drug Knowledge

Pharmacotherapeutics

Insulin therapy is indicated for all patients with type 1 DM, and those patients with type 2 DM whose hyperglycemia cannot be controlled properly by diet, exercise, weight reduction, and/or oral antidiabetic drugs. Regular insulin, like all insulins, is administered subcutaneously. Regular insulin is the only insulin that is also administered by the intravenous route. Regular insulin can also be administered through an implantable insulin pump.

Subcutaneous insulin therapy for type 1 DM consists frequently of daily injections of mixtures of regular insulin (short-acting) with intermediate-acting insulins; multiple doses of regular insulin before each meal in association with one or two daily doses of long-acting insulin may also be used. Combining the two types of insulin allows for rapid adjustment to elevated glucose levels as well as for prolonged control, such as all day or overnight (Fig. 41-3). Some premixed combinations are also available.

Regular insulin may be used on a "sliding scale," where the dose is based on blood glucose levels, according to guidelines provided in a specific medication order. Sliding scale insulin may be utilized before meals and at bedtime or every 4 to 6 hours. It is ordered frequently for hospitalized diabetic patients during times when insulin needs may be greatest; for example, with fever, infection, or after surgery or trauma.

Pharmacokinetics

Regular insulin, like all insulins, is destroyed by gastric acids and must be given subcutaneously. The subcutaneous route usually produces slow, steady absorption. The rate of absorption is affected by the site of administration. The most rapid absorption occurs when administration is into the abdominal subcutaneous layer (as much as 50% faster than other routes). The next most rapid is the arm, followed by the thigh, and finally the buttocks.

When regular insulin is administered via IV infusion, some of the drug is absorbed into the plastic tubing set, usually between 20% and 30%. Up to 80% loss has occasionally been reported. Close monitoring of the therapeutic effect is necessary, because it is not possible to determine the exact amount that will be lost and never received by the patient.

Regular insulin has a quick onset and a short duration of action. This is why it can be administered to a patient several times a day. In comparison to regular insulin, other forms of insulin have slower onsets but longer durations of action (Table 41-2). Insulin deteriorates if exposed to excessive heat or light. Regular insulin is stable at room temperature for 1 month. For longer storage, place insulin in the refrigerator.

Insulin is filtered at the glomerulus with most of the dose (98%) reabsorbed in the proximal renal tubule. Slightly more than half of the reabsorbed insulin is metabolized and excreted; the remaining insulin is returned to the venous blood. Renal function impairment occurs commonly in diabetic patients because of the vascular insufficiency. Renal function impairment reduces the amount of insulin excreted, thus reducing the amount of insulin required.

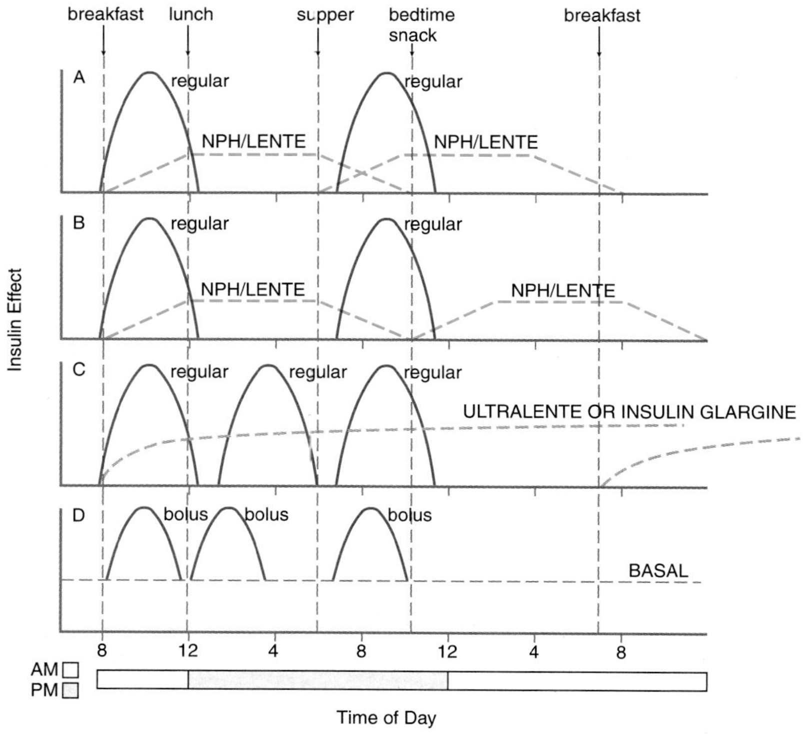

Figure 41-3. (**A**) A typical "split-mixed" regimen consisting of twice-daily injections of a mixture of regular and intermediate-acting insulin. (**B**) A variation in which the evening dose of intermediate-acting insulin is delayed until bedtime to increase the amount of insulin available the next morning. (**C**) A regimen that incorporates ultralente insulin or insulin glargine. (**D**) Patterns of insulin administration with a regimen of continuous subcutaneous insulin infusion.

TABLE 41-2 Summary of Selected Antidiabetic Drugs

Drug (Trade) Name	Selected Indications	Route and Dosage Range	Pharmacokinetics
Protein Hormone Injectable Hypoglycemics			
Short Acting			
Regular insulin (Humulin R, Novolin R, Regular Iletin I; *Canadian:* Novolin ge Toronto)	*All insulin preparations*, Types 1 and 2 diabetes mellitus	*Adult and child:* SC, dosages determined and adjusted depending on plasma glucose, diet, activity, and health status	*Onset:* 30–60 min *Duration:* 6–8 h $t_{1/2}$: Varies with preparation
Rapid Acting			
insulin lispro (Humalog)			*Onset:* 10–15 min *Duration:* 3.5–4.5 h $t_{1/2}$: 1 h
insulin aspart (Novolog)			*Onset:* 5–10 min *Duration:* 3–5 h $t_{1/2}$: 1.5 h
Intermediate Acting			
isophane insulin suspension, NPH (Humulin N, NPH Iletin I, *Canadian:* Novolin ge)			*Onset:* 1–1.5 h *Duration:* 24 h $t_{1/2}$: Unknown
insulin zinc suspension, Lente (Humulin L, Lente Iletin I, Lente L, Novolin L)			*Onset:* 1–2.5 h *Duration:* 24 h $t_{1/2}$: Unknown
Long Acting			
insulin zinc suspension, extended, Ultralente (Humulin U Ultralente; *Canadian:* Novolin ge)			*Onset:* 30 min *Duration:* 24 h $t_{1/2}$: Unknown
glargine (Lantus)			
Combination			
Isophane insulin suspension (NPH) and insulin injection (70% NPH and 30% regular insulin) (Novolin 70/30)			*Onset:* 30 min *Duration:* 24 h $t_{1/2}$: Unknown
Oral Hypoglycemics			
Sulfonylureas			
glyburide (Diabeta; *Canadian:* Albert Glyburide)	**All oral hypoglycemics** type 2 diabetes mellitus	*Adult:* PO, initially 2.5–5 mg with breakfast; maintenance, 1.25–20 mg/d *Child:* Safety and efficacy not determined	*Onset:* 1–2 h *Duration:* 24 h $t_{1/2}$: 10 h
glipizide (Glucotrol)		*Adult:* PO, initial, 5 mg before breakfast; then increase in increments of 2.5–5 mg not to exceed 15 mg/d *Child:* Safety and efficacy not determined	*Onset:* 1–1.5 h *Duration:* 10–16 h $t_{1/2}$: 2–4 h
chlorpropamide (Diabenese; *Canadian:* Apo-Chlorpropamide)		*Adult:* PO, 100–250 mg/d; maximum dose is 750 mg/d *Child:* PO, 100–250 mg/d; maximum dose is 750 mg/d	*Onset:* 1 h *Duration:* 60 h $t_{1/2}$: 36 h
tolazamide (Tolinase)		*Adult:* PO, 400 mg q8h; 1,200–1,800 mg/d in three divided doses is the suggested therapeutic range	*Onset:* Variable *Duration:* 12–24 h $t_{1/2}$: 7 h

(continued)

TABLE 41-2 Summary of Selected Antidiabetic Drugs (Continued)

Drug (Trade) Name	Selected Indications	Route and Dosage Range	Pharmacokinetics
tolbutamide (Orinase; *Canadian:* Apo-Tolbutamide)		*Adult:* PO, 0.25–3 g/d in single or divided doses *Child:* Safety and efficacy not determined	*Onset:* 1 h *Duration:* 6–12 h $t_{1/2}$: 7 h
Acetohexamide (Dymelor; *Canadian:* Dimelor)		*Adult:* PO, 250 mg–1.5 g /d *Child:* Safety and efficacy not determined	*Onset:* 1 h *Duration:* 12–24 h $t_{1/2}$: 6–8 h
Meglitinides			
repaglinide (Prandin)		*Adult and child:* PO, 0.5–4 mg before meals; maximum dose is 16 mg/d	*Onset:* Rapid *Duration:* Unknown $t_{1/2}$: 1 h
nateglinide (Starlix)		*Adult and child:* PO, 120 mg tid (60 mg tid if A_{1C} is near therapeutic goal), 1–30 min before meals	*Onset:* Rapid *Duration:* Unknown $t_{1/2}$: 1.5 h
Biguanides			
metformin (Glucophage)		*Adult:* 500–3,000 mg/d in divided doses *Child:* Safety and efficacy not determined	*Onset:* 2–2.5 h *Duration:* 10–16 h $t_{1/2}$: 1.5–6.2 h
Alpha-glucosidase Inhibitors			
acarbose (Precose; *Canadian:* Prandase)		*Adult:* PO, 50–100 mg tid with the first bite of each main meal *Child:* Safety and efficacy not determined	*Onset:* < 30 min *Duration:* 4–6 h $t_{1/2}$: 2 h
miglitol (Glyset)		*Adult and child:* PO, initial dose of 25 mg tid at first bite of meal; may start at 25 mg/d if GI effects are severe. Maintenance dose of 50 mg/tid; maximum dose of 100 mg tid	*Onset:* Rapid *Duration:* Unknown $t_{1/2}$: 2 h
Thiazolidinediones			
rosiglitazone (Avandia)		*Adult and child:* PO, 4 mg/d as single dose or divided into two doses; may increase to maximum of 8 mg/d after 8 wks	*Onset:* Rapid *Duration:* Unknown $t_{1/2}$: 3–4 h
pioglitazone (Actos)		*Adult and child:* PO, 15–30 mg/d as single dose; may increase to maximum of 45 mg/d	*Onset:* Rapid *Duration:* Unknown $t_{1/2}$: 3–7 h
Glucose Elevating Agents			
glucagon	Reverse severe hypoglycemia resulting from insulin overdosage	*Adult:* SC, IM, IV, 0.5–1.0 mg; dose may be repeated once or twice *Child:* (up to 20 kg): 0.5 mg	*Onset:* IM, 8–10 min; IV, 1 min *Duration:* IM, 19–32 min; IV, 9–20 min $t_{1/2}$: 3–10 min

Pharmacodynamics

Insulin is the principal hormone required for proper glucose use in normal metabolic processes. Most of the body's cells require insulin to facilitate entry of glucose. Insulin's effects are tissue specific; namely, membrane transport of glucose (and some other amino acids and ions) into muscle, adipose, and connective tissue cells and into leukocytes. Nerve tissues, erythrocytes, kidney epithelium (tubules), and cells of the brain, intestines, liver, and retina are the exceptions to the insulin requirement.

Injected insulin mimics the effect of endogenous insulin. Serum glucose level is regulated by insulin control over the metabolism of carbohydrates, fats, and proteins. At the cellular level, insulin increases the cell membrane permeability to glucose, amino aids, and fatty acids and maintains a constant glucose level by changing glycogen into glucose. In addition, insulin converts excess glucose into glycogen and promotes the storage of fat by combining alpha-glycerophosphate (a product of glucose metabolism) with fatty acids to form triglycerides. Consequently, one effect of insulin on metabolism is weight gain.

Contraindications and Precautions

Changes in insulin purity, strength, brand, type, or species source may result in the need for dosage adjustment.

Adverse Effects

Hypoglycemia, the most common adverse effect of insulin therapy, may result from an excessive insulin dose or increased physical activity without eating. Another condition marked by subjective signs (e.g., trembling, apprehension, sweating, and headache) of hypoglycemia but with clinical signs, such as glucosuria and hyperglycemic glucose levels, also may occur. This condition is known as the **Somogyi effect** (Fig. 41-4), which is characterized by blood glucose levels that are normal at bedtime, low at midnight, and high before breakfast. Counterregulatory hormones released by the body in response to a low blood glucose level direct the liver to release glucose to restore the glucose level to normal (it often releases too much glucose). Another effect is known as the **dawn phenomenon**, in which the blood glucose level, which is normal until about 3 AM, begins to rise because of the early morning release of growth hormone and cortisol, which triggers the release of stored glucose from the liver.

An adverse effect marked by decreased subcutaneous fat caused by repeated insulin injections into the same site also may occur. This condition is known as **lipodystrophy** (also called lipoatrophy).

Drug Interactions

Table 41-3 gives a discussion of significant drug interactions.

Assessment of Relevant Core Patient Variables

Health Status

The nurse should assess patients for allergies and for immunocompromised state and should determine whether the patient is just beginning insulin therapy or whether he or she will only be using insulin intermittently. Human insulin is preferred for these patients.

It is important for the nurse to complete a thorough history and physical assessment from which to establish a baseline. Current drug history, including information on all prescription and over-the-counter (OTC) drugs, including dietary supplements and herbal products should be solicited from the patient or family. A careful review of this information may identify drugs that can alter the action of insulin. It is important for the nurse to assess for complications related to DM, such as neuropathy, nephropathy, or retinopathy as well as the patient's ability to perform psychomotor skills such as self-blood glucose monitoring or self-injection of insulin.

An assessment of psychosocial aspects of DM, such as role changes and presence of financial concerns may help to ascertain the patient's ability to cope with a chronic illness that involves significant changes in lifestyle.

It is important for the nurse to assess the integumentary system and to inquire into the patient's general health practices, especially in regard to the skin. For example, lipoatrophy or lipodystrophy at injection sites may adversely affect insulin absorption and pharmacotherapeutic effects, color and temperature of the lower

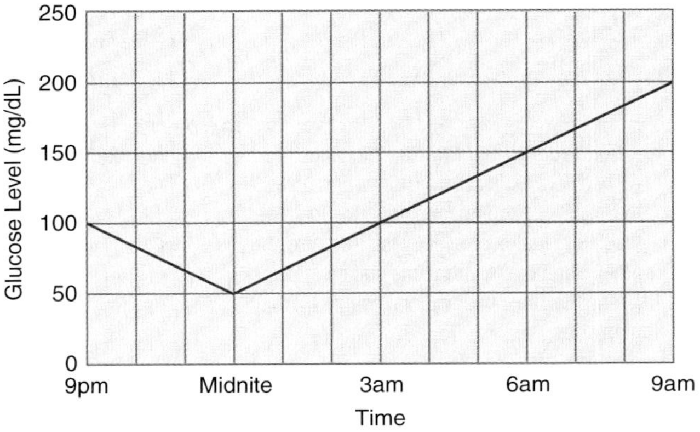

A Somogyi effect

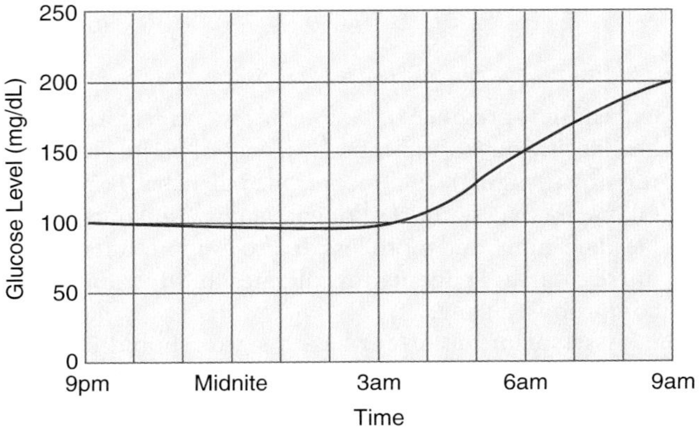

B Dawn phenomenon

Figure 41-4. Blood glucose levels characteristic of unusual phenomena, (**A**) the Somogyi effect and (**B**) the dawn phenomenon. In the Somogyi effect, the blood glucose level dips around midnight but rises significantly in the morning before breakfast. In the common problem known as the dawn phenomenon, the blood glucose level is stable until about 3 AM but begins rising after dawn. These kinds of problems illustrate why diabetic drug dosages are tailored to meet the individual patient's needs. They present the health care practitioner with challenges and opportunities to mix insulins and adjust dosage regimens to benefit the patient.

TABLE 41-3 Agents That Interact With Regular Insulin

Interactants	Effect and Significance	Nursing Management
acetazolamide, AIDS antivirals, calcitonin, corticosteroids, diazoxide, diltiazem, thiazide diuretics, dobutamine, epinephrine, estrogens (including oral contraceptives), isoniazid, lithium carbonate, morphine sulfate, niacin, phenothiazines, phenytoin, nicotine, thyroid hormones	Decreased hypoglycemic effect of insulin	Monitor plasma glucose and A1C levels. Observe for hyperglycemic complications
ACE inhibitors, alcohol, beta blockers, calcium, chloroquine, clofibrate, guanethidine, lithium carbonate, MAO inhibitors, mebendazole, octreotide, pentamidine, phenylbutazone, pyridoxine, salicylates, sulfinpyrazone, sulfonamides, tetracyclines	Increased hypoglycemic effect of insulin	Monitor blood glucose level. Observe for hypoglycemic complications.

extremities, presence of callous/ulcers on feet, delayed healing of wounds, indicating evidence of peripheral neuropathy (possibly), and uncontrolled diabetes. Periodontal disease may occur resulting in gingival inflammation, bleeding gums, and tooth loss. It also is important for the nurse to assess patients for allergies and for immunocompromised state.

Assessment of current health status should include medication and methods used for monitoring blood glucose. When the patient has been receiving regular insulin at home, the nurse should determine the type, amount, usual time of administration, and who administers it, and what sites are used. It is important to determine the frequency of hypoglycemic reactions and how the patient or family handles these reactions. This information helps to assess knowledge, usual practices, and teaching needs.

It is important to obtain baseline and periodic assessments of blood glucose levels, blood cell counts, electrolytes (especially potassium), blood lipid levels (e.g., cholesterol and triglycerides), and A_{1C} levels. The nurse should assess the patient's knowledge of diabetes and basics of self-care, including meal patterns, incidences of hypo-/hyperglycemia, exercise patterns, blood glucose monitoring, and skin and foot care. Assess insulin injection sites (e.g., abdomen, thighs, and arms) for abscess formation or allergy.

Life Span and Gender

The nurse should assess for pregnancy. Human insulin is preferred for use during gestation (both in gestational diabetes and in women who have diabetes prior to pregnancy). Human insulin is also recommended for women with diabetes who are considering pregnancy. Insulin is ranked in Food and Drug Administration (FDA) pregnancy category B. The nurse should also assess for lactation. Although the hormone does not pass into breast milk, lactation may decrease insulin requirements despite the increase in caloric intake necessitated by it.

Type 1 DM can occur at any age. It is important for the nurse to adjust care to meet the patient's chronologic and developmental age. Infants and toddlers require low dosages of insulin. Usually, a multiple-injection regimen of mixed short- and intermediate-acting insulins is used to maintain a serum glucose level of 100 to 200 mg/dL. Hypoglycemia may occur because of the unpredictable food intake and activity levels in preschool-age children. Hypoglycemia may manifest as a seizure. The brain and spinal column do not develop normally without an adequate and available source of glucose. Thus, it is important to avoid hypoglycemia in infants and young children because of its potentially damaging effects on growth and development.

Growth spurts during adolescence may cause a substantial increase in insulin requirements. Periodic determinations of A_{1C} levels will reflect the overall consistency of diabetic control. Frequent monitoring of glucose by CBGM will help to maintain a consistent blood glucose level. Usually a multiple-injection regimen of mixed short- and intermediate-acting insulins is used to maintain a normal serum glucose level. Adolescents with type 1 or 2 DM may resist medication, especially insulin injections. They may delay or omit their insulin dosages to fit in socially or to control their weight.

Changes in the diet and activity level of the elderly pose challenges to control of blood glucose levels. Diet and weight loss (if necessary) are considered the treatments of choice in the elderly diabetic patient. Dietary challenges in the elderly include the presence of ill-fitting dentures, difficulty in chewing and swallowing, decreased ability and interest in cooking, age-related changes in taste perception, reluctance to change long-established eating patterns, limited finances, and reliance on others for meals. Furthermore, decreased motor coordination and visual acuity may impair the patient's ability to perform self-monitoring of blood glucose levels and self-injection of insulin. Older adults may have impaired vision, decreased motor coordination, and/or other health problems that affect their ability to perform needed tasks for diabetic control, such as CBGM, self-administration of insulin, and managing diet and exercise. Drugs taken for other disorders (e.g., thiazide diuretics, corticosteroids, and estrogens) may cause hyperglycemia, which complicates diabetic control and requires higher dosages of the antidiabetic medication.

Lifestyle, Diet, and Habits

Exercise increases the permeability of the cell membrane to glucose, decreasing the need for insulin to transport glucose into the cell. Therefore, it is important for the nurse to determine the activity and exercise patterns of the patient. This can be accomplished by asking about the patient's usual activity level, occupation, amount and type of recreational activities, and daily exercise patterns. The nurse should also assess the patient's typical eating habits, because this will also alter the individual response to regular insulin.

It is also important to assess the patient's typical alcohol intake because consuming alcohol may cause hypoglycemia or hyperglycemia. Nutritionally alcohol has no value, although if consumed, it must be included in the fat allowances of the diabetic diet plan. Patients taking insulin and consuming alcohol may need to adjust the insulin dosage because alcohol potentiates the hypoglycemic effect of insulin.

Environment

The nurse should note the environment in which regular insulin will be administered. Insulin is most commonly self-administered by the patient in the home or occupational setting. Therefore, patient education is a primary nursing concern. It is important to evaluate the technical skills (e.g., insulin injection) that will be used by the patient for self-care at home. The nurse should evaluate the patient's desire for compliance with the prescribed diabetic regimen and should determine whether there is a need for follow-up care at home.

Proper needle disposal is a growing concern because of the large number of patients administering medications with syringes in the home-care setting. The Environmental Protection Agency's current guidelines suggest syringes, lancets, and other sharp objects be placed in a hard plastic or metal container with a screw-on or other tight-fitting lid. Patients should check local regulations regarding sharps disposal.

Culture

Before administering insulin, it is advisable to note the patient's ethnic background. Human regular insulin would be preferred in patients whose religion forbids pork products.

Nursing Diagnoses and Outcomes

- Risk For Ineffective Individual Coping or Risk for Compromised Family Coping related to the chronicity of diabetes, the complexity of self-care regimens, and an uncertain future

  Desired outcome: The patient will verbalize feelings regarding the disease process of diabetes, identify at least two methods to cope with diabetes, describe stressful situations and several methods of stress reduction and identify appropriate resources.
- Deficient Knowledge related to diagnosis of diabetes mellitus

  Desired outcome: Knowledge deficit is a significant obstacle for diabetic patients to overcome, and significant learning and lifestyle changes (e.g., diet, exercise, drug therapy) must be accomplished to control and manage the disease. The desired outcome of the nursing diagnosis and process is the patient's initiation of the necessary lifestyle changes and participation in the treatment regimen. An evaluative measure of the effectiveness of the nursing process is the patient's ability to express verbally an understanding of the pharmacologic management of DM.
- Fear (patient, family) related to insulin injections

  Desired outcome: The patient (or family) will state brand, type, onset, peak, duration and dose of insulin, demonstrate techniques for administration of insulin, and verbalize recommendations for site rotation, storage of insulin, and disposal of syringes.
- Imbalanced Nutrition: More Than Body Requirements related to weight gain secondary to insulin therapy

  Desired outcome: The patient will verbalize the value of decreasing weight to help control blood sugar and state an intent to follow a prescribed meal plan in which caloric intake is sufficient to decrease weight.
- Risk for Infection related to alterations in circulation and hyperglycemia

  Desired outcome: The patient will identify situations contributing to infection and practice appropriate health behaviors to avoid infection.
- Anxiety related to change in self-concept and change or threat to health status

  Desired outcome: The patient will identify and utilize resources available to promote positive adaptation to chronic illness.
- Risk for Injury related to changes in neuromuscular and sensory systems (e.g., peripheral and/or autonomic neuropathy)

  Desired outcome: The patient will describe and demonstrate accurate administration of insulin, proper techniques for CBGM, and appropriate foot care procedures.

Planning and Intervention

Maximizing Therapeutic Effects

The nurse should store opened vials of regular insulin at room temperature. Extra supplied should be stored in the refrigerator, but not the freezer. Extreme temperatures (under 2°C or over 30°C) should be avoided to prevent loss of maximum function.

The nurse should administer regular insulin with an insulin syringe into an appropriate subcutaneous site. Regular insulin should be administered about 30–60 minutes before eating. To promote regular absorption, one anatomic location should be selected for regular insulin injections (i.e., the abdomen). Serial locations within that anatomic location should be used to rotate the exact injection site. This is sometimes known as intrasite rotation. The nurse should **not** rotate injection sites by using the arm one day, the stomach the next day, and the thigh the next day, because this will substantially change the absorption of the insulin and the blood glucose levels of the patient. If the patient routinely receives regular insulin in the morning and in the evening, one anatomic site may be selected for each time of day (e.g., use the abdomen for all morning injections and the thighs for all evening injections).

The nurse should monitor carefully the blood sugar levels of patients receiving regular insulin intravenously because of varying absorption of the drug into the plastic.

Minimizing Adverse Effects

The nurse should avoid administering cold insulin. This will help to limit local irritation (e.g., lipodystrophy) at the injection site. Intrasite rotation of injection sites will also help prevent lipodystrophy. This is especially important in infants and children.

The nurse should assess the current blood sugar level of the patient prior to administering regular insulin. Caution is necessary if the blood glucose level is below 70 mg/dL prior to administration of regular insulin. Usually the dose is withheld until the blood sugar level has risen to normal levels. The nurse should consult with the physician or nurse practitioner prior to administering regular insulin if the blood sugar is low.

The patient should be monitored closely for hypoglycemic reactions, especially near the peak action time of the insulin (see Table 41-2). Reassess the patient's blood glucose level if signs or symptoms of hypoglycemia occur. It is also possible that if the regular insulin dose is too low for the patient's current metabolic needs, hyperglycemia may occur. Monitor the patient for signs and symptoms of this and reevaluate blood glucose levels as appropriate.

Providing Patient and Family Education

In addition to the information provided within this section, which is specific to insulin therapy, see also the accompanying display, Patient and Family Education Common to Antidiabetic Drugs.

Discussing Diet

- The nurse should stress the importance of following the diet recommended by the health care provider, which is based on the diet available in printed form from the ADA.
- The nurse also needs to emphasize the importance of eating after insulin dosing. The patient should be warned that hypoglycemia might occur from the omission of a meal or food's not being absorbed in the usual manner because of postponing a meal.
- It is important to counsel the patient not to take any nonprescription or over-the-counter (OTC) preparations, including herbs or alcohol, without first consulting the health care provider, because these may interact with the effectiveness of regular insulin.

Understanding Activity and Rest

- The patient and family need to understand that a vital part of glucose control is physical exercise and activity. These are helpful in lowering the blood glucose level and increasing insulin sensitivity. In addition, exercise and activity are keys to weight reduction and control, cardiovascular fitness, circulation, and a general feeling of well being.
- When working with the patient to identify important blood glucose management strategies, the nurse may suggest incorporating an exercise program into the treatment regimen.
- The nurse and patient need to recognize that physical activity should occur after meals. Exercise before meals increases the risk of hypoglycemia because glucose crosses over the cell membrane of the active muscle cell without insulin.
- Exercise when diabetes is in poor control (blood glucose exceeding 250 mg/dL or if ketonuria is present) acts as a stressor, releasing the insulin-antagonistic counter-regulatory hormones (i.e., epinephrine, glucagon, cortisol, growth hormone, and somatostatin). In such cases, the nurse should teach the patient to avoid exercise.

Recognizing the Role of Stress

- The nurse should teach the patient and family that stress, both physiologic (e.g., illness, surgery, and trauma) and psychological (e.g., death in the family, divorce, and job changes), might change insulin requirements because the hormones released in stressful situations are insulin antagonistic.
- In cases of stress, the nurse should urge the patient to consult the health care provider in case a change is needed in the insulin dosage or regimen.

Monitoring the Blood Glucose Level

- Generally, most diabetic patients learn to test their own blood (urine in acute illness for sugar and acetone) to measure the level of circulating glucose. Various kits and devices are commercially available for this task.
- When blood sugar is elevated, some patients will use a "sliding scale" of very small doses of regular insulin supplements to "cover" the increase.
- Typically, blood is monitored periodically (e.g., before meals and bedtime) and regular insulin is given according to the degree of glucose detected (see the

Patient and Family Education Common to Antidiabetic Drugs

Management of diabetes mellitus (DM)—perhaps more than any other chronic disease process—requires substantial and ongoing self-care activity on the part of the patient or caregiver. For example, people with diabetes need to know what diabetes is and why treatment is necessary, how to administer and store insulin, test blood glucose several times a day, adjust their insulin dosages, and how and when to take oral medications if they suffer type 2 diabetes. In addition, they must continually consider lifestyle choices related to the food eaten, occupational and leisure activities, how to take precautions when traveling, and demands on their time and energy. Research has shown that when patients with diabetes practice appropriate self-care, blood glucose levels improve resulting in fewer hospitalizations and complications.

The importance of 1) complying with dietary instructions, 2) scheduling and keeping follow-up appointments, 3) implementing a regular and consistent exercise program, and 4) regularly monitoring parameters indicative of blood sugar control (e.g., capillary blood-glucose monitoring [CBGM], fasting blood-glucose levels [FBG], glycosylated hemoglobin [A_{1c}]) as well as renal function and other blood chemistry values cannot be overemphasized.

- The nurse should emphasize that insulin, diet, and exercise comprise the primary forms of treatment for Type 1 DM, and that diet, exercise, and, sometimes, antidiabetic medication are the primary forms of treatment for Type 2 DM; caloric restriction and weight loss are essential in the treatment of the obese diabetic patient. The nurse should stress the importance of regular physical activity because exercise has marked beneficial effects on muscle insulin sensitivity and weight loss/control. It also is important to teach the patient to modify treatment for exercise or illness.
- The nurse should carefully review diabetic dietary guidelines with the patient and family, including instructions on when to take the drug in relationship to meals, and how to select the proper foods at each meal.
- The nurse needs to emphasize that drug therapy is not a substitute for diet control, exercise, and weight loss.
- It is important to caution the patient against the consumption of alcohol because of its hypoglycemic or hyperglycemic effects with insulin and other antidiabetic drugs as well as the possibility of a disulfiram-like reaction when combined with some sulfonylureas.
- The nurse needs to teach the patient how to self-monitor blood glucose levels and when and how to test the urine for sugar and acetone.
- The nurse should inform patients and their families that keeping blood sugar levels as near normal as possible may help reduce the risk of developing acute or chronic diabetic complications.
- It is important to teach the patient to recognize and report symptoms of hypoglycemia (e.g., fatigue, excessive hunger, diaphoresis, and numbness or tingling of extremities), or hyperglycemia (e.g., excessive thirst or urination, urinary glucose, or ketones) to the health care provider.
- It is important to teach the patient with diabetes how to practice proper foot care.
- The nurse should caution the patient with type 1 diabetes that if the blood glucose level is more than 240 mg/dL and moderate or greater levels of urinary ketones are present, it is essential to notify the health care provider.
- The nurse should educate patients with type 2 diabetes and their families in the prevention and recognition of HHS. HHS is a syndrome of severe hyperglycemia and profound dehydration in the patient with type 2 diabetes that has a slow and subtle onset. Ketosis usually does not occur because typically there is enough insulin present to prevent excessive fat catabolism. The hyperosmolar state causes water to be lost from the body cells including the brain accounting for the signs and symptoms of dehydration and altered level of consciousness. Risk factors for HHS include any condition that results in fluid loss; for instance, therapy with diuretics (especially thiazides), decreased fluid intake, infection or illness, and hypertonic tube feeding. Older patients with type 2 diabetes are at a greater risk for developing HHS due to their diminished thirst sensation, and especially if they live alone or are cognitively impaired. Preventive measures include maintenance of adequate hydration and adherence to medications and meal plan, "sick day" management, and avoidance of drugs and situations that can exacerbate hyperglycemia.
- No educational program is complete without educational materials (audio, visual, or printed) for reference and review. Materials should include information about adverse and toxic drug effects, dosage (amount and timing of doses), possible drug interactions, and principles of safe storage for drugs and equipment.
- The nurse should encourage the patient to carry some type of medical identification (e.g., MedicAlert bracelet) and to inform all health care providers of current drug therapy.

The ADA has information available in Spanish and also an African-American Program that offers special posters and printed materials aimed at those groups of the U.S. population.

accompanying display, Balancing Act: Insulin and Diabetes).

- As a general rule, insulin coverage is calculated at about 1 U per 25 mg/dL over 180 mg/dL.

Administering Insulin

- Most patients with type I DM administer their own insulin with disposable needle and syringe injection devices (see the accompanying display, Insulin Delivery Devices). The nurse should teach the patient to perform aseptic technique, select the appropriate type of insulin, mix insulin properly (if necessary), administer insulin correctly by subcutaneous injection, rotate sites serially in an anatomic location (intrasite rotation) and store insulin carefully (see the accompanying display, Insulin Administration). If an acute infection is present or there is decreased resistance to infection, the needles should not be reused.
- Manufacturers of disposable syringes recommend a single use. Some patients, however, prefer to reuse a syringe until its needle becomes dull, usually up to 3 or 4 times. Reuse effectively reduces the cost of injections, and this may be important for patients with limited financial resources. Most insulin preparations have bacteriostatic additives that inhibit growth of bacteria commonly found on the skin. If reuse is planned, the needle must be carefully recapped after each use. Aseptic technique should be followed. The patient who reuses a syringe should be taught to

Critical Thinking Scenario

Balancing act: insulin and diabetes

Your neighbor Mr. F is a 58-year-old African-American man who asks you what he can do for his aching muscles. He mentions that he has had type 2 diabetes for 6 years and that he now takes insulin. When you ask what he thinks is causing his aching muscles, he tells you that he left his desk job for a position painting houses and office buildings. This job involves more physical exertion. When you inquire further, he tells you that he is also getting palpitations at work and becoming increasingly sweaty, weak, and shaky by midmorning, which he blames on the stress of the new job. He adds that he has to be at work very early so he has been eating smaller breakfasts and that he hasn't been checking his blood glucose level during the day, because he does not feel comfortable checking it at his new job. You learn that his current insulin regimen is 20 U of NPH insulin in the morning and 10 U at night to keep his blood glucose level under control.

1. After analyzing all of this information, how do you account for Mr. F.'s symptoms?
2. What kind of help do you think you can give Mr. F.?

inspect the skin around the injection sites for unusual redness or signs of infection.

- The nurse should teach the patient thoroughly about safe insulin administration. It is important to stress that needles or syringes should never be shared with anyone else, because this may cause transmission of blood-borne infections (e.g., hepatitis B or C, HIV).
- Nearly as important as learning about injection techniques is learning about safe and proper disposal of insulin injection equipment. The EPA recommends that insulin needles and lancets be discarded whole in opaque, puncture-resistant containers to avoid the hazards of exposed or broken needles, and the lid should be taped on tightly before disposing of it in the trash. For example, a plastic milk container or a coffee can is preferable to a glass jar, which can break.

Explaining Other Safety Measures

- The nurse should encourage patients to wear diabetic identification, such as a MedicAlert bracelet, so that appropriate treatment can be given if complications, such as diabetic coma, occur away from home.
- The nurse also should caution the patient that changing the kind of insulin normally used may affect blood glucose control and should be done only under the supervision of the health care professional.
- The nurse can advise the patient always to carry a spare vial of each type of insulin used and to pay attention to the expiration date stamped on the vial.
- There are many other aspects to diabetic care and management of outpatient insulin, oral hypoglycemic, or antidiabetic drug therapy. The patient and family may obtain additional detailed information from publications available from the ADA and local support groups specializing in diabetes. The nurse may obtain additional detailed information from textbooks about diabetes, nursing textbooks, specialty journals, and particularly the ADA and local support groups specializing in diabetes.

Ongoing Assessment and Evaluation

Specific assessment and evaluation criteria may include the patient's verbal willingness to adhere to recommended drug therapy and management techniques for DM and blood glucose levels that remain within normal limits as specified by the health care provider.

Nursing management of drug therapy is considered successful if the patient experiences few episodes of hypoglycemia or hyperglycemia, demonstrates the ability to perform correctly the technical tasks necessary for managing diabetes at home, follows the ADA diet and incorporates it into the lifestyle, incorporates an exercise regimen to attain or maintain normal body weight, and recognizes situations in which knowledge deficit may require guidance of a diabetic professional for additional information or follow-up care.

Fasting blood glucose and glycosylated hemoglobin (A_{1C}) levels are valuable in monitoring the patient's response to therapy. It is important to monitor response to all diabetic therapies by periodic measurements of fasting blood glucose and A_{1C} levels, with a goal of decreasing these levels toward the normal range. During initial dose titration, fasting glucose can be used to determine the therapeutic response. Thereafter, monitor both fasting glucose and A_{1C}. Measurements of A_{1C} may be especially useful for evaluating long-term control (about 90 days). ■

DRUGS CLOSELY RELATED TO P REGULAR INSULIN

Rapid-acting Insulins

The pharmacodynamically rapid-acting (rDNA) insulins aspart (NovoLog) and lispro (Humalog), compared with regular insulin, have a faster onset of glucose-lowering activity (10–15 minutes), an earlier peak glucose-lowering effect (1 to 2 hours), and a shorter duration of action (3.5 hours) after SC administration. The rapid onset of action allows patients more flexibility in taking insulin and preparing and consuming meals. Lispro is well suited for use in implantable pumps, because its short duration of action mimics endogenous insulin more closely than regular insulin.

COMMUNITY-BASED CONCERNS

Insulin Delivery Devices

INSULIN INFUSION PUMP*

An insulin pump is a small (2 × 3-in) precise computerized device that consists of a reservoir filled with insulin. The reservoir is connected by an infusion set (a thin plastic tube) to an SC catheter or needle. The catheter is changed every 2 to 3 days. An insulin pump can be programmed to deliver a basal infusion of insulin (microdoses; ~0.1 U) 24 hours a day. Continuous delivery of insulin helps maintain blood glucose concentrations between meals and overnight. Insulin dosing adjustments require little or no patient effort. When the patient eats, a predetermined bolus dose of insulin is delivered that is matched to the estimated caloric intake. The bolus mode requires the patient to determine the dose and push a button to administer insulin before or after each meal. Pump devices help patients achieve tighter blood glucose control, thus minimizing potential complications. The pumps have an alarm system if insulin delivery is interrupted.

JET INJECTORS**

Jet injectors deliver insulin transcutaneously without a needle. A fine stream of insulin directed at high speed and pressure penetrates the skin. The dose of insulin is controlled by a dial-a-dose mechanism similar to that used in insulin pens. An advantage to this method is a more rapid absorption of regular human insulin. Their use is limited, however, by size (about 8 oz) and expense. Other limitations include pain or bruising at the injection site and the potential for a decreased amount of absorbed insulin.

INSULIN PENS***

Pen devices are unique because they combine the insulin container and the syringe into a single modular unit. Although insulin pens are available in a variety of types and styles—for example, prefilled or reusable—generally, they have a characteristic design—the patient must attach a needle, prime the pen, dial the dose, and depress a plunger to deliver the dose. The convenient insulin delivery can add lifestyle flexibility (i.e., they are pocket sized and easy to carry) and may lead to improved glycemic control.

FUTURE INSULIN DELIVERY DEVICES

The "Innovo" by Novo-Nordisk Pharmaceuticals is a new insulin-delivery device. It is the size of a pager, advertised as a "doser" rather than an injectable pen. The top half of the device is a miniature screen that displays the dose amount and elapsed time since the last dose. All doses can be dialed in 1-U increments up to 70 U. The device includes a compartment for an insulin-syringe cartridge. In the future, insulin may be delivered by implanted, intranasal, transdermal, inhalation, or oral systems. Implantable insulin pumps are currently under development in the United States. The intranasal route of insulin administration has been demonstrated to be effective in clinical trials. However, some concerns over this method include low intranasal insulin bioavailability (8%), nasal irritation, loss of olfactory sense, and the effects of nasal congestion on insulin absorption. Transdermal insulin appears to be effective (70% absorbed into bloodstream), but slow.

Inhaled Therapeutic System and Pfizer Inc. are currently developing a device for inhaled insulin to treat both type 1 and type 2 diabetes. This portable aerosol delivery system—about the size of a flashlight—is similar to an asthma inhaler. It delivers a dose of insulin in a dry powder through the mouth, directly into the lungs, where it enters the blood to act as a rapid acting insulin. Two multicenter clinical trials—one for type 1 patients and one for type 2 patients—have demonstrated that the inhaled insulin worked as well as injected insulin in achieving overall blood glucose control as measured by the hemoglobin A_{1c}. Phase 3 clinical trials of this drug are expected to begin soon.

Generex Biotechnology Corporation has announced that it has completed a significant series of short-term clinical trials of Oralgen (Canada-Oralin), its proprietary insulin formulation that is administered to the oral cavity using a lightweight, hand-held spray device. Andrew Lewin conducted the trials at the National Research Institute of Los Angeles. The primary aim of the studies was to examine the effect of using Oralgen in treating patients with type 2 diabetes. Tests were conducted under a study protocol that called for patients to be challenged with a high calorie meal following administration of Oralgen in combination with administering metformin hydrochloride, an oral antihyperglycemic drug in wide use in treating patients with type 2 diabetes versus placebo. Test results demonstrated that glucose control in patients who received Oralgen product was superior in most circumstances to the results obtained in patients who received the placebo. According to Lewin, "after an examination of the oral insulin preparation compared to placebo in sixteen Type 2 diabetic patients . . . the oral insulin preparation was well absorbed and lowered the plasma glucose. The oral insulin was well tolerated and there were no side effects in this short-term trial." Oralgen is continuing clinical testing in long-term trials (McCann, 2001).

BLOOD GLUCOSE MONITORING DEVICES

Newer blood glucose meters may offer alternate sites for testing such as blood drawn from the thigh, forearm, or upper arm using a lancet (e.g., One-Touch Ultra, FreeStyle) or an all-inclusive system that incorporates the meter and sampler into a single unit (e.g., At-Last).

The *GlucoWatch Biographer* is a wristwatch-like device for patients with diabetes (>18 years old) that automatically, and painlessly, checks blood sugar levels every 20 minutes by sending tiny electric currents through the skin. The device works by having the patient slide a thin plastic sensor onto the watch back each time it is trapped on; small electric currents then extract fluid from the skin and measure its glucose content. This occurs every 20 minutes for 12 hours. GlucoWatch supplements rather than replaces the routine finger (or arm/thigh in newer blood glucose meters) sticks because it sometimes gives false readings. An alarm sounds if blood sugar reaches dangerous levels—either too high or too low—even when the patient is asleep.

*Some patients may find the pump complicated to use. The individual needs to be very motivated and adherent to therapy. The pump is not automatic; the user must decide how much insulin to give.

**The patient must possess sufficient coordination and visual acuity to attach and detach a needle for injection. Some newer pens have larger numbers for ease of reading; others have an audible click as the dose is dialed.

***Sometimes pens continue to deliver insulin after removal of the pen needle from the skin. This dribbling of insulin from the pens, which has been attributed to air in the insulin cartridges, has the potential to cause insulin underdosing. Pen manufacturers suggest leaving the needle in the skin for at least 5 seconds to ensure complete delivery of the insulin dose into the subcutaneous tissue (Campbell, 2000).

Insulin Administration

ADA Guidelines for Preparing and Administering a Subcutaneous Dose of Insulin

- Check the type of insulin and the expiration date
- Inspect the solution for visible changes (e.g., solid clumps) that indicate deterioration of the drug.
- If possible, verify *D*ose, *E*xpiration date, *C*oncentration, *T*ype, *S*pecies source (*DECTS*) with another individual (nurse if in health care setting).
- Wash hands.
- Cleanse injection site and insulin vial by wiping with alcohol.
- If using suspension (cloudy solution), roll gently between palms of hand to resuspend the insulin.
- Inject an amount of air into the vial (each vial if using two) that is equal to the dose of insulin.
- When mixing two types of insulin in one syringe, the clear insulin should be drawn into the syringe first; do not mix insulins if 1) they are from a different species source (e.g., bovine, porcine), or 2) their purity level is different, or 3) they are produced by different manufacturers.
- Eliminate air bubbles from the syringe to ensure an accurate dose.
- Injection sites—in their order of rapidity of absorption—include the 1) abdomen (excluding 2 in around the umbilicus), 2) subcutaneous tissue of the upper arm, 3) anterior and lateral aspects of the thigh, and 4) buttocks.*
- Insulin injections are made into SC tissue so it is not necessary to aspirate for blood routinely before injecting the insulin.
- The needle angle during the injection (45 to 90 degrees) should be individualized to avoid IM injection; the needle length is usually ⅝ in. Gently pinch a skin fold to determine the angle that will deliver an SC injection.

Other Considerations

- Insulin vials in current use may be stored at room temperature; avoid exposure to direct sunlight and high temperatures. Some potency of product may be lost after 30 days.
- Spare insulin vials should be stored in the refrigerator. No potency is lost when stored in the refrigerator.
- Prefilled syringes:
  Are stable up to 30 days when stored in the refrigerator.
  Filled with an insulin suspension (cloudy solution) should preferably be stored with the needle pointed up (vertical position) to avoid clumping of suspended insulin molecules in the needle.
  Insulin combinations inappropriate for pre-filling and storage:
  aspart insulin with crystalline zinc preparations
  regular insulin mixed with lente or ultralente insulins
  glargine insulin mixed with any other type of insulin
- Adaptive equipment—several products are available for patients with diabetes who are visually or functionally impaired. Some of the commonly-used assistive devices include:
  Syringe magnifiers to enlarge the measurements on the syringe barrel.
  Needle guides to help direct the needle into the vial stopper.
  Vial stabilizers mounted on a surface to hold the vial in place during needle insertion.
  Insertion aids add bulk to the syringe for patients unable to hold a small syringe.
  Dose-measuring devices assist the visually impaired patient to draw up the recommended insulin dosage into a syringe.
  "Talking" blood glucose meters produce audible test results with tactile guides for test strip insertion.

*Site selection influences absorption; it is recommended that rotation of insulin injection sites take place within the same anatomic area.

MEMORY CHIP

Regular Insulin

- Used primarily to treat type 1 diabetes mellitus; only type of insulin used for intravenous administration, in external insulin pumps, and for "sliding scale" coverage for hypoglycemia
- Most common adverse effect: hypoglycemia
- Most serious adverse effects: anaphylaxis and hypersensitivity
- Maximizing therapeutic effects: protect insulin from excessive heat and light to avoid deterioration
- Minimizing adverse effects: use the same type and brand of syringe to avoid dosage errors; rotate injection sites to prevent tissue damage
- Most significant patient education: thorough patient teaching regarding dosage, administration techniques for subcutaneous injection, delivery devices, diet and exercise, and capillary blood glucose testing; wear medical alert tag identifying diabetic condition treated with insulin to alert emergency medical personnel

Although their pharmacologic actions are quite similar, their chemical characteristics differ in that insulin lispro contains zinc. They are normally used in regimens along with an intermediate- or long-acting insulin. In patients with type 1 DM, insulin lispro is used in regimens that include a longer acting insulin. In patients with type 2 DM, however, insulin lispro may be used without a longer-acting insulin when used in combination therapy with sulfonylureas. It may also be used in combination with sulfonylureas in adults and children. Unlike regular insulin, rapid-acting insulins (e.g., insulin lispro, insulin aspart) should be administered 10–15 minutes before a meal because of their onset of action. Adverse effects and patient education are similar to those for regular insulin.

Regular [Concentrated] Iletin II

Regular [Concentrated] Iletin II, like regular insulin, has no additives to prolong onset or duration of action. Unlike regular insulin, its higher concentration (500 U/mL) extends its duration of activity to 24 hours. Furthermore, it is given SC, more rarely as an IM injection but never IV. It is used in patients who have developed marked insulin resistance. It is usually given once daily. Some patients may, however, require doses 2 or 3 times a day. Hypoglycemia may occur 18 to 24 hours after an injection. Concentrated insulin is a pregnancy category C drug.

DRUGS SIGNIFICANTLY DIFFERENT FROM P REGULAR INSULIN

Insulin is available in a variety of forms with the different forms made by the addition of zinc or protamine with a buffer. These modifications delay the absorption of the insulin from a subcutaneous site, resulting in a later onset of action, peak action, and an extended duration of action. Thus, insulin preparations may be rapid-, short-, intermediate-, or long-acting based on their duration of action. NPH, Lente, Ultralente, and glargine differ from regular insulin primarily in terms of type. NPH and Lente are considered intermediate acting and Ultralente and glargine are long-acting insulins. They are cloudy in appearance, administered subcutaneously once or twice daily, and never used for sliding scale coverage or in implantable pumps. Because these insulins are suspensions and tend to separate inside the vial, they must be mixed by rolling the vial between the palms of both hands before withdrawing the mixture into the insulin syringe. Excessive agitation should be avoided to prevent precipitation (especially for porcine and human insulins) or loss of potency.

NPH and Lente

NPH and Lente insulins are intermediate-acting insulins that contain protamine and zinc to prolong their duration of action. Onset of action is 1 to 4 hours, peak action occurs in 6 to 10 hours, and duration of action is up to 24 hours. These insulins are mixed frequently with regular insulin and given twice daily.

NPH (isophane insulin suspension) insulin is the most widely used intermediate-acting insulin. It contains protamine and a small amount of zinc. Occasionally a white precipitate called flocculation may appear as frosting that adheres to the vial. Why this occurs is unknown although vigorous mixing of the vial is thought to be a contributing factor. Flocculation decreases the potency of the insulin; if present, the insulin should be discarded. NPH insulin may be mixed with regular insulin; premixed solutions of NPH and regular insulin are available in ratios of 70:30 and 50:50. Use of premixed insulin is especially useful for patients who are visually impaired or have difficulty with fine motor skills (hand coordination); this may reduce the number of errors that might typically occur when using the standard mixing technique. A limiting factor to the premixed solutions is that the patient's insulin requirements must match the fixed ratio of the premixed preparations.

Lente insulin (insulin zinc suspension) is an intermediate-acting preparation of 30% short-acting insulin zinc suspension (Semilente) and 70% long-acting insulin zinc suspension (Ultralente). Lente insulins may not be mixed with non-Lente insulins.

Nursing interventions specific for intermediate-acting insulins (e.g., NPH insulin, Lente insulin) include observing patients for adequate nutritional intake and monitoring for hypoglycemia during mid-to-late afternoon (after an early morning dose) as the lengthy peak action time produces additional risks for hypoglycemic reactions. The onset of hypoglycemia with the intermediate-acting insulins is insidious and more prolonged. Adverse effects, nursing actions, and patient education are also similar to those for regular insulin.

Ultralente

Long-acting Ultralente suspension contains higher levels of zinc to greatly prolong the duration of action. Onset of action is 4 to 6 hours after injection with peak effect occurring at approximately 18 hours. This type of insulin is not excreted entirely from the body for 36 or more hours. Ultralente insulin is used in combination with multiple injections of regular insulin to provide a basal level of insulin that mimics normal basal insulin production by the pancreas.

Glargine

Insulin glargine (rDNA) is characterized by a chemical structure that regulates its release from the SC tissue into the circulation, providing a relatively constant glucose-lowering effect with no pronounced peak of action over a 24-hour period. Glargine must not be diluted or mixed with any other insulin or solution because it may result in a delayed onset of action.

C ORAL HYPOGLYCEMIC/ ANTIDIABETIC MEDICATIONS

There are currently five chemical classes of oral antidiabetic agents available for the treatment of type 2 DM. They are the sulfonylureas (eight drugs), meglitinides (one drug), biguanides (one drug), alpha-glucosidase inhibitors (two drugs), and thiazolidinediones (four drugs).

There is a documented cardiovascular risk with treatment of type 2 DM with the oral hyperglycemic drugs—especially the sulfonylureas.

C SULFONYLUREAS

The **sulfonylureas**—until the mid-1990s—were the single class of oral antidiabetic agents available to manage type 2 DM. The sulfonylureas are classified as first- or second-generation. In comparison, the first generation sulfonylureas (e.g., acetohexamide, chlorpropamide, tolazamide, and tolbutamide) are associated with a greater potential for drug interactions.

The sulfonylureas reduce serum glucose indirectly by enhancing the production of insulin and stimulating its release from pancreatic beta cells. They also help to inhibit hepatic glycogenolysis and gluconeogenesis. Furthermore, they increase the number of insulin receptors in peripheral tissue and increase their insulin sensitivity. First-generation sulfonylureas exert a greater effect on insulin release; second-generation drugs have their maximal effect on cellular receptors.

Research performed in the 1970s demonstrated a higher rate of cardiovascular death in patients who received a first generation sulfonylurea than patients treated with placebo or insulin. No comparable studies have refuted this observation; the question of whether treatment with sulfonylureas is associated with increased cardiovascular mortality is still unresolved.

The prototype, glyburide, is a second-generation sulfonylurea that is similar structurally to a first-generation drug, acetohexamide, and to another second-generation drug, glipizide.

NURSING MANAGEMENT OF THE PATIENT RECEIVING GLYBURIDE

Core Drug Knowledge

Pharmacotherapeutics

Glyburide is a potent second-generation oral sulfonylurea that is used as an adjunctive treatment to lower blood glucose levels in patients with type 2 DM in whom hyperglycemia cannot be controlled by diet and exercise alone (see Table 41-2).

Combination administration of a sulfonylurea and insulin has been used with some success in patients with type 2 DM whose disease is difficult to control with diet and sulfonylurea therapy alone. One such method is the "BIDS" system—*B*edtime *I*nsulin (usually NPH) in combination with a *D*aytime (morning only or morning and evening) *S*ulfonylurea.

Pharmacokinetics

Administered orally, glyburide is absorbed rapidly and completely from the GI tract. The onset of action occurs within 2 hours, with a maximal decrease in serum glucose occurring within 3 to 4 hours. Like the other sulfonylureas, glyburide is highly protein bound by nonionic binding, which differs from the ionic protein binding observed with first-generation sulfonylureas. Displacement of sulfonylurea agents from protein-binding sites will result in greater hypoglycemic response.

Glyburide is metabolized completely in the liver to two metabolites, both of which are only weakly active. Both unchanged drug and metabolites are excreted equally in the urine and feces. The elimination half-life of the drug is 10 hours, and the duration of action is 24 hours in patients with normal renal function.

The two forms of glyburide—micronized and nonmicronized—differ in their bioavailability. Patients transferring to micronized glyburide from conventional glyburide or other oral hypoglycemic agents should have their dosages adjusted.

Pharmacodynamics

The hypoglycemic action of glyburide results from the stimulation of pancreatic beta cells, leading to increased insulin secretion. Sulfonylureas are ineffective with nonfunctional beta cells (type 1 DM) or the number of viable beta cells is low (as in severe cases of type 2 DM).

Prolonged administration of glyburide produces extrapancreatic effects that contribute to its hypoglycemic activity. These effects include reduced basal hepatic glucose production and enhanced peripheral sensitivity to insulin secondary to an increase in insulin receptors and/or to changes in the events that follow insulin-receptor binding. These actions are characterized by an interindividual variability.

Contraindications and Precautions

Glyburide is contraindicated in patients with a known hypersensitivity to the sulfa drugs as the sulfonylureas are related chemically to the antimicrobial sulfonamides, although they do not demonstrate any of this activity. Sulfonylureas should not be used in type 1 DM and should be used cautiously in individuals with renal or hepatic disease.

Adverse Effects

Glyburide and other sulfonylureas are generally well tolerated. The primary adverse effect associated with glyburide (and the other sulfonylureas) is hypoglycemia. Renal or hepatic insufficiency may elevate drug blood levels; hepatic insufficiency may also diminish gluconeogenic capacity, both of which increase the risk of serious hypoglycemic reactions. Hypoglycemia may be manifested as hunger, pallor, nausea, fatigue, perspiration, headache, palpitations, numbness, paresthesias, tremors, muscle weakness, blurred vision, irritability, mental confusion, tachycardia, and alterations in consciousness. Hypoglycemia may result from excessive dosage, but it also could be due to other factors, such as altered hepatic metabolism and renal excretion, improper diet, excessive physical activity, when alcohol is ingested (especially first-generation sulfonylureas), or when more than one glucose-lowering drug is used. The hypoglycemia induced by glyburide (and other first- and second-generation sulfonylureas) may be severe and will require immediate reevaluation and adjustment of the drug dosage and the patient's lifestyle (e.g., diet and activity). GI effects may include anorexia, nausea, vomiting, heartburn, and metallic taste in the mouth. Elderly, debilitated, or malnourished patients, and those with adrenal or pituitary insufficiency are particularly susceptible to the hypoglycemic action of glucose-lowering drugs. Hypoglycemia may be difficult to recognize in the elderly and in patients taking adrenergic blocking drugs.

Signs of allergic reactions to glyburide therapy can include maculopapular rash, urticaria, pruritus, and erythema. These reactions are usually mild, but if they persist or become severe, the drug should be discontinued. Photosensitivity reactions also may occur with sulfonylureas. Rarely, blood dyscrasias occur (e.g., leukopenia, thrombocytopenia, pancytopenia, agranulocytosis, aplastic anemia, hemolysis) that may lead to hemolytic anemia. These effects are mild and typically subside following cessation of the drug.

Hyponatremia and the syndrome of inappropriate secretion of antidiuretic hormone (SIADH) have occurred in patients receiving sulfonylureas. Signs and symptoms of SIADH include water intoxication characterized by mental confusion, nausea, anorexia, dizziness, decreased sodium concentration, increased urinary osmolality, and decreased serum osmolality.

Drug Interactions

As with other first- and second-generation sulfonylureas, a synergistic drug interaction occurs between glyburide (which stimulates insulin release) and the "insulin sensitizers," metformin, and rosiglitazone (which improve tissue use of insulin). Hypoglycemia may occur. Some of the sulfonylureas may cause a disulfiram-like reaction when combined with alcohol. Early signs and symptoms of a disulfiram-like reaction include flushing, throbbing pain in the head and neck, shortness of breath, nausea and vomiting, thirst, chest pain, palpitations, syncope and vertigo, blurred vision, anxiety, sweating, and weakness. Later signs include arrhythmias, respiratory depression, seizures, and possibly death (Table 41-4).

Concomitant use of some alternative therapies (e.g., juniper berries, ginseng, garlic, fenugreek, coriander, dandelion root, or celery) increases the risk of hypoglycemia.

Assessment of Relevant Core Patient Variables

Health Status

Assessments to be made before therapy with the sulfonylureas are similar to those necessary with insulin. Glyburide undergoes hepatic metabolism and renal excretion. Impairment in these functions can result in elevated serum concentrations and increase the risk for hypoglycemia. Hepatic disease can reduce gluconeogenic capacity. Consequently, glyburide and other sulfonylureas should be used cautiously in patients with type 2 DM and hepatic or renal impairment. Renal and hepatic function (especially bilirubin, cholesterol, aspartate transaminase [AST], and alanine transaminase [ALT]) should be monitored frequently in these patients. Thyroid hormone increases the GI absorption of glucose and stimulates gluconeogenesis and glycogenolysis. Patients with both thyroid disease and DM must be treated for both diseases.

To detect or prevent possible adverse drug interactions, additional assessment activities by the nurse should include a review of all other drugs—prescription and OTC including herbal products and dietary supplements—used by the patient. Assessment of current health status should include diet, activity, and methods used for monitoring blood glucose. If hypoglycemic reactions occur, it is important to determine their frequency and how the patient or family handles these reactions. This information helps to assess knowledge, usual practices, and teaching needs.

It is important to assess the patient's knowledge, attitude, and physical condition in relation to diabetes, the prescribed treatment plan, and evidence of complications. Assessment data should also include past manifes-

TABLE 41-4 Agents That Interact With Glyburide

Interactants	Effect and Significance	Nursing Management
antacids (MG+ salts)	Increased glyburide serum levels due to increased glyburide absorption	Monitor blood glucose level for hypoglycemia.
sulfonamides, chloramphenicol, phenylbutazone, salicylates, clofibrate, anticoagulants, fluconazole, H_2-antagonists (e.g., cimetidine), MAOIs, probenecid, sulfonamides, tricyclic antidepressants	Increased risk for hypoglycemia	Monitor blood glucose level for hypoglycemia. Teach patient to recognize signs of hypoglycemia, and to carry food with sugar to eat if necessary.
diazoxide, beta blockers, cholestyramine, hydantoins, thiazide diuretics, rifampin	Decreased hypoglycemic effect	Monitor blood glucose level for hyperglycemia. Monitor A_{1C} levels.
digitalis	Increased serum digitalis levels	Monitor serum digitalis levels and heart rate and rhythm. Observe for symptoms of digitalis toxicity.
alcohol	Disulfiram-like reaction with some sulfonylureas. May cause hypoglycemia or hyperglycemia	Avoid concomitant use.

tations of diabetic complications, present health status, and potential problem areas.

Temporary use of insulin may be necessary during periods of physiologic stress (e.g., systemic infection, trauma, surgery, or fever) in patients receiving oral antidiabetic drugs; stress can induce alterations in glucose regulation that can be controlled only with exogenously administered insulin.

Life Span and Gender

The nurse should assess the patient for pregnancy or lactation. Glyburide is in FDA pregnancy category B. Animal reproduction studies have shown adverse fetal effects, and therefore, insulin is recommended to maintain blood glucose levels during pregnancy. Prolonged severe neonatal hypoglycemia may occur if glyburide is administered near the time of delivery. It is not known whether glyburide is excreted in breast milk. However, because of the possibility of hypoglycemia in breastfed infants, lactating women should avoid use of glyburide.

It also is important to note the age of the patient before administering glyburide. Safety and efficacy have not been established in children. Although the FDA has not approved any of the oral hypoglycemic and antihyperglycemic drugs for use in children with type 2 DM, the ADA states that a number of pediatric diabetologists use oral antidiabetic agents in children and adolescents with type 2 DM because of a greater patient compliance and convenience for the patient's family (McEvoy, Litvak, & Welsh, 2001).

Elderly patients may be more susceptible to the hypoglycemic effects of glyburide because of age-related decline in renal function that slows down the drug excretion; it may be necessary to administer the drug cautiously at a reduced initial dosage. Hypoglycemic reactions may be more difficult to recognize in elderly individuals.

Lifestyle, Diet, and Habits

It is a good idea to assess the patient's willingness or ability to adhere to strict drug therapy. Patients should take their pills daily and at the same time each day. It is important to note the patient's weight and typical alcohol consumption before therapy is initiated. Obese patients (more than 20% over ideal body weight) may not respond to glyburide. Concomitant alcohol use increases the rate of glyburide metabolism and may cause a disulfiram-like reaction.

Environment

The nurse should be aware of the environment in which glyburide will be administered. Glyburide is most commonly self-administered by the patient in the home setting. Therefore, patient education regarding use and adverse effects is a primary nursing concern. The nurse should tell the patient to avoid consuming alcohol and medicinal preparations that contain alcohol. Concomitant use may result in an increased risk of hypoglycemia or a disulfiram-like reaction of nausea and vomiting with some sulfonylureas. The nurse should focus the care plan on the patient's response to the disease process and treatment plan. It is important that the plan include preparation of the patient and family for self-care at home.

Nursing Diagnoses and Outcomes

- Ineffective Health Maintenance related to glyburide-induced nausea, vomiting, abdominal pain, and disulfiram-like reaction secondary to alcohol ingestion

  Desired outcome: The patient will follow ADA dietary guidelines and avoid consuming alcohol.
- Imbalanced Nutrition: More Than Body Requirements related to weight gain secondary to glyburide/sulfonylurea therapy

  Desired outcome: The patient will follow ADA dietary guidelines and not experience a weight gain.
- Ineffective Protection related to leukopenia secondary to bone marrow depression associated with glyburide use

  Desired outcome: The patient will be free from infection while taking glyburide.

Planning and Intervention

Maximizing Therapeutic Effects

When sulfonylureas are prescribed, the nurse should review with the patient the prescribed diabetic regimen, stressing the importance of dietary control, regular exercise, good general hygiene include foot care and monitoring practices (e.g., CBGM). The nurse should provide the patient with oral and written information amount and timing of the doses to be taken. For example, glyburide, like insulin, should be administered before meals, particularly with the first main meal of the day. In addition, glyburide should be stored in a tightly capped container at room temperature. It also is necessary for the nurse to review all drugs—prescription, OTC, and herbal or dietary supplements—to assess the risk for adverse drug reactions.

During the first several weeks of treatment, the nurse should monitor the patient closely for glucose imbalance and for the incidence of infections (especially sore throat).

Throughout treatment it is important to analyze the results of blood and urine tests to determine glucose balance and renal function. Other body systems such as GI, central nervous, cardiovascular, and hepatic should be monitored to assess for diabetic complications or adverse drug effects.

Minimizing Adverse Effects

The nurse should advise the patient that OTC preparations or alcohol should be avoided without first consulting the health care provider. It also is important to caution the patient that there is an increased risk of hypoglycemia if glyburide is taken with some alternative therapies, dietary supplements, or herbs.

Providing Patient and Family Education

- The nurse should demonstrate how to accurately perform and interpret CBGM; encourage the patient and family to return the demonstration.
- Self-monitoring of blood glucose levels may help to promote compliance by allowing the patient to view the effects of diet, exercise, and antidiabetic medications on glucose levels.
- It is important to discuss the importance of regular follow-up visits to the health care provider for measurements of blood glucose, weight, blood pressure, and eye examinations.
- The nurse should demonstrate proper foot care such as inspecting the foot for lesions and trimming toenails; have the patient and family perform a demonstration of the skill.
- The nurse should promote early recognition and treatment of problems by observing for signs and symptoms of hypo- or hyperglycemia, HHNC, DKA, foot ulcers, peripheral vascular disease, urinary tract infections, and vision changes.
- The nurse should stress to the patient that diabetes is a disease that requires considerable adaptation in activities of daily living.
- It is important to alert the patient and family to the signs and symptoms of diabetes out of control such as hyperglycemia, polydipsia, polyphagia, and polyuria. Persistent hyperglycemia may indicate a need to adjust some aspect of the treatment program such as diet or antidiabetic medication.
- The nurse should advise the patient and family that behavior such as irritability, confusion, nervousness, weakness, hunger may signal hypoglycemia. Appropriate treatment is consumption of approximately 15 g of a rapidly acting carbohydrate (e.g., orange juice, milk, or a few bites of candy). Caution the patient and family about consuming so much sugar that hyperglycemia occurs.
- It is important to caution the patient to avoid OTC medications and herbal or dietary supplements without first consulting the health care provider. Drug interactions or adverse reactions may occur; for example, nasal decongestants may cause "hypoglycemic" symptoms of tachycardia and nervousness, antitussive elixirs may contain alcohol and sugar and affect blood glucose levels.
- Patients who receive oral hypoglycemic or antihyperglycemic drugs must adhere to a health regimen similar to that required of patients with diabetes who are receiving insulin. The prescribed diet and medication, a regular schedule of activity, exercise, and rest, and the avoidance of infection and stress need to be maintained for normal glucose levels.

(Also see the previous display, Patient and Family Education Common to Antidiabetic Drugs.)

Ongoing Assessment and Evaluation

The nurse should interview the patient and family and observe for therapeutic and adverse responses to antidiabetic drugs and compliance with prescribed treatments. When assessing the success of nursing management, the nurse should be alert for adverse drug effects (especially GI) and should appropriately refer the patient to the health care provider for reevaluation of pharmacotherapy if pertinent symptoms are identified. Control of diet and body weight is crucial to a successful therapeutic outcome with oral hypoglycemic or antihyperglycemic medications. Blood tests monitoring glucose levels (e.g., fasting, 2-hour postprandial, and A_{1C}) are as important for patients taking exogenous insulin. The nurse should review the patient's hepatic and renal function periodically, particularly if there is pre-existing liver or kidney impairment. Additionally, cardiovascular function should be assessed at regular intervals. Other ongoing assessment and evaluation is similar to that for regular insulin. ■

DRUGS CLOSELY RELATED TO GLYBURIDE

Differences exist among the sulfonylureas in the duration of their hypoglycemic effects.

MEMORY CHIP

Glyburide

- Oral hypoglycemic that stimulates insulin release and increases peripheral tissue sensitivity to insulin effects; used as adjunct with dietary restrictions to treat type 2 diabetes mellitus. Is available commercially combined with metformin to manage type 2 diabetes (e.g., Glucovance).
- Significant contraindications: severe hepatic or renal impairment; allergy to sulfa drugs
- Most common adverse effects: nausea, epigastric fullness, heartburn
- Most serious adverse effect: hypoglycemia
- **Lifespan alert: older adults may be at greater risk for hypoglycemia related to drug accumulation from age-related decline in hepatic and renal functions.**
- Maximizing therapeutic effects: daily dosage of >10 mg should be divided into two doses and taken 30 minutes before the meal
- Minimizing adverse effects: avoid taking glyburide with certain alternative dietary therapies, supplements, or herbs because of increased risk for hypoglycemia
- Most significant patient education: signs and symptoms of out-of-control diabetes, such as hyperglycemia, polydipsia, polyphagia, and polyuria; dietary restrictions for serum glucose control and weight loss

First-Generation Sulfonylureas

Acetohexamide (Dymelor) is reduced in the liver to potent metabolites significantly more active (2.5 times) than the parent compound. It has significant uricosuric activity and is associated with an unpredictable incidence of hepatotoxicity.

Chlorpropamide (Diabinese) has the longest half-life and highest incidence of adverse effects. It may cause a disulfiram-like effect when combined with alcohol, and respiratory difficulties and congestive heart failure when given to individuals with cardiac problems. Chlorpropamide stimulates antidiuretic hormone release. SIADH with water retention and dilutional hyponatremia has occurred after administration to individuals with type 2 DM (especially those with congestive heart failure or hepatic cirrhosis). Approximately 80% of the drug is metabolized; its metabolite activity is unknown, however. Individuals taking chlorpropamide who become hypoglycemic—because of its long half-life, which is prolonged in renal disease—require close and careful supervision. Hospitalization and IV glucose may be necessary to manage the hypoglycemia. An unlabeled use (200 to 500 mg/day) is the treatment of diabetes insipidus.

Tolazamide (Tolinase) may produce a mild diuresis. Tolbutamide (Orinase) is the shortest-acting sulfonylurea. It is metabolized rapidly to an inactive metabolite and is useful for patients with kidney disease.

Second-Generation Sulfonylureas

Therapeutically, effective doses and serum concentrations of the second-generation sulfonylureas are lower because of their higher inherent potency.

Glimepiride (Amaryl), like the other sulfonylureas, improves glycemic control by stimulating the pancreatic beta cells to produce more insulin. It is thought to have fewer adverse effects and more "insulin-sparing effects" because of action at different cellular receptors than other sulfonylureas. Glimepiride is the first sulfonylurea with FDA approval for concomitant use with insulin. It has a once-daily dosing schedule.

Glipizide (Glucotrol) is the only sulfonylurea whose absorption is impaired by food in the stomach. It is most effective taken 30 minutes before a meal. Glipizide is associated with a reduction in very low-density lipoprotein triglyceride concentrations and plasma low-density lipoprotein cholesterol concentrations. High-density lipoprotein cholesterol concentrations generally do not appear to be changed during therapy. Concurrent administration with insulin has been used with some success in patients with type 2 DM who are difficult to control with diet and sulfonylurea therapy alone.

DRUGS SIGNIFICANTLY DIFFERENT FROM GLYBURIDE

Repaglinide (Prandin) is not a sulfonylurea; it is in a new chemical class—the meglitinides. The meglitinides are hypoglycemic agents; they share many of the pharmacologic actions and adverse effects of the sulfonylureas. They increase release of insulin from the pancreas; this effect is glucose-dependent and diminishes at low blood glucose concentrations.

In lowering blood glucose levels, repaglinide has a mechanism of action much like that of the sulfonylureas. It stimulates the secretion of insulin from the pancreatic beta cells by binding to the beta cell sites. In contrast to the sulfonylureas, this agent is absorbed rapidly and undergoes minimal renal excretion, making it suitable for elderly patients or others with decreased kidney function. Peak action occurs with one hour of ingestion and is metabolized completely in 3 to 4 hours after each dose. Administered orally before each meal, repaglinide is effective in lowering postprandial glucose levels as the amount of insulin released from the pancreas increases during and just after a meal, mimicking the normal blood glucose response to eating. Because of its rapid elimination in contrast to the sulfonylureas, repaglinide does not cause the beta cells to continuously release insulin for long periods of time. Therefore, insulin levels return to normal before the next meal. The number of meals eaten is equivalent to the number of doses taken; for example, if a meal is missed, the corresponding dose of medication also is skipped. Conversely, however, a dose is added when an extra meal or large snack is taken.

Nateglinide (Starlix) is a meglitinide that may be used alone or in combination therapy with metformin. It lowers blood glucose by stimulating insulin secretion from the pancreas within 20 minutes following oral administration; the extent of pancreatic insulin release is glucose dependent and diminishes at low glucose levels. Used prior to meals, there is a rapid rise in plasma insulin with peak levels occurring within 1 hour and a fall to baseline by 4 hours. Nateglinide is metabolized predominantly by the CYP450 system and rapidly and completely eliminated renally. Nateglinide is contraindicated in pregnancy (category C) and lactation. It should be used with caution in chronic hepatic disease and its safety and efficacy in children is not established. Although infrequently occurring, hypoglycemia is the most common adverse reaction. Drug interactions potentiating the hypoglycemic effect of nateglinide include nonsteroidal anti-inflammatory drugs (NSAIDs), salicylates, and nonselective beta-adrenergic blockers. Drugs reducing the hypoglycemic effect of nateglinide include thiazides, corticosteroids, thyroid products, and sympathomimetics.

BIGUANIDE ANTIHYPERGLYCEMICS

The biguanide antihyperglycemics reduce fasting and postprandial blood glucose, enhance insulin sensitivity at postreceptor levels, lower triglyceride and cholesterol levels, and stimulate insulin-mediated glucose clearance. The biguanides (e.g., metformin) are not hypoglycemic agents; rather they are antihyperglycemic or "insulin sensitizer" agents. They act by reducing glyconeogenolysis (reduces hepatic glucose production) and enhancing insulin-stimulated glucose transport in adipose tissue and skeletal muscle. Thus, insulin resistance is lessened.

The prototype biguanide antihyperglycemic drug is metformin (Glucophage).

NURSING MANAGEMENT OF THE PATIENT RECEIVING METFORMIN

Core Drug Knowledge

Pharmacotherapeutics

Metformin is used as an adjunct to diet and exercise to lower blood glucose in type 2 DM (see Table 41-2). Metformin does not stimulate insulin secretion; rather, it suppresses hepatic glucose production while enhancing insulin sensitivity in the muscle and subsequent glucose uptake. Thus, for individuals without some residual functioning pancreatic islet cells, metformin is ineffective.

In addition, it lowers triglyceride levels and promotes weight loss. Metformin may be used in combination with a sulfonylurea when either drug alone is ineffective in controlling glucose levels in type 2 DM.

Drug labeling includes warnings on lactic acidosis and also the potential risk of cardiovascular death, which is increased with other oral hypoglycemics as well.

Another biguanide, phenformin, was withdrawn from the U.S. market in 1977 because of an unacceptable risk of lactic acidosis. It is now available under FDA "Investigational New Drug" status and may be used only in patients with type 2, nonketotic DM who meet a number of qualifying conditions. Phenformin also is available under a separate IND clearance for some selective dermatologic conditions.

Pharmacokinetics

Administered in oral tablet form, metformin is absorbed slowly and incompletely from the GI tract; its bioavailability is between 50% and 60%. It is distributed rapidly into peripheral body tissues and fluids and peak serum levels are achieved in 2 to 3 hours after administration. Following oral administration, 90% of the absorbed drug is eliminated renally within the first 24 hours, with a plasma elimination half-life of 6.2 hours; half-life is longer in patients with impaired renal function. Food slightly delays and decreases the extent of its absorption. Metformin does not bind to plasma proteins and does not undergo hepatic metabolism or biliary excretion as no metabolites have been identified. Largely unchanged, metformin is excreted by the kidneys. Tubular secretion is the major route of elimination because renal clearance is significantly greater (3.5 times) than creatinine clearance.

Pharmacodynamics

Metformin decreases hepatic glucose production, decreases intestinal absorption of glucose, and improves insulin sensitivity. It does this by increasing peripheral glucose uptake and use in skeletal muscle and adipose tissue by increasing transport of glucose across the cell membrane.

Unlike the sulfonylureas, metformin rarely causes hypoglycemia because it does not stimulate insulin secretion. In fact, insulin secretion remains unchanged whereas fasting insulin levels and day long plasma insulin response may actually decrease. In addition, it lowers triglyceride levels and promotes weight loss. Clinically, metformin lowers fasting and postprandial hyperglycemia, demonstrating more of an antihyperglycemic action than a hypoglycemic action.

Contraindications and Precautions

Metformin is contraindicated in patients with hepatic disease, alcoholism, acute or chronic metabolic acidosis, and renal impairment (creatinine clearance less than 40 mL/minute) because these conditions can precipitate lactic acidosis.

Adverse Effects

Minor, but common, side effects of metformin include GI disturbances such as anorexia, nausea and vomiting, abdominal discomfort, dyspepsia, flatulence, diarrhea, and a metallic taste sensation. These adverse effects tend to decline with continued use and can be minimized by initiating therapy with lower doses of metformin.

Serious side effects are rare and usually occur in individuals with impaired renal or liver function. Lactic acidosis is the most serious side effect and carries a mortality rate of nearly 50%. Although rare, it is a metabolic complication that can occur from metformin accumulation and may also occur in association with a number of pathophysiologic conditions, including DM and whenever there is significant tissue hypoperfusion and hypoxemia. An increased anion gap, elevated blood lactate levels, decreased blood pH, and electrolyte disturbances characterize **lactic acidosis.** When metformin is implicated as the cause of lactic acidosis, plasma levels generally exceed 5 μg/mL. Lactic acidosis is less likely to result from metformin than with the other biguanide, phenformin, because of its different pharmacokinetics. Other serious adverse effects associated with metformin include asymptomatic vitamin B12 deficiency or megaloblastic anemia.

Drug Interactions

There is a synergistic drug interaction between metformin, which improves insulin use, and the sulfonylureas, which stimulate insulin production. Metformin may react with contrast media used for radiographic procedures (Table 41-5).

Assessment of Relevant Core Patient Variables

Health Status

Assessments to be made before therapy with the biguanide hypoglycemic, metformin, are similar to those necessary with insulin. Assessment of current health status should include diet, activity, medication, and methods used for monitoring blood glucose. If the antidiabetic/

TABLE 41-5 Agents That Interact With Metformin

Interactants	Effect and Significance	Nursing Management
cimetidine	Increased risk for hypoglycemia	Monitor blood glucose levels.
sulfonylureas	Synergistic reaction between metformin and sulfonylurea that improves insulin use; may increase risk for hypoglycemia	Monitor blood glucose levels. Observe for hypoglycemic complications.
glucocorticoids, alcohol	Increased risk of lactic acidosis	Monitor serum lactate levels.

anti-hyperglycemic drug prescribed is the biguanide, metformin, the nurse should determine whether any precautions to its use apply, the usual time of administration, and who administers it.

If used concomitantly with a sulfonylurea, hypoglycemic reactions may occur. One example of this is the combination drug of glyburide and metformin—Glucovance. If hypoglycemic reactions occur, it is important to determine their frequency and how the patient or family handles these reactions. This information helps to assess knowledge, usual practices, and teaching needs. It is important to assess the patient's knowledge, attitude, and physical condition in relationship to diabetes, the prescribed treatment plan, and evidence of complications. Assessment data also should include past manifestations of diabetic complications, present health status, and potential problem areas.

The patient receiving metformin should have periodic renal and hepatic function tests. Metformin's half-life is prolonged, and its excretion is decreased in patients with impaired renal function, especially those with decreased creatinine clearance. Hepatic function impairment may increase the risk of lactic acidosis. The patient also should have periodic blood tests because megaloblastic anemia may be an adverse effect of therapy.

Weight loss may occur during therapy with metformin, perhaps as a result of the drug's anorexic and lipid-lowering effects. In contrast, sulfonylureas and insulin tend to cause weight gain. An overweight diabetic patient with abnormal lipid levels is the ideal candidate for metformin.

Life Span and Gender

The nurse should assess whether the patient is pregnant or breastfeeding. Metformin is in FDA pregnancy risk category B. Animal studies demonstrate metformin excretion into breast milk, but studies in lactating women have not been performed. It is important to determine the age of the patient before administering metformin. Safety and efficacy in children have not been established. Age-related changes in renal function account for altered pharmacokinetics; metformin should be used cautiously in elderly patients because of the prevalence of decreased renal function in this age group. In general, elderly patients are better able to tolerate lower doses of metformin.

Lifestyle, Diet, and Habits

The nurse should ask patients about their typical diet and exercise habits and about alcohol intake. Hypoglycemia is more common when metformin is administered concomitantly with other oral hypoglycemic agents or when there is deficient caloric intake or strenuous exercise. The nurse should caution patients against excessive alcohol intake while taking metformin, because alcohol use increases the risk for lactic acidosis.

Environment

The nurse should note the environment in which metformin will be administered. Metformin is an oral drug that is easily self-administered in the home setting.

Culture

In controlled clinical studies of metformin in individuals with type 2 DM, the antihyperglycemic effect was comparable among whites, African Americans, and Hispanics.

Nursing Diagnosis and Outcome

- Imbalanced Nutrition: Less Than Body Requirements related to anorexia secondary to and adverse GI effects of weight loss, diarrhea, and anorexia from metformin

  Desired outcome: The patient will ingest daily nutritional requirements in accordance with activity level and metabolic needs and relate the importance of good nutrition.

Planning and Intervention

Maximizing Therapeutic Effects

There is no fixed dosage regimen with metformin for the management of hyperglycemia in type 2 DM. The dosage is individualized on the basis of both effectiveness and tolerance, while not exceeding the maximum recommended daily dose of 2,550 mg/day. Fasting plasma glucose and A_{1C} (glycosylated hemoglobin) are used to identify the minimum effective dose of metformin, either when used as monotherapy or in combination with a sulfonylurea.

Minimizing Adverse Effects

Adverse GI effects during initiation of metformin therapy appear to be dose related. Taking the drug at mealtimes and using gradual dosage increments will minimize these effects. The nurse should advise the patient not to take any OTC preparations, including dietary and herbal supplements, without first consulting the health care provider.

The nurse should caution patients against the use of alcohol, because this may increase the risk of lactic acidosis. Because the liver is responsible for removing lactate from the system, individuals with a history of heavy alcohol abuse and/or binge drinking should not use metformin. Metformin should be withheld temporarily when patients undergo any procedure using iodinated contrast dye due to its renal excretion.

Providing Patient and Family Education

See the previous display, Patient and Family Education Common to Antidiabetic Drugs.

Ongoing Assessment and Evaluation

Periodic screening for hematologic changes is recommended during therapy with metformin, as asymptomatic vitamin B_{12} deficiency or megaloblastic anemia may occur (see also the "Ongoing Assessment and Evaluation" section within the "Insulin" discussion). ■

MEMORY CHIP

P Metformin

- Oral antihyperglycemic that increases peripheral tissue sensitivity to the effects of insulin and decreases hepatic glucose production. Is available commercially combined with glyburide to manage type 2 diabetes (e.g., Glucovance)
- Significant contraindications: serious hepatic or renal function impairment
- Most common adverse effects: nausea, diarrhea, abdominal bloating, flatulence, and anorexia; GI adverse effects appear to be dose related
- Most serious adverse effects: lactic acidosis and hypoglycemia
- **Life span alert: older adults may be at greater risk for lactic acidosis from age-related decline in renal function**
- Maximizing therapeutic effects: individualize the dosage on the basis of both the effect and tolerance while not exceeding the maximum recommended daily dose
- Minimizing adverse effects: daily dosage of > 2g should be divided into three doses taken at each meal; the drug should be taken with food to decrease adverse GI effects
- Most significant patient education: dietary restrictions for serum glucose control and weight loss

DRUG CLOSELY RELATED TO P METFORMIN

Phenformin, which was removed from the market because of its high risk for causing lactic acidosis, is available for treating selected patients with type 2 DM as an IND monitored by the FDA.

C ALPHA-GLUCOSIDASE INHIBITORS

Alpha-glucosidase inhibitors (also known as starch blockers) provide a unique mechanism of action for patients with type 2 DM. This drug class does not enhance insulin secretion. Rather, the antihyperglycemic activity results from a significant reduction in postprandial glucose levels.

The alpha-glucosidase inhibitors competitively inhibit enzymes in the small intestine that enable oligosaccharides to be broken down. In essence, the alpha-glucosidase inhibitors delay the digestion and absorption of carbohydrates, thus allowing the beta cell enough time to augment insulin release in response to plasma glucose levels. This results in a small rise in postprandial blood glucose concentration.

The prototype alpha-glucosidase inhibitor is acarbose (Precose).

NURSING MANAGEMENT OF THE PATIENT RECEIVING P ACARBOSE

Core Drug Knowledge

Pharmacotherapeutics

Acarbose effectively lowers postprandial serum glucose when administered alone or in combination with insulin, metformin, or a sulfonylurea. Alpha-glucosidase inhibitors are suitable alternative antidiabetic drugs for patients with type 2 DM who have mild to moderate hyperglycemia and who are at risk for hypoglycemia or lactic acidosis (see Table 41-2).

Pharmacokinetics

Acarbose is administered orally. It undergoes exclusive metabolism within the GI tract—principally by intestinal bacteria but also by digestive enzymes. Systemic absorption is about 35%, mostly as metabolites. One metabolite has alpha-glucosidase inhibitory activity. Plasma half-life of acarbose is about 2 hours. The small amount of acarbose that is absorbed undergoes virtually complete renal excretion.

Pharmacodynamics

The action of the alpha-glucosidase inhibitors (e.g., acarbose) is antihyperglycemic. These agents inhibit alpha-glucosidase enzymes in the brush border of the small intestine and inhibit pancreatic alpha-amylase leading to a reduction in carbohydrate-mediated postprandial blood glucose elevation. Inhibition of these enzyme systems reduces the rate of digestion of complex carbohydrate and the subsequent absorption of glucose.

The antihyperglycemic action of acarbose results from a competitive, reversible inhibition of pancreatic alpha amylase and membrane-bound intestinal alpha-glucosidase hydrolase enzymes. Pancreatic alpha amylase hydrolyzes complex starches to oligosaccharides in the lumen of the small intestine, whereas the membrane-bound intestinal alpha-glucosidases hydrolyze oligosaccharides, trisaccharides, and disaccharides to glucose and other monosaccharides in the small intestine. In diabetic patients, this enzyme inhibition delays glucose absorption and lowers postprandial hyperglycemia, subsequently reducing the A_{1C} level.

Contraindications and Precautions

Acarbose is contraindicated in patients with diseases of the bowel (e.g., inflammatory bowel disease, absorptive disorders, colonic ulceration, and history of bowel obstruction). It should be used cautiously in patients with hiatal hernia or other conditions that might be exacerbated by increased formation of gas due to drug effects of acarbose.

Adverse Effects

Adverse effects of acarbose are primarily GI in nature, and include flatulence, diarrhea, and abdominal distention. These occur because the delay in carbohydrate absorption increases fermentation and formation of intestinal gases.

Drug Interactions

Monotherapy with acarbose does not cause hypoglycemia, whereas combination therapy with agents that increase insulin levels may. Patients receiving acarbose in combination with insulin or a sulfonylurea should be observed closely for hypoglycemia.

Assessment of Relevant Core Patient Variables

Health Status

Assessments to be made before therapy with the alpha-glucosidase inhibitors are similar to those necessary with insulin. In addition, 1-hour postprandial blood glucose and serum transaminase levels should be obtained. It is important to assess for the presence of conditions that preclude the use of alpha-glucosidase inhibitors such as inflammatory bowel disease, colonic irritation, absorption disorders, or any condition that may cause intestinal obstruction.

The nurse should stress the importance of notifying the health care provider if unusual fatigue or muscle pain, difficulty breathing, GI distress, dizziness, lightheadedness, or irregular heartbeat occurs as these symptoms may indicate the onset of lactic acidosis, which is often insidious.

Assessment of current health status should include diet, activity, medication, and methods used for monitoring blood glucose. If the antidiabetic/antihyperglycemic drug prescribed is an alpha-glucosidase inhibitor, the nurse should determine whether any precautions to its use apply, the usual time of administration, and who administers it. If used concomitantly with a sulfonylurea, hypoglycemic reactions may occur. If hypoglycemic reactions occur, it is important to determine their frequency and how the patient or family handles these reactions. This information helps to assess knowledge, usual practices, and teaching needs.

It is important to assess the patient's knowledge, attitude, and physical condition in relation to diabetes, the prescribed treatment plan, and evidence of complications. Assessment data should also include past manifestations of diabetic complications, present health status, and potential problems areas.

There is a direct correlation between plasma concentrations of acarbose and the degree of renal impairment. Long-term study of acarbose use in significant renal impairment has not been done. Consequently, treatment with acarbose for patients with significant renal function impairment (serum creatinine exceeding 2 mg/dL) is not recommended. Some acarbose treatment studies (phase III U.S. clinical trials) have disclosed elevated liver transaminase levels. Higher dosages of acarbose may increase this incidence. Consequently, the drug is contraindicated in patients with chronic liver diseases.

Life Span and Gender

The nurse should assess whether the patient is pregnant or breastfeeding. Acarbose is in FDA pregnancy risk category B. Animal data reveal that acarbose and its metabolites are distributed into breast milk and cross the placental barrier.

Lifestyle, Diet, and Habits

The nurse should assess the patient's willingness to adopt necessary lifestyle changes. Caloric restriction, weight loss, and exercise are essential for the proper treatment of the patient who has type 2 DM and who takes acarbose.

Environment

The nurse should note the environment in which acarbose will be administered. Acarbose is an oral drug that is easily self-administered in the home setting.

Culture

It is a good idea to note the patient's culture and ethnic background before administering acarbose. Japanese women weighing less than 60 kg and receiving dosages exceeding 100 mg three times daily demonstrated liver enzyme abnormalities during phase III clinical drug trials of acarbose in the United States (Hebel, 2000).

Nursing Diagnosis and Outcome

- Diarrhea related to adverse effects of acarbose therapy

Desired outcome: The patient will describe contributing factors when known, explain rationales for interventions, and report less frequent diarrhea.

Planning and Intervention

Maximizing Therapeutic Effects

Dietary caloric restriction, weight loss, and exercise are important in maintaining the efficacy of acarbose therapy.

Minimizing Adverse Effects

To avoid possible undesired drug interactions, the nurse should caution the patient not to take any OTC drug preparations (including herbs and alcohol) without consulting the health care provider.

Providing Patient and Family Education

- The nurse should tell the patient that acarbose inhibits the absorption of regular cane sugar (e.g., candy or orange juice). If a hypoglycemic reaction occurs, the patient must use oral glucose tablets to increase blood glucose levels.

Also see the previous display, Patient and Family Education Common to Antidiabetic Drugs.

Ongoing Assessment and Evaluation

See the "Ongoing Assessment and Evaluation" section within the "Insulin" discussion. ■

MEMORY CHIP

Acarbose

- Alpha-glucosidase inhibitor antidiabetic that delays carbohydrate digestion and glucose absorption from the small intestine; lowers blood glucose levels after eating.
- Drug may be used with insulin, glyburide, or metformin to manage type 2 diabetes
- Significant contraindication: inflammatory bowel disease
- Most common adverse effects: flatulence, abdominal cramping, diarrhea, hypoglycemia (if combined with oral hypoglycemic)
- Most serious adverse effects: elevated serum aminotransferases—ALT, AST (especially in dosages >150 mg/d), and hyperbilirubinemia
- **Lifespan alert: GI adverse effects may be especially troublesome to the elderly patient with diabetes; low doses initially (e.g., 25 mg) may lessen this**
- Maximizing therapeutic effects: dietary caloric restriction, weight loss, and exercise
- Minimizing adverse effects: patients must not take OTC drug preparations without consulting the health care provider
- Most significant patient education: if hypoglycemia occurs, dextrose must be used; absorption of sucrose (e.g., candy or table sugar) is inhibited and ineffective

DRUG CLOSELY RELATED TO ACARBOSE

Miglitol (Glyset) is an alpha-glucosidase inhibitor that delays the digestion of ingested carbohydrates. Miglitol is used for treating type 2 DM. The manufacturer claims the drug is especially effective in Hispanics and African Americans with type 2 DM. Miglitol inhibits membrane-bound intestinal alpha-glucosidase; the primary physiologic effect is a reduction in postprandial glucose and glycosylated hemoglobin levels. Miglitol does not enhance insulin secretion, and overdoses will not result in hypoglycemia.

Like acarbose, the actions of miglitol are additive to those of the sulfonylureas in mediating a hypoglycemic effect. Protein binding of miglitol is negligible (less than 4%), and the plasma half-life is about 2 hours. Miglitol undergoes renal excretion essentially unchanged. Patients with impaired renal function may experience an accumulation of miglitol. Miglitol is contraindicated in patients with significant renal impairment (creatinine clearance exceeding 2 mg/dL).

The most commonly observed adverse effects are GI symptoms, such as abdominal pain, diarrhea, and flatulence. Each dose should be administered with the first bite of each main meal. Dosage should be adjusted in accord with glycosylated hemoglobin levels, which should be determined at 3-month intervals. The maximum recommended miglitol dosage is 100 mg orally three times daily.

Miglitol is in FDA pregnancy risk category B. It is excreted into breast milk and should not be given to lactating women. Safety and efficacy in children have not been established.

THIAZOLIDINEDIONE ANTIHYPERGLYCEMICS

The action of the thiazolidinedione oral antihyperglycemic drugs are similar to those of the biguanides; they are antihyperglycemic and "insulin sensitizers." These drugs specifically target insulin resistance, which is thought to be central to the development of type 2 DM. They appear to lower blood sugar primarily by enhancing the activity of endogenous insulin rather than by stimulating insulin secretion.

The thiazolidinediones act primarily by decreasing insulin resistance. They improve sensitivity to insulin in muscle and adipose tissue, inhibit hepatic gluconeogenesis, and enhance insulin action by opening up the insulin receptors in the liver and skeletal muscle. When this occurs, insulin resistance is reversed and the body is able to utilize circulating insulin effectively. A secondary action of the thiazolidinediones is that they decrease the production and release of glucose from the liver. Because these agents are not hypoglycemic agents, they will not generally lower blood glucose to levels less than normal. When used in combination with insulin or sulfonylureas, the potential for hypoglycemia exists.

Thiazolidinedione antidiabetic drugs include rosiglitazone and pioglitazone. The prototype thiazolidinedione is rosiglitazone.

NURSING MANAGEMENT OF THE PATIENT RECEIVING ROSIGLITAZONE

Core Drug Knowledge

Pharmacotherapeutics

Rosiglitazone is indicated as an adjunct to diet and exercise to lower blood glucose in patients with type 2 DM and for use in insulin-treated (dosages exceeding 30 U/day in multiple injections), patients with type 2 DM who are controlled inadequately (measured by A_{1c}) with insulin (see Table 41-2).

Pharmacokinetics

Rosiglitazone is absorbed rapidly after oral administration with a bioavailability of 99%. Peak plasma concentrations occur within 2 to 3 hours. Protein binding is extensive (over 99%), primarily to serum albumin. Rosiglitazone undergoes extensive hepatic metabolism, primarily by conjugation. Half-life is 3 to 4 hours. Excretion is urinary (64%) and fecal (23%).

Pharmacodynamics

Rosiglitazone lowers the blood glucose level by improving target cell response to insulin. Rosiglitazone decreases hepatic glucose output and increases insulin-dependent glucose use in skeletal muscle. Its mechanism of action depends on insulin. It binds to nuclear receptors that regulate the transcription of several insulin-responsive genes that control glucose and lipid metabolism. The decrease in systemic and local tissue lipid availability is thought to contribute to its antidiabetic effects.

Contraindications and Precautions

Rosiglitazone should not be given to patients exhibiting clinical evidence of active liver disease or increased serum transaminase or aminotransferase levels (ALT or AST more than 2.5 times the upper limits of normal). It is recommended that patients treated with rosiglitazone undergo periodic monitoring of liver enzymes. Hepatic enzymes should be measured before the initiation of therapy in all treated patients. In patients with normal baseline liver enzymes, it is recommended that liver enzymes be monitored every 2 months for the first 12 months and periodically thereafter.

Rosiglitazone should be used with caution in patients with cardiovascular disease, particularly hypertension and congestive heart failure, because fluid retention and edema may occur.

Adverse Effects

In general, rosiglitazone therapy is well tolerated, possibly because the drug produces few adverse effects. Adverse effects include fluid retention, headache, and weight gain. Mild changes in blood lipid levels have been observed. Plasma volume expansion may occur with rosiglitazone therapy. As a result, small decreases in hemoglobin, hematocrit, and neutrophil counts (within the normal range) have occurred.

Drug Interactions

Rosiglitazone monotherapy does not induce a risk of hypoglycemia; combination therapy with insulin may. In vitro drug metabolism studies suggest that rosiglitazone does not inhibit any of the major P450 enzymes at clinically relevant concentrations. In vitro data demonstrate that rosiglitazone is metabolized predominantly by the CYP450 microsomal enzyme system (Table 41-6).

Assessment of Relevant Core Patient Variables

Health Status

Assessment of current health status should include diet, activity, medication, and methods used for monitoring blood glucose. The nurse also should review blood studies, particularly those associated with hepatic function. Rosiglitazone should be used with caution in patients with hepatic dysfunction. If the antidiabetic drug prescribed is an "insulin sensitizer" thiazolidinedione, the nurse should determine whether any precautions to its use apply, the usual time of administration, and who administers it. If used concomitantly with insulin or a sulfonylurea, hypoglycemic reactions may occur. If hypoglycemic reactions occur, it is important to determine their frequency and how the patient or family handles

TABLE 41-6 Agents That Interact With Rosiglitazone

Interactants	Effect and Significance	Nursing Management
insulin, sulfonylureas, repaglinide	Increased risk for hypoglycemic effects	Monitor blood glucose level for hypoglycemia. Anticipate need for dosage adjustment.
oral contraceptives	May reduce plasma levels of contraceptive by one third; may resume ovulation in premenopausal anovulatory women	Advise patient to use a back-up form of birth control.

these reactions. This information helps to assess the patient's knowledge, usual practices, and teaching needs. It is important to assess the patient's knowledge, attitude, and physical condition in relationship to diabetes, the prescribed treatment plan, and evidence of complications. Assessment data should also include past manifestations of diabetic complications, present health status, and potential problem areas.

Life Span and Gender

The nurse should assess whether the patient is pregnant or breastfeeding. Rosiglitazone is in FDA pregnancy category B. It is unknown whether it is excreted in human breast milk. Insulin-resistant, premenopausal, anovulatory diabetic women taking rosiglitazone are at risk for resuming ovulation with this drug therapy and be at risk for pregnancy.

Lifestyle, Diet, and Habits

The nurse should assess the patient's ability and willingness to adopt necessary lifestyle changes. Calorie restriction, weight loss, and exercise are essential for the proper treatment of the patient with type 2 DM.

Nursing Diagnosis and Outcome

- Ineffective Sexuality Patterns related to resumption of ovulation and compromise of oral contraceptive effectiveness secondary to rosiglitazone

  Desired outcome: The patient will identify appropriate modifications in sexual practices in responses to changes in fertility and oral contraceptive ineffectiveness.

Planning and Intervention

Maximizing Therapeutic Effects

Rosiglitazone may be administered either with or without meals and still be effective.

Minimizing Adverse Effects

It is important to monitor liver enzyme levels monthly for the first 6 months of rosiglitazone therapy and every 2 months for the remainder of the first year. Patients with elevated enzymes should stop rosiglitazone therapy.

Providing Patient and Family Education

- The nurse should instruct patients on the importance of returning for follow-up blood work.
- It also is important to teach patients to report signs of early liver impairment (i.e., nausea, vomiting, malaise, and dark urine).

Also see the previous display, Patient and Family Education Common to Antidiabetic Drugs.

Ongoing Assessment and Evaluation

See the section, "Ongoing Assessment and Evaluation" within the "Insulin" discussion. ■

DRUGS CLOSELY RELATED TO P ROSIGLITAZONE

Pioglitazone

Use of pioglitazone (Actos) can cause resumption of ovulation in women taking oral contraceptives and in patients with polycystic ovary disease. Female patients should be counseled to consider an alternative method of contraception or referred to their health care provider for consideration of a dosage increase in the oral contraceptive.

C GLUCOSE ELEVATING AGENTS

Glucagon is a hyperglycemic polypeptide hormone produced by the alpha cells of the pancreatic islets of Langerhans. Its physiologic effect is generally the opposite of that of insulin. Glucagon is the body's first line of defense against hypoglycemia. Whether endogenous or exogenous, it reduces the effectiveness of insulin and some commonly used drugs.

The main stimulus to glucagon secretion is a decrease in intracellular glucose concentrations that usually occurs as a result of a drop in serum blood sugar. Diabetic patients have been shown to have high levels of glucagon, although the cause-effect relationship is uncertain. Theoretically, glucagon

MEMORY CHIP

P Rosiglitazone

- Oral antidiabetic that increases insulin sensitivity and decreases hepatic gluconeogenesis. It is used adjunctively with dietary restrictions to treat type 2 diabetes mellitus.
- Significant contraindication: do not use if AST>2.5 times upper limits of normal
- Most common adverse effects: upper respiratory tract infection, sinusitis, headache, edema, fatigue, and diarrhea
- Most serious adverse effect: increased liver enzyme levels
- **Life span alert: drug causes weight gain and increased HDL cholesterol, which may be problematic for the obese elderly patient with type 2 diabetes**
- Minimizing adverse effects: measure liver function tests—baseline, every 2 months for 1 year, then periodically—to monitor for hepatotoxicity
- Most significant patient education: report signs of early liver impairment.

imbalances could contribute to many of the diabetic patient's problems with glucose metabolism.

NURSING MANAGEMENT OF THE PATIENT RECEIVING GLUCAGON

Core Drug Knowledge

Pharmacotherapeutics

Most commonly, glucagon is used in unconscious diabetic patients to reverse the severe hypoglycemia resulting from insulin overdosage. Glucagon is effective in hypoglycemia only if liver glycogen is available. Glucagon also is used to induce intestinal relaxation before radiographic examinations. Unlabeled uses for glucagon include propranolol (beta-adrenergic antagonist) overdose and cardiovascular emergencies.

Pharmacokinetics

Glucagon has a plasma half-life of 3 to 6 minutes. The hormone undergoes hepatic metabolism and is excreted in urine and bile.

Pharmacodynamics

Glucagon increases blood glucose levels by stimulating glycogenolysis in the peripheral tissues, exerts a positive inotropic and chronotropic effect on the heart by increasing cyclic adenosine monophosphate, and relaxes the GI smooth muscle. After parenteral injection of glucagon, the maximum hyperglycemic effect occurs within 30 minutes. The duration of action is about 1 to 2 hours. GI smooth muscle relaxation occurs within 15 minutes and lasts for approximately 30 minutes. The mechanism by which glucagon relaxes GI smooth muscle is not known.

Contraindications and Precautions

A hypersensitivity to glucagon contraindicates its use. Glucagon causes insulin release and is contraindicated in insulinoma. It causes catecholamine release and is contraindicated in pheochromocytoma. It should be used cautiously in pregnancy and lactation.

Adverse Effects

Glucagon may cause nausea and vomiting, hypokalemia in overdosage, and hypersensitivity reactions of urticaria, respiratory distress, and hypotension.

Drug Interactions

Glucagon increases the hypoprothrombinemic effect of oral anticoagulants and may cause bleeding. The interaction appears to be dose related.

Assessment of Relevant Core Patient Variables

Health Status

After emergency use of glucagon, the nurse should assess the patient's level of adherence to the therapeutic regimen and the patient's level of understanding of the disease and its treatment.

Life Span and Gender

The nurse should note whether the patient is pregnant or breastfeeding. Glucagon crosses the placental barrier and enters breast milk.

Lifestyle, Diet, and Habits

The nurse should review the patient's adherence to the diabetic treatment plan. It is important to assess whether the patient is administering the drug and monitoring blood glucose correctly, and whether he or she is complying with the prescribed dietary and exercise regimens. Adherence to the treatment plan will help to prevent episodes of hypoglycemia.

Environment

The nurse should be aware of the environment in which glucagon will be administered. Glucagon is usually administered as an emergency treatment. It may be administered in any setting (e.g., hospital, home, or extended care settings) as required. The nurse should carefully review the home environment for reasonable uniformity from day to day with regard to diet, insulin or oral antidiabetic medications, activity, and exercise. A review of the timing of medications (e.g., insulin, oral hypoglycemic, or oral antihyperglycemic) is also advisable as this may help to reduce the incidence and frequency of hypoglycemic reactions.

Nursing Diagnosis and Outcome

- Risk for Injury related to aspiration secondary to the adverse glucagon effects of nausea and vomiting
  Desired outcome: Aspiration of gastric contents will not result from glucagon treatment during a hypoglycemic episode.

Planning and Intervention

Maximizing Therapeutic Effects

Glucagon is administered IM, SC, or IV. The drug is dispensed in a powder form and must be reconstituted to a concentration of 1 mg/mL using the diluent supplied by the manufacturer. Reconstituted glucagon should be used immediately, although refrigerated solution may be kept for 48 hours. The solution should be clear after dilution; otherwise, it should be discarded. A dose of 0.5 to 1.0 mg is usually effective. Doses exceeding 2 mg should be reconstituted with sterile water and used immediately.

Patients with type 1 DM demonstrate a poorer response to glucagon therapy than do patients with type 2 DM. Supplemental carbohydrates should be administered as soon as possible to restore liver glycogen and prevent secondary hypoglycemia.

Following glucagon administration, the nurse should observe the patient be closely for response to the drug;

consciousness should resume quickly. An additional dose may be administered if the patient's response is inadequate or incomplete after 20 minutes.

The nurse should evaluate the abilities of the patient and family to prepare and administer glucagons in case of any emergency. To prevent severe hypoglycemia, patients and family members should be informed of symptoms suggesting mild hypoglycemia and how to treat it appropriately, such as routinely carrying sugar, candy, or another rapidly absorbable carbohydrate to consume at the first warning of an impending reaction.

Minimizing Adverse Effects

Adverse effects of glucagon include nausea and vomiting. Advise the patient and family members to become familiar with the technique of preparing glucagon before an emergency arises. Dosage to use is 1 mg (1 U) for adults and half the adult dose (0.5 mg or 0.5 U) for pediatric patients weighing less than 44 lb or 20 kg.

Providing Patient and Family Education

- The nurse should inform patients and family members of the following measures to prevent hypoglycemic reactions due to insulin:
  1. Reasonable uniformity from day to day with regard to diet, insulin, and exercise
  2. Careful adjustment of the insulin program so that the type (or types) of insulin, dose, and time (or times) of administration are suited to the individual patient.
  3. Frequent testing of the blood or urine for glucose so that a change in insulin requirements can be foreseen
  4. Routine carrying of sugar, candy, or other readily absorbable carbohydrate by the patient so that it may be taken at the first warning of an oncoming reaction.
- The nurse should convey the importance of early recognition and treatment of hypoglycemic episodes by explaining that immediate use of rapidly acting carbohydrates, such as simple sugars (e.g., milk, orange juice, or candy) may prevent hypoglycemia from progressing to coma. It is important to inform family members to arouse the patient as quickly as possible because prolonged hypoglycemia may result in damage to the CNS.
- The nurse should advise patients to inform their physician when hypoglycemic reactions occur so that the treatment regimen may be adjusted if necessary.
- The nurse should urge the patient to obtain a glucagon emergency kit and to learn the correct techniques for administering injections in case complications prevent the patient from swallowing sugar or neurologic effects prevent oral intake.
- It is important to advise the patient and family members to become familiar with the technique of preparing glucagon before an emergency arises. Instruct patients to use 1 mg (1 U) for adults and half the adult dose (0.5 mg [0.5 U]) for pediatric patients weighing less than 44 lb (20 kg).
- It is a good idea to inform the patient and family that glucagon or IV glucose should awaken the patient sufficiently so that oral carbohydrates may be taken.

Ongoing Assessment and Evaluation

Blood glucose levels should be monitored before, during, and after glucagon administration, and the patient's emergency supply of glucagon should be restored as soon as possible. Survival and return to normal function are signs of effective nursing management. ■

DRUGS SIGNIFICANTLY DIFFERENT FROM GLUCAGON

Diazoxide

Administered orally, diazoxide (Proglycem), produces a prompt, dose-related increase in blood glucose levels. Its hyperglycemic effects occur because it inhibits insulin release from the pancreas and has an extrahepatic effect. Its clinical indications are hyperinsulinism due to an inoperable islet cell cancer, islet cell hyperplasia, or an extrapancreatic cancer. Diazoxide administered intravenously will quickly lower blood pressure in a hypertensive emergency. See chapter 30 for a discussion of this use of the drug.

Diazoxide is absorbed rapidly. Onset of action occurs within 1 hour. It is highly protein bound (more than 90%),

MEMORY CHIP

Glucagon

- Glucose-elevating agent that accelerates hepatic glyconeogenesis, increasing blood glucose levels
- Significant contraindications: insulinoma and pheochromocytoma
- Most common adverse effects: nausea, vomiting, generalized allergic reactions, including urticaria, respiratory distress, and hypotension
- Most serious adverse effect: hypokalemia
- Maximizing therapeutic effects: use the diluent provided in preparation of glucagons for parenteral injection (SC, IM, or IV). Reconstituted glucagons should be clear, watery, and used immediately. Any unused portion should be discarded. Provide supplemental carbohydrates as soon as possible after drug injection to restore liver glycogen and prevent secondary hypoglycemia.
- Minimizing adverse effects: teach the patient and family members preparation and administration techniques for glucagons before an emergency arises
- Most significant patient education: teach the patient and family members measures to prevent hypoglycemic reactions due to insulin; convey importance of early recognition and treatment of hypoglycemic episodes

has an 8-hour duration of effect, and has a half-life that ranges from 20 to 36 hours. Diazoxide undergoes hepatic metabolism and renal elimination. Diazoxide is in FDA pregnancy risk category C.

The most common adverse effects from oral dosing are: sodium and fluid retention, hyperglycemia, and glycosuria. In some patients, congestive heart failure may develop secondary to sodium and fluid retention.

Other adverse effects can include dizziness and weakness, peripheral edema of the hands, GI discomfort (e.g., nausea, vomiting, anorexia, abdominal pain, and constipation), and taste alterations.

The usual dosage of diazoxide (adult or child) is 1 mg/kg every 8 hours initially. Neonates may be given 3.3 mg/kg every 8 hours initially. The maximum dosage is 15 mg/kg/day. The total daily dose is divided equally, and administration times also are evenly spaced within the 24 hour day.

Glucose

Glucose, a monosaccharide, is absorbed directly from the intestine, resulting in a rapidly increased blood glucose concentration. It is indicated for managing hypoglycemia. The dosage is 10 to 20 g orally, repeated in 10 minutes if necessary. An occasional adverse effect is nausea. Glucose is not absorbed from the buccal mucosa. It must be swallowed to be effective. It should be used with caution in children younger than 2 years of age. Intravenous glucose (dextrose) is also used to treat hypoglycemia. Solutions with a concentration of 25% dextrose are used in neonates and infants and solutions of 50% dextrose are used in other age groups.

CHAPTER SUMMARY

- DM is primarily a disorder of carbohydrate metabolism, although it is associated with derangements of protein and fat metabolism and a series of vascular disorders. In the United States, diabetes is the most common endocrine disorder and the third leading cause of death.
- The patient with type 1 DM has an absolute insulin deficiency, cannot maintain a normal blood glucose level, and depends on exogenous insulin for survival.
- The patient with type 2 DM has a relative insulin deficiency (secondary to insulin resistance) and does not need exogenous insulin for survival. However, this patient may need insulin to achieve glucose balance during times of stress, such as illness, or to achieve maximum control of blood sugar.
- All insulins manage hyperglycemia by promoting cellular glucose uptake and metabolism. Insulins vary in peak, onset, and duration of action; they are similar in absorption, distribution, metabolism, and excretion.
- Hypoglycemia is the most common adverse effect of insulin therapy.
- Nursing care of the patient receiving insulin therapy calls for balancing diet, exercise, and insulin requirements; preventing and monitoring for complications of therapy; and teaching the patient how to do the same.
- One class of the available antidiabetic/oral hypoglycemic drugs includes the sulfonylureas; they vary in pharmacokinetics and hypoglycemic potency. Other drug classes similar in action are the meglitinides, the thiazolidinedione "insulin sensitizers," the biguanides, and the "starch blocker" alpha-glucosidase inhibiters.
- Sulfonylureas are used to treat hyperglycemia in type 2 DM. The most common adverse effects of the sulfonylureas are hypoglycemia and drug failure. Patient education for the sulfonylureas should focus on the importance of diet and exercise and the prevention of adverse drug effects.
- Glucagon is a protein made by the pancreas that is used in the emergency treatment of severe hypoglycemia. It regulates the rate of glucose production through glycogenolysis, gluconeogenesis, and lipolysis.
- **Glycosylated hemoglobin** provides a quantitative index of relatively long-term metabolic control. It can be used as a retrospective index of glucose control.

QUESTIONS FOR STUDY AND REVIEW

1. What are the three pancreatic islet peptide hormones that affect glucose metabolism? What are their effects?
2. What effect does glucagon have on glucose metabolism? What effect does it have on the effect of insulin?
3. What effects do the "stress hormones" (cortisol, epinephrine, growth hormone, somatostatin) have on glucose metabolism?
4. How do the characteristics of type 1 and type 2 DM compare?
5. What are the acute and chronic complications of diabetes?
6. Why must insulin be injected?
7. What effect would be expected from too much insulin? How would this be recognized?
8. What type of effects may insulin produce at the injection site? How common are these effects?
9. What is the mechanism of action for the following oral hypoglycemic drugs: sulfonylureas, biguanides, alpha-glucosidase inhibitors, and thiazolidinediones? Which type of diabetic patient benefits from each of these drug therapies?
10. What common adverse effects occur with sulfonylureas, biguanides, alpha-glucosidase inhibitors, and thiazolidinediones?
11. What interaction occurs between the sulfonylureas and ethyl alcohol?
12. Identify the clinical use for glucagons. Explain its mechanism of action and necessary patient and family education for proper use.

NEED MORE HELP?

Chapter 41 of the study guide for *Drug Therapy in Nursing* contains exercises and activities to reinforce your understanding of the concepts presented in this chapter. For additional information see the text's accompanying website at *http://www.connection.lww.com.*

REFERENCES AND BIBLIOGRAPHY

American Diabetes Association. (2000a). Consensus statement: Type 2 diabetes in children and adolescents. *Diabetes Care, 23*(3), 381–389.

American Diabetes Association. (2000b). Panel issues recommendations for Type 2 diabetes testing in children. *Pediatrics, 105*, 671–680.

American Diabetes Association. (2000c). Position statement: Standards of medical care for patients with diabetes mellitus. *Diabetes Care, 23*, (Suppl. 1), S32–S42.

American Diabetes Association. (2000d). Report of the expert committee on the diagnosis and classification of diabetes mellitus. *Diabetes Care, 23*, (Suppl. 1), S4–S19.

American Diabetes Association Website. (2001). http:\\www.diabetes.org/main/application/commercwf.

An, A. & Deng, E. (2000). A review of current treatment options for Type 2 diabetes mellitus. *Pharmacy Times, 64*(10), 86–99.

Balasubramanyan, A. (2000). *Role of beta-cell dysfunction in the pathogenesis of Type 2 diabetes and its link to obesity.* Presented at the

60th Scientific Sessions of the American Diabetes Association, San Antonio, TX.

Balasubramanyan, A. (June 11, 2000). *The physiology and biochemistry of exercise: Implications for diabetes.* Presented at the 60th Scientific Sessions of the American Diabetes Association, San Antonio, TX.

Bektas, A., Hughes, J. N., Warram, J. H., Krolewski, A. S., & Doria, A. (2001). Type 2 diabetes locus on 12q15: Further mapping and mutation screening of two candidate genes. *Diabetes, 50*(1), 204–208.

Beyzarov, E. P. (2000). ADA releases statement on newest Type 2 DM patients. *Drug Topics, 144*(6), 44.

Bloomgarden, Z. T. (2000). *Insulin sensitizers for Type 1 and Type 2 diabetes.* Presented at the 60th Scientific Sessions of the American Diabetes Association, San Antonio, TX.

Boyko, E. J., Fujimoto, W. Y., Leonetti, D. L., & Newell-Morris, L. (2000). Visceral adiposity and risk of Type 2 diabetes: A prospective study among Japanese Americans. *Diabetes Care, 23*(4), 465–471.

Caffrey, R. M., & Flaherty, T. (2000). Insulin delivery options in 2000. *Pharmacy Times, 66*(11), 74–83.

Campbell, K. (2000). Update on insulin injection devices. *U.S. Pharmacist, 25*(5), 44–64.

Campbell, R. K., & White, J. R. (2000). Strategies for insulin therapy in Type 2 diabetes. *U.S. Pharmacist, 25*(11), 101–112.

Chernin, T. (1999). Management of Type 1 diabetes mellitus in children and adolescents. *Pharmacy Times, 65*(10), 20–31.

Cohen, M. (2000). Reuse of syringes and needles in diabetes care. *U.S. Pharmacist, 25*(11), 59–62.

Diabetes Control and Complications Trial Research Group. (1993). The effect of intensive treatment of diabetes on the development of long-term complications in insulin-dependent diabetes mellitus. *New England Journal of Medicine, 329,* 977–986.

Everhart, W. H. (2000). Diabetes treatment. An evolution in progress. *Pharmacy Times, 67*(3), 36–40.

Fauci, A., Braunwald, E., Wilson, J. D., Martin, J. B., Hauser, S. L., Longo, D. L., Kasper, D. L., & Isselbachter, K. J. (Eds.). (1999). *Harrison's online.* New York: McGraw-Hill, Inc.

Garber, A. J. (1996). Magnesium utilization survey in selected patients with diabetes. *Clinical Therapeutics, 18*(2), 285–294.

Goran, M. I. (2000). Diet does not account for ethnic differences in children's risk of Type 2 diabetes. *American Journal of Clinical Nutrition, 71,* 725–732.

Hardman, J. G., Limbird, L. E., Molinoff, P. B., & Ruddon R. (Eds.). (1996). *Goodman & Gilman's pharmacological basis of therapeutics* (9th ed.). New York: McGraw-Hill.

Hebel, S., et al. (2001). *Drug Facts and Comparisons.* St. Louis: Facts and Comparisons.

Markowitz, J. S. (1998). Herbal medicines assuming a larger role in psychiatric care. *Drug Topics, 142*(17), 50–53.

Irwin, M. L., Mayer-Davis, E. J., Addy, C. L., Pate, R. R., Durstine, J. L., Stolarcyzk, L. M., & Ainsworth, B. E. (2000). Moderate-intensity physical activity and fasting insulin levels in women: The cross-cultural activity participation study. *Diabetes Care, 23*(4), 449–457.

Jick, S. S. (1999). Frequency of liver disease in Type 2 diabetic patients treated with oral antidiabetic agents. *Diabetes Care, 22*(12), 2067–2071.

Jovanovic, L. (2000). *The diabetic pregnancy: A clinical challenge.* Presented at the Symposium of the Diabetes and Pregnancy Council: 60th Scientific Sessions of the American Diabetes Association, San Antonio, TX.

Judd, R. L., & Raman, P. (1999). Pharmacological management of Type 2 diabetes mellitus: Current and future therapies. *Pharmacy Times, 65*(10), 85–94.

Kim, K. Y., An, A., & Deng, E. (1999). Advances in the treatment of Type 2 diabetes mellitus: Focus on insulin resistance. *Pharmacy Times, 65*(6), 78–88.

Kim, K. Y., & Nace, A. (2001). Controlling diabetes through counseling. *Pharmacy Times, 67*(3), 36–40.

King, D. S., & Wofford, M. R. (2000). Obesity and new-onset diabetes mellitus. *Drug Topics, 144*(2), 69–78.

Kitabvchai, A. E., Umpierrez, G. E., Murphy, M. B., Barrett, E. J., Kreisberg, R. A., Malone, J. I., & Wall, B. M. (2001). Management of hyperglycemic crises in patients with diabetes. *Diabetes Care, 24*(1), 131–144.

Konzem, S. L. (2000). Optimization of treatment of Type 2 diabetes in the elderly. *U.S. Pharmacist, 25*(11), 32–49.

McCann, J. (2001). Alternatives to injectable insulin; other new d rugs on the way. *Drug Topics, 145*(7), 40.

McEvoy, G. K., Litvak, K., & Welsh Jr., O. H. (Eds.). (2001). *Drug Information.* Bethesda: American Hospital Formulary Service.

Oki, J. C. (2000). Alcohol and diabetes mellitus. *U.S. Pharmacist, 25*(11), 71–78.

Schwetschenau, K. H. (2000). An overview of Type 2 diabetes. *Pharmacy Times, 66*(6), 20–26.

Rajan, A. S. (2000). *Advances in pancreas and islet transplantation.* Presented at the 60th Scientific Sessions of the American Diabetes Association, San Antonio, TX.

Rajan, A. S. (2000). Psychosocial aspects in diabetes education an d management. Presented at the 60th Scientific Sessions of the American Diabetes Association, San Antonio, TX.

Semb, S. (2000). Diabetes care: Competencies for patient teaching. *CME Resource, 64*(4), 49–85.

White, J. R., & Campbell, R. K. (1999). Insulin sensitizers: New options for treating Type 2 diabetes. *U.S. Pharmacist, 24*(11), 124–134.

Zagaria, A. E. (2000). Gestational diabetes mellitus: Risks, complications, and therapeutic outcomes. *U.S. Pharmacist, 25*(11), 50–56.

Zimmet, P. (2000). The global scope of diabetes and obesity-an epidemic in progress: Paradise lost. Presented at the 60th Scientific Sessions of the American Diabetes Association, San Antonio, TX.

Chapter 42

DRUGS AFFECTING MEN'S HEALTH AND SEXUALITY

KEY TERMS

androgens
benign prostatic hypertrophy
erectile dysfunction
follicle-stimulating hormone
luteinizing hormone
male pattern baldness

Learning Objectives

At the completion of this chapter the student will:

1. Identify common health problems of men that are treated with drug therapy.
2. Identify core drug knowledge about drugs that affect men's health and sexuality.
3. Identify core patient variables relevant to drugs that affect men's health and sexuality.
4. Relate the interaction of core drug knowledge and core patient variables for drugs that affect men's health and sexuality.
5. Generate a nursing plan of care from the interactions between core drug knowledge and core patient variables for drugs that affect men's health and sexuality.
6. Describe nursing interventions to maximize therapeutic and minimize adverse effects of drugs that affect men's health and sexuality.
7. Determine key points for patient and family education related to drugs that affect men's health and sexuality.

Androgens

testosterone

(short-acting, long-acting, transdermal system, methyltestosterone, fluoxymesterone)

Anabolic steroids

oxymethalone
stanozolol
oxandrolone
nandrolone phenpropionate
nandrolone decanoate

Drugs to treat erectile dysfunction

sildenafil

alprostadil
yohimbine

Drugs to treat BPH

finasteride

Alpha-1 blockers

prazocin
terazocin
doxazocin
tamsulosin

Drugs to treat male pattern baldness

minoxidil

finasteride

The symbol C indicates the **drug class**.

Drugs in bold type marked with the symbol P are **prototypes**.

Drugs in blue type with no symbol are **closely related** to the prototype.

Drugs in **red** type with no symbol are **significantly different** from the prototype.

Drugs in **black** type with no symbol are **also used in drug therapy**; no prototype.

Men's health and sexuality differ from women's. Men, over their lifetime, experience unique health problems. Some problems may be directly related to deficiencies of the male sex hormone testosterone; others may be indirectly related to changing hormone levels. Additionally, changes in the cardiovascular (e.g., peripheral vascular disease, ischemic heart disease), neurologic (e.g., neuropathies), and endocrine (e.g., diabetes mellitus) systems are responsible for other health problems in men.

This chapter discusses drug therapy used to treat insufficient testosterone, erectile dysfunction, benign prostatic hypertrophy (BPH), and male pattern baldness. It discusses the prototype male sex hormone testosterone. The prototype for treating erectile dysfunction is sildenafil (Viagra). The prototype drug for treatment of BPH is finasteride (Proscar, Propecia). The prototype drug for treating male pattern baldness is minoxidil (Rogaine, Minoxidil for Men).

In addition, this chapter briefly discusses prostatic cancer. Chapters 45 and 46 present a fuller discussion of the drugs used in the treatment of prostatic cancer.

PHYSIOLOGY

HORMONES

Androgens are naturally occurring or synthetic steroidal compounds that produce the masculinization and tissue-building properties of testosterone, the main male sex hormone. Other androgens include dihydrotestosterone, androstenedione, and dehydroepiandrosterone. During puberty, the pituitary gland secretes large volumes of **follicle-stimulating hormone** (FSH) and **luteinizing hormone** (LH). The predominant effect of FSH is believed to be formation of sperm cells. LH in males stimulates the interstitial cells of the testes, which produce approximately 95% of testosterone. Interstitial cell development is influenced by interstitial cell-stimulating hormone (ICSH). Therefore, increased production of ICSH stimulates the production of testosterone.

Testosterone is responsible for the normal growth and development of the male sex organs. It also is responsible for development and maintenance of the male secondary sexual characteristics, such as hair distribution (beard, pubic area, chest, and axilla), hair texture and color (more deeply pigmented, heavier, and sometimes curly), laryngeal enlargement and vocal cord thickening (voice deepening), and alterations in body musculature and fat distribution. Testosterone also causes retention of sodium, potassium, and phosphorus and decreased urinary excretion of calcium. In addition, it stimulates the growth of skeletal muscle tissue and enhances the growth of long bones in prepubescent boys—the growth spurt of adolescence. The ossification (hardening) process of the epiphyseal growth plates, which stops the growth of the long bones, also occurs with prolonged elevation of testosterone levels. Testosterone also is reported to stimulate the production of red blood cells by enhancing the production of erythropoietin-stimulating factor. The adult man produces approximately 7 to 8 mg of testosterone daily. In women, the adrenal cortex and the ovaries secrete androgens, including testosterone, although in much smaller amounts than are found in men.

PENIS

The male penis has a dermal layer of smooth muscle, under which is loose connective tissue. This pliable connective tissue allows the skin of the penis to move without distorting the underlying structures. This important characteristic allows for erection of the penis. Beneath the connective tissue is a dense network of elastic fibers that encircle the internal structures of the penis. Most of the shaft of the penis is composed of three cylindric columns of erectile tissue, which consists of a maze of vascular channels incompletely separated by partitions of elastic connective tissue and smooth muscle fibers. In the nonaroused state, the arterial branches are constricted, and the muscular partitions are tense. These two events restrict blood flow into the erectile tissue. The parasympathetic system innervates the penile arteries. Normal erection involves the release of nitric oxide, secondary to sexual stimulation, in the erectile tissue of the penis. The nitric oxide activates an intermediary enzyme that boosts cyclic guanosine monophosphate (cGMP), a substance that mediates the action of certain hormones. By some unknown mechanism, cGMP stimulates smooth muscle, producing relaxation and an inflow of blood into the erectile tissue.

URETHRA AND PROSTATE

Passing through the penis is the urethra, which, in men, transports both urine and semen. The prostate gland is a small muscular rounded organ that encircles the proximal portion of the urethra as it leaves the urinary bladder. The ejaculatory duct joins the urethra in the prostate (Fig. 42-1). The prostate gland is very small until puberty, when it begins to grow as a result of hormonal changes. The growth of the prostate gland slows after age 20 years, but continues throughout the rest of the man's life. The primary hormone in the prostate cell that affects growth of the prostate is dihydrotestosterone (DHT). A special enzyme, 5-alpha reductase, converts testosterone to DHT.

PATHOPHYSIOLOGY

HORMONAL PROBLEMS

If a male is deficient in endogenous sex hormones, he will not experience normal sexual development. The primary sex organs will not mature, secondary sexual characteristics will not develop, reproduction will not be possible, and the normal growth spurt of adolescence will not happen. If the level of endogenous hormones drops after puberty has occurred and the sexual organs and reproductive system have matured, secondary sexual characteristics may diminish. Ability to reproduce, despite developed organs, will be

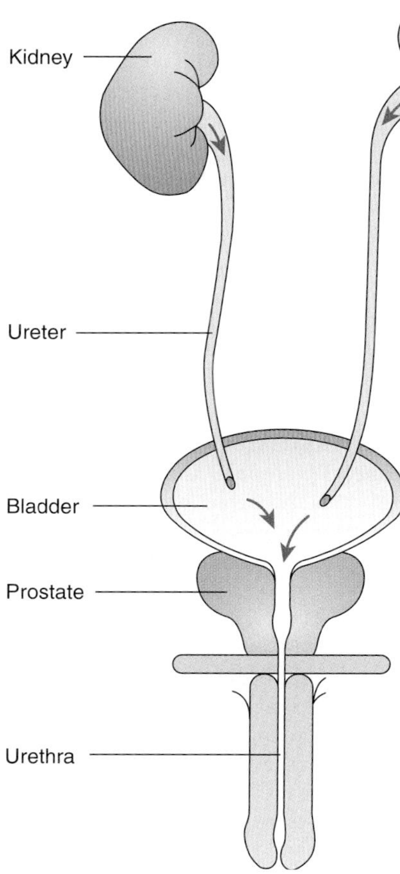

Figure 42-1. Normal urine flow.

diminished. A man may not create enough sperm to impregnate a woman.

ERECTILE DYSFUNCTION

Erectile dysfunction is the inability to achieve or maintain an erection in at least every three of four attempts at intercourse. Erectile dysfunction affects 10 to 30 million men in the United States and more than 140 million men worldwide (Philpot & Morley, 2000). It may be a temporary or chronic problem. Erectile dysfunction may result from the use of drug therapy, alcohol, trauma, or illness that affects either the autonomic nervous system or the central nervous system (CNS). Physical causes, such as vascular changes or neural alterations, may produce this problem. Emotions also may affect male sexual performance. Severe stress, emotional problems, depression, anxiety, or fear of impaired performance may all result in sexual dysfunction. Almost 90% of men older than age 50 years have an organic cause for erectile dysfunction; in younger men most cases of erectile dysfunction stem from psychogenic problems. Vascular disease is the most common physical cause of erectile dysfunction, and atherosclerosis of the penile artery is the primary cause for more than half of men older than age 50 years. Men with diabetes have a high risk for erectile dysfunction because of a combination of vascular disease and neuropathy.

BENIGN PROSTATIC HYPERTROPHY

Prostatic enlargement that is not caused by cancer is called **benign prostatic hypertrophy or hypoplasia (BPH)**. BPH occurs spontaneously in men as they age, and incidence rises after men turn age 40. By age 80 almost 80% of men will have BPH. The exact cause of BPH is not well understood. Although testosterone levels fall with aging, DHT (the primary hormone in the prostate) levels remain fairly constant. DHT is the hormone primarily responsible for prostate growth. Additionally, the small amount of estrogen in the man may also affect prostate growth because decreasing testosterone levels no longer offset the effects of estrogen (Fig. 42-2).

BPH first affects the urethra as the enlarged prostate tightens around it. The pressure of the gland against the urethra is like a clamp on a garden hose, making passage of fluid more difficult. The man has difficulty initiating a stream or stopping the flow of urine (dribbling). This pressure on the urethra from the prostate causes the man's bladder to thicken. Initially the bladder is irritable and contracts even when it contains only a small amount of urine; thus, he has frequent urination and nocturia. As the prostate continues to place pressure on the bladder, the bladder weakens, with poor contraction during urination. Eventually, the bladder can no longer empty completely, causing urinary retention. Urinary tract infections may result. Complete inability to void may also occur.

MALE PATTERN BALDNESS

The adult has two major types of hair: vellus hair and terminal hair. *Vellus hair* is the fine "peach fuzz" located over much of the body surface. *Terminal hair* is heavy, more deeply pigmented, and sometimes curly. It is located mostly on the head. Hair follicles may alter the structure of the hair on the body in response to circulating hormones. In men, decreasing levels of sex hormones can affect the scalp, causing a shift from terminal hair to vellus hair production beginning at the temples and the crown of the head. An alteration of the

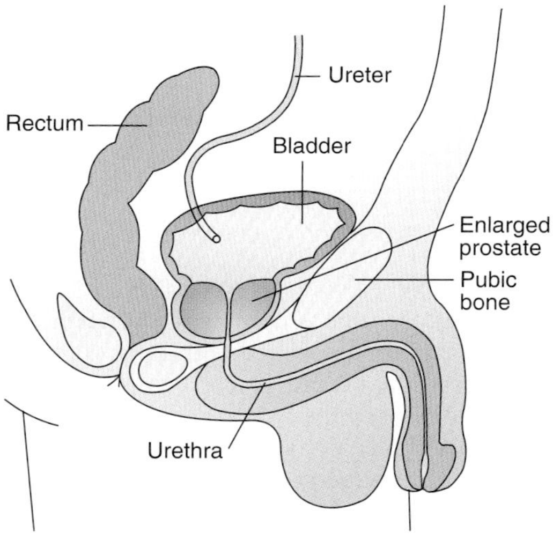

Figure 42-2. Urine flow with benign prostatic hypertrophy.

receptors for testosterone and other male sex hormones may also induce hair loss.

Male pattern baldness, also referred to as androgenetic alopecia, is baldness of the vertex of the scalp. Women may also have hair loss related to decreased sex hormone levels. Hair loss in women is different from hair loss in men in that the loss is diffuse or there may be thinning of the frontoparietal areas.

PROSTATE CANCER

Prostatic cancer is a malignant metastasizing cancer and the second most common cause of cancer deaths in men. One in five men in the United States will develop prostate cancer, which is not caused by BPH. Prostate cancer usually originates in one of the secretory glands. As the cancer grows, it produces a nodular lump on the prostatic surface. During a digital examination, this lump can be palpated through the rectal wall. If diagnosis is not made until after the cancer has metastasized, the prognosis for survival decreases, as metastasis rapidly involves the lymphatic system, lungs, bone marrow, liver, or adrenal glands.

Prostate cancer treatment varies for each affected man. Treatment options include surgical intervention, radiation therapy, cryotherapy, and hormonal therapy (antiandrogen antineoplastics and gonadotropin-releasing hormone analogs). Drugs used to treat prostatic cancer are discussed in chapters 45 and 46.

C ANDROGENS

The prototype male sex hormone is testosterone. When testosterone is administered exogenously as a drug, it may be given in different forms. These differences may relate to the onset or duration of action or to the route of administration (oral, buccal, parenteral, topical, and subdermal implants). Drugs similar to testosterone are the anabolic steroids, which include oxymethalone (Anadrol-5), stanozol (Winstrol), oxandrolone (Oxandrin), nandrolone phenopropionate (Durabolin, Hybolin Improved), and nandrolone decanoate (Deca-Durabolin, Hybolin Decanoate-50, Hybolin Decanoate-100, Neo-Durabolic, and Androlone-D 200).

NURSING MANAGEMENT OF THE PATIENT RECEIVING P TESTOSTERONE

Core Drug Knowledge

Pharmacotherapeutics

In males, testosterone is used as replacement therapy for hypogonadism associated with low or no endogenous testosterone (Table 42-1). Boys with low or no testosterone before puberty need testosterone treatment to develop secondary sexual characteristics and must continue it after puberty to maintain them. Men who develop a deficiency of testosterone after puberty require testosterone to maintain sexual characteristics. Testosterone may also be given to males with delayed puberty (puberty that is expected to occur but much later than normal) to stimulate the onset of puberty. These patients must be carefully selected and have a clear familial pattern of delayed puberty that is not secondary to a pathologic disorder. Brief treatment with conservative doses may be justified if these patients are having serious emotional problems as a result of delayed puberty. Testosterone is also used in the treatment of erectile dysfunction and male climacteric symptoms when these conditions are secondary to androgen deficiency.

In women, testosterone may be used as secondary treatment in advanced, inoperable metastatic breast cancer if the woman is 1 to 5 years postmenopause.

Short-acting testosterone is known by the trade names Histerone, Tesamone, and Testandro. Short-acting testosterone is available in an aqueous suspension or in an oil for injection. Long-acting testosterone is known by the trade names Andro L.A. 200, Delatestryl, Durathate-200, Everone 200, depAndro100, DepAndro200, Andropository-200, Depotest 100, Depo-Testosterone, Duratest-100, and Duratest-200.

Testosterone implantable pellets have the trade name Tesopel. Transdermal patches of testosterone have the trade names Testoderm and Androderm. Oral forms of testosterone are methyltestosterone and fluoxymesterone. Trade names for these are Android-10, Android-25, Oreton Methyl, Testred, Virilon, and Halotestin.

Pharmacokinetics

Natural testosterone undergoes a high first-pass effect and is not used orally. The form of testosterone that is used orally is a synthetic androgen and is less extensively metabolized than natural testosterones. The synthetic form of testosterone also has a longer half-life. The synthetic androgens are also available as buccal tablets. They are absorbed directly into the bloodstream, bypassing the gastrointestinal (GI) tract and the first-pass effect. These buccal androgens have approximately twice the potency of oral androgens. Peak serum level from buccal administration occurs in 1 hour compared with 2 hours for oral administration. Testosterone esters are less polar than free testosterone. Testosterone esters in oil are given intramuscularly. These testosterone esters will be slowly absorbed, allowing for dosing intervals of 2 to 4 weeks.

In the plasma, testosterone is about 98% bound to a specific testosterone-estradiol binding globulin. The amount of binding globulin determines the percentages of free and bound testosterone. The concentration of free testosterone determines half-life. Inactivation of testosterone occurs mostly in the liver. The conjugates and metabolites of testosterone are eliminated in the urine and feces. Testosterone crosses the placenta and enters the breast milk.

Pharmacodynamics

The effects of testosterone on males are the same as the effects of endogenous testosterone. In females, the drug causes masculinization. In addition, increased

TABLE 42-1 Summary of Selected Drugs Used to Treat Men's Health Problems

Drug (Trade) Name	Selected Indications	Route and Dosage Range	Pharmacokinetics
Androgens			
testosterone			
testosterone (short-acting; Histerone, Tesamone)	*Males:* replacement therapy in hypogonadism, delayed puberty, impotence secondary to androgen deficiency	Male hypogonadism (initiation of puberty), IM 40–50 mg/m^2 dose/mo or 50–400 mg/dose q 2–4 wk; androgen replacement, IM, 25–50 mg two to three times per week	*Onset:* Slow *Duration:* 1–3 d $t_{1/2}$: 10–100 min
testosterone (long-acting; Delatest, Everone, Andronate, Depo, Duratest; *Canadian:* Scheinpharm Testone - CYP)	*Males:* replacement therapy in hypogonadism, delayed puberty *Females:* palliation of inoperable breast cancer	*Adult:* hypogonadism (initiation of puberty), IM, 50–400 mg q 2–4 wk; androgen replacement, IM, 25–50 mg q2–4 wk *Females:* IM, 200–400 mg q2–4 wk	*Onset:* Slow *Duration:* 2–4 wk $t_{1/2}$: Up to 8 d
testosterone, transdermal (Testoderm, Androderm)	*Males:* primary hypogonadism, hypogonadotropic hypogonadism	*Adult:* Patch, 4–6 mg/d applied to scrotal skin (Testoderm); 5 mg/d applied to nonscrotal skin (Androderm)	*Onset:* Rapid *Duration:* 24 h $t_{1/2}$: 10–100 min
methyltestosterone (Android, Oreton, Testred, Virilon, Metandren)	*Males:* hypogonadism, androgen deficiency, impotence, postpubertal cryptorchidism *Females:* breast cancer	*Males:* PO, 10–50 mg/d *Females:* PO, 50–200 mg/d	*Onset:* 2 h *Duration:* 24 h $t_{1/2}$: 2.5–3 h
fluoxymesterone (Halotestin)	*Males:* hypogonadism *Females:* inoperable breast cancer	*Males:* PO, 5–20 mg/d *Females:* PO, 10–40 mg/d in divided doses	*Onset:* 2 h *Duration:* 24 h $t_{1/2}$: 9.2 h
Drugs to Treat Erectile Dysfunction			
sildenafil (Viagra)	Erectile dysfunction	PO: usual dose 50 mg once/d, may use 25–100 mg based on effectiveness and tolerance	*Onset:* <30 minutes *Duration:* up to 4 hours $t_{1/2}$: 4 h
alprostadil (Caverject, Edex, Muse)	Erectile dysfunction	Intracavernosal injection: initial dose 2.5 μg; titrate upward by first another 2.5 μg, then by 5–10 μg until desired effect achieved; give no more than 3 times/week. Intraurethral: 125–1000 μg; use smallest effective dose; no more than 2 doses in 24 hours	*Onset:* Intracavernosal—rapid Intraurethral—5–10 min *Duration:* Intracavernosal—up to 1 h *Intraurethral*—30–60 min $t_{1/2}$: Unknown
Drugs to Treat Benign Prostatic Hypertrophy (BPH)			
finasteride (Proscar) (Propecia)	BPH Male pattern baldness	PO: 5 mg/d PO: 1 mg/d	*Onset:* <2 h *Duration:* 24 h $t_{1/2}$: 6 h
Alpha-1 blockers			
tamsulosin (Flomax)	BPH	PO: 0.4 mg/d about 30 min after the same meal daily	*Onset:* Varies *Duration:* 24 h $t_{1/2}$: 9–13 h
Drug to Treat Male Pattern Baldness			
minoxidil (Rogaine, Minoxidil for Men)	Male pattern baldness	Topically to affected area of scalp—1 mL bid	*Onset:* ≥4 mo *Duration:* 3–4 mo after discontinuing effective dosing $t_{1/2}$: Unknown

testosterone levels in women will slow the growth of advanced breast cancers, which are estrogen dependent.

Contraindications and Precautions

Testosterone is contraindicated for patients with serious cardiac, hepatic, or renal disease because edema with or without congestive heart failure (CHF) may be a complication in these patients. It is also contraindicated in those hypersensitive to the drug and in men with carcinomas of the breast or prostate. Although it is not normally used in premenopausal women, it is a pregnancy category X drug because it will cause masculinization of the genitalia in the female fetus.

Caution must be used when administering testosterone to the following patients:

- Young males with delayed puberty because of testosterone's adverse effect on bone maturation
- Males with preexisting gynecomastia (breast enlargement) because testosterone may compound the gynecomastia problem
- Elderly men because they may be at increased risk for prostatic hypertrophy and prostatic carcinoma
- Patients with BPH because they may develop acute urethral obstruction
- Patients with acute intermittent porphyria (a group of disorders that result from a disturbance in porphyrin [nitrogen-containing organic compounds in protoplasm] metabolism) because androgens have precipitated attacks of this condition
- Patients with a history of myocardial infarction (MI) or coronary artery disease (CAD) because testosterone may promote hypercholesterolemia

Adverse Effects

Most adverse effects are related to high doses of the drug. In males, the most common adverse effects include gynecomastia, excessive frequency and duration of penile erections, decreased ejaculatory volumes, and oligospermia (low sperm counts).

In females, the most common adverse effects are adrenergic and include amenorrhea and other menstrual irregularities (if given prior to menopause), inhibition of gonadotropin secretion, and virilization, including deepening of the voice and clitoral enlargement. Clitoral enlargement is not reversible after therapy ends.

Other effects related to the actions of testosterone on the body may occur. They include hypercalcemia, particularly in immobile patients and those with metastatic breast cancer; retention of sodium, chloride, water, potassium, calcium, and inorganic phosphates; hypercholesterolemia; and edema. In addition, rash, acne, seborrhea, and hirsutism may occur. Prostatic hypertrophy, prostatic cancer, and urethral obstruction are also possibilities. Other potential adverse effects include hepatitis (life-threatening), hepatocellular carcinoma (prolonged use of high doses), premature closing of the long bones, dizziness, headache, sleep disorders, fatigue, changes in libido, and polycythemia.

Drug Interactions

No significant drug interactions are associated with natural testosterone. With the synthetic forms, anticoagulation effect is increased if anticoagulants are given with either floxymesterone or methyltestosterone. Coadministration of methyltestosterone and imipramine may result in paranoid-like symptoms.

Assessment of Relevant Core Patient Variables

Health Status

The nurse should assess for existing serious heart, kidney, or liver disease, because these are contraindications for therapy. The nurse also needs to know whether the patient has an established hypersensitivity to testosterone. He or she should determine whether male patients have carcinoma of the breast or prostate, because these are contraindications, or whether they have gynecomastia or BPH, as these conditions require precautions. Assessing for a history of MI, CAD, or acute intermittent porphyria is important, because all these factors require caution in use of testosterone. Because of testosterone's effects on bone growth, only those with expert training and knowledge of the drug and its effects on bone growth should prescribe it.

Life Span and Gender

The nurse should carefully consider age-related assessment data for possible related problems with the use of testosterone. When testosterone is used in prepubescent boys to treat hypogonadism or delayed onset of puberty, premature closure of the long bones may lead to stunted growth. Caution also is necessary when testosterone is used in elderly men. Testosterone is not normally used in premenopausal females because it is likely to produce masculinization. If a woman is prescribed testosterone, the nurse must assess the patient for pregnancy. Testosterone will cause masculinization of the female fetus, as characterized by clitoromegaly, abnormal vaginal development, and fusion of the genital folds to form a scrotal-like structure. These effects are most likely if testosterone is given during the first trimester. If significantly large amounts of the drug are given to a male fetus, adverse effects are possible. It is not known whether testosterone crosses into breast milk, but because of the rare use of testosterone in young women the information is not critical.

Lifestyle, Diet, and Habits

Although anabolic steroids are more frequently abused for enhancement of athletic performance, testosterone has also been abused for this purpose. This is not a safe and effective use for this drug. The nurse should verify that the patient is not abusing testosterone.

Environment

Testosterone may be administered in any setting.

Nursing Diagnoses and Outcomes

- Delayed Growth and Development related to potential for early epiphyseal closure secondary to drug therapy
  Desired outcome: *The patient will attain normal height while receiving drug therapy.*
- Ineffective Sexuality Patterns related to effect of drug therapy
  Desired outcome: *The male patient will develop normal male sexual organs and characteristics. The female patient will not experience excessive masculinization during therapy.*
- Excess Fluid Volume related to potential effects of drug therapy
  Desired outcome: *The patient will not experience enough increase in fluid volume to become edematous during drug therapy.*
- Potential Complication: Hypercalcemia related to drug therapy, immobility, or diagnosis of breast cancer
  Desired outcome: *The patient will not develop hypercalcemia.*

Planning and Intervention

Maximizing Therapeutic Effects

The nurse administers the drug at regular intervals to maintain therapeutic testosterone levels. He or she adjusts the dose upward when giving testosterone to treat hypogonadism and induce puberty. At the end of the growth spurt, the patient should remain on a maintenance dose.

Some nursing actions specific to the route of administration can maximize the therapeutic effect of testosterone. When administering testosterone as Testaderm transdermal patches, the nurse places the patches on clean, dry, scrotal skin that has been dry shaved for optimal skin contact. He or she does not use chemical depilatories. The patient should wear these transdermal patches for 22 to 24 hours before replacing them.

The nurse does not place Testaderm TTS patches on the scrotum. Rather, he or she places them on clean dry skin on the arm, back, or upper buttocks. The skin area should not be oily, damaged, or irritated. The patient wears these patches for 24 hours and then replaces them.

The nurse places Androderm transdermal patches on the back, abdomen, upper arms, or thighs. He or she avoids placing them on the scrotum or over bony areas such as the shoulder and hip. These patches stay in place for 7 days before replacement.

The nurse places buccal tablets between the gum and the cheek. They should be allowed to dissolve, never be swallowed.

The nurse agitates the suspension vial to mix the drug thoroughly before drawing it into a syringe and administering it IM.

Minimizing Adverse Effects

Every 6 months, radiographs should be taken to assess bone age when treating prepubescent boys. Radiographs help to document bone maturation and the effect of testosterone on the epiphyseal centers.

Some nursing actions can minimize the adverse effects of testosterone. The nurse monitors serum cholesterol levels and liver function periodically. He or she checks hemoglobin and hematocrit levels periodically for polycythemia during treatment with high doses. The nurse monitors serum and urine calcium levels in women receiving testosterone for disseminated breast cancer. In women receiving testosterone for palliative treatment of metastasized breast cancer, the nurse must monitor the disease progression closely, because occasionally the drug may accelerate the disease process.

When administering by IM injection, the nurse injects deep into the gluteal muscle to prevent inflammation and pain at the administration site. He or she never administers the drug intravenously.

The nurse discards used transdermal patches by folding them and putting them in trash in an appropriate manner or by flushing them down the toilet. Active drug remains after use so that accidental application or ingestion by children would be dangerous.

The nurse assesses for signs of adverse effects and contacts the health care provider if adverse effects are noted, especially severe masculinization in women or edema or jaundice in either sex. Dosage adjustments or cessation of therapy may be indicated.

Providing Patient and Family Education

- The nurse teaches the patient and family the rationale for use of the drug, including therapeutic effects and potential adverse effects.
- The nurse instructs the patient and family about proper administration technique. If drug administration will be IM, the patient requires teaching related to safe handling and disposal of needles and syringes. If the patient will be using transdermal patches, he or she requires instruction about how to dispose of used patches.
- The nurse reviews the importance of scheduling and keeping follow-up appointments for radiographs and blood tests.
- For patients taking buccal tablets, the nurse teaches them to place the tablet between gum and cheek and not to swallow it. He or she reminds these patients not to eat, drink, or smoke while the tablet is in place because doing so will alter absorption of the drug.
- The nurse must alert patients to notify the health care provider if swelling of the extremities (edema), jaundice, or prolonged painful erection develops. Women should notify the health care provider if they develop

hoarseness, deepening of the voice, menstrual irregularities, acne, or facial hair growth.

Ongoing Assessment and Evaluation

Monitoring for adverse effects throughout therapy is necessary, as is regular monitoring of blood test results and bone growth as noted previously. Therapy is considered effective if development of male sex organs and male sexual characteristics occurs normally or if males maintain secondary male sexual characteristics without adverse effects. If given to women with breast cancer, testosterone therapy is considered effective if discomfort from the malignant tumor is minimized and the disease advances no further. ■

DRUGS CLOSELY RELATED TO P TESTOSTERONE

The anabolic steroids include oxymethalone, stanozolol, oxandrolone, nandrolone phenpropionate, and nandrolone decanoate. They are derived from testosterone and, like testosterone, have both anabolic and androgenic effects. Unlike testosterone, the anabolic effects of anabolic steroids are much stronger than the androgenic effects. In fact, their two major actions are to promote body tissue-building processes and reverse catabolic or tissue-depleting processes. Anabolic steroids are indicated for treating certain anemias because they stimulate erythropoiesis. They are also used prophylactically to decrease the frequency and severity of attacks of hereditary angioedema (characterized by episodic edema of the abdominal viscera, extremities, face, and airway). Anabolic steroids are also used to control metastatic breast cancer in women.

An abuse or addiction syndrome has been recognized with the chronic use of anabolic steroids to improve athletic performance (see the accompanying display, Athletes and Testosterone). The use of these drugs to improve athletic performance is questionable because of the accompanying serious possibly adverse effects, which may be irreversible. Serious adverse effects include peliosis hepatitis (blood-filled cysts replace normal liver cells and sometimes spleen cells, which can be associated with liver failure), liver tumors (possibly malignant), and blood lipid changes (which may be significant) associated with an increased risk of atherosclerosis (resulting from decreased high-density lipoprotein and sometimes increased low-density lipoprotein). In females, masculinization effects similar to those produced by (short-acting) testosterone occur with use. Like testosterone, anabolic steroids are in pregnancy category X because of the possibility of fetal masculinization.

MEMORY CHIP

P Testosterone

- Used as hormone replacement therapy in male hypogonadism that is associated with low or absent endogenous testosterone
- Most significant contraindication: serious cardiac, hepatic, or renal disease because edema with or without CHF may be a complication
- Most common adverse effects: gynecomastia, excessive frequency and duration of penile erections, decreased ejaculatory volumes, and oligospermia; masculinization in females
- Most serious adverse effect: life-threatening hepatitis
- **Lifespan alert: pregnancy category X drug; prepubescent boys may have premature closing of long bones**
- Maximizing therapeutic effects: administer at regular intervals; place transdermal patches appropriately on skin (varies by trade preparation)
- Minimizing adverse effects: radiographs every 6 months to determine bone maturation and the effect on the epiphyseal growth centers when treating prepubescent boys; safe disposal of used transdermal patches
- Most significant patient education: notify health care provider if swelling of the extremities (edema), jaundice, or painful, continued erection develop

C DRUGS USED TO TREAT ERECTILE DYSFUNCTION

Agents to treat erectile dysfunction work to mimic the body's natural methods of achieving an erection. The prototype is sildenafil (Viagra). A drug closely related to sildenafil is alprostadil (Caverject, Edex, Muse). A drug significantly different from sildenafil is yohimbine (Aphrodyne, Dayto Himbin, Yocon, Yohimex).

NURSING MANAGEMENT OF THE PATIENT RECEIVING P SILDENAFIL

Core Drug Knowledge

Pharmacotherapeutics

Sildenafil is used in the treatment of erectile dysfunction. It is administered orally, usually 1 hour before sexual activity. Sildenafil is effective only with accompanying sex-

COMMUNITY-BASED CONCERNS

Athletes and Testosterone

Nurses perform a significant service when they teach patients or community groups about pitfalls of unorthodox drug use:

- Athletes have used and abused testosterone and anabolic steroids in an effort to increase muscle mass. These drugs have not been shown to be effective for this purpose.
- Serious potential adverse effects include early closure of epiphyseal growth plates, which stunts normal growth; edema (with or without CHF); and male gynecomastia.
- Increase in weight and muscle size is partially the result of water retention.

ual stimulation. It is effective in erectile dysfunction after a radical prostatectomy, but only if either a bilateral or unilateral nerve-sparing procedure has been performed (Feng, Huang, Kaptein, Kaswick, & Aboseif, 2000). Effectiveness if only one nerve is not cut (unilateral sparing) may be true only for men younger than 55 years of age (Zagaja, Mhoon, Aikens, & Brendler, 2000).

Pharmacokinetics

Sildenafil is rapidly absorbed. Maximum plasma concentrations are reached within 30 to 120 minutes (most frequent peak time is 60 minutes) of oral dosing when taken on an empty stomach. When taken with a high-fat meal, absorption is delayed, so that approximately 60 extra minutes are needed to reach peak plasma levels. A high-fat meal also reduces peak serum concentrations by 29%.

Sildenafil is metabolized by two hepatic microsomal isoenzymes. The primary isoenzyme involved in metabolism is CYP3A4. A second isoenzyme with a more minor effect on metabolism is CYP2C9. Through these pathways, sildenafil is converted into an active metabolite that is further metabolized. The metabolite has pharmacologic properties similar to the parent drug and accounts for about 20% of sildenafil's pharmacologic effect. The metabolite of sildenafil is excreted primarily in the stool and to a small extent in the urine. Men older than 65 years have a reduced sildenafil clearance and elevated free plasma concentrations that are about 40% greater than in younger men.

Pharmacodynamics

Sildenafil inhibits the isoenzyme (phosphodiesterase [PDE] type 5) that metabolizes cGMP. The decreased metabolism of cGMP allows it to remain active longer, increasing smooth muscle relaxation and inflow of blood. These circumstances allow for an improved and more sustained erection. Because sildenafil works at the end of a cascade of events that produce erection, starting with sexual stimulation releasing nitric oxide, sildenafil is not effective in normal doses without sexual stimulation. Men must continue sildenafil treatment to maintain improvement in erectile function (Christiansen, Guirguis, Cox, & Osterloh, 2000).

Contraindications and Precautions

Sildenafil is contraindicated if the patient is currently using nitrates, because its vasodilating effects potentiate the hypotensive effects of nitrates. Sildenafil is also contraindicated if the patient has hypersensitivity to any component of the tablet.

The American College of Cardiology and the American Heart Association recommend caution when sildenafil is prescribed to patients with the following cardiovascular problems: coronary ischemia, CHF, hypotension, or a history of MI, cerebrovascular accident (stroke), or life-threatening arrhythmias within the last 6 months. These professional groups also recommend that any patients with significant cardiac risk factors or known cardiac disease should undergo an exercise stress test prior to beginning any treatment for erectile dysfunction.

Adverse Effects

Adverse effects from sildenafil are generally transient and mild to moderate in nature. The most common adverse effects are facial flushing, headache, nasal congestion, and heartburn (Moreira, Brannigan, Spitz, Orejuela, Lipschultz, & Kim, 2000). Other adverse effects are diarrhea, urinary tract infections, blue-tinged vision and light sensitivity, or blurred vision, dizziness, and rash.

Although some cardiovascular system–related deaths have been reported in patients taking sildenafil since the drug has been marketed, research and statistical analysis have found that sildenafil is not responsible for causing an excessive number of cardiovascular deaths. The anecdotal reports of deaths are believed to be caused by preexisting cardiac risk factors (i.e., hypertension, diabetes mellitus, smoking, and depression) and the cardiovascular "work" or effort involved in sexual intercourse. Based on these incidents of cardiovascular deaths, however, precaution must be used with patients who have current cardiovascular problems because they may have greater risk of cardiovascular adverse effects from sildenafil (see Contraindications and Precautions above).

Overdosing produces adverse effects similar to those associated with normal dosing but at an increased rate of incidence. Standard supportive measures for drug overdose should be used. Renal dialysis is not helpful because little of the drug is excreted renally.

Drug Interactions

The CYP3A4 isoenzyme and, to a lesser degree, the CYP2C9 isoenzyme, mediate sildenafil metabolism. Any drug that inhibits these systems may produce a drug interaction with sildenafil and decrease its clearance, raising plasma levels as a result. Strong CYP3A4 inhibitors (i.e., ketoconazole, itraconazole, erythromycin, and cimetidine) have been shown to increase the plasma levels of sildenafil as much as 200%. It is probable that any drug that induces CYP3A4, such as rifampin, will therefore increase the metabolism of sildenafil, subsequently decreasing plasma levels of sildenafil. This has not been definitively proven (see Table 42-2). Nitrates interact with sildenafil, increasing both vasodilation and hypotension.

A drug-food interaction occurs when a patient takes sildenafil with a high-fat meal, delaying the rate of absorption and reducing peak serum levels.

Assessment of Relevant Core Patient Variables

Health Status

The nurse reviews the patient's medication history to determine whether the patient is taking nitrates, because this is a contraindication for use of sildenafil. He or she

TABLE 42-2 Agents That Interact With Sildenafil

Interactants	Effect and Significance	Nursing Management
nitrates	Sildenafil potentiates the vasodilating effect of nitric oxide from nitrates, resulting in a significant and potentially fatal decrease in blood pressure (BP).	Teach patient that he should not use any nitrate while taking sildenafil.
amlodipine	In hypertensive patients, produces mean additional BP reduction of 7–8 mg.	Monitor the patient's BP. In most cases, this drop is not clinically significant.
beta blockers, nonspecific	Beta blockers increase the level of sildenafil's active metabolite; this is not believed to be clinically significant.	None
cimetidine	Coadministration increases the plasma concentrations of sildenafil by more than 50%.	Monitor for adverse effects; a decreased dose may be indicated; consider starting dose of 25 mg.
diuretics	Diuretics increase the level of sildenafil's active metabolite; this is not believed to be clinically significant.	None
erythromycin	A single dose of 100 mg of sildenafil administered with erythromycin at steady state (500 mg bid for 5 days) resulted in a 182% increase in sildenafil's peak concentration.	Monitor for adverse effects; a decreased dose may be indicated; consider starting dose of 25 mg.

assesses for any of the cardiovascular problems that require cautious use of sildenafil: coronary ischemia, CHF, hypotension, or a history of MI, cerebrovascular accident, or life-threatening arrhythmias within the last 6 months. The nurse must verify that the patient is not allergic to any component of sildenafil prior to beginning drug therapy. He or she should also assess for hepatic cirrhosis, which decreases metabolism of sildenafil and increases blood level of active sildenafil. Such patients may need a decreased dose. Although only a small portion of sildenafil is excreted renally, severe renal impairment does increase the maximum concentration that is in the blood. A decreased dose may also be indicated in this situation.

Life Span and Gender

The nurse must inquire about the patient's age. Men aged 65 years or older show increased circulating levels of sildenafil, which is most likely the result of decreased metabolism from normal age-related changes in the liver. They may require a decreased dose. Sildenafil is not approved for use in women.

Lifestyle, Diet, and Habits

A high-fat meal eaten prior to the use of sildenafil will decrease the rate of absorption and reduce the maximum blood level achieved by drug therapy by about 29%. If the patient states that the drug is not always effective, the nurse should assess his dietary intake. Decreasing dietary fat may increase the effectiveness of the drug therapy without a need for an increased dose.

Environment

Sildenafil is self-administered in the home.

Culture

Although most research on sildenafil has been performed on white men, it has also been studied in Asian men and found to be effective and well tolerated in this population (Tan, Moh, Mendoza, Gans, Albano, de la Cruz, et al., 2000).

Nursing Diagnoses and Outcomes

- Sexual Dysfunction related to erection dysfunction
  Desired outcome: *Use of sildenafil will allow the patient to experience normal expression of sexuality.*
- Risk for Injury related to adverse effects of drug therapy.
  Desired outcome: *The patient will not experience adverse effects from sildenafil, or effects will be mild, transient, and well-tolerated.*

Planning and Intervention

Maximizing Therapeutic Effects and Minimizing Adverse Effects

Nursing strategies to maximize the therapeutic effects and minimize the adverse effects of sildenafil are related to the patient education that is provided.

Providing Patient and Family Education

- Sildenafil is not effective without sexual stimulation and arousal.
- The patient should take sildenafil about 1 hour prior to sexual activity.
- The patient should not take nitrates (e.g., nitroglycerin, isosorbide) if also taking sildenafil.
- Sexual activity increases the risk of cardiovascular problems, such as MI, for people with known cardio-

vascular risks. If a patient experiences any symptoms of cardiovascular problems during sexual intercourse (e.g., angina, dizziness, nausea), he must stop the sexual activity. He should discuss any problems experienced with his physician.

- The patient must avoid high-fat meals prior to the use of sildenafil. (See the accompanying display, Effectiveness of Sildenafil.) ■

DRUG CLOSELY RELATED TO SILDENAFIL

A drug closely related to sildenafil is alprostadil, which is also used to treat erectile dysfunction. Unlike sildenafil, which is administered orally, alprostadil is administered by injection into the dorsal lateral aspect of the proximal third of the penis, or by intraurethral pellets. Alprostadil, administered by IV infusion, is used as palliative treatment for infants with patent ductus arteriosus until surgery can be performed. Unlabeled uses of alprostadil include activity in the performance of diagnostic peripheral arteriography and in the treatment of atherosclerosis, gangrene, and pain related to peripheral vascular disease. Alprostadil produces various pharmacologic effects; the most important are relaxation of smooth muscle, vasodilation of the arteries in the erectile tissue, and inhibition of platelet aggregation. Erection is achieved by the combination of relaxation of smooth muscles in the penis and vasodilation. An erection should occur within 5 to 20 minutes after administration. Unlike sildenafil, sexual arousal is not a prerequisite to the effectiveness of alprostadil.

In a recent study, about 40% of the men who used intracavernous injection to treat erectile dysfunction and then used sildenafil considered that the sildenafil response (i.e., quality of erection) was inferior. Some men prefer to continue with intracavernous alprostadil in addition to sildenafil or to use it as an alternative to sildenafil (McMahon, Samali, & Johnson, 2000).

Absorption occurs from the urethra for both forms of administration. With the intraurethral technique, urination should precede drug administration. The residual urine then disperses the medicated pellet, allowing absorption through the urethral mucosa. Little alprostadil enters the general circulation. Alprostadil is rapidly converted to compounds that are further metabolized prior to excretion. Metabolism occurs in the first pass through the lung by way of enzymatic oxidation, and almost all the drug is metabolized. This finding accounts for the very low systemic concentration of alprostadil. Excretion of the metabolites occurs primarily through the kidneys.

Contraindications to alprostadil use are those conditions that might predispose the patient to priapism (erection lasting more than 6 hours). These conditions include sickle cell anemia or trait, multiple myeloma, and leukemia. Alprostadil is also contraindicated in patients with anatomic deformations of the penis (e.g., angulation, cavernosal fibrosis) or penile implants (intracavernosal placement), if sexual activity is inadvisable or contraindicated for the man, and for sexual intercourse with a pregnant woman unless a condom is used. Vasodilation from the drug's action may be harmful to the pregnancy.

The most common adverse effect for both routes is penile pain, which is usually mild or moderate. The most common adverse effects that are solely related to intraurethral administration are urethral pain and burning. Vaginal burning, itching, or both can occur in the female partner of the man using intraurethral administration of alprostadil. Other adverse effects that may occur with the intracavernosal administration route are penile fibrosis, injection site hematoma, prolonged erection, and penile rash or edema. Priapism may occur, although it is not common. Hemodynamic changes (decrease in blood pressure and an increase in heart rate) may result from pharmacodynamics. These changes are not clinically significant.

Patient education on the administration technique is important. It is essential for the nurse to assess the patient's technique prior to using the drug on his own at home.

MEMORY CHIP

Sildenafil

- Used to treat erectile dysfunction in men
- Most significant contraindication: current use of nitrates
- Most common adverse effects: facial flushing, headache, nasal congestion, and heartburn
- Most serious adverse effect: may increase risk of cardiovascular death in patients with current cardiovascular problems
- Most significant patient education: sexual stimulation and arousal are needed for drug effectiveness; take 1 hour before engaging in sexual activity

Critical Thinking Scenario

Effectiveness of sildenafil

Joe Rosenbaum is 64 years old and takes sildenafil for erectile dysfunction. He returns to the clinic for follow-up. On assessment, you learn that the drug therapy appears to be effective and that Mr. Rosenbaum is tolerating it well without apparent adverse effects. You ask whether he has any other concerns or questions. He hesitates, and then laughingly says, "The only thing is, this pill doesn't seem to be as helpful if we've gone out to a restaurant for dinner. I guess it likes my wife's cooking better." What questions might you ask Mr. Rosenbaum to help determine a possible cause of this variation in sildenafil's effectiveness?

DRUG SIGNIFICANTLY DIFFERENT FROM SILDENAFIL

Yohimbine, while a recognized drug, has no approved FDA indications. It has several unlabeled uses, however, for which it is prescribed. Its unlabeled uses are as a sympatholytic and mydriatic. It may have activity as an aphrodisiac. It has been used successfully in treating erectile dysfunction with vascular or diabetic origins, but related data are scanty. In some men whose sexual dysfunction is related to the use of selective serotonin reuptake inhibitors, yohimbine may be helpful in improving sexual function/desire.

Yohimbine is taken orally, three times a day. It is an alkaloid with chemical similarities to the drug reserpine. Yohimbine is believed to have properties similar to *Rauwolfia* alkaloids. It is primarily an alpha-2 adrenergic blocker of presynaptic alpha-2 receptors, which causes release of norepinephrine. Its effect on the peripheral autonomic nervous system is to increase parasympathetic (cholinergic) activity and decrease sympathetic (adrenergic) activity, thus producing erection. Yohimbine has a stimulating effect on mood and may increase anxiety, although mostly at high doses. Yohimbine is contraindicated in renal disease. All major adverse effects occur in the CNS (e.g., nervousness, irritability, tremor, dizziness, headache, and skin flushing). Reportedly the drug exerts no significant influence on cardiac stimulation. Its exact effect on blood pressure is not known.

DRUGS TO TREAT BENIGN PROSTATIC HYPERTROPHY

As discussed earlier, 5-alpha reductase (specifically type II) converts testosterone into the androgen 5-alpha dihydrotestosterone (DHT). Because the prostate gland depends on DHT for growth, interference with this process is helpful in the treatment of BPH. Surgical intervention is one option. Transurethral resection of the prostate (TURP) is the most common surgical intervention, although a prostatectomy or radical prostatectomy may be performed.

The prototype drug for treatment of BPH is finasteride (Proscar). Drugs significantly different from finasteride are the alpha-1 blockers, which include prazosin (Minipres), terazosin (Hytrin), doxazosin (Cardura), and tamsulosin (Flomax).

NURSING MANAGEMENT OF THE PATIENT RECEIVING FINASTERIDE

Core Drug Knowledge

Pharmacotherapeutics

Finasteride is used to treat BPH and androgenetic alopecia (male pattern baldness); the dose for male hair loss is much smaller than is used for BPH. Two separate trade names are used to differentiate these preparations. Proscar is the trade name of finasteride used in BPH. Propecia is the trade name when used for male pattern baldness. Therapeutic effect for BPH is seen within 6 to 12 months of treatment, although it sometimes occurs earlier. Daily usage for more than 3 months is needed to see therapeutic effects when treating baldness. The therapeutic effects are reversed for both BPH and hair loss if the patient stops drug therapy.

Pharmacokinetics

Finasteride is well absorbed after oral administration. Food does not affect its absorption. Finasteride is highly protein bound, at rates of about 90%. It is extensively metabolized in the liver through oxidative pathways. The inactive metabolites are excreted in the bile and feces (see Table 42-1).

Pharmacodynamics

Finasteride specifically inhibits the steroid 5-alpha reductase and consequently blocks the peripheral conversion of testosterone to DHT. The results are significant decreases in serum and tissue DHT concentrations. Finasteride reduces prostatic DHT by as much as 90% and circulating levels of DHT between 60 and 80%. Finasteride also decreases DHT prostate-specific antigen (PSA) levels between 41% and 71%. In addition, finasteride increases testosterone level because testosterone is no longer converted to DHT. These changes improve BPH-related symptoms, increase maximum urinary flow rates, and decrease prostate size.

In men with male pattern hair loss, DHT is found in increased amounts in the scalp. Finasteride decreases scalp and serum DHT concentrations in these men. Finasteride does not appear to affect body hair.

Contraindications and Precautions

Finasteride is contraindicated in women and children. It is a pregnancy category X drug because it will cause abnormalities of the external genitalia in the male fetus. Because of these risks, pregnant women or women who may become pregnant should not handle crushed or broken finasteride tablets. Finasteride is also contraindicated if hypersensitivity to the drug or any of its components exists. Caution should be used if the patient has impaired liver function, because finasteride is metabolized extensively in the liver.

Adverse Effects

Finasteride is generally well tolerated; adverse effects are usually mild and transient. Adverse effects that occur in less than 4% of patients taking finasteride include erectile dysfunction, decreased libido, and decreased volume of ejaculate. Sexual adverse effects resolved with continued treatment in more than 60% of patients who reported these effects (Drug Facts & Comparisons, 2000). Overdose of finasteride has not been associated with adverse effects.

Drug Interactions

Finasteride will decrease PSA levels by about 50%. A decrease in PSA level will occur even if the patient also has prostate cancer. This reduction does not suggest a beneficial effect of finasteride on prostate cancer but rather an effect of the drug.

Assessment of Relevant Core Patient Variables

Health Status

Prior to administering the drug, the nurse should verify that the patient has the clinical indications for receiving finasteride. He or she should assess patients with BPH for prostate cancer before beginning and periodically throughout therapy.

Life Span and Gender

Finasteride is not given to women or children.

Environment

The nurse should be aware of the environment in which the medication will be administered. Finasteride may be administered in any environment but is most frequently self-administered in the home.

Nursing Diagnoses and Outcomes

- Risk for Sexual Dysfunction related to drug therapy
  Desired outcome: If the patient experiences sexual dysfunction, it will resolve with continued drug therapy.
- Impaired Urinary Elimination related to BPH
  Desired outcome: Following drug therapy with finasteride, the patient will have no or fewer lower urinary tract symptoms from BPH.

Planning and Intervention

Minimizing Adverse Effects

To minimize adverse effects from occurring in the female nurse, the nurse, if pregnant or in the childbearing years, should not handle crushed or broken finasteride tablets. Absorption is more likely to occur in these circumstances, and the drug is pregnancy category X. When the drug is given at home, the nurse teaches the patient and family how to handle the drug to minimize risks.

Providing Patient and Family Education

- The nurse teaches the patient the following:
- Rationale for drug use
- Possible adverse effects of the drug (impotence and decreased libido) and that these are usually transient
- That volume of ejaculate may decrease with the use of finasteride but does not interfere with normal sexual function
- The nurse should warn female family members capable of having children or currently pregnant not to handle broken or crushed finasteride. (See the accompanying display, Saw Palmetto and Benign Prostatic Hypertrophy.)

Focus on Research

Saw palmetto and benign prostatic hypertrophy (BPH)

Gerber, G. S. (2000). Saw palmetto for the treatment of men with lower urinary tract symptoms. *Journal of Urology, 163*(5), 1408–1412.
Marks, L. S., Partin, A. W., Epstein, J. I., Tyler, V. E., Simon, I., Macairan, M. L., Chan, T. L., et al. (2000). Effects of a saw palmetto herbal blend in men with symptomatic benign prostatic hyperplasia. *Journal of Urology, 163*(5), 1451–1456.
Wilt, T., Ishani, A., Stark, G., MacDonald, R., Mulrow, C., & Lau, J. (2000). *Serenoa repens* for benign prostatic hyperplasia. *Cochrane Database System Review,* (2), CD001423.

The Studies

Saw palmetto, also known as *Serenoa repens,* is an herb sold over the counter with claims it improves a man's prostate health and decreases the urinary symptoms of BPH. Several studies have been done to determine if saw palmetto is indeed a safe and effective therapy for BPH. Two reviews of the literature (Gerber, 2000; Wilt et al., 2000) were conducted with the aim of determining mechanisms of action and effectiveness of saw palmetto. An additional new small clinical study also examined the effects of this herb.

Clinical studies reported in the literature suggest that saw palmetto does positively affect urinary flow rates and lower urinary tract symptoms in men with mild to moderate BPH when compared with placebo. The literature also suggests that saw palmetto produces similar improvements in urinary symptoms and flow rate when compared with finasteride. Saw palmetto appears safe and to have few to no adverse effects. Long-term efficacy, safety, and ability to prevent BPH complications, however, have not been determined.

Research studies have demonstrated various potential mechanisms of action of saw palmetto. These include 5-alpha reductase inhibition, adrenergic receptor antagonism, intraprostatic androgen receptor blockade, and prostate epithelial contraction.

Nursing Implications

Americans are widely using alternative medicines and complementary therapies. People are self-treating with herbs for various problems. Frequently, people do not tell their doctors or nurses that they are using herbs. Nurses need to be aware that their male patients may be using saw palmetto to treat symptoms of BPH. The nurse should ask whether the patient uses saw palmetto when obtaining a drug history so that the drug history is complete. Patients may seek information on the safety and efficacy of this herb from nurses. Although the nurse would not prescribe saw palmetto (unless he or she is a nurse practitioner), patient teaching can include that this herb appears to be safe and effective if the patient has mild to moderate symptoms of BPH. Nurses should caution patients that more research needs to be done in a large controlled clinical drug study to fully determine the long-term effects and safety of saw palmetto. They should teach patients not to randomly substitute this herb for any prescribed medication. Nurses should encourage patients seeking assistance for symptoms of BPH to discuss the use of saw palmetto as one treatment option with either the physician or nurse practitioner.

Ongoing Assessment and Evaluation

The nurse should monitor the patient for improvement in BPH-related symptoms and increased ease of urination. If used for male pattern baldness, increased hair growth and decreased hair loss indicate effectiveness. Throughout therapy, the nurse monitors men with BPH for prostate cancer. PSA levels require monitoring throughout therapy. The nurse carefully evaluates any

MEMORY CHIP

Finasteride

- Used to treat BPH and male pattern baldness
- Most significant contraindication: use in women and children
- Most common adverse effects: altered sexual function (effects are mild and transient)
- **Lifespan alert: pregnancy category X**
- Most significant patient education: women should not handle crushed or broken tablets

man on finasteride whose PSA levels increase; this development may be related to noncompliance or to prostate cancer. ■

DRUGS SIGNIFICANTLY DIFFERENT FROM FINASTERIDE

The alpha-1 blockers include prazosin (Minipres), terazosin (Hytrin), doxazosin (Cardura), and tamsulosin (Flomax). These drugs benefit patients with BPH by relaxing prostatic smooth muscle and relieving the lower urinary tract symptoms of BPH. Although a review of clinical drug trials shows that all the alpha adrenergic receptor antagonists are similar in their efficacy in symptom relief and urodynamic improvement (Clifford & Farmer, 2000), the FDA has approved only terazosin, dosazosin, and tamsulosin for this usage. One recent study suggests that tamsulosin may be safer than the other alpha-1 blockers for older men and patients with hypertension who have impaired blood pressure regulation. This study also suggests that terazosin may be more effective in improving lower urinary tract symptoms than the other alpha-1 blockers (Tsujii, 2000), although other studies have not supported this possibility.

Alpha-1 blockers have a rapid onset of action, producing a therapeutic response within weeks (regardless of the presence of prostatic enlargement or bladder outlet obstruction). This is in contrast to finasteride, which takes longer to achieve therapeutic effects and alleviates only those symptoms associated with a significantly large prostate. Except for tamsulosin, alpha-1 blockers are also used to treat hypertension (see Chapter 30 for more information). Tamsulosin is similar to finasteride in that neither drug lowers blood pressure and therefore neither is associated with the cardiovascular adverse effects (e.g., dizziness, postural hypotension) that are linked with the other alpha blockers. Both are associated, however, with an increased risk of sexual dysfunction; tamsulosin is associated with ejaculatory dysfunction, and finasteride is associated with decreased libido and erectile dysfunction.

DRUGS TO TREAT MALE PATTERN BALDNESS

Male pattern baldness may respond to drug therapy with topical minoxidil (Rogaine, Minoxidil for Men), which is the prototype drug. A drug significantly different from minoxidil is finasteride (Propecia), previously discussed.

NURSING MANAGEMENT OF THE PATIENT RECEIVING MINOXIDIL

Core Drug Knowledge

Pharmacotherapeutics

Minoxidil is used topically in the treatment of androgenetic alopecia. Although men primarily use minoxidil, women also may use it. Minoxidil is effective in male pattern baldness of the vertex and in women with diffuse hair loss or thinning of the frontoparietal areas. It is not effective in patients who have predominantly frontal hair loss. Topical minoxidil is available as an over-the-counter (OTC) medication.

Pharmacokinetics

Topical minoxidil has poor absorption from normal intact scalp. Decreased integrity of the epidermal barrier from conditions such as inflammation, excoriations of the scalp, scalp psoriasis, or severe sunburn may increase systemic absorption. Possibly, these abnormal scalp conditions may increase absorption enough to pose a risk for increased adverse effects.

Pharmacodynamics

The exact mode of action for topical minoxidil is unknown. Oral minoxidil was originally developed to be a peripheral vasodilator used in the treatment of hypertension. Hair growth was found to be an adverse effect of the drug when used orally (see chapter 30 for more information on peripheral vasodilators used in hypertension). Topical applications require at least 4 months of twice-daily application before the patient can expect evidence of hair growth. About 60% of patients who use the product experience hair growth. Patients who are responsive to drug therapy need to continue the drug to maintain therapeutic effects. There are reports that the balding process will return 3 to 4 months after stopping drug therapy.

Contraindications and Precautions

The only contraindication to topical minoxidil is hypersensitivity to any component of the drug. Topical minoxidil is classified as a pregnancy category C drug, because no adequate and well-controlled studies in pregnant women have been conducted. Thus, women must avoid use during pregnancy. Safety and efficacy in children younger than 18 years have not been established.

Adverse Effects

The most common adverse effects of topical minoxidil are irritant dermatitis and allergic contact dermatitis. Other dermatologic effects are eczema, local erythema, pruritus, dry skin/scalp flaking, and exacerbation of hair loss/alopecia. From any systemic absorption the adverse effects of orally administered minoxidil are possible. These include edema, chest pain, blood pressure changes (increases or decreases), and pulse changes (increases or decreases).

Topical minoxidil contains alcohol. If the drug gets into the eyes, mouth, or mucous membranes or onto sensitive skin, burning or irritation may develop. Overdosage is unknown with topical applications of minoxidil.

Drug Interactions

Topical minoxidil should not be used in conjunction with other topical agents (e.g., corticosteroids, retinoids, petrolatum) known to enhance cutaneous drug absorption.

Assessment of Relevant Core Patient Variables

Health Status

The nurse must verify that the patient has male pattern baldness and does not have predominantly frontal hair loss, because topical minoxidil is not effective for frontal hair loss. If given to women, the hair loss must be diffuse or identified as thinning of the frontoparietal area for the drug to be effective. The nurse should ensure that the patient has a normal, healthy scalp prior to beginning and throughout therapy. A nonintact scalp will promote systemic absorption, and adverse effects may be more prominent, especially in patients with a history of heart disease. The nurse must monitor these patients closely for any problems with tachycardia or fluid retention.

Life Span and Gender

Topical minoxidil is used primarily in men, although it may be used in women. If female patients, the nurse must assess for pregnancy and intention to become pregnant, because use of minoxidil in pregnancy is to be avoided. The nurse must ensure that the patient is older than 18 years of age, because the drug's safety for children has not been established.

Environment

The nurse should be aware of the environment in which minoxidil will be administered. Topical minoxidil is self administered in the patient's home.

Nursing Diagnoses and Outcomes

- Situational Low Self-Esteem related to hair loss
  Desired outcome: The patient's self-esteem will improve related to hair growth from drug therapy.
- Risk for Injury related to adverse effects of drug therapy
  Desired outcome: The patient will not experience adverse effects of drug therapy.

Planning and Intervention

Maximizing Therapeutic Effects and Minimizing Adverse Effects

Nursing actions to maximize the therapeutic effect and to minimize the adverse effects are related to patient education.

Providing Patient and Family Education

- The nurse teaches the patient receiving topical minoxidil the purpose and possible adverse effects of the drug.
- The nurse teaches the patient to administer the drug using this technique:
  - Dry the hair and scalp before application.
  - Apply 1 mL to the total affected areas of the scalp twice daily, once in the morning and once at night.
  - Wash hands after applying the drug.
  - Do not apply if scalp is irritated or sunburned, because these circumstances may increase the risk of adverse effects.
  - Do not try to make up for any missed doses. Resume normal administration schedule instead.
  - Do not use more than the prescribed amount twice a day.
  - Twice daily use for 4 months or longer may be needed to see results. Fine, soft colorless hair that is barely visibly may be the first hair to grow. Over time, the new hair will be the same color and thickness as the other hair on the scalp.
- Keep medication out of eyes and mouth; avoid applying to sensitive skin on the face. If accidental exposure occurs, flush the area with large amounts of cool tap water. Consult with the physician if irritation continues.
- Do not use along with other topical medications on the scalp.
- If no response to treatment occurs in 4 months or more, consult with the physician about the appropriateness of continuing therapy.

MEMORY CHIP

Minoxidil (topical)

- Used topically to promote growth of hair in male pattern baldness
- Use for 4 months or more required to see effect
- Is an over-the-counter drug
- Most common adverse effects: irritation and dermatitis at application site
- Most serious adverse effects: edema and tachycardia
- Most significant patient education: use bid; do not increase dosage or frequency; do not use if scalp is irritated or sunburned

Ongoing Assessment and Evaluation

The nurse should assess the patient's scalp periodically to determine whether irritation has developed. The patient will usually do this personally during therapy. Topical minoxidil treatment is effective when hair growth has occurred with no adverse effects. ■

CHAPTER SUMMARY

- Testosterone is the main male sex hormone. Insufficient testosterone will prevent the growth spurt of adolescence and the development of secondary male sex characteristics. Lack of testosterone after development of secondary sex characteristics will cause them to diminish.
- Exogenous testosterone is used when endogenous levels are low. Exogenous testosterone will cause the same effects on the body as endogenous testosterone.
- One problem affecting male sexuality is erectile dysfunction. This problem may result from multiple factors, such as stress, adverse effects of drug therapy, and cardiovascular or neurologic impairments.
- When erectile dysfunction is a recurring problem, drug therapy may be used. Drug therapy used in erectile dysfunction includes sildenafil, alprostadil, and occasionally yohimbine. Sildenafil has the advantage of being a drug taken orally that is very effective. Sildenafil requires sexual stimulation for effectiveness.
- A common problem of the older man is BPH. The exact cause of BPH is unknown, although excessive growth of the prostate is believed to be caused primarily by elevated levels of DHT (the primary hormone in the prostate cells). Overgrowth of the prostate places pressure on the urethra and the bladder, causing lower urinary tract symptoms.
- Drug therapy is one type of treatment for BPH. Drug therapy for BPH includes finasteride, which decreases the size of the prostate over time, and alpha-1 blockers, which relax the smooth muscle of the bladder and decrease difficulties in voiding.
- Male pattern baldness is another men's health issue. Changing testosterone levels or alterations in the male sex hormone receptors may be related to this problem.
- Topical minoxidil can be effective in promoting hair growth for male pattern baldness. This drug is available OTC. Women may also use minoxidil.

QUESTIONS FOR STUDY AND REVIEW

1. What effects does testosterone have on the male?
2. What is the main risk when administering testosterone to induce the growth spurt of puberty?
3. How does sildenafil act to help the man achieve an erection?
4. Why should women not handle broken or crushed finasteride?
5. Topical minoxidil is poorly absorbed into the systemic circulation. What is the advantage of this factor?

NEED MORE HELP?

Chapter 42 of the study guide for *Drug Therapy in Nursing* contains exercises and activities to reinforce your understanding of the concepts presented in this chapter. For additional information see the text's accompanying website at *http://www.connection.lww.com*.

REFERENCES AND BIBLIOGRAPHY

Blanker, M. H., Bohnen, A. M., Groeneveld, F. P., Bernsen, R. M., Prins, A., & Ruud Bosch, J. L. (2000). Normal voiding patterns and determinants of increased diurnal and nocturnal voiding frequency in elderly men. *Journal of Urology, 164*(4), 1201–1205.

Boyle, P., Robertson, C., Lowe, F., & Roehrborn, C. (2000). Meta-analysis of clinical trials of permixon in the treatment of symptomatic benign prostatic hyperplasia. *Urology, 55*(4), 533–539.

Christiansen, E., Guirguis, W. R., Cox, D., & Osterloh, I. H. (2000). Long-term efficacy and safety of oral Viagra (sildenafil citrate) in men with erectile dysfunction and the effect of randomised treatment withdrawal. Sildenafil Multicentre Study Group. *International Journal of Impotence Research, 12*(3), 177–182.

Clifford, G. M., & Farmer, R. D. (2000). Medical therapy for benign prostatic hyperplasia: A review of the literature. *European Urology, 38*(1), 2–19.

DeBusk, R., Drory, Y., Goldstein, I., Jackson, G., Kaul, S., Kimmel, S. E., Kostis, J. B., et al. (2000). Management of sexual dysfunction in patients with cardiovascular disease: recommendations of the Princeton Consensus Panel. *American Journal of Cardiology, 86*(2A), 62F–68F.

Enid, J. F. (2000). Sildenafil citrate: Current clinical experience. *International Journal of Impotence Research, 12,* (Suppl. 4), S62-6.

Feng, M. I., Huang, S., Kaptein, J., Kaswick, J., & Aboseif, S. (2000). Effect of sildenafil citrate on postradical prostatectomy erectile dysfunction. *Journal of Urology, 164*(6), 1935–1938.

Giuliano, F., Montorsi, F., Mirone, V., Rossi, D., & Sweeney, M. (2000). Switching from intracavernous prostaglandin E1 injections to oral sildenafil citrate in patients with erectile dysfunction: Results of a multicenter European study. The Sildenafil Multicenter Study Group. *Journal of Urology, 164*(3 Pt 1), 708–11.

Kovac, J., & Mensa, J. (1999). Sexual activity and the cardiovascular system in health and disease. Use of sildenafil in heart patients [in Czech]. *Vnitrni Lekarstvi, 45*(10), 610–613.

Lepor, H., Jones, K., & Williford, W. (2000). The mechanism of adverse events associated with terazosin: An analysis of the Veterans Affairs cooperative study. *Journal of Urology, 163*(4), 1134–1137.

McMahon, C. G., Samali, R., & Johnson, H. (2000). Efficacy, safety and patient acceptance of sildenafil citrate as treatment for erectile dysfunction. *Journal of Urology, 164*(4), 1192–1196.

Mediconsult.com. *Educational materials on BPH* [On-line]. Available: http://www.mediconsult.com/mc/mcsite.nsf/con . . . /bph~Educational+Material.

Medina, P., Segarra, G., Vila, J. M., Domenech, C., Martinez-Leon, J. B., & Lluch, S. (2000).

Effects of sildenafil on human penile blood vessels. *Urology, 56*(3), 539–543.

Michel, M. C., Mehlburger, L., Schumacher, H., Bressel, H. U., & Goepel, M. (2000). Effect of diabetes on lower urinary tract symptoms in patients with benign prostatic hyperplasia. *Journal of Urology, 163*(6), 1725–1729.

Michelakis, E., Tymchak, W., & Archer, S. (2000). Sildenafil: From the bench to the bedside. *Canadian Medical Association Journal, 163*(9), 1171–1175.

Moreira, S. G. Jr., Brannigan, R. E., Spitz, A., Orejuela, F. J., Lipshultz, L. I., & Kim, E. D. (2000). Side-effect profile of sildenafil citrate (Viagra) in clinical practice. *Urology, 56*(3), 474–476.

Muirhead, G. J., Wulff, M. B., Fielding, A., Kleinermans, D., & Buss, N. (2000). Pharmacokinetic interactions between sildenafil and saquinavir/ritonavir. *British Journal of Clinical Pharmacology, 50*(2), 99–107.

Mydlo, J. H., Volpe, M. A., & MacChia, R. J. (2000). Results from different patient populations using combined therapy with alprostadil and sildenafil: predictors of satisfaction. *BJU International, 86*(4), 469–473.

Palmer, J. S., Kaplan, W. E., & Firlit, C. F. (2000). Erectile dysfunction in patients with spina bifida is a treatable condition. *Journal of Urology, 164*(3 Pt 2), 958–961.

Philpot, C. D., & Morley, J. E. (2000). Health issues unique to the aging man. *Geriatric Nursing, 21*(5), 234–241.

Roehrborn C. G., Bruskewitz, R., Nickel, G. C., Glickman, S., Cox, C., Anderson, R., Kandzari, S., et al. (2000). Urinary retention in patients with BPH treated with finasteride or placebo over 4 years. Characteristics of patients and ultimate outcomes. The PLESS Study Group. *European Urology, 37*(5), 528–536.

Reuters Medical News. (2000, Nov. 20). *Herbal remedy PC-SPES active against advanced prostate cancer* [On-line]. Available: http://nurses.medscape.com/reuters/prof/2000/11/11.20/20001117drgd003.html.

Tan, H. M., Moh, C. L., Mendoza, J. B., Gans, T., Albano, G. J., de la Cruz, R., Chye, P. L., & Sam, C. C. (2000). Asian sildenafil efficacy and safety study (ASSESS-1): A double-blind, placebo-controlled, flexible-dose study of oral sildenafil in malaysian, singaporean, and filipino men with erectile dysfunction (1). *Urology, 56*(4), 635–640.

Tsujii, T. (2000). Comparison of prazosin, terazosin and tamsulosin in the treatment of symptomatic benign prostatic hyperplasia: A short-term open, randomized multicenter study. BPH Medical Therapy Study Group. Benign prostatic hyperplasia. *International Journal of Urology, 7*(6), 199–205.

Zagaja, G. P., Mhoon, D. A., Aikens, J. E., & Brendler, C. B. (2000). Sildenafil in the treatment of erectile dysfunction after radical prostatectomy. *Urology, 56*(4), 631–634.

Chapter 43

DRUGS AFFECTING WOMEN'S HEALTH AND SEXUALITY

KEY TERMS

estrogen
follicle-stimulating hormone
gonadotropin-releasing hormone
luteinizing hormone
menopause
osteoporosis
Paget disease
progestin
proliferative phase
secretory phase

Learning Objectives

At the completion of this chapter the student will:

1. Identify core drug knowledge about drugs that affect women's health and sexuality.
2. Identify core patient variables relevant to drugs that affect women's health and sexuality.
3. Relate the interaction of core drug knowledge to core patient variables for drugs that affect women's health and sexuality.
4. Compare the risks and benefits of hormone replacement therapy in postmenopausal women.
5. Generate a nursing plan of care from the interactions between core drug knowledge and core patient variables for drugs that affect women's health and sexuality.
6. Describe nursing interventions to maximize therapeutic and minimize adverse effects of drugs that affect women's health and sexuality.
7. Determine key points for patient and family education for drugs that affect women's health and sexuality.

Estrogens

conjugated estrogen
synthetic conjugated estrogens, A
oral contraceptives
clomiphene
gonadotropins
human chorionic gondadotropin
gonadotropin-releasing hormone
androgen-estrogen combinations
synthetic androgens

Progestins

progesterone
megestrol acetate
oral contraceptives
levonorgestrel implants
intrauterine progesterone contraceptive system
mifepristone

Oral contraceptives

Bisphosphonates

alendronate
etidronate
tiludronate
pamidronate
risendronate
raloxifene

The symbol C indicates the **drug class**.
Drugs in bold type marked with the symbol P are **prototypes**.
Drugs in blue type with no symbol are **closely related** to the prototype.
Drugs in **red** type with no symbol are **significantly different** from the prototype.
Drugs in **black** type with no symbol are **also used in drug therapy**; no prototype.

The female sex hormones are responsible for the normal development and maintenance of adult female sexual characteristics. If endogenous hormone levels are insufficient, sexual characteristics will fail to develop. If endogenous levels are low after the development of female sexual characteristics, the woman may be unable to become pregnant or maintain a pregnancy. If levels of sex hormones become low enough, masculinization may occur. Additionally, research has shown that low levels of female sex hormones contribute to some common women's health problems. This chapter presents the use of female sex hormones as replacement drug therapy when endogenous levels are absent or insufficient. It discusses two classes of female sex hormones: estrogens and progestins. The prototype estrogen is conjugated estrogen (Premarin), and the prototype progestin is progesterone (Prometrium, Progesterone).

This chapter also presents drug therapy used in the treatment of osteoporosis, a common health problem in postmenopausal women. The prototype drug is alendronate (Fosamax).

PHYSIOLOGY

The female sex hormones are responsible for the production of female sexual characteristics, development of the female reproductive system, and maintenance of pregnancy. The two types of female sex hormones are **estrogen** and **progestin.** Both are steroidal compounds that the ovaries begin to secrete at puberty and that the placenta secretes during pregnancy. The adrenal cortex also secretes estrogen and progestin, but in much smaller amounts.

ESTROGEN

The female body produces six different estrogens but only three in significant amounts: estradiol, estrone, and estriol. Estradiol is the most potent and the major estrogen secreted by the ovaries. In addition to promoting and maintaining female organs and secondary sexual characteristics (i.e., distribution of body hair, high-pitched voice), estrogen affects the release of pituitary gonadotropins, causes capillary dilation, and promotes fluid retention. It also enhances protein anabolism, promotes thinning of cervical mucus, inhibits or facilitates ovulation, and prevents postpartum breast pain. Estrogen also maintains the tone and elasticity of the urogenital structures and stimulates growth of axillary and pubic hair and pigmentation of the nipples and genitals.

Estrogen promotes growth during the adolescent growth spurt; continued elevated levels of estrogen terminate growth by stimulating closure of the epiphyses of the long bones. This results because estrogen stimulates the osteoblasts in the bone to produce bone faster than the epiphyseal cartilage can expand. As estrogens cause a faster epiphyseal closure than androgens, women are generally shorter than men by adulthood. Indirectly, estrogen contributes to strengthening the skeleton by conserving calcium and phosphorus and encouraging bone formation. After puberty, estrogen is important in maintaining normal bone density and composition. The organic and mineral components of bone are continuously being recycled and renewed throughout life; this process is called bone remodeling.

PROGESTIN

Progestins, which include progesterone and its derivatives, are the other female sex hormones. Progesterone is the primary endogenous progestational substance. The progestins change the proliferative endometrium into a secretory endometrium. Through positive feedback, they also inhibit or facilitate the secretion of pituitary gonadotropins. Doing so either prevents follicular maturation and ovulation or promotes maturation for the primed follicle. Progestins also inhibit spontaneous uterine contractions and contractions of other smooth muscles throughout the body. They may also demonstrate some anabolic or androgenic activity.

MENSTRUAL CYCLE

Much of the secretion of the female sex hormones is cyclic, and these cyclic changes comprise the menstrual cycle. **Gonadotropin-releasing hormone** (GRH), which is secreted by the hypothalamus and then perfused throughout the anterior pituitary, stimulates the release of **follicle-stimulating hormone** (FSH) and **luteinizing hormone** (LH). During puberty, the pituitary gland secretes large volumes of FSH and LH to initiate and establish the menstrual cycle. These hormones stimulate the development of the ovarian follicles and the release of the ovum from the mature follicle (Fig. 43-1). As the follicles grow, they produce estrogen. Estrogen increases the vascularity of the uterine lining, preparing it for implantation of a fertilized egg. This phase of the menstrual cycle is termed the **proliferative phase.** The rapidly rising estrogen levels further stimulate GRH, encouraging further release of LH. The high levels of LH trigger the rupture of the mature follicle, and ovulation occurs.

After ovulation, the follicle is transformed into the corpus luteum, which secretes much progesterone and estrogen. This phase is known as the **secretory phase** of the menstrual cycle. In response to the rising levels of estrogen and progesterone, the endometrial glands continue to grow, the arteries of the endometrium become spiraled, and the endometrium prepares for implantation of a fertilized egg. When estrogen and progesterone have reached critical levels, they create a negative feedback on further release of GRH and indirectly on release of FSH and LH. If fertilization does not occur, the corpus luteum disintegrates, estrogen and progesterone levels fall, and the endometrial tissue sloughs off in the menses. As the levels of estrogen and progesterone continue to decline, GRH is again secreted, reinitiating the process. If fertilization occurs, the corpus luteum remains and continues to secrete estrogen and progesterone for the first month of pregnancy. By the second month, the placenta has developed, and it becomes the major source of estrogen and progesterone to maintain the pregnancy.

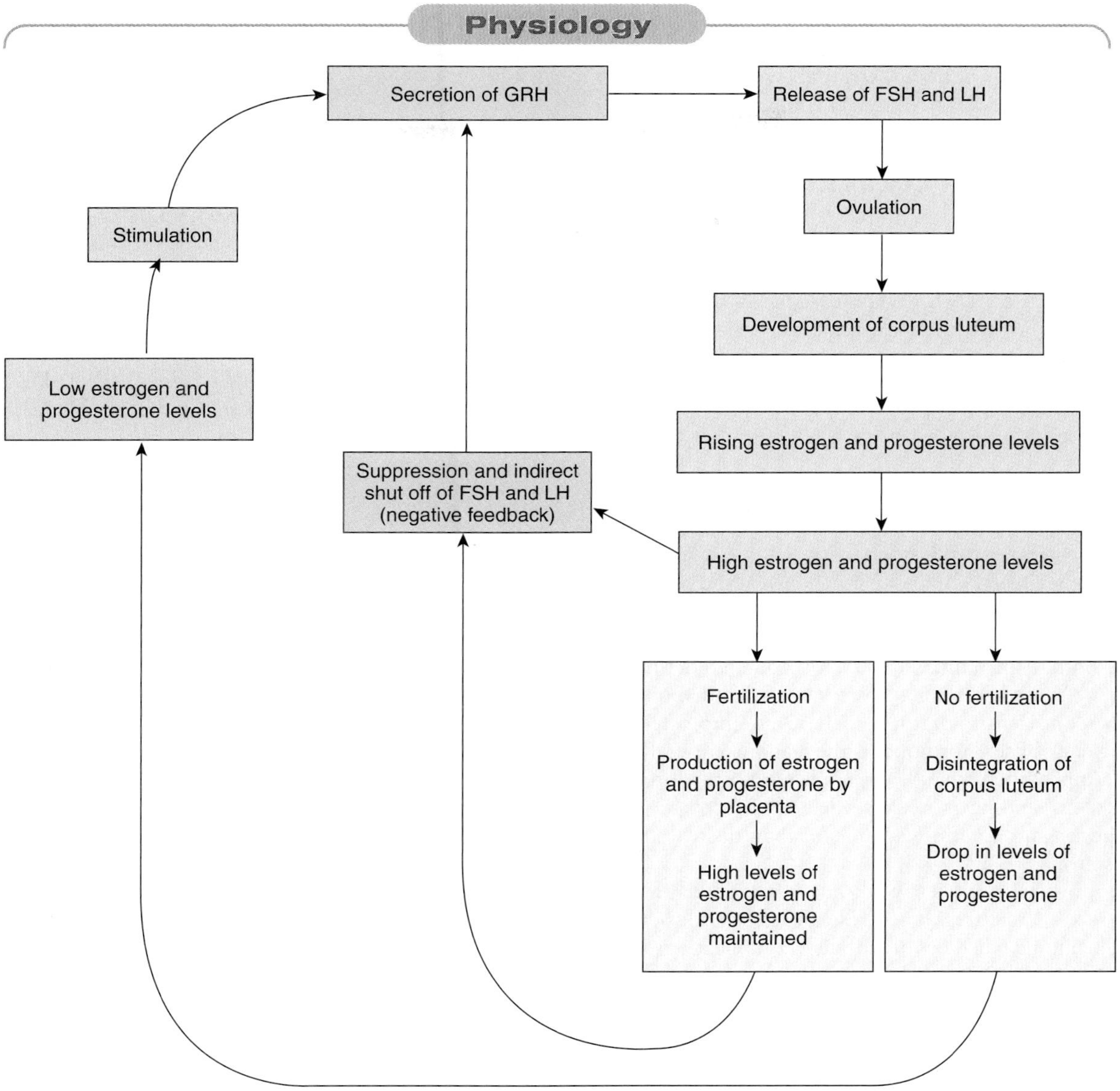

Figure 43-1. Menstrual cycle and fertility. In the *proliferative phase* of the menstrual cycle gonadotropin-releasing hormone (GRH) is secreted by the hypothalamus and perfused through the anterior pituitary, which stimulates release of both follicle-stimulating hormone (FSH) and luteinizing hormone (LH). In response, estrogen production is stimulated in preparation for implantation of a fertilized egg. Then the *secretory phase* of the menstrual cycle begins, during which rising estrogen levels stimulate GRH, which stimulates release of more LH, which in turn prompts ovulation and the formation of the corpus luteum. Estrogen and progesterone levels continue to rise in preparation for implantation of a fertilized egg. When estrogen and progesterone levels peak, they halt additional release of GRH and indirectly, FSH and LH. When fertilization does not occur, the corpus luteum is sloughed off, and estrogen and progesterone levels fall. GRH is again secreted to continue the cycle. When fertilization occurs, the corpus luteum remains to provide estrogen and progesterone until the second month of pregnancy when the placenta is developed and becomes the major source of estrogen and progesterone to maintain the pregnancy.

PATHOPHYSIOLOGY

If a woman is deficient in endogenous sex hormones, she will not experience normal sexual development. The primary sex organs will not mature, secondary sexual characteristics will not develop, reproduction will not be possible, and the normal growth spurt of adolescence will not happen. If levels of endogenous hormones drop after puberty has occurred and the sexual organs and reproductive system have matured, secondary sexual characteristics may diminish. Ability to reproduce, despite developed organs, will be diminished, and the woman may be unable to carry a pregnancy to term.

When a woman's estrogen levels drop during **menopause,** the ending of the monthly ovarian cycles, she experiences several changes. A vasomotor response is typical. The woman will experience periods of hot flashes not related to physical exertion and perfuse periodic sweating, even at night, which may awaken women from sleep. The menstrual periods become irregular because the frequency and quality of ovulation decrease. In addition, vaginal secretions diminish, the drier vagina may be uncomfortable, and intercourse may become uncomfortable or painful.

The loss of estrogen from menopause appears to affect the cardiovascular system negatively, placing postmenopausal women at increased risk for cardiovascular disease and myocardial infarction (MI). For example, the risk for coronary artery disease (CAD) increases twofold after menopause, and heart disease is the primary cause of death for postmenopausal women. The exact effect of estrogen on the cardiovascular system is still being researched. (Also see Chapter 28 for drugs to treat angina.)

In postmenopausal women, the loss of estrogen and its positive effects on bone remodeling contribute to the development of osteoporosis. **Osteoporosis,** characterized by low bone mineral density, is a loss in bone mass sufficient to compromise normal function. Osteoporosis occurs when the body fails to form enough new bone, reabsorbs too much of the old bone, or both. Approximately 20% of women older than 50 years in the United States have osteoporosis, and about 50% have low bone density that may deteriorate into osteoporosis. Deficiency of sex hormones is the leading cause of osteoporosis. Approximately 80% of people with osteoporosis are women. This finding is because decreased estrogen levels occur sooner and are more significant than decreased levels of testosterone.

Osteoporosis produces weak bones and leads to an increased risk of fractures. Fractures can have serious complications, including pain, loss of mobility, complications related to immobility, and death. Bone changes in postmenopausal women may also be related to decreased physical activity. Heavily stressed bones, such as develop with regular weight-bearing exercise (e.g., walking, running), are stronger and thicker; bones not subjected to ordinary stresses become thin and brittle. Moderate physical activity and weight bearing are essential for bone remodeling. Other than decreased estrogen levels, osteoporosis may result from corticosteroid excess (e.g., Cushing disease), hyperthyroidism, hyperparathyroidism, immobilization, bone malignancies, and genetic disorders. Risk factors for osteoporosis include Asian or white race, family history of osteoporosis, smoking, eating disorders, excessive alcohol intake, low dietary calcium, eating disorders, and use of steroid medications.

Deficiencies of estrogen may possibly be related to dementia and decreased cognitive function. In healthy aging women, hormone-replacement therapy (HRT) has been shown to have small but inconsistent effects on cognitive function, including enhancement of verbal memory, abstract reasoning, and information processing. Epidemiologic studies have suggested that HRT protects against the development of clinically diagnosed Alzheimer disease. Controlled experimental studies, however, have found that estrogen therapy has not been able to prevent further cognitive decline in women who already have Alzheimer disease. More research is needed on the effect of estrogen on mental function and Alzheimer disease (Hogervorst, Williams, Budge, Riedel, & Jolles, 2000).

ESTROGENS

The many different types of estrogen differ by indications (with most being used for HRT), route of administration, and pharmacokinetics. Conjugated estrogen (Premarin) is the prototype. Other estrogens are estradiol (Estrace, Fem-Patch, Vivelle, Vivelle-Dot, Climara, Alora, Estraderm, Delestrogen, Gynogen, Valergen) [oral, transdermal, in oil for IM injection, vaginal cream, and vaginal ring], estrone (Kestrone) (IM injection), esterified estrogens (Estratab, Menest) (oral), estropipate (Ortho-Est, Ogen, estropipate) (oral), ethinyl estradiol (Estinyl) (oral), estradiol hemihydrate (Vagifem) (vaginal tablets), and estradiol cypionate (dep-Gynogen, Depo-Estradiol Dypionate, DepoGen) (IM injection). Drugs closely related to conjugated estrogen are oral contraceptives and synthetic conjugated estrogens, A (Cenestin).

Several drugs that affect female sexuality are significantly different from conjugated estrogen. These are clomiphene (Clomid, Milophene, Serophene), the gonadotropins (follitropin alfa [Gonal-F], follitropin beta [Follistim], urofollitropin [Fertinex], and menotropins [Pergonal, Humegon, Repronex]), human chorionic gonadotropin (hCG) (A.P.L., Chorex-5, Profasi, Choron 10, Gonic, Pregnyl), gonad-releasing hormones (gonadorelin acetate [Lutrepulse], nafarelin acetate [Synarel], and histrelin acetate [Supprelin]), androgen-estrogen combination drugs (DepAndrogyn, Depo-Testadiol, Duratestrin, Valertest No. 1, Premarin with Methyltestosterone, Estratest), and synthetic androgens (danzal) (Danocrine).

NURSING MANAGEMENT OF THE PATIENT RECEIVING CONJUGATED ESTROGEN

Core Drug Knowledge

Pharmacotherapeutics

Conjugated estrogen is used primarily as HRT in female hypogonadism, female castration, and primary ovarian failure. Estrogen replacement therapy is also used in menopausal women to treat moderate to severe vasomotor responses (hot flashes). Other uses in menopause include treatment of atrophic vaginitis, vaginal dryness, painful intercourse, mood swings, and loss of tone in genitourinary muscles. Another use is in postmenopausal women who have evidence of bone loss (osteoporosis) to reduce further bone loss and to improve bone density (Table 43-1). Conjugated estrogen is also used to treat abnormal uterine bleeding resulting from hormonal imbalance with no organic pathology. Additionally, conjugated estrogen is used as palliative therapy in advanced prostatic cancer, men with metastatic breast cancer, and selected women with breast cancer who do not have an estrogen-dependent tumor.

TABLE 43-1 Summary of Selected Estrogens

Drug (Trade) Name	Selected Indications	Route and Dosage Range	Pharmacokinetics
conjugated estrogen (Premarin; *Canadian:* Congest)	Hormone replacement therapy	*Adult:* PO, 0.3–7.5 mg/d cyclically (3 wk on, 1 wk off)	*Onset:* Slow *Duration:* 24 h $t_{1/2}$: Unknown
estradiol, transdermal (Vivelle, Estraderm, Climara)	Female hypogonadism Vasomotor symptoms associated with menopause Hormone replacement therapy	*Adult:* 0.05 mg applied to skin once or twice weekly (brand dependent)	*Onset:* Slow *Duration:* 3–7 d $t_{1/2}$: Unknown
estradiol, oral (Estrace)	Hormone replacement therapy Inoperable breast cancer	*Adult:* PO, 1–2 mg/d *Adult:* 10 mg tid; prostatic cancer 1–2 mg tid	*Onset:* Slow *Duration:* Unknown $t_{1/2}$: Unknown
estradiol valerate in oil (Gynogen, Delestrogen, Estra-L, Valergen, Dioval)	Hormone replacement therapy Prostate cancer	*Adult:* IM, 10–20 mg q4wk *Adult:* IM, 30 mg q1–2wk	*Onset:* Slow *Duration:* 4 wk $t_{1/2}$: Unknown
diethylstilbestrol (DES; *Canadian:* Honvol)	Female breast cancer (inoperable) Prostate cancer	*Adult:* PO, 15 mg/d *Adult:* PO, 1–3 mg/d	*Onset:* Rapid *Duration:* 24 h $t_{1/2}$: Unknown
Selected Non-estrogens			
clomiphene (Clomid, Milophene)	Ovulatory failure	*Adult:* PO, 50–100 mg/d for 5 d	*Onset:* 5–8 d *Duration:* 6 wk $t_{1/2}$: 5 d
menotropins (Pergonal, Humegon)	Ovulation stimulation Spermatogenesis stimulation	*Adult:* IM, 75 IU/d for 7–12 d, follow with hCG *Adult:* IM, 75–150 IU three times a week, pretreat and cotreat with human chorionic gonadotropin	*Onset:* Slow *Duration:* Months $t_{1/2}$: Unknown
chorionic gonadotropins (Choron, Pregnyl)	Hypogonadotropic Hypogonadism (males) Ovulation stimulation Spermatogenesis stimulation	*Adult:* 500–4,000 USP three times a week *Adult:* 5,000–10,000 USP 1 d after last menotropin dose *Adult:* Pretreatment, IM, 5,000 IU three times a week for 4–6 mo; cotreatment, 2,000 IU two times a week with menotropins	*Onset:* Unknown *Duration:* Unknown $t_{1/2}$: Unknown after pretreatment with menotropins

Pharmacokinetics

Absorption from the gastrointestinal (GI) tract is complete. Estrogen binds to specific receptor proteins in tissues that are responsive to estrogen (female genital organs, breasts, hypothalamus, pituitary). Metabolism occurs primarily in the liver. While circulating through the liver, estrogen is degraded to less active estrogenic compounds. Some estrogens are excreted into the bile and then reabsorbed from the intestines and returned to the liver. The estrogen conjugates are water soluble and are excreted through the kidneys, with minimal resorption. Conjugated estrogen crosses the placenta and enters the breast milk.

Pharmacodynamics

Estrogen stimulates the development of the female sex organs and secondary female sexual characteristics when given to females with insufficient endogenous estrogen (hypogonadism). Estrogen also stimulates the long-bone growth spurt of adolescence; when estrogen levels reach a certain level, they trigger closure of the epiphyseal plates to stop growth. Other actions of estrogen include facilitation or inhibition of ovulation (depending on dose), increased fluid retention, protein anabolism, conservation of calcium and phosphorus, stimulation of bone formation, and maintenance of tone and elasticity of urogenital structures.

When given during and after menopause, conjugated estrogen reduces hot flashes. It also increases vaginal secretions, improves urogenital tone, and reduces irritability and emotional lability.

When given to postmenopausal women for treating or preventing osteoporosis, estrogen significantly increases spinal bone mineral density. Bone loss in women taking HRT is rare (Greendale, et al., 2000). Increased bone mass is likely to assist in preventing fractures of the hip, wrist, and spine.

As previously stated, research on the exact effects of estrogen on the cardiovascular system is ongoing. Although oral estrogen has a procoagulant effect and increases the risk of venous thromboembolism, this risk is not a significant concern for most healthy women. Conversely, estrogen has also been found to have a cardioprotective action. Several large observational studies, including the Framingham Heart Study and the Nurses' Health Study, have shown that HRT protects against postmenopausal cardiovascular disease. Several animal studies also confirm estrogen's cardioprotective effect. The Postmenopausal Estrogen/Progestin Intervention (PEPI) trial, a large prospective randomized clinical trial, evaluated cardiovascular risk factors. The PEPI trial proved that estrogen, with or without concomitant progestin, decreased low-density lipoprotein (LDL) cholesterol and total cholesterol levels, increased high-density lipoprotein (HDL) cholesterol level, and promoted vasodilation and fibrinolysis. Thus, the use of estrogen (sometimes with progestin) as postmenopausal HRT decreased several known risk factors for CAD. Investigators hypothesized that the incidence of CAD and cardiovascular events, such as MI, would decrease with HRT; however, the Heart and Estrogen/Progestin Replacement Study (HERS) did not support this theory. Postmenopausal women who currently had CAD but no history of venous thromboembolism were treated with estrogen and progestin. The HERS trial failed to demonstrate a beneficial effect of oral HRT on cardiovascular events in older women with advanced CAD. In fact, the incidence of cardiovascular events increased by 50% in the first year for women receiving estrogen and progestin. The incidence of cardiovascular events decreased considerably over the next 2 years, so that HRT ended being more effective than a placebo in preventing MI and other deaths from CAD (Grady, Wenger, Herrington, Khan, Furberg, Hunninghake, et al., 2000; McPherson, 2000). It may be that the pattern of early increase and then later reduction in risk results from real but opposing effects of HRT. The initial increase in risk for women with pre-existing coronary heart disease may stem from prothrombic effects of oral estrogen. The women who were most at risk from this effect of estrogen suffered an adverse cardiovascular event. The women who were not at great risk from the prothrombic effects of estrogen were eventually protected by estrogen's ability to lower LDL levels and decrease other risk factors (Herrington, Reboussin, Klein, Sharp, Shumaker, Snyder, et al., 2000) (see the accompanying display, Hormone Replacement Therapy and Cardiovascular Benefits Versus Risks).

Estrogen's effects on atherosclerosis are also being determined. Examination of data from the HERS trial indicates that treatment with an oral conjugated estrogen plus progestin was not associated with a significant decrease in the incidence of peripheral arterial events in postmenopausal women with preexisting coronary heart disease (Hsia, Simon, Lin, Applegate, Vogt, Hunninghake, et al., 2000). Another study currently under way is

Focus on Research

Hormone replacement therapy and cardiovascular benefits versus risks

Blakely, J. A. (2000). The Heart and Estrogen/Progestin Replacement Study revisited: Hormone replacement therapy produced net harm, consistent with the observational data. *Archives of Internal Medicine, 160*(19), 2897–2900.
Bush, T. L. (2000). Preserving cardiovascular benefits of hormone replacement therapy. *Journal of Reproductive Medicine, 45* (Suppl 3), 259–273.
Espeland, M. A., Marcovina, S. M., Miller, V., Wood, P. D., Wasilauskas, C., Sherwin R., Schrott, H., & Bush, T. L. (1998). Effect of postmenopausal hormone therapy on lipoprotein (a) concentration. PEPI Investigators. Postmenopausal Estrogen/Progestin Interventions. *Circulation, 97*(10), 979–986.
Seed, M., Sands, R. H., McLaren, M., Kirk, G., & Darko, D. (2000). The effect of hormone replacement therapy and route of administration on selected cardiovascular risk factors in post-menopausal women. *Family Practice, 17*(6), 497–507.
Wells, G., & Herrington, D. M. (1999). The Heart and Estrogen/Progestin Replacement Study: What have we learned and what questions remain? *Drugs and Aging, 15*(6), 419–422.

The Studies

The effect of HRT on the cardiovascular system of postmenopausal women is not clearly understood. No consensus has been yet reached on the role HRT should play in treating and preventing CAD in postmenopausal women. Research clearly shows that HRT, either estrogen alone, or estrogen with progestin, decreases the risk factors for heart disease, such as decreasing levels of LDL, total cholesterol, and fibrinogen, and increasing levels of HDL. This was shown in the landmark PEPI study and again in a more recent smaller study of shorter duration. Although combinations of estrogen and progestin have fewer effects on decreasing the risk factors than estrogen alone, cardiovascular risk factors are reduced significantly. This appears to be true whether the drug therapy is oral or transdermal. Researchers believe that this reduction of cardiovascular risk factors should diminish postmenopausal risk of CAD. Apparently contradictory is the finding from the HERS group. In that study, HRT was used in postmenopausal women with coronary heart disease. Although overall HRT had no effect on heart disease, initially cardiovascular incidents, including MI, increased. This finding has caused some researchers to suggest that women with or at high risk for coronary heart disease should not receive HRT. Furthermore, they suggest that women without coronary heart disease may also be at greater risk of harm than benefit from HRT. Most researchers still believe that HRT has an important role in preventing coronary heart disease and should be used.

Nursing Implications

The issue of whether HRT therapy should be used in postmenopausal women to treat or prevent cardiovascular disease is still being studied. Recommendations in this area are likely to change over the next few years, as more data from clinical trials become known. At this time, it appears that the use of *HRT, as primary prevention* of postmenopausal coronary heart disease (before the woman has heart disease), *is appropriate* and should decrease the woman's risk of death from cardiovascular disease. The use of *HRT as secondary prevention* of postmenopausal coronary heart disease (after the woman has heart disease) *does not* appear *appropriate,* and may increase the woman's risk of death from cardiovascular disease.

Nurses must be knowledgeable regarding current and ongoing research in this area so that they may provide appropriate patient education and assist patients in making informed decisions regarding HRT. This is especially important because the popular press and other news media may headline a finding (either positive or negative) related to HRT but fail to provide enough information to give the new information perspective.

the Estrogen Replacement and Atherosclerosis (ERA) study, a clinical trial that is examining the effect of either estrogen alone or estrogen with progestin on the progression of coronary arthrosclerosis. The ERA study is the only study that examines the effect on the coronary vessels by using coronary angiography. When the ERA trial is completed, more information will be known about the effectiveness of HRT in slowing progression or causing regression of defined coronary atherosclerosis (Herrington et al., 2000).

When given alone, estrogen is known to increase the risk for endometrial cancer. The risk of developing endometrial cancer increases approximately 120% for every 5 years of estrogen replacement therapy. The addition of progestin to estrogen therapy decreases the risk of endometrial cancer (see Progesterone).

Long-term use of HRT (i.e., more than 5 years) may slightly increase the risk of breast cancer. Unfortunately, the use of progestin, added to prevent endometrial cancer, appears to be responsible for the increased risk of breast cancer (American Cancer Society, web page). The PEPI trial (Greendale, Wells, Marcus, & Barrett-Connor, 1999) showed that women receiving HRT with estrogen alone had a slight increase in mammographic density (a risk factor for breast cancer). The increase in mammographic density, however, occurred at a much greater rate when estrogen was combined with progestin. More research is still needed to confirm the effects of estrogen and estrogen combined with progesterone on risk for breast cancer.

Contraindications and Precautions

Estrogen is contraindicated in patients with breast cancer because it stimulates the growth of breast cancer cells. It may be used in appropriately selected patients, however, receiving treatment for metastatic disease. It is also contraindicated in the following conditions:

- Estrogen-dependent neoplastic diseases
- Undiagnosed abnormal genital bleeding
- Active thrombophlebitis or thromboembolic disorders
- History of thrombophlebitis, thrombosis, or thromboembolic disorders associated with previous estrogen use (except when used in treating breast or prostatic malignancy)
- Known or suspected pregnancy (estrogen is a pregnancy category X drug because of known adverse effects on the developing fetus)

Conjugated estrogen should be administered with caution to breast-feeding women, because estrogen has been shown to decrease the quantity and quality of breast milk and may be excreted into it. Safety and efficacy in children have not been established. Cautious use must be observed in patients with incomplete bone growth because of the epiphyseal closure that accompanies estrogen use. Caution also is necessary in patients for whom some degree of fluid retention may cause complications, such as those with epilepsy, migraine headaches, cardiac dysfunction, or renal dysfunction. Caution should also be used in patients with renal insufficiency or metabolic bone diseases associated with hypercalcemia.

Adverse Effects

Postmenopausal estrogen use has been associated with some serious and significant adverse effects. Estrogen use increases the risk of endometrial cancer. How much the risk increases appears to depend on dose and duration of therapy; high doses given over long periods create the greatest risk. Estrogen use may also increase the risk of breast cancer in some women, especially if they have previously had or have a familial history of breast cancer. As already noted, some research indicates that the increased risk of breast cancer is related to the administration of progesterone. Postmenopausal women with no history of breast cancer who receive conjugated estrogen as replacement therapy may not have a significantly higher risk of developing breast cancer, although the research results are still somewhat contradictory. Postmenopausal women who receive estrogen have a twofold to threefold increase in the risk of developing gallbladder disease.

The use of estrogen during early pregnancy may cause teratogenic effects in the fetus. Use of conjugated estrogen in patients with breast cancer and bone metastases may cause severe hypercalcemia. The rate of thromboembolic disease (such as that which occurs with estrogen oral contraceptives) is potentially increased in postmenopausal users of conjugated estrogen, especially if they are receiving large doses or have preexisting CAD.

Most adverse effects of estrogen therapy are related to the effect of estrogen on the body and may be dose related. Common adverse effects include breakthrough bleeding, changes in menstrual flow, dysmenorrhea, premenstrual-like syndrome, headache, nausea, vomiting, bloating, abdominal cramps, chloasma (dark patchy pigmentation to skin), and photosensitivity. Other adverse effects include cholestatic jaundice, colitis, acute pancreatitis, steepened corneal curvature, intolerance to contact lenses, migraine headaches, dizziness, mental depression, pain at injection site, edema, changes in libido, and breast tenderness, enlargement, or secretion.

Drug Interactions

No significant drug interactions are associated with conjugated estrogen.

Assessment of Relevant Core Patient Variables

Health Status

Before the patient begins estrogen therapy, the nurse should assess his or her blood pressure (for hypertension) and breasts (for masses). The patient should also undergo a pelvic examination and a Papanicolaou test to rule out cervical cancer. It is important to determine whether the patient has breast cancer, undiagnosed genital bleeding, active thrombophlebitis or thromboembolic disorders, or a history of thrombophlebitis, thrombosis, or thromboembolic disorders associated with previous estrogen use (except in palliative treatment of breast or prostatic cancer). These conditions are contraindications to use of conjugated estrogen.

Other assessment data to look for in the patient are a personal or family history of breast cancer, a history of benign breast tumors, early menarche, a first pregnancy late in life, or never having been pregnant. These factors are considered to increase the risk of breast cancer with estrogen replacement therapy.

It is also important to determine whether the patient has a metabolic bone disease associated with hypercalcemia or renal insufficiency, because these conditions mandate cautious use of estrogen. The nurse should also determine whether the patient has a condition that might be adversely affected by fluid retention, such as epilepsy, migraine headaches, cardiac dysfunction, or renal insufficiency.

Life Span and Gender

The nurse must check the patient's age. The use of parenteral conjugated estrogen in premature infants has been associated with the development of a fatal "gasping syndrome" because of the benzyl alcohol in the preparation. The nurse must assess whether long-bone growth has been completed. If the patient is prepubescent, the nurse will need to monitor growth throughout therapy to prevent premature closing of the epiphyses.

The nurse should assess for possible pregnancy, which is a contraindication for therapy. Use of conjugated estrogen during pregnancy may promote congenital defects, including heart and limb reduction defects. Male fetuses exposed to conjugated estrogen through maternal use may develop genitourinary structural problems and, later, abnormal semen. Use of estrogen to treat threatened or habitual miscarriage has not been proved effective. The nurse should also assess the patient's menopausal or postmenopausal status.

Lifestyle, Diet, and Habits

If a woman has been assessed and is overweight, not physically active, or calcium deficient, consumes alcohol, or smokes, she is still a candidate for estrogen therapy. Smoking has not been found to interfere with the positive effects of estrogen on bone mineral density in postmenopausal women. Alcohol consumption, calcium intake, physical activity, and body weight also have not been found to interfere with the positive effects of estrogen.

Environment

Conjugated estrogen may produce photosensitivity. Patients who are outdoors frequently need to take precautions against the sun's ultraviolet rays until tolerance to the drug is determined. The nurse needs to be aware of the environment in which estrogen will be administered. Oral conjugated estrogen may be administered in any setting, including the home by the patient. Parenteral conjugated estrogen (IM or IV) is administered in a hospital setting.

Nursing Diagnoses and Outcomes

- Ineffective Sexuality Patterns related to therapy for female hypogonadism or lack of intrinsic estrogen
  Desired outcome: The patient will develop normal sex organs and secondary sexual characteristics while using estrogen drug therapy.
- Risk for Delayed Growth and Development related to intrinsic estrogen deficiency and early hypophysis closing from estrogen replacement therapy
  Desired outcome: The patient will achieve normal growth and development while using drug therapy.
- Impaired Physical Mobility related to osteoporosis
  Desired outcome: The patient will not experience osteoporosis and its complications because of the preventive effects of estrogen replacement therapy.
- Decisional Conflict related to risks versus benefits of postmenopausal estrogen replacement therapy
  Desired outcome: The patient will make an informed decision about estrogen replacement therapy after considering personal risks versus benefits.

Planning and Intervention

Maximizing Therapeutic Effects

Several nursing actions are geared toward maximizing the therapeutic effects of estrogen. The nurse should administer conjugated estrogens cyclically (3 weeks of daily administration, 1 week off) to simulate the normal cycling of endogenous estrogen (except when given for carcinomas or postpartum breast engorgement). The drug should remain refrigerated before reconstitution (IV or IM use); after reconstitution, the solution can remain refrigerated for up to 60 days. The solution should not be used if it darkens or if precipitation occurs.

Minimizing Adverse Effects

To minimize adverse effects of estrogen therapy, the nurse must monitor for signs of thrombophlebitis and thromboembolus. The estrogen dosage should remain as low as possible to minimize the chances for development of endometrial or breast cancer but still achieve the desired therapeutic effects. The duration of therapy should be minimized in postmenopausal women to decrease the risks of cancer. The nurse should not administer IV conjugated estrogen with other agents. (An exception is in emergencies in which a separate drug infusion has already been started. In such cases, the nurse should inject the drug into the IV tubing as close to the angiocatheter insertion site as possible.) The nurse must protect the patient from ultraviolet light until it is determined whether the patient will experience photosensitivity.

Providing Patient and Family Education

- The nurse should teach patients and their families about the therapeutic purpose of estrogen. He or she should provide and clarify information on risks versus benefits of postmenopausal therapy so that the patient can make an informed choice regarding drug therapy.
- The nurse should provide instruction on how to take estrogen cyclically, unless the patient is taking it for palliative cancer treatment or postpartum breast engorgement.
- The nurse should instruct the patient on the signs and symptoms of thrombophlebitis and thromboembolism (pain in groin or calves, sharp chest pain or sudden shortness of breath, sudden severe headache, dizziness or fainting, vision or speech disturbance, weakness or numbness in arm or leg). He or she should urge the patient to notify the physician or nurse practitioner at once if these occur.
- The nurse also should teach the patient to notify the physician or nurse practitioner if he or she experiences any of the following: abnormal vaginal bleeding, missed menstrual period or suspected pregnancy, lumps in the breast, severe abdominal pain, yellowing of the skin or eyes, or severe depression.
- The nurse should educate the patient to avoid prolonged exposure to the sun and to use sunblock and appropriate clothing in the sun because photosensitivity may occur.
- In addition, the nurse should emphasize the importance of returning for follow-up care and physical examinations while receiving estrogen therapy (see the accompanying display, Pros and Cons of Estrogen Replacement Therapy).

Critical Thinking Scenario

Pros and cons of estrogen replacement therapy

Marsha Robbins, a 52-year-old woman, is going through menopause. She is trying to decide whether to start estrogen replacement therapy after menopause. She says to you, "How can I decide? It seems both good and bad things can happen to me if I take estrogen." While interviewing Ms. Robbins, you learn that she has had hypertension for 5 years. She does not currently have CAD or peripheral artery disease. Both her parents had cardiovascular problems, and her father died of an MI. She has no personal or family history of breast cancer or benign breast tumors. Her menstrual history was normal up to the start of menopause. She has two adult children, 31 and 29 years old. She does not drink milk or exercise regularly. Her cholesterol levels are borderline high.

Analyze the potential risks versus the benefits of HRT for Ms. Robbins. What information would you offer to help her make an informed choice regarding this therapy?

Ongoing Assessment and Evaluation

If the patient is a prepubescent girl, the nurse should evaluate for normal sexual development with therapy and should monitor the patient's growth as appropriate. Checking for evidence of early epiphyseal closure is essential. The nurse should monitor the postmenopausal woman for development of endometrial or breast cancer. Therapy is considered effective when normal growth and sexual development occur, bone mineral density increases, or cardiovascular disease does not occur, and the patient does not show any serious adverse effects from the drug therapy. ■

DRUGS CLOSELY RELATED TO P CONJUGATED ESTROGEN

Oral contraceptives are combinations of estrogen and progesterone and are discussed in the section on estrogen-progestin combination drugs. Synthetic conjugated estrogens (Cinestin) are very similar to conjugated estrogen.

MEMORY CHIP

P Conjugated Estrogen

- Used as HRT when endogenous levels of estrogen are low (premenopausal)
- Used to treat moderate to severe symptoms of menopause
- Used to prevent and treat postmenopausal osteoporosis and prevent coronary heart disease
- Used in treating abnormal uterine bleeding resulting from hormonal imbalance, advanced prostatic cancer (palliative), metastatic breast cancer in men, and selected breast cancer (non–estrogen dependent tumors) in women
- Significant contraindications: most breast cancers, estrogen-dependent cancers, thrombophlebitis or thromboembolic disorders (active or history of), undiagnosed abnormal genital bleeding
- Most common adverse effects: menstrual cycle problems (breakthrough bleeding, changes in menstrual flow, dysmenorrhea, premenstrual-like syndrome, headache, nausea, vomiting, bloating, abdominal cramps, chloasma, and photosensitivity)
- Most serious adverse effects: thromboembolic events, increased risk of endometrial cancer; may cause breast cancer
- **Life span alert: pregnancy category X drug**
- Maximizing therapeutic effects administer cyclically
- Minimizing adverse effects: monitor bone growth for early epiphyseal growth plate closure (prepubescent girls); monitor for thrombophlebitis or thromboembolism
- Most significant patient education: report signs and symptoms of thrombophlebitis or thromboembolism at once; assess benefits versus risks of postmenopausal HRT

terone is produced. Progesterone changes the endometrium from its proliferative phase into its secretive stage. When levels of progesterone (in combination with estrogen) are high enough, a signal is sent to the pituitary gonadotropins to stop producing FSH and LH, thus preventing further ovulation. Progesterone is necessary to increase the endometrial receptivity for implantation of an embryo if pregnancy occurs. Once implanted, progesterone helps to maintain the pregnancy. If pregnancy does not occur, the corpus luteum will disintegrate, progesterone levels will fall, the pituitary gonadotropins will be stimulated, and more FSH and LH will be produced, creating ovulation again. Progesterone also inhibits spontaneous uterine contractions and contractions of other smooth muscles in the body, but, because of its potential teratogenic effects, use to prevent spontaneous abortion (miscarriage) is not recommended. Progesterone has some anabolic or androgenic activity, although such function is minor.

Progesterone is known to decrease the risk of endometrial cancer in postmenopausal women receiving estrogen. Recent research indicates that progesterone may increase the risk of breast cancer when given to postmenopausal women (Greendale, et al, 1999; Pike & Ross, 2000). Progesterone or other progestins need to be added to HRT but in such a way as to decrease the risk to breast tissue. Theorists have suggested that this could be accomplished by administering progesterone through routes that will minimize the systemic levels of progesterone (such as vaginally) or by giving progesterone orally for 10 days every third to fourth month of estrogen replacement therapy (Pike & Ross, 2000). Progesterone does not affect bone mineral density.

Contraindications and Precautions

Progesterone is contraindicated in patients with hypersensitivity to progestins. It is also contraindicated for patients with thrombophlebitis, thromboembolic disorder, cerebral hemorrhage, or a history of any of these conditions. Further contraindications include impaired liver function or disease, carcinoma of the breast or genital organs, undiagnosed vaginal bleeding, or missed abortion. Progesterone is a pregnancy category D drug, and its use during pregnancy has led to fetal abnormalities, including masculinization of the female fetus. It does pass into breast milk, although the effect on the infant remains undetermined.

Caution should be used in patients with pathologies that may be adversely affected by fluid retention (epilepsy, migraine headaches, asthma, cardiac dysfunction, or renal dysfunction). Patients who have a history of depression should be observed carefully for signs of this disorder while taking progesterone. Photosensitivity may occur with use of this drug. The benzyl alcohol that some of these products contain may produce a fatal gasping syndrome if given to premature infants.

Adverse Effects

Common adverse effects include breakthrough bleeding, spotting, change in menstrual flow, amenorrhea, changes in cervical secretions, breast tenderness, changes in weight, and nausea. Research indicates that progesterone and other progestins may increase the risk of breast cancer in postmenopausal women receiving HRT (Greendale, et al., 1999). Other uncommon but serious adverse effects include sudden partial or complete loss of eyesight, thrombophlebitis, mental depression, and cholestatic jaundice. Progesterone is irritating at the injection site; the aqueous form is especially painful.

Drug Interactions

No known drug interactions are associated with progesterone. Progesterone, however, may affect results of the following laboratory tests: hepatic function tests, coagulation tests (decrease in prothrombin and factors VII, VIII, IX, and X), thyroid tests, metyrapone tests, and endocrine function tests.

Assessment of Relevant Core Patient Variables

Health Status

The nurse should assess for a history of or current thrombophlebitis, thromboembolic disorder, and cerebral hemorrhage; impaired liver function or disease; mental depression; or undiagnosed vaginal bleeding, because these are contraindications to use of progesterone. Prior to treatment, a complete physical examination is required, including assessment of the breasts and pelvic organs. A Papanicolaou test should be performed. The nurse should also assess the patient's menstrual cycles for irregularities. All vaginal bleeding should be diagnosed carefully before therapy starts.

Life Span and Gender

The nurse should assess the patient for pregnancy or intention to become pregnant, because progesterone is associated with genital and congenital abnormalities when exposure occurs in the first 4 gestational months. Genital abnormalities include masculinization of the genital organs in the female fetus and hypospadias in the male fetus. Congenital abnormalities include congenital heart defects and limb reduction defects. If the patient is in the later stages of pregnancy, progesterone might be used to halt premature labor. The nurse should assess whether the patient is breast-feeding, because progesterone's effects on the infant are unknown. Progesterone may be added to postmenopausal HRT.

Environment

The nurse should caution patients about ultraviolet light exposure. He or she must be aware of the environment in which progesterone will be administered. Progesterone may be administered in any environment, including the home, if the patient or family member has learned correct administration of an IM injection.

Nursing Diagnoses and Outcomes

- Disturbed Body Image related to potential breakthrough bleeding, spotting, changes in menstrual flow, weight gain, or breast tenderness secondary to adverse effects of drug therapy

  Desired outcome: The patient will not experience significant adverse effects from drug therapy to alter body image.
- Risk for Injury related to loss of vision, onset of thrombotic disorders, and depression secondary to adverse effects of drug therapy

  Desired outcome: The patient will not suffer an injury related to adverse effects of drug therapy.

Planning and Intervention

Maximizing Therapeutic Effects

The dosing schedule varies based on the clinical indication for using progesterone. In treatment of amenorrhea, the drug should be administered for 6 to 8 consecutive days. For treating dysfunctional uterine bleeding, the drug should be administered daily for 6 days. The best dosing schedule when progesterone is used in HRT is currently unknown.

Minimizing Adverse Effects

There are a few nursing actions to minimize the adverse effects of progesterone therapy. The nurse should not administer the drug to any woman who is in the first 4 months of pregnancy to avoid risk of injury to the fetus. Postmenopausal dosage should be minimized to the smallest effective dose to decrease risk of endometrial cancer yet cause minimal increased risk to breast tissue. Assessment throughout therapy for signs and symptoms of endometrial or breast cancer is essential. The nurse should not give progesterone to patients with a history of or active thrombophlebitis, thromboembolic disorders, breast cancer, or cerebral hemorrhage, because these conditions are possible adverse effects of therapy. Therapy must be discontinued at the first sign of any of these conditions. The nurse must carefully monitor patients who may be adversely affected by fluid retention. Therapy also must be discontinued if excessive fluid retention places them at risk in their primary disease or disorder.

Providing Patient and Family Education

- The nurse should instruct patients and their families on progesterone's therapeutic and adverse effects.
- The nurse should instruct patients how to perform breast self-examination.
- The nurse should teach patients to notify the health care provider if they suspect that they are pregnant or if sudden loss of vision, severe headache, or numbness in an arm or leg occurs.
- If the patient is using the vaginal gel form of progesterone, ideally, this is the only intravaginal therapy she should be using. If she requires other intravaginal therapy, administration should be at least 6 hours before or after progesterone gel. If indicated, the nurse should discuss with the patient how to time her self-administration of intravaginal therapies.

Ongoing Assessment and Evaluation

The nurse should monitor premenopausal women for return of normal menstrual flow and cessation of abnormal bleeding. If amenorrhea or dysfunctional uterine bleeding is corrected without adverse effects, the drug therapy has been effective. In postmenopausal women, the nurse should assess throughout therapy for signs or symptoms of endometrial or breast cancer. Combination therapies of estrogen and progestin (such as progesterone) are effective in the postmenopausal woman if they prevent or treat osteoporosis, decrease cardiovascular risk factors, prevent thromboembolic incidents, and avoid endometrial cancer, breast cancer, and other serious adverse effects. ■

DRUGS CLOSELY RELATED TO PROGESTERONE

Megestrol (Megace) is a progestin-like progesterone and shares many of progesterone's qualities and characteristics. Pharmacotherapeutic effects appear to be the major

MEMORY CHIP

Progesterone

- Used to treat amenorrhea to help produce normal menstrual cycles, to stop dysfunctional uterine bleeding, or as part of postmenopausal HRT
- Used in combination with estrogen in oral contraceptives to prevent pregnancy
- Significant contraindications: breast cancer, thrombophlebitis, thromboembolism
- Most common adverse effects: menstrual irregularities (e.g., breakthrough bleeding, spotting, change in menstrual flow, amenorrhea, changes in cervical secretions, breast tenderness, changes in weight)
- Most serious adverse effects: possible increased risk of breast cancer; sudden partial or complete loss of eyesight (uncommon)
- Minimizing adverse effects: in premenopausal women, verify that the patient is not pregnant; in postmenopausal women, perform follow up care to assess for endometrial or breast cancer
- Most significant patient education: in premenopausal women—report serious adverse effects at once; in postmenopausal women—perform breast self-examination

differences between the drugs. Unlike progesterone, megestrol is used as palliative treatment for patients with advanced breast or endometrial cancer (tablet form) or to increase appetite in patients with acquired immunodeficiency syndrome (AIDS) (suspension form). Exactly how megestrol increases appetite in patients with AIDS who have anorexia and cachexia is unknown. Weight gain, however, is not related to water retention. Megestrol is not used as part of HRT in postmenopausal women. Its contraindications are similar to those of progesterone. Safety and efficacy of megestrol acetate therapy in children have not been established.

The oral contraceptives—estrogen-progestin combination drugs—also are closely related to progesterone and are discussed fully in the section on estrogen-progestin combination drugs.

DRUGS SIGNIFICANTLY DIFFERENT FROM P PROGESTERONE

Levonorgestrel Implant and Intrauterine Progesterone Inserts

Levonorgestrel implants (Norplant system) and intrauterine progesterone inserts (Progestasert) are unique forms of progesterone. Their main effects on the body and reproductive system are the same as those of progesterone. Like progesterone in combined estrogen-progestin oral contraceptives, these drugs are used solely for contraception—to prevent pregnancy. The major difference is in their routes of administration and lengths of effectiveness.

Levonorgestrel implants consist of six flexible closed capsules made of a synthetic material (Silastic). Each capsule contains 36 mg of levonorgestrel. The capsules are implanted subdermally in the midportion of the upper arm, about 8 to 10 cm above the antecubital space, in a fan-like pattern. Diffusion of levonorgestrel through the capsules provides continuous, slow release of progesterone to prevent pregnancy for up to 5 years. The capsules may be removed at any time to reverse the contraceptive effect. A new set of capsules may be placed after 5 years if the woman desires continued contraceptive protection.

Intrauterine progesterone inserts are T-shaped units filled with progesterone. They are placed in the uterine cavity for 1 year; the system must be replaced 1 year after insertion. The exact mechanism of action is unknown. It is believed that the progesterone inhibits the survival of sperm or alters the uterine environment to prevent implantation. Suppression of endometrial tissue proliferation is one progestational influence of the insert on the endometrium.

Adverse effects of the intrauterine progesterone inserts are unique to the administration route and may be severe. They include increased risk for septic abortion or congenital anomalies if pregnancy does occur, increased risk of pelvic inflammatory disease, device embedment in the endometrium, perforation of the uterine wall or cervix by the device, endometritis, vaginitis, midcycle spotting, increased menstrual flow, pain, cramping, and amenorrhea.

Mifepristone

Mifepristone (Mifeprex) is used to end an early pregnancy (defined as 49 days or less from the start of the last menstrual period). It competes with progesterone for binding at the progesterone-receptor sites and is a progesterone antagonist. Mifepristone inhibits the activity of endogenous and exogenous progesterone, resulting in termination of pregnancy. Mifepristone also has some antiglucocorticoid and weak antiandrogenic effects. Compensatory elevation of adrenocorticotropic hormone (ACTH) and cortisol levels have been observed in some patients. Animal studies have indicated some antiandrogenic effects with large doses, but no studies have been done on this effect in humans. Mifepristone is rapidly absorbed. It is highly protein bound and metabolized by the CYP450-3A4 pathway in the liver. Most mifepristone is excreted in the feces.

Mifepristone, although effective for the vast majority of women who use it, may result in an incomplete medical abortion, necessitating surgical intervention. Mifepristone may also fail to initiate an abortion or produce significant vaginal bleeding; either of these two events may also require a surgical procedure. Between 1% and 5% of women will require a surgical procedure related to any of these potential problems. For this reason, the FDA has established very specific and unique requirements in the United States for use of mifepristone. Although it is a prescription drug, mifepristone is not available in pharmacies. Instead it is distributed directly to physicians who have the knowledge and skill necessary to determine the duration of a patient's pregnancy through menstrual history and clinical examination and to detect an ectopic pregnancy. Ultrasonographic scanning should be used if the duration of pregnancy is uncertain or if ectopic pregnancy is suspected. Physicians must be able to provide surgical intervention in cases of incomplete abortion or severe bleeding, or they must have pre-established plans to provide such care through others. Some states allow nurse practitioners or nurse midwives who work closely with physicians to be authorized prescribers of mifepristone.

Drug therapy with mifepristone should not be used if the patient cannot or is unwilling to return to the physician's office for two follow-up visits. It also should not be administered to patients who do not have adequate access in the following 2 weeks to medical facilities equipped to provide emergency treatment of incomplete abortion, blood transfusion, and emergency resuscitation. The prescriber must give the patient the FDA Written Medication Guide for mifepristone and discuss the information thoroughly. The Medication Guide contains FDA-approved information written especially for patients. Medication Guides accompany drugs that the FDA has determined pose a serious risk; however, appropriate patient education reduces the risk. The patient must sign an agreement prior to receiving treatment.

After the patient meets all the baseline requirements, she swallows three tablets of mifepristone in the physician's or provider's office. This is considered Day 1. At Day 3 the woman returns to the provider's office to determine whether she is still pregnant. If medical abortion is incomplete, the woman is to take two tablets of misoprostol. (This is a different drug. Misoprostol is a synthetic prostaglandin E_1 analog. Although it is used to prevent gastric ulcers resulting from use of nonsteroidal anti-inflammatory drugs (NSAIDS), it also is known to have abortifacient properties, producing uterine contractions. See Chapter 37 for more information on anti-ulcer properties.) In clinical trials, about 44% of women who took misoprostol following mifepristone expelled the products of conception within 4 hours; about 63% expelled them within 24 hours after the misoprostol dose. The patient returns to the provider's office at Day 14 to verify complete ending of the pregnancy. Although bleeding itself is not proof of termination of the pregnancy, lack of bleeding indicates that the therapy was ineffective in creating a medical abortion. If the pregnancy has not been completely terminated, surgical intervention to end the pregnancy is recommended. Pregnancies that are carried to term after use of mifepristone may result in fetal deformities.

Contraindications for using mifepristone are a pregnancy that has lasted longer than 49 days since the start of the last menstrual period; confirmed or suspected ectopic pregnancy; intrauterine device (IUD) in place (must be removed prior to drug therapy); chronic adrenal failure; concurrent long-term corticosteroid therapy; bleeding disorders or use of anticoagulant drugs; allergy to mifepristone, misoprostol, or other prostaglandins; and inherited porphyrias (rare inherited disturbances in porphyrin metabolism that may cause hemolytic anemia and splenomegaly).

The most common adverse effects of mifepristone are heavy vaginal bleeding, abdominal pain, and uterine cramping. Most women will have vaginal bleeding or spotting for 9 to 16 days after pregnancy; some women will bleed for 30 days or more. Vaginal bleeding may be severe enough to warrant blood transfusions, treatment with vasoconstrictor or uterotonic drugs, surgical intervention, or IV fluids. Other common adverse effects include nausea, vomiting, and diarrhea. Pelvic pain, fainting, headache, dizziness, and muscle weakness may also occur, but they are rare. Reported adverse effects decrease after day 3 and are rare by day 14 except for complaints of bleeding and spotting.

Specific drug or food interactions with mifepristone have not been studied. But as the CYP3A4 pathway metabolizes this drug, other drugs that are metabolized by or inhibit metabolism from this pathway may produce a drug interaction if taken concurrently.

Pregnancy can reoccur after treatment with mifepristone. The patient should resume contraception after verification that the pregnancy has been completely eliminated or before resuming sexual activity.

C ORAL CONTRACEPTIVES

The oral contraceptives are closely related to both estrogen and progestin because they contain varying amounts of these drugs in combination. A very few oral contraceptives contain progestins only. Oral contraceptives are given to prevent pregnancy; the patient's cultural beliefs may affect their use. Combination oral contraceptives inhibit ovulation by suppressing the gonadotropins FSH and LH. In addition, oral contraceptives alter the quality of cervical and other mucus in the female genital tract (inhibiting sperm penetration) and change the characteristics of the endometrium (reducing the likelihood of implantation). These drug effects may also assist in preventing pregnancy.

Oral contraceptives differ in the type and relative strength (potency) of their components and as to whether estrogen or progesterone activity dominates. Their ultimate effect is related to combined activity. Progestin-only oral contraceptives prevent pregnancy in a way not clearly understood. It is known that they alter the cervical mucus and exert a progestational effect on the endometrium, which apparently produces cellular changes that render the endometrium hostile to implantation of a fertilized egg. In some patients, the effects of progestin also prevent ovulation.

There are three types of combination oral contraceptives:

- Monophasic: the dose of estrogen and progestin remains the same throughout the entire cycle.
- Biphasic: the amount of estrogen remains the same, but the amount of progestin rises in the second half of the cycle.
- Triphasic: estrogen amounts remain the same or may vary throughout the cycle, whereas progestin varies throughout the cycle.

Some serious adverse effects may occur with oral contraceptive use. These effects are usually related to high doses of estrogen in the drug. Oral contraceptives should be prescribed with the smallest effective dose of estrogen possible for the patient; thus, high-dose estrogen formulations are prescribed infrequently, usually only when a lower dose has been ineffective. Dose-related serious adverse effects include thromboembolism, stroke, MI, hepatic lesions, and gallbladder disease. The risk of cardiovascular and cerebrovascular effects is substantially increased in women age 35 years or older with other risk factors (e.g., smoking, uncontrolled hypertension, hypercholesterolemia, elevated LDL, obesity, diabetes). Mortality rates associated with circulatory disease have been shown to increase substantially in smokers older than 35 years and nonsmokers older than 40 years.

In addition, a decrease in glucose tolerance has been observed in a small percentage of patients on estrogen-progestin combination drugs; the mechanism appears to be related to estrogen dose. Elevated blood pressure may be related to use of oral contraceptives; this development is believed to result from estrogen and progesterone effects. Other adverse effects are related to the dosage of estrogen and progestin and reflect the individual adverse effects of these drugs. Lower doses minimize these effects, which include breakthrough bleeding (transitory), spotting, amenorrhea during and after treatment, breast tenderness, nausea and vomiting (usually transitory), steepening of the corneal curvature, contact lens intolerance, weight gain or loss, edema, migraine, elevated triglyceride levels, and depression.

For greatest effectiveness, the woman should take the oral contraceptive every day (or for 21 days and then off for 7 days, depending on the drug formulation) at the same time every day, such as with a meal or at bedtime. Patients may follow several regimens for beginning a cycle. The patient should refer to the package insert with each preparation. If the woman misses a dose, she should take the next dose as quickly as possible; a woman may take two tablets on the same day. The woman should make up two missed pills over 2 days. If she misses three consecutive pills, she should begin a new cycle the day after she missed the last pill or 7 days after taking the last pill. She should use another form of birth control as a backup for at least 7 consecutive days and preferably for the rest of the new cycle.

If a woman misses a menstrual period, she should be evaluated for pregnancy. Oral contraceptives should be withheld until pregnancy is ruled out because of possible damage to the fetus if the woman takes the drug during early pregnancy.

Non-breast-feeding mothers may begin use of oral contraceptives 4 to 6 weeks after delivery even if they have not resumed spontaneous menstrual periods. Oral contraceptives are not recommended in breast-feeding women, although they may be used carefully if absolutely necessary.

C BISPHOSPHONATES

The drug class bisphosphonates affects normal and abnormal bone resorption. The prototype is alendronate (Fosamax). Drugs closely related to alendronate are risedronate, tiludronate, etidronate, and pamidronate. See Table 43-3 for more information. A significantly different drug is raloxifene.

NURSING MANAGEMENT OF THE PATIENT RECEIVING P ALENDRONATE

Core Drug Knowledge

Pharmacotherapeutics

Alendronate is used to treat and prevent osteoporosis in postmenopausal women. It is also used in the treatment of patients with **Paget disease.** Paget disease is an idiopathic bone disease characterized by chronic, focal areas of bone destruction complicated by concurrent excessive bone repair. The result is thick but weak bones that may fracture or bend under stress.

Pharmacokinetics

Alendronate is absorbed orally. Food and beverages other than plain water can decrease its absorption and bioavailability by about 40%. After absorption, alendronate is stored in the skeleton and does not appear to be metabolized. It is excreted in the urine as it is slowly released from the skeleton.

Pharmacodynamics

The major action of alendronate is to inhibit normal and abnormal bone resorption. Alendronate is a highly selective and potent inhibitor of bone resorption, which

TABLE 43-3 Summary of Selected Drugs Used to Treat Bone Resorption

Drug (Trade) Name	Selected Indications	Route and Dosage Range	Pharmacokinetics
P alendronate (Fosamax)	Treat/prevent postmenopausal osteoporosis Paget disease	PO, 10 mg/d PO, 40 mg/d for 6 mo	*Onset:* Slow *Duration:* Days $t_{1/2}$: Unknown
etidronate (Didronel)	Paget disease Hypercalcemia of malignancy	PO, 5–10 mg/kg/d not to exceed 6 months IV, 7.5 mg/kg/d for 3 successive d diluted in at least 250 mL sterile normal saline	*Onset:* Slow for PO, rapid for IV *Duration:* Days $t_{1/2}$: 6 h in plasma; >90 d in bone
pamidronate (Aredia)	Paget disease	IV, 30 mg diluted in 500 mL normal saline or 0.45% saline, infuse over 4 h for 3 consecutive d	*Onset:* Rapid *Duration:* Days $t_{1/2}$: biphasic in plasma 1.6 h, then 27.3 h
	Hypercalcemia of malignancy	IV, 60–90 mg as a single-dose infusion diluted in 1 L normal saline, 0.45% saline, or 5% dextrose. Infuse 60 mg over 4 h, 90 mg over 24 h	From bone up to 300 d
	Breast cancer with bone metastases	IV, 90 mg over 4 h every 3 to 4 wk in at least 500 mL	
risedronate (Actonel)	Paget disease	PO, 30 mg/d for 2 mo	*Onset:* Rapid *Duration:* Days $t_{1/2}$: Multiphasic, 1.5 to 220 h
tiludronate (Skelid)	Paget disease	PO: 400 mg active tiludronate/d (comes in 240 mg tablets each with 200 mg active drug) for 2 mo	*Onset:* Rapid *Duration:* Unknown $t_{1/2}$: Unknown

occurs following recruitment, activation, and polarization of osteoclasts. The exact mechanism of antiresorptive action is not fully understood but may be related to the inhibition of hydroxyapatite crystal dissolution or its action on bone resorbing cells. Reduction of abnormal bone resorption is responsible for reductions in serum calcium and phosphate concentrations. Alendronate has been found to significantly increase bone-mineral density (BMD) in patients with osteoporosis. Evidence of increased BMD is seen after 3 months of use and continues throughout therapy. Alendronate thus appears to reverse the progression of osteoporosis.

Contraindications and Precautions

Alendronate is contraindicated if the patient is hypocalcemic or hypersensitive to the drug or any of its components. Caution is necessary if the patient has mild to moderate renal insufficiency because this drug is likely to reduce elimination, leading to a slightly increased accumulation of alendronate in the bone. Alendronate is not recommended for patients with severe renal insufficiency. It is a pregnancy category C drug. Animal studies show increases in maternal and fetal hypocalcemia and deaths; no studies have been done on pregnant women. Alendronate is used in pregnancy only if benefits outweigh risks. Although it is unknown whether alendronate enters breast milk, alendronate should not be given to breast-feeding mothers based on the fetal risks determined from results of animal studies. Safety and efficacy in children have not been established.

Adverse Effects

When given to treat osteoporosis, the most common adverse effect of alendronate is abdominal pain; musculoskeletal pain is also fairly common. Other adverse effects are flatulence, acid regurgitation, esophageal ulcer, abdominal distention, gastritis, headache, rash, and erythema (rare). When given to treat Paget disease, alendronate increases the risk of upper GI symptoms; otherwise, the adverse effects are similar to use for osteoporosis.

Overdosage with alendronate will produce hypocalcemia, hypophosphatemia, and upper GI adverse effects. Administering milk or antacids to bind with the alendronate may be helpful. Dialysis is not beneficial. Otherwise, care is directed at treating the symptoms of overdosage.

Drug Interactions

Drug interactions between alendronate and some other drugs are known to occur. Because of potential interactions, recommendations are for the patient to wait at least 30 minutes after taking alendronate before taking any other drug (Table 43-4).

Assessment of Relevant Core Patient Variables

Health Status

The nurse should assess whether the patient has hypocalcemia or other disturbances in mineral metabolism, such as phosphate or vitamin D deficiency. These imbalances require correction prior to starting drug therapy with alendronate, as alendronate may cause additional slight decreases in serum calcium and phosphate levels. The nurse must verify that the patient has a clinical indication (i.e., treatment or prevention of osteoporosis, Paget disease) for use of alendronate prior to beginning therapy. As a family history of osteoporosis increases a woman's risk of developing osteoporosis, the nurse should also assess for this. The nurse must also assess for severe renal insufficiency, as this condition may necessitate a dose reduction.

Life Span and Gender

Alendronate is used in postmenopausal women to treat or prevent osteoporosis; it may be used as treatment for all patients with Paget disease. The nurse must assess the patient for pregnancy or intention to become pregnant, because alendronate is a pregnancy category C drug. He or she must assess the patient's lactation status, because administration to breast-feeding mothers must be avoided. Use of this drug in children requires caution, because safety and efficacy have not been established. Older adults require no precautions or dosage adjustments.

Lifestyle, Diet, and Habits

The nurse should review the patient's normal eating habits, because food and beverages (e.g., coffee, orange juice, mineral water) will decrease absorption of alen-

TABLE 43-4 Agents That Interact With Alendronate

Interactants	Effect and Significance	Nursing Management
ranitidine	IV ranitidine doubles alendronate's bioavailability. Clinical significance is unknown.	Monitor for therapeutic and adverse effects.
calcium supplements, antacids	Products with calcium and other multivalent ions interfere with absorption of alendronate.	Separate doses of alendronate and calcium or antacids by 2 h.
aspirin	Coadministration increases risk of adverse effects in upper gastrointestinal system.	Monitor for adverse effects. If severe adverse effects develop, discontinue aspirin.

dronate. He or she must assess the patient's calcium and vitamin D intake to verify that amounts are adequate. Patients who have a history of eating disorders, such as excessive dieting, have an increased risk for osteoporosis. The nurse must assess for normal weight-bearing exercise, because this helps to prevent osteoporosis. He or she also must ask the patient about consumption of cigarettes and alcohol, because these factors increase the risk of osteoporosis.

Environment

The nurse must be aware of the setting in which alendronate will be administered. Alendronate is normally self-administered in the home, although it could be given in any setting.

Culture

Asian and white women are at increased risk of osteoporosis.

Nursing Diagnoses and Outcomes

- Risk for Injury related to fractures from osteoporosis or Paget disease
  Desired outcome: The patient using drug therapy will have no fractures.
- Potential Complication: Electrolyte Imbalance related to drug therapy with alendronate
  Desired outcome: The patient will not experience electrolyte imbalance.
- Potential Complication: Altered GI Function related to adverse effects of drug therapy with alendronate
  Desired outcome: The patient will experience either no or minimal adverse effects.

Planning and Intervention

Maximizing Therapeutic Effects and Minimizing Adverse Effects

Nursing actions to maximize therapeutic effects are related to patient education. To minimize adverse effects from hypocalcemia, the nurse must take measures to correct pre-existing hypocalcemia before treatment. He or she should monitor electrolyte levels throughout therapy as indicated. Other actions to minimize adverse effects are related to patient education.

Providing Patient and Family Education

- The nurse should teach the patient to take alendronate at least 30 minutes before eating, drinking any beverage other than plain water, or taking any other medication. The patient should swallow the medicine with 6 to 8 ounces (180 to 240 mL) of plain water, which will improve absorption of the drug.
- The nurse should instruct the patient not to lie down for at least 30 minutes after swallowing alendronate to decrease adverse GI effects.
- The nurse must encourage the patient to take supplemental calcium and vitamin D if dietary intake is inadequate to meet the needs of the bones. Calcium or vitamin D will decrease absorption of alendronate, however, if either is taken at the same time as alendronate. The nurse should instruct the patient to take alendronate at least 1 hour before taking calcium or vitamin D.
- The nurse should encourage the patient to make lifestyle changes that will be beneficial for bone health such as engaging in weight-bearing exercise (e.g., walking as tolerated and permitted by the patient's physical condition), limiting or stopping cigarette smoking, and limiting or stopping alcohol use.

Ongoing Assessment and Evaluation

The nurse must verify throughout therapy that the patient is not experiencing hypocalcemia or other adverse effects from drug therapy. Therapy is effective when adverse effects are absent or minimal, bone mass density increases, and bone resorption and bone formation decrease. ■

DRUGS CLOSELY RELATED TO ALENDRONATE

The other bisphosphonates are etidronate (Didronel), tiludronate (Skelid), pamidronate (Aredia), and risedronate (Actonel). They all act primarily on bone to prevent bone resorption. Unlike alendronate, they are not used in the treatment or prevention of osteoporosis; their therapeutic indication is for treatment of Paget disease. Tiludronate and risedronate are used like alendronate for patients with Paget disease who have alkaline phosphatase levels at least two times greater than the upper limit of normal, or who are symptomatic or at risk for future complications. Oral etidronate is used in the treatment of symptomatic Paget disease, and pamidronate is used in the treatment of moderate to severe Paget disease.

MEMORY CHIP

Alendronate

- Used to treat or prevent osteoporosis in postmenopausal women; also used to treat Paget disease
- Prevents bone resorption
- Significant contraindication: hypocalcemia
- Most common adverse effects: GI problems
- Most serious adverse effect: hypocalcemia (uncommon)
- **Life span alert: used in postmenopausal women**
- Most significant patient education: take medication at least 30 minutes before eating, drinking, or taking other medication; take with plain water only

Additional therapeutic uses for these drugs are treatment and prevention of heterotopic ossification (formation of bone in abnormal location) after total hip replacement or spine injury (oral etidronate); treatment of moderate to severe hypercalcemia of malignancy, with or without bone metastasis (pamidronate, parenteral etidronate); and breast cancer/ multiple myeloma in conjunction with standard chemotherapy (pamidronate). Unlabeled uses include treatment of postmenopausal osteoporosis (etidronate, pamidronate, risedronate) and hyperparathyroidism (pamidronate); prevention of glucocorticoid-induced osteoporosis (pamidronate); reduction of bone pain in patients with prostate cancer (pamidronate); and treatment of hypercalcemia from immobilization (pamidronate).

Pharmacokinetics, pharmacodynamics, and adverse effects for all these drugs are similar to those of alendronate.

DRUG SIGNIFICANTLY DIFFERENT FROM ALENDRONATE

Like alendronate, raloxifene (Evista) is prescribed to prevent osteoporosis in postmenopausal women. It reduces resorption of bone and decreases overall bone turnover. Unlike alendronate, however, raloxifene works as a selective estrogen receptor modulator. Raloxifene is actually an estrogen antagonist, because it blocks estrogen from attaching itself to the estrogen-receptor sites. It produces some effects of estrogen. These include its estrogen-like effects on bone (increasing bone mass density) as well as on lipids (decreases in total and LDL cholesterol levels). Raloxifene does not share estrogen's effects on the uterus or the breasts.

Raloxifene is rapidly absorbed after oral dosing. It has an extensive first pass metabolism, although the CYTP450 pathways do not appear to metabolize it. The metabolites that are formed have a long half-life. The drug is highly protein bound. Raloxifene is excreted in the feces. It may cause fetal harm if given to pregnant women. It is a pregnancy category X drug and its use is therefore contraindicated in pregnant women. Raloxifene is also contraindicated if the woman has a history of or active venous thromboembolic events (deep vein thrombosis, pulmonary embolism, retinal vein thrombosis). Precaution should be used if coadministering raloxifene with other highly protein-bound drugs, such as clofibrate, indomethacin, ibuprofen, or diazepam. Raloxifene may decrease the binding of these drugs, allowing for more free and active drug.

Common adverse effects of ralozifene are hot flashes and leg cramps. Ralozifene increases the risk of venous thromboembolic events, especially during the first 4 months of treatment. To minimize this risk, patients should discontinue use of raloxifene at least 72 hours prior to an expected prolonged immobilization (e.g., a planned surgical event requiring immobilization or bed rest). Raloxifene also should be discontinued throughout periods of prolonged immobilization and bed rest. Patients should resume therapy only when fully ambulatory. If patients are traveling, the nurse must advise them to avoid prolonged sitting in the same position.

The nurse must teach patients to take supplemental calcium and Vitamin D if their dietary intake is inadequate. Similar to the case in the use of alendronate, the nurse must encourage the patient to do weight-bearing exercises and to decrease alcohol consumption and cigarette smoking to promote bone density.

CHAPTER SUMMARY

- Women need adequate levels of sex hormones to develop and maintain the sexual and reproductive organs, create and maintain the secondary sexual characteristics, induce and stop the growth spurt of adolescence, and to achieve and maintain pregnancy.
- Estrogen and progestin are the primary female sex hormones.
- Estrogen causes capillary dilation, promotes fluid retention, enhances protein anabolism, contributes to strengthening the skeleton, and maintains normal bone density and composition.
- Progestins are composed of progesterone and its derivatives. They regulate, through stimulation or inhibition, the secretion of pituitary gonadotropins. This, in turn, regulates the development of the ovarian follicle. Progestins also inhibit spontaneous uterine contractions.
- Decreased levels of female sex hormones (primarily estrogen) that result from menopause increase the risk of cardiovascular disease and osteoporosis. Cardiovascular disease is the primary cause of death for postmenopausal women. Osteoporosis affects women more than men, because levels of male sex hormones (testosterone) fall more gradually and occur at a later age than the decline of estrogen in women.
- Postmenopausal HRT to treat or prevent cardiovascular disease and osteoporosis may contain estrogen alone or estrogen and a progestin. HRT is not without risks. Benefits versus risks for each individual patient should be considered before therapy is initiated. Research is still being conducted about the role HRT should play in managing current and potential health problems in postmenopausal women.
- Most oral contraceptives are combinations of estrogen and progestin. They may have serious adverse effects, but it has been found that these are usually related to higher doses of estrogen in the drugs. Oral contraceptives should be prescribed with the smallest effective dose of estrogen possible for the patient.

QUESTIONS FOR STUDY AND REVIEW

1. Describe the positive effects of estrogen therapy on postmenopausal women.
2. Explain why progesterone can be used to treat amenorrhea and abnormal uterine bleeding.
3. What are the serious adverse effects that may result from estrogen therapy?
4. What is the benefit of using the selective estrogen receptor modulator, raloxifene, instead of conjugated estrogen to treat postmenopausal osteoporosis?
5. What teaching points regarding missed pills would you review with a patient who was starting oral contraceptives?
6. What unique instructions about drug administration do you need to give to a patient who is to receive alendronate for osteoporosis?

NEED MORE HELP?

Chapter 43 of the study guide for *Drug Therapy in Nursing* contains exercises and activities to reinforce your understanding of the concepts presented in this chapter. For additional information see the text's accompanying website at *http://www.connection.lww.com*.

REFERENCES AND BIBLIOGRAPHY

American Cancer Society: Breast Cancer Resource Center [On-line]. Available: http://www3.cancer.org/cancerinfo/load_cont.asp?st=pr&ct=5&language=english

Blakely, J. A. (2000). The heart and Estrogen/Progestin replacement study revisited: Hormone replacement therapy produced net harm, consistent with the observational data. *Archives of Internal Medicine, 160*(19), 2897–2900.

Bush, T. L. (2000). Preserving cardiovascular benefits of hormone replacement therapy. *Journal of Reproductive Medicine, 45,* (3 Suppl.), 259–273.

Espeland, M. A., Marcovina, S. M., Miller, V., Wood, P. D., Wasilauskas, C., Sherwin, R., Schrott, H., & Bush, T. L. (1998). Effect of postmenopausal hormone therapy on lipoprotein (a) concentration. PEPI Investigators. Postmenopausal Estrogen/Progestin Interventions. *Circulation, 97*(10), 979–986.

Grady, D., Wenger, N. K., Herrington, D., Khan, S., Furgerg, C., Hunninghake, D., Vittinghoff, E., & Hulley, S. (2000). Postmenopausal hormone therapy increases risk for venous thromboembolic disease. The Heart and Estrogen/Progestin Replacement Study. *Annals of Internal Medicine, 132*(9), 689–696.

Greendale, G. A., Reboussin, B. A., Sie, A., Singh, H. R., Olson, L. K., Gatewood, O., Bassett, L. W., Wasilauskas, C., Bush, T., & Barrett-Connor, E. (1999). Effects of estrogen and estrogen-progestin on mammographic parenchymal density. Postmenopausal Estrogen/ Progestin Interventions (PEPI) Investigators. *Annals of Internal Medicine, 130*(4 Pt 1), 262–269.

Greendale, G. A., Wells, B., Marcus, R., & Barrett-Connor, E. (2000). How many women lose bone mineral density while taking hormone replacement therapy?: Results from the Postmenopausal Estrogen/ Progestin Interventions trial. *Archives of Internal Medicine, 160*(20), 3065–3071.

Grodstein, F., Stampfer, M. J., Manson, J. E., Colditz, G. A., Willett, W. C., Rosner, B., Speizer, F. E., & Hennekens, C. H. (1996). Postmenopausal estrogen and progestin use and the risk of cardiovascular disease. *New England Journal of Medicine, 335*(7), 453-4–61.

Grodstein, F., Stampfer, M. J., Colditz, G. A., Willett, W. C., Manson, J. E., Joffe, M., Rosner, B., Fuchs, C., Hankinson, S. E., Hunter, D. J., Hennekens, C. H., & Speizer, F. E. (1997). Postmenopausal hormone therapy and mortality. *New England Journal of Medicine, 336*(25), 1769–1775.

Herrington, D. M. (1999). The HERS trial results: paradigms lost? Heart and Estrogen/Progestin Replacement Study. *Annals of Internal Medicine, 131*(6), 463–466.

Herrington, D. M., Reboussin, D. M., Klein, K. P., Sharp, P. C., Shumaker, S. A., Snyder, T. E., & Geisinger, K. R. (2000). The estrogen replacement and atherosclerosis (ERA) study: Study design and baseline characteristics of the cohort. *Controlled Clinical Trials, 21*(3), 257–285.

Hsia, J., Simon, J. A., Lin, F., Applegate, W. B., Vogt, M. T., Hunninghake, D., & Carr, M. (2000). Peripheral arterial disease in randomized trial of estrogen with progestin in women with coronary heart disease: The Heart and Estrogen/Progestin Replacement Study. *Circulation, 102*(18), 2228–2232.

Hogervorst, E., Williams, J., Budge, M., Riedel, W., & Jolles, J. (2000). The nature of the effect of female gonadal hormone replacement therapy on cognitive function in post menopausal women: A meta-analysis. *Neuroscience, 101*(3), 485–512.

Jacobs, H. S. (2000). Postmenopausal hormone replacement therapy and breast cancer. *Medscape Womens Health, 5*(4), E2.

McPherson, R. (2000). Is hormone replacement therapy cardioprotective? Decision making after the heart and estrogen/progestin replacement study. *Canadian Journal of Cardiology, 16,* (Suppl. A), 14A–19A.

Pike, M. C., & Ross, R. K. (2000). Progestins and menopause: epidemiological studies of risks of endometrial and breast cancer. *Steroids, 65*(10-11), 659–664.

Sawaya, G. F., Grady, D., Kerlikowske, K., Valleur, J. L., Barnabei, V. M., Bass, K., Snyder, T. E., Pickar, J. H., Agarwal, S. K., & Mandelblatt, J. (2000). The positive predictive value of cervical smears in previously screened postmenopausal women: The Heart and Estrogen/Progestin Replacement Study (HERS). *Annals of Internal Medicine, 133*(12), 942–950.

Seed, M., Sands, R. H., McLaren, M., Kirk, G., & Darko, D. (2000). The effect of hormone replacement therapy and route of administration on selected cardiovascular risk factors in post menopausal women. *Family Practice, 17*(6), 497–507.

The Writing Group for the PEPI. (1996a). Effects of hormone replacement therapy on endometrial histology in postmenopausal women. The Postmenopausal Estrogen/Progestin Interventions (PEPI trial). *Journal of the American Medical Association, 275*(5), 370–375.

The Writing Group for the PEPI. (1996b). Effects of hormone therapy on bone mineral density: Results from the Postmenopausal Estrogen/ Progestin Interventions (PEPI trial). *Journal of the American Medical Association, 276*(17), 1430–1432.

University of Maryland Medicine. *Osteoporosis* [On-line]. Available: http://umm.drkoop.com/conditions/ency/article/000360.htm

U.S. Food and Drug Administration Center for Drug Evaluation and Research. *Mifeprex (mifepristone) Tablets Label* [On-line]. Available: http://www.fda.gov/cder/foi/label/2000/20687lbl.htm

U.S. Food and Drug Administration Center for Drug Evaluation and Research. *Mifepristone Medication Guide* [On-line]. Available: http://www.fda.gov/cder/drug/infopage/mifepristone/medguide.htm

Wells, G., & Herrington, D. M. (1999). The Heart and Estrogen/ Progestin Replacement Study: What have we learned and what questions remain? *Drugs and Aging, 15*(6), 419–422.

Chapter 44

DRUGS AFFECTING UTERINE MOTILITY

KEY TERMS

antepartum
intrapartum
oxytocics
postpartum
tocolytics
uterine tetany

Learning Objectives

At the completion of this chapter the student will:

1. Identify core drug knowledge about drugs that affect uterine motility.
2. Identify core patient variables relevant to drugs that affect uterine motility.
3. Relate the interaction of core drug knowledge to core patient variables for drugs that affect uterine contraction.
4. Generate a nursing plan of care from the interactions between core drug knowledge and core patient variables for drugs that affect uterine motility.
5. Describe nursing interventions to maximize therapeutic effects and minimize adverse effects for drugs that affect uterine motility.
6. Determine key points for patient and family education for drugs that affect uterine motility.

Oxytocics

- **oxytocin**
- ergonovine maleate
- methylergonovine
- carboprost
- dinoprostone
- misoprostol

Tocolytics

- **ritodrine**
- terbutaline
- magnesium sulfate
- indomethacin

The symbol (C) indicates the **drug class**.

Drugs in bold type marked with the symbol (P) are **prototypes**.

Drugs in blue type with no symbol are **closely related** to the prototype.

Drugs in **red** type with no symbol are **significantly different** from the prototype.

Drugs in **black** type with no symbol are **also used in drug therapy**; no prototype.

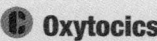

For labor and delivery of the fetus, normal uterine function is necessary. Normal uterine function consists of labor contractions beginning between 38 and 42 weeks of gestation. The contractions must be regular and strong enough to facilitate delivery of the fetus. At times, labor occurs prematurely, and stopping the uterine contractions is desirable. This chapter examines two classes of drugs that are used when the uterus does not function normally:

- **Oxytocics:** uterine stimulants used to initiate or augment a contractile pattern of labor
- **Tocolytics:** uterine relaxants used to stop labor contractions that occur before completion of the 37th week of gestation
- Oxytocin (Pitocin, Syntocin) is the prototype oxytocic drug. The prototype tocolytic drug is ritodrine.

PHYSIOLOGY

CONTRACTIONS AND RELATED CHANGES

Most women progress through pregnancy with contractions beginning between 38 and 42 gestational weeks. The onset of labor begins the **intrapartum** period of pregnancy. The induction of labor is related to oxytocin, a hormone that is produced in the hypothalamus, stored in the posterior pituitary, and released into the circulatory system. Once the pituitary releases oxytocin, oxytocin binds to cell-membrane receptors on target tissues, primarily the uterine myometrium (muscle cells) and the mammary epithelium. The fetus may also secrete some oxytocin during labor. Oxytocin receptors are also located in the decidua, which is the endometrium (or lining) of the uterus. Although the exact mechanism of oxytocin in labor is unknown, endogenous oxytocin stimulates the myometrial cells of the uterus, initiating uterine contractions (Fig. 44-1). The myometrial cells increase in sensitivity as pregnancy progresses, because the number of oxytocin receptors doubles just before labor. Estrogen may have a role in the creation of additional oxytocin receptors. The oxytocin receptors that are located in the endometrium increase during labor and reach peak levels at birth. If the number of oxytocin receptors is limited, the response of the uterus to oxytocin will be diminished. Oxytocinase, produced by the placenta, rapidly degrades oxytocin, which allows circulating oxytocin to restimulate the oxytocin receptors.

Endogenous oxytocin also has some vasopressive (i.e., vascular constriction) and antidiuretic (i.e., increased water resorption from the glomerular filtrate) effects. Oxytocin is also necessary for the letdown of breast milk. Additionally, oxytocin is believed to have an intricate role in the creation and maintenance of maternal behavior (e.g., bonding with the infant, caring for the infant).

In addition to the necessary number of oxytocin receptors and the amount of available oxytocin, contraction of uterine muscle also depends on oxygenation and glucose. Oxygen and glucose are required to provide the energy needed for muscle contraction. If these two elements are inadequate, the uterine contractions will be too weak or too few to advance labor and progress to delivery. For example, if the woman in labor has pathophysiology that impairs her respiratory status (e.g., a chronic respiratory disease), she may be unable to fully oxygenate the uterus. Conversely, if the woman has had a prolonged labor, she may have exhausted her glucose reserves.

Prostaglandins also have a role in preparing the uterus for labor and delivery. Prostaglandin E_2 (PGE_2) leads to sensitization of the myometrium to oxytocin. PGE_2 primarily plays a role in assisting with cervical ripening (by which the cervix becomes softened, yielding, and dilated to allow for the passage of the fetus in vaginal delivery) without affecting uterine contractions. PGE_2, however, is capable of initiating uterine contractions and may interact with oxytocin to increase uterine contractility.

Physiology

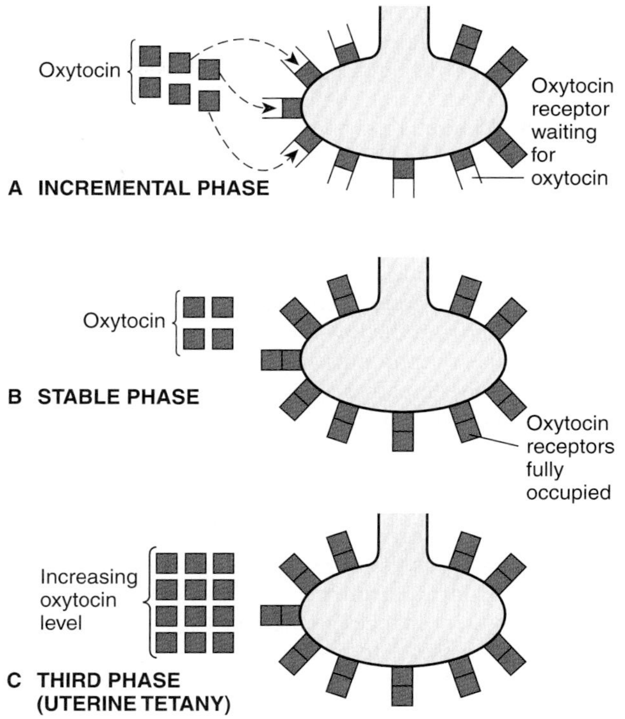

Figure 44-1. Phases of oxytocin activity. Oxytocic drug therapy is usually initiated to mimic the role of natural oxytocin in prompting or augmenting labor. Oxytocin undergoes three phases of activity. (**A**) In the incremental phase, oxytocin levels rise, and oxytocin receptors are stimulated, producing increased intensity and frequency of uterine contractions. (**B**) In the stable phase, receptor sites are occupied with oxytocin, so no further oxytocin effects occur until a receptor site opens again. (**C**) In the third phase—uterine tetany—oxytocin levels continually rise. Uterine contractions increase in number while the force of the contractions decreases. In such instances, the uterus experiences hyperstimulation.

SYSTEMIC CHANGES IN LABOR

Systemic changes initiated in the **antepartum** period (pregnancy before labor starts) continue into the intrapartum period. When labor contractions begin, the child-bearing woman and her fetus exhibit additional physiologic alterations. The stress produced by uterine contractions affects many maternal systemic responses.

The woman experiences significant cardiovascular system changes. Blood pressure remains close to the antepartal baseline, except during uterine contractions. With contractions during the first stage of labor, the systolic pressure may increase by 35 mm Hg, while the diastolic pressure may increase by 25 mm Hg. During the second stage of labor, with bearing-down efforts, blood pressure increases even more. Pulse rate may increase because of the pain of labor contractions but should return to antepartal baselines. The bearing-down efforts (pushing against a closed glottis) of the second stage also increase intrathoracic pressure, which interrupts venous return from the lower extremities. This in turn decreases cardiac output, pulse pressure, and blood pressure. When the patient breathes again, the intrathoracic pressure decreases, helping cardiac output, pulse pressure, and blood pressure return to baseline values. Immediately after birth, cardiac output increases 80% above prelabor values; within the first hour after delivery, it will decrease by approximately 50%. Most child-bearing women can adapt to these cardiovascular changes successfully without requiring drug therapy.

During the intrapartum period, the woman experiences respiratory system changes because oxygen demand and consumption increase. The respiratory rate increases above pregnancy rates because of uterine contractions. This hyperventilation causes the level of $PaCO_2$ to fall; consequently, respiratory alkalosis develops.

As labor progresses, the contracting uterus increases muscular activity and oxygen requirements, which produces a mild metabolic acidosis. This mild metabolic acidosis continues, so that during the second stage of labor and by the time of birth, the acid-base balance remains as metabolic acidosis uncompensated by respiratory alkalosis. The acid-base imbalances created by labor are quickly reversed after delivery because respiratory rates return to prepregnancy values and lactic acid production decreases. By 24 hours after birth, acid-base status is similar to prepregnancy levels.

The major labor adaptation in the hemopoietic system is the development of leukocytosis above pregnancy levels. The child-bearing patient's white blood cell count may be between 25,000 and 30,000 mm^3. Although an elevated white blood cell count is normally considered a sign of infection, laboratory assessment that shows an elevation of the white blood cells in the woman who has just delivered must not routinely be considered a sign of infection. This leukocytosis most likely results from labor stress, heavy exertion, and the opened healing placental site.

Profuse perspiration and hyperventilation alter fluid and electrolyte balance during labor. Most women are not permitted to eat or drink as labor progresses to prevent nausea, vomiting, and possible aspiration. Generally, healthy women having uncomplicated vaginal deliveries do not require IV fluids during labor but merely do not have any food or drink during this period. If labor is long, the woman may experience dehydration and electrolyte imbalance. She may require hydration through the administration of IV fluids.

Compensation within the renal system because of decreased oral intake and increased insensible water loss includes the excretion of more concentrated urine. The increasing uterine muscular activity leads to a breakdown of proteins and the presence of a trace of protein in the urine. As the fetal head descends in the pelvis, it extends pressure against the bladder walls and the urethra. The woman may not be sensitive to bladder filling.

The gastrointestinal (GI) system experiences a reduction or cessation of gastric motility and absorption of solid foods as labor begins. Gastric emptying time is prolonged, and more than 25 mL of gastric contents remains in the stomach regardless of when the woman consumed her last meal. Gastric acidity increases, and more than 50% of laboring women have a gastric pH below 2.5. Most circulating blood shifts away from the GI system to more vital maternal organs during labor.

The healthy fetus can progress through a normal labor and delivery with no adverse effects. The labor process produces a stressful physiologic state in the fetus with each contraction, but fetal compensatory mechanisms generally allow the fetus to respond successfully to those events.

Fetal acid-base status in labor depends on the maternal contractile pattern and the fetus's ability to compensate for contraction-produced decreases in oxygen. Oxygen/carbon dioxide exchange between the mother and the fetus occurs primarily between contractions when the blood flow is not impeded. In women who are laboring efficiently, the contractions occur at intervals that allow the intervillous spaces in the placenta to refill with oxygenated blood between contractions; this maintains an adequate oxygen supply to the fetus. The healthy fetus thus maintains a pH above 7.25. The two main indicators of fetal well-being and adequate fetal compensation during labor are a stable fetal heart rate (FHR) and the presence of fetal movements. The mature FHR ranges within a baseline of 120 to 160 beats/min.

PATHOPHYSIOLOGY

Occasionally, uterine function proceeds abnormally, causing failure of labor to occur or failure of labor to progress. The two main categories of unique obstetric situations that require medical intervention with drug administration to initiate the onset of contractions include labor that does not begin at term and a pregnancy that is detrimental to the patient or her fetus.

Stimulation of uterine contractions using drugs before a spontaneous labor is called induction of labor. Specific maternal and fetal conditions that may require induction of labor include the following:

- Diabetes
- Preeclampsia
- Premature rupture of the membranes
- Fetal demise
- Renal disease
- Postterm pregnancy
- Chorioamnionitis (inflammation of the membrane covering the fetus)
- Isoimmunization (response of an Rh-negative mother when exposed to Rh-positive blood from her infant)
- Intrauterine fetal growth retardation
- Mild abruptio placentae with no fetal distress

Before induction is initiated, the patient's cervix is assessed using the Bishop scoring system, and the fetus is assessed for evidence of maturity. The Bishop scale is a prelabor scoring system used to assist in predicting patient success if labor is induced. The system consists of five assessment parameters:

1. Cervical dilation
2. Cervical effacement
3. Fetal station
4. Cervical consistency
5. Cervical position

Each parameter is scored on a scale of 0 to 3. The higher the score, the greater is the likelihood that induction will lead to a vaginal delivery. The favorable cervix is described as one that is anterior, soft, at least 50% effaced and 2 cm dilated, with the fetal station at +1 or lower. These findings are equal to a Bishop score of 9.

Drugs may be administered to increase uterine contractions if labor is spontaneous but labor patterns are dysfunctional, particularly when labor patterns are not strong or rhythmic enough to spur delivery. This type of labor needs augmentation with drug therapy that increases uterine contractions.

Another obstetric event usually requiring drug therapy is premature labor. The parturitional (child-birthing) process is now known to begin long before clinically detected preterm labor. Increases in gap junctions, oxytocin receptors, and enhanced uterine contractility accompany the parturitional process. If labor begins before completion of the 37th gestational week, drug therapy may be used (in addition to conservative methods of bed rest in side-lying position, hydration, and sedation) to stop the uterine contractions and prolong the pregnancy. None of the currently used drug therapies appears to alter the fundamental process of parturition. The goal of drug therapy is to secure some additional time before delivery to administer drugs to the mother. The purpose of this delay is to help promote fetal respiratory function and to allow time to transfer the mother, if necessary, to a hospital capable of providing acute medical care to the mother and neonatal intensive care to the newborn. Corticosteroids are administered to improve neonatal outcomes. "Corticosteroid administration reduces the odds of neonatal death by 63 percent, the odds of respiratory distress syndrome (RDS) by 30 percent, and the odds of intraventricular hemorrhage (IVH), a risk factor for cerebral palsy, by 46 percent. These effects of corticosteroids are greatest when the pregnancy is prolonged for at least 24 hours; the benefits continue for at least 7 days. The impact of corticosteroid therapy appears to differ according to gestational age. After the 28th week, both the incidence of death and RDS are significantly reduced. Between 24 and 28 weeks, the incidence of death and IVH are significantly reduced. Although the incidence of RDS is not significantly reduced, the severity of disease is." (Dr. Steve Carilis; testimony to the FDA on atosifan 1998) (See chapter 40 for a complete discussion of corticosteroids.)

OXYTOCICS

Oxytocic drugs are synthetic forms of the endogenous posterior pituitary hormone oxytocin. They produce uterine contractions and milk ejection for breast-feeding. The prototype oxytocic drug is oxytocin (Pictocin, Syntocin). Drugs closely related to oxytocin are ergonovine maleate (Ergotrate Maleate) and methylergonovine (Methergine). Drugs significantly different from oxytocin are carboprost (Hemabate), dinoprostone (Prepidil, Cervidil), and misoprostol (Cytotec).

NURSING MANAGEMENT OF THE PATIENT RECEIVING OXYTOCIN

Core Drug Knowledge

Pharmacotherapeutics

Oxytocin is given by IV drip infusion to initiate or augment (improve) labor contractions when there are significant fetal or maternal reasons to do so. Examples of such reasons include Rh problems, maternal diabetes, preeclampsia near term, premature rupture of membranes, or uterine inertia. IV oxytocin may also be used to treat incomplete or inevitable spontaneous abortion during the second trimester. IV infusion or IM injection of oxytocin is used to control postpartum bleeding or hemorrhage. Oxytocin should be dosed to mimic the release of endogenous oxytocin, which is about 2 to 3 mU/min in spontaneous labor. The dose of oxytocin should achieve adequate uterine contractility while minimizing maternal and fetal adverse effects. The dose should be low initially, no more than 1 to 2 mU/min. The dose requires slow upward titration in increments of 1 to 2 mU/min. Most women (with cervical ripening) will develop adequate labor patterns with 4 to 8 mU/min of oxytocin. The necessary dosage to achieve adequate labor is generally lower if labor is being augmented. The desired contractile pattern is described as consisting of one contraction every 2 to 3 minutes, with durations of 40 to 90 seconds per contraction and an intensity of 40 to 90 mm Hg for internal uterine monitoring or firm to palpation for external monitoring. In some other established protocols, called high-dose active management protocols, oxytocin is initiated at a higher rate and titrated with higher doses of the drug; dose changes may be as frequent as every 15 minutes. The use of these high-dose protocols is controversial (Clayworth, 2000).

Pharmacokinetics

Onset of action occurs almost immediately after IV administration. Steady state plasma levels are reached in approximately 40 minutes with continuous IV infusion, during which maximum uterine contraction occurs. Physiologic steady state is achieved when there is no further uterine response to increased oxytocin infusion because the receptor sites are already bound with oxytocin and are temporarily unavailable. Elimination is through the liver, kidneys, and mammary glands and by the enzyme oxytocinase (Table 44-1).

TABLE 44-1 Summary of Selected Uterine Motility Drugs

Drug (Trade) Name	Selected Indications	Route and Dosage Range	Pharmacokinetics
Oxytocics			
oxytocin (Pitocin, Syntocinon; nasal spray, Syntocinon)	Antepartum: to induce or augment uterine contractions Postpartum: to control postpartum bleeding or hemorrhage (parenteral)	*Adult:* IV (induction or augmentation of labor), 1–2 mU/min, through infusion pump, and should be increased by this amount at 30–60 or 40–60 min intervals; do not exceed 20 mU/min; IV (treatment of incomplete or spontaneous abortion), infusion of 10-U oxytocin with 500-mL physiologic saline solution or 5% dextrose in physiologic saline infused at a rate of 10–20 mU/min; (control of postpartum uterine bleeding), IV drip, add 10–40 U to 1,000 mL of a nonhydrating diluent: run at a rate to control uterine atony; IM, 10 U after delivery of placenta; (initial milk letdown)	*Onset:* IV, immediate; IM, 3–5 min; nasal, varies *Duration:* IV, 60 min; IM, 2–3 h; nasal, 20 min $t_{1/2}$: 1–6 min
ergonovine maleate (Ergotrate Maleate)	Prevention and treatment of postpartum and postabortal hemorrhage due to uterine atony	*Adult:* IM, 0.2 mg, severe bleeding may require repeat dosing q2–4 h; IV, 0.2 mg in emergency situations	*Onset:* IM, 7–8 min; IV, immediate *Duration:* IM, 3 h; IV, 45 min $t_{1/2}$: 0.5–2 h
methylergonovine (Methergine)	Routine management after delivery of the placenta Treatment of postpartum atony and hemorrhage; subinvolution of the uterus	*Adult:* IM, 0.2 mg after delivery of the placenta, after delivery of the anterior shoulder, or during puerperium; may be repeated q2–4 h; IV, same dosage as IM, infuse slowly over at least 60 seconds, monitor BP very carefully because severe hyper-tensive reaction can occur; oral, 0.2 mg tid or qid daily in the puerperium for up to 1 wk	*Onset:* IM, 2–5 min; IV, immediate; oral, 5–10 min *Duration:* IM, 3 h; IV, 1–3 h; oral, 3 h $t_{1/2}$: 30 min
Tocolytics			
ritodrine (Yutopar)	Management of preterm labor in selected patients ≥ 20 wk gestation	*Adult:* IV, 0.05 mg/min initially; gradually increase by 0.05 mg/min q10min until desired result is attained; usual effective dosage between 0.15 and 0.35 mg/min continued for at least 12 h after uterine contractions cease	*Onset:* Rapid *Duration:* Unknown $t_{1/2}$: 1.7–2.6 h
terbutaline sulfate (Brethaire, Brethine, Bricanyl)	Unlabeled use: inhibition of premature labor	*Adult:* IV, initially 10 μg/min; titrate upward to a maximum of 80 μg/min; maintain at minimum effective dosage for 4 h; oral, 2.5 mg q4–6 h daily as maintenance therapy	*Onset:* IV, unknown oral, 30 min *Duration:* IV, unknown oral, 4–8 h $t_{1/2}$: Unknown
Others			
carboprost (Hemabate)	Termination of pregnancy 13–20 wk Evacuation of the uterus in instance of missed abortion or intrauterine fetal death in the second trimester Postpartum hemorrhage due to uterine atony that does not respond to conventional methods	*Adult:* (Abortion) IM, 250 μg at 1½ to 3½ h intervals; may be increased to 500 μg; do not exceed 12 mg total dose or continuous administration over 2 d; (postpartum hemorrhage) IM, 250 μg as one dose; multiple doses at 15–90 min intervals may be used; do not exceed a total dose of 2 mg	*Onset:* 15 min *Duration:* Unknown $t_{1/2}$: 8 h

TABLE 44-1 Summary of Selected Uterine Motility Drugs (Continued)

Drug (Trade) Name	Selected Indications	Route and Dosage Range	Pharmacokinetics
dinoprostone (Prostaglandin E_2)	Termination of pregnancy 12–20 wk Evacuation of the uterus in missed abortion or intrauterine fetal death up to 28 wk gestational age Management of nonmetastatic gestational trophoblastic disease (benign hydatidiform mole) Initiation of cervical ripening before induction of labor	*Adult:* (Abortion) Intravaginal, one suppository (10 mg); additional suppositories may be given at 3–5 h intervals; (cervical ripening) intravaginal gel, 0.5 mg dose; repeat dose may be given if no response in 6 h	*Onset:* 10 min *Duration:* 2–3 h $t_{1/2}$: 2.5–5 min
magnesium sulfate	Unlabeled use: inhibition of premature labor; seizure prevention and control in pre-eclampsia and eclampsia	*Adult:* IM, 4–5 g of a 50% solution q4h as necessary; IV, 4 g of a 10%–20% solution; do not exceed 1.5 mL/min of a 10% solution; IV infusion, 4–5 g in 250-mL 5% dextrose; do not exceed 3 mL/min	*Onset:* IV, immediate; IM, 60 min *Duration:* IV, 30 min; IM, 3–4 h $t_{1/2}$: Unknown

Pharmacodynamics

Synthetic exogenous oxytocin has the same effects on the body as natural endogenous oxytocin. It stimulates uterine contractions and milk letdown for breast-feeding. Although the endogenous hormone has a known effect on milk production, exogenous oxytocin is not administered for this purpose.

Response to oxytocin therapy has three phases (see Fig. 44-1):

1. Incremental phase: uterine activity increases evenly as the dose of oxytocin increases.
2. Stable phase: uterine activity remains constant even if the oxytocin dose increases, because the myometrial receptor sites are already fully bound with oxytocin. Because the sites are full, they cannot be receptive to more effects from the oxytocin. As half-life and elimination of oxytocin occur, the uterus will again have open receptors and be responsive to increases in oxytocin. The uterus will shift periodically between the incremental and stable phases.
3. Hyperstimulation: this third phase of uterine response is possible from oxytocin, although it indicates adverse effects from the drug. If the dose continually increases, the frequency of contractions will increase, but the uterine pressure will decrease so that the contractions are less effective. This results in hyperstimulation of the uterus with uterine fibrillation and prolonged contraction. This condition is known as **uterine tetany**. The American College of Obstetricians and Gynecologists (ACOG) has defined hyperstimulation as a "persistent pattern of more than 5 contractions in 10 minutes, contractions lasting 2 minutes or more, or contractions of normal duration occurring within 1 minute of each other" (ACOG, 1995).

Oxytocin therapy also has vasopressive and antidiuretic effects. Oxytocin affects the cardiovascular system by initially decreasing blood pressure. With prolonged oxytocin administration, baseline blood pressure may increase by 30%. Cardiac output and stroke volume also increase. Oxytocin doses of 20 mU/min or above have antidiuretic effects when administered over a prolonged period. Although the antidiuretic effects are weak, fatal water intoxication has occurred with the use of oxytocin. (Water intoxication occurs when retention of water and sodium is excessive, resulting in abdominal cramps, dizziness, lethargy, nausea, vomiting, convulsions, and coma.)

Contraindications and Precautions

Oxytocin is contraindicated in significant cephalopelvic (fetal head to maternal pelvis) disproportion and with unfavorable fetal positions or presentations that must be converted before delivery (e.g., transverse lies). It is also contraindicated in the following conditions:

- Obstetric emergencies in which the benefit:risk ratio for either mother or fetus favors cesarean section
- Fetal distress without signs of imminent delivery
- Prolonged use in uterine inertia or severe toxemia
- Hypertonic or hyperactive uterine patterns
- Failure of adequate uterine activity to achieve satisfactory progress
- Contraindication of vaginal delivery (e.g., invasive cervical carcinoma, active genital herpes, cord presentation or prolapse, total placenta previa, vas previa)
- Hypersensitivity to the drug

Oxytocin must be administered very cautiously if cyclopropane anesthesia is used, because maternal sinus bradycardia with abnormal atrioventricular rhythms and hypotension may result. Water intoxication is pos-

cardiogram [ECG] changes), hyperventilation, and weakness may all occur. Sinus bradycardia may occur after discontinuation of the drug. A few patients experience impaired liver functioning. Transient leukopenia or agranulocytosis may occur if infusions are given for longer than 2 to 3 weeks; leukocyte count will return to normal after discontinuation of the drug.

Overdosage symptoms are signs of excessive beta-adrenergic stimulation. They include tachycardia, palpitations, cardiac arrhythmias, hypotension, dyspnea, nervousness, tremor, nausea, and vomiting. In instances of overdose, the drug should be discontinued and an appropriate beta blocker, such as propranolol, should be given as an antidote. Ritodrine is dialyzable.

Drug Interactions

Concomitant use of ritodrine and atropine may produce systemic hypertension. Corticosteroid use with ritodrine may lead to pulmonary edema. Diazoxide, general anesthetics, magnesium sulfate, and meperidine may all potentiate the cardiovascular effects of ritodrine, especially arrhythmias and hypotension. Use of other sympathomimetics may produce additive or potentiated effects with ritodrine. Beta blockers will inhibit the action of ritodrine (see Table 44-2).

IV administration of ritodrine is associated with transient elevations of blood glucose and insulin levels. These levels usually return to normal in 48 to 72 hours, even with continued infusion. Elevated levels of free fatty acids and cyclic adenosine monophosphate have also been reported with ritodrine use. Serum potassium levels will decrease but return to baseline within 24 hours of stopping administration of ritodrine.

Assessment of Relevant Core Patient Variables

Health Status

The nurse must determine whether the patient has any conditions that contraindicate therapy. These conditions may include hypovolemia, cardiac arrhythmias associated with tachycardia or digitalis toxicity, uncontrolled hypertension, pheochromocytoma, or bronchial asthma already treated with beta agonists or steroids. Assessment of the patient's pulse rate and blood pressure is important for the nurse to perform. A baseline ECG should be performed to rule out undiagnosed maternal heart disease prior to beginning an IV infusion of ritodrine. The nurse should determine whether the patient is sensitive to sulfites or receiving beta blockers or corticosteroids.

Life Span and Gender

The nurse should ask whether the woman's pregnancy is 20 weeks or more, because pregnancy of less than 20 weeks is a contraindication. The nurse should try to determine the stage of labor; if the patient is in advanced labor, safety and efficacy of ritodrine are not established. Ritodrine crosses the placenta, but fetal abnormalities have not been found in women receiving the drug after the 20th week of gestation. Infants born before 36 weeks' gestation, although a minority of births account for most perinatal deaths and half of all neurologically handicapped infants. By delaying or preventing preterm birth, ritodrine should promote an increase in neonatal survival. Still, although long-term effects on the child are believed to be nondetrimental, they are not definitely known. Risk versus benefit of ritodrine use must be considered for each patient.

Environment

The nurse should be aware of the environment required to administer ritodrine. Ritodrine must be given in a hospital labor and delivery suite where the mother and fetus can be monitored continually while the IV solution is infused. Undiluted ritodrine may be stored at room temperature and should be protected from excessive heat (above 30°C or 86°F).

Nursing Diagnoses and Outcomes

- Decreased Cardiac Output related to potential adverse effects of drug therapy
  Desired outcome: Cardiac output will remain stable to support the vital functions of the patient and fetus.
- Excess Fluid Volume, pulmonary edema, related to potential adverse effects of drug therapy
  Desired outcome: The patient's fluid volume will remain within normal limits.

Planning and Intervention

Maximizing Therapeutic Effects

The nurse should begin drug therapy as soon as possible after diagnosis. Ritodrine is administered by IV infusion. The nurse dilutes about 150 mg of ritodrine in 500 mL of 5% dextrose in water. He or she starts an initial dose of 0.05 mg/min (or 0.17 mL/min or 10 drops/min using a microdrip, 60 drops/mL tubing if diluted according to recommendation) and increases the dose by 0.05 mg/min every 10 minutes until contractions have stopped. The nurse should continue the IV infusion for 12 hours after cessation of uterine contractions.

Minimizing Adverse Effects

The nurse should monitor the patient's pulse rate and blood pressure closely throughout therapy. The patient should lie on her left side during infusion to help minimize the risk of hypotension and to promote circulation to the fetus. The nurse must also closely monitor the patient's fluid status and avoid fluid overload. Related measures include monitoring intake and output, assessing peripheries for edema, and auscultating breath sounds for rales and rhonchi every hour. If pulmonary edema develops, the nurse must discontinue drug administration and notify the health care provider or nurse midwife immediately. He or she should seek orders to manage the edema by diuretic therapy.

If the patient demonstrates signs of adverse effects, such as palpitations, tachycardia, hypotension, or nervousness, the dosage should be decreased. A beta blocker, such as propranolol, should be available as an antidote in case of overdosage. If the patient is diabetic or receives potassium-depleting diuretics, the nurse should monitor the serum glucose and potassium levels carefully. See the accompanying display, Maternal Monitoring and Ritodrine.

Administration of ritodrine infusions should be through an IV infusion controller or pump to keep the dosage rate accurate. If the patient requires other IV drugs, they nurse may piggyback them onto the ritodrine line so long as control of the infusion rate of ritodrine is separate and unaffected. A secondary IV administration site is preferable to maintain integrity of the ritodrine line. Because of the risk of pulmonary edema, the nurse usually should avoid diluting ritodrine with saline (i.e., 0.9% sodium chloride solution or lactated Ringer solution) and Hartmann solution; he or she should use a dextrose solution instead. The nurse should not administer ritodrine after 48 hours of dilution or if the solution is discolored or has precipitates.

Providing Patient and Family Education

- The nurse should educate the patient and family about the therapeutic and adverse effects of the drug.
- The nurse should explain to the patient the rationale for lying on her left side.
- The nurse should instruct the patient to notify the nurse immediately if she experiences swelling in her hands or feet, shortness of breath, palpitations, or chest pain. See the accompanying display, Teaching About Drugs That Affect Uterine Function.

Ongoing Assessment and Evaluation

The nurse should monitor the maternal heart rate, FHR, and the maternal blood pressure and fluid status throughout therapy. Ritodrine drug therapy is considered effective when the premature contractions decrease in intensity and frequency, premature birth is avoided, and the woman and fetus do not incur adverse effects. ■

Critical Thinking Scenario

Maternal monitoring and ritodrine

Susan Hartmann, who is 30 weeks pregnant, has diabetes that is well controlled with oral hypoglycemics. She begins preterm labor, and ritodrine is ordered for her.

If you were the nurse, discuss which laboratory values you would monitor most closely. Explain the rationale for your choices.

DRUG CLOSELY RELATED TO RITODRINE

Like ritodrine, terbutaline (Brethine, Bricanyl) is a beta agonist and therefore works similarly in the body. Unlike ritodrine, the primary use of terbutaline is as a bronchodilator. Use of terbutaline to stop preterm labor is unlabeled. Terbutaline is considered a pregnancy category B drug. Adverse effects are similar to those of ritodrine. Terbutaline may be

COMMUNITY-BASED CONCERNS

Teaching About Drugs That Affect Uterine Function

Prenatal teaching should include the following:

- Signs of preterm labor
- Rationale for not giving ritodrine to stop preterm labor before 20-weeks' gestation (spontaneous abortion may be related to fetal defects; ritodrine's effects on fetus less than 20 weeks are unknown)
- Rationale regarding use of oxytocin (these should focus on medical indications, not convenience of delivery)

MEMORY CHIP

Ritodrine

- Used to control preterm labor after 20-weeks' gestation
- Beta-receptor agonist (stimulant) that selectively prefers the receptors in the uterine smooth muscle; antidote: beta blockers
- Significant contraindications: before the twentieth week of pregnancy; when continuation of the pregnancy is hazardous to the woman or fetus; preexisting maternal medical conditions that would be seriously affected by the pharmacologic properties of a beta agonist
- Most common adverse effects: (almost 100%) maternal and fetal tachycardia; maternal blood pressure changes
- Most serious adverse effects: maternal—pulmonary edema, hypotension, cardiac arrhythmias
- Maximizing therapeutic effects: continue IV infusion for 12 hours after cessation of uterine contractions
- Minimizing adverse effects: monitor maternal pulse rate, blood pressure, fluid status, and fetal heart rate; decrease infusion rate if adverse effects are present
- Most significant patient education: importance of left side-lying position during infusion

given either orally, by IV, or by subcutaneous continuous infusion (see Table 44-1). The use of terbutaline in preterm labor, although widespread in clinical practice, is still considered controversial. Terbutaline does not appear to have any benefits over ritodrine; for control of preterm labor the two drugs are equally efficacious. Terbutaline, like ritodrine, will prolong gestation for 24 to 48 hours but does not decrease neonatal morbidity or mortality (Higby & Suiter, 1999). The results of one meta-analysis (which is a comparison of multiple research studies on the same topic) found oral terbutaline, used as maintenance tocolytic therapy after successful treatment of preterm labor, did not reduce the incidence of recurrent preterm labor or preterm delivery. It also did not improve perinatal or neonatal outcomes (Sanchez-Ramos, Kaunitz, Gaudier, & Kelke, 1999; Gyetvai, Hannah, Hodnett, & Ohlsson, 1999). A second meta-analysis stated that the available studies failed to share enough factors in regard to treatment offered and definition of outcome variables to allow adequate comparison. Recommendations are that further well-designed, large, randomized trials are still needed to evaluate the efficacy of oral tocolytics (Meirowitz, Ananth, Smulian, & Vintzelios, 1999). The literature is contradictory as to whether continuous subcutaneous infusion of terbutaline has long-term effectiveness in preventing recurrent preterm labor (Lam, Bergauer, Jacques, Coleman, & Stanziano, 2000; Guinn, Goepfert, Owen, Wenstrom, Hauth, 1998).

Further discussion of terbutaline's respiratory function is found in Chapter 36.

DRUGS SIGNIFICANTLY DIFFERENT FROM P RITODRINE

Magnesium Sulfate

Magnesium is a trace mineral involved in multiple chemical reactions within the body. Therefore, the pharmacotherapeutics of magnesium sulfate are diverse, and more potential therapeutic uses are under consideration. Oral magnesium sulfate preparations are used in laxatives and antacids (see chapter 37). Oral and IV forms of magnesium sulfate are often given to correct electrolyte imbalances (e.g., hypomagnesemia). IV magnesium is effective for suppressing ventricular ectopy and is a first-line therapy for torsades de pointes. It may also be useful in treating patients with congestive heart failure or acute myocardial infarction. Magnesium sulfate is the drug of choice to treat or prevent seizures associated with preeclampsia, eclampsia, and pregnancy-induced hypertension. Magnesium sulfate is also used to control hypertension, encephalopathy, and convulsions in children with acute nephritis. Magnesium sulfate has been found to have some effectiveness as a tocolytic similar to ritodrine. Unlike ritodrine, however, it is not a first-line agent for uterine relaxation, because this use of the drug is still considered unlabeled. IV magnesium may be useful in treating asthma and chronic lung disease that have been unresponsive to conventional therapy with beta agonists. Magnesium may also have a role in the prevention and treatment of vascular headaches, although this possibility is still being researched (Swain & Kaplan-Machlis, 1999).

Magnesium sulfate acts as a CNS and muscular depressant, producing peripheral neuromuscular blockade. It prevents or controls convulsions by blocking neuromuscular transmission and by decreasing the amount of acetylcholine freed at the end plate by the motor nerve impulse. Secondarily, magnesium sulfate relaxes smooth muscle, decreasing uterine contractions and blood pressure. The effectiveness of magnesium sulfate as a tocolytic is controversial. It appears to inhibit myometrial contractility, but unlike other drugs used as tocolytics, magnesium sulfate does not appear to significantly prolong pregnancy (Gyetvai, et al., 1999; Higby & Suiter, 1999). Although magnesium sulfate is a pregnancy category A drug (meaning that it does not create fetal structural defects), its use carries some risk to the fetus. Magnesium sulfate has not been proven to decrease neonatal morbidity or mortality; in fact, some research has shown that magnesium sulfate increases infant mortality (Higby & Suiter, 1999).

Adverse effects are usually associated with elevated serum levels or magnesium intoxication (Table 44-3). A serum level of 10 to 12 mg/dL is associated with toxicity. The most common maternal adverse effects are as follows:

- Headache
- Hyporeflexia
- Weakness
- Thirst
- Flushing
- Burning at infusion site

The most life-threatening maternal adverse effects are as follows:

- Circulatory collapse
- Respiratory depression
- Pulmonary edema

The most common fetal/neonatal adverse effects are as follows:

- Heart rate changes
- Neonatal hypotonia
- Neonatal respiratory depression (possibly serious)

TABLE 44-3 Correlation of Serum Levels and Effects of Magnesium Sulfate

Serum Level (mEq/L)	Effect
1.5–3	Normal level
4–7	Therapeutic level for preeclampsia/eclampsia/convulsions
7–10	Loss of deep tendon reflexes, hypotension, loss of consciousness
13–15	Respiratory paralysis
16–25	Cardiac conduction altered (lengthened PR interval, QRS widening, prolonged QT interval arrhythmias)
25	Cardiac arrest

Other maternal adverse effects from magnesium toxicity are sweating, hypotension, flaccid paralysis, hypothermia, and cardiac depression. IV infusion, especially for prolonged periods (more than 24 hours), may produce hypermagnesemia in the newborn, including neuromuscular or respiratory depression. Overdosage produces a sharp drop in the blood pressure, respiratory paralysis, and ECG changes (increased PR interval, increased QRS complex, and prolonged QT interval). Heart block and asystole may also occur. Serum levels need to be monitored closely when the patient is receiving magnesium sulfate to prevent overdosage and adverse effects from therapy. Calcium gluconate will antagonize the effects of magnesium toxicity and is the antidote for overdosage.

Magnesium sulfate may be administered by IM, IV, or IV infusion (see Table 44-1). An IV pump should be used to regulate the flow of magnesium sulfate infusion. Dosing is accomplished by first using a loading dose and then a maintenance dose. The IV route is preferred for initial stabilization; after that, an oral dose may be used for maintenance. The goal is to maintain a therapeutic serum level without causing adverse effects. The therapeutic level varies based on the clinical indication for the therapy. It is 5 to 8 mg/dL in preterm labor, and 4 to 8 mg/dL in pregnancy-induced hypertension.

In addition to using an IV pump, several other nursing actions can minimize adverse effects. The nurse should assess for signs of magnesium toxicity by monitoring the serum magnesium levels and the patient's clinical response to drug administration. The nurse should use continuous maternal cardiac monitoring and continuous fetal monitoring while the patient is receiving IV magnesium sulfate. He or she should place the patient on bed rest in the left lateral recumbent position to prevent hypotension and to maximize blood flow to the fetus. The patient must receive nothing orally to eat or drink (e.g., remain NPO) during stabilization to help prevent nausea and vomiting. The nurse should document uterine activity, cervical changes, and maternal-fetal responses with each change in dose. He or she must implement safety measures or seizure precautions if the drug is used to prevent or treat seizures associated with pregnancy-induced hypertension. Finally, the nurse should always keep calcium gluconate at the bedside to use as an antidote if magnesium toxicity occurs.

Indomethacin

Indomethacin is an NSAID that suppresses uterine activity by inhibiting prostaglandin synthesis. It has been shown effective in stopping premature labor, but its use as a tocolytic is very limited because of concerns over fetal safety. Indomethacin appears to increase the risk of necrotizing enterocolitis, intercranial hemorrhage, and patent ductus arteriosus. These serious effects severely limit the use of this and other prostaglandin inhibitors in the treatment of preterm labor. Use of the drug for treating preterm labor is not recommended. For additional information about the other uses of indomethacin see Chapter 25.

CHAPTER SUMMARY

- Drug therapy may be used when labor does not occur at term, does not bring about delivery effectively, or begins preterm.
- Oxytocin is given by IV drip infusion to initiate or augment (improve) labor contractions when there are significant fetal or maternal reasons to do so. It is also used to control postpartum bleeding or hemorrhage.
- Response to oxytocin therapy has three phases: incremental phase, stable phase, and hyperstimulation. The hyperstimulation phase is undesirable and indicates that administration of oxytocin has been excessive.
- Adverse effects of oxytocin are dose related.
- The nurse requires an accurate understanding of the physiology involved in producing contractions, the core drug knowledge (most specifically the pharmacokinetics, pharmacodynamics, and adverse effects of oxytocin), and the relevant core patient variables to be able to make sound professional judgments in managing patients receiving oxytocin therapy.
- The nurse is responsible for determining the maternal and fetal response to oxytocin therapy (frequency of contractions, progress of labor, and fetal tolerance) and to titrate the dose, per the physician's or nurse-midwife's orders, based on this assessment.
- The nurse must stop the infusion of oxytocin if hyperstimulation of the uterus occurs.
- Tocolytic drugs are used to stop preterm labor. Although they are effective for short-term use, they have not decreased the number of preterm births, neonatal morbidity, or neonatal mortality.
- Ritodrine is a beta-receptor agonist (stimulant) that selectively prefers the receptors in the uterine smooth muscle. Stimulation of these receptors inhibits contractility of uterine smooth muscle. Infusions will decrease intensity and frequency of uterine contractions. Beta-blocking compounds will stop the effects of ritodrine.
- Dose-related maternal and fetal tachycardia and changes in maternal blood pressure occur in nearly all patients receiving ritodrine. Adverse effects reflect stimulation of the beta receptors.
- Drugs that alter uterine motility are potentially dangerous to the woman and fetus. Infusions of these drugs should be regulated with IV controllers or pumps. These patients need close monitoring for signs of adverse effects throughout therapy.

QUESTIONS FOR STUDY AND REVIEW

1. Why should the nurse titrate oxytocin slowly upward with dosage adjustments every 40 to 60 minutes?
2. Define the three phases of oxytocin response.
3. Which adverse effect of oxytocin is most dangerous to the pregnant woman?
4. What nursing assessments should be made to minimize adverse effects from oxytocin?
5. How does ritodrine stop preterm labor?
6. If the patient develops tachycardia, palpitations, and nervousness while on ritodrine infusion, what action should the nurse take?

NEED MORE HELP?

Chapter 44 of the study guide for *Drug Therapy in Nursing* contains exercises and activities to reinforce your understanding of the concepts presented in this chapter. For additional information see the text's accompanying website at *http://www.connection.lww.com.*

REFERENCES AND BIBLIOGRAPHY

American College of Obstetricians and Gynecologists. (1995). *Dystocia and the augmentation of labor.* (Technical Bulletin Number 217). Washington, D.C.: Author.

American College of Obstetricians and Gynecologists. (1999). *Induction of labor.* (Practice Bulletin Number 10). Washington, D.C.: Author.

American College of Obstetricians and Gynecologists (ACOG) news release. October 27,2000. *ACOG writes FDA on safety of misoprostol* [On-line]. Available: http:www.acog.com/from{_}home/publications/press{_}releases/nr10-27-00.htm

Association of Women's Health, Obstetric and Neonatal Nurses. (1998). *Standards and guidelines for professional nursing practice in the care of women and newborns* (5th ed.). Washington, D.C.: Author.

Bishop, E. H. (1964). Pelvic scoring for elective induction. *Obstetric Gynecology, 24*(2), 266–268.

Cook, C. M., Spurrett, B., & Murray, H. (1999). A randomized clinical trial comparing oral misoprostol with synthetic oxytocin or syntometrine in the third stage of labour. *Australian and New Zealand Journal of Obstetrics and Gynaecology, 39*(4), 414–419.

Clayworth, S. (2000). The nurse's role during oxytocin administration. *MCN American Journal of Maternal Child Nursing, 25*(2), 80–85.

El-Refaey, H., Nooh, R., O'Brien, P., Abdalla, M., Geary, M., Walder, J., & Rodeck, C. (2000). The misoprostol third stage of labour study: A randomised controlled comparison between orally administered misoprostol and standard management. *British Journal of Obstetrics and Gynaecology, 107*(9), 1104–1110.

Food and Drug Administration Center for Drug Evaluation and Research Advisory Committee for Reproductive Health Drugs. (April 20, 1998). Sponsor Presentation: R. W. Johnson Pharmaceutical.Research Institute for NDA 20-797 Antocin (Atosiban Injection) for Use in the Management of Premature Labor. http://www.fda.gov/ohrms/dockets/ac/98/transcpt/3407tl.rtf.

Guinn, D. A., Goepfert, A. R., Owen, J., Wenstrom, K. D., & Hauth, J. C. (1998). Terbutaline pump maintenance therapy for prevention of preterm delivery. *American Journal of Obstetrics and Gynecology, 179*(4), 874–878.

Gyetvai, K., Hannah, M. E., Hodnett, E. D., & Ohlsson, A. (1999). Tocolytics for preterm labor: a systematic review. *Obstetrics and Gynecology, 94*(5 Pt. 2), 869–877.

Higby, K., & Suiter, C. R. (1999). A risk-benefit assessment of therapies for premature labour. *Drug Safety, 21*(1), 35–56.

Hoffmeyr, G. J., & Gulmezoglu, A. M. (2000). Vaginal misoprostol for cervical ripening and labour induction in late pregnancy (Cochrane Review). In *The Cochrane Library,* Issue 3, 2000. Oxford: Update Software.

Kamitomo, M., Sameshima, H., Ikenoue, T., & Nishibatke, M. (2000). Fetal cardiovascular function during prolonged magnesium sulfate tocolysis. *Journal of Perinatal Medicine, 28*(5), 377–382.

Katz, V. L., Farmer, R. M., Deean, C. A., & Carpenter, M. E. (2000). Use of misoprostol for cervical ripening. *Southern Medical Journal, 93*(9), 881–884.

Lam, F., Elliot, J., Jones, J. S., Katz, M., Knuppel, R. A., Morrison, J., Newman, R., Phelan, J., & Willcourt, R. (1998). Clinical issues surrounding the use of terbutaline sulfate for preterm labor. *Obstetrical and Gynecological Survey, 53,* (Suppl. 11), S85–S95.

Lam, F., Bergauer, N., Jacques, D., Coleman, S., & Stanziano, G. (2000). The clinical and cost-effectiveness of treating recurrent preterm labor with subcutaneous terbutaline. *Obstetrics and Gynecology, 95*(4 Suppl 1), S39.

Main, D. M., Main, E. K., & Moore D. H. 2nd. (2000). The relationship between maternal age and uterine dysfunction: A continuous effect throughout reproductive life. *American Journal of Obstetrics and Gynecology, 182*(6), 1312–1320.

McDonald, S., Prendiville, W. J., & Elbourne, D. (2000). *The Cochrane Database System Review,* 2:CD000201.

McNamara, H., & Johnson, N. (1995). The effect of uterine contractions on fetal oxygen saturation. *British Journal of Obstetrics and Gynaecology, 102*(8), 644–647.

Meirowitz, N. B., Ananth, C. V., Smulian, J. C., & Vintzileos, A. M. (1999). Value of maintenance therapy with oral tocolytics: a systematic review. *Journal of Maternal and Fetal Medicine, 8*(4), 177–83.

Moutquin, J. M., Sherman, D., Cohen, H., Mohide, P. T., Hochner-Celnikier, D., Fejgin, M., Liston, R. M., Dansereau, J., Mazor, M., Shalev, E., Boucher, M., Glezerman, M., Zimmer, E. Z., & Rabinovici, J. (2000). Double-blind, randomized, controlled trial of atosiban and ritodrin in the treatment of preterm labor: a multicenter effectiveness and safety study. *American Journal of Obstetrics and Gynecology, 182*(5), 1191–1199.

Ngai, S. W., Chan, Y. M., Lam, S. W., & Lao, T. T. (2000). Labour characteristics and uterine activity: misoprostol compared with oxytocin in women at term with prelabor rupture of the membranes. *British Journal of Obstetrics and Gynaecology, 107*(2), 222–227.

Renfrew, M. J., Lang, S., & Woolridge, M. (2000). Oxytocin for promoting successful lactation. *Cochrane Database System Review,* (2): CD000156.

Romero, R., Sibai, B. M., Sanchez-Ramos, L., Valenzuela, G. J., Veille, J. C., Tabor, B., Perry, K. G., Varner, M., Goodwin, T. M., Lane, R., Smith, J., Shangold, G., & Creasy, G. W. (2000). An oxytocin receptor antagonist (atosiban) in the treatment of preterm labor: a randomized, double-blind, placebo-controlled trial with tocolytic rescue. *American Journal of Obstetrics and Gynecology, 182*(5), 1173–1183.

Sanchez-Ramos, L., Kaunitz, A. M., Gaudier, F. L., & Delke, I. (1999). Efficacy of maintenance therapy after acute tocolysis: a meta-analysis. *American Journal of Obstetrics and Gynecology, 181*(2), 484–490.

Simpson, K. R., & Poole, J. H. (1998). *Cervical ripening and induction and augmentation of labor, practice symposia.* Washington, DC: Association of Women's Health, Obstetric and Neonatal Nurses.

Swain, R., & Kaplan-Machlis, B. (1999). Magnesium for the next millennium. *Southern Medical Journal, 92*(11), 1040–1047.

Tan, B. P., & Hannah, M. E. (2000). Oxytocin for prelabor rupture of membranes at or near term. *Cochrane Database System Review,* (2):CD000157.

Tan, B. P., & Hannah, M. E. (2000). Prostaglandins versus oxytocin for prelabor rupture of membranes at term. *Cochrane Database System Review,* (2):CD000159.

Terrone, D. A., Rinehart, B. K., Kimmel, E. S., May, W. L., Larmon, J. E., & Morrison, J. C. (2000). A prospective, randomized, controlled trial of high and low maintenance doses of magnesium sulfate for acute tocolysis. *American Journal of Obstetrics and Gynecology, 182*(6), 1477–1482.

Vivil-De Gracia, P., Simiti, E., & Lora, Y. (2000). Intrapartum fetal distress and magnesium sulfate. *International Journal of Gynaecology and Obstetrics, 68*(1), 3–6.

Walley, R. L., Wilson, J. B., Crane, J. M., Matthews, K., Sawyer, E., & Hutchens, D. (2000). A double- blind placebo controlled randomised trial of misoprostol and oxytocin in the management of the third stage of labour. *British Journal of Obstetrics and Gynaecology, 107*(9), 1111–1115.

Wing, D. A., Fassett, M. J., & Mishell, D. R. (2000). Mifepristone for preinduction cervical ripening beyond 41 weeks' gestation: A randomized controlled trial. *Obstetrics and Gynecology, 96*(4), 543–548.

Unit XII

Antineoplastic Drugs

Chapter 45

CELL CYCLE-SPECIFIC DRUGS

KEY TERMS

adjuvant therapy
cell cycle
cell cycle-specific
cell cycle-nonspecific
chemotherapy
consolidation therapy
cytokinesis
first-order kinetics
G0 phase
G1 phase
G2 phase
generation time
growth fraction
induction therapy
intensification
irritant
maintenance
mitosis
M phase
nadir
neoadjuvant therapy
palliative therapy
radiation recall
salvage therapy
S phase
vesicant

Learning Objectives

At the completion of this chapter the student will:

1. Identify core drug knowledge about cell cycle-specific drugs.
2. Understand the goals of treatment and strategies used in chemotherapy.
3. Identify the phases of the cell life cycle and describe what happens at each phase.
4. Differentiate a normal from a malignant cell.
5. Identify the different routes administration for the various chemotherapeutic agents.
6. Describe precautions and practices to ensure safety, minimize exposure, and deal with untoward effects of chemotherapy to the patient, health care provider, and the environment.
7. Explain the difference between a cell cycle-specific and a cell cycle-nonspecific chemotherapeutic agent.
8. Identify core patient variables relevant to cell cycle-specific drugs.
9. Relate the interaction of core drug knowledge to core patient variables for cell cycle-specific drugs.
10. Generate a nursing plan of care from the interactions between the core drug knowledge and core patient variables for cell cycle-specific drugs.
11. Describe nursing interventions to maximize therapeutic and minimize adverse effects for cell cycle-specific drugs.
12. Gain an understanding of the potential impact of herbal medicine on chemotherapy.
13. Determine key points for patient and family education for cell cycle-specific drugs.

Antimetabolites

5-fluorouracil (5-FU)
methotrexate

Mitotic inhibitors

Vinca alkaloids

vincristine
vinblastine

Podophyllotoxins

etoposide
teniposide

Taxanes

paclitaxel
docetaxel

Camptothecines

topotecan
irinotecan

Miscellaneous cell cycle-specific drugs

hydroxyurea
L-asparaginase

The symbol (C) indicates the **drug class**.
Drugs in bold type marked with the symbol (P) are **prototypes**.
Drugs in blue type with no symbol are **closely related** to the prototype.
Drugs in red type with no symbol are **significantly different** from the prototype.
Drugs in black type with no symbol are **also used in drug therapy**; no prototype.

Chemotherapy is the term that describes the use of cytotoxic agents to destroy cancer cells. The goals of chemotherapy are cure, control, and palliation. Chemotherapy dates back to the 1500s when heavy metals were used to treat cancers and severe toxicities and limited cures were reported. Since then, a vast spectrum of chemotherapeutic drugs has been discovered to achieve these goals.

Chemotherapy is a vital part of the cancer armamentarium. Unlike surgery and radiation, which are other cancer treatment modalities, chemotherapy is distinguished for its systemic effect. The chemotherapeutic drugs are transported by the bloodstream to different parts of the body, although most of these drugs do not cross the blood-brain barrier and therefore cannot reach the central nervous system (CNS).

Chemotherapy plays an important role in cancer therapy. It is the primary treatment for some cancers (see the accompanying display, Role of Chemotherapy in Various Cancers) or serves as an adjunct to other treatment modalities: surgery, radiation, and the biologic response modifiers. Chemotherapeutic agents may be administered as single agents or in combination regimens. They are used in various treatment strategies as follows:

- **Adjuvant treatment:** This therapy involves a short course of high-dose drug therapy (usually a combination of drugs) administered after radiation or surgery to destroy residual tumor cells.
- **Induction therapy:** This term commonly describes treatment of hematologic cancers. It refers to the use of high-dose drug therapy (usually a combination of drugs) to induce a complete response when initiating a curative regimen.
- **Consolidation therapy:** This is chemotherapy that is given after induction therapy has achieved a complete remission; the regimen is repeated to increase cure rate or prolong patient survival.
- **Intensification:** After complete remission is achieved, the same agents used for induction therapy are given at higher (intensified) doses, or different drugs are given also at high doses to effect a better cure rate or longer remission.
- **Maintenance:** This therapy involves using single or combination, low-dose cytotoxic drugs on a long-term basis in patients who are in complete remission to delay regrowth of residual cancer cells.
- **Neoadjuvant therapy:** This therapy involves the use of adjuvant chemotherapeutic drugs during the preoperative or perioperative periods.
- **Palliative therapy:** This therapy involves the use of chemotherapeutic drugs to control symptoms, provide comfort, and improve patient's quality of life symptoms if cure is not achievable.
- **Salvage therapy:** This therapy involves the use of a potentially curative high-dose drug regimen that is given to a patient whose symptoms have recurred or whose treatment by another regimen has failed.

The practitioner needs to be equipped with a clear knowledge of cell physiology, cancer pathophysiology, routes of administration for chemotherapeutic drugs, safety guidelines for handling chemotherapeutic drugs, classifications of antineoplastic drugs, and the therapeutic and adverse effects (toxicities) of antineoplastic drugs so that patient needs can be anticipated early. Armed with this knowledge and set of skills, the nurse is able to manage the patient efficiently in any clinical setting and educate him/her to perform self-care measures in the home environment.

Role of Chemotherapy in Various Cancers

Primary Treatment

Chemotherapy is the primary treatment for the following localized cancerous neoplasms:

Burkitt's lymphoma
CNS lymphomas
Hodgkin disease (of childhood and some adult stages)
Embryonal rhabdomyosarcoma
Wilms tumor
Small-cell lung cancer
Large-cell lymphomas

Future as a Primary Treatment

Chemotherapy holds promise as a future primary treatment for the following cancers:

Breast cancer
Esophageal cancer
Non–small-cell lung cancer
Nasopharyngeal cancer and other cancers of the head and neck
Pancreatic cancer
Prostate cancer
Cervical carcinoma
Gastric carcinoma

Treatment Before Surgery

Sometimes chemotherapy is the treatment used to shrink a tumor so that surgery can be less extensive and therefore less mutilating. Some cancers for which chemotherapy is used as a pretreatment include the following:

Soft-tissue sarcomas
Laryngeal cancer
Anal carcinoma
Bladder cancer
Breast cancer
Osteogenic sarcoma

PHYSIOLOGY

A knowledge of cellular kinetics and the life span of the **cell cycle** is needed to understand how chemotherapy works. The cell is the basic structure of the human organism. It is capable of reproducing itself. The process by which this occurs is called cell division, wherein two new daughter cells are formed. The time span over which the cell reproduces is called the cell cycle. The cell cycle has five phases. All cells, whether normal or abnormal, progress through the different phases of the cell cycle, which are G_0, G_1, S, G_2, and M. The complete cycle is illustrated in Figure 45-1.

Physiology

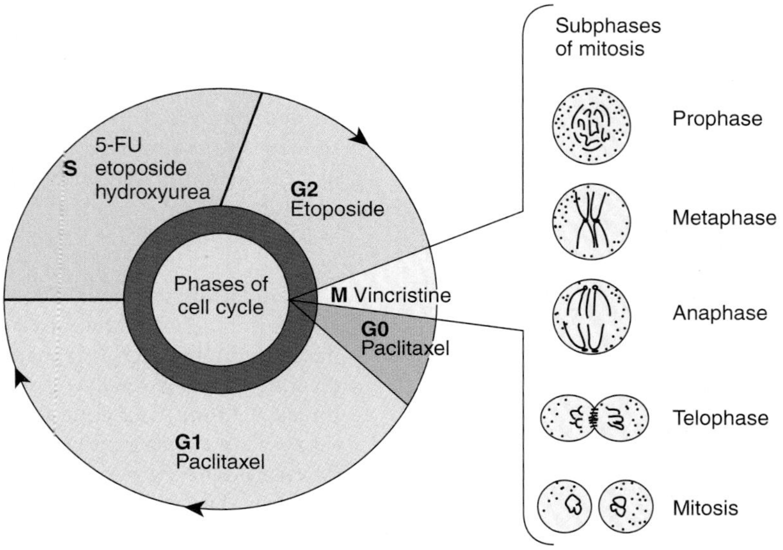

Figure 45-1. Cell cycle. The cell cycle has five phases through which it passes in reproducing itself. The phases represented include G_0 (resting, nonreproductive phase), G_1 (waiting for reproductive stimulus), S (stimulus received; DNA and RNA assembled), G_2 (mitotic spindles constructed and RNA synthesized), and M (mitosis; cell division). Antineoplastic drugs with actions that occur in a particular phase of the cycle are known as cell cycle-specific drugs. Among these drugs are 5-fluorouracil, which affects the S phase of the cell cycle; vincristine, which affects the M phase (mitosis); etoposide, which affects the S and G_2 phases; paclitaxel, which affects the G_0 and possibly the G_1 phases; and hydroxyurea, which affects the S phase.

The cell cycle is the cornerstone of cell cycle division and proliferation. Both normal and malignant cells undergo this process that might last for approximately 25 to 30 hours. In the first phase, **Gap 0** (G_0), a cell can stay in a dormant or latent state for months or even years until stimulated to move forward in the cycle. Because certain cells divide more rapidly than others, some rest in the G_0 phase for a brief period of time, whereas others bypass the G_0 phase and enter the second phase, the **Gap 1** (G_1) phase, directly if the body needs the immediate production of a certain cell. During **Gap 1,** the cell synthesizes RNA and the proteins needed for DNA synthesis. The time a cell spends in this phase varies and can last from hours to days, depending on the cell type.

After RNA and protein syntheses occur, the cell then enters the third phase, the **synthesis (S) phase.** During the S phase, ribonucleic acid (RNA), proteins, and enzymes necessary for deoxyribonucleic acid (DNA) synthesis are formed. DNA contains the genetic code necessary for the growth and replication of the cell. DNA is an essential nucleic acid composed of deoxyribose, a phosphate, and four nitrogenous bases: adenine, guanine, cytosine, and thymine. Adenine and guanine are purines, and cytosine and thymine are pyrimidines. Chemical reactions occur between the two purines and between the two pyrimidines, leading to the formation of the double-stranded DNA helix, which serves as the genetic template of the cell. Generally the synthesis phase lasts 8 to 12 hours.

The cell then enters the fourth phase, **Gap 2** (G_2), when more RNA and protein syntheses take place in preparation for mitosis. In this phase, the cellular apparatus, called the mitotic spindle, is constructed and RNA synthesis occurs. The G_2 phase lasts for approximately 2 hours. After the G_2 phase, the cell is ready to undergo cell division in the **M phase.**

The fifth phase of the cell cycle is the M phase, which consists of the following orchestrated subphases: prophase, metaphase, anaphase, and telophase (see Fig. 45-1). As the cell progresses through these subphases, the cytoplasm and nucleus divide so that replication of the cell results in the birth of two daughter cells. Mitosis involves the duplication of genetic material (chromosomes) and distribution of this material into the two daughter cells as the nucleus divides. **Cytokinesis** is the actual division of the remainder of the cell (cytoplasm) into the new daughter cells. Each of these two new daughter cells will either pass through a new reproductive cycle or become arrested in G_0 performing other cellular activities.

The length of time needed to complete the cell cycle, which varies with each type of cell, is called **generation time.** Tumors consisting of cells that have a short generation time or rapid mitotic rate are most sensitive to antineoplastic agents. Tumors that have cancer cells with a long generation time or slow mitotic rate are often resistant to chemotherapy.

It is not clearly understood how the body maintains normal cellular homeostasis. What has been postulated is that the body possesses a feedback system that signals a cell to enter the G_1 phase of the cell life cycle in response to cell death. In individuals with cancer, this feedback system is dysfunctional, and the cancer cell enters the cell life cycle independently of the body's feedback system.

PATHOPHYSIOLOGY

Every cell in the body has a genetically programmed clock that directs the timing of its reproductive activity. Cancer is a disease in which the cells fail to respond to the homeostatic mechanism that controls the normal cellular birth and death processes.

Four basic features differentiate the cancer cell from the normal cell:

- Uncontrolled cell proliferation
- Decreased cellular differentiation
- Inappropriate ability to invade surrounding tissue
- Ability to establish new growth at ectopic sites

Although cancer cells have the same chemical structures as normal cells and undergo the same phases of the cell life cycle, the critical change appears to be in their altered response to mechanisms that control growth and differentiation. Cell production in a cancer is not proportional to cell loss; production of new cells occurs at a faster rate than is needed to compensate for the loss of cells.

CELLULAR KINETICS OF CHEMOTHERAPY DRUGS

Most chemotherapy drugs exert cytotoxic activity primarily on macromolecular synthesis or function. This means that they interfere either with the synthesis of DNA, RNA, or proteins or with the appropriate functioning of the preformed molecule. When this interference happens, a proportion of the cells die. Chemotherapy works on the principle of **first-order kinetics.** This means that the number of tumor cells killed by an antineoplastic drug(s) is proportional to the dose used. The proportion of cells killed after chemotherapy administration is a constant percentage of the total number of malignant cells present. Figure 45-2 gives a visual explanation of the cell kill theory. For example, if a tumor containing 1 million (1,000,000) cells is exposed to a chemotherapeutic drug that has a 90% cell kill rate, the first dose of chemotherapy will destroy 90% (900,000) of the cancer cells, and 100,000 cells will survive. The second dose will kill another 90% of the remaining cells (90,000 cells), and 10,000 cells will survive. Because only a portion of the cells die, expected doses of chemotherapy must be repeated to reduce the population of cancer cells until just one cell remains. Hopefully, the body's immune response will kill the final cell.

ROUTES OF CHEMOTHERAPY ADMINISTRATION

As advances in chemotherapy occur, variations in the routes of administration continue to evolve. The choice of drug route depends on the therapeutic intent. Drug administration through peripheral and central lines are the most commonly used methods to administer chemotherapy. Alternate routes of drug delivery to specific sites within the body using devices or catheters are becoming more popular in clinical practice. Recently, additional oral cytotoxic agents have been discovered, which makes it very convenient to patients to receive treatment at home less expensively. This route presents different challenges for the clinician. Table 45-1 lists the different methods of drug delivery, traditional and alternate routes, and the practice implications for the nurses who participate in the care of patients using these various routes and treatment modalities in cancer therapy.

HANDLING AND PROPER DISPOSAL OF CHEMOTHERAPY

Over the past decade, more health care professionals than ever before have handled chemotherapy agents. The mutagenic and carcinogenic effects known to occur in laboratory

Physiology

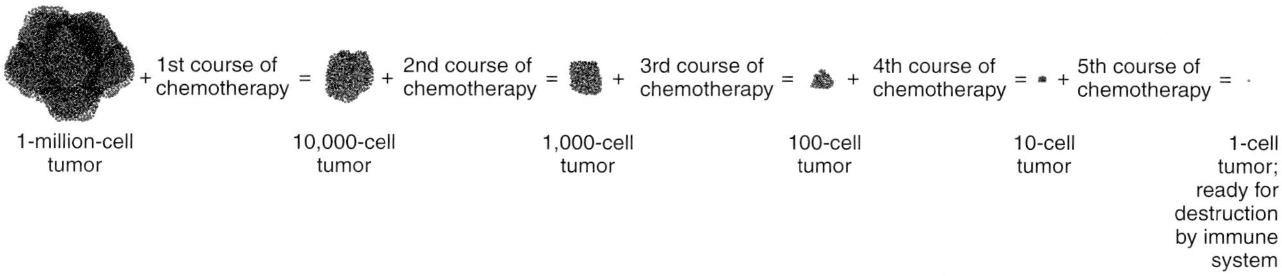

Figure 45-2. Cell kill theory. A set percentage of cells is killed after each dose of chemotherapy. The percentage killed is dependent upon the drug therapy. In the above example, each course of chemotherapy kills 90% of cells in a cancerous tumor.

TABLE 45-1 Administration Routes for Antineoplastic Drugs

Route	Advantages	Disadvantages	Potential Complications	Nursing Implications
Oral	Ease of administration	Inconsistency of absorption	Drug-specific complications	Evaluate compliance with medication schedule. Teach patient handling techniques.
Subcutaneous, Intramuscular	Ease of administration Decreased side effects	Requires adequate muscle mass and tissue for absorption Pain	Infection, bleeding	Evaluate platelet count (>50,000). Use smallest needle gauge possible. Prepare injection site with an antiseptic solution. Assess injection site for signs and symptoms of infection.
IV	Consistent absorption Required for vesicants	Sclerosing of veins over time	Infection, phlebitis	Check for blood return before and after administration of drugs
Intra-arterial*	Increased doses to tumor with decreased systemic toxic effects	Requires surgical procedure or special radiography for device placement	Bleeding, embolism	Monitor for signs and symptoms of bleeding. Monitor partial thromboplastin time, prothrombin time.
External pump	With intra-arterial port, patient freedom increased	Patient lies flat for 3–7 d during drug infusion	Pump occlusion, malfunction	Extensive patient education is needed.
Internal (implanted) pump	Greater mobility	Cost-effective only with long-term therapy (i.e., 3–6 mo)	Pump occlusion malfunction	Specialized nursing skills is needed.
Intrathecal,* intraventricular	More consistent drug levels in cerebrospinal fluid	Requires lumbar puncture or surgical placement of reservoir or implanted pump for drug delivery	Headaches, confusion, lethargy, nausea and vomiting, seizures	Observe site for signs of infection. Monitor functioning of reservoir or pump. Assess patient for headache or signs of increased intracranial pressure.
Intraperitoneal*	Direct exposure of intra-abdominal metastases to drug	Requires placement of Tenckhoff catheter or intraperitoneal port	Abdominal pain, abdominal distention, bleeding, ileus, intestinal perforation, infection	Warm chemotherapy solution to body temperature. Check patency of catheter or port. Instill solution according to protocol—infuse, dwell, and drain or continuous infusion.
Intrapleural	Sclerosing of pleural lining to prevent recurrence of effusions	Requires insertion of a thoracotomy tube	Pain, infection	Monitor for complete drainage from pleural cavity before instillation of drug. Following instillation, clamp tubing and reposition patient every 10–15 min for 2 h Attach tubing to suction for 18 h. Assess patient for pain or anxiety. Provide analgesia and emotional support.

TABLE 45-1 **Administration Routes for Antineoplastic Drugs** (Continued)

Route	Advantages	Disadvantages	Potential Complications	Nursing Implications
Intravesicular	Direct exposure of bladder surfaces to drug	Requires insertion of Foley catheter	Urinary tract infections, cystitis, bladder contracture, urinary urgency, allergic drug reactions	Maintain sterile technique when inserting Foley catheter. Instill solution, clamp catheter for 1 h, and unclamp to drain.

*Note: Specialized nursing education may be required for certain administration methods. Refer to individual state nurse practice acts and agency policies and procedures.

Data from: Oncology Nursing Society. (1998) *Cancer chemotherapy guidelines and recommendation for practice.* Pittsburgh: Oncology Nursing Press, Inc.

treatment recipients have raised great concern regarding the potential long-term risks to those health care professionals exposed to antineoplastic drugs. The teratogenic risks especially for health care professionals of childbearing age are another concern.

Conflicting research findings regarding the suspected and unknown potential long-term effects on individuals exposed to chemotherapeutic agents led to the establishment of advisory bodies that address exposure issues and recommend safe practice techniques for the handling and disposal of these drugs. These advisory bodies are as follows:

- Occupational Safety and Health Administration (OSHA)
- American Society of Hospital Pharmacy (ASHP)
- Oncology Nursing Society (ONS)
- National Study Commission on Cytotoxic Exposure

The identified advisory bodies maintain that if professionals follow the recommendations given while handling and disposing of these drugs, teratogenic risk is unlikely. The questioned potential risk to health care professionals who handle chemotherapy and the body excreta of patients who have received these agents is unknown. Therefore, it is imperative that professionals know the precautions recommended and implement them to minimize their potential exposure. Exposure to chemotherapy is through the following routes: skin and mucous membrane absorption, inhalation, and ingestion.

Skin and mucous membrane absorption and inhalation can occur during the following activities

1. Opening a chemotherapy vial or ampule
2. Eliminating air from a syringe filled with chemotherapy
3. Disposing of IV bags, bottles, syringes, and tubing used in the administration of these agents
4. Disposing of the body excreta of patients who have received these drugs

Ingestion can occur through hand-to-mouth contact with the following:

1. Food
2. Cosmetics
3. Cigarettes
4. Equipment contaminated with chemotherapy

The recommendations made by these advisory bodies serve as guidelines, and therefore institutional policies for chemotherapy handling, administration, and disposal may vary. It is important that employees be familiar with their own institution's policies and procedures and use them as precautionary measures to minimize their potential exposure.

RECOMMENDATIONS TO MINIMIZE EXPOSURE DURING PREPARATION, TRANSPORT, DISPOSAL, AND STORAGE OF CHEMOTHERAPEUTIC AGENTS

To minimize exposure during preparation, transport, disposal and storage of chemotherapeutic agents, the nurse should adhere to the following recommendations:

1. Prepare these agents using a Class II or class III Biological Safety Cabinet (also referred to as a vertical laminar airflow hood). These cabinets contain high-efficiency particulate air filters that pull and filter air away from the face of the person preparing the drug. It is recommended that these cabinets remain functioning 24 hours a day, 7 days a week, be vented to the outside; be cleaned daily with a 70% alcohol solution, and be serviced every 6 months to ensure performance.
2. Wear long-sleeve, nonabsorbent gowns with elastic at the wrists and back closure during drug preparation.
3. Wear a plastic mask and goggles in settings without biologic safety cabinets, such as a physician's office.
4. Use a plastic absorbent pad to cover the work surface preparation area so that any droplet contamination is absorbed.
5. Prime IV lines for chemotherapy administration with 5% dextrose in water (D_5W) or normal saline before the actual drug administration. Do not prime with the chemotherapy drug.
6. Use hydrophobic filter needles to draw antineoplastic drugs from vials and ampules.
7. Use a sterile gauze pad to purge air from a chemotherapy-filled syringe, connect and disconnect IV tubing containing antineoplastic drugs, open chemotherapy vials and ampules; remove syringes from IV lines used for IV push administration, and remove empty chemotherapy bags or bottles from IV spikes.

8. Use a needleless delivery system or Luer-Lok lock connection to prevent accidental disconnection.
9. Use powder free latex gloves at least 0.007-in thickness when handling chemotherapy agents and the body excreta of patients who have received these drugs within a 48-hour period. Personnel who have latex allergy should use alternative products made with nitrile.
10. Wash hands before and after handling antineoplastic agents.
11. Never store food or beverages in a refrigerator used for chemotherapy storage.
12. Avoid eating, drinking, applying cosmetics, or chewing gum in the drug preparation vicinity.
13. Transport chemotherapeutic drugs in sealed bags to prevent spillage. Spill kits should be readily available to personnel who have been properly instructed in chemotherapy handling and exposure procedures.
14. Dispose of all chemotherapy waste in impervious, leakproof containers.
15. Instruct patients who have chemotherapy at home to store the drugs in areas where proper temperature will be maintained, and away from the reach of children.
16. Cover the toilet with a waterproof shield or pad before flushing.
17. All equipment contaminated with antineoplastic drugs must be disposed of in distinctly labeled hazardous waste receptacles. These chemotherapy wastes should be disposed in Environmental Protection Agency permitted landfill waste sites or incinerators.

MANAGEMENT OF CHEMOTHERAPY SPILLS

To manage spills of chemotherapeutic agents, the nurse should adhere to the following recommended sequence:

1. Don a pair of powder-free latex gloves.
2. Place an absorbent pad over the spill to contain it.
3. Rinse the absorbed spill area with water.
4. Clean the area with a detergent.
5. Dispose of all equipment used as chemotherapy waste.

To expedite the handling of a spill and to minimize undue patient and employee exposure, it is recommended that well-equipped chemotherapy spill kits be readily available (see the accompanying display for suggested requirements, Contents of a Chemotherapy Spill Kit).

Contents of a Chemotherapy Spill Kit

1	Gown with cuffs and back closure*
1 pair	Shoe covers
2 pairs	Gloves
1 pair	Utility gloves
1 pair	Chemical splash goggles
1	Rebreather mask†
1	Disposable dust pan (to collect broken glass)
1	Plastic scraper (to scoop materials into dust pan)
2	Plastic-backed absorbable towels
1 each	250-mL and 1-L spill control pillows
2	Disposable sponges (to clean up spill, to clean up floor after spill removal)
1	Container for sharps
2	Large, heavy duty waste disposal bags for cleaning soiled area

*Made of water nonpermeable fabric.

†To meet National Institute of Occupational Safety and Health standards.

From "Controlling occupational exposure to hazardous drugs". (1995) OSHA Instruction CPL2-2.20B. Washington, D.C.: Author. (© 1995), 21-1–21-34.

MEASURES FOR ACCIDENTAL EXPOSURE WITH CHEMOTHERAPY

The nurse should implement the following measures to manage accidental exposure with chemotherapy:

1. Eye contact: Immediately rinse the affected eye(s) with copious amounts of water for no less than 15 minutes.
2. Skin contact: Immediately wash the area with soap and water.
3. Clothing contact: Immediately remove the article(s) of clothing and wash any areas in which skin contact occurred with soap and water. Soiled clothing should be placed in a plastic bag until laundered and then washed twice separately from all other clothing. After laundering twice, the machine should be put through a separate wash rinse cycle.
4. Bed linen contact: Immediately remove the linen and place in a contaminated linen receptacle; then clean the mattress using a 70% alcohol solution. Once the alcohol dries, the bed may be remade with clean linens.

CLASSIFICATION OF ANTINEOPLASTIC DRUGS

Antineoplastic drugs are classified according to their mode of action and the phase of the cell cycle in which the drug is active. However, it is always the rapidly dividing cells that are most sensitive to these drugs. Chemotherapeutic drugs that are most effective during a particular phase of the cycle are known as **cell cycle** (or cell-phase) **specific,** whereas drugs that act independently of a specific cell cycle (or cell phase) are **cell cycle nonspecific.** This classification is not absolute; it is likely that the cytotoxic mechanisms of the drugs involve more than one mechanism. Multiple intracellular sites might be implicated and not confined to specific cycle events.

This chapter discusses the cell cycle-specific group of drugs (Table 45-2), the prototype or a representative drug from each classification, and the nursing management for each drug. Chapter 46 discusses the cell cycle-nonspecific group of drugs. The cell cycle-specific drugs consist of the antimetabolites (prototype, 5-fluorouracil) and mitotic inhibitors. These drugs exert the greatest tumor kill when given as a continuous infusion or in divided doses with a short cycle. The mitotic inhibitors are subdivided into the Vinca alkaloids (prototype,

TABLE 45-2 Summary of Selected C Cell Cycle–Specific Antineoplastic Drugs

Drug (Trade) Name	Selected Indications	Route and Dosage Range	Pharmacokinetics
Antimetabolites			
P 5-fluorouracil (5-FU, Adrucil)	Carcinoma of colon, rectum, stomach, pancreas, breast, and ovary; hepatocellular carcinoma	*Adult:* IV, 12–15 mg/kg daily for 4 d/wk (maximum daily dose: 800 mg), then 6 mg/kg on days 6, 8, 10, and 12; maintenance, repeat first course every	*Onset:* IV, immediate *Duration:* IV, 6 h $t_{1/2}$: IV, 18–20 min
	Skin cancer, superficial basal cell cancer	*Adult:* Topical, apply sufficient drug to cover affected area bid	*Onset:* Minimal absorption in topical use *Duration:* Unknown $t_{1/2}$: Unknown
cytarabine (Ara-C)	Acute myelocytic leukemia, acute lymphocytic leukemia (ALL), Hodgkin disease, non-Hodgkin lymphoma	*Adult:* IV, 100 mg/m² d by continuous infusion for 7 d; then 100 mg/m²q 12h for 1–3 wk; intrathecal, 20–30 mg/m²	*Onset:* Rapid *Duration:* 12–18 h $t_{1/2}$: 1–3 h
floxuridine (FUDR)	Gastrointestinal (GI) adenocarcinoma with metastasis to liver, gallbladder, or bile ducts	*Adult:* Intra-arterial only, 0.1–0.6 mg/kg/d	*Onset:* Immediate *Duration:* 3 h $t_{1/2}$: 20 h
fludarabine (Fludara)	Chronic lymphocytic leukemia, non-Hodgkin lymphoma (investigational)	*Adult:* IV, 25 mg/m² d for 5 d, every 28 d	*Onset:* Rapid *Duration:* Unknown $t_{1/2}$: 10 h
6-mercaptopurine (Purinethol)	Acute leukemia, chronic myelogenous leukemia (CML)	*Adult and Child:* PO (induction and consolidation), 2.5 mg/kg/d; maintenance, 1.5–2.5 mg/kg/d	*Onset:* Varies *Duration:* Unknown $t_{1/2}$: 20–50 min
methotrexate (Mexate, Folex)	Hodgkin disease; lymphomas; acute lymphoblastic and myelocytic leukemia; CNS metastasis; carcinoma of ovary, lung, cervix, testicle, breast; sarcomas; epidermoid carcinoma of head and neck	*Adult:* Trophoblastic neoplasms, PO/IM, three to five cycles of 15–30 mg/d for 5 d; leukemia maintenance, IV, 2.5 mg/kg every 14 d or 15 mg/m² PO/IM two times a wk; lymphoma, PO, 10–25 mg/d	*Onset:* PO, varies; IV rapid *Duration:* Unknown $t_{1/2}$: 2–4 h
6-thioguanine (Tabloid)	Acute myelocytic leukemia, chronic granulocytic leukemia	*Adult:* PO, 1–3 mg/kg/d	*Onset:* Slow *Duration:* 8 h $t_{1/2}$: 11 h
Vinca Alkaloids			
P vincristine (Oncovin)	Acute lymphocytic leukemia (ALL), Hodgkin and non-Hodgkin lymphoma, CML, sarcomas, breast and small-cell lung cancers	*Adult:* IV, 1.4 mg/m²/wk *Child:* 2.0 mg/m²/wk; total single dose of 2 mg is seldom exceeded	*Onset:* Varies *Duration:* Not available $t_{1/2}$: 5 min, then 2–3 h, then 85 h
vinblastine (Velban)	Hodgkin disease, lymphocytic and histiocytic lymphomas, mycosis fungoides, advanced testicular cancer, breast cancer, squamous cell carcinoma of head and neck, Kaposi sarcoma	*Adult:* IV, 0.1 mg/kg–6 mg/m² weekly; continuous infusion, 1.4–1.8 mg/d for 5 d	*Onset:* Slow *Duration:* Unknown $t_{1/2}$: 3.7 min, then 16 h, then 24.8 h
vinorelbine (Navelbine)	Non–small-cell lung cancer, breast cancer combination with cisplatin	*Adult:* IV, 30 mg/m² weekly or in	*Onset:* Slow *Duration:* Unknown $t_{1/2}$: 22–66 h

(*continued*)

TABLE 45-2 Summary of Selected Cell Cycle–Specific Antineoplastic Drugs (Continued)

Drug (Trade) Name	Selected Indications	Route and Dosage Range	Pharmacokinetics
Podophyllotoxins			
etoposide (VePesid)	Refractory testicular tumors	*Adult:* IV, testicular cancer, 50–100 mg/m² d for 5 d every 3–4 wk or 100 mg/m² on days 1, 3, and 5	*Onset:* IV, 30 min; PO 30–60 min *Duration:* IV/PO, 20–30 h $t_{1/2}$: 4–11 h
	Small-cell lung cancer Other cancers	*Adult:* IV, 35 or 50 mg/m² d for 5 d every 3–4 wk *Adult:* PO, twice the IV dose	
teniposide (VM-26, Vumon)	Childhood acute lymphoblastic leukemia	*Adult:* IV, 165 mg/m² with cytarabine 300 mg/m² two times a wk for eight to nine doses	*Onset:* 30 min *Duration:* Unknown $t_{1/2}$: 5 h
Taxanes			
paclitaxel (Taxol)	Metastatic carcinoma of the breast, ovary, small-cell lung cancer	*Adult:* IV, 135–175 mg/m² over 24 h every 3 wk	*Onset:* Rapid *Duration:* 6–12 h $t_{1/2}$: 5.3–17.4 h
docetaxel (Taxotere)	Same as paclitaxel	*Adult:* IV, 60–100 mg/m² every 3 wk	*Onset:* Unknown *Duration:* Unknown $t_{1/2}$: 11 h
Camptothecines			
topotecan (Hycamtin)	Metastatic carcinoma of the ovary	*Adult:* IV, 1.5 mg/m² for 5 days every 3 wk	*Onset:* Unknown *Duration:* Unknown $t_{1/2}$: 3 h
irinotecan (Camptosar, CPT11)	Metastatic carcinoma of the colon or rectum in patients whose disease has progressed or recurred after 5-FU therapy	*Adult:* IV, 125 mg/m²/wk × 4wk fld. By 2wk rest	*Onset:* Unknown *Duration:* Unknown $t_{1/2}$: 6 h
Miscellaneous			
hydroxyurea (Hydrea)	CML, malignant melanoma, inoperable carcinoma of ovary, squamous-cell carcinoma of head and neck (excluding lip)	*Adult:* PO, for CML, 20–30 mg/kg as continuous therapy; for solid tumors, 80 mg/kg every 3 d or 20–30 mg/kg/d	*Onset:* Varies *Duration:* 18–20 h $t_{1/2}$: 2–3 h
L-asparaginase (Elspar)	ALL, CLL, Hodgkin disease, lymphosarcoma	*Adult:* IV/IM, 200 IU/kg for 28 d; dosage varies with protocol	*Onset:* IM, varies; IV 30–40 min *Duration:* Unknown $t_{1/2}$: 8–30 h

*Note: Antineoplastic drug dosages are calculated specifically for each patient based on his/her body surface area (BSA). The BSA is calculated from height and weight measurements and determined by using a nomogram as illustrated in Chapter 7 or by using an electronic conversion calculator. There is a separate nomogram for the adult and pediatric populations.

vincristine), the podophyllotoxins (prototype, etoposide), and the taxanes (prototype, paclitaxel). A new category of cell cycle-specific drugs called camptothecines (prototype, topotecan) and a miscellaneous group of antineoplastic drugs, such as the prototype drug hydroxyurea and L-asparaginase, are also included in this chapter.

ANTIMETABOLITES

Antimetabolites are synthetically produced to mimic the naturally produced metabolites, purines, pyrimidines, and folates, which are essential for DNA and RNA synthesis. This substitution results in cell death. Antimetabolites exert their cytotoxic activity during the S phase of the cell's life cycle. Because of this, they are most effective against tumors that have a high **growth fraction.** The growth fraction of a cell is the fraction of the cell population that is in any phase of the cell cycle. Relatively quiescent cells found in such organs like the pancreas and the uterus have low growth fractions, whereas rapidly proliferating cells, such as those of the gastrointestinal (GI) mucosal epithelium and the hair follicles, have high growth fractions. The drugs in this category include 5-fluorouracil (5-FU), cytarabine (ARA-C), floxuridine (FUDR), fludarabine (Fludara), 6-mercaptopurine (Purinethol), methotrexate (MTX), thioguanine (6-thioguanine), gemcitabine (Gemzar), and capecitabine (Xeloda). The drug 5-FU, a pyrimidine antagonist that is a mainstay in chemotherapy, is discussed as the representative antimetabolite drug.

NURSING MANAGEMENT OF THE PATIENT RECEIVING 5-FLUOROURACIL

Core Drug Knowledge

Pharmacotherapeutics

The drug 5-FU interferes in the synthesis of DNA and, to a lesser extent, inhibits the formation of RNA. It has proven to be clinically effective against a wide spectrum of solid tumors, particularly malignant GI tumors. It is indicated for the palliative management of carcinoma of the colon, breast, liver, ovary, pancreas, rectum, and stomach. It has been used in combination with cisplatin and most often with levamisole or leucovorin.

Preclinical studies show that the cytotoxic activity can be potentiated by reduced folates, such as leucovorin calcium. However, the health care provider should be vigilant in monitoring for severe adverse effects resulting from this combination. Dosage adjustments (see Table 45-2) are imperative for patients who are poorly nourished or poor risks.

In addition to the common IV route for administration, 5-FU is also given by intra-arterial infusion into the hepatic artery through a surgically implanted pump. The goal of this type of delivery is to supply a high concentration of the drug directly to the tumor and surrounding area while sparing the normal tissues from toxic effects of the antineoplastic drug. A topical form of 5-FU is also available and has been curative for basal cell carcinomas and other malignant skin cancers.

Pharmacokinetics

After infusion, 5-FU distributes into tumors, intestinal mucosa, bone marrow, liver, and tissues throughout the body. It diffuses readily across the blood-brain barrier and distributes into cerebrospinal fluid (CSF) and brain tissue. The drug is extensively metabolized in the liver and excreted by the kidneys and lungs. The mean half-life of elimination from plasma is about 16 minutes, with a range of 8 to 20 minutes. The clearance of 5-FU is significantly lower in women than in men, whereas age has no significant effect on clearance in either gender.

Pharmacodynamics

During the S phase, 5-FU exerts its maximum cytotoxic effects. It acts as a "false" antimetabolite causing a thymine deficiency. This deficiency deprives the cell of DNA and RNA, which are essential for cell division and growth. The result is unbalanced growth and death of the cell. The deprivation of DNA and RNA is most marked in rapidly growing cells that take up 5-FU at a faster rate.

Contraindications and Precautions

5-Fluorouracil is a pregnancy category D drug. It is not known whether it is excreted in human milk and caution should be exercised by women when breast-feeding. The drug has demonstrated mutagenic and teratogenic properties. The use of 5-FU is contraindicated in patients with poor nutritional status, depressed bone marrow function, and any known serious infection. This drug should not be administered to patients who have a known sensitivity to the drug. Because 5-FU is known for its toxicity, patients who are poor risks should be monitored vigilantly. Death from toxicity can result even in patients who are in relatively good condition. Patients with familial pyrimidinemia should not receive 5-FU because of the potential for severe neurotoxicity.

Adverse Effects

Myelosuppression, evidenced by anemia, leukopenia, and thrombocytopenia, is the dose-limiting side effect of 5-FU. **Nadir** is the period during which the maximum cytotoxic effect of the drug is exerted on the bone marrow causing the lowest blood cell count. The white blood cell (WBC) nadir occurs within 10 to 14 days after the drug is given; recovery is within 21 days.

Other dose-dependent toxicities are nausea, vomiting, diarrhea, and stomatitis. GI ulceration and hemorrhage can lead to death. Cutaneous changes can also occur: alopecia (thinning of the hair); hyperpigmentation of the skin, hands, and vein along the site of infusion; brittle and cracking nails; maculopapular rash; and painful, erythematous desquamation and fissures of the palms and soles.

Patients may also develop acute cerebellar syndrome (which may persist after the drug is stopped) characterized by headache, disorientation, and nystagmus. Photophobia and ocular changes, such as increased lacrimation and blurred vision, may occur.

Drug Interactions

5-fluorouracil is incompatible with diazepam, droperidol, metoclopramide, ondansetron, and other chemotherapeutic drugs such as cytarabine, gallium nitrate, methotrexate, and vinorelbine. Leucovorin calcium may enhance the toxicity of 5-FU. Some drug-laboratory test interferences can occur with 5-FU administration, such as increased 5-hydroxyindoleacetic acid (5-HIAA) excretion and plasma albumin levels may decrease as a result of protein malabsorption (Table 45-3).

Assessment of Relevant Core Patient Variables

Health Status

Before treatment begins, the nurse should assess the patient's hematologic profile. She should also document baseline neurologic status. Because GI alterations may occur with 5-FU dosing, the nurse should check the patient's oral mucosa, bowel elimination patterns, and

TABLE 45-3 Agents That Interact With 5-Fluorouracil

Interactants	Effect and Significance	Nursing Management
thiazide diuretics: hydrochlorothiazide, chlorothiazide, chlorthalidone, benzthiazide, metolazone	Possible blood abnormalities	Notify physician for possible dose modification. Monitor hematopoetic status of the patient.
cimetidine	Increased pharmacologic effect of 5-fluorouracil (5-FU)	Same as above.
leucovorin	Potentiates toxicity of 5-FU	Same as above.

dietary habits. The nurse should review the patient's drug and hypersensitivity history, especially to 5-FU. Because of potential cutaneous changes, the nurse should assess the condition of the patient's skin, nails, and hair.

Life Span and Gender

The nurse should explore reproductive goals of the patient and assess women of childbearing age for pregnancy and lactation. Chemotherapy with 5-FU may cause fetal harm when administered to pregnant women. The drug has been found to be mutagenic and teratogenic in laboratory animals. It is not known whether 5-FU is excreted in the breast milk; therefore, breastfeeding may be hazardous. The nurse should explore the benefit versus risk factors for children. The safety and efficacy of 5-FU in children are not established.

Lifestyle, Diet, and Habits

One adverse effect of 5-FU is skin sensitivity to the sun. The nurse should ask the patient whether he or she engages in activities that cause undue exposure to the sun and methods of sun protection. The nurse should assess the patient's feelings regarding hair loss and its impact on the patient's sexuality and body image. The possibility and actuality of hair loss can be very distressing to the patient. Hair loss, which is the major visible reminder that the patient is undergoing chemotherapy, may seriously affect the patient's sexuality and body image. The impact may be greater on the patient who has an active social and work life. Because of the deleterious effects on the GI mucosa, the nurse should obtain information on normal dietary intake and eating patterns, which might necessitate dietary modifications.

Environment

The drug is given in both inpatient and ambulatory care settings. In some situations, 5-FU may be given as a continuous infusion through an ambulatory pump in the home setting. In these instances, the nurse should explore whether the patient or significant other is ready to take on this responsibility and knows how to troubleshoot should problems with the pump arise.

Nursing Diagnoses and Outcomes

- Risk for Infection related to drug-induced bone marrow suppression

  Desired outcome: The patient will be free from infection and exercise caution to avoid exposure to sources of infection.
- Risk for Injury: Bleeding related to drug-induced bone marrow suppression

  Desired outcome: The patient will attain pretreatment hematologic status and learn to recognize, monitor, and manage situations that might induce bleeding.
- Imbalanced Nutrition: Less than Body Requirements related to drug-induced nausea, vomiting, stomatitis, and diarrhea

  Desired outcome: The patient will maintain adequate nutrition with good emetic control and less frequent passage of stools. Oral mucosa will remain intact, and the patient will not experience pain or discomfort in the GI mucosa.
- Disturbed Body Image related to loss of cutaneous integrity evidenced by alopecia and changes in skin and nails

  Desired outcome: The patient will develop coping strategies (use of wigs, hair covering) to enhance appearance that may be distorted because of hair loss. In addition, cutaneous integrity will be sustained.
- Disturbed Sensory Perception related to ocular changes, photophobia, cerebellar ataxia

  Desired outcome: The patient will be free from adverse effects resulting from oculomotor dysfunction.

Planning and Intervention

Maximizing Therapeutic Effects

The daily dose of 5-FU should not exceed 800 mg. The dosage should be reduced if the patient has impaired liver function or poor nutritional status. The drug should be protected from light and should be inspected for precipitates before infusion. The solution should be stored at controlled temperature. If a precipitate due to low temperature storage is noted, the solution can be restabilized by heating it to 140°F, shaking it vigorously, and allowing it to cool down to body temperature before administration. A slight discoloration may happen after storage, which does not affect its potency and safety.

Minimizing Adverse Effects

The nurse should closely monitor the patient because hematologic and GI toxicities can be fatal despite dosage reductions. A differential count should be obtained before each drug course. Treatment should be withheld if laboratory test values are below safe levels. The drug should not be administered to patients with familial pyrimidinermia because of incidence of severe neurotoxicity.

If any of the following conditions occur, the drug should be discontinued:

- Stomatitis and esophagopharyngitis (first visible sign)
- Leukopenia (WBC less than 3,500) or a rapidly dropping WBC, thrombocytopenia (platelet count less than 100,000)
- Intractable vomiting
- Diarrhea
- GI ulceration and bleeding
- Bleeding from any site

Providing Patient and Family Education

- The nurse should follow the guidelines described in the accompanying display, General Patient and Family Education for Chemotherapy.
- The nurse needs to explain that 5-FU, like most chemotherapeutic drugs with a narrow margin of safety, is highly toxic.
- The nurse should give troubleshooting instructions, if an alternative access device or an ambulatory infusion device is used at home. The patient should also know whom to call in case of problems.
- The nurse should explain that nausea and vomiting may occur 3 to 6 hours after drug therapy is administered; the nurse should provide appropriate antiemetic regimen.
- If loose stools exceed normal bowel patterns by more than three movements daily, the nurse should instruct the patient to observe the stools and notify the health care provider if stools are black or if blood is visible.
- Mouth sores may develop 5 to 8 days after drug administration. The nurse should offer helpful strategies such as practicing daily oral hygiene after meals and at bedtime, brushing with a soft toothbrush, avoiding commercial mouthwashes, and gently flossing with unwaxed dental floss. If bleeding occurs, flossing should be stopped until bleeding subsides.
- The nurse should caution the patient not to use aspirin or any pain-relieving drugs containing aspirin without consulting the health care provider.
- The nurse should teach the patient to self assess for signs and symptoms of potential infection, check temperature, and report temperature spikes higher than 101°F.
- The nurse should suggest that the patient apply moisturizers to the lips and avoid irritating, very hot, cold, or spicy foods and beverages. Bland, cool, soft foods, such as yogurt, custards, gelatins, and puddings, may be less irritating choices.
- The nurse should help the patient to understand that drug therapy produces photosensitivity. The nurse should instruct the patient to avoid the sun or protect the skin by applying a sunscreen (SPF 15 or more) and wearing protective clothing.
- The nurse should encourage the patient to express his or her concerns about the impact of cutaneous changes to body image and assist in developing strate-

COMMUNITY-BASED CONCERNS

General Patient and Family Education for Chemotherapy

The nurse plays a pivotal role in providing adequate information to assist the patient/family with the new roles so that treatment outcomes will be achieved. After diagnosis, the treatment modality is discussed and chosen. For most cancers, chemotherapy plays a significant benefit. The talking points for the nurse when called on to educate patients, irrespective of the type of chemotherapeutic agent used, include:

- Instruct patient about the significant side effects and reportable signs and symptoms of the chemotherapeutic agent(s).
- Emphasize self-management measures to be undertaken to prevent or decrease the side effects:

  Practice good personal hygiene, wash hands frequently, and avoid sources of infection

  Maintain dietary intake of food and fluids. Refer to dietician for consultation.

  Avoid trauma or injury and potential sources of bleeding by shaving with an electric razor, avoiding aspirin and other nonsteroidal anti-inflammatory drugs, and avoiding unnecessary injections, use of rectal thermometers, and venipunctures.

  Check urine, stool, skin for signs of bleeding.

  Practice good oral hygiene, use of soft toothbrush, noncommercial (i.e., alcohol-based) mouthwashes, use of lubricants.

  Schedule appointments for blood tests and follow-up visits for chemotherapy and related medications.
- If the patient goes to other physicians, dentists, or another health care provider, patient should inform them of chemotherapy treatment.
- Teach patients the importance of relaxation techniques and other forms of complementary medicine from which they might benefit.
- Referrals to other agencies and support groups might be helpful. Provide patient with a list of these resources.
- Instruct patients in the importance of maintaining a balance between rest and exercise to avoid fatigue.
- Explain to patient that some of side effects of treatment are reversible and are thus not a sign of disease progression.
- If patients are using chemotherapy drugs at home, teach the patient how to properly handle, store, and dispose of the agents and related materials.
- Teach patient to accept a "new" baseline especially in activities and responsibilities imposed by demands of disease and treatment. Teach patients to learn how to delegate and ask for assistance with activities of daily living.

gies to minimize the emotional impact. The nurse might offer cosmetic strategies such as wearing nail polish to cover darkened, dry brittle nails and using wigs, hats, and scarves to hide hair loss.

- The nurse should instruct the patient to notify the physician if any visual disturbances or confusion occur.
- The nurse should advise women of childbearing potential of the potential for harm to the fetus and methods of contraception.

Ongoing Assessment and Evaluation

The main adverse effects of 5-FU therapy are alterations in the patient's hematopoietic system and GI functions. Therefore, the nurse should closely monitor the patient's complete blood counts (CBCs) during each cycle to make sure that bone marrow recovery has occurred before another dose of the drug is given. Likewise, the nurse should assess the patient's nutritional status. Stomatitis or other problems related to the gastric mucosa should be under control to avoid putting the patient at risk for poor nutrition. ■

MEMORY CHIP
5-Fluorouracil

- Indicated for the treatment of carcinoma of the colon, rectum, breast, stomach, and pancreas
- Significant contraindications: poor nutritional status, decreased bone marrow reserve or a potentially serious infection
- Most common adverse effects: alopecia and other cutaneous changes, such as photosensitivity, and increased pigmentation of the skin
- Dose-limiting effects: mainly on the bone marrow manifested by myelosuppression and the gastrointestinal mucosa, causing nausea, vomiting, diarrhea and stomatitis
- **Life span alert: advise women of child-bearing age of the potential for harm to the fetus and so that they practice contraception. It is not known whether the drug is excreted in breast milk; therefore, explain that breast-feeding is not advised.**
- Maximizing therapeutic effects: potentiate antineoplastic activity of 5-FU by reduced folates such as the addition of leucovorin calcium
- Minimizing adverse effects: monitor CBC and assess for signs and symptoms of myelosuppression, which include infection and bleeding
- Most significant patient education: teach patient good oral care and to monitor for signs and symptoms of stomatitis and infection. Advise patient of the possibility of transient alopecia reversed after chemotherapy is finished.

DRUG SIGNIFICANTLY DIFFERENT FROM 5-FLUOROURACIL

Methotrexate (MTX) is a folate antimetabolite that induces folate depletion, leading to the inhibition of purine synthesis resulting in arrests of DNA, RNA, and protein synthesis. It is indicated in the management of trophoblastic neoplasm; acute leukemia; meningeal leukemia; breast carcinoma; head, neck, and lung neoplasms; Burkitt lymphoma; osteosarcoma; lymphosarcoma, and mycosis fungoides. It may be given in a variety of doses and schedules through various routes of administration such as oral, intramuscular, intravenous, intrathecal (in preservative free solution) and intra-arterial. A small portion is metabolized in the liver; the drug is excreted in the urine mostly as unchanged drug. Because the drug is secreted by the renal tubules, certain drugs that follow the same pathway such as salicylates, sulfonamides, phenytoin, and penicillin may compete with MTX excretion resulting in its accumulation and increased toxicity to the patient. It is therefore advisable that these drugs should be discontinued 2 days prior to and restarted 2 days after MTX therapy. MTX toxicity includes nausea and vomiting, diarrhea, cumulative myelosuppression, photosensitivity, rashes, and acute hepatotoxicity manifested by elevated liver enzyme levels. With high dose regimens, the following important considerations should be undertaken:

- Emetogenic potential is high; initiate appropriate antiemetic regimen.
- Monitor specific gravity, urine output, and urinary pH. Administer sodium bicarbonate and hydrate the patient to maintain urinary alkalinization of over 7 and urinary output at more than 100 mL/hour.
- Obtain orders for leucovorin rescue. Leucovorin is given to bypass the inhibitor action of MTX and supplies the form of folic acid needed by the normal cells for DNA synthesis. Leucovorin is usually initiated 24 hours after MTX according to a prescribed schedule based on serum MTX and creatinine levels. It is important that no doses of leucovorin are missed, which may increase toxicity.
- Monitor MTX levels for 72 hours until the nontoxic level of less than 0.1 micromolar is reached.

MITOTIC INHIBITORS

The mitotic inhibitors interfere with the formation of the mitotic spindle, causing metaphase arrest. They are primarily known as M-phase active, but they may also have some activity in the G_2 and S phases. These drugs are the vinca alkaloids, the podophyllotoxins, and the taxanes.

VINCA ALKALOIDS

Vinca alkaloids are extracts of the periwinkle plant. They bind to microtubular proteins, which are key to forming the mitotic spindle of the dividing cells. This binding arrests mitosis and eventually causes cell death. The vinca alkaloids act mainly in the M phase. However, high doses of the vinca alkaloids vincristine (Oncovorin, Oncovin, Vincasar PFS) and vinblastine (Velban, VLB) can also disrupt RNA and protein synthesis. Drugs in this category include vincristine, vinblastine, and vinorelbine (Navelbine). The drug vincristine is discussed as the representative Vinca alkaloid drug.

NURSING MANAGEMENT OF THE PATIENT RECEIVING P VINCRISTINE

Core Drug Knowledge

Pharmacotherapeutics

The major clinical use of vincristine is in treating acute lymphoblastic leukemia. It is used in combination therapy for Hodgkin disease, non-Hodgkin malignant lymphomas, rhabdomyosarcoma, neuroblastoma, and Wilms tumor. The recommended dosage of vincristine for an adult is discussed in Table 45-2. For children weighing less than 10 kg, or with body surface areas (BSAs) of less than 1 square meter, the dose is 0.05 mg/kg per week.

Pharmacokinetics

Following IV administration, vincristine binds extensively to both the plasma proteins and the blood elements, particularly the platelets. There is poor penetration across the blood-brain barrier. Vincristine is metabolized by the hepatic system, and 70% of the drug is excreted in the bile or feces. A small fraction is excreted in the urine.

Pharmacodynamics

The mechanism of action of vincristine is attributed to mitotic inhibition, causing an arrest of cell division in metaphase stage of mitosis. The drug interferes with intracellular tubulin fraction. The depolymerized tubulin proteins do not allow the spindle proteins to assemble, and cell division is halted in the metaphase.

Contraindications and Precautions

Vincristine is a pregnancy category D drug. Neurotoxicity from vincristine may be more pronounced in patients with underlying neurologic problems. Vincristine is contraindicated in patients with the demyelinating form of Charcot-Marie-Tooth syndrome, a neurologic disease characterized by absence of deep tendon reflexes. Because liver disease may alter the elimination of vincristine, dosage modifications may be needed in patients with elevated bilirubin levels. Care must be taken to prevent accidental contamination of the eyes, because the drug can cause severe eye irritation, including corneal ulceration if given under severe pressure. If eye contamination happens, the eyes must be washed immediately and thoroughly.

Vincristine is administered by IV only. Given intrathecally, vincristine may be fatal. Drug delivery may be by IV push directly over 1 minute or given by IV sidearm through a running IV line. It can also be given by continuous infusion but only through a central line. Vincristine is a **vesicant.** Vesicants are extremely acidic drugs that may cause significant and undesired tissue damage when accidental infiltration occurs. Therefore, extravasation precautions should be exercised during their infusion, as discussed later in this chapter.

Adverse Effects

The most common dose-limiting adverse effect with vincristine is neurologic. This effect is marked by motor, sensory, and autonomic neuropathy. Signs and symptoms of these neurologic deficits include loss of deep tendon reflexes, numbness and tingling of the hands and feet, myalgias, weakness, and jaw pain. Constipation, which is a forerunner of paralytic ileus, can be serious and bothersome to the patient. The neurotoxic signs and symptoms appear weeks or months after drug administration and are long lasting and slow to resolve. The severity of the neurotoxicity is related to the cumulative dose of the drug.

Drug Interactions

The toxicity of vincristine may be potentiated by drugs acting on the peripheral nervous system. It has been reported that vincristine increases the cellular uptake of MTX (high dose) in cancer cells. When given concomitantly with digoxin, vincristine may decrease the serum digoxin levels and the subsequent effects of digoxin. Mitomycin used together with vincristine may cause acute pulmonary reactions (Table 45-4).

Assessment of Relevant Core Patient Variables

Health Status

Careful consideration should be given if vincristine is administered to patients with preexisting neuromuscular disease or when other neurotoxic drugs are given. Clin-

TABLE 45-4 Agents That Interact With P Vincristine

Interactants	Effect and Significance	Nursing Management
digoxin	Decreased serum level and therapeutic effect	Monitor digoxin level.
methotrexate (MTX)	Increased cellular uptake of MTX when given sequentially	Notify physician for dosage modification. Monitor for signs and symptoms of neurotoxicity.

ical evaluation, including a thorough history and physical examination, may be needed for dose adjustments. The nurse should monitor the patient's hematologic profile. Concurrent use of drugs that cause constipation, such as narcotic analgesics and cholinergic drugs, should also be taken into account.

Life Span and Gender

Vincristine may have a potential impact on sexual function. The nurse should explore the sexual patterns of the patient. The nurse should assess women of childbearing age for pregnancy and lactation. Vincristine may cause fetal harm, so pregnant patients should be apprised of this if the drug is used in pregnancy. It is unknown whether vincristine is excreted in breast milk. Because of the potential for adverse effects in breast-feeding infants, the patient should decide either to stop breast-feeding or to stop drug therapy, taking into account the potential therapeutic effects of the drug on the mother. The nurse should note the patient's age and developmental status. Vincristine therapy may cause azoospermia and amenorrhea in postpubertal patients, although recovery occurs after therapy is completed. Potential motor and sensory dysfunction associated with vincristine pose an increased risk to elderly patients.

Lifestyle, Diet, and Habits

Before drug administration, the nurse should determine the patient's sensory, motor, and perceptual functions, because of the potential dysfunctions associated with vincristine. The nurse should consider bowel elimination patterns and food and fluid intake.

Environment

The nurse should be aware of the environment in which the drug will be administered. Vincristine may be given in an inpatient or ambulatory care setting.

Nursing Diagnoses and Outcomes

- Disturbed Sensory Perception related to perceptual neuropathies as evidenced by absent deep tendon reflexes, numbness, weakness, and myalgias.

  Desired outcome: The patient will be able to function safely without injury. Optimal sensory and perceptual function will be maintained.
- Risk for Constipation related to adverse effects of vincristine

  Desired outcome: The patient will have a regular bowel elimination pattern and will pass soft stools.
- Risk for Infection and bleeding related to bone marrow depression

  Desired outcome: Bone marrow recovery will be attained ; rare and mild myelosuppression might occur. The patient will verbalize and also implement self-care measures to prevent infection.
- Impaired Skin Integrity related to potential for vesicant extravasation

  Desired outcome: The skin will remain intact without cutaneous breakdown. The patient and health care provider will be able to recognize signs and symptoms of suspected extravasation and initiate prompt measures that will prevent further tissue damage.
- Disturbed Body Image related to drug-induced hair loss

  Desired outcome: The patient will be accepting of change in physical appearance and will develop strategies to cope with hair loss.
- Ineffective Sexuality Patterns: impotence related to adverse effects of vincristine

  Desired outcome: The patient will have increased understanding of reversible effect of drug and will exhibit behavior change that will result in more satisfying sexual functioning.

Planning and Intervention

Maximizing Therapeutic Effects

Before each drug administration, the nurse should monitor the patient's CBC to ensure that it is within safe limits. The drug is light-sensitive and should be protected from light. It should also be refrigerated. The bolus should be given through a new or and patent free-flowing IV access, noting patient's response during and after drug instillation. If the drug is given as a continuous infusion, a central line should always be used. Oncovin is only given intravenously. Intrathecal administration can result in death.

Minimizing Adverse Effects

The occurrence of peripheral neuropathies is a major concern with vincristine therapy. The toxicity to the nerve fibers can induce severe motor, sensory, and autonomic deficits. The nurse should assess the patient before each cycle for significant changes. The nurse should report any changes in perceptual or sensory functioning and consult the health care provider immediately regarding dosage modifications or discontinuation of the drug.

Because vincristine has vesicant properties, careful attention should be given to prevent extravasation (see the accompanying display, Managing Peripheral Extravasation). The nurse should be thoroughly familiar with appropriate antidotes and protocols for the use of vesicants. (Table 45-5).

Providing Patient and Family Education

- The nurse should follow the guidelines described in General Patient and Family Education for Chemotherapy.
- The nurse should discuss and explain precautionary measures to the patient to lessen further insult to the hematologic and cutaneous systems.
- The nurse should advise the patient to promptly report problems resulting from the IV infusion, for

Managing Peripheral Extravasation

Extravasation is the inadvertent infiltration of the chemotherapeutic drug into the subcutaneous tissues surrounding the site of infusion. Because a vesicant drug is very acidic, it can cause severe damage depending on the tissue it infiltrates, the amount of drug the tissue absorbs, and the length of the tissue's exposure to the infiltrated drug.

Extravasation over joint spaces, tendons, or neuromuscular bundles increases the risk of tissue damage. When a drug extravasates, the patient typically complains of pain, burning, or discomfort at the injection site. Sometimes pain might be a delayed reaction with other signs, such as reddening of the skin and blistering, which may progress to severe tissue involvement. The best cure for extravasation is prevention.

The nurse should be familiar with the institutional policies for managing extravasation. Although specific protocols for managing extravasation may vary among health care settings, general guidelines for managing extravasation include the following:

- Stop the infusion immediately and restart the infusion at a new site.
- Apply warm or cold compresses as indicated to the extravasation site, and if prescribed, administer a local antidote, such as hyaluronidase, to minimize any tissue damage.
- Notify the health care provider.
- Rest and elevate the affected extremity for 48 hours.
- Apply a sterile dressing that allows the extravasation area to remain visible. Avoid any pressure to the site.
- Obtain a photograph of the site for baseline comparisons
- Document the following: patient's name, date and time of extravasation, name of drug, approximate volume of infiltrate, needle gauge, site of extravasation, symptoms reported by the patient and assessed by the nurse, nursing measures implemented, name of health care provider notified, patient education provided, and nurse's signature.
- Consult physician regarding need for referral to plastic surgeon, if appropriate.

FLOWSHEET FOR SUSPECTED/ACTUAL CHEMOTHERAPY EXTRAVASATION

addressograph stamp

Date: ____________ Date extravasation occurred: ____________

INITIAL EVALUATION (Day 0)

DESCRIPTION OF EXTRAVASATION
Name and Volume of drug given: ____________
IV site location: (indicate on diagram and describe):
____
Needle type and gauge: ____________
Patient complaints: ____________
Physician notified (name): ____________
R.N. (name): ____________

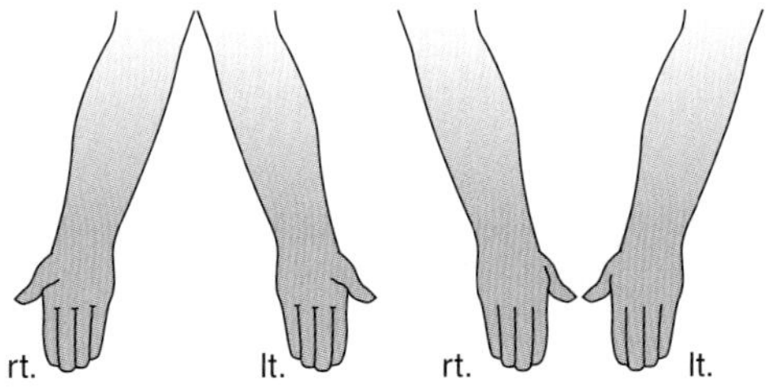

INITIAL INTERVENTIONS
Date
________ Antidote admin. (specify) ________
________ Cold compresses
________ Warm compresses
________ 1% Hydrocortisone cream applied
________ Baseline photo

ADDITIONAL INTERVENTIONS
Date
________ Dermatology Consult
________ Plastic Surg. Consult
________ Wound care (described)
____
____
________ Follow-up photo

PATIENT TEACHING
Date
________ Extravasation fact card given and reviewed
________ Follow-up schedule reviewed

example, pain, redness, swelling, or blistering at the infusion site.

- The nurse should instruct the patient and caregiver to observe and monitor the infusion site for early extravasation and cutaneous reactions.
- The nurse should teach the patient and caregiver how to care for a suspected extravasation at home until medical attention can be obtained, if needed.
- The nurse should discuss methods for coping with adverse effects, for example, a metallic taste sensation during drug administration, nausea or appetite loss, constipation accompanied by cramping (report to health care provider who can order laxatives or stool softeners).
- The nurse should encourage the patient to maintain adequate nutrition. A high-fiber diet and plenty of fluids should be consumed to help relieve constipation.
- The nurse should instruct the patient to avoid injury related to drug-related altered sensory and perceptual changes manifested by muscle weakness and neuropathy, numbness of the fingers and toes, tingling sensation, or absence of deep tendon reflexes that may be temporary or permanent.

TABLE 45-5 Common Vesicants and Known Antidotes

Vesicant	Antidote	Nursing Management
vincristine (Oncovin, Vincasar PFS) vinorelbine (Navelbine) vinblastine (Velban) vindesine (Eldisine)		Apply warm compress to extravasation site for 15–20 min at least qid for the first 2 d.
cisplatin (Platinol)	Isotonic sodium	Rapid administration of antidote is crucial.
mechlorethamine hydrochloride (nitrogen mustard)	Thiosulfate	Prepare antidote as prescribed. (example: 4-mL 10% sodium (nitrogen mustard) Inject solution through IV cannula–2-mL solution for each mL of vesicant extravasated.
Others: dactinomycin (Actinomycin) daunorubicin (Cerubidine) doxorubicin (Adriamycin) epirubicin (Ellence) idarubicin (Idamycin) fluorouracil (5-FU, rare vesicant potential), mitomycin (Mitomycin-C) mitoxantrone (Novantrone)	No known antidotes	Institute comfort measures. Apply cold compresses as indicated. Teach about infection prevention.

- The nurse should review strategies for taking care of hair and skin with the patient, because thinning or loss of hair may occur 2 or 3 weeks after treatment. The nurse should teach the patient techniques to provide gentle care by avoiding heat or chemical irritants, and wearing wigs or hair coverings. The nurse can help the patient recognize that hair will regrow within a few months after therapy stops.
- The nurse should emphasize to the patient and caregiver to schedule and keep appointments for laboratory tests and medical checkups.
- The nurse should explore with the patient and significant other sexuality issues and discuss strategies to maintain sexual health. Reassure the patient that impotency should it occur, is usually reversible after drug is discontinued.

Ongoing Assessment and Evaluation

Acute elevation of uric acid may occur during induction of remission for leukemic patients. Uric acid levels should be measured during the first 3 to 4 weeks of treatment and measures undertaken to prevent the occurrence of uric acid nephropathy. Daily assessment of the patient's bowel function and motor and sensory functions is necessary. ■

DRUG CLOSELY RELATED TO VINCRISTINE

Vinblastine (Velban) is another vinca alkaloid derived from the periwinkle plant. Although its chemical structure, pharmacokinetics, and mechanism of action are similar to those of vincristine, this drug has markedly more clinical indications from vincristine. Like vincristine in its efficacy in treating malignant lymphomas and Hodgkin disease, vinblastine is also used for chemotherapy in mycosis fungoides, testicular carcinoma, Kaposi sarcoma, choriocarcinoma, and breast cancer.

The toxicity profile of vinblastine differs from that of vincristine. The dose-limiting toxicity of vinblastine is myelosuppression, whereas that of vincristine is neurotoxicity. Vincristine is considered more potent than vinblastine, because it rarely affects the bone marrow. The mildly myelosuppressive action of vincristine makes it more attractive for combination chemotherapy than vinblastine.

MEMORY CHIP

Vincristine

- Primarily indicated for acute leukemia and for other cancers such as hodgkin's disease, breast cancer, neuroblastoma, and multiple myeloma
- Significant contraindications: demyelating form of CharcotMarie syndrome
- Most common adverse effect: tissue necrosis if the drug, which is a vesicant, accidentally extravasates
- Most serious adverse effects: neurotoxic deficits manifested by paresthesias, myalgias, loss of deep tendon reflexes, and jaw pain. Paralytic ileus as evidenced by constipation may also occur.
- **Life span alert: caution elderly patients regarding the potential for motor and sensory deficits that may compromise their safety and sensory acuity. Vincristine may cause fetal harm or risk to mothers who are breast-feeding. Apprise patients of these side effects.**
- Maximizing therapeutic effects: the drug is light sensitive; protect it from light. Infuse it slowly over approximately 1 minute.
- Minimizing adverse effects: always assess bowel elimination pattern because of the danger of paralytic ileus.
- Ensure good vascular access and monitor for signs and symptoms of extravasation.
- Most significant patient education: instruct the patient to obtain a prescription for a prophylactic stool regimen.

PODOPHYLLOTOXINS

The podophyllotoxins were isolated from the mandrake plant (May crab apple). Examples of drugs in this group are etoposide (VP-16) and teniposide (VM-26), which are semisynthetic derivatives. They act in the premitotic, G2, and S phases and interfere with topoisomerase II enzyme reaction. The drug etoposide is discussed as the representative podophyllotoxin drug.

NURSING MANAGEMENT OF THE PATIENT RECEIVING ETOPOSIDE

Core Drug Knowledge

Pharmacotherapeutics

Etoposide is the prototype drug of the subgroup of alkaloids called podophyllotoxins. This drug is used in combination therapy for refractory testicular tumors and small-cell lung cancer. Etoposide is also available in an oral formulation (see Table 45-2). The recommended dose for oral use is twice the IV dose rounded to the nearest 50 mg.

Pharmacokinetics

Etoposide binds to serum albumin and becomes extensively bound to tissues (see Table 45-2).

It is predominantly excreted in the urine and to a lesser extent in the bile. About 30%% of the drug is excreted unchanged. The drug's half-life is 4 to 11 hours.

Pharmacodynamics

Etoposide acts by inhibiting a DNA enzyme called topoisomerase II, causing breaks in the double strands of protein-linked DNA. This action inhibits DNA synthesis in the S and G_2 phases so that cells do not enter mitosis and prophase.

Contraindications and Precautions

Etoposide should not be given to patients with a known hypersensitivity to this drug or teniposide, the other podophyllotoxin derivative. The drug should never be administered by IV push because of the danger of hypotension. It should be infused over 30 to 60 minutes or longer depending on the volume of the infusion. If the patient is taking warfarin concomitantly with etoposide, the patient's prothrombin time should be monitored closely. Etoposide is a pregnancy category D drug and should not be used in pregnant women.

Adverse Effects

Hypersensitivity or anaphylactic-like reactions manifested by hypotension, chills, fever, facial flushing, bronchospasm, dyspnea, and tachycardia can occur during an etoposide infusion. However, these are not related to any cardiorespiratory pathology but rather to the rapid infusion of the drug itself. These can be ameliorated by stopping the infusion and giving the patient IV fluids, corticosteroids, antihistamines, and volume expanders as ordered.

The major dose-limiting effect of etoposide is myelosuppression manifested primarily by granulocytopenia, which nadirs (reaches its lowest count) in 7 to 14 days, and has a platelet nadir in 9 to 16 days after parenteral administration. Recovery is noted in 20 days. When given orally, the nadir granulocyte counts appear between 21 and 28 days, with recovery in 35 days. The other adverse effects of note are mild to moderate nausea and vomiting, which can be controlled by antiemetics. GI toxicities are more pronounced with the oral form of the drug. Hepatic toxicity shown by elevated liver enzyme levels is a result of administering higher than recommended doses.

Drug-induced alopecia is reversible on discontinuation of the drug. Patients who have had radiation therapy might get **radiation recall** characterized by erythematous rash in the irradiated area. This condition may progress to desquamation, vesicle formation, and permanent hyperpigmentation of the affected area.

Etoposide is classified as an **irritant.** As such, it may produce pain, urticaria, redness, and inflammation along the vein path in which the drug is infusing. Unlike vesicants, irritants do not generally cause tissue damage.

Drug Interactions

Etoposide has a synergistic effect with cisplatin. It is incompatible with gallium nitrate and MTX (Table 45-6).

Assessment of Relevant Core Patient Variables

Health Status

The nurse should assess the patient for prior extensive myelosuppressive chemotherapy or irradiation to marrow-bearing areas of the skeleton. This is important to know so that dose reduction can be considered to avoid the potential for more severe myelosuppression. The patient's CBC should be determined before and during therapy. The patient's renal and hepatic functions should also be monitored so that dose adjustments may be made in cases of system dysfunctions.

Life Span and Gender

The nurse should document the age and gender of the patient. The safety and efficacy of etoposide have not been established in children. The nurse should explore the sexual patterns and reproductive goals of the patient. The nurse should assess women of childbearing age for pregnancy. This drug has mutagenic, carcinogenic, and teratogenic properties.

Lifestyle, Diet, and Habits

Alopecia affects 20% to 90% of patients. The nurse should explore the impact on the patient's sexuality and body image with the patient. Hair loss could be complete and may have more of a distressing impact on socially active, working, or female patients.

Environment

The nurse should be aware of the environment in which the drug will be administered. Etoposide can be given in an acute care or ambulatory setting where the necessary clinical support is available should hypotension or an anaphylactic reaction develop.

Nursing Diagnoses and Outcomes

- Risk for Injury related to etoposide-induced hypotension or anaphylactic reaction
  Desired outcome: The patient will not experience hypotension or anaphylactic reaction.
- Risk for Infection related to bleeding resulting from bone marrow suppression
  Desired outcome: The patient will recover adequate hematologic function. The patient will undertake self-care measures to prevent infection and bleeding.
- Imbalanced Nutrition: Less than Body Requirements related to nausea, vomiting, and anorexia from drug therapy
  Desired outcome: The patient will maintain proper nutritional status and good emetic control.
- Disturbed Body Image related to drug-induced alopecia
  Desired outcome: The patient will implement coping strategies to alleviate feelings associated with loss of hair.
- Sexual Dysfunction related to disease process and drug therapy
  Desired outcome: The patient will increase knowledge about the effects of chemotherapy on sexual function and will continue functioning without interfering with sexual patterns and reproductive goals.
- Impaired Skin Integrity resulting from irritation to infusion site and possible radiation recall
  Desired outcome: The patient's skin will remain intact without breakdown from irritant chemotherapy. Patient will demonstrate competence in wound management if radiation recall occurs.

Planning and Intervention

Maximizing Therapeutic Effects

The stability of the drug depends on the concentration. It should be diluted in 5% dextrose for injection or in 0.9% sodium chloride solution. Etoposide is stable in a glass container for 96 hours and for 48 hours in plastic at a concentration of 0.2 mg/mL.

Minimizing Adverse Effects

Because of dose-limiting myelosuppression, WBC counts should be monitored prior to chemotherapy and at expected nadir. The patient receiving etoposide therapy should be observed closely for hypotension or anaphylactic reactions. The drug should be given by slow infusion, never by rapid infusion, over 30 to 60 minutes and possibly longer, depending on the volume of the infusion. Cardiopulmonary resuscitation equipment should

TABLE 45-6 Agents That Interact With Etoposide

Interactants	Effect and Significance	Nursing Management
warfarin	Increases prothrombin time (PT)	Monitor PT closely. Monitor for signs of increased bleeding.
gallium-nitrate and methotrexate	Incompatible combinations	Avoid combined therapy.

be present at the patient's bedside. During drug administration, the nurse should help allay the patient's fears about possible anaphylactic reactions by staying with the patient and infusing the solution slowly through a patent IV line to prevent hypotension and chemical phlebitis. Warm compresses should be applied to the affected site. The patient's hepatic and renal function should be monitored before and during therapy. The nurse needs to assess for signs and symptoms of infection and teach the patient to monitor and self-report the same. If the oral formulation of etoposide is given, adequate antiemetics should be given.

Providing Patient and Family Education

- The nurse should follow the guidelines described in General Patient and Family Education for Chemotherapy.
- The nurse should focus education for patients receiving etoposide on the importance of minimizing risks related to infection and injury, which are major concerns of patients with cancer.
- The nurse should discuss what to expect during the infusion (metallic taste, which may last a while but can be relieved by sucking on hard candy). If the oral formulation is used, the drug should be taken on a full stomach.
- The nurse should explain to the patient that an allergic reaction may occur during infusion or after it; this is signaled by facial flushing, shortness of breath, or a feeling of faintness.
- The nurse should assist the patient explore ways to manage adverse effects of mild nausea, loss of appetite, and mouth sores, which may develop in 4 to 7 days.
- The nurse should offer helpful oral hygiene practices, such as brushing the teeth at least four times daily with a soft brush and avoiding commercial mouthwashes containing alcohol, which can be irritating to the mucous lining.
- The nurse should provide nutritional guidelines, such as taking antiemetics as prescribed, eating many small meals rather than a few full meals, and avoiding highly seasoned food.
- The nurse should explain the importance of regular laboratory examinations, such as blood tests at certain intervals, to detect any decreases in blood counts (usually within 1 to 2 weeks after treatment).
- The nurse should stress guidelines for avoiding infection resulting from bone marrow suppression.
- The nurse should demonstrate methods to cope with hair loss and with tingling in the hands and feet.
- The nurse should teach the patient how to avoid injury resulting from drug-related neuropathy.
- The nurse should instruct the patient to contact the health care provider about serious adverse effects, such as a temperature over 100.5°F, excessive vomiting, painful mouth sores with inability to eat or drink for 24 hours, black stools, uncontrolled bleeding.
- The nurse should discuss with the patient and patient's significant other both reproductive goals and birth control because of the possible mutagenic and teratogenic properties of the drug.

Ongoing Assessment and Evaluation

Prior to each subsequent dose of drug therapy, the WBC and platelet counts should be checked; platelet levels less than 50,000/mm^3 or an absolute neutrophil count less than 500/mm^3 are indications for withholding the drug until the bone marrow recovers sufficiently. ■

DRUG CLOSELY RELATED TO P ETOPOSIDE

Teniposide (VM-26, Vumon) and etoposide possess basic similarities in terms of their pharmacologic makeup, toxicities, and clinical applications. The structures of etoposide and teniposide differ only by the substitution of a methyl group (etoposide) for the thenylidene (teniposide) on the glycopiranoside sugar. They are both extracted from the American mandrake plant *Podophyllum peltatum.*

For teniposide administration, only non-diethylhexylphthalate (DEHP) containers, such as glass or polyolefin plastic containers, can be used. This prevents the leaching of

MEMORY CHIP

P Etoposide

- Indicated for the treatment of testicular carcinoma, small-cell and non–small-cell lung cancer, lymphoma, Hodgkin disease, and multiple myeloma
- Significant contraindications: known hypersensitivity to etoposide or to any podophyllotoxin derivative
- Most common adverse effect: hypersensitivity or anaphylaxis evidenced by orthostatic hypotension, chills, dyspnea, or bronchospasm (wheezing) when given rapidly
- Dose-limiting effect: Myelosuppression
- **Life span alert: radiation recall may happen. The safety and efficacy of VP-16 have not been established in children**
- Maximizing therapeutic effects: always infuse slowly over 30–60 minutes; never by IV push
- Minimizing adverse effects: monitor results of complete blood count before chemotherapy and at expected nadir, approximately 10–14 days after the drug dose. Monitor for signs and symptoms of myelosuppression, which include infection and bleeding.
- Most significant patient education: forewarn the patient that the infusion causes a metallic taste. Advise the patient that sucking on hard candy may alleviate the metallic taste.

DEHP from polyvinyl containers into the solution. Administration with heparin is contraindicated because heparin causes a precipitate to form.

TAXANES

The taxanes cause mitotic arrest by promoting the formation of abnormal spindle fibers and mitotic asters. Paclitaxel (Taxol), the first drug in this category was isolated from the bark of the Pacific yew *Taxus brevifolia*. Because the demand exceeded the supply available, a semisynthetic form was developed. Docetaxel (Taxotere) is the other taxane, a semisynthetic derivative of the European yew, *Taxus baccata*. The drug paclitaxel is discussed as the representative taxane drug.

NURSING MANAGEMENT OF THE PATIENT RECEIVING PACLITAXEL

Core Drug Knowledge

Pharmacotherapeutics

The most significant cytotoxic activity of paclitaxel has been in treating ovarian and breast cancers. It is approved for use after failure of first-line or subsequent therapy in metastatic ovarian cancer. In breast cancer, it is given to patients who have metastatic breast cancer that has progressed or relapsed during anthracycline-based therapy and for the adjuvant treatment of node-positive breast cancer administered sequentially to standard doxorubicin-containing combination chemotherapy. Significant activity has been observed in clinical studies in a diverse range of solid tumors that are refractory to conventional chemotherapy. It has recently been approved for the second-line treatment of AIDS-related Kaposi sarcoma. Several administration regimens are used, such as 1-, 3-, 6-, and 24-hour infusions with varying doses (see Table 45-2).

Pharmacokinetics

Paclitaxel crosses the placenta and enters breast milk. The liver is the principal organ responsible for paclitaxel metabolism. The drug is excreted into the bile; less than 10% of the intact drug is excreted in the urine.

Pharmacodynamics

Paclitaxel inhibits the normal dynamic reorganization of the microtubular network during interphase and mitosis. Microtubules are cellular elements that appear to play an important role in the initiation of DNA synthesis, mitosis, and other cellular functions. The interference with the microtubules prevents depolymerization, which triggers apoptosis or cell death in rapidly dividing cells. It also prevents transition from the G_0 phase to the S phase by blocking cellular response to protein growth factors.

Contraindications and Precautions

Paclitaxel is a pregnancy category D drug. Patients who have a history of hypersensitivity to drugs formulated in Cremophor EL should not be challenged with paclitaxel because of the possibility of hypersensitivity reaction.

Adverse Effects

About 10% of patients experience a hypersensitivity reaction. This occurs during the first 10 minutes of the infusion, especially in patients who are new to the drug. The reaction is caused by the Cremophor diluent used in paclitaxel preparation and is manifested by dyspnea, hypotension, tachycardia, wheezing, and chest pain.

Myelosuppression is dose limiting; neutrophils nadir at day 11, and platelets nadir by day 8. Fever is associated with low counts. Neurotoxicity is another significant problem that generally begins 2 or 3 days postinfusion. Patients complain of numbness, tingling, and pain in the hands and feet, which may progress to painful paresthesias, loss of deep tendon reflexes, arthralgia, and diffuse myalgia. The GI manifestations are mucositis, diarrhea, mild nausea and vomiting, and elevated liver enzyme levels. The cutaneous reactions are alopecia, facial flushing, and chemical phlebitis.

Paclitaxel has weak vesicant properties. It also appears to be cardiotoxic: bradyarrhythmias, including heart block, have been reported. Severe conduction abnormalities have been observed in fewer than 1% of patients receiving paclitaxel, in some cases, necessitating pacemaker insertion.

Drug Interactions

The most significant drug interaction is between paclitaxel and cisplatin. When given in combination, it can cause synergistic myelosuppression and neurotoxicity. Table 45-7 presents other drugs that might have significant interactions with paclitaxel. Additionally, paclitaxel infusion needs to be administered in glass or polyolefin containers with polyethylene-lined administration sets. Polyvinyl chloride containers or tubing causes leaching of the plasticizer DEHP into the fluid and should not be used. An inline filter of less than 0.22 μm should also be used because particulates can form.

Assessment of Relevant Core Patient Variables

Health Status

Before administering the first dose of paclitaxel, the nurse should ensure that baseline CBC, electrocardiographic, and vital signs are recorded. The nurse should assess the hepatobiliary function, particularly serum bilirubin levels. Patients with existing neuropathies resulting from diabetes mellitus or alcohol ingestion could experience potentiated neurotoxicity resulting from paclitaxel administration. The nurse should investigate hypersensitivity to other drugs with a Cremophor base.

TABLE 45-7 Agents That Interact With Paclitaxel

Interactants	Effect and Significance	Nursing Management
quinidine, cyclosporine, quinine, verapamil	Reversal of multidrug resistance	Administer medications as ordered.
cisplatin (CDDP)	Myelosuppression more severe when CDDP is given before paclitaxel	Give paclitaxel first when these two drugs are ordered sequentially.
ketoconazole	Inhibits metabolism of paclitaxel	Monitor for paclitaxel toxicity.

Life Span and Gender

The nurse should assess women of childbearing age for pregnancy and lactation. This drug is believed to be embryotoxic; therefore, its use should be avoided in pregnancy. It may be excreted in milk; breast-feeding should be stopped while on paclitaxel therapy. The clinical efficacy of paclitaxel in children has not been evaluated.

Lifestyle, Diet, and Habits

The nurse should discuss the impact of alopecia and other adverse effects on the patient's sexuality, body image, and activities of daily living. The resultant alopecia, which may include loss of eyebrow, eyelash, pubic, and axillary hair, may be devastating to a patient who leads an active social life. Similarly limiting are the neurotoxic effects of pain, burning, sensory loss, paresthesia, and loss of deep tendon reflexes. These symptoms might be more pronounced in patients with a history of alcohol abuse.

Environment

The nurse should be aware of the environment in which paclitaxel will be administered. It may be administered either on an inpatient or outpatient basis. However for precautionary measures, it is not unusual to administer the first paclitaxel dose in an inpatient setting because severe reactions manifested by hypotension, bronchospasm, tachycardia, and chest pain can occur. In any setting where the drug is given, resuscitation equipment and adequate supportive drugs should always be present so that prompt intervention can be implemented if necessary.

Nursing Diagnoses and Outcomes

- Risk for Injury related to hypersensitivity or anaphylactic reactions from paclitaxel
  Desired outcome: The patient will not suffer any injury resulting from hypersensitivity reaction to the paclitaxel.
- Risk for Infection and bleeding related to bone marrow depression
  Desired outcome: The patient will be free from infection and bleeding evidenced by normal vital signs and recovery from neutropenia and anemia as shown in the blood counts.
- Disturbed Sensory Perception related to neuropathy
  Desired outcome: The patient will be able to function safely within limitations of lessened perceptual and sensory acuity due to paclitaxel.
- Imbalanced Nutrition: Less than Body Requirements related to drug-induced nausea, vomiting, and diarrhea
  Desired outcome: The patient will maintain adequate nutritional intake and be able to gain adequate emesis/diarrhea control.
- Impaired Skin Integrity and Disturbed Body Image related to drug-induced alopecia
  Desired outcome: The patient will understand that the loss of hair is reversible and will initiate strategies to minimize body image distortion from alopecia.

Planning and Intervention

Maximizing Therapeutic Effects

Paclitaxel is an important drug in combination with cisplatin. The cytotoxicity from these two drugs are sequence dependent; for optimal results, paclitaxel should be given first. Dose-intensity regimens of 250 mg/m^2 of paclitaxel have been given combined with a colony-stimulating factor, such as filgrastin. The use of this growth factor is critical because it accelerates bone marrow recovery and prevents severe nadirs from occurring. It is given subcutaneously at a dose of 5 μg/kg every day for 10 days starting 1 day after the chemotherapy is given (see the accompanying display, Implementing Paclitaxel Therapy).

Critical Thinking Scenario

Implementing paclitaxel therapy

Mrs. A. S., a 55-year-old woman with diagnosed breast cancer, is going to receive paclitaxel for the first time. The dose that is prescribed is 175 mg/m^2 to be given as a 3-hour infusion every 3 weeks for four cycles.

1. Describe the nursing responsibilities before the start of the infusion.
2. Because neutropenia is a major adverse effect of paclitaxel therapy, what are the main points to include in the teaching plan?

COMMUNITY-BASED CONCERNS

Home Therapy With Hydroxyurea

Some patients receive hydroxyurea (Hydrea) at home. They need to learn about safe, effective self-care. Some considerations to cover in patient education include the following:

- Because hydroxyurea is taken PO, problems with swallowing capsules can present difficulties. To counteract swallowing problems, hydroxyurea capsules can be mixed with applesauce, water, or juice and swallowed in liquid form.
- Taken in large doses, hydroxyurea may cause moderate drowsiness; patients should be cautioned to prevent risk of injury.
- Early side effects of nausea, vomiting, diarrhea, and loss of appetite may interfere with drug effectiveness. Antiemetic medications should be taken as prescribed. In some cases, taking hydroxyurea before bedtime helps to decrease nausea.
- The health care provider should be notified if foods or liquids cannot be retained for more than 24 hours after taking hydroxyurea.
- If the physician recommends blood testing, appointments should be scheduled so that the blood count can be monitored closely. A temporary decrease may occur within 7 to 14 days after treatment, but the blood counts will recover.
- Ways to prevent infection include avoiding people who have colds or any infection during the drug therapy period and avoiding injury, such as cuts from razor blades or kitchen knives.
- The health care provider should be notified if a severe skin rash or facial redness develops, although a less severe rash may occur in 1 to 2 weeks after treatment.
- Because hydration is important for therapeutic effect, the patient should drink plenty of fluids to prevent any problems with kidney function.
- Proper handling of cytotoxic agents particularly avoidance of contact with skin should be observed.

sure that they are within safe treatment parameters. If the patient is receiving concomitant radiation therapy, the nurse should check the oral mucosa to ensure that severe reactions, which can cause pain and difficulty with food intake, do not compromise the patient. Because radiation recall may occur with concomitant treatment, dermatologic changes should be reported to the health care provider and managed appropriately. ■

DRUG SIGNIFICANTLY DIFFERENT FROM HYDROXYUREA

L-asparaginase (Elspar) belongs to the miscellaneous group of drugs that are cell cycle-phase specific. The inhibitory action of this drug is in the postmitotic (i.e., G_1) phase of the cell cycle. It is indicated in patients with acute lymphocytic leukemia. In this condition, the tumor cells depend on exogenous asparagine for survival. Normal cells are able to synthesize asparagine and are less affected by depletion of this enzyme. When L-asparaginase is administered to the leukemic patient, the serum asparagine is hydrolyzed to nonfunctional aspartic acid and ammonia, depriving malignant cells of the required amino acid. This causes rapid inhibition of DNA and RNA synthesis.

L-asparaginase does not appear to cross the blood-brain barrier and is not excreted in the urine. It is administered by the intramuscular or IV routes. Patients receiving this drug should be treated in the hospital because of the frequency of anaphylactic reactions. Toxicity is more common in adults than in children.

In addition to anaphylaxis, other common side effects are hepatotoxicity, which occurs in most patients, and decreased clotting factors, which may lead to bleeding problems, such as intracranial hemorrhage and fatal bleeding associated with low fibrinogen. Bone marrow depression is rare and transient. Mild to severe CNS effects manifested by somnolence, lethargy, drowsiness, and feeling of malaise have been noted. These are usually reversible with discontinuation of drug.

MEMORY CHIP

Hydroxyurea

- Indicated for managing hematologic cancers, such as acute blastic or chronic myelogenous leukemia. It is used in combination chemotherapy or with radiation and has shown some clinical efficacy against malignant melanoma, ovarian cancer, and head and neck tumors.
- Significant contraindication: depressed bone marrow reserve
- Most common adverse effects: gastrointestinal effects manifested by anorexia, nausea and vomiting, stomatitis, and diarrhea or constipation
- Most serious adverse effects: bone marrow depression including leukopenia, anemia, and thrombocytopenia. Rapid decrease in white blood cell counts may occur within a short period, which is the desired effect for leukemia patients.
- Minimizing adverse effects: monitor the patient's blood count before, during, and after treatment. If anemia occurs, the patient may receive blood transfusion without interrupting treatment cycles. Premedicate the patient with the appropriate antiemetic regimen.
- Most significant patient education: hydroxyurea is administered orally. If the patient has difficulty swallowing, instruct the patient to empty the contents of the capsule into a glass of water, mix and drink immediately. The contents may not be dissolved completely because of the drug formulation. Advise the patient on careful handling of a cytotoxic agent particularly to avoid contact with the skin or mucous membrane.

HERBAL MEDICINE AND CHEMOTHERAPY

Plants and herbs for medicinal purposes have been used in the Eastern and Western cultures for thousands of years. In the United States, the use of herbal medicine is increasingly pop-

TABLE 45-8 Agents With Potential Interactions With St. John's Wort

Chemotherapeutic agents	Antiemetic agents
anastrozole (Arimidex)	dolasetron (Anzemet)
cyclophosphamide (Cytoxan)	granisetron (Kytril)
docetaxel (Taxotere)	ondansetron (Zofran)
etoposide (VP-16)	
ifosfamide (Ifex)	
paclitaxel (Taxol)	
teniposide (VM-26)	
tretinoin (retinoic acid)	
vinblastine (Velban)	
vincristine (Oncovin)	

ular. Herbs are marketed as nutritional supplements, therefore their content and efficacy do not have to pass through the standard rigorous requirements of the Food and Drug Administration. Because of the lack of quality control, the purity of these products is of concern. Studies have shown that some herbs are contaminated with heavy metals. For these reasons, nurses should ask patients about the use of herbs and the possibility of discontinuing them when they initiate therapy with antineoplastic agents. *St. John's Wort,* commonly known as "nature's Prozac," have been studied and potential interactions with certain chemotherapy (Table 45-8) have been found.

CHAPTER SUMMARY

- All cells, normal and malignant, progress through the different phases of the cell life cycle.
- Health care workers can be exposed to chemotherapy through the following routes: skin and mucus membrane absorption, inhalation, and ingestion.
- In general, antineoplastic drugs are most effective on cells in the proliferative phases.
- Cell cycle-specific drugs exert their cytotoxicity at a particular phase(s) of the cell cycle and cause no significant harm during the remaining phases.
- The major toxicities of antineoplastic drugs are seen on rapidly dividing cells, such as the bone marrow, GI mucosa, hair follicles, and gonadal cells.
- Hypersensitivity, anaphylactic reactions, and extravasations are the most common immediate reactions associated with chemotherapy administration.
- The major teaching points that a nurse should emphasize to a patient receiving chemotherapy are to 1) practice good body and oral hygiene; 2) eat a nutritious diet and drink plenty of fluids; 3) protect oneself from injury especially cuts to the skin; 4) avoid possible sources of infection, such as people with colds, chickenpox, and herpes, and avoid handling animal excrement; and 5) pace your activities of daily living to provide adequate rest and exercise.
- Medicinal herbs have the potential to interact with chemotherapeutic drugs and their consumption should be discussed with health care provider before initiating treatment.

QUESTIONS FOR STUDY AND REVIEW

1. What are the goals of chemotherapy?
2. What are the different strategies undertaken in the use of chemotherapeutic agents?
3. What are the basic features of a malignant cell?
4. How do you clean up a chemotherapy spill?
5. How are health care workers exposed to chemotherapy?
6. Why is vincristine preferred over vinblastine for combination chemotherapy?
7. What are the nursing measures to take when an extravasation occurs?
8. What causes hypotension during an etoposide infusion?
9. What are the signs and symptoms of a hypersensitivity reaction?
10. Before starting a paclitaxel infusion, for what should the nurse check?
11. What are examples of neoplastic agents that may potentially interact with St. John's wort?

NEED MORE HELP?

Chapter 45 of the study guide for *Drug Therapy in Nursing* contains exercises and activities to reinforce your understanding of the concepts presented in this chapter. For additional information see the text's accompanying website at *http://www.connection.lww.com.*

REFERENCES AND BIBLIOGRAPHY

Allegra, C. J., & Green, J. L. (1997). Antimetabolites. In V. T. De Vita, S. Hellman, & S. A. Rosenberg (Eds.). *Cancer: Principles and practice of oncology* (5th ed.) Philadelphia: Lippincott-Raven.

Baquiran, D. C. (2001). *Lippincott's cancer chemotherapy handbook* (2nd ed.), Philadelphia, Pa: Lippincott Williams & Wilkins.

Berg, D. (1998a). Irinotecan hydrochloride: Drug profile and nursing implications of a topoisomerase-I inhibitor in patients with advanced colorectal cancer. *Oncology Nursing Forum, 25,* 543.

Berg, D. (1998b). Managing the side effects of chemotherapy for colorectal cancer. *Seminars in Oncology, 25,* (Suppl. 11), 53–59

Camp-Sorrell, D. (1997). Chemotherapy: toxicity management. In S. L. Groenwald SL, M. H. Frogge, M. Goodman, C. H. Yarbro (Eds) (1997). *Cancer Nursing Principles and Practice.* (4th ed., pp. 387–389). Boston: Jones and Bartlett.

Camptosar (irinotecan HCI) prescribing information. (1996). Kalamazoo, MI: Upjohn Pharmaceuticals.

Cassileth, B. (1999). Evaluating complementary and alternative therapies for cancer patients. *CA: A Cancer Journal for Clinicians, 49,* 362–375.

DeVita, V. T., Hellman, S. & Rosenberg, S. A. (1997). *Cancer: principles and practice of oncology* (5th ed.). Philadelphia: Lippincott-Raven.

Dorr, R. T., & Von Hoff, D. D. (1994). *Cancer chemotherapy handbook* (2nd ed.), Norwalk, CT: Appleton and Lange.

Eisenberg, D. M., Kessler, R. C., Foster, C., Norlock, P. E., Calkins, D. R., & Delbanco, T. L. (1993). Unconventional medicine in the United States, prevalence, costs and patterns of use. *New England Journal of Medicine, 328,* 246–252.

Eisenberg, D. M., Davis, R. B., Ettner, S. L., Appel, S., Wilkey, S., Van Rompay, M., & Kessler, R. C. (1998). Trends in alternative medicine use in the United States 1990–1997. *Journal of the American Medical Association, 280*(18), 1569–1575.

Groenwald, S., Forgge, M., Goodman, M., & Yarbro, C. (1995). *Comprehensive cancer nursing review* (2nd ed.). Boston: Jones and Bartlett.

Guy, J. L., & Ingram, B. A. (1996). Medical oncology: The agents. In R. McCorkle, M. Grant, M. Frank-Stromborg, & S. B. Baird (Eds.). *Cancer nursing: A comprehensive textbook* (2nd ed., pp. 359–394). Philadelphia: W. B. Saunders.

Lederle Laboratories. (1997). *Methotrexate package insert.* Pearl River, NY: Author.

Oncology Nursing Society. (1998). *Cancer chemotherapy guidelines: Recommendations for the management of extravasation, hypersensitivity and anaphylaxis.* Pittsburgh: Oncology Nursing Press.

Sasson, Z., Morgan, C., Wang, B., Thomas, G., Mackenzie, B., & Platts, M. (1994). 5-fluorouracil related toxic myocarditis: Case reports and pathologic confirmation. *Canadian Journal of Cardiology, 10*(8), 861–864.

Tatro, D. S. (1999). Drug interactions with herbal products. In R. M. Short & T. H. Burnham (Eds.), *Facts and comparisons: The review of natural products.* St. Louis: Facts and Comparisons.

Smith Kline Beecham Oncology. (1996). *Hycamtin package insert.* Philadelphia, PA: Author.

Chapter 46

CELL CYCLE-NONSPECIFIC DRUGS

KEY TERMS

acute emesis
alkylating agent
antitumor antibiotics
cell cycle-nonspecific
combination chemotherapy
delayed emesis
disease flare
emetogenics
hormones
hormone antagonists
liposomes
nitrosureas
radiomimetic
tumor burden

Learning Objectives

At the completion of this chapter the student will:

1. Differentiate a cell cycle-specific from a cell cycle-nonspecific agent.
2. Identify core drug knowledge about cell cycle-nonspecific drugs.
3. Differentiate cell cycle-nonspecific drugs by their mechanism of action.
4. Identify core patient variables relevant to cell cycle-nonspecific drugs.
5. Relate the interaction of core drug knowledge to core patient variables for cell cycle-nonspecific drugs.
6. Generate a nursing plan of care based on the above interactions between core drug knowledge and core patient variables for cell cycle-nonspecific drugs.
7. Describe the nursing interventions to maximize therapeutic and minimize adverse effects of cell cycle-nonspecific drugs.
8. Determine key points for patient and family education for cell cycle-nonspecific drugs.
9. State the rationale for using a combination of drugs in chemotherapy.
10. Identify the characteristics of drugs that are useful for combination chemotherapy.

Alkylating agents
- **cyclophosphamide** (P)
- cisplatin

Nitrosureas
- **carmustine** (P)
- streptozocin

Antitumor antibiotics
- **doxorubicin** (P)
- bleomycin

Hormones and hormone antagonists

Adrenal corticosteroids
- betamethasone
- dexamethasone
- prednisone

Estrogens
- diethylstilbestrol
- estradiol

Antiandrogens
- bicalutamide
- flutamide
- nilutamide

Aromatase inhibitor
- anastrazole

Androgens
- testolactone
- fluoxymesterone

Progestins
- megestrol acetate
- medroxyprogesterone

Gonadotropin-releasing hormone analogues
- goserelin acetate
- leuprolide

Antiestrogens
- **tamoxifen** (P)

The symbol (C) indicates the **drug class**.
Drugs in bold type marked with the symbol (P) are **prototypes**.
Drugs in blue type with no symbol are **closely related** to the prototype.
Drugs in **red** type with no symbol are **significantly different** from the prototype.
Drugs in **black** type with no symbol are **also used in drug therapy**; no prototype.

Cancer chemotherapy alters the phase or phases of the cell's life cycle. As discussed in Chapter 45, the antineoplastic drugs are classified according to their cytotoxic activity in the cell cycle. Drugs that are effective at specific phases in the cell's life cycle are classified as cell cycle-specific. Drugs that are effective through all phases of the cell cycle and are not limited to a specific phase are classified as **cell cycle-nonspecific**. This chapter focuses on the cell cycle-nonspecific antineoplastic drugs.

Cell cycle-nonspecific drugs act on cells that are in the proliferative and nonproliferative phases of the cell cycle. They directly affect the deoxyribonucleic acid (DNA) molecule and do not display any specificity for cells that are dividing. They are considered more toxic than the cell cycle-specific drugs because their destructive action does not differentiate between normal and malignant cycling cells. Additionally, their toxicities are felt throughout the cell cycle. Included in the cell cycle-nonspecific class of drugs are the alkylating agents, antitumor antibiotics, and the hormonal drugs (hormones and hormone antagonists). Nonspecific agents are given in bolus doses because they cause death independently of the proliferative state of the cell. These agents also reduce the number of cells that make up a tumor, which is known as the **tumor burden.**

This chapter also focuses on the important role of cell cycle-specific or cell cycle-nonspecific drugs in combination therapy for malignant neoplasms. The combination of a cell cycle-nonspecific and a cell cycle-specific drug can kill cells that are slowly dividing and those that are actively dividing. Cell cycle-nonspecific drugs can also help recruit cells into a more actively dividing state, which then makes them more sensitive to cell cycle-specific drugs. The rationale for implementing combination therapy and designing effective single drug combinations is also discussed. Finally, some of the most common drug combinations in clinical use today are included.

C ALKYLATING AGENTS

The **alkylating agents** attack malignant cells in any phase of the cell cycle, including (for some agents) the resting phase. They exert their toxic effects through the transfer of their alkyl groups to various intracellular components, including nuclear DNA. Once the nucleotides have been alkylated, abnormal base pairing may occur, which in turn leads to DNA breakage or scission, and to cross-linking. The damaged DNA molecule cannot replicate itself, and cell death results. The alkylating drugs are described as **radiomimetic**, so named because they mimic the actions of radiation therapy on the cells.

The alkylating drugs, the first modern chemotherapeutic agents, are a product of the secret wartime gas programs in World Wars I and II. The exposure of seamen to mustard gas in World War II led to the discovery that alkylating drugs cause marrow and lymphoid hypoplasia, which led to their use in treating hematopoietic neoplasms, such as Hodgkin disease and lymphocytic lymphoma.

Alkylating agents include cyclophosphamide (Cytoxan) and cisplatin (Cisplatinum, CDDP). The prototypical alkylating agent is cyclophosphamide (Cytoxan). Table 46-1 summarizes these drugs.

NURSING MANAGEMENT OF THE PATIENT RECEIVING P CYCLOPHOSPHAMIDE

Core Drug Knowledge

Pharmacotherapeutics

Cyclophosphamide (Cytoxan) has a broad spectrum of antitumor activity. It plays a major role in the treatment of hematologic malignancies such as Hodgkin disease, non-Hodgkin lymphoma, and multiple myeloma. It is the only alkylating agent effective against acute as well as chronic leukemias. Cytoxan is an important component of regimens used in stem cell transplantation. It is also effective against solid tumors such as those associated with breast cancer, small-cell lung cancer, and endometrial cancer, and with ovarian tumors. Cyclophosphamide is given intravenously or orally.

Pharmacokinetics

Cyclophosphamide and its metabolites are well distributed throughout the body, including the brain and cerebrospinal fluid. The drug also distributes into breast milk and saliva. The majority of the drug is metabolized in the liver and about 60% binds extensively to plasma protein. It is exclusively excreted by the kidneys; however, because of avid tubular reabsorption, only about 60% of the drug and a larger amount of its metabolites appear in the urine.

Pharmacodynamics

Cyclophosphamide is a nitrogen mustard derivative, the most widely used alkylating agent. During extensive first-pass hepatic metabolism, it undergoes hydroxylation and is converted into a cytotoxic agent with a wide clinical utility in the treatment of various tumors. It is particularly effective with leukemias because the lymphocytes are very sensitive to this drug's effects.

Contraindications and Precautions

Patients with severely compromised bone marrow function and with known hypersensitivity to the drug should not be treated with cyclophosphamide. If the patient has poor renal or hepatic function, dose modification should be considered.

Adverse Effects

The dose-limiting toxicity associated with this drug (at high dosage) is leukopenia, which nadirs within 2 weeks with recovery after 3 to 4 weeks. At standard doses, it is more platelet sparing. At very high doses, cyclophosphamide has a propensity for inducing sterile hemorrhagic cystitis. This problem is manifested by hematuria, pain, and burning on urination caused by the irritation

TABLE 46-1 Summary of Selected Cell Cycle–Nonspecific Antineoplastic Drugs

Drug (Trade) Name	Selected Indications	Route and Dosage Range	Pharmacokinetics
Alkylating Agents			
cyclophosphamide (Cytoxan; *Canadian:* Procytox)	Neck, genitourinary, advanced ovarian, and cervical cancers; also recurrent brain tumors in children	*Adult:* IV, single agent 360 mg/m^2 on d 1 every 4 wk, depending on platelet count; in combination with cyclophosphamide, 300 mg/m^2 on d 1 every 4 wk	*Onset:* Rapid *Peak:* 1 h *Duration:* Unknown $t_{1/2}$: 4–6 h
cisplatin (Platinol, CDDP)	Testicular cancer and other genitourinary tumors (bladder, prostate, metastatic ovarian, cervical, and endometrial)	*Adult:* IV, low level, 20–49 mg/mg^2; moderate level, 50–75 mg/m^2; and high level, 75–120 mg/m^2 or 3 mg/kg over 20–30 min or continuous 24-h infusion	*Onset:* 8–10 h *Peak:* 18–23 d *Duration:* 20–35 d $t_{1/2}$: 25–49 min; then 58–73 h
carboplatin (Paraplatin)	Ovarian cancer	*Adult:* IV, 360 mg/m^2 on d 1 given q 4 wk	*Onset:* Rapid *Peak:* Unknown *Duration:* 48–96 h $t_{1/2}$: 1.1–2h, then 2.6–5.9 h
ifosfamide (Ifex)	Testicular cancer	*Adult:* 1–2 g/d × 5 d	*Onset:* Rapid *Peak:* Unknown *Duration:* Unknown $t_{1/2}$: 3–10 h for low dose; 13.8 h for high dose
busulfan (Myeleran)	Chronic granulocytic leukemia	*Adult:* PO, 4–8 mg/d until WBC decreases by half, then maintenance doses up to 4 mg/d	*Onset:* 0.5–2 h *Peak:* 2–3 h *Duration:* 4 h $t_{1/2}$: Unknown
chlorambucil (Leukeran)	Hodgkin disease, chronic lymphocytic leukemia, non-Hodgkin lymphoma, breast and ovarian cancer	*Adult:* 0.1–0.2 mg/kg for 3–6 wk then a maintenance dose not to exceed 0.1 mg/kg/d	*Onset:* Varies *Peak:* 1 h *Duration:* 15–20 h $t_{1/2}$: 1 h
mechlorethamine (nitrogen mustard, Mustargen)	Lung cancer, chronic lymphocytic leukemia, chronic myelocytic leukemia, Hodgkin disease, lymphosarcoma, malignant effusions	*Adult:* IV, 0.4 mg/kg; intracavitary, 0.2–0.4 mg/kg	*Onset:* Immediate *Peak:* Seconds *Duration:* Minutes $t_{1/2}$: Minutes
melphalan (Alkeran)	Multiple myeloma	*Adult:* PO, 0.25 mg/kg/d × 7 d, followed by 3 wk drug free, then maintenance dose of 2 mg/d; IV, 16 mg/m^2 q 3 wk × 4 doses then q 4 wk	*Onset:* Varies (PO), Rapid (IV) *Peak:* 2 h (PO), 1 h (IV)
Nitrosureas			
carmustine (BCNU)	Palliative therapy of brain tumors, multiple myeloma, Hodgkin disease, and non-Hodgkin lymphoma as single-drug or combination therapy	*Adult:* IV, 150–200 mg/m^2 q 6 wk as a single dose or given in 2 d in divided doses as a slow infusion over 1–2 h	*Onset:* Immediate *Peak:* 15 min *Duration:* Unknown $t_{1/2}$: 15–30 min
streptozocin (Zanosar)	Pancreatic cancer, colon cancer, carcinoid tumors	*Adult:* IV, 500 mg/m^2 d for 5 d every 6 wk or 1 g/m^2 wk for 2 wk; dosages not to exceed 1.5 g/m^2 wk	*Onset:* Varies *Peak:* Unknown *Duration:* 24 h $t_{1/2}$: 35 min

TABLE 46-1 Summary of Selected Cell Cycle–Nonspecific Antineoplastic Drugs (Continued)

Drug (Trade) Name	Selected Indications	Route and Dosage Range	Pharmacokinetics
lomustine (CCNU)	Hodgkin disease, brain tumors	*Adult:* 130 mg/m² q 6 wk	*Onset:* 10 min *Peak:* 5 h *Duration:* 48 h $t_{1/2}$: 16–72 h
Antitumor Antibiotics			
doxorubicin (Adriamycin)	Hematologic cancers (leukemias, Hodgkin disease, lymphomas, multiple myeloma); solid tumors (breast, ovarian, prostate, stomach, thyroid, liver, small-cell lung, and head and neck cancers)	*Adult:* IV, 60–75 mg/m² as single injection every 21 d; alternate schedule, 30 mg/m² on each of 3 successive d 4 wk; administered by slow IV push through a free-flowing IV line over 3–5 min or as a continuous 24-h infusion through a central venous access device	*Onset:* Rapid *Peak:* 2 h *Duration:* 24–36 h $t_{1/2}$: 12 min; then 3.3 h
doxorubicin HCl liposome (Doxil)	AIDS-related Kaposi sarcoma	*Adult:* IV, 20 mg/m² q 3 wk	*Onset:* Unknown *Peak:* Unknown *Duration:* Unknown $t_{1/2}$: 55 h
bleomycin (Blenoxane)	Lymphomas, squamous cell carcinoma, and testicular cancers	*Adult:* IV/IM/SC, 10–20 U/m² weekly or twice weekly	*Onset:* Immediate *Peak:* IV, 10–20 min; IM/SC, 30–60 min *Duration:* Unknown $t_{1/2}$: 2 h
daunorubicin hydrochloride (Cerubidine, DNR,)	Acute myelogenous leukemia, acute lymphocytic leukemia	*Adult:* 30–60 mg/m²/d for 3 d IV *Child:* 25–45 mg/m² IV	*Onset:* Slow *Peak:* Unknown *Duration:* 8 d $t_{1/2}$: 20 h
daunorubicin citrate liposome (Daunoxome)	Advanced AIDS related Kaposi sarcoma	*Adult:* IV 40 mg/m² q 2 wk	*Onset:* Unknown *Peak:* Unknown *Duration:* Unknown $t_{1/2}$: 5.9–43.6 h
dactinomycin (Actinomycin, Cosmegen)	Testicular cancer, Ewing sarcoma trophoblastic tumor, rhabdomyosarcoma, trophoblastic neoplasms	*Adult:* 500 μg/d for a maximum 5 d *Child:* 15 μg/d to a max of 500 μg/d for 5 d	*Onset:* Rapid *Peak:* Unknown *Duration:* 9 d $t_{1/2}$: 36 h
idarubicin (Idamycin)	Acute myeloid leukemia	*Adult:* 12 mg/m² d × 3 d in combination with cytarabine	*Onset:* Rapid *Peak:* Minutes *Duration:* Unknown $t_{1/2}$: 6–9.4 h
mitoxantrone (Novantrone)	Acute monocytic leukemia, acute myelocytic leukemia, acute promyelocytic leukemia, breast cancer	*Adult:* 12 mg/m² d × 2–3 d in combination with cytosine arabinoside	*Onset:* Varies *Peak:* 10–14 d *Duration:* 28 d $t_{1/2}$: 5.8 d (median)
pentostatin (Nipent)	Alfa-interferon refractory hairy cell leukemia	*Adult:* IV, 4 mg/m² q other week	*Onset:* Rapid *Peak:* 11 min *Duration:* Unknown $t_{1/2}$: 5.7 h
plicamycin (Mithramycin)	Testicular tumors, severe hypercalcemia	*Adult:* IV, 25–30 μg/kg/d for 8–10 doses; severe hypercalcemia: 25 μg/kg/d × 3–4 d	*Onset:* Rapid *Peak:* 4 h *Duration:* Unknown $t_{1/2}$: Unknown

(continued)

TABLE 46-1 Summary of Selected Cell Cycle–Nonspecific Antineoplastic Drugs (Continued)

Drug (Trade) Name	Selected Indications	Route and Dosage Range	Pharmacokinetics
Hormones and Hormone Antagonists			
Adrenocorticosteroids			
prednisone (Meticorten; *Canadian:* Apo-Prednisone)	Adjunct for palliation of symptoms in acute leukemia, Hodgkin disease, lymphoma, complications of cancer such as thrombocytopenia, hypercalcemia	Individualize dosage depending on severity of condition and patient's response	*Onset:* Varies *Peak:* 1–2 h *Duration:* 1–1.5 d $t_{1/2}$: 3.5 h
Androgens			
fluoxymesterone (Halotestin)	Advanced breast cancer in premenopausal women	*Adult*: 10–40 mg/d PO in divided doses	*Onset:* Rapid *Peak:* 2 h *Duration:* Unknown $t_{1/2}$: 9.5 h
testolactone (Teslac)	Advanced breast cancer	*Adult:* PO, 250 mg qid	*Onset:* Rapid *Peak:* Unknown *Duration:* Unknown $t_{1/2}$: Unknown
Estrogens			
diethylstilbestrol diphosphate (Stilphostrol; *Canadian:* Hanvol)	Inoperable prostate cancer, postmenopausal metastatic breast cancer	*Adult:* PO, 50 mg tid increasing to 200 mg with maximum daily dose no greater than 1 g; IV, 0.5 g for 5 d, then 0.25–0.50 g once or twice wk	*Onset:* Rapid *Peak:* Unknown *Duration:* Unknown $t_{1/2}$: Not available
estradiol (Estinyl)	Advanced breast cancer in postmenopausal women, prostate cancer	*Adult:* Breast cancer: PO, 0.5 mg/d initially, gradually increased to 3 mg/d in three divided doses; prostate cancer:, PO 0.15–2 mg/d	*Onset:* Slow *Peak:* Days *Duration:* Unknown $t_{1/2}$: Unknown
Progestins			
medroxyprogesterone (Provera, Depo-Provera)	Advanced endometrial carcinoma	*Adult:* IM 400–800 mg twice/wk; PO 200–300 mg/d	*Onset:* Slow, weeks *Peak:* Unknown *Duration:* Unknown $t_{1/2}$: Unknown
megestrol acetate (Megace)	Advanced endometrial carcinoma, breast cancer	*Adult:* PO 40–320 mg/d	*Onset:* Slow *Peak:* Weeks *Duration:* Unknown $t_{1/2}$: Unknown
Antiandrogens			
bicalutamide (Casodex)	Advanced prostate cancer	*Adult:* PO, 500 mg once daily	*Onset:* Slow *Peak:* 31.3 h *Duration:* Days $t_{1/2}$: 5.8 d
flutamide (Eulexin)	Advanced prostate cancer	*Adult:* PO 250 mg q8h	*Onset:* Varies *Peak:* 2 h *Duration:* 72 h $t_{1/2}$: 6 h
nilutamide (Nilandron)	Advanced breast cancer in postmenopausal women with disease progression after tamoxifen	*Adult:* PO 300 mg/d × 30 d, then 150 mg/d	*Onset:* Varies *Peak:* Unknown *Duration:* Unknown $t_{1/2}$: Unknown

TABLE 46-1 Summary of Selected Cell Cycle-Nonspecific Antineoplastic Drugs (Continued)

Drug (Trade) Name	Selected Indications	Route and Dosage Range	Pharmacokinetics
Gonadotropin-releasing hormone (GnRH) analogues			
goserelin (Zoladex)	Advanced prostatic cancer, advanced breast cancer, endometriosis	*Adult:* SC 3.6 mg q 28 d	*Onset:* Slow *Peak:* 12–15 d *Duration:* Unknown $t_{1/2}$: 4.2 h
leuprolide (Lupron), Lupron Depot	Advanced prostatic cancer	*Adult:* SC, 1 mg/d *Depot:* 7.5 mg IM monthly q28–33d	*Onset:* Slow *Peak:* Unknown *Duration:* Unknown $t_{1/2}$: Unknown
Aromatase Inhibitors			
anastrozole (Arimidex)	Advanced breast cancer in post-menopausal women whose disease progressed after tamoxifen therapy	*Adult:* PO, 1 mg daily	*Onset:* Rapid *Peak:* Unknown *Duration:* Unknown $t_{1/2}$: 7 d
Antiestrogens			
tamoxifen (Nolvadex; *Canadian:* Apo-Tamoxifen)	Breast cancers	*Adult:* PO, 20–40 mg/d	*Onset:* Varies *Peak:* 4–7 h *Duration:* Unknown $t_{1/2}$: 7–14 h

of the bladder wall by *acrolein*, a metabolic by-product of cyclophosphamide. Other adverse effects of high dose therapy (120 to 270 mg/kg) include syndrome of inappropriate antidiuretic hormone (SIADH) and cardiomyopathy in the form of congestive heart failure and hemipericardium secondary to hemorrhagic myocarditis and myocardial necrosis. Hypersensitivity has also been observed in both untreated and pretreated patients. Cyclophosphamide is a pregnancy category D drug. Reproductive effects such as amenorrhea, gonadal suppression, sterility, and ovarian fibrosis can occur. Secondary malignancies have been reported with drug use. Other adverse effects include cutaneous problems manifested by alopecia, transverse ridging, and hyperpigmentation of the nails. Nausea, vomiting, and anorexia may also occur. On rapid infusion of the drug, patients may complain of dizziness, nasal stuffiness, and rhinorrhea.

Drug Interactions

Table 46-2 notes the effects of cyclophosphamide on other drugs. It is compatible with other common antineoplastics such as melphalan, paclitaxel, vinorelbine, idarubicin, cisplatin,and bleomycin.

Assessment of Relevant Core Patient Variables

Health Status

The nurse should assess any organ system that could be potentially compromised by dosing with cyclophosphamide. Before initiating treatment, baseline tests to determine sufficient hematopoietic and renal function should be performed. Cytoxan should not be given to patients who have impaired renal function, myelosuppression, or a known hypersensitivity to the drug. Patients who have had prior radiation to the pelvis or bladder are at increased risk of hemorrhagic cystitis.

Life Span and Gender

The nurse should document the age and developmental status of the patient. Cyclophosphamide can cause secondary malignancies, which generally occur at a later part of the patient's life span. The incidence of bladder and skin cancers has been reported in patients receiving prolonged (12% of patients on drug for 12 years) low-dose therapy. Patients should be counseled about this long-term risk. Pediatric populations may be at an increased risk with lower single and total doses; the exact etiology of this is unclear. It is believed to result from the rate of administration versus the age of administration.

Because of possible reproductive side effects, the nurse should discuss the reproductive goals of patients with child-bearing potential and who are considering high-dose therapy. The nurse should also assess the woman of child-bearing age for pregnancy and explore contraceptive methods, because cyclophosphamide is a pregnancy category D drug.

Lifestyle, Diet, and Habits

Activities of daily living should be assessed because of the importance of frequent diuresis and mobility to ameliorate the potential adverse effects of drug admin-

TABLE 46-2 Agents That Interact With Cyclophosphamide

Interactants	Effect and Significance	Nursing Management
doxorubicin	Potentiates doxorubicin-induced cardiotoxicity	Dose modification is advised. Monitor cardiac function.
succinylcholine	Prolongs neuromuscular blocking activity	Administer with caution.
digoxin	Decreases pharmacologic effect	Digoxin dosage may need to be increased.
halothane and nitrous oxide	When used in conjunction, has produced mortality	Notify anesthesia department.
corticosteroids	Decreases conversion of cyclophosphamide to its active metabolites, decreasing activity	Notify health care provider for dose adjustment.

istration. The nurse should assess the daily dietary habits and elimination patterns of patients taking oral formulation of the drug. It is important that the metabolites of the drug be excreted during the day and do not stagnate to erode the bladder wall.

Environment

The nurse should be aware of the environment in which the drug will be administered. High-dose intravenous cyclophosphamide therapy is usually given in an acute care facility where patients may be adequately managed for potential major and acute toxicities, such as severe nausea and vomiting and hemorrhagic cystitis. However, pretreatment hydration with vigorous oral intake may be accomplished in the home setting if the patient and caregiver are well instructed and adhere to the hydration regimen.

Nursing Diagnoses and Outcomes

- Risk for Infection related to bone marrow suppression
  Desired outcome: The patient will be free from infection and exercise caution to avoid exposure to sources of infection.
- Risk for Injury associated with bone marrow depression and related bleeding and hypersensitivity reaction (or anaphylaxis)
  Desired outcome: The patient will attain pretreatment hematologic status, learn to monitor and manage situations that may induce bleeding, and recognize and immediately report signs and symptoms associated with a hypersensitivity reaction.
- Imbalanced Nutrition: Less than Body Requirements related to nausea, vomiting, and taste alterations
  Desired outcome: The patient will experience adequate emetic control using pharmacologic and nonpharmacologic measures.
- Impaired Urinary Elimination related to cyclophosphamide-induced nephrotoxicity
  Desired outcome: The patient will maintain fluid balance and be free from signs and symptoms of hemorrhagic cystitis as evidenced by adequate fluid intake and output. In addition, renal function will not be compromised as shown by normal renal and blood count values and absence of hematuria, pain, and dysuria.
- Impaired Skin Integrity and Disturbed Body Image related to alopecia and changes in skin pigmentation and nail condition.
  Desired outcome: The patient will be able to recognize and report any changes in the skin and integuments and will undertake measures to enhance appearance and body image.

Planning and Intervention

Maximizing Therapeutic Effects

Before administering Cytoxan, the nurse ensures that the test results disclose good renal function and adequate hematopoietic reserves to achieve the intended therapeutic effects.

Minimizing Adverse Effects

Hemorrhagic cystitis can be ameliorated by a vigorous hydration regimen of at least 2 to 3 L/day and in high-dose therapy, the administration of the uroprotectant agent, mesna. The nurse should prehydrate the patient orally and intravenously with at least 1 to 2 L of normal saline solution with potassium and magnesium additives several hours before and after the infusion. The nurse should monitor urine output vigilantly to reflect an output of at least half of the intake. Mannitol diuresis may be implemented to increase urine output. Aminoglycoside antibiotics should be avoided to prevent compromising renal function.

Providing Patient and Family Education

- The nurse should emphasize prevention of major toxicities resulting from cyclophosphamide.
- The nurse should encourage the patient to drink large amounts of fluid as directed to induce diuresis. Some of the pretreatment hydration can be accomplished at home, but understanding the reason for doing so will promote the patient's adherence to the regimen the night before drug administration. Additional hydration will be given in the hospital to augment previous oral intake.

- The nurse should advise the patient of temporary and reversible hair loss. The nurse should refer the patient to a wig specialist before treatment is initiated. The nurse should educate the patient to refrain from using chemical treatments on the hair and vigorous brushing of the hair. The nurse should teach the patient to use mild shampoos and if the patient has long hair, suggest that it be cut before chemotherapy starts to avoid the trauma of seeing the gradual loss of hair.
- The nurse should review signs and symptoms of a hypersensitivity reaction with the patient to alleviate the patient's anxiety. The nurse should ask the patient for other known sensitivity to drugs and determine whether the patient is asthmatic.
- The nurse should instruct the patient to notify the health care provider about other serious adverse effects. Signs and symptoms to report include lower volume of urine or less frequent urination than usual; a fever of 100.5°F or higher; excessive vomiting, diarrhea, inability to keep food and fluids down for more than 24 hours; and the presence of black stools, red rash, or unusual bruising, which are signs of bleeding.
- The nurse should reassure the patient that nausea and vomiting may be relieved with antiemetic drug therapy and that the patient should request these agents when needed. The nurse should teach nonpharmacologic measures such as relaxation and always ask the patient to initiate practices that have helped alleviate these symptoms in the past. Good emesis management is important because either acute or delayed emesis has distressing effects on physical and psychological functioning.
- The nurse should counsel the patient about the long-term risks of secondary malignancies (e.g., bladder and skin cancers) associated with prolonged low-dose cyclophosphamide therapy.
- If patients are taking oral formulation of the drug, the nurse should instruct the patient to ingest the drug early in the morning on an empty stomach, to drink at least 10 to 12 glasses of water daily, and to empty the bladder frequently. These practices will ensure that the metabolites of the drug are excreted during the day and do not stagnate to erode the bladder wall.
- The nurse should discuss the need for sperm/egg banking with patients who are on high-dose therapy and are considering having children in the future.

Ongoing Assessment and Evaluation

When patients undergo subsequent courses of chemotherapy, the nurse needs to assess parameters to ensure adequate renal function and hematopoietic reserve. The nurse should assess the patient's hematologic status every week during the first months of therapy and until maintenance therapy is set, and then at intervals of 2 to 3 weeks. For high-dose regimens, the nurse should also monitor cardiac function. Dose modification should be considered in patients with impaired renal, hematologic, and hepatic function. ■

DRUG SIGNIFICANTLY DIFFERENT FROM CYCLOPHOSPHAMIDE

Cisplatin (Cisplatinum, CDDP) is a widely used heavy metal that acts as a bifunctional alkylating agent. It produces intrastrand and interstrand linking in DNA through covalent bonds with the platinum molecule, leading to the breaking of DNA strands during cell replication. It is clinically used in almost every solid tumor and lymphoma. The pharmacokinetics show rapid distribution of the drug to the tissues after IV infusion. Most of it bonds to protein. The drug is believed to be metabolized in the liver and excreted in the urine.

The major dose-limiting adverse effects of cisplatin are nephrotoxicity for individual doses and neurotoxicity for cumulative doses. Pretreatment hydration and forced diuresis are required to prevent neurotoxicity. Peripheral neuropathy is common and painful. Cumulative ototoxicity is also common. Cisplatin belongs to a group of antineoplastic drugs called **emetogenics**, which have high potential for causing severe nausea and vomiting (see the accompanying display, Ranking Chemotherapeutic Drugs According to Emetogenic Potential). The risk factors that predispose the patient's tolerance to this distressing problem are illustrated in the accompanying display, Risk Factors for Nausea and Vomiting. Patients on cisplatin can suffer from acute emesis. **Acute emesis** refers to vomiting within 24 hours after chemotherapy. In cisplatin therapy, severe nausea and vomiting occur within 1 to 4 hours after treatment and usually last for 24 hours. The drugs that have the highest therapeutic index for this emetic pattern are the *serotonin receptor antagonists*. Four agents are currently available: dolasetron,

MEMORY CHIP

Cyclophosphamide

- Indicated for testicular, ovarian, and bladder cancers
- Significant contraindications: severe bone marrow depression, serious infections, nursing mothers, and women and men with child-bearing potential
- Most common adverse effect: hemorrhagic or nonhemorrhagic cystitis
- Dose-limiting effect: leukopenia
- **Lifespan alert: patients on long-term therapy should be counseled about risks of secondary malignancy.**
- Maximizing therapeutic effects: ensure that patient has adequate bone marrow reserve and good renal function
- Minimizing adverse effects: promote vigorous hydration and diuresis to prevent cystitis
- Most significant patient education: instruct the patient to drink plenty of fluids and empty the bladder every 2 hours

Ranking Chemotherapeutic Drugs According to Emetogenic Potential

The following antineoplastic drugs are listed according to their emetogenic potential. Highly emetogenic drugs begin the list; mildly emetogenic drugs complete it.

Cisplatin
Dacarbazine
Streptozocin
Nitrogen mustard
Hexamethylmelamine
Actinomycin D
Cyclophosphamide*
Carboplatin*
Lomustine
Carmustine
Anthracyclines
Ifosfamide
Cytosine arabinoside
Procarbazine
Taxanes
Mitomycin-C
Etoposide
Methotrexate
Irinotecan
Topotecan
Gemcitabine
Bleomycin
Vinca alkaloids
5-Fluorouracil
Hormones
Chlorambucil

*Late onset of nausea and vomiting.

granisetron, ondansetron, and troposetron. *Corticosteroids* such as dexamethasone and methylprednisolone are also effective. Other drugs commonly used to control nausea and vomiting, such as *phenothiazines, butyrophenones, cannabinoids, dopamine antagonists,* and *substituted benzamides,* are rated as having lower therapeutic effects. **Delayed emesis** (nausea and vomiting 24 hours after chemotherapy) have also been noted and may persist for up to 5 days after treatment. The mechanism for delayed emesis is unclear. Although it is not as distressing as acute emesis, it may severely affect a patient's food intake and prolong hospitalization. The accompanying display presents the American Society of Clinical Oncologists (ASCO) guidelines for managing chemotherapy-induced emesis.

Cisplatin therapy causes potassium and magnesium wasting. Foods that are known to increase absorption of magnesium include dairy products. High amounts of milk, cheese, or other calcium-rich foods should be limited when eating foods high in magnesium. Calcium and magnesium compete to gain entrance into the intestines, so a calcium-rich food increases the body's requirements for magnesium. Examples of these foods are nuts, chocolate, whole wheat breads and cereals, instant coffee and tea, oatmeal, beans, and peas. Needles or administration sets containing aluminum should not

Risk Factors for Nausea and Vomiting

Anxiety, expectations of severe side effects, and previous chemotherapy experience are predisposing factors to the adverse effects of nausea and vomiting. Certain patient characteristics and prognostic factors also affect the incidence of nausea and vomiting:

- Age: younger patients experience nausea and vomiting more than older patients.
- Gender: a higher incidence of nausea and vomiting in women is thought to result from administration of more highly emetogenic drugs to women than to men and lower alcohol consumption among women.
- Alcohol intake: high alcohol consumption has a positive effect on emetic control.
- Performance status and motivation: patients who have a better physical, emotional, and functional status have a better tolerance of emesis.
- History of motion sickness or severe emesis during pregnancy: these patients are more susceptible to chemotherapy-induced episodes of nausea and vomiting.

Guidelines for Managing Chemotherapy-Induced Emesis

1. Determine the emetogenic potential of the drug: high, intermediate, or low.
2. When combination agents are given, give the antiemetic appropriate for the chemotherapeutic agent with the highest risk.
3. For acute emesis, the agents with the highest therapeutic index are the serotonin antagonists. At equivalent doses, they have the same safety and efficacy profiles and can be used interchangeably.
4. The oral route is as effective and safe as the intravenous route.
5. For acute emesis with high-risk agents, the combination of a serotonin antagonist with a corticosteroid is recommended. A corticosteroid is suggested for patients treated with intermediate emetic risk agents, whereas for low-risk agents, no antiemetic is needed. Antiemetics should be given for each day of the chemotherapy.
6. For delayed emesis, in patients receiving high-risk cisplatin, a corticosteroid plus metoclopramide or plus a serotonin antagonist is recommended. For high-risk agents without cisplatin, a corticosteroid as a single agent, a corticosteroid plus metoclopramide, or plus a serotonin antagonist are suggested regimens.
7. For intermediate and low-risk agents, no preventive agent for delayed emesis is recommended.
8. Prevention of chemotherapy-induced emesis by using the most active antiemetic agents appropriate for the drug to prevent acute or delayed emesis is suggested. Such regimens should be used with the **first** chemotherapy treatment to avoid the patient's "anticipating" poor emetic response on subsequent cycles. If anticipatory emesis occurs, behavioral therapy with systematic desensitization is effective and suggested.

Adapted from Gralla, R. J., Osoba, D., Kris, M. G., et al. (1999). American Society of Clinical Oncologists Recommendations for the Use of Antiemetics: Evidence-Based, Clinical Practice Guidelines. *Journal of Clinical Oncology, 17*(9), 2971.

be used, because these will result in precipitate formation or loss of drug potency.

NITROSUREAS

The **nitrosureas** are alkylating drugs, which are frequently classified separately because they also have additional mechanisms of cytotoxicity. Like the alkylating agents, they cause breaks and cross-linking in DNA strands. They also inhibit the repair of DNA. Nitrosureas are highly lipid soluble. As such, they cross the blood-brain barrier. They have broad clinical activity in treating leukemias and some solid tumors. Examples of frequently used nitrosureas are carmustine and streptozocin, which are discussed in this chapter. Carmustine is the prototype of the nitrosureas.

NURSING MANAGEMENT OF THE PATIENT RECEIVING CARMUSTINE

Core Drug Knowledge

Pharmacotherapeutics

Carmustine (BCNU) is a nitrosurea used in the palliative therapy of brain tumors, multiple myeloma, Hodgkin disease, and non-Hodgkin lymphoma. It may be administered as a single drug or in combination with other antineoplastics. It is given as a slow infusion to prevent severe pain and burning over the IV site.

Pharmacokinetics

After IV administration, carmustine is rapidly degraded. Most of the drug is excreted by the renal system in 96 hours, and about 10% is excreted by the respiratory system as carbon dioxide. This drug crosses the blood-brain barrier because of its high lipid solubility.

Pharmacodynamics

The mechanism of action of carmustine is similar to that of an alkylating drug. It alkylates DNA and RNA, thereby blocking synthesis and repair. It also inhibits essential enzymes by carbamoylation of the amino acids.

Contraindications and Precautions

This drug is contraindicated in patients who are hypersensitive to it. It should be used cautiously in those with impaired respiratory or bone marrow function. Accidental skin contamination can cause hyperpigmentation and brown discoloration of the affected area. The drug should be dispensed in glass. Plastic containers should be avoided. Carmustine is a pregnancy category D drug.

Adverse Effects

The major toxic effect of carmustine is bone marrow suppression, which occurs 6 weeks after drug administration. This delayed suppression is cumulative and is manifested as thrombocytopenia and leukopenia. Nausea and vomiting occur frequently. Pulmonary toxicity associated with prolonged therapy and cumulative doses of more than 1,400 mg/m^2 are other adverse effects. The patient may complain of local reactions, such as intense pain and discomfort in the vein used for drug administration, flushing of the skin, and suffusion of the conjunctiva within 2 hours and lasting for 4 hours after administration of the drug.

Drug Interactions

When given concomitantly with other drugs, carmustine exhibits certain effects, as shown in Table 46-3.

Assessment of Relevant Core Patient Variables

Health Status

Because the major carmustine-induced toxicities are related to bone marrow function and pulmonary functions, the nurse should assess patients for adequate bone marrow reserve and pulmonary function. Patients at risk are those with a history of lung disease, patients receiving greater than 1,400 mg/m^2 of carmustine, and children treated with cumulative doses of 770 to 1,800 mg/m^2 and cranial irradiation.

Life Span and Gender

If the patient is on prolonged therapy, the nurse should regularly perform pulmonary assessments to monitor the occurrence of pulmonary dysfunction and disease. The onset of pulmonary problems is usually delayed and chronic. Pulmonary fibrosis has been reported to occur up to 15 years later in adolescent patients receiving cumulative doses of as high as 1,800 mg/m^2 concomitantly with irradiation. Among adults, the same has been noted with prolonged therapy and large cumulative doses. The nurse should assess women of childbearing

TABLE 46-3 Agents That Interact With Carmustine

Interactants	Effect and Significance	Nursing Management
cimetidine	Increased toxicity and myelosuppression	Monitor blood counts.
digoxin, phenytoin	Decreased serum level	Measure serum level. Consult health care provider about dose modification if needed.

age for pregnancy and lactation because carmustine is a pregnancy category D drug. It is not known if carmustine is excreted in milk, so breast-feeding women should be cautioned.

Lifestyle, Diet, and Habits

The nurse needs to forewarn patients about the acute onset of nausea and vomiting associated with carmustine therapy. The nurse should assess the impact that nausea and vomiting will have on the patient's activities of daily living and diet. Nausea and vomiting usually occur 2 to 4 hours after drug administration. Because the signs and symptoms of myelosuppression are delayed, the nurse should explore the patient's activities of daily living that might expose the patient to risks of infection and bleeding.

Environment

The nurse should be aware of the environment in which carmustine will be administered. It is usually given in an acute care setting so that medical and nursing support are easily available should a hypersensitivity reaction or anaphylaxis occur.

Nursing Diagnoses and Outcomes

- Pain related to discomfort of drug administration
  Desired outcome: The patient will be free from discomfort along the infusion site.
- Risk for Infection and injury especially bleeding related to bone marrow suppression
  Desired outcome: The patient will take steps to prevent exposure to potential sources of infection and bleeding, minimize risks of infection and bleeding, comply with requirements for periodic blood counts.
- Impaired Gas Exchange related to drug-related pulmonary fibrosis
  Desired outcome: The patient will learn to recognize and report signs and symptoms of respiratory dysfunction. The patient will comply with the need to have pulmonary function tests during the course of treatment.
- Imbalanced Nutrition: Less than Body Requirements due to drug-induced nausea and vomiting
  Desired outcome: The patient will recognize emetic episodes and ask for antiemetics as needed. The patient will learn how to manage dietary intake and patterns to ensure adequate nutritional intake.
- Sexual Dysfunction related to mutagenic and teratogenic properties of the drug
  Desired outcome: The patient will be accepting of the impact of carmustine on reproductive and sexual functions. The patient will take steps to participate in counseling and accept emotional support to cope with these effects and achieve a satisfying sexual experience.

Planning and Intervention

Maximizing Therapeutic Effects

After reconstitution, the solution is stable in a glass container for 24 hours at 4°C or for 8 hours at 25°C. when protected from light.

Minimizing Adverse Effects

The nurse must monitor hematologic indices regularly, especially because myelotoxicity is delayed. The nurse should also monitor renal, hepatic, and pulmonary function tests to abrogate any impending problems that might compromise the host. If long-term therapy is planned, the health care provider should discuss the possible use of a venous access device (such as an implanted port through which to deliver the drug). During drug administration, the patient may experience intense discomfort. The nurse must exercise care to use a large vein for infusion if a port is not used. To minimize the pain, the nurse should slow the infusion, and prolong the duration of administration. An ice compress can also help relieve the pain. The nurse can control nausea and vomiting, which may occur within 2 hours of the treatment, with an adequate antiemetic regimen.

Providing Patient and Family Education

Once the patient can be treated safely in an outpatient setting, the nurse should develop an education plan that includes both the patient and significant caregivers.

- The nurse should teach patients about general adverse effects and adverse signs and symptoms specific to carmustine therapy, including infection and bleeding (which might have delayed onset) and pulmonary fibrosis if they are going to be on long-term therapy.
- The nurse should inform patients about IV drug delivery and signs and symptoms to report that might signal possible extravasation.
- The nurse should discuss the potential for nausea and vomiting and provide the appropriate antiemetic regimen.
- The nurse should review reportable problems, such as inability to eat or drink for more than 24 hours and respiratory problems.
- The nurse should explain the need for regular blood counts and pulmonary testing.
- The nurse should advise the patient to avoid taking aspirin or drugs that contain aspirin unless prescribed by the health care provider and to report signs of bleeding, such as black stools, bloody gums, bruises, and red rash.
- The nurse should ask patients for concurrent drugs and potential drug interactions with phenytoin (Dilantin) or cimetidine if they are taking these drugs.
- The nurse may need to discuss the patient's concerns and the impact of the adverse effects on her reproductive, sexual functions, and quality of life.

- The nurse should teach patients which problems to report more urgently to the health care team. The nurse should make sure the patient has phone numbers or beeper numbers to access when appropriate.

Ongoing Assessment and Evaluation

The nurse should closely monitor complete blood counts every week for 6 weeks to ensure that blood counts are adequate before retreatment. The nurse may need to monitor pulmonary function tests during the course of therapy so that appropriate management of patients at risk for pulmonary toxicity may be instituted. ■

DRUG CLOSELY RELATED TO P CARMUSTINE

Streptozocin (Zanosar) is another drug that belongs to the nitrosurea group. It is the product of the organism *Streptomyces achromogenes*. It is well known for its efficacy in treating malignant islet cell tumors of the pancreas. Streptozocin is given intravenously. Patients may complain of pain and burning during the infusion. The nurse may relieve this discomfort by slowing the infusion, increasing the volume used for dilution, and increasing the total volume of the primary IV infusion.

The most frequently reported adverse effect is severe nausea and vomiting. Other GI reactions are hepatotoxicity manifested by an increase in liver enzyme and bilirubin levels, hypoalbuminemia, and jaundice. The development of renal toxicity is dose limiting and may be fatal. The mechanism of nephrotoxicity is unclear. Early manifestations include hypophosphatemia, glycosuria, proteinuria, azotemia, and renal tubular acidosis. Patients with preexisting renal disease are at risk. The nurse should closely monitor renal functions and the hematopoietic and hepatic functions at baseline and periodically during therapy so that the patient's organ systems are not severely compromised. Additionally, streptozocin has shown diabetogenic activity evidenced by altered glucose metabolism, decrease in insulin levels, and elevated fasting blood glucose levels. This is thought to result from an increased uptake of the drug into the islets. Clinical trials suggest that this activity can be reduced by pharmacologic intervention with nicotinamide.

MEMORY CHIP

P Carmustine

- Indicated for the treatment of brain tumors, multiple myelomas, Hodgkin and non-Hodgkin lymphomas, and malignant melanoma
- Significant contraindications: poor pulmonary function, which places the patient at risk of developing pulmonary toxicity, and known hypersensitivity to the drug
- Most common adverse effects: acute nausea and emesis
- Dose-limiting effect: delayed myelosuppression
- Most serious adverse effect: pain and burning at the site during drug infusion
- Maximizing therapeutic effects: after reconstitution, solution is stable in a glass container for 24 hours at 4°C or for 8 hours at 25°C when protected from light.
- Minimizing adverse effects: to decrease pain and burning during drug administration, infuse the IV slowly over 1 to 2 hours, increase the primary IV volume, and apply an ice pack over the site
- Most significant patient education: instruct patient to comply with the prescribed hematologic monitoring

C ANTITUMOR ANTIBIOTICS

Most **antitumor antibiotics** are isolated from fermented broths of various *Streptomyces* bacteria. The focal point for their cytotoxicity is the DNA. Antitumor antibiotics interfere with DNA-directed ribonucleic acid (RNA) synthesis by intercalating between the base pairs of DNA, binding to DNA, and changing the normal structure of the DNA and RNA chains. This action prevents the normal duplication and separation of these chains resulting in the inhibition of DNA and RNA synthesis. The antitumor antibiotics are dactinomycin, bleomycin, doxorubicin, daunorubicin, mitomycin, idarubicin, pentostatin, and the liposomal version of doxorubicin and daunorubicin (see Table 46-1). Several of these antibiotics also induce double-stranded DNA breaks, as such are considered topoisomerase II inhibitors. These include doxorubicin, daunorubicin, idarubicin, which are anthracycline-based (i.e., red-pigmented), as well as a mitoxantrone synthetic anthracenedione structurally similar to the anthracyclines. Their major dose-limiting toxicity is cardiotoxicity. Daunorubicin was the original prototype for the antitumor antibiotic class; however, doxorubicin (Adriamycin) is currently the most useful and popular antitumor antibiotic. Therefore, doxorubicin is discussed as the representative drug.

NURSING MANAGEMENT OF THE PATIENT RECEIVING P DOXORUBICIN HCL

Core Drug Knowledge

Pharmacotherapeutics

Doxorubicin was isolated from the soil fungus *Streptomyces peucetius var caesius*. Although doxorubicin is the most recently discovered anthracycline, it has gained the distinction of being the most commonly prescribed. It has wide clinical activity, particularly against hematologic cancers, such as the leukemias, Hodgkin disease, various lymphomas, and multiple myeloma, and solid tumors, such as carcinoma of the breast, ovary, prostate, stomach, thyroid, liver, and small-cell lung and head and neck cancers.

Doxorubicin may be used as a single drug or in combination with other drugs, such as vinblastine, cyclophosphamide, and paclitaxel. Dose adjustments are necessary for patients who have poor bone marrow reserve due to age, prior therapy, and neoplastic marrow infiltration. Dose reductions are also recommended for patients with liver function impairment as evidenced by elevated serum bilirubin levels and transaminases.

Pharmacokinetics

Doxorubicin is rapidly distributed in body tissues. It is metabolized in the liver and is primarily excreted in the bile. A small percentage is excreted in the renal system and may produce reddish discoloration of the urine. The pharmacokinetic profile of doxorubicin appears in Table 46-1. Recent advances in pharmaceutical technology led to the approval by the Food and Drug Administration (FDA) of two anthracycline antibiotics, daunorubicin and doxorubicin to be encapsulated in **liposomes**. Liposomes are microscopic spheric vesicles that encapsulates the drug molecules. This novel drug formulation enhances the therapeutic indices of the drug by increasing the concentration, delaying clearance, retarding metabolism, decreasing the volume of distribution of the drug and shifting its distribution to the diseased tissues with increased capillary permeability.

Pharmacodynamics

Doxorubicin acts mainly by intercalation between specific base pairs within the cancer cell's DNA. This results in the blocking of the synthesis of new RNA or DNA, or DNA strand scission. Normal proliferating cells are also affected by doxorubicin, which accounts for such adverse effects as myelosuppression, alopecia, and stomatitis.

Contraindications and Precautions

Doxorubicin is contraindicated in severe congestive heart failure (CHF) or any existing cardiomyopathy or marked myelosuppression from irradiation or chemotherapy. Precautions should be observed in patients with hepatic insufficiency because active metabolite concentrations may be increased. Doxorubicin is a pregnancy category D drug.

Adverse Effects

The adverse effects of doxorubicin may be grouped into acute, chronic, and local reactions. Acute toxicities include nausea, vomiting, bone marrow suppression, and mucositis. Alopecia is reversible, and other cutaneous reactions noted are hyperpigmentation of the nailbeds and dermal creases.

Cardiotoxicity is chronic and is the major toxicity that limits its usage. It is cumulative and may manifest in weeks or months after the initial treatment. Cardiomyopathy may range from insignificant electrocardiographic changes to more serious complications, such as CHF. Signs and symptoms include dyspnea, ankle swelling, palpitations, and exhaustion. Doxorubicin shows an affinity for the myocytes, which are the cells of the heart muscle. The damaged myocytes are not easily replaced because they have a slow mitotic rate. In turn, the decreased number of myocytes and the ensuing interstitial edema weaken the pumping capacity of the heart muscle. The resultant heart failure can be fatal.

Local adverse effects include the cutaneous effects that can have devastating consequences to the patient. These include extravasation injury and radiation recall reaction. Anthracyclines such as doxorubicin are thought of as the most dreaded vesicants. Extravasation is especially problematic because anthracyclines bind to nucleic acids, causing destructive and prolonged tissue injuries. They form free radicals that are toxic to the tissues and especially impede wound healing. The DNA doxorubicin complex is retained and recirculates in the tissues, setting up a pattern for continuous tissue damage (Refer to Chapter 45 for extravasation management).

Radiation recall is exhibited as erythematous changes that appear at a previously irradiated site. The phenomenon can occur weeks or months—even years—after radiation but appears more frequently with shorter time intervals and high-dose chemotherapy. These reactions are manifested by erythema (redness), blisters, hyperpigmentation, edema (swelling), vesicle formation, exfoliation (skin loss), and sometimes ulcer formation. They can occur in the skin, lung, heart, and gastrointestinal (GI) tract.

Drug Interactions

The drug interactions are summarized in Table 46-4. Doxorubicin should not be admixed with the following drugs in solution because of incompatibility: aminophylline, cephalothin sodium, dexamethasone sodium phosphate, diazepam, hydrocortisone, furosemide, heparin, and fluorouracil.

Assessment of Relevant Core Patient Variables

Health Status

The risk of cardiotoxicity in patients receiving doxorubicin can be potentiated by certain factors. These factors are concurrent therapy with cyclophosphamide and mediastinal irradiation. The nurse should ensure that initial cardiac evaluations, which might include an electrocardiogram (ECG) and a multigated radionuclide angiogram, are made to establish a safe baseline for treatment. Before initiating treatment, the nurse should obtain a careful history to ascertain that the patient does not have existing cardiomyopathy or hepatic insufficiency that might put him or her at risk for treatment.

TABLE 46-4 **Agents That Interact With Doxorubicin**

Interactants	Effect and Significance	Nursing Management
digoxin	Decreased serum levels and therapeutic effect of digoxin.	Monitor serum digoxin levels.
heparin	Precipitate formation if mixed together.	Administer doxorubicin and heparin separately.
barbiturates	Increased plasma clearance of doxorubicin.	Notify health care provider for dosage considerations.

Life Span and Gender

The nurse should document the age and gender of the patient. The risk for cardiac damage increases with age. Age influences cardiac tolerance to anthracycline therapy. Children and the elderly are more susceptible to adverse cardiac effects at lower cumulative doses. Children, especially, suffer more from the synergistic cardiotoxicities of mediastinal irradiation and doxorubicin. However, they have a better chance of recovering from CHF-related problems than adults. Women, especially those younger than 50 years, are more likely to experience nausea and vomiting. The nurse should assess the woman of child-bearing age for pregnancy and explore her reproductive goals. Doxorubicin is a pregnancy category D drug and its potential effect on fertility is not known.

Lifestyle, Diet, and Habits

The nurse should assess the client for adequate nutritional intake. Malnutrition, particularly in children, potentiates cardiotoxicity. The nurse should also assess the patient anxiety related to the impact of chemotherapy-related nausea and vomiting, which can substantially impair one's quality of life.

Environment

The nurse should be aware of the environment in which the drug will be administered. Doxorubicin is given either in an inpatient or outpatient setting because of the need for monitoring adverse effects, especially the potential for extravasation that needs prompt medical attention and patient education.

Nursing Diagnoses and Outcomes

- Risk for Infection related to bone marrow suppression
  Desired outcome: The patient will be free from infection and will exercise caution to avoid exposure to sources of infection.
- Risk for Injury related to cardiotoxicity and bone marrow depression and associated bleeding
  Desired outcome: The patient will not suffer from any acute or chronic cardiotoxicity and will be able to recognize and promptly report any of its clinical manifestations. In addition, the patient will attain pretreatment hematologic status. Patient will learn to monitor and manage situations that may induce bleeding.
- Imbalanced Nutrition: Less than Body Requirements related to nausea, vomiting, and taste alterations
  Desired outcome: The patient will remain adequately nourished because emesis control will be achieved by pharmacologic and nonpharmacologic means.
- Impaired Skin Integrity related to possible extravasation and radiation recall
  Desired outcome: The patient will recognize and report signs and symptoms that suggest an extravasation or recall reaction. Ideally, the patient will receive the doxorubicin dose without vascular or tissue damage.

Planning and Intervention

Maximizing Therapeutic Effects

Recent advances in drug development have made possible the use of cardioprotectants in conjunction with anthracycline therapy. One such drug is dexrazoxane (Zinecard). Dexrazoxane is a potent intracellular chelating drug that interferes with iron-mediated free radical generation thought to be responsible for anthracycline-induced cardiotoxicity. It is indicated to reduce the severity and incidence of cardiomyopathy associated with doxorubicin in women with metastatic breast cancer who have received a cumulative dose of 300 mg/m^2 and who in their health care provider's opinion would benefit from continuing treatment with doxorubicin. The recommended dose of dexrazoxane to the doxorubicin is at a ratio of 10:1 (e.g., dexrazoxane 500 mg to doxorubicin 50 mg). It should be given by slow IV push or rapid IV infusion before administering doxorubicin. The total elapsed time from the beginning of the dexrazoxane infusion to the initiation of doxorubicin should not be more than 30 minutes. The side effects of the drug using the recommended dose are mild; however, it could add to the myelotoxic effects of doxorubicin.

Minimizing Adverse Effects

Prior to initiating therapy, the nurse should carefully assess the patient's cardiac and hematopoietic functions, because of the major impact of doxorubicin on the systems involved. The nurse should implement strategies for modifying the risk for cardiotoxicity with regard to dose administration and scheduling. The recommended maximum cumulative lifetime dose of doxorubicin is 550 mg/m^2. However, if the patient has had myocardial irradiation or prior cytotoxic drugs, the cumulative lifetime dose should be lowered to 400 mg/m^2. Modifying the dose and dosing schedule of the patient can ameliorate the cardiotoxic adverse effects. Multiple, daily doses rather than large single boluses of the drug can minimize cardiac damage.

Dose adjustment for patients who had or who are receiving concurrent radiation therapy or cyclophosphamide (Cytoxan) is advocated to a reduced cumulative dose of 400 mg/m^2. With regard to extravasation, prevention is the key. This requires that medical and nursing personnel be skilled in venous access techniques, perform meticulous monitoring during drug administration, and know prompt actions to undertake in case extravasation occurs. Large veins should be used with a new peripheral line for vesicant administration. Extravasation can occur with a good venous return and without the usual initial complaint of stinging at the injection site (see the display Managing Peripheral Extravasation in Chapter 45).

Providing Patient and Family Education

- The nurse should reassure the patient that reddish urine after doxorubicin injection is a harmless and expected response to the drug. This may happen within 1 to 2 days postinfusion.
- The nurse should explain that a significant fraction of patients who receive this drug complain of acute nausea and vomiting. The nurse should reassure the patient that proper antiemetics will be available and the patient should ask for them if needed. The nurse should carefully review nonpharmacologic interventions, such as relaxation techniques, with the patient and caregiver.
- The nurse should review signs and symptoms of extravasation. If a suspected extravasation occurs, the nurse should provide and review a teaching card with directions for caring for an extravasation site, so that the patient can best participate in care. The nurse should reassure the patient that adequate monitoring and follow-up, through telephone triage by the nurse, will be undertaken even in the home setting.
- The nurse should discuss the signs and symptoms of other adverse effects, particularly cardiotoxicity and bone marrow depression, with the patient and encourage appropriate precautions. For example, the nurse should encourage the patient to keep appointments for cardiac function tests and caution against taking aspirin or drugs that contain aspirin, which may promote bleeding during bone marrow suppression.
- The nurse should remind the patient who has had irradiation that recall reactions manifested by redness, blistering, and hyperpigmentation can occur with a delayed onset.

Ongoing Assessment and Evaluation

The nurse should advise the patient who continues on doxorubicin to have periodic examinations of cardiac functions as ordered. The use of radionuclide ventriculography or echocardiography are useful methods to detect impending myocardial damage. The nurse should look for any significant changes in the ECG readings that might indicate potential problems such as irreversible cardiac damage. The practitioner should also assess the patient frequently for weight gain, presence of ankle edema, dyspnea, elevated blood pressure, and nonproductive cough, which are typical clinical signs of CHF. ■

DRUG SIGNIFICANTLY DIFFERENT FROM DOXORUBICIN

Bleomycin (Blenoxane) is an antitumor antibiotic. Unlike doxorubicin, it is not an anthracycline, nor is it a cell cycle-nonspecific drug. It is used in treating lymphomas, squamous-cell carcinoma, and testicular cancers. It is given by IV, subcutaneous, or intramuscular routes. The recommended dosage is expressed in either units or milligrams (1 U = 1 mg). Bleomycin is known for its pulmonary toxicity. For this reason, this drug has been used in a more limited way. The early clinical features are dyspnea and rales, which might progress to pneumonitis and pulmonary fibrosis and might be fatal.

The treatment of bleomycin-induced toxicity consists of discontinuing the drug and administering corticosteroids. The practitioner should review pulmonary function tests and chest radiographs at baseline and periodically thereafter to monitor adequate pulmonary reserve. The nurse should

MEMORY CHIP

Doxorubicin HCl

- Indicated for the treatment of acute leukemias, soft tissue and bone sarcoma, Hodgkin and non-Hodgkin lymphoma, breast and ovarian cancers, bronchogenic carcinoma
- Significant contraindication: severe bone marrow suppression
- Most common adverse effects: alopecia and nausea with vomiting
- Most serious adverse effects: cardiac damage, bone marrow depression, and extravasation
- Maximizing therapeutic effects: administer dexrazoxane cardioprotectant therapy, if indicated
- Minimizing adverse effects: maintain maximum lifetime dose of 550 mg/m^2; if patient is receiving radiation or concurrent myelotoxic therapy, dose is 400 mg/m^2
- Most significant patient education: warn patient of the appearance of red urine discoloration after administration (harmless) and of the reality of alopecia, which is reversible.

advise the patient to notify the health care provider—especially the anesthesiologist—that he or she has received bleomycin therapy, because pulmonary toxicity is enhanced by a high intraoperative fraction of inspired oxygen.

Other adverse effects are cutaneous toxicity, which is often seen as urticaria or erythematous swelling and phlebitis at the injection site due to the irritant properties of bleomycin. Following drug administration, patients may complain of fever and chills. Patients may also have nausea and vomiting, general weakness, and rare instances of hypotension. These symptoms are considered to be an idiosyncratic reaction similar to anaphylaxis and noted rarely and mostly in lymphoma patients. This problem could be prevented by administering a test dose of 2 U of bleomycin before the first two treatments. Premedication with acetaminophen and diphenhydramine are also helpful.

HORMONES AND HORMONE ANTAGONISTS

The **hormones** and **hormone antagonists** (antihormones) are a diverse group of drugs that are beneficial in treating neoplasms. Their use predates the first chemotherapeutic agent (nitrogen mustard) as the oldest form of cancer treatment. Hormones are hormonal or hormone-like drugs that inhibit tumor proliferation by blocking or antagonizing the naturally occurring substances that stimulate tumor growth.

Some hormones alter the cellular environment and affect the permeability of the cell membrane in ways that will affect cell growth. This group (see Table 46-1) consists of adrenocorticosteroids, androgens, estrogens, progestins, antiestrogens, antiandrogens, gonadotropin inhibitors, and aromatase inhibitors. Hormonal therapy is recognized mostly for its efficacy in treating neoplasms that originate from tissues in which growth is hormonally mediated. Of note are prostate and breast cancers. The clinical responsiveness of breast tumors to hormonal manipulations was demonstrated more than 100 years ago. Over time, hormonal treatment of breast cancer has been accomplished by ablative surgery (oophorectomy, adrenalectomy, and hypophysectomy) or pharmacologically by using hormonal and antihormonal therapy.

ADRENOCORTICOSTEROIDS

In addition to the cytotoxic effects of hormones, adrenocorticosteroids are used for their palliative benefits. For example, adrenocorticosteroids such as betamethasone, dexamethasone, and prednisone have anti-inflammatory properties and are useful in reducing the edema and associated symptoms in brain tumors. Adrenocortical steroids are effective in leukemias and lymphomas because of their suppressant effect on lymphocytes. Many of their side effects are an extension of their normal physiologic activity and are considered beneficial and palliative like increased appetite and a feeling of well-being. Some of their adverse effects are glucose intolerance, peptic ulceration, manic psychosis, and suppression of cellular immunity which predisposes patients to be prone to infection.

ANDROGENS, ESTROGENS, AND PROGESTINS

Androgens, estrogens, and progestins are used to treat cancers of tissues that have specific hormone receptors, for example, mammary tissue and the prostate gland. Because these drugs have a greater degree of specificity for these tissues, their effects will inhibit proliferation of the tumor.

Androgens

Androgens control the growth and development of the male sex organs and maintain secondary sex characteristics. This group affects the release of various endogenous hormones, namely testosterone, follicle-stimulating hormone (FSH), and luteinizing hormone (LH). The two androgenic agents are fluoxymestrone and testolactone used palliatively for androgen-responsive recurrent breast cancer in postmenopausal women. These drugs are well tolerated although they may exhibit side effects similar to those produced by the estrogens, including fluid retention, hypercalcemia, and liver impairment. Their most profound side effect is virilization in women manifested by hirsutism, alopecia, acne, clitoral hypertrophy, and increased libido.

Estrogens

Estrogens are necessary for the development and maintenance of secondary sexual characteristics, control the female menstrual cycle, and affect the maturation of long bones. They diffuse through the membrane of the estrogen-responsive cells and bind to and activate receptors in the cell nucleus. It is believed that they change the hormonal milieu of the cells, making them less conducive to growth. Estrogen-responsive (ER) cells are located in the reproductive system, breast, pituitary, hypothalamus, liver, and bone. However, not all of the tumors that arise in these organs are estrogen sensitive. In many patients, after the initial hormonal manipulation, even as the estrogen receptor-sensitive cells are being destroyed, the ER-negative cells continue to proliferate. Therefore, the response is neither complete nor permanent. Diethylstilbestrol (DES) and estradiol are estrogens. Both are given orally to treat advanced prostate adenocarcinoma and metastatic breast cancer. Estradiol is also available as a vaginal cream that is well absorbed through the skin and mucous membranes. The adverse effects of these agents include gynecomastia, voice changes, hirsutism, change in libido, fluid retention, nausea, vomiting, and thrombophlebitis. During the first 2 weeks of DES therapy, hypercalcemia has been reported in women with breast cancer and bone metastases. Deaths from cardiovascular events or thromboembolic adverse effects have also been reported with long-term use of DES and higher doses.

Progestins

Progestins are natural or synthetic substances that affect the actions of progesterone, a steroid that counteracts the actions of estrogens. Megestrol acetate (Megace) is a progestin indicated for treating carcinoma of the breast, endometrium, and renal carcinoma. It is also used for the treatment of anorexia and cachexia associated with cancer. Medroxyprogesterone is the other agent used in patients with advanced endometrial cancer. They are contraindicated during pregnancy because they have been found to cause fetal genital abnormalities.

ANTIANDROGENS

Antiandrogens compete with testosterone for androgen receptor binding sites on target cells. The most frequently used antiandrogenic agents are bicalutamide (Casodex), flutamide (Eulexin), and nilutamide (Nilandron). These agents are used for advanced stages of prostate cancer. Side effects are gynecomastia, diarrhea, hot flashes, breast pain, impotence, loss of libido, and abnormal liver function test results. The nurse should monitor the patient's liver function if the patient is on prolonged therapy.

GONADOTROPIN-RELEASING HORMONE ANALOGS

The gonadotropin-releasing hormone (GnRH) analogs are goserelin acetate (Zoladex) and leuprolide (Lupron). LH and FSH are gonadotropins that stimulate hormone secretion by the gonads. They play an important role in the maturation of the germ cell. GnRH regulates the release of these hormones from the pituitary gland. Goserelin inhibits the secretion of gonadotropin. When patients are on prolonged therapy with this drug, their serum testosterone level is decreased to a level equivalent to that associated with surgical castration. This drug is an alternative treatment for males with advanced prostatic cancer who do not wish to undergo orchiectomy or estrogen therapy. It is also used in advanced breast cancer. Goserelin is well tolerated. In men, the adverse effects are hot flashes, sexual dysfunction, and decreased erections. Women suffer from decreased bone mineral density, vaginal bleeding, and breast tenderness. Goserelin is available as a preloaded, disposable syringe with a 14-gauge needle that is injected subcutaneously into the upper abdominal wall. The other drug, leuprolide, has similar indications and also causes chemical orchiectomy in men who have metastatic prostate cancer. The drug has fewer side effects. It is available in three formulations: a subcutaneous injection, a depot suspension, and a suspension given intramuscularly. With both these medications, it is important that the nurse teach the patient the correct technique for drug administration appropriate to the drug formulation and emphasize to the patient the importance of adhering to the dosage schedule.

AROMATASE INHIBITOR

Anastrozole is a nonsteroidal aromatase inhibitor that is also considered an antiestrogen, similar to tamoxifen. Many breast cancers have estrogen receptors; the growth of these tumors are stimulated by estrogen. In postmenopausal women, the main source of estrogen is from the conversion of adrenal androgen to estrogen (primarily estradiol) by an enzyme called aromatase. Anastrozole (Arimidex) inhibits aromatase that is required for this conversion. It is indicated for the treatment of postmenopausal women who have advanced breast cancer that has progressed after tamoxifen therapy. It is given orally and is well tolerated. The nurse should discuss the patient's reproductive goals and warn patients that this drug can cause fetal harm.

ANTIESTROGENS

Antiestrogens are first-line therapy for treating breast cancer in postmenopausal women. They act as agonists by binding to the estrogen receptors in the target cells, making the estrogen unavailable to the tumor. Tamoxifen, which is the most widely recognized, and anastrozole, which is also an inhibitor, belong to this category. Several drugs are in development. Tamoxifen (Nolvadex) is the prototypical antiestrogen drug.

NURSING MANAGEMENT OF THE PATIENT RECEIVING TAMOXIFEN

Core Drug Knowledge

Pharmacotherapeutics

Tamoxifen (Nolvadex) is indicated as a first-line drug for treating advanced breast cancer in postmenopausal women. It is used in adjuvant therapy for the treatment of axillary node-negative breast cancer in women after mastectomy or segmental mastectomy, axillary dissection, and breast irradiation. In premenopausal women with metastatic breast cancer, tamoxifen is an alternative to oophorectomy and irradiation. It is the only drug approved for use in reducing the incidence of breast cancer in high-risk women.

Pharmacokinetics

Tamoxifen is well absorbed, highly protein bound, and extensively metabolized in the liver after oral administration. It undergoes enterohepatic circulation, prolonging blood levels. It is taken up by tissues, such as the lung, uterus, breast, brain, pancreas, and liver. It has a half-life of 7 to 14 days. Most tamoxifen is excreted in the bile and feces.

Pharmacodynamics

Tamoxifen is a potent nonsteroidal antiestrogenic drug. It is also considered the prototype selective estrogen receptor modulator (SERM), a concept involving pharmacologic agents often called "designer drugs" that produce estrogenic effects, alone or combined with antiestrogenic effects at various sites in a woman's body. These sites include the breast, endometrium, cardiovascular, brain, and bone. Tamoxifen competes with estrogen for binding sites in tissues high in estrogen receptors, such as breast tissue. This mechanism deprives estrogen-sensitive tumors of estrogen. It may also stimulate the production of transforming growth factor-beta, which inhibits the growth of most breast cancer and other epithelioid cells.

Other favorable consequences of tamoxifen treatment have been reported, namely, an increase in bone mineral density in postmenopausal women and a reduction in cholesterol levels, which may account for a lower incidence of fatal myocardial infarction in women receiving adjuvant tamoxifen.

Contraindications and Precautions

Tamoxifen is contraindicated in patients with known hypersensitivity. Precautions should be observed when administering the drug to patients with myelosuppression and in pregnancy and lactation. Tamoxifen is a pregnancy category D drug. An increased incidence of endometrial changes, including hyperplasia, polyps, and endometrial cancer, has been reported with long-term tamoxifen therapy.

Adverse Effects

The lack of short-term toxicity of tamoxifen is emphasized. The vast majority of patients on drug experience no toxicity whatsoever. However, these common side effects have been reported to occur infrequently: hot flashes, particularly in premenopausal women and mild nausea, which is transient and unaccompanied by vomiting. The severity of hot flashes diminishes with continued use of the drug. Other less common adverse effects are headache, light-headedness, weight gain, vaginal bleeding and discharge, menstrual irregularities, fluid retention, visual side effects, and skin rash, all of which are reported in fewer than 1% to 2% of patients. Increased bone and tumor pain and a local **disease flare** have been observed; they indicate a positive tumor response. Hypercalcemia may occur but is infrequent. Data from long-term studies have clearly established the serious long-term effects of tamoxifen use including endometrial cancer, thromboembolic events, and cataract formation requiring cataract surgery. Patients on long-term therapy should be monitored regularly.

Drug Interactions

Drug-laboratory test interactions have been reported, including elevated serum calcium and thyroxin levels with tamoxifen therapy. Other interactions are discussed in Table 46-5.

Assessment of Relevant Core Patient Variables

Health Status

Even though the adverse effects of tamoxifen are fairly mild, the nurse needs to evaluate baseline hematopoietic test results, particularly platelet counts, to make sure that bone marrow function is adequate. Adverse hematopoietic reactions are transient and uncommon, usually exhibited by thrombocytopenia. The nurse should assess the tumor receptor status of the patient because the measurement of ERs provides important information for planning treatment. The nurse should also screen the patient for a history of thrombophlebitis or endometrial cancer, which may modify the treatment plan. A baseline vision test may also be necessary.

Life Span and Gender

One of the most important issues confronting women receiving hormonal therapy is its impact on their sexual and reproductive health. The nurse should explore these concerns and discuss the various changes associated with tamoxifen therapy. The nurse can explain that tamoxifen is a promising therapy for breast cancer and is the preferred adjuvant treatment for postmenopausal women with nodal involvement and ER-positive tumors. The nurse should assess the patient for pregnancy and explore the contraceptive practices of the patient because the drug can cause fetal harm.

Lifestyle, Diet, and Habits

Women taking tamoxifen experience no limitations in their functional capacities. Lifestyle considerations are not a big issue, except for possible physical changes, such as hot flashes, menstrual irregularities, weight gain, and vaginal bleeding. The nurse might explore how these changes could effect the woman's lifestyle. Although visual side effects are rare, the nurse should caution patients about driving and performing tasks requiring acuity.

Environment

The nurse should be aware of the environment in which the drug will be administered. Tamoxifen is a fairly mild oral drug that does not usually require close monitoring. Patients take this drug at home and are instructed to have periodic checkups with their health care provider.

TABLE 46-5 Agents That Interact With P Tamoxifen

Interactants	Effect and Significance	Nursing Management
oral anticoagulants	Increased risk of bleeding	Monitor prothrombin time. Notify health care provider for dose modifications. Monitor for signs of bleeding.
bromocriptine	Increased serum levels	Monitor tamoxifen serum levels.

Hematologic screenings can be done at an accredited laboratory and findings sent to the health care provider for comparison with baseline values.

Nursing Diagnoses and Outcomes

- Pain related to discomfort produced by a flare reaction to drug therapy
  Desired outcome: The patient will learn to recognize the signs and symptoms of a flare reaction and appreciate it as a positive tumor response to tamoxifen therapy.
- Sexual Dysfunction resulting from drug therapy
  Desired outcome: The patient will be aware of the physical changes to reproductive and sexual functions. The patient will be accepting of these changes and will explore ways to enhance sexual and reproductive health.
- Risk for Infection and bleeding related to suppression of bone marrow
  Desired outcome: The patient will learn to recognize and report symptoms related to infection and bleeding and will implement measures to prevent unnecessary risks or injury that will compromise the hematopoietic and immune systems.
- Risk for Impaired Skin Integrity related to skin rash and pedal edema.
  Desired outcome: The patient will report the appearance of skin rash and monitor peripheral edema from fluid retention. The patient will take steps to reduce edema from the fluid retention such as eating a low salt diet.
- Disturbed Sensory Perception (Vision and Balance) related to adverse effects of drug therapy
  Desired outcome: The patient will recognize and report changes in visual acuity and other related symptoms, such as headache, dizziness, and lightheadedness, to the caregiver. The patient will take the necessary precautions to avoid injury resulting from altered visual acuity.
- Risk for Injury related to drug-induced hypercalcemia
  Desired outcome: The patient will be knowledgeable about clinical manifestations of hypercalcemia, such as nausea, vomiting, constipation, decreased urine, malaise, and loss of muscle tone. The patient will also know to report these signs and symptoms immediately to the health care provider who might consider the need for hospitalization The patient's calcium level will normalize.

Planning and Intervention

Maximizing Therapeutic Effects

Tamoxifen is very effective in treating metastatic breast tumors identified as ER positive. This criterion is an important determinant in the patient's response to tamoxifen therapy. The nurse should ensure that the necessary testing is done to determine patient's ER status.

Minimizing Adverse Effects

As discussed in a previous section, tamoxifen's toxicity profile is mild or rare. The nurse should ensure monthly monitoring of blood counts, annual Papanicolaou smears, and regular visual function tests, if these mild or rare adverse effects occur and if there are deviations from the baseline eye examinations. The most usually noted changes are those related to the menopausal symptoms that are very bothersome especially to premenopausal women. The nurse should teach these patients to implement comfort measures such as: wearing absorbent cotton clothing, lowering the thermostat at home, avoiding caffeine and spicy foods, and exercising regularly. The nurse may need to discuss the patient's concerns and the impact of the adverse effects on her reproductive, sexual functions, and quality of life. The occurrence of a disease flare is actually a positive sign of tumor response to the therapy. Nurses should advise the patient about the initial bone pain and tumor pain, including an increase in tumor size that might be experienced. If these symptoms are bothersome, the nurse can obtain a prescription for pain medication.

Providing Patient and Family Education

- The nurse should instruct the patient to report signs and symptoms of flare reaction to the health care provider and if these are distressful, obtain the necessary supportive medications for the patient.
- The nurse should teach the patient to recognize and report changes in visual acuity and other related symptoms, such as headache, dizziness, and lightheadedness. If ordered, emphasize the importance of periodic vision check-ups.
- The nurse should remind the patient to report immediately if clinical manifestations of hypercalcemia, such as nausea, vomiting, constipation, decreased urine, malaise, and loss of muscle tone are experienced which may require hospitalization.
- The nurse should teach the patient to recognize and report the appearance of skin rash and peripheral edema.
- The nurse should educate the patient regarding changes in reproductive or sexual function, for example, irregular or missed menstrual periods or unscheduled vaginal bleeding.
- The nurse should reassure the patient that all of the above symptoms are mild and rarely occurring adverse effects of tamoxifen therapy. These symptoms do not usually require discontinuing the drug.
- The nurse should counsel the patient about contraception and that the drug can cause fetal harm.
- The nurse should advise the patient on long-term use to have annual pelvic examination and Papanicolaou screening and to note and report unusual vaginal bleeding.

Ongoing Assessment and Evaluation

Throughout treatment, the nurse should monitor the patient's blood count regularly. Although hypercalcemia is uncommon, the nurse should evaluate serum calcium levels during therapy to make sure that appropriate measures are initiated to correct this condition. The nurse should also assess the patient's vision because of the possibility for corneal changes and decreased visual acuity. ■

COMBINATION THERAPY

Many antineoplastic drugs are dose limiting because of their overall cytotoxicity. The limits imposed by toxicities on the different organ systems led to the use of combination drugs to achieve better therapeutic outcomes. **Combination chemotherapy** involves using two or more drugs proven effective against a tumor type. Its development is one of the major advances in cancer therapy in the last 20 years (see the accompanying display, Combination Therapy for Patients with Breast Cancer). It is considered superior to single-drug therapy because of higher tumor response rates and increased duration of remissions. The effectiveness of a particular antineoplastic drug is measured by objective criteria and tumor response (see the accompanying display, Rating Tumor Response).

Many regimens in current use have proved to increase the response rate two to four times (Table 46-6). Two or more drugs can be administered simultaneously or in a preplanned sequence (see the accompanying displays, Making Decisions Related to Combination Chemotherapy and Implementing MAID Therapy). In combination therapy, the response rates and survival are more dramatic because they accomplish the following:

- Maximum cell kill within the range of toxicity tolerated by the host
- A broader range of coverage of resistant cell lines in the heterogenous tumor population
- Minimal or slow development of new resistant cell groups

When designing successful drug combinations, the choice of drug combinations follows these principles:

MEMORY CHIP

Tamoxifen

- Indicated for advanced breast cancer in postmenopausal women and cancers of tissues having specific hormone receptors, such as the prostate gland
- Significant contraindications: allergy to the drug, pregnancy, and lactation
- Most common adverse effect: occurrence of hot flashes, especially among premenopausal women
- Most serious adverse effects: risk of endometrial cancer and thromboembolic events associated with long-term therapy
- Maximizing therapeutic effects: instruct the patient to take his/her pills bid, in the morning and evening. Drug should not be discontinued without consulting the physician or nurse
- Minimizing adverse effects: teach the patient to regulate the home environment to a cooler temperature, wearing loose, cotton, layered clothing (for hot flashes); to eat small, frequent meals and to stay away from spicy foods (for nausea and vomiting); to notify the physician immediately if symptoms of muscle weakness, pain and swelling of legs and ankles, mental confusion, and constipation are noted
- Most significant patient education: counsel women about the possible risks of endometrial cancer and to have regular gynecologic check-ups

Focus on Research

Combination therapy for patients with breast cancer

Sledge, G. (2000). Update of the National Surgical Adjuvant Breast and Bowel Project (NSABP-28). Highlights of the 2000 NIH Consensus Conference on Adjuvant therapy for breast cancer. pp. 4–5

The Study

Results were presented of the third interim analysis of a phase III trial, NSABP B-28 using adriamycin and cyclophosphamide (AC) with or without sequential paclitaxel in 3,060 patients with node-positive breast cancer. Patients were randomized into two treatment arms that consisted of the following regimens: adriamycin 60 mg and AC 600 mg given every 21 days for four cycles or AC with paclitaxel 225 mg/m^2 over 3 hours every 21 days × four cycles. Tamoxifen 20 mg daily for 5 years was given concurrently with chemotherapy in patients > 50 years old and in patients < 50 years old with estrogen receptor or progesterone receptor–positive tumors in both arms. Toxicities reported among the first treatment group consisted of granulocytopenia (8%), febrile neutropenia (7%), nausea (6%), and infection (3%). Patients receiving paclitaxel with AC manifested neurosensory problems (15%), arthralgias/myalgias (12%), neuromotor disorders (7%), and granulocytopenia on day 1 (5%). The study concluded that patients receiving paclitaxel following the AC regimen did not benefit in terms of disease-free and overall survival rates compared with those receiving AC alone. Although there appeared to be a trend that patients who did not receive tamoxifen benefited from the addition of paclitaxel, the difference for either disease-free or overall survival was not statistically significant.

Nursing Implications

Nurses play a pivotal role in teaching patients and helping them understand risks and benefits of treatment. To do this, the nurse should have a thorough knowledge of the drugs involved, including their side effects and appropriate symptom management. The nurse should also be versed in the design and goals of the treatment plan, to clarify issues and respond to patients learning needs, thus helping the patient make an informed decision.

Rating Tumor Response

How well a tumor responds to chemotherapy can be rated by the categories below.

Complete Response

All evidence of tumor (physical examination and radiologic studies) has disappeared and no new lesions have developed. Response must last for at least 4 weeks. The patient must have no cancer-related symptoms and all abnormal biochemical parameters must have returned to normal.

Partial Response

The sum of the product of the diameters of measured lesions decreases 50% or more for at least 4 weeks without cancer-related symptoms or weight or performance deteriorations. If there is no change in tumor size but the biochemical parameters decline by 80% or more, the patient is considered stable.

Stable Disease

Patients who do not meet the criteria for partial response but who are without signs and symptoms of progressive disease for at least 3 months comprise this category.

Progressive Disease

An increase exceeding 25% in the total area of the bidimensionally measured lesions, the appearance of new lesions, or greater or significant deterioration that cannot be attributed to treatment or medical conditions is considered disease progression.

Critical Thinking Scenario

Making decisions related to combination chemotherapy

Ms. J. M. is a 30-year-old patient with recurrent cancer of the tongue. The patient is being admitted to the hospital to start a combination treatment with cisplatin and paclitaxel. The prescribed dosage is paclitaxel 135 mg/m^2 by IV continuous infusion over 24 hours and cisplatin 75 mg/m^2 by IV piggyback one time.

1. Explain how you would sequence the delivery of these two drugs, and propose the rationale for this sequence.
2. Identify and prioritize the important nursing considerations to keep in mind when faced with this drug combination.

- Selected drugs should be proven partially effective against the tumor when used alone.
- Ideally, the drugs used in combination are best if they do not have overlapping toxicities.
- The dosage and schedule of the various drugs should be maximized.
- Drugs should be administered at consistent intervals.
- Drugs that can produce synergy should be selected.

TABLE 46-6 Common Combination Regimens

Acronym	Regimen	Indications
ABVD	Doxorubicin, bleomycin, vinblastine with dacarbazine	Hodgkin lymphoma
AC	Doxorubicin, cyclophosphamide	Breast cancer
BEP	Bleomycin, etoposide, cisplatin	Testicular cancer
BIP	Bleomycin, ifosfamide, cisplatin, mesna	Cervical cancer
CAF	Cyclophosphamide, doxorubicin, fluorouracil	Breast cancer
CAP	Cyclophosphamide, doxorubicin, cisplatin	Non–small-cell lung cancer
CHOP	Cyclophosphamide, doxorubicin, vincristine	Non-Hodgkin lymphoma
CHOP-BLEO	Add bleomycin to CHOP	Non-Hodgkin lymphoma
CMF	Cyclophosphamide, methotrexate, fluorouracil	Breast cancer
CP	Cyclophosphamide, cisplatin	Ovarian cancer
DHAP	Cisplatin, cytarabine, dexamethasone	Hodgkin lymphoma
EAP	Etoposide, doxorubicin, cisplatin	Gastric cancer
EC	Etoposide, carboplatin	Small-cell lung cancer
FAC	Fluorouracil, doxorubicin, cyclophosphamide	Breast cancer
FAM	Fluorouracil, doxorubicin, mitomycin	Gastric cancer
FAMTX	Fluorouracil, doxorubicin, methotrexate, leucovorin	Gastric cancer
ITP	Ifosfamide, taxol, cisplatin	Genitourinary cancer
IVAC	Ifosfamide, vincristine, doxorubicin, cyclophosphamide	Multiple myeloma
ICE	Ifosfamide, carboplatin, etoposide	Lung cancer
MAID	Mesna, adriamycin (doxorubicin), ifosfamide, dacarbazine	Sarcoma
MOPP	Mechlorethamine, vincristine, procarbazine	Hodgkin lymphoma
MVAC	Vincristine, doxorubicin, cyclophosphamide	Lung cancer
MVP	Mitomycin, vinblastine, cisplatin	Lung cancer

Critical Thinking Scenario

Implementing MAID Therapy

T. M. is a 53-year-old woman who was admitted for chemotherapy for a sarcoma on her right leg. The oncologist has just ordered for the patient to receive the MAID regimen. Because this is the patient's first treatment, she has a lot of questions to ask. Some of the questions are:

1. Which drugs are included in MAID?
2. Name three important clinical considerations for this treatment.

CHAPTER SUMMARY

- Cell cycle-nonspecific drugs exert their cytotoxic activity irrespective of the phase(s) of the cell life cycle.
- Cell cycle-nonspecific drugs are considered more toxic than cell cycle-specific drugs.
- Alkylating drugs are radiomimetic.
- The nitrosureas are alkylating agents that are highly lipid soluble.
- The antitumor antibiotics that are considered both as anthracyclines and topoisomerase II inhibitors are daunorubicin, doxorubicin, and idarubicin. Mitoxantrone is a synthetic anthracenedione.
- The most feared adverse effect of anthracycline therapy is cardiotoxicity.
- Some prognostic factors relating to a patient's tolerance to acute emesis are age, gender, and method of drug administration.
- The different groups of hormones used in cancer therapy are the adrenal corticosteroids, androgens, antiandrogens, estrogens, antiestrogens, gonadotropin-releasing hormone analogs, progestins, and aromatase inhibitors.
- Combination chemotherapy is superior to single-drug therapy, because it kills a maximum number of cancer cells within a toxicity range tolerated by the patient; it provides a broader range of coverage of resistant cells in the heterogenous tumor population; and it is characterized by minimal or slow development of new resistant cancer cells.

QUESTIONS FOR STUDY AND REVIEW

1. What are anthracyclines, and which of the antitumor antibiotics are they?
2. Which cell cycle-nonspecific drugs are highly lipid soluble? What can they do?
3. What are the different groups of drugs used to control acute emesis?
4. What is the role of dexrazoxane in anthracycline therapy? How is it administered?
5. What are the characteristics of drugs that are useful for combination therapy?
6. Why is combination chemotherapy superior to single-drug therapy?

NEED MORE HELP?

Chapter 46 of the study guide for *Drug Therapy in Nursing* contains exercises and activities to reinforce your understanding of the concepts presented in this chapter. For additional information see the text's accompanying website at *http://www.connection.lww.com.*

REFERENCES AND BIBLIOGRAPHY

Allen, T. M. (1997). Liposomes: Opportunities in drug delivery. *Drugs, 54,* (Suppl. 4), 8–14.

American Society of Hospital Pharmacists. (1990). Technical assistance bulletin on handling cytotoxix and hazardous drugs. *American Journal of Hospital Pharmacy, 47,* 1033–1049.

Armstrong, T., Rust, D., & Kohts, J. (1997). Neurologic pulmonary, and cutaneous toxicities of high-dose chemotherapy. *Oncology Nursing Forum, 24,* (Suppl. 1), 23–39.

Baquiran, D. C. (2001). *Lippincott's cancer chemotherapy handbook* (2nd ed.). Philadelphia: Lippincott Williams & Wilkins.

DeForni, M., & Armand, J. (1994). Cardiotoxicity of chemotherapy. *Current Opinions in Oncology, 6,* 340–344.

DeVita, V. T., Hellman, S., & Rosenberg, S. A. (1997). *Cancer: Principles and practice of oncology* (5th ed.). Philadelphia: Lippincott-Raven.

Gralla, R. J., Osoba, D., Kris, M. G., Kirkbride, P., Hesketh, P. J., et al. (1999). Recommendations for the use of antiemetics: Evidence-based, clinical practice guidelines. *Journal of Clinical Oncology, 17*(9), 2971.

Fisher, B., Constantino, J. P., Redmond, C., et al. (1994). Endometrial cancer in tamoxifen-treated breast cancer patients: Findings from the National Surgical Adjuvant Breast and Bowel Project (NSABP) B-14. *Journal of the National Cancer Institute, 86,* 527–537.

Joint Commission on Accreditation of Healthcare Organizations. (2000). *Patient and family education, Accreditation Manual for Hospitals* (Vol. 1). Oak Brook, IL: Author.

Lamb, M. (1995). Effects of cancer on the sexuality and fertility of women. *Seminars in Oncology Nursing, 11*(2), 120–127.

Lipshultz, S., Sanders, S., Gorin, A., Krischer, J., Sallan, S., & Colan, S. (1994). Monitoring for anthracycline cytotoxicity. *Pediatrics, 93*(3), 433–437.

National Study Commission on Cytotoxic Exposure. (1987). *Recommendations for handling cytotoxic agents.* Providence, RI: Author.

Occupational Safety and Health Administration. (1986). *Work practice guidelines for personnel dealing with cytotoxic (antineoplastic) drugs.* (OSHA Instruction Publication #8-1.1). Washington D.C.: Department of Labor.

Oncology Nursing Society. (1998). *Cancer chemotherapy guidelines: Recommendations for practice.* Pittsburgh: Oncology Nursing Press.

Pritchard, K. I. (2001). Selective estrogen receptor modulators in the prevention and treatment of breast cancer. *Clinical Oncology Updates, 3*(4), 1–15.

Wilkes, G. M., Ingwersen, K., & Burke, M. B. (1999). *1999 oncology nursing drug handbook.* Sudbury, MA: Jones and Bartlett.

Drugs used in the management of infections are called **antimicrobials** or **anti-infectives.** The first effective antimicrobial drug was penicillin. Since its introduction, morbidity and mortality from infections have continued to decline. However, as we grow in our knowledge of how specific types of microbes work and how to eradicate them, the microbes also continue to develop ways to mutate or secrete enzymes that make current antimicrobials ineffective.

This chapter focuses on the basics of antimicrobial therapy including classification of antimicrobial drugs, selective toxicity, antimicrobial resistance, general considerations of antimicrobial therapy, and monitoring antimicrobial therapy. Although this chapter discusses all antimicrobial drugs, the reader will note a bias toward antibiotics because these drugs have multiple mechanisms of action, require more specificity to the microbe and have a higher incidence of resistance. Additional information on specific antimicrobial agents is discussed in individual chapters.

CLASSIFICATION OF ANTIMICROBIAL DRUGS

Two popular ways to classify antimicrobial drugs are by susceptible organism or by mechanism of action.

CLASSIFICATION BY SUSCEPTIBLE ORGANISM

A **microbe** is a unicellular or small multicellular organism. Those that are disease producing are called **pathogens**. Types of microbes include bacteria, viruses, protozoa, some algae and fungi, and some worms. Drugs used for the treatment of infection can be classified according to the type of microbe they affect. The major classifications include **antibacterial** drugs, **antiviral** drugs, **antifungal** drugs, **antiprotozoan** drugs, and **anthelmintic** agents. Antibacterial drugs are subdivided into narrow-spectrum, broad-spectrum, or antimycobacterial drugs. As the name implies, a narrow-spectrum drug is effective against a few types of bacteria whereas a broad-spectrum drug is effective against many types of bacteria. The antiviral classification also has a subdivision: antiretroviral agents. The accompanying display, Classifications of Antimicrobial Drugs by Susceptible Organism, outlines these classifications.

Classifications of Antimicrobial Drugs by Susceptible Organism

Antibacterial drugs

Narrow-spectrum
Broad-spectrum
Mycobacterium

Antiviral drugs

Antiretroviral

Antifungal drugs

Antiparasitic drugs

Anthelmintic drugs

CLASSIFICATION BY MECHANISM OF ACTION

Antimicrobial drugs work in six different ways. They include:

- Inhibition of bacterial cell wall synthesis
- Inhibition of protein synthesis
- Inhibition of nucleic acid synthesis
- Inhibition of metabolic pathways (antimetabolites)
- Disruption of cell membrane permeability
- Inhibition of viral enzymes

These classifications and examples of antibiotics for each group are outlined in Table 47-1. In addition to their mechanism of action as already listed, antibiotic drugs are further classified as bacteriocidal or bacteriostatic. Antibiotics that actually kill bacteria are called **bacteriocidal.** They are less dependent on defense mechanisms of the body. Examples include beta-lactam antibiotics such as the penicillins and cephalosporins or aminoglycosides. **Bacteriostatic** drugs have an inhibition effect on bacteria that will be reversible on removal of the drug unless the host defense mechanisms have eradicated the organism. Sulfonamides, erythromycin, and tetracyclines are examples of bacteriostatic drugs.

Inhibition of Bacterial Cell Wall Synthesis

Unlike human cells, bacteria have rigid cell walls containing complex macromolecules, which are formed through biosynthetic pathways. The osmotic pressure within the cell is very high and relies on the integrity of the cell wall to resist the absorption of water. Without the rigid cell wall, the bac-

TABLE 47-1 Classification of Antimicrobial Drugs by Mechanism of Action

Antibiotics	Mechanism of Action
Penicillins Cephalosporins Vancomycin	Inhibit cell wall synthesis
Aminoglycosides Chloramphenicol Clindamycin Erythromycin Tetracyclines	Inhibit protein synthesis
Fluoroquinolones Rifampin	Inhibit nucleic acid synthesis
Polymyxins Polyene antimicrobials Imidazole antifungal agents	Disrupt cell membrane permeability
Sulfonamides Trimethoprim	Work as an antimetabolite
Acyclovir Saquinavir	Inhibit viral enzymes

teria would absorb water, swell, and then lyse. There are several antimicrobial drugs that weaken this cell wall, allowing the cell to absorb water with resultant bacterial death. Penicillins and cephalosporins bind to specific proteins that are located within the bacterial cytoplasmic membrane. Binding to these proteins results in inhibition of transpeptidase, which is an enzyme involved in the final step of cell wall synthesis. The result is decreased cell wall synthesis. These antibiotics also activate autolytic enzymes that are destructive to the cell wall. Another antibiotic, vancomycin, interferes with bacterial cell wall synthesis by inhibiting the synthesis of precursors of murein or by preventing the formation of linear peptidoglycan chains. These are polysaccharides and polypeptides that are cross linked to form the bacterial cell wall.

Inhibition of Protein Synthesis

Both human and bacterial cells require ribosomes to synthesize protein for use by the cell. However, there is a structural difference between ribosomes from human cells and those from bacterial cells. Thus, many of the commonly used antimicrobial drugs are able to disrupt bacterial protein synthesis while leaving the human protein synthesis alone.

Tetracyclines bind to the 30S ribosomal subunit and block the attachment of aminoacyl-tRNA. Aminoglycoside antibiotics also interact with the 30S ribosomal subunit but with different receptors, and this binding blocks the formation of the 70S initiation complex.

Erythromycin and clindamycin inhibit the formation of the initial complex and interfere with translocation reactions by binding to the 50S subunit of bacterial ribosomes. Chloramphenicol also binds to the 50S ribosomal subunit and inhibits peptidyl transferase activity.

Tetracycline and chloramphenicol do not have absolute selective toxicity. They are able to inhibit protein synthesis in some human cells as well.

Inhibition of Nucleic Acid Synthesis

Many bacteria use enzymes for replication that do not exist in human cells. For instance, fluoroquinolones inhibit deoxyribonucleic acid (DNA) gyrase, an enzyme needed for bacterial DNA replication. Although human cells contain an enzyme that functions in the same manner, the human enzyme is not affected by fluoroquinolones.

Inhibition of Metabolic Pathways (Antimetabolites)

Nucleic acid synthesis is dependent on folic acid, which acts as a coenzyme in many biosynthetic reactions. Humans obtain folate in the diet, but many microorganisms must synthesize folate. Sulfonamides inhibit bacterial folate synthesis by acting as an antimetabolite of the precursor to folate, paraaminobenzoic acid, or PABA. Similarly, trimethoprim is an antimetabolite of folic acid that selectively inhibits dihydrofolate reductases of bacteria and protozoa.

Disruption of Cell Membrane Permeability

The chemical composition of the cellular membrane in microbes is different than in human cells. This difference permits the selective toxicity of polymyxins, polyene antimicrobials, and imidazole antifungal agents. The polymyxins disrupt the bacterial cell membranes by insertion into the lipid bilayer and form artificial pores. The polyene antimicrobials bind to membrane components that are present only in microbial cells. The imidazole antifungal agents act as selective inhibitors of enzymes involved in the synthesis of sterols that are essential components of fungal membranes.

Inhibition of Viral Enzymes

The replication of viruses requires multiple enzymatic activity. Nucleoside analogs, such as acyclovir, and protease inhibitors, such as saquinavir, interrupt important enzymes required for viral replication.

SELECTIVE TOXICITY

An important principle of antimicrobial therapy is **selective toxicity**, which is the ability to suppress or kill an infecting microbe without injury to the host. Selective toxicity is achievable because the drug accumulates to a higher level in a microbe than in human cells; a specific action of a drug on cellular structures or biochemical processes is unique to the microbe; or an action of a drug on biochemical processes is more critical to the microbe than to host cells. Understanding selective toxicity has made antimicrobial drugs safe and effective in the management of infection in humans.

ANTIMICROBIAL RESISTANCE

Despite the large number of antimicrobial agents available, pharmaceutical companies are constantly looking for new ways to eradicate old microbes. This is due to antimicrobial resistance. Please note that the resistance is derived from the microbe—not the patient.

CONTRIBUTING FACTORS

Antimicrobial resistance may occur for several reasons: production of drug-inactivating enzymes, changes in receptor structure, changes in drug permeation and transport, development of alternative metabolic pathways, emergence of drug-resistant microbes, or facilitation of the development of resistance.

Production of Drug-Inactivating Enzymes

This is a common mechanism that causes resistance to many beta-lactam antibiotics. The microbe synthesizes hydrolytic beta-lactamase enzymes that are specific for certain penicillin and cephalosporin structures. To date, more than 100 beta-lactamases have been identified. Pathogens such as *Staphylococcus aureus, Haemophilus,* and *Escherichia coli* have specificity to affect penicillins but not cephalosporins. *Pseudomonas aeruginosa* and *Enterobacter* species have a broader spectrum and may affects cephalosporins as well as penicillins. When these enzymes affect the beta-lactam structure, the antibiotic becomes inactivated.

Changes in Receptor Structure

Bacteria contain molecules that act as targets, or receptors, for antimicrobial drugs. These molecules may undergo changes in their structure. This results in the microbe's becoming less susceptible to the toxic action of the antibiotic. For example, alteration in penicillin-binding proteins (PCB) decreases the affinity for binding beta-lactam antibiotics except in high drug concentrations that may not be achievable.

Changes in Drug Permeation and Transport

The antimicrobial action of many drugs depends on their ability to penetrate the cell membranes of an organism and reach effective intracellular concentrations. The organism's defense starts in the efficiency of the cell wall. Although the antibiotics may eventually reach the intracellular structures, the bacteria are able to hydrolyze the antibiotic as it slowly enters the cell. Another defense mechanism of the organism is the production of an efflux pump that effectively extrudes certain drugs, such as tetracycline, from the cell.

Development of Alternative Metabolic Pathways

Some bacteria are affected by antibiotics, such as sulfonamides, that act as antimetabolites interrupting their metabolic pathway for replication. In the case of sulfonamides, the antibiotic inhibits dihydropteroate synthase, the enzyme necessary to metabolize folic acid. Resistant bacteria may produce levels of PABA (the precursor to folic acid) high enough to overcome the inhibition of dihydropteroate synthase. Additionally, certain bacteria are able to utilize preformed folic acid from their environment, thus bypassing the inhibitory actions of the sulfonamides.

Emergence of Drug-Resistant Microbes

All antimicrobials have the ability to promote the emergence of drug-resistant microbes. However, resistance is more likely to occur in broad-spectrum drugs. The use of antimicrobials promotes the potential for drug resistance to occur, they do not directly cause the resistance. Drug-resistant microbes are developed in two ways: spontaneous mutation and conjugation.

Spontaneous Mutation

Spontaneous mutation is exactly as the name infers. It is a change in the genetic composition of the microbe that may just be a random occurrence, or the microbe may have mutated by acquiring DNA from an external source. The resistance developed is drug-specific.

Conjugation

Conjugation is a form of sexual reproduction in which two individual microbes join in temporary union to transfer genetic material. An important element of conjugation is a structure composed of DNA called a plasmid. Essentially, the plasmid can hold additional information, which codes for proteins that can sometimes be utilized by the host. Because polymerases work nonspecifically, information can be transcribed from them and utilized by any host, including bacterial hosts. DNA on plasmids can code for any protein. Among the many things plasmids can code for is for the ability of conjugation. Most plasmids that have this ability are considered F positive (F+) and are said to have the **F factor**. (F = fertility). For the plasmid to propagate, it must come in contact with another plasmid with the F factor. Conjugation may occur between two members of the same species or between different species.

For drug resistance to occur, the plasmid must come in contact with another plasmid that not only has the F factor but also possesses information necessary to deactivate an antibiotic. These two DNA segments together are known as **R factor** (R = resistance). More and more of our body's natural flora contain R factor. Thus, bacteria with F factor may combine with bacteria with R factor and transfer antibiotic resistance to the invading pathogen. Conjugation frequently results in multiple drug resistance.

Facilitation of the Development of Resistance

There are several factors that facilitate the development of resistance. Low drug concentrations in tissues that are too low to kill resistant organisms contribute to the development of resistance. This may occur due to an improper dose of drug or improper length of time between doses. Insufficient duration of therapy may allow resistant organisms to repopulate and re-establish an infection. Patients frequently stop their antibiotic when they feel better "to save some if it comes again." Treatment must be continued beyond clinical improvement, especially is there is any problem with host defenses.

Prophylactic use of antibiotics may also contribute to the development of resistant organisms. Prophylactic use of antimicrobial drugs means that the drug is given to prevent an infection rather than treating an infection. This practice increases the risk for the development of resistant microbes, therefore, antimicrobial prophylaxis should be reserved for appropriate indications. They include:

- Exposure to sexually transmitted diseases
- Recurrent urinary tract infections
- Neutropenia
- Surgery
- Bacterial endocarditis

COMMON ANTIBIOTIC-RESISTANT MICROBES

Although any microbe may become drug resistant, there are four important microbes to consider: methicillin-resistant *Staphylococcus aureus* (MRSA), penicillin-resistant *Strepto-*

coccus pneumoniae, vancomycin-resistant *Enterococci,* and multiple drug-resistant *Mycobacterium tuberculosis* (TB).

Methicillin-Resistant *Staphylococcus aureus* (MRSA)

The abbreviation MRSA is commonly used for this infection, however, it is somewhat misleading. In actuality, the pathogen is widely resistant to all of the antistaphylococcic penicillins, not just methicillin. In MRSA, there is an alteration of penicillin binding proteins, reducing the ability of penicillins to inhibit cell wall synthesis except in very high drug concentrations that may not be achievable. Many strains of MRSA are also resistant to aminoglycosides, tetracyclines, erythromycin, and clindamycin.

Closely related to MRSA is methicillin-resistant *Staphylococcus epidermidis* (MRSE). MRSE frequently colonizes the nasal passages of health care workers resulting in nosocomial infections, especially in critical care units.

Vancomycin is the drug of choice in the management of MRSA and MRSE. Because vancomycin is also used for many other drug-resistant microbes, vancomycin-resistance is emerging. New drugs such as linezolid (Zyvox) and dalfopristin/quinupristin (Synercid) have been developed to treat vancomycin-resistant microbes.

Penicillin-Resistant *Streptococcus pneumoniae*

Penicillins have successfully treated pneumococcal infections such as otitis media in children, community-acquired pneumonia, or meningitis in the past. Because of their frequent use in children and the elderly, strains of penicillin-resistant *Streptococcus* are emerging. To decrease the frequency of penicillin-resistant streptococcus pneumoniae, the Centers for Disease Control and Prevention (CDC) has suggested stopping the use of penicillins or cephalosporins as prophylaxis for otitis media and to immunize patients over the age of 65 or those over the age of 2 who have an increased risk for pneumococcal infections.

Vancomycin-Resistant *Enterococci* (VRE)

Enterococci are generally treated with a combination of either penicillins or cephalosporins with an aminoglycoside. The penicillin or cephalosporin damages the bacterial cell wall and allows the aminoglycoside to penetrate the cell. Strains of *Enterococci* have developed resistance to penicillin, gentamicin, and vancomycin. Potential drugs for VRE include teicoplanin (Targocid), minocycline (Minocin), ciprofloxacin (Cipro) or quinupristin/dalfopristin (Synercid).

Multiple Drug-Resistant Tuberculosis (TB)

Multiple drug-resistant TB is increasing in frequency. Although some of the bacilli are inherently resistant, others develop resistance over the long course of treatment, which can be as long as 2 years. The cause of multiple drug-resistant TB is inadequate drug therapy. This includes a duration of therapy that is too short; a dose that is too low, or more commonly patient compliance that is only intermittent. To decrease the incidence of multiple drug-resistant TB, drug therapy is implemented at the onset of therapy, followed by a decrease in the number of drugs, but never less than four are given at any time.

GENERAL CONSIDERATIONS OF ANTIMICROBIAL THERAPY SELECTION

The most important factor in the management of infections is to match the "drug with the bug." Each pathogen has a "drug of choice" and "alternative drugs" (Table 47-2).

TABLE 47-2 Antimicrobial Drugs of Choice for Selected Pathogens

Pathogen	Drugs of Choice	Alternates
Gram-positive bacteria		
Bacillus anthracis	penicillin G	erythromycin, ciprofloxacin, tetracyclines
Clostridium dificile	metronidazole	PO vancomycin
Clostridium perfringens	penicillin G	metronidazole, clindamycin
Clostridium tetani	penicillin G	tetracyclines
Clostridium diphtheriae	erythromycin	penicillin G
Enterococcus (UTI)	ampicillin or amoxicillin	fluoroquinolones, nitrofurantoin
Enterococcus (severe infections)	penicillin G	vancomycin + gentamicin, quinupristin/dalfopristin
Staphylococcus aureus MRSA	penicillinase-resistant penicillin vancomycin	cephalosporins, amoxicillin-clavulanic acid, vancomycin, fluoroquinolones, trimethoprim-sulfamethoxazole
Streptococcus pyogenes	penicillin G or V	clindamycin, erythromycin, vancomycin
Streptococcus viridans	penicillin G ± gentamicin	cephalosporins, vancomycin
Streptococcus bovis	penicillin G	cephalosporins, vancomycin
Streptococcus, anaerobic	penicillin G	cephalosporins, vancomycin, clindamycin
Streptococcus pneumoniae	penicillin G or V	cephalosporins, vancomycin, fluoroquinolones, erythromycin

(continued)

TABLE 47-2 Antimicrobial Drugs of Choice for Selected Pathogens (Continued)

Pathogen	Drugs of Choice	Alternates
Gram-negative bacteria		
Bacteroides	metronidazole or clindamycin	imipenem or meropenem, amoxicillin-clavulanic acid
Bordetella pertussis	erythromycin	trimethoprim-sulfamethoxazole
Campylobacter jejuni	erythromycin, azithromycin	fluoroquinolones, gentamicin, tetracyclines
Escherichia coli (UTI)	trimethoprim-sulfamethoxazole	fluoroquinolones, ampicillin or amoxicillin
Escherichia coli (GI)	cefotaxime, ceftizoxime, cefepime	ampicillin ± gentamicin
Enterobacter	imipenem or meropenem	trimethoprim-sulfamethoxazole, gentamicin, ciprofloxacin, cefotaxime
Gardnerella vaginalis	metronidazole	topical or PO clindamycin
Haemophilus influenzae (URI)	trimethoprim-sulfamethoxazole	cefuroxime, amoxicillin-clavulanic acid, fluoroquinolones
H. influenzae (other)	cefotaxime or ceftriaxone	cefuroxime, chloramphenicol, meropenem
Legionella species	azithromycin, fluoroquinolones, erythromycin ± rifampin	doxycycline ± rifampin, trimethoprim-sulfamethoxazole
Klebsiella pneumoniae	cefotaxime, ceftizoxime	imipenem or meropenem, gentamicin, tobramycin, amikacin
Neisseria gonorrhoeae	ceftriaxone, cefixime, ciprofloxacin, ofloxacin	cefotaxime, penicillin G, spectinomycin
Neisseria meningitidis	penicillin G	cefotaxime, chloramphenicol, fluoroquinolones
Proteus mirabilis	ampicillin	cephalosporins, ticarcillin, trimethoprim-sulfamethoxazole
Pseudomonas aeruginosa (UTI)	ciprofloxacin	piperacillin, ceftazidime, imipenem or meropenem, carbenicillin, ticarcillin, gentamicin
P. aeruginosa (other)	ticarcillin, mezlocillin, or piperacillin + tobramycin, gentamicin, or amikacin	ceftazidime, gentamicin, or amikacin, imipenem or meropenem, aztreonam
Salmonella	ceftriaxone, cefotaxime, fluoroquinolones	trimethoprim-sulfamethoxazole, chloramphenicol, ampicillin, amoxicillin
Serratia	imipenem or meropenem	gentamicin, amikacin, cefotaxime, fluoroquinolones, trimethoprim-sulfamethoxazole
Shigella	fluoroquinolones	trimethoprim-sulfamethoxazole, ampicillin, ceftriaxone, azithromycin
Mycobacteria		
Mycobacterium tuberculosis	INH, rifampin, pyrazinamide ± ethambutol and spectinomycin	cycloserine, ethionamide, kanamycin, ciprofloxacin, ofloxacin, levofloxacin
M. leprae	dapsone + rifampin	minocycline, ofloxacin, clarithromycin
Mycobacterium avium complex	clarithromycin ± rifampin ± ethambutol ± ciprofloxacin	rifampin, amikacin
Chlamydiae		
Chlamydia trachomatis		
Trachoma	azithromycin	tetracycline (PO plus topical)
Pneumonia	erythromycin (PO or IV)	sulfonamides
Urethritis, cervicitis	doxycycline or azithromycin	sulfonamides
Mycoplasma		
Mycoplasma pneumoniae	erythromycin or tetracycline	fluoroquinolones
Ureaplasma urealyticum	erythromycin	tetracyclines, clarithromycin, ofloxacin
Rickettsia		
Rocky Mountain spotted fever, typhus, Q fever	doxycycline	fluoroquinolones, chloramphenicol
Spirochetes		
Lyme disease	doxycycline or amoxicillin	ceftriaxone, cefotaxime, penicillin G
Syphilis	penicillin G	tetracyclines, ceftriaxone

Several factors must be considered when choosing the drug of choice or an alternative:

1. Identification of the pathogen
2. Drug susceptibility
3. Drug spectrum
4. Drug dose
5. Period of time to affect the pathogen
6. Site of infection
7. Patient assessment

IDENTIFICATION OF THE PATHOGEN

It is important to note that drugs to eradicate an infection must be specific to the type of pathogen involved. Thus, an antiviral agent will not eradicate bacteria nor will an antibacterial agent eradicate fungi.

The first step in the identification of the pathogen is viewing a Gram-stained preparation under a microscope. A sample of the contaminant is obtained from body fluids, sputum, blood or exudates. Visualization under the microscope shows the shape of the pathogen that aids in its identification (Fig. 47-1). A **Gram stain** is a simple test done with a dye and a glass slide. The Gram stain indicates whether the pathogen is gram-positive or gram-negative type. Gram-positive bacterial absorb Gram stain and are often aerobic. Aerobic bacteria need a fresh and continuous supply of oxygen to reproduce. Gram-negative bacteria do not absorb Gram stain and tend to be anaerobic. They are much more difficult to eradicate because anaerobic bacteria can reproduce in an environment that is oxygen free. There are drugs that affect only gram-positive microbes, some that affect only gram-negative microbes, and some that will affect both but not to the same extent. In some cases, the contaminant must be grown out in a culture medium for identification.

DRUG SUSCEPTIBILITY

To choose the right drug for the infection, a drug susceptibility test is optimal. However, it is not always required. The site of infection is frequently a clue to the causative agent. For instance, *E. coli* most frequently causes urinary tract infections. The health care practitioner would then choose a drug that has the ability to eradicate *E. coli*. This is called "**empiric therapy**." When multiple microbes may be the causative agent, empiric therapy may be started, but a culture of the infected area should be done prior to the initiation of antimicrobial agents, because their use may make identification of the microbe difficult. It is important for the nurse to check the sensitivity test result of a patient receiving empiric therapy and notify the health care provider immediately if the current antibiotic is rated as "resistant."

The most common test to identify drug susceptibility is called a culture and sensitivity. A sample of the exudate, body fluids, or serum is sent to the laboratory. The **culture** determines the identity of the microbe and the **sensitivity** determines which antimicrobial agent will be therapeutic. Sensitivity testing can be done by a disk-diffusion test or broth dilution procedure.

Disc Diffusion Test

This is the most commonly performed test to determine drug susceptibility. In the disc diffusion method, a disc containing a standardized amount of an antimicrobial agent is placed on an agar plate inoculated with the infecting organism. The plate is placed in an incubator and the bacterial lawn is allowed to grow. A growth inhibition zone will appear around the antibiotics that affect the microbe (Fig. 47-2). The diameter of the visible growth inhibition zone correlates with the minimum inhibitory concentration (MIC), which is the lowest concentration of an antibiotic that prevents visible growth of a microbe. Antibiotics are rated as sensitive (S) if they have an effect on the organism and resistant (R) if they do not.

Broth Dilution Procedure

In the broth dilution procedure, the bacteria are inoculated into the liquid medium containing graduated concentrations, of the test antimicrobial for direct determination of the MIC (Fig. 47-3). In addition to the MIC, the broth dilution procedure determines the minimum bacterial concentration (MBC), that is the lowest concentration that will kill more than 99.9% of the original inoculum of the microbe. Because the broth dilution procedure demonstrates both MIC and MBC, it is particularly helpful in the management of difficult infections.

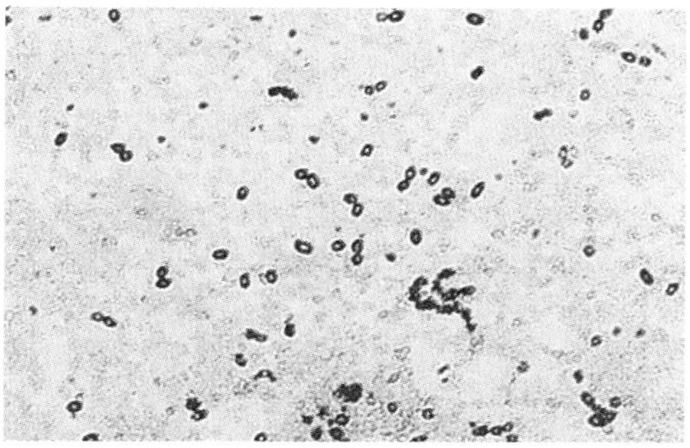

Figure 47-1. Gram-stained slide. This slide contains a type of Gram-positive bacilli.

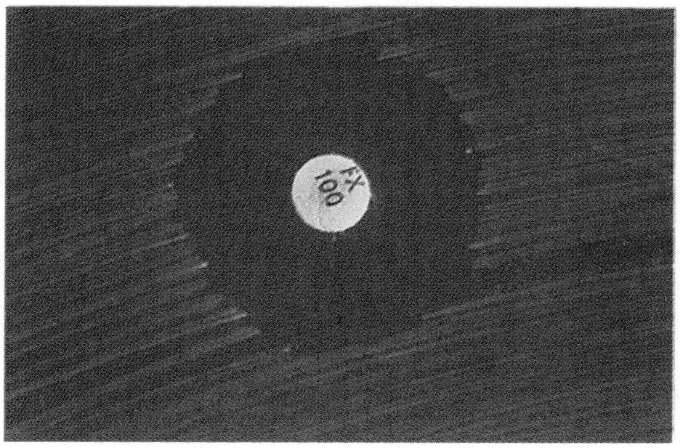

Figure 47-2. Disc diffusion test. In the disc diffusion test, samples of antibiotics are placed on a plate of the infecting organism. The antibiotic is "sensitive" if there is a bacteria-free zone around the antibiotic and "resistant" if the bacteria remain around the antibiotic.

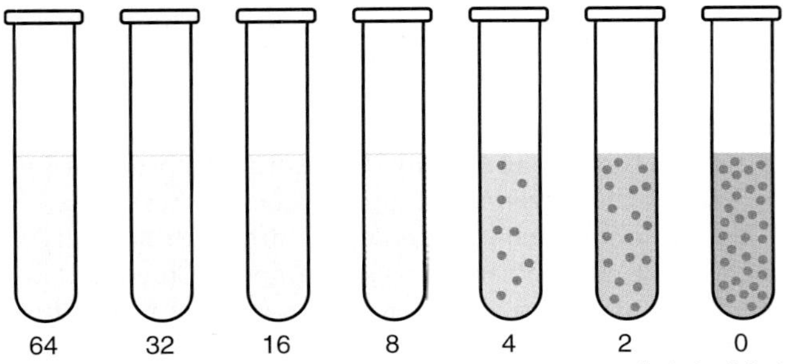

Figure 47-3. Broth dilution procedure. Bacteria are inoculated into a liquid medium containing graduated concentrations of the test antimicrobial. A clear test tube indicates that the concentration of the antimicrobial is sufficient to eradicate the microbe.

DRUG SPECTRUM

It is important to choose a drug with the narrowest **spectrum**. The benefit of a narrow spectrum antimicrobial agent is that it limits the potential for adverse effects such as suprainfection. A **suprainfection** is one that occurs during the course of treatment for a primary infection. For example, an antibiotic suppresses all susceptible microbes including bacteria that may keep other microbes "in check." This allows nonsusceptible microbes to proliferate because they no longer have other microbes secreting toxins in their proximity and they no longer need to compete for available nutrients. Two consequences may occur: secondary infections and the development of drug-resistant microbes.

An alternative to the use of broad-spectrum antimicrobials is combination therapy. Combination therapy is used frequently for an initial severe infection in which the pathogen is unknown. Once the pathogen is known, the appropriate drug can be administered. Another use for combination therapy is an infection that is caused by more that one pathogen. This is known as a mixed infection. Combination therapy is also used to prevent the development of resistant microbes. For instance, drug resistance occurs frequently in the management of TB as a result of the duration of treatment. When multiple drugs are given at the same time, the bacterium is less likely to be able to become resistant to all of the drugs employed. Another benefit of combination therapy is an enhanced antibacterial action. For instance, some bacteria are susceptible to an aminoglycoside when the aminoglycoside can enter the cell. For the aminoglycoside to enter the cell, it may be given with penicillin or a cephalosporin that destroys the cell wall.

Although there are many benefits to combination therapy, there are also disadvantages. These include an increased risk for toxic or allergic reactions, an increased risk for the development of resistant bacteria, and an increased risk for suprainfection.

DRUG DOSE

It is also important to choose the antimicrobial agent with the lowest effective dose. The dose of the antimicrobial agent is adjusted to affect the MIC at the site of infection. Pediatric doses are calculated as mg/kg per day.

DURATION

It is equally important to choose the antimicrobial agent that takes the shortest period of time to affect the pathogen. The drug must remain at the site of infection at drug concentrations equal to or greater than MIC. The duration is dependent on the type of pathogen, the site of infection, and the presence or absence of host defenses. The duration is generally 7 to 10 days but may be extended to 30 days or more for infections such as prostatitis.

It is important for the nurse to instruct the patient to take the medication until all the medication is gone. Early cessation of therapy may result in re-infection with the pathogen's having become more drug resistant.

SITE OF INFECTION

To be effective, a drug must be able to reach the site of infection at a concentration greater than the MIC. This is a particular problem when the infection is in the meninges, because many drugs do not cross the blood-brain barrier. Another difficult site is within an abscess, because there is poor vascularity and the presence of pus impedes drug concentrations. Specific types of infections such as endocarditis are difficult to treat because the vegetative bacteria are hard to penetrate.

Infections that occur in foreign objects such as pacemakers or prosthetic joints are also difficult to treat. When a foreign object enters the body, the immune system attempts to destroy the object by phagocytosis. When the phagocytes are busy attacking the foreign object, they are less able to attack bacteria that are multiplying at the site. Frequently, the infected foreign object must be removed to eradicate the bacterial infection.

PATIENT ASSESSMENT

Health care providers need to evaluate the individual patient before starting antimicrobial drugs. Important core patient variables include health status, life span, gender, environment, and culture.

Health Status

The type of antimicrobial agent chosen must reflect the immune status of the patient. It is important to remember that most antimicrobial agents cannot eradicate infection without the assistance of the immune response. Immunocompetent patients may receive either bacteriocidal or bacteriostatic drugs because their immune system can function with adequate response from phagocytic cells such as macrophages and neutrophils. Immunocompromised patients should receive drugs that are quickly bacteriocidal because their immune response is limited.

The patient must also be assessed for previous allergic responses to a particular drug class. When the patient states she or he has an allergy to a certain drug, it is important to find out what symptoms occurred when they took the drug. Many patients think that nausea, diarrhea, or headaches reflect an "allergy" to a certain drug. Allergic symptoms reflect an antigen-antibody reaction and include symptoms such as rash, itching, hives, periorbital swelling, and shortness of breath.

Life Span and Gender

Infants and the elderly are the most vulnerable populations for drug toxicity. In the infant, the liver and kidneys are still immature and may have difficulty metabolizing or excreting the drug, which results in accumulation. Although the same process is true in the elderly, it is related to the advanced maturity of their liver and kidneys, which may not be functioning at an optimal level.

Health care providers may request a lower dose of an antimicrobial agent for these two populations to minimize the risk for toxicity.

During pregnancy, antimicrobial drugs may cross the placenta and cause damage to the developing fetus. For instance, tetracycline binds to developing teeth produces a gray mottled discoloration.

Most antimicrobial agents enter breast milk resulting in injury to the nursing child. For example, sulfonamide drugs may cause kernicterus in the neonate.

Environment

The severity of the infection may influence the environment in which the antimicrobial is administered. The highest serum drug concentration is achieved when the antimicrobial is administered intravenously.

Another aspect to consider for IV therapy is the potential for severe adverse effects. For instance, amphotericin b, a powerful antifungal agent, causes an infusion reaction when administered. For that reason, most patients receiving amphotericin b will be admitted to a facility that employs licensed nurses to monitor its administration.

Culture

Certain cultures have genetic factors that are influenced by antimicrobial therapy. For example, some cultures have a predisposition to glucose-6-phosphate deficiency (G-6-PD). This deficiency tends to lyse red blood cells. Patients with this deficiency should not receive antimicrobials such as sulfonamides, which may induce red blood cell lysis.

MONITORING ANTIMICROBIAL THERAPY

Successful antimicrobial therapy is reflected in the eradication of the infection. Some antimicrobial agents have the ability to induce toxic adverse effects. Serum drug levels should be monitored for drugs that have a high potential for severe adverse effects. In addition, serum peak and trough levels may be drawn. A peak level is drawn 30 to 45 minutes after IV administration or 1 hour after IM administration. The goal is to keep the serum drug level within the therapeutic margin.

For patients receiving long-term or high-dose antimicrobial therapy, other laboratory testing may be indicated. For instance, if an antimicrobial is known to cause anemia, then serial complete blood counts (CBC) should be monitored.

The very young and the very old should also be monitored closely. Immature or advanced maturity may affect liver and kidney functioning. Appropriate testing would include hepatic and renal function tests.

The bottom line for patient monitoring is that it must be individualized depending on the type of pathogen, site of infection, potential for inducing adverse effects during therapy, and the patient care variables associated with each patient.

CHAPTER SUMMARY

- Bacteriocidal drugs kill bacteria whereas bacteriostatic drugs inhibit bacterial growth but rely on the immune system to eradicate the pathogen.
- Antimicrobial therapy is effective because of the principle of selective toxicity: the ability of the drug to harm the pathogen without injuring the host.
- Drug resistance is an ever-present danger to the effective management of infection.
- Prophylactic use of antimicrobial drugs must be limited to appropriate indications to decrease the potential development of drug-resistant microbes.
- There are four major drug-resistant pathogens in the United States: methicillin-resistant Staphylococcus aureus (MRSA), penicillin-resistant Streptococcus pneumoniae, vancomycin-resistant Enterococci (VRE), and multiple drug-resistant Mycobacterium tuberculosis.
- The most important principle in the management of infection is to use the right drug for the right bug.
- A culture determines the pathogen whereas a sensitivity test determines the susceptibility of the pathogen to a particular antibiotic.
- The antimicrobial agent with the narrowest spectrum, at the lowest dose, that needs to be taken for the shortest period of time to affect the pathogen should be used.
- Narrow-spectrum drugs affect only a few microorganisms, whereas broad-spectrum drugs affect many microorganisms.
- The minimum inhibitory concentration (MIC) is defined as the minimum concentration of an antibiotic to completely suppress bacterial growth.
- The minimum bactericidal concentration (MBC) is defined as the concentration that decreases 99.9% of the initial inoculum.
- The drug of choice to eradicate a particular pathogen may need to be changed to an alternate choice because of specific core patient variables such as health status, life span, gender, environment, and culture.
- The most important element of patient education is to advise the patient to complete the entire course of therapy with the prescribed dose and the prescribed intervals.

QUESTIONS FOR STUDY AND REVIEW

1. What is the most important principle of antimicrobial therapy?
2. How are antimicrobials classified?
3. How do most antimicrobials work?
4. What is the principle of selective toxicity?
5. How does a suprainfection occur?

NEED MORE HELP?

Chapter 47 of the study guide for *Drug Therapy in Nursing* contains exercises and activities to reinforce your understanding of the concepts presented in this chapter. For additional information see the text's accompanying website at *http://www.connection.lww.com.*

REFERENCES AND BIBLIOGRAPHY

Ambrose, P. G., Owens, R. C., & Grasela, D. (2000). Antimicrobial pharmacodynamics. *Medical Clinics of North America, 84*(6), 1431–1446.

Arnold, G. J. (1999). Avoiding inappropriate drug prescribing: fundamental principles for rational medication management. *Clinical Nurse Specialties, 13*(6), 289–295.

Burgess, D. S. (1999). Pharmacodynamic principles of antimicrobial therapy in the prevention of resistance, *Chest, 115,* (3 Suppl.), 19S–23S.

Cassell, G. H., & Mekalanos, J. (2001). Development of antimicrobial agents in the era of new and reemerging infectious diseases and increasing antibiotic resistance, *Journal of the American Medical Association, 285*(5), 601–605.

Drug Facts and Comparisons. (2000). St. Louis: Facts and Comparisons Division.

Gay, K., Baughman, W., Miller Y, et al. (2000). The emergence of *Streptococcus pneumoniae* resistant to macrolide antimicrobial agents: A 6-year population-based assessment. *Journal of Infectious Diseases, 182*(5), 1417–1424.

Hardman, J. G., Limbird, L. E., Molinof, P. B., Ruddon, R. W., & Gilman, A. (Eds.). (1997). *Goodman and Gilman's the pharmacological basis of therapeutics* (9th ed.). New York: McGraw-Hill.

Hessen, M. T., & Kaye, D. (2000). Principles of selection and use of antibacterial agents. In vitro activity and pharmacology. *Infectious Diseases Clinics of North America, 14*(2), 265–279.

Katzung, B. (1998). *Basic and clinical pharmacology* (7th ed.). Stamford: Appleton & Lange

Kaye, K. S., Fraimow, H. S., & Abrutyn, E. (2000). Pathogens resistant to antimicrobial agents. Epidemiology, molecular mechanisms, and clinical management. *Infectious Diseases Clinics of North America, 14*(2), 293–319.

Mandell, L. A., Ball, P., & Tillotson, G. (2001). Antimicrobial safety and tolerability: Differences and dilemmas. *Clinical Infectious Diseases, 32,* (Suppl. 1), S72–S79.

Porth, C. (1998). *Pathophysiology: Concepts of altered health states* (5th ed.). Philadelphia: Lippincott Williams & Wilkins.

Steinberg, I. (2000). Clinical choices of antibiotics: judging judicious use. *American Journal of Managed Care, 6,* (23 Suppl.), S1178–S1188.

Chapter 48

ANTIBIOTICS AFFECTING THE BACTERIAL CELL WALL

KEY TERMS

beta-lactam
beta-lactamases
cell envelope
cephalosporinases
penicillinases
penicillin-binding proteins (PBPs)

Learning Objectives

At the completion of this chapter the student will:

1. Identify the antibiotic drug classes that affect the bacterial cell wall, and name at least one drug in each class.
2. Describe the primary therapeutic uses for each antibiotic drug class that affects the bacterial cell wall.
3. Identify core drug knowledge pertaining to antibiotics that affect the bacterial cell wall.
4. Identify core patient variables pertaining to antibiotics that affect the bacterial cell wall.
5. Relate the interaction of core drug knowledge to core patient variables for antibiotics that affect the bacterial cell wall.
6. Generate a nursing plan of care from the interactions between core drug knowledge and core patient variables for antibiotics that affect the bacterial cell wall.
7. Describe nursing interventions to maximize therapeutic and minimize adverse effects for antibiotics that affect the bacterial cell wall.
8. Determine key points for patient and family education for antibiotics that affect the bacterial cell wall.

Penicillins

Narrow spectrum penicillins

penicillin G

penicillin V

procaine penicillin

benzathine penicillin

Aminopenicillins (broad spectrum penicillins)

ampicillin

amoxicillin

bacampicillin

Extended spectrum penicillins (antipseudomonal penicillins)

carbenicillin indanyl

mezlocillin

piperacillin

Penicillinase-resistant penicillins (antistaphylococcal penicillins)

cloxacillin

dicloxacillin

methicillin

nafcillin

oxacillin

Beta-lactamase inhibitors

clavulanic acid

tazobactam

sulbactam

bacitracin

Monobactam antibiotics

aztreonam

Carbapenems

imipenem

meropenem

Cephalosporins

cefazolin

First generation

(cefadroxil, cephalexin, cephradine, cephalothin, cephapirin)

Second generation

(cefaclor, cefprozil, loracarbef, cefuroxime, cefamandole, cefoxitin, cefonicid, cefotetan, cefmetazole)

Third generation

(cefixime, cefpodoxime, ceftibuten, cefoperazone, cefotaxime, ceftizoxime, ceftriaxone, ceftazidime)

Fourth generation

(cefepime)

Vancomycins

vancomycin

The symbol C indicates the **drug class**.

Drugs in bold type marked with the symbol P are **prototypes**.

Drugs in blue type with no symbol are **closely related** to the prototype.

Drugs in **red** type with no symbol are **significantly different** from the prototype.

Drugs in **black** type with no symbol are **also used in drug therapy**; no prototype.

Drugs affecting the bacterial cell wall include the penicillins, monobactams, carbapenems, cephalosporins, and vancomycin. The prototype drugs discussed in this chapter include penicillin G for the penicillin drug class; aztreonam for the monobactam drug class; imipenem for the carbapenem drug class; cefazolin for the cephalosporin drug class; as well as vancomycin, which is the only drug in its class.

In addition to explaining how these drugs work, this chapter discusses nursing management related to evaluating the patient's condition, monitoring the patient's response, and teaching the patient and family about antibiotic therapy.

PHYSIOLOGY

Bacteria are surrounded by a rigid cell wall that is responsible for maintaining the integrity of the internal cellular environment. The interior of the cell has a high osmotic pressure. If the bacterial cell wall is not intact, the internal osmotic pressure will draw fluid into the cell until it bursts.

Even when the cell wall is breached by an antibiotic, bacterial death may not occur because of bacterial resistance. Bacterial resistance occurs for two reasons: the drug is unable to reach binding sites within the cell, or the bacteria produced an enzyme that inactivated the drug.

BACTERIAL CELL ENVELOPE

Drugs that affect the bacterial cell wall must be able to penetrate the cell wall to bind to molecular targets on the cytoplasmic membrane within the cell. Gram-positive bacteria have only two layers to its **cell envelope**: a thick cell wall and cytoplasmic membrane. Despite the thickness of this cell wall, many drugs are capable of penetrating this wall and attaching to the targets on the cytoplasmic membrane. Gram-negative bacteria have an additional outer membrane to its cell envelope and the cell wall is much thinner. Although the cell wall can be penetrated easily, the outer membrane cannot. Only drugs that can pass through the very small pores of the outer membrane can reach the target sites on the cytoplasmic membrane (Fig. 48-1).

BACTERIAL ENZYMES

Beta-lactamases are enzymes that disrupt the beta-lactam ring. This inactivates **beta-lactam** drugs such as penicillins or cephalosporins because their antibiotic activity is derived from activity of the beta-lactam ring. Enzymes that affect penicillins are called **penicillinases**, whereas enzymes that affect cephalosporins are called **cephalosporinases**.

PATHOPHYSIOLOGY

Bacteria may cause infections in any body organ, structure, or fluid. In addition to the original bacterial infection, the loss of certain "good" bacteria may also result in a superinfection, such as those caused by *Candida*.

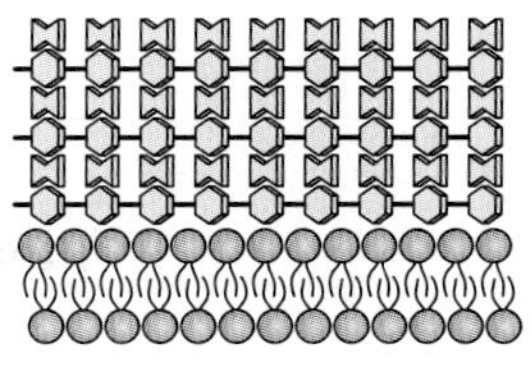

The lipid bilayer cell membrane of most of the Gram-positive bacteria is covered by a porous **peptidoglycan layer** which does not exclude most antimicrobial agents.

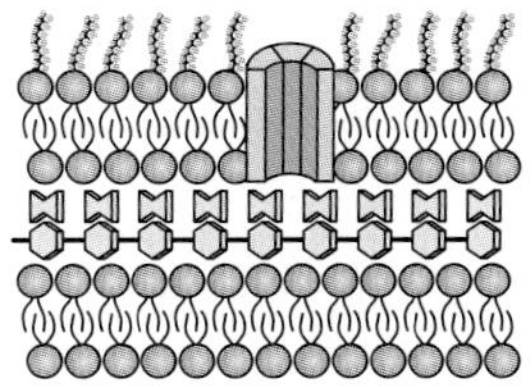

Gram-negative bacteria are surrounded by two membranes. The outer membrane functions as an efficient permeability barrier because it contains lipopolysaccharides **(LPS)** and porins.

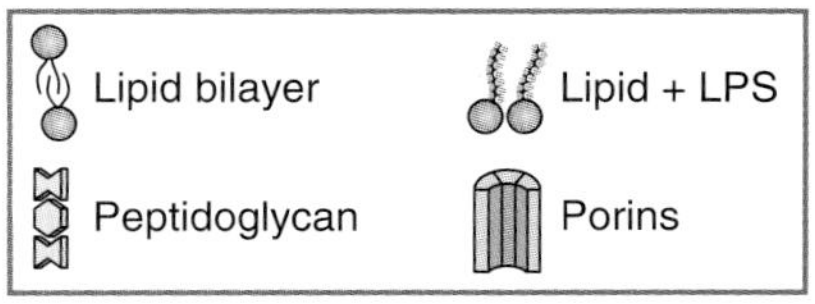

Figure 48-1. Bacterial cell envelope.

PENICILLINS

Penicillins were the first antibiotics introduced for clinical use. Alexander Fleming derived them from *Penicillium* molds in 1929. Subsequent versions of penicillin have been developed to decrease the adverse effects of the drug and to modify its ability to act on resistant bacteria. The emergence of penicillin was so important that the Nobel Prize was awarded to its inventors. Penicillins are also called beta-lactam antibiotics because their chemical structure contains a beta-lactam ring that is essential for antibacterial activity. All penicillins contain the essential beta-lactam ring; however, addition of a side chain to specific types of penicillins influences pharmacokinetic properties, binding capabilities, penicillinase resistance, and resistance to stomach acids. Penicillins are classified as narrow-spectrum penicillins, aminopenicillins (broad-spectrum penicillins), extended-spectrum penicillins, and penicillinase-resistant penicillins. Penicillin G is the first penicillin with clinical uses and is the prototype for the penicillin class. It is a narrow-spectrum penicillin.

NURSING MANAGEMENT OF THE PATIENT RECEIVING PENICILLIN G

Core Drug Knowledge

Pharmacotherapeutics

Penicillin G is indicated for use in infections caused by susceptible gram-positive bacteria, anaerobes, and spirochetes. These include *Streptococcus*, non–penicillinase-producing *Staphylococci*, and *Treponema pallidum*. Although penicillin G is generally ineffective for gram-negative bacteria, it is indicated for use in a few gram-negative infections such as *Neisseria meningitidis*, and non–penicillinase-producing strains of *N. gonorrhoeae*. Clinically, these bacteria cause infections such as pneumonia, pharyngitis, tonsillitis, endocarditis, and scarlet fever. Other clinical uses include therapy for tetanus, anthrax, meningitis, syphilis, diphtheria, rat bite fever, and fusospirochetal infections.

Penicillin G may also be used as prophylaxis in special patient populations to prevent bacterial endocarditis prior to procedures likely to produce temporary bacteremia, such as dental procedures. These patients include those with prosthetic heart valves, mitral valve prolapse, most congenital heart diseases, and those with acquired valvular heart disease. It may also be used as prophylaxis in patients with recurrent rheumatic fever or rheumatic heart disease.

Penicillin G may sometimes be used for gram-negative infections.

Pharmacokinetics

Penicillin G is absorbed rapidly from the GI tract but is unstable in gastric acid. This means that the amount of penicillin G that is actually absorbed with any given dose varies with the acidity of stomach contents. The development of more stable penicillins, such as penicillin V, has led prescribers to discontinue using oral penicillin G.

There are four forms of parenteral penicillin G commercially available as salts of potassium, sodium, benzathine, and procaine. The potassium and sodium salts are referred to as the aqueous and crystalline forms of the drug and may be administered intravenously or intramuscularly. Benzathine and procaine penicillin are referred to as repository forms of penicillin as they provide tissue depots from which the drug is absorbed over several hours (procaine penicillin) or over days (benzathine penicillin). As such, benzathine and procaine penicillins are administered only intramuscularly.

Penicillin G is bound to plasma proteins and circulates in the blood to be released at various tissue sites. The average peak drug effect is 4 hours after administration. Penicillin G crosses the placenta and is secreted in breast milk. It does not penetrate the blood-brain barrier very well except in the presence of meningeal inflammation, making it of limited use in treating meningitis.

Penicillin G is rapidly cleared unchanged from the plasma by the kidneys (glomerular filtration and renal tubular secretion). Because this rapid clearance of the drug makes it somewhat difficult to maintain therapeutic levels, around-the-clock administration is needed for therapy to be truly effective (Table 48-1).

Pharmacodynamics

Penicillin G inhibits the third and final stage of bacterial cell wall synthesis by binding to specific **penicillin-binding proteins** (PBPs) located inside the bacterial cell wall. After binding with specific PBPs, penicillin inhibits transpeptidase, an enzyme that is responsible for the development of cross-bridges within the cell wall. These cross-bridges give the cell wall its strength. Additionally, penicillin also affects autolytic enzymes (autolysins) that promote active cell wall destruction. The relationship between PBPs and autolysins is unclear, but it is possible that penicillin interferes with an autolysin inhibitor. As the cell wall weakens, the internal osmotic pressure of the bacteria changes allowing the cell to swell then burst. The body's immune system completes the process of fighting the infection and cleans up debris from ruptured bacteria.

Penicillin has selective toxicity to bacteria because the human cell does not use the biochemical process that the bacteria use to form a cell wall, thus protecting the human cells from destruction.

Contraindications and Precautions

Penicillin G is contraindicated in the presence of known allergies to penicillin, cephalosporins, or imipenem. Penicillin sensitivity tests are available if the patient's history of allergy is unclear and penicillin is the drug of choice. Caution should be exercised in the presence of renal disease, pregnancy, and lactation.

Adverse Effects

The most serious adverse effect to penicillin G is allergic reaction: rash, fever, and wheezing, and possibly anaphylaxis and death. More common adverse effects of penicillin therapy involve the gastrointestinal (GI) tract: nausea, vomiting, diarrhea, abdominal pain, glossitis, stomatitis, gastritis, sore mouth, and furry tongue. These effects are primarily related to the loss of normal flora (naturally occurring bacteria in the body) and subsequent opportunistic infections. Other adverse effects include superinfections (e.g., yeast infections) and local pain or inflammation at the injection site. Other, less common, effects include lethargy, hallucinations, anemia, thrombocytopenia, nephritis, and sodium overload (especially true with the sodium salt of penicillin G).

Drug Interactions

The effectiveness of penicillin G is decreased if it is taken concurrently with tetracyclines. Parenteral aminoglycosides (amikacin, gentamicin, kanamycin, neomycin, netilmicin, streptomycin, tobramycin) are inactivated when these drugs are administered with penicillin G (Table 48-2).

Oral probenecid may be given with IV penicillin G because it slows the excretion of the drug by competing with the penicillin molecule for excretion sites in the renal tubule. The result is that penicillin levels stay higher for a longer time for greater effect. When the supply of penicillin G is adequate, probenecid is not required. However, when supplies of penicillin G are low, probenecid can be used to prolong the duration of action of IV penicillin. In 1999, the main supplier of IV peni-

TABLE 48-1 Summary of Selected Penicillins and Other Beta-Lactam Antibiotics

Drug (Trade) Name	Selected Indications	Route and Dosage Range	Pharmacokinetics
Penicillins			
penicillin G (Pfizerpen, Pentids, Wycillin, Bicillin; *Canadian:* Falapen)	Pneumococcal infections Streptococcal infections (Group A) Bacterial endocarditis Diphtheria Neurosyphilis Congenital syphilis	Penicillin G is administered IV as penicillin G potassium or sodium and IM as penicillin G potassium, sodium, procaine, or benzathine. Dosages highly individualized by disorder. *Adult:* IM, 300,000–8 million units qd in divided doses; IV, 6–20 million units qd by continuous or intermittent infusion (q2–4 hours) *Child:* IM/IV, 25,000–250,000 units/kg/d in divided doses	*Onset:* IM, rapid; IV, rapid *Duration:* Varies $t_{1/2}$: 30–60 min
penicillin G benzathine (Bicillin, Bicillin Long-Acting)	Streptococcal Early syphilis Syphilis of > 1 y duration	*Adult:* IM, 1.2 million U q4wk *Adult:* IV, 2.4 million U in one single dose *Adult:* Parenteral, 2.4 million U once weekly for 3 wk *Child:* >27 kg, parenteral, 900,000–1.2 million U in one dose; >27 kg, 300–600,000 U in one dose	*Onset:* IM, slow *Duration:* 1–4 wk $t_{1/2}$: 30–60 min
penicillin G procaine (Wycillin)	Pneumococcal infections Staphylococcal infections	*Adult/Child:* IM, 600,000–1.2 million U/d in one or two doses for 10 d–2 wk	*Onset:* IM, slow *Duration:* 15–20 h $t_{1/2}$: 30–60 min
penicillin V (Pen-Vee-K, V-Cillin K; *Canadian:* Nadopen)	Fusospirochetal infections Streptococcal infections	*Adult:* PO, 250–500 mg q6–8 h *Adult:* PO, 125–250 mg q6–8 h for 10 d *Child:* PO, 25–50 mg/kg/d q6–8h	*Onset:* Rapid *Duration:* Varies $t_{1/2}$: 30–60 min
Aminopenicillins			
ampicillin (Omnipen; *Canadian:* Apo-Ampi)	Septicemia	*Adult:* IV, 150–200 mg/kg/d for 3 d, then IM q3–4h *Child:* Same as adult	*Onset:* PO, 30 min; IM, 15 min; IV, immediate *Duration:* 6–8 h $t_{1/2}$: 1–2 h
	Bacterial meningitis	*Adult:* IV, 150–200 mg/kg/d by continuous infusion and then IM injections q3–4h *Child:* Same as adult	
	Respiratory/soft-tissue infections	*Adult:* PO, 40 kg or more; IV or IM, 250–500 mg q6h; <40 kg, IV or IM, 25–50 mg/kg at 6–8 h intervals; <20 kg, PO, 50 mg/kg/d in equal doses q6–8h	
amoxicillin (Amoxil; *Canadian:* Gen-Amoxicillin)	URI, GU infections	*Adult:* PO, 250–500 mg q8h *Child:* Same as adult	*Onset:* Varies *Duration:* 6–8 h $t_{1/2}$: 1–1.4 h
	Lower respiratory tract infections	*Adult:* PO, 500 mg q8h *Child:* Same as adult	
bacampicillin (Spectrobid; *Canadian:* Penglobe)	URI, UTI	*Adult:* PO, 400 mg q12h *Child:* PO, 25 mg/kg/d in two doses q12h	*Onset:* Varies *Duration:* 8–10 h $t_{1/2}$: 1.5 h
	Lower respiratory tract infections	*Adult:* PO, 800 mg q12h *Child:* 50 mg/kg/d in two doses q12h	

(*continued*)

TABLE 48-1 Summary of Selected Penicillin and Other Beta-Lactam Antibiotics (Continued)

Drug (Trade) Name	Selected Indications	Route and Dosage Range	Pharmacokinetics
Extended-Spectrum Penicillins			
carbenicillin (Geopen, Geocillin)	UTI	*Adult:* PO, 382–764 mg PO qid *Child:* PO, 30–50 mg/kg/d in divided doses q6h	*Onset:* Varies *Duration:* 6–8 h $t_{1/2}$: 60–70 min
	UTI due to *Pseudomonas*, *Enterococcus*, or prostatitis	PO, 764 mg qid	
ticarcillin (Ticar)	Bacteremia, septicemia Intraabdominal infections Intraabdominal abscess Bone and joint infections Gynecologic infections Lower respiratory tract meningitis Skin and skin structure infections Pulmonary infection secondary to complications of cystic fibrosis	*Adult and child* ≥ 40 kg: IV/IM, 200–300 mg/kg/d in divided doses q4–6h *Child* <40 kg (serious infection): IM/IV, 200–300 mg/kg/d in divided doses q4–6h *Child* <40 kg (uncomplicated infection): IM/IV, 50–100 mg/kg/d in divided doses q6–8h	*Onset:* IM/IV, rapid *Duration:* 4–6 h $t_{1/2}$: 0.8–1.4 h
	Uncomplicated UTI	*Adult and child* ≥ 40 kg: IM/IV, 1 g q6h *Child* ≥1 mo and <40 kg: IM/IV, 50–100 mg/kg in divided doses q6–8h	
	Complicated UTI	*Adult and child:* IV, 150–200 mg/kg in equally divided doses q4–6 h	
piperacillin (Zosyn, Pipracil)	Lower respiratory tract infections Skin and skin structure infections Bone and joint infections Intraabdominal infections Gynecologic infections Bacteremia Septicemia	*Adult:* IV, 3–4 g infusion over 20–30 min q4h *Child:* Although safety and efficacy in children have not been fully established, pediatric patients have received 76–100 mg/kg/day IV or IM in divided doses q4h	*Onset:* IV, rapid *Duration:* 4–6 h $t_{1/2}$: 0.7–1.3 h
mezlocillin (Mezlin)	Same as piperacillin	*Adult:* IM/IV, 3g q4h or 4 g q6h *Child:* IV, 50 mg/kg over 30 min q4h or IM q4h	*Onset:* IM, rapid; IV, immediate *Duration:* 8–10 h $t_{1/2}$: 50–55 min
	Endocarditis due to *Pseudomonas aeruginosa* or *Serratia sp.*	*Adult:* IV, 5 g IV q8h in combination with an aminoglycoside	
	Uncomplicated UTI	*Adult:* IM/IV, 1.5–2g q6h	
	Complicated UTI	*Adult:* 3 g IV q6h	
	Uncomplicated gonorrhea	*Adult:* IM/IV, 1–2 g as a single dose with probenecid	
Penicillinase-Resistant Penicillins			
cloxacillin (Tegopen; *Canadian:* Apo-Cloxi)	Infections due to penicillinase-producing staphylococci	*Adult:* PO, 250 mg q6h up to 500 mg q6h in severe infection *Child:* PO, 50 mg/kg/d in equally divided doses q6h up to 100 mg/kg/d in equally divided doses q6h in severe infections	*Onset:* Varies *Duration:* 6–8 h $t_{1/2}$: 30–90 min
dicloxacillin (Dynapen)	Infections due to penicillanase-producing staphylococci	*Adult and Child* >40 kg: PO, 125 mg q6h; up to 250 mg q6h in severe infections *Child:* <40 kg; PO, 12.5–25 mg/kg/d in equally divided doses q6h; up to 25 mg/kg/d in equally divided doses q6h in severe infections	*Onset:* Varies *Duration:* 4–6 h $t_{1/2}$: 30–60 min
methicillin (Staphcillin)	Infections due to penicillinase-producing staphylococci. Initiation of treatment in any infection suspected to be staphylococcal	*Adult:* IV or IM, 1–2 g q4–6h *Child:* IM or IV, 100–300 mg/kg/d q4–6h	*Onset:* IM, rapid; IV, immediate *Duration:* IM, 4 h; IV, 2 h $t_{1/2}$: 20–30 min

TABLE 48-1 Summary of Selected Penicillin and Other Beta-Lactam Antibiotics (Continued)

Drug (Trade) Name	Selected Indications	Route and Dosage Range	Pharmacokinetics
nafcillin (Unipen)	Infections due to penicillinase-producing staphylococci Infections caused by group A beta-hemolytic streptococci, *Streptococcus viridans*	*Adult:* IV, 0.5–2 g q4h *Child:* IV, 50–100 mg/kg/d in equally divided doses q6h; for severe infections 100–200 mg/kg/d *Adult:* IM, 500 mg q4–6h *Child:* IM, 50–100 mg/kg/d in equally divided doses q6h; for severe infections 100–200 mg/kg/d *Adult:* PO, 0.25–1 g q4–6h *Child:* PO, 50–100 mg/kg/d in divided doses q6h	*Onset:* PO, varies; IM, rapid; IV, immediate *Duration:* PO and IV, 4 h; IM, 4–6 h $t_{1/2}$: 1 h
oxacillin (Prostaphlin)	Infections due to penicillinase-producing staphylococci Infections caused by streptococci	*Adult and child* >40 kg: IM/IV, 0.25–2 g q4–6h; maximum daily dose is 12 g *Child* <40 kg: IM/IV, 50–100 mg/kg/d in equally divided doses q4–6h *Adult and child* >40 kg: PO, 0.5–1 g q4–6 h *Child* <40 kg: PO, 50–100 mg/kg/d in equally divided doses q4–6h	*Onset:* PO, varies; IM/IV, rapid *Duration:* PO/IM, 4–6 h; IV, length of infusion $t_{1/2}$: 0.5–1 h
Monobactams			
aztreonam (Azactam)	Moderately severe systemic infection *Pseudomonas aeruginosa* Urethritis Endocervicitis Proctitis Gonorrhea	*Adult:* IV, 0.5–2 g IV q6–12h *Infant and child* ≥ 1 mo of age: IV, 30 mg/kg q6–8h; for patients with cystic fibrosis, 50 mg/kg q6–8 h *Infant and child* ≥ 1 mo of age: IV, 50 mg/kg q4–6h *Adult:* IM, 1 g as a single dose	*Onset:* IM, varies; IV, rapid *Duration:* 6–8 h $t_{1/2}$: 1.5–2 h
Carbapenems			
imipenem/cilastatin (Primaxin)	Mild infection Lower respiratory tract infection	*Adult:* IV, 250–500 mg q6h to a maximum of 2 g/d *Adult:* IM, 500 or 750 mg q12h depending on severity of infection	*Onset:* IM, unknown; IV, immediate *Duration:* 6–8 h $t_{1/2}$: 1 h

TABLE 48-2 Agents That Interact With Penicillin G

Interactants	Effect and Significance	Nursing Management
aminoglycosides	GI absorption of penicillins may be impaired by aminoglycosides.	Avoid combination therapy if possible. Administer at least 2 h apart. Tailor dose of penicillin as needed.
food	GI absorption of penicillins are impaired by the presence of food.	Administer at least 1 h before or 2 h after meals.
oral contraceptives	Penicillins may suppress intestinal flora, which provide an enzyme essential for enterohepatic recirculation for certain oral contraceptives. This may result in a decreased contraceptive plasma level.	Advise patients taking oral contraceptives to use an additional method of birth control while taking penicillins.
tetracyclines	The bacteriostatic action of tetracyclines may impair the bactericidal activity of penicillins.	Avoid combination therapy.

cillin G in the United States voluntarily recalled the drug due to a production problem. The Food and Drug Administration approved another manufacturer to produce IV penicillin G through the drug shortage allocation program. Currently, probenecid is still prescribed due to a shortage of penicillin G.

Assessment of Relevant Core Patient Variables

Health Status

The nurse should take a careful health history to assess for any known reactions to antibiotics. It is important for the nurse to examine the skin for any rash or lesions to provide a baseline to avoid misdiagnosis of an allergic reaction. The nurse should also assess the respiratory status of the patient as a baseline for possible wheezing associated with an allergic reaction.

For patients with a questionable history of allergic reaction to penicillin, a skin test may be performed to determine current allergic status. Because the skin test itself may cause an anaphylactic response in susceptible patients, it should be done only in a setting that can respond to the potential emergency. In rare situations, a penicillin allergic patient may need to be administered penicillin. In these rare cases, the patient is administered penicillin according to a desensitization schedule. Desensitization does not always stop an allergic response, therefore, it must be done in an acute care setting. Epinephrine and respiratory support must be immediately available for either skin testing or desensitization.

For elderly patients or patients with kidney disease, the nurse should evaluate kidney function (including blood urea nitrogen [BUN] and creatinine clearance) to determine baseline functioning. Patients with decreased kidney functioning may need a reduced dose of penicillin G. For long-term therapy, baseline liver function tests should also be performed. In addition, the nurse should assess for previously prescribed drugs that may interact with penicillin to cause undesired effects.

When penicillin G is used for gram-negative infections, culture and sensitivity tests should always be performed to be sure that the causative bacteria are sensitive to penicillin G.

Life Span and Gender

The nurse should document the method of birth control used by a woman of child-bearing age, because an antibiotic, such as penicillin G, can counteract the effects of an oral contraceptive. The nurse should assess a woman of child-bearing age for pregnancy and lactation. Pregnant and lactating women should be given penicillin G with caution because diarrhea and superinfections may occur in the fetus or infant. The nurse should note if the patient is elderly because these patients may need reduced dosages due to decreased kidney function.

Lifestyle, Diet, and Habits

The nurse should instruct patients self-administering penicillin G to administer the drug around the clock to ensure drugs levels stay within a therapeutic range. The nurse should assess the patient's daily schedule to ensure that the patient who is self-administering penicillin G can do so around the clock and complete the therapy as prescribed. This will ensure that drug levels remain within therapeutic range.

Environment

The nurse should be aware of the environment in which the drug will be administered. Whether administered at home or in an acute care setting, penicillin G solution should be mixed and stored in a refrigerator between 2°C and 8°C (36°F and 46°F) for up to 7 days. It should never be frozen. Commercially prepared infusion solutions may be kept at room temperature for 24 hours. Oral penicillin does not require specific environmental requirements.

Nursing Diagnoses and Outcomes

- Risk for Injury related to drug-related allergic reactions
  Desired outcome: The patient will recognize symptoms of allergy and contact the prescriber immediately to minimize ill effects.
- Imbalanced Nutrition: Less than Body Requirements related to drug-induced GI effects, such as diarrhea, GI upset, altered taste sensation, or superinfection
  Desired outcome: The patient will maintain consistent body weight and consult prescriber about persistent adverse effects that affect nutritional status.
- Diarrhea related to drug therapy
  Desired outcome: The patient will avoid dehydration, maintain fluid intake, and contact prescriber about persistent diarrhea.
- Risk for Infection related to overgrowth of nonsusceptible organisms.
  Desired outcome: The patient will report signs of superinfection to the health care provider.

Planning and Intervention

Maximizing Therapeutic Effects

The nurse should review culture and sensitivity reports to make sure that penicillin G is appropriate for the patient, especially for gram-negative infections. It is also important for the nurse to administer penicillin G as prescribed, spaced evenly around the clock to increase effectiveness. For oral preparations, the nurse should administer the dose on an empty stomach. Optimally, drug therapy should continue for at least 7 to 10 days but may continue for 2 weeks.

In acute care settings, the nurse should retrieve the antibiotic from the refrigerator approximately 15 minutes before administration, and the IV site should be evaluated for signs of phlebitis before and after administration.

IM penicillin should be administered deep into the muscle mass. The nurse should be sure to aspirate prior to administration, to avoid accidental injection into the vasculature. The nurse should also assess landmarks for IM administration to avoid injection into a nerve.

Minimizing Adverse Effects

The nurse should provide small, frequent meals; mouth care; and ice chips for the patient to suck if stomatitis and sore mouth are problems. The nurse should also monitor the patient to ensure adequate fluids are given to replace fluid lost with an adverse effect such as diarrhea. It is especially important to monitor intake and output. The nurse should notify the health care provider if a significant change in intake:output ratio develops because this may be the first indication of kidney dysfunction.

With parenteral administration of penicillin (IM or IV), the patient should be monitored for a minimum or 30 minutes. Epinephrine and respiratory support should be immediately available whenever parenteral penicillin is administered.

Providing Patient and Family Education

- The nurse should explain the importance of wearing some form of identification (e.g., Medic Alert necklace or bracelet) to alert health care personnel of their penicillin allergy in an emergency.
- The nurse should stress the importance of completing the full course of antibiotics, explaining the purpose of the drug and stating that it may not work for other types of infection.
- The nurse should emphasize the need to take penicillin G exactly as prescribed at evenly spaced intervals around the clock. The nurse should instruct the patient that oral drugs should be taken on an empty stomach 1 hour before or 2 hours after a meal.
- The nurse should instruct the patient to take missed doses as soon as remembered but not at the time that the next dose is scheduled.
- If the patient must mix the solution, the nurse should instruct the patient to do so just prior to administration. When premixed solutions are used, they should be kept in the refrigerator and retrieved approximately 15 minutes before administration.
- If no improvement occurs within 3 days, the patient should be advised to contact the health care provider.
- Because any patient may develop a sensitivity to penicillin G at any time, the nurse should discuss the signs and symptoms of allergic reaction and instruct the patient to stop the drug and call the health care provider if a rash, welts, itching, or shortness of breath develops.
- The nurse should advise the patient who has any type of allergic reaction to penicillin to never take any other drug with a name containing the ending "cillin."
- The nurse should also review common adverse effects and home interventions that may relieve discomfort. Patients who experience abdominal cramps or GI distress may try eating small, frequent meals. To relieve a sore mouth or throat, sucking on ice chips may help. If diarrhea occurs, the nurse should teach the patient to increase fluids and contact the health care provider if symptoms do not resolve in 24 hours.
- The nurse should also teach the patient about other adverse effects, such as a change in tongue color, fatigue, easy bruising, or vaginal discharge. The nurse should instruct the patient to report these signs and symptoms of superinfection to the health care provider immediately.
- The nurse should advise women of child-bearing age to use a backup method of birth control for the duration of therapy.
- The nurse should also explain the importance of sterile technique if IV therapy is administered at home by family members.

Ongoing Assessment and Evaluation

The nurse should monitor for signs of allergic reactions and for resolution of the presenting symptoms of infection (e.g., fever, lethargy, or hot and reddened or inflamed skin). Failure of these symptoms to resolve may indicate a treatment failure. The nurse also needs to monitor for signs of superinfection and notify the health care provider immediately to arrange for treatment. For patient comfort, the nurse may provide warm compresses and gentle massage to painful or swollen injection sites and observe for signs of phlebitis or abscess formation.

The nurse should monitor patients receiving parenteral sodium penicillin G for potential fluid overload. This is especially important in patients with cardiac disease or hypertension. The nurse should monitor patients receiving potassium penicillin G for signs of hyperkalemia that may result in cardiac arrhythmias. The nurse should arrange for periodic electrolyte studies for patient receiving either preparation.

By the completion of therapy, the patient should be free of the initial infection. The patient's nutritional status should be adequate and any adverse drug effects resolved. ■

DRUGS CLOSELY RELATED TO PENICILLIN G

Other Narrow-Spectrum Penicillins

In addition to penicillin G, other narrow-spectrum penicillins include penicillin V, procaine penicillin, and benzathine penicillin.

MEMORY CHIP

Penicillin G

- Used for infections caused by gram-positive bacteria, anaerobes, and spirochetes. Also used as prophylaxis to prevent bacterial endocarditis.
- Significant contraindications: hypersensitivity to penicillin, cephalosporins, or imipenem
- Most common adverse effects: nausea, vomiting, diarrhea
- Most serious adverse effect: hypersensitivity
- **Life span alert: Elderly patients may need reduced dosage because of decreased kidney function.**
- Maximizing therapeutic effects: Oral preparations should be given on an empty stomach. When using for gram-negative infections, be sure a culture and sensitivity are done before administration.
- Minimizing adverse effects: Monitor intake and output as it may be the first sign of kidney dysfunction. Blood levels may become toxic if the kidneys cannot excrete penicillin.
- Most significant patient education: Take the medication exactly as prescribed until the entire prescription is completed, despite the absence of symptoms. Monitor for signs and symptoms of allergic response and stop the medication if any occur

Penicillin V

Penicillin V (Pen-Vee-K, V-cillin-K), is the acid-stable form of penicillin G. It has replaced the need for oral penicillin G. It is indicated for the same infections as penicillin G and for prophylaxis in dental and upper respiratory procedures for patients who are immunocompromised or who are prone to bacterial endocarditis.

Contraindications, precautions, drug interactions, and adverse effects are the same as those associated with penicillin G.

Penicillin V should be given only to a patient on an empty stomach, 1 hour before or 2 to 3 hours after meals with a full glass of water. The nurse needs to advise the patient to continue the drug for the full course of the drug therapy, usually 7 to 10 days. The nurse should also advise the patient not to save the drug for self-medication at a later date nor to share the drug with any other person (see the accompanying display, Implementing Penicillin V Therapy.)

Procaine Penicillin

Procaine penicillin is the procaine salt of penicillin G. Because it is given by IM injection only, its use has been limited by the advent of IV antibiotics or newer broad-spectrum IM antibiotics. This drug must be stored in the refrigerator. Because it is viscous, it must warm at room temperature for approximately 15 minutes before being injected. Patients may react to procaine with confusion or agitation. This response is sometimes mistaken for a penicillin allergy.

Benzathine Penicillin

Benzathine penicillin is the benzathine salt of penicillin G. It has low solubility and provides an IM reservoir for low levels of penicillin over a long time. It can be detected in serum for up to 12 weeks after injection. It is used primarily for treating syphilis and preventing rheumatic fever.

Critical Thinking Scenario

Implementing penicillin V therapy

You have a patient who has been taking penicillin V for 2 days to "cure" an infection. You find out that this antibiotic was left over from an upper respiratory infection for which it had been prescribed 2 years earlier. The patient states that he stopped the drug when he felt better and kept it around just in case he got sick again. Describe how you would explain the dangers of taking antibiotics in this manner in a way that will make sense to the patient and lead to his adherence to antibiotic therapy in the future.

Aminopenicillins (Broad-Spectrum Penicillins)

Aminopenicillins include ampicillin, amoxicillin, and bacampicillin. The aminopenicillins have a slightly altered side chain, that makes them effective against many gram-negative microorganisms, including *Haemophilus influenzae*, *Escherichia coli*, *Salmonella*, *Shigella*, and indole-positive *Proteus mirabilis*. Aminopenicillins are ineffective against most infections caused by *Staphylococcus aureus* because they are easily inactivated by penicillinase produced by this species.

The benefits of these drugs include their higher oral absorption, higher serum levels, and longer half-lives (amoxicillin and bacampicillin). Within this group, ampicillin is the only drug that may be administered orally and intravenously.

Because these drugs are available for oral use and are effective against some of the most serious pediatric infections, they are frequently used in treating otitis media, upper respiratory infections, tonsillitis, skin infections, and pneumonia in children. Aminopenicillins should be used only for infections that are not sensitive to penicillin G or penicillin V because they have a broader spectrum of activity and therefore pose a greater opportunity for resistant strains to develop and adverse effects to occur.

The nurse should teach parents or other caregivers to follow storage and administration instructions exactly, to discard left over drug and not save it for later use, to be alert to the frequent occurrence of rash or diarrhea, and to watch for superinfections.

Extended-Spectrum Penicillins (Antipseudomonal Penicillins)

This group of penicillins, including carbenicillin indanyl, mezlocillin, piperacillin, and ticarcillin, are even broader in spectrum than the aminopenicillins. They are effective against all of the organisms susceptible to the aminopenicillins plus *Pseudomonas aeruginosa*, *Enterobacter*, *Bacteroides fragilis*, many *Klebsiella*, as well as *Proteus vulgaris*, *Proteus morganii*, and *Proteus rettgeri*. Like the aminopenicillins, extended-spectrum penicillins are easily inactivated by penicillinase produced by *Staphylococcus aureus*. They are available for oral or parenteral administration.

When given to combat *Pseudomonas*, extended-spectrum penicillins are frequently given concurrently with aminoglycoside antibiotics. Although this combination is highly effective, the nurse must remember to administer these two antibiotics at least 2 hours apart to avoid an antagonist drug-drug interaction.

The extended-spectrum penicillins should be reserved for use in serious infections by susceptible organisms. Again, the nurse should caution patients to take oral preparations on an empty stomach, to complete the full course, and to monitor for side effects.

Penicillinase-Resistant Penicillins (Antistaphylococcal Penicillins)

With the use of penicillins over the years, more bacterial species are developing the enzyme penicillinase to counteract the effects of penicillin. The penicillinase-resistant drugs were developed, which allowed them to remain effective against bacteria that are resistant to penicillin. Although the penicillinase-resistant antibiotics are highly effective against strains of *Staphylococcus*, they are inactive against many other bacteria that secrete penicillinase, especially gram-negative bacteria. Culture and sensitivity tests are mandatory when using a penicillinase-resistant drug. The drugs in this group include cloxacillin and dicloxacillin, which are oral preparations, and methicillin, nafcillin, and oxacillin, which are IV preparations.

Certain strains of *Staphylococcus* are resistant to the drugs in this class. A patient infected with these strains of *Staphylococci*, for example, may have an infection known as methicillin-resistant *Staphylococcus aureus* (MRSA). A resistance to methicillin implies resistance to any drug in this class. Methicillin is used infrequently because it can cause interstitial nephritis, whereas nafcillin and oxacillin are equally effective and do not have this adverse effect. The oral use of these drugs is now recommended for treating all gram-positive infections, because *Staphylococcus* is almost entirely penicillin resistant. Again, the nurse should urge the patient should to complete the full course of drug therapy, to take oral drugs on an empty stomach, and not to self-medicate with this drug at another time.

DRUGS SIGNIFICANTLY DIFFERENT FROM PENICILLIN G

Beta-Lactamase Inhibitors

Resistance to beta-lactams may occur because of the bacteria's ability to produce beta-lactamase. Clavulanic acid, tazobactam, and sulbactam are bound with other beta-lactam antibiotics to act as competitive "suicide" inhibitors of bacteria's beta-lactamases. They accomplish this by binding to the enzyme's active site, thus allowing the antibiotic to reach its target site. Clavulanic acid, tazobactam, and sulbactam do not alter the actions of the beta-lactam antibiotics. They simply prevent penicillins from being destroyed. On their own, they exhibit only weak antibacterial effects. Table 48-3 presents common combination drugs.

Bacitracin

Bacitracin is an oral, parenteral, and topical polypeptide antibiotic. It is active principally against gram-positive bacteria. Thus, it is combined frequently with drugs such as neomycin and polymyxins, which are active against gram-negative bacteria. The most common use of bacitracin is as a topical agent to prevent superficial skin and eye infections following minor injuries. It is available as a cream or ointment as well as ophthalmic drops or ointment.

Oral bacitracin is designated as an orphan drug for the treatment of pseudomembranous colitis caused by *Clostridium difficile*. IM bacitracin is used rarely because of the risk of serious nephrotoxicity. However, IM bacitracin may be used in the treatment of infants with pneumonia or empyema. Oral or parenteral bacitracin is used only in clinical situations in which less toxic drugs have not been effective.

Bacitracin is bacteriostatic, but it may also be bacteriocidal. Whether it is bacteriostatic or bacteriocidal depends on the antibiotic concentration and the specific susceptibility of the organism. It inhibits bacterial cell wall synthesis by preventing transfer of mucopeptides into the growing cell wall.

To avoid systemic absorption of bacitracin, it should not be applied to serious burns, deep wounds, animal bites, over large areas of the body, or into a perforated tympanic membrane. Although topical bacitracin has few adverse effects, ophthalmic bacitracin may cause blurred vision that resolves spontaneously.

MONOBACTAM ANTIBIOTICS

Aztreonam is a monobactam with a mechanism of activity similar to penicillin because it inhibits bacterial cell wall synthesis. It is used in the management of infections caused by gram-negative aerobic bacteria. These organisms include *Klebsiella*, *Pseudomonas*, *Proteus*, *Serratia*, *Shigella*, *Salmonella*, and *Neisseria* species. It has no activity against gram-positive bacteria or anaerobes. The structure of aztreonam is significantly different from other beta-lactam antibiotics, thus, there is little cross-sensitivity and may be given safely to penicillin-allergic patients.

TABLE 48-3 Common Penicillin Combination Drugs

ampicillin + sulbactam = Unasyn
amoxicillin + clavulanic acid = Augmentin
ticarcillin + clavulanic acid = Timentin
piperacillin + tazobactam = Zosyn

Aztreonam is administered IV or IM and is eliminated by renal tubular secretion. Half-life is prolonged in patients with renal failure. It is widely distributed throughout the body, including the central nervous system (CNS).

Hypersensitivity is the only contraindication to aztreonam therapy. Common adverse effects include vertigo and headache. Serious, but rare, adverse effects include GI distress with possible superinfection, hepatotoxicity, seizures, and blood dyscrasias including neutropenia.

Significant drug-drug interactions include synergistic effects when given with aminoglycosides and other beta-lactam antibiotics. Potential antagonistic effects may occur when given with cefoxitin or imipenem. Toxic aztreonam levels may occur with concomitant administration of probenecid.

When given intravenously, the nurse should check frequently for signs of thrombophlebitis at the IV insertion site. For long-term therapy, the nurse should monitor laboratory studies, such as complete blood count (CBC), liver function test (LFT), prothrombin time (PT), partial thromboplastin time (PTT), and platelet count.

CARBAPENEMS

Like monobactams, carbapenems are chemically different from penicillins but retain the beta-lactam ring structure. Imipenem and meropenem are the two carbapenems approved for use in the United States.

Imipenem (Primaxin) and meropenem (Merrem) are a very broad-spectrum antibiotics with activity against gram-positive cocci, gram-negative cocci and bacilli, and anaerobes. They are the most effective beta-lactam antibiotics for use against anaerobes. Meropenem is useful in the management of nosocomial infections that are resistant to to other antibiotics.

Imipenem is rapidly inactivated by renal dehydropeptidase 1, thus, it is always administered with cilastatin, an inhibitor of this enzyme. Cilastatin-imipenem increases the plasma half-life of imipenem and inhibits the formation of a potentially nephrotoxic metabolite.

Meropenem is not degraded by renal dipeptidases, thus is given as a single agent.

Hypersensitivity is the only contraindication for the administration of imipenem and meropenem. Potential adverse effects of imipenem and meropenem include GI distress and skin rash. In patients with high plasma levels, confusion, encephalopathy, or seizures may occur. There is also a potential for cross-sensitivity for patients who have penicillin allergy.

Drug interactions include synergistic effects with aminoglycosides and antagonistic effects with beta-lactam antibiotics. Seizure activity may occur when given concurrently with ganciclovir. Potential toxicity may occur with imipenem or meropenem when given with probenecid.

The nurse should administer imipenem or meropenem over 30 to 60 minutes. Meropenem should not be added to solutions containing other medications.

CEPHALOSPORINS

The cephalosporins were first introduced in the 1960s. They are similar to the penicillins in structure and in activity and are also considered beta-lactam antibiotics. Four generations of cephalosporins have been introduced, each group with its own spectrum of activity. Selection of an antibiotic from this class depends on the sensitivity of the involved organism, the route of choice, and sometimes the cost of therapy. Cephalosporins are popular therapeutic agents and are the most commonly prescribed antibiotics today. For that reason, bacteria resistant to cephalosporins are appearing in increasing numbers. Cefazolin (Ancef, Kefzol), a first-generation agent, is the prototypical cephalosporin.

NURSING MANAGEMENT OF THE PATIENT RECEIVING CEFAZOLIN

Core Drug Knowledge

Pharmacotherapeutics

Cefazolin can be used to treat many kinds of infections: skin, bone, heart, blood, respiratory tract, GI tract, sinuses, ear, and urinary tract. It is used to treat respiratory infections caused by *Streptococcus pneumoniae*, *Staphylococcus aureus*, *Klebsiella*, *H. influenzae*, and group A beta-hemolytic streptococci; skin infections caused by *Staphylococcus aureus* and strains of streptococci; GI infections caused by *E. coli, P. mirabilis, Klebsiella,* sensitive strains of *Enterobacter*, and enterococci; biliary tract infections caused by *E. coli, P. mirabilis, Staphylococcus aureus,* and streptococci; septicemia caused by *S. pneumoniae*, *Staphylococcus aureus*, *E. coli*, *P. mirabilis*, and *Klebsiella*; bone and joint infections caused by *S. aureus*; and endocarditis caused by *S. aureus* and beta-hemolytic streptococci. Cefazolin is also used for perioperative prophylaxis in surgeries involving the GI or GU tracts, bone, and skin.

Pharmacokinetics

Cefazolin is rapidly absorbed after IM injection. Peak effect occurs within 1.5 to 2 hours. It is also administered IV, with immediate onset and peak effect in 5 minutes. Only two of the first-generation cephalosporins are available exclusively for oral use: cephalexin and cefadroxil.

Cefazolin is widely distributed to body fluids and tissues, including bone. It does not cross the blood-brain barrier, but it does cross the placenta and enters breast milk. It is excreted unchanged in the urine (Table 48-4).

Pharmacodynamics

Cefazolin, like penicillin G, has no direct effect on the body. Cefazolin produces its bactericidal effects by binding with PBPs, which results in disruption of cell wall synthesis. Like penicillin, it also activates autolysins, which results in additional damage to the cell wall, allowing the cell to swell and then burst from the osmotic pressure within the cell. Like penicillins, it is

TABLE 48-4 Summary of Selected Cephalosporins

Drug (Trade) Name	Selected Indications	Route and Dosage Range	Pharmacokinetics
First-Generation Cephalosporins			
cefazolin (Kefzol)	Moderate to severe infections	*Adult:* IM or IV, 500 mg–1 g q6–j8h *Child:* IM or IV, 25–50 mg/kg/d in three or four equal doses	*Onset:* IM, 30 min; IV, immediate *Duration:* 6–12 h $t_{1/2}$: 90–120 min
	Life-threatening infections	*Adult:* IM or IV, 1–2 g q6h; maximum 12 g/d *Child:* IM or IV, 100 mg/kg/d; maximum 6 g/d	
cefadroxil (Duricef; *Canadian:* Ultracef)	UTI	*Adult:* PO, 1–2 g/d in single or two divided doses; for complicated UTIs, use 2 g/d in two divided doses. *Child:* PO, 30 mg/kg/d in divided doses q12h	*Onset:* Varies *Duration:* 12–24 h $t_{1/2}$: 78–96 min
	Dermatologic infection	*Adult:* PO, 1 g/d in single or divided doses *Child:* PO, 30 mg/kg/d in divided doses q12h	
cephalexin (Keflex; *Canadian:* Apo-Cefelex)	Skin and skin-structure infections	*Adult:* PO, 500 mg q12h *Child:* PO, 25–50 mg/kg/d in divided doses	*Onset:* Varies *Duration:* 6–12 h $t_{1/2}$: 50–80 min
	Otitis media	*Child:* PO, 75–100 mg/kg/d in four divided doses	
cephradine (Velosef)	Respiratory tract infections and community-acquired pneumonia	*Adult:* PO, 250–500 mg q6h or 500–1000 mg q12h *Child >9 months of age:* PO, 25–50 mg/kg/d in divided doses q6–12h	*Onset:* PO, varies; IM, 20 *Duration:* 6–12 h $t_{1/2}$: 48–80 min
	Haemophilus influenzae otitis media	*Adult:* PO, 75–100 mg/kg/d in divided doses q6–12h; do not exceed 4 g/d *Child:* Not recommended	
	UTI	*Adult:* 500 mg PO q12h; for more severe infections, up to 1 g PO q12h may be administered *Child:* Not recommended	
	Cesarean section prophylaxis	*Adult:* IV, 1 g IV once the umbilical cord is clamped, followed by 1 g IV or IM 6 h and 12 h after the first dose	
	Surgical prophylaxis	*Adult:* IM/IV, 1 g $^{1}/_{2}$–1$^{1}/_{2}$ hours before surgery, followed by 1 g IM or IV q4–6h	
cephapirin (Cefadyl)	Generalized infections	*Adult:* IM/IV 500 mg–1 g q4–6h *Child:* IV, 40–80 mg/kg IV in four divided doses; not indicated for children <3 months of age.	*Onset:* IM, 10 min; IV, rapid *Duration:* 4–6 h $t_{1/2}$: 24–36 min
	Surgical prophylaxis	*Adult:* IV, 1–2 g just before surgery, during surgery, and every 6 h postoperatively for 24 h	
Second-Generation Cephalosporins			
cefaclor (Ceclor; *Canadian:* Apo-Cefaclor)	Lower respiratory tract infections Upper respiratory infections	*Adult:* PO, 250–500 mg q8h *Child:* PO, 20–40 mg/kg/d in divided doses q8h	*Onset:* Varies *Duration:* 6–12 h $t_{1/2}$: 30–60 min
cefprozil (Cefzil)	Pharyngitis/tonsillitis Dermatologic infections	*Adult:* PO, 250–500 mg q12h *Child:* PO, 7.5–15 mg/kg q12h	*Onset:* Varies *Duration:* 12–24 h $t_{1/2}$: 78 min
loracarbef (Lorabid)	Pharyngitis/tonsillitis Pneumonia	*Adult:* PO, 200–400 mg q12h *Child:* PO, 15–30 mg/kg/d in divided doses q12h	*Onset:* Varies *Duration:* 12 h $t_{1/2}$: 60 min
cefuroxime (Ceftin; *Canadian:* Cefuroxime Axetil)	Uncomplicated UTIs Uncomplicated gonorrhea Bacterial meningitis	*Adult:* PO, 125–250 mg q12h *Child:* PO, 15 mg/kg q12h *Adult:* IM or IV, 1.5 g with 1 g of oral probenecid *Child:* IV, 200–240 mg/kg/d in divided doses q6–8h	*Onset:* PO, varies; IM, 20 min; *Duration:* 8–12 h $t_{1/2}$: 1–2 h

(*continued*)

TABLE 48-4 Summary of Selected Cephalosporins (Continued)

Drug (Trade) Name	Selected Indications	Route and Dosage Range	Pharmacokinetics
cefamandole (Mandol)	Acute UTI Severe infections Perioperative prophylaxis	*Adult:* IM or IV, 0.5–2 g q4–6h *Adult:* IM or IV, 1–2 g 1/2–1 h before initial incision; 1–2 g q6h for 24 h after surgery. *Child:* IM or IV, 50–100 mg/kg/d, starting 1/2–1 h before initial incision and continue for 24 h after surgery	*Onset:* Varies *Duration:* 6–8 h $t_{1/2}$: 30–60 min
cefoxitin (Mefoxin)	Uncomplicated gonorrhea Lower respiratory tract infection	*Adult:* IM or IV, 1–2 g q4–6h with 1 g oral probenecid *Child:* >3 mo, IM or IV, 80–160 mg/kg/d in divided doses q4–6h	*Onset:* IM, 5–10 min; IV, immediate *Duration:* 6–8 h $t_{1/2}$: 45–60 min
cefonicid (Monocid)	Perioperative prophylaxis cesarean section (after cord is clamped)	*Adult:* IM or IV, 1 g, 1 h before initial incision; 1 g/d for 24 h after surgery	*Onset:* IM, 1 h; IV, immediate *Duration:* 24 h $t_{1/2}$: 4.5–5.8 h
cefotetan (Cefotan)	UTI, other infections, and severe infections	*Adult:* IM or IV, 1–2 g q12h	*Onset:* IM, 30–60 min; IV, 15–20 min *Duration:* 12 h $t_{1/2}$: 3–4.5 h
cefmetazole (Zefazone)	Vaginal hysterectomy Cholecystectomy	*Adult:* IV, 2-g single dose 30–90 min before surgery or 1 g dose 30–90 min before surgery and repeated 8 and 16 h later *Adult:* IV, 1-g dose 30–90 min before surgery and repeated 8 and 16 h later *Child:* Safety not established	*Onset:* IV, rapid *Duration:* 6–12 h $t_{1/2}$: 1.2 h
Third-Generation Cephalosporins			
cefixime (Suprax)	Uncomplicated UTI Otitis media	*Adult:* PO, 400 mg/d as a single tablet *Child:* PO, 8 mg/kg/d suspension as a single dose	*Onset:* Varies *Duration:* 24 h $t_{1/2}$: 3–4 h
cefpodoxime (Vantin)	Lower respiratory infection Upper respiratory infection	*Adult:* PO, 200–400 mg q12h; continue for 7–14 d *Child:* PO, 5 mg/kg per dose q12h; continue for 10 d	*Onset:* Varies *Duration:* 12 h $t_{1/2}$: 120–180 min
ceftibuten (Cedax)	Acute bacterial otitis media Pharyngitis and tonsillitis	*Adult:* PO, 400 mg/d for 10 d *Child:* PO, 9 mg/kg for 10 d to a maximum dose of 400 mg/d	*Onset:* Rapid *Duration:* 24 h $t_{1/2}$: 30–60 min
cefoperazone (Cefobid)	Respiratory tract infections Dermatologic infections UTI	*Adult:* IM or IV, 2–4 g/d in equal divided doses q12h *Child:* Not established	*Onset:* IM, 1 h; IV, 5–10 min *Duration:* 6–12 h $t_{1/2}$: 1.75–2.5 h
cefotaxime (Claforan)	Gonorrhea Disseminated infection	*Adult:* IM/IV, 1 g q6–8h *Child:* IV, IM (for both indications): 50–180 mg/kg/d in four to six divided doses	*Onset:* IM, 1 h; IV, 5–10 min *Duration:* 4–12 h $t_{1/2}$: 1 h
ceftizoxime (Cefizox)	Gonorrhea Uncomplicated UTI	*Adult:* IM, single 1-g dose *Adult:* IV, 500 mg q12h *Child:* >6 mo, IM or IV, 50 mg/kg q6–8h	*Onset:* IM, 30 min; IV, rapid *Duration:* 6–12 h $t_{1/2}$: 84–114 min

TABLE 48-4 Summary of Selected Cephalosporins (Continued)

Drug (Trade) Name	Selected Indications	Route and Dosage Range	Pharmacokinetics
ceftriaxone (Rocephin)	Gonorrhea Meningitis	*Adult:* IM, single 250 mg *Adult:* IV or IM, 100 mg/kg/d in divided doses q12h *Child:* IV or IM, same as above	*Onset:* IM, 30 min; IV, rapid *Duration:* 12–24 h $t_{1/2}$: 5–10 h
ceftazidime (Fortaz, Tazicef, Tazidime)	Aminoglycoside-resistant infections	*Adult and child* >12: IM/IV, 1 g q8–12h *Child* 1 mo–12 yrs: IV, 30–50 mg/kg q8h; IV, 30 mg/kg q12h	*Onset:* IM, 30 min; IV, rapid *Duration:* 6–12 h $t_{1/2}$: 110–120 min
Fourth-Generation Cephalosporins			
cefepime (Maxipime)	UTI due to *Escherichia* or *Klebsiella* Skin and soft tissue infections Staphylococcal and streptococcal infections Pneumonia	*Adult:* IV: 0.5–2 g q12h IM: 0.5–1 g q12h *Child:* Not recommended	*Onset:* IV, immed; IM, 30 min *Duration:* 10–12 h $t_{1/2}$: 2–2.3 h

most effective against cells undergoing active growth and division.

Contraindications and Precautions

Cefazolin is contraindicated in anyone with a known allergy to cephalosporins. Caution must be used in patients with renal failure and in pregnant or lactating patients. Because of the structural similarities between cephalosporins and penicillins, patients with one type of drug allergy may experience a cross-sensitivity with the other. Cephalosporin hypersensitivity occurs in 5% to 10% of patients with penicillin allergy. Patients with a history of severe allergic reactions to penicillins should not receive cephalosporins.

Adverse Effects

Hypersensitivity reactions occur frequently with cephalosporin drugs. Although severe immediate reactions are rare, hypersensitivity presents most frequently with a maculopapular rash that develops several days after the onset of therapy.

Other common adverse effects of cefazolin involve the GI tract. Nausea, vomiting, diarrhea, anorexia, abdominal pain, and flatulence are common side effects. Pseudomembranous colitis, a potentially dangerous disorder, has also been reported with cefazolin. The drug should be discontinued immediately at any sign of violent, bloody diarrhea and abdominal pain.

CNS symptoms include headache, dizziness, lethargy, and paresthesias. Nephrotoxicity is also associated with the use of cefazolin, most particularly with patients who have a predisposing renal insufficiency. Superinfections are also common with cephalosporin use. As with the penicillins, this reaction is related to the destruction of normal flora bacteria. Thrombophlebitis or an abscess at the injection site are potential adverse effects of IV administration.

Serum sickness-like reactions, such as erythema multiforme or skin rashes accompanied by polyarthritis, arthralgia, and fever, may occur following a second course of therapy.

Symptoms resolve after discontinuation of the drug.

Drug Interactions

There is an increased risk of nephrotoxicity when cefazolin is given concurrently with aminoglycoside antibiotics. Patients receiving oral anticoagulants may experience increased bleeding when also given cefazolin. Like penicillin, cefazolin may have prolonged effects when given concurrently with probenecid. Table 48-5 discusses agents that interact with cefazolin. A disulfiram-like reaction may occur in patients taking cephalosporins with a chemical structure similar to disulfiram. These include cefamandole (Mandol), cefonicid (Monocid), cefoperazone (Cefobid), and cefotetan (Cefotan).

Effect on Test Results

False-positive results may occur in tests of urine glucose using Benedict solution, Fehling solution, and Clinitest tablets. Blood glucose monitoring is recommended is recommended in patients with diabetes who are receiving this drug. False-positive results have also been noted in direct Coombs tests and measurements of urinary 17-ketosteroids. These tests should be avoided in patients receiving any cephalosporins. A disulfiram-like reaction may occur in patients taking cephalosporins with a chemical structure similar to disulfiram. These include cefamandole (Mandol), cefonicid (Monocid), cefoperazone (Cefobid), and cefotetan (Cefotan).

Assessment of Relevant Core Patient Variables

Health Status

The nurse should follow the same guidelines for evaluating the health status of a patient receiving penicillin.

TABLE 48-5 Agents That Interact With Cefazolin

Interactants	Effect and Significance	Nursing Management
aminoglycosides	Increased risk of nephrotoxicity, although the mechanism of action is unknown.	Monitor aminoglycoside levels frequently. Monitor kidney function closely. Reduce dosage or discontinue one or both drugs if signs of kidney dysfunction occur.
oral anticoagulants	Some cephalosporins may have a warfarin-like activity and anti-platelet effects. This results in an augmentation of the action of oral anticoagulants and an increased risk of bleeding.	Advise patients of the signs and symptoms of overanti-coagulation. Monitor oral anticoagulant levels. Reduce oral anticoagulant dosage accordingly.

Life Span and Gender

The nurse should document the age of the patient and, if appropriate, assess for pregnancy and lactation. Cefazolin should be used cautiously and the dosage adjusted in elderly patients who have any degree of renal insufficiency. Adjusted dosage recommendations are based on creatinine clearance levels. Cefazolin is not recommended for infants younger than 1 month because of their immature renal and hepatic functioning.

Lifestyle, Diet, and Habits

The nurse should assess the patient's lifestyle and dietary practices to ensure that the drug can be taken consistently, completely, and on an empty stomach, if possible. The nurse should assess for the patient's use of alcoholic beverages. While all cephalosporins will not cause a disulfiram-like reaction, it is preferable to refrain from drinking alcohol while on cephalosporin therapy.

Environment

The nurse should be aware of the environment in which the drug will be administered. After dilution, cefazolin can be kept at room temperature for 24 hours or in a refrigerator between 2°C and 8°C (36°F and 46°F) for 96 hours. In acute care settings, the nurse should retrieve the antibiotic from the refrigerator and let it warm at room temperature for about 15 minutes before administering it. The IV site should be evaluated for signs of phlebitis before and after drug administration. Premixed solutions should be kept in the refrigerator and retrieved approximately 15 minutes before administration as well.

Nursing Diagnoses and Outcomes

- Diarrhea related to drug effects
  Desired outcome: The patient will avoid dehydration, maintain fluid intake, and contact the prescriber if diarrhea persists.
- Imbalanced Nutrition: More or Less than Body Requirements related to GI effects, alteration in taste, superinfections
  Desired outcome: The patient will maintain body weight and contact the prescriber if persistent adverse effects impact nutritional status.
- Risk for Infection related to overgrowth of nonsusceptible organisms.
  Desired outcome: The patient will report signs of superinfection to the health care provider.

Planning and Intervention

Maximizing Therapeutic Effects

The nurse should review culture and sensitivity tests to evaluate the efficacy of treatment. Oral suspensions of cephalosporins should be kept in the refrigerator. The nurse should be sure that the patient receives injections of cefazolin as prescribed around the clock for increased effectiveness. The nurse should monitor the site of infection and presenting signs and symptoms throughout the course of drug therapy. Failure of the signs and symptoms of infection to resolve may indicate the need to repeat culture and sensitivity testing. For optimal effect, drug therapy should continue for at least 2 days after all signs and symptoms resolve.

Minimizing Adverse Effects

Cefazolin may be taken with food or fluids to decrease GI distress. The nurse should provide small, frequent meals; mouth care; and ice chips to suck on if stomatitis and sore mouth are problems. The nurse should also monitor the patient's hydration status and ensure that adequate fluids are given to replace fluid lost with diarrhea. The nurse should also evaluate the patient for CNS effects and use safety precautions, such as elevation of side rails.

IM administration of cefazolin should be deep into a large muscle. The nurse should forewarn the patient that the injection may be uncomfortable. The patient receiving IM cefazolin should be monitored for an abscess at the injection site. IV administration may be as an IV push or IV piggyback. The nurse should administer IV cefazolin exactly as prescribed by the health care provider. The patient receiving IV cefazolin should also be monitored for the possibility of thrombophlebitis.

The patient receiving combination therapy with aminoglycoside antibiotics should be monitored (serum blood urea nitrogen and creatinine levels) frequently for nephrotoxicity. The patient receiving oral anticoagulants in addition to cefazolin should receive instructions to monitor for signs of blood loss, for example, bleeding gums and easily bruised skin. Dosages of the oral anticoagulant may need reduction.

Providing Patient and Family Education

- Because cefazolin and the other cephalosporins are similar to penicillins, the nurse should follow the same guidelines for providing patient and family education to a patient receiving penicillin.
- In addition, the nurse should inform patients about possible interactions between cephalosporins and alcohol, urging the patient to refrain from drinking alcohol for 72 hours after drug therapy stops.
- The nurse can also educate patients on hidden sources of alcohol, such as over-the-counter cough and cold preparations.

Ongoing Assessment and Evaluation

The nurse must monitor the patient for any signs of superinfection and notify the provider immediately to arrange for treatment if superinfection does occur. The nurse should also monitor for signs of allergic or serum sickness-like reactions (fever, hives, swollen glands, neutropenia, arthralgia, and edema). The nurse needs to implement comfort measures as needed and monitor for signs of phlebitis, abscess formation, and other complications. By the completion of therapy, the patient should be free of the presenting infection. The patient will be adequately nourished and adverse effects will be resolved. ■

MEMORY CHIP

Cefazolin

- Used for infections caused by gram-positive bacteria, anaerobes, and spirochetes. Also used as prophylaxis in patients having GI or GU surgery.
- Significant contraindication: hypersensitivity to cephalosporins or penicillin
- Most common adverse effects: nausea, vomiting, diarrhea
- Most serious adverse effect: hypersensitivity
- **Life span alert: Cefazolin should be used cautiously and the dosage adjusted in elderly patients who have any degree of renal insufficiency.**
- Maximizing therapeutic effects: when using for gram-negative infections, be sure culture and sensitivity are made before administration.
- Minimizing adverse effects: inject IM preparations into a large muscle mass. Be sure IV preparations are administered according to the healthcare prescriber's orders, either IV push or IV piggyback.
- Most significant patient education: Take the medication exactly as prescribed until the entire prescription is completed, despite the absence of symptoms. Monitor for signs and symptoms of allergic response and stop the medication if any should occur.

DRUGS CLOSELY RELATED TO CEFAZOLIN

First-Generation Cephalosporins

Similar to cefazolin are these other first-generation cephalosporins: oral cefadroxil and cephalexin; cephradine, which is available in oral, IV, and IM preparations; and cephalothin and cephapirin, which are available for IM and IV administration only. All of these drugs cover basically the same spectrum of pathogens. They are most active against gram-positive bacterial, especially staphylococci and nonenterococcal streptococci. They have minor activity against gram-negative bacteria. Most first-generation cephalosporins are destroyed by beta-lactamases and have minimal ability to concentrate in the cerebrospinal fluid (CSF). Oral forms are not affected by food. They are best taken with food to decrease the GI upset that accompanies their use.

Second-Generation Cephalosporins

Second-generation cephalosporins include cefaclor, cefprozil, and loracarbef, which are available for oral administration; cefuroxime, which is available in oral, IM, or IV preparations; cefamandole, cefoxitin, cefonicid, and cefotetan, which are available for IM or IV administration; and cefmetazole, which is available for IV administration only. These drugs are less sensitive to destruction by beta-lactamases than first-generation drugs but still cannot achieve significant concentrations in the CSF to be effective.

The second-generation cephalosporins have broader coverage against gram-negative bacteria. This occurs because they have an increased ability to penetrate the gram-negative cell envelope and an increased affinity for PBPs of gram-negative bacteria.

In addition to the same uses as first-generation cephalosporins, second-generation cephalosporins are used to treat lower respiratory tract infections caused by *Bacteroides*; dermatologic infections caused by *Staphylococcus epidermidis*, *Bacteroides*, *Clostridium*, *Peptococcus*, *Peptostreptococcus*; urinary tract infections (UTIs) caused by *M. morganii*, *Proteus vulgaris*; uncomplicated gonorrhea caused by *Neisseria gonorrhoeae*; intra-abdominal infections caused by *E. coli*, *Klebsiella*, *Bacteroides*, *Clostridium*; gynecologic infections caused by *E. coli*, *N. gonorrhoeae*, *Bacteroides*, *Clostridium*, *Peptococcus*, *Peptostreptococcus*; and septicemia caused by *Bacteroides*.

Cefotetan and cefmetazole may induce two additional adverse effects. They may induce bleeding tendencies or disulfiram-like reactions. Cefotetan and cefmetazole have been associated with the reduction of prothrombin levels by interfering with vitamin K metabolism. This may induce bleeding tendencies. Patients receiving these drugs should be monitored for signs and symptoms of bleeding. The nurse should advise the patient to stop the drug immediately if any signs of bleeding occur and notify the health care provider. The nurse should also advise the patient to avoid aspirin, other nonsteroidal anti-inflammatory drugs, or other anticoagulants throughout therapy.

Patients who consume alcohol during therapy with cefotetan and cefmetazole may experience a disulfiram-like reaction. Symptoms include flushing, shortness of breath, nausea and vomiting, chest pains, palpitations, dizziness and faintness, confusion, sweating, blurred vision, and possibly respiratory depression, seizures, and unconsciousness. The nurse should advise patients who take these cephalosporins to avoid alcohol for 72 hours after the completion of therapy.

Third-Generation Cephalosporins

Third-generation cephalosporins include the oral drugs cefixime, cefpodoxime, and ceftibuten and the IM and IV drugs cefoperazone, cefotaxime, ceftizoxime, ceftriaxone, and ceftazidime. These drugs are highly resistant to destruction by beta-lactamases as well have highly effective against gram-negative aerobes. Ceftazidime is especially effective for bacterial strains resistant to aminoglycosides and is also effective against *P. aeruginosa*. This generation of cephalosporins is used for more severe infections or in immunocompromised patients. The exception is ceftriaxone, which is the drug of choice for gonorrhea. With the exception of cefoperazone and cefixime, third-generation cephalosporins can penetrate the blood-brain barrier to treat CNS infections caused by *E. coli*, *H. influenzae*, *Neisseria meningitidis*, *S. pneumoniae*, and *Klebsiella pneumoniae*. They are also effective against *Serratia marcescens* and *Citrobacter*.

Cefoperazone, a third-generation cephalosporin, is similar to the second-generation cephalosporins cefotetan and cefmetazole. It, too, may also induce bleeding tendencies. The nurse should educate the patient as described in the the section on second-generation cephalosporins.

Cefamandole, another third-generation cephalosporin, may induce a disifulram-like reaction similar to cefotetan and cefmetazole. The nurse should advise patients receiving cefamandole to refrain from alcohol intake for 72 hours after the completion of therapy.

Fourth-Generation Cephalosporin

Cefepime is the first fourth-generation cephalosporin. It is active against both gram-positive and gram-negative organisms. It has a greater spectrum than third-generation drugs and is more active against organisms such as *Pseudomonas aeruginosa* or *Enterobacteriaceae* that have developed resistance to third-generation drugs and has good penetration into the CSF. Like third-generation cephalosporins, cefepine is highly resistant to destruction by beta-lactamases.

VANCOMYCIN

Vancomycin (Vancocin) is a complex and unusual tricyclic glycopeptide antibiotic. It is the only drug in its class. The use of vancomycin is limited by its ability to produce toxic effects. Because of its toxicity, vancomycin is used only when other antibiotics fail to resolve an infection. It has been touted as able to eradicate most gram-positive pathogens; however, the emergence of vancomycin-resistant enterocolitis (VRE) has become problematic.

NURSING MANAGEMENT OF THE PATIENT RECEIVING VANCOMYCIN

Core Drug Knowledge

Pharmacotherapeutics

Vancomycin is used in treating bacterial septicemia, endocarditis, bone and joint infections, and pseudomembranous colitis caused by *Clostridium difficile*. It is effective for most strains of *Staphylococcus aureus* and *Staphylococcus epidermidis*; streptococci, including enterococci; *Corynebacterium*; and *Clostridium*. Vancomycin is exceptionally effective for treating gram-positive infections in penicillin-allergic patients. It is also used for penicillin- and methicillin-resistant staphylococcal infections.

Vancomycin is used with aminoglycosides to combat *Streptococcus faecalis* and methicillin-resistant organisms. However, this synergism also increases possible toxicity.

Gram-negative bacteria and mycobacteria are resistant to vancomycin. Vancomycin is not used in treating meningitis because of poor penetration into CSF.

Pharmacokinetics

Oral bioavailability of vancomycin is extremely low; therefore, it is generally administered intravenously. Oral administration is used in treating some GI infections, such as pseudomembranous colitis. Some patients, especially those with renal impairment, have developed detectable vancomycin serum levels following oral administration.

After intravenous administration, plasma concentrations reach a peak approximately 1 hour after infusion. In patients with normal renal function, vancomycin has a serum half-life of 4 to 6 hours, but in elderly patients or those with renal impairment, half-life can be as long as 146 hours.

Vancomycin is distributed widely into most body tissues and fluids, including pericardial, pleural, ascitic, synovial, and the meninges if they are inflamed. It is not known whether any metabolism takes place. Excretion is mainly by glomerular filtration with only small amounts excreted in the feces. With oral administration, excretion is mainly fecal.

Pharmacodynamics

Vancomycin is bactericidal because it inhibits cell wall synthesis by altering the cell's permeability. Vancomycin also inhibits the synthesis of ribonucleic acid (RNA). Because of this dual mechanism of action, resistance to vancomycin has been limited to strains of group D *Streptococcus*. There is no direct effect on the body.

Contraindications and Precautions

Vancomycin is contraindicated for patients with a hypersensitivity to it and for pregnant patients. Although it is excreted into breast milk, vancomycin is not contraindicated for breast-feeding women. Breast-feeding neonates and infants, however, should have vancomycin concentration monitoring to avoid potential toxicities. It is used with caution in patients with renal disease, such as renal failure or renal impairment. It should also be used with caution in patients receiving other drugs with the potential for nephrotoxicity, such as aminoglycosides.

Oral vancomycin should be used with caution in patients with inflammatory bowel disease because this disorder increases the absorption of oral vancomycin, thereby increasing the risk for toxicity.

Adverse Effects

The most serious toxicities caused by vancomycin are ototoxicity and nephrotoxicity. Ototoxicity can take the form of cochlear toxicity (tinnitus, hearing loss) or vestibular toxicity (ataxia, vertigo, nausea and vomiting, nystagmus).

Nephrotoxicity can also occur with vancomycin, although its incidence has decreased. Besides elevated serum concentrations, nephrotoxicity is more likely to occur in patients receiving other nephrotoxic drugs, such as aminoglycosides. Cases of interstitial nephritis, a hypersensitivity reaction, have been reported.

Vancomycin can cause histamine release, resulting in anaphylactoid reactions. Symptoms include fever, chills, sinus tachycardia, and pruritus. Paresthesias, flushing, rash, or redness in the face, neck, upper body, arms, or back are also symptoms of histamine release. In some cases, hypotension occurs. Because of the presenting symptoms, this histamine-release reaction is often called the "red man" or "red neck" syndrome. Other adverse reactions include phlebitis or other injection site reactions, leukopenia, and thrombocytopenia.

Drug Interactions

Orally administered vancomycin should be avoided in patients receiving antihyperlipidemic drugs. Vancomycin should be used with caution in combination with other drugs that have potential nephrotoxic or ototoxic effects and in patients receiving nondepolarizing muscle relaxants. Table 48-6 presents drugs that interact with vancomycin.

Assessment of Relevant Core Patient Variables

Health Status

The nurse should assess the patient for contraindications or precautions to the use of vancomycin, including other drugs with potential nephrotoxicity and ototoxicity. Lower doses of vancomycin are recommended for

TABLE 48-6 Agents That Interact With Vancomycin

Interactants	Effect and Significance	Nursing Management
antihyperlipidemic drugs cholestyramine colestipol	These antihyperlipidemic agents are anion-exchange resins and can bind with vancomycin, resulting in a decreased effectiveness.	Separate administration of these drugs by 3–4 h. Monitor efficacy of vancomycin therapy.
nephrotoxic drugs aminoglycosides amphotericin B bacitracin cisplatin cyclosporine polymyxin B	Parenteral vancomycin with other nephrotoxic drugs can lead to additive risks for nephrotoxicity.	Monitor renal function closely. Consider lower doses of vancomycin.
nondepolarizing muscle relaxants atracurium gallamine metocurine pancuronium pipecuronium tubocurarine vecuronium	Vancomycin may affect presynaptic and postsynaptic myoneural function and act synergistically with nondepolarizing muscle relaxants. This may result in additive neuromuscular blockade.	Avoid this combination when possible. When given, monitor neuromuscular function closely, and be prepared to initiate mechanical ventilation.
ototoxic drugs aminoglycosides salicylates ethacrynic acid furosemide paromomycin	Parenteral vancomycin with other ototoxic drugs can lead to additive risks for ototoxicity.	Monitor sensory/hearing functions closely. Consider lower doses of vancomycin.

patients with renal dysfunction or in patients receiving other ototoxic or nephrotoxic drugs. The nurse should also assess gross hearing in patients with preexisting hearing impairment. Periodic audiograms may be necessary during therapy. For patients with expected long-term therapy, a baseline CBC and hepatic and renal function tests should be performed, and the nurse should consult with the health care provider about any laboratory abnormalities before vancomycin therapy begins.

Life Span and Gender

The nurse should explore the contraceptive method of the woman of child-bearing age and assess for pregnancy and lactation. Vancomycin should not be given to the pregnant woman and should be given cautiously to the breast-feeding woman. The nurse should note if the patient is elderly because such patients are at a higher risk of toxicity and drug accumulation secondary to age-related decreases in renal function.

Environment

The nurse should be aware of the environment in which the drug will be administered. Vancomycin is generally administered in an inpatient setting. This is because of the potentially serious toxicities and the need to monitor closely vancomycin serum concentrations.

Nursing Diagnoses and Outcomes

- Risk for Injury related to drug-induced histamine-release reactions

  Desired outcome: The patient will experience no preventable reaction related to vancomycin.
- Disturbed Sensory Perception (auditory) related to drug-induced ototoxicity

  Desired outcome: The patient will report any unusual auditory sensations and have periodic audiograms to detect early ototoxicity.
- Excess Fluid Volume related to nephrotoxicity from drug therapy

  Desired outcome: The patient will remain normovolemic throughout therapy.

Planning and Intervention

Maximizing Therapeutic Effects

The nurse should ensure that the patient receives the full course of vancomycin as prescribed, divided around the clock to increase effectiveness. The nurse should also coordinate the administration of drugs to decrease potential drug-drug interactions. In addition, culture and sensitivity results should be monitored to be sure that vancomycin is the drug of choice for this patient.

Minimizing Adverse Effects

The nurse should administer vancomycin over at least 60 minutes. This will diminish effects such as flushing, tachycardia, hypotension, or rashes that occur when administration is too fast.

Ototoxicity after IV administration is believed to be associated with serum concentration ranges above 60 to 80 μg/mL, which may occur when doses are too large or infused too rapidly. Too-rapid IV administration of vancomycin may also lead to red man syndrome. In addition, the nurse must take care to avoid extravasation because vancomycin is extremely irritating to tissues.

Peak and trough levels are terms associated with serum concentration measurements. The nurse should obtain the peak serum level 1 hour after the initiation of the infusion and the trough serum level 30 minutes before beginning the next infusion. The risk for nephrotoxicity is minimized if trough serum concentrations are kept below 10 μg/mL, although nephrotoxicity can still occur in patients with therapeutic concentrations.

Providing Patient and Family Education

- The nurse should advise the patient of the importance of completing therapy.
- The nurse should explain the potential adverse effects and need for periodic blood monitoring.
- The nurse should advise the patient to report symptoms such as tinnitus, hearing loss, vertigo, or nausea and vomiting.
- The nurse should also teach the patient the importance of accurate intake and output measurements.

Ongoing Assessment and Evaluation

Elderly patients may need vancomycin concentration monitoring because of a higher risk of toxicity and drug accumulation secondary to age-related decreases in renal function.

MEMORY CHIP

Vancomycin

- Used for serious gram-positive infections, especially *Clostridium difficile* and methicillin-resistant *Staphylococcus aureus.*
- Significant contraindications: hypersensitivity and pregnancy
- Most common adverse effects: histamine release resulting in "red-man" syndrome
- Most serious adverse effects: ototoxicity and nephrotoxicity
- **Life span alert: Elderly patients may need vancomycin concentration monitoring because of a higher risk of toxicity and drug accumulation secondary to age-related decreases in renal function.**
- Maximizing therapeutic effects: Obtain culture and sensitivity before administration
- Minimizing adverse effects: Administer over 60 minutes
- Most significant patient education: Need for periodic CBC when taking for prolonged period or high doses. Need to advise the health care team for changes in hearing.

The nurse must monitor for signs of ototoxicity. Factors that may increase the risk of developing ototoxicity include excessive dose, serum concentrations above 60 μg/mL, prolonged exposure to the drug, multiple ototoxic drugs, dehydration, noise, and bacteremia. The nurse should assess for symptoms, such as ataxia and nystagmus, that may indicate ototoxicity. The nurse should also monitor intake and output to assess for potential nephrotoxicity.

For patients receiving long-term or high-dose therapy, the nurse should coordinate periodic audiometric testing and serial CBCs, LFTs, and kidney function tests. As with other potent antibiotics, the nurse should monitor for signs of superinfection. At the end of therapy, the patient should be free of the presenting infection and any adverse effects resolved. ■

CHAPTER SUMMARY

- Penicillins are classified as narrow spectrum, penicillinase-resistant, aminopenicillins (broad spectrum), and extended-spectrum (antipseudomonal) penicillins. They are also known as a beta-lactam antibiotic.
- Penicillins may be inactivated by beta-lactamases, an enzyme produced by the bacteria. Use of penicillinase-resistant penicillins, or penicillins in combination with drugs such as clavulanic acid, tazobactam, and sulbactam decreases the effects of penicillinase.
- Penicillins are most effective against gram-positive bacteria since they have difficulty penetrating the gram-negative cell envelope.
- Penicillins are the safest antibiotics available, except in patients with a hypersensitivity to penicillin.
- Penicillins can be administered orally, intramuscularly, or intravenously.
- Patients with a questionable history of penicillin allergy should receive skin testing prior to administration.
- Patients with a hypersensitivity to one penicillin should be considered allergic to all penicillins.
- Patients with a documented penicillin allergy should wear a medic-alert necklace or bracelet.
- Imipenem is also a beta-lactam antibiotic. It has the broadest spectrum of activity of all antibiotics.
- Monobactam and carbapenem antibiotics are also beta-lactam antibiotics
- Cephalosporin antibiotics are the most widely used antibiotic today.
- Cephalosporin antibiotics are structurally similar to penicillins. Between 5% and 10% of patients with a hypersensitivity to penicillin will also react to cephalosporins.
- Cephalosporin antibiotics are grouped according to "generations."
- As cephalosporin generations progress, there is increasing activity against gram-negative bacteria and anaerobes, increasing resistance to destruction by beta-lactamases, and increasing ability to reach the CSF.
- Most of the cephalosporins are administered parenterally. Only 11 of 23 cephalosporins currently on the market may be given orally.
- Cefotetan and cefmetazole, both second-generation cephalosporins and cefoperazone, a third-generation cephalosporin, may induce bleeding tendencies.
- Cefotetan and cefamandole, both second-generation cephalosporins and cefoperazone, a third-generation cephalosporin, may induce a disulfiram-like reaction during therapy when combined with alcohol.
- Vancomycin is very effective against most gram-positive infections, however, its use is limited by its potential to cause severe adverse effects.
- Vancomycin is the drug of choice for pseudomembranous colitis caused by *C. difficile,* infections caused by methicillin-resistant *Staphylococcus aureus* and serious infections in penicillin allergic patients.

QUESTIONS FOR STUDY AND REVIEW

1. How do penicillins work?
2. Why are most penicillins ineffective against gram-negative bacteria?
3. Why are there four classifications of penicillins?
4. Why are clavulanic acid, tazobactam, and sulbactam added to some penicillin preparations?
5. What is the difference between the generations of cephalosporins?
6. What classes of antibiotics are called beta-lactam antibiotics? Why?
7. Why is vancomycin reserved for serious infections?

NEED MORE HELP?

? Chapter 48 of the study guide for *Drug Therapy in Nursing* contains exercises and activities to reinforce your understanding of the concepts presented in this chapter. For additional information see the text's accompanying website at *http://www.connection.lww.com.*

REFERENCES AND BIBLIOGRAPHY

Anonymous. (2000). Update: penicillin G availability, *MMWR Morbidity and Mortality Weekly Report, 49*(3), 61–71.

Bryan, C. S. (1999). Treatment of pneumococcal pneumonia: The case for penicillin G., *American Journal of Medicine, 107*(1A), 63S–68S.

CCIS System. (2001). *Computerized Clinical Information System.* Denver, CO: Micromedex.

Clinical Drug Monographs [CDRom]. (2001). Gold Standard Media.

Drug Facts and Comparisons. (2000). St. Louis: Facts and Comparisons Division

Hardman, J. G., Limbird, L. E., Molinof, P. B., Ruddon, R. W., & Gilman, A. (Eds.). (1997). *Goodman and Gilman's the pharmacological basis of therapeutics* (9th ed.). New York: McGraw-Hill.

Karch, A. (2001). *2001 Lippincott's nursing drug guide.* Philadelphia: Lippincott Williams & Wilkins

Katzung, B. (1998). *Basic and clinical pharmacology* (7th Ed.), Stamford: Appleton & Lange

Marchese, A., Schito, G. C., & Debbia, E. A. (2000). Evolution of antibiotic resistance in gram-positive pathogens. *Journal of Chemotherapy, 12*(6), 459–462.

Marshall, W. F., & Blair, J. E. (1999). The cephalosporins. *Mayo Clinic Proceedings, 74*(2), 187–195.

McCracken, G. H., Jr. (1999). Prescribing antimicrobial agents for treatment of acute otitis media, *Pediatric Infectious Disease Journal, 18*(12), 1141–1146.

Massova, I., & Mobashery, S. (1999). Structural and mechanistic aspects of evolution of beta-lactamases and penicillin-binding proteins. *Current Pharmaceutical Design, 5*(11), 929–937.

Porth, C. (1998). *Pathophysiology: Concepts of altered health states* (5th ed.). Philadelphia: Lippincott Williams & Wilkins.

Tatro, D. (Ed.). (2000). *Drug interaction facts* (6th ed.). St. Louis: Facts and Comparisons.

Chapter 49

ANTIBIOTICS AFFECTING PROTEIN SYNTHESIS

KEY TERMS

azotemia
cylindruria
hyposthenuria
nephrotoxicity
ototoxicity
peak and trough
proteinuria
pyuria
xeroderma
xerophthalmia

Learning Objectives

At the completion of this chapter the student will:

1. Identify core drug knowledge pertaining to drugs affecting protein synthesis.
2. Identify core patient variables pertaining to drugs affecting protein synthesis.
3. Relate the interaction of core drug knowledge to core patient variables for drugs affecting protein synthesis.
4. Generate a nursing plan of care from the interactions between core drug knowledge and core patient variables for drugs affecting protein synthesis.
5. Describe nursing interventions to maximize therapeutic and minimize adverse effects for drugs affecting protein synthesis.
6. Determine key points for patient and family education for drugs affecting protein synthesis.

Aminoglycosides
- **gentamicin**
- amikacin
- kanamycin
- neomycin
- netilmicin
- tobramycin
- paromomycin
- streptomycin

Lincosamides
- **clindamycin**
- lincomycin

Macrolide antibiotics
- **erythromycin**
- azithromycin
- clarithromycin
- troleandomycin
- dirithromycin

Oxazolidinones
- **linezolid**

Streptogramins
- **quinupristin/dalfopristin**

Tetracyclines
- **tetracycline**
- doxycycline
- minocycline
- demeclocycline

Miscellaneous antibiotics that affect protein synthesis
- **chloramphenicol**
- spectomycin

The symbol C indicates the **drug class**.

Drugs in bold type marked with the symbol P are **prototypes**.

Drugs in blue type with no symbol are **closely related** to the prototype.

Drugs in **red** type with no symbol are **significantly different** from the prototype.

Drugs in **black** type with no symbol are **also used in drug therapy**; no prototype.

Drugs affecting protein synthesis include aminoglycoside agents, lincosamide agents, macrolide agents, oxazolidinone, streptogramins, tetracyclines, and miscellaneous antibiotics.

The prototype drugs discussed in this chapter include the aminoglycoside prototype gentamicin, the lincosamide prototype clindamycin, the macrolide prototype erythromycin, the oxazolidinone prototype linezolid, the streptogramin prototype quinupristin/dalfopristin, the tetracycline prototype tetracycline, as well as the miscellaneous antibiotics chloramphenicol and spectinomycin.

In addition to explaining how these drugs work, this chapter discusses nursing management related to evaluating the patient's condition, monitoring the patient's response, and teaching the patient and family about antibiotic therapy.

PHYSIOLOGY

The process of protein synthesis is divided into two sections: transcription and translation. Initially, transcription occurs within the nucleus by producing messenger ribonucleic acid (mRNA). This mRNA migrates from the nucleus to the cytoplasm. During this step, mRNA goes through different types of maturation including one called splicing when the noncoding sequences are eliminated. The coding mRNA sequence can be described as a unit of three nucleotides called a codon.

Translation occurs in the cytoplasm. The ribosome binds to the mRNA at the start codon (AUG) that is recognized only by initiator tRNA (transfer ribonucleic acid). The ribosome proceeds to the elongation phase of protein synthesis. During this stage, complexes, which are composed of an amino acid linked to tRNA, sequentially bind to the appropriate codon in mRNA by forming complementary base pairs with the tRNA anticodon. The ribosome moves from codon to codon along the mRNA. Amino acids are added one by one, translated into polypeptidic sequences dictated by DNA and represented by mRNA. At the end, a release factor binds to the stop codon, terminating translation and releasing the complete polypeptide from the ribosome. Figure 49-1 illustrates the process of protein synthesis.

AMINOGLYCOSIDES

The aminoglycosides are extremely effective antibiotics for treating severe infections. Their general use, however, is limited because of the potential for serious adverse effects. As newer aminoglycosides are developed, older drugs are used less frequently, although each has a specific organism against which it is still the most effective drug. Aminoglycosides include gentamicin, amikacin, kanamycin, netilmicin, neomycin, tobramycin, paromomycin, and streptomycin. Gentamicin (Garamycin) is the prototype drug for the aminoglycoside family.

NURSING MANAGEMENT OF THE PATIENT RECEIVING GENTAMICIN

Core Drug Knowledge

Pharmacotherapeutics

Clinically, gentamicin is useful for urinary tract infections (UTIs), such as pyelonephritis; gynecologic infections; peritonitis; endocarditis; pneumonia; bacteremia

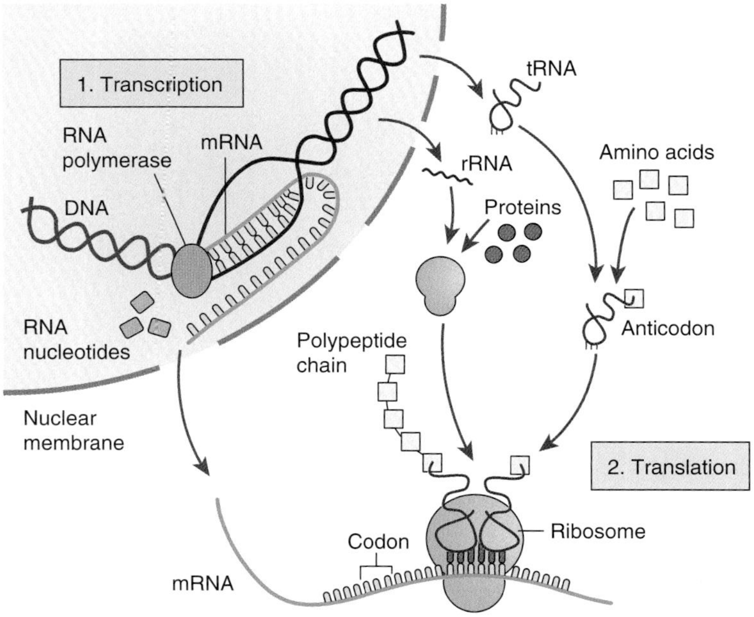

Figure 49-1. Protein synthesis.

and sepsis; respiratory infections, including those associated with cystic fibrosis; osteomyelitis; and foot and other soft-tissue infections associated with diabetes.

Gentamicin is effective in the management of gram-negative bacilli. Susceptible organisms include *Pseudomonas aeruginosa*, *Proteus mirabilis*, *Escherichia coli*, *Klebsiella*, *Enterobacter* species, *Serratia* species, *Citrobacter*, and the staphylococci. Gentamicin must be transported across the cell membrane in order to enter the cell and disrupt protein synthesis. This process is oxygen dependent, therefore, gentamicin and other aminoglycosides are ineffective in the management of anaerobes. Gentamicin is not considered useful in treating meningitis unless it is administered intrathecally in the presence of inflamed meninges.

Gentamicin is also indicated for topical treatment of susceptible eye or skin infections caused by susceptible organisms, as an orphan drug indication on impregnated polymethylmethacrylate (PMAA) beads on surgical wire for treating chronic osteomyelitis, and as a liposome injection for treating disseminated *Mycobacterium avium-intracellulare* infection.

Pharmacokinetics

Parenteral gentamicin is widely distributed through the body in extracellular fluids; however, it does not penetrate appreciably into the central nervous system (CNS). It crosses the placenta and is secreted in breast milk. Gentamicin concentrates in the kidney reaching levels 50 times higher than serum. It also concentrates in the endolymph and perilymph of the inner ear. These higher concentrations of gentamicin are associated with its major adverse effects—**nephrotoxicity** and **ototoxicity**. Parenteral gentamicin is excreted unchanged in urine whereas oral gentamicin is excreted unchanged in feces (Table 49-1).

Because of its poor oral absorption, gentamicin is usually reserved for parenteral or topical use. It may, however, be given orally to exert a local effect on the gastrointestinal (GI) tract to decrease bacteria before surgical or invasive procedures.

Pharmacodynamics

Gentamicin, like all antibiotics, has no direct effect on the body. It exerts its effect by entering the bacterial cell and binding to the 30S ribosomes. This leads to a misreading of the protein formation information within the cell. The cell then produces amino acids that do not link correctly. The result is a change in metabolic function that in turn prevents bacterial reproduction and weakens the cell wall, leading to cell wall rupture and death. Many strains of bacteria are resistant to the aminoglycosides and do not allow them to enter the cell. Because of this, aminoglycosides are often given with synergistic antibiotics to increase their effectiveness or to alter the cell wall so that the aminoglycoside can enter.

Contraindications and Precautions

Gentamicin is contraindicated during pregnancy and lactation. It is also contraindicated in patients with known allergy to any aminoglycoside. It is used cautiously in patients with renal or hepatic disease, dehydration, preexisting hearing loss, myasthenia gravis, parkinsonism, and infant botulism.

Adverse Effects

Many serious side effects are associated with gentamicin, limiting its usefulness. The most well-known adverse effects are nephrotoxicity, ototoxicity, and neuromuscular blockade.

In the CNS, gentamicin therapy may induce confusion, depression, disorientation, numbness, tingling, and weakness. Leukemoid reactions and depressed bone marrow are potential adverse effects in the hematologic system. GI symptoms include nausea, vomiting, diarrhea, weight loss, stomatitis, and hepatic toxicity. Gentamicin may induce palpitations, hypotension, and hypertension in the cardiovascular system. Hypersensitivity reactions include purpura, rash, urticaria, and exfoliative dermatitis. Other adverse effects, such as superinfections, fever, apnea, and joint pain, may also occur.

Drug Interactions

Gentamicin may interact with other drugs that are known to be ototoxic, nephrotoxic, or neurotoxic. These drugs include acyclovir, amphotericin B, other aminoglycosides, cisplatin, cyclosporine, vancomycin, ethacrynic acid, and furosemide. Gentamicin may also interact with anesthetics, nondepolarizing neuromuscular blockers, succinylcholine, citrate-anticoagulated blood, indomethacin, and penicillins (Table 49-2).

Assessment of Relevant Core Patient Variables

Health Status

In assessing the health status of the patient taking gentamicin, the nurse should elicit a thorough health history, particularly the renal history. Because gentamicin is excreted unchanged by glomerular filtration, patients with renal dysfunction or dehydration are at risk for nephrotoxicity. The nurse should also evaluate patients for a history of hearing impairment and eighth cranial nerve impairment because these patients have an increased risk of ototoxicity. The nurse should investigate any history of myasthenia gravis or parkinsonism and botulism in infants. Gentamicin may cause severe neuromuscular weakness lasting hours to days because of its potential curare-like effect, and it may aggravate muscle weakness in patients with these disorders.

The nurse should perform a baseline gross hearing test prior to administration of gentamicin. The nurse should

TABLE 49-1 Summary of Selected Aminoglycoside Antibiotics

Drug (Trade) Name	Selected Indications	Route and Dosage Range	Pharmacokinetics
gentamicin (Garamycin; *Canadian:* Alcomicin)	Gram-negative infections Staphylococcal infections	*Adults:* IM/IV, 3–5 mg/kg/d in divided doses *Child:* 6–7.5 mg/kg in divided doses *Infants and neonates:* 7.5 mg/kg in divided doses q8h	*Onset:* Rapid *Duration:* 6–8 h $t_{1/2}$: 2–3 h
amikacin (Amikin)	Gram-negative infections Staphylococcal infections	*Adult:* IM/IV, 15 mg/kg/d *Child:* Same as adults *Neonate:* IM/IV 10 mg/kg initially then 7.5 mg/kg q12h	*Onset:* IM, varies; IV, immediate *Duration:* 6–8 h $t_{1/2}$: 2–3 h
kanamycin (kantrex)	*Escherichia coli* and other infectious agents Suppression of intestinal flora	*Adult:* IM, 15 mg/kg/d; IV, dilute 500-mg vial with 100–200 mL sterile diluent per day PO, 1 g every hour for 4 h then 1 g q6h for 36–72 h	*Onset:* IM/IV, rapid *Duration:* 8–12 h $t_{1/2}$: 2–3 h
netilmicin (Netromycin)	Complicated urinary tract infections Septicemia Intra-abdominal infections	*Adult:* IM/IV, 4–6.5 mg/kg q8–12h *Child:* (6 wk–12 years): IM/IV, 5.5–8 mg/kg q8–12h *Neonate:* (<6 wk): 4–6.5 mg/kg q12h	*Onset:* IM, rapid; IV, immediate *Duration:* 12–16 h $t_{1/2}$: 2.0–2.5 h
neomycin (Mycifradin Sulfate)	Preoperative suppression of intestinal bacteria	*Adult:* 1 g at 19, 18 and 9 h before surgery	*Onset:* PO, varies *Duration:* 6–8 h $t_{1/2}$: 3 h
	Hepatic coma	*Adult:* 4–12 g/d	
tobramycin (Nebcin; *Canadian:* Tomycine)	Gram-negative infections especially *Pseudomonas* staphylococcal infections, burns Soft tissue wounds	*Adult and Child:* 3–5 mg/kg every 12 h *Neonate:* (<1 week): IM/IV: up to 4 mg/kg every 12 h	*Onset:* Rapid *Duration:* 8–12 h $t_{1/2}$: 2–3 h
streptomycin	Nontuberculosis infections	*Adult:* IM, 1–2 g/d in divided doses *Child:* IM, 20–40 mg/kg/d q12h	*Onset:* Rapid *Duration:* 8–12 h $t_{1/2}$: 2.5 h
	Tuberculosis	*Adult:* IM, 15 mg/kg 2–3 times a week (max 1.5 g per dose)	
paromomycin (Humatin)	Intestinal amebiasis	*Adult and Child:* 25–35 mg/kg/d in three divided doses	*Onset:* Poorly absorbed *Duration:* Excreted $t_{1/2}$: Unchanged in feces
	Hepatic coma	*Adult:* 4 g/d in divided doses	

also evaluate laboratory test results indicating the renal and hepatic function of the patient.

Life Span and Gender

It is important for the nurse to evaluate women for potential pregnancy. Although gentamicin is not absolutely contraindicated during pregnancy, it has been found to be ototoxic to the fetus. The nurse should evaluate neonates (younger than 1 month) and patients older than 65 years frequently because they have increased risk for nephrotoxicity due to decreased renal function.

Lifestyle, Diet, and Habits

The nurse should assess the nutritional status of the patient. Patients on restricted oral intake or patients who eat poorly have an increased risk for hypomagnesemia during gentamicin therapy. Dehydrated patients have an increased risk for nephrotoxicity.

Environment

The nurse should be aware of the environment in which gentamicin will be administered and if appropriate assess the home or living environment for potential risk factors. Parenteral gentamicin is usually administered in the acute hospital setting, however, it may also be given in the home environment by a home health care nurse. Oral gentamicin may be given in any environment.

In the hospital setting, the nurse should store gentamicin in the refrigerator and be sure that it does not freeze. Before administration, gentamicin solution should be inspected for discoloration or particulates. After administration, any unused solution should be discarded.

TABLE 49-2 Agents That Interact With Gentamicin

Interactants	Effect and Significance	Nursing Management
ototoxic, nephrotoxic, and neurotoxic drugs: acyclovir, amphotericin B, aminoglycosides, cisplatin, cyclosporine, vancomycin, ethacrynic acid, furosemide, prostaglandin synthetase inhibitors	Risk of ototoxicity, nephrotoxicity, and neurotoxicity and neurotoxic effects is increased when these drugs are coadministered with gentamicin.	Avoid these combinations if possible. Monitor serum concentrations Conduct baseline hearing test before coadministration begins. Monitor for hearing change daily. Monitor intake and output. Conduct baseline kidney function tests. Monitor kidney function tests for prolonged therapy. Reduce dose of one or both drugs as needed.
indomethacin	Indomethacin may increase serum aminoglycoside concentrations in premature infants receiving indomethacin for patent ductus arteriosus.	Monitor serum gentamicin levels. Monitor for signs of toxicity.
neuromuscular blockers and citrate-anticoagulated blood	The actions of neuromuscular blockers and citrate-anticoagulated blood may be enhanced, resulting in protracted neuromuscular blockade.	Mark patient's chart and arrange for extended monitoring and support of the patient following anesthesia. Monitor respirations and other vital signs.
extended penicillins: carbenicillin, ticarcillin	Extended penicillins may inactivate aminoglycosides.	Avoid combination therapy if possible. Administer at least 2 h apart.
penicillin and cephalosporins	Synergistic bacterial action when coadministered.	This is a beneficial interaction.

Nursing Diagnoses and Outcomes

- Risk for Injury related to potential drug-related allergic reactions or neuromuscular blockade or bone marrow suppression
  Desired outcome: The patient will remain free of injury and will contact the prescriber if unusual adverse effects occur.
- Diarrhea related to drug effects
  Desired outcome: The patient will avoid dehydration, maintain fluid intake, and contact the health care provider if diarrhea persists.
- Imbalanced Nutrition: Less than Body Requirements related to drug-induced GI effects or superinfection
  Desired outcome: The patient will maintain body weight and report to the health care provider any persistent adverse effects that affect nutritional status.
- Risk for Injury related to CNS effects
  Desired outcome: The patient will remain free of injury and contact the provider if confusion, disorientation, or depression occur.
- Disturbed Sensory Perception related to potential ototoxicity
  Desired outcome: The patient will report sensory or perceptual changes to the prescriber.
- Excess Fluid Volume related to potential nephrotoxicity
  Desired outcome: The patient will report any weight gain exceeding 3 lb to the health care prescriber.

Planning and Intervention

Maximizing Therapeutic Effects

The nurse should make sure that patients receive the full course of gentamicin as prescribed at around-the-clock intervals; coordinate the administration of drugs to decrease potential drug interactions; and evaluate culture and sensitivity reports to make sure that gentamicin is the appropriate drug.

Because gentamicin may be inactivated by extended penicillins, such as carbenicillin or ticarcillin, the nurse must administer these drugs at least 2 hours apart to ensure the efficacy of gentamicin.

Minimizing Adverse Effects

To reduce the occurrence of adverse effects, it is imperative to maintain blood levels of gentamicin within a therapeutic margin that is very narrow. To do this, **peak and trough** drug levels are monitored throughout therapy. Blood for peak levels is drawn 30 minutes after IV administration and 1 hour after IM administration. Blood for trough levels is drawn just prior to the next dose.

Safety measures should be instituted to protect the patient if CNS effects occur. Small, frequent meals can be arranged for patients with GI effects and frequent mouth care and ice chips can be offered to relieve stomatitis and sore mouth.

The nurse should also monitor the hydration status of the patient to minimize potential renal toxicity from gentamicin. The nurse should monitor the patient for gentamicin-induced diarrhea because diarrhea may also cause dehydration.

If a patient receiving gentamicin requires surgery, that gentamicin has been given should be indicated prominently on the chart. Remember that gentamicin may interact with neuromuscular blocking agents commonly used during surgery, which results in a prolongation of neuromuscular blockade. The patient will require extended monitoring and support after surgery to detect and intervene for problems should they occur.

Providing Patient and Family Education

- It is important that patients understand that they should not take gentamicin or any other aminoglycoside antibiotic if they have ever had a reaction to a drug with a generic name that ends in the suffixes -mycin or -micin.
- Patients should be advised that they should not take this drug if they are pregnant or breast-feeding.
- The nurse should advise the patient to take oral gentamicin on an empty stomach, 1 hour before or 2 hours after any meal or other drugs. Patients should also be instructed to take forgotten doses as soon as they remember, not to double the dose, and to contact the prescriber if symptoms do not improve in 3 days.
- The nurse should teach the patient how to identify, report, and manage signs and symptoms of allergic reaction and adverse effects, especially those that may signal nephrotoxicity or ototoxicity.
- The nurse should teach the patient how to recognize superinfection or CNS effects such as confusion, depression, numbness, tingling, or weakness and explain the importance of contacting the health care provider if any of these symptoms occur.
- The nurse should help the patient develop strategies for minimizing GI upset and oral soreness.
- The nurse should show patients how to use gentamicin eye drops correctly, making sure to stress the importance of keeping the dropper portion of the bottle from touching the eye to avoid contamination.

Ongoing Assessment and Evaluation

The nurse should coordinate the care of the patient to ensure other potentially nephrotoxic or ototoxic drugs are not added to the treatment plan. The primary health care provider should be notified if this occurs. Another important role of the nurse is to monitor peak and trough levels of gentamicin. Although it is commonly believed that maintaining gentamicin serum concentrations within traditional ranges minimizes the risk of nephrotoxicity, some patients may still develop nephrotoxicity. Acute tubular necrosis is the most common gentamicin-induced nephrotoxicity. The nurse should monitor for **azotemia** (excessive urea levels in the blood), decreased creatinine clearance, **hyposthenuria** (loss of the ability to concentrate urine), **pyuria** (increased white blood cell count), **proteinuria**, and **cylindruria** (cells or casts in the urine).

The nurse should also evaluate for signs of ototoxicity. Gentamicin may induce both cochlear and vestibular damage to the inner ear. Cochlear damage, a high-frequency hearing loss, may be preceded by high-pitched tinnitus. Cochlear damage may be subtle, therefore, the nurse should coordinate referrals for audiologic testing for patients who receive repeated or prolonged courses of gentamicin therapy. Vestibular damage is characterized by a headache followed by vertigo, dizziness, or nausea. To avoid permanent ototoxic damage, the drug should be withdrawn at the first sign of tinnitus or persistent headache.

The nurse should also evaluate patients for signs of neuromuscular blockade, such as muscle weakness, especially the respiratory muscles.

Because of potential irritation associated with IM injection of gentamicin, the nurse needs to observe the injection site regularly.

When therapy ends, the presenting infection should be resolved. The patient should be adequately nourished and hydrated and free from adverse drug effects. ■

DRUGS CLOSELY RELATED TO P GENTAMICIN

Amikacin

Amikacin (Amikin) is a parenteral aminoglycoside with a broader spectrum of activity for gram-negative bacilli than gentamicin. Another difference is that is induces lower bacterial resistance. In many hospitals, amikacin has replaced gentamicin as the first-line treatment of systemic infection because of an increased resistance to gentamicin. Its contraindications, adverse effects, drug interactions, and patient management are similar to gentamicin.

MEMORY CHIP

P Gentamicin

- Used for serious gram-negative infections
- Significant contraindications: hypersensitivity, pregnancy, and breast-feeding
- Most common adverse effects: nausea, vomiting, diarrhea, and weight loss
- Most serious adverse effects: nephrotoxicity, ototoxicity, and neuromuscular blockade
- Maximizing therapeutic effects: administer at least 2 hours before or after extended infusions of penicillins
- Minimizing adverse effects: monitor peak and trough levels throughout therapy
- Most significant patient education: teach the patient the signs and symptoms of both nephrotoxicity and ototoxicity and also the importance of contacting the health care provider immediately if any symptoms should occur

Kanamycin

Kanamycin (Kantrex) is used orally to reduce ammonia-forming bacteria in hepatic coma and to decrease GI flora as an adjunctive therapy. Its use for systemic infections is limited by the number of bacteria that is resistant to it. Its contraindications, adverse effects, drug interactions, and patient management are similar to those of gentamicin.

Neomycin

Neomycin (Mycifradin Sulfate) has the highest risk for toxicity of all the aminoglycosides. Because of its high toxicity, it is never administered parenterally. It is available orally to decrease GI flora as a bowel preparation for surgery. Because it is not absorbed from the GI tract, it frequently causes superinfection within the bowel. Neomycin is also available in over-the-counter drugs as a topical antibiotic. Contraindications, adverse effects, drug interactions, and patient management are the same as those for gentamicin.

Netilmicin

Netilmicin (Netromycin) has essentially the same spectrum of action as gentamicin. Netilmicin induces less resistance than gentamicin and is less likely to produce ototoxicity. Contraindications, adverse effects, drug interactions, and patient management are the same as gentamicin.

Tobramycin

Tobramycin (Nebcin) is similar to gentamicin in its antibacterial spectrum; however, it is more active than gentamicin against *Pseudomonas*. It is given parenterally, topically to treat superficial ophthalmic infections, or by nebulization. Tobramycin has a low therapeutic index. Use of ideal body weight for determining the mg/kg/dose appears to be more accurate than dosing on the basis of total body weight. Peak and trough levels should be closely monitored in patients with serious infections or in disease states known to significantly alter aminoglycoside pharmacokinetics such as cystic fibrosis, burns, or major surgery. Contraindications, adverse effects, drug interactions, and patient management are the same as those of gentamicin.

DRUGS SIGNIFICANTLY DIFFERENT FROM P GENTAMICIN

Paromomycin

Paromomycin (Humatin) is an aminoglycoside antibiotic with broad-spectrum antibacterial and amebicidal activity. It is used for extraintestinal amebiasis and tapeworm infestation and to reduce ammonia-forming bacteria in hepatic coma. It is poorly absorbed from the GI tract and thus is used only for intestinal forms of amebiasis and helminths.

Paromomycin is contraindicated in patients with renal failure or intestinal obstruction. Adverse GI effects of paromomycin include anorexia, nausea, vomiting, gastric burning and pain, abdominal cramps, and diarrhea.

The only significant drug-drug interaction with paromomycin is succinylcholine. When given in combination, paromomycin may potentiate the neuromuscular effects of succinylcholine.

The nurse should coordinate follow-up appointments for the patient. Stool cultures should be done weekly for 6 weeks after therapy then monthly for 2 years.

Streptomycin

Streptomycin is a parenteral aminoglycoside. It is used as part of combination therapy for active tuberculosis or treatment of streptococcal or enterococcal endocarditis. As a single agent, it is used for mycobacterial infections, plague, tularemia, and brucellosis. In addition to ototoxicity and nephrotoxicity, streptomycin may induce neurotoxicity.

C LINCOSAMIDES

The lincosamides include clindamycin (Cleocin, Cleocin Pediatric) and lincomycin (Lincocin). They are very toxic drugs, so their use must be monitored and limited to situations with infections by bacteria with known sensitivity. Although lincomycin was the first drug developed in this class, it is rarely used. Clindamycin is discussed as the prototype lincosamide.

NURSING MANAGEMENT OF THE PATIENT RECEIVING P CLINDAMYCIN

Core Drug Knowledge

Pharmacotherapeutics

Clindamycin is active against a wide range of aerobic gram-positive cocci and several anaerobic gram-negative and gram-positive organisms. Many species of streptococci, except enterococci, and staphylococci are extremely susceptible. Most anaerobes, both gram positive and gram negative, are also susceptible. Clindamycin is indicated for treating serious to life-threatening infections caused by susceptible strains of anaerobes; streptococci; staphylococci; pneumococci, including septicemia; and acute hematogenous osteomyelitis. Topical forms are used to treat acne vulgaris. A vaginal preparation is available for treating bacterial vaginosis.

Pharmacokinetics

The oral absorption of clindamycin varies greatly depending on the presence of food in the stomach. Peak levels are achieved in about 1 or 2 hours. Given IM, clindamycin is rapidly absorbed within 20 to 30 minutes with peak levels occurring at 1 to 3 hours. IV administration produces a peak effect within minutes. Topical clindamycin is only minimally absorbed.

Clindamycin crosses the placenta and enters breast milk and cerebrospinal fluid (CSF). It is readily carried to most body tissues. Metabolized in the liver, it is excreted through the bile and urine (Table 49-3).

Pharmacodynamics

Clindamycin is either bacteriostatic or bactericidal, depending on its concentration at the site of action and on the specific susceptibility of the organism being treated. It enters the bacterial cell and binds to bacterial ribosomes, suppressing protein synthesis and leading to cell death in susceptible bacteria. No direct effect on the body occurs.

Contraindications and Precautions

Clindamycin is contraindicated in pregnancy and lactation and in patients with a known allergy to lincosamides, history of asthma or other allergies, allergy to tartrazine (found in several oral preparations), or hepatic or renal dysfunction. Caution should be exercised in patients with a history of antibiotic-associated colitis, regional enteritis, or ulcerative colitis.

Adverse Effects

The most common adverse effects to clindamycin are nausea and vomiting and abdominal pain from oral delivery. Diarrhea, abdominal cramps, and abdominal tenderness may suggest antibiotic-associated colitis, also known as pseudomembranous colitis or *Clostridium difficile* colitis.

Thrombocytopenia, neutropenia, and eosinophilia have been reported during clindamycin therapy. Sore throat or fever may indicate neutropenia.

Maculopapular rash, erythema, and pruritus can develop from systemic or topical use of clindamycin. Pathologic dryness of the skin (**xeroderma**), conjunctiva (**xerophthalmia**), or mucous membranes is the most common effect of topical application. Alcohol in some topical formulations may irritate the eyes, mucous membranes, or abraded skin if allowed to come into contact with them.

Hypersensitivity reactions range from skin rashes and urticaria to anaphylactoid reactions. After injection, pain, abscess, and phlebitis are relatively common.

Drug Interactions

Neuromuscular blockers, aluminum salts, erythromycin, and pyrimethamine interact with clindamycin (Table 49-4). Topical preparations containing benzoyl peroxide, tretinoin, salicylic acid, or other topical preparations for acne, when used with clindamycin preparations, can cause a cumulative irritant effect, leading to excessive drying and peeling of the skin.

Assessment of Relevant Core Patient Variables

Health Status

The nurse should assess patients for allergy or predisposition to allergy to lincosamides. Some preparations contain tartrazine dye, which can precipitate bronchial asthma or other allergic reactions in sensitive patients. Patients sensitive to clindamycin may also be sensitive to doxorubicin.

Next, the nurse should investigate any history of GI disease because clindamycin predisposes patients to the overgrowth of nonsusceptible organisms and hence may induce pseudomembranous colitis.

Any previous renal or hepatic disease may be explored because the half-life of clindamycin is prolonged in patients with hepatic dysfunction, and toxicity can occur. Baseline hepatic and renal function test results should be evaluated before beginning therapy. For patients with severe renal impairment, dose reduction should be considered.

Patients on long-term therapy should have a baseline complete blood count (CBC) because of the drug's potential to induce blood dyscrasias.

TABLE 49-3 Summary of Selected Lincosamide Antibiotics

Drug (Trade) Name	Selected Indications	Route and Dosage Range	Pharmacokinetics
clindamycin (Cleocin; *Canadian:* Dalacin-c)	Serious infections from streptococci, pneumococci, and staphylococci	*Adult:* PO, 150–450 mg q6h; IM/IV, 600 mg–2.7 g q6–12h up to 4.8 g/d for life-threatening infections *Child:* PO, 8–12 mg/kg/d in three divided doses; 10 kg, maximum of 37.5 mg tid; IM/IV, 15–40 mg/kg q6–12h up to 40 mg/kg/d for severe infection	*Onset:* PO, varies; IM, 20–30 min; IV, immediate *Duration:* 8–12 h $t_{1/2}$: 2–3 h
lincomycin (Lincocin)	Serious infections from streptococci, pneumococci, and staphylococci	*Adult:* PO, 500 mg q8h; IM, 600–1,200 mg/d; IV, 600–1,000 mg q8–12 h	*Onset:* PO, varies; IM, 20–30 min; IV, immediate *Duration:* PO, 6–8 h; IM, 0.5 h; IV, 14 h $t_{1/2}$: 5 h

TABLE 49-4 Agents That Interact With Clindamycin

Interactants	Effect and Significance	Nursing Management
antibiotics erythromycin chloramphenicol	Coadministration antagonizes the effects of clindamycin.	Avoid coadministration.
aluminum salts or kaolin	Marked decreased GI absorption of lincosamides if taken with these.	Administer absorbent antidiarrheal product 2 h before or 3–4 h after administering oral clindamycin.
neuromuscular blockers	Lincosamides potentiate the action of neuromuscular blockers, resulting in increased neuromuscular blockade, respiratory depression, and extended paralysis.	Mark patient's chart with warning of the drug combination. Arrange for extended monitoring and support of patient after surgery or procedure. Monitor respiration and other vital signs.
opiate agonists	Coadministration enhances the effect of opiates, resulting in increased respiratory depression.	Monitor respiration and other vital signs.
pyrimethamine	Synergistic effects in treating toxoplasmic encephalitis in patients with AIDS.	This is a beneficial interaction.

Life Span and Gender

The nurse should explore the benefits versus potential risks with the pregnant or lactating woman. In general, clindamycin is prescribed for pregnant or lactating women only if the benefits outweigh the potential risks.

The nurse should assess the growth and developmental level of the child or infant. Clindamycin should be used cautiously in children. Neonates younger than 1 month (and premature infants) have a prolonged plasma half-life for clindamycin, probably because of an immature hepatic system.

Lifestyle, Diet, and Habits

The nurse should assess the patient's lifestyle to determine the likelihood that the patient will take the drug around the clock.

Environment

The nurse should be aware of the environment in which gentamicin will be administered and, if appropriate, assess the home or living environment for potential risk factors. Parenteral solutions of clindamycin must be used within 24 hours of reconstitution. Oral or topical clindamycin may be administered in any environment.

Nursing Diagnoses and Outcomes

- Risk for Injury related to allergic reactions
  Desired outcome: The patient will stop drug therapy and immediately report symptoms of allergic reaction to the prescriber.
- Diarrhea related to drug effects
  Desired outcome: The patient will avoid dehydration and report persistent diarrhea to the provider.
- Imbalanced Nutrition: Less than Body Requirements related to drug-related GI effects, alteration in taste, superinfections
  Desired outcome: The patient will maintain body weight and report persistent symptoms affecting nutritional status.
- Risk for Injury related to possible blood dyscrasias
  Desired outcome: The patient will remain injury free throughout drug therapy.

Planning and Intervention

Maximizing Therapeutic Effects

The nurse should make sure that the patient receives the full course of clindamycin as prescribed at around-the-clock intervals for maximal effectiveness. The nurse should also coordinate the administration of drugs to decrease potential undesired interactions. Culture and sensitivity reports may be reviewed periodically to confirm that clindamycin is the appropriate drug for the patient.

Minimizing Adverse Effects

Clindamycin should be administered with food to reduce minor gastric distress. For patients with additional GI effects, the nurse should provide small, frequent meals as tolerated; frequent mouth care; and ice chips to suck if stomatitis and sore mouth are problems. It is also important to keep this drug out of the reach of children to avoid accidental overdose.

Providing Patient and Family Education

- The patient should understand that they should not take clindamycin or any other lincosamide antibiotic if they have ever had a reaction to a drug with a generic name that ends in the suffixes -mycin and -micin.

- The nurse should advise pregnant or breast-feeding patients to avoid clindamycin.
- The nurse should discuss general dosage and safe storage recommendations.
- The nurse should advise the patient to take clindamycin on an empty stomach.
- The patient should be urged to contact the prescriber if clindamycin therapy does not improve symptoms in 3 days.
- The nurse must teach the patient to recognize and report symptoms of allergic reaction and superinfection characterized by sore throat, easy bruising or bleeding, and fatigue.
- Patients of child-bearing age taking birth control pills should be advised to use a backup method of contraception while taking clindamycin.
- The nurse should advise patients using clindamycin lotion that dry skin may occur. Instruct the patient to drink lots of fluids and keep the skin moisturized.

Ongoing Assessment and Evaluation

The nurse should monitor the patient for the onset of diarrhea. If it occurs, the prescriber should be notified immediately because this may be the presenting sign of pseudomembranous colitis. The nurse should obtain an order for the stool to be evaluated for white blood cells (WBCs), blood, and mucus. The nurse should also coordinate a proctoscopy to be performed.

During therapy, the nurse should monitor for potential procedures that would require the use of neuromuscular blocking agents. Should a procedure be scheduled, the nurse should note prominently on the patient's chart the current use of clindamycin. After the procedure, the patient should be monitored and supported for an extended period after the discontinuation of the neuromuscular blocker.

The nurse should also monitor for sore throat and fever, which may be signs of thrombocytopenia, neutropenia, or eosinophilia.

By the completion of therapy, the patient should be free of the presenting infection. The patient will have maintained adequate nutrition, and any adverse effects will have been resolved. ■

DRUG CLOSELY RELATED TO CLINDAMYCIN

Lincomycin is an oral and parenteral lincosamide antibiotic. It is used for serious staphylococcal and streptococcal infections. Lincomycin is usually reserved for patients who cannot take penicillins or clindamycin. It is not a drug of choice because it has been associated with severe or fatal colitis. Like clindamycin, lincomycin is used with caution in patients with asthma, liver disease, GI disease, colitis, and tartrazine sensitivity. Adverse effects, drug interactions, and patient management are similar to those of clindamycin.

MEMORY CHIP

Clindamycin

- Used for serious infections caused by gram-positive cocci and both gram-positive and gram-negative anaerobes.
- Significant contraindications: hypersensitivity, pregnancy, breast-feeding, and renal or hepatic dysfunction
- Most common adverse effects: nausea, vomiting, abdominal pain, rash, and pruritus
- Most serious adverse effect: pseudomembranous colitis
- Maximizing therapeutic effects: administer at evenly spaced intervals
- Minimizing adverse effects: give with food to minimize GI distress
- Most significant patient education: teach the patient the signs and symptoms of superinfection, especially pseudomembranous colitis and explain the importance of contacting the health care provider immediately should any symptom occur.

MACROLIDE ANTIBIOTICS

The macrolide antibiotics are characterized by molecules made up of large-ring lactones. They are bacteriostatic or bactericidal in susceptible bacteria. Macrolide antibiotics include erythromycin, azithromycin, clarithromycin, troleandomycin, and dirithromycin. Erythromycin is the first macrolide discovered and is the prototype for this class.

NURSING MANAGEMENT OF THE PATIENT RECEIVING ERYTHROMYCIN

Core Drug Knowledge

Pharmacotherapeutics

Erythromycin is commonly used in treating Legionnaire disease, *Mycoplasma pneumoniae* pneumonia, and as an alternative to beta-lactam antibiotics in patients who are allergic to penicillin. Erythromycin may have benefits in hypomotility conditions, such as diabetic gastroparesis, because of its actions of increased gastric motility and emptying.

Erythromycin is generally more effective against gram-positive organisms than against gram-negative organisms because of its ability to penetrate into gram-positive organisms. Gram-positive organisms susceptible to erythromycin include *Staphylococcus aureus*, *Streptococcus agalactiae*, *Streptococcus pyogenes*, *Streptococcus pneumoniae*, *Streptococcus viridans* species, and *Corynebacterium diphtheriae*.

Other susceptible organisms include *Chlamydia trachomatis*, *Entamoeba histolytica*, *Listeria monocytogenes*, *Borrelia burgdorferi* (the causative agent in Lyme disease), *Mycoplasma pneumoniae*, *Treponema pallidum*, and *Ureaplasma urealyticum*.

Pharmacokinetics

Erythromycin base (E-Mycin, Ery-Tab) is easily inactivated by gastric acid, therefore several formulations have been developed to overcome this problem. Erythromycin stearate (Erythrocin) is the most likely to yield to gastric acid destruction. Erythromycin estolate (Ilosone) is more acid stable, dissociates in the upper intestine and releases an inactive ester that is absorbed and hydrolyzed in the blood to produce free erythromycin. Erythromycin ethylsuccinate (EES, EryPed) is absorbed first then hydrolyzed in the blood to free erythromycin. The newest formulation of oral erythromycin is encapsulated pellets that are small enough to pass through the pyloric sphincter independent of gastric emptying and are absorbed as the base. None of the oral forms, however, allows complete absorption. The drug reaches peak levels 1 to 4 hours after administration. Erythromycin is also available for IV use as erythromycin lactobionate or erythromycin gluceptate. Administration of IV erythromycin is painful and is used only when high serum levels of erythromycin are required. When given IV, erythromycin peak effect occurs within 1 hour. Erythromycin is also available in an ophthalmic preparation.

Erythromycin crosses the placenta and is secreted in breast milk. It does not cross the blood-brain barrier. It is metabolized in the liver and excreted in the bile and urine. Table 49-5 has additional information.

Pharmacodynamics

No direct effect on the body occurs with erythromycin. The macrolides are bactericidal or bacteriostatic. They exert their effect by inhibiting RNA-dependent protein

TABLE 49-5 Summary of Selected Macrolide Antibiotics

Drug (Trade) Name	Selected Indications	Route and Dosage Range	Pharmacokinetics
erythromycin (E-Mycin, Ilosone, EES, Erythrocin stearate; *Canadian:* Apo-Erythro)	Urethral, endocervical, or rectal infections Syphilis Legionnaire disease Rheumatic fever Bacterial endocarditis *Mycoplasma* infections Bronchitis Pharyngitis Skin infections	*Adult:* PO, 250–500 mg q6h (maximum 4g) *Child:* PO, 30–50 mg q6–12h (maximum 100 mg/kg in divided doses) (*Note:* EES dosage is slightly higher)	*Onset:* 1–2 h *Duration:* 6–8 h $t_{1/2}$: 3–5 h
azithromycin (Zithromax)	Lower respiratory tract infection Nongonococcal urethritis and cervicitis Skin infections Acute otitis media Pharyngitis/tonsillitis *Helicobacter pylori* infection *Mycobacterium avium* (prevention or treatment)	*Adult:* PO, 500 mg/d on first day, then 250 mg for days 2 through 5 *Child:* 6 mo–2 y, PO, 10 mg/kg on day 1, then 5 mg/kg on days 2–5; >6 mo, PO, 10 mg/kg as single dose (not to exceed 500 mg) first day; then 5 mg/kg (not to exceed 250 mg) once daily for 4 d *Adult:* PO, 500 mg q12h	*Onset:* Rapid *Duration:* 24 h $t_{1/2}$: 11–48 h
clarithromycin (Biaxin)	Respiratory infections Skin infections	*Adult:* PO, 250–500 mg q12h for 7–14 d *Child:* PO, 7.5 mg/kg bid to maximum of 500 mg bid	*Onset:* Rapid *Duration:* 8–12 h $t_{1/2}$: 3–7 h
troleandomycin (Tao)	Respiratory trace infections	*Adult:* PO, 250–500 mg q6h *Child:* PO, 125–250 mg q6h	*Onset:* Rapid *Duration:* 8–12 h $t_{1/2}$: 8–10 h
dirithromycin (Dynabac)	Bronchitis Skin infections Pharyngitis/tonsillitis Community-acquired pneumonia	*Adult:* 500 mg qd; duration depends on disorder *Child:* Not recommended	*Onset:* Rapid *Duration:* 24 h $t_{1/2}$: 2–36 h

synthesis at the chain elongation step. This action can prevent the cell from dividing, or it can cause cell death depending on the sensitivity of the bacteria and the concentration of the drug.

Contraindications and Precautions

Erythromycin is contraindicated in patients who are allergic to it. Caution should be used in any patient with hepatic insufficiency because the ability to break down erythromycin for excretion may be compromised. Caution should be exercised during pregnancy or lactation and in patients with impaired hearing, biliary function, GI disease, and cardiac arrhythmias. Ocular preparations are contraindicated in patients with viral, fungal, or mycobacterial infections of the eye.

Adverse Effects

Adverse effects suggesting allergic reaction to erythromycin include urticaria, maculopapular rash, erythema, and interstitial nephritis. Pruritus is a possible reaction to topical application of erythromycin.

The most common adverse effects related to erythromycin are GI in nature. They include nausea or vomiting, abdominal pain, and diarrhea. These effects are often dose related and may occur regardless of the route of administration.

Rare potential adverse effects include hepatotoxicity, pseudomembranous colitis, QT interval prolongation and ventricular tachycardia of the torsade de pointes type, tinnitus, and reversible hearing loss.

Drug Interactions

Erythromycin interacts with many agents, among which are antihistamines, benzodiazepines, carbamazepine, corticosteroids, cyclosporine, digoxin, food, oral anticoagulants, and theophylline (Table 49-6).

Assessment of Relevant Core Patient Variables

Health Status

In assessing patients' health status before administering erythromycin, the nurse explores any history of hypersensitivity to erythromycin or other macrolide antibiotic (because of the risk of cross-sensitivity).

The nurse should also assess for hepatic or biliary dysfunction. Moreover, hepatic function should be monitored in patients receiving prolonged treatment. The estolate salt of erythromycin should not be used in patients with hepatic disease because of the potential for hepatotoxicity.

TABLE 49-6 Agents That Interact With Erythromycin

Interactants	Effect and Significance	Nursing Management
benzodiazepines	Macrolide antibiotics may decrease the metabolism of certain benzodiazepines, resulting in an increased CNS depression and prolonged effects of benzodiazepines.	Monitor patients for increased CNS depression Ensure safety precautions for patients. Reduce dosage of benzodiazepines as necessary.
carbamazepine	Macrolide antibiotics may decrease the metabolism of carbamazepine, resulting in accumulation and toxicity of carbamazepine.	Avoid if possible. Monitor carbamazepine levels closely. Reduce dose of carbamazepine as necessary.
corticosteroids	The pharmacologic and toxicologic properties of corticosteroids may be increased when administered with erythromycin.	Monitor for therapeutic and toxic effects of corticosteroids. Reduce dosage of corticosteroids as necessary.
cyclosporine	Macrolide antibiotics may decrease the metabolism of cyclosporine, resulting in accumulation and renal toxicity.	Avoid this combination. Monitor cyclosporine levels closely. Reduce dose of cyclosporine as necessary.
digoxin	Increased serum levels of digoxin, leading to risk of toxicity.	Monitor digoxin levels carefully, and adjust dosage as needed during and after completion of macrolide therapy.
food	GI absorption of nonenteric-coated erythromycin tablets may be decreased by food.	Administer 1 h before or 2 h after meals.
oral anticoagulants	The total body clearance of oral anticoagulants is reduced by an unknown interaction with erythromycin. Hemorrhage has been reported.	Reduce oral anticoagulant dosage. Monitor for signs of bleeding.
theophylline	Macrolides inhibit the metabolism of theophylline. Theophylline reduces the bioavailability and increases the renal clearance of macrolides. These actions result in increased efficacy of theophylline and decreased efficacy of macrolides.	Monitor theophylline levels closely. Monitor for treatment failure of macrolides.

The nurse should review the patients' GI history, particularly because the normal flora of the colon may allow an overgrowth of *Clostridium* organisms. A toxin produced by *C. difficile* is a primary cause of antibiotic-associated colitis. Patients who develop diarrhea while taking or soon after taking erythromycin should be evaluated for the potential of antibiotic-associated pseudomembranous colitis.

Another assessment area the nurse should consider is hearing because erythromycin may cause a reversible loss of hearing, and patients with preexisting hearing impairment may be at greater risk.

In addition, the nurse should explore any possibility cardiovascular disorder, specifically a history of torsades de pointes, because IV administration of erythromycin at a rate above 15 mg/min may place patients with such a history at risk for this arrhythmia.

Life Span and Gender

The nurse should evaluate the woman for pregnancy and lactation. Erythromycin should be used with caution in breast-feeding women because it is excreted into breast milk at about 50% of maternal plasma concentrations. This may induce diarrhea and superinfection in the infant. The nurse should consider the developmental level of the patient. Erythromycin lactobionate injection may contain benzyl alcohol as a preservative, which can cause toxicity in neonates.

Lifestyle, Diet, and Habits

The nurse should assess the patient's dietary habits to determine the likelihood that the patient will take erythromycin stearate at least 1 hour before or 2 hours after meals.

Environment

The nurse should be aware of the environment in which the drug will be administered. Oral or ophthalmic erythromycin may be given in any environment, whereas IV infusion should be given in a monitored setting.

Nursing Diagnoses and Outcomes

- Risk for Injury related to possible allergic reactions
  Desired outcome: The patient will stop drug therapy and report any signs of allergy reaction immediately to the prescriber.
- Diarrhea related to drug-induced GI upset
  Desired outcome: The patient will avoid dehydration, maintain fluid intake, and contact the prescriber if diarrhea persists.
- Risk for Infection related to potential for superinfection following drug therapy
  Desired outcome: The patient will contact the provider if any signs of superinfection occur, for example, sore throat or fever.

Planning and Intervention

Maximizing Therapeutic Effects

The nurse should reconstitute erythromycin with sterile water only. Diluents containing preservatives or organic salts should not be used. Prepared infusion solutions that are stored at room temperature must be used within 8 hours. Prepared solution that are refrigerated must be used within 24 hours.

The nurse should evaluate culture and sensitivity reports to verify that erythromycin is the drug of choice. Moreover, the nurse must administer erythromycin as prescribed, at around-the-clock intervals to increase effectiveness. Because food interferes with drug absorption, the nurse should administer erythromycin stearate at least 1 hour before or 2 hours after meals. Other formulations of erythromycin may given without regard to meals. If GI irritation occurs, however, erythromycin may be administered with food. Each dose should be administered with a full glass of water, not with fruit juice.

Minimizing Adverse Effects

The nurse should provide small, frequent meals; mouth care; and ice chips to suck if stomatitis and sore mouth are problems. Additionally, regular monitoring is needed to ensure adequate hydration with fluids provided to replace fluid lost with diarrhea. Because erythromycin can be very irritating to veins, it is important to administer IV infusions over 30 to 60 minutes. If pain persists, the nurse should reduce the rate of infusion. If pain persists, ice may be applied and the prescriber notified.

Providing Patient and Family Education

- The nurse should encourage patient to take the complete course of antibiotics.
- The nurse should explain safe drug handling and storage.
- The nurse should explain the importance of taking erythromycin around the clock to maintain a therapeutic drug level.
- The nurse should teach the patient the potential adverse effects and the measures to alleviate their discomfort.
- The nurse should advise patients to take erythromycin on an empty stomach, unless GI distress is unbearable.
- The nurse should advise the patient to contact the health care provider if there is no improvement in 3 days.

Ongoing Assessment and Evaluation

The nurse should monitor for signs of allergic reactions, resolution of presenting signs and symptoms of infection, signs of superinfection, and for patients receiving IV erythromycin, signs of phlebitis, or abscess formation. By the conclusion of therapy, the patient should be free of the presenting infection. The patient will have an adequate nutritional status, and adverse effects will have been resolved. ■

MEMORY CHIP

Erythromycin

- Used for infections caused by gram-positive organisms. Less effective for gram-negative organisms.
- Significant contraindication: hypersensitivity
- Most common adverse effect: GI distress
- Most serious adverse effects: hepatotoxicity, QT prolongation, pseudomembranous colitis, and ventricular tachycardia
- Maximizing therapeutic effects: administer on an empty stomach, unless GI distress is pronounced
- Minimizing adverse effects: provide small, frequent meals
- Most significant patient education: complete the entire course of medication, even when feeling better

DRUGS CLOSELY RELATED TO ERYTHROMYCIN

Azithromycin

Azithromycin (Zithromax) is a semisynthetic macrolide antibiotic that is similar in structure to erythromycin. Azithromycin is generally active against organisms that are also usually susceptible to erythromycin. It is not clear whether azithromycin, like erythromycin, is effective in treating diabetic gastroparesis. Azithromycin produces less GI intolerance than does erythromycin. It is unique in that it can reach exceptionally high levels in tissues, thus increasing its efficacy and duration of action. For this reason, it is administered only once a day.

Absorption of azithromycin *capsules* is decreased in the presence of food and should be given on an empty stomach. The absorption of azithromycin *suspension* is increased in the presence of foods, so much so that the serum concentration may be too high. For that reason, the suspension should be taken on an empty stomach. Conversely, azithromycin *tablets* have an increased absorption when given with a meal with high-fat content and may be given with or without food.

Because azithromycin is not metabolized, it should be used cautiously in patients with hepatic disease. Adverse effects, drug interactions and patient management is similar to those for erythromycin.

Clarithromycin

Clarithromycin (Biaxin) is an oral macrolide antibiotic similar to erythromycin and azithromycin. Like azithromycin, clarithromycin penetrates tissues to a greater degree than erythromycin. Clarithromycin is generally active against organisms that are usually susceptible to erythromycin. These include most staphylococcal and streptococcal strains. In addition, clarithromycin is active against *Moraxella catarrhalis*, *Mycoplasma pneumoniae*, *Legionella* species, and *Chlamydia pneumoniae*. Clarithromycin inhibits *Mycobacterium avium* at concentrations achievable in lung tissue and is active against *Borrelia burgdorferi*, the cause of Lyme disease. Combined with omeprazole, clarithromycin is useful for *Helicobacter pylori*-associated peptic ulcer disease.

Clarithromycin is administered orally as a tablet or suspension. It is administered without regard to meals. To prepare the oral suspension, the nurse should tap the bottle several times to loosen the powder, then add 55-mL distilled or purified water to bottles labeled as containing 125 mg/5 mL or 250 mg/5 mL, respectively, of clarithromycin. The preparation should be shaken vigorously before each administration. This drug is stable at room temperature for up to 14 days.

Clarithromycin is contraindicated during pregnancy. It is unknown whether clarithromycin passes into breast milk. It is used cautiously in patients either hepatic or renal insufficiency because it is partially renally excreted.

Adverse effects, drug interactions, and patient management are similar to those associated with erythromycin.

Troleandomycin

Troleandomycin (Tao), a synthetic macrolide, is available only in oral form. It is associated with serious hepatic effects only when there is a treatment failure with other macrolides. It should not be used in any patient with hepatic impairment. Adverse effects, drug interactions, and patient management are similar to those of erythromycin.

Dirithromycin

Dirithromycin (Dynabac), a newer oral macrolide, is also similar to erythromycin but is pharmacokinetically more effective. Additionally, it does not affect the microsomal enzyme system. Dirithromycin's spectrum of activity is similar to that of erythromycin, and once-daily dosing is possible because of the extensive tissue distribution of the active dirithromycin metabolite, erythromycylamine. Adverse effects, drug interactions, and patient management are similar to those of erythromycin.

OXAZOLIDINONES

Oxazolidinones are the first new class of antibiotics developed specifically for treatment of methicillin-resistant *Staphylococcus aureus* (MRSA) infections. Linezolid (Zyvox) is the prototype for this new class of drugs.

NURSING MANAGEMENT OF THE PATIENT RECEIVING LINEZOLID

Core Drug Knowledge

Pharmacotherapeutics

Linezolid is approved for use in the treatment of bacteremia associated with vancomycin-resistant *Enterococcus faecium* or *E. faecalis* (VRE); complicated skin infections and nosocomial or community-acquired pneumonia caused by MRSA; and bacteremia associated with nosocomial or community-acquired pneumonia caused by penicillin-susceptible *Streptococcus pneumoniae*. Many hospitals require approval by the Infectious Disease committee prior to administration of linezolid.

Pharmacokinetics

Linezolid is available in both oral and parenteral formulations. Oral linezolid is 100% bioavailable. This means that the IV and oral forms are interchangeable without making dosage adjustments. Oral linezolid is rapidly absorbed from the GI tract and is widely distributed. Food delays the absorption but does not decrease peak plasma concentrations. Linezolid is partly metabolized in the liver and excreted in urine. The half-life is approximately 5 hours.

Pharmacodynamics

Linezolid attacks bacteria by blocking the early stages of the process bacteria use to make proteins, while other antibiotics act at later stages of protein synthesis. This unique mechanism of action suggests that bacteria may not be able to develop resistance as quickly and that cross resistance between linezolid and other antibiotics is less likely to occur.

Contraindications and Precautions

The only contraindication for linezolid is hypersensitivity. Linezolid oral suspension should be used with caution in those patients with phenylketonuria because the linezolid oral suspension is formulated with aspartame, which supplies roughly 20-mg phenylalanine per each 5-mL suspension. Other linezolid products do not contain phenylalanine. Linezolid is given cautiously to patients with pre-existing blood dyscrasias because it may induce bone marrow suppression. For the same reason, it should be given cautiously to patients receiving other drugs known to induce bone marrow suppression. Because linezolid is a nonselective inhibitor of monoamine oxidase (MAO), it should be used with caution in patients with hypertension, untreated hyperthyroid disease, severe cardiac disease, cerebrovascular disease, or pheochromocytoma. These patients have an increased risk for poor sequelae because linezolid-induced MAO inhibition will reduce the metabolism of pressor amines, which may increase blood pressure in these individuals. Linezolid is classified as a pregnancy category C drug.

Adverse Effects

Linezolid is generally well tolerated. The most common adverse effects associated with linezolid therapy are diarrhea, headache, nausea, and vomiting. Events were usually mild to moderate in intensity and limited in duration. Serious adverse effects include thrombocytopenia, elevated hepatic enzyme levels, and pseudomembranous colitis. Hypertension is another potentially serious adverse effect in special populations, as already mentioned. As with other antibiotics, superinfections may occur.

Drug Interactions

Because linezolid is a reversible, nonselective MAO inhibitor, most potential drug interactions are related to this action of the drug. Table 49-7 presents potential drug interactions.

Food and dietary interactions with nonselective MAO inhibitors can be serious. Foods containing tyramine should be avoided but so also should beverages containing caffeine or ethanol.

Assessment of Relevant Core Patient Variables

Health Status

The nurse should elicit a complete history from the patient focusing on pre-existing medical conditions that require cautious use of linezolid. The nurse should also evaluate the patient's current medications for drugs that may interact with linezolid. The nurse should communicate positive findings to the health care provider prior to the administration of linezolid.

The nurse should review the culture and sensitivity report to establish that linezolid is an appropriate therapy. For patients requiring therapy longer than 14 days, the nurse should obtain a baseline CBC and liver function tests.

Life Span and Gender

The nurse should assess the patient for potential pregnancy or breast-feeding as linezolid is a pregnancy category C drug and is not approved for use in children.

Lifestyle, Diet, and Habits

The nurse should ask the patient about dietary intake, focusing on foods that are rich in tyramine. The nurse should evaluate the use of caffeine from coffee, tea, or carbonated beverages. The nurse should also evaluate for potential alcohol abuse, because alcohol consumption during therapy increases the risk for a hypertensive crisis.

Because linezolid may interact with many OTC medications, the nurse should assess for self-medicating of coughs, colds, allergies, or weight loss.

Environment

The nurse should be aware of the environment in which linezolid will be administered. Parenteral linezolid should be administered in an acute hospital setting. Oral linezolid may be administered in any setting.

Nursing Diagnoses and Outcomes

- Deficient Fluid Volume related to nausea, vomiting and diarrhea from linezolid therapy

  Desired outcome: The patient will remain well hydrated throughout therapy.
- Risk for Injury related to thrombocytopenia and pseudomembranous colitis

  Desired outcome: The patient will remain free from injury and contact the health care provider immediately if any signs of bleeding or abdominal pain occur.

TABLE 49-7 Agents That Interact With Linezolid

Interactants	Effect and Significance	Nursing Management
entacapone tolcapone	Monoamine oxidase (MAO) and catechol-O-methyltransferase (COMT) are the two major enzymes involved in the metabolism of catecholamines. It is theoretically possible that the coadministration of entacapone or tolcapone with linezolid would result in inhibition of normal catecholamine metabolism.	Do not administer linezolid within 14 d of entacapone or tolcapone administration.
levodopa	Concomitant use of nonselective MAO inhibitors (MAOIs) such as linezolid with levodopa can result in hypertensive crisis.	Do not administer linezolid within 14 d of levodopa administration.
MAOIs and drugs that possess MAOI-like activity • isocarboxazid • phenelzine • tranylcypromine • selegiline • furazolidone • procarbazine	Coadministration of these drugs with linezolid may result in hypertensive crisis, convulsions, or death.	Do not administer linezolid within 14 d of these drugs.
meperidine	When meperidine is given in combination with a MAOI, accumulation of serotonin may occur and may lead to severe cardiovascular and/or neurologic adverse reactions.	Avoid administration of meperidine within 14 d of linezolid therapy. Morphine is the preferred agent in emergency situations.
selective serotonin reuptake inhibitors (SSRIs)	SSRIs potentiate the action of serotonin by inhibiting its neuronal reuptake. Because monoamine oxidase type A deaminates serotonin, administration of a nonselective MAOI concurrently with an SSRI can lead to a serious reaction known as "serotonin syndrome."	Avoid coadministration of these drugs.
serotonin-receptor agonists • naratriptan • rizatriptan • sumatriptan • zolmitriptan	The MAO type A enzyme metabolizes serotonin. Non-selective MAOIs increase the plasma concentrations of these drugs and some of their active metabolites, thus increasing levels of serotonin. This interaction could lead to "serotonin syndrome."	Do not administer linezolid within 14 d of serotonin-receptor agonists.
Sympathomimetics or psychostimulants with sympathomimetic actions • phenylephrine • phenylpropanolamine • pseudoephedrine • amphetamine • dexfenfluramine, • dextroamphetamine, • fenfluramine, • methylphenidate	Linezolid has been noted to enhance the pressor response of these drugs, resulting in a rise in systolic blood pressure.	Avoid these drugs in combination if possible. Monitor blood pressure during linezolid therapy. Teach the patient to avoid OTC medications used for coughs, colds, or weigh loss.
tryptophan tyrosine	When used concomitantly with tryptophan, linezolid may cause the "serotonin syndrome."	Do not coadminister these drugs

- Risk for Injury related to hypertensive crisis

  Desired outcome: The patient will remain normotensive by adhering to antihypertensive therapy and limiting foods or beverages with tyramine, caffeine, or alcohol.

Planning and Intervention

Maximizing Therapeutic Effects

The nurse should administer linezolid at evenly spaced intervals throughout the day.

Minimizing Adverse Effects

To avoid hypertensive crisis, the nurse should monitor the patient's intake of food or beverages containing tyramine, caffeine, or alcohol.

Providing Patient and Family Education

- The nurse should explain the importance of taking linezolid exactly as prescribed for the entire course of treatment, regardless if the patient feels better.
- The nurse should explain the need for periodic laboratory tests if therapy is anticipated to last longer than 14 days.
- The nurse should explain dietary restrictions, focusing on food or beverages containing tyramine, caffeine, or alcohol.
- The nurse should explain the importance of refraining from use of OTC drugs that may interact with linezolid.
- The nurse should explain that linezolid may interact with many types of prescription medications. The patient should contact the health care professional before taking any other medications, even those prescribed by another health care professional.
- The nurse should teach the signs and symptoms of thrombocytopenia and pseudomembranous colitis. Advise the patient to contact the health care provider immediately if any symptoms occur.

Ongoing Assessment and Evaluation

The nurse should monitor for efficacy of treatment and the resolution of the presenting infection. The nurse should also monitor for signs and symptoms of thrombocytopenia and pseudomembranous colitis and advise the health care provider if any occur. The nurse should monitor the patient's intake of foods or beverages containing tyramine, caffeine, or alcohol. The nurse should coordinate serial CBC and liver enzyme tests should therapy persist after 14 days.

By the end of therapy, the presenting infections should be resolved and any adverse effects should be resolved. ■

MEMORY CHIP

Linezolid

- Used for infections caused by vancomycin-resistant *Enterococcus faecium* or *E. faecalis* (VRE), methicillin-resistant *Staphylococcus aureus* (MRSA), and penicillin-susceptible *Streptococcus pneumoniae.*
- Significant contraindication: hypersensitivity
- Most common adverse effects: nausea, vomiting, headache, and diarrhea
- Most serious adverse effects: thrombocytopenia and pseudomembranous colitis
- Maximizing therapeutic effects: administer at evenly spaced intervals
- Minimizing adverse effects: monitor the patient's intake of foods or beverages containing tyramine, caffeine, or alcohol
- Most significant patient education: teach the patient dietary restrictions and the importance of not taking any medications, including OTC medications, without the health care providers' approval.

STREPTOGRAMINS

Streptogramins are the newest class of antibiotics, specifically designed to eradicate "superbugs" resistant to other antibiotics. Quinupristin and dalfopristin are the only streptogramins approved for use in the United States by the Food and Drug Administration; they are marketed as a combination drug quinupristin/dalfopristin (Synercid).

NURSING MANAGEMENT OF THE PATIENT RECEIVING QUINUPRISTIN/DALFOPRISTIN

Core Drug Knowledge

Pharmacotherapeutics

Quinupristin/dalfopristin is indicated for the treatment of serious or life-threatening infections associated with vancomycin-resistant *Enterococcus faecium* (VREF) bacteremia and for complicated skin and skin-structure infections due to *Staphylococcus aureus* and *Streptococcus pyogenes.* In many hospitals, the prescribing of quinupristin/dalfopristin requires Infectious Diseases Committee approval in an attempt to avoid inducing resistance. See the accompanying display, Explaining the Drug Selection Process.

Pharmacokinetics

Quinupristin/dalfopristin is administered by IV administration only. Both drugs are converted to several active major metabolites with excretion primarily through bile. The onset is rapid, duration is unknown, and the elimination half-life is approximately 1 hour.

Critical Thinking Scenario

Explaining the drug selection process

Georgia James, age 64, is admitted to your unit with a diagnosis of pneumonia. She has just completed her first dose of IV gentamicin when her granddaughter arrives. The granddaughter comes to the nurses' station and is very upset. She states in a very loud voice, "Why is my grandmother getting gentamicin? I saw on the Internet that there is a new type of drug for pneumonia called syner-something. Why isn't she getting the strongest kind of medication?" How would you handle this situation?

Pharmacodynamics

Quinupristin/dalfopristin inhibits bacterial protein synthesis by irreversibly blocking ribosome functioning. When used as a single agent, these drugs are bacteriostatic. When used in combination quinupristin/dalfopristin has up to 16 times the activity of each agent alone.

Contraindications and Precautions

The only contraindication to use of quinupristin/dalfopristin is hypersensitivity. It should be used cautiously in patients with decreased hepatic function.

Adverse Effects

Serious adverse effects include pseudomembranous colitis, superinfection, and hepatotoxicity. Common adverse effects include injection site reaction, injection site pain, nausea, vomiting, diarrhea, thrombophlebitis, arthralgias/myalgias, rash, pruritus, and hyperbilirubinemia.

Drug Interactions

Quinupristin/dalfopristin is a potent inhibitor of CYP3A4, a cytochrome of P450. Drugs metabolized through this pathway, such as cyclosporine, midazolam, and nifedipine may have increased serum concentrations. Table 49-8 presents additional drugs metabolized through this pathway.

Assessment of Relevant Core Patient Variables

Health Status

The nurse should elicit a complete medical history to evaluate for potential contraindications or precautions to the administration of quinupristin/dalfopristin. The nurse should be especially alert for a history of liver dysfunction. The nurse should evaluate the patient's current medications for drugs that are metabolized through the CYP3A4 enzyme system. Be sure to communicate any positive findings to the health care provider prior to administration.

The nurse should coordinate baseline liver function and bilirubin tests to be drawn prior to the administration of quinupristin/dalfopristin. The nurse should also coordinate liver function and bilirubin tests to be done twice weekly for the first week of therapy and once weekly thereafter.

Life Span and Gender

The nurse should evaluate the patient for pregnancy and lactation. Dalfopristin/qinupristin is a pregnancy category B. It is unknown whether quinupristin/dalfopristin is secreted into breast milk. The nurse should consider the benefits versus potential risks ratio for the pediatric patient. Dalfopristin/qinupristin has not been approved for use in children, however, in emergency situations it has been administered.

Environment

The nurse should be aware of the environment in which the drug will be administered. Quinupristin/dalfopristin should be administered in an acute hospital setting. The nurse should review the policy of the parent institution to be sure that approval by the Infectious Disease Committee is documented if needed.

Nursing Diagnoses and Outcomes

- Pain related to IV administration
  Desired outcome: The patient will inform the nurse immediately should pain at the injection site occur.
- Diarrhea related to potential pseudomembranous colitis
  Desired outcome: The patient will remain well hydrated throughout therapy and report any diarrhea immediately.
- Risk for Injury related to potential superinfection or hepatotoxicity
  Desired outcome: The patient will remain free of injury throughout therapy.
- Risk for Impaired Skin Integrity related to rash or pruritus.
  Desired outcome: The patient will report itching or rash immediately to minimize potential for infection.

Planning and Intervention

Maximizing Therapeutic Effects

Qinupristin/dalfopristin should not be administered with any other medications through a y-site unless compatibility with both the drug and diluent are established. The line should be flushed before and after administration with 5% dextrose and water (D_5W) to minimize venous irritation. *DO NOT FLUSH* the IV line with saline or heparin after administration of dalfopristin/quinupristin because this procedure is not compatible with these solutions.

TABLE 49-8 Agents That Interact With Quinupristin/Dalfopristin

Interactants	Effect and Significance	Nursing Management
Drugs metabolized via cytochrome CYP3A4 • alfentanil • alprazolam • carbamazepine • cyclosporine • delavirdine • diazepam • diltiazem • disopyramide • dofetilide • donepezil • erythromycin • ethinyl estradiol • felodipine • fexofenadine • indinavir • lidocaine • lovastatin • methylprednisolone • midazolam • nevirapine • nifedipine • norethindrone • quinidine • ritonavir • saquinavir • simvastatin • tacrolimus • triazolam • trimetrexate • verapamil • vinca alkaloids • zonisamide	Quinupristin/dalfopristin inhibits cytochrome P450 3A4 and decreases the elimination rate of drugs metabolized by this enzyme, resulting in an increased risk of toxicity and adverse effects.	Avoid these drugs in combination with dalfopristin/quinupristin Monitor for toxicity of interactants if coadministration with quinupristin/dalfopristin is unavoidable

Minimizing Adverse Effects

Because injection site problems are very common with the administration of quinupristin/dalfopristin, they should be administered in a peripherally inserted central catheter (PICC) or central line whenever possible. If administered peripherally, it should be diluted in 250-mL D_5W and infused over 1 hour.

Providing Patient and Family Education

Because quinupristin/dalfopristin is used for serious life-threatening infections, the patient may not be able to comprehend patient teaching at the onset of therapy. When appropriate, teaching should include:

- The nurse should encourage the patient to verbalize any pain during infusion.
- The nurse should teach the patient the potential adverse effects associated with quinupristin/dalfopristin such as arthralgias/myalgias, rash, or pruritus.
- The nurse should advise the patient to report feeling warm, cough, congestion, or rash because superinfection may occur.
- The nurse should advise the patient to report any diarrhea immediately to avert pseudomembranous colitis, if possible.

Ongoing Assessment and Evaluation

During infusion, the nurse should monitor the IV site for signs of infiltration, edema, or phlebitis. The nurse should question the patient regarding pain at the injection site. During therapy, the nurse should monitor for signs and symptoms of hyperbilirubinemia or hepatotoxicity. The nurse should also monitor for the onset of diarrhea. Pseudomembranous colitis may develop from a toxin produced by *Clostridium difficile*. Therefore, this diagnosis should be considered in any patient who complains of diarrhea after administration of quinupristin/dalfopristin.

At the completion of therapy, the presenting infection should be resolved. The patient will have maintained adequate nutrition, have normal liver function and bilirubin test results, and any adverse effects will be resolved. ■

TETRACYCLINES

The tetracyclines were developed as semisynthetic antibiotics based on the structure of a common soil mold. They are broad-spectrum antibiotics because of their effects on both gram-positive and gram-negative bacteria. These drugs have a common four-ring structure, hence the first syllables of their name. Over the years, major resistance has developed to tetracyclines and less toxic and more effective drugs have been discovered. Still, tetracyclines are effective against discrete organisms for which they remain the drug of choice. Tetracyclines include tetracycline, doxycycline, minocycline, and demeclocycline. The prototype tetracycline is tetracycline.

NURSING MANAGEMENT OF THE PATIENT RECEIVING TETRACYCLINE

Core Drug Knowledge

Pharmacotherapeutics

Oral tetracycline (Sumycin) is indicated in treating infections caused by *Rickettsia* species; *Mycoplasma pneumoniae*; agents of psittacosis, ornithosis, lymphogranuloma venereum, and granuloma inguinale; and *Borrelia recurrentis*. It is also used to treat *Haemophilus influenzae*, *Pasteurella pestis*, *Pasteurella tularensis*, *Bartonella bacilliformis*, *Bacteroides* species, *Vibrio comma*, *Vibrio fetus*, *Brucella* species, *Escherichia coli*, *Enterobacter aerogenes*, and *Shigella*. *Acinetobacter calcoaceticus*, *Haemophilus ducreyi*, *Klebsiella*, *Diplococcus pneumoniae*, *Staphylococcus aureus* may also be treated with tetracycline. Its use is also indicated when penicillin is contraindicated in susceptible infections; for treating acne; and for uncomplicated GU infections caused by *Chlamydia trachomatis*.

Tetracycline is also available as an ophthalmic drug to treat superficial ocular lesions due to susceptible microorganisms and as a prophylactic drug of ophthalmia neonatorum caused by *Neisseria gonorrhoeae* and *C. trachomatis*. A topical preparation is also available to treat acne vulgaris and minor skin infections due to susceptible organisms.

Pharmacokinetics

Tetracycline is administered orally because it is no longer available for parenteral administration. In the fasting state, tetracycline is about 75% to 77% absorbed. Absorption takes place mainly in the stomach and upper intestine. As the dosage is increased, the percentage absorbed decreases. Absorption is decreased in the presence of food, iron preparations, and antacids containing calcium, magnesium, and aluminum salts.

Tetracycline is widely distributed into body fluids, including CSF. Tetracycline tends to concentrate in bone, liver, tumors, spleen, and teeth. It crosses the placenta and is distributed into breast milk. Tetracycline is about 65% bound to plasma protein and does not appear to undergo hepatic metabolism; however, it undergoes enterohepatic circulation and is excreted in the feces by way of the bile. The primary excretion route is the kidney. The serum half-life of tetracycline is between 6 and 12 hours in adults with normal renal function but is greatly increased in patients with severely impaired renal function (Table 49-9). About 60% of a dose is excreted unchanged from both routes.

Tetracycline periodontal fibers are inserted into periodontal pockets. The fiber releases tetracycline in vitro at a rate of approximately 2 μg/cm per hour. Tetracycline is released at this continuous rate for 10 days at concentrations far exceeding inhibitory concentrations for most periodontal organisms.

Pharmacodynamics

The tetracyclines are bacteriostatic; they inhibit or retard the growth of bacteria but do not kill them. They retard bacterial growth by inhibiting protein synthesis in sensitive bacteria and preventing cell division and replication. Like other antibiotics, their effect on the body is indirect.

Contraindications and Precautions

Tetracycline is contraindicated in patients with a known allergy to tetracyclines or to tartrazine (specific oral preparations contain tartrazine) and during pregnancy and lactation. Tetracycline should be used with caution in children younger than 8 years and in patients with hepatic and renal dysfunction. The oph-

MEMORY CHIP

Quinupristin/Dalfopristin

- Used for vancomycin-resistant *Enterococcus faecium* bacteremia and for complicated skin and skin-structure infections due to *Staphylococcus aureus*
- Significant contraindication: hypersensitivity
- Most common adverse effects: injection site pain, swelling, or phlebitis
- Most serious adverse effect: hepatotoxicity
- Maximizing therapeutic effects: do not use saline or heparin to flush the solution because they are not compatible with this drug
- Minimizing adverse effects: administer through PICC or central line whenever possible
- Most significant patient education: teach the patient about the potential for injection site adverse effects and about the importance of notifying the nurse if injection site pain should occur.

TABLE 49-9 Summary of Selected Tetracycline Antibiotics

Drug (Trade) Name	Selected Indications	Route and Dosage Range	Pharmacokinetics
tetracycline (Sumycin; *Canadian:* Apo-Tetra)	Various infections of varying severities (e.g., *Rickettsiae, Mycoplasma pneumoniae, Haemophilus ducreyi, Escherichia coli, Streptococcus pneumoniae, Staphylococcus aureus, Klebsiella, H. influenzae, Vibrio cholerae, Neisseria gonorrhoeae, Treponema pallidum,* and more)	*Adult:* PO, 500 mg bid or 250 mg qid *Child:* (≥8 y) PO, 25–50 mg/kg in four equal doses	*Onset:* PO, varies *Duration:* Varies $t_{1/2}$: 6–12 h
doxycycline (Vibramycin; *Canadian:* Apo-Doxy)	Same as above and for antidiuretic hormone-secreting tumors	*Adult:* PO, 200 mg initially; maintenance, 100 mg/d; IV, 200 mg/d initially, then 100–200 mg depending on infection *Child:* (8 y) PO, 4.4 mg/kg divided in two doses initially; maintenance, 2.2 mg/kg in one or two doses per day; IV, 4.4 mg/kg on first day in one or two infusions depending on infection	*Onset:* PO, varies; IV rapid *Duration:* 24–36 h $t_{1/2}$: 15–25 h
minocycline (Minocin; *Canadian:* Alti-Minocycline)	Same as tetracycline and *Neisseria meningitidis*	*Adult:* PO, 200 mg initially followed by 100 mg q12h; IV, 200 mg followed by 100 mg q12h not to exceed 400 mg/d *Child:* (>8 y) PO, 4 mg/kg initially, followed with 2 mg/kg q12h; IV, 4 mg/kg followed by 2 mg/kg q12h	*Onset:* PO, varies; IV, rapid *Duration:* 24–36 h $t_{1/2}$: 11–18 h
demeclocycline (Declomycin)	Same as tetracycline	*Adult:* PO, 600 mg in four doses of 150 mg each *Child:* >8 y, PO, 6–12 mg/kg in two to four doses	*Onset:* Varies *Duration:* 18–20 h $t_{1/2}$: 12–16 h

thalmic preparation is contraindicated if the patient has fungal, mycobacterial, or viral ocular infections.

Adverse Effects

The major adverse effects of tetracycline therapy involve the GI tract and include nausea, vomiting, diarrhea, abdominal pain, glossitis, dysphagia, damage to the teeth, and, in rare cases, hepatic toxicity and fatty liver. Like other broad-spectrum antibiotics, tetracycline has a high potential to cause superinfections.

Patients with kidney dysfunction are at risk for azotemia. Dermatologic effects include photosensitivity and rash. Local pain and a stinging sensation with topical or ocular application are also fairly common. Other less frequently seen effects include hemolytic anemia and bone marrow depression. Hypersensitivity reactions have been reported to range from urticaria to anaphylaxis, including intracranial hypertension.

Drug Interactions

The effectiveness of penicillin G decreases if it is taken concurrently with tetracyclines. If this combination is used, the dosage of the penicillin will need to be increased. There is a possibility of decreased effectiveness of oral contraceptives if taken with tetracycline. Patients on oral contraceptives should be advised to use an additional form of birth control while receiving tetracycline. For more information on drug interactions, see Table 49-10.

Assessment of Relevant Core Patient Variables

Health Status

The nurse should follow the same guidelines for evaluating health status as those for a patient receiving penicillin. The nurse should assess for known allergies to any drug with a name ending in the suffix -cycline. Additionally, the nurse should closely evaluate the renal/hepatic status of patients prescribed tetracycline. It should be avoided by anuric patients, and the dosage should be decreased in patients with renal insufficiency. If renal impairment exists, even usual doses may lead to excessive systemic accumulation of tetracycline, resulting in liver toxicity.

If the dermatologic preparation of tetracycline is being used, the status of the affected area should be noted and recorded carefully to allow a baseline to evaluate the drug's effects.

Life Span and Gender

The nurse should evaluate the woman for potential pregnancy, because tetracycline is a pregnancy category D. Because the tetracyclines have an affinity for developing teeth and bones, women in the second and third trimesters of pregnancy should not take this drug. In babies born to mothers who took tetracyclines during pregnancy, mottled and discolored primary teeth may develop. The nurse should note if the child is younger than 8 years, in which case tetracycline should be avoided to prevent damage to the developing secondary teeth.

TABLE 49-10 Agents That Interact With Tetracycline

Interactants	Effect and Significance	Nursing Management
antacids aluminum salts bismuth salts calcium salts iron salts magnesium salts zinc salts	Tetracyclines form an insoluble chelate with antacids, decreasing absorption and serum levels of either or both.	Avoid simultaneous administration. Separate administration by 3–4 h.
digoxin	In some patients, digoxin is metabolized by bacteria in the GI tract. Tetracycline may reverse the process by altering GI flora, allowing more digoxin to be absorbed and increasing digoxin levels.	Monitor digoxin levels. Monitor patients for signs of digoxin toxicity.
milk and dairy products	Foods such as milk and dairy products contain calcium, which forms poorly absorbed chelates with tetracyclines.	Administer tetracycline at least 1 h before or 2 h after meals.
methoxyflurane	Tetracycline may induce biotransformation and impairment of renal excretion of toxic metabolites of methoxyflurane, resulting in an increased risk of nephrotoxicity.	Avoid this combination.
oral contraceptives	Tetracyclines may suppress intestinal flora, which provides an enzyme essential for enterohepatic recirculation for certain oral contraceptives. This may result in a decreased contraceptive plasma level.	Advise patients taking oral contraceptives to use an additional method of birth control while taking tetracyclines.
penicillins	The bacteriostatic action of tetracyclines may impair the bactericidal activity of penicillins.	Avoid combination therapy.
urinary alkalinizers	This combination may alter tubular reabsorption of tetracycline, resulting in a decreased absorption of tetracycline.	Separate administration of these drugs by 3–4 h. Monitor for efficacy of tetracycline therapy. Tetracycline dosage may need to be increased.

Lifestyle, Diet, and Habits

Because many over-the-counter (OTC) drugs contain elements that may decrease the absorption of tetracycline, the nurse should obtain an OTC drug history from the patient or an appropriate caregiver. The nurse should explore the dietary habits of the patient because tetracycline is not absorbed effectively if taken with food or dairy products.

Environment

The nurse should assess for the patient's potential to be outdoors while taking tetracycline. Because this drug causes photosensitivity, the patient should be taught to avoid direct sunlight, and if going outdoors is unavoidable, the patient should be encouraged to wear sunscreen that is rated at least as a sun protection factor (SPF) #15 and appropriate cover-up clothing, hat, and sunglasses.

Nursing Diagnoses and Outcomes

- Risk for Injury related to potential superinfection or allergic drug reaction

  Desired outcome: The patient will experience no new infection and no preventable allergic reaction related to tetracycline.
- Diarrhea related to drug induced GI effects

  Desired outcome: The patient will report any incidence of diarrhea and follow the health care provider's recommendation.
- Imbalanced Nutrition: Less than Body Requirements related to adverse GI effects of nausea, vomiting, diarrhea, and altered taste

  Desired outcome: The patient will maintain dietary intake to provide adequate nutrition.
- Risk for Impaired Skin Integrity related to drug-induced photosensitivity

  Desired outcome: The patient will dress appropriately and take adequate precautionary measures while outdoors to avoid unnecessary sunburn.

Planning and Intervention

Maximizing Therapeutic Effects

To judge the efficacy of ongoing treatment, the nurse should evaluate results of initial culture and sensitivity tests done on the infection site. The nurse should make sure that the patient receives tetracycline as prescribed, divided around the clock to increase effectiveness. To maximize absorption, oral preparations should be administered on an empty stomach either 1 hour before or 2 hours after any meals or other drugs. It is optimal to continue drug therapy for at least 7 to 10 days.

Minimizing Adverse Effects

The nurse should provide small, frequent meals; mouth care; and ice chips or sugarless candy to suck if stomatitis and sore mouth are problems. The nurse should also monitor the patient to ensure that adequate fluids are given to replace fluid lost with diarrhea. Patients should also be reminded of the potential for photosensitivity and the need to wear protective clothing and a sunscreen with a minimum 15 SPF.

The nurse should caution patients about taking outdated tetracycline. The shelf life of tetracycline is limited, and ingestion of outdated tetracycline has been associated with the development of nausea, vomiting, and renal failure. This is thought to be a result of the effects of degradation products.

Providing Patient and Family Education

- The nurse should explain that tetracycline is one drug in a class of drugs. It is important that patients understand that they should not take this drug if they have ever had a reaction to a drug with a name that ends with the suffix -cycline.
- The nurse should advise women of child-bearing age that tetracycline should not bet taken during pregnancy or breast feeding.
- The nurse should explain that tetracycline is prescribed for a particular infection and should not be used to self medicate or treat any other infection.
- The nurse should also emphasize that this drug should not be given to any other person, especially if he or she is a child, and to keep it out of the reach of children.
- The nurse should advise the patient to complete the full course of drug therapy, even if the patient feels better, and to avoid taking any outdated tetracycline because it may cause liver damage.
- The nurse should advise the patient to take tetracycline on an empty stomach, with water and not dairy products. Patients should also be instructed to take forgotten doses as soon as they remember but not if it is almost time for the next dose.
- The nurse should instruct the patient to call the health care provider if the symptoms do not improve in 3 days.
- The nurse should explain the potential adverse effects of tetracycline and potential remedies for these discomforts. The importance of contacting the provider if the symptoms persist should also be emphasized. Measures to relieve GI upset include taking small, frequent meals if the patient experience GI distress and increasing fluid intake for diarrhea. Patients with a sore mouth or throat should be advised to suck on ice chips or hard candy.
- The nurse should also teach the patient signs and symptoms of superinfections, such as discoloration of the tongue, fatigue, easy bruising, or vaginal discharge in women. The nurse should caution the patient about the potential for photosensitivity and the importance of staying out of direct sunlight and wearing sunscreen.
- The nurse should advise women who use oral contraceptives to use a back-up method of contraception while taking tetracycline.

Ongoing Assessment and Evaluation

The nurse should monitor the site of infection and compare it with presenting signs and symptoms throughout the course of drug therapy. Failure to resolve these signs and symptoms may indicate a treatment failure. The nurse should also monitor the patient for completion of the full course of therapy.

It is also important to monitor renal status to detect and prevent hepatotoxicity and to observe for any signs of superinfections and notify the provider immediately if they occur.

At the end of therapy, the patient should be free of the presenting infection. The patient will have maintained adequate nutrition, and any adverse effects will be resolved. ■

DRUGS CLOSELY RELATED TO TETRACYCLINE

Doxycycline

Doxycycline (Vibramycin) is a new type of tetracycline. It has the same pharmacotherapeutics as tetracycline and is used specifically for bacterial enteritis and Lyme disease. It is better absorbed than tetracycline, even in the presence of food and dairy products. It is excreted mainly through feces, unlike the other tetracyclines. Its half-life is longer than tetracycline, allowing for twice-daily dosing. Contraindi-

MEMORY CHIP

Tetracycline

- Used for *Rickettsia*, *Mycoplasma pneumoniae*, chlamydia, and acne
- Significant contraindications: pregnancy, breast-feeding, and in children under the age of 8
- Most common adverse effects: discoloration of teeth, nausea, vomiting, and photosensitivity
- Most serious adverse effect: azotemia
- Maximizing therapeutic effects: administer at evenly spaced intervals on an empty stomach
- Minimizing adverse effects: give frequent small meals and increase mouth care when GI distress is present
- Most significant patient education: teach the patient to complete the entire course of medication, despite feeling better. Teach the patient to keep medication out of the reach of children.

cations, adverse effects, drug interactions, and patient management are similar to tetracycline.

Minocycline

Minocycline (Minocin) is another of the newer tetracyclines. Like doxycycline, minocycline has a long half-life. In addition to the uses of other TCNs, minocycline is also used to treat meningococcal carrier states of *Neisseria meningitidis*.

Minocycline may cause dizziness, lightheadedness, or vertigo. Patients should be cautioned to assess for these symptoms before driving a motor vehicle or performing hazardous tasks. Contraindications, other adverse effects, drug interactions, and patient management are similar to those of tetracycline.

Demeclocycline

Demeclocycline (Declomycin) is used for treating antidiuretic hormone (ADH)-secreting tumors. It inhibits the renal actions of ADH. For that reason, it has also been associated with the appearance of the diabetes insipidus syndrome (polyuria, polydipsia, and weakness) in patients on long-term therapy. This syndrome is nephrogenic, dose dependent, and reversible on discontinuation of the drug.

Demeclocycline is also associated with an increased risk for exaggerated sunburn reactions. This is characterized by severe burns on exposed surfaces. Patients at highest risk are taking moderate to high doses of demeclocycline. Patients must be advised to remain indoors and to take precautions when outdoor activity is unavoidable. Contraindications, other adverse effects, drug interactions, and patient management are similar to tetracycline.

MISCELLANEOUS ANTIBIOTICS THAT AFFECT PROTEIN SYNTHESIS

Miscellaneous antibiotics include chloramphenicol and spectinomycin. Chloramphenicol is the prototypical miscellaneous antibiotics. In 1947, chloramphenicol was isolated from *Streptomyces venezuelae* and used to treat large outbreaks of typhus. It is now available synthetically as chloramphenicol, chloramphenicol palmitate, or chloramphenicol sodium succinate.

NURSING MANAGEMENT OF THE PATIENT RECEIVING CHLORAMPHENICOL

Core Drug Knowledge

Pharmacotherapeutics

Chloramphenicol is a true broad-spectrum antibiotic. It is active against a wide range of gram-positive and gram-negative bacteria, many anaerobic bacteria, *Chlamydia*, *Mycoplasma* species, and *Rickettsia*. However, it is inactive against fungi.

Chloramphenicol is reserved for use in serious infections against which other antibiotics have been ineffective or in patients who cannot take safer drugs due to resistance or allergies. It is the drug of choice for treating meningitis caused by *Streptococcus pneumoniae*, *Neisseria meningitidis*, or *Haemophilus influenzae*. It is also used in treating brain abscesses, rickettsial infections, and acute typhoid fever.

Pharmacokinetics

Chloramphenicol palmitate is hydrolyzed in the GI tract to chloramphenicol; chloramphenicol sodium succinate is hydrolyzed to free chloramphenicol in vivo. Free chloramphenicol is rapidly absorbed from the GI tract. Peak action occurs within 1 to 3 hours. Peak concentrations rise with repeated administration. Plasma concentration levels of chloramphenicol are increased in patients with hepatic and renal dysfunction and in premature or newborn infants with immature systems. The goal is to keep plasma concentrations below 25 μg/mL to decrease the risk for adverse hematologic effects.

Chloramphenicol is widely distributed throughout most body tissues and fluids, with highest concentrations in the liver and kidneys. Chloramphenicol can reach significant CSF concentrations, especially in patients with inflamed meninges. In adults with adequate renal and hepatic function, the plasma half-life for chloramphenicol is 1.5 to 4.1 hours.

Following oral administration, between 5% and 15% of chloramphenicol is excreted unchanged in the urine by glomerular filtration, and the remainder is excreted by tubular secretion, mostly as inactive metabolites. Small amounts are excreted unchanged in the bile and feces. A higher proportion (about 30%) is excreted unchanged following IV dosage, but this varies considerably in neonates and children.

Pharmacodynamics

Chloramphenicol is usually bacteriostatic but may be bactericidal in high concentrations or against more susceptible organisms, such as *H. influenzae* and *S. pneumoniae*. It works by inhibiting the protein synthesis of bacterial cells. Chloramphenicol also inhibits mitochondrial protein synthesis in both bacterial and human cells. In humans, the protein synthesis of rapidly proliferating cells, such as erythrocytes, may be affected. This may explain the mechanism of reversible bone marrow depression associated with chloramphenicol therapy.

Contraindications and Precautions

Chloramphenicol should not be given to patients who have had known toxic reactions to the drug because some fatal reactions have occurred. It should not be used systemically for minor infections because of the potential for serious toxicity. Chloramphenicol is also contraindicated in breast-feeding women because it can induce bone marrow suppression in breast-feeding infants.

Chloramphenicol should be given with extreme caution to pregnant women, infants, and children. Other patients at high risk for chloramphenicol therapy include patients with hepatic disease, renal impairment, or those with glucose 6-phosphate dehydrogenase deficiency (G6PD deficiency) and those with acute intermittent porphyria.

Chloramphenicol should be used with caution in patients with bone marrow depression or patients who have received cytotoxic drug therapy or radiation therapy. Chloramphenicol can cause a dose-related bone marrow depression and an idiosyncratic aplastic anemia.

Chloramphenicol should be used with caution in patients with dental disease. Chloramphenicol can cause myelosuppression, and there may be an increased risk of infection. Dental work should be performed prior to initiating chloramphenicol therapy or deferred until blood counts return to normal.

Ophthalmic or topical chloramphenicol should not be used continuously because it could lead to overgrowth of nonsusceptible organisms, including fungi. The drug should be discontinued if superinfection occurs. Prolonged or repeated use of topical chloramphenicol should be avoided because it could be absorbed systemically, resulting in marrow hypoplasia, aplastic anemia, and possibly death.

Otic preparations of chloramphenicol should not be used in the presence of a tympanic membrane perforation. Ototoxicity may occur if chloramphenicol enters the middle ear.

Adverse Effects

A serious and potentially life-threatening adverse effect of chloramphenicol is "gray-baby" syndrome. It is seen in premature infants or newborns receiving chloramphenicol. This syndrome is characterized by failure to feed, abdominal distention, possible vomiting, progressive blue-gray skin, and vasomotor collapse. The infant may also have irregular breathing.

Other serious and potentially life-threatening adverse effects of chloramphenicol are blood dyscrasias. These include aplastic anemia, hypoplastic anemia, thrombocytopenia, pancytopenia, and granulocytopenia. These adverse effects have all occurred following short-term or long-term therapy as a result of bone marrow depression.

Bone marrow toxicity may or may not be be dose related. Irreversible bone marrow depression, a type of nondose-related toxicity, can result in aplastic anemia, which has a high mortality rate. This type of aplasia or hypoplasia can develop months after the drug has been discontinued or from a single dose. Reversible bone marrow depression usually is dose related and is characterized by anemia, reticulocytopenia, leukopenia, or thrombocytopenia.

Other adverse effects, which may be dose related, are optic neuritis, which can cause blindness, and peripheral neuritis. Patients with either of these effects should have immediate discontinuation of the drug.

Other adverse neurotoxic effects include headache, mild depression, confusion, and delirium, but these reactions are usually mild. Patients should be monitored for other signs of peripheral neuropathy.

GI effects are usually minimal during therapy with chloramphenicol but can include nausea, vomiting, diarrhea, dysgeusia, glossitis, stomatitis, pruritus ani, or enterocolitis. Adverse GI symptoms should be reported immediately because they can indicate more severe reactions, such as superinfection.

Maculopapular rash and urticaria can occur from either systemic administration or topical application of chloramphenicol. Topical use can also cause pruritus and burning, vesicular dermatitis, or maculopapular rash. Adverse reactions indicate the discontinuation of the drug. Transient burning or itching of the eye following ophthalmic application can occur. Repeated or prolonged use of eye or topical preparations should be discouraged.

Drug Interactions

Chloramphenicol interacts with oral hypoglycemics, oral anticoagulants, hydantoins, iron salts, and vitamin B_{12}. Chloramphenicol may also interact with antibiotics, such as penicillins, cephalosporins, aminoglycosides, and erythromycin. Table 49-11 discusses potential interactions.

Assessment of Relevant Core Patient Variables

Health Status

Because therapeutic benefits generally do not outweigh the risks for chloramphenicol therapy, the nurse should assess the culture and sensitivity findings to evaluate the efficacy of chloramphenicol.

The nurse should evaluate the patient for risks that would increase the potential for severe toxicities. This includes patients with recent cytotoxic or radiation therapy, anemia, bone marrow depression, hepatic disease, renal impairment, acute intermittent porphyria, or G6PD deficiency. Patients with recent cytotoxic or radiation therapy are at risk for blood dyscrasias. Administration of chloramphenicol will increase the risk for these dyscrasias. Patients with acute intermittent porphyria or G6PD deficiency may have exacerbations of these conditions with chloramphenicol therapy.

The nurse should also evaluate the patient for the use of other drugs, such as oral hypoglycemics, oral anticoagulants, or antiseizure agents, which may interact with chloramphenicol. Other drugs to consider are those with a high risk for hematologic, hepatic, or nephrotoxicity because these conditions will increase the risk for adverse effects with chloramphenicol therapy.

Prior to initiating therapy, the nurse should evaluate baseline laboratory test results, including CBC and hepatic and renal function. Abnormal findings in these tests should be communicated to the health care provider immediately. The nurse should perform a baseline

TABLE 49-11 Agents That Interact With Chloramphenicol

Interactants	Effect and Significance	Nursing Management
antibiotics aminoglycosides cephalosporins penicillins	The bactericidal effects of penicillins, cephalosporins, and aminoglycosides can be affected by the bacteriostatic action of chloramphenicol.	Avoid concurrent administration of these drugs.
erythromycin	Chloramphenicol can displace erythromycin from binding sites on the 50 S subunits of bacterial ribosomes, resulting in subtherapeutic levels of erythromycin.	Concurrent use of these drugs is not recommended.
oral anticoagulants dicumarol warfarin	Chloramphenicol may interfere with hepatic metabolism of the anticoagulant and possibly the hypoprothrombinemic effect. This results in an increased risk of bleeding.	Monitor anticoagulation parameters closely. Adjust oral anticoagulant dose as needed.
oral hypoglycemic agents acetohexamide chlorpropamide glipizide glyburide tolazamide tolbutamide	Chloramphenicol may reduce hepatic clearance of oral hypoglycemics, resulting in clinical hypoglycemia.	Monitor blood glucose concentrations. Teach patient signs and symptoms of hypoglycemia.
hydantoins ethotoin mephenytoin phenytoin	Chloramphenicol alters metabolism of hydantoins, resulting in an increased risk for hydantoin toxicity.	Monitor serum concentration of hydantoins. Adjust hydantoin dosage as needed.
iron salts ferrous fumerate ferrous gluconate ferrous sulfate iron dextran iron polysaccharide	Chloramphenicol decreases iron clearance and erythropoiesis due to bone marrow toxicity. This may result in iron overload and anemia.	Choose another antibiotic if bone marrow suppression occurs. Monitor CBC. Monitor serum iron levels. Adjust iron dosage as needed.
vitamin B_{12}	Although the mechanism of action is unknown, chloramphenicol may decrease the hematologic effects of vitamin B_{12} in patients with pernicious anemia.	Monitor patient's clinical response to vitamin B_{12}. Consider alternative antibiotic therapy.

neurologic examination because chloramphenicol may induce adverse CNS effects. For patients receiving topical chloramphenicol, the nurse should perform a baseline dermatologic assessment because chloramphenicol may cause a rash or pruritus.

Life Span and Gender

The nurse should evaluate the woman for pregnancy. Chloramphenicol is contraindicated for pregnant women who are near term because it may cause bone marrow depression or gray baby syndrome in the neonate. The nurse should determine whether the patient is breastfeeding. Chloramphenicol is contraindicated for use with nursing mothers. Because it is excreted into breast milk, there is a risk of inducing bone marrow depression in the infants.

The nurse should assess the developmental status of the infant. Premature infants and neonates have hepatic systems that have difficulty with conjugation or excretion of the drug, resulting in gray baby syndrome. This syndrome can affect children up to 2 years of age. However, infants receiving chloramphenicol within the first 48 hours of life are at highest risk. Chloramphenicol should be discontinued at the first signs of this syndrome, because it can be fatal in a matter of a few hours.

Environment

The nurse should be aware of the environment in which the drug will be administered. Administration of chloramphenicol must occur in a setting where appropriate serum level and patient monitoring can be undertaken. The nurse should evaluate the patient daily to discontinue therapy at the first sign of adverse reactions.

Nursing Diagnoses and Outcomes

- Risk for Injury related to drug-induced adverse effects, such as blood dyscrasias, gray baby syndrome, and CNS effects, including optic or peripheral neuritis, headache, depression, confusion, or delirium

Desired outcome: Regular and careful monitoring will protect the patient from permanent drug-related adverse effects.

- Risk for Impaired Skin Integrity, rash and pruritus, related to topical drug use

  Desired outcome: The nurse and patient will observe for and report signs of unusual skin reaction and contact the health care provider.

Planning and Intervention

Maximizing Therapeutic Effects

Oral chloramphenicol should be administered on an empty stomach 1 hour before or 2 hours after meals. However, for patients with GI distress, chloramphenicol may be administered with meals.

Minimizing Adverse Effects

Although adverse effects may occur when therapeutic concentrations are within normal limits, they are more likely to occur if they are high. The nurse should monitor plasma concentrations at least weekly or more often in patients with hepatic or renal impairment. Peak levels should be in the range of 10 to 20 μg/mL, whereas trough levels should be 5 to 10 μg/mL.

The nurse should avoid IM injections because they may cause bleeding, bruising, or hematomas due to thrombocytopenia secondary to chloramphenicol-induced bone marrow depression.

Providing Patient and Family Education

- The nurse should explain the importance of completing therapy.
- The nurse should point out the potential adverse effects and the need for periodic blood monitoring and daily assessment.
- The nurse should teach the patient the importance of measuring intake and output accurately.
- The patient should be advised to report any symptoms experienced to the health care team immediately.

Ongoing Assessment and Evaluation

Serum concentrations and patients' responses to systemic chloramphenicol therapy are unpredictable. For patients receiving systemic therapy, the nurse should coordinate the serial monitoring of chloramphenicol plasma concentrations.

The nurse should assess patients on chloramphenicol therapy for signs of anemia and bone marrow depression. These include bleeding, easy bruising, or fatigue. Serial CBCs should be monitored throughout therapy.

The nurse should also monitor for signs of hepatic or renal insufficiency. For long-term or high-dose therapy or for patients with a history of hepatic or renal insufficiency, serial hepatic and renal function tests should be done. In addition to increasing the risk for toxicities, adults with impaired hepatic function have had reactions similar to gray baby syndrome.

Other important assessments by the nurse are GI and CNS effects. Although GI effects occur infrequently, they may be an indication of a more serious problem, such as superinfection. In the CNS, the nurse should monitor for optic or peripheral neuritis, headache, depression, confusion, or delirium.

For patients receiving topical chloramphenicol, the nurse should monitor for signs such as rash, itching, or burning sensation with administration.

Because most adverse effects require discontinuation of therapy, the nurse's assessment of the patient on a daily basis and communication of findings to the health care provider are the most important aspects of chloramphenicol therapy. ■

DRUG SIGNIFICANTLY DIFFERENT FROM CHLORAMPHENICOL

Spectinomycin is related to the aminoglycosides but is somewhat different structurally. Spectinomycin is usually given as a one-time injection followed by other antibiotic therapy to treat acute gonorrheal urethritis and prostatitis in men and acute gonorrheal cervicitis and proctitis in women. It is also a prophylactic treatment after known recent exposure to gonorrhea. Spectinomycin is active against a number of other gram-negative bacteria, although it is inferior to other antibiotics commonly used to treat these organisms. It is contraindicated in patients with a known hypersensitivity to the drug. Soreness at the injection site is the most common adverse effect. Other serious adverse effects are limited because the drug is only given once.

MEMORY CHIP
Chloramphenicol

- Used for serious gram-positive or gram-negative infections, especially brain abscesses or meningitis
- Significant contraindications: hypersensitivity and breast-feeding
- Most common adverse effects: headache, nausea, vomiting, and diarrhea
- Most serious adverse effects: blood dyscrasias, "gray-baby" syndrome
- Maximizing therapeutic effects: administer oral preparations on an empty stomach
- Minimizing adverse effects: monitor peak and trough levels throughout therapy
- Most significant patient education: teach the patient the signs and symptoms of bone marrow suppression and the importance of contacting the health care provider immediately if any symptoms should occur.

CHAPTER SUMMARY

- Drugs that inhibit protein synthesis may be bacteriocidal or bacteriostatic.
- Gentamicin is the prototype for aminoglycoside drugs.
- Gentamicin is used for serious infections caused by gram-negative bacilli.
- Gentamicin use is limited by its potential for adverse effects, especially nephrotoxicity, ototoxicity and neuromuscular blockade.
- Gentamicin is generally given parenterally but may be given orally to exert a local effect on the GI tract because oral drugs are more poorly absorbed.
- Drugs similar to gentamicin include amikacin, kanamycin, netilmicin, and tobramycin.
- Clindamycin, the lincosamide prototype, is used for infections caused by gram-positive cocci as well as many gram-negative or gram-positive anaerobes.
- Clindamycin is reserved for the treatment of serious infections that have not responded to less toxic antibiotics.
- Clindamycin therapy is limited by its potential for adverse effects, especially pseudomembranous colitis.
- Macrolides, such as erythromycin, are used in treating an array of infections caused by gram-positive organisms. It is less effective against gram-negative organisms.
- Erythromycin is used for patients with a hypersensitivity to penicillin.
- Erythromycin has a spectrum of activity similar to those of penicillins and cephalosporins.
- Oxazolidinones and streptogrammins are the newest classes of antibiotics developed to manage "superbugs" that do not respond to vancomycin.
- The prototype oxazolidinone is linezolid (Zyvox).
- The unique mechanism of action of linezolid may reduce the emergence of resistance.
- Quinupristin/dalfopristin, the prototype streptogrammin, is a combination drug that is 16 times more potent that each drug alone.
- The tetracyclines have been used for many types of infections in the past so that resistance is now a problem.
- Tetracyclines remain useful in the treatment of *Rickettsiae, Mycoplasma pneumoniae*, chlamydia, and acne.
- Chloramphenicol is used for serious gram-positive or gram-negative infections that have not responded to less toxic antibiotics.
- Chloramphenicol passes the blood-brain barrier and is useful in the treatment of brain abscesses or meningitis.
- Chloramphenicol therapy is limited by its potential for adverse effects, especially bone marrow suppression.

QUESTIONS FOR STUDY AND REVIEW

1. List disadvantages of TCN therapy.
2. Why are aminoglycosides only used in serious infections?
3. What are the most serious adverse effects to chloramphenicol therapy?
4. After a patient receives erythromycin for 10 days for a severe skin infection, the patient develops a vaginal yeast infection. Describe why this occurred.
5. A patient who is taking clindamycin at home calls you to report violent, watery, and bloody diarrhea. Explain the probable cause for these symptoms. What advice would you give to this patient?
6. Compare the differences between quinupristin/dalfopristin and linezolid in the management of VRE and MRSA.

NEED MORE HELP?

Chapter 49 of the study guide for *Drug Therapy in Nursing* contains exercises and activities to reinforce your understanding of the concepts presented in this chapter. For additional information see the text's accompanying website at *http://www.connection.lww.com*.

REFERENCES AND BIBLIOGRAPHY

Andes, D. R., & Craig, W. A. (1999). Pharmacokinetics and pharmacodynamics of antibiotics in meningitis, *Infectious Diseases Clinics of North America, 13*(3), 595–618.

Begg, E. J., Barclay, M. L., & Kirkpatrick, C. J. (1999). The therapeutic monitoring of antimicrobial agents, *British Journal of Clinical Pharmacology, 47*(1), 23–30.

CCIS System. (2001). Computerized Clinical Information System. Denver, CO: Micromedex.

Clemett, D., & Markham, A. (2000). Linezolid. *Drugs, 59*(4), 815–827.

Clinical Drug Monographs [CDRom]. (2001). Gold Standard Media.

Diekema, D. I., & Jones, R. N. (2000). Oxazolidinones: A review. *Drugs, 59*(1), 7–16.

Dresser, L. D., & Rybak, M. J. (1998). The pharmacologic and bacteriologic properties of oxazolidinones, a new class of synthetic antimicrobials. *Pharmacotherapy, 18*(3), 456–462.

Drug Facts and Comparisons. (2000). St. Louis: Facts and Comparisons Division

Ford, C., et al. (1999). Oxazolidinones: A new class of antimicrobials, on line at *http://www.medscape.com/SCP/IIM/1999/v16.n07/m3362. ford/m3362.ford-01.html.*

Forge, A., & Schacht, J. (2000). Aminoglycoside antibiotics. *Audiology and Neurootology, 5*(1), 3–22.

Hardman, J. G., Limbird, L. E., Molinof, P. B., Ruddon, R. W., & Gilman, A. (Eds.). (1997). *Goodman and Gilman's pharmacological basis of therapeutics* (9th ed.). New York: McGraw-Hill.

Russell, N. E., & Pachorek, R. E. (2000). Clindamycin in the treatment of streptococcal and staphylococcal toxic shock syndromes. *Annals of Pharmacotherapy, 34*(7–8), 936–939.

Sills, M. R., & Boenning, D. (1999). Chloramphenicol. *Pediatrics in Review, 20*(10), 357–358.

Tatro, D. (Ed.). (2000). *Drug interaction facts* (6th ed.). St. Louis: Facts and Comparisons

von Eiff, C., & Peters, G. (1999). Comparative in-vitro activities of moxifloxacin, trovafloxacin, quinupristin/dalfopristin and linezolid against staphylococci. *Journal of Antimicrobial Chemotherapy, 43*(4), 569–573.

Zuckerman, J. M. (2000). The newer macrolides: Azithromycin and clarithromycin. *Infectious Disease Clinics of North America 14*(2), 449–462.

Chapter 50

MISCELLANEOUS ANTIBIOTICS

KEY TERMS

arthropathy
fluoroquinolones
postantibiotic effect

Learning Objectives

At the completion of this chapter the student will:

1. Identify core drug knowledge pertaining to miscellaneous antibiotic agents.
2. Identify core patient variables pertaining to miscellaneous antibiotic agents.
3. Relate the interaction of core drug knowledge to core patient variables for miscellaneous antibiotic agents.
4. Generate a nursing plan of care from the interactions between core drug knowledge and core patient variables for miscellaneous antibiotic agents.
5. Describe nursing interventions to maximize therapeutic and minimize adverse effects for miscellaneous antibiotic agents.
6. Determine key points for patient and family education for miscellaneous antibiotic agents.

Fluoroquinolones

ciprofloxacin
enoxacin
gatifloxacin
levofloxacin
lomefloxacin
moxifloxacin
norfloxacin
ofloxacin
sparfloxacin
trovafloxacin
alatrofloxacin

Polymyxin B

The symbol indicates the **drug class**.
Drugs in bold type marked with the symbol are **prototypes**.
Drugs in blue type with no symbol are **closely related** to the prototype.
Drugs in **red** type with no symbol are **significantly different** from the prototype.
Drugs in **black** type with no symbol are **also used in drug therapy**; no prototype.

Miscellaneous antibiotics are those that have a mechanism of action other than disrupting the cell wall or protein synthesis of bacteria. These drugs include the fluoroquinolones, rifampin, metronidazole, and polymyxin B. This chapter discusses the fluoroquinolones and polymyxin B. Rifampin, the prototype for drugs affecting leprosy, is discussed in Chapter 52. Metronidazole is used most frequently to manage protozoan infections and thus is discussed in Chapter 55.

FLUOROQUINOLONES

The **fluoroquinolones** are a relatively new, synthetic, broad-spectrum class of antibiotics. Drugs within this class include ciprofloxacin, enoxacin, gatifloxacin, levofloxacin, lomefloxacin, moxifloxacin, norfloxacin, ofloxacin, sparfloxacin, trovafloxacin, and alatrofloxacin. The prototype drug for this class is ciprofloxacin (Cipro).

NURSING MANAGEMENT OF THE PATIENT RECEIVING CIPROFLOXACIN

Core Drug Knowledge

Pharmacotherapeutics

Ciprofloxacin is most active against aerobic gram-negative organisms, such as *Escherichia coli*, *Proteus mirabilis*, *Klebsiella pneumoniae*, *Enterobacter cloacae*, *Proteus vulgaris*, *Proteus rettgeri*, *Morganella morganii*, *Citrobacter freundii*, *Staphylococcus aureus*, *Staphylococcus epidermidis*, and group D streptococci.

Ciprofloxacin also has been used extensively for the treatment of serious gram-negative infections; however, resistance has developed in strains of *Pseudomonas aeruginosa* and *Serratia marcescens*. It is generally active against aerobic gram-positive organisms, but resistance has been noted in *Staphylococcus aureus* and *Pneumococcus*. For this reason, ciprofloxacin should be used cautiously in skin infections. Ciprofloxacin also is useful in treating sexually transmitted diseases, bacterial conjunctivitis, otitis externa, and in combination with other agents against mycobacterial infections. An unlabeled use of ciprofloxacin is treatment of cystic fibrosis with pulmonary exacerbations. It is not active against anaerobic organisms. Table 50-1 summarizes selected fluoroquinolones.

Pharmacokinetics

Ciprofloxacin is available in oral, parenteral, and topical formulations. Topical formulations include both otic and ophthalmic preparations. Oral preparations are absorbed rapidly from the gastrointestinal (GI) tract and undergo minimal first-pass metabolism. In healthy, fasting adults, 50% to 85% is absorbed, and peak serum concentrations are reached in 0.5 to 2.3 hours. Ciprofloxacin is distributed widely into most tissues because protein binding is low. Penetration into cerebrospinal fluid is minimal when the meninges are not inflamed. Ciprofloxacin is eliminated through renal and nonrenal routes. Renal excretion accounts for 15% to 50% of unchanged drug, whereas fecal excretion accounts for 20% to 40% of the dose. IV administration of ciprofloxacin has an onset of action within 10 minutes and peak effects within 30 minutes. Ciprofloxacin as a topical preparation has an onset of 5 minutes.

Pharmacodynamics

Ciprofloxacin, like other antibiotics, has no direct effect on the body but acts on the bacterial cell. Ciprofloxacin is bactericidal. It inhibits deoxyribonucleic acid (DNA) gyrase, an enzyme needed for bacterial DNA replication. Although human cells contain an enzyme that functions in the same manner, the enzyme is not affected by bactericidal concentrations of ciprofloxacin. Both rapid- and slow-growing organisms are inhibited by ciprofloxacin. In addition, ciprofloxacin exhibits a prolonged **post-antibiotic effect**; organisms may not resume growing for 2 to 6 hours after exposure to ciprofloxacin, despite undetectable drug levels. Ciprofloxacin is concentrated within human neutrophils, which may explain its effectiveness in treating mycobacterial infections.

Contraindications and Precautions

Ciprofloxacin is contraindicated in patients who are pregnant or lactating and in patients with a known allergy to any fluoroquinolone. Oral and parenteral ciprofloxacin is contraindicated for children under the age of 18, although topical ciprofloxacin may be used in children.

Caution should be used in patients with GI disease (especially colitis), renal dysfunction, hepatic dysfunction, and in patients who are dehydrated. Because ciprofloxacin can stimulate the central nervous system (CNS), it should be used with caution in patients with CNS disorders (e.g., seizures) or cerebrovascular disease (e.g., cerebral arteriosclerosis).

Adverse Effects

Ciprofloxacin is generally well tolerated. The most significant adverse reaction is **arthropathy** (joint disease). This often irreversible adverse reaction tends to occur in children under 18 years old. The most common adverse reactions are GI effects, including nausea and vomiting, diarrhea, and abdominal pain. These effects occur more frequently in elderly adults or in instances of high dosages.

For the most part, CNS reactions, such as headache and restlessness, occur in only 1% to 2% of patients. Other CNS effects that occur in fewer than 1% of patients include dizziness, vertigo, insomnia, nightmares, hallucinations, confusion, agitation, drowsiness, anxiety, malaise, depression, paresthesia, and increased intracranial pressure. In predisposed patients, seizures may occur.

Cardiovascular adverse effects, such as palpitations, atrial flutter, premature ventricular contractions, syncope, angina, myocardial infarction, cardiac arrest, and

TABLE 50-1 Summary of Selected Fluoroquinolones

Drug (Trade) Name	Selected Indications	Route and Dosage Range	Pharmacokinetics
ciprofloxacin (Cipro; *Canadian:* Ciloxin)	Uncomplicated UTI	*Adult:* PO 250 mg bid × 7–14 d IV: 200 mg q12h	*Onset:* PO, varies; IV 10 min
	Complicated UTI	*Adult:* PO 500 mg bid 10–21 d IV: 40 mg q12h	*Duration:* 4–5 h $t_{1/2}$: 3.5–4 h
	Respiratory, bone, joint infections	*Adult:* PO 500 mg q12h IV: 400 mg q12h	
	Severe skin infections	*Adult:* PO 750 mg q12h	
	Infectious diarrhea	*Adult:* PO 500 mg bid 5–7 d	
	Ophthalmic	*Adult:* 1–2 gtt qd-bid	
	Otic	*Adult:* 4 gtt tid-qid	
		Child: Not recommended	
enoxacin (Penetrex)	Uncomplicated UTI	*Adult:* PO 200 mg bid × 7 d	*Onset:* PO, varies;
	Complicated UTI	*Adult:* PO 400 mg bid × 14 d	*Duration:* 4–5 h
	(STD)	*Adult:* PO 400 mg once	$t_{1/2}$: 4–6 h
		Child: Not recommended	
gatifloxacin (Tequin)	Pneumonia	*Adult:* PO/IV 400 mg qd 7–14 d	*Onset:* PO, varies; IV rapid
	Sinusitis	*Adult:* PO/IV 400 mg qd 10 d	*Duration:* 18–24 h
	Chronic bronchitis	*Adult:* PO/IV 400 mg qd 7–10 d	$t_{1/2}$: 7–14 h
	Uncomplicated UTI	*Adult:* PO 200 mg qd × 3 d PO/IV 400 mg single dose	
	Complicated UTI, nephritis	*Adult:* PO/IV 400 mg qd 7–10 d	
		Child: Not recommended	
levofloxacin (Levaquin)	Pneumonia, skin infections	*Adult:* PO/IV 500 mg qd for 7–14 d	*Onset:* Varies
	Sinusitis	*Adult:* PO/IV 500 mg qd 10–14 d	*Duration:* 3–5 h
	Chronic bronchitis	*Adult:* PO/IV 500 mg qd × 7 d	$t_{1/2}$: 4–7 h
	UTI, nephritis	*Adult:* PO/IV 250 mg qd × 10 d	
		Child: Not recommended	
lomefloxacin (Maxaquin)	Lower respiratory tract infections, uncomplicated UTI	*Adult:* PO 400 mg qd × 10 d	*Onset:* Varies *Duration:* 8–10 h
	Complicated UTI	*Adult:* PO 400 mg qd × 14 d	$t_{1/2}$: 8 h
	Prophylaxis	*Adult:* PO 400 mg 2–6 h prior to surgery	
		Child: Not recommended	
moxifloxacin (Avelox)	Pneumonia, sinusitis	*Adult:* PO 400 mg qd × 10 d	*Onset:* varies
	Chronic bronchitis	*Adult:* PO 400 mg qd × 5 d	*Duration:* unknown
		Child: Not recommended	$t_{1/2}$: 12–13.5 h
norfloxacin (Noroxin; *Canadian:* Apo-Norflox)	Uncomplicated UTI	*Adult:* PO 400 mg q 12 h × 7–10 d	*Onset:* varies
	Complicated UTI	*Adult:* PO 400 mg q 12 h × 10–21 d	*Duration:* unknown
	STD	*Adult:* 800 mg single dose	$t_{1/2}$: 3–4.5 h
	Prostatitis	*Adult:* PO 400 mg q 12 h for 28 d	
		Child: Not recommended	
ofloxacin (Floxin; *Canadian:* Apo-Oflox)	Uncomplicated UTI	*Adult:* PO/IV 200 mg bid for 3 d	*Onset:* varies
	Complicated UTI, lower respiratory tract infections, skin infections	*Adult:* PO/IV 200 mg bid for 10 d	*Duration:* 9 h $t_{1/2}$: 5–10 h
	Prostatitis	*Adult:* PO/IV 300 mg bid for 6 wk	
	Uncomplicated gonorrhea	*Adult:* PO/IV 400 mg single dose	
	Cervicitis, urethritis	*Adult:* PO/IV 300 mg bid for 7 d	
		Child: Not recommended	
sparfloxacin (Zagam)	Lower respiratory tract infections, sinusitis, bronchitis, skin infections	*Adult:* PO 400 mg first day, then 200 mg qd for 7–10 d	*Onset:* slow *Duration:* 8–12 h
		Child: Not recommended	$t_{1/2}$: 16–20 h

TABLE 50-1 Summary of Selected Fluoroquinolones (Continued)

Drug (Trade) Name	Selected Indications	Route and Dosage Range	Pharmacokinetics
trovafloxacin (Trovan)	Pneumonia	*Adult:* PO/IV, 200–300 mg qd for 10–14 d	*Onset:* rapid *Duration:* 24 h $t_{1/2}$: 9–13 h
alatrofloxacin (Trovan IV)	Sinusitis Bronchitis Complicated intraabdominal infections, gynecologic infections Skin infections Complicated skin infections UTI Chronic prostatitis Gonorrhea	*Adult:* PO, 200 mg qd for 10 d *Adult:* PO, 200 mg qd for 7–10 d *Adult:* IV, 300 mg first day followed by 200 mg PO qd for 7–10 d *Adult:* PO, 100 mg qd for 7–10 d *Adult:* PO/IV, 200 mg first day followed by 200 mg qd for 10–14 d *Adult:* PO, 100 mg qd for 3 d *Adult:* PO, 200 mg qd for 28 d *Adult:* PO, 100 mg single dose *Child:* Not recommended	

cerebral thrombosis, have been reported with ciprofloxacin, but they occur infrequently.

Photosensitivity may occur with ciprofloxacin. However, this adverse effect occurs more frequently with other fluoroquinolones. Tendon rupture has been reported with ciprofloxacin therapy. Ruptures have occurred unilaterally and bilaterally and have involved the Achilles tendon, shoulder, and hands. Other adverse reactions include rash, fever, eosinophilia, and interstitial nephritis.

Adverse reactions with ophthalmic ciprofloxacin usually are associated with local effects, such as burning or discomfort. Other adverse effects to ophthalmic ciprofloxacin include lid margin crusting, crystals, scales, foreign body sensation, pruritus, conjunctival hyperemia, or a bad taste following administration.

Drug Interactions

Potential drug interactions include those with compounds that contain various salts (e.g., aluminum, calcium, iron, magnesium, or zinc). Because ciprofloxacin is bound by various cations (e.g., calcium, magnesium, iron, or zinc), administration with food that contains cations can reduce bioavailability significantly (Table 50-2). Ciprofloxacin, in combination with over-the-counter (OTC) preparation/herbal supplement St. John's wort, increases the potential for severe photosensitivity reactions. Ciprofloxacin may bind to birth control pill–receptor sites, thus increasing the risk for conception.

Assessment of Relevant Core Patient Variables

Health Status

The nurse should elicit a patient history to evaluate for preexisting GI disease, renal or hepatic dysfunction, CNS disorder, pregnancy, or lactation. Any positive finding should be communicated to the health care provider. The nurse also should assess for any known reactions to antibiotics.

Physical examination should include an examination of the skin for any rash or lesions to provide a baseline for comparison should an allergic reaction be suspected or misdiagnosed. For the same reason, the nurse should assess respiratory status, checking breath sounds for wheezing. Patients with preexisting renal or hepatic disease should have baseline blood tests performed to document current functioning. Patients with preexisting anemias or proposed long-term therapy should have a baseline complete blood count. Patients with preexisting cardiac disorders should have a baseline electrocardiogram.

Life Span and Gender

The nurse should assess the patient for pregnancy and lactation. Because ciprofloxacin crosses the placenta and enters breast milk, pregnant or breast-feeding women should not take ciprofloxacin. It also is important to note the patient's age before administering fluoroquinolone. Fluoroquinolone antibiotics have caused arthropathies, such as cartilage deterioration, when administered to immature animals. Although similar consequences of therapy have not been demonstrated in humans, ciprofloxacin should not be used in patients younger than 18 years. However, the use of ciprofloxacin ophthalmic solution is approved for use in children. Elderly patients should be monitored carefully for renal or hepatic dysfunction and receive reduced dosages of ciprofloxacin as needed.

Lifestyle, Diet, and Habits

It is important to assess the patient's typical food, caffeine, and OTC drug use. The nurse should caution the patient that food or caffeine may interrupt the action of ciprofloxacin. Patients with frequent dyspepsia should be reminded that antacids may decrease the absorption

TABLE 50-2 Agents That Interact With Ciprofloxacin

Interactants	Effect and Significance	Nursing Management
antacids	Concurrent administration of antacids and ciprofloxacin may decrease the absorption of ciprofloxacin.	Avoid concurrent use. Administer antacids if needed 6 h before or 2 h after ciprofloxacin.
azlocillin	The clearance of ciprofloxacin may be decreased by azlocillin. This may result in increased adverse effects or toxicity.	Monitor plasma drug levels of ciprofloxacin. Monitor for signs of adverse effects or toxicity.
caffeine	Ciprofloxacin may inhibit the hepatic metabolism of caffeine.	Monitor for excessive CNS stimulation or cardiovascular effects. Restrict caffeine intake if needed.
didanosine	The magnesium and aluminum cations in the buffers of didanosine decrease GI absorption of ciprofloxacin.	Avoid concurrent use. Administer didanosine if needed 6 h before or 2 h after ciprofloxacin.
food	Food interferes with the absorption of ciprofloxacin.	Administer on an empty stomach. Lengthen time interval between milk and ciprofloxacin as much as possible.
hydantoins	The mechanism of action is unclear, but ciprofloxacin may reduce serum phenytoin concentrations. This may result in seizure activity.	Monitor serum phenytoin levels. Adjust phenytoin dose as needed.
salts aluminum calcium iron magnesium zinc	GI absorption of ciprofloxacin may be decreased by the formation of iron-ciprofloxacin complex.	Avoid coadministration.
sucralfate	GI absorption of ciprofloxacin may be decreased by sucralfate.	Avoid concurrent use. Administer sucralfate if needed 6 h before or 2 h after ciprofloxacin.
theophyllines	Ciprofloxacin inhibits the hepatic metabolism of theophyllines. This may result in theophylline toxicity.	Monitor for theophylline levels. Observe for signs of toxicity. Adjust theophylline dose as needed.

of ciprofloxacin. Some vitamins also may decrease the absorption of ciprofloxacin. The safest advice would be to take any vitamin therapy at least 2 hours before or after administration of ciprofloxacin.

Environment

The nurse should be aware of the setting in which ciprofloxacin will be administered. Ciprofloxacin may be given as an oral, parenteral, or topical ophthalmic and otic preparation. In acute care settings, parenteral ciprofloxacin should be administered over 60 minutes through a large vein to minimize discomfort and reduce the risk of venous irritation.

In the home, the patient should take ciprofloxacin every 12 hours on an empty stomach. The nurse should advise patients using the ophthalmic or otic solutions not to contaminate the tip of the dispenser by contact with the eye, ear, fingertips, or other surface.

Nursing Diagnoses and Outcomes

- Diarrhea related to adverse drug effects
  Desired outcome: The patient will avoid dehydration, maintain fluid intake, and contact the prescriber if diarrhea persists.
- Imbalanced Nutrition: More or Less Than Body Requirements related to GI effects, alteration in taste, and superinfections
  Desired outcome: The patient will maintain body weight and contact the prescriber if persistent adverse effects alter nutritional status.
- Risk for Injury related to drug-induced dizziness, confusion, and other CNS effects
  Desired outcome: The patient will remain free of injury and contact the prescriber about persistent CNS disturbances.

Planning and Intervention

Maximizing Therapeutic Effects

The nurse should ensure that the patient receives the full course of ciprofloxacin as prescribed around the clock to increase effectiveness. The nurse also should coordinate the administration of drugs to decrease potential drug-drug interactions.

The nurse should review culture and sensitivity reports to confirm that the causative bacteria are sensitive to ciprofloxacin.

Minimizing Adverse Effects

The nurse should institute safety measures to protect the patient if CNS effects occur. For patients with adverse GI effects, the nurse should provide small, frequent meals as tolerated.

Frequent mouth care and sucking on ice chips may relieve stomatitis and sore mouth.

Providing Patient and Family Education

- One of the most important features of patient and family education is for the nurse to teach the patient that ciprofloxacin is one drug within a class of drugs. The patient needs to understand that neither ciprofloxacin nor any other drug having a suffix of "oxacin" (in the fluoroquinolone class) should be taken if the patient ever had a reaction to it or them.
- The nurse should advise patients who are pregnant or breast-feeding not to take ciprofloxacin.
- It is important to explain that ciprofloxacin is prescribed for a particular infection and should not be used to self-medicate or treat any other infection or any other person, especially not a child.
- The nurse should instruct patients to call the health care provider if their symptoms do not improve within 3 days.
- It is important to instruct patients to complete the full course of drug therapy, even when they feel better.
- The nurse should advise the patient to take ciprofloxacin every 12 hours. A forgotten dose can be taken as soon as it is remembered, but not if it is almost time for the next dose.
- The nurse should teach the patient symptoms of an allergic reaction (i.e., rash, welts, itching, or shortness of breath) to ciprofloxacin and instruct him or her to stop taking the drug at once and notify the health care provider if these symptoms occur.
- It is important to advise patients who experience GI upset to eat small, frequent meals and to increase their fluid intake, particularly if they have diarrhea. For patients with a sore mouth or throat, sucking on ice chips may provide relief.
- It is important to caution the patient about possible photosensitivity and encourage the patient to avoid sunlight or ultraviolet light, to wear appropriate clothing, and to apply a sunscreen with a sun protection factor of at least 15 if exposure is unavoidable.
- The nurse should advise the patient of signs and symptoms of a superinfection, such as discoloration of the tongue, fatigue, easy bruising, or vaginal discharge in women. In addition, the patient needs to know that ciprofloxacin may cause CNS disturbances or cardiovascular symptoms, and that the patient should contact the health care provider immediately if these adverse reactions occur.
- The nurse should tell the patient to report any tendon pain to the health care provider immediately because of the potential for tendon rupture as an adverse effect of ciprofloxacin therapy (see the accompanying display, Thinking Globally About Fluoroquinolones).
- It is important to inform women who use oral contraceptives to use a backup method of contraception during ciprofloxacin therapy because of the possibility of decreased effectiveness of birth control pills while taking ciprofloxacin.

Ongoing Assessment and Evaluation

Antibiotic therapy can result in superinfection or suprainfection with nonsusceptible organisms. Because overgrowth of candidal organisms can occur with ciprofloxacin therapy, the nurse should monitor patients closely during treatment. In addition, patients who develop diarrhea while taking, or soon after taking, ciprofloxacin should be considered for differential diagnosis of antibiotic-associated pseudomembranous colitis. ■

> **Critical Thinking Scenario**
>
> **Thinking globally about fluoroquinolones**
>
> Keri H., age 25, came to your clinic after a weekend of skiing in the mountains with a complaint of chest pain, cough, and shortness of breath. She is diagnosed with pneumonia and is started on ciprofloxacin 500 mg bid. Five days after starting the medication, Keri calls the clinic and asks, "Can I come back and get seen again? My chest pain and cough are gone but I am limping and my left heel hurts. I guess I must have done something while I was skiing, but I don't remember hurting myself." How would you respond to Keri?

DRUGS CLOSELY RELATED TO CIPROFLOXACIN

Enoxacin

Enoxacin (Penetrex) is very similar to ciprofloxacin except it has a narrower spectrum of activity. It diffuses into the cervix, Fallopian tubes, and myometrium at levels 1 to

> **MEMORY CHIP**
>
> **Ciprofloxacin**
>
> - Used for infections caused by aerobic gram-negative organisms
> - Significant contraindications: hypersensitivity, children, pregnancy, or breast-feeding
> - Most common adverse effects: GI
> - Most serious adverse effect: arthropathy (in children under 18 years old)
> - Maximizing therapeutic effects: complete the full course of antibiotic therapy
> - Minimizing adverse effects: provide small, frequent meals for GI distress
> - Most significant patient education: importance of completion of therapy and for women to use a back-up method of contraception

2 times, and into the kidneys and prostate at levels two to four times those seen in plasma. For that reason, it only is approved for the treatment of urinary tract infections and uncomplicated cervical and urethral gonorrhea. Contraindications, adverse effects, and drug interactions are the same as those listed for ciprofloxacin. Lower dosages of enoxacin may be given to older patients because the mean peak plasma levels are 50% higher in these patients compared with young adult patients.

Gatifloxacin

Gatifloxacin (Tequin) is a new type of fluoroquinolone. It was designed with a unique 8-methoxy structure that appears to enhance bactericidal action and decrease the rate of the development of resistance of gram-positive bacteria. Gatifloxacin is effective in the treatment of patients with respiratory infections, such as acute exacerbation of chronic bronchitis, acute sinusitis, and community-acquired pneumonia. It also is approved for the treatment of urinary tract infections and gonorrhea. It is available in bioequivalent 400 mg oral and IV formulations. Oral preparations require once-a-day dosing.

Contraindications, adverse effects, and drug interactions are similar to those for ciprofloxacin. Photosensitivity reactions occur less frequently with gatifloxacin than with other fluoroquinolones. Prolongation of the QT interval and torsades de pointes associated with sparfloxacin does not occur with gatifloxacin.

Levofloxacin

Levofloxacin (Levaquin) may be more active than other fluoroquinolones against pneumococci and certain "atypical" respiratory pathogens. It is indicated for acute maxillary sinusitis, acute bacterial exacerbation of chronic bronchitis, community-acquired pneumonia, uncomplicated skin and skin structure infections, complicated urinary tract infections, acute pyelonephritis, cystitis, prostatitis, and sexually transmitted diseases such as urethral and cervical gonorrhea, nongonococcal urethritis and cervicitis, and for mixed infections of the urethra and cervix. It is administered orally or parenterally. Oral preparations require once-a-day dosing.

Food has little effect on absorption, so levofloxacin can be taken without regard to meals.

Although levofloxacin has less affinity for cations than do many other fluoroquinolones, patients should be cautioned about taking antacids, vitamin and mineral supplements, and sucralfate 2 hours before or 2 hours after levofloxacin administration.

Significant precautions include patients with CNS disorders that predispose them to seizure activity and kidney failure. Severe renal impairment dictates a necessity for dosage reduction. Like gatifloxacin, levofloxacin has a relatively low incidence of photosensitization and QT prolongation. Unlike other fluoroquinolones, interaction studies have shown few or no problems with drugs such as theophylline, warfarin, digoxin, and cyclosporine.

Lomefloxacin

Lomefloxacin (Maxaquin) is used in the treatment of lower respiratory tract infections, such as bronchitis, and urinary tract infections. It also may be given as a preoperative prophylaxis to patients undergoing transurethral procedures or transrectal prostate biopsy. Lomefloxacin is a once-a-day oral preparation. Contraindications, adverse effects, and drug interactions are similar to those for ciprofloxacin. Lomefloxacin may induce serious photosensitivity reactions. It should be discontinued at the first sign of rash, redness, or burning sensation on the skin.

Moxifloxacin

Moxifloxacin (Avelox) is another 8-methoxy fluoroquinolone similar to gatifloxacin. It is indicated for treatment of acute exacerbations of chronic bronchitis, acute sinusitis, and pneumonia. It is especially efficacious in eradicating pathogens known to cause acute bacterial infections that cause exacerbations of chronic bronchitis. An important consideration for moxifloxacin is that to date, as a new drug, no organisms have been shown to be resistant to it. Moxifloxacin is being investigated currently for use in the management of tuberculosis. Moxifloxacin is administered once a day for 5 to 10 days. Contraindications, adverse effects, and drug interactions are similar to those listed for ciprofloxacin. In addition, significant prolongation of the QT segment has been reported with moxifloxacin. It should be avoided in patients who have conditions or are taking medications known to prolong the QT interval, or in patients with a predisposition to arrhythmias.

Norfloxacin

Norfloxacin (Noroxin) is used to treat urinary tract infections, prostatitis, and urethral or endocervical gonorrhea. It is very similar to ciprofloxacin with the same antimicrobial spectrum.

Contraindications, adverse effects, and drug interactions are the same as those listed for ciprofloxacin.

Ofloxacin

Ofloxacin (Floxin) is available in oral, parenteral, and topical formulations. It is very similar to ciprofloxacin in antimicrobial spectrum, pharmacotherapeutics, and adverse effects. However, ofloxacin is considered to be less efficacious. Drug interactions also are similar to ciprofloxacin with the exception that ofloxacin does not affect theophylline levels.

Sparfloxacin

Sparfloxacin (Zagam) is an oral fluoroquinolone indicated for community-acquired pneumonia and acute bacterial exacerbations of chronic bronchitis. It is less active than ciprofloxacin against *Pseudomonas aeruginosa* and some other gram-negative bacilli. Because of its long half-life, sparfloxacin can be administered once daily. It is administered as two 200-mg tablets the first day, followed by one tablet daily for 9 additional days.

Sparfloxacin may cause potentially treatment-limiting photosensitivity reactions as well as QT prolongation. Torsades de pointes have been reported in patients receiving sparfloxacin who were also receiving disopyramide or amiodarone. As is the case with levofloxacin, severe renal impairment dictates a necessity for dosage reduction.

Trovafloxacin and Alatrofloxacin

Trovafloxacin (Trovan) and alatrofloxacin are two different names for the same active drug. Trovafloxacin is the generic name for the oral tablets, whereas alatrofloxacin is the IV prodrug, which metabolizes into trovafloxacin. Trovafloxacin is a once-a-day drug that is highly effective against resistant organisms, including anaerobic bacteria, and penetrates the CSF to a greater degree than other fluoroquinolones. Trovafloxacin is the first fluoroquinolone to be approved for oral surgery prophylaxis.

Trovafloxacin is metabolized by conjugation, which decreases the potential for cytochrome-based drug interactions and theoretically may induce fewer adverse effects compared with those of other fluoroquinolones. However, significant interactions may occur with aluminum-magnesium antacids, iron, sucralfate, and IV morphine. Trovafloxacin has been associated with elevation of hepatic enzymes, hepatitis, and fatal hepatotoxicity. Additionally, acute pancreatitis may be induced by trovafloxacin therapy.

POLYMYXIN B

Polymyxin B is an older antibiotic that is completely different from the fluoroquinolones. It has a spectrum of activity that is limited to gram-negative bacteria with the exception of *Proteus* and *Neisseria* species. Polymyxin B binds to gram-negative bacterial cell membrane phospholipids. This binding increases the permeability of the cell membrane, which results in loss of metabolites essential to bacterial existence.

Polymyxin B is administered commonly as either a topical, ophthalmic, or an otic drug. It rarely is used systemically because of its potential for causing nephrotoxicity or neurotoxicity. It frequently is used in combination with other drugs such as trimethoprim B (Polytrim) or bacitracin and neomycin (Neosporin). It also is used in combination with neomycin alone as a urinary tract irrigant.

CHAPTER SUMMARY

- Fluoroquinolones are broad-spectrum antibiotics that inhibit an enzyme needed for bacterial DNA replication.
- Ciprofloxacin is the prototype fluoroquinolone.
- Oral ciprofloxacin may be used as an alternative to other IV medications.
- Fluoroquinolones should not be used in children, during pregnancy, or while breast-feeding due to the potential for development of arthropathies in children.
- Additional fluoroquinolone drugs include enoxacin, gatifloxacin, levofloxacin, lomefloxacin, moxifloxacin, norfloxacin, ofloxacin, sparfloxacin, and trovafloxacin.
- Polymyxin B is another type of miscellaneous antibiotic.

QUESTIONS FOR STUDY AND REVIEW

1. How do fluoroquinolone drugs, such as ciprofloxacin, inhibit bacteria?
2. In addition to hypersensitivity, which other contraindications are associated with ciprofloxacin use?
3. Why is it important that patients take ciprofloxacin on an empty stomach?
4. Why is polymyxin B rarely used in its parenteral form?

NEED MORE HELP?

Chapter 50 of the study guide for *Drug Therapy in Nursing* contains exercises and activities to reinforce your understanding of the concepts presented in this chapter. For additional information see the text's accompanying website at *http://www.connection.lww.com*.

REFERENCES AND BIBLIOGRAPHY

Ball, P. (1999). New fluoroquinolones: Real and potential roles. *Current Infectious Disease Report, 1*(5), 470–479.

Bertino, J., & Fish, D. (2000). The safety profile of the fluoroquinolones, *Clinical Therapy, 22*(7), 798–817; discussion 797.

CCIS System. (2001). *Computerized Clinical Information System*. Denver, CO: Micromedex.

Clinical Drug Monographs [CDRom]. (2001). Gold Standard Media.

Drug Facts and Comparisons. (2000). St. Louis: Facts and Comparisons Division.

Garcia-Rodriguez, J. A. (2000). The role of fluoroquinolones in respiratory tract infections: Community acquired pneumonia. *International Journal of Antimicrobial Agents, 16*(3), 281–285.

Grasela, D. M. (2000). Clinical pharmacology of gatifloxacin, a new fluoroquinolone. *Clinical Infectious Diseases 2*, (Suppl 2), S40–S44.

Hardman, J. G., Limbird, L. E., Molinof, P. B., Ruddon, R. W., & Gilman, A. (Eds.). (1997). *Goodman and Gilman's the pharmacological basis of therapeutics* (9th ed.). New York: McGraw-Hill.

Hooper, D. C. (2000). Mechanisms of action and resistance of older and newer fluoroquinolones, *Clinical Infectious Diseases 2*, (Suppl. 2), S24–S28.

Karch, A. (2001). *2001 Lippincott's nursing drug guide*. Philadelphia: Lippincott Williams & Wilkins.

Katzung, B. (1998). Basic and clinical pharmacology (7th ed.). Stamford: Appleton & Lange.

Morden, N. E., Berke, E. M. (2000). Topical fluoroquinolones for eye and ear. *American Family Physician*, 62(8), 1870–1876.

Porth, C. (1998). *Pathophysiology: Concepts of altered health states* (5th ed.), Philadelphia: Lippincott Williams & Wilkins.

Schentag, J. J. (2000). Clinical pharmacology of the fluoroquinolones: Studies in human dynamic/kinetic models. *Clinical Infectious Diseases*, 2(Suppl.), S40–S44.

Tatro, D. (Ed.). (2000). *Drug interaction facts* (6th ed.). St. Louis: Facts and Comparisons.

Chapter 51

DRUGS FOR TREATING URINARY TRACT INFECTIONS

KEY TERMS

acute pyelonephritis
crystalluria
cystitis
para-aminobenzoic acid (PABA)
prostatitis
recurrent infection
reinfection
relapse
sulfonamides
urethritis

Learning Objectives

At the completion of this chapter the student will:

1. Identify core drug knowledge about drugs that are used for treating urinary tract infections.
2. Identify core patient variables relevant to drugs that are used for treating urinary tract infections.
3. Relate the interaction of core drug knowledge to core patient variables for drugs that are used for treating urinary tract infections.
4. Generate a nursing plan of care from the interactions between core drug knowledge and core patient variables for drugs that are used for treating urinary tract infections.
5. Describe nursing interventions to maximize therapeutic and minimize adverse effects for drugs that are used for treating urinary tract infections.
6. Determine key points for patient and family education for drugs that are used for treating urinary tract infections.

DRUGS FOR TREATING URINARY TRACT INFECTIONS

Sulfonamides

SMZ-TMP
sulfisoxazole
sulfasalazine
fosfomycin

Urinary tract antiseptics

methenamine
nitrofurantoin
nalidixic acid
cinoxacin

Urinary tract analgesic

phenazopyridine

The symbol C indicates the **drug class**.

Drugs in bold type marked with the symbol P are **prototypes**.

Drugs in blue type with no symbol are **closely related** to the prototype.

Drugs in **red** type with no symbol are **significantly different** from the prototype.

Drugs in **black** type with no symbol are **also used in drug therapy**; no prototype.

A urinary tract infection (UTI) is a clinical condition caused by microorganisms infecting structures within the urinary system. It is the most common cause of infection in the United States affecting more than 7 million individuals yearly. Females are more likely to have UTIs than males because of their short urethra and the potential for contamination of the vaginal vestibule with fecal flora. Men have protection from UTIs because of the length of the urethra and the antibacterial properties of the prostatic fluid. After 50 years of age, however, men become more prone to UTIs because of prostatic hypertrophy and the potential for obstruction. Several disorders can be classified as UTIs. These include cystitis, acute urethral syndrome, prostatitis, and acute pyelonephritis.

This chapter discusses drugs used in the management of UTIs. These include sulfonamide antibiotics, urinary tract antiseptics, and urinary tract analgesics. The prototypical sulfonamide is sulfamethoxazole-trimethoprim (SMZ-TMP) (Bactrim, Septra). Urinary tract antiseptics include methenamine (Hiprex, Urex), nitrofurantoin (Furadantin, Macrodantin, Macrobid), nalidixic acid (NegGram), and cinoxacin (Cinobac). The only urinary analgesic is phenazopyridine (Pyridium). In addition, this chapter discusses nursing management related to evaluating the patient's condition, monitoring for adverse effects, and teaching the patient and family about agents for UTI.

PHYSIOLOGY

Normally, several host defenses protect an individual from a UTI. The urinary bladder is lined with a mucin layer that acts as a barrier against bacterial invasion. This layer also secretes protective substances that eventually become part of the mucin layer. Elderly and postmenopausal women produce less mucin, so they are at a higher risk for UTI.

Another host defense is the washout phenomenon. The ureters assist the movement of urine out of the renal pelvis to the bladder by peristaltic movement. During micturition, bacteria are washed out of the ureters and bladder. Interruption of outflow, such as urethrovesicular reflux (in which urine from the urethra backs up into the bladder) or vesicoureteral reflux (in which urine from the bladder backs up into the ureters) can increase the risk of UTI by introducing bacteria into the renal system. Obstruction of the outflow results in stasis of urine, which acts as a medium for microbial growth. Functional obstructions, such as neurogenic bladder, constipation, or infrequent voiding, can also increase the risk for UTIs.

Immune mechanisms provide another host defense. These include immunoglobulin A, which provides an antibacterial defense, and phagocytic blood cells, which remove bacteria from the urinary tract. Alterations in the immune system increase the risk for UTIs.

PATHOPHYSIOLOGY

Urinary tract infections are generally classified as complicated or uncomplicated. UTIs are also divided into upper and lower UTIs. Upper UTIs are commonly associated with symptoms such as fever, nausea and vomiting, and flank or back pain. Lower UTIs are associated with symptoms such as dysuria (painful urination), hematuria (blood in urine), urgency, and frequency. It is important to use these distinctions as guidelines only because studies have indicated that a patient may have an upper UTI while exhibiting only lower tract symptoms (Fig. 51-1).

UTIs can be acute, **recurrent** or chronic. Acute UTI is also known as the "initial infection." Recurrent UTIs are those caused by **relapse** or **reinfection.** A relapse is caused by the same organism as the initial infection. A reinfection is caused by a new organism. Chronic infections are those that need prophylactic pharmacotherapy because of the frequency of UTIs.

CYSTITIS

Cystitis is an infection of the lower urinary tract caused by introduction of a pathogen into the bladder. This results in redness, inflammation, irritation, and edema of the bladder mucosa, with multiple submucosal hemorrhages and sometimes pus. Symptoms may include urgency and frequency, incontinence, dysuria, hematuria, burning or a feeling of warmth on urination, bladder cramps or spasms, perineal itching, suprapubic discomfort, mild backache, or a low-grade fever. Nosocomial bladder infections, which are infections acquired in the hospital, are frequently caused by instrumentation and urinary catheterization. More commonly, bladder infections occur in the community. Factors that increase the risk of community-acquired UTIs include

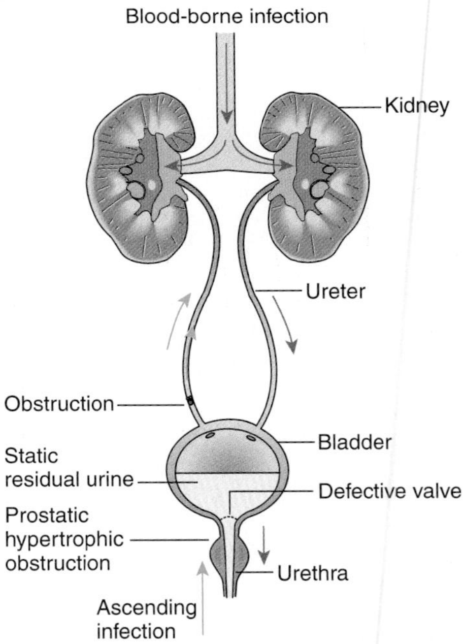

Figure 51-1. Urinary tract infections (UTIs) result from various causes: blood-borne infections that cycle through the renal system; ascending infection from external or other sources; stagnant urine (urinary stasis) caused by immobility or obstructions that allow microorganisms to colonize; defective valves that may allow infected urine to flow backward; and other problems.

pregnancy, diaphragm with spermicide use, sexual intercourse, and delayed postcoital micturition. Complications include chronic cystitis or acute pyelonephritis.

ACUTE URETHRAL SYNDROME

Acute urethral syndrome is also known as **urethritis.** It is characterized by redness, irritation, and edema of the urethral mucosa. Urethral discharge may also be evident. Common pathogens include *Ureaplasma*, *Chlamydia*, and *Trichomonas vaginalis* infections. In women, urethritis is associated with irritation by chemicals in feminine deodorants, suppositories, bubble baths, and spermicidal gels. In postmenopausal women, it is commonly caused by tissue changes related to low estrogen levels. Complications include chronic urethritis, cystitis, periurethral abscess, urethral stricture or fistula, pyelonephritis, and in men, prostatitis or epididymitis.

PROSTATITIS

Prostatitis is usually associated with urethritis or cystitis. Organisms can infect the prostate gland through the bloodstream or by ascending from the urethra. Symptoms include fever, chills, dysuria, urethral discharge, and a boggy, tender prostate. Diagnosis may be made by massaging the prostate, which results in a urethral discharge filled with white blood cells in the prostatic secretions. Complications include chronic prostatitis, epididymitis, and pyelonephritis.

ACUTE PYELONEPHRITIS

Acute pyelonephritis is an infection of the kidneys and renal pelvis. Infection can occur by way of the bloodstream or ascending organisms from the bladder. Approximately 80% of cases of pyelonephritis are caused by a uropathogenic strain of *Escherichia coli* that have specific fimbriae that attach to the epithelial cells of the kidney. When microorganisms invade the kidney, an inflammatory process is initiated, resulting in local edema. As the edema subsides with treatment, fibrosis and scar tissue develop. This may lead to impaired tubular reabsorption and diminished renal function.

Predisposing factors are urinary tract instrumentation, catheterization, pregnancy, vesicoureteral reflux, and neurogenic bladder. Symptoms include acute onset of chills and fever, flank pain, hematuria, general malaise or fatigue, headache, and costovertebral angle tenderness.

SULFONAMIDES

Sulfonamides are the mainstay of treatment for UTIs. They have similar structures, functions, and therapeutic indications. Sulfonamides are categorized as short acting, intermediate acting, topical, and long acting, although the long-acting sulfonamides are not available for use in the United States because of their ability to cause Stevens-Johnson syndrome. Table 51-1 presents a selection of drugs used in treating UTIs. Sulfamethoxazole-trimethoprim is a combination of a sulfonamide and another antibacterial drug. Sulfamethoxazole-trimethoprim, often abbreviated as SMZ-TMP, is the prototype sulfonamide.

NURSING MANAGEMENT OF THE PATIENT RECEIVING SULFAMETHOXAZOLE-TRIMETHOPRIM

Core Drug Knowledge

Pharmacotherapeutics

Sulfamethoxazole-trimethoprim has a broad range of therapeutic uses. It is indicated for uncomplicated UTIs and systemic infections caused by susceptible organisms. SMZ-TMP is frequently used for respiratory infections caused by *Haemophilus influenzae* or *Streptococcus pneumoniae.* It is an alternative treatment for *Legionella pneumophila.* SMZ-TMP is used for prophylaxis and treatment of *Pneumocystis carinii* pneumonia. Gastrointestinal (GI) infections treated with SMZ-TMP include shigellosis and salmonella. SMZ-TMP concentrates in prostate and vaginal fluids and thus is an effective treatment for infections at these sites. SMZ-TMP is also effective for sexually transmitted diseases, such as acute gonococcal urethritis and oropharyngeal gonorrhea.

Pharmacokinetics

Sulfamethoxazole-trimethoprim is completely absorbed following oral administration. It is metabolized in the liver to inactive by-products and excreted primarily in the urine. Peak plasma levels generally occur within 4 hours. After IV administration of SMZ-TMP, peak plasma levels occur in approximately 1 hour, and the half-life is age dependent. SMZ-TMP is well distributed throughout the body and crosses the blood-brain barrier and the placenta and is excreted in breast milk.

Pharmacodynamics

Sulfamethoxazole-trimethoprim inhibits microorganisms by interfering with the synthesis of folic acid (folate). Folate is necessary for the microorganism's biosynthesis of DNA, RNA, and proteins. SMZ, which is structurally similar to **para-aminobenzoic acid (PABA)**, displaces PABA and blocks the synthesis of dihydrofolic acid (Fig. 51-2). TMP interferes with microbial production of tetrahydrofolic acid. This results in the formation of nonfunctional folate. SMZ-TMP is bacteriostatic in that it inhibits the formation of new bacteria but has no effect on already formed bacteria. The presence of necrotic tissue, pus, or serum interferes with the action of SMZ-TMP because these materials contain PABA.

Contraindications and Precautions

Sulfamethoxazole-trimethoprim is contraindicated in patients with hypersensitivity to sulfonamides, deficiency of G6PD or other folate deficiency disorders, porphyria (porphobilinogen in urine), urinary obstruction, term pregnancy, infants younger than 2 months (except for treating congenital toxoplasmosis), and lactating

TABLE 51-1 Summary of Selected Drugs to Treat Urinary Tract Infections

Drug (Trade) Name	Selected Indications	Route and Dosage Range	Pharmacokinetics
Sulfonamides			
Sulfamethoxazole-trimethoprim (SMZ-TMP; Bactrim) Single strength (SS): 80 mg TMP/400 mg SMZ; double strength (DS): 160 mg TMP/800 mg SMZ; pediatric suspension: 40 mg TMP/200 mg SMZ per tsp (5 mL)	UTIs, otitis media, acute bronchitis, skin or soft tissue infections	*Adult:* 1 DS or 2 SS or 4 tsp suspension q 12 h for 10–14 d *Alternate:* 6 tablets at one time *Child >2 mo:* Up to 10 kg: 1 tsp; 11–20 kg: 2 tsp or 1 SS tab; 21–30 kg: 3 tsp or 1.5 SS tab; 31–40 kg: 4 tsp or 2 SS tab or 1 DS tab for 10–14 d	*Onset:* Varies *Duration:* 6–12 h $t_{1/2}$: 8–12 h
	Diarrhea or shigella	Same dose as above but stop after 5 days	
	PCP	*Adult and child:* 15–20 mg/kg TMP and 75–100 mg/kg SMZ in 24 h in divided doses every 6 h for 14–21 d	
	PCP prophylaxis	*Adult:* 1 DS every day *Child:* 150 $mg/m^2/d$ TMP with 750 $mg/m^2/d$ SMZ in equally divided doses 2 ×/d on 3 consecutive days per week	
sulfisoxazole (Novosoxazole; *Canadian:* Novo-Soxazole)	UTIs, chancroid trachoma, nocardiosis, meningococcal meningitis, inclusion conjunctivitis, and others	*Adult:* PO, 4–8 g/d in four to six divided doses *Child:* >2 y, PO, 25–30 mg/kg AM and PM	*Onset:* Varies *Duration:* Unknown $t_{1/2}$: 4.5–7.8 h
sulfasalazine (Azulfidine; *Canadian:* Alti-Sulfasalazine)	UTIs, ulcerative colitis	*Adult:* PO, 3–4 g/d in evenly divided doses; maintenance, 2 g/d (500 mg qid) *Child:* (>2 y): PO, 20–30 mg/kg/d in four divided doses	*Onset:* 1 h *Duration:* 6–12 h $t_{1/2}$: 5–10 h
fosfomycin (Monurol)	UTIs	*Adult and child:* (>12 y): 3 g PO, one time only	*Onset:* Rapid *Duration:* Unknown $t_{1/2}$: 4–8 h
Urinary Tract Antiseptics			
methenamine (Hiprex, Urex; *Canadian:* Dehydral)	UTIs	*Adult:* PO, 1 g > qid *Child:* (6–12 y): PO, 500 mg qid; <6 y, PO 50 mg/kg in 3 divided doses	*Onset:* Rapid *Duration:* Unknown $t_{1/2}$: 3–6 h
nitrofurantoin (Furadantin, Macrodantin, Macrobid; *Canadian:* Apo-Nitrofurantoin)	UTIs	*Adult:* 50–100 mg qid 10–14 d; suppressive history: 50–100 mg PO hs. *Child:* (> 1 mo): 5–7 mg/kg/d in 4 divided doses; suppressive history: 1 mg/kg/d	*Onset:* Rapid *Duration:* Unknown $t_{1/2}$: 20–60 min
nalidixic acid (NegGram)	UTIs	*Adult and child:* >12 y: PO, 1 gm qid 1–2 wk; prolonged therapy, 2 g/d *Child:* (3 mo–12 y): 55 mg/kg/d in four divided doses; prolonged therapy, 33 mg/kg/d	*Onset:* Varies *Duration:* Unknown $t_{1/2}$: 1–2.5 h
cinoxacin (Cinobac)	UTIs	*Adult and child:* (>12 y): PO, 1 g/d in four divided doses, 7–14 d *Child:* < 12 y: Not recommended	*Onset:* 2 h *Duration:* 10–12 h $t_{1/2}$: 1–1.5 h
Urinary Tract Analgesic			
phenazopyridine (Pyridium; *Canadian:* Phenazo)	UTIs	*Adult:* PO 200 mg tid after meals *Child:* (6–12 y): 12 mg/kg/d in three divided doses	*Onset:* Rapid *Duration:* Unknown $t_{1/2}$: Unknown

Physiology

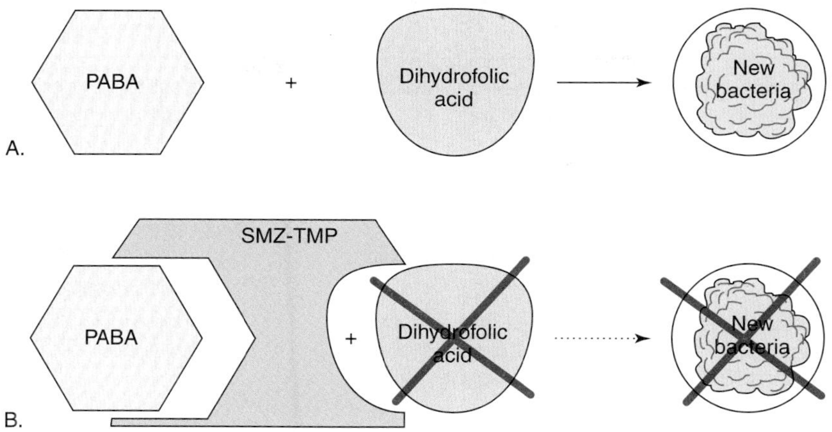

Figure 51-2. Simplified mechanism of action of SMZ-TMP. SMZ-TMP interferes with the formation of folic acid, which is needed to create the DNA and RNA for new microorganisms. SMZ-TMP displaces para-aminobenzoic acid (PABA) and blocks the synthesis of dihydrofolic acid. Both PABA and dihydrofolic acid are needed for new bacteria to form.

mothers. Patients with hypersensitivity to thiazide diuretics or sulfonylureas may have a cross sensitivity to sulfonamides because of the related sulfa structures of these drugs.

Use in pregnant women at term, in children younger than 2 months, and mothers nursing infants younger than 2 months is contraindicated because sulfonamides may promote kernicterus (staining of certain areas of the brain by bilirubin) in the newborn by displacing bilirubin from plasma proteins.

Patients with G6PD deficiency may develop dose-related hemolytic anemia. SMZ-TMP is used cautiously in patients with hepatic or renal failure.

Adverse Effects

Sulfamethoxazole-trimethoprim is well tolerated in routine use. In immunocompromised patients, however, SMZ-TMP produces a higher incidence of adverse effects. Although nausea, vomiting, and diarrhea occur most frequently with SMZ-TMP, there are three classic potential adverse reactions to this drug: hematologic effects (such as anemia), allergic reactions, and crystalluria.

Hematologic effects are related to SMZ-TMP's direct action on bone marrow. SMZ-TMP can induce megaloblastic anemia in patients with folate deficiency. Other blood dyscrasias, such as hemolytic anemia, agranulocytosis, leukopenia, thrombocytopenia, and aplastic anemia, may occur. Patients at high risk for folate deficiency are elderly adults, patients with long-term alcoholism, patients with malabsorption disorders, and patients with malnutrition.

Allergic reactions are common. SMZ-TMP is associated with several cutaneous reactions, including urticaria, maculopapular rashes, pruritus, contact dermatitis, and erythema nodosum. More severe reactions, such as Stevens-Johnson syndrome and exfoliative dermatitis, have been reported. Photosensitivity reactions may also occur and can continue for months after discontinuing the drug. Immunocompromised patients have a higher risk for photosensitive cutaneous eruptions. The mechanism for this increase in cutaneous eruptions is not clear.

Although the newer sulfonamides are much more soluble, sulfonamides in general have low solubility. As the urine volume and pH value drop, these drugs may crystallize in the renal tubules. This condition, called **crystalluria**, results in severe renal damage. To avoid crystalluria, patients should be instructed to maintain hydration by drinking at least 1.5 L of water/day.

Other potential adverse reactions may affect the central nervous system (CNS). Effects such as drowsiness, dizziness, and ataxia may occur. Additionally, depression and psychosis have been reported rarely.

Drug Interactions

Certain sulfonamides are highly bound to serum proteins. When given in combination with other drugs that are also protein-bound, sulfonamides may displace those drugs from their binding sites and enhance their action. This occurs most frequently with drugs such as oral hypoglycemics, phenytoin, oral anticoagulants, and the antineoplastic drug methotrexate. The action of sulfonamides may be diminished when administered with local anesthetics, such as procaine, that are derived from PABA (Table 51-2).

Foods that can acidify the urine (e.g., cranberry juice) should be avoided. When the urine pH falls, the sulfonamides may precipitate and cause crystalluria.

TABLE 51-2 Agents That Interact With Sulfamethoxazole-Trimethoprim (SMZ-TMP)

Interactants	Effect and Significance	Nursing Management
oral anticoagulants dicumarol warfarin	Sulfonamides inhibit the hepatic metabolism of oral anticoagulants, resulting in an increased risk for hemorrhage.	Monitor anticoagulant activity closely. Consult with prescriber about adjusting dose as needed.
cyclosporine	Although the mechanism is unknown, sulfonamides may increase the risk of nephrotoxicity associated with cyclosporine.	Monitor cyclosporine levels. Monitor serum creatinine frequently. Avoid coadministration if possible.
hydantoins	Sulfonamides inhibit the hepatic metabolism of hydantoins, resulting in an increased risk for toxicity.	Monitor hydantoin levels. Consult with prescriber about adjusting dose as needed.
methotrexate	Sulfonamides may displace methotrexate from protein binding sites and decrease renal clearance of drug. This results in an increased risk for methotrexate-induced bone marrow suppression.	Monitor closely for signs of hematologic toxicity. Consult with prescriber about adjusting dose as needed.
oral hypoglycemics	Sulfonamides inhibit the hepatic metabolism of oral hypoglycemics, resulting in hypoglycemia.	Monitor blood glucose level. Consult with prescriber about adjusting dose as needed.
zidovudine	Sulfonamides inhibit renal clearance of zidovudine, resulting in an increased effect of zidovudine in clients with impaired hepatic function.	Monitor zidovudine level. Consult with prescriber about adjusting dose as needed.

SMZ-TMP may produce false-positive results when testing for proteinuria with sulfosalicylic acid tests. This is significant because SMZ-TMP can cause a true proteinuria with associated nephrotoxicity. It may also give a false-positive result when testing for urine urobilinogen.

Assessment of Relevant Core Patient Variables

Health Status

The nurse should carefully assess for potential hypersensitivity to sulfonamides and other contraindications for drug therapy. Cross sensitivity may also occur with chemically related drugs, such as the thiazide or loop diuretics and the oral sulfonylureas. SMZ-TMP should not be administered to patients with hepatic or renal dysfunction, porphyria, blood dyscrasias, or G6PD deficiency. Patients with folate deficiency should be monitored closely.

When therapy is anticipated to last more than 2 weeks, baseline complete blood counts should be done to establish a baseline value.

Life Span and Gender

The nurse should evaluate the patient's possible pregnancy or breast feeding status. To avoid inducing kernicterus, SMZ-TMP and the other sulfonamides should not be administered to pregnant or lactating women, nor should they be given to infants younger than 2 months.

Lifestyle, Diet, and Habits

The nurse should ask the patient about dietary intake of foods and fluids that acidify the urine because many drugs are affected by urine's pH, and acidic urine increases the risk for crystalluria. The nurse should determine whether the patient has a condition that contraindicates an increased fluid intake because increasing fluids decreases the potential for crystalluria.

Environment

The nurse should evaluate the amount of time the patient spends outdoors because photosensitivity may occur. The patient should avoid direct sunlight; if going outdoors is unavoidable, the patient should be encouraged to wear sunscreen with a minimum #15 skin protective factor and appropriate clothing.

Nursing Diagnoses and Outcomes

- Pain related to altered comfort level (nausea, vomiting, diarrhea, dizziness, or headache) from adverse effects of SMZ-TMP

  Desired outcome: The patient will develop strategies to cope with pain and take the drug as directed for the full course of therapy.
- Risk for Injury related to drug-induced hypersensitivity reactions, liver or kidney dysfunction, or blood dyscrasias

  Desired outcome: By the end of therapy, the patient will be free from avoidable drug therapy-related injuries and infection.
- Risk for Impaired Tissue Integrity related to drug-induced photosensitivity

  Desired outcome: The patient will take measures to protect his or her skin from prolonged sun exposure.

Planning and Intervention

Maximizing Therapeutic Effects

The nurse should administer SMZ-TMP 1 hour before or 2 hours after a meal with a full glass of water to enhance the absorption of the drug. Patients who experience adverse GI effects may take the drug with food.

Minimizing Adverse Effects

Unless contraindicated, the patient's fluid intake should increase by 1.5 L/day. Increasing fluid intake will decrease the potential for crystalluria and decrease the ability of bacteria to multiply because of dilution of the urine. The patient should take precautions before exposure to the sun. The IM route of administration should be avoided. When administering by the IV route, the nurse should infuse the drug slowly, over 60–90 minutes. After completion of the infusion, the nurse should flush all lines to remove any residual SMZ-TMP.

Providing Patient and Family Education

- The nurse should teach the patient the optimal way to take SMZ-TMP, advising the patient to take it 1 hour before or 2 hours after a meal. However, if the patient becomes nauseated, vomits, or cannot eat, the drug may be taken with meals to minimize discomfort.
- The nurse should teach interventions to decrease the risk of adverse effects. The patient should avoid foods that may acidify the urine and drink at least 1.5 L of water a day. The patient should also wear sunscreen and protective clothing when outside. These interventions will decrease the risk for crystalluria and photosensitivity reactions, respectively.
- The nurse should explain the potential adverse effects of SMZ-TMP and advise the patient to contact the health care provider immediately if a skin rash, fever, sore throat, blood in the urine, easy bruising, or nose bleeds develop.

See the accompanying display, Teaching Strategies for Sulfamethoxazole-Trimethoprim (SMZ-TMP) Therapy.

Ongoing Assessment and Evaluation

The nurse should monitor patients for signs of hematologic dysfunction, such as sore throat, fever, bruising, or bleeding. The nurse should also carefully monitor intake and output of hospitalized patients. Optimally, the patient should maintain an output of 1,500 mL daily. The nurse should monitor urine pH as well. Urine pH below 5.5 may potentiate crystalluria. Patients with acidic urine may need sodium bicarbonate to neutralize the urine. With prolonged therapy, the nurse should monitor kidney function and perform periodic urine testing to check for crystals. For patients receiving parenteral SMZ-TMP, the nurse should monitor the IV site for signs of phlebitis. ■

Critical Thinking Scenario

Teaching strategies for sulfamethoxazole-trimethoprim (SMZ-TMP) therapy

Melissa Hawthorne, a 25-year-old graduate student, comes to the campus health clinic with a complaint of dysuria and urinary frequency and urgency. She is diagnosed with a UTI and given a prescription for SMZ-TMP.

1. Prepare some instructions related to drug therapy for Melissa, explaining the rationale for the instructions.
2. How would you vary the instructions if Melissa were 78 years old or had a history of congestive heart failure?

DRUG CLOSELY RELATED TO SULFAMETHOXAZOLE-TRIMETHOPRIM

Sulfisoxazole

Of the short-acting sulfonamides, sulfisoxazole (Novasoxazole) is the most frequently used. Sulfisoxazole is highly soluble, which minimizes the risk for crystalluria. Sulfisoxazole may be administered orally and parenterally. High plasma levels are possible, making sulfisoxazole appropriate for a variety of systemic infections, such as nocardiosis and chancroid.

MEMORY CHIP

Sulfamethoxazole-Trimethoprim (SMZ-TMP)

- Used for UTI, prophylaxis and treatment of *Pneumocystis carinii* pneumonia, infection by *Legionella, shigella, salmonella, Haemophilus influenzae*, or *Streptococcus pneumoniae*
- Significant contraindications: hypersensitivity, patients with deficiencies in G-6-PD or other folates, porphyria, urinary obstruction, term pregnancy just ready to deliver, and infants younger than 2 months old
- Most common adverse effects: nausea, vomiting, diarrhea
- Most serious adverse effects: hematopoietic effects, crystalluria, Stevens-Johnson syndrome
- **Life span alert: To avoid inducing kernicterus, this drug should not be given to pregnant or breast-feeding women nor to infants younger than 2 months old.**
- Maximizing therapeutic effects: administer 1 hour before or 2 hours after a meal
- Minimizing adverse effects: increase fluids by 1.5 L/day to avoid crystalluria
- Most significant patient education: teach the patient management strategies to avoid photosensitivity and crystalluria

DRUGS SIGNIFICANTLY DIFFERENT FROM P SULFAMETHOXAZOLE-TRIMETHOPRIM

Sulfasalazine

Sulfasalazine (Azulfidine), another short-acting sulfonamide, is given as an enteric-coated tablet for treating ulcerative colitis. Within the colon, sulfasalazine splits into its components aminosalicylic acid and sulfapyridine, which are the active antimicrobial metabolites. Its action begins in the bowel lumen instead of systemically. Its potential adverse effects and adverse reactions are similar to those of other sulfonamides.

Other Antibiotic Classes

There are several different classes of antibiotics that may also be used to manage UTIs.

Aminoglycoside drugs such as gentamicin, tobramycin, and amikacin are used for infections that originated in the urinary tract but have become systemic. This is known as urosepsis. These drugs are all administered IV.

Cephalosporins may be given orally or parenterally. Oral drugs include cephalexin, cephradine, and cefadroxil. Ceftazidime and ceftriazone may be given orally or parenterally. Although these drugs are effective, they offer no clear advantage over less expensive drugs.

The fluoroquinolones ciprofloxacin, norfloxacin, and ofloxacin are very effective in the management of UTIs. Ciprofloxacin and ofloxacin may be given both orally and parenterally. Fluoroquinolones have a broad spectrum of activity that affects most microbes that cause UTIs. Many providers use these drugs as first-line agents, despite their expense. Other providers use these drugs after treatment fails with SMZ-TMP.

The penicillin drugs ampicillin, amoxicillin, and amoxicillin-clavulanate may also be administered. Ampicillin may be given orally or parenterally. Other parenteral penicillin drugs include ticarcillin, mezlocillin, and piperacillin. Penicillins are useful for most microbes that cause UTI; however, some *Escherichia coli* resistance has been reported.

Tetracycline drugs are most useful in the management of UTI caused by *Chlamydia*. There is a high incidence of resistance with other causative microbes. Both tetracycline and doxycycline are effective.

Fosfomycin

Fosfomycin (Monurol) is classified as a miscellaneous antibiotic. It works by inhibiting an enzyme, pyruvyl transferase, which is critical in the synthesis of bacterial cell walls. The drug is distributed to the kidneys, bladder wall, prostate, and seminal vesicles. Fosfomycin has been shown to cross the placenta; however, it is unknown whether it enters breast milk. It is not metabolized and excretion occurs through both urine and feces.

Fosfomycin is administered for acute UTI as a one-time dose. Fosfomycin is administered orally without regard to meals. The nurse should advise the patient to place the entire contents of a sachet containing the equivalent of 3-g fosfomycin into 3 to 4 oz (½ cup) of water then stir to dissolve it. It is best not to use hot water. The patient should take the medication immediately after dissolving the powder.

Fosfomycin is a pregnancy category B drug. It is not recommended for children under the age of 12.

The most frequent adverse effects with fosfomycin therapy are asthenia, diarrhea, dizziness, dyspepsia, headache, nausea and vomiting, rash, and vaginitis. Although rare, serious adverse effects such as angioedema, aplastic anemia, asthma exacerbation, cholestatic jaundice, hepatic necrosis, and toxic megacolon have been reported.

C URINARY TRACT ANTISEPTICS

Urinary tract antiseptics are drugs that work by a local action because high serum levels are not achievable. Because of their local action, there are few systemic effects. There is no true prototype, so each drug will be discussed separately here.

Methenamine (Hiprex, Urex) is indicated for suppressing or eliminating bacteriuria (bacteria in urine) associated with chronic cystitis and other chronic UTIs. It is effective against both gram-positive and gram-negative organisms. In fact, the only resistance to methenamine comes from organisms such as *Proteus vulgaris* and *Pseudomonas aeruginosa*, which raise urine pH.

In acidic urine, methenamine is hydrolyzed to ammonia and formaldehyde in the bladder. Therefore, it is not useful in patients with upper UTIs and indwelling catheters. Because methenamine must be hydrolyzed into its components to be effective, it does not work for upper UTIs because the time through the upper urinary tract is insufficient for this to occur. Additionally, patients with indwelling catheters have a constant outflow of urine, again negating the time needed for hydrolization to occur.

Methenamine is contraindicated with patients with hepatic dysfunction because ammonia is also a product of its hydrolization and may elevate serum ammonia levels. Methenamine should not be give concurrently with sulfamethizole because they form an insoluble precipitate in acid urine.

Adverse reactions are minimal. The most common are nausea, vomiting, and anorexia. Methenamine may also cause bladder irritation, dysuria, hematuria, and crystalluria when administered as long-term prophylaxis.

Nitrofurantoin (Furadantin, Macrodantin, Macrobid) is another synthetic urinary tract antiseptic. Its mechanism of action is uncertain but is presumed to interfere with several bacterial enzyme systems. Although nitrofurantoin has a broad spectrum of activity, it is not an effective systemic drug because it does not achieve high blood levels because of the rapid excretion by the kidneys. It is highly effective against gram-negative and gram-positive organisms in the urinary system because high concentrations are found in urine. Resistant microbes include *Enterobacter*, *Klebsiella*, *Proteus*, and *Pseudomonas*.

Nitrofurantoin is administered in two formulations: microcrystalline nitrofurantoin (Furadantin) and macrocrystalline nitrofurantoin (Macrodantin, Macrobid). Although both types of nitrofurantoin have equal therapeutic efficacy, macrocrystalline nitrofurantoin is absorbed more slowly and induces less GI distress.

Contraindications include patients with renal impairment and infants younger than 1 month as well as pregnant women at term. As previously mentioned, nitrofurantoin has high concentrations in urine but low concentrations in blood. In the presence of kidney dysfunction, there is a decreased concentration in urine and increased concentration in blood. This results in decreased efficacy of treatment and an increased risk for toxic adverse effects. Nitrofurantoin is contraindicated for infants younger than 1 month due to the possibility of hemolytic anemia. It should also be used with caution in the elderly (due to decreased renal function) and in patients with G-6-PD deficiency, anemia, vitamin B deficiency, diabetes mellitus, or electrolyte abnormalities.

The most common adverse reactions are anorexia, nausea, and vomiting. Other adverse reactions include abdominal pain, diarrhea, parotitis, and pancreatitis. Hepatic reactions, including hepatitis, have occurred. Nitrofurantoin may induce an asthma attack in patients with a history of asthma. As with other urinary tract antiseptics, nitrofurantoin may cause hematopoietic effects, especially in patients with folate deficiency.

Nitrofurantoin has potentially serious adverse reactions. Peripheral neuropathy is one of the most serious toxic effects; however, it is reversible if detected early. Permanent damage may result if the drug is not discontinued. Peripheral neuropathy may be enhanced in debilitating diseases, such as diabetes mellitus, anemia, and vitamin B deficiency.

Nitrofurantoin is also associated with acute and chronic pulmonary reactions. Acute reactions are manifested by sudden onset of fever, cough, chills, myalgias, and dyspnea. As with other drugs, the effects are reversible if the drug is discontinued. Subacute pulmonary reactions develop over time with many of the same symptoms; however, diffuse interstitial pulmonary fibrosis may be irreversible in some patients. Subacute pulmonary reactions occur most frequently with patients on therapy longer than 6 months.

Nalidixic acid (NegGram) is an oral quinolone agent that is effective against gram-negative bacteria. Gram-positive microbes are generally resistant to it. It is indicated for use only in UTIs because it concentrates in the urine and achieves low concentrations in serum. Resistance to nalidixic acid may develop rapidly during treatment.

Nalidixic acid appears to work by interfering with DNA polymerase, thereby inhibiting bacterial DNA synthesis. It is orally administered and well absorbed, however, serum concentration levels are too low for antibacterial effects. It is metabolized by the liver into one metabolite, hydroxy nalidixic acid, which is renally excreted.

Contraindications include cerebral arteriosclerosis or seizure disorders, hepatic dysfunction, and patients with G-6-PD deficiency. Patients with severe cerebral arteriosclerosis or a history of seizure disorders may be at increased risk of toxicity, especially seizures. Hemolytic anemia may occur in patients with G6PD deficiency.

Nalidixic acid achieves therapeutic levels in urine in patients with moderate to severe renal impairment. However, patients with a creatine clearance less than 10 mL/min may be at increased risk of toxicity.

Adverse effects include drowsiness, weakness, headache, dizziness, vertigo, photosensitivity, visual impairment, abdominal pain, nausea and vomiting, diarrhea, rash, pruritus, urticaria, angioedema, and arthralgia. In patients with long-term therapy, nalidixic acid may induce blood dyscrasias.

Nalidixic acid interacts with multiple drugs. It can displace anticoagulants such as warfarin from binding sites resulting in an increased anticoagulant effect. The following agents may substantially interfere with the absorption of nalidixic acid: antacids containing magnesium, aluminum, or calcium; sucralfate or divalent or trivalent cations such as iron; multivitamins containing zinc; and didanosine chewable/buffered tablets or the pediatric powder for oral solution. These agents should not be taken within 2 hours before or 2 hours after nalidixic acid administration.

Cinoxacin (Cinobac) is another urinary tract antiseptic that works in much the same way as nalidixic acid. It is also used for acute or recurrent UTIs caused by susceptible gram-negative organisms. Like nalidixic acid, cinoxacin works by interfering with DNA polymerase.

Cinoxacin is contraindicated for use in patients with severe hepatic or renal dysfunction. The adverse effect profile is the same as that of nalidixic acid, however, they occur less frequently.

The only significant drug interaction is probenecid. Probenecid blocks the excretion of cinoxacin resulting in increased serum concentrations and decreased urine concentrations.

C URINARY ANALGESIC

Phenazopyridine (Pyridium) is used frequently for UTIs but does not itself have any antibacterial activity. It is excreted in the urine where it exerts a topical analgesic effect. It is indicated for the symptomatic relief of pain, burning, frequency, and urgency due to the irritation of the urinary tract mucosa. The precise mechanism of action is not known. Phenazopyridine is contraindicated for patients with known hypersensitivity or renal insufficiency. Adverse reactions include headache, rash, pruritus, and gastrointestinal disturbances. Hematologic reactions are possible with overdose. Phenazopyridine is an azo dye, which will discolor the patient's urine orange or red. It is important to inform the patient to expect this change in urine color.

CHAPTER SUMMARY

- A UTI is caused by microorganisms infecting any structure within the urinary system.
- UTI is the most frequent type of infection in the United States.
- Sulfamethoxazole-trimethoprim (SMZ-TMP) is the prototype sulfonamide, which is the drug class most commonly used to treat UTI.

- Many other drug classes may be used to treat UTI. These include aminoglycosides, cephalosporins, fluoroquinolones, penicillins, tetracyclines, and fosfomycin.
- Urinary tract antiseptics work directly in the urinary tract and have minimal systemic activity. These drugs include methenamine, nitrofurantoin, nalidixic acid, and cinoxacin.
- Phenazopyridine has no antimicrobial effects. It is used as a urinary analgesic in combination with antimicrobial drugs.

QUESTIONS FOR STUDY AND REVIEW

1. In addition to UTI, which other diseases or disorders are treated with SMZ-TMP?
2. Why are sulfonamides ineffective against organisms that do not synthesize their own folate?
3. What is the difference between antibiotics used in the management of UTI and urinary tract antiseptics?

NEED MORE HELP?

? Chapter 51 of the study guide for *Drug Therapy in Nursing* contains exercises and activities to reinforce your understanding of the concepts presented in this chapter. For additional information see the text's accompanying website at *http://www.connection.lww.com.*

REFERENCES AND BIBLIOGRAPHY

Brown, P. D. (1999). Antibiotic selection for urinary tract infection: New microbiologic considerations. *Current Infectious Diseases Report, 1*(4), 384–388.

CCIS System. (2001). *Computerized Clinical Information System.* Denver, CO: Micromedex.

Clinical Drug Monographs [CDRom]. (2001). Gold Standard Media.

Drug Facts and Comparisons. (2000). St. Louis: Facts and Comparisons.

Hardman, J. G., Limbird, L. E., Molinof, P. B., Ruddon, R. W., & Gilman, A. (Eds.). (1997). *Goodman and Gilman's the pharmacological basis of therapeutics,* (9th ed.). New York: McGraw-Hill.

Holten, K. B., & Onusko, E. M. (2000). Appropriate prescribing of oral beta-lactam antibiotics. *American Family Physician, 62*(3), 611–620.

Hooton, T. M. (2000). Pathogenesis of urinary tract infections: An update. *Journal of Antimicrobial Chemotherapy, 46,* (Suppl. A), 1–7.

Karch, A. (2001). *2001 Lippincott's nursing drug guide.* Philadelphia: Lippincott Williams & Wilkins.

Katzung, B. (1998). *Basic and clinical pharmacology* (7th Ed.). Stamford: Appleton & Lange.

Porth, C. (1998). *Pathophysiology: Concepts of altered health states* (5th ed.). Philadelphia: Lippincott Williams & Wilkins.

Ross, A. M. (2000). UTI antimicrobial resistance: Tricky decisions ahead? British Journal of General Practice, 50(457), 612–613.

Stein, G. E. (1999). Comparison of single-dose fosfomycin and a 7-day course of nitrofurantoin in female patients with uncomplicated urinary tract infection. *Clinical Therapeutics, 21*(11), 1864–1872.

Tatro, D. (Ed.). (2000). *Drug interaction facts* (6th ed.). St. Louis: Facts and Comparisons.

Warren, J. W., Abrutyn, E., Hebel, J. R., et al. (1999). *Guidelines for antimicrobial treatment of uncomplicated acute bacterial cystitis and acute pyelonephritis in women* [On-line]. Available: http://www.idsociety.org/pg/toc.htm.

Chapter 52

DRUGS FOR TREATING MYCOBACTERIAL INFECTIONS

KEY TERMS

chemoprophylaxis
Ghon complex
leprosy
Hansen Disease
Mycobacteria
Mycobacterium avium complex (MAC)
M. tuberculosis
M. leprae
M. avium

Learning Objectives

At the completion of this chapter the student will:

1. Identify core drug knowledge about drugs that are used for treating mycobacterial infections.
2. Identify core patient variables relevant to drugs that are used for treating mycobacterial infections.
3. Relate the interaction of core drug knowledge to core patient variables for drugs that are used for treating mycobacterial infections.
4. Generate a nursing plan of care from the interactions between core drug knowledge and core patient variables for drugs that are used for treating mycobacterial infections.
5. Describe nursing interventions to maximize therapeutic and minimize adverse effects for drugs that are used for treating mycobacterial infections.
6. Determine key points for patient and family education for drugs that are used for treating mycobacterial infections.

Drugs for treating *M. tuberculosis*

- **isoniazid**
- rifampin
- ethambutol
- pyrazinamide
- streptomycin

Drugs for treating *M. leprae*

- **rifampin**
- rifabutin
- rifapentine
- dapsone
- clofazimine

The symbol C indicates the **drug class**.
Drugs in bold type marked with the symbol P are **prototypes**.
Drugs in blue type with no symbol are **closely related** to the prototype.
Drugs in **red** type with no symbol are **significantly different** from the prototype.
Drugs in **black** type with no symbol are **also used in drug therapy**; no prototype.

This chapter discusses pharmacologic management of mycobacterial infections. **Mycobacteria** are slow-growing microbes that require prolonged treatment, generally with multiple medications. Many of the antimycobacterial drugs may be used for more than one type of infection.

Although there are many *Mycobacterium* species, this chapter focuses on three species: *M. tuberculosis, M. leprae,* and *M. avium*. The prototype drug for treating *M. tuberculosis* is isoniazid (INH) and the prototype for *M. leprae* is rifampin. The drugs of choice for *M. avium* are clarithromycin or azithromycin, both macrolide drugs that are covered in Chapter 49.

PATHOPHYSIOLOGY

TUBERCULOSIS

Tuberculosis (TB) is a mycobacterial infection that is found most frequently in the lungs; however, it may invade any organ of the body. There are two types of TB: *Mycobacterium tuberculosis hominis* (human) and *Mycobacterium tuberculosis bovis* (bovine). Human TB is an airborne disease spread by tiny, invisible particles called droplet nuclei. Bovine TB is spread through the gastrointestinal (GI) system after drinking milk from infected cows. In the United States, bovine TB is very rare because of strict monitoring of dairy herds and widespread pasteurization of milk. Symptoms of active TB include night sweats, cough, low-grade fever, fatigue, weight loss, and anorexia.

Human TB can become a devastating disease, although the bacteria itself are not particularly virulent. The damage to the human host is a result of a hypersensitivity response evoked by the bacteria. Untreated TB may result in death, whereas inadequately treated TB may result in multiple drug-resistant TB.

Human TB is subdivided into primary or reactivated TB. Primary TB occurs in a person not previously exposed to the TB bacillus. After the droplet nuclei are inhaled, it passes through the upper airways and implants in an area of rich oxygenation, such as the apices of the lungs or upper area of the lower lobes. After implantation, the bacillus is engulfed by macrophages. The combination of bacillus and macrophages becomes a gray-white granulomatous lesion called Ghon focus. As the center of this lesion becomes necrotic, it drains into the lung lymph system and creates caseous granulomas. The combination of the primary lung lesion and lymph node granulomas is referred to as **Ghon complex.** At this time, the patient will have a positive reaction to the screening test for TB, the purified-protein derivative (PPD). This is a solution that is placed intradermally on the forearm of the patient. A positive reaction is more than 10 mm of induration at the site of injection or 5 mm of induration for an immunocompromised patient.

The body's hypersensitive response to Ghon complex is to "wall off" the bacillus, and the patient remains asymptomatic. A small percentage of people with primary TB will develop active TB and become symptomatic. People with the highest risk for developing active TB at this time are those with chronic diseases and immunosuppressed patients.

Reactivated TB results from activation of previously healed primary lesions. This may occur as the body's defenses decline as the patient ages or acquires other diseases that weaken the immune system.

The standard criterion for the diagnosis of pulmonary TB is identification of the TB bacillus in a sputum culture. Three samples are usually obtained for an acid-fast stain. Another strong indication of active TB is identification of caseation and inflammation on a chest radiograph. Multiple-drug therapy is used for active TB because of the duration of therapy and the potential for drug resistance.

Patients with primary active or reactive TB require multiple drug therapy for 6 to 12 months. Therapy is based on the susceptibility of the infecting organism and the immunocompetence of the patient. Immunocompromised patients need a longer duration of therapy due to their reduced ability to fight infections.

Treatment of TB is divided into two phases: induction phase and continuation phase. For most patients, four drugs are administered daily during the induction phase with the goal to render the sputum noninfectious. During the continuation phase, at minimum, two drugs are administered daily with the goal to eliminate all intracellular bacilli. The World Health Organization advocates TB treatment with Direct Observed Treatment Short-course (DOTS). See the accompanying display, The Five Elements of the DOTS Strategy.

Patients who have been exposed to TB but have not developed active TB may benefit from chemoprophylaxis. **Chemoprophylaxis** should be considered for patients younger than 35 years with a positive PPD, patients who are or have been in close contact with people with active TB, seroconversion from negative to positive PPD within the past 1 to 2 years, history of untreated or inadequately treated TB, chest radiograph indicating TB lesions but no evidence of active TB, and those with special risk factors. Special risk factors include diabetes mellitus, prolonged corticosteroid therapy, immunosuppression therapy, end-stage renal disease, preexisting lung disorders, chronic malnutrition, and positive human immunodeficiency virus or acquired immunodeficiency syndrome. INH is given as chemoprophylaxis for 6 months or up to 12 months in an immunocompromised patient.

The Five Elements of the DOTS Strategy

- Government commitment to sustained TB control activities
- Case detection by sputum smear microscopy among symptomatic patients self-reporting to health services
- Standardized treatment regimen of 6 to 8 months for at least sputum smear–positive cases, with DOTS for at least the initial 2 months
- A regular, uninterrupted supply of all essential anti-TB drugs
- A standardized recording and reporting system that allows assessment of treatment results for each patient and the TB control program performance overall

LEPROSY

Leprosy (Hansen disease) is a chronic infectious disease caused by *M. leprae*, an acid-fast, rod-shaped bacillus. The disease mainly affects the skin, the peripheral nerves, mucosa of the upper respiratory tract, and the eyes.

There are two classifications of leprosy: paucibacillary leprosy (PB) and multibacillary leprosy (MB). It can be classified on the basis of skin-smear results or clinical manifestations. In the classification based on skin smears, patients showing negative smears at all sites are grouped as PB, whereas those showing positive smears at any site are grouped as having MB. However, in practice, most health care providers use clinical criteria for classifying and deciding the appropriate treatment regimen for individual patients, particularly in view of the nonavailability or nondependability of the skin-smear services. The clinical system of classification includes the use of number of skin lesions and nerves involved as the basis for grouping leprosy. Patients with fewer than five lesions are diagnosed with PB leprosy and patients with six or more lesions are diagnosed with MB leprosy. The correct classification is important because the treatment regimens differ between the two types of leprosy. Like TB, leprosy must be treated with a multiple drug regimen for a prolonged period of time. Drugs used in the management of leprosy include rifampin, dapsone, clofazimine, ofloxacin, and minocycline.

MYCOBACTERIUM AVIUM COMPLEX

***Mycobacterium avium* complex (MAC)** is the term used to describe an opportunistic infection caused by two similar types of bacteria named *M. avium* and *M. avium–intracellulare*. Because these bacteria are so similar, they are referred to together as a "complex." However, *M. avium* is the predominant infective organism seen in most MAC infections in people with acquired immunodeficiency syndrome (AIDS).

M. avium and *M. intracellulare* are very common. They are found in water, soil, dust, and food, and almost everyone has them in their body. A healthy immune system will control MAC, but immunocompromised people can develop a MAC infection. MAC can be localized or disseminated (sometimes called DMAC). It often occurs in the lungs, intestines, bone marrow, liver, and spleen. Symptoms of MAC include high fevers, chills, diarrhea, weight loss, stomach aches, fatigue, and anemia. When MAC disseminates, it can cause blood infections, hepatitis, pneumonia, and other serious problems.

MAC bacteria can mutate and develop resistance to pharmacotherapy. As with other mycobacterial infections, a combination of antibacterial drugs are used to manage MAC. Immunocompromised patients are started on MAC prophylaxis when their T-cell count drops below 50. Once a immunocompromised patient develops a MAC infection, treatment must continue for life to avoid recurrence. The drugs of choice for MAC prophylaxis and treatment are azithromycin and clarithromycin. These drugs are discussed in chapter 49. Additional drugs that may be used for MAC include rifampin, rifabutin, and clofazimine, which are presented in this chapter with discussion of TB and leprosy.

C ANTITUBERCULAR DRUGS

Antitubercular drugs are divided into two major categories: first- and second-line drugs. First-line drugs are those with efficacy for treatment combined with manageable toxicities. First-line drugs include isoniazid, rifampin, ethambutol, pyrazinamide, and streptomycin. Because TB can easily become drug resistant, combination therapy with three to four drugs is common.

Isoniazid is frequently referred to as INH, an abbreviation related to its clinical structure. Isoniazid is included in all therapeutic options, except in INH-resistant TB. For that reason, INH is the prototype for antitubercular drugs.

NURSING MANAGEMENT OF THE PATIENT RECEIVING P ISONIAZID

Core Drug Knowledge

Pharmacotherapeutics

Isoniazid is an antibacterial drug used to treat or prevent TB infection and other susceptible mycobacterial infections. Organisms generally considered susceptible to INH therapy include *M. avium*, *M. bovis*, *M. intracellulare*, *M. kansasii*, *M. szulgai*, and *M. xenopi*. In unlabeled use, INH has treated severe tremors associated with multiple sclerosis.

Pharmacokinetics

Isoniazid is administered orally and intramuscularly. It is absorbed rapidly from the GI tract with peak serum levels attained within 12 hours. It is distributed into all body tissues and fluids and crosses the blood-brain barrier to achieve therapeutic levels in the cerebrospinal fluid (CSF). It also crosses the placenta and is distributed into breast milk. INH is metabolized in the liver to inactive metabolites. About 75% of the drug and its metabolites are excreted in the urine and the rest in the feces, saliva, and sputum (Table 52-1).

Pharmacodynamics

Isoniazid is bactericidal or bacteriostatic, depending on the drug concentration within an infected site and the susceptibility of the organism. It works by disrupting the synthesis of the bacterial cell wall. Some patients have experienced adverse effects after ingesting tyramine-containing foods. This suggests that INH may inhibit plasma monoamine oxidase, although this action has not been documented. INH has no direct effect on the body.

Contraindications and Precautions

Isoniazid is contraindicated in patients with acute hepatic disease and patients with a history of INH-induced hepatic disease. INH should be used with caution in patients with chronic hepatic disease, alcoholism, or severe renal impairment because elimination of the drug can be prolonged, increasing the likelihood of adverse reactions.

TABLE 52-1 Summary of Selected Antimycobacterial Drugs

Drug (Trade) Name	Selected Indications	Route and Dosage Range	Pharmacokinetics
isoniazid (Laniazid; *Canadian:* Isotamine)	TB in conjunction with other drug therapy, prophylaxis of TB	*Adult:* PO, active TB, 5 mg/kg/d up to 300 mg in single dose; prophylaxis, 300 mg/d in single dose *Child:* PO, active TB, 10–20 mg/kg/d; prophylaxis, 10 mg/kg/d in single dose	*Onset:* Varies *Duration:* 24 h $t_{1/2}$: 1–4 h
rifampin (Rifadin; *Canadian:* Rofact)	TB in conjunction with other drug therapy, prophylaxis of TB	*Adult:* PO or IV, 600 mg in single daily dose until improvement occurs; direct observed treatment (DOTS) 10 mg/kg 2 × wk *Child:* 10–20 mg/k not to exceed 600 mg qd	*Onset:* PO, varies; IV, rapid *Duration:* 6 h $t_{1/2}$: 3–5.1 h
	Leprosy	*Adult:* PO or IV 600 mg 1 × month for 6–24 mo *Child:* not recommended	
	Mycobacterium avium complex (MAC)	*Adult:* 600 mg PO or IV in combination with other antimycobacterials *Child:* 10–20 mg/kg PO or IV in combination with other antimycobacterials	
clofazimine (Lamprene)	Leprosy	*Adult:* 50 mg qd self-administered 300 mg q month if supervised *Child:* 1 mg/kg/d	*Onset:* 1 h *Duration:* Unknown $t_{1/2}$: Terminal 8 days, tissue 70 days
dapsone (Avlosulfon)	Leprosy	*Adult:* PO, 100 mg qd *Child:* 1–2 mg/kg/d	*Onset:* 2 h *Duration:* Unknown $t_{1/2}$: 30 h
ethambutol (Myambutol; *Canadian:* Etibi)	TB in conjunction with other drug therapy, prophylaxis of TB	*Adult:* PO, mg/kg/d as single oral dose; retreatment, 25 mg/kg/d reduced after 60 d to 15 mg/kg/d once daily *Child:* Not recommended for children younger than 13 y	*Onset:* Rapid *Duration:* 20–24 h $t_{1/2}$: 3.3 h
pyrazinamide	TB in conjunction with other drug therapy, prophylaxis of TB	*Adult:* PO, 15–30 mg/d once daily *Child:* Same	*Onset:* Rapid *Duration:* 9.5 h $t_{1/2}$: 9–10 h
rifabutin (Mycobutin)	TB, leprosy, MAC	*Adult:* 300 mg PO qd, may be given 150 mg bid to decrease GI distress *Child:* Not approved	*Onset:* 1 h *Duration:* Unknown $t_{1/2}$: 16–69 h
rifapentine (Priftin)	TB	*Adult and child:* (> 12 y); 600 mg 2 × wk for 2 mo, then 1 × week for 4 mo *Child:* Not recommended	*Onset:* 5–6 h *Duration:* Unknown $t_{1/2}$: 13 h
streptomycin	TB in conjunction with other drug therapy, prophylaxis of TB	*Adult:* IM, 15 mg/kg with a maximum of 1 g/d; reduce to 25–30 mg/kg or maximum of 1.5 g two to three times a week *Child:* IM, 20–40 mg/kg/d in divided doses q6–12h to a maximum of 1 g/d; reduce to 25–30 mg/kg two to three times a week	*Onset:* Rapid *Duration:* 24 h $t_{1/2}$: 2.5 h

INH should also be given with caution to patients with diabetes mellitus, malnutrition, or alcoholism. INH can cause peripheral neuropathy due to pyridoxine antagonism or increased excretion of pyridoxine. These patients have a higher risk for this adverse effect. Pyridoxine (vitamin B_6) may be given concurrently with INH to decrease the risk for this adverse effect.

INH should be used with caution in patients with a seizure disorder. INH may cause neurotoxicity and result in seizures. It also may produce an acneiform rash or exacerbate preexisting acne.

Data are conflicting about INH use during pregnancy; it is classified as pregnancy category C. Because of the multidrug regimen to combat TB, studies have not been able to elicit the exact risk of INH to the fetus. INH appears to be safe for use during lactation.

Adverse Effects

The major adverse effect of INH therapy is hepatitis. In addition to hepatitis, elevated hepatic enzyme levels (aspartate transaminase, alanine transaminase), bilirubinemia, and jaundice have been reported.

of INH.

before or 2 hours after administering INH.

Another frequent adverse effect is peripheral neu- cause interstitial nephritis or CNS toxicity resulting in

fatal anaphylactoid reactions, although the incidence is low.

Because of its potential adverse effects to the liver, rifampin is used cautiously in patients with a history of hepatic dysfunction or in patients known to have alcoholism. It is also used cautiously with patients taking other medications known to be hepatotoxic.

Adverse Effects

Rifampin may cause adverse effects similar to those of INH, especially hepatic injury. Additionally, rifampin can discolor bodily fluids, such as urine, saliva, tears, and sputum.

Wearers of soft contact lenses should be cautioned that the lenses may be permanently discolored.

Although rifampin is generally well tolerated, it may cause GI disturbances such as nausea and vomiting, anorexia, flatulence, cramps, and diarrhea. Rarely, rifampin may induce pseudomembranous colitis or pancreatitis.

High-dose therapy may induce a flu-like syndrome with fever, chills, headache, and fatigue. Other adverse effects that can be induced by high-dose therapy include leukopenia, hemolysis with anemia, shortness of breath, shock, and renal failure.

Drug Interactions

Rifampin is a potent inducer of the cytochrome P450 hepatic enzyme system and its subsets. This may result in the reduction of plasma concentrations of other drugs metabolized by the P450 enzyme system. When these drugs are given concurrently with rifampin, their dosage may need to be increased. In some cases, the drugs are contraindicated for concurrent use (Table 52-3).

Assessment of Relevant Core Patient Variables

Health Status

The nurse should assess for diseases or disorders that contradict the use rifampin or require strict monitoring during therapy, especially those that increase the risk for hepatotoxicity. The nurse should assess for any medications that may interact with rifampin or other drugs known to be hepatotoxic. Any positive findings should be communicated to the health care provider prior to initiation of therapy.

The nurse should pay special attention to patients with a diagnosis of human immunodeficiency virus (HIV) or AIDS.

Many drugs used to treat these disorders are contraindicated for use with rifampin. Additionally, patients with HIV or AIDS need therapy for a longer duration, increasing the problem of compliance.

The nurse should arrange for baseline laboratory tests prior to administration of rifampin. These tests include a CBC and hepatic and renal studies.

Life Span and Gender

Rifampin is a pregnancy category C, so it is important to evaluate the patient's possible pregnancy status. The drug may be used in children less than 1 month of age.

Lifestyle, Diet, and Habits

The nurse should assess for the consumption of alcohol and explain the increased risk for hepatoxicity when alcohol consumption is combined with rifampin therapy. Because rifampin can discolor body fluids red-orange, the nurse should suggest that soft contact lens wearers change to a different type of contacts or regular glasses throughout therapy. Dietary changes are not needed.

Environment

Rifampin can be given in any environment. It is most frequently used in the home environment. Intravenous rifampin is given most frequently administered in an acute care hospital. The nurse should be aware of the environment in which the drug will be administered. It is important to explore with the patient any factors in the home setting that may affect compliance with drug therapy.

Nursing Diagnoses and Outcomes

- Risk for Injury related to hepatic injury
  Desired outcome: The patient will remain free of injury and contact the health care provider if signs such as yellow skin, itching, or fatigue occur.
- Imbalanced Nutrition: Less than Body Requirements related to potential nausea, vomiting, anorexia, and diarrhea
  Desired outcome: The patient will have balanced nutrition throughout therapy.
- Ineffective Protection related to potential leukopenia or hemolysis with anemia
  Desired outcome: The patient will remain without superinfection throughout therapy.

Planning and Intervention

Maximizing Therapeutic Effects

The nurse should administer intravenous rifampin by slow infusion over 3 hours. Oral rifampin should be given 1 hour before or 2 hours after a meal to avoid decreasing its absorption. The nurse should promote compliance with oral rifampin by explaining the importance of taking the medication daily.

Minimizing Adverse Effects

The nurse should evaluate the patient for contraindications of its use and should avoid administration of rifampin to a patient with signs of hepatotoxicity.

Providing Patient and Family Education

- The nurse should explain the potential effect of rifampin to the liver. Patients should be advised to contact the health care provider immediately if they

TABLE 52-3 Agents That Interact With Rifampin

Interactants	Effect and Significance	Nursing Management
protease inhibitors, non-nucleoside reverse transcriptase inhibitors	Rifampin increases the metabolism of the antiretroviral drugs resulting in decreased plasma concentrations.	Concurrent use is not recommended.
Drugs affected by induction: • anticoagulants • beta-blockers • oral contraceptives • corticosteroids • cyclosporine • digitoxin • disopyramide • doxycycline • estrogens • haloperidol • hydantoins • nifedipine • quinine derivatives • sulfonylurea agents • theophyllines • tricyclic antidepressants • zolpidem	Increased hepatic microsomal enzyme metabolism (induction) by rifampin results in decreased action of interactant drugs.	Monitor for efficacy of interactant drugs. Adjust interactant drug dosages as needed. Consult prescriber about choosing an alternate drug in place of the interactant as needed.
azole antifungal agents	Rifampin may induce the metabolism of azole antifungal drugs resulting in decreased action of azole antifungal drugs. Additionally, azole antifungal drugs interfere with the absorption of rifampin resulting in decreased serum rifampin levels.	Monitor for efficacy of azole antifungal drugs. Monitor for efficacy of rifampin. Consult with prescriber about adjusting drug dosages as needed.
benzodiazepines	The oxidative metabolism of benzodiazepines may be increased resulting in decreased pharmacologic effects.	Monitor for efficacy of benzodiazepine drugs. Consult with prescriber about adjusting benzodiazepine drug dosages as needed.
buspirone, verapamil	Rifampin induces first-pass metabolism of these drugs resulting in decreased plasma concentration.	Monitor for efficacy of interactants. Consult with prescriber about adjusting dosages of interactants as needed.
isoniazid	Rifampin may cause an alteration in the metabolism of isoniazid. Hepatotoxicity may occur at a rate higher than with either agent alone.	Monitor for signs of hepatotoxicity. Monitor liver function studies. Discontinue as needed.
macrolide antibiotics	The metabolism of rifampin may be inhibited while the metabolism of macrolide antibiotics may be increased, resulting in decreased antimicrobial effects and increased GI adverse effects.	Monitor for efficacy of macrolide antibiotics. Monitor for adverse GI effects of macrolide antibiotics. Consult with prescriber about using azithromycin or dirithromycin as alternative drugs because they do not undergo metabolism.
methadone	Rifampin stimulates the metabolism of methadone, resulting in a decreased efficacy of methadone.	Monitor the patient for signs of narcotic withdrawal.
morphine	Rifampin stimulates the metabolism of morphine resulting in a decreased efficacy of morphine.	Monitor the patient's clinical response to morphine. Administer an alternative analgesic as needed.

experience anorexia, nausea, fatigue, malaise, jaundice, cola-colored urine, or pale stools. The nurse should also explain that many drugs increase the risk for hepatic damage and to contact the health care provider before taking any new drugs, even those prescribed by another provider. The nurse should explain that alcohol consumption may also increase the risk for hepatic damage.

- The nurse should advise patients with soft contact lenses to consult their ophthalmologist for an alternate form of contacts or glasses. Assure the patient that the discoloration of body fluids is not harmful.
- Because compliance is always difficult when the medication needs to be taken for a prolonged period of time, the nurse should explain the importance of

consistently taking the medication, despite the fact the patient will not feel different.

- The nurse should explain the importance of consistent follow-up visits to ensure eradication of the *Mycobacterium* as well as monitoring for adverse effects.

Ongoing Assessment and Evaluation

The nurse should ask patients whether they have experienced any symptoms suggestive of hepatic dysfunction. Periodic testing of hematopoietic, renal, and hepatic function should also be arranged.

By the end of therapy, the *Mycobacterium* should be eradicated and the patient should be free from any adverse effects from rifampin therapy. ■

DRUGS CLOSELY RELATED TO RIFAMPIN

Rifabutin

Rifabutin (Mycobutin) is an oral antimycobacterial agent that is a derivative of rifamycin. It is used for prophylaxis or treatment of TB and MAC. *M. leprae* is also considered to be susceptible to rifabutin, but it is not a labeled indication. Like rifampin, rifabutin inhibits mycobacterial RNA synthesis.

Rifabutin is administered orally and is rapidly absorbed. Absorption can be slowed in the presence of a high-fat meal. It is metabolized in the liver. Excretion is predominantly in the urine, with approximately 30% in feces and 5% through the biliary pathway.

The most serious adverse effects of rifabutin are uveitis and blood dyscrasias. Like rifampin, rifabutin may cause discoloration of body fluids. Common adverse effects include rash, nausea, abdominal pain, and dyspepsia. Less frequently reported adverse reactions to rifabutin include seizures, taste perversion, nonspecific T-wave changes on electrocardiography, and myalgia. Rifabutin may cause hepatitis and elevated hepatic enzyme levels, but those adverse effects occur most frequently in patients with disseminated disease.

Rifabutin appears to be a less potent hepatic enzyme inducer than rifampin, although similar drug-drug interactions may still occur. Rifabutin does not interfere with the metabolism of INH. Rifabutin is contraindicated for concurrent use with nonnucleoside reverse transcriptase inhibitors, hard-gel formulation saquinavir, or ritonavir. It can be given cautiously with other antiretroviral agents, but the dosage of those other agents may need to be increased.

MEMORY CHIP

Rifampin

- Used for the management of acute TB and leprosy; also used in the management of other mycobacterial infections
- Significant contraindication: hypersensitivity
- Most common adverse effects: discoloration of body fluids, GI disturbances
- Most serious adverse effect: hepatotoxicity
- Maximizing therapeutic effects: administer on an empty stomach
- Minimizing adverse effects: evaluate the patient for potential drug-drug interactions
- Most significant patient education: teach patients the importance of compliance and the need to contact the health care provider if any signs of hepatic dysfunction occur

Rifapentine

Rifapentine (Priftin) is very similar to rifampin. Although many mycobacteria are considered susceptible to rifapentine, its only approved use is in the management of TB. The major difference between rifapentine and rifampin is rifapentine's extended half-life that allows for twice a week dosing. Contraindications, precautions, adverse effects, and drug interactions are the same as rifampin.

DRUGS SIGNIFICANTLY DIFFERENT FROM RIFAMPIN

Dapsone

Dapsone (Avlosulfon) is a synthetic sulfone that is chemically similar to sulfonamides. It is used as an antimicrobial for leprosy, *Pneumocystis carinii* pneumonia (PCP), and prophylaxis of malaria. It is also used as an immunosuppressive agent for systemic lupus erythematosus and as a dermatologic agent in a variety of integumentary disorders. In the management of leprosy, dapsone is used in combination with other drugs such as rifampin and clofazimine (discussed later in this chapter). In the past, dapsone was the mainstay of therapy for leprosy. Now there is significant resistance when used as monotherapy.

Dapsone works by inhibiting folic acid synthesis in susceptible organisms. Although the mechanism of dapsone in integumentary disorders is unknown, it has been suggested that it may act as an immunomodulator. Dapsone is orally administered and almost completely absorbed from the GI tract. It is widely distributed throughout the body, crosses the placenta, and enters into breast milk. Dapsone is metabolized in the liver. Approximately 20% of the drug is excreted unchanged in the urine, whereas 70% to 85% is excreted as metabolites. A small amount can be detected in the feces.

Hypersensitivity is the only contraindication to the use of dapsone. Caution is used in patients with sulfonamide hypersensitivity, but there is no direct cross-sensitivity. Dapsone is also used with caution in cases of severe anemia, deficiency glucose 6-phosphate dehydrogenase (G6PD) deficiency or methemoglobin reductase deficiency because hemolytic anemia can occur.

Dapsone can induce serious adverse effects including hemolytic anemia, aplastic anemia, agranulocytosis, methemoglobinemia, acute tubular necrosis, and hepatotoxicity. More common adverse effects include fever, myalgias, headache, chills, fatigue, malaise, rash, and urticaria.

Probenecid may reduce renal excretion of dapsone resulting in an increased risk for toxicity and adverse effects. Patients receiving other hemolytic agents such as folic acid antagonists should be closely monitored because concurrent use increases the potential for hematopoietic adverse effects.

Clofazimine

Clofazimine (Lamprene) is used as an antimycobacterial and antiinflammatory agent. It is bacteriocidal against *M. tuberculosis* and *M. leprae*, although its action against *M. leprae* is very slow. It is bacteriostatic against *M. avium–intracellulare.*

Clofazimine works by binding to mycobacterial DNA thus inhibiting reproduction and growth. As an antiinflammatory agent, it inhibits neutrophil motility and enhances the phagocytic activity of the polymorphonuclear cells and macrophages.

Clofazimine is insoluble in water and is incompletely absorbed from the GI tract. The extent of absorption varies with the individual and with the form of the drug administered. Clofazimine concentrates and can crystallize in mesenteric lymph nodes, adipose tissue, adrenals, liver, lungs, gallbladder, bile, and spleen. It crosses the placenta and enters breast milk. Clofazimine is excreted unchanged in feces.

The only contraindication to clofazimine therapy is hypersensitivity. Precautions include pre-existing GI disease and hepatic dysfunction.

Common GI adverse effects to clofazimine include anorexia, diarrhea, nausea and vomiting, or colicky or burning abdominal pain. GI toxicity can include hepatitis (with elevated hepatic enzyme levels) or jaundice. Rare, but serious adverse effects include splenic infarction, GI obstruction or ileus, and any type of GI bleeding. Clofazimine can cause dark, black, or tarry stools that may be misinterpreted as GI hemorrhage.

Clofazimine can cause long-lasting discoloration of the skin. In white people, the skin may be bronze or dark tan. This effect may last months after clofazimine is discontinued. Like rifampin, clofazimine may discolor body fluids.

Miscellaneous Drugs

Other drugs used in the management of leprosy include ofloxacin, a fluoroquinolone antibiotic, and minocycline, a tetracycline antibiotic. These drug classes are discussed in chapters 51 and 49, respectively.

CHAPTER SUMMARY

- The most common mycobacteria are *M. tuberculosis, M. leprae, M. avium* and *M. intracellulare.*
- INH, the prototype for antitubercular drugs, is used for both prophylaxis and treatment of acute active TB.
- Other first-line drugs for TB include rifampin, ethambutol, pyrazinamide, and streptomycin.
- Rifampin is the prototype drug for the management of leprosy (Hansen disease).
- Other medications useful for leprosy include rifabutin, rifapentine, dapsone, clofazimine, ofloxacin, and minocycline.
- *M. avium* and *M. intracellulare* are the causative agents of *Mycobacterium avium complex* (MAC), a condition that frequently afflicts immunocompromised patients.
- Azithromycin and clarithromycin are the drugs of choice for MAC prophylaxis and treatment.
- Additional drugs used in the management of MAC include rifampin, rifabutin, and clofazimine.

QUESTIONS FOR STUDY AND REVIEW

1. What type of patient has the highest risk for developing chemically induced hepatitis from INH therapy?
2. What is the difference between chemoprophylaxis and active TB therapy?
3. Why does multiple drug-resistant TB occur?
4. What are the obstacles to successful drug therapy with rifampin?
5. Why is compliance an issue when treating mycobacterial infections?

NEED MORE HELP?

Chapter 52 of the study guide for *Drug Therapy in Nursing* contains exercises and activities to reinforce your understanding of the concepts presented in this chapter. For additional information see the text's accompanying website at *http://www.connection.lww.com.*

REFERENCES AND BIBLIOGRAPHY

Anonymous. (1999). Rifapentine—a long-acting rifamycin for tuberculosis., *Medical Letter on Drugs & Therapeutics, 41*(1047), 21–22.

Bradford, W. Z., & Daley, C. L. (1998). Multiple drug-resistant tuberculosis. *Infectious Diseases Clinics of North America, 12*(1), 157–172.

CCIS System. (2001). *Computerized Clinical Information System.* Denver, CO: Micromedex.

Clinical Drug Monographs. [CDRom]. (2001). Gold Standard Media.

Drug Facts and Comparisons. (2000). St. Louis: Facts and Comparisons Division.

Fajardo, T. T., Abalos, R. M., dela Cruz, E. C., et al. (1999). Clofazimine therapy for lepromatous leprosy: a historical perspective. *International Journal of Dermatology, 38*(1), 70.

Gourevitch, M. N., Hartel, D., Selwyn P. A., et al. (1999). Effectiveness of isoniazid chemoprophylaxis for HIV-infected drug users at high risk for active tuberculosis. *AIDS, 13*(15), 2069–2074.

Haimanot, R. T., & Melaku, Z. (2000). Leprosy. *Current Opinion in Neurology, 13*(3), 317–322.

Hardman, J. G., Limbird, L. E., Molinof, P. B., Ruddon, R. W., & Gilman, A. (Eds.). (1997). *Goodman and Gilman's pharmacological basis of therapeutics* (9th ed.). New York: McGraw-Hill.

Heymann, S. J., Sell, R., & Brewer, T. F. (1998). The influence of program acceptability on the effectiveness of public health policy: A study of directly observed therapy for tuberculosis *American Journal of Public Health, 88*(3), 442–445.

Ji, B., & Grosset, J. H. (1999). Drugs and regimens for preventive therapy against tuberculosis, disseminated Mycobacterium avium complex infection and leprosy. *International Journal of Leprosy and Other Mycobacterial Diseases, 67,* (Suppl. 4), S45–S55.

Karch, A. (2001). *2001 Lippincott's nursing drug guide.* Philadelphia: Lippincott Williams & Wilkins.

Katzung, B. (1998). *Basic and clinical pharmacology* (7th Ed.), Stamford: Appleton & Lange.

Martinjak-Dvorsek, I., Gorjup, V., Horvat, M., et al. (2000). Acute isoniazid neurotoxicity during preventive therapy. *Critical Care Medicine, 28*(2), 567–568.

Narita, M., Stambaugh, J. J., Hollender, E. S., et al. (2000). Use of rifabutin with protease inhibitors for human immunodeficiency virus-infected patients with tuberculosis. *Clinical Infectious Diseases, 30*(5), 779–783.

Ormerod, L. P. (1999). Directly observed therapy (DOT) for tuberculosis: why, when, how and if? *Thorax, 54,* (Suppl. 2), S42–S45.

Porth, C. (1998). *Pathophysiology: Concepts of altered health states* (5th ed.). Philadelphia: Lippincott Williams & Wilkins.

Tatro, D. (Ed.). (2000). *Drug interaction facts* (6th ed.), St. Louis: Facts and Comparisons

Temple, M. E., & Nahata, M. C. (1999). Rifapentine: Its role in the treatment of tuberculosis. *Annals of Pharmacotherapeutics, 33*(11), 1203–1210.

Wright, J. (1998). Current strategies for the prevention and treatment of disseminated Mycobacterium avium complex infection in patients with AIDS. *Pharmacotherapy, 18*(4), 738–747.

Chapter 53

DRUGS FOR TREATING VIRAL AND FUNGAL DISEASES

KEY TERMS

Candida
cryptococcosis
cytomegalovirus
dermatophytes
dimorphic fungi
herpes simplex virus
herpes zoster
respiratory syncytial virus
phosphorylation
tinea

Learning Objectives

At the completion of this chapter the student will:

1. Identify core drug knowledge about drugs that are used in treating viral and fungal infections.
2. Identify core patient variables relevant to drugs that are used in treating viral and fungal infections.
3. Relate the interaction of core drug knowledge to core patient variables for drugs that are used in treating viral and fungal infections.
4. Generate a nursing plan of care from the interactions between core drug knowledge and core patient variables for drugs that are used in treating viral and fungal infections.
5. Describe nursing interventions to maximize therapeutic and minimize adverse effects for drugs that are used in treating viral and fungal infections.
6. Determine key points for patient and family education for drugs that are used in treating viral and fungal infections.

Antivirals

- **acyclovir**
- cidofovir
- famciclovir
- ganciclovir
- penciclovir
- valacyclovir
- vidarabine
- ribavirin
- idoxuridine
- trifluridine
- docosanol
- interferons (alfa, beta, gamma)
- amantadine
- foscarnet
- rimantadine
- oseltamivir
- zanamivir

Antifungals

Polyenes

- **amphotericin B**
- nystatin
- flucytosine
- griseofulvin

Azoles

- **fluconazole**
- itraconazole
- miconazole
- ketoconazole
- clotrimazole

Topicals

- butenafine
- ciclopirox olamine
- naftifine
- terbinafine
- tolnaftate

The symbol C indicates the **drug class**.

Drugs in bold type marked with the symbol P are **prototypes**.

Drugs in blue type with no symbol are **closely related** to the prototype.

Drugs in **red** type with no symbol are **significantly different** from the prototype.

Drugs in black type with no symbol are **also used in drug therapy**; no prototype.

Viral and fungal diseases affect people throughout the life span. In healthy people, these diseases may be considered an annoyance; in immunocompromised people, these diseases may be deadly.

Viruses are responsible for many infectious disorders ranging from the common cold to life-threatening meningitis. In contrast to the advances that have been made in the pharmacologic treatment of bacterial disease, few antiviral drugs have been developed. Viruses have no metabolic enzymes of their own; they can replicate only within a living host cell by using the metabolic processes of the host. Most drugs used to eliminate a virus also may do significant harm to the host. However, a few antiviral drugs have been developed that can target the invading virus yet leave the host intact. These drugs have a narrow spectrum of activity, and each drug has specific clinical applications.

Fungal infections, like viral infections, also can be life threatening to immunocompromised patients. Fungal infections may be divided into three categories:

- Systemic infections
- Dermatophytic (skin) infections
- Mucous membrane infections (e.g., candidiasis)

Systemic infection, such as aspergillosis, cryptococcosis, blastomycosis, and histoplasmosis, can present serious medical problems. The most common superficial (i.e., dermatophytic and mucous membrane–related) are tinea and *Candida*.

This chapter has two areas of focus. The first part of the chapter discusses antiviral drugs and their prototype acyclovir. The second part discusses two classes of antifungal drugs: polyenes (prototype, amphotericin B) and azoles (prototype, fluconazole), as well as an additional group of drugs, the topical antimycotics, which are used to treat superficial mycoses. This arbitrary division is made to assist the student in focusing on each specific group of disorders caused by these different microbes.

PHYSIOLOGY

VIRAL REPRODUCTION

There are five steps in the reproduction of virus in humans—adsorption, penetration, uncoating, replication, and transcription (the change of ribonucleic acid [RNA] to deoxyribonucleic acid [DNA]), all of which precede assembly and release. During the adsorption step, the virus attaches itself to receptor sites on the host cell surface. Once attached, the virus releases enzymes that allow penetration of the cell. After entering the cell, the protein coat of the virus dissolves and releases viral genetic material. The virus then synthesizes new messenger RNA and, using host ribosomes, synthesizes viral proteins. The viral nucleic acids and proteins are assembled into mature viruses that are then released by budding off from infected cells or by lysis of the infected cell (Fig. 53-1).

FUNGAL GROWTH

Fungi can be separated into two groups—yeasts and molds. The yeasts are single-celled organisms, approximately the size of a red blood cell, that reproduce by a budding process. The buds separate from the parent cell and mature into identical daughter cells. Molds produce long, hollow, branching filaments called hyphae. The term **dimorphic fungi** refers to the ability of a limited number of fungi that are capable of growing as yeasts at one temperature and as molds at another. Reproduction for most fungi may be sexual or asexual.

Fungi can produce disease in humans only if they can grow at the temperature of the infected body site. Fungi that cannot grow at core body temperature are called **dermatophytes**. Infections caused by this type of fungi are contained at the cutaneous level of the body. They are called superficial mycoses, as opposed to systemic mycoses, which are serious, deep-tissue, fungal infections caused by organisms capable of growth at core body temperature.

The normal body has yeast colonies on the skin, mucous membranes, and gastrointestinal (GI) tract. Intact immune mechanisms and competition for nutrients, provided by the bacterial flora, normally keep colonizing fungi in check. Alteration of either of these components by disease states or antibiotic therapy can upset the balance, permitting fungal overgrowth and opportunistic infections.

PATHOPHYSIOLOGY

SELECTED VIRAL INFECTIONS

Herpes Simplex

Herpes simplex virus (HSV) has two manifestations—type 1 (HSV-1) and type 2 (HSV-2). Both types of virus cause similar effects. HSV-1 is associated generally with herpes labialis (cold sores or fever blisters), signs of which occur on or near the lips. HSV-2 may cause herpes labialis and herpes genitalis (genital lesions). The virus is characterized by the formation of painful vesicles, which rupture and form a crust.

The virus is spread by direct contact with fluid from active lesions. Self-inoculation may occur to other parts of the body when fluid from active lesions is placed on parts of the body that have a break in the skin. In between outbreaks, the virus remains in a latent stage in sensory nerve ganglions. Recurrence may be triggered by infections, sun exposure, or stress. Outbreaks are preceded by a burning or tingling sensation along the nerve and at the site of infection.

Herpes Zoster

Herpes zoster is an acute unilateral and segmental inflammation of the dorsal root ganglia caused by infection with the herpesvirus varicella zoster, which also causes chickenpox. This infection usually occurs in adults and produces localized vesicular skin lesions confined to a dermatome and severe neuralgic pain in peripheral areas innervated by the nerves arising in the inflamed root ganglia.

Physiology

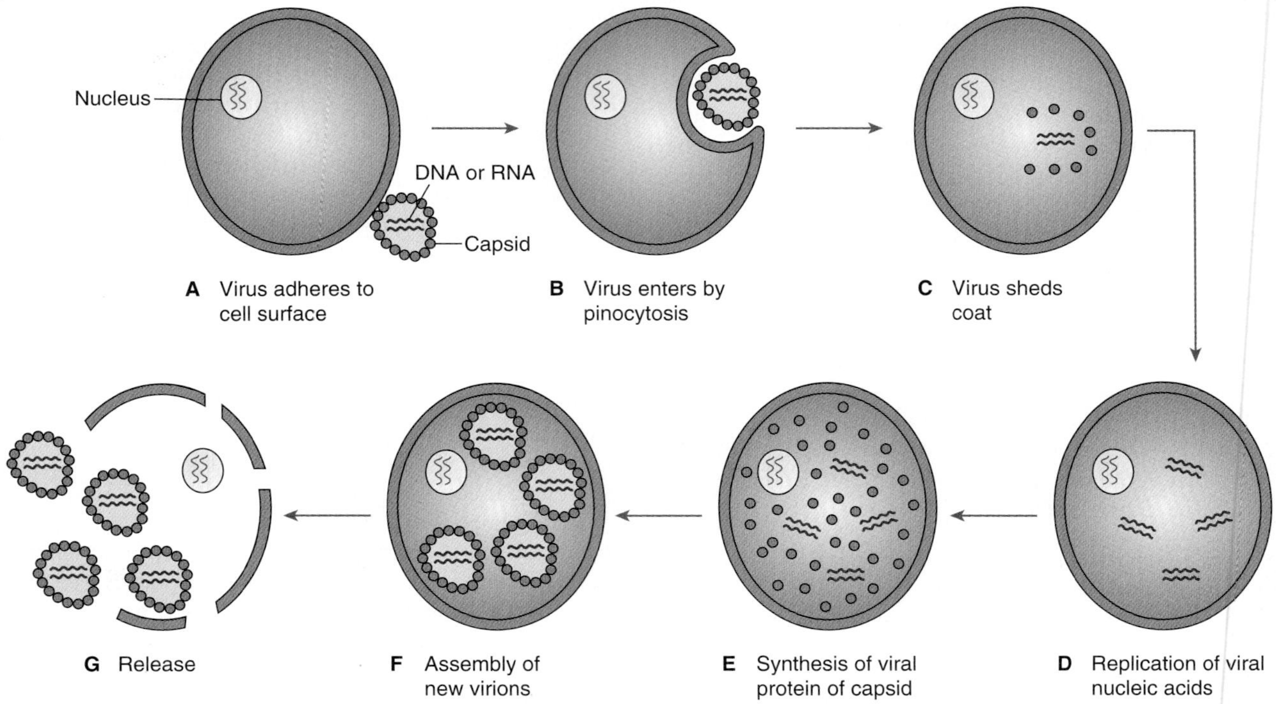

Figure 53-1. Viral replication. Viruses replicate in a series of steps: adsorption, penetration, uncoating, replication and transcription, and assembly and release (APURA). By adsorption (**A**), the virus adheres to receptors on the host cell surface. Then by pinocytosis promoted by enzyme activity, the virus penetrates (**B**) the cell wall. Once inside the cell, the virus uncoats (**C**), shedding its protein cover and allowing the genetic material RNA to be replicated (**D**) and changed to DNA. Next, new viral proteins are synthesized (**E**) and assembled (**F**) into new viruses, which are then released (**G**). Antiviral drugs interfere with the various stages of replication to limit or stop the viral disease process. (Adapted with permission from Swonger, A. K., & Matejski, M. P. [1991]. *Nursing pharmacology* [2nd ed.]. Philadelphia: J.B. Lippincott.)

Onset of herpes zoster is characterized by fever and malaise. Within 2 to 4 days, severe deep pain, pruritus, and paresthesia or hyperesthesia develop, usually on the trunk and occasionally on the arms and legs. The pain may be continuous or intermittent and usually lasts from 1 to 4 weeks. Up to 2 weeks after the first symptoms, small, red, nodular skin lesions erupt on the painful areas.

After the initial outbreak, the virus retreats back to the dorsal root ganglia but may recur. Pain and neuralgia may persist after the lesions resolve, especially in elderly patients.

Cytomegalovirus

Cytomegalovirus (CMV) is a type of herpesvirus. CMV infection is extremely prevalent—approximately 80% of the population demonstrates evidence of infection. In most individuals, infection is asymptomatic. However, in some individuals, such as those with acquired immunodeficiency syndrome (AIDS) and bone marrow transplant recipients, CMV infection is associated with severe and usually fatal disease. CMV infection during pregnancy can be hazardous to the fetus, possibly leading to stillbirth, brain damage, and other birth defects or to neonatal illness.

Although CMV most frequently causes retinitis, it also can cause illness in the lungs, throat, brain, kidneys, gallbladder, liver, and colon. In immunocompromised patients, CMV prophylaxis is started when the CD4+ T-cell count measures less than 50.

Respiratory Syncytial Virus

The **respiratory syncytial virus** (RSV) is a major cause of respiratory illness in all age groups. In adults, it tends to cause mild cold symptoms; in school-aged children, it can cause a cold and bronchial cough; and in infants and toddlers, it can cause bronchiolitis (inflammation of the smaller airways of the lungs) or pneumonia. Reinfection throughout life is common.

The highest rates of RSV illness occur in infants 2 to 6 months old, with a peak at 2 to 3 months. RSV infection is often carried home by a school-aged child and passed to a younger one, especially an infant.

RSV is especially dangerous in infants younger than 1 year and in children with asthma, other lung disorders, or heart disease. It is a major cause of hospitalization of children in the winter months. The symptoms of bronchiolitis include a hacking cough and wheezing on exhalation. In addition, there is typically fever and a cloudy nasal drainage; the infant often is irritable and oral intake decreases, sometimes to the point of dehydration.

Influenza-A

Influenza-A is one of three types of influenza viruses that cause infection in humans. It is the only type that can be affected by current antiviral agents. The virus attacks both the upper and lower respiratory tracts. It is transmitted directly by respiratory droplet or indirectly by contact with a contaminated object. Influenza virus is difficult to control because it undergoes constant antigenic changes, which limits the ability of individuals to develop long-term immunity and the development of vaccines.

Influenza has a sudden, acute onset with fever and chills, marked malaise, headache, general muscle aching, sore throat, unproductive cough, and nasal congestion. It may be self-limiting or may progress to pneumonia. Elderly patients, patients with chronic diseases, and immunocompromised patients should be immunized yearly.

SELECTED FUNGAL INFECTIONS

Tinea (Ringworm)

Tinea is not a worm infection as the name suggests; rather, it is a fungal infection caused by mold-like fungi called dermatophytes. Tinea lives on the dead tissues on the skin and any structures that grow from the skin (e.g., hair or nails).

Tinea can affect most skin sites, depending on the specific fungal type. The descriptive terms in the following list refer to the location of the infection and not to which specific type of fungus is involved:

- Tinea pedis—athlete's foot
- Tinea cruris—jock itch
- Tinea capitis—ringworm of the scalp
- Tinea corporis—ringworm of the body
- Tinea unguium—ringworm of the nails

A slightly different type of tinea infection is known as tinea versicolor. This chronic, noninflammatory infection is characterized only by patchy, hypopigmented discoloration of the skin.

The classic features of tinea are itching, redness on the skin, and a circular patchy lesion that spreads along its borders and clears at the center. In time, it may appear as a ring or a series of rings around a clear center, hence its common name, ringworm. These particular characteristics may not always be seen in every infected person; lack of certain signs or symptoms or the presence of additional signs or symptoms depends on which site is infected and how advanced the disease is. On the palms of the hands or soles of the feet, redness may be the only sign. Sometimes there may be deep-seated blisters on the soles of the feet that, with time, dry and end up as brown crusts. There may be thick, white scales between the toes. Nails can turn thick and white and eventually crumble if untreated. On the scalp, there may be hair loss as the hairs break off at their shafts.

Candidiasis

Candida is a yeastlike fungus that is almost always present as part of the normal population of organisms in the mouth, skin, intestinal tract, and vagina. The immune system and other organisms in the mucous membranes normally prevent it from growing in colonies. However, in immunocompromised patients, deterioration of the immune system can lead to candidal colonization; most outbreaks occur when the CD4+ T-cell count falls below 400.

Human immunodeficiency virus (HIV)-infected infants and children are particularly prone to serious and extensive candidal infections. Other factors that can promote growth of *Candida* in healthy individuals include use of broad-spectrum antibiotics (alters the natural population of organisms in the mouth and vagina); use of topical and systemic corticosteroids; diabetes; ill-fitting dentures; drugs or conditions that alter saliva flow; radiation therapy; cancer; chemotherapy; nutritional deficiency in iron, folate, vitamin B_{12}, or zinc; oral contraceptives with a high estrogen content; pregnancy; poor oral or dental hygiene; smoking; stress; depression; and use of antihistamines.

Aspergillosis

Aspergillus is a fungus commonly found in soil, water, and decaying vegetation. It has been cultured from unfiltered air, ventilation systems, contaminated dust dislodged during hospital renovation and construction, horizontal surfaces, food, and ornamental plants. It has been recognized increasingly as a cause of severe illness and mortality in highly immunocompromised patients, such as those undergoing chemotherapy or those having transplantation of bone marrow or vital organs.

Aspergillus infection, which is airborne, may be acquired by inhaling the fungal spores. In severely immunocompromised patients, primary *Aspergillus* pneumonia results from local lung tissue invasion. Colonization of the lower respiratory tract by *Aspergillus* in patients with preexisting lung disease, such as chronic obstructive lung disease, cystic fibrosis, or inactive tuberculosis, has predisposed patients to invasive pulmonary or disseminated infection. After pulmonary invasion, the fungus may disseminate through the bloodstream to involve multiple organs. The most reliable technique for diagnosis is a lung biopsy, although the fungus may be cultured from sputum or from specimens acquired by bronchoalveolar lavage.

Cryptococcosis

Cryptococcosis, which usually manifests itself as cryptococcal meningitis, is the most serious of the fungal infections in immunocompromised patients. Cryptococcosis rarely occurs when the CD4+ T-cell count is over 100 and is most likely when the count drops below 50. It is caused by a yeast-like organism, *Cryptococcus neoformans*. This fungus is not restricted geographically and is common in the environment, especially in soil containing bird droppings. Exposure occurs when contaminated sources become airborne and are inhaled.

In people with intact immune systems, the fungus may form inactive fungal nodules in the lungs, which may be visible on x-ray films and can later produce active infection when the immune response decreases. As cryptococcosis progresses, either from the original infection or a later reactivation, it can take three forms (more than one of which may be present):

- Central nervous system (CNS)
- Pulmonary
- Disseminated

Meningitis, inflammation of the membranes surrounding the spinal cord or brain, is the most common manifestation of cryptococcal infection.

Blastomycosis

Blastomycosis is a chronic infection characterized by a granulomatous and suppurative lesion. It is caused by inhalation of the dimorphic fungus *Blastomyces dermatitidis*. Blastomycosis is endemic in eastern parts of the United States, but it also is seen throughout Canada and Central America.

Two basic forms of blastomycosis are recognized: pulmonary and chronic cutaneous. Most infections originate in the lungs and then disseminate to any organ but usually to the skin and bones. In chronic cutaneous blastomycosis, the initial skin lesion presents as one or more subcutaneous nodules that eventually ulcerate. They are most common on exposed skin, such as that of the face, hands, wrist, and lower leg. Diagnosis is usually made by direct culture, agents that contain potassium hydroxide, special stains, and measurement of complement-fixing antibodies to various antigens.

Histoplasmosis

Histoplasmosis is a fungus infection that affects the lungs or other organs by dissemination. The disease is acquired by inhaling fungal spores. Outbreaks may occur in groups who have been exposed to bird or bat droppings or recently disturbed contaminated soil found in chicken coops or caves. Person-to-person spread of histoplasmosis does not occur. Although anyone can get histoplasmosis, it more often infects immunocompromised patients. Infection usually results in increased resistance to further infection, although the immunity is not complete. Symptoms vary from mild to severe, ranging from flulike illness to serious lung infection.

There are four clinical forms of histoplasmosis. The most common is acute pulmonary histoplasmosis. Patients with this form of the infection experience a flulike cough, chest pains, dyspnea, fever, weight loss, and hemoptysis. The symptoms may resolve spontaneously. In children, primary histoplasmosis can lead to disseminated infection. Therefore, children who have HIV and histoplasmosis should receive suppressive therapy for life. The second form of histoplasmosis is chronic pulmonary histoplasmosis, which may develop after acute infection; this form resembles pulmonary tuberculosis. The third form is termed acute disseminated histoplasmosis. Patients with this form may develop hepatosplenomegaly, fever, and prostration. This type of histoplasmosis is usually fatal. The last form of histoplasmosis is termed chronic disseminated histoplasmosis, which may present a diagnostic problem because of the extremely varied presentation. Like the acute form, it also may be fatal.

Coccidioidomycosis

Coccidioidomycosis (valley fever) is primarily a disease of the lungs, which is common in the southwestern United States and northwestern Mexico. It is caused by the fungus *Coccidioides immitis,* which grows in soil. The fungal spores become airborne when the soil is disturbed by wind, construction, farming, and other activities. Within the lung, the spore changes into a larger, multicellular structure called a spherule. The spherule grows and bursts, releasing endospores, which develop into other spherules. Person-to-person transmission does not occur.

Most cases of coccidioidomycosis are mild. It is thought that more than 60% of infected people have either no symptoms or experience flulike symptoms and never seek medical attention. Of those patients seeking medical care, the most common symptoms are fatigue, cough, chest pain, fever, rash, headache, and joint aches. Some people develop erythema nodosum, which produces painful red bumps that gradually turn brown.

Disseminated disease occurs in less than 0.5% of patients. In patients with disseminated disease, spores may be found in lymph nodes and meningeal, spleen, liver, kidney, and adrenal tissues. Meningitis is the most frequent cause of death. Patients at risk for disseminated disease are immunocompromised and include patients who have undergone organ transplantation, and those with lymphoma, HIV infection, adrenal corticosteroid therapy, and diabetes. Disseminated disease also occurs more frequently in men, in African Americans and Filipinos, and in pregnant women during the third trimester.

ANTIVIRAL DRUGS

The largest group of antiviral drugs are nucleoside analogues, initially developed as antitumor drugs but used as antiviral drugs for more than 30 years. They have relatively selective toxicity to viruses because viral DNA polymerases are more sensitive to inhibition by these drugs than human polymerases. Antiviral drugs in the nucleoside analogue subclass include acyclovir, cidofovir, famciclovir, ganciclovir, penciclovir, valacyclovir, vidarabine, ribavarin, idoxuridine, and trifluridine. Other antiviral drugs include docosanol, the interferons, amantadine, foscarnet, oseltamivir phosphate, rimantadine, and zanamivir. The prototype nucleoside analogue antiviral drug is acyclovir (Zovirax).

NURSING MANAGEMENT OF THE PATIENT RECEIVING ACYCLOVIR

Core Drug Knowledge

Pharmacotherapeutics

Acyclovir is an oral, parenteral, and topical antiviral agent. Its antiviral spectrum is limited to the herpesviruses, including herpes simplex, herpes zoster, Epstein-

Barr virus, and CMV. Acyclovir is not active against HIV. Clinically, use of acyclovir is limited to treating herpes simplex, herpes genitalis, and herpes zoster infections (Table 53-1).

Pharmacokinetics

After topical application, there is minimal percutaneous absorption, and no drug is detected in the blood or urine. After oral administration, acyclovir is absorbed poorly from the GI tract with a bioavailability of approximately 20%. Peak serum concentrations occur in about 1.5 to 2 hours. Acyclovir distributes extensively, with the highest concentrations in the kidneys, liver, and intestines. Cerebrospinal fluid (CSF) concentrations are about 50% of plasma. Acyclovir crosses the placenta and enters the breast milk. Acyclovir is metabolized minimally. Approximately 70% is eliminated by the kidneys unchanged. Half-life in patients with normal renal function is about 2.5 hours. In patients with impaired renal function, the half-life may extend to 20 hours.

Pharmacodynamics

To be active, acyclovir must undergo **phosphorylation**, a process by which a phosphate combines with an organic compound. In an infected cell, acyclovir is converted by the viral enzyme thymidine kinase. Fully active acyclovir triphosphate competes for a position in the DNA chain of the herpesvirus. Once incorporated, it terminates DNA synthesis. Uninfected cells show only minimal phosphorylation of acyclovir; thus, there is only a small amount of uptake into these cells. Acyclovir only is effective against actively replicating viruses; it does not eliminate the latent herpesvirus. Acyclovir has only indirect effects on the body by eliminating the viral infection.

Contraindications and Precautions

Acyclovir should be used with caution in patients with ganciclovir hypersensitivity because acyclovir has a similar chemical structure. It also should be given with caution to women who are pregnant or breast-feeding.

IV acyclovir should be used with caution in patients with renal disease and preexisting neurologic disorders, especially seizures. Systemic acyclovir is excreted primarily by glomerular filtration and tubular secretion. Therefore, renal toxicity may occur in patients with renal disease. Patients with preexisting neurologic disorders have an increased risk for the development of tremors and myoclonus.

Adverse Effects

Acyclovir is well tolerated. Common adverse effects to acyclovir include lightheadedness, anorexia, nausea, vomiting, abdominal pain, and headache. More serious adverse effects include confusion, tremors, hallucinations, seizures, or coma. IV acyclovir may be nephrotoxic. Acyclovir nephrotoxicity appears to result from crystallization of the drug in the nephron, which can lead to renal tubular obstruction.

Drug Interactions

Acyclovir may interact with probenecid and zidovudine. There is also an increased risk for nephrotoxicity when given concurrently with other drugs known to cause nephrotoxicity (Table 53-2).

Assessment of Relevant Core Patient Variables

Health Status

The nurse should elicit a patient history to evaluate for preexisting renal dysfunction, dehydration, pregnancy, or breast-feeding. The nurse also should assess for any concurrent drugs known to be nephrotoxic. Any positive finding should be communicated to the health care provider. Physical examination should include a dermatologic inspection to verify that the patient has active lesions and does not have a secondary bacterial infection (acyclovir will not affect bacterial pathogens). Immunocompromised patients and patients with preexisting renal dysfunction should have baseline renal function tests documented. For patients with preexisting neurologic disorders, the nurse should complete a baseline neurologic assessment.

Life Span and Gender

The nurse should determine whether the patient is pregnant or breast-feeding. Acyclovir is assigned to pregnancy category C and should be used with caution during pregnancy. Breast milk concentrations of acyclovir are greater than serum concentrations; therefore, it should be given cautiously to nursing mothers.

It also is a good idea to note the patient's age before administering acyclovir. Although acyclovir is not contraindicated for use with elderly patients, these patients should be monitored closely for the onset of nephrotoxicity because renal function diminishes with age.

Lifestyle, Diet, and Habits

The nurse should be aware of the patient's economic status. Oral acyclovir therapy is expensive. It is one of the drugs approved for reimbursement in many statewide AIDS programs. Patients may qualify for medical assistance from county, state, or federal funds or receive their drugs from local health departments. The nurse should refer patients with financial problems to the hospital or clinic's social service department.

Environment

The nurse should be aware of the environment in which acyclovir will be administered. Acyclovir is most frequently given in the outpatient community setting. The nurse should caution patients to take acyclovir only when active lesions are present to avoid inducing acyclovir-resistant virus. However, some immunocompromised

TABLE 53-1 Summary of Selected Antiviral Drugs

Drug (Trade) Name	Selected Indications	Route and Dosage Range	Pharmacokinetics
acyclovir (Zovirax; *Canadian:* Apo-Acyclovir)	Herpes simplex Herpes genitalis Herpes zoster	*Adult:* IV, 5–10 mg/kg infused over 1 h, q8h (15 mg/kg/d) for 7 d; PO (initial genital herpes), 200 mg q4h while awake (1,000 mg/d) for 10 d; PO (chronic suppressive therapy), 400 mg bid for up to 12 mo; topical, apply sufficient quantity to cover all lesions six times per day for 7 d; 1.25 cm (1/2 in) ribbon of ointment covers 2.5 cm^2 (4 in^2) surface area q3h *Child:* IV (> 12 y), adult dosage; IV (<12 y), 250–500 mg/m^2 infused over 1 h, q8h (750 mg/m^2/d); PO, safety not established	*Onset:* IV, immediate; PO, varies *Duration:* IV, 8 h; PO, unknown $t_{1/2}$: 2.5–5 h
cidofovir (Vistide)	CMV retinitis in AIDS patients	*Adult:* IV, 5 mg/kg IV infused over 1 h once wk for 2 consecutive wk during induction (5 mg/kg once every 2 wk for maintenance); probenecid must be administered PO with each dose, 2 g PO 3 h before cidofovir and 1 g at 2 h and 8 h after infusion *Child:* Safety and efficacy not established for children younger than 12 y	*Onset:* Rapid *Duration:* 24 h $t_{1/2}$: 1 h
famciclovir (Famvir)	Acute herpes zoster	*Adult:* PO, 500 mg q8h for 7 d *Child:* Safety and efficacy not established	*Onset:* Varies *Duration:* 24 h $t_{1/2}$: 2 h
	Recurrent genital herpes	*Adult:* PO, 125 mg bid for 5 d	
ganciclovir (DHPG, Cytovene)	CMV infections (retinitis, colitis, esophagitis) in immunocompromised patients	*Adult:* IV, 5 mg/kg given at a constant rate over 1 h, q12h for 14–21 d (maintenance: 5 mg/kg given over 1 h once daily, 7 d/wk or 6 mg/kg/d 5d per wk; PO, 1,000 mg tid with food or 500 mg six times daily q3h with food while awake *Child:* Safety and efficacy not established	*Onset:* IV, slow; PO, slow *Duration:* Unknown $t_{1/2}$: 2–4 h; PO, 4.8 h
	Prevention of CMV infection in transplant patients	*Adult:* IV, 5 mg/kg over 1 h q12h for 7–14 d, then 5 mg/kg/d once daily for 7 d or 6 mg/kg/d once daily for 5 d	
penciclovir (Denavir)	Herpes labialis	*Adult:* Topical, apply thin layer to affected area q2h while awake. Therapy continues for 4 d	Not generally absorbed systemically
valacyclovir (Valtrex)	Initial or recurrent genital herpes	*Adult:* PO, 500 mg bid for 5 d *Child:* Safety and efficacy not established	*Onset:* Rapid *Duration:* 3 h $t_{1/2}$: 2.5–3.3 h
	Herpes zoster	*Adult:* PO, 1 g tid for 7 d, most effective if started within 48 h of onset of symptoms	
ribavirin (Virazole)	RSV infection	*Adult and Child:* Aerosol, dilute to 20 mg/mL and deliver for 12–18 h/d for at least 3 but not more than 7 d	*Onset:* Slow *Duration:* Unknown $t_{1/2}$: 9.5 h
vidarabine (Vira-A)	Acute keratoconjunctivitis and recurrent epithelial keratitis due to HSV-1 and HSV-2	*Adult:* Apply eye drops an additional 7 d after reepithelialization has occurred; do not administer for more than 21 d at a time	Not generally absorbed systemically
idoxuridine (IDU)	Herpes simplex keratitis	*Adult:* Ophthalmic preparation, thin strip of 0.5% ointment to conjunctiva of affected eye q4h while awake, continuing treatment for 5–7 d after healing appears complete; or instill 1 drop 0.1% solution qh by day and q2h at night until condition improves, then reduce dose to 1 drop q2h by day and q4h by night, continuing treatment for 5–7 d after healing appears complete; do not administer for more than 21 d at a time	Not generally absorbed systemically

TABLE 53-1 Summary of Selected Antiviral Drugs (Continued)

Drug (Trade) Name	Selected Indications	Route and Dosage Range	Pharmacokinetics
trifluridine (Viroptic)	Primary keratoconjunctivitis and recurrent epithelial keratitis from HSV-1 and HSV-2	*Adult:* Ophthalmic preparation, instill 1 drop of 1% solution into the affected eye q2h while awake, up to a maximum daily dosage of 9 drops; continue therapy until corneal ulcer has completely reepithelialized and then treat for an additional 7 d with 1 drop q4h while awake up to a maximum daily dosage of 5 drops; do not administer for more than 21 d at a time	Not generally absorbed systemically
amantadine (Symmetrel; *Canadian:* Gen-Amantadine)	Prevention and treatment of influenza A virus	*Adult: Prevention,* PO, 200 mg/d or 100 mg bid for 10 d after exposure, for up to 90 d if vaccination is impossible and exposure is repeated; *Treatment,* PO, same dose as above, start treatment as soon after exposure as possible, continue for 24–48 h after symptoms are gone *Child:* Not recommended for children younger than 1 y; *Prevention,* PO, 1–9 y, 2–4 mg/lb/d in two to three divided doses, not to exceed 150 mg/lb/d; 9–12 y, 100 mg bid; *Treatment,* same as above, start as soon after exposure as possible, continue for 24–48 h after symptoms are gone	*Onset:* 36–48 h *Duration:* Unknown $t_{1/2}$: 15–24 h
	Parkinson disease	*Adult:* (younger than 65 y) PO, 100 mg bid (up to 400 mg/d) when used alone, reduce in patients receiving other antiparkinson drugs; older than 65 y, PO, 100 mg once a day	
foscarnet (Foscarvir)	CMV retinitis in patients with AIDS Cyclovir-resistant HSV infections in immunocompromised patients	*Adult:* IV induction, 60 mg/kg q8h for 2–3 wk; maintenance, 90–120 mg/kg *Adult:* IV, 40 mg/kg q8–12h for 2–3 wk or until healed	*Onset:* Immediate *Duration:* Unknown $t_{1/2}$: 1.4–3 h
rimantadine (Flumadine)	Prophylaxis and treatment of influenza A virus infection in adults Prophylaxis of influenza A virus infection in children	*Adult:* PO, prophylaxis, 100 mg/d bid; treatment, same dose as above; start treatment as soon after exposure as possible; continue for 7 d *Child:* PO, older than 10 y, prophylaxis and treatment, same as adult; younger than 10 y, prophylaxis only, 5 mg/kg qd, do not exceed 150 mg/d	*Onset:* Slow *Duration:* Unknown $t_{1/2}$: 25.4 h
oseltamivir (Tamiflu)	Influenza types A and B	*Adult* (>18 y): 75 mg PO bid for 5 d *Child* (<18 y): Not recommended	*Onset:* Rapid *Duration:* 6–10 h $t_{1/2}$: 1–3 h
zanamivir (Relenza)	Influenza types A & B	*Adult and child* (>12 y): two blister-pack inhalations bid at least, 2 h apart	*Onset:* 1 h *Duration:* 24 h $t_{1/2}$: 2.5–5.1 h
docosanol (Abreva)	HSV	*Adult and child:* apply cream 5 times/d	*Onset:* Rapid *Duration:* Unknown $t_{1/2}$: Unknown

patients with frequent and severe outbreaks may be placed on a prophylactic regimen. Acyclovir should be protected from light and moisture in the home environment.

Intravenous acyclovir may be administered in acute care settings to patients with a severe outbreak. Reconstituted acyclovir should be used within 12 hours. The nurse should administer the infusion over 60 minutes.

Nursing Diagnoses and Outcomes

- Disturbed Thought Processes related to drug-induced confusion, hallucinations, or seizures

TABLE 53-2 Agents That Interact With Acyclovir

Interactants	Effect and Significance	Nursing Management
probenecid	Probenecid inhibits renal tubular secretion of acyclovir. This may increase the risk for adverse effects, especially nephrotoxicity.	Do not coadminister if possible. Monitor for adverse effects. Decrease dosage of acyclovir as needed.
zidovudine	Although the mechanism of action is unknown, these drugs in combination may induce severe drowsiness and lethargy.	Monitor for adverse effects. Decrease dosage of acyclovir as needed. Discontinue as needed.

Desired outcome: The patient will be free of thought aberrations related to drug therapy.

- Acute Pain related to drug-induced headache
  Desired outcome: Drug-related pain will subside after administration of acetaminophen.
- Imbalanced Nutrition: Less than Body Requirements related to acyclovir-related anorexia, nausea and vomiting, or abdominal pain
  Desired outcome: The patient will remain within an acceptable weight range.
- Excess Fluid Volume related to adverse effects of drug therapy, such as nephrotoxicity
  Desired outcome: The patient will have an adequate fluid intake and output profile.

Planning and Intervention

Maximizing Therapeutic Effects

The nurse should administer acyclovir tablets or capsules with a full glass of water. The drug can be administered with or without food. It is important to administer the drug at regular intervals.

Minimizing Adverse Effects

Oral acyclovir is well tolerated. However, for patients who report GI complaints, the nurse should administer the drug with food. It is important to advise the patient to drink at least eight 8-oz glasses of water a day.

To minimize potential nephrotoxicity, the nurse should ensure that the patient is well hydrated. The nurse should administer IV acyclovir over 60 minutes. It is best to use an infusion pump to ensure the correct timing of administration. The nurse should monitor the patient's urine output for 2 hours after the infusion and notify the health care provider if urine output is less than 500 mL/g of acyclovir administered.

Providing Patient and Family Education

- One of the most important points to stress with patients is that they should not take this drug if they have ever had a reaction to any drug with a name that ends in "vir."
- The nurse also should advise patients to notify the prescriber if they are pregnant or breast-feeding.
- Another important point to explain is that acyclovir is prescribed for a particular infection and should not be used to self-medicate or treat any other infection.
- The nurse should emphasize that this drug does not prevent the transmission of infection to another person and does not cure the infection.
- The nurse should instruct patients to complete the full course of drug therapy, even if the lesions resolve. If patients are taking 200-mg tablets, the nurse should advise them to take the drug every 4 hours (five times a day). For patients who have difficulty taking pills, the drug may be taken in 400-mg doses three times a day. The nurse should consult with the prescriber, however, to be sure the alternate method is acceptable.
- It is important to advise patients to keep the drug away from light and moisture, and to instruct them to take forgotten doses as soon as they remember, but not if it is time for the next dose.
- The nurse should inform patients of the importance of remaining well hydrated while taking this drug.
- It is especially important that patients learn to recognize the symptoms of an allergic reaction to acyclovir. Patients should stop taking the drug and contact their health care provider if a rash, welts, itching, or shortness of breath occurs.
- The nurse should explain the potential adverse effects of acyclovir and the potential remedies for these discomforts. If patients experience CNS effects, such as confusion, tremors, hallucinations, or coma or in patients who have signs of nephrotoxicity, such as weight gain or decreased urinary output, the prescriber should be contacted immediately.
- Because autoinoculation is possible with herpetic lesions, it is important to teach patients to wear a glove or finger cot when applying topical acyclovir. The nurse should explain the importance of washing the hands after each application, even when barriers are used. The drug should be applied to cover the lesions every 3 hours, six times a day for 7 days.
- The nurse should advise patients to contact the health care provider if the lesions turn red, become hot, or exude purulent material, all of which are indications of a secondary bacterial infection.
- The nurse should instruct the patient to self-administer acetaminophen should headache occur. For per-

sistent pain, unrelieved by acetaminophen, the patient should contact the health care provider.
- The nurse should instruct the patient to consume frequent small meals if GI distress occurs. If weight loss persists, the patient should contact the health care provider.

Ongoing Assessment and Evaluation

The nurse should monitor for the effectiveness of therapy, making sure to document new lesions and assess for possible secondary bacterial infections. The nurse also should monitor for adverse effects, such as lethargy, tremors, headache, change in mental status, and GI complaints.

For immunocompromised and elderly patients, it is important to monitor renal function to detect early nephrotoxicity. Periodic renal function tests should be done for patients on long-term therapy. Hospitalized patients receiving IV acyclovir also should be monitored closely for developing nephrotoxicity. The nurse should measure and monitor intake and output to ensure adequate hydration. The nurse also should monitor for the development of phlebitis when administering IV acyclovir. By the completion of therapy, herpetic lesions and any adverse effects should be resolved. ■

DRUGS CLOSELY RELATED TO ACYCLOVIR

Cidofovir

Cidofovir (Vistide) is an IV drug indicated for treating CMV retinitis in patients with AIDS. Cidofovir gel has been effective for topical treatment of acyclovir-resistant mucocutaneous HSV infections in AIDS patients. Cidofovir may also be used in patients with ganciclovir resistance.

Cidofovir use is limited by its serious potential toxic effects. Major adverse effects with cidofovir therapy include renal impairment, granulocytopenia, metabolic acidosis, uveitis, and ocular hypotony. To minimize possible nephrotoxicity, IV normal saline solution and oral probenecid must be used before and after each cidofovir dose. Renal function tests should be completed before each dose of cidofovir. Neutrophil counts also should be monitored throughout therapy. Cidofovir therapy is contraindicated in patients taking other nephrotoxic agents.

Famciclovir

Famciclovir (Famvir) is an oral antiviral agent used as an alternative to acyclovir in treating acute herpes zoster and recurrent episodes of genital herpes. In patients with chronic hepatitis B virus (HBV), famciclovir has decreased HBV, DNA, and aminotransferase activity. Famciclovir is converted rapidly to penciclovir after oral administration.

Famciclovir has a similar spectrum of activity to acyclovir but a longer duration of action. Thus, famciclovir can be taken three times a day compared with oral acyclovir, which requires five doses per day. Despite the bioavailability and duration of action advantages of famciclovir, acyclovir possesses a higher affinity for thymidine kinase, the enzyme that promotes phosphorylation. Adverse effects and drug interactions are the same as those seen with acyclovir.

Ganciclovir

Ganciclovir (DHPG, Cytovene) is an antiviral agent used in treating CMV infections, especially retinitis, colitis, and esophagitis, in immunocompromised patients. It also is used to prevent CMV infection in transplant patients. Its spectrum of activity also includes HSV-1 and HSV-2, herpesvirus type 6, Epstein-Barr virus, varicella zoster virus, and HBV.

Like acyclovir, ganciclovir works by terminating DNA synthesis. It is administered IV, orally, and by intravitreal implantation. After implantation, ganciclovir is released at a steady rate over 5 to 8 months. After oral administration, ganciclovir is absorbed poorly from the GI tract. Bioavailability is increased when administered with a high-fat meal. Following IV administration, distribution into body tissues and fluids is extensive, including significant intraocular penetration. Ganciclovir crosses the placenta and the blood-brain barrier.

Ganciclovir is not indicated for use in neonates and children and should not be taken during pregnancy and lactation. It must be used with caution in patients with bone marrow depression, dehydration, neutropenia, hematologic disease, thrombocytopenia, renal disease or impairment, or recent radiation therapy. There is also a possibility of cross-sensitivity with acyclovir.

Ganciclovir can cause significant hematologic toxicity. Granulocytopenia, neutropenia, and thrombocytopenia have all occurred during ganciclovir therapy. Ganciclovir is moderately nephrotoxic. Slight-to-moderate increases in serum

MEMORY CHIP

Acyclovir

- Used for the management of herpes simplex, herpes zoster, Epstein-Barr virus, and cytomegalovirus
- Significant contraindication: hypersensitivity or cross sensitivity to ganciclovir
- Most common adverse effects: nausea, vomiting, anorexia, light-headedness, abdominal pain, and headache
- Most serious adverse effects: seizures and renal dysfunction
- Maximizing therapeutic effects: administer the drug at regular intervals
- Minimizing adverse effects: ensure hydration to avoid nephrotoxicity
- Most significant patient education: acyclovir treats the symptoms of the disease; it does not cure it or prevent its transmission to another person

creatinine and azotemia have occurred. Elevated liver function test results also may occur during therapy with ganciclovir and are generally reversible. Liver function tests should be performed routinely.

Adverse effects, which occur most commonly with IV administration of ganciclovir, include diaphoresis, pruritus, pneumonia, chills, sepsis, and phlebitis. Adverse effects seen with intravitreal administration of ganciclovir may induce bacterial endophthalmitis, retinal detachment, vitreous hemorrhage, cataracts, corneal opacification, hyphema, floaters, ocular pain, posterior chamber inflammation, macular abnormalities, spikes of increased intraocular pressure, optic disc/nerve changes, and uveitis.

Ganciclovir is teratogenic, carcinogenic, and mutagenic and has been shown to cause aspermatogenesis in animals. Human data on spermatogenesis are not available.

Penciclovir

Penciclovir (Denavir) is a topical antiviral agent used to treat herpes labialis. Penciclovir is the active metabolite of famciclovir. It works by inhibiting viral DNA. Penciclovir is applied every 2 waking hours. Like ganciclovir, penciclovir may produce testicular toxicity according to animal studies. Adequate human studies, however, are not available.

Valacyclovir

Valacyclovir (Valtrex) is an ester of acyclovir. This oral drug was developed to improve acyclovir's oral bioavailability. Improved bioavailability means less frequent dosing is required for valacyclovir than for acyclovir. Valacyclovir is the drug of choice in treating genital herpes, either as a first episode or as a recurrent episode. It also is the drug of choice in treating herpes zoster. Compared with acyclovir, it demonstrates earlier pain reduction or cessation of pain in treating herpes zoster.

The adverse effects and drug interactions of valacyclovir are similar to those of acyclovir. In immunocompromised patients with high-dose and long-term therapy, valacyclovir also may induce thrombotic thrombocytopenic purpura/hemolytic uremia syndrome.

Vidarabine

Vidarabine (Vira-A) is an ophthalmic antiviral drug with activity against HSV-1 and HSV-2, varicella zoster virus, CMV, vaccinia, and HBV. Although the IV formulation of vidarabine was discontinued by the manufacturer in October 1992, it is the most effective and least toxic of the topical nucleoside analogues.

Corticosteroids, especially ophthalmically administered steroids, should be avoided in patients receiving ophthalmic vidarabine in treating herpes simplex keratitis because they can increase the spread of infection. In addition, vidarabine may increase possible adverse ocular effects of the corticosteroids, such as increased intraocular pressure, glaucoma, and cataracts.

Ophthalmic doses of vidarabine are very small, and the risk of adverse systemic effects is very low. Hypersensitivity reactions, such as pruritus, erythema, swelling, ocular pain or burning, or foreign body sensation, may occur. Ophthalmic administration should not be continued for longer than 21 days. Too frequent application can damage the cornea.

Ribavarin

Ribavirin (Virazole) is a synthetic nucleoside aerosol antiviral drug. It is used as a primary agent to treat respiratory syncytial virus infections. Ribavirin currently is being investigated for use in treating herpes zoster, herpes genitalis, varicella, and HCV.

Ribavirin should be administered using the SPAG-2 aerosol generator. The nurse should be thoroughly familiar with the use of this device before administering ribavirin. Solutions placed in the SPAG-2 reservoir should be discarded every 24 hours and before adding newly reconstituted solutions. Reconstituted solutions may be stored at room temperature for 24 hours.

Ribavirin is one of the few drugs that is indicated for use in children. Ribavirin is teratogenic and embryotoxic in animals; therefore, it is contraindicated for use in adults because of its potential for producing testicular lesions and teratogenic effects. It is considered a pregnancy category X drug. Pregnant health care workers should not administer aerosolized ribavirin because it can disperse into the immediate bedside area. Additionally, ribavirin should not be given concurrently with zidovudine because it blocks the action of zidovudine.

Idoxuridine

Idoxuridine (IDU) is an ophthalmic antiviral drug used to treat herpes simplex keratitis. Idoxuridine should not be coadministered with boric acid–containing solutions; coadministration can result in a precipitate formation that can cause irritation. Adverse effects associated with idoxuridine therapy include eye irritation, pain, pruritus, inflammation, or edema of the eyes or eyelids. Photophobia and corneal clouding also may occur.

Idoxuridine should be administered by applying a thin strip of 0.5% ophthalmic ointment to the conjunctiva of the affected eye(s) every 4 hours during waking hours. Idoxuridine also may be administered as 0.1% ophthalmic solution, 1 drop every hour by day and every 2 hours at night until the condition improves. At this point, the dose can be reduced to 1 drop every 2 hours by day and every 4 hours at night. For both dosage forms, treatment should be continued for 5 to 7 days after healing appears complete.

Trifluridine

Trifluridine (Viroptic) is an ophthalmic antiviral preparation indicated for use in primary keratoconjunctivitis and recurrent epithelial keratitis due to HSV-1 and HSV-2. There are no significant interactions between trifluridine and other drugs. Adverse effects include mild transient burning or stinging on instillation, palpebral edema, epithelial keratopathy, irritation, keratitis sicca, hyperemia, and increased intraocular pressure.

To administer correctly, the nurse should instill 1 drop of 1% solution into the affected eye(s) every 2 hours during waking hours, up to a maximum daily dose of nine drops. This therapeutic regimen should continue until the corneal ulcer has completely reepithelialized. At this point, it is important to treat for an additional 7 days with one drop every 4 hours during waking hours up to a maximum daily dosage of five drops.

DRUGS SIGNIFICANTLY DIFFERENT FROM P ACYCLOVIR

Docosanol

Docosanol (Abreva) is an over-the-counter (OTC) topical cream for recurrent oral-facial herpes simplex episodes. Docosanol works by inhibiting fusion between the plasma membrane and the HSV envelope, thereby preventing viral entry into cells and subsequent viral replication. Other antivirals, such as acyclovir, work by inhibition of viral DNA replication and carry a risk of mutating the virus. Because docosanol does not act directly on the virus, it is unlikely it will produce drug resistant mutants of HSV. Docosanol has minimal adverse effects, headache is the most common. Successful therapy occurs when the drug is applied at the earliest sign of infection.

Interferons

The interferons are a family of glycoproteins that affect many types of viral illness. They are administered parenterally, either subcutaneously or intramuscularly. Although pharmacologically similar, each is used for specific viral illnesses. There are three main classes of interferons: interferon alfa, interferon beta, and interferon gamma, each of which is discussed briefly next in this chapter. The interferons are presented in depth in Chapter 33.

Interferon Alfa

Interferon alfa is an immunomodulator. The name interferon alfa actually refers to at least three compounds that differ slightly in their amino acid sequence:

- Interferon alfa-2a (Roferon-A)
- Interferon alfa-2b (Intron-A)
- Interferon alfa-n3 (Alferon N)

Interferon alfa is approved for treatment of hairy cell leukemia, AIDS-related Kaposi sarcoma, condylomata acuminatum, chronic HBV, and chronic hepatitis C virus (HCV). It also has been used investigationally for treating renal cell carcinoma, bladder carcinoma, chronic myelogenous leukemia, and lymphomas.

Interferon Beta

Interferon beta-1b is a form of native human interferon beta prepared by recombinant DNA technology. It is similar to interferon alfa or gamma in chemistry and adverse effects but differs in efficacy. Interferon beta-1b is used primarily for treating relapsing or remitting multiple sclerosis (MS) to decrease both the number and severity of attacks of multiple sclerosis (MS). It has also been tested in cutaneous T-cell lymphoma, HCV C, HIV infection, Kaposi sarcoma, malignant melanoma, and renal cell carcinoma.

Interferon Gamma

Interferon gamma-1b is a parenteral recombinant DNA drug that is essentially identical to natural gamma interferon. It is indicated for use in treating chronic granulomatous disease, an inherited disorder of phagocytic oxidative metabolism. Many patients with this disorder develop life-threatening infections. Since the development of interferon gamma-1b, these patients have experienced a significant decrease in the number and severity of infections.

Amantadine

Amantadine (Symmetrel) is a synthetic antiviral agent used for the prophylactic or symptomatic treatment of influenza A virus, especially in high-risk patients. It also is used to relieve the symptoms of Parkinson disease.

As an antiviral, amantadine appears to block the uncoating of the virus particle and subsequent release of viral nucleic acid into the host cell. Amantadine also may interfere with penetration of the cell wall by adsorbed virus. In treating Parkinson disease, amantadine appears to potentiate CNS dopaminergic responses. It may release dopamine and norepinephrine from storage sites and inhibit the reuptake of dopamine and norepinephrine.

Amantadine is administered orally and is well absorbed from the GI tract. It crosses the blood-brain barrier and the placenta; distributes into tears, saliva, and nasal secretions; and is excreted into breast milk. About 90% of amantadine is excreted in the urine by way of glomerular filtration and tubular secretion.

Amantadine should be given with caution to patients with congestive heart failure, peripheral edema, seizure disorders, eczema, and history of psychosis. These conditions may be exacerbated by amantadine therapy. Patients with renal impairment, elderly patients, and pregnant women also should be given amantadine with caution because these conditions increase the risks for adverse effects. Abrupt withdrawal of amantadine should be avoided in patients with Parkinson disease because this may precipitate symptoms of increased rigidity, confusion, urinary retention, or bulbar palsy.

Amantadine has many potential adverse effects. In the GI system, amantadine may cause nausea and vomiting, diarrhea, constipation, anorexia, and xerostomia. CNS effects include dizziness, anxiety, impaired coordination, insomnia, and nervousness. Other CNS effects that occur less commonly are headache, irritability, nightmares, depression, ataxia, confusion, somnolence/drowsiness, agitation, fatigue, and hallucinations. Patients with a history of psychosis may experience an exacerbation of symptoms, including abnormal thinking, weakness, amnesia, slurred speech, and hyperkinesia. In rare cases, amantadine has been associated with more serious effects, including increased frequency of seizures, suicidal ideation, and neuroleptic malignant syndrome.

Adverse cardiovascular effects include orthostatic hypotension and peripheral edema. Livedo reticularis, a persistent purplish network-patterned discoloration of the skin, is a frequent adverse reaction of patients taking amantadine for Parkinson disease. It is believed to be caused by abnormal capillary permeability associated with peripheral vasoconstriction, which results in decreased skin temperature and peripheral blood flow. Amantadine also may cause adverse reactions in the eyes. Diffuse, white, subendothelial corneal opacification may occur. Other ophthalmic adverse reactions include corneal edema, light sensitivity, and optic nerve palsy.

Amantadine should not be used with CNS stimulants, alcohol (ethanol), opiate agonists, hydrochlorothiazide, and triamterene. Nervousness, irritability, insomnia, seizures, or cardiac arrhythmias may occur in combination with CNS stimulants. Ethanol use with amantadine may increase CNS effects, such as dizziness, confusion, light-headedness, fainting, or orthostatic hypotension. Use of opiate agonists may increase the incidence of adverse effects. Hydrochlorothiazide or triamterene, used in conjunction with amantadine, can reduce renal clearance of amantadine, with subsequent increase in plasma amantadine concentrations and possible toxicity.

Foscarnet

Foscarnet (Foscavir) is an IV antiviral agent that is structurally unrelated to other antiviral agents. Foscarnet currently is indicated for treating CMV retinitis in patients with AIDS. It is also being investigated for treatment of CMV disease, herpes simplex, and varicella zoster infection in HIV-infected patients. Its mechanism of action is similar to that of acyclovir and ganciclovir, yet it does not require phosphorylation before becoming activated.

Foscarnet therapy should be given with caution to patients with anemia, dehydration, renal impairment, and electrolyte imbalances. Patients who have cardiac disease, are receiving other drugs that influence serum electrolytes, or have a preexisting seizure disorder or other neurologic disease require close monitoring during treatment. Foscarnet is assigned to pregnancy category C and should therefore be used with caution during pregnancy.

Foscarnet has an extensive and serious adverse reaction profile. Up to 33% of patients on foscarnet therapy acquire anemia, granulocytopenia, or leukopenia. Electrolyte imbalances, such hypocalcemia, hypophosphatemia or hyperphosphatemia, hypomagnesemia, and hypokalemia also may occur. GI disturbances, such as anorexia, abdominal pain, nausea, and vomiting may occur in 30% of patients. Up to 33% of patients will acquire significant renal impairment, resulting in azotemia or necrosis. Patients with renal impairment also are at high risk for developing seizures. Other CNS effects include headache, peripheral neuropathy, and anxiety.

Foscarnet should be given with caution in combination with other drugs known to be nephrotoxic, such as acyclovir, aminoglycosides, amphotericin B, cisplatin, cyclosporine, gold compounds, lithium, nonsteroidal anti-inflammatory drugs, penicillamine, pentamidine, rifampin, and vancomycin. Foscarnet, in combination with ciprofloxacin, increases the risk for seizures, whereas the combination of foscarnet and zidovudine increases the risk for anemia.

Rimantadine

Rimantadine (Flumadine) is an oral antiviral agent. It is indicated for the prophylaxis and treatment of influenza A virus infections in adults and for prophylaxis only in children. Rimantadine is related chemically and structurally to amantadine, but it does not produce the CNS effects seen with amantadine and does not have therapeutic value in treating Parkinson disease.

Rimantadine is contraindicated for use in infants and neonates. It should be used cautiously in elderly patients and in patients with hepatic or renal dysfunction. Delaying the metabolism or excretion of rimantadine may increase the risk for toxic effects.

Rimantadine has a much better adverse effects profile than amantadine does. The most common adverse effects reported are nausea, vomiting, insomnia, dizziness, anorexia, xerostomia, abdominal pain, headache, asthenia, nervousness, and fatigue.

Clearance of rimantadine is reduced by concurrent administration of cimetidine. Decreased serum concentration may occur with coadministration of acetaminophen and aspirin.

Oseltamivir Phosphate

Oseltamivir phosphate (Tamiflu) is a neuraminidase inhibitor used for the management of influenza A and B virus. Influenza A and B viruses contain the viral enzyme neuraminidase on their surfaces that facilitates the release of newly formed virus particles from infected cells. This allows for infection of adjacent cells. Neuraminidase inhibitors, such as oseltamivir, appear to inhibit the release of viruses from infected cells, thus reducing spread to adjacent cells and limiting tissue damage and the duration of symptoms.

Oseltamivir is an oral agent for use in patients who have been symptomatic for no more than 2 days. The effectiveness of the drug depends on how early the treatment is initiated. Oseltamivir also is thought to be effective for prevention of influenza, however, this is not a labeled use.

Oseltamivir is a pregnancy category C agent and is not indicated for children under the age of 18. The most common adverse effects to oseltamivir are nausea and vomiting, bronchitis, insomnia, and vertigo. Nausea and vomiting can be reduced by administration with milk, a snack, or a meal. No significant drug-drug interactions have been identified. Oseltamivir is converted extensively into oseltamivir carboxylate by the liver then excreted renally.

It is important for the nurse to encourage patients in especially at-risk populations, such as the elderly or immunocompromised patients, that they should continue to receive a yearly influenza vaccine.

Zanamivir

Zanamivir (Relenza) is the second neuraminidase inhibitor. Its mechanism of action is the same as that of oseltamivir. Zanamivir is an orally inhaled agent that is approved for use in adults and children older than 12 years of age. It is a pregnancy category B. Like oseltamivir, the effectiveness of the drug is directly related to the quickness of the initiation of treatment.

Adverse effects with zanamivir include headache, dizziness, nausea, diarrhea, and respiratory effects such as sinusitis, bronchitis, cough, nasal symptoms, and infections. Because zanamivir is administered by oral inhalation, it is more likely to have respiratory adverse effects, however, it is less likely to cause systemic reactions. This is especially important for patients with asthma who may experience bronchospasm after use of zanamivir. The nurse should instruct the patient to have a fast-acting inhaled bronchodilator, such as albuterol, available when administering zanamivir.

Zanamivir is supplied on a Rotadisk containing four blisters of a powder mixture. The Rotadisk is loaded into a Diskhaler, the blister is punctured, and the patient inhales through the mouthpiece. The actual amount of drug delivered to the respiratory tract depends on the ability of the patient to inhale adequately. Approximately 10% of zanamivir is absorbed systemically. It is excreted renally as unchanged drug. Like oseltamivir, zanamivir should not substitute for yearly influenza vaccine in high risk populations.

ANTIFUNGAL DRUGS

Antifungal drugs generally are assigned to four groups—polyenes, azoles, fluorinated pyrimidines, and miscellaneous drugs. Although polyenes and azoles have different chemical structures, both groups work by altering cell membrane permeability. Fluorinated pyrimidines, such as flucytosine, block nucleic acid synthesis, whereas griseofulvin, classified as a miscellaneous drug, disrupts microtubule function. Because polyenes and azoles are prescribed commonly, they are discussed in depth in this chapter. In addition, antifungal topical drugs for treating superficial mycoses are discussed in this chapter.

POLYENE ANTIFUNGAL DRUGS

Polyene antimicrobials include amphotericin B and nystatin. These drugs have high affinity for fungal infections. Unfortunately, they also have the ability to induce severe adverse effects. Amphotericin B (Fungizone) is the prototype polyene antifungal drug.

NURSING MANAGEMENT OF THE PATIENT RECEIVING AMPHOTERICIN B

Core Drug Knowledge

Pharmacotherapeutics

Amphotericin B is an IV antifungal agent used to treat progressive and potentially fatal systemic fungal or protozoal infections. It has a wide spectrum of activity against many fungi, including *Aspergillus fumigatus*, *Blastomyces dermatitidis*, *Candida albicans*, *Candida guilliermondii*, *Candida tropicalis*, *Coccidioides immitis*, *Cryptococcus neoformans*, *Histoplasma capsulatum*, *Rhodotorula* species, and *Sporothrix schenckii*. Certain protozoan infections also are sensitive to amphotericin B, including *Leishmania braziliensis*, *Leishmania donovani*, *Leishmania mexicana*, *and Naegleria fowleri*.

Amphotericin B is available in lipid-complex and nonlipid-complex formulations. Liposomal amphotericin B is indicated for treating invasive fungal infections in patients refractory to or intolerant of conventional amphotericin B therapy. In addition to its IV formulation, amphotericin B is also available as a topical cream, lotion, or ointment for superficial use (Table 53-3).

Pharmacokinetics

Amphotericin B, given PO, is absorbed poorly from the GI tract. Because of its poor GI absorption, it may be given orally when GI tract sterilization is required to rid the tract of fungal colonies. Distribution of amphotericin B is limited; it crosses the placenta and may pass into breast milk. Low concentrations are achieved in aqueous humor, pleural, pericardial, peritoneal, and synovial fluids. Because CSF concentrations are approximately 3% of those in serum, amphotericin B must be given intrathecally to achieve fungistatic concentrations within the CSF.

The metabolism of amphotericin B is unknown. It is presumed that the drug enters the tissues of the body and is released slowly over time. Amphotericin B can be detected for up to 4 weeks in blood and 4 to 8 weeks in urine after discontinuation of therapy. The initial half-life is approximately 24 hours, followed by a second elimination phase with a half-life of about 15 days. The drug is excreted in the urine.

Pharmacodynamics

Amphotericin B works by binding to membrane sterols in fungal cell membranes. This binding appears to form pores or channels and results in increased cell permeability, cell leakage, and death. Because human cells also contain sterols, damage to the host's cells also may occur. At low concentrations, amphotericin B is fungistatic; higher concentrations may induce fungicidal activity.

Contraindications and Precautions

Amphotericin B can cause anemia, hypokalemia, and hypomagnesemia. The nurse should administer the drug cautiously to patients with any of these conditions because parenteral therapy with amphotericin B can cause significant renal electrolyte loss. For patients with preexisting renal impairment, the nurse should administer amphotericin B at a lower dose and should monitor the patient for signs of nephrotoxicity. Amphotericin B is assigned to pregnancy category B and should be used with caution during pregnancy and lactation.

TABLE 53-3 Summary of Selected Antifungal Drugs

Drug (Trade) Name	Selected Indications	Route and Dosage Range	Pharmacokinetics
Polyene Antifungal Drugs			
amphotericin B (Fungizone, Fungizone, Intravenous, Abelcet [lipid complex formula])	Progressive and potentially fatal systemic fungal or protozoal infections (*Aspergillus, Blastomyces,* coccidioidomycosis, histoplasmosis, sporotrichosis, mucormycosis)	*Adult:* IV (sporotrichosis), 20 mg per injection, up to 9 mo; IV (aspergillosis), total dose of 3.6 g, treat up to 11 mo; IV (other infections in adult or child), administer over 6 h at a concentration of 0.1 mg/mL, usual dose is 0.25 mg/kg/d not to exceed 1.5 mg/kg/d	*Onset:* 20–30 min *Duration:* 20–24 h $t_{1/2}$: 24 h initially and, then 15 d; Abelcet, 173.4 h
	Aspergillosis in patients refractory to, or intolerant of, conventional therapy (Abelcet)	*Adult:* IV (Abelcet), 5 mg/kg/d given as single infusion at 2.5 mg/kg/h	
	Cutaneous and mucocutaneous mycotic infections caused by *Candida* species	*Adult:* Topical, apply liberally to candidal lesions two to four times daily, treat for 2–4 wk based on response	
nystatin (Mycostatin, Nilstat, Nystex; *Canadian:* Candistatin)	*Candida*—oropharyngeal, cutaneous, mucocutaneous, vulvovaginal, intestinal	*Adult:* PO, 500,000–1,000,000 U tid, continued for at least 48 h after clinical cure; PO suspension, 400,000–600,000 U qid (½ dose in each side of mouth, retain the drug as long as possible before swallowing); troche, dissolve 1–2 tablets in mouth four to five times daily up to 14 d; vaginal preparation, 1 tablet (100,000 U) intravaginally qd for 2 wk; topical, apply to affected area two to three times daily until healing is complete *Child:* Oral suspension (infants), 200,000 U qid (100,000 in each side of mouth); oral suspension (premature and low-birth-weight infants), 100,000 U qid	Not generally absorbed systemically
flucytosine (5-FC, 5-fluorocytosine, Ancobon)	Serious infections caused by susceptible strains of *Candida, Cryptococcus*	*Adult:* PO, 50–150 mg/kg/d q6h	*Onset:* Varies *Duration:* 10–12 h $t_{1/2}$: 2–5 h
griseofulvin (Fulvicin P/G, Fulvicin U/F, Grifulvin V, Gris-Peg, Grisactin, Grisactin Ultra, Grisovin-FP)	Superficial dermatophyte infections (ringworm)–tinea corporis, tinea barbae, tinea capitis, tinea ungulum Tinea pedis and tinea cruris only when unresponsive to topical therapy	*Adult:* PO, 250–500 mg bid for 2 wk, up to 18 mo	*Onset:* 4 h *Duration:* 2 d $t_{1/2}$: 9–24 h
Azole Antifungal Drugs			
fluconazole (Diflucan; *Canadian:* Apo-Fluconazole)	Esophageal, oropharyngeal, vulvovaginal candidiasis	*Adult:* PO/IV, 200 mg on first day, followed by 100 mg/d as indicated *Child:* PO/IV, 6 mg/kg on the first day, followed by 3 mg/kg once daily; treat for a minimum of 3 wk and at least 2 wk after resolution	*Onset:* PO, unknown; IV, immediate *Duration:* Unknown $t_{1/2}$: 20–21 h
	Systemic mycoses (cryptococcal meningitis)	*Adult:* PO/IV, 400 mg on first day, followed by 200 mg qd; 400 mg qd may be needed; continue treatment for 10–12 wk *Child:* PO/IV, 12 mg/kg on first day, followed by 6 mg/kg once daily, continue treatment for 10–12 wk	
itraconazole (Sporanox)	Blastomyces dermatitidis, histoplasma capsulatum, aspergillosis	*Adult:* PO, 200 mg qd, increase dose in 100-mg increments to a maximum 400 mg qd; give doses over 200 mg/d in divided doses; continue treatment for a minimum of 3 mo and	

TABLE 53-3 Summary of Selected Antifungal Drugs (Continued)

Drug (Trade) Name	Selected Indications	Route and Dosage Range	Pharmacokinetics
		until clinical parameters and laboratory tests indicate that the active fungal infection has subsided *Child:* Safety and efficacy not established	
	Onychomycosis	*Adult:* PO, 200 mg bid for 1 wk, followed by 3-wk rest period; repeat	
miconazole (Monistat I.V., Micatin, Monistat 3, Monistat 7, Monistat-Derm, Monistat Dual Pak)	Severe systemic fungal infections: coccidioidomycosis Candidiasis Cryptococcosis Petriellidiosis Paracoccidioldo-mycosis Vulvovaginal candidiasis	*Adult:* IV (dosage varies with organism involved), 1,800–3,600 mg for 3 to >20 wk *Adult:* 600–1,800 mg for 1–20 wk *Adult:* 1,200–2,400 mg for 3–12 wk *Adult:* 600–3,000 mg for 5–20 wk *Adult:* 200–1,200 mg for 2–16 wk *Adult:* Vaginal suppositories, insert 1 suppository intravaginally once daily hs for 3 or 7 d (depending on drug dosage regimen); repeat course as necessary	*Onset:* IV, rapid; vaginal and topical, not systemically absorbed *Duration:* IV, unknown; vaginal and topical, not systemically absorbed $t_{1/2}$: IV, 21–24 h; vaginal and topical, not systemically absorbed
	Tinea pedia, tinea cruris, tinea corporis, cutaneous candidiasis, tinea versicolor	*Adult:* Topical, apply to affected areas bid	
ketoconazole (Nizoral; *Canadian:* Apo-Ketoconazole)	Systemic fungal infections: candidiasis, chronic mucocutaneous candidiasis, oral thrush, candiduria, blastomycosis, coccidioidomycosis, histoplasmosis, chromomycosis, paracoccidioldomycosis	*Adult:* PO, 200 mg qd, up to 400 mg/d; treat from 3 wk to 6 mo, depending on infecting organism and site *Child:* PO, >2 y, 3.3–6.6 mg/kg/d as a single dose; <2 y, safety and efficacy not established	*Onset:* PO, varies; topical, slow, not appreciably systemically absorbed *Duration:* Unknown $t_{1/2}$: 8 h
	Dermatophytosis; tinea corporis, tinea cruris, tinea versicolor	*Adult:* Topical, apply daily to affected area; may be treated twice daily; continue treatment for at least 2 wk *Child:* Topical, >2 y, same as adult; <2 y, safety and efficacy not established	
clotrimazole (Mycelex, Lotrimin)	Oropharyngeal candidiasis	*Adult:* Troche, administer 1 troche five times daily for 14 d	*Onset:* Unknown *Duration:* Unknown $t_{1/2}$: Unknown
	Vulvovaginal candidiasis	*Adult:* Vaginal cream, 1 applicator (5 g/d) hs for 7–14 d; vaginal tablet, one 100-mg tablet intravaginally hs for 7 d, or two 100-mg tablets intravaginally hs for 3 d, or one 500-mg tablet intravaginally one time	
	Tinea pedia, tinea cruris, tinea corporis, candidiasis, tinea versicolor	*Adult:* Topical, apply to affected area bid for 1–4 wk	
Topical Drugs for Superficial Mycoses			
butenafine (Mentax)	Tinea pedis, tinea corporis, tinea cruris	*Adult:* Topical, apply to affected area once daily for 4 wk	Not generally absorbed systemically
ciclopirox olamine (Loprox)	Tinea pedis, tinea cruris, tinea corporis, tinea versicolor	*Adult:* Topical, apply to affected area as directed twice daily	Not generally absorbed systemically
naftifine (Naftin)	Tinea pedis, tinea cruris, tinea corporis	*Adult:* Topical, massage into area bid; do not use longer than 4 wk	Not generally absorbed systemically

(*continued*)

TABLE 53-3 Summary of Selected Antifungal Drugs (Continued)

Drug (Trade) Name	Selected Indications	Route and Dosage Range	Pharmacokinetics
terbinafine (Lamisil)	Onychomycosis	*Adult:* PO, 250 mg/d; topical, apply to area bid up to 4 wk *Child:* 20 kg, PO, 62.5 mg/d *Child:* 20–40 kg, PO, 125 mg/d	*Onset:* 24 h *Duration:* 90 d $t_{1/2}$: 100 h
tolnaftate (Aftate, Genaspor, Tinactin, Ting)	Tinea pedis, tinea cruris, tinea corporis, tinea versicolor, onychomycosis, chronic fungal scalp infections, and prophylactically for tinea pedis	*Adult:* Topical, apply bid for 2–3 wk, up to 6 wk	Not generally absorbed systemically

Adverse Effects

Amphotericin B has an extensive adverse effects profile. In fact, some clinicians refer to it as "amphoterrible." Nephrotoxicity occurs in more than 80% of patients receiving IV amphotericin B. Nephrotoxicity is manifested in many forms, including renal insufficiency, azotemia, hyposthenuria, renal tubular acidosis, and frank renal failure.

Administration of IV amphotericin B may induce infusion-related reactions, such as headache, chills, fever, rigors, hypotension, bronchospasm, and nausea and vomiting. Slowing the rate of administration is not helpful. However, the severity of these symptoms usually diminishes with subsequent doses of amphotericin B.

Electrolyte abnormalities also may occur with amphotericin B therapy. These include hypokalemia, hypomagnesemia, hypochloremia, and hypocalcemia. Patients with preexisting cardiac problems may have exacerbations of their disorders when electrolyte abnormalities occur.

A normocytic, normochromic anemia occurs in most patients receiving amphotericin B. This reaction is believed to be caused by a suppressive effect on erythropoietin production. Transfusions are not usually necessary, and the anemia resolves on discontinuation of therapy. Leukopenia and thrombocytopenia also may occur.

Less frequent adverse effects from amphotericin B consist of ventricular fibrillation, hypertension, cardiac arrest (primarily in situations when infusion is too rapid), hypersensitivity, peripheral neuropathy, and seizures.

Intrathecal amphotericin B can cause blurred vision and in some cases, difficulty in urination. Polyneuropathy or paresthesias can occur in some patients, which are exhibited by numbness, tingling, pain, or weakness. Arachnoiditis, an inflammation of the arachnoid membrane, also is possible.

Drug Interactions

Amphotericin B should not be coadministered with drugs known to be nephrotoxic or hemotoxic, such as antineoplastic agents, cyclosporine, tacrolimus, or aminoglycosides (Table 53-4). It should not be used with drugs that may be affected by electrolyte imbalances, such as corticosteroids, digitalis glycosides, and thiazide diuretics. Other drugs that interact with amphotericin B include neuromuscular blocking agents, imidazoles, and flucytosine.

Assessment of Relevant Core Patient Variables

Health Status

The nurse should elicit a patient history to evaluate for preexisting renal dysfunction, cardiac disease, electrolyte imbalance, or anemia. The nurse also should assess for use of diuretics or for any concurrent drugs known to be nephrotoxic. The nurse should communicate any positive findings to the prescriber.

The nurse should perform a complete physical examination, especially assessing the renal system. For patients with preexisting cardiac disease, a baseline electrocardiogram should be performed. Baseline laboratory values should include complete blood count (CBC), complete metabolic profile (e.g., Sequential Multiple Analysis [SMA]-20), and renal function tests.

Life Span and Gender

The nurse should assess for pregnancy and lactation. Amphotericin B may be given during pregnancy. However, because of the potential adverse effects, it should be given only when absolutely needed. It should not be given to breast-feeding women because of its potential effects on the infant.

It is important to note the patient's age before administering amphotericin B. Safety of amphotericin B has not been demonstrated in children and older adults. When given to these patients, the nurse should closely monitor them. Elderly patients are more likely to have decreased renal function, which may increase the risk for nephrotoxicity.

Lifestyle, Diet, and Habits

It is important to assess fluid intake in patients on amphotericin B therapy. The nurse should make sure that patients on amphotericin B therapy are kept well

TABLE 53-4 Agents That Interact With Amphotericin B

Interactants	Effect and Significance	Nursing Management
antineoplastic agents	Coadministration of antineoplastic agents and amphotericin B increases the risks for renal toxicity, bronchospasm, and hypotension.	Monitor for adverse effects. Monitor renal function tests. Adjust dosage of antineoplastic agents if needed.
corticosteroids	Concurrent use may cause potential hypokalemia.	Do not coadminister unless needed for control of adverse reactions.
digitalis glycosides	Amphotericin B may induce hypokalemia, which increases the risk for digitalis glycoside toxicity.	Monitor electrolytes. Monitor for signs of digitalis toxicity. Replace electrolytes as needed.
flucytosine	Coadministration of flucytosine and amphotericin B have a synergistic effect, which increases the risk for flucytosine toxicity.	Monitor drug levels. Monitor for flucytosine toxicity. Adjust drug dosages as needed.
hemotoxic agents	Concurrent use increases the risk for anemia, neutropenia, and thrombocytopenia.	Monitor drug levels closely. Monitor for signs of blood dyscrasias. Adjust drug dosages as needed.
imidazoles	Coadministration of imidazoles and amphotericin B has antagonistic effects, resulting in subtherapeutic levels.	Monitor for efficacy of therapy. Adjust drug dosages as needed.
nephrotoxic agents	Concurrent use increases the risk for nephrotoxicity.	Monitor drug levels closely. Monitor for signs of renal impairment. Monitor intake and output. Adjust drug dosages as needed.
neuromuscular blocking agents	Amphotericin B-induced hypokalemia may enhance the curariform effect of skeletal muscle relaxants.	Monitor electrolytes. Replace electrolytes as needed. Monitor for prolonged action of neuromuscular blocking agents. Secure airway if prolonged activity is suspected.
thiazide diuretics	Coadministration may increase electrolyte losses.	Monitor electrolytes. Replace electrolytes as needed. Adjust drug dosages as needed.
zidovudine	Coadministration increases the risk of myelosuppression and nephrotoxicity.	Monitor renal function tests. Monitor CBC. Adjust drug dosages as needed.

hydrated. This may minimize the potential for nephrotoxicity.

Environment

The nurse should note the environment in which amphotericin B will be administered. Amphotericin B should be administered in an acute care environment. The nurse should be familiar with administration of IV amphotericin B. The drug should not be reconstituted with a bacteriostatic agent in the solution because this may lead to precipitation. Before administration, the nurse should document vital signs. The nurse should administer a test dose of amphotericin B (1 mg in 20 to 50 mL of 5% dextrose in water [D_5W] over 30 minutes) to assess for possible hypersensitivity and potential infusion reaction.

Nursing Diagnoses and Outcomes

- Risk for Injury related to infusion reaction or to electrolyte imbalance imposed by drug therapy

  Desired outcome: The patient will remain free from injury during drug administration or respond without injury to electrolyte replacement therapy.
- Altered Protection related to drug-induced leukopenia and thrombocytopenia

  Desired outcome: The patient will remain free from opportunistic infections resulting from leukopenia and thrombocytopenia.
- Excess Fluid Volume related to renal dysfunction resulting from drug therapy

  Desired outcome: The patient will have an appropriate ratio of intake to output.
- Acute Pain related to infusion reaction

  Desired outcome: The patient will have a decrease in pain after administration of analgesic drug, such as meperidine (Demerol).
- Ineffective Breathing Patterns due to drug-induced bronchospasm

  Desired outcome: The patient will maintain adequate oxygenation.

- Ineffective Cardiopulmonary Tissue Perfusion related to cardiac arrest or arrhythmias resulting from drug therapy
  Desired outcome: The patient will remain adequately perfused.
- Disturbed Sensory Perception: Visual due to drug-related blurred vision
  Desired outcome: The patient will regain adequate vision after therapy concludes.
- Risk for Injury related to drug effects of numbness, tingling, or weakness
  Desired outcome: The patient will remain injury free throughout therapy.

Planning and Intervention

Maximizing Therapeutic Effects

Patients may desire to stop amphotericin B therapy if they have infusion reactions. The nurse should prepare the patient for the possibility of this reaction. The nurse also should provide comfort measures, such as extra blankets, diversion therapy, or warm fluids to offset the discomfort of this reaction.

Minimizing Adverse Effects

The nurse should be prepared for the possibility of an infusion reaction. Administering preordered drugs, such as hydrocortisone, meperidine, and ibuprofen, before the initiation of therapy has been shown to be effective in preventing an infusion reaction. Varying success in preventing an infusion reaction has been demonstrated by using dantrolene. The nurse also should coordinate the administration of amphotericin B with possible blood transfusions. Infusion-related reactions can be more severe if administration occurs shortly after platelet or granulocyte transfusions.

The nurse should administer amphotericin B in a central line if possible. It is important to make sure there is an in-line filter on the IV administration set. The nurse can place the solution on an infusion pump and deliver over 4 to 6 hours.

Providing Patient and Family Education

- The nurse should describe and explain the possibility of an infusion reaction and the importance of notifying staff immediately if symptoms occur.
- The nurse also should explain possible adverse effects of amphotericin B and the need for serial blood tests. Because the adverse effects of amphotericin B can induce severe complications, it is important to explain the necessity of reporting any change in baseline that may occur.
- Another important area to discuss with patients and family is the importance of an accurate fluid intake and output record. It will be necessary to enlist the assistance of patients and their families to document fluid intake and output as needed.
- The nurse should inform patients using topical amphotericin B to report any skin irritation. It also is important to advise these patients to avoid occlusive dressings.
- The nurse should instruct the patient to immediately report symptoms of altered protection, such as easy bruising, sore throat, or fatigue to the health care provider.
- It is important to instruct patients with CNS symptoms, such as numbness, tingling, or weakness, to report them to the health care provider.

Ongoing Assessment and Evaluation

During the first dose of amphotericin B, the nurse should take vital signs every 15 minutes. This also is a good time to evaluate the patient for possible infusion reactions. Should a reaction occur, the nurse should stop the infusion, call for another nurse to stay with the patient, and contact the health care provider immediately. The nurse also should monitor the IV site during administration for signs of thrombophlebitis because amphotericin B is very irritating to tissues.

Throughout therapy, the nurse should coordinate the collection of laboratory tests, including a CBC, SMA-20, and renal function tests. The nurse should weigh the patient daily and evaluate intake and output every shift.

It is important to monitor patients with preexisting cardiac disease for exacerbation of their symptoms. Fluid overload and electrolyte imbalances place these patients at high risk for a cardiac event.

The nurse should monitor for adverse effects that may place the patient at increased risk for injury. For patients with sensory-perceptual disturbances or numbness, tingling, and weakness, the nurse should be sure the patient understands the need for assistance to and from the bed. The nurse should be sure to keep the bed in the low position and the side rails up at all times.

The nurse should use strict aseptic technique for patients receiving amphotericin B. Most patients will have anemia related to the therapy, which will increase their risk for infection.

By the end of therapy, the fungal infection should be resolved. In addition, all adverse effects should be identified and appropriate intervention should be started. ■

DRUG SIMILAR TO AMPHOTERICIN B

Nystatin (Mycostatin) is an antifungal antibiotic that is nearly identical to amphotericin B in structure. It is available in topical, vaginal, and oral formulations. Nystatin is not used for systemic fungal infections because of its poor absorption from the GI tract and its potential for toxicity. It is used to treat oropharyngeal, cutaneous, mucocutaneous, and vulvovaginal candidiasis. Like amphotericin B, it may be given orally when GI tract sterilization is required

MEMORY CHIP

Amphotericin B

- Used for severe systemic fungal or protozoal infections
- Significant contraindication: hypersensitivity
- Most common adverse effects: infusion reactions, electrolyte abnormalities, and anemia
- Most serious adverse effect: nephrotoxicity
- Maximizing therapeutic effects: prepare the patient for the possibility of an infusion reaction so the patient does not cease therapy
- Minimizing adverse effects: do not administer with other nephrotoxic drugs to minimize the potential for nephrotoxicity
- Most significant patient education: discuss the potential for an infusion reaction and the need for close monitoring of the hematopoietic and renal systems

to rid the GI tract of fungi. A liposomal formulation of nystatin is undergoing clinical investigation and has been well tolerated after systemic administration. Liposomal nystatin may have activity against *Aspergillus*, although its present place as an antifungal agent is an orphan drug for salvage therapy in patients not responding to lipid-based amphotericin B formulations and/or other antifungals.

Some formulations of nystatin, such as its oral suspension, contain methylparaben and propylparaben. Therefore, these products should be used with caution in patients with paraben hypersensitivity. In addition, some formulations of nystatin oral suspension contain sucrose, which may cause hyperglycemia, especially in the diabetic patient.

Adverse effects from nystatin are infrequent. Oral doses of nystatin can cause mild and transient nausea and vomiting, diarrhea, and abdominal pain. Topical and vaginal forms of nystatin may produce skin irritation, rash, or urticaria.

The oral suspension of nystatin is called a "swish and swallow" drug. The nurse should advise the patient to swish the solution throughout the mouth and then swallow or spit the drug as directed by the prescriber. When nystatin troches are prescribed, the nurse should advise the patient to allow them to dissolve completely in the mouth and not to chew or swallow the drug. This may take up to 30 minutes.

DRUGS SIGNIFICANTLY DIFFERENT FROM AMPHOTERICIN B

Flucytosine

Flucytosine (5-FC) is an oral antifungal drug. Historically, it has been used in combination with amphotericin B in treating cryptococcal meningitis. However, since the release of fluconazole in 1990, flucytosine use has declined significantly.

Flucytosine acts as an antimetabolite, interfering with pyrimidine metabolism and eventually disrupting both RNA and protein synthesis. It also may disrupt DNA synthesis. Flucytosine itself does not possess antineoplastic activity.

Flucytosine is assigned to pregnancy category C and is contraindicated for use during pregnancy and breast-feeding. It is not metabolized; over 90% is excreted by glomerular filtration as unchanged drug. Therefore, it is used cautiously in patients with preexisting renal impairment. It also is used with caution in patients with preexisting bone marrow depression, recent radiation therapy or cytotoxic drug therapy, dental disease, or a history of a hematologic disease because these patients are most susceptible to flucytosine's myelosuppressive effects. In patients with hepatic disease, flucytosine can cause hepatitis or jaundice.

Flucytosine can induce serious adverse effects. Flucytosine toxicity involves the rapidly proliferating tissues, such as the bone marrow and the lining of the GI tract. Therefore, frequent hematologic adverse effects include anemia, leukopenia, and thrombocytopenia. GI adverse effects include abdominal pain, diarrhea, nausea, vomiting, and anorexia. Other adverse effects caused by flucytosine include hepatic dysfunction, photosensitivity, and CNS effects, such as dizziness, headache, and light-headedness. It is important to monitor patients who are concurrently taking other drugs also known to cause hematologic toxicity, nephrotoxicity, or hepatotoxicity.

Griseofulvin

Griseofulvin (Grisactin, Fulvicin-U/F) is an antifungal drug used in treating superficial dermatophytic infections, such as ringworm and tinea. It is available in a microsize or ultramicrosize formulation. These different formulations are meant to increase the bioavailability of, and to decrease the GI intolerance to, the drug.

Griseofulvin works by disrupting the mitotic spindle structure of the fungal cell, thereby stopping cell division. It also may cause defective DNA that is unable to replicate. It is very effective for superficial mycoses because it is deposited in keratin precursor cells, which creates an unfavorable environment for fungal infection. Infected skin, cells, and hair are then replaced slowly by tissue that is not infected by the dermatophyte. Griseofulvin therapy lasts until the infected area has completely regrown. This may take 6 to 12 months in treating tinea unguium.

Griseofulvin is contraindicated during pregnancy and breast-feeding. It should be given with caution to patients with hepatic dysfunction, porphyria, or systemic lupus erythematosus because the drug may exacerbate these conditions.

Griseofulvin has a moderate adverse effect profile. Common adverse effects include nausea, vomiting, flatulence, and epigastric distress. CNS effects may include headache, fatigue, dizziness, insomnia, confusion, psychotic symptoms, and paresthesias of the hands and feet. Integumentary adverse effects may include maculopapular rash, urticaria, and photosensitivity. In addition, hepatitis, elevated hepatic enzymes, granulocytopenia, and leukopenia have occurred after high-dose or long-term therapy.

Griseofulvin interacts with several drugs. Most importantly, it interacts with oral contraceptives by decreasing their effectiveness. Therefore, the nurse should advise women taking birth control pills to use another method of contraception during griseofulvin therapy. Griseofulvin also may decrease the effectiveness of warfarin. The nurse should closely monitor prothrombin time if griseofulvin is either added to or discontinued from warfarin therapy. Barbiturates can decrease the antifungal activity of griseofulvin. Finally, griseofulvin may increase the adverse effects of alcohol when taken concurrently.

C AZOLE ANTIFUNGAL DRUGS

The azole antifungal drugs have two subgroups: imidazoles and triazoles. These two groups differ slightly in their chemical structures, but they have the same clinical applications. Azole antifungal drugs can be used for both superficial mycoses and more serious systemic mycoses. Drugs within the azole antifungal class include fluconazole, itraconazole, miconazole, ketoconazole, and clotrimazole. Fluconazole (Diflucan) is the prototype azole antifungal drug.

NURSING MANAGEMENT OF THE PATIENT RECEIVING P FLUCONAZOLE

Core Drug Knowledge

Pharmacotherapeutics

Fluconazole has a wide spectrum of antifungal activity. It is the drug of choice for esophageal and oropharyngeal candidiasis and is used to suppress vulvovaginal candidiasis. It is used for primary fungal prophylaxis in immunocompromised patients with a CD4+ T cell count less than 200 and as prophylaxis against coccidioidomycosis, cryptococcosis, and histoplasmosis in patients with a CD4+ T-cell counts below 50.

Although amphotericin B is usually the drug of choice for systemic mycoses, especially cryptococcal meningitis, fluconazole is used as an alternative drug to treat these conditions (see Table 53-3 for more information).

Pharmacokinetics

Fluconazole is administered orally and IV. The pharmacokinetics of both oral and IV fluconazole are similar. GI absorption is rapid and almost complete. Oral bioavailability is more than 90% in fasting adults, and peak serum concentrations are attained within 1 to 2 hours after oral administration.

Fluconazole is distributed widely into body tissues and fluids. Saliva, sputum, nail, blister, and vaginal secretion concentrations are approximately equal to plasma concentrations. High concentrations also can be achieved in the cornea, aqueous humor, and vitreous body following IV administration. Fluconazole distributes well into the CSF and achieves CSF concentrations that are 50% to 94% of plasma concentrations, regardless of the degree of meningeal inflammation. Fluconazole crosses the placenta and enters breast milk. Elimination is mainly renal; about 60% to 80% of a dose is excreted in the urine unchanged and 11% as metabolites. Small amounts of fluconazole are excreted in the feces. Elimination of the drug can be impaired in elderly patients.

Pharmacodynamics

Fluconazole works directly by altering the fungal cell membrane. Fluconazole inhibits ergosterol synthesis, a cytochrome P450 enzyme that is an essential component of the fungal membrane. Inhibition of ergosterol synthesis results in increased cellular permeability, causing leakage of cellular contents. Other proposed antifungal effects of fluconazole include inhibition of endogenous respiration, interaction with membrane phospholipids, and inhibition of the transformation of yeasts to molds. There are no direct effects on the body.

Contraindications and Precautions

There are no absolute contraindications with fluconazole. It should be used with caution during pregnancy and in patients with preexisting hepatic and renal dysfunction.

Adverse Effects

The most common adverse effects of fluconazole are diarrhea, nausea, vomiting, abdominal pain, headache, and dizziness. Mild elevations in levels of alanine transaminase, aspartate transaminase, alkaline phosphatase, and bilirubin may occur. These abnormalities usually return to pretreatment levels after completion of therapy. Rarely, hepatotoxicity has been reported.

Other symptoms that have occurred during fluconazole therapy include alopecia and exfoliative skin disorders, such as Stevens-Johnson syndrome. These conditions occur most frequently in HIV-infected patients and patients with a concurrent malignancy who are taking multiple drugs. A direct causative relationship has not been determined. Rarely, fluconazole therapy may induce hypokalemia, eosinophilia, and thrombocytopenia.

Drug Interactions

There are many potential drug-drug interactions involving fluconazole. Although no longer available in the U.S. market, astemizole, cisapride, and terfenadine may induce fatal arrhythmias when given concurrently with fluconazole. Fluconazole also may interact with anticoagulants, benzodiazepines, hydantoins, oral contraceptives, sulfonylurea agents, tricyclic antidepressants, and zidovudine (Table 53-5).

Assessment of Relevant Core Patient Variables

Health Status

The nurse should elicit a patient history to evaluate for preexisting renal or hepatic dysfunction, pregnancy, or breast-feeding. It is important to communicate any positive findings to the health care provider. The nurse also should assess for any known reactions to azole antifungal agents.

The nurse should perform a complete physical examination, documenting signs and symptoms of the

TABLE 53-5 Agents That Interact With P Fluconazole

Interactants	Effect and Significance	Nursing Management
anticoagulants	Fluconazole may decrease the metabolism of anticoagulants such as warfarin. This may increase the anticoagulant activity and result in toxicity	Monitor prothrombin time at least every 2 d. Monitor patient for signs of bleeding. Adjust anticoagulant dosage as needed.
benzodiazepines	Metabolism of certain benzodiazepines and first-pass effect of triazolam may be decreased resulting in increased CNS depression	Monitor for CNS depression. Adjust dosage of benzodiazepines. Avoid use of itraconazole or ketoconazole.
buspirone	Inhibition of the CYP3A4 isozyme by azole antifungal agents may result in increased plasma buspirone concentrations resulting in an increased risk for adverse effects.	Avoid concurrent use if possible. Monitor for buspirone adverse effects.
cyclosporin tacrolimus	Fluconazole may inhibit cyclosporine or tacrolimus hepatic metabolism. This may induce toxicity and increase the risk for nephrotoxicity.	Monitor cyclosporine or tacrolimus levels. Monitor serum creatinine levels. Adjust cyclosporine or tacrolimus dosage as needed.
hydantoins	Fluconazole may decrease the metabolism of hydantoins, such as phenytoin. This may result in toxicity of hydantoins.	Monitor hydantoin levels. Monitor patient for sign of toxicity. Adjust hydantoin dosage as needed.
losartan	Fluconazole may inhibit the metabolism of losartan resulting in an increased antihypertensive effect and risk for adverse effects.	Monitor the blood pressure daily. Monitor the patient for adverse effects to losartan.
oral contraceptives	Concurrent use with oral contraceptives containing ethinyl estradiol/levonorgestrel may decrease serum concentration of the oral contraceptives.	Advise women taking ethinyl estradiol or levonorgestrel BCP to use another method of contraception.
rifamycins	Rifamycins may induce the metabolism of fluconazole. This may decrease plasma concentration of fluconazole and decrease antifungal activity.	Monitor for therapeutic efficacy of fluconazole. Adjust the dose of fluconazole as needed.
sulfonylureas	Although the mechanism of action is unclear, fluconazole may increase the hypoglycemic effects of sulfonylurea agents.	Monitor blood glucose levels daily. Adjust dose of sulfonylurea agent as needed.
tricyclic antidepressants	Fluconazole may inhibit the metabolism of TCA drugs resulting in an increase in therapeutic and adverse effects.	Monitor the patient's clinical response to tricyclic agents (TCA) agents. Adjust dosage of TCA as needed.
zidovudine	Coadministration of zidovudine and fluconazole increases the area under the curve (AUC) of zidovudine.	Monitor for toxic effects of zidovudine. Monitor renal function.

fungal infection. For patients with preexisting anemia, renal, or hepatic disease or patients expected to be on long-term therapy, the nurse should obtain baseline CBC, renal, and hepatic function tests to determine current functioning.

Life Span and Gender

The nurse should determine whether the patient is pregnant or breast-feeding. Fluconazole is assigned to pregnancy category C and should, therefore, be used with caution during pregnancy. It has high concentrations in breast milk.

It is important to note the patient's age before administering fluconazole. Although there is a dosage schedule for children, the safety of fluconazole has not been demonstrated in children younger than 13 years. However, drug therapy has been successful and complications have not occurred in neonates treated with IV fluconazole in emergency treatment situations. With this in mind, the nurse should closely monitor children throughout therapy. Elderly patients are more likely to have decreased renal and hepatic function, which may increase the risk for toxicities.

Lifestyle, Diet, and Habits

The nurse should assess whether fluconazole is causing gastric distress in the patient. Fluconazole absorption and bioavailability are not affected by food or changes in gastric pH. Therefore, the nurse should encourage patients who experience GI distress to take the drug with food.

The nurse should ask questions to uncover information about alcohol ingestion and other substance use (e.g., drugs and tobacco). Fluconazole may elevate hepatic enzymes. The nurse should caution the patient to refrain from alcohol ingestion throughout therapy because this increases the risk of hepatotoxicity. As with other drugs used as prophylaxis against opportunistic diseases in immunocompromised patients, the nurse should discuss potential substance abuse (other drugs, alcohol, tobacco) with the patient. The nurse should explain how a healthy lifestyle decreases the risk for opportunistic diseases.

It also is important to determine which type of OTC pain reliever the patient generally uses. The nurse should advise the patient to use aspirin instead of acetaminophen for relief of minor discomforts because acetaminophen has the potential to damage the liver or kidneys.

Environment

The nurse should be aware of the environment in which fluconazole will be administered. Fluconazole is administered orally and IV. The oral preparation is used in the home environment, often as long-term prophylaxis for fungal infections in immunocompromised patients. The nurse should be sure to explain the importance of follow-up visits to assess the efficacy of therapy and to evaluate the patient for possible adverse effects.

Intravenous therapy is usually reserved for patients unable to tolerate or take fluconazole orally and is administered in the hospital setting. Prior to administration, the nurse should visually inspect the solution for particulate matter and discoloration. Do not administer unless the solution is clear. Fluconazole should be administered with an infusion pump at a rate not to exceed 200 mg/h.

Nursing Diagnoses and Outcomes

- Acute Pain related to fluconazole-induced headache
  Desired outcome: The patient will self-administer aspirin to relieve headache.
- Altered Protection related to adverse effects of blood dyscrasias and Stevens-Johnson syndrome
  Desired outcome: The patient will report signs and symptoms of these adverse reactions immediately to the health care provider.
- Disturbed Body Image from drug-related alopecia
  Desired outcome: The patient will verbalize concerns of changes in body image to the health care provider and develop coping strategies.
- Imbalanced Nutrition: Less Than Body Requirements related to adverse effects of nausea, vomiting, and abdominal pain
  Desired outcome: The patient will remain within acceptable weight parameters throughout therapy.
- Risk for Injury related to elevated hepatic enzymes and hypokalemia resulting from drug therapy
  Desired outcome: The patient will remain injury free throughout therapy.

Planning and Intervention

Maximizing Therapeutic Effects

The nurse should administer fluconazole in evenly divided intervals throughout the day.

Minimizing Adverse Effects

The nurse should carefully screen patients for preexisting disorders, which may increase the risk of adverse reactions. In the hospitalized patient, the nurse should contact the primary health care provider if any drugs known to interact or increase the risk of adverse effects are added to the drug profile. The nurse can administer an antiemetic or antidiarrheal agent, if prescribed, for adverse GI effects.

Providing Patient and Family Education

- It is important that patients understand that they should not take this drug if they have ever had a reaction to any drug whose name includes the ending "azole."
- The nurse should advise patients to notify the health care provider if they are pregnant or breast-feeding.
- It is important to explain that fluconazole is prescribed for a particular infection and should not be used to self-medicate or treat any other infection.
- Unless specified by the doctor, the nurse should caution that this drug should not be used in children younger than 13 years.
- The nurse should teach the patient about the need to complete the full course of drug therapy, even if the infection resolves. Patients should be instructed to take forgotten doses as soon as they remember but not if it is time for the next dose.
- The nurse should remind patients of the importance of remaining well hydrated while taking this drug.
- The nurse should explain potential adverse effects of fluconazole and potential remedies for these discomforts. It is important to advise patients to contact the health care provider immediately if they experience darkening of their urine, yellowing of the eyes or skin, unusual bruising or bleeding, skin rash (including inside the mouth), redness, blistering, peeling, or loosening of the skin. This is especially important for patients taking fluconazole as a prophylaxis for opportunistic diseases (see the accompanying display, Fluconazole and Chronic Candidiasis).
- The nurse should explain the decreased effectiveness of oral contraceptives and should suggest that patients use an alternative form of contraception while taking fluconazole.
- The nurse should advise patients taking sulfonylureas to monitor their blood glucose frequently and to notify the health care provider in the event of frequent episodes of hypoglycemia.

Critical Thinking Scenario

Fluconazole and chronic candidiasis

Janice Wind is a 40-year-old woman infected with HIV. She has been diagnosed with esophageal candidiasis, for which fluconazole therapy has been prescribed. This is her third episode of esophageal candidiasis for which she will receive prolonged therapy. Assume you are Ms. Wind's nurse.

1. Identify the assessments and evaluations you would find valuable before initiating therapy.
2. Propose or construct a patient-teaching plan. Which features would you include?
3. Develop some questions about the effects of therapy to explore with Ms. Wind when she returns to the clinic in 6 weeks for a follow-up evaluation.

- It is important to advise patients taking anticoagulants to have blood tests performed frequently to detect altered prothrombin times. They should contact the health care provider if they experience easy bruising or bleeding.
- It is also important to advise patients of signs and symptoms of secondary bacterial infections that may occur with superficial mycoses. The nurse should advise patients to contact the health care provider if the affected skin becomes red and hot or exudes pus.
- The nurse should assure patients with alopecia that the condition is temporary. Patients may choose to wear a wig if they wish.

Ongoing Assessment and Evaluation

The nurse should monitor the effectiveness of therapy. When treating superficial mycoses, the nurse should be sure to document new lesions and assess for possible secondary bacterial infections. In the hospital setting, the nurse also should monitor for hepatic or renal dysfunction. It is important to monitor intake and output carefully; the nurse can enlist the patient and family to document intake and output not observed by the nurse.

Throughout therapy, the nurse should arrange for serial blood testing to evaluate renal, hepatic, and hematopoietic function. For suspected electrolyte imbalance, it is important to review SMA-20 test results.

The nurse should monitor the patient for GI distress, headache, dizziness, and exfoliative skin disorders. It is important to ensure the safety of the patient experiencing CNS effects by keeping the bed in the low position and the side rails up at all times. The nurse should be sure the patient understands the need to ask for ambulatory assistance if experiencing dizziness to avoid injury. By the end of therapy, the patient should be without symptoms of fungal infection. In addition, adverse reactions should be controlled. ■

DRUGS CLOSELY RELATED TO P FLUCONAZOLE

Itraconazole

Itraconazole (Sporanox) is an oral triazole antifungal drug that is related closely to ketoconazole. Itraconazole is active against many of the same fungi as ketoconazole and fluconazole but has greater activity against *Aspergillus*. Currently, itraconazole is approved for treating *Blastomyces dermatitidis*, *Histoplasma capsulatum*, and onychomycosis. It is under investigation for treating dermatophytic skin infections unresponsive to topical therapy. Itraconazole also is available for IV use as an alternative to IV amphotericin B. Itraconazole's oral bioavailability may increase to 90% to 100% when given with a meal or a cola beverage. Like ketoconazole, it requires an acidic environment for solubility. Itraconazole appears to have fewer adverse effects compared to ketoconazole. However, significant drug interactions are associated with this drug. Concomitant administration of itraconazole and pimozide or quinidine is contraindicated. A new warning listed for this drug is that life-threatening cardiac arrhythmias and/or sudden death have occurred in patients using quinidine, pimozide, or quinidine concomitantly with itraconazole.

Miconazole

Miconazole (Monistat I.V., Micatin) is an imidazole-type antifungal agnet. When miconazole was first released, it was hoped it would replace amphotericin B as a parenteral antifungal agent. Unfortunately, it was found to be less efficacious and caused major toxicities. Although micona-

MEMORY CHIP

P Fluconazole

- Used for treatment of candidiasis and prophylaxis for fungal diseases in immunocompromised patients
- Most common adverse effects: nausea, vomiting, diarrhea, abdominal pain, headache, and dizziness
- Most serious adverse effect: Stevens-Johnson syndrome
- Maximizing therapeutic effects: administer adjunct medications for nausea and diarrhea
- Minimizing adverse effects: do not give with any drugs that increase the potential for adverse effects
- Most significant patient education: watch for signs and symptoms of adverse effects and call the health care provider immediately if any occur

zole is still marketed in a parenteral formulation, it is used most commonly topically and intravaginally. It is the active ingredient in many OTC antifungal formulations.

Ketoconazole

Ketoconazole (Nizoral) is an imidazole antifungal agent. In addition to its antifungal activity, ketoconazole possesses actions that may make it useful in other types of conditions. For example, ketoconazole has been used successfully for treating advanced prostate cancer. When used in higher doses, ketoconazole can inhibit sterol synthesis in humans, including the synthesis of aldosterone, cortisol, and testosterone. Ketoconazole also is a potent inhibitor of thromboxane synthesis and has been used clinically to prevent adult respiratory distress syndrome in patients at high risk for this syndrome.

When given orally, the bioavailability of ketoconazole is affected by the pH of the stomach. It should not be given concurrently with agents that increase gastric pH such as food, antacids, histamine-2 blockers, and omeprazole. It also should be given with caution with other agents that induce or inhibit the P450 isoenzymes.

Clotrimazole

Clotrimazole (Mycelex, Lotrimin) is another imidazole antifungal drug. It is not orally absorbed and is too toxic for IV administration. It is marketed in various forms, including vaginal suppositories and cream, topical lotion and cream, and oral solution and lozenges. It is active against a wide variety of fungi, yeast, and dermatophytes; certain gram-positive bacteria; and superficial fungal infections. These include dermatophytosis, vaginal and oral candidiasis, and tinea infections. The ability of formulations to reach subcutaneous tissues is poor. Therefore, clotrimazole is not indicated for treatment of subcutaneous mycoses.

C TOPICAL DRUGS FOR SUPERFICIAL MYCOSES

Superficial mycoses involving the skin are the most frequent fungal infections. There are many topical drugs to treat this type of infection. Generally speaking, the drug is chosen according to the prescriber's preference. Azole topical drugs, such as butoconazole, clotrimazole, econazole, ketoconazole, miconazole, oxiconazole, sulconazole, and terconazole, are frequently prescribed. Additional topical drugs include butenafine, ciclopirox olamine, naftifine, terbinafine, and tolnaftate.

Butenafine

Butenafine (Mentax) is a new topical antifungal drug indicated for treating tinea pedis, tinea corporis, and tinea cruris. It currently is under investigation for treatment of onychomycosis. Butenafine is similar to tolnaftate (discussed later in this chapter); however, it also is effective against *Candida*, whereas tolnaftate is not. There are no significant drug interactions or adverse effects identified at this time.

Ciclopirox Olamine

Ciclopirox olamine (Loprox) is a broad-spectrum antifungal drug used to treat both dermatophytes and *Candida*. It is used primarily for tinea pedis, tinea cruris, tinea corporis, and tinea versicolor. It works by blocking transport of amino acids into the fungal cell, thus altering the cell membrane to allow leakage of intracellular material. Ciclopirox olamine also is manufactured as a nail lacquer (Penlac) for the topical treatment of mild-to-moderate onychomycosis of the fingernails and toenails without lunula involvement in immunocompetent patients.

Ciclopirox olamine is absorbed deeper into the dermal layers than other topical drugs. However, it is not significantly absorbed systemically. There are no significant drug-drug interactions. Potential adverse effects include irritation, pruritus at the application site, redness, pain, burning, and worsening of clinical signs or symptoms.

Naftifine

Naftifine (Naftin) is a topical allylamine antifungal drug. It is used primarily for tinea pedis, tinea cruris, and tinea corporis. Naftifine is believed to interfere with sterol biosynthesis but with a different mechanism than azoles. There are no significant interactions with naftifine. Adverse effects include burning, stinging, dryness, erythema, pruritus, local irritation, and rash.

Terbinafine

Terbinafine (Lamisil) is administered either orally or topically. Its topical formulation is now available OTC. Terbinafine is pharmacologically similar to naftifine. Oral terbinafine is highly effective for treating onychomycosis because of its fungicidal activity and ability to concentrate within the nail. In fact, it has been found to be superior to griseofulvin and itraconazole for treating onychomycosis.

Oral terbinafine should be given with caution to patients with hepatic and renal insufficiency and during breast-feeding. The most common adverse effects are GI, followed by elevated hepatic enzyme levels, urticaria, pruritus, and occasionally a distorted sense of taste (dysgeusia). Rare but serious adverse effects include symptomatic idiosyncratic hepatobiliary dysfunction (including cholestatic hepatitis), serious skin reactions, severe neutropenia, and allergic reactions (including anaphylaxis).

Tolnaftate

Tolnaftate (Aftate, Genaspor, Tinactin, Ting) is used primarily for tinea pedis, tinea cruris, tinea corporis, and tinea versicolor. Tolnaftate also is used for onychomycosis, in chronic fungal scalp infections, and prophylactically for tinea pedis. There are no significant drug interactions with tolnaftate, and the only adverse reaction is mild skin irritation.

CHAPTER SUMMARY

- Viral and fungal diseases range from annoying disorders to life-threatening infections.
- Fungal infections are either systemic or dermatophytic, or occur in the mucous membranes.
- There are few effective antiviral drugs because eradicating the virus also may severely damage the host.
- Acyclovir is the prototype nucleoside analogue drug used to treat viral infections.
- Two major classes of antifungal drugs are polyenes and azoles.
- Amphotericin B is the prototype polyene antifungal and is the drug of choice for most systemic fungal infections.
- Amphotericin B may induce severe adverse effects, including infusion reactions.
- Fluconazole is the prototype azole antifungal drug.
- Fluconazole may be used as an alternative to IV amphotericin B.
- Topical forms of azole drugs also are useful in the treatment of superficial mycoses. Additional topical antifungal drugs include butenafine, ciclopirox olamine, naftifine, terbinafine, and tolnaftate.

QUESTIONS FOR STUDY AND REVIEW

1. Why are there so few effective antiviral drugs?
2. How does acyclovir work to fight herpes infections?
3. Acyclovir should be given cautiously to patients with which types of diseases or disorders?
4. Why is ribavirin not generally used in adults?
5. What are the indications for amantadine therapy?
6. What are the potential serious adverse effects of foscarnet therapy?
7. What special instructions should be given to immunosuppressed patients regarding oseltamivir or zanamivir?
8. Why is amphotericin B sometimes referred to as "amphoterrible"?
9. What significant adverse effects are associated with fluconazole therapy?

NEED MORE HELP?

Chapter 53 of the study guide for *Drug Therapy in Nursing* contains exercises and activities to reinforce your understanding of the concepts presented in this chapter. For additional information see the text's accompanying website at *http://www.connection.lww.com.*

REFERENCES AND BIBLIOGRAPHY

Anonymous. (1999). Aronex pharmaceuticals announces preliminary results of a phase III clinical trial for Nyotran. June 29, 1999a. Available at: http://www.aronex-pharm.com.

Balzarini, J., Naesens, L., Clercq, E. (1998). New antivirals—mechanism of action and resistance development. *Current Opinion in Microbiology, 1*(5), 535–546.

CCIS System. (2001). *Computerized Clinical Information System.* Denver, CO: Micromedex.

Clinical Drug Monographs. [CDRom]. (2001). Gold Standard Media.

Colacino, J. M., Staschke, K. A., Laver, W. G. (1999). Approaches and strategies for the treatment of influenza virus infections. *Antivir Chemistry and Chemotherapeutics, 10*(4), 155–185.

DiDomenico, B. (1999). Novel antifungal drugs. *Current Opinion in Microbiology, 2*(5), 509–515.

Drug Facts and Comparisons. (2000). St. Louis: Facts and Comparisons.

Gigolashvili, T. (1999). Update on antifungal therapy. *Cancer Practice, 7*(3), 157–159.

Hardman, J. G., Limbird, L. E., Molinof, P. B., Ruddon, R. W., & Gilman, A. (Eds.). (1997). *Goodman and Gilman's the pharmacological basis of therapeutics,* (9th Ed.). New York: McGraw-Hill.

Karch, A. (2001). *2001 Lippincott's nursing drug guide.* Philadelphia: Lippincott Williams & Wilkins.

Katzung, B. (1998). *Basic and clinical pharmacology* (7th ed.). Stamford: Appleton & Lange.

Lomaestro, B. M., & Piatek, M. A. (1998). Update on drug interactions with azole antifungal agents. *Annals of Pharmacotherapeutics, 32*(9), 915–28.

Porth, C. (1998). *Pathophysiology: Concepts of altered health states* (5th ed.). Philadelphia: Lippincott Williams & Wilkins.

Sheehan, D. J., Hitchcock, C. A., & Sibley, C. M. (1999). Current and emerging azole antifungal agents. *Clinical Microbiology Review, 12*(1), 40–79.

Tatro, D. (Ed.). (2000). *Drug interaction facts* (6th ed.). St. Louis: Facts and Comparisons.

Tyring, S. K. (1998). Advances in the treatment of herpesvirus infection: The role of famciclovir. *Clinical Therapeutics, 20*(4), 661–670.

Chapter 54

DRUGS FOR TREATING HIV AND AIDS

KEY TERMS

CD4+ T cells
enzyme immunoassay
enzyme-linked immunosorbent assay
highly active antiretroviral therapy (HAART)
HIV RNA
nucleoside reverse transcriptase inhibitors (NRTI)
nonnucleoside reverse transcriptase inhibitors (NNRTI)
polymerase chain reaction
protease inhibitors (PI)
provirus
viral load
Western blot

Learning Objectives

At the completion of this chapter the student will:

1. Describe the parameters that govern the choice of antiretroviral agents.
2. Identify core drug knowledge about drugs that are used in treating human immunodeficiency virus (HIV) infection and acquired immunodeficiency syndrome (AIDS).
3. Identify core patient variables relevant to drugs that are used in treating HIV infection and AIDS.
4. Relate the interaction of core drug knowledge to core patient variables for drugs that are used in treating HIV infection and AIDS.
5. Generate a nursing plan of care from the interactions between core drug knowledge and core patient variables for drugs that are used in treating HIV infection and AIDS.
6. Describe nursing interventions to maximize therapeutic and minimize adverse effects for drugs that are used in treating HIV infection and AIDS.
7. Determine key points for patient and family education for drugs that are used in treating HIV infection and AIDS.

Nucleoside reverse transcriptase inhibitors

zidovudine
didanosine
zalcitabine
stavudine
lamivudine
abacavir

Protease inhibitors

saquinavir
ritonavir
lopinavir
indinavir
nelfinavir
amprenavir

Non-nucleoside reverse transcriptase inhibitors

nevirapine
delavirdine
efavirenz

Nucleotide analogue reverse transcriptase inhibitor

adefovir

The symbol C indicates the **drug class**.

Drugs in bold type marked with the symbol P are **prototypes**.

Drugs in blue type with no symbol are **closely related** to the prototype.

Drugs in **red** type with no symbol are **significantly different** from the prototype.

Drugs in black type with no symbol are **also used in drug therapy**; no prototype.

Human immunodeficiency virus (HIV) is transmitted from person to person through sexual contact, by blood, or perinatally. Patients with the HIV virus have HIV infection. Acquired immunodeficiency syndrome (AIDS) is diagnosed when the CD4+ count of patients with HIV is less than 200; when patients with HIV infection develop opportunistic diseases, such as thrush, *Pneumocystis carinii* pneumonia (PCP), or *Mycobacterium avium* complex (MAC); in the presence of pulmonary tuberculosis (TB), recurrent pneumonia, or invasive cervical cancer in a patient with HIV disease; or when there is no other reason for immune impairment.

Pharmacotherapy for HIV infection and AIDS has changed dramatically since AIDS was first identified in 1982, and it continues to evolve. Recommended pharmacotherapy for HIV and AIDS is highly individualized. However, providers agree that multiple drug therapy, called **highly active antiretroviral therapy (HAART)** or a "cocktail," is the only way to control the progression of the disease. Because of the staggering impact of HIV infection and AIDS-related illnesses, the Food and Drug Administration (FDA) has "fast-tracked" new drugs and new drug classes; nurses and other health care professionals are encouraged to keep abreast of rapid pharmacotherapeutic changes for HIV infection by reviewing the most current information presented in nursing and medical journals.

This chapter presents the drug classes currently used in treating HIV infection and AIDS, which include:

- Nucleoside reverse transcriptase inhibitors (NRTIs; prototype, zidovudine)
- Protease inhibitors (PIs; prototype, saquinavir)
- Nonnucleoside reverse transcriptase inhibitors (NNRTIs; prototype, nevirapine)
- Nucleotide analogue reverse transcriptase inhibitor (prototype, adefovir)

In addition to explaining how each of these drug classes works to affect HIV infection and AIDS, this chapter addresses the core drug knowledge, core patient variables, nursing management, potential nursing diagnoses, and patient education related to the administration of anti-HIV agents. This chapter also reviews current treatment recommendations for common opportunistic diseases associated with HIV infection and AIDS.

PHYSIOLOGY

CD4+ T-CELL FUNCTION

CD4+ T cells are necessary for normal immune function. The CD4+ cell recognizes foreign antigens and infected cells and helps activate the antibody-producing B lymphocytes. CD4+ T cells also induce cell-mediated immunity in which cytotoxic CD8+ T cells and natural killer cells directly destroy foreign antigens. Phagocytic monocytes and macrophages also are influenced by CD4+ T cells. Figure 54-1 illustrates normal CD4+ T-cell function. Chapter 33 presents a more thorough review of immune system physiology.

HUMAN IMMUNODEFICIENCY VIRUS

Human immunodeficiency virus (HIV) is like all other viruses in structure. The ribonucleic acid (RNA) is surrounded by core proteins, which are surrounded by a protein shell called a capsid. The capsid is then surrounded by a lipid bilayer envelope. The envelope contains glycoproteins that are used to attach to host cells. The two glycoprotein subunits, gp41 and gp120, are attached to each other and embedded in the lipid bilayer (Fig. 54-2).

The HIV virus is called a retrovirus. The difference between a virus and a retrovirus is the genetic material. Like all viruses, HIV is an obligate parasite; it cannot replicate unless it is inside a living cell. Retroviruses have positive-sense single-stranded RNA and thus must transcribe their RNA into DNA to replicate. This process is completed by an enzyme called reverse transcriptase.

PATHOPHYSIOLOGY

HIV infection begins by gp120, a surface protein on the HIV viral envelope, binding to cells that have a CD4+ protein receptor site. These cells include CD4+ T cells, monocytes, macrophages, and certain nerve cells. Once bound, the genetic material of the virus enters the cell. In the cell, viral RNA is transcribed into a single strand of viral DNA with the assistance of reverse transcriptase, an enzyme made by HIV. This DNA strand replicates itself, becoming double-stranded viral DNA. At this point, viral DNA can enter the cell's nucleus and, using an enzyme called integrase, splice itself into the genome, becoming a permanent part of the cell's genetic structure. This action results in two major problems. First, because all genetic material is replicated during cellular division, all daughter cells from the infected cell also will be infected. Second, because the genome now contains viral DNA, the cell's genetic codes can direct the cell to make HIV. Production of the new virus then occurs by translation-transcription of the code from integrated DNA into RNA. Some of the RNA enters the genome and the rest is messenger RNA that codes HIV proteins. This complex process results in long strands of **HIV RNA**, which must be cut into viable lengths. Late in the life cycle, when the newly formed virus separates from the cell, these HIV proteins are cleaved into small proteins by the enzyme protease. HIV protease is critical for viral infectivity and replication. It has been shown that HIV **provirus** (the virus before it exits the cell) manufactured without protease is noninfectious. Figure 54-3 represents HIV replication.

The HIV virus has an affinity for CD4+ T cells. The virus destroys these important cells responsible for normal immune function, which effectively strips the person of protection against common organisms.

Originally, researchers believed that after initial infection, viral replication remained dormant until stimulated by an unknown event. Now researchers have discovered that viral replication is never dormant; new viruses are produced from the time of infection. At the initial stage of infection, the **viral load** (the amount of virus in the body) is exceptionally high.

Physiology

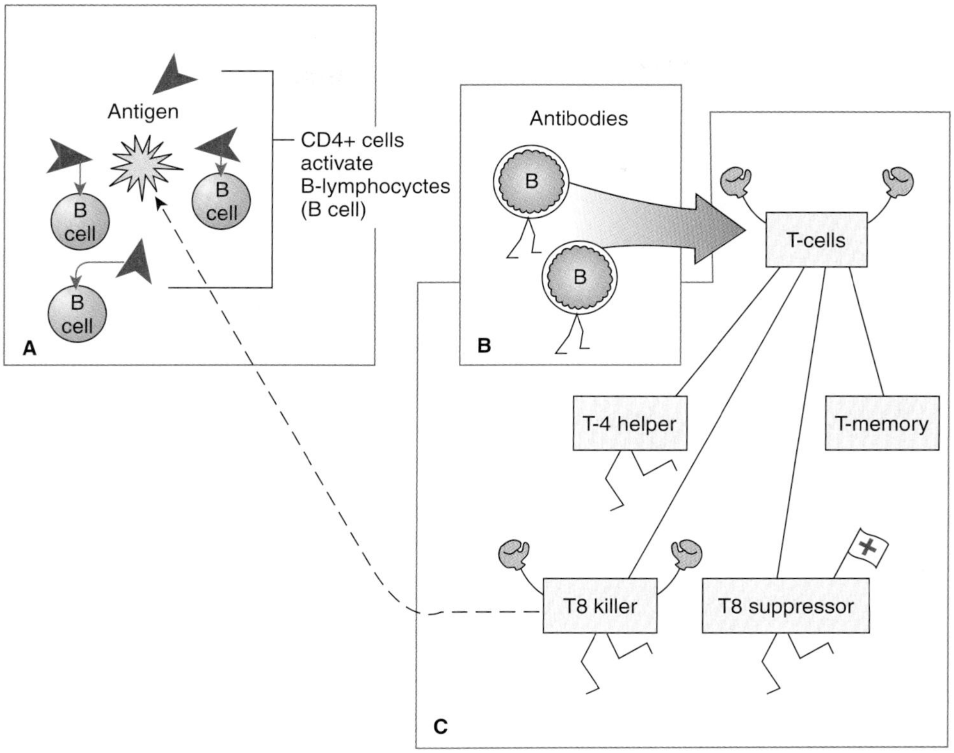

Figure 54-1. CD4+ cell function. CD4+ cells are the cells needed for normal immune functioning. (**A**) The CD4+ cells are the macrophages that recognize antigens (foreign substances) and signal the defenses needed to dispel them. (**B**) In beginning the defense against the antigen, the CD4+ cells activate the antibody-producing B lymphocytes, which in turn call forth the various T cells. (**C**) The T cells proliferate and differentiate to serve different functions. Cells known as T4-helper cells release lymphokines, which enhance macrophage and monocyte activity; T8 killer cells directly attack and destroy the antigen; T8 suppressor cells help to stop the immune response when appropriate; and T-memory cells are stored for future use against returning antigens.

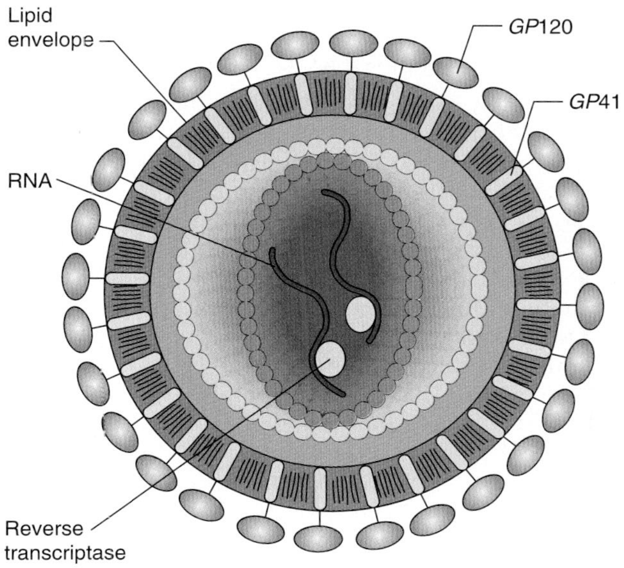

Figure 54-2. Structure of the HIV virus.

There are two reasons for this to occur. First, as a new virus entering the host, the immune system is not yet sensitized to the foreign antigen and the immune response is suboptimal. Second, because the immune system has not yet been affected by the virus, there are many CD4+ cells to invade.

During this initial stage, the patient may experience an acute retroviral syndrome that includes fever, pharyngitis, rash, myalgia or arthralgia, diarrhea, and headache. Although these symptoms are common in HIV infection, they may be dismissed initially by the patient as "the flu." After the immune system responds to the viral insult, the viral load decreases and the patient may become asymptomatic for a long period of time.

HIV infection eventually induces symptoms in every body system. In addition to those already mentioned, common symptoms associated with HIV infection include lymphadenopathy, hepatosplenomegaly, thrush, and weight loss. Neurologic symptoms, such as meningoencephalitis or aseptic meningitis, peripheral neuropathy, radiculopathy, facial palsy, Guillain-Barré syndrome, brachial neuritis, cognitive impairment, or psychosis, also may occur.

Physiology

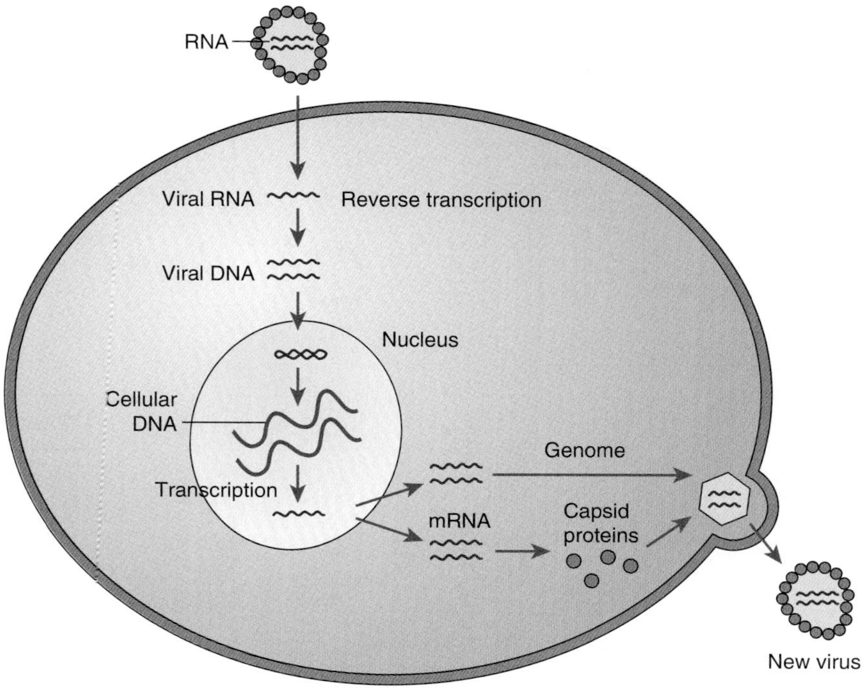

Figure 54-3. HIV replication. HIV is a retrovirus. The genetic code of a retrovirus is contained in single-stranded RNA instead of double-stranded DNA. When HIV enters a CD4+ cell (one of the mainstay cells of the immune system), it uses the enzyme known as reverse transcriptase (RT) to convert its RNA to DNA. Then the HIV's DNA enters the nucleus of the CD4+ cell, combines with that cell's DNA, and transmits instructions to duplicate the original HIV organism. The newly assembled HIV cells then leave the cell and infect other CD4+ cells.

DIAGNOSIS OF HIV INFECTION

Infection with HIV is diagnosed commonly by the **enzyme immunoassay (EIA)** or **enzyme-linked immunosorbent assay (ELISA)** test. The EIA detects antibodies produced in response to infection and is based on the light absorbance of antigen-antibody complexes. If the patient tests positive with the EIA test, a **Western blot (WB)** assay test is administered. This test allows identification of antibodies to specific viral antigens.

The **polymerase chain reaction (PCR)** test detects the presence of the virus rather than the antibody to the virus as in the EIA and WB tests. This is helpful in diagnosing HIV infection in newborns of HIV-infected mothers because infants have circulating maternal antibodies for approximately 15 months.

LABORATORY TESTS

CD4+ T-CELL COUNT

CD4+ T-cell counts are an indication of the current immunologic status of the patient. In the healthy patient, CD4+ range is 800 to 1,200 cell/mm^3. As HIV infection progresses, the CD4+ T-cell count decreases. Although individualized, most health care providers consider initiating pharmacotherapy when the CD4+ T-cell count falls below 500. Initiation of pharmacotherapy prophylaxis for opportunistic diseases is also based on the CD4+ T-cell count.

VIRAL LOAD (HIV RNA) COUNT

The HIV RNA counts are reported as copies per milliliter (mL). Viral load of HIV RNA indicates the risk of disease progression. There are three tests currently used to measure viral load—branched-chain DNA (bDNA), reverse transcriptase (RT)-PCR (quantitative polymerase chain reaction), and nucleic acid sequence-based amplification (NASBA). The RT-PCR is the only test for determining prognosis and for monitoring the response to therapy approved by the Food and Drug Administration (FDA).

Viral load testing is the essential parameter in the decision to initiate or change antiretroviral therapies. The viral load test should be performed at the time of diagnosis and every 3 to 4 months thereafter in an untreated patient. It also should be performed immediately before initiation of antiretroviral therapy and again 2 to 8 weeks later.

When the therapy proves to be effective, the patient should have repeat testing of the viral load every 3 to 4 months to evaluate the continuing efficacy of therapy. The goal is to have the viral load undetectable (i.e., less than 50 copies/mL) within 6 months.

MONITORING TESTS

When assessing the need to change antiretroviral therapy, CD4+ T-cell counts and viral load counts should be evaluated at the same time. The goal of antiretroviral therapy is to increase the CD4+ T-cell count and decrease the viral load burden. If the CD4+ T-cell count continues to decrease, or the viral load burden increases despite therapy, a change in pharmacotherapy should be considered.

RESISTANCE ASSAYS

Resistance assays are used as an adjunct to guide antiretroviral therapy. Genotyping assays detect drug resistance mutations that are present in the relevant viral genes, such as reverse transcriptase and protease. Phenotyping assays measure the ability of viruses to grow in various concentrations of antiretroviral drugs. These tests are most useful in cases of antiretroviral therapy failure or a suboptimal response to therapy.

PRINCIPLES OF DRUG THERAPY FOR HIV INFECTION

The Department of Health and Human Services and the Henry J. Kaiser Family Foundation sponsored the Panel on Clinical Practices for the Treatment of HIV infection. The principles established by the panel should be used for all drug classes in treating HIV infection. See the accompanying display, Principles of Drug Therapy for HIV Infection.

It is important for the nurse to recognize that early antiretroviral therapy has many potential benefits for the HIV-infected patient:

- Control of viral replication and mutation
- Reduction of viral burden
- Prevention of progressive immunodeficiency
- Potential maintenance of a normal immune system
- Delayed progression to AIDS and prolongation of life
- Decreased risk of selection of resistant virus
- Decreased risk of drug toxicity

It is equally important for the nurse to recognize that early antiretroviral therapy also has potential risks:

- Reduced quality of life from adverse drug effects
- Earlier development of drug resistance
- Limited future choices of antiretroviral agents
- Risk of dissemination of drug-resistant virus
- Unknown long-term toxicity of certain drugs
- Unknown duration of effectiveness of current antiretroviral therapies

NUCLEOSIDE REVERSE TRANSCRIPTASE INHIBITOR DRUGS

The **nucleoside reverse transcriptase inhibitors (NRTIs)** were the first class of drugs approved by the FDA to treat HIV infection and AIDS. Although more potent drug classes have emerged, nucleoside analogues continue to be crucial

COMMUNITY-BASED CONCERNS

Principles of Drug Therapy for HIV Infection

When patients or patient groups ask about drug therapy for HIV, the nurse can explain the following points:

- Ongoing HIV replication leads to immune system damage and progression to AIDS. HIV infection is always harmful and true long-term survival free from clinically significant immune dysfunction is unusual.
- Plasma HIV RNA levels indicate the magnitude of HIV replication and its associated rate of CD4+ T-cell destruction; CD4+ T-cell counts indicate the extent of HIV-induced immune damage already suffered. Regular periodic measurements of plasma HIV RNA levels and CD4+ T-cell counts are necessary to determine the risk of disease progression in an HIV-infected individual and to determine when to initiate or modify antiretroviral treatment regimens.
- Because rates of disease progression differ among individuals, treatment decisions should be individualized by level of risk indicated by plasma HIV RNA levels and CD4+ T-cell counts.
- The use of potent combination antiretroviral therapy to suppress HIV replication below the limits of detection of sensitive plasma HIV RNA assays narrows the potential for selection of antiretroviral-resistant HIV variants, which is the major factor limiting the ability of antiretroviral drugs to inhibit virus replication and delay disease progression. Therefore, maximum achievable suppression of HIV replication should be the goal of therapy.
- The most effective means to accomplish durable suppression of HIV replication is the simultaneous initiation of combinations of effective anti-HIV drugs with which the patient has not been treated previously and that are not cross-resistant with antiretroviral agents with which the patient has been treated previously.
- Each antiretroviral drug used in combination-therapy regimens should always be used according to optimal schedules and dosages.
- The available effective antiretroviral drugs are limited in number and mechanism of action, and cross-resistance between specific drugs has been documented. Therefore, any change in antiretroviral therapy increases future therapeutic constraints.
- Women should receive optimal antiretroviral therapy regardless of pregnancy status.
- The same principles of antiretroviral therapy apply to both HIV-infected children and adults, although the treatment of HIV-infected children involves unique pharmacologic, virologic, and immunologic considerations.
- People with acute primary HIV infections should be treated with combination antiretroviral therapy to suppress virus replication to levels below the limit of detection of sensitive plasma HIV RNA assays.
- HIV-infected people, even those with viral loads below detectable limits, are considered infectious and should be counseled to avoid sexual and drug-use behaviors that are associated with transmission of HIV and other infectious pathogens.

drugs in the pharmacologic management of HIV infection and AIDS (see Figure 54-3). Zidovudine was first synthesized as an antineoplastic drug in the 1960s. In 1985, it was found to inhibit the in vitro infectivity of HIV type-1 (HIV-1). Drugs within the NRTI class besides zidovudine include didanosine, zalcitabine, stavudine, lamivudine, abacavir, and the combination drugs lamivudine/zidovudine and abacavir/zidovudine/lamivudine. Zidovudine (AZT, ZDV, Compound S, Retrovir) is the prototype for the NRTIs.

NURSING MANAGEMENT OF THE PATIENT RECEIVING P ZIDOVUDINE

Core Drug Knowledge

Pharmacotherapeutics

Zidovudine is a synthetic nucleoside antiviral drug. Zidovudine is active against other retroviruses and some bacteria, but its sole indication is for treating HIV in adults and children and preventing transmission of HIV to the fetus in pregnant, HIV-infected women. The parameters to start antiretroviral therapy are controversial, complex, and constantly changing. Symptomatic patients should begin therapy regardless of laboratory values. Recommendations for asymptomatic patient treatment is a CD4+ count below 500 or plasma HIV-RNA levels above 10,000 (Table 54-1).

Pharmacokinetics

Zidovudine is administered orally or parenterally. Following oral administration, zidovudine is absorbed rapidly from the gastrointestinal (GI) tract. The half-life of zidovudine is about 1 hour in patients with normal renal function and increases to 1.4 to 2.9 hours in patients with renal dysfunction. Hepatic dysfunction also causes a moderate prolongation of zidovudine half-life.

Zidovudine crosses the blood-brain barrier and the placenta. Rapid metabolism into triphosphate occurs in the liver where the drug is changed into an inactive metabolite. Both active drug and inactive metabolite are excreted by glomerular filtration and tubular secretion. Patients with hepatic or renal dysfunction have reduced clearance rates.

Pharmacodynamics

Direct pharmacodynamics occur within the virus. After zidovudine is metabolized into triphosphate, it incorporates into the DNA of the virus. This effectively stops the building process. The resulting DNA is incomplete and cannot create a new virus. Zidovudine also is active against the Epstein-Barr virus and hepatitis B virus, and it has some antibacterial activity against Enterobacteriaceae, but bacterial resistance develops rapidly.

Contraindications and Precautions

Administration of zidovudine is contraindicated in patients with hypersensitivity to any of its components. In addition, the drug is assigned to pregnancy category C and is contraindicated during the first 14 weeks of pregnancy. Because safety and efficacy are uncertain in neonates and infants (up to 3 months), zidovudine is contraindicated in these populations. However, it is used in pregnant women after 14 weeks gestation and in children younger than 3 months who are born to HIV-positive mothers. Zidovudine should be given with caution to patients with preexisting bone marrow depression, folate deficiency, or vitamin B_{12} deficiency. Patients with these disorders are at increased risk for severe hematologic toxicity. It is also given with caution to patients who have recently received cytotoxic drugs or radiation therapy because zidovudine may induce myelosuppression. Because of the risk for myelosuppression, patients with dental disease are also given zidovudine with caution.

Zidovudine should be used with caution in patients with hepatic or renal disease. The drug is metabolized in the liver to an inactive metabolite. In patients with impaired hepatic function, zidovudine can accumulate. Both zidovudine and its inactive metabolite are excreted in the urine. Zidovudine can accumulate in patients with renal impairment, causing an increased risk of toxicity. It is not known if zidovudine is excreted into breast milk. However, there has been a report of a nursing infant's becoming infected from an HIV-positive mother through breast milk. Therefore, mothers with HIV are encouraged not to breast-feed.

Adverse Effects

The most serious adverse effects of zidovudine therapy are anemia, granulocytopenia, and thrombocytopenia. These effects may indicate bone marrow depression. Signs of anemia can develop in 2 to 4 weeks, and signs of granulocytopenia can develop in 6 to 8 weeks. Discontinuation of the drug usually resolves anemia and granulocytopenia.

Although zidovudine actually can produce an increase in platelet count, drug-induced thrombocytopenia can occur as well. Initial increases in platelet count usually occur within 1 to 2 weeks and can continue for 4 to 7 weeks of therapy.

Adverse GI effects of zidovudine therapy include nausea and vomiting, diarrhea, abdominal pain, dyspepsia, and anorexia. Esophageal ulceration also has occurred in patients treated with zidovudine. Another adverse effect is myopathy. Because myopathy also may be a component of HIV infection, it may be overlooked as an adverse effect. Discontinuation of zidovudine can provide some improvement, but rapid worsening can occur when the drug is readministered. Cardiomyopathy also has been reported.

Several effects on the central nervous system (CNS) have been reported during zidovudine therapy. These include headache, seizures, somnolence, paresthesias, agitation, restlessness, and insomnia. Other adverse effects that have been described include nail discolora-

TABLE 54-1 Summary of Selected Nucleoside Reverse Transcriptase Inhibitors

Drug (Trade) Name	Selected Indications	Route and Dosage Range	Pharmacokinetics
zidovudine (AZT, Compound S Retrovir, ZDV; *Canadian:* Apo-Zidovudine)	HIV infection	*Adult:* PO, 300–1,200 mg/d in divided doses *Child:* 3 mo–12 y, PO, 180 mg/m^2 q6h; maximum dose, 200 mg 16h *Adult:* IV, 1–2 mg/kg, by infusion over 1 h at a constant rate, q4h around the clock *Child:* Safety and efficacy of parenteral therapy in children 12 years of age and younger not established	*Onset:* Rapid *Duration:* Unknown $t_{1/2}$: 30–60 min *Onset:* Rapid *Duration:* Unknown $t_{1/2}$: 30–60 min
didanosine (ddI, Videx)	HIV infection	*Adult:* PO, ≥75 kg, 300 mg q12h; 50–74 kg, 200 mg q12h; 35–49 kg, 125 mg q12h *Child:* PO, body surface area 1.1–1.4 m^2, 100 mg q12h; body surface area 0.8–1.0 m^2, 75 mg q12h; body surface area 0.5–0.7 m^2, 50 mg PO q12h; body surface area up to 0.4 m^2, 25 mg q12h	*Onset:* Rapid *Duration:* Unknown $t_{1/2}$: 1.6 h
zalcitabine (ddC, Hivid)	HIV infection	*Adult:* PO, 0.75 mg q8h *Child:* <13 y, safety and efficacy not established	*Onset:* Rapid *Duration:* Unknown $t_{1/2}$: 1–3 h
stavudine (d4T, Zerit)	HIV infection	*Adult:* PO, ≥60 kg, 40 mg q12h; <60 kg, 30 mg q12h *Child:* PO, <30 kg, 2 mg/kg/d divided into two doses given q12h	*Onset:* Rapid *Duration:* Unknown $t_{1/2}$: 30–60 min
lamivudine (3TC, Epivir)	HIV infection	*Adult and child:* PO ≥ 12 y weighing > 50 kg (110 lb), 150 mg bid in combination with ZDV; <50 kg (110 lb), 2 mg/kg bid in combination with ZDV *Child:* PO, 3 mo–12 y, 4 mg/kg bid (up to a maximum of 150 mg twice a day) in combination with ZDV	*Onset:* Slow *Duration:* Unknown $t_{1/2}$: 5–7 h
abacavir (ABC, Ziagen)	HIV infection	*Adult:* PO, 300 mg bid *Child:* 3 mo–16 y, 8 mg/kg bid	*Onset:* 0.7 h *Duration:* Unknown $t_{1/2}$: 1.5 h
Combination Drugs			
3TC/ZDV (Combivir)	HIV infection	*Adult:* PO, 150 mg/300 mg tablet bid	*Onset:* Slow *Duration:* Unknown $t_{1/2}$: 5–7 h
3TC/ZDV/ABC (Trizivir)	HIV infection	*Adult:* PO, >50 kg 150 mg/300 mg/300 mg tablet bid	*Onset:* Rapid *Duration:* Unknown $t_{1/2}$: 1.5 h

tion, rash, taste disturbance, and elevated hepatic enzymes.

As a class, NRTI drugs may induce lactic acidosis and severe hepatomegaly with steatosis (fatty degeneration). Although the actual incidence is low, the mortality with these adverse effects is extremely high. Patients may complain of fatigue, nausea, vomiting, abdominal pain, weight loss, or dyspnea. Evaluation shows lactic acidosis with elevated levels of creatine phosphokinase (CPK), alanine aminotransferase (ALT), and/or lactate dehydrogenase (LDH), and abdominal computed tomography (CT) scans or liver biopsy often shows steatosis. The initial clinical manifestations of lactic acidosis are variable and may include nonspecific gastrointestinal symptoms without dramatic elevation of hepatic enzymes, and in some cases dyspnea. All NRTIs have been implicated, although these adverse effects occur most frequently with stavudine and didanosine.

Drug Interactions

The most significant drug interaction with zidovudine is ganciclovir, which may induce life-threatening hematologic toxicity. Other drug interactions with zidovudine include acetaminophen, interferon beta-1b, probenecid, rifampin, trimethoprim, and valproic acid.

Additionally, drugs that increase the risk for bone marrow suppression, such as adriamycin, dapsone, flucytosine, vincristine, and vinblastine, should be coadministered with caution. The rate and extent of zidovudine absorption may be decreased by fatty meals (Table 54-2).

TABLE 54-2 Agents That Interact With Zidovudine

Interactants	Effect and Significance	Nursing Management
acetaminophen	Enhanced nonhepatic or renal clearance of zidovudine (ZDV) may occur. This may result in subtherapeutic levels of ZDV.	Avoid coadministration if interaction is suspected. Increase dose of ZDV.
food	The rate and extent of ZDV absorption may be decreased by fatty meals.	Administer ZDV at least 1 h before meals.
ganciclovir	Although the mechanism of action is unclear, ganciclovir in combination with ZDV may induce life-threatening hematologic toxicity.	Avoid coadministration.
interferon beta-1b	Interferon beta may inhibit the glucuronidation of ZDV. This may increase ZDV serum concentrations and induce toxic effects.	Monitor ZDV serum concentration levels. Consider decreased ZDV dose.
probenecid	Probenecid appears to inhibit ZDV glucuronidation. This may increase ZDV serum concentration levels and induce toxic effects.	Monitor for systemic symptoms, such as malaise, myalgia, and fever. Consider decreased ZDV dose.
rifampin/rifabutin	Rifampin may increase hepatic metabolism of ZDV, resulting in decreased serum concentration.	Consider increasing ZDV dose if interaction is suspected.
trimethoprim	The pharmacologic effects of ZDV may be increased in patients with impaired hepatic function who receive trimethoprim.	Monitor ZDV serum concentration. Consider decreased ZDV dose.
valproic acid	First-pass glucuronide metabolism of ZDV may be decreased.	Consider ZDV dose adjustment when starting, changing, or stopping valproic acid.

Assessment of Relevant Core Patient Variables

Health Status

The nurse should assess the patient for hypersensitivity to zidovudine and for early pregnancy. It also is important to assess the patient for preexisting hepatic or renal dysfunction. The nurse also should review the patient's current pharmacotherapies for drugs that are potentially myelosuppressive, nephrotoxic, or directly toxic to red blood cells. Any positive findings should be communicated to the health care provider.

Prior to initiation of therapy, the nurse should perform a complete physical examination. It is important to document this baseline status because drug therapy may be discontinued or modified based on changes from baseline. Laboratory tests should include a complete blood count (CBC), chemistry profile, CD4+ T-lymphocyte count, and plasma HIV-RNA measurement.

Life Span and Gender

The nurse should assess the patient for pregnancy and lactation. Zidovudine is the only drug that has been shown to reduce the risk of perinatal HIV transmission. It is administered antenatally after 14 weeks' gestation and continued throughout pregnancy, intravenously during the intrapartum period, and to the newborn for the first 6 weeks of life. This regimen reduces the risk of perinatal transmission between 70% and 80%.

Zidovudine should not be given during lactation to prevent adverse effects to zidovudine in the neonate. In addition, HIV-infected women are advised not to breast-feed to avoid potential postnatal transmission to an infant who may not be infected.

It is important to note the age of the infant before administering zidovudine. Zidovudine is approved for use in HIV-infected infants older than 3 months. However, children younger than 15 months should have confirmatory evaluation of HIV infection (a positive PCR test result). HIV antibody test findings may reflect maternal antibodies and not infant-induced antibodies.

Lifestyle, Diet, and Habits

It is important for the nurse to assess the patient's understanding of HIV transmission, and to explain that despite drug therapy, the patient can still transmit HIV to others. Compliance is another issue that the nurse must assess. Even when zidovudine is taken exactly as directed, resistance may develop. However, resistance develops much more quickly when serum concentrations are suboptimal, which can be caused by either missing doses during the day or by intermittent use of the drug.

The nurse also should assess the patient's typical dietary habits. Zidovudine should be taken 1 hour before meals. It is important to avoid fatty foods because they decrease the drug's absorption. The nurse should outline a high-carbohydrate, moderate-protein, and low-fat diet.

It is important to investigate whether the patient has a problem or a potential problem with substance abuse. HIV infection is prevalent among IV drug abusers. Once the diagnosis of HIV infection is made, some patients may view behavior changes as "too late." Although HIV infection has been considered to be unmanageable in the past, resulting in ultimate death, new drug classes and polytherapy have decreased the severity of symptoms and have been proven to prolong life significantly. The nurse should explain the toll drug abuse takes on the body and the need for the patient to establish a healthy lifestyle.

The nurse should be aware of the patient's economic status. The cost of zidovudine is prohibitive. Many patients do not have insurance or other resources to obtain this expensive drug. Patients may qualify for medical assistance through county, state, or federal funds or receive their drugs from local health departments. The nurse should refer patients with financial problems to the hospital's or clinic's social worker.

Environment

The nurse should be aware of the setting in which zidovudine will be administered. Zidovudine is administered most frequently in an outpatient setting. Because HIV infection is treated routinely with complicated polytherapy, the nurse should assess the patient's ability to understand complex instructions. It is important that the nurse be explicit—verbally and in writing—concerning the instructions for taking which drug at what time of day.

Intravenous zidovudine is stable for 24 hours at room temperature and for 48 hours when refrigerated. The drug should be infused over 1 hour. Prior to infusion, the nurse should examine the solution for particulate matter and discoloration. If either is present, the solution should not be administered. All preparations of zidovudine should be protected from light during infusion.

Nursing Diagnoses and Outcomes

- Acute Pain related to headache from drug effects
  Desired outcome: The patient will self-medicate with analgesics such as acetaminophen.
- Altered Protection related to anemia and granulocytopenia
  Desired outcome: The patient will remain free of opportunistic diseases related to blood dyscrasias.
- Imbalanced Nutrition: Less Than Body Requirements related to GI distress
  Desired outcome: The patient will maintain adequate weight.
- Disturbed Sleep Pattern: Insomnia related to CNS adverse effects
  Desired outcome: The patient will obtain adequate sleep throughout drug therapy.
- Disturbed Thought Processes related to adverse CNS effects
  Desired outcome: The patient will remain oriented and able to communicate effectively with others.
- Diarrhea related to adverse drug effects
  Desired outcome: The patient will avoid dehydration and contact the prescriber if diarrhea persists.
- Risk for Injury related to adverse drug effects
  Desired outcome: The patient will remain injury free throughout therapy.

Planning and Intervention

Maximizing Therapeutic Effects

The nurse should administer zidovudine 1 hour before meals. It also is important to make sure the patient receives 600 mg/day in divided doses—200-mg tablets tid or 300-mg tablets bid. The nurse should make sure the patient is on a low-fat diet.

Minimizing Adverse Effects

Intramuscular injections should not be administered to patients receiving zidovudine; they may cause bleeding, bruising, or hematomas due to thrombocytopenia secondary to zidovudine-induced bone marrow depression.

Providing Patient and Family Education

- The nurse should explain the importance of adherence to the therapeutic regimen. As previously mentioned, the instructions should be clear and in writing.
- The nurse should explain the importance of periodic blood monitoring to ensure the efficacy of therapy.
- It is important to advise patients about potential adverse effects. The nurse should stress the importance of contacting the health care provider for signs of anemia or bone marrow depression, such as bleeding, easy bruising, or fatigue. The nurse also should explain that adverse effects, such as GI distress or headache, may resolve spontaneously after 3 to 4 weeks of therapy. Headaches may be treated with acetaminophen. Persistent problems should be reported to the health care provider.
- The nurse should instruct patients to advise the health care provider if any other drugs are prescribed by another prescriber. The nurse should explain that many drugs may alter the way zidovudine works, and other drugs may increase the risk for adverse effects from zidovudine therapy.
- The nurse should advise the patient to postpone any dental work if myelosuppression is suspected.
- The nurse should instruct patients with sleep disturbance to attempt relaxation techniques or warm baths to facilitate sleep.
- The nurse should explain the importance of contacting the health care provider should the patient have difficulty thinking or experience memory problems.

Ongoing Assessment and Evaluation

The nurse should perform a physical examination at each encounter with the patient. Laboratory data should be obtained every 2 to 4 weeks. Once HIV-RNA levels are undetectable and the CD4+ count is stable, follow-up visits should occur every other month.

The nurse should monitor for signs of adverse effects symptomatic of anemia, bone marrow depression, or nephrotoxicity. The nurse also should monitor for signs of myelosuppression or myalgias. Symptoms of myalgia include proximal muscle weakness or elevations of creatinine kinase values.

The nurse should monitor for the need to change pharmacotherapy. Considerations for change in pharmacotherapy are highlighted in the accompanying display, Factors That Precipitate Changes in Pharmacotherapy. It is important for the nurse to remember that changes in therapy based on blood analysis may be necessary because the patient may remain asymptomatic.

The patient should have a stable CD4+ count and a declining or undetectable HIV-RNA count throughout therapy. The patient should be free of opportunistic infections and signs of anemia or bone marrow suppression. ■

MEMORY CHIP

Zidovudine

- Used for management of HIV and AIDS
- Significant contraindications: hypersensitivity, first 14 weeks of pregnancy
- Most common adverse effects: nausea, headache, rash, fever, and abdominal pain
- Most serious adverse effects: anemia, granulocytopenia, and thrombocytopenia; bone marrow suppression; lactic acidosis; and hepatomegaly with steatosis
- Maximizing therapeutic effects: administer 1 hour before meals
- Minimizing adverse effects: avoid IM injections due to thrombocytopenia
- Most significant patient education: signs and symptoms of anemia and importance of notifying the health care provider immediately

DRUGS CLOSELY RELATED TO ZIDOVUDINE

Didanosine

Didanosine (ddI, Videx) was approved in 1996 as a first-line drug in treating HIV disease. It was approved relatively quickly under the compassionate-use protocols and expanded-access programs. For this reason, long-term effects of didanosine are not well documented. Didanosine is similar to zidovudine. However, its active metabolite has a much longer half-life, which allows for twice-daily dosing.

Didanosine is inactivated in an acidic environment. To overcome this problem, the oral drug is available in a buffered powder form, which decreases gastric pH. Unfortunately, this buffering agent may decrease the absorption of other drugs, such as the fluoroquinolones, dapsone, indinavir, and azole antifungals.

The adverse effect profile of didanosine includes GI problems similar to those seen with zidovudine. Two potentially serious adverse effects associated specifically with didanosine are pancreatitis and peripheral neuropathy. Patients with prior episodes of pancreatitis, active alcohol abuse, or coadministration of other drugs that may cause pancreatitis have an even higher risk for the development of pancreatitis. Didanosine should be discontinued at the first signs or symptoms of pancreatitis, such as anorexia, nausea, vomiting, and abdominal pain.

In addition, didanosine should not be given with other drugs known to cause pancreatitis, such as asparaginase, azathioprine, estrogens, ethanol, furosemide, methyldopa, nitrofurantoin, pentamidine, sulfonamides, sulindac, tetracyclines, thiazide diuretics, and valproic acid. Additionally, it should not be given with drugs known to cause peripheral neuropathy, such as chloramphenicol, cisplatin, dapsone, ethambutol, ethionamide, hydralazine, isoniazid (INH), lithium, metronidazole, nitrous oxide, phenytoin, and vincristine.

Didanosine should be given on an empty stomach, because administration with food may decrease serum concentrations by as much as 50%.

Factors that Precipitate Changes in Pharmacotherapy

- Less than a 0.5 to 0.75 $\log_{10}$ reduction in plasma HIV-RNA by 4 weeks following initiation of therapy, or less than a 1 $\log_{10}$ reduction by 8 weeks
- Failure to suppress plasma HIV-RNA to undetectable levels within 4 to 6 months of initiating therapy
- Repeated detection of virus in plasma after initial suppression to undetectable levels, suggesting the development of resistance
- Any reproducible significant increase, defined as threefold or greater, from the nadir of plasma HIV-RNA not attributable to intercurrent infection, vaccination, or test methodology except as already noted
- Undetectable viremia in the patient receiving double nucleoside therapy
- Persistently declining CD4+ T-cell numbers, as measured on at least two separate occasions
- Clinical deterioration

(*Adapted from* Guidelines for the Use of Antiretroviral Agents in HIV-Infected Adults and Adolescents, US Health and Human Services, January 2001.)

Zalcitabine

Zalcitabine (ddC, Hivid) is the third agent to be approved by the FDA solely for use in treating HIV. It was approved for use only in conjunction with zidovudine. Zalcitabine is excreted largely unchanged by the kidneys. It should be used with caution, and dosages should be reduced in patients with impaired renal function. Zalcitabine has a very short half-life and requires three-times-daily dosing.

Like didanosine, the major adverse effects of zalcitabine are pancreatitis and peripheral neuropathy; therefore, these drugs should not be given together. Additionally, zalcitabine may cause stomatitis. In addition to drugs that cause pancreatitis or peripheral neuropathy, zalcitabine should not be given with aminoglycosides, amphotericin B, or foscarnet because these drugs reduce zalcitabine's renal clearance and may increase its toxicity. Zalcitabine's absorption is decreased by approximately 25% when coadministered with antacids; therefore, antacids should not be administered concomitantly with this nucleoside.

Stavudine

Stavudine (d4T, Zerit) was initially approved by the FDA for use in patients who are intolerant of other antiretroviral agents. Subsequent studies have shown that stavudine induces a slower rate of disease progression than zidovudine.

Stavudine is safe and well tolerated, its absorption and serum concentrations are not affected by meals, and its half-life allows for twice-daily dosing. It is excreted by the kidneys; therefore, a reduced dose should be considered for patients with decreased renal function.

The major clinical adverse effect of stavudine is peripheral neuropathy. The drug should be discontinued in patients with symptoms of neuropathy, such as tingling, burning, pain, or numbness in the distal extremities. Stavudine may induce elevations in hepatic transaminases. Therefore, baseline studies should be done for patients with a history of hepatic dysfunction or alcoholism.

Lamivudine

Lamivudine (3TC, Epivir) is a potent RT inhibitor. It also is highly active against the hepatitis B virus. Its FDA approval was delayed due to the observation that resistance to the drug develops rapidly. Like stavudine, it is safe and well tolerated, it has a long half-life, and it is administered twice a day. It is renally excreted; therefore, patients with significant renal impairment should be given reduced doses. Food decreases the rate but not the extent of oral absorption; therefore, lamivudine may be administered with or without food.

Abacavir

Abacavir (ABC, Ziagen) is an oral, synthetic antiretroviral agent. It may be significantly more potent than some other reverse transcriptase inhibitors. Abacavir is available in tablet and suspension formulas. It has excellent bioavailability and wide-spread distribution, including the cerebral spinal fluid.

Hypersensitivity is a common adverse effect of abacavir. Reintroduction after a hypersensitivity reaction has resulted in fatal hypotension. Abacavir should be discontinued if any signs of hypersensitivity occur. These include fever, skin rash, fatigue, GI symptoms, and respiratory symptoms, such as pharyngitis, dyspnea, or cough.

Patients receiving abacavir should refrain from alcohol intake. Alcohol increases the plasma levels of abacavir by 41%, which increases the risk for adverse effects.

PROTEASE INHIBITORS

Protease inhibitors are the second major class of drugs used in treating HIV infection and AIDS. Their arrival has changed the opinion of many experts as to the ultimate fatality of HIV and AIDS. The PIs represent the most potent anti-HIV drugs known. However, their potency and activity vary widely among individual patients. Drugs within the PI class include saquinavir, ritonavir, lopinavir, indinavir, nelfinavir, amprenavir, and a combination drug lopinavir/ritonavir. Saquinavir, the first FDA-approved PI, is the prototype for this class. There are two formulations of this drug—saquinavir mesylate (Invirase, HGC [hard gel capsule]) and saquinavir (Fortovase, SGC [soft gel capsule]).

NURSING MANAGEMENT OF THE PATIENT RECEIVING SAQUINAVIR

Core Drug Knowledge

Pharmacotherapeutics

Saquinavir is an agent for treatment of HIV infection in adults. It is approved for use in combination with RT inhibitors. Combination therapy allows for reduced dosage and helps to limit the incidence of adverse events. Saquinavir demonstrates activity against both HIV-1 and HIV-2 and is effective in acutely and chronically infected cells (Table 54-3).

Pharmacokinetics

Saquinavir is administered orally. It is only about 4% bioavailable after oral dosing due to poor absorption combined with extensive first-pass metabolism. A high-calorie, high-fat meal can significantly increase the bioavailability of saquinavir. The bioavailability of saquinavir administered as the soft gel, Fortovase, has not been determined.

Metabolism occurs in the liver and is affected by the P450 enzyme system; the isozyme CYP3A4 is responsible for about 90% of the initial biotransformation. The metabolites of saquinavir have not been identified and appear to play little part in antiviral activity. The serum half-life of saquinavir is 1 to 2 hours. Renal elimination of saquinavir is negligible; only 1% is excreted in urine, whereas 88% is excreted in feces.

Pharmacodynamics

Saquinavir is a competitive inhibitor of HIV protease, an enzyme involved in replicating HIV. During the later stages of the HIV growth cycle, integrated DNA is translated into polyproteins to become immature budding particles. Protease is responsible for packaging these polyproteins into mature virions. Virions produced without protease render the virus noninfectious. Protease also activates reverse transcriptase. Thus, PIs indirectly decrease viral replication by blocking reverse transcriptase. PIs also inhibit replication of HIV in the macrophages, major reservoirs of HIV.

Contraindications and Precautions

Saquinavir is contraindicated for patients with hypersensitivity to any of its components. Saquinavir is not approved for use in infants, children, or adolescents younger than 16 years. Saquinavir is assigned to pregnancy category B; its safety for use during pregnancy and lactation has not been established.

TABLE 54-3 Summary of Selected Protease Inhibitors

Drug (Trade) Name	Selected Indications	Route and Dosage Range	Pharmacokinetics
saquinavir mesylate (Invirase)	HIV infection	*Adult and child>16:* PO, 600 mg tid	*Onset:* Slow *Duration:* Unknown $t_{1/2}$: 7–12 h
saquinavir (Fortovase)	HIV infection	*Adult and child>16:* 1200 mg tid	*Onset:* Slow *Duration:* Unknown $t_{1/2}$: 7–12 h
ritonavir (Norvir)	HIV infection	*Adult:* PO, 600 mg bid *Child:* 600 mg/m² bid	*Onset:* Rapid *Duration:* Unknown $t_{1/2}$: 3–5 h
indinavir (Crixivan)	HIV infection	*Adult:* PO, 800 mg tid *Child:* Dosage not established	*Onset:* Rapid *Duration:* Unknown $t_{1/2}$: 2–3 h
nelfinavir (Viracept)	HIV infection	*Adult:* PO, 750 mg tid *Child:* 2–12 y: 20–30 mg/kg tid	*Onset:* Rapid *Duration:* Unknown $t_{1/2}$: 3.5–5 h
amprenavir (Agenerase)	HIV infection	*Adult and child>50 kg:* PO, 1200 mg bid *Child 4–12 years old or<50 kg:* 20 mg/kg tid	*Onset:* 1–2 h *Duration:* Unknown $t_{1/2}$: 7–9.5 h
Combination Drug			
lopinavir/ritonavir (Kaletra)	HIV infection	*Adult and child>6 mo:* 400 mg/100 mg tablet bid or 5 mL bid	*Onset:* Unknown *Duration:* Unknown $t_{1/2}$: 5–6 h

Saquinavir use has not been investigated in patients with baseline liver function tests more than five times the upper limit of normal. Therefore, saquinavir should be administered with caution to patients with hepatic disease because metabolism of saquinavir is largely hepatic. Some patients with hemophilia A and B have experienced bleeding episodes during saquinavir therapy. Although a direct causal relationship has not been established, these patients should be monitored closely.

Adverse Effects

In general, few adverse effects have been reported with saquinavir therapy. However, it is difficult to discern adverse effects thought to occur only with saquinavir, because it often is given with other agents. The most common adverse effects are diarrhea, abdominal discomfort, nausea, and vomiting. Other adverse effects include headache, flatulence, vasovagal syncope, lethargy, and dizziness. Saquinavir may induce hyperglycemia. Patients with preexisting diabetes mellitus are at risk for losing glycemic control.

HIV-infected patients with hemophilia (type A or B) may be at increased risk for bleeding. Episodes of spontaneous skin hematomas and hemarthrosis, in some cases requiring additional doses of factor VIII, have been reported.

As with all other antiretroviral agents, antimicrobial resistance can develop after continued use. Resistance to saquinavir may appear more slowly than with other PIs. Additionally, saquinavir does not appear to have cross-resistance to other PIs. Combining saquinavir therapy with reverse transcriptase inhibitors enhances the suppression of viral replication and limits the emergence of viral resistance. Because resistance emerges by different mechanisms, there is no cross-resistance between saquinavir and reverse transcriptase inhibitors.

As a class, PIs also have been associated with an unusual adverse reaction involving the deposition of fatty-like tissue at the base of the posterior neck ("buffalo hump") and the abdominal area ("protease paunch"). The syndrome is associated with peripheral lipodystrophy, central adiposity, female breast enlargement, hyperlipidemia, and insulin resistance. Although the long-term consequences of fat redistribution are unknown, substantial increases in triglycerides or cholesterol are of concern because of the possible association with cardiovascular events and pancreatitis.

Drug Interactions

Saquinavir interacts with ketoconazole, ritonavir, ergot alkaloids, and rifamycins. Other drugs that interact with saquinavir include simvastatin, lovastatin, midazolam, and triazolam. Drugs that induce CYP3A4 may reduce serum saquinavir concentration, resulting in treatment failure (Table 54-4).

TABLE 54-4 Agents That Interact With Saquinavir

Interactants	Effect and Significance	Nursing Management
P450 inhibitors grapefruit juice ritonavir	Coadministration of P450 inhibitors may result in a substantial increase of saquinavir steady-state levels.	These interactions may be used purposefully to increase the bioavailability of saquinavir. Monitor for adverse effects or toxicity.
P450 inhibitors ergot alkaloids rifamycins	Coadministration of saquinavir with these agents may increase their plasma concentrations, resulting in increased risk of adverse effects, such as cardiac arrhythmias.	Do not coadminister these drugs.
CYP3A4 inducers phenobarbital phenytoin dexamethasone carbamazepine	Coadministration of CYP3A4 inducers may result in a reduction in serum plasma levels of saquinavir.	Avoid coadministration of these drugs. Monitor for therapy failure.
CYP3A4 inhibitors calcium channel blockers clindamycin dapsone itraconazole ketoconazole quinidine ranitidine triazolam	Coadministration of CYP3A4 inhibitors may result in an increase in serum plasma levels of saquinavir.	Monitor for adverse effects and toxicity.
NNRTIs	Coadministration may lower level of saquinavir.	Do not coadminister.

Assessment of Relevant Core Patient Variables

Health Status

The nurse should assess the patient for hypersensitivity to saquinavir. It also is important to assess for preexisting hepatic dysfunction or hemophilia. Patients receiving rifampin or rifabutin for TB should delay the use of saquinavir until rifampin or rifabutin has been deleted from the treatment regimen. The nurse also should review the patient's current pharmacotherapies for other drugs that may react with saquinavir. It is important to communicate positive findings to the health care provider.

Before therapy begins, the nurse should perform a complete physical examination. It is important to document this baseline status because drug therapy may be discontinued or modified based on changes from baseline. Laboratory tests should include CBC, chemistry profile, lipid profile, CD4+ T-lymphocyte count, and plasma HIV-RNA measurement. For patients with preexisting hepatic disorders, liver function tests also should be performed.

Life Span and Gender

The nurse should assess the patient for pregnancy or lactation. Although studies have not shown saquinavir to induce teratogenicity in rats, women of childbearing age should be warned that studies on humans have not been conducted.

It is unknown whether saquinavir is excreted into breast milk. However, HIV-infected women are advised not to breast-feed to avoid potential postnatal transmission to an infant who may not be infected. It is important to note the patient's age before administering saquinavir. Saquinavir has not been studied in patients younger than 16 years or older than 65 years.

Lifestyle, Diet, and Habits

The nurse should assess the patient's ability or willingness to comply with drug therapy. Compliance with the saquinavir drug regimen is crucial. Viral load may increase dramatically when saquinavir is not taken as directed, and as with other anti-HIV drugs, resistance is more likely when drugs are taken indiscriminately. The development of viral resistance to this PI will eliminate the entire potent class of these drugs from the patient's therapeutic strategy because cross-resistance to other PIs does occur. The nurse should vigorously discourage nonadherence and drug holidays.

The nurse should be aware of the patient's dietary and substance use habits. The nurse should administer saquinavir within 2 hours of a high-calorie, high-fat meal. This may increase the low bioavailability of saquinavir by sevenfold. As with zidovudine, the nurse should discuss potential substance abuse with the patient. The nurse should explain how a healthy lifestyle complements pharmacotherapy of HIV infection.

It is important to assess the patient's financial status. The cost of saquinavir is prohibitive. Many patients do not have insurance or other resources to obtain this expensive drug. Patients may qualify for medical assistance through county, state, or federal funds or receive their drugs from local health departments. The nurse should refer patients with financial problems to the hospital's or clinic's social worker.

Environment

It is important to be aware of the setting in which saquinavir will be administered. Saquinavir is administered most frequently in an outpatient setting. HIV infection is treated routinely with complicated polytherapy. Therefore, the nurse should assess the patient's ability to understand complex instructions. It is important that the instructions be explicit—both verbally and in writing—concerning which drug to take at which time of the day. Saquinavir capsules should be stored at room temperature in a tightly closed bottle.

Nursing Diagnoses and Outcomes

- Acute Pain related to headache from adverse drug effect
  Desired outcome: The patient will self-medicate with analgesics such as acetaminophen.
- Imbalanced Nutrition: Less Than Body Requirements related to GI distress
  Desired outcome: The patient will maintain body weight and report any persistent symptoms affecting nutritional status to the prescriber.
- Disturbed Thought Processes related to adverse CNS effects
  Desired outcome: The patient will remain oriented and able to communicate effectively with others.
- Diarrhea related to adverse GI effects
  Desired outcome: The patient will avoid dehydration and report persistent diarrhea to the health care provider.

Planning and Intervention

Maximizing Therapeutic Effects

The nurse should administer saquinavir capsules within 2 hours after eating a high-calorie, high-fat meal, tid in divided doses. It is important not to miss any dose because it may affect viral load.

Minimizing Adverse Effects

The nurse should give small, frequent meals when GI distress is problematic. The nurse can administer acetaminophen for complaints of headache.

Providing Patient and Family Education

- The nurse should explain the importance of adherence to drug therapy. As previously mentioned, it is important to make sure that the instructions are clear and in writing.
- The nurse should explain the importance of periodic blood monitoring to ensure the efficacy of therapy.
- The nurse should advise patients about potential adverse effects. The nurse should also explain that adverse effects, such as GI distress or headache, may spontaneously resolve after 3 to 4 weeks of therapy. The nurse should tell patients that persistent problems should be reported to the health care provider.
- It is important to instruct patients to advise the health care provider if any other drugs are ordered by another prescriber. The nurse should explain that many drugs may alter the way saquinavir works and that other drugs may increase the patient's risk for adverse effects from saquinavir therapy.
- The nurse should instruct the patient to use over-the-counter (OTC) antidiarrheal agents should diarrhea occur. If persistent, the patient should contact the health care provider.
- The nurse should explain the importance of contacting the health care provider should the patient have difficulty thinking or experience memory problems.

Ongoing Assessment and Evaluation

Patients should have periodic examinations and blood monitoring. This is important to assess for potential progression of the disease, treatment failure, or the emergence of drug resistance. CD4+ T-cell counts and HIV RNA should be assessed every 3 months. The nurse should monitor for the need to change pharmacotherapy (see the previous display, Factors that Precipitate Changes in Pharmacotherapy, and the accompanying display, Changing Therapy From Zidovudine to Saquinavir).

The nurse should monitor patients with hemophilia for signs of bleeding and for clinical signs, particularly those evident in laboratory test results, if necessary. It also is important to monitor patients for the development of hepatic dysfunction. For patients with preexist-

Critical Thinking Scenario

Changing therapy from zidovudine to saquinavir

Mark Williams is 24 years old. He has had diagnosed HIV for the last 5 years. He is currently taking zidovudine 300 mg bid and lamivudine 150 mg bid. His last visit to the clinic where you practice was 3 months ago. At that time, his CD4+ T-cell count was 375 and his viral load was 3,450. Today's laboratory values indicate a CD4+ T-cell count of 200 and a viral load of 15,000.

1. Consider what assessments should be made at this time. Mark's drug therapy is changed to saquinavir (Invirase).
2. Propose which assessments to make now, and develop a patient education checklist.
3. Discuss other therapy that you think should be initiated at this time.

ing hepatic disorders, the nurse should monitor liver function test results.

The patient should be evaluated for fat redistribution and hypertriglyceridemia or hypercholesterolemia. Should these adverse effects occur, the patient should be evaluated for cardiovascular events and pancreatitis. Potential interventions include dietary modifications or discontinuation of PIs.

The patient should have a stable CD4+ count and a declining or undetectable HIV-RNA count throughout therapy. The patient should have a stable lipid panel. The patient should also be free of opportunistic infections and signs of hepatic dysfunction or bleeding. ■

DRUGS CLOSELY RELATED TO SAQUINAVIR

Ritonavir

Ritonavir (RTV, Norvir) is an oral PI used to treat HIV infection. Its oral bioavailability is greater than that of other PIs. The prolonged absorption and half-life of ritonavir allow for twice-daily dosing. Ritonavir may be used either as monotherapy or in combination with an NRTI. Ritonavir has a complex set of drug interactions and may be the least tolerated of the PIs currently available. It should be kept refrigerated and taken with meals. To minimize adverse effects, lead-in dosing should be administered according to the following schedule:

- Day 1: 300 mg bid
- Days 2 and 3: 400 mg bid
- Day 4: 500 mg bid

Of the currently available PIs, ritonavir appears to have the greatest incidence of adverse effects. Mild-to-moderate adverse effects reported include asthenia; headache; GI effects, including nausea, diarrhea, vomiting, anorexia, abdominal pain, and taste perversion; and neurologic disturbances, including circumoral and peripheral paresthesia.

MEMORY CHIP

Saquinavir

- Used for the management of HIV and AIDS
- Significant contraindications: hypersensitivity, children <16 years old
- Most common adverse effects: diarrhea, abdominal discomfort, and nausea and vomiting
- Most serious adverse effects: cardiovascular events and pancreatitis resulting from fat redistribution
- Maximizing therapeutic effects: administer within 2 hours of a high-fat, high-calorie meal
- Minimizing adverse effects: small frequent meals to decrease GI distress
- Most significant patient education: refrain from taking any medication that is not prescribed by the health care provider treating the patient for HIV

Ritonavir has an extensive drug-drug interaction profile. It increases drug levels of many drugs, which in turn increases the risk for adverse effects or toxicity. These drugs include alprazolam, amiodarone, bepridil, bupropion, clorazepate, clozapine, diazepam, encainide, estazolam, flecainide, flurazepam, meperidine, midazolam, piroxicam, propoxyphene, propafenone, quinidine, rifampin, triazolam, zolpidem, and ergot alkaloids.

Ritonavir also may decrease drug levels of ethinyl estradiol (a common component found in birth control pills), theophylline, clarithromycin, sulfamethoxazole, and zidovudine. The nurse should monitor patients receiving these drugs for treatment failure. In addition, it is important to caution women to use another method of contraception besides birth control pills while taking ritonavir.

Lopinavir

Lopinavir (Kaletra) is a new PI for adults and children. Each lopinavir capsule contains 133 mg of a drug called ABT-378 and 33 mg of ritonavir. One of the most important attributes of lopinavir is its potency. Because of the addition of ritonavir, lopinavir reaches high serum drug levels. This allows for lopinavir to be effective against some PI-resistant viruses and may result in longer suppression of viral load. The high potency of lopinavir also may cause problems. People who develop resistance to lopinavir are more likely to become cross-resistant to other PIs, which may limit options for future therapy. To avoid the development of resistance, lopinavir should not be used alone.

Lopinavir is contraindicated for patients who have had a previous reaction to ritonavir. It is also contraindicated for patients taking dihydroergotamine, ergotamine, lovastatin, midazolam, pimozide, rifampin, simvastatin, and triazolam. Patients with hemophilia or diabetes mellitus should use lopinavir with caution because the drug might interfere with blood clotting or worsen diabetes. It should also be used with caution in pregnant women as it has not been studied in this population. Women should also be cautious of breast-feeding while taking lopinavir because it may be passed through breast milk and may harm the infant.

Lopinavir is generally well tolerated. The most common side effects reported are diarrhea, shortness of breath, nausea, abdominal pain, headache, and vomiting. Increases in levels of cholesterol, triglycerides, and liver enzymes may also occur.

There are multiple drug-drug interactions that may occur with lopinavir. They include amprenavir, atorvastatin, efavirenz, birth control pills (ethinyl estradiol), indinavir, itraconazole, ketoconazole, methadone, nelfinavir, nevirapine, rifabutin, and saquinavir. Because ritonavir suppresses a liver enzyme used to break down dozens of drugs, it may boost the blood levels of street drugs such as Ecstasy (3,4-methylenedioxymethamphetamine, MDMA) or heroin.

Indinavir

Indinavir (Crixivan) is an oral PI indicated for treating HIV infection. Indinavir, in combination with other reverse transcriptase inhibitors, may reduce HIV counts to undetectable levels. Indinavir is a very complex drug; a 21-step, 1-year process is required simply to produce the drug. This complexity may limit supplies.

Indinavir also has a complicated dosing regimen—800 mg every 8 hours with the patient fasting. High-fat and high-protein meals result in a significant decrease in the drug's bioavailability.

Indinavir is generally well tolerated. Mild adverse events reported are abdominal discomfort, nausea, and headache. The formation of indinavir crystals in the urine is a concern in some patients. The precipitation of indinavir in the renal collecting ducts is associated with flank pain, hematuria, dysuria, urinary frequency, and nausea. This complication may be limited and treated by increased daily fluid intake. Indinavir administration also is associated with elevations in liver transaminase and bilirubin levels. For this reason, the nurse should obtain baseline liver function test results before the initiation of indinavir therapy.

Like ritonavir, indinavir also inhibits cytochrome P450, although not as significantly. Drugs not recommended for coadministration with indinavir include rifampin, triazolam, midazolam, and ergot alkaloids. Other drug interactions include the NRTIs, didanosine, and ketoconazole. Because of its buffering system, didanosine should be administered at least 2 hours before or after administration of indinavir to avoid reducing indinavir absorption. Although ketoconazole may increase indinavir levels, no changes in dosage recommendations are necessary.

Nelfinavir

Nelfinavir (Viracept) is another oral PI. It is touted as having the best side-effect profile of all the anti-HIV drugs. Another benefit of nelfinavir is that the resistance to nelfinavir that may develop is not cross sensitive with other PIs. The major adverse effect of nelfinavir is diarrhea, which may be controlled with loperamide or other antidiarrheals. Nelfinavir also is associated with elevations in ALT, aspartate aminotransferase, and CPK levels. Drug interactions are similar to those for indinavir.

Amprenavir

Amprenavir (Agenerase) is the newest drug in the PI class. Like other PIs, it works at the end of the replication cycle and inhibits the production of viable virions. It can be taken with or without food, but high-fat meals should be avoided. Antacids should be avoided within 1 hour of taking amprenavir. Researchers are excited about amprenavir because it may not be cross-resistant with other PIs.

Amprenavir is related structurally to sulfa. Therefore, patients with a sulfa allergy should not take this medication. Amprenavir also contains vitamin E. Because vitamin E thins the blood, patients taking anticoagulants should be monitored carefully.

The major adverse effects of amprenavir are nausea, vomiting, diarrhea, headache, stomach pains/gas, rash, and numbing sensations on the skin, particularly around the mouth. Amprenavir may induce a severe, life-threatening allergic reaction called Stevens-Johnson Syndrome.

Amprenavir interacts with many drugs. The drugs bepridil, lovastatin, midazolam, simvastatin, triazolam, and ergot derivatives should not be taken with amprenavir as the interactions can be life threatening.

Patients taking amiodarone, lidocaine, phenobarbital, phenytoin, quinidine, tricyclic antidepressants (such as amitriptyline), warfarin and rifampin should have drug levels monitored frequently.

NON-NUCLEOSIDE REVERSE TRANSCRIPTASE INHIBITORS (NNRTIs)

The NNRTIs comprise the third class of drugs used to treat HIV infection. Although they work at the same site as NRTIs, their mechanism of action is very different. NRTIs constrain HIV replication by their incorporation into the elongating strand of viral DNA, which causes chain termination. NNRTIs do not incorporate into viral DNA; instead, they inhibit replication directly by binding noncompetitively to reverse transcriptase. This action blocks HIV replication by preventing the conversion of RNA to DNA. Nevirapine, delavirdine, and efavirenz are drugs within the NNRTI class. The prototype for the NNRTI class of drugs is nevirapine (Viramune).

NURSING MANAGEMENT OF THE PATIENT RECEIVING NEVIRAPINE

Core Drug Knowledge

Pharmacotherapeutics

Nevirapine is indicated for use in treating HIV infection in combination with NRTIs. Resistant virus emerges rapidly and uniformly when nevirapine is administered as monotherapy (Table 54-5).

Pharmacokinetics

Nevirapine is absorbed readily after oral administration. Following administration, nevirapine has an absolute bioavailability between 91% and 93%. Nevirapine absorption is not dependent on food or fasting. It also is not affected by buffers, so it can be administered concurrently with the nucleoside reverse transcriptase didanosine. Peak plasma concentrations occur within 4 hours after a single 200-mg dose. The drug is distributed widely in the body, crosses the blood-brain barrier and placenta, and enters breast milk.

Nevirapine is an inducer of hepatic cytochrome P450 metabolic enzymes. It is biotransformed extensively in the liver into several metabolites. Nevirapine and its metabolites are eliminated mainly in the urine.

Pharmacodynamics

The direct pharmacodynamic effects are on the virus. Nevirapine inhibits HIV reverse transcriptase. It binds directly to reverse transcriptase, causing disruption of the enzyme's catalytic site. This results in the blockage of RNA- and DNA-dependent DNA polymerase activities.

TABLE 54-5 Summary of Selected Non-Nucleoside Reverse Transcriptase Inhibitors

Drug (Trade) Name	Selected Indications	Route and Dosage Range	Pharmacokinetics
nevirapine (Viramune)	HIV infection	*Adult:* PO, 200 mg bid *Child:* Dosage not established	*Onset:* Rapid *Duration:* Unknown $t_{1/2}$: 45 h single dose, then 25–30 h, multiple dosing
delavirdine (Rescriptor)	HIV infection	*Adult:* PO, 400 mg tid *Child:* Dosage not established	*Onset:* Rapid *Duration:* Unknown $t_{1/2}$: 2–11 h
efavirenz (Sustiva)	HIV infection	*Adult:* PO, 600 mg at hs *Child >3 y:* PO, 10–15 kg, 200 mg at hs; 15–20 kg, 250 mg at hs; 20–25 kg, 300 mg at hs; 25–32.5 kg, 350 mg at hs; 32.5–40 kg, 400 mg at hs; >40 kg, 600 mg at hs	*Onset:* Rapid *Duration:* Unknown $t_{1/2}$: 52–76 h

Contraindications and Precautions

Nevirapine is contraindicated for patients with hypersensitivity to any of its components. A pregnancy category C drug, it is contraindicated during pregnancy because adequate safety studies have not been completed.

Nevirapine should be given with caution to patients with hepatic or renal insufficiency. Nevirapine is metabolized by the liver, so patients with hepatic impairment are more likely to have increased serum concentrations of nevirapine. In addition, nevirapine is excreted through the kidneys, so patients with renal insufficiency may also have an increased risk for elevated serum concentrations of nevirapine.

Adverse Effects

Common adverse effects to nevirapine therapy include fever, headache, nausea, vomiting, and maculopapular rash. The rash, common to all NNRTI drugs, usually consists of mild-to-moderate erythematous, cutaneous eruptions, with or without pruritus and may be located on the trunk, face, and extremities. Severe and life-threatening skin reactions (including Stevens-Johnson syndrome) also have occurred, however.

Elevated hepatic enzyme levels are common in patients receiving nevirapine. Furthermore, nevirapine can cause life-threatening liver injury. Other adverse drug effects include abdominal pain, hepatitis, paresthesias, and ulcerative stomatitis. Antimicrobial resistance also can occur during therapy with nevirapine. Although this develops most rapidly when nevirapine is used as monotherapy, it also may occur with polytherapy.

Drug Interactions

Nevirapine is an inducer of the cytochrome P450 enzyme. Concomitant administration of nevirapine with drugs that are metabolized extensively by this enzyme may require dosage adjustments. Additionally, because of this effect, nevirapine should not be used in combination with PIs. Nevirapine might decrease the plasma concentrations of certain highly metabolized sedatives and hypnotics due to induction of cytochrome P450 enzymes.

In addition, nevirapine is metabolized hepatically by the CYP3A isoenzyme. Coadministration of nevirapine with drugs that increase the activity of CYP3A would be expected to increase the clearance of nevirapine, thereby decreasing nevirapine plasma concentrations. Nevirapine also may alter the effectiveness of hormonal contraceptives; therefore, the nurse should encourage women to use a different type of contraceptive while taking nevirapine (Table 54-6).

Assessment of Relevant Core Patient Variables

Health Status

The nurse should assess the patient for hypersensitivity to nevirapine and for pregnancy or lactation. The nurse also should assess the patient for preexisting hepatic or renal dysfunction. Nevirapine should not be administered to patients taking PIs. It is important to review the patient's current pharmacotherapies for other drugs that may react with nevirapine. The nurse should communicate positive findings to the health care provider.

Before the initiation of therapy, the nurse should perform a complete physical examination. It is important to document this baseline status because drug therapy may be discontinued or modified based on changes from baseline. Laboratory tests should include CBC, chemistry profile, CD4+ T-lymphocyte count, and plasma HIV-RNA measurements. For patients with preexisting hepatic or renal disorders, the nurse may need to coordinate baseline hepatic and renal function tests.

Life Span and Gender

It is important to note the age of the patient before administering nevirapine. Nevirapine is not indicated for use in children or infants. The nurse should assess the

TABLE 54-6 Agents That Interact With Nevirapine

Interactants	Effect and Significance	Nursing Management
CYP3A enzyme inducers calcium-channel blockers carbamazepine clonazepam cyclosporine dexamethasone disopyramide erythromycin ethosuximide fentanyl lidocaine lovastatin pravastatin prednisone quinine rifampin sertraline tamoxifen trazodone vinblastine vincristine warfarin	Coadministration of nevirapine with CYP3A inducers may result in reduction of serum concentration of nevirapine.	Monitor for treatment failure.
CYP3A enzyme inhibitors phenobarbital phenytoin rifampin rifabutin	Coadministration of nevirapine with CYP3A inhibitors may result in an increase of serum concentration of nevirapine.	Monitor for adverse effects and toxicity.
P450 inducers alprazolam clorazepate diazepam estazolam flurazepam midazolam triazolam zolpidem	Coadministration of nevirapine with P450 inducers may result in reduction of serum concentration of these drugs.	Monitor serum concentrations. Monitor for therapy failure.
hormonal contraceptives	Nevirapine may decrease plasma concentrations of hormonal contraceptives.	Advise patient to use another method of contraception.
protease inhibitors	Nevirapine may lower serum concentration of protease inhibitors when coadministered.	Do not coadminister these classes of drugs.

patient for pregnancy. Nevirapine may be used during pregnancy if necessary, but the patient should be cautioned about the lack of information for potential effects on the fetus.

Lifestyle, Diet, and Habits

As with other anti-HIV drugs, resistance is more likely when drugs are taken indiscriminately. Therefore, the nurse needs to assess the patient's understanding of the importance of taking the drug as directed. The nurse also should assess for potential substance abuse by the patient and explain that a healthy lifestyle complements pharmacotherapy of HIV infection.

It is important to assess the patient's financial status. The cost of nevirapine is prohibitive, and the availability is limited. Many patients do not have insurance or other resources to obtain this expensive drug. Patients may qualify for medical assistance through county, state, or federal funds or receive their drugs from local health departments. The nurse should refer patients with financial problems to the hospital's or clinic's social worker.

Environment

The nurse should note the setting in which nevirapine will be administered. Nevirapine is administered most frequently in an outpatient setting. It is always administered as polytherapy. Therefore, the nurse should assess the patient's ability to understand complex instructions. It is important that the instructions be explicit—verbally and in writing—concerning which drug to take at which time of day. The nurse should tell the patient to store nevirapine at room temperature in a tightly closed container and to discard any unused drug after the expiration date.

Nursing Diagnoses and Outcomes

- Acute Pain, headache, related to adverse drug effects
  Desired outcome: The patient will self-medicate with analgesics such as acetaminophen.
- Imbalanced Nutrition: Less Than Body Requirements related to GI distress
  Desired outcome: The patient will maintain adequate weight and nutrition and notify the health care provide about persistent GI symptoms.
- Altered Protection related to drug-related rash
  Desired outcome: The patient will report any rash to the health care provider.
- Disturbed Thought Processes related to CNS adverse effects
  Desired outcome: The patient will remain oriented and able to communicate effectively with others.

Planning and Intervention

Maximizing Therapeutic Effects

The nurse should administer nevirapine in divided doses throughout the day. For missed doses, it is important that the patient take the drug as soon as remembered unless it is time for the next dose.

Minimizing Adverse Effects

The nurse should administer nevirapine by dose escalation (200 mg daily for 2 weeks, then 200 mg twice daily). Using dose escalation may decrease the incidence of rash. However, it is especially important never to double the dose of nevirapine to avoid adverse effects.

Providing Patient and Family Education

- The nurse should explain the importance of compliance with drug therapy. As previously mentioned, it is important to make sure the instructions are clear and in writing.
- The nurse should explain the importance of periodic blood monitoring to ensure the efficacy of therapy.
- The nurse should teach signs of potential adverse effects to patients. It is important to inform patients that the most common adverse reaction to nevirapine is rash. The nurse also should instruct patients to monitor for signs of hepatic dysfunction, such as fatigue, jaundice, and nausea or vomiting. It is important to tell patients to contact their health care provider immediately if signs of hepatic dysfunction or rash occur.
- The nurse should instruct patients to advise their health care provider if any other drugs are prescribed by another prescriber. It is important to explain that many drugs may alter the way nevirapine works and that other drugs may increase the risk for adverse effects from nevirapine therapy.
- The nurse should instruct patients with GI distress to eat frequent small meals. For persistent symptoms and weight loss, the patient should contact the health care provider.
- The nurse should instruct the patient to take acetaminophen for headaches, but to report persistent headache pain to the health care provider.
- The nurse should explain the importance of contacting the health care provider should the patient have difficulty thinking or experience memory problems.

Ongoing Assessment and Evaluation

It is important that patients have periodic examinations and blood monitoring. This is important to assess for potential progression of the disease, treatment failure, or the emergence of resistance. CD4+ T-cell counts and HIV RNA should be assessed every 3 months. The nurse should monitor for the need to change pharmacotherapy.

The nurse should monitor for a diffuse, maculopapular erythematous rash involving the trunk, face, and extremities. This may occur most often within the first month of dosing. A more severe integumentary reaction is Stevens-Johnson syndrome. It is characterized by aching joints and muscles; redness, blistering, peeling, or loosening of skin; and unusual tiredness or weakness accompanied by fever. It is important to advise the health care provider immediately if these symptoms occur.

The nurse also should monitor for signs of liver dysfunction. Periodic liver function tests should be evaluated. It is important to interrupt treatment if moderate or severe liver function test abnormalities develop. Treatment may be restarted after elevated levels have returned to baseline. It is important to restart treatment at half the previous dosage and if abnormal liver test results recur, nevirapine therapy should be discontinued permanently.

The patient should have a stable CD4+ count and a declining or undetectable HIV-RNA count throughout therapy. The patient should be free of opportunistic infections and signs of rash or hepatic dysfunction. ■

MEMORY CHIP

Nevirapine

- Used for the management of HIV and AIDS
- Significant contraindication: hypersensitivity
- Most common adverse effects: fever, headache, nausea, and vomiting and rash
- Most serious adverse effects: Stevens-Johnson syndrome and hepatotoxicity
- Maximizing therapeutic effects: administer in equally divided doses throughout the day
- Minimizing adverse effects: dose escalation over a 2-week period
- Most significant patient education: explain the symptoms of hepatotoxicity and the importance of contacting the health care provider immediately

DRUGS CLOSELY RELATED TO NEVIRAPINE

Delavirdine

Delavirdine (Rescriptor) was approved by the FDA in 1997. It is indicated for combined use with NRTIs. Resistance to delavirdine develops differently than resistance to other antiretrovirals, which may slow the development of resistance to the other antiretrovirals. It has not yet been studied in combination with PIs and therefore these drugs should not be coadministered.

Delavirdine is metabolized by the cytochrome P450 system. Delavirdine inhibits cytochrome P450 enzymes. It is contraindicated for use with terfenadine, astemizole, alprazolam, midazolam, cisapride, rifabutin, and rifampin. Delavirdine increases the levels of clarithromycin, dapsone, rifabutin, ergot alkaloids, quinidine, warfarin, indinavir, and saquinavir. Drugs that decrease delavirdine levels include phenytoin, rifabutin, rifampin, carbamazepine, and phenobarbital. When coadministering delavirdine with antacids or the NRTI didanosine, the nurse should separate administration by at least 1 hour. Like nevirapine, rash is the most common adverse effect of delavirdine use. Other adverse effects include headache, nausea, diarrhea, fatigue, and elevated hepatic enzyme levels.

Efavirenz

Efavirenz (Sustiva) is the newest NNRTI. Efavirenz may be given in combination with PIs. However, dosage adjustments must be considered with saquinavir, amprenavir, and indinavir. Efavirenz decreases the levels of saquinavir and amprenavir when given in combination. If given concurrently with indinavir, the indinavir dose must be increased to 1000 mg every 8 hours.

Efavirenz can be taken with or without food. However, taking it at the same time as eating a fatty meal is not recommended, because the fat can cause drug levels in the body to become too high. The major adverse effects from efavirenz are on the CNS and include dizziness, sleeplessness, intense dreams, altered mood, and anxiety. These side effects are worst during the first 2 to 4 weeks of treatment. There have been reports of severe anxiety, depression, and difficulty concentrating in people starting efavirenz. Patients should be advised to assess its affects before attempting tasks that require concentration. Like other NNRTI drugs, efavirenz may cause a rash. The rash is milder than with other NNRTIs and usually goes away on its own. Potential drug interactions with efavirenz are similar to other NNRTI drugs.

NUCLEOTIDE ANALOGUE REVERSE TRANSCRIPTASE INHIBITOR

At the present time there is only one drug in this class, adefovir dipivoxil (Preveon). In the United States, this drug is not FDA-approved because of its potential adverse effect on the kidneys. However, it may be obtained through studies and early access programs. Other potential uses for adefovir include hepatitis B and cytomegalovirus (CMV).

Like the NRTIs, adefovir interrupts the ability of reverse transcriptase to convert the virus' RNA into DNA. A key benefit to the use of adefovir is that it works against several strains of HIV that are already resistant to zidovudine, zalcitabine, or didanosine.

Adefovir reduces the amount of the amino acid carnitine in the body. Therefore, patients need to take a daily supplement of 500 mg of carnitine. Other common adverse effects include nausea, vomiting, and anorexia. The carnitine supplement also may induce nausea.

The most serious adverse effect is the potential injury to the kidneys. Approximately 40% of patients have renal function abnormalities after 6 months of therapy. Patients should have renal function tests monitored monthly while on this medication.

PROPHYLAXIS FOR OPPORTUNISTIC INFECTIONS

Patients with HIV infection are at increased risk for a multitude of opportunistic diseases. Many of these diseases must be treated on an individual basis, and routine prophylaxis is not recommended. However, several diseases do have recommendations for ongoing prophylaxis. These diseases and recommendations for prophylaxis are discussed below and in Table 54-7.

PNEUMOCYSTIS CARINII PNEUMONIA

Patients should start prophylaxis therapy for PCP when their CD4+ T-cell count is less than 200 cells/μL; when they experience unexplained fever exceeding 100°F for more than 2 weeks; or when they have a history of oropharyngeal candidiasis.

The drug treatment of choice is sulfamethoxazole-trimethoprim (SMZ-TMP). Patients who experience non-life-

TABLE 54-7 Strongly Recommended Preventive Regimens for Opportunistic Diseases

Infection	Indication	First Choice	Alternate
Pneumocystis carinii pneumonia	CD4+ count <200/μL or oropharyngeal candidiasis	Trimethoprim-sulfamethoxazole (SMZ-TMP)	• Dapsone plus pyrimethamine **or** • Dapsone plus leucovorin **or** • Dapsone plus pyrimethamine plus leucovorin • Aerosolized pentamidine • Atovaquone
Mycobacterium tuberculosis	Tuberculin skin test (TST) reaction ≥ 5 mm; prior positive TST result without treatment; or contact with case of active TB	Isoniazid plus pyridoxine	Rifabutin plus pyrazinamide **or** Rifampin
Toxoplasma gondii	IgG antibody to Toxoplasma and CD4+ count <100/μL	(SMZ-TMP)	• Dapsone plus pyrimethamine plus leucovorin • Atovaquone plus leucovorin with or without pyrimethamine
Mycobacterium avium complex (MAC)	CD4+ count <50/μL	Azithromycin **or** clarithromycin	• Rifabutin • Azithromycin plus rifabutin
Varicella zoster virus (VZV)	Significant exposure to chicken-pox or shingles for patients who have no history of either condition or, if available, negative antibody to VZV	VZV immune globulin	

threatening adverse drug effects should continue SMZ-TMP therapy if clinically feasible. If SMZ-TMP cannot be tolerated, alternative prophylactic regimens include dapsone, dapsone plus pyrimethamine plus leucovorin, and aerosolized pentamidine administered monthly by the Respirgard II nebulizer or atovaquone.

Children born to HIV-infected mothers should receive prophylactic SMZ-TMP therapy beginning at 4 to 6 weeks of age. Therapy should be discontinued if they are subsequently found not to be infected with HIV. Children with a history of PCP, however, should receive lifelong prophylaxis to prevent recurrent disease.

For additional information on SMZ-TMP, see Chapter 50. Pentamidine and pyrimethamine are discussed in Chapter 55.

TUBERCULOSIS

Patients with a diagnosis of HIV infection should have a baseline tuberculin skin test (TST). Depending on the progression of the disease at the time of diagnosis, the TST results may be negative. Clinical evaluation for the potential of TB is needed to determine if anergy testing should be done at this time.

All HIV-infected patients who have positive TST results (exceeding 5 mm) should undergo chest radiography. For patients with positive TST findings and normal chest x-ray findings, prophylaxis with INH and pyridoxine should be initiated and continued for 9 months. Another first-line choice is rifampin and pyrazinamide given for 2 months. Alternative therapy includes rifabutin plus pyrazinamide for 2 months or rifampin alone for 4 months.

Any HIV-infected patients who are in close contact with people who have active TB should be started on prophylaxis therapy with isoniazid regardless of TST results. Infants of HIV-infected mothers should have a TST between 9 and 12 months. These children should be retested every 2 to 3 years. Additional information on isoniazid may be found in Chapter 52.

TOXOPLASMA GONDII

Patients infected with HIV should be tested for immunoglobulin G antibody to Toxoplasma soon after the diagnosis of HIV infection to detect latent infection with *Toxoplasma gondii.* Prophylaxis therapy should be initiated for patients with IgG antibody to Toxoplasma and a CD4+ T-cell count lower than 100 cells/μL. The drug of choice is SMZ-TMP. If unable to tolerate SMZ-TMP, the patient may receive alternative prophylaxis therapy with dapsone, pyrimethamine, and leucovorin in combination, or atovaquone with or without pyrimethamine plus leucovorin.

The nurse should counsel patients to avoid raw or undercooked meat, particularly undercooked pork, lamb, or venison. It also is important to caution patients to wash their hands after touching raw meat, gardening, or changing a cat's litter box. Patients with cats should be advised to change the litter box daily.

MYCOBACTERIUM AVIUM COMPLEX

Prophylaxis for MAC should be initiated when the patient's CD4+ T-cell count falls below 50 cells/μL. The drugs of choice are azithromycin or clarithromycin. In addition to MAC protection, these drugs also offer protection against respiratory bacterial infections.

For patients who cannot tolerate azithromycin or clarithromycin, rifabutin is the alternative. It is important to remember that rifabutin interacts with almost all anti-HIV agents; therefore, it should be administered cautiously. Additional information on azithromycin and clarithromycin is located in Chapter 49.

VARICELLA ZOSTER VIRUS (VZV)

Varicella zoster virus immune globulin should be administered to patients with significant exposure to chickenpox or shingles, who have had no history of exposure to either disorder. It also should be administered to patients with a negative antibody to VZV. Five vials (1.25 mL each) are administered at one time, ideally within 48 hours of exposure.

BACTERIAL RESPIRATORY INFECTIONS

Streptococcus pneumoniae and *Haemophilus influenzae* are very common in the community, and there is no effective way to limit exposure to these bacteria. For patients with a CD4+ T-cell count exceeding 200 cells/μL, pneumococcal vaccine should be administered. For patients with a CD4+ T-cell count under 200 cells/μL, pneumococcal vaccine may be administered, but the humoral response is likely to be diminished. Additional information on pneumococcal vaccine may be found in Appendix G.

HEPATITIS B

HIV-positive patients should be tested for antibodies to hepatitis B virus. If negative, the hepatitis B vaccine should be administered. This vaccine is administered in three doses, with the second dose given 1 month after the initial dose and the last dose given 6 months after the initial dose.

HEPATITIS A

HIV-positive patients should be tested for antibodies to hepatitis A virus. If negative, or the patient has chronic hepatitis C, the hepatitis A vaccine should be administered. This vaccine is administered in two doses.

CANDIDA

Routine primary prophylaxis is not recommended because of the effective treatment for acute disease, the low mortality associated with mucosal candidiasis, the potential for resistant *Candida* organisms to develop, the possibility of drug interactions, and the cost of prophylaxis.

However, some experts believe prophylaxis should be initiated when the CD4+ T-cell count is below 50 cells/μL. The drug of choice is fluconazole, which is discussed in Chapter 53.

MISCELLANEOUS DISORDERS

Patients with a CD4+ T cell count less than 100/μL who live in a geographic area in which *Histoplasma capsulatum* endemic should receive itraconazole daily. Patients with a CD4+ T-cell count below 50 should receive prophylaxis for *Cryptococcus neoformans* and CMV. Cryptococcus is treated with fluconazole daily. Itraconazole is the alternative therapy. Cytomegalovirus is managed with oral ganciclovir three times daily. Acyclovir is not effective and valacyclovir is contraindicated because of an unexplained trend toward increased mortality when used with patients who have AIDS. Ganciclovir is discussed in Chapter 53.

CHAPTER SUMMARY

- HIV infection and AIDS are chronic diseases affecting the immune system
- HIV is diagnosed by positive results to EIA, ELISA, WB, or PCR tests.
- HIV infection is monitored by CD4+ T-cell counts and HIV-RNA counts.
- Pharmacotherapy for asymptomatic patients has benefits and risks. Patients should be informed of both before starting therapy.
- Pharmacotherapy should be considered for all symptomatic patients. For asymptomatic patients, drug therapy should be considered when the CD4+ T-cell count is less than 500 cells/μL or the HIV-RNA count is over 10,000.
- Resistance develops in all classes of anti-HIV agents, especially when the therapeutic regimen is not followed.
- Absorption of individual anti-HIV agents is enhanced either by administration with food or on an empty stomach (fasting).
- All anti-HIV drugs may produce adverse effects that decrease the quality of the patient's life.
- Most anti-HIV drugs have numerous drug-drug interactions that may increase or decrease their effectiveness.
- Anti-HIV agents include NRTIs, PIs, and NNRTIs.
- Opportunistic diseases develop as HIV progresses. Many opportunistic diseases have recommended prophylactic regimens.

QUESTIONS FOR STUDY AND REVIEW

1. How is HIV infection diagnosed?
2. Why do patients with HIV infection have an increased risk for opportunistic diseases?
3. What information is gained from CD4+ T-cell counts and viral load counts?
4. What is the rationale for highly active antiretroviral therapy (HAART)?
5. Which adverse effects of zidovudine (AZT, ZDV) therapy may indicate a need to stop therapy?
6. Before initiation of zidovudine therapy, what laboratory tests should be completed?
7. What assessments and interventions should be made in light of lifestyle, diet, and habits for the patient taking zidovudine?
8. How do PIs inhibit HIV replication?
9. Why is therapeutic adherence critically important with saquinavir therapy?
10. How do NNRTIs differ in action from NRTIs?

NEED MORE HELP?

? Chapter 54 of the study guide for *Drug Therapy* in Nursing contains exercises and activities to reinforce your understanding of the concepts presented in this chapter. For additional information see the text's accompanying website at *http://www.connection.lww.com.*

REFERENCES AND BIBLIOGRAPHY

Acosta, E. P., Kakuda, T. N., Brundage, R. C., et al. (2000). Pharmacodynamics of human immunodeficiency virus type 1 protease inhibitors, *Clinical Infectious Diseases, 30,* (Suppl. 2), S151–S159.

Baxter, J. D., et al. (1999). CPCRA 046 Study Team. A pilot study of the short-term effects of antiretroviral management based on plasma genotypic antiretroviral resistance testing (GART) in patients failing antiretroviral therapy [Abstract LB8]. In 6th Conference on Retroviruses and Opportunistic Infections, Chicago, Illinois.

Centers for Disease Control and Prevention. (1999). USPHS/IDSA Guidelines for the prevention of opportunistic infections in persons infected with human immunodeficiency virus. U.S. Department of Health and Human Services. *Morbidity and Mortality Weekly Report, 48*(No. RR-10), 1–67.

CCIS System. (2001). *Computerized Clinical Information System.* Denver, CO: Micromedex.

Clinical Drug Monographs [CDRom]. (2001). Gold Standard Media.

Deeks, S. G., & Volberding, P. (June, 1997). Antiretroviral therapy for HIV disease: A review of the clinical pharmacology, safety, efficacy, and resistance patterns of each currently available drug. Available: http://www.HIVinsite.ucsf.edu.

Drug Facts and Comparisons. (2000). St. Louis: Facts and Comparisons Division

Durant, J., et al. (1999). Drug-resistance genotyping in HIV-1 therapy: The VIRADAPT randomized controlled trial. *Lancet, 353,* 2195–2199.

Eron, J. J., Jr. (2000) HIV-1 protease inhibitors. *Clinical Infectious Diseases, 30,* (Suppl. 2), S160–S170/

Fish, D. N. (July, 1997). HIV drug interaction: Monitoring update. Online Available: http://www.medscape.com/mon_hs/HIVManagement.fish/fish/html July, 1997

Foster, R. H., & Faulds, D. (1998). Abacavir. *Drugs 55,* 729–736.

Hardman, J. G., Limbird, L. E., Molinof, P. B., Ruddon, R. W., & Gilman, A. (Eds.). (1997). *Goodman and Gilman's the pharmacological basis of therapeutics* (9th Ed.). New York: McGraw-Hill.

Karch, A. (2001). *2001 Lippincott's nursing drug guide.* Philadelphia: Lippincott Williams & Wilkins.

Katzung, B. (1998). *Basic and clinical pharmacology* (7th ed.). Stamford: Appleton & Lange.

Perry, C. M. & Noble, S. (1998). Saquinavir soft-gel formulation. A review of its use in patients with HIV infection. *Drugs 55*(3), 461–486.

Porth, C. (1998). *Pathophysiology: Concepts of altered health states* (5th.), Philadelphia: Lippincott Williams & Wilkins.

Powderly, W. G., et al. (1999). Predictors of optimal virological response to potent antiretroviral therapy. *AIDS, 13,* 1873–1880.

O'Brien, W. A. (2000). Resistance against reverse transcriptase inhibitors, *Clinical Infectious Diseases, 30,* (Suppl. 2), S185–192.

Report of the NIH Panel to define principles of therapy of HIV infection (1998). *Morbidity and Mortality Weekly Recommendations & Reports 47*(NO RR-5), 1–41.

Staszewski, S., et al. (1999). Determinants of sustainable CD4 lymphocyte count increases in response to antiretroviral therapy. *AIDS, 13,* 951–956.

Tatro, D. (Ed.). (2000). *Drug interaction facts* (6th ed.). St. Louis: Facts and Comparisons.

Vella, S., & Palmisano, L. (2000). Antiretroviral therapy: State of the HAART. *Antiviral Research, 45*(1), 1–7.

Vittinghoff, E., et al. (1999). Combination antiretroviral therapy and recent declines in AIDS incidence and mortality, *Journal of Infectious Diseases, 179,*717–720.

Chapter 55

DRUGS FOR TREATING PARASITES

KEY TERMS

amebiasis
arthropods
cestodes
ectoparasites
giardiasis
helminths
malaria
nematodes
parasite
Pneumocystis carinii pneumonia
protozoa
toxoplasmosis
trematodes
trichomoniasis

Learning Objectives

At the completion of this chapter the student will:

1. Describe the guidelines that govern the choice of antiparasitic drugs.
2. Identify core drug knowledge about drugs used to treat parasitic infections.
3. Identify core patient variables relevant to drugs used to treat parasitic infections.
4. Relate the interaction of core drug knowledge and core patient variables to drugs used to treat parasitic infections.
5. Generate a nursing plan of care from the interactions between core drug knowledge and core patient variables for drugs used to treat parasitic infections.
6. Describe nursing interventions to maximize therapeutic actions and minimize adverse effects for drugs used to treat parasitic infections.
7. Determine key points for patient and family education for drugs that are used in the treatment of parasitic infections.
8. Explain the modifications needed to prevent parasitic reinfection.

Antimalarials

chloroquine
hydroxychloroquine
mefloquine
primaquine
pyrimethamine
quinine sulfate

Antibacterial agents
sulfonamides
atovaquone/proguanil

Antiprotozoans

Drugs affecting ameblasis, giardiasis, trichomoniasis, and toxoplasmosis

metronidazole
iodoquinol
paromomycin
quinacrine

Drugs affecting *Pneumocystis carinii* pneumonia

pentamidine
atovaquone

Antihelminthics

mebendazole
albendazole
thiabendazole
diethylcarbamazine
niclosamide
paraziquantel
piperazine
pyrantel
oxaminiquine

Antiectoparasitics

lindane
crotamiton
permethrin
ivermectin

The symbol (C) indicates the **drug class**.
Drugs in bold type marked with the symbol (P) are **prototypes**.
Drugs in blue type with no symbol are **closely related** to the prototype.
Drugs in **red** type with no symbol are **significantly different** from the prototype.
Drugs in **black** type with no symbol are **also used in drug therapy**; no prototype.

A **parasite** is an organism that must live on other organisms to survive. The parasitic diseases are commonly grouped into those caused by helminths, arthropods, and unicellular organisms, such as **protozoa**. Protozoan infections include malaria, amebiasis, giardiasis, *Pneumocystis carinii* pneumonia, toxoplasmosis, and trichomoniasis. **Helminths** (worms) are grouped into three categories: **nematodes** (roundworms), **trematodes** (flukes), and **cestodes** (tapeworms). **Ectoparasites** are vectors of disease, such as ticks, mosquitoes, and biting flies, and **ectoparasites** that infect external body surfaces. Arthropods include mites (scabies), chiggers, lice (pediculosis), and fleas.

Pharmacologic intervention for parasitic infections must be specific not only to the type of parasite but also to the stage of its life cycle. Some parasites have simple life cycles, and some have extremely complex life cycles. Thus, many parasitic diseases are treated with a combination of drugs to eradicate all stages of the parasite.

This chapter discusses the appropriate drug or drugs used to eradicate the most common parasitic diseases. Antiparasitic drugs are divided into four drug families: antimalarials, antiprotozoan drugs, anthelminthic drugs, and antiectoparasitic drugs. The antiprotozoan drugs used in treating *Pneumocystis carinii* pneumonia, a common complication of acquired immunodeficiency syndrome (AIDS), are discussed separately within the antiprotozoan drug class section.

The prototype drugs discussed in this chapter include the antimalarial chloroquine, the antiprotozoans metronidazole and pentamidine, the anthelminthic mebendazole, and the antiectoparasitic lindane. In addition to explaining how these drugs work, this chapter discusses nursing management related to evaluating the patient's condition, administering antiparasitic drugs, monitoring the patient's response, and teaching the patient and family about antiparasitic therapy.

PATHOPHYSIOLOGY

MALARIA

Malaria is caused by protozoan parasites of the genus *Plasmodium*. There are four species of *Plasmodium* that produce disease in humans—*P. falciparum, P. vivax, P. ovale*, and *P. malariae*. *P. falciparum* is the most widespread and dangerous of the four. Because *P. falciparum* can destroy up to 60% of circulating red blood cells (RBCs) and induce serious adverse complications such as toxic encephalopathy, it is fatal in about 1% of all cases. That 1% accounts for more than 95% of all malaria-caused deaths worldwide.

The complex life cycle begins when a female Anopheles mosquito bites a human whose blood contains the sexual forms of the malaria parasite (gametocytes). Within the now-infected mosquito, the gametocyte completes a maturation process and becomes a sporozoite that is stored in the salivary glands. When the mosquito next feeds, the sporozoites inoculate another human host.

Once in the human host, the asexual life cycle begins. The first stage of asexual development, the exoerythrocytic phase, occurs in the liver. During this phase, the form of the *Plasmodium* is called a tissue schizont. At the end of the phase, the *Plasmodium*, now in a form called a merozoite, is released from the liver into the bloodstream.

The second stage of asexual development, the erythrocytic phase, begins when the merozoites are released into the blood stream. The merozoites invade the erythrocytes and develop into erythrocytic schizonts. They, in turn, develop more merozoites within the RBCs. At the end of the phase, the RBCs rupture, releasing the merozoites and pyrogenic substances into the bloodstream to invade new RBCs. The release of merozoites into the bloodstream initiates the symptoms of fever, shivering, joint pain, and headache. With *P. vivax* and *P. ovale*, merozoites may reinvade the liver tissue and develop a dormant hepatic stage (hypnozoite), which is responsible for subsequent relapses.

The cycle of invasion, multiplication, and RBC rupture is repeated many times. After a few cycles, some of the asexual parasites develop into sexual forms (gametocytes), which remain in the bloodstream. When a mosquito bites a human with gametocytes in the blood, the cycle begins again (Fig. 55-1). Because of its complex life cycle, malaria is frequently treated with combination drug therapy.

PARASITIC DISEASES

Amebiasis

Amebiasis is most frequently caused by the microorganism *Entamoeba histolytica*, which is passed from host to host by ingestion of fecally contaminated food or water. It also is transmitted by vectors such as flies. Amebic disease is present worldwide, but it is most common in those tropical areas where crowded living conditions and poor sanitation exist. Africa, Latin America, Southeast Asia, and India have significant health problems associated with this disease. In the United States, amebiasis is seen with increased frequency among homosexual men.

Ingested in its cyst form, the microorganism has thick walls that are resistant to stomach acids. In the intestine, the cysts change into a sexually active organism called a trophozoite. The trophozoite produces active amebiasis. The active disease organisms may remain in the intestine (intestinal amebiasis), or the trophozoites may penetrate the intestinal wall and produce abscesses in other tissues and organs (extraintestinal amebiasis). Symptoms may be mild or severe. Mild symptoms include mucoid diarrhea, flatulence, fatigue, weight loss, and colicky abdominal pain. Severe disease may be marked with frequent foul-smelling stools tinged with mucus and blood, fever to 105°F, tenesmus (painful but unsuccessful straining to defecate), generalized abdominal tenderness, and vomiting.

Giardiasis

Giardiasis is a common disease caused by a flagellated protozoan, *Giardia lamblia*. It is transmitted by fecal contamination. Hikers who drink unfiltered water or travelers to foreign countries where the water supply is impure are most susceptible. Animal reservoirs for the parasites include beavers and dogs.

Giardiasis is more prevalent in children than in adults, possibly because many individuals seem to have a lasting im-

Physiology

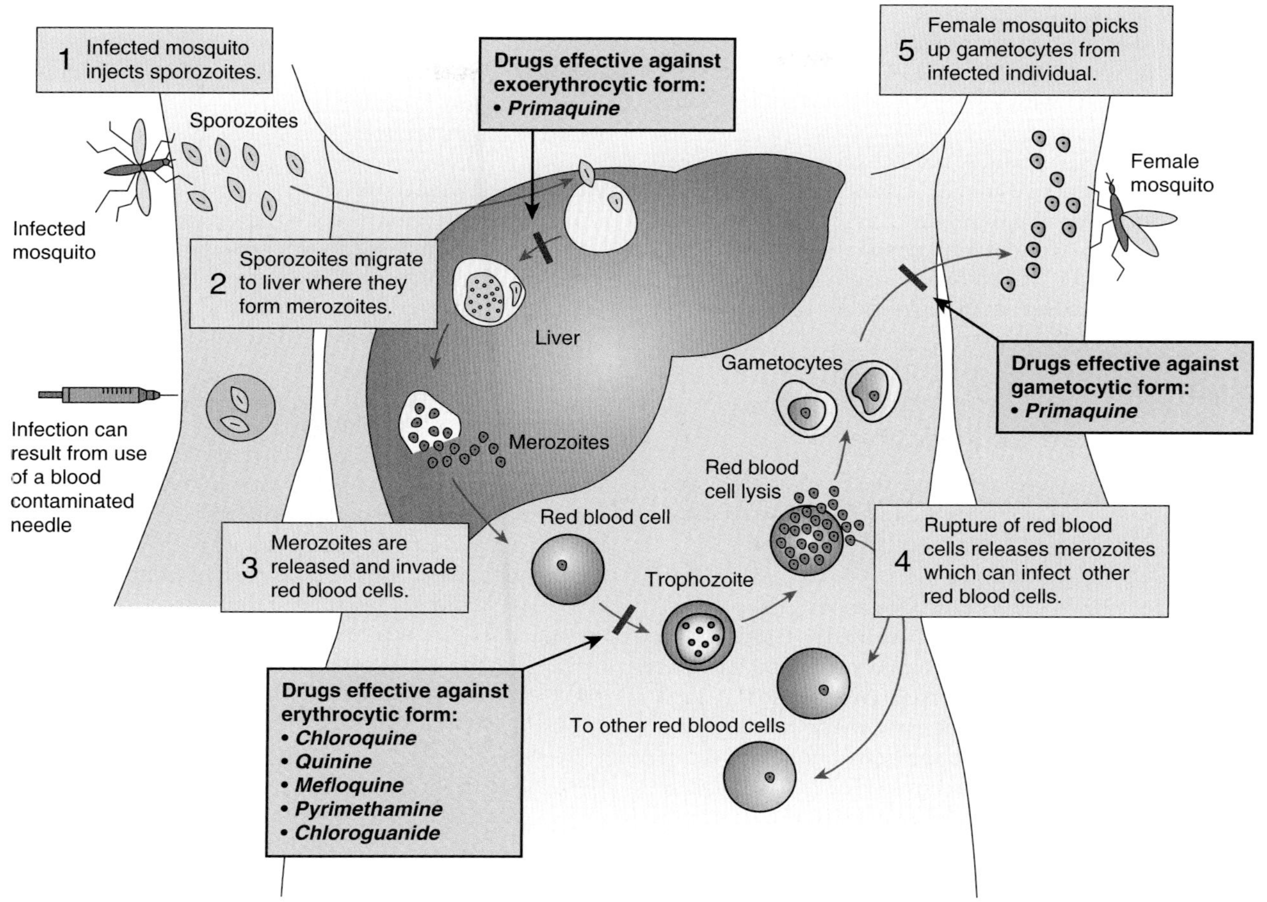
1 Infected mosquito injects sporozoites.
Sporozoites
Infected mosquito
Drugs effective against exoerythrocytic form:
• Primaquine
2 Sporozoites migrate to liver where they form merozoites.
Liver
Infection can result from use of a blood contaminated needle
Merozoites
3 Merozoites are released and invade red blood cells.
Red blood cell
Trophozoite
Drugs effective against erythrocytic form:
• Chloroquine
• Quinine
• Mefloquine
• Pyrimethamine
• Chloroguanide
5 Female mosquito picks up gametocytes from infected individual.
Female mosquito
Gametocytes
Drugs effective against gametocytic form:
• Primaquine
Red blood cell lysis
4 Rupture of red blood cells releases merozoites which can infect other red blood cells.
To other red blood cells

Figure 55-1. Life cycle of the malarial parasite and the sites of action of antimalarial drugs. (Courtesy of Mycek, M. J., Harvey, R. A., and Champe, P. C. [1997]. *Pharmacology*, [2nd ed.]. Philadelphia: Lippincott-Raven.)

munity after infection. The disease is common in children's day-care centers, especially those in which diapering is done. This disease also afflicts many homosexual men, both HIV-positive and HIV-negative individuals. This presumably results from sexual transmission.

Giardia affects only the intestinal system, resulting in acute or chronic diarrhea and possibly malabsorption syndrome. The acute phase may last days to weeks; however, the chronic phase may last years. Symptoms include diarrheal, soft, or steatorrheal stools with mucus but without blood. Abdominal cramps, vomiting, flatulence, and weight loss also may occur.

Trichomoniasis

Trichomoniasis is an infection of the vagina caused by the parasite *Trichomonas vaginalis*. Both sexual partners are generally infected although both may not be symptomatic. Symptoms of trichomoniasis include a thin, yellow, frothy and malodorous discharge. The vagina may be inflamed as well as a "strawberry" cervix, which is very friable and bleeds easily.

Toxoplasmosis

Toxoplasmosis is caused by a parasite found in a variety of animals, especially cats and birds.

Infection results from ingestion of oocysts from cat feces, ingestion of cysts in raw or undercooked meat, congenital transmission, or transmission during blood transfusion.

In adults, the disease is usually mild with symptoms such as fever, malaise, headache, lymphadenopathy, and sore throat. However, toxoplasmosis is very dangerous to immunocompromised patients. The infection may affect the lungs, heart, and liver, but usually it affects the brain. Patients may succumb to meningoencephalitis.

Congenital toxoplasmosis may result in damage to the eyes (retinochoroiditis) and brain (encephalitis) of the fetus or other congenital anomalies.

PNEUMOCYSTIS CARINII PNEUMONIA

An opportunistic lung infection, ***Pneumocystis carinii* pneumonia** (PCP) is caused by a parasite of uncertain classification. The parasite's life cycle is similar to that of a protozoan; however, recent analysis indicates that *P. carinii* may be a fungus. The microorganism is found in a variety of domesticated and wild animals, and transmission is thought to be airborne. Although contact with *P. carinii* is worldwide, only debilitated or immunosuppressed and immunodeficient patients develop symptoms. Because PCP infection occurs so frequently in patients with AIDS, it is used as a diagnostic criterion for the disease.

Symptoms of PCP include abrupt onset, high fever, tachypnea, nonproductive cough, shortness of breath, and cyanosis. As the disease rapidly progresses, patients have symptoms similar to those of adult respiratory distress syndrome. Untreated PCP has an exceptionally high mortality rate. Patients who recover are at high risk for recurrence.

HELMINTHIC INFECTIONS

Intestinal Nematode Infections

The common intestinal nematodes are the giant roundworm, pinworm, threadworm, whipworm, and pork roundworm.

Ascariasis (Giant Roundworm)

Ascariasis is endemic in areas known for poor hygiene or sanitation and those where human feces are used as fertilizer. Ascariasis is transmitted by ingesting fecally contaminated food or drinks. Once ingested, the worm eggs migrate to the small bowel where they hatch, releasing larvae. The motile larvae migrate from the small bowel to the heart and lungs, to the esophagus, and back to the small bowel. They can survive up to 5 years and reach a length of 30 cm. Symptoms include low-grade fever, nonproductive cough, blood-tinged sputum, wheezing, dyspnea, and substernal pain.

Enterobiasis (Pinworm)

Enterobius vermicularis is the most common helminthic infection in the United States. Children are infected more frequently than adults. Transmission occurs by contact with eggs in food, water, or bed linens. Adult worms inhabit the cecum and adjacent bowel areas. Female worms migrate through the anus to the perianal skin and deposit large numbers of eggs, especially at night. In a few hours, infection can be transmitted to others or remain in the host. The most common symptoms are rectal itching and vulvar itching.

Strongyloidiasis (Threadworm)

Strongyloidiasis results from infection with *Strongyloides stercoralis*. The infection is potentially serious in adults because the worm can multiply within the host. In its filariform larvae cycle, the parasites penetrate the skin from soil, enter the bloodstream, and travel to the lungs. From the lungs, they escape the alveoli and ascend the bronchial tree to the glottis where they are swallowed and propelled to the small intestine to mature into adult threadworms. The mature worm embeds itself in the mucosa where eggs are laid and hatched. The larvae disseminate into the lungs and most other tissues, causing local inflammation and granulomas. Symptoms include skin reactions, such as inflammation, petechiae, and urticaria, and intestinal reactions, such as diarrhea, abdominal pain, and flatulence. Pulmonary symptoms include dry cough, throat irritation, dyspnea, wheezing, and hemoptysis. Hyperinfection syndrome caused by intense dissemination of larvae to the lungs and other tissues can result in complications, such as pleural effusion, pericarditis, and myocarditis. Additional problems include perforation of the colon and peritonitis, gram-negative septicemia, and shock leading to death.

Trichuriasis (Whipworm)

Trichuriasis infection is acquired by ingesting an infected egg. Human-to-human transmission is not possible. Worms attach to the mucosa of the large intestine by means of their anterior whip-like end. Symptoms include abdominal cramps, tenesmus, diarrhea, flatulence, nausea, vomiting, and weight loss.

Trichinosis (Pork Roundworm)

Trichinella spiralis is the parasite that causes trichinosis. The infection is transmitted by ingesting encysted larvae in inadequately cooked meat, especially pork. Gastric juices liberate the encysted larvae, which migrate to the intestines where they mature, mate, and produce eggs that hatch into new larvae. These larvae are distributed through the body and enter skeletal muscle tissues, producing an inflammatory response. Eventually, the larvae become reencysted and remain within the tissues. Symptoms include diarrhea, cramps, and malaise. As the infection progresses, patients may experience muscle pain, tenderness, fever, periorbital and facial edema, and conjunctivitis.

Blood and Tissue Nematode Infections

Filarial infections are among the more serious and debilitating helminthiases associated with blood and tissue nematodes. There are two forms of filarial infections. The first form is caused by two microbes, *Wuchereria bancrofti* and *Brugia malayi*. Both microbes are transmitted by mosquitoes.

Bancroftian filariasis also is known as elephantiasis because the helminths migrate to the lymphatic system, causing lymphadenopathy and resultant edema of the extremities. Brugian filariasis also affects the lymphatic system. In this infection, microfilariae are produced and circulated in the bloodstream.

The second type of filariasis also is known as onchocerciasis or river blindness. The adult helminths reside in subcutaneous nodules and migrate to the eye, causing ocular lesions and eventual loss of vision.

Cestode Infections

Cestodes cause taeniasis infections. Tapeworm infections are transmitted in contaminated raw or improperly cooked fish (*Diphyllobothrium latum*), beef (*Taenia saginata*), and pork (*Taenia solium*). The adult tapeworm consists of a head (scolex) that attaches to the intestinal wall and segments called proglottids. The proglottids contain tapeworm eggs and are expelled in feces. Beef and fish tapeworms do not cause serious illness. Pork tapeworms, however, produce larvae that enter the bloodstream and invade other body tissues. Symptoms include nausea, vomiting, diarrhea, fatigue, hunger, and dizziness.

Trematode Infections

Trematodes cause schistosomiasis, which is a leading cause of morbidity and mortality in parasitic diseases. The vector of schistosomiasis is a specific snail. There are three major types of schistosomes. Each migrates to a specific part of the human host and produces clinical symptoms specific to each type.

ECTOPARASITIC INFECTIONS

Common ectoparasitic infections include scabies and pediculosis (lice).

Scabies

Scabies is a skin inflammation caused by *Sarcoptes scabiei*. The mite is barely visible with the naked eye and is transmitted by contact with an infected individual or infested bedding. Characteristic lesions consist of generalized excoriations with small pruritic vesicles, pustules, and burrows. The infestations occur on the sides of the fingers and the palms, wrists, elbows, and around the axillae. The head and neck are usually spared in adults. Diagnosis is made by identifying the parasite or its ova or feces microscopically. Treatment includes all family members and close contacts, which helps to prevent reinfestation.

Pediculosis

Pediculosis infestations occur on the scalp (pediculosis capitis), trunk (pediculosis corporis), or pubic areas (pediculosis pubis). Transmission is by direct contact with lice, particularly those on hats, combs, and body hair. Symptoms include pruritus with excoriation, nits on hair shafts, and lice on skin or clothes.

ANTIMALARIAL DRUGS

Drug therapy for malaria has three distinct categories: suppressive therapy (prophylaxis), treatment of an acute attack (clinical cure), and prevention of a relapse (radical cure). Some drugs may be used in more than one category. All antimalarials are called schizonticides. They are further divided into tissue schizonticides or blood schizonticides. Blood schizonticides affect the erythrocytic state of the schizont replicating in the RBCs of the human host. Tissue schizonticides affect schizonts that have invaded the liver. Some antimalarial drugs, such as the prototype chloroquine, have multiple actions; it is both a blood schizonticide and a gametocytocide.

Drugs within the antimalarial class include chloroquine (Aralen), hydroxychloroquine (Plaquenil Sulfate), mefloquine (Lariam), primaquine, pyrimethamine (Daraprim), and quinine (Quinamin).

NURSING MANAGEMENT OF THE PATIENT RECEIVING CHLOROQUINE

Core Drug Knowledge

Pharmacotherapeutics

Chloroquine is indicated to suppress or treat acute attacks of malaria due to *P. vivax*, *P. malariae*, *P. ovale*, and susceptible strains of *P. falciparum*. It does not prevent relapses because it is not effective against exoerythrocytic forms of the parasite, nor will it prevent infections caused by *P. vivax* or *P. malariae* when administered as a prophylactic. In addition to its use in treating malaria, chloroquine also is used to treat extraintestinal amebiasis, rheumatoid arthritis, and discoid lupus erythematosus.

Pharmacokinetics

Chloroquine is absorbed rapidly and completely from the gastrointestinal (GI) system. The drug concentrates in the erythrocytes (RBCs), liver, spleen, kidney, lung, melanin-containing tissues, and leukocytes (white blood cells). It penetrates the central nervous system (CNS) and crosses the placenta. Although chloroquine action peaks rapidly, its half-life is between 70 and 120 hours. About 70% of chloroquine is excreted unchanged by the kidneys. Any unabsorbed drug is excreted in feces. Small amounts of chloroquine have been detected in urine for months and even years after treatment stops (Table 55-1).

Pharmacodynamics

Chloroquine, a 4-aminoquinoline, is classified as a blood schizonticide. In treating malaria, the direct effects are on the parasite. Chloroquine is taken up by plasmodia residing within the RBCs of the human host. It is thought that chloroquine increases blood pH and upsets phospholipid metabolism, thereby interrupting the synthesis of ribonucleic acid (RNA) and deoxyribonucleic acid (DNA). The drug's action in treating amebiasis is unknown. In patients with rheumatoid arthritis, chloroquine antagonizes histamine and serotonin, thereby inhibiting prostaglandin synthesis. The result is an anti-inflammatory effect.

Contraindications and Precautions

Chloroquine is contraindicated for patients with a hypersensitivity to any 4-aminoquinoline, such as hydroxychloroquine. Chloroquine also is contraindicated for patients with preexisting eye disease because the drug can cause corneal opacities, keratopathy, or retinopathy. Retinopathy can lead to blindness and can progress even after the drug is discontinued.

Chloroquine is used with caution in patients with various preexisting disorders. In patients with psoriasis or porphyria, chloroquine has precipitated severe attacks. Because chloroquine concentrates in the liver,

TABLE 55-1 Summary of Selected Antimalarial Drugs

Drug (Trade) Name	Selected Indications	Route and Dosage Range	Pharmacokinetics
chloroquine (Aralen)	Suppression of malaria	*Adult:* PO, 300-mg base once a week on the same day for 2 wk before exposure and continuing until 4–6 wk after exposure *Child:* PO, 5 mg base PO once a week on the same day for 2 wk before exposure and continuing until 4–6 wk after exposure	*Onset:* Rapid *Duration:* Week $t_{1/2}$: 70–120 h
	Acute malaria attack	*Adult:* PO, 600-mg base initially, then 300-mg base 6 h later and on days 2 and 3 *Child:* PO, 10-mg base/kg initially, then 5-mg base/kg 6 h later and on days 2 and 3 *Adult:* IM, 160–200 mg base initially and 6 h later if needed; not to exceed 800 mg base/d *Child:* IM, 5 mg base/kg mg base initially and 6 h later if needed	
	Amebiasis	*Adult:* PO, 1 g (600-mg base)/d for 2 d, then 500 mg (300-mg base)/d for 2–3 wk *Child:* PO, not recommended *Adult:* IM, 200–250 mg (160–200-mg base) daily for 10–12 d	
atovaquone/proguanil (Malarone)	Treatment of malaria	*Adult:* PO single dose of four tablets (total daily dose 1 g atovaquone/400 mg proguanil hydrochloride) for 3 consecutive days.	*Onset:* Rapid *Duration:* Unknown $t_{1/2}$: 3 d
	Prophylaxis	Malarone is one tablet (250 mg atovaquone/100 mg proguanil hydrochloride) per day for adults *Child:* Based on weight of child	
hydroxychloroquine (Plaquenil Sulfate)	Suppression of malaria	*Adult:* PO, 310-mg base/wk on the same day each week, beginning 2 wk before exposure and continuing for 6–8 wk after leaving the malaria area. If suppressive therapy does not begin before exposure, the initial loading dose is doubled and given in two doses 6 h apart *Child:* 5-mg base/kg/wk, then the same dosage regimen as adults	*Onset:* Rapid *Duration:* Unknown $t_{1/2}$: 50 d
	Acute malaria attack	*Adult:* PO, initial dose (day 1), 620-mg base; dose 2 (6 h after dose 1), 310 mg; dose 3 (day 2), 310 mg; dose 4 (day 3) 310 mg *Child:* PO, same as adult in the following amounts, respectively: 10 mg/kg base, 5 mg/kg, 5 mg/kg, 5 mg/kg	
mefloquine (Lariam)	Suppression of malaria	*Adult:* PO, 250 mg once weekly for 4 wk, then 250 mg every other week; CDC recommends a single dose taken weekly starting 1 wk before exposure and for 4 wk after exposure *Child:* PO, 15–19 kg 1/4 tablets; 20–30 kg 1/2 tablet; 31–45 kg 3/4 tablet; more than 45 kg 1 tablet; CDC recommends a single dose taken weekly starting 1 wk before exposure and for 4 wk after exposure	*Onset:* Delayed *Duration:* Varies $t_{1/2}$: 15–23 d
	Acute malaria attack	*Adult:* PO, 5 tablets (1,250 mg) as a single dose	
primaquine	Malaria	*Adult:* PO, begin treatment during the last week of or after a course of suppression with chloroquine or a comparable drug, then 26.3 mg (15-mg base)/d for 14 d *Child:* PO, 0.5 mg/kg/d (0.3-mg base/kg) for 14 d, maximum, 15-mg base/dose	*Onset:* Rapid *Duration:* Unknown $t_{1/2}$: 3.7–9.6 h

TABLE 55-1 Summary of Selected Antimalarial Drugs (Continued)

Drug (Trade) Name	Selected Indications	Route and Dosage Range	Pharmacokinetics
pyrimethamine (Daraprim)	Suppression of malaria	*Adult:* PO, 25 mg once weekly for at least 6–10 wk *Child:* <4 y, PO, 6.25 mg once weekly for 6–10 wk; 4–10 y, PO, 12.5 mg once weekly for 6–10 wk	*Onset:* Unknown *Duration:* Unknown $t_{1/2}$: 56–148 h
	Acute treatment of malaria	*Adult:* PO, 25 mg/d for 2 d *Child:* PO, 4–10 y, 25 mg/d for 2 d	
	Toxoplasmosis	*Adult:* PO, initially 50–75 mg/d with 1–4 g of sulfapyridine; continue for 1–3 wk; dosage of each drug may then be decreased by half and continued for an additional 4–5 wk *Child:* PO, 1 mg/kg/d divided into two equal daily doses; after 2–4 d, reduce to half and continue for approximately 1 mo	
quinine (Quinamin)	Chloroquine-resistant malaria	*Adult:* PO, 650 mg q8h, for 5–7 d *Child:* PO, 25 mg/kg/d in divided doses q8h for 5–7 d	*Onset:* Varies *Duration:* Varies $t_{1/2}$: 4–5 h
	Chloroquine-sensitive malaria	*Adult:* PO, 600 mg q8h for 5–7 d *Child:* PO, 10 mg/kg/d in divided doses q8h for 5–7 d	

it can produce toxic effects in patients with hepatic disease or alcoholism or in patients using other hepatotoxic drugs concurrently.

Chloroquine should be given with caution to patients with GI disorders, blood dyscrasias, dental disease, and neurologic disorders. Patients with these disorders may have exacerbations of disease because of the actions and potential adverse effects of chloroquine. Chloroquine should be given with extreme caution to infants and children because of potentially fatal toxicities.

Adverse Effects

Potential adverse effects of chloroquine may affect the cardiovascular, GI, hematologic, integumentary, and neurologic systems. The most frequent adverse effects are hypotension, cardiac changes reflected on an electrocardiogram (ECG), nausea, vomiting, diarrhea, and abdominal pain.

Infrequent but important potential adverse effects include blurred vision, difficulty focusing and changes in accommodation, irreversible retinal damage, tinnitus and reduced hearing in patients with preexisting auditory damage, headaches or psychic stimulation, convulsive seizures, and neuromyopathy.

Potential adverse hematologic effects include agranulocytosis, aplastic anemia, pancytopenia, neutropenia, and thrombocytopenia. Potential integumentary effects are pruritus, skin discoloration, skin eruption, and hair bleaching or loss.

Drug Interactions

Chloroquine may interact with cimetidine, digoxin, penicillamine, and rabies vaccine. With kaolin and magnesium-containing antacids, its absorption is decreased. Most patients will remember any prescription drugs they are taking, but they may forget to mention over-the-counter (OTC) drugs, such as cimetidine or antacids. Therefore, the nurse must remember to assess the patient's use of OTC drugs as well. See Table 55-2 for more information.

Assessment of Relevant Core Patient Variables

Health Status

Before administering chloroquine, the nurse should assess for anemia, porphyria, psoriasis, ocular disease, neurologic disorders, liver and kidney diseases, and other conditions that contraindicate using the drug or that require close monitoring. Next, the nurse should review the patient's drug history to identify substances that may interact with chloroquine and advise the patient to consult with the prescriber before taking any OTC drugs.

Because chloroquine may affect the eyes, the nurse should arrange for the patient to have a complete baseline ophthalmologic examination, including visual acuity, slit-lamp, and fundoscopic examinations. Similarly, because chloroquine may affect reflexes, muscle strength, and hearing, the nurse should perform a physical examination and document baseline measurements of these factors. Additional baseline studies include laboratory results related to liver function, kidney function, and complete blood count (CBC).

Life Span and Gender

In general, chloroquine may be administered to children to prevent or treat malaria. However, careful monitoring is needed because of the drug's potential for fatal toxicity in children. The nurse should assess the patient for pregnancy or lactation. Breast-feeding women need to know that chloroquine enters breast milk. Although chloroquine is assigned to pregnancy risk category C,

TABLE 55-2 Agents That Interact With P Chloroquine

Interactants	Effect and Significance	Nursing Management
cimetidine	The metabolism of aminoquinolines may be decreased, resulting in the pharmacologic effects of aminoquinolines being increased.	Monitor for possible aminoquinoline toxicity.
digoxin	Serum levels of digoxin may be increased. The actions of digoxin may be enhanced, or toxicity may develop.	Monitor patients on combined therapy for sign and symptoms of digoxin toxicity. Monitor serum digoxin level.
kaolin magnesium antacids	Kaolin and antacids containing magnesium may decrease the absorption and therapeutic effect of aminoquinolines. The antacid activity may also be decreased.	Administer doses of chloroquine and kaolin or antacids containing magnesium at least 2 h apart.
penicillamine	Serum levels of penicillamine may be increased. This may induce hematologic, renal, or skin reactions to penicillamine.	During concurrent use of penicillamine and chloroquine, monitor patient closely for adverse effect to penicillamine. Avoid concurrent use if possible.
rabies vaccine	When the rabies vaccine is administered intradermally, chloroquine may interfere with the antibody response.	Use the IM route for rabies vaccine if concurrent use is indicated.

most prescribers believe the benefits of chloroquine therapy outweigh the risks associated with malaria.

Lifestyle, Diet and Habits

The nurse should determine the patient's willingness or ability to arrange activities and lifestyle to accommodate weekly therapy for suppression.

Environment

It is important to assess the patient's understanding of the need for prophylactic *drug therapy*. People traveling to areas where malaria is endemic should begin drug prophylaxis 2 weeks before the trip and continue therapy for 4 to 6 weeks after returning. In addition to pharmacologic prophylaxis, the patient should implement activities that decrease exposure to disease-bearing mosquitoes.

Nursing Diagnoses and Outcomes

- Acute Pain: headache and itching related to drug therapy
  Desired outcome: The patient will use acetaminophen and take soothing oatmeal baths to relieve drug-related discomforts.
- Risk for Deficient Fluid Volume related to drug-induced fluid losses from nausea, vomiting, diarrhea, and anorexia
  Desired outcome: The patient will maintain adequate hydration despite the effects of drug therapy and minimize GI upset by taking the drug with food.
- Altered Protection related to possible agranulocytosis, aplastic anemia, neutropenia, and thrombocytopenia resulting from drug therapy
  Desired outcome: The patient will report signs and symptoms of blood abnormalities (bruising, unexplained fatigue) to the prescriber immediately.
- Disturbed Sensory Perception, Auditory and Visual related to potential tinnitus, hearing loss, retinopathy, and blurred vision related to drug therapy
  Desired outcome: The patient will report problems with hearing or vision to the prescriber immediately.
- Risk for Injury: cardiovascular toxicity, neuromyopathy, or seizures related to drug therapy
  Desired outcome: The patient will remain free of injury throughout therapy with chloroquine.

Planning and Intervention

Maximizing Therapeutic Effects

The patient taking chloroquine on a weekly basis for prophylaxis should take the drug on the same day each week, usually by mouth. An IM injection is given when the oral route is not possible. In such situations, the nurse or patient injects the drug into a large muscle mass, making sure to aspirate to avoid hitting a blood vessel. The IM route is unsuitable for children because of the risk for toxic effects. For children, the bitter-tasting tablets may be pulverized and mixed with a pleasantly flavored preparation, such as chocolate syrup or grape jam.

Minimizing Adverse Effects

The patient may take chloroquine with meals to minimize GI discomfort. After taking the drug, the patient may need to change positions slowly to minimize symptoms of dizziness or light-headedness, which signify a hypotensive response. The patient who experiences pruritus (itching) may be soothed by an oatmeal bath because antihistamines are ineffective in such cases. To relieve a headache, the patient may take acetaminophen. Patients with blood dyscrasias or myelosuppression should postpone dental work or other procedures that increase the risk of infection. Patients with these disorders have a higher risk for infection. The nurse should double-check pediatric doses to prevent toxicity.

Providing Patient and Family Education

- The nurse should teach the patient how to take chloroquine to prevent or treat malaria.
- Prophylactic chloroquine therapy should begin about 2 weeks prior to scheduled travel and should continue for about 4 to 6 weeks after the patient leaves the malaria area.
- The nurse also should tell the patient to wear cover-up clothing as a barrier to mosquitoes (see the accompanying display, Stop Malaria Before It Starts!).
- It is important to explain that if a fever develops within 2 months of a trip to a malaria area, the patient should notify the health care provider immediately.
- The nurse should point out potential adverse effects of chloroquine. For example, chloroquine use may discolor urine (red or brown). In addition, itching, nausea or vomiting, dizziness, and headaches may occur. Periodic ophthalmologic and audiometric examinations should be scheduled by patients on prolonged therapy because the drug can cause vision and hearing problems. The patient also should be instructed to contact the health care provider immediately if fever, sore throat, easy bruising, unusual fatigue, or problems with hearing or eyesight develop.
- The nurse also should caution the patient to avoid alcohol while taking chloroquine.
- The nurse should caution the patient to notify the health care provider if nausea, vomiting, or diarrhea is persistent.

Ongoing Assessment and Evaluation

The nurse needs to monitor for episodes of misty or foggy vision, difficulty reading and complaints that words tend to disappear, and visual field changes (e.g., seeing half an object, light flashes or streaks, or pigmentation changes). The patient's gross hearing, reflexes, and muscle strength should also be evaluated throughout therapy. Additional assessments include checking for irritability, excitability, and personality or behavioral changes and signs and symptoms of anemia and hepatic or renal dysfunction. Symptomatic patients or patients at high risk for hemolytic anemia should have periodic blood analyses, and seizure precautions should be instituted as needed.

Patients who exhibit signs of toxicity may complain of headache, drowsiness, visual disturbances, nausea, or vomiting. These symptoms may be quickly followed by cardiovascular collapse, convulsions, and respiratory or cardiac arrest. Patients suspected of experiencing toxicity should go to an emergency department. ■

COMMUNITY-BASED CONCERNS

Stop Malaria Before It Starts!

In addition to prophylactic pharmacotherapy instructions, the nurse should include the following when educating the patient about malaria:

- Be sure to use mosquito netting. Check for holes in the net.
- Always sleep in screened areas. Spray the area with permethrin-containing insecticide before the sun sets.
- Wear protective clothing. Use 30-mL DEET (N,N-diethyl meta-toluamide) in 250 mL of water to impregnate cotton garments.
- Minimize nocturnal exposure; long-sleeved clothing and long pants should be worn if outdoors after sunset
- DEET insect repellents should be applied to exposed skin. Refined lemon eucalyptus oil also may be used on the skin.

DRUGS CLOSELY RELATED TO P CHLOROQUINE

Hydroxychloroquine

Hydroxychloroquine (Plaquenil Sulfate) is very similar to chloroquine but is less toxic. Although it may be used to treat malaria, it is used more commonly to treat rheumatoid arthritis and lupus erythematosus. Higher dosages are needed for treating rheumatoid arthritis.

The pharmacokinetics and pharmacodynamics of hydroxychloroquine are the same as those of chloroquine except it is unknown whether it enters breast milk. Because the drugs are so similar and chloroquine does enter breast milk, the safest course is to refrain from its use in patients who are breast-feeding.

Hydroxychloroquine has the same extensive adverse effects profile as chloroquine. Like chloroquine, the most common adverse effects to hydroxychloroquine are GI in nature. Patients should take hydroxychloroquine with food to minimize these effects.

MEMORY CHIP

P Chloroquine

- Used primarily for malaria; secondarily for amebiasis, rheumatoid arthritis, and lupus
- Significant contraindications: preexisting eye diseases
- Most common adverse effects: hypotension, nausea, vomiting, diarrhea, and abdominal pain
- Most serious adverse effects: retinopathy and aplastic anemia
- Maximizing therapeutic effects: administer medication on the same day each week
- Minimizing adverse effects: administer with meals to decrease potential GI effects
- Most significant patient education: begin prophylaxis 2 weeks before entering any area where malaria is endemic and continue for 4 to 6 weeks after leaving the area

Mefloquine

Mefloquine (Lariam), a 4-quinolinemethanol derivative, is related chemically to quinine. Mefloquine is the drug of choice for chloroquine-resistant and multidrug-resistant *P. falciparum*. Because it is the only drug available for treating these parasites, it is reserved for these conditions to avoid inducing resistance. As a blood schizonticide, it prevents the replication of erythrocytic parasites but has no action on exoerythrocytic parasites. Its mechanism of action is unknown, but it may work by raising intravascular pH in parasite acid vesicles, causing death.

Mefloquine is given orally, despite its variable absorption, because of its irritation to tissues. It is distributed widely, crosses the placenta, and may enter breast milk. It is highly bound to plasma proteins and concentrates in blood erythrocytes.

Mefloquine is contraindicated in known hypersensitivity. In cases of overwhelming acute *P. falciparum* infections, the patient should receive an IV antimalarial treatment initially, followed by oral mefloquine. Mefloquine is contraindicated for use in patients with seizure disorders or psychiatric disturbances. It also is contraindicated during pregnancy due to its potential teratogenic and embryotoxic effects.

The most common adverse effects to mefloquine when used in suppressive therapy are vomiting, dizziness, syncope, and extrasystoles. When used for acute malaria, the most common symptoms are similar to the disease itself, and include nausea, vomiting, fever, headache, myalgias, and chills. Additional adverse effects include diarrhea, skin rash, abdominal pain, fatigue, loss of appetite, tinnitus, alopecia, sinus bradycardia, and ECG changes. Neuropsychiatric adverse effects include vertigo, visual disturbances, and psychotic manifestations such as hallucinations, nightmares, confusion, anxiety, severe mood swings, and depression.

There are several significant drug-drug interactions with mefloquine. Concurrent use of beta-blockers or quinine can result in ECG abnormalities or cardiac arrest. Coadministration with chloroquine or quinine increases the risk for seizure activity. Concurrent use with valproic acid may decrease valproic acid concentrations, resulting in loss of seizure control.

Primaquine

Primaquine is an 8-aminoquinoline. It is classified as a tissue schizonticide. The exact mechanism of action is uncertain, although it is believed it interferes with the function of plasmodial DNA. Primaquine is the only tissue schizonticide available for the radical cure of *P. vivax* and *P. ovale*. In addition to the destruction of exoerythrocytic (tissue) forms, primaquine prevents the development of erythrocytic (blood) forms, which cause relapses in *P. vivax*. Primaquine also is gametocidal for all four plasmodia species.

Because of its potential toxicity, primaquine is not used as a first-line drug except for chloroquine-resistant malaria. Toxicity may occur when primaquine is given concurrently with other antimalarial drugs such as quinacrine.

Primaquine is contraindicated for patients with known sensitivity. Patients with iodoquinol hypersensitivity may have cross sensitivity to primaquine. It is administered cautiously to African Americans and ethnic groups of the Eastern Mediterranean region where G6PD deficiency is most prevalent due to its association with hematologic effects. Patients with preexisting hematologic conditions are at risk for developing hemolytic anemia and methemoglobinemia.

Symptoms such as dark urine, anorexia, pallor, unusual tiredness or weakness, or back, leg, or abdominal pain may indicate the patient is developing hemolytic anemia. Bluish fingernails, lips, or skin, dizziness, breathing difficulty, or unusual tiredness or weakness may indicate methemoglobinemia. This occurs most frequently with high-dose therapy. Immediate discontinuation of primaquine is necessary if any of these adverse reactions occur.

Pyrimethamine

Pyrimethamine (Daraprim) is a folic acid antagonist that blocks the protozoal enzyme dihydrofolic reductase. This results in a blockage of folic acid metabolism. Like chloroquine and hydroxychloroquine, pyrimethamine is a blood schizonticidal and has some tissue schizonticidal activity. However, its blood schizonticidal activity is slower that that of the 4-aminoquinoline compounds.

Pyrimethamine is used for the prophylaxis of malaria due to susceptible strains of plasmodia. It may be used concurrently with fast-acting antimalarials, such as chloroquine, for transmission control and suppressive care but should not be used alone for an acute attack. In combination with antibiotics, it may be used for acute malaria. In combination with a sulfonamide or clindamycin, it also may be used for toxoplasmosis.

Pyrimethamine is administered orally. Distribution is mainly into kidneys, lungs, liver, and spleen, with concentrations in blood erythrocytes. It crosses the placenta and enters breast milk. Metabolism produces several unidentified metabolites that all are excreted in the urine. Urine excretion of this agent can persist for up to 30 days.

Pyrimethamine should be used cautiously in patients with anemia, folate deficiency, and bone marrow suppression. It is used cautiously for patients with preexisting anemia because folic acid antagonism can potentiate anemias, especially megaloblastic anemia. Bone marrow suppression may result in myelosuppression leading to leukopenia, agranulocytosis, or thrombocytopenia. Some clinicians routinely prescribe folinic acid when treating toxoplasmosis because higher doses of pyrimethamine are necessary. Routine CBCs are also prudent. High doses of pyrimethamine may precipitate seizures.

Pyrimethamine should be used with extreme caution during the first 14 to 16 weeks of pregnancy. Possible interference with folic acid metabolism could cause birth defects. If its use cannot be avoided, concurrent use of folinic acid is recommended. Use during breast-feeding should be avoided as it may interfere with the infant's folic acid metabolism.

Common GI complaints with pyrimethamine include anorexia, nausea, vomiting, abdominal pain, and diarrhea. As with other antimalarials, taking the medication with food may decrease these symptoms.

Potential dermatologic reactions include urticaria, toxic epidermal necrolysis, exfoliative dermatitis, and Stevens-Johnson syndrome. Pyrimethamine should be discontinued at the first sign of rash.

CNS effects related to pyrimethamine therapy include weakness, ataxia, tremor, and, rarely, respiratory failure. In those patients with preexisting seizure disorders, pyrimethamine may precipitate seizures, especially in patients on high-dose therapy.

Drug-drug interactions include other bone marrow depressants or folate antagonists because of the potential for the development of blood dyscrasias. Bone marrow depression may be more likely to occur with sulfonamide combination therapy. Other drugs that can interact with pyrimethamine in this manner include carbamazepine, clozapine, chloramphenicol, phenothiazines, procainamide, antiretroviral agents, antineoplastic agents, or antithyroid agents. Folic acid (vitamin B_9) can interfere with the action of pyrimethamine and therefore, should not be used concomitantly with pyrimethamine.

Quinine Sulfate

Quinine sulfate has been used in the treatment of malaria for 170 years. Quinine is significantly more toxic than chloroquine. It is active against the asexual erythrocytic forms of *Plasmodium*. It does not provide a radical cure for malaria because it is not effective against exoerythrocytic forms of malaria.

Although the exact mechanism of action is unknown, quinine elevates the pH of parasitic acid vesicles and may upset molecular transport and phospholipase activity. Quinine is administered orally and distributes widely into liver, lungs, kidneys, and spleen, with some distribution into the cerebrospinal fluid (CSF). Although it crosses the placenta and enters breast milk, the American Academy of Pediatrics considers quinine compatible with breast-feeding.

Quinine should not be used for patients with a known allergy to quinidine. Patients with quinidine hypersensitivity may have cross sensitivity to quinine. Quinine is classified as pregnancy category X. Quinine can cause congenital malformation and has been associated with stillbirths. In addition to the potential effects on the fetus, quinine stimulates the release of insulin and may induce hypoglycemia in pregnant women.

Quinine should not be used for patients with optic neuritis or tinnitus because it can exacerbate these conditions. Even at therapeutic dosages, quinine may cause cinchonism (tinnitus, headache, nausea, vertigo, and vision impairment).

Quinine should be used cautiously for patients with a deficiency of glucose-6-phosphotate dehydrogenase (G6PD), or those with myasthenia gravis, or cardiac arrhythmias. Patients with G6PD deficiency have a higher risk of developing hemolytic anemia. Quinine produces neuromuscular blockade exacerbating muscular weakness and can cause respiratory distress and dysphagia in myasthenic patients. Patients with cardiac arrhythmias may be at risk of developing quinine-induced dysrhythmias. Patients treated with quinine have shown prolonged Q-T intervals.

Quinine has several important drug-drug interactions. High doses of quinine can affect the clearance of digitalis glycosides and require dosage adjustment to avoid digoxin toxicity.

Alkalinization of the urine by acetazolamide can decrease the renal clearance of quinine resulting in an increased risk of toxicity. Conversely, rifampin has been shown to significantly accelerate quinine clearance and reduce its half-life. Higher doses of quinine may be required in patients receiving rifampin.

Quinine can increase the hypoprothrombinemic effects of warfarin. The patient should have close monitoring for signs and symptoms of bleeding. Additionally, the possibility of cinchonism is increased if quinine and quinidine are administered concomitantly.

Finally, quinine should not be used concomitantly with mefloquine because additive cardiac effects can produce arrhythmias and seizures.

DRUGS SIGNIFICANTLY DIFFERENT FROM CHLOROQUINE

Antibacterials

A different drug class altogether, antibacterial drugs are used in conjunction with antimalarial drugs to treat malaria. Tetracycline and doxycycline are used to eradicate *Plasmodium* in the erythrocytic stage. They are not considered first-line drugs because they work very slowly. Tetracycline is used in conjunction with quinine in the treatment of *P. falciparum*. Doxycycline is an alternative regimen for *P. falciparum* prophylaxis in patients who cannot tolerate mefloquine. It is not used in the treatment of acute malaria. Clindamycin also is used to eradicate plasmodium in the erythrocytic stage. Like tetracycline, it is used in conjunction with quinine in the treatment of *P. falciparum*. These three drugs are discussed in Chapter 49.

Sulfonamides

Sulfonamides also are used in the management of malaria. They are generally combined with pyrimethamine. The most common drug combination is pyrimethamine and sulfadoxine (Fansidar). Fansidar is given concurrently with quinine to treat chloroquine-resistant *P. falciparum*. Sulfonamides are discussed in Chapter 50.

Atovaquone/proguanil

Malarone is the trade name for a combination of atovaquone and proguanil hydrochloride. Atovaquone is currently marketed in the United States under the trade name Mepron for PCP. Proguanil was approved in the United States in 1948 for use in malaria. Because it was not widely used in this country, it ceased to be marketed here in the 1970s. The advantage of Malarone is that it is effective in regions where resistance to other antimalarial drugs has developed. Another unique feature of Malarone is that is is not metabolized. It is eliminated by biliary excretion.

Malarone therapy should be started 1 or 2 days before entering a malaria-endemic area and continued daily during the stay and for 7 days after return. It should be taken at the same time each day with food or milk to increase its bioavailability. In the event of vomiting, a repeat dose should be taken within 1 hour of dosing.

Among adults who received Malarone for treatment of malaria, the side effects included abdominal pain, nausea, vomiting, and headache. Among pediatric patients, vomiting and itching were reported adverse reactions. In study subjects given Malarone for prevention of malaria, the most commonly reported side effects were headache and abdominal pain.

ANTIPROTOZOAN DRUGS

Antiprotozoan drugs treat many human infections, including amebiasis, giardiasis, trichomoniasis, toxoplasmosis, and opportunistic infections such as PCP. The most frequently used drugs are metronidazole, iodoquinol, quinacrine hydrochloride, pentamidine, and atovaquone. Some drugs are effective for many types of infections, whereas others are effective for only one or two types of infections (see the accompanying display, Drugs Used for Protozoan Infections). Because of the increase in protozoan infections in the United States, many new antiprotozoan drugs are being developed. Investigational drugs such as albendazole, diloxaride furoate, and dehydroemetine are obtainable only from the Centers for Disease Control and Prevention (CDC) in Atlanta, Georgia.

DRUGS AFFECTING AMEBIASIS, GIARDIASIS, TRICHOMONIASIS, AND TOXOPLASMOSIS

Metronidazole is the prototype antiprotozoan drug for treating amebiasis, giardiasis, and trichomoniasis. In addition to its antiprotozoan effects, metronidazole has antibacterial effects and is extremely effective against the anaerobic bacteria that cause intra-abdominal infections and *Helicobacter pylori*, which is a cause of peptic ulcer disease.

NURSING MANAGEMENT OF THE PATIENT RECEIVING METRONIDAZOLE

Core Drug Knowledge

Pharmacotherapeutics

Metronidazole (Flagyl) is a synthetic antibacterial and antiprotozoan drug. As an antiprotozoan drug, it is used in treating *T. vaginalis*, amebiasis, and giardiasis. As an antibacterial drug, it is extremely effective against anaerobic infections. It also is useful in treating Crohn disease, antibiotic-associated diarrhea, and rosacea.

Pharmacokinetics

Metronidazole can be administered orally, IV, and topically. About 90% of metronidazole is absorbed orally, with food delaying but not interfering with absorption. Minimal amounts of metronidazole are absorbed systemically when used as an intravaginal drug. Both IV and oral metronidazole are distributed widely into most body tissues and fluids, including CSF. Metronidazole is metabolized in the liver. It crosses the placenta and enters breast milk (Table 55-3).

Pharmacodynamics

There are no direct effects on the human body. Metronidazole is taken up readily by anaerobic organisms and cells. Its selectivity for anaerobic bacteria results from the ability of these organisms to reduce metronidazole to its active form intracellularly because the electron transport proteins necessary for this reaction are found only in anaerobic bacteria. Metronidazole acts against anaerobic bacteria by inhibiting DNA synthesis, which causes bacterial cell death.

Contraindications and Precautions

Major precautions are taken when using metronidazole in patients who are alcohol dependent or pregnant. Metronidazole enters fetal circulation rapidly. A theoretical risk remains for the fetus. Most prescribers prefer to postpone using metronidazole until after the first trimester.

Because of the capacity for a disulfiram-like (i.e., nausea, vomiting, headache, and chest pain) interaction, ingestion of metronidazole and alcohol should be separated by at least 1 day. Patients with hepatic dysfunction should be monitored for toxicity resulting from decreased clearance and possible accumulation of metronidazole. Dosage reduction may be necessary for patients with severe hepatic dysfunction. Because metronidazole can cause leukopenia, the drug should be used with caution in patients with active or previous bone marrow depression.

Adverse Effects

The most frequent adverse effects to metronidazole are nausea and vomiting, dry mouth (xerostomia), altered sense of taste (dysgeusia), anorexia, and abdominal pain. Other consequences of xerostomia include periodontal disease and dental caries. Some patients report discolored urine (reddish brown) while taking metronidazole.

Intravenous metronidazole contains 28 mEq of sodium per gram of metronidazole. This may promote water retention and exacerbate preexisting congestive heart failure (CHF) or peripheral edema. Oral pre-

Drugs Used for Protozoan Infections

Amebiasis: metronidazole, iodoquinol, paromomycin, diloxanide furoate, chloroquine
Giardiasis: metronidazole, quinacrine
Pneumocytosis: pentamidine, atovaquone, sulfamethoxazole-trimethoprim
Schistosomiasis: praziquantel, oxamniquine, metrifonate
Toxoplasmosis: metronidazole, pyrimethamine with sulfonamides
Trichomoniasis: metronidazole

TABLE 55-3 Summary of Selected Antiprotozoan Drugs

Drug (Trade) Name	Selected Indications	Route and Dosage Range	Pharmacokinetics
metronidazole (Flagyl; *Canadian:* Apo-Metronidazole)	Anaerobic bacterial infection	*Adult:* IV, 15 mg/kg infused over 1 h, then 7.5 mg/kg infused over 1 h every 6 h for 7–10 d; not to exceed 4 g/d *Child:* IV, not recommended	*Onset:* PO, varies; IV, rapid *Duration:* Variable $t_{1/2}$: 6–8 h
	Amebiasis	*Adult:* PO, 750 mg tid for 5–10 d *Child:* PO, 35–50 mg/kg in three divided doses for 10 d	
	Trichomoniasis	*Adult:* PO, 2 g at one time for 250 mg tid for 7–10 d	
	Bacterial prophylaxis	*Adult:* IV, 15 mg/kg infused over 30–60 min and completed about 1 h before surgery, then 7.5 mg/kg infused over 30–60 min at 6 to 12-h intervals after initial dose during the day of surgery	
	Gardnerella vaginalis	*Adult:* PO, 500 mg bid for 7 d	
	Antibiotic-associated pseudomembranous colitis	*Adult:* PO, 1–2 g/d for 7–10 d	
	Inflammatory papules, pustules, and erythema of rosacea	*Adult:* Topical, apply and rub in a thin film twice daily, morning and evening, to entire affected areas after washing *Adult and child:* IM/IV, 4 mg/kg once a day for 14 d by deep IM injection or IV infusion over 60 min *Adult and child:* Inhalational, 300 mg once every 4 wk administered by nebulizer (e.g., Respirgard II)	
pentamidine (NebuPent, Pentam 300; *Canadian:* Pentacarinate)	PCP	*Adult and child:* Inhalational, 300 mg once every 4 wk with Respirgard nebulizer; IM/IV 4 mg/kg once daily for 14 d by deep IM injection or IV infusion over 60 min	*Onset:* Inhalation, rapid; IM, slow *Duration:* 6–8 wk $t_{1/2}$: 6.5–9.5 h
atovaquone (Mepron)	PCP	*Adult:* PO, 750 mg, tid for 21 d	*Onset:* Varies *Duration:* 3–5 d $t_{1/2}$: 2–3 d
iodoquinol (Yodoxin; *Canadian:* Diodoxaquin)	Amebiasis	*Adult:* PO, 650 mg tid before meals for 20 d *Child:* PO, 40 mg/kg/d in three divided doses before meals for 20 d, not to exceed 1.95 g/d	*Onset:* Minimal absorption *Duration:* Unknown $t_{1/2}$: Unknown
quinacrine (Atabrine)	Malaria	*Adult and children* (>8 y): PO, 200 mg with 1 g sodium bicarbonate every 6 h for 5 doses; then 100 mg every 8 h for 6 d. The maximum dose is 2.8 g in 7 d *Children* (4–8 y): PO, 200 mg every 8 h; then 100 mg every 12 h for 6 d *Children* (1–4 y): PO, 100 mg every 8 h; then 100 mg daily for 6 d	*Onset:* Unknown *Duration:* 4–6 wk $t_{1/2}$: 5 d
	Giardiasis	*Adult:* PO, 100 mg tid for 5–7 d *Child:* PO, 7 mg/kg/d in 3 divided doses for 5 d	
quinacrine	Cestodiasis	*Adults and children* (>14 y): PO, 4 doses of 200 mg given 10 min apart with 600 mg of sodium bicarbonate given with each dose *Children* (11–14 y): PO, 600 mg in 3–4 divided doses given 10 min apart with 300 mg of sodium bicarbonate given with each dose *Children:* (5–10 y): PO, 400 mg in 3–4 divided doses given 10 min apart with 300 mg of sodium bicarbonate given with each dose	

parations of metronidazole do not contain this large amount of sodium and can be used without jeopardy.

Other frequent adverse effects include CNS effects, such as dizziness, light-headedness, and headache. CNS toxicity has occurred and is exhibited as ataxia, mood changes, encephalopathy, or clumsiness. High dosages and prolonged use of metronidazole are associated with peripheral neuropathy and seizures.

As noted previously, patients receiving metronidazole and drinking alcoholic beverages may experience disulfiram-like adverse effects. The flavor of alcoholic beverages also may be altered as well.

Vaginal candidiasis occurs in some women because metronidazole can suppress natural bacteria, leading to an overgrowth of *Candida* organisms. Candidal overgrowth may also occur in the mouth. Symptoms include glossitis, stomatitis, and furry tongue.

Thrombophlebitis can occur from IV metronidazole and is characterized as pain, redness, and swelling at the injection site. The potential for this adverse effect can be minimized by avoiding prolonged use of indwelling IV catheters.

Less common potential adverse effects include visual impairment, photophobia, and ocular motility disorders. Rare reports of optic neuritis have occurred. Additionally, using metronidazole may lead to blood dyscrasias and leukopenia. Pancreatitis is another serious, but rare, adverse reaction.

Drug Interactions

As mentioned, metronidazole interferes with the metabolism of ethanol (alcohol) resulting in disulfiram-like effects, such as nausea, vomiting, and abdominal cramps. Patients taking disulfiram have reported psychotic reactions with concomitant use of metronidazole. Metronidazole may interact with barbiturates, anticoagulants, ethanol, and disulfiram (Table 55-4).

Assessment of Relevant Core Patient Variables

Health Status

Before administering metronidazole, the nurse should assess the patient for potential medical conditions that contraindicate or require close monitoring, such as alcoholism, cardiac disease, dental disease, hepatic disease, seizure disorders, and bone marrow depression.

A baseline neurologic assessment should be performed because metronidazole may cause CNS toxicity or exacerbate peripheral neuropathy and seizure disorders. In addition, a baseline visual acuity assessment may be needed. Other important assessments include liver function tests, because metronidazole is metabolized in the liver, and a complete blood count (CBC), particularly for patients with a history of bone marrow depression or severe anemia. The patient's drug history needs to be reviewed to identify drugs that may interact with metronidazole.

Life Span and Gender

The nurse should assess women for possible pregnancy because metronidazole is not recommended in the first trimester. Metronidazole enters breast milk and is not recommended for use in children or infants.

Lifestyle, Diet, and Habits

It is important to determine the patient's typical intake of alcohol. Patients should be cautioned to refrain from alcohol ingestion for 48 hours after completing metronidazole therapy. They should also be reminded that many OTC products contain alcohol, so they should

TABLE 55-4 Agents That Interact With Metronidazole

Interactants	Effect and Significance	Nursing Management
anticoagulants	Hepatic metabolism of anticoagulants may be decreased by metronidazole, resulting in enhanced effects of the anticoagulant. This may induce hemorrhage.	Monitor patients more frequently, and teach them to recognize signs and symptoms of bleeding. Notify the prescriber who may need to prescribe a lower dose of anticoagulant.
barbiturates	Barbiturates may induce a faster elimination of metronidazole, resulting in therapeutic failure of metronidazole.	Observe for treatment failure in patients receiving a barbiturate concurrently with metronidazole. If necessary, the metronidazole dose may need to be increased accordingly. Alternatively, the prescriber may order a higher initial metronidazole dose.
disulfiram	The coadministration of disulfiram and metronidazole may result in an acute psychosis or confusional state. The mechanism of the interaction is unclear.	Monitor patients closely for signs of confusion. Discontinue both agents if symptoms occur. Avoid coadministration.
ethanol	Metronidazole can inhibit alcohol dehydrogenase and other alcohol-metabolizing enzymes. This can lead to an accumulation of drug in the blood and the development of disulfiram-like side effects.	Caution patient to avoid ethanol during therapy and 1–2 d after therapy stops.

avoid taking OTC drugs without consulting their health care provider.

Environment

The nurse should be aware of the setting in which metronidazole will be administered. Hospitalized patients usually receive metronidazole by IV infusion. The nurse should monitor the patient's cardiovascular and respiratory status frequently because IV metronidazole may promote fluid retention, leading to an exacerbation of CHF or peripheral edema. The nurse also needs to monitor the IV site frequently for signs of thrombophlebitis.

Nursing Diagnoses and Outcomes

- Risk for Deficient Fluid Volume: Anorexia, nausea, vomiting, and diarrhea related to drug administration
  Desired outcome: The patient will maintain adequate hydration throughout therapy.
- Risk for Disturbed Sensory Perception: Drug-induced dizziness, vertigo, syncope, and ataxia
  Desired outcome: The patient will compensate for sensory-perceptual disturbances by moving slowly and carefully to prevent accidents and asking for help with ambulation as needed.
- Disturbed Thought Processes: Acute confusional state related to potential disulfiram-like interaction
  Desired outcome: The patient will refrain from alcohol consumption for 48 hours after completing drug therapy.
- Risk for Injury: Potential teratogenic effects related to drug administration
  Desired outcome: The patient will act to prevent conception while taking metronidazole.

Planning and Intervention

Maximizing Therapeutic Effects

To avoid reinfection, patients taking metronidazole for *Trichomonas* infection need to understand that a sexual partner must be treated at the same time. To avoid early cessation of therapy, advise the patient that the drug may discolor the urine and reassure the patient this discoloration is harmless.

Minimizing Adverse Effects

Because some patients will downplay their intake of ethanol or neglect to mention they take disulfiram because of the social stigma attached to alcoholism, the nurse needs to emphasize the importance of potential adverse effects resulting from the interaction of ethanol and metronidazole.

To minimize possible GI irritation, metronidazole may be administered with meals. Patients who experience dry mouth can use sugar-free hard candies or ice chips to moisten the mouth. Sugar-containing products tend to promote dental caries in an environment that is already friendly to decay-causing organisms. IV metronidazole needs to be infused slowly over 1 hour.

Providing Patient and Family Education

- The nurse should create teaching plans that focus on explaining the potential adverse effects (e.g., GI upset, altered taste, discolored urine), adapting to adverse effects (taking drug with meals to relieve GI upset), and identifying which effects to report to the health care provider. For example, candidal overgrowth, ataxia, easy bruising or bleeding may represent adverse effects that require immediate intervention.
- The nurse must discuss the importance of refraining from ethanol or disulfiram during metronidazole therapy.
- The importance of sex partners being treated simultaneously for trichomonal infections must be stressed, as should the importance of follow-up stool examinations for patients taking metronidazole for giardiasis.
- The nurse should emphasize the need for birth control measures for women on long-term therapy.

Ongoing Assessment and Evaluation

When administering intravenous metronidazole, the nurse needs to monitor for thrombophlebitis and signs of edema or CHF. When administering oral metronidazole, the nurse should monitor all patients for oral candidiasis (white spots in the mouth), and women for symptoms of vaginal candidiasis.

Additional evaluative assessments include monitoring for signs and symptoms of peripheral neuropathy (numbness and tingling of the extremities) and CNS toxicity (mood changes and irritability).

For patients on prolonged therapy, the nurse should arrange for periodic CBCs and liver function tests, as well as tests for visual acuity. The nurse should remind the patient to schedule frequent dental checkups.

For patients with giardiasis, the nurse should arrange testing three stool specimens, taken several days apart. Three negative stool test results indicate success of metronidazole therapy. ■

DRUGS SIGNIFICANTLY DIFFERENT FROM METRONIDAZOLE

Iodoquinol

Iodoquinol (Yodoxin) is an oral antiprotozoan agent used in the treatment of intestinal amebiasis by exerting its action directly in the large intestine, although the exact mechanism of action in unknown. Iodoquinol is active against both the trophozoite and encysted forms of the parasite. It can be used alone in mild cases or in asymptomatic carriers. In more severe cases, it should be used in combination with other amebicidal drugs.

MEMORY CHIP

Metronidazole

- Used for *Trichomonas vaginalis*, amebiasis, giardiasis, and anaerobic infections
- Significant contraindications: alcohol dependency and pregnancy
- Most common adverse effects: nausea, vomiting, xerostomia, and dysgeusia
- Most serious adverse effect: blood dyscrasias
- Maximizing therapeutic effects: treat both partners at the same time
- Minimizing adverse effects: assess alcohol intake closely
- Most significant patient education: reinforce the need to refrain from alcohol intake during therapy

Adverse effects associated with iodoquinol include mild GI disturbances, skin disorders, discoloration of hair and nails, thyroid enlargement, fever, chills, headache, vertigo, and malaise. Neurotoxicity from iodoquinol may induce optic neuritis, optic atrophy, and peripheral neuropathy.

Protein-bound serum iodine levels may increase during iodoquinol treatment and therefore interfere with certain thyroid function tests. These effects may persist for up to 6 months after therapy discontinues.

Paromomycin

Paromomycin (Humatin) is not an antiprotozoan drug; it is an aminoglycoside antibiotic with broad-spectrum antibacterial and amebicidal activity. Paromomycin is used for extraintestinal amebiasis and tapeworm infestation. It is absorbed poorly from the GI tract and thus is used only for intestinal forms of amebiasis and helminths.

Adverse GI effects of paromomycin include anorexia, nausea, vomiting, gastric burning and pain, abdominal cramps, and diarrhea. The only significant drug-drug interaction with paromomycin is succinylcholine. When given in combination, paromomycin may potentiate the neuromuscular effects of succinylcholine.

Quinacrine

Quinacrine (Atabrine) is an oral antiprotozoan agent used most commonly in the treatment of giardiasis. It also has been used in the treatment of malaria and cestodiasis, although more efficacious drugs are currently used for those disorders. Quinacrine is absorbed readily from the GI tract and concentrates primarily in the liver. Quinacrine is metabolized and excreted slowly. It may be detected in the urine up to 2 months after therapy has been discontinued.

Due to high concentrations of quinacrine in the liver, it should be used with caution in patients with hepatic disease, other hepatotoxic drugs, or alcoholism. Quinacrine should be used with caution in patients with psoriasis and porphyria because it can exacerbate these conditions. Quinacrine should be administered with caution to patients with renal disease with severe renal impairment, cardiac disease, G6PD deficiency, or to infants (younger than 1 year). Quinacrine should be used with caution in patients with a history of psychosis or in patients over the age of 60 years because the drug can cause a transient psychosis. Other potential neuropsychiatric disturbances include nightmares, restlessness, confusion, anxiety, irritability, euphoria, aggressive behavior, nervousness, and emotional change.

When small doses of quinacrine are taken, potential adverse effects include mild headache, dizziness, and GI disturbances. Large doses of quinacrine can produce adverse effects such as severe headache and GI disturbances including nausea and vomiting, abdominal pain or cramps, and mild diarrhea. Other adverse side effects during therapy with quinacrine include blood dyscrasias, hepatitis (and elevated hepatic enzymes), aplastic anemia, pancytopenia, fainting, seizures, and retinopathy.

Quinacrine may induce integumentary adverse effects such as urticaria, black and blue skin and nail discoloration, exfoliative dermatitis, and contact dermatitis. It temporarily imparts a yellow color to the urine and skin.

Quinacrine may potentiate the toxicity of aminoquinolines such as primaquine and chloroquine. Quinacrine is metabolized extensively in the liver. Therefore, it should be given cautiously with other drugs that may induce hepatotoxicity, such as acetaminophen.

DRUGS AFFECTING *PNEUMOCYSTIS CARINII* PNEUMONIA

Drugs used to treat PCP include pentamidine isethionate, atovaquone, and sulfamethoxazole-trimethoprim (SMZ-TMP). SMZ-TMP is not an antiprotozoan drug, but an antibiotic that is covered in Chapter 50. Patients at high risk for PCP (low T-cell count or high viral load count) and those unable to take SMZ-TMP (also known as cotrimoxazole) should be maintained on a prophylactic dosage of pentamidine. Atovaquone is used for treating acute PCP infection. The prototype antiprotozoan drug for prophylaxis and treatment of PCP is pentamidine isethionate.

NURSING MANAGEMENT OF THE PATIENT RECEIVING PENTAMIDINE ISETHIONATE

Core Drug Knowledge

Pharmacotherapeutics

Historically, pentamidine (Pentam 300) was used only for trypanosomiasis (African sleeping sickness) and leishmaniasis. Currently, pentamidine is an important therapeutic drug for prophylaxis and treatment of PCP.

Pharmacokinetics

Pentamidine is absorbed readily and binds to body tissues. It is sequestered in the liver and kidney and eliminated unchanged by the kidneys. Pentamidine can be detected in the urine up to 8 weeks after therapy has ended (see Table 55-3).

Pharmacodynamics

Pentamidine is administered by inhalation or parenterally. Its action is unclear but appears to interfere with nucleotide, phospholipid, and protein synthesis of the parasite. It causes local tissue damage when given IM. Therefore, it usually is given IV. For prophylaxis, pentamidine is delivered by inhalation through an aerosol device to the alveoli where *P. carinii* lodges.

Contraindications and Precautions

Pentamidine is contraindicated for use in patients with a history of an anaphylactic reaction to it. However, once the diagnosis of PCP is established, there are no absolute contraindications. The drug is given with caution to patients with asthma; hematologic disorders; cardiac, hepatic, and renal diseases; and diabetes mellitus.

Adverse Effects

Sudden severe effects may develop after a single dose of pentamidine. Patients should be lying down and monitored closely during administration. Equipment for emergency resuscitation should be readily available.

The most frequent adverse effects from pentamidine are cough and bronchospasm, especially in patients with asthma. Another frequent adverse reaction to pentamidine is a sudden, severe hypotension.

Thrombocytopenia, leukopenia, or anemia are potential hematologic problems; arrhythmias, tachycardia, torsades de pointes, or other adverse cardiac effects may occur as well. Pentamidine is toxic to pancreatic cells. After receiving IV pentamidine, patients with diabetes mellitus can become acutely hypoglycemic immediately after the infusion. Additionally, pentamidine may precipitate pancreatitis. Pentamidine also can cause elevations in aspartate transaminase (AST), alanine transaminase (ALT), bilirubin, and alkaline phosphatase. Patients with preexisting hepatic diseases are more vulnerable to these effects. Pentamidine can cause azotemia or acute renal insufficiency as well.

Drug Interactions

Concomitant use of other drugs associated with bone marrow suppression, electrolyte imbalance, pancreatitis, or nephrotoxicity may cause additive effects. Pentamidine also may interact with drugs that have similar adverse effects (Table 55-5).

Assessment of Relevant Core Patient Variables

Health Status

The nurse should assess for concurrent drug use that is potentially nephrotoxic. Baseline measurements should

TABLE 55-5 Agents That Interact With Pentamidine

Interactants	Effect and Significance	Nursing Management
Bone Marrow Suppressants		
antineoplastic agents azathioprine carbamazepine clozapine cotrimoxazole phenothiazines zidovudine	Concomitant use of bone marrow suppressants and pentamidine has the potential to cause additive hemotoxicity.	Monitor for sore throat, easy bruising, or bleeding. Monitor CBC and platelet counts.
Diuretics		
loop diuretics thiazide diuretics	Diuretics and pentamidine can produce similar toxicities.	Monitor for hypokalemia, hypomagnesemia, and pancreatitis. Monitor serum electrolyte and amylase levels.
Drugs That May Cause Nephrotoxicity		
aminoglycosides amphotericin B cyclosporine vancomycin	Drugs associated with nephrotoxicity and pentamidine have the potential for causing additive renal toxicity.	Monitor for nephrotoxicity, hypokalemia, hypomagnesemia, and bone marrow depression.
Drugs That May Cause Pancreatitis		
azathioprine didanosine estrogens furosemide tetracycline valproic acid	Drugs associated with pancreatitis and pentamidine have the potential for causing additive pancreatic toxicity.	Monitor for signs of pancreatitis. Monitor amylase levels.

be obtained and then reviewed. These include vital signs (especially blood pressure), CBC, hepatic and renal function values, and glucose and amylase levels.

Administration of aerosolized pentamidine to patients with a history of asthma should be closely monitored because the drug may induce bronchospasm and acute asthma.

Lifestyle, Diet, and Habits

It is important to assess lifestyle because patients at risk for PCP and diseases associated with compromised immune function include IV drug abusers, men who have sex with men, and people with multiple sex partners. Immunocompromised patients may be taking multiple drugs, placing them at risk for potential hematologic, renal, and hepatic toxicities. Because pentamidine also may affect these systems, patients should be monitored closely for adverse effects.

Environment

The nurse should note the environment in which pentamidine will be administered. Many patients receive IV or aerosolized pentamidine therapy at home.

Nursing Diagnoses and Outcomes

- Altered Protection: Risk for drug induced leukopenia, thrombocytopenia, and anemia
  Desired outcome: The patient will report any signs and symptoms of blood abnormalities (i.e., unusual fatigue, fever and infection, and bruising).
- Risk for Deficient Fluid Volume related to drug-induced nausea, vomiting, and anorexia
  Desired outcome: The patient will remain adequately hydrated throughout therapy.
- Risk for Injury: Hypoglycemia, hyperglycemia, or acute renal failure related to drug therapy and bronchospasm, cough, hypotension, or cardiovascular complications related to drug administration
  Desired outcome: The patient will remain free of injury or complications related to pentamidine administration.

Planning and Intervention

Maximizing Therapeutic Effects

Intravenous pentamidine should be protected from the light and used within 24 hours of preparation. It should not be mixed with other drugs because of incompatibilities, nor should it be mixed with saline solutions because a precipitate will form. When pentamidine is administered by inhalation, a bronchodilator may be given before treatment to reduce bronchospasm and increase drug effectiveness.

Minimizing Adverse Effects

The nurse should administer pentamidine with the patient lying down. Baseline vital signs are obtained initially and monitored continuously during the infusion, and then every 2 hours after the infusion until blood pressure stabilizes. Patients receiving pentamidine should not receive IM injections because they may cause bleeding, bruising, or hematomas due to thrombocytopenia secondary to pentamidine-induced bone marrow depression. Pentamidine should not be administered at bedtime because resultant hypoglycemia may occur when the patient cannot respond to the symptoms.

Appropriate respiratory precautions must be taken to protect health care staff from contact with cough-induced organisms, such as *Mycobacterium*.

Providing Patient and Family Education

- The nurse should make sure that the patient and family understand the therapeutic and adverse effects of pentamidine and the importance of monthly treatments for PCP prophylaxis. In addition, they need to realize that PCP infection is still possible despite pentamidine prophylaxis.
- The nurse should urge the patient to contact the prescriber if fever or respiratory difficulties occur. Other conditions for which the patient should contact the prescriber include nausea, vomiting, or diarrhea that do not subside; persistent urinary frequency, inability to void, continual hunger and thirst, or unexplained weight loss; and abdominal pain, leg cramps, fever, sore throat, unexplained bruising, or extreme fatigue.
- The nurse should emphasize the need for frequent small meals despite the patient's anorexia.

Ongoing Assessment and Evaluation

Care of hospitalized patients includes monitoring blood urea nitrogen, serum creatinine, serum calcium, and blood glucose levels; CBC and platelet counts; and liver function test results (including bilirubin, alkaline phosphatase, AST, and ALT levels) on a daily basis. ECGs should be scheduled at regular intervals throughout therapy. It is important to measure daily fluid intake and output. ■

DRUGS SIGNIFICANTLY DIFFERENT FROM P PENTAMIDINE

Oral atovaquone is indicated for the acute treatment of mild-to-moderate *P. carinii* in patients who are intolerant to cotrimoxazole. Atovaquone is roughly equivalent to IV pentamidine but less effective than cotrimoxazole in the treatment of PCP.

Atovaquone is unique in the management of *P. carinii* because it can kill *Pneumocystis* organisms rather than inhibiting their growth. Besides *Pneumocystis*, atovaquone is active against other protozoans including *Plasmodium* species, *Toxoplasma gondii*, *Entamoeba histolytica*, *Trichomonas vaginalis*, *Leishmania* species, and *Microsporidia*. The antiprotozoan activity of atovaquone is probably related to its

MEMORY CHIP

Pentamidine

- Used for prophylaxis and management of PCP
- Significant contraindication: previous anaphylactic reactions to the drug
- Most common adverse effects: cough and bronchospasm
- Most serious adverse effects: cardiac abnormalities, renal failure, and bone marrow suppression
- Maximizing therapeutic effects: protect from light and administer within 24 hours of preparation
- Minimizing adverse effects: monitor blood pressure throughout administration
- Most significant patient education: contact the health care provider if fever or respiratory difficulties occur; PCP may occur despite prophylactic treatment

ability to selectively inhibit mitochondrial electron transport, leading to inhibition of pyrimidine synthesis.

Atovaquone is absorbed poorly from the GI tract. Because it is a highly lipophilic compound, administering it with a fatty meal will improve its absorption. Because many patients who are treated with atovaquone have advanced HIV, it often is difficult to distinguish adverse effects caused by atovaquone from those caused by underlying medical conditions. At this time, no life-threatening effects are attributable to atovaquone.

ANTHELMINTHIC DRUGS

As discussed previously, helminthic infections result from cestodes, nematodes, and trematodes. The most commonly used anthelminthic drugs are mebendazole, thiabendazole, niclosamide, pyrantel pamoate, diethylcarbamazine, oxamniquine, and praziquantel (see the accompanying display, Which Drug for Which Worm?).

Of all the drugs in the class, the prototype for treating most helminths is mebendazole (Vermox). Mebendazole is indicated for the treatment of cestodes and nematodes, such as pinworm, whipworm, common roundworm, common hookworm, and American hookworm. It also is used for treating enterobiasis. Mebendazole is usually the drug of choice in helminthic infections because of the frequency of mixed infections.

Which Drug for Which Worm?

Most antihelminthic agents are effective against many types of helminths; only a few have limited application. The following helminths are controlled by the following drugs:

- Intestinal nematodes: mebendazole, thiabendazole, albendazole, ivermectin, pyrantel
- Blood and tissue nematodes: diethylcarbamazine, ivermectin
- Trematodes: praziquantel, oxamniquine
- Cestodes: praziquantel, niclosamide

NURSING MANAGEMENT OF THE PATIENT RECEIVING MEBENDAZOLE

Core Drug Knowledge

Pharmacotherapeutics

Mebendazole is an oral, broad-spectrum, synthetic anthelminthic drug. It is particularly effective against susceptible GI nematodes, such as whip worms, pinworms, and hookworms. Along with pyrantel pamoate, it is considered the drug of choice for treating infections caused by these nematodes.

Pharmacokinetics

Mebendazole is absorbed minimally from the GI tract because of significant first-pass metabolism. It is metabolized to an inactive metabolite. Approximately 10% of the drug is excreted unchanged in the urine, and the remainder is excreted in the feces (Table 55-6).

Pharmacodynamics

Direct pharmacodynamics occur in the parasite. Mebendazole is a broad-spectrum anthelmintic available in chewable tablets. It selectively damages cytoplasmic microtubules in the absorptive and intestinal cells of the helminth but not in the host. This microtubular deterioration is irreversible and leads to disruption of absorptive and secretory functions of the cells that are essential to the helminth's survival. Efficacy varies as a function of such factors as preexisting diarrhea and GI transit time, degree of infection, and helminth strains.

Contraindications and Precautions

Mebendazole is contraindicated in patients with hypersensitivity to the drug, and it is used with caution in patients with inflammatory bowel disease, hepatic disease, and during pregnancy, especially in the first trimester. In patients with Crohn disease or ulcerative colitis, drug absorption, and therefore the risk for toxicity, is increased. Mebendazole is metabolized primarily by the liver and can accumulate in patients with hepatic impairment, increasing the risk for adverse effects. Because it is not known whether mebendazole is excreted in breast milk, the drug is used with caution in breast-feeding mothers. It has not been evaluated for use in children younger than 2 years old.

Adverse Effects

Because of its poor absorption, mebendazole rarely causes systemic toxicity, except in patients with diseases that increase absorption of drugs from the bowel. Transient abdominal pain, diarrhea, dizziness, headache, and fever are common. However, these symptoms may result from expulsion of worms rather from the drug. Other reported adverse effects include blood abnormalities, such as leukopenia, thrombocytopenia, and eosinophilia. Integumentary effects include pruritus, rash, and flushing. In the renal system, hematuria and crystalluria are

TABLE 55-6 Summary of Selected Antihelminthic Drugs

Drug (Trade) Name	Selected Indications	Route and Dosage Range	Pharmacokinetics
mebendazole (Vermox)	Trichuriasis, ascariasis, hookworm infections	*Adult:* PO, 100 mg bid for 3 consecutive d *Child:* >2 y, same as adults; <2 y, safety and efficacy not established	*Onset:* Under 2 h *Duration:* 48 h $t_{1/2}$: 3–9 h
	Enterobiasis	*Adult:* PO, 100 mg once; if not cured in 3 wk, a second dose may be given	
diethylcarbamazine (Hetrazan)	Ascariasis	*Adult:* PO, 13 mg/kg/d for 7–10 d *Child:* PO, 6–10 mg/kg tid for 7–10 d	*Onset:* 1 h *Duration:* Variable $t_{1/2}$: 8 h
	Filariasis	*Adult:* PO, 6–10 mg/kg tid pc for 3–4 weeks	
niclosamide (Niclocide)	Beef or fish tapeworm	*Adult:* PO, 2 g as a single dose *Child:* 11–34 kg, PO, 1 g as a single dose; > 34 kg, 1.5 g as a single dose	*Onset:* Minimal absorption *Duration:* Unknown $t_{1/2}$: Unknown
	Dwarf tapeworm	*Adult:* PO, 2 g daily for 7 d *Child:* 11–34 kg, PO, 1 g as a single dose; >34 kg, 1.5 g on day 1, then 1 g for the next 6 d	
oxamniquine (Vancil)	Strains of *S. mansoni*	*Adult:* PO, 12–15 mg/kg as a single dose *Child:* 30–40 kg, PO, 500 mg; 41–60 kg, 750 mg; 61–80 kg, 1,000 mg; 81–100 kg, 1,250 mg	*Onset:* Rapid *Duration:* 24 h $t_{1/2}$: 1–2.5 h
praziquantel (Biltricide)	Schistosomiasis	*Adult:* PO, 60 mg/kg in three equally divided doses as a 1-day treatment with 4–6 h between doses *Child:* Safety and efficacy not established	*Onset:* Rapid *Duration:* Unknown $t_{1/2}$: 0.8–1.5 h
	Clonorchiasis and opisthorchiasis	*Adult:* PO, 75 mg/kg in three equally divided doses as a 1-day treatment *Child:* Safety and efficacy not established	
pyrantel pamoate (Antiminth; *Canadian:* Combantrin)	Pinworm and roundworm infections	*Adult:* PO, 11 mg/kg as a single dose; maximum dose of 1 g *Child:* >2 y, PO, same as adults; <2 y, safety and efficacy not established	*Onset:* Poorly absorbed *Duration:* Unknown $t_{1/2}$: Unknown
thiabendazole (Mintezol)	Enterobiasis	*Adult:* <150 lb and child >30 lb, PO, 10 mg/kg per dose, >150 lb, PO, 1.5 g/dose; maximum daily dose, 3 g two doses/day for 1 d; repeat in 7 d to reduce risk of reinfection	*Onset:* Rapid *Duration:* 24 h $t_{1/2}$: 1.2 h

possible. In addition, mebendazole may elevate liver enzyme levels.

Drug Interactions

Mebendazole may interact with anticonvulsant drugs, such as carbamazepine and the hydantoins. Although the mechanism of interaction is unknown, the pharmacologic effects may be decreased, resulting in failure to eradicate the helminth. However, no special precautions appear necessary. If an interaction is suspected, dosage may need increasing.

Assessment of Relevant Core Patient Variables

Health Status

The nurse must assess the patient for potential medical conditions that contraindicate or require close monitoring during therapy. Additional assessments should be made to prepare for potential drug interactions. Helminth specimens should be collected to ensure that mebendazole is therapeutic. A baseline CBC is needed because mebendazole may cause blood abnormalities.

Patients with a history of Crohn disease or ulcerative colitis should be monitored closely. Patients in whom the bowel lumen is no longer intact may absorb mebendazole in toxic quantities.

Life Span and Gender

The nurse should assess for pregnancy, lactation, and the age of the patient before administering mebendazole. Laboratory studies show that even one dose of mebendazole is teratogenic and embryotoxic. Therefore, it should not be given during pregnancy. Because it has not been adequately tested in children younger than 2 years of age, it should not be given to them nor to breastfeeding women.

Environment

The nurse should evaluate the patient's close contacts because helminthic infections are highly contagious. Ideally, all family members are treated simultaneously, and care is taken to disinfect clothing and bedding.

Nursing Diagnoses and Outcomes

- Acute Pain related to headache, abdominal discomfort, rash, and perianal itching from drug therapy
  Desired outcome: The patient will adopt measures to help tolerate therapy, including taking acetaminophen for headache and taking with food if GI distress occurs.
- Risk for Deficient Fluid Volume related to drug-induced diarrhea
  Desired outcome: Unless contraindicated, the patient will maintain fluid intake to prevent dehydration.

Planning and Intervention

Maximizing Therapeutic Effects

Anthelminthic tablets may be crushed and mixed with applesauce or other food. Chewing the drug offers the greatest effectiveness as does taking the drug with fatty foods, such as milk, cheese, or ice cream. All family members and close patient contacts should be treated at the same time to avoid reinfection.

Minimizing Adverse Effects

Mebendazole may be given with small, frequent meals if GI distress occurs. The nurse can recommend soothing oatmeal baths to relieve pruritus or rash because antihistamines are not effective. Relaxation techniques or acetaminophen may be used to manage headaches or constant distress. Unless contraindicated, fluid intake may be increased to at least eight 8-oz glasses of fluid daily to minimize the potential for crystalluria.

Providing Patient and Family Education

- The nurse should provide information about potential adverse drug effects, such as anemia and other blood problems signaled by sore throat, fever, and fatigue. In addition, the importance of contacting the prescriber if serious adverse effects occur should be stressed. The nurse can explain that minor adverse effects, such as itching, may be relieved with oatmeal baths.
- The nurse should urge the patient to follow the instructions of the prescriber; printed directions may be given if appropriate.
- To prevent treatment failure, the nurse should encourage the patient to complete the full course of drug therapy.
- To prevent future infections, the nurse should urge the patient to wear shoes and wash all fruits and vegetables well before eating. Moreover, it is important to teach the patient about hygiene (e.g., laundering infested bedclothes and undergarments daily) and other measures that help to prevent reinfection.

Ongoing Assessment and Evaluation

Evaluation of nursing care includes monitoring for eradication of the helminth and for complications of therapy, such as dehydration in instances of severe nausea and vomiting; sore throat, fever, and easy bruising; and hematuria or crystalluria. Periodic CBC counts and liver function tests should be performed for patients at risk for hematologic or hepatic effects and for patients on long-term therapy. ■

DRUGS CLOSELY RELATED TO MEBENDAZOLE

Albendazole

Albendazole (Albenza) is not available routinely in the United States and is not approved by the Food and Drug Administration. However, it can be obtained from the CDC in Atlanta. It is well absorbed from the GI tract and relatively free of adverse effects. Like mebendazole, it is teratogenic and has not been tested for use in children. In most clinical trials, it has been shown to be more efficacious than mebendazole in treating intestinal and systemic nematodes. In limited trials, it has been effective against systemic cestode infections, which have been historically refractory to chemotherapy.

Thiabendazole

Thiabendazole (Mintezol) is a vermicidal drug related structurally to mebendazole. It has more limited usefulness than mebendazole because of its potential toxicity. The precise mechanism of action is not clear. It inhibits specific enzymes in the helminth and is used to treat pinworm, roundworm,

MEMORY CHIP

Mebendazole

- Used for management of helminthic infections
- Significant contraindication: hypersensitivity
- Most common adverse effects: abdominal pain, diarrhea, dizziness, and headache
- Most serious adverse effect: blood dyscrasias
- Maximizing therapeutic effects: treat all family members at the same time
- Minimizing adverse effects: small frequent meals to decrease GI effects
- Most significant patient education: wash all clothing and bed linens at the same time the whole family is being treated

threadworm, and hookworm infections. It is the drug of choice for strongyloidiasis.

Because thiabendazole is better absorbed from the bowel, adverse effects are more common than with mebendazole. It is used with caution in children weighing less than 15 kg, in patients with hepatic or renal dysfunction, and in patients with severe dehydration, malnutrition, or anemia.

DRUGS SIGNIFICANTLY DIFFERENT FROM MEBENDAZOLE

Pyrantel Pamoate

Like mebendazole, pyrantel pamoate (Antiminth) is used to treat pinworm and roundworm infections. Unlike mebendazole, pyrantel pamoate exhibits a selective depolarizing neuromuscular blocking action. This results in spastic paralysis of worms.

Pyrantel is administered as an oral suspension that is absorbed poorly from the GI tract. Because of its poor absorption, it is well tolerated by patients older than 2 years. It is metabolized in the liver and excreted mainly in feces and secondarily in urine.

Pyrantel is used with caution in patients who have liver dysfunction, anemia, or both and in patients who are malnourished or dehydrated. Its safety has not been proved during pregnancy nor for children younger than 2 years of age. Pyrantel and piperazine are mutually antagonistic and should not be given together.

Piperazine

Another drug used in treating roundworms and pinworms is piperazine. It differs from mebendazole in its mechanism of action, working by hyperpolarization of the parasite's membranes, which produces flaccid paralysis. The parasites are not killed by the drug but are expelled from the host by normal peristalsis.

Also unlike mebendazole, piperazine may be used during pregnancy. However, it has the potential for producing neurotoxicity and is contraindicated in patients who have seizures. It is an antagonist to pyrantel.

Diethylcarbamazine

Diethylcarbamazine (Hetrazan) is the only drug currently used for suppressing and curing bancroftian and brugian filariasis. It works in two ways. First, it decreases muscular activity and causes eventual paralysis of the microfilariae. It also causes changes in the parasite's surface, which make it more susceptible to the host's immune responses.

Common adverse effects include nausea and vomiting, anorexia, and headache. Another type of reaction caused by the dying microfilariae is called the Mazzotti reaction. This is characterized by severe itching, papular rash, tachycardia, and an intense headache. Rapid drug-induced death of *Onchocerca volvulus* microfilariae in the eye can result in permanent loss of vision.

Praziquantel

Praziquantel (Biltricide) is used in treating schistosomes: flukes and tapeworms. It increases the helminths' permeability to calcium, which causes contracture and paralysis of the helminth.

Adverse effects are minimal, the most common include malaise, headache, dizziness, and abdominal discomfort. Patients should be warned not to drive a car or operate machinery on the day of treatment and the day after. In extensive animal trials, praziquantel has not exhibited mutagenicity, carcinogenicity, or teratogenicity. However, prescribers advise breast-feeding women to refrain from nursing on the day of treatment and for 72 hours thereafter.

Oxamniquine

Oxamniquine (Vansil) is a tetrahydroquinoline derivative that is effective against *Schistosoma mansoni* infections, although it is ineffective against other helminths. Its selectivity restricts its use. It is thought to act through a reaction that affects the macromolecules of the parasite.

Administered orally, oxamniquine is absorbed readily from the GI tract. Absorption is slowed by the presence of food, yet the drug is better tolerated after a meal. The major adverse effects are dizziness, drowsiness, nausea, and diarrhea. Oxamniquine should be given with caution to patients with preexisting seizure disorders because convulsions have been associated with its use. It is contraindicated in pregnancy.

Niclosamide

Niclosamide (Niclocide) differs from mebendazole in its therapeutic effects and mechanism of action. Used to treat cestodes, it inhibits oxidative phosphorylation in the cestodal mitochondria. The scolex and proximal segments are killed on contact with the drug. The scolex of the tapeworm, loosened from the gut wall, may be digested in the intestine and may not be identified in the feces even after extensive purging. Niclosamide affects the cestodes of the intestine only. It has no effect in cysticercosis. Niclosamide is indicated for treating beef, fish, and dwarf tapeworms.

A laxative is given before administration to purge the bowel of all dead segments. Digestion of the segments may liberate the eggs and lead to cysticercosis. The most common adverse effects are abdominal distress, anorexia, nausea, and vomiting.

ANTIECTOPARASITIC DRUGS

Antiectoparasitic drugs include lindane, crotamiton, and permethrin. These are topical drugs with local action. Although they can eradicate the parasite, they have minimal effect on the pruritus that frequently accompanies ectoparasitic infections. The prototype drug for treating ectoparasitic diseases is lindane (Kwell).

NURSING MANAGEMENT OF THE PATIENT RECEIVING LINDANE

Core Drug Knowledge

Pharmacotherapeutics

Lindane is used in treating scabies and pediculosis. Topical lindane is absorbed systemically and contraindicated for patients with known seizure disorders and for individuals with a known hypersensitivity. CNS toxicity may precipitate seizures. Lindane should not be used where there is a skin rash, abrasion, or inflammation because systemic absorption may be enhanced, which increases the possibility of CNS toxicity. Ectoparasites and infections affected by lindane include *S. scabiei* (scabies and its eggs), pediculosis capitis, pediculosis corporis, and *Phthirus pubis* (crab louse).

Pharmacokinetics

Lindane is absorbed slowly and incompletely through intact skin, through the GI tract when ingested, and through mucous membranes when inhaled. Following topical administration, some lindane is absorbed systemically. Absorption is greater through damaged skin (Table 55-7). It is stored in body fats, metabolized in the liver, and excreted in urine and feces.

Pharmacodynamics

Direct effects of lindane are in the parasite. Lindane is a topical scabicide. It is absorbed through the exoskeleton of parasites, presumably causing excessive CNS stimulation and resulting in convulsion and death. If absorbed systemically, lindane is a CNS stimulant, producing adverse effects similar to those of dichlordiphenyltrichloroethane (DDT), a potent insecticide.

Contraindications and Precautions

Lindane is contraindicated for patients with known seizure disorders and for individuals with a known hypersensitivity. CNS toxicity may precipitate seizures. Lindane should not be used where there is a skin rash, abrasion, or inflammation because systemic absorption may be enhanced, which increases the possibility of CNS toxicity. Lindane also is contraindicated for children younger than 2 years of age. These children have more permeable skin, and there may be high systemic absorption. Caution should be used with this drug in children between 2 and 10 years of age because of an increased risk of toxicity. Lindane therapy during pregnancy is questionable because of the potential for serious adverse CNS effects. Lindane is not recommended for use while breast-feeding because it is secreted into the breast milk. An alternative form of feeding should be used for at least 2 days.

Adverse Effects

Adverse effects to lindane seldom occur. Too frequent or incorrect applications can produce skin irritation, such as a maculopapular rash or contact dermatitis. Although pruritus may occur, it may be due to an acquired sensitivity to mites. Lindane has the potential for serious adverse CNS effects, ranging from dizziness, nervousness, and restlessness to seizures. However, this occurs more frequently in children and patients with broken or damaged skin.

TABLE 55-7 Summary of Selected Antiectoparasitic Drugs

Drug (Trade) Name	Selected Indications	Route and Dosage Range	Pharmacokinetics
lindane (Kwell, Scabene)	Scabies and pediculosis	*Adult and child:* Topical cream, apply cream to clean, dry skin from the neck to the toes, and rub in well; leave on skin for 8–12 h; wash skin well *Adult and child:* Topical shampoo, wash and dry the hair and allow to cool; apply shampoo to dry hair and rub into the scalp; allow shampoo to remain in place for 4 min; use enough water to work up a good lather; rinse thoroughly and towel dry; use a fine-toothed comb when hair is thoroughly dry	*Onset:* Rapid *Duration:* 3 h $t_{1/2}$: 18 h
crotamiton (Eurax)	Scabies	Same as above	*Onset:* Unknown *Duration:* Unknown $t_{1/2}$: Unknown
permethrin (Elimite, Nix)	Pediculosis	Same as above	*Onset:* 10 min *Duration:* Unknown
ivermectin (Stromectol)	Onchocerciasis Strongyloidiasis Scabies	*Adult and child* (>15 kg): PO, 150 µg/kg 1 h after breakfast *Adult and child* (>15 kg): PO, 200 µg/kg 1 h after breakfast *Adult and child* (>15 kg): PO, 150–200 µg/kg	*Onset:* Well absorbed *Duration:* Unknown $t_{1/2}$: 16–35 h

Drug Interactions

Oils may enhance absorption; therefore, simultaneous use of creams, ointments, or oils should be avoided.

Assessment of Relevant Core Patient Variables

Health Status

The nurse should assess the patient for potential medical conditions, such as damaged skin or seizure disorders, that contraindicate lindane therapy or require close monitoring. Before therapy begins, a baseline assessment of the integumentary and neurologic systems should be conducted for patients at risk with these conditions.

Life Span and Gender

The patient's pregnancy status needs to be determined, and breast-feeding mothers should be advised to use an alternative form of feeding for 72 hours after using lindane. It is important to note the patient's age before administering lindane. Children younger than 2 years of age should not use lindane because the permeability of their skin puts them at risk for CNS toxicity.

Lifestyle, Diet, and Habits

The patient's use of creams, ointments, or oils should be determined and the patient cautioned to refrain from their use during lindane therapy.

Environment

The nurse should be aware of the setting in which lindane will be administered. Because lindane is routinely used at home, the patient needs to understand clearly how to use it to avoid increased absorption and the possibility of CNS toxicity.

Nursing Diagnoses and Outcomes

- Risk for Injury related to potential CNS toxicity from systemic absorption of lindane
  Desired outcome: The patient will identify the signs and symptoms of toxicity and report them immediately to the health care provider and implement measures to prevent a reinfection with lice.
- Risk for Impaired Skin Integrity: Rash and pruritus related to drug therapy
  Desired outcome: The patient will self-medicate with OTC diphenhydramine.

Planning and Intervention

Maximizing Therapeutic Effects

Lindane is for external use only, and the patient should be encouraged to use it exactly according to directions.

Minimizing Adverse Effects

The patient needs to follow the directions for using lindane carefully to avoid potential adverse effects. The drug needs to be kept out of the reach of children who may ingest it accidentally.

Providing Patient and Family Education

- The nurse should emphasize the potential adverse effects of lindane, and should tell the patient to contact the prescriber if any occur.
- The nurse should provide directions so that the patient uses lindane correctly.
- It is important to cover the following teaching points about lindane cream:
  - Cleaning and drying the skin
  - Applying the cream from the neck to the toes
  - Leaving the cream on the skin for 8 to 12 hours and then washing the skin well
- The nurse should cover the following teaching points about lindane shampoo:
  - Washing, drying, and cooling the hair
  - Applying shampoo to dry hair and rubbing into the scalp
  - Allowing the shampoo to remain in place for 4 minutes
  - Adding enough water to work up a lather
  - Rinsing thoroughly and towel drying
  - Using a fine-toothed comb to remove remaining nits from thoroughly dry hair
- Additional patient teaching may focus on preventing reinfection by washing all contaminated clothing and bed linens in hot water to kill the mite or lice nits (eggs) and not sharing hats, brushes, or combs. If the problem continues, lindane may be reapplied after 1 week.

Ongoing Assessment and Evaluation

Patients with a history of seizure disorders should be monitored for signs of seizure activity. Likewise, patients undergoing recurrent treatment should be monitored for signs of neurotoxicity. After-treatment evaluations consist of monitoring for signs of successful treatment or failure by reinfection. The patient should remain free from adverse effects and should be able to express the importance of contacting the prescriber if adverse effects occur. The patient should be free from infection. See the accompanying display, Home Care Concerns in Antiectoparasitic Therapy. ■

DRUGS CLOSELY RELATED TO P LINDANE

Crotamiton

Crotamiton (Eurax) is a scabicidal and antipruritic drug used for treating *S. scabiei* (scabies) and relieving pruritus. The drug can be used with caution during pregnancy, and the only contraindication to its use is hypersensitivity. Pediatric safety has not been established. Crotamiton should not

Critical Thinking Scenario

Home care concerns in antiectoparasitic therapy

After treatment and recovery from status epilepticus, your patient, J. Colone, is discharged home on phenytoin (Dilantin) therapy. One of your assignments as a student nurse is to accompany the visiting nurse who will visit with Mr. Colone to assess his progress. When you arrive, you learn by surprise that the whole family is being treated for head lice. Examine your concerns about Mr. Colone's current situation. In addition to teaching him about drug therapy, what other points will you emphasize in the teaching plan? What is especially important for Mr. Colone to know?

be applied in the eyes or mouth because it may cause irritation. It should not be applied to acutely inflamed skin or raw or weeping surfaces until the acute inflammation resolves. The only adverse reaction is a potential rash.

Crotamiton should be applied from the chin to the toes after taking a routine bath or shower. A second application is advisable 24 hours later. A cleansing bath should be taken 48 hours after the last application. Clothing and bed linens should be changed the second day. Contaminated clothing and bed linen may be dry-cleaned or washed in very hot water.

Permethrin

Permethrin (Elimite) is a synthetic drug active against lice, ticks, mites, and fleas. It acts on nerve cell membranes to disrupt the sodium channel current. The result is paralysis of the pests. Permethrin is used in treating head lice and their nits. Head lice infestation is often accompanied by pruritus, erythema, and edema, which may be exacerbated temporarily with permethrin treatment. However, hypersensitivity is the only contraindication for its use.

Patients should be instructed to wash, rinse, and towel dry hair. Then they can apply enough permethrin to saturate the hair and scalp, leave the preparation in place for 10 minutes, and rinse with water. A single treatment is usually sufficient; however, if live lice are observed after 7 days, a second treatment may be given.

MEMORY CHIP

Lindane

- Used for scabies and pediculosis
- Significant contraindications: hypersensitivity and preexisting seizure disorders
- Most common adverse effects: skin irritation and pruritus
- Most serious adverse effect: seizures
- Maximizing therapeutic effects: apply as directed
- Minimizing adverse effects: keep out of reach of children
- Most significant patient education: it is important to use the right instructions because each formulation is different

DRUGS SIGNIFICANTLY DIFFERENT FROM LINDANE

Ivermectin (Stromectol) is an oral drug used in the management of onchocerciasis or strongyloidiasis. It is an anthelminthic drug that also is used as an antiectoparasitic drug. Although not FDA-approved for the treatment of scabies, ivermectin has been used successfully to treat this condition. Ivermectin is used only in cases of treatment failure with topical agents.

Ivermectin should not be used during pregnancy or in women who breast-feed. It should be given cautiously to patients with severe illness such as hepatic, cardiovascular, renal, or pulmonary diseases.

CHAPTER SUMMARY

- Parasites include protozoa, helminths, and arthropods.
- Helminths include cestodes, nematodes, and trematodes.
- Arthropods include ectoparasites, such as scabies and lice.
- Pharmacologic intervention for parasites must be specific not only to the type of parasite, but also to the stage of its life cycle.
- Chloroquine is the prototypical antimalarial drug. Additional drugs used in treating malaria include hydroxychloroquine, mefloquine, primaquine, pyrimethamine, and quinine.
- Metronidazole is the prototypical antiparasitic drug. Additional antiprotozoan drugs include iodoquinol, paromomycin, and quinacrine.
- PCP occurs most often in immunocompromised patients. Drug treatment for PCP includes pentamidine, atovaquone, and TMP-SMZ.
- Mebendazole is the prototypical anthelminthic drug. The choice of anthelmintic therapy, however, depends on the type of helminth. Other anthelminthic drugs include albendazole (in clinical trial), thiabendazole, pyrantel pamoate, piperazine, diethylcarbamazine, praziquantel, oxamniquine, and niclosamide.
- Lindane is the prototypical antiectoparasitic drug. Drugs closely related to lindane include crotamiton and permethrin.

QUESTIONS FOR STUDY AND REVIEW

1. Why should patients with chloroquine therapy continue to have their eyes examined after completing therapy?
2. Why is chloroquine used cautiously in children?
3. What baseline evaluations should be done for a patient on long-term antimalarial therapy?
4. Why would an patient with alcoholism need to be monitored closely during antiparasitic therapy?
5. Why should the nurse take respiratory protective measures during the administration of inhaled pentamidine?
6. How can the nurse intervene to minimize potential severe adverse effects from the administration of pentamidine?
7. What are the major causes of treatment failure with lindane?

NEED MORE HELP?

Chapter 55 of the study guide for *Drug Therapy in Nursing* contains exercises and activities to reinforce your understanding of the concepts presented in this chapter. For additional information see the text's accompanying website at *http://www.connection.lww.com*.

REFERENCES AND BIBLIOGRAPHY

Badalamenti, S., Jameson, J. E., Reddy, K. R. (1999). Amebiasis. *Current Treatment Options in Gastroenterology, 2*(2), 97–103.

CCIS System. (2001). *Computerized Clinical Information System*. Denver, CO: Micromedex.

Chan, C., Montaner, J., Lefebvre, E. A., et al. (1999). Atovaquone suspension compared with aerosolized pentamidine for prevention of *Pneumocystis carinii* pneumonia in human immunodeficiency virus-infected subjects intolerant of trimethoprim or sulfonamides. *Journal of Infectious Diseases, 180*(2), 369–376.

Chouela, E. N., Abeldano, A. M., Pellerano, G., et al. (1999). Equivalent therapeutic efficacy and safety of ivermectin and lindane in the treatment of human scabies. *Archives of Dermatology, 135*(6), 651–655.

Clinical Drug Monographs [CDRom]. (2001). Gold Standard Media

Common Parasitic Worm Infections [Online], June, 1998. Available: http://www.medscape.com/adis/DTP/1998/vII.no1/atp1101.03/dtp1101.03.html.

Dorsey, G., Gandhi, M., Oyugi, J. H., et al. (2000) Difficulties in the prevention, diagnosis, and treatment of imported malaria. *Archives of Internal Medicine, 160*(16), 2505–2510.

Droogan, J. (1999). Treatment and prevention of head lice and scabies, *Nursing Times, 95*(29), 44–45.

Drug Facts and Comparisons. (2000). St. Louis: Facts and Comparisons Division.

Gogtay, N. J., Desai, S., Kamtekar, K. D., et al. (1999). Efficacies of 5- and 14-day primaquine regimens in the prevention of relapses in Plasmodium vivax infections. *Annals of Tropical Medicine and Parasitology, 93*(8), 809–812.

Hardman, J. G., Limbird, L. E., Molinof, P. B., Ruddon, R. W., & Gilman, A. (Eds.). (1997). *Goodman and Gilman's pharmacological basis of therapeutics* (9th ed.). New York: McGraw-Hill.

Karch, A. (2001). *2001 Lippincott's nursing drug guide*. Philadelphia: Lippincott Williams & Wilkins.

Katzung, B. (1998). *Basic and clinical pharmacology* (7th ed.). Stamford: Appleton & Lange.

Porth, C. (1998). *Pathophysiology: Concepts of altered health states* (5th ed.). Philadelphia: Lippincott Williams & Wilkins.

Tatro, D. (Ed.). (2000). *Drug interaction facts* (6th ed.). St. Louis: Facts and Comparisons.

van Agtmael, M. A., Eggelte, T. A., van Boxtel, C. J. (1999). Artemisinin drugs in the treatment of malaria: From medicinal herb to registered medication. *Trends in Pharmacology, 20*(5), 199–205.

White, N. J. (1999). Delaying antimalarial drug resistance with combination chemotherapy. *Parasitologia, 41*(1–3), 301–308.

Appendix **A**

SUPPLEMENTAL CANADIAN DRUG INFORMATION

Narcotic, Controlled Drugs, Benzodiazepines and Other Targeted Substances

Table I summarizes the requirements for prescribing, dispensing and record keeping for narcotic, controlled drugs, benzodiazepines and other targeted substances. This information is not intended to present a comprehensive review; the reader is therefore encouraged to seek additional and confirmatory information (e.g., Controlled Drugs and Substances Act, Narcotic Control Regulations, Controlled Drugs Regulations, Benzodiazepines and Other Targeted Substances Regulations).

Table I—Narcotic, Controlled Drugs, Benzodiazepines and Other Targeted Substances Summary

Classification and Description	Legal Requirements
Narcotic Drugs*	
• 1 narcotic (e.g., cocaine, codeine, hydromorphone, morphine) • 1 narcotic + 1 active non-narcotic ingredient (e.g., Cophylac, Empracet-30, Tylenol No. 4) • All narcotics for parenteral use (e.g., fentanyl, pethidine) • All products containing diamorphine (hospitals only), hydrocodone, oxycodone, methadone or pentazocine • Dextropropoxyphene, propoxyphene (straight) (e.g., Darvon-N, 642)	• Written prescription required. • Verbal prescriptions not permitted. • Refills not permitted. • Written prescription may be prescribed to be dispensed in divided portions (part-fills). • For part-fills, copies of prescriptions should be made in reference to the original prescription. Indicate on the original prescription: the new prescription number, the date of the part-fill, the quantity dispensed and the pharmacist's initials. • Transfers not permitted. • Record and retain all documents pertaining to all transactions in a manner that permits an audit. • Sales reports required except for dextropropoxyphene, propoxyphene. • Report any loss or theft of narcotic drugs as well as forged prescriptions within 10 days to the Office of Controlled Substances at the address indicated on the forms.

(continued)

Table I—Narcotic, Controlled Drugs, Benzodiazepines and Other Targeted Substances Summary (Continued)

Classification and Description	Legal Requirements
Narcotic Preparations*	
• Verbal prescription narcotics: 1 narcotic + 2 or more active non-narcotic ingredients in a recognized therapeutic dose (e.g., Cophylac Expectorant, Darvon-N Compound, Fiorinal with Codeine, 692, 282, 292, Tylenol No. 2 and No. 3) • Exempted codeine compounds: contain codeine up to 8 mg/solid dosage form or 20 mg/30 mL liquid + 2 or more active non-narcotic ingredients (e.g., Atasol-8, Robitussin with Codeine).	• Written or verbal prescriptions permitted. • Refills not permitted. • Written or verbal prescriptions may be prescribed to be dispensed in divided portions (part-fills). • For part-fills, copies of prescriptions should be made in reference to the original prescription. Indicate on the original prescription: the new prescription number, the date of the part-fill, the quantity dispensed and the pharmacist's initials. • Transfers not permitted. • Exempted codeine compounds when dispensed pursuant to a prescription follow the same regulations as for verbal prescription narcotics. • Record and retain all documents pertaining to all transactions in a manner that permits an audit. • Sales reports not required. • Report any loss or theft of narcotic drugs as well as forged prescriptions within 10 days to the Office of Controlled Substances at the address indicated on the forms.
Controlled Drugs*	
• Part I e.g., amphetamines (Dexedrine) methylphenidate (Ritalin) pentobarbital (Nembutal) secobarbital (Seconal, Tuinal) preparations: 1 controlled drug + 1 or more active noncontrolled drug(s) (Cafergot-PB)	• Written or verbal prescriptions permitted. • Refills not permitted for verbal prescriptions. • Refills permitted for written prescriptions if the prescriber has indicated in writing the number of refills and dates for, or intervals between, refills. • Written or verbal prescriptions may be prescribed to be dispensed in divided portions (part-fills). • For refills and part-fills, copies of prescriptions should be made in reference to the original prescription. Indicate on the original prescription: the new prescription number, the date of the repeat or part-fill, the quantity dispensed and the pharmacist's initials. • Transfers not permitted. • Record and retain all documents pertaining to all transactions in a manner that permits an audit. • Sales reports required except for controlled drug preparations. • Report any loss or theft of controlled drugs as well as forged prescriptions within 10 days to the Office of Controlled Substances at the address indicated on the forms.
• Part II e.g., barbiturates (amobarbital, phenobarbital) butorphanol (Stadol NS) diethylpropion (Tenuate) nalbuphine (Nubain) phentermine (Ionamin) preparations: 1 controlled drug + 1 or more active noncontrolled ingredient(s) (Fiorinal, Neo-Pause, Tecnal)	• Written or verbal prescriptions permitted. • Refills permitted for written or verbal prescriptions if the prescriber has authorized in writing or verbally (at the time of issuance) the number of refills and dates for, or intervals between, refills. • Written or verbal prescriptions may be prescribed to be dispensed in divided portions (part-fills). • For refills and part-fills, copies of prescriptions should be made in reference to the original prescription. Indicate on the original prescription: the new prescription number, the date of the repeat or part-fill, the quantity dispensed and the pharmacist's initials.
• Part III e.g., anabolic steroids (methyltestosterone, nandrolone decanoate)	• Transfers not permitted. • Record and retain all documents pertaining to all transactions in a manner that permits an audit. • Sales reports not required. • Report the loss or theft of controlled drugs as well as forged prescriptions within 10 days to the Office of Controlled Substances at the address indicated on the forms.

Table I—Narcotic, Controlled Drugs, Benzodiazepines and Other Targeted Substances Summary (Continued)

Classification and Description	Legal Requirements
Benzodiazepines and Other Targeted Substances*	
e.g., alprazolam (Xanax) bromazepam (Lectopam) chlordiazepoxide (Librium) clobazam (Frisium) ethchlorvynol lorazepam (Ativan) mazindol meprobarnate oxazepam (Serax)	• Written and verbal prescriptions permitted. • Refills for written or verbal prescriptions permitted if indicated by prescriber. • Part-fills permitted as per prescriber's instructions. • For refills or part-fills of prescriptions, the following information should be recorded: date of the repeat or part-fill, prescription number, quantity dispensed and the pharmacist's initials. • Transfer of prescriptions permitted except a prescription that has been already transferred. • Sales reports not required. • Report any loss or theft of benzodiazepines and other targeted substances within 10 days to the Office of Controlled Substances at the address indicated on the forms.

* The products noted are examples only.
Reprinted with permission from *Compendium of Pharmaceuticals and Specialties*, 36th ed., Canadian Pharmacists Association, Ottawa, 2001.

Immunization Schedules for Infants and Children

The following is an overview of routine immunization schedules for infants and children. This information is not intended to present a comprehensive review; the reader is therefore encouraged to seek additional and confirmatory information.

Few measures in preventive medicine are of such proven value and as easy to implement as routine immunization against infectious diseases. Immunization carried out as recommended in the following schedules (Tables I, II and III) will provide good basic protection for most children against the diseases shown.

Both live and inactivated polio vaccines have been used in Canada with equal success in preventing the occurrence of paralytic poliomyelitis, but inactivated vaccine is now used by all jurisdictions in Canada.

Varicella vaccine is now recommended by Health Canada's National Advisory Committee on Immunization (NACI) for healthy children aged 12 months or older. However, each province/territory is to establish its own routine childhood varicella immunization program. (At presstime, only Prince Edward Island had included varicella vaccine as part of their routine immunization schedule funded by the province.)

Following a standard schedule ensures complete and adequate protection. However, modifications to the recommended schedule may be necessary because of missed appointments or intercurrent illness. Interruption of a recommended series does not require starting the series over again, regardless of the interval elapsed.

Similar vaccines are now available from different manufacturers but they may not be identical. It is therefore essential for the user to read the manufacturer's package insert. The user is encouraged to consult the *Canadian Immunization Guide*, 5th ed., for further information.

(*continued*)

Routine Immunization Schedules	Age/Timing	DTaP[a]	IPV[a]	Hib[a,b]	MMR	Td[c]	Hep B[d,g] (3 doses)
Table I— Infants and Children	2 months old	X	X	X			Infancy
	4 months old	X	X	X			
	6 months old	X	X[e]	X			or
	12 months old				X		
	18 months old	X	X	X	X[f] or		
	4–6 years old	X	X		X[f]		Preadolescence[g]
	Grade 3–7						(9–13 yrs)
	14–16 years old					X	
Table II— Children <7 Years of Age Not Immunized in Early Infancy	1st visit	X	X	X	X[h]		
	2 months after 1st visit	X	X	X[i]	X[f]		
	2 months after 2nd visit	X	X[e]				
	6–12 months after 3rd visit	X	X	X[i]			
	4–6 years of age	X[j]	X[j]				Preadolescence[g]
	14–16 years of age					X	(9–13 yrs)
Table III— Children ≥7 Years of Age Not Immunized in Early Infancy	1st visit	N/A	X	N/A	X	X	
	2 months after 1st visit		X		X[f]	X	
	6–12 months after 2nd visit		X			X	Preadolescence[g]
	10 years after 3rd visit					X	(9–13 yrs)

Legend: DTaP = diphtheria, tetanus and pertussis (acellular) vaccine, Hep B = recombinant hepatitis B vaccine series, Hib = Haemophilus influenzae b conjugate vaccine, IPV = inactivated polio vaccine, MMR = measles, mumps and rubella vaccine, N/A = not applicable, Td = tetanus and diphtheria toxoid, "adult type".

[a] Diphtheria, tetanus, pertussis, polio and Haemophilus influenzae b are commonly administered as one injection for the 2, 4, 6 and 18 month doses in Table I. Diphtheria, tetanus, pertussis and polio are commonly administered as one injection for the 4 to 6 year old dose in Table I.

[b] Hib schedule shown is for PRP-T (e.g., Act-HIB) or HbOC (e.g., HibTITER) vaccine. If PRP-OMP is used (e.g., PedVax HIB), give at 2, 4 and 12 months of age.

[c] Td (tetanus and diphtheria toxoid), a combined, adsorbed "adult type" preparation for use in persons ≥7 years of age, contains less diphtheria toxoid than preparations given to younger children and is less likely to cause reactions in older persons.

[d] Hepatitis B vaccine can be routinely given to infants or pre-adolescents, depending on the provincial/territorial policy; three doses at 0-, 1- and 6- month intervals are preferred. The second dose should be administered at least 1 month after the first dose, and the third dose should be administered at least 4 months after the first dose, and at least 2 months after the second dose.

[e] This dose is not needed routinely, but can be included for convenience.

[f] A second dose of MMR is recommended, at least 1 month after the first dose given. For convenience, options include giving it with the next scheduled vaccination at 18 months of age or with school entry vaccinations at 4–6 years of age (depending on the provincial/territorial policy), or at any intervening age that is practicable.

[g] Alternatively, adolescents 11 to 15 years of age may be given a two dose regimen of adult formulation Recombivax HB• (10 mcg/dose). The second dose is administered 4 to 6 months after the first dose.

[h] Delay until subsequent visit if child is <12 months of age.

[i] Recommended schedule and number of doses depend on the product used and the age of the child when vaccination is begun (see the current *Canadian Immunization Guide* or the product monograph for specific recommendations). Not required past age 5.

[j] Omit these doses if the previous doses of DTaP and polio were given after the 4th birthday.

Adapted from *Canadian Immunization Guide*, 5th edition, Health Canada, 1998.

Reference:

1. National Advisory Committee on Immunization. Canadian immunization guide, 5th ed. Ottawa, ON: Health Canada, 1998.

Appendix **B**

DIAGNOSTIC IMAGING AGENTS

The number of medical test procedures that rely on diagnostic imaging agents is legion. The kinds of pharmacologic agents used for testing, however, can be quantified. Common imaging agents include radiopaque contrast agents, such as barium sulfate; ionic iodinated imaging agents, such as diatrizoate meglumine; nonionized iodinated imaging agents, such as metrizamide; oral cystographic compounds, such as iocetamic acid; provocative agents, such as arginine; and skin testing agents, such as coccidioidin.

Radiopaque contrast agents highlight and provide contrast among internal structures. Iodinated imaging agents and cystographic compounds are composed of iodine compounds with radiopaque properties. Provocative agents provoke measurable responses that are an indication of disease or its absence. Skin testing agents help in identifying allergic responses and other disorders.

As technology advances, more patients will undergo testing procedures with these agents. Nurses must be prepared to administer and monitor some of these agents and provide care for patients receiving them. Like therapeutic drugs, these diagnostic agents require special administration methods, produce adverse effects, and call for careful patient education. This of course requires a firm understanding of the interrelationship between *core drug knowledge* related to diagnostic drugs and *core patient variables* specific to the testing procedures. A summary of various pharmacologic test agents follows.

Drug (Trade) Name	Indications	Nursing Management
Imaging Agent		
barium sulfate suspensions (Baro-CAT, Prepcat, Entrobar) concentrated suspensions (Tomocat) powder (Baroflave) powder for suspension (Barosperse, Anatrast, Tonopaque)	GI diagnostics	Do not administer if obstruction of GI tract is suspected. Keep the patient fasting (NPO) for 8 h for oral, administration. Provide mouth care for NPO patients. Administer cathartic or enema posttest as ordered. Assess GI status posttest; document passage of stool. Keep patient well hydrated to expel barium. Monitor for constipation, intestinal cramping, distention, diarrhea, and bowel obstruction.

(*continued*)

Continued

Drug (Trade) Name	Indications	Nursing Management
Ionic Iodinated Imaging Agents		
diatrizoate meglumine (Gastrografin) diatrizoate sodium (Hypaque Sodium)	GI diagnostics, discography, urography, angiography, angiocardiography, arteriography, aortography, ventriculography, venography, venacavography, computed tomography (CT)	Assess for allergy to iodine, iodine compounds, foods that contain iodine, or dye allergy. Assess patient history of: bronchial asthma; renal, hepatic, or thyroid diseases; sickle cell disease. Notify the provider of any positive allergy or history before administering the drug. Monitor fluid and electrolyte status. Have emergency equipment available for possible allergic reactions. Monitor extravasation from injection site.
ethiodized oil (Ethiodol)	Hysterosalpingography	Same as diatrizoate meglumine. When injected into lymph nodes, monitor for compromised pulmonary function. Monitor for infection in the insertion site and delayed wound healing.
iodamide meglumine (Renovue-Dip, Renovue-65)	Urography, pyelography, CT	Same as diatrizoate meglumine.
iodipamide meglumine (Cholografin Meglumine)	Cholecystography, cholangiography	Same as diatrizoate meglumine.
iophendylate	Lumbar, thoracic, and total columnar myelography	Same as diatrizoate meglumine. Keep patient in a flat position for 24 h after test procedure. Monitor for signs of meningeal irritation or subarachnoid bleeding.
iothalamate meglumine iothalamate sodium (Conray)	Cholangiography, urography, pyelography, cystourethrography, arthrography, angiography, angiocardiography, arteriography, aortography, CT, cholangiopancreatography, cystography	Same as diatrizoate meglumine.
Nonionized Iodinated Imaging Agents		
metrizamide (Amipaque)	Myelography, angiocardiography, arteriography, ventriculography, CT, cisternography	Assess for history of iodine sensitivity. Assess for the following: seizure disorder, local or systemic infection, pheochromocytoma, multiple sclerosis, sickle cell anemia, severe cardiovascular disease, impaired hepatic function, active alcoholism. Notify the provider of any positive history prior to administering the drug. Assess pretest and posttest fluid and electrolyte balance. Monitor for CNS effects after test.
iopamidol (Isovue)	Urography, angiography, angiocardiography, arteriography, aortography, ventriculography, venography	Same as for metrizamide.
iohexol (Omnipaque)	Urography, myelography, angiography, angiocardiography, arteriography, aortography, ventriculography, venography, CT	Same as for metrizamide. After intrathecal administration, elevate the head of the bed 45 degrees.
ioversol (Optiray)	Urography, angiography, arteriography, aortography, ventriculography, venography, CT	Same as for metrizamide.
ioxaglate meglumine (Hexabrix)	Urography, arthrography, angiography, angiocardiography, arteriography, aortography, ventriculography, venography, hysterosalpingography, CT	Same as for metrizamide.

Continued

Drug (Trade) Name	Indications	Nursing Management
Oral Cholecystographic Compounds		
iocetamic acid (Cholebrine)	Cholecystography	Assess for allergy to iodine, iodine compounds, or foods that contain iodine. Assess for allergy to dyes (FD&C yellow dye No. 5). Assess for the following: bronchial asthma, hyperuricemia, renal disease, hepatic impairment, GI absorption diseases, cardiovascular disease, and thyroid diseases. Administer high-fat diet the day before the test. Administer the contrast medium as ordered. Keep the patient NPO, except for water, after administration of contrast medium. Administer laxative or enema as ordered. Keep patients well hydrated, especially those with hyperuricemia.
iopanoic acid (Telepaque)	Cholecystography, cholangiography	Same as iocetamic acid.
ipodate calcium (Oragrafin calcium) ipodate sodium (Oragrafin sodium, Bilivist)	Cholecystography, cholangiography	Same as iocetamic acid.
tyropanoate sodium (Bilopaque)	Cholecystography, cholangiography	Same as iocetamic acid.
Provocative Drugs		
arginine	Evaluate pituitary growth hormone reserve	Assess for allergy or hypersensitivity reactions. Assess for sickle cell anemia and renal disease. Notify the provider of any positive history before administration of the test. Administer through an indwelling catheter to prevent extravasation. Draw blood sample at 30 min before and again immediately before the test. Draw blood sample at the initiation of the injection and at 30-min intervals for 2½ h thereafter.
corticotropin (ACTH)	Evaluate adrenal function	Assess for porcine protein sensitivity. Notify provider of positive allergic response prior to administration of the drug. Advise low-carbohydrate diet for 48 h prior to day of testing. Keep patient NPO 12 h before test. Restrict patient's activity 12 h before test. Withhold the following medications: amphetamines, calcium gluconate, corticosteroids, estrogens, lithium, and spironolactone.
cosyntropin	Assist in diagnosing adrenocortical insufficiency	Assess for allergy to corticotropin or cosyntropin. Notify the provider of any positive allergy history before administration of the drug. The following drugs may interfere with test results: cortisone, hydrocortisone, estrogens, and spironolactone. Draw blood specimen 30–60 min after administration of cosyntropin.
edrophonium (Tensilon)	Assist in the diagnosis of myasthenia gravis Differentiate between cholinergic crisis and myasthenic crisis Evaluate therapy	Withhold the following medications: anticholinergics, muscle relaxants, prednisone, procainamide, and quinidine. Have 1-mg atropine available to reverse possible severe cholinergic reactions.

(*continued*)

Continued

Drug (Trade) Name	Indications	Nursing Management
		Interpretation timing: myasthenia gravis diagnosis 45 s after administration; differentiation between cholinergic crisis and myasthenic crisis—1 min after administration; and evaluation of treatment—1 min after administration.
gonadorelin (Factrel)	Evaluate anterior pituitary function	Withhold the following medications: androgens, estrogens, gonadotrophins, and glucocorticoids. Avoid interacting drugs: digoxin, dopamine antagonists, levodopa, phenothiazines, and spironolactone. Draw blood sample every 15 min for the first hour, then at 2 h postadministration.
histamine phosphate	Evaluate production of hydrochloric acid Assist in diagnosing pheochromocytoma	Ensure NPO status for 12 h before test. Allow no smoking for 8 h before test. Withhold the following medications: adrenaline blockers, alcohol, antacids, anticholinergics, cimetidine, corticosteroids, and reserpine. Have epinephrine available for severe hypotension. Monitor blood pressure and pulse rate closely.
metyrapone	Evaluate hypothalamic-pituitary function	Same as gonadorelin.
pentagastrin (Peptavlon)	Evaluate gastric acid secretion Assist in diagnosing Zollinger-Ellison syndrome	Assess for the following: allergies, pancreatic disease, biliary disease, and hepatic disease. Notify the provider of any positive history before administration of the test. Do not use in patients with acute bleeding or penetrating ulcers. Place a nasogastric tube for the procedure. Obtain gastric acid specimen 60 min after administration of pentagastrin.
secretin	Assist in diagnosing pancreatic exocrine disorders and gastrinoma	Assess for the following: allergies, asthma, anticholinergic therapy, inflammatory bowel disease, and vagotomy. Notify the provider of any positive history before administration of the test. Assist in the insertion of a double-lumen catheter. Administer test dose if the patient has a history of asthma or allergies; continue test if no reaction after 1 min. For pancreatic disorders: obtain gastrin and duodenal secretion samples taken during the first 60 min after secretin injection. For gastrinoma: draw blood sample during the first 30 min after secretin injection.
thyrotropin	Assist in diagnosing low thyroid reserve and subclinical hypothyroidism Differentiate between primary and secondary hypothyroidism Detect thyroid cancer Evaluate treatment	Assess for a history of: angina pectoris, cardiac failure, hypopituitarism, adrenal cortical suppression, corticosteroid therapy, coronary thrombosis, untreated Addison disease, and hypersensitivity to thyrotropin. Notify the provider of any positive history before administration of the test. Monitor for signs of hypersensitivity reaction. Monitor for nausea, vomiting, headache, fever, tachycardia, and ventricular fibrillation.
tolbutamide sodium	Assist in diagnosing diabetes mellitus, insulinoma, pancreatic carcinoma, acute pancreatitis	Assess for a history of hypersensitivity to tolbutamide or other sulfonylureas, and identify current drug therapy that may enhance the hypoglycemic effect of tolbutamide. Notify the provider of any positive history before administration of the test. Monitor for signs and symptoms of hypoglycemia. Have IV glucose on hand for severe hypoglycemia. Draw blood for baseline glucose level and serial glucose levels as ordered after administration.

Continued

Drug (Trade) Name	Indications	Nursing Management
xylose	Assist in diagnosing malabsorptive conditions	Assess for a history of impaired renal function, thyroid dysfunction, pernicious anemia, and iron-deficiency anemia. Notify the provider of any positive history before administration of the test. To avoid inaccurate results, assess for vomiting or diarrhea, gastric stasis, bacterial infections, and cardiovascular dysfunction. Encourage fluid intake before and after procedure.
Skin Testing Drugs		
coccidioidin	Assist in the diagnosis of coccidiomycosis Evaluate cell-mediated immune status	Assess for diagnosis of coccidioidal erythema nodosum or allergy to mercury. Notify the provider of any positive history before administration of the test. Assess for an allergy to mercury. Administer by intradermal injection being sure to produce a wheal. Repeat the test in another location (at least 5 cm away) if no wheal appears. Assess for induration at the injection site 24 h later. False-positive results may be reported if assessed after 48 h. A positive test result is an area of induration.
histoplasmin	Assist in diagnosing histoplasmosis	Assess for a history of histoplasmosis or previous positive test results. Notify the provider of any positive history before administration of the test. Do not use more than 0.1 mL for testing because larger doses may cause necrosis and ulceration. Have epinephrine available in case of severe reaction. Administer by intradermal injection being sure to produce a wheal. Repeat the test in another location (at least 5 cm away) if no wheal appears. Assess for induration at the injection site 48–72 h later.
penicilloylopolylysine (PPL)	Assist in assessing risk for hypersensitivity reaction with the administration of penicillin	Assess for a history of penicillin or cephalosporin allergy. Monitor these patients closely. Notify the provider of any positive history before administration of the test. Administer the scratch test first. If no reaction, or questionable reaction to the scratch test, administer the intradermal test. A positive result will be itching or increased size of the wheal within 15 min.
mumps	Assess cell-mediated immunity	Assess for previous hypersensitivity to the test. Assess for allergy to avian protein or to thimerosal because these patients have a higher risk for an anaphylactic reaction to the test. Notify the provider of any positive history before administration of the test. Administer by intradermal injection, being sure to produce a wheal. Repeat the test in another location (at least 5 cm away) if no wheal appears. Assess for induration at the injection site 48–72 h later. In immunocompromised patients, a positive test result is any amount of induration.

(*continued*)

Continued

Drug (Trade) Name	Indications	Nursing Management
		In immunocompetent patients, a positive test result is 5 mm or more of induration.
tuberculin	Assist in diagnosing tuberculosis Evaluate cell-mediated immune status	Assess for previous positive test results. Notify the provider of any positive history before administration of the test. Administer by intradermal injection, being sure to produce a wheal. Repeat the test in another location (at least 5 cm away) if no wheal appears. To avoid false-positive results, do not administer in an area of atopic dermatitis, sun-damaged skin, or ultraviolet treatment. Assess for induration at the injection site 48–72 h later. In immunocompromised patients, a positive test result is 5 mm or more of induration. In immunocompetent patients, a positive test result is 10 mm or more of induration.

Appendix **C**

ENZYME OR DÉBRIDEMENT THERAPY

Enzymes are composed of proteins and similar substances. Having catalytic action, they are used to slow or speed organic processes, replace or supplement deficient enzymes, break down proteins (such as blood clots) and débride wounds, and increase absorption and distribution.

The nurse administering enzyme therapy and caring for a patient receiving enzyme therapy is responsible for understanding the enzyme's action and effects (core drug knowledge); assessing the patient's health history and physical condition (core patient variables); and planning and implementing associated patient education.

Drug (Trade) Name	Indications	Nursing Management
Enzymes		
alglucerase (Ceredase)	Replacement of glucosylceramidase in patients with Gaucher disease (a congenital disorder of lipid metabolism)	Assess the patient's health history for an immune-deficiency disease, unusual or allergic reaction to alglucerase, other drugs, foods, dyes, or preservatives. Determine whether the patient is pregnant, trying to get pregnant, or breast-feeding. Monitor for fever, chills, or stomach discomfort; nausea, vomiting; pain, burning, swelling, or irritation at the injection site.
chymopapain (Chymodiactin)	Decreases intradisk pressure and relieves compressive symptoms in patients with vertebral disk herniation	Use in the lumbar region only. Assess the patient for papaya sensitivity, spondylolisthesis, spinal stenosis, progressive paralysis, spinal cord tumor, and previous injection of chymopapain. Administer pretreatment with H1 and H2 blockers to reduce the severity of possible anaphylactic reaction. Monitor for anaphylaxis, erythema, pilomotor erection, urticaria, conjunctivitis, vasomotor rhinitis, angioedema, back pain/spasm, and transverse myelitis/myelopathy.

(*continued*)

Continued

Drug (Trade) Name	Indications	Nursing Management
desoxyribonuclease and fibrinolysin (Elase)	Attacks protein (DNA) component of purulent exudates Attacks fibrin of blood clots and fibrinous exudates	Replenish at least once daily because significant activity is lost after 24 h.
hyaluronidase (Wydase)	Adjunct therapy to increase the absorption and dispersion of other injected drugs or during urography to improve reabsorption of radiopaque agents Antidote for extravasation	Change needle after each injection when used for extravasation. Monitor for urticaria and anaphylactic-like reactions.
imiglucerase (Cerezyme)	DNA recumbent enzyme used for Gaucher disease	Assess the patient's health history for an unusual or allergic reaction to imiglucerase and other drugs, foods, dyes, or preservatives; pregnancy or plans for pregnancy; breast-feeding. Monitor for fever, chills, or stomach discomfort; nausea; vomiting.
pancreatin (Donnazyme)	Used as a pancreatic enzyme supplement for conditions in which pancreatic enzymes are deficient or absent, such as cystic fibrosis, chronic pancreatitis, pancreatectomy, gastrointestinal bypass surgery, and ductal obstruction from neoplasm	Administer PO with meals. Advise the patient to refrain from keeping drug in the mouth prior to swallowing because it may cause mucosal irritation and stomatitis. Do not give concurrently with antacids or iron salts. Give with caution during pregnancy, breast-feeding, or in porcine hypersensitivity. Monitor for maculopapular rash (sign of porcine hypersensitivity).
pancrelipase (Cotazym, Creon, Ilozyme, Pancrease, Viokase)	Same as pancreatin Has 12 times the lipolytic activity, 4 times the proteolytic activity, and 4 times the amylolytic activity of pancreatin	Administer pancrelipase orally. Products are not interchangeable. Administer delayed-release capsules containing enteric-coated spheres, microspheres, or microtablets by opening and mixing the contents with liquids or soft food. Advise patient not to chew or crush to avoid destruction of enteric coating. The enteric coating will dissolve if in contact with food with a pH greater than 6. Powder drug form may be administered with liquids or mixed with food. Avoid inhaling the powder.
pegademase bovine (Adagen)	Replacement in patients with adenosine deaminase (ADA) deficiency	Give with caution in patients with thrombocytopenia or coagulopathy. Monitor for headache; also monitor injection site. Do not coadminister with vidarabine.
thrombin (Thrombinar, Thrombostat)	Used during surgery to control incisional or surgical bleeding	Avoid parenteral administration because intravascular clots may be fatal. Do not administer to pregnant patients or to patients with bovine hypersensitivity. Before applying, sponge away blood from the surface to which thrombin is to be applied. Apply as a dry powder, spray, or with a saturated absorbable gelatin sponge. Prepare spray and saturated absorbable gelatin sponge as directed by the manufacturer. To avoid disturbing the clot after applying thrombin, do not sponge the area.

Continued

Drug (Trade) Name	Indications	Nursing Management
Débridement Agents		
collagenase (Santyl)	Débridement of chronic dermal ulcers and severe burns	Apply topically once daily for inpatients and every other day for outpatients. Débride wound before each administration. Monitor for systemic bacterial infections.
dextranomer (Debrisan)	Cleansing of exudative wounds. Treatment of decubitus or leg ulcers.	Débride and clean wound before applying bid. Paste is easier to apply than beads. Apply dressing and seal on all four sides. Remove by irrigation.
sutilains (Travase)	Used as an adjunct agent for wound care, causing biochemical débridement of lesions	Keep in mind that a moist environment is needed for optimal enzymatic activity. Use with caution in wounds communicating to major body cavities and wounds containing exposed major nerves or nerve tissue. Apply $\frac{1}{2}$ in. beyond the tissue being débrided. Cover with moist loose dressings. Repeat three to four times daily as needed.

Appendix D

ENTERAL AND NUTRITIONAL SUPPLEMENTS

Vitamins and minerals are substances that the body requires for essential metabolic reactions. The body cannot synthesize enough of these components to meet all of its needs. Therefore, vitamins and minerals must be obtained from animal and vegetable sources ingested as food. In a well-balanced diet, humans take in all they need. Only small amounts of vitamins and minerals are needed because they function as coenzymes that activate the protein portion of enzymes, which catalyze a great deal of biochemical activity.

Vitamins are either water soluble and excreted in the urine or fat soluble and capable of being stored in adipose tissue. Additional *core drug knowledge* includes specific uses of enteral nutrition. Enteral nutrition treats vitamin or mineral deficiencies, supplements the diet when needed, and provides specific therapeutic effects related to vitamin or mineral activity.

Enteral nutrients are classified in pregnancy category C and are contraindicated in cases of allergy to components of the vitamin or mineral, such as colorants, additives, or preservatives. Adverse effects to anticipate from enteral nutrition include nausea, diarrhea, and sometimes toxic reactions, particularly in instances of overdose.

Core patient variables should be assessed. The health history should disclose any condition that would contraindicate using enteral nutrition. The physical examination should include a skin evaluation, respiratory status, pulse rate, and blood pressure. Each enteral drug should be checked for special administration needs. The patient or family should be cautioned to avoid additional supplements in OTC products because overdose can occur. Patients also should be cautioned to avoid using mineral oil if they are taking fat-soluble vitamins.

Nutritional Component	Purpose	Nursing Management
Fat-Soluble Vitamins		
vitamin A (Aquasol A, Del-Vi-A)	Treats severe deficiency, maintains adequate levels during periods of growth or stress	Administer PO or IM. Protect IM vial from light. Watch for hypervitaminosis A: cirrhotic-like liver syndrome with CNS effects, GI drying, rash, and liver changes. Liver damage may be permanent.

Continued

Nutritional Component	Purpose	Nursing Management
calcitriol D-3 (Calcijex, Rocaltrol)	Manages hypocalcemia in patients on renal dialysis; reduction of elevated parathyroid; may help treat psoriasis	Administer orally. Monitor serum calcium levels before and during therapy. Discontinue if patient does not respond or if hypercalcemia occurs.
vitamin D	Treats severe vitamin D deficiency Maintains adequate vitamin levels during periods of growth or stress Possibly useful for hypocalcemic tetany and hypoparathyroidism	Administer as prescribed. Encourage balanced diet and exposure to sunlight. Do not use with mineral oil. Monitor calcium levels before administration and periodically during therapy.
vitamin E (Aquasol E, Vita-Plus E, Softgels)	Reduces toxic effects of oxygen on the lung and retina in certain premature infants Treats severe vitamin E deficiency Maintains adequate levels of vitamin E during periods of stress and growth	Do not administer IV. Instruct patient to report fatigue, weakness, nausea, headache, blurred vision, diarrhea. If above adverse effects occur, vitamin therapy should stop immediately.
phytonadione (Mephyton)	Treats hypoprothrombinemia due to anticoagulants, hemorrhagic disease of the newborn, hypoprothrombinemia in adults Maintains adequate levels during periods of stress and growth	Administer PO or IM. To prevent hemorrhagic disease of newborn, administer 0.5–1 mg within 1 h of birth, or give 1–5 mg IM to the mother before delivery. Monitor prothrombin time carefully before and frequently during therapy. Instruct patient to watch for signs of increased bleeding or bruising. Administer by deep IM injection if given parenterally.
ascorbic acid, vitamin C (Cebid, Vita-C, Cevalin, N'ice Vitamin C Drops)	Treats severe deficiency—scurvy Maintains adequate levels during periods of stress or growth Enhances wound healing, burn healing	Monitor combination and OTC products for vitamin C content. Be forewarned; many patients receive more than the recommended dose. Administer PO and if necessary, IM, slow IV, or SC depending on patient's condition. Keep in mind that dose may decrease effectiveness of anticoagulant therapy and increase adverse effects to oral contraceptives.
cyanocobalamin, vitamin B_{12} (Ener-B)	Treats severe deficiency Maintains adequate levels during periods of stress or growth May treat cyanide toxicity associated with sodium nitroprusside	Monitor patient for mouth sores or skin breakdown. Do not give to patient with cobalt sensitivity.
niacin, vitamin B_3 (Nicotinic Acid)	Prevents and treats pellagra, niacin deficiency, hyperlipidemia in patients not responsive to diet therapy Maintains adequate B3 levels during periods of stress or growth	Advise patient that he or she may feel sensation of warmth and flushing on administration, but sensation usually subsides within 24 h. Monitor serum lipid levels in patients being treated for hyperlipidemia. Encourage proper diet and exercise. Advise patient that adverse effects of nausea, abdominal pain, and diarrhea may occur and that taking vitamin with meals may relieve these problems.
pyridoxine, vitamin B_6 (Nestrex, Beesix)	Treats severe deficiency Also treats isoniazid toxicity and vitamin B deficiency syndrome Maintains adequate levels during periods of stress or growth	Avoid administering to patients taking levodopa because serious toxic effect may result. Monitor for adverse effects, such as sensory neuropathic syndrome marked by unsteady gait and somnolence. Provide safety measures if this occurs.
riboflavin, vitamin B_2	Treats severe B_2 deficiencies Maintains adequate levels during periods of stress or growth	Monitor patient for response to treatment. Warn patient that this drug may discolor urine yellow-orange; explain that the discoloration will subside when therapy discontinues.

(*continued*)

Continued

Nutritional Component	Purpose	Nursing Management
thiamine, vitamin B_1 (Thiamilate, Biamine)	Treats severe B_1 deficiencies (e.g., beriberi) Maintains adequate levels during periods of stress or growth	Do not mix in alkaline solutions. Advise patient that this vitamin changes composition of sweat and body odor. Warn patient that a warm and flushing sensation may accompany administration but that sensation will subside quickly.
Minerals		
calcium (Calciday, Chooz, Dicarbosil, Oystercal, Tums)	Treats severe calcium deficiency Maintains calcium levels Reduces gastric acid levels Helps cardiac contraction in arrest situations	Administer with meals to avoid food and drug interactions and decrease GI effects. Avoid combination with digoxin, thiazide, oral contraceptives (toxicity may occur). Keep in mind that calcium may decrease absorption of atenolol, iron, quinolones, tetracyclines. Avoid combining with high-fiber diets, oxalate, or zinc because these combinations may decrease absorption. Combining with milk or dairy products may increase the risk of hypercalcemia. Monitor calcium levels in acute situations; also monitor for signs of hypercalcemia, hypophosphatemia. Caution patient to avoid OTC multiple combination products that may increase risk of hypercalcemia.
iron, ferrous fumarate, gluconate, and sulfate (Feostat, Feosol, Fer-in-sol)	Treats severe deficiency Maintains normal iron levels during periods of growth or stress Treats iron deficiency anemia Supplements epoetin therapy	Avoid administering iron with tetracycline (both poorly absorbed), antacids, cimetidine, vitamin C, chloramphenicol (decreases iron absorption). If appropriate, tell patient that absorption of levodopa, methyldopa, penicillamine, quinolones are decreased if taken with iron. Administer with food to relieve GI upset. Other adverse effects may include anorexia, vomiting, constipation, green or dark stools. Dilute liquid form, and have patient drink it through a straw to decrease dental staining. Keep out of reach of children. Serious toxicity can occur if accidentally ingested.
magnesium, citrate and hydroxide (Citrate of Magnesia, Milk of Magnesia)	Decreases gastric acidity when used as antacid Relieves mild constipation Evacuates colon when used before rectal/bowel examinations	Caution patients to read labels of OTC products carefully for magnesium content. Forewarn patients that diarrhea may occur. When administering magnesium, recognize that combination with the following drugs will decrease their absorption: digoxin, penicillamine, aminoquinolones, nitrofurantoin, and tetracyclines. Administer these drugs at least 2 h apart.
phosphorus (Neutra-Phos)	Dietary supplement for periods of growth or stress	Avoid using phosphorus if patient is on a sodium- or potassium-restricted diet. Reconstitute powdered drug form before administering. Monitor potassium level if patient is receiving potassium or using potassium-sparing diuretics. Caution patient that antacids, calcium vitamin D products may decrease phosphorus levels. Explain that adverse effects may include GI upset, diarrhea, dizziness, seizures, confusion, muscle cramps. Advise patient to stop taking drug and report excessive diarrhea.
zinc (Orazinc, Verazinc, Zincate)	Supplements diet to treat or prevent zinc deficiency Speeds healing	Administer with food if GI upset occurs. Avoid high-fiber diets, calcium, and phosphates in combination; administer at least 2 h apart.

Continued

Nutritional Component	Purpose	Nursing Management
	Treats rheumatoid arthritis, Wilson's disease, and common cold	Encourage patients to check OTC products to avoid zinc overdose. Caution patients that adverse effects may include nausea, vomiting, and diarrhea.
Enteral Supplements		
Contain: amino acids carbohydrates fats electrolytes vitamins trace elements	Supplement intake for anorectic patient, those with impaired swallowing or those with digestive or absorptive disorders	Check placement of feeding tube prior to administration. Check order for continuous or intermittent administration. Check for residual per institution's protocol. Monitor for signs of aspiration. Check glucose. Monitor for signs of electrolyte imbalance.

Appendix E

PARENTERAL NUTRITION

Parenteral nutrition (PN) is administration through a central or other IV line of essential proteins, amino acids, carbohydrates, vitamins, minerals, trace elements, lipids, and fluid. PN is used to improve or stabilize the nutritional status of cachetic or debilitated patients who cannot take or absorb oral nutrition to maintain their nutritional status. The exact composition of the PN solution is determined after a nutritional assessment and takes into account *core drug knowledge* related to the parenteral solution and *core patient variables* of the patient's current health status, age, and metabolic needs.

PN is contraindicated in anyone with known allergies to any of the solution's components. Many multiple combination products are available and a solution that is suitable for any patient can be given. Adverse effects that may accompany PN include mechanical problems (related to the IV line, such as pneumothorax, infections, air emboli, or emboli related to protein or lipid aggregations), infections related to the nutrient-rich solution and invasive administration, metabolic imbalances related to the composition of the solution, gallstone development (especially in children), and nausea (associated with administering lipids).

Before PN begins, a nutritional assessment should be performed with additional assessments made periodically during therapy. Core patient variables to include in the assessment are the patient's height, weight, dietary and medical histories, current illness, and current drug therapy regimens. Daily assessments include daily weights, fractional urine analyses, blood glucose levels every 6 to 8 hours, vital signs, strict intake and output, condition of the infusion pump and insertion site (checked at every shift), neurologic status, and blood chemistry values (to evaluate the effectiveness of therapy).

Parenteral solutions should be refrigerated until ready to be administered. Just before administration, the solution's components should be checked against the prescribed components. Then, the solution should be inspected for abnormalities, such as precipitates, cloudiness, or color changes. The solution should not hang for more than 24 hours after which it should be replaced. In most cases, inline filters are recommended to decrease the opportunity for bacteria or aggregates to be infused with the solution.

PN is used during pregnancy in patients whose conditions limit nutritional intake. Elderly patients should be assessed carefully when receiving PN because they may not tolerate the increased volume or concentrated glucose solutions. Extreme caution must be used when giving intralipids to premature infants in whom hepatic clearance is decreased. PN should be discontinued slowly by gradually reducing the infusion rate over several hours. PN should not be discontinued, however, until an alternate source of nutrition has been established.

Patient and family education materials should focus on why PN is being given, the need for monitoring both the patient and the infusion equipment (pump and line) regularly, signs and symptoms to report to the health care provider—particularly chest pain, difficulty breathing, pain at the injection site, fever, and flulike symptoms. Many patients now receive PN at home and must deliver their own infusions. These patients need special instructions in maintaining sterile technique and recognizing warning signs of infection or emboli to be reported immediately. Information about typical PN formulas follows.

PN Component*	Purpose	Nursing Management
Typical Central PN Solution (1L)		
Provides 1,350 total nonprotein calories in 1,250-mL volume of solution with 25% dextrose concentration, 5% amino acid concentration, and osmolarity of 1900 mOsm/L		
Actual concentration and components of any PN solution are determined by the patient's current status and nutritional needs.		
10% amino acids	Provides 50 g protein for growth and healing	*Dosage:* 500 mL Monitor blood pressure, cardiac output, blood chemistries, urine analyses to determine effect of intravascular protein pull.
50% dextrose	Provides 850 kcal for energy	*Dosage:* 500 mL Monitor blood glucose level. Evaluate injection site for signs of infection or irritation.
20% fat emulsion	Provides 500 fat calories, ready energy	*Dosage:* 250 mL Monitor for emboli; signs include shortness of breath, chest pain, deep leg pain, neurologic changes. Monitor for signs of increased vascular workload, especially in very young and very old patients.
sodium chloride	Provides sodium and chloride needed for various chemical reactions within the body	*Dosage:* 40 mEq Monitor cardiac rhythm and serum electrolyte levels.
calcium gluconate	Provides essential calcium for muscle contraction, blood clotting, and numerous chemical reactions	*Dosage:* 4.8 mEq Monitor cardiac rhythm, muscle strength, and serum electrolyte levels.
magnesium sulfate	Provides magnesium for various chemical reactions within the body	*Dosage:* 8 mEq Monitor blood pressure and serum electrolyte levels.
potassium phosphate	Provides needed potassium for nerve functioning and muscle contraction	*Dosage:* 9 mMol Monitor blood pressure, cardiac rhythm, muscle function, and serum electrolyte levels.
multivitamins	Provides essential vitamins to maintain cell integrity and promote healing	*Dosage:* 10 mL Monitor for signs of vitamin deficiency or toxicity.
trace elements zinc 3 mg copper 1.2 mg manganese 0.3 mg chromium 12 µg selenium 20 µg	Provides small amounts of elements essential for various chemical reactions in the body and maintenance of cell integrity and healing	Periodically monitor blood chemistry findings to determine adequacy of elemental replacement.
Typical Peripheral Parenteral Nutrition Solution (1 L)		
Provides 840 total nonprotein calories in 1,250-mL volume of solution with 10% dextrose concentration, 4.25% amino acid concentration, and osmolarity of 900 mOsm/L.		
Actual concentration and components of any PN solution are determined by the patient's current status and nutritional needs.		
8.5% amino acids	Provides 41 g protein for growth and healing	*Dosage:* 500 mL Monitor blood pressure, cardiac output, blood chemistries, urine analyses to determine effect of intravascular protein pull.

(continued)

Continued

PN Component*	Purpose	Nursing Management
20% dextrose	Provides 340 calories for energy	*Dosage:* 500 mL Monitor blood glucose level. Evaluate injection site for signs of infection or irritation.
20% fat emulsion	Provides 500 fat calories, ready energy	*Dosage:* 250 mL Monitor for emboli; signs include shortness of breath, chest pain, deep leg pain, neurologic changes. Monitor for signs of increased vascular workload, especially in very young and very old patients.
sodium chloride	Provides sodium and chloride needed for various chemical reactions within the body	*Dosage:* 40 mEq Monitor cardiac rhythm and serum electrolyte levels.
calcium gluconate	Provides essential calcium for muscle contraction, blood clotting, and numerous chemical reactions	*Dosage:* 4.8 mEq Monitor cardiac rhythm, muscle strength, and serum electrolyte levels.
magnesium sulfate	Provides magnesium for various chemical reactions within the body	*Dosage:* 8 mEq Monitor blood pressure and serum electrolyte levels.
potassium phosphate	Provides needed potassium for nerve functioning and muscle contraction	*Dosage:* 9 mMol Monitor blood pressure, cardiac rhythm, muscle function, and serum electrolyte levels.
multivitamins	Provides a combination of essential vitamins to maintain cell integrity and promote healing	*Dosage:* 10 mL Monitor for signs of vitamin deficiency or toxicity.
trace elements zinc 3 mg copper 1.2 mg manganese 0.3 mg chromium 12 μg selenium 20 μg	Provides small amounts of elements essential for various chemical reactions in the body and maintenance of cell integrity and healing	Periodically monitor blood chemistry findings to determine adequacy of replacement.

*Multiple combination preparations are available commercially. Each preparation varies in the concentration of one or more components and should be checked carefully before administering.

Appendix **F**

ANTIDOTES

Antidotes are usually given in emergency situations for which the nurse must be prepared with sufficient knowledge (*core drug knowledge*) of their uses and administration. Specific antidotes react chemically with or block the receptor sites of specific toxins. This decreases the toxic effect or, in many cases, reverses the effect of the poison. There are generally no contraindications for using antidotes, although they are appropriate only in potentially serious or life-threatening situations when their benefits clearly outweigh the risk of their use. Antidotes are drugs and, as such, produce adverse effects, which vary with the antidote.

Before an antidote is administered, the nursing assessment should focus on *core patient variables* and include a careful history of the time and amount of exposure to the toxin. In many situations, timing is crucial to treatment. The physical assessment should include vital signs, orientation, and blood chemistries appropriate to the toxin and the antidote. Supportive measures should be readily available, including life support, IV fluids to counteract shock, ventilating devices, and so forth. Patient and family education, which may occur after the situation stabilizes, should cover reasons for the antidote, adverse effects to expect, and drugs and other products to avoid after receiving the antidote. In cases of accidental overdose, the nurse should help the patient and family determine ways to prevent accidents in the future.

Antidote (Trade) Name	Poison	Nursing Management
acetylcysteine (Mucomyst, Mucosil, Mucomyst 10 IV)	*acetaminophen:* Prevents or minimizes hepatic injury after acetaminophen overdose	Administer 140 mg/kg PO as a loading dose followed by 70 mg/kg q4h starting 4 h after loading dose. IV dose is available if oral route is not. Begin treatment within 24 h of overdose. Empty stomach by gastric lavage, and use activated charcoal if feasible to decrease absorption of acetaminophen. Obtain blood chemistries and measure acetaminophen levels before antidote administration and daily until blood chemistry returns to nontoxic levels. Provide supportive care for electrolyte imbalances, hypoglycemia, and clotting problems related to hepatic injury. (*continued*)

Continued

Antidote (Trade) Name	Poison	Nursing Management
aminocaproic acid (Amicar)	Management of acute bleeding syndromes resulting from fibrinolysis	Dilute drug per manufacturer's recommendation. Use cautiously in patients with cardiac, renal, or hepatic disease. Monitor fibrinogen levels.
atropine	*anticholinesterases* (organophosphorus insecticides) and *muscarine/mushroom* poisoning	Administer 2–3 mg IM or IV, and repeat until signs of atropine toxicity disappear. Provide ventilatory support and cardiac massage as needed. Monitor vital signs continually until they stabilize.
calcium chloride, calcium gluconate	*calcium channel blocker:* overdose	Administer 4.6–16 mEq IV. Monitor vital signs continually. Monitor serum calcium levels. Be prepared to provide life support and to counteract hypotension and bradycardia as appropriate.
activated charcoal (Antidose-Aqua, CharcoAid, LiquiChar)	*various poisons:* (including chemicals and drugs, such as acetaminophen, benzodiazepines, and others)	Administer 30–100 g or 1 g/kg PO (5–10 times the amount of toxin ingested) as an emergency treatment to absorb toxic substances from the GI tract and inhibit GI absorption. Administer as soon as possible after ingestion. Induce emesis before giving to conscious patient only. Have life support equipment on standby. Give only to conscious patients.
deferoxamine (Desferal)	*iron:* acute or chronic toxicity	*Adult:* Administer 1 g IM followed by 0.5 g IM q4h; then 0.5 IM q4–12 h based on patient's response. *Child:* Administer 50 mg/kg IM or IV q6h. Monitor neurologic status periodically. Anticipate common adverse effects: skin rash and pain at injection site. Stop drug administration and reevaluate if patient reports impaired vision.
dexrazoxane (Zinecard)	*doxorubicin:* reduces incidence and severity of cardiotoxicity associated with chemotherapy with doxorubicin	Administer IV as prescribed; dexrazoxane: doxorubicin ratio should be 10 : 1. Administer by slow IV push or rapid IV drip. Do not mix with other drugs. Use special caution when handling and disposing of dexrazoxane.
digoxin immune fab (Digibind)	*digoxin:* overdose or toxicity (life threatening)	Administer in an amount determined by serum digoxin level or amount of digoxin ingested. If this information is unobtainable, give 800 mg IV (20 vials). Monitor serum digoxin levels before and periodically during therapy. Monitor cardiac response continually. Keep life-support equipment on hand at all times. Do not redigitalize patient until digoxin has cleared the system (several days to 1 week). Teach patient to report palpitations, dizziness, muscle cramps.
dimercaprol (BAL in oil)	acute and chronic *mercury* poisoning; *arsenic* and *gold* poisoning; *lead* poisoning in combination with edetate disodium	Administer 2.5–5 mg/kg q4–6 h IM; continue for up to 10 d. Administer this chelating agent by deep IM injection only. Monitor for severe nausea and vomiting because medication may be needed. Advise patient to report severe headache or weakness and tingling in the hands and feet.
edetate calcium disodium (Calcium Disodium Versenate) edetate disodium (Disotate, Endrate)	*lead* poisoning, *calcium* overdose, *digitalis* toxicity	*Adult (lead):* Administer 5 mL IV undiluted bid for up to 5 d or 35 mg/kg IM bid; *(calcium or digitalis)* 50 mg/kg/d IV for 5 consecutive d then 2 free d followed by another antidote series.

Continued

Antidote (Trade) Name	Poison	Nursing Management
		Child (lead): Administer 35 mg/kg IM bid for 3–5 d followed by a 2-d rest before repeating antidote therapy; *(calcium or digitalis)* 40 mg/kg/d IV. Prepare a schedule of drug administration days and rest days. Monitor electrolytes and BUN before and periodically during therapy. Monitor cardiac rhythm if treating digitalis overdose. Instruct patient to report pain at injection site or difficulty voiding.
flumazenil (Romazicon)	*benzodiazepine* (to reverse serious adverse effects completely or partially)	Administer 0.2 mg IV; wait 45 s and repeat at 60-s intervals until effect is apparent. Administer 0.2 mg IV and give repeated doses of 0.3 mg IV to a maximum of 3 mg for acute overdose. Inject into running IV line. Monitor clinical response and sedation carefully. Have life-support equipment on standby. Teach patient to avoid OTC drugs and alcohol for at least 18–24 h after receiving this drug.
glucagon	*insulin* overdose/shock (counteracts hypoglycemia)	Administer 0.5–1.0 mg SC, IV, or IM; repeat 1 to 2 times until response is apparent. Monitor skin, color, orientation, and vital signs. Evaluate blood glucose levels and adjust dosage accordingly. Teach diabetic patients, family members, and caregivers how to recognize signs of hypoglycemia and how to administer glucagon by injection.
leucovorin calcium (Wellcovorin)	*methotrexate*	Administer 12–15 g/m^2 PO, IM, or IV followed by 10 mg/m^2 PO q6h for 72 h as rescue drug to reverse toxic effects of high-dose methotrexate therapy on normal cells. Begin rescue within 24 h of methotrexate administration. Arrange for fluid loading and urine alkylinization to decrease methotrexate toxicity. Give drug orally if possible. Be sure to have life-support equipment on standby.
mesna (Mesnex)	*ifosfamide* (reacts chemically with urotoxic ifosfamide and used prophylactically to prevent hemorrhagic cystitis from ifosfamide therapy)	Administer mesna at 20% of the ifosfamide dose as a single IV dose at the time of each ifosfamide injection; repeat at 4 h and 8 h. Prepare within 6 h of use. Discard any unused portion. Record times of injection to ensure accurate timing of dose. Monitor patient for signs of hemorrhagic cystitis.
methylene blue (Urolene Blue)	*cyanide* or *nitrite* poisoning (converts ferrous iron of reduced hemoglobin to the ferric form, producing methemoglobin)	Inject 1–2 mg/kg IV slowly over several minutes; avoid SC injection. Monitor blood chemistries. Keep life-support equipment on standby.
nalmefene (Revex) naloxone (Narcan) naltrexone (Re Via)	*opioid* overdose (to block opioid receptors and displace the opioid from the receptor)	Administer nalmefene 0.5 mg/70 kg IV, then 0.5 mg/70 kg IV 2–5 min later (maximum dose 1.5 mg/70 kg). Administer naloxone 0.4–2.0 mg IV; repeat at 2- to 3-min intervals (maximum dose 10 mg). Administer naltrexone 50 mg/24 h PO (maintenance program for narcotic withdrawal). Keep life-support equipment on standby. Monitor patient continually. Anticipate common adverse effects of dizziness and drowsiness. Advise patient to avoid opiate-containing drugs, including analgesics and cough and cold medicines, for several weeks after receiving this drug.

(*continued*)

Continued

Antidote (Trade) Name	Poison	Nursing Management
neostigmine (Prostigmin)	*nondepolarizing neuromuscular junction blockers*	Administer atropine sulfate 0.6–1.2 mg IV before giving neostigmine. Administer neostigmine 0.5–2.0 mg IV by slow injection; repeat as needed (maximum dose 5 mg). Monitor patient continually. Keep life-support equipment on standby.
penicillamine (Cuprimine Depen)	*copper* (chelating agent that forms inactive complex with copper, leading to rapid urinary excretion)	Administer 1 g/d PO in divided doses qid (up to two doses may be needed). Monitor patient for potentially lethal myasthenic syndrome and bone marrow depression. Arrange for blood chemistries prior to and at least every 2 wk during therapy. Administer antidote on an empty stomach at least 30–60 min before meals and at least 2 h after evening meal.
physostigmine (Antilirium)	*anticholinergics*, including *tricyclic antidepressants* and *diazepam* overdoses	Administer 2 mg IM or IV slowly 1 mg/min or less. Keep atropine on standby in case of cholinergic crisis. Monitor patient response carefully.
pralidoxime chloride (Protopam Chloride)	*organophosphate pesticides* and *chemicals with anticholinesterase activity*	Administer 1–2 g IV as a 15–30-min infusion; repeat in 1 h; give additional doses as needed. Administer 2–4 mg atropine IV concomitantly with pralidoxime. Give antidote as soon as possible after exposure to poison. Maintain airway and have life-support equipment on standby.
protamine sulfate	*heparin* (heparin antagonist that treats heparin overdose)	Administer in amount determined by heparin dose; 1 mg IV neutralizes 90 USP U heparin from lung sources or 115 USP U heparin from intestinal sources. Monitor coagulation studies to adjust dosage and to detect heparin rebound response to protamine sulfate. Have life-support equipment on standby.
pyridoxine (Nestrex, Beesix)	*isoniazid* (competitively blocks isoniazid effects in cases of toxicity)	Administer 4 g IV followed by 1 g IM every 30 min. Monitor injection sites for signs of irritation. Have life-support equipment on standby.
succimer (Chemet)	*lead* (chelates lead in the system)	Administer 10 mg/kg PO q8h for 5 d then 10 mg/kg PO q12h for 2 wk. Obtain serum lead levels before therapy. Ensure adequate hydration during therapy. Also ensure that patient completes full 19-d course of therapy.
vitamin K (Mephyton, Aquamephyton)	*oral anticoagulant* (overdosages) (treats prothrombin deficiency)	Administer 2.5–10 mg IM, SC, or PO; repeat in 12–48 h if needed. Because adequate coagulation will take time, protect patient from injury or invasive procedures. Monitor coagulation studies. Have plasma or whole blood on standby if patient does not respond as anticipated.

Appendix G

IMMUNIZATIONS

People develop immunity to disease either naturally or by receiving biologic drugs, such as vaccines. These formulations provide preformed antibodies to specific antigens, which provide passive immunity, or they stimulate the body to produce antibodies to an injected antigen, which provide active immunity. Passive immunity does not provide long-term protection and must be repeated as needed. Active immunity provides long-term protection against various antigens.

The nurse who is administering a biologic product should have an understanding of *core drug knowledge* related to these preparations. For example, most must be injected and are metabolized within the RES system. If at all possible, they should not be used during pregnancy or given when the patient has an acute infection. Specific formulations may be associated with allergies to other drugs and should not be used if the patient has these allergies. In addition, biologic drugs should be used with caution in instances of immunosuppression and chronic illness, after blood transfusions, and in combination with other biologic drugs. Adverse effects associated with these drugs include pain and swelling at the injection site, fever, flulike symptoms, lethargy, and fatigue.

Before administering a biologic formulation, the nurse should review *core patient variables*—for example, the patient's health and medical history—for any condition that contraindicates using the vaccine or for any condition suggesting the need for extra caution. Physical assessment should include temperature, respiratory status, pulse rate, and blood pressure. The biologic drug should be injected using sterile technique into the site recommended by the manufacturer. The patient or caregivers should receive information on comfort measures (analgesics and antipyretics, warm compresses to the injection site), a written record of the drug/vaccine given, and the dates on which to return for repeated immunizations.

Product (Trade) Name	Action and Purpose	Nursing Management
Immunoglobulins		
cytomegalovirus immune globulin (CytoGam)	Attenuation of CMV associated with kidney transplantation	Administer 150 mg/kg IV within 72 h; then 100 mg/kg at 2, 4, 5, and 8 wk after transplantation; then 50 mg/kg at 12 and 16 wk. Give to seronegative recipient of seropositive kidney.

(*continued*)

Continued

Product (Trade) Name	Action and Purpose	Nursing Management
hepatitis B immune globulin (H-BIG, H-BIGIV, Hyper-Hep)	Provides passive immunity after exposure to hepatitis B Adjunct to hepatitis B vaccine when rapid protection is desired Prophylaxis against hepatitis B infection after liver transplant	*Perinatal exposure:* Administer 0.5 mL IM within 12 h after birth; repeat at 3 and 6 mo. *Percutaneous exposure:* Administer 0.06 mL/kg IM within 7 d, repeat at 28–30 d, or administer at same time as hepatitis B vaccine if needed. Avoid administering to patient with history of allergy to gammaglobulins. Inject IM into gluteal or deltoid region. Have epinephrine handy for possible anaphylactic reaction. Provide comfort; injection site will be painful. Give patient written record of injection and follow-up injection schedule as needed.
immune globulin intramuscular (Gamastan, Gammar)	Provides passive immunity through injection of preformed antibodies Prophylaxis after exposure to hepatitis A, measles, varicella, and rubella; also for patient with immunodeficiency Treats ITP, CLL, Kawasaki syndrome, bone marrow transplant, pediatric HIV infection	Do not give to patient with allergy to gammaglobulin. Refrigerate vials. Provide comfort measures for painful injection site. Give patient written record of injection and follow-up injection schedule as needed.
lymphocyte immune globulin, antithymocyte globulin (Atgam)	Management of allograft rejection in renal transplants Treats aplastic anemia Possibly useful for other transplants	*Adult transplant:* Administer 1–3 mg/kg/d IV. *Child transplant:* Administer 5–25 mg/kg/d IV. Administer 10–20 mg/kg/d IV for 8–14 d for aplastic anemia. Refrigerate; solution is stable for up to 12 h after reconstitution.
rabies immune globulin (Hyperab, Imogam)	Passive protection against rabies in non-immunized patients exposed to rabies	Administer 20 IU/kg IM. Infuse wound area if possible. Give in conjunction with rabies vaccine. Refrigerate vial of solution.
Rh_0(d) immune globulin (Gamulin Rh, HypRho D, RhoGAM)	Prevents Rh_0 factor sensitization; prevents hemolytic disease of the newborn in subsequent pregnancies; prevents Rh_0 sensitization in Rh_0-negative patients infused with Rh_0-positive blood	*Postpartum prophylaxis:* Administer 1 vial IM or IV within 72 h of delivery. *Antepartum prophylaxis:* Administer 1 vial IM or IV at 28 wks' gestation and 1 vial within 72 h of delivery. Determine Rh_0 status of parents before giving. Administer within 72 h of Rh_0 incompatible delivery, abortion, miscarriage or transfusion. Provide comfort measures for painful injection site. Teach patient about drug, and explain implications for future pregnancies.
Rh_0(d) immune globulin micro-dose (HypRh$_0$ Mini-Dose, MICRh$_0$GAM, Mini-Gamulin Rh)	Used for transfusion error	Multiply volume of blood administered by hematocrit of donor unit, and divide this volume by 15 to obtain the number of vials needed.
tetanus immune globulin (Hyper-Tet)	Provides passive immunity to tetanus; useful at time of injury	Administer 250 U IM. Do not give IV. Care for wound. Reduce pediatric dosage based on child's weight.
varicella-zoster immune globulin	Passive immunity for immunosuppressed patients with significant exposure to varicella (chickenpox)	Administer 125 U/10 kg IM to a maximum of 625 U within 96 h of exposure to chickenpox. Do not give to patients who are not immunosuppressed.
Antitoxins and Antivenins		
diphtheria antitoxin	Prevents or treats diphtheria	Administer 20,000–120,000 U IM or by slow IV infusion immediately at first sign of symptoms. Warm product before using.

Continued

Product (Trade) Name	Action and Purpose	Nursing Management
tetanus antitoxin	Prophylaxis in patients with untended wound for 24 h; also treats active tetanus	Administer 1,500–5,000 U IM or SC. To treat active tetanus, use 50,000–100,000 U partly IV and partly IM. Perform sensitivity test to equine products. Use only if immune globulin is unavailable.
antivenin (crotalidae) polyvalent	Neutralizes venom of pit vipers, rattlesnakes, copperheads	Administer 20–40 mL IV, up to 100–150 mL IV in severe cases. Remove venom at once. Obtain rare antivenins from CDC.
antivenom (micrurus fulvius)	Neutralized coral snake venom	Administer 30–50 mL by slow IV infusion. Flush with up to 100 mL IV fluids after infusing antivenin.
black widow spider antivenin	Treats black widow spider bites	Administer 2.5 mL IM or IV in 10–50 mL saline solution over 15 min. Give supportive care and muscle relaxants as indicated.
Bacterial Vaccines		
BCG (TICE BCG)	Prevents tuberculosis	Administer 0.2–0.3 mL percutaneously. Refrigerate and protect vaccine from light. Keep the vaccination site clean until reaction occurs.
Haemophilus b conjugate vaccine (HibTITER, PedvaxHIB, ProHIBIT)	Stimulates immune response to *Haemophilus b* in children 2 mo-5 y	Administer 0.5 mL IM in three injections given once every 2 mo for 2–6 mo old; two injections given once every 2 mo for 7–11 mo old; one injection for 12–16 mo old. Do not give to child with fever or active infection. Provide comfort measures for injection site and febrile response. Provide parent with vaccination record and dates for follow-up.
meningococcal polysaccharide vaccine (Menomune-A/C/Y/W-135)	Prevents meningitis in patients at risk	Administer 0.5 mL SC after reconstitution with diluent provided.
cholera vaccine	Immunity against cholera (for travelers)	Administer 0.2–0.3 mL SC or IM with a booster of 0.5 mL at 10 y. Do not give within 3 wk of yellow fever vaccine.
pneumococcal vaccine polyvalent (Pneumovax 23, Pnu-Immune 23)	Immunity and prophylaxis against pneumococcal pneumonia or bacteremia in adults or children at risk	Administer 0.5 mL SC or IM in the deltoid muscle or lateral midthigh as one dose (but not to children younger than 2 y). Exercise caution with pregnant or chronically ill patients. Provide comfort measures for pain at injection site and possible reaction. Provide a written record of the immunization.
typhoid vaccine (Vivotif Berna)	Active immunity against typhoid fever	Administer two doses of 0.5 mL SC at 4-wk intervals; give booster dose every 3 y for continued exposure. Do not give during acute illness. Provide comfort measures for injection site and flulike response. Provide written record of immunization and dates for booster follow-up.
Viral Vaccines		
hepatitis A vaccine, inactivated (VAQTA)	Active immunity of patients older than 2 mo against hepatitis A virus	*Adult:* Inject 5 U/mL IM as a single dose. *Child:* Inject 25 U/0.5 mL IM with a repeated dose in 6–18 mo. Do not give during acute illness. Give injection in deltoid muscle and provide comfort measures (e.g., analgesics, warm compresses). Provide written record of immunization and dates for booster follow-up.
hepatitis A vaccine, inactivated (Havrix)	Active immunity of people older than 2 y against hepatitis A virus	*Adult:* Administer 1,440 EL U IM. *Child:* Administer two doses of 360 EL U each IM.

(*continued*)

Continued

Product (Trade) Name	Action and Purpose	Nursing Management
		Do not give during acute infection. Give injection in deltoid muscle and provide comfort measures (e.g., analgesics, warm compresses). Provide written record of immunization and dates for booster follow-up.
hepatitis B vaccine (Energix-B, Recombivax-HB)	Active immunity to infection caused by all subtypes of hepatitis B	*Adult:* Administer 1 mL IM followed by 1 mL IM at 1 mo and 6 mo after initial dose. *Child:* Energix-B, give 0.5 mL IM followed by 0.5 mL at 1 mo and 6 mo; Recombivax-HB, give 0.25 mL IM followed by 0.25 mL IM at 1 mo and 6 mo. Avoid immunization during any active infection and use caution with compromised patients. Shake container well before withdrawing solution. Inject deltoid muscle in adults, anterolateral thigh muscle in children. Provide comfort measures for pain and reactions. Provide written record of immunization and dates for booster follow-up.
influenza virus vaccine (Fluogen, Fluzone, Flu-Shield)	Stimulates active immunity to influenza virus antigens in people at high risk for developing complications from influenza	Administer according to patient's age: 6–35 mo, 0.25 mL IM repeated in 4 wk; 3–6 y, 0.5 mL IM repeated in 4 wk, older than 6 y, 0.5 mL IM. Do not give to anyone allergic to chicken eggs, feathers, chicken dander. Do not administer with other vaccines or to patients with acute respiratory infections. Monitor for toxicity if combined with theophylline or warfarin. Provide comfort measures and written record of immunization.
measles (rubeola) virus vaccine (Attenuvax)	Stimulates active immunity in those never infected with measles	Administer 0.5 mL SC in the upper, outer arm, and repeat if first given before age 15 mo. Do not give to patients with acute infection or anaphylactic reaction to neomycin. Use caution in patients allergic to chicken products. Do not administer within 1 mo of any live virus vaccine. Refrigerate vaccine and protect it from light. Provide comfort measures. Provide written record of immunization.
mumps virus vaccine, live (Mumpsvax)	Stimulates active immunity to mumps virus in patients older than 12 y	Administer 0.5 mL SC in the upper, outer arm. Do not give to patients with acute infection or anaphylactic reaction to neomycin. Use caution in patients allergic to chicken products. Do not administer within 1 mo of any live virus vaccine. Refrigerate vaccine and protect it from light. Provide comfort measures. Provide written record of immunization.
poliovirus vaccine, live, oral, trivalent—OPV, TOPV, Sabin (Orimune)	Stimulates active immunity to prevent poliomyelitis caused by poliovirus types 1, 2, and 3	Administer 0.5 mL PO at 2, 4, and 18 mo of age; *older children:* two doses of 0.5 mL PO given 8 wk apart and a third dose 6–12 mo later. *Adults:* follow dose schedule for older children if necessary. Do not administer to patients sensitive to streptomycin or neomycin or to patients with persistent vomiting or diarrhea or with immunosuppression. Refrigerate or freeze vaccine; thaw before use. Caution unimmunized adults about risk of exposure to children receiving TOPV.

Continued

Product (Trade) Name	Action and Purpose	Nursing Management
		Provide comfort measures. Provide written record of immunization.
poliovirus vaccine inactivated—IPV, Salk (Ipol)	Stimulates active immunity; given to patients unwilling or unable to take oral vaccine	*Child:* Administer 0.5 mL SC at 2, 4, and 18 mo with booster at time of entry to elementary school. *Adult:* Seldom administered but if needed, inject 0.5 mL SC, two doses given at 1–2 mo intervals and a third dose given 6–12 mo later. See other management measures for live vaccine above.
rabies vaccine (HDCV, Imovax Rabies)	Preexposure rabies immunization for patients at high risk Postexposure antirabies regimen given with rabies immunoglobulin	*Preexposure:* Administer 1 mL IM on d 0, 7, 21, and 28. *Postexposure:* Give 1 mL IM on d 0, 3, 7, 21, 28. Refrigerate vaccine. If titer values are low, booster may be needed.
rubella virus vaccine, live (Meruvax II)	Stimulates active immunity against the rubella virus	Inject total contents of reconstituted vial SC in the upper outer aspect of arm. Do not give to pregnant patients or those with allergy to neomycin or immune deficiency. Defer vaccine in cases of acute infection. Do not administer within 1 mo of other live vaccines or 3 mo of blood transfusion. Refrigerate and protect vaccine vials from light. Provide comfort measures. Provide written record of immunization.
varicella virus vaccine, live (Varivax)	Stimulates active immunity against the chickenpox virus	Administer 0.5 mL SC as a single dose in children 1–12 y; inject 0.5 mL SC in the deltoid area to children 13 y and older. Avoid in patients with allergy to neomycin or gelatin. Do not give salicylates for up to 6 wk after vaccine. Do not administer while child has acute infection. Provide comfort measures and record of immunization.
yellow fever vaccine (YF-Vax)	Immunity for travelers to areas where yellow fever is endemic	Administer 0.5 mL SC and booster dose every 10 y. Administer with caution in patients allergic to chicken or egg products.
diphtheria and tetanus toxoids, combined, adsorbed (DT, Td)	Active immunity of patients older than 7 y against diphtheria and tetanus	Administer 2 doses of 0.5 mL IM at 4–8-wk intervals, then 0.5 mL IM at 6–12 mo and booster every 10 y. Do not give to treat acute tetanus or diphtheria or during acute infection. Administer IM only. Provide comfort measures and record of immunization with dates for follow-up immunizations.
diphtheria and tetanus toxoids and whole cell pertussis vaccine, adsorbed—DTwP (Tri-Immunol)	Active immunity in children 6 wk to 7 y against diphtheria, tetanus, pertussis	Administer 0.5 mL IM on three occasions at 4–8-wk intervals, then booster 1 y after third injection and booster needed in 4–6 y. Do not give to treat acute tetanus, diphtheria, or whooping cough. Do not administer to anyone older than 7 y. Use with caution if patient has history of adverse reaction to early injections. Provide comfort measures and record of immunization with dates for follow-up immunizations.
diphtheria and tetanus toxoids and acellular pertussis vaccine, adsorbed—DTwP (Acel-Imune, Infanrix, Tripedia)	Stimulates active immunity against diphtheria, tetanus, and pertussis (fourth and fifth doses in a series of immunizations)	Administer as fourth dose in series: 0.5 mL IM at 18 mo or 6 mo after last dose of DTwP; then administer fifth dose in series: 0.5 mL IM at 4–6 y.

(*continued*)

Continued

Product (Trade) Name	Action and Purpose	Nursing Management
		Do not give to treat acute tetanus, diphtheria, or whooping cough. Do not administer to anyone older than 7 y. Use with caution if patient has history of adverse reaction to early injections. Provide comfort measures. Provide written record of immunization and dates for follow-up immunizations.
diphtheria and tetanus toxoids and whole cell pertussis vaccine with *H. influenzae B* conjugate vaccine—DTwp-HIB (Tetramune)	Stimulates active immunity against diphtheria, tetanus, pertussis, and *H. influenzae B* in children 2 mo–5 y	Administer in three doses of 0.5 mL IM at 2-mo intervals with a fourth dose at 15 mo. Do not give to treat acute tetanus, diphtheria, *H. influenzae B,* or whooping cough. Do not administer to patient older than 5 y. Use with caution if patient has history of adverse reaction to early injections. Provide comfort measures, record of immunization, and dates for follow-up immunizations.
H. influenzae B conjugated vaccine hepatitis B surface antigen (Comax)	Stimulates active immunity to *H. influenzae B* and hepatitis B	Administer only to children of HBsAg-negative mothers. Do not give to adults or to children with febrile illnesses. Administer IM only. Provide comfort measures. Provide written record of immunization and dates for follow-up immunizations.
H. influenza B conjugated vaccine tetanus toxoid (ActHIB, OmniHIB)	Stimulates active immunity to *H. influenzae B* and tetanus in children at 2 mo–5 y	Administer 0.5 mL IM at 2, 4, and 6 mo and then at 12–15 mo. Do not give to treat acute *H. influenzae B* infection. Do not give to children older than 5 y. Administer IM only. Provide comfort measures, record of immunization, and dates for follow-up immunizations.
measles, mumps, rubella vaccine, live (MMR-II)	Stimulates active immunity to measles, mumps, and rubella in children older than 15 mo	Administer 0.5 mL SC in the upper outer aspect of the arm. Provide booster immunization at entry into school (5–6 y) and at entry into junior high school (12–13 y). Do not give to pregnant patients or those with allergy to neomycin or immunosuppression. Give cautiously to patient with allergy to eggs, chickens, or chicken feathers. Do not give within 1 mo of other live vaccines or 3 mo of blood transfusion. Refrigerate and protect vaccine from light. Provide comfort measures, record of immunization, and dates for follow-up immunizations.

Recommended Childhood Immunization Schedule United States, January–December 2001

Vaccines[1] are listed under routinely recommended ages. [Bars] indicate range of recommended ages for immunization. Any dose not given at the recommended age should be given as a "catch-up" immunization at any subsequent visit when indicated and feasible. (Ovals) indicate vaccines to be given if previously recommended doses were missed or given earlier than the recommended minimum age.

<table>
<tr><th>Age ▶
Vaccine ▼</th><th>Birth</th><th>1 mo</th><th>2 mos</th><th>4 mos</th><th>6 mos</th><th>12 mos</th><th>15 mos</th><th>18 mos</th><th>24 mos</th><th>4–6 yrs</th><th>11–12 yrs</th><th>14–18 yrs</th></tr>
<tr><td>Hepatitis B</td><td colspan="3">[Hep B #1]</td><td></td><td></td><td></td><td></td><td></td><td></td><td></td><td></td><td></td></tr>
<tr><td></td><td></td><td colspan="3">[Hep B #2]</td><td colspan="4">[Hep B #3]</td><td></td><td></td><td>(Hep B)</td><td></td></tr>
<tr><td>Diphtheria, tetanus, pertussis</td><td></td><td></td><td>DTaP</td><td>DTaP</td><td>DTaP</td><td></td><td colspan="2">[DTaP]</td><td></td><td>(DTaP)</td><td colspan="2">[Td]</td></tr>
<tr><td>H. influenzae type B</td><td></td><td></td><td>Hib</td><td>Hib</td><td>Hib</td><td colspan="2">[Hib]</td><td></td><td></td><td></td><td></td><td></td></tr>
<tr><td>Inactivated polio</td><td></td><td></td><td>IPV</td><td>IPV</td><td colspan="4">[IPV]</td><td></td><td>IPV</td><td></td><td></td></tr>
<tr><td>Pneumococcal conjugate</td><td></td><td></td><td>PCV</td><td>PCV</td><td>PCV</td><td colspan="2">[PCV]</td><td></td><td></td><td></td><td></td><td></td></tr>
<tr><td>Measles, mumps, rubella</td><td></td><td></td><td></td><td></td><td></td><td colspan="2">[MMR]</td><td></td><td></td><td>MMR</td><td>(MMR)</td><td></td></tr>
<tr><td>Varicella</td><td></td><td></td><td></td><td></td><td></td><td colspan="3">[Var]</td><td></td><td></td><td>(Var)</td><td></td></tr>
<tr><td>Hepatitis A</td><td></td><td></td><td></td><td></td><td></td><td></td><td></td><td></td><td colspan="4">[Hep A-in selected areas]</td></tr>
</table>

Approved by the Advisory Committee on Immunization Practices (ACIP), the American Academy of Pediatrics (AAP), and the American Academy of Family Physicians (AAFP).

Appendix **H**

ANTIEMETIC DRUGS

Stimulation of the chemoreceptor trigger zone (CTZ) in the brain stimulates the vomiting center (VC). When the VC is stimulated, vomiting occurs. The VC may also be directly stimulated by conditions such as GI irritation, motion sickness, and vestibular neuritis. Increased activity of neurotransmitters, for example, dopamine in the CTZ and acetylcholine in the VC, appears to have an important role in inducing vomiting. Serotonin also has a role in vomiting, and special serotonin receptors are located in the CTZ. The release of serotonin from the small intestine during chemotherapy stimulates these receptors and therefore stimulates vomiting. Nurses administering antiemetic drugs need an understanding of *core drug knowledge* related to these drugs.

The nurse should be knowledgeable regarding why the drug is prescribed and how it works prior to administering it. The nurse should also determine whether the pharmacokinetics of the drug may be altered by any disease processes, or whether the drug has contraindications or precautions relevant to administration. Assess for drug interactions with other current medications while administering antiemetics. Appropriate dosage should be determined for each drug relevant to the patient's age and weight.

The nurse needs to determine core patient variables relevant to antiemetic drug therapy. Assess the patient's health status and life span to determine whether there are conditions that may prohibit the use of the drug. Determine whether the patient's lifestyle, diet, or habits are contributing to the nausea and vomiting. It may be helpful to place the patient on clear liquids or only ice chips to promote the antiemetic effect and minimize additional nausea and vomiting. If vomiting is severe and prolonged, the patient may need to be NPO and receive IV fluids during antiemetic drug therapy. A quiet environment with dimmed lighting is often helpful as an adjunct therapy to control nausea and vomiting.

To maximize the therapeutic effects of antiemetics, administer through an appropriate route on a regular basis. When severe nausea is anticipated as a result of a procedure or drug therapy, such as antineoplastic therapy, the prophylactic use of antiemetics is often recommended.

Drug (Trade) Name	Indications	Nursing Management
Antidopaminergics		
chlorpromazine (Thorazine) perphenazine (Trilafon) prochlorperazine (Compazine) promethazine (Phenergan) thiethylperazine (Torecan) metoclopramide (Reglan)	Nausea and vomiting Chlorpromazine and perphenazine are also used for relieving intractable hiccups	Limit use in children with prolonged vomiting of known etiology due to possible adverse effects. Anticipate drowsiness and caution patients not to drive or perform activities requiring mental alertness until effects of the antiemetic drug are known. Teach patients to avoid alcohol and other CNS depressants due to possible additive effects. Administer by whichever route is recommended, depending on the drug.
Anticholinergics		
cyclizine (Marezine) meclizine (Antivert) buclizine (Buculadin-S Softabs) dimenhydrinate (Dramamine) diphenhydramine (Benadril) trimethobenzamide (Tigan) scopolamine (Transderm-Scop)	Nausea and vomiting Diphenhydramine and scopolamine only indicated for motion sickness Meclizine and dimenhydrinate also used for vertigo	Use with caution in patients with glaucoma, obstructive disease of the GI or GU tract, and elderly men with possible prostatic hypertrophy. Caution patients about additive effects with alcohol and other CNS depressants. Teach patients to wash hands after handling scopolamine transdermal disks because temporary dilation of the pupil and blurred vision are possible if drug comes in accidental contact with the eyes. Safety and efficacy in children have not been established.
Selective Serotonin Receptor Antagonists		
ondansetron (Zofran) granisetron (Kytril)	Nausea and vomiting associated with initial and repeated courses of chemotherapy and radiation therapy. Ondansetron also used to prevent postoperative nausea and vomiting, also an unlabeled use for granisetron	Little is known about the dosing of ondansetron in children 3 y or younger. Dosage recommendations are available for children 4–18 y. Safety and efficacy for children younger than 2 y have not been established for granisetron. Dosage recommendations are available for children 2–16 y. These drugs may be administered PO or by IV infusion. Stable under normal lighting conditions for storage, protect from excessive light.
dolasetron (Anzemet)	Dolasetron is used to prevent nausea and vomiting associated with chemotherapy	Administer orally (100 mg) before chemotherapy. It can be mixed in juice for children. It is given with caution to patients with potential cardiac problems from electrolyte imbalances and patients taking antiarrhythmic drugs.
Miscellaneous		
diphenidol (Vontrol)	Nausea and vomiting related to postoperative status, malignant neoplasms, or labyrinthine disorders	Because drug has weak peripheral anticholinergic effect, use with care in patients sensitive to these effects. Administer orally.
benzquinamide (no other names)	Nausea and vomiting associated with surgery and anesthesia Prophylactic use reserved for patients in whom emesis would cause harm or endanger outcome of surgery	Administer preferably by IM route because IV route may cause sudden increases in blood pressure and transient arrhythmias. Safety and efficacy in pregnancy and children have not been established.
hydroxyzine (Vistaril)	Nausea and vomiting (unlabeled use)	Administer by deep IM into a large muscle. The Z-tract method is often recommended to minimize tissue irritation.
phosphorated carbohydrate solution (Emetrol)	Nausea associated with flu, pregnancy, food indiscretions, and emotional upsets	Do not administer to patient with fructose intolerance. Safe for children with flu or fever. Administer 10–20 mL g15min until distress subsides but no more than 5 doses. Do not dilute because the optimal pH for functioning may be destroyed.
Cannabinoids		
dronabinol (Marinol) nabilone (Cescamet)	Treatment of nausea and vomiting associated with cancer chemotherapy	Administer 1–3 h before chemotherapy begins with last dose 1 h after chemotherapy is completed. Monitor for tachycardia, hypotension and dysphoria.
Glucocorticoids		
dexamethasone (Decadron) methyl-prednisolone (Solu-Medrol)	Treatment of nausea and vomiting associated with cancer chemotherapy	Administer intravenously just prior to chemotherapy. Adverse effects are rare due to short duration of treatment.

Appendix **I**

THERAPEUTIC AND TOXIC LEVELS OF SELECTED DRUGS

In evaluating the effects of drug therapy, nurses always need to keep an eye on the drug concentration in the patient's blood or serum. The following table identifies therapeutic and toxic concentrations commonly established for adults. These ranges are presented in conventional measures and SI units.

The Systeme Internationale (SI) is helpful to understand because, as with the metric system, it has been adopted by most countries in an effort to standardize clinical data in the world community and across all disciplines. The SI is structured on biologic substances reacting in the human body on a molar basis. Like the conventional system, the SI uses the kilogram as a measure of mass or weight and the meter as a measure of length. Unlike the conventional system, the SI uses the mole as a measure of volume.

A mole is the amount of a chemical compound whose weight in grams equals its molecular weight. Thus, the concentration of a solution is expressed in moles, millimoles, or micromoles per liter (mol/L, mmol/L, μmol/L, respectively) instead of in grams or milligrams per milliliter (mL) or deciliter (dL). Although a few laboratory values are the same in conventional and SI units, many differ dramatically, and normal values in both systems vary depending on laboratory methods, equipment calibrations, and other reference sources.

Quantifying the amount of drug in blood plasma or serum is helpful to healthcare professionals because it informs drug dosages and dosage adjustments, identifies inadequate and therapeutic responses, and diagnoses drug toxicity.

Drug	Blood Component*	Conventional Units	SI Units
acetaminophen	P		
therapeutic		0.2–0.6 mg/dL	13–40 μmol/L
toxic		>5.0 mg/dL	>300 μmol/L
barbiturate, therapeutic: see *phenobarbital*	S		
bromide, toxic	S		
as bromide ion		>20 mg/dL	>15 mmol/L
as sodium bromide		>150 mg/dL	>15 mmol/L
		>15 mEq/L	>15 mmol/L

Continued

Drug	Blood Component*	Conventional Units	SI Units
carbamazepine, therapeutic	P	4.0–10.0 mEq/L	17–42 μmol/L
chlordiazepoxide	P		
therapeutic		0.5–5.0 mg/L	2–17 μmol/L
toxic		>10.0 mg/L	>33 μmol/L
chlorpropamide, therapeutic	P	76–250 mg/L	270–900 μmol/L
citrate (as citric acid)	B	1.2–3.0 mg/dL	60–160 μmol/L
corticotropin (ACTH)	P	20–100 pg/mL	4–22 pmol/L
cyanocobalamin (vit. B_{12})	S	200–1000 pg/mL	150–750 pmol/L
desipramine, therapeutic	P	50–200 ng/mL	170–700 nmol/L
diazepam	P		
therapeutic		0.1–0.25 mg/L	350–900 nmol/L
toxic		>1.0 mg/L	>3510 nmol/L
digoxin, therapeutic	P	0.5–2.2 ng/mL 0.5–2.2 μg/L	0.6–2.8 nmol/L 0.6–2.8 nmol/L
diphenylhydantoin, therapeutic	P	10–20 mg/L	40–80 μmol/L
doxepin, therapeutic	P	50–200 ng/mL	180–720 nmol/L
epinephrine (radioenzymatic procedure)	P	31–95 pg/mL	170–520 pmol/L
estrogens (as estradiol)	S		
female		20–300 pg/mL	70–1100 pmol/L
peak production		200–800 pg/mL	750–2900 pmol/L
male		<50 pg/mL	<180 pmol/L
ethchlorvynol, therapeutic	P	>40 mg/L	>280 μmol/L
ethosuximide, therapeutic	P	40–110 mg/L	280–780 μmol/L
folate (as pteroylglutamic acid)	S	2–10 ng/mL	4–22 nmol/L
fructose	P	≤10 mg/dL	≤0.55 mmol/L
glucagon	S	50–100 pg/mL	50–100 ng/L
glucose	P	70–110 mg/dL	3.9–6.1 mmol/L
glutethimide	P		
therapeutic		<10 mg/L	<46 μmol/L
toxic		>20 mg/L	>92 μmol/L
gold	S	300–800 μg/dL	15.0–40.0 μmol/L
imipramine, therapeutic	P	50–200 ng/mL	180–710 nmol/L
insulin	P, S	5–20 μU/mL 5–20 mU/L 0.20–0.84 μg/L	35–145 pmol/L 35–145 pmol/L 35–145 pmol/L
iron	S		
male		80–180 μg/dL	14–32 μmol/L
female		60–160 μg/dL	11–29 μmol/L
isoniazid	P		
therapeutic		<2.0 mg/L	<15 μmol/L
toxic		>3.0 mg/L	>22 μmol/L
lithium, therapeutic	S	0.50–1.50 mEq/L	0.50–1.50 mmol/L
magnesium	S	1.8–3.0 mg/dL 1.6–2.4 mEq/L	0.80–1.20 mmol/L 0.80–1.20 mmol/L

(*continued*)

Continued

Drug	Blood Component*	Conventional Units	SI Units
meprobamate	P		
therapeutic		<20 mg/L	<90 µmol/L
toxic		>40 mg/L	>180 µmol/L
methsuximide, therapeutic	P	10–40 mg/L	50–210 µmol/L
norepinephrine (radioenzymatic procedure)	P	215–475 pg/mL (at rest for 15 min)	1.27–2.81 nmol/L
phenobarbital, therapeutic	P	2–5 mg/dL	85–215 µmol/L
phenylbutazone, therapeutic	P	<100 mg/L	<320 µmol/L
potassium	S	3.5–5.0 mEq/L	3.5–5.0 mmol/L
primidone	P		
therapeutic		6–10 mg/L	25–45 µmol/L
toxic		>10 mg/L	>46 µmol/L
procainamide	P		
therapeutic		4.0–8.0 mg/L	17–34 µmol/L
toxic		>12 mg/L	>50 µmol/L
propoxyphene, toxic	P	>20 mg/L	>5.9 µmol/L
propranolol hydrochloride (inderal), therapeutic	P	50–200 ng/mL	190–770 nmol/L
pyruvate (as pyruvic acid)	B	0.3–0.9 mg/dL	35–100 µmol/L
quinidine	P		
therapeutic		1.5–3.0 mg/L	4.6–9.2 µmol/L
toxic		>6.0 mg/L	>18.5 µmol/L
salicylate (salicylic acid)	S	Toxic >20 mg/dL	>1.45 mmol/L
sulfonamides, all as sulfanilamide, therapeutic	B	10.0–15.0 mg/dL	580–870 µmol/L
theophylline, therapeutic	P	10.0–20.0 mg/L	55–110 µmol/L
thiocyanate (nitroprusside toxicity)	P	10 mg/dL	1.75 mmol/L
thyroxine (T4)	S	4–11 µg/dL	51–142 nmol/L
trimethadione, therapeutic	P	<50 mg/L	<350 µmol/L
trimipramin, therapeutic	P	50–200 ng/ml	170–680 nmol/L
vitamin B_2 (riboflavin)	S	2.6–3.7 µg/dL	70–100 nmol/L
vitamin B_6 (pyridoxal)	B	20–90 ng/mL	120–540 nmol/L
vitamin B_{12} (cyanocobalamin)	P, S	200–1000 pg/mL	150–750 pmol/L
vitamin E (alpha-tocopherol)	P, S	0.78–1.25 mg/dL	18–29 µmol/L

*P = plasma; B = blood; S = serum.

Appendix J

DRUGS THAT MAY CAUSE PHOTOSENSITIVITY

Antidepressants

clomipramine (*Anafranil*)
isocarboxazid (*Marplan*)
maprotiline (*Ludiomil*)
mirtazapine (*Remeron*)
paroxetine (*Paxil*)
sertraline (*Zoloft*)
TRICYCLIC AGENTS, eg, *Elavil, Asendin, Norpramin, Sinequan, Tofranil, Aventyl, Vivactil, Surmontil*
venlafaxine (*Effexor*)

Antihistamines

cetirizine (*Zyrtec*)
cyproheptadine (*Periactin*)
dimenhydrinate (*Dramamine*)
diphenhydramine (*Benadryl*)
hydroxyzine (*Atarax, Vistaril*)
loratadine (*Claritin*)

Antimicrobials

amantadine (*Symmetryl*)
azithromycin (*Zithromax*)
dapsone
griseofulvin (*Fulvicin, Grisactin*)
isoniazid
*nalidixic acid (*NegGram*)
QUINOLONES, eg, *Cipro, Penetrex, Raxar, Levaquin, *Maxaquin, Noroxin, Floxin, *Zagam*

Antimicrobials (cont.)

sulfasalazine (*Azulfidine*)
*SULFONAMIDES, eg, *Gantrisin, Bactrim, Septra,* etc. .
TETRACYCLINES, eg, **Declomycin, Vibramycin, Minocin, Terramycin*

Antiparasitics

*bithionol (*Bitin*)
chloroquine (*Aralen*)
mefloquine (*Lariam*)
pyrvinium pamoate (*Povan, Vanquin*)
quinine

Antipsychotics

chlorprothixene (*Taractan, Tarasan*)
haloperidol (*Haldol*)
*PHENOTHIAZINES, eg, *Compazine, Mellaril, Stelazine, Phenergan, Thorazine,* etc.
risperidone (*Risperdal*)
thiothixene (*Navane*)

Cancer Chemotherapy

*dacarbazine (*DTIC*)
fluorouracil (5-FU)
methotrexate (*Mexate*)
procarbazine (*Matulane, Natulan*)
vinblastine (*Velban, Velbe*)

Cardiovasculars (see also Diuretics)

ACE INHIBITORS, eg, *Capoten, Vasotec, Monopril, Accupril, Altace, Univasc*
*amiodarone (*Cordarone*)
cerivastatin (*Baycol*)
diltiazem (*Cardizem*)
disopyramide (*Norpace*)
fluvastatin (*Lescol*)
losartan (*Hyzaar*)
lovastatin (*Mevacor*)
nifedipine (*Procardia*)
pravastatin (*Pravachol*)
quinidine (*Quinaglute*, etc.)
simvastatin (*Zocor*)
sotalol (*Betapace*)

Diuretics

acetazolamide (*Diamox*)
amiloride (*Midamor*)
furosemide (*Lasix*)
metolazone (*Diulo, Zaroxolyn*)
*THIAZIDES, eg, *HydroDiuril, Naturetin,* etc.

*Hypoglycemic Sulfonylureas

acetohexamide (*Dymelor*)
chlorpropamide (*Diabinese*)
glimepiride (*Amaryl*)
glipizide (*Glucotrol*)
glyburide (*DiaBeta, Micronase*)

*Hypoglycemic Sulfonylureas (cont.)

tolazamide (*Tolinase*)
tolbutamide (*Orinase*)

NSAIDs

All nonsteroidal anti-inflammatory drugs, eg, ibuprofen (*Motrin*), naproxen (*Anaprox, Naprosyn*), ketoprofen (*Orudis*), piroxicam (*Feldene*), diclofenac (*Voltaren*), etodolac (*Lodine*), nabumetone (*Relafen*), oxaprozin (*Daypro*), celecoxib (*Celebrex*)

Sunscreens

*benzophenones (*Aramis, Clinique,* etc.)
cinnamates (*Aramis, Estee Lauder,* etc.)
dioxybenzone (*Solbar Plus,* etc.)
oxybenzone (*Eclipse, PreSun, Shade,* etc.)

Sunscreens (cont.)

PABA (*PreSun,* etc.)
*PABA esters (*Block Out, Sea & Ski, Eclipse,* etc.)

Miscellaneous

acitretin (*Soriatane*)
alitretinoin (*Panretin*)
benzocaine
benzoyl peroxide (*Oxy 10,* etc.)
carbamazepine (*Tegretol*)
chlordiazepoxide (*Librium,* etc.)
coal tar, eg, *Tegrin, Zetar,* etc. .
CONTRACEPTIVES, oral
estazolam (*ProSom*)
*etretinate (*Tegison*)
felbamate (*Felbatol*)
gabapentin (*Neurontin*)
gold salts (*Myochrysine, Ridaura, Solganal*)
hexachlorophene (*pHisoHex,* etc.)

Miscellaneous (cont.)

interferon alfa-2b (*Intron A*)
interferon beta-1b (*Betaseron*)
*isotretinoin (*Accutane*)
masoprocol (*Actinex*) Note: This drug does not cause photosensitivity but is used to treat solar keratoses; patients should avoid sun exposure.
olsalazine (*Dipentum*)
*PERFUME OILS, eg, bergamot, citron, lavender, sandalwood, cedar, musk, etc.
*PSORALENS
ribavirin
ropinirole (*Requip*)
selegiline (*Deprenyl, Eldepryl*)
St. John's wort
*tretinoin (*Retin-A, Renova, Vitamin A Acid*)
zolpidem (*Ambien*)

* Items with an asterisk are more likely to cause photosensitivity reactions. Individual sensitivity varies widely. Overall, the drugs in this table cause reactions in less than one percent of patients. Tell them that if they get an unusual "sunburn", allergic, or eczematous reaction in skin areas exposed to light, to let their pharmacist or physician know.

References: Pharmacist's Letter Research Staff. Knoben JE, Anderson PO. Handbook of Clinical Drug Data, 9th ed, 1999. Medical Letter 1995;37(945):35.

Users of this document are cautioned to use their own professional judgment and consult any other necessary or appropriate sources prior to making clinical judgments based on the content of this document.

PHARMACIST'S LETTER ® PRESCRIBER'S LETTER ®

Pharmacist's Letter/Prescriber's Letter • P.O. Box 8190, Stockton, CA 95208 • Phone: 209-472-2240 • Fax: 209-472-2249

ANSWERS TO QUESTIONS FOR STUDY AND REVIEW

UNIT I: PRINCIPLES AND PROCESS OF NURSING MANAGEMENT IN DRUG THERAPY

Chapter 1. Nursing Management in Drug Therapy

1-1. Core patient variables are assessed in several ways: the patient interview, the physical assessment, and the medical record. Data on some of the variables can be obtained from more than one source.

1-2. Core drug knowledge contains basic pharmacologic facts about the drug. The nurse needs to know this information to administer drugs safely, to determine interactions with core patient variables, to devise strategies to maximize therapeutic effect and minimize adverse effects, and to educate patients and their families.

1-3. Learning about a prototype drug gives the nurse information about a group of drugs instead of just one drug. This simplifies learning and helps the nurse organize drug information logically.

Chapter 2. Pharmaceuticals: Development, Safeguards, and Delivery

2-1. The *United States Pharmacopeia* (USP) and the *National Formulary* (NF) are compendia of drugs available in the United States. The drugs are listed by their official names.

2-2. When administering drug therapy, the nurse must understand how body tissues process or absorb, distribute, metabolize, and eliminate a drug (pharmacokinetics) and the effect of that drug on body tissues and systems (pharmacodynamics).

2-3. Drugs are named to describe their organic structure (chemical structure), their chemical composition (chemical name), their general properties derived from their chemical components (generic name), and their desired effect as intended by the manufacturer (trade name).

2-4. Drugs are classified according to chemical composition, physiologic effect, or therapeutic use. Organizing a multitude of drugs into family groups—drug classes—with similar characteristics facilitates learning about an individual drug within the group. A general characteristic of the drug class is likely to apply to a single drug within the class.

2-5. The 1938 Food, Drug, and Cosmetic Act prohibited the marketing of new drugs before they had been properly tested for safety. It further stipulated that pharmaceutical companies had to submit an investigational new drug exemption to the government for review of a drug's safety before it could sell the product. The Durham-Humphrey Amendment provided further safety. This amendment distinguished between legend drugs (requiring a prescription) and over-the-counter drugs (not requiring a prescription) and required that labels of legend drugs carry the legend: "Caution—Federal law prohibits dispensing without a prescription." It further specified certain drugs that could not be refilled without a new prescription from the health care provider. The Canadian Narcotics Council Act (1961) regulated possession, sale, manufacture, production, and distribution of narcotics.

2-6. Clinical trials proceed after extensive animal testing proves the safety and efficacy of a new drug. There are four phases to a clinical trial. Phase I establishes optimal dosage range and pharmacokinetics. Phase II closely monitors study participants for the drug's effectiveness and adverse effects. Phase III begins if no serious adverse effects have been identified in phase II. Double-blind studies (neither the investigator nor the study subject knows whether the drug being administered is a placebo or the new drug being studied) establish the drug's clinical effectiveness, safety, and dosage range. Phase IV consists of postmarketing studies. Some drugs make it through all phases of clinical trials without problems; not until they are used in the general population do severe adverse effects show up. Examples of this are felbamate and aplastic anemia, troglitazone and hepatic failure.

2-7. Controlled substances are drugs defined and categorized according to their abuse potential and dependence-producing liability. The 1970 Controlled Substance Act requires an accounting of all controlled drugs on a special record and an accounting of all discarded or wasted medication. Another licensed nurse must countersign the special record. Furthermore, all controlled substances must be kept under double lock. Only authorized people have access to the keys.

2-8. The FDA pregnancy categories (A, B, C, D, X) are a classification system related to the effects of drugs on the unborn fetus. The category helps health care providers recommend drugs on a risk-versus-benefit basis. Drugs in categories A through D could be used in life-threatening situations. Drugs in category X (e.g., thalidomide) should be avoided during pregnancy.

2-9. All patients should be taught not to share drugs with anyone else, to follow directions for use that appear on the drug label, to avoid drinking alcohol with any prescription or OTC drug, and not to take a drug after its expiration date.

2-10. The patient teaching plan for drug therapy should include drug name and reason for use; the dosage (amount, frequency, duration of therapy, what to do about a missed dose or a double dose); administration route; special directions or procedures (for drug administration, drug stability, storage, disposal); minor adverse effects and reportable serious adverse effects; drug interactions (among drugs and foods); effects of other disease states on drug therapy; and self-monitoring techniques.

Chapter 3. Drug Preparations and Administration

3-1. The most frequently used drug administration route is the enteral route for oral drugs.

3-2. An enteric coating prevents the drug from breaking down in the stomach and thus prevents GI irritation and inactivation of the drug by stomach acid. Sustained release may also occur with enteric coating.

3-3. The parenteral route may be recommended for a patient who is unable to swallow, is confused and uncooperative with oral medications, is unconscious, or may have a physiologic need to keep the GI tract empty to prepare for diagnostic tests, surgery, or rest the tract. The drug may have a high first-pass effect when administered orally, which eliminates most of the active drug, or the drug may be inactivated by gastric acid.

3-4. The greatest risk for rapid drug toxicity is the intravenous route, especially in cases of continuous intravenous infusion.

UNIT II: CORE DRUG KNOWLEDGE

Chapter 4. Pharmacotherapeutics and Pharmacokinetics

4-1. Factors that may influence absorption are drug solubility, ionization, drug concentration, blood flow, surface conditions, absorptive site, and contact time.

4-2. First-pass phenomenon occurs when drugs entering the body by the enteral route first go through the portal circulation to the liver before being presented to the general circulation. This metabolic process usually involves extensive drug breakdown.

4-3. Most drugs, medications, environmental pollutants, food additives, packing materials, dyes, and contaminants are in a class of substances described as "xenobiotic," which means alien to the organism. Introduction of xenobiotic substances, specifically drugs, into the organism requires the host to initiate a process known as drug metabolism, by which the body attempts to neutralize or detoxify the substance. The resultant actions may effect many changes in the original material before its secretion or excretion. The outcome of these transforming metabolic processes is known as biotransformation.

4-4. Differences in individual drug responses occur for several reasons. Individual responses and susceptibilities to drugs usually result from the balance or imbalance produced from the bioactivation of the drug to toxic metabolites and their subsequent detoxification. Such imbalances may be genetically determined or acquired and may be systemwide or tissue specific. Other factors, such as physiology, chronobiology, environment, and pathologic and other problems may modify a person's response to drug therapy as well.

4-5. In elderly patients, clearance (rate of drug removal from the body) is reduced. Specifically, hepatic clearance of many drugs is reduced; most likely from a decrease in liver size and function, decreased function of the nephron and decreased blood flow. In frail elderly patients, a reduction in hepatic enzyme capacity also may contribute to this reduced clearance. In chronic illness, especially with multiorgan dysfunction, patients are often exposed to multiple drugs (polypharmacy). The resultant complex of interactions between drugs and poorly responsive organ systems may produce unpredictable adverse effects.

Chapter 5. Pharmacodynamics

5-1. The three mechanisms are known as the pharmaceutical phase, the pharmacokinetic phase, and the pharmacodynamic phase.

5-2. A drug agonist is a drug capable of combining with receptors to initiate a drug action. Agonist drugs work directly to alter the biologic functional properties of the receptor to which they bind. They possess affinity and intrinsic activity (efficacy). In short, agonists are molecules that stimulate receptors. Drug antagonists attach to cell receptors (by affinity); they do not effect a response (known as efficacy), however. An antagonist opposes or resists the action of other agents, structures, diseases, or physiologic processes that would neutralize or impede its action or effect. Antagonistic drugs prevent receptor stimulation; they may also be called receptor blockers because they "block" the receptor from binding to agonist molecules.

Chapter 6. Adverse Effects and Drug Interactions

6-1. Drugs can interact with other drugs to alter drug binding in the GI tract, GI motility, GI pH, intestinal flora, drug metabolism (enzyme induction or inhibition), protein binding displacement, and renal excretion (glomerular filtration, renal tubular secretion).

6-2. Symptoms of a drug allergy include redness, swelling rash, wheals (hives), itching, and possibly wheezing and breathing problems.

6-3. Ototoxicity is characterized by damage to the eighth cranial nerve. It involves vestibular and cochlear functions of the ear. Signs and symptoms include tinnitus, hearing loss, and problems with balance. It may or may not be reversible.

UNIT III: CORE PATIENT VARIABLES

Chapter 7. Life Span: Children

7-1. In the infant and especially the neonate, immature liver function affects drug distribution. The neonate's immature liver produces fewer plasma proteins, especially albumin, with which drugs bind. Pharmacologic effects of drugs result from unbound or free drug. In the neonate and infant, more free drug is available because less drug is bound to the fewer plasma proteins. This state results in increased blood levels of drugs, resulting in more side effects and toxicity.

7-2. Body surface area is the external surface of the body expressed in square meters. The ratio of body surface area to weight is inversely proportional to length.

7-3. An increased dose for some drugs may be given because the drug is diluted as a result of the higher body water content of the infant.

7-4. No. Some drugs have adverse effects only in children and are contraindicated in them. Other drugs do not have enough clinical studies to determine what effect they will have on a child. Extreme caution must be used if these drugs are administered.

7-5. Vastus lateralis or rectus femoris.

7-6. If the past experiences were unpleasant, the child would more likely be fearful and anxious about this interaction or drug therapy. In children, parents and sometimes other family members are normally responsible for seeing that the child receives the appropriate drug therapy at home. This is why it is crucial to include them in the planning and education relevant to drug therapy. Children also need to be involved, at an age-appropriate level, in their drug therapy.

Chapter 8. Life Span: Pregnant or Breastfeeding Women

8-1. A drug assigned to FDA pregnancy category X should not be used because it is almost sure to harm the fetus. The benefits of drug therapy cannot compensate for the risk to the fetus.

8-2. Drugs that have low molecular weight and are lipophilic and nonprotein bound will pass through the placenta's lipid membrane easily.

8-3. Gestational weeks 3 through 8 mark the period of organogenesis, which is when all major fetal organ systems are developing. Teratogenic exposure during this period may cause major malformations that are usually recognized at birth.

8-4. Physiologic changes in the renal system that increase drug excretion rates include that renal blood flow increases 40% to 50%. This increases filtration through the glomerulus about 50% and contributes to increased excretion rates.

8-5. Lipophilic or fat soluble drugs will pass into breast milk due to the high fat content in breast milk.

Chapter 9. Life Span: Older Adults

9-1. Liver function and metabolism are impaired because of decreased mass of the liver, decreased hepatic blood flow and hepatic tissue perfusion, and changes in the phases of metabolism.

9-2. Normal renal function decreases with aging. Drugs that depend on renal elimination are not excreted as quickly in the older adult. This leads to elevated circulating active drug levels, which places the patient at risk for adverse effects or drug toxicity.

9-3. Polypharmacy is the simultaneous use of multiple prescription and over-the-counter drugs by one person, and it puts the patient at increased risk for drug interactions, adverse effects, and nonadherence with drug therapy. Polypharmacy occurs frequently in older adults because they often experience multiple health problems related to organ and body system deterioration with advanced age.

9-4. Adverse drug effects often mimic many changes, which frequently occur naturally with advanced age.

9-5. Activity will affect absorption and distribution of some drugs. Dietary habits will indicate whether a patient will be able to swallow oral tablets or pills. Quality of life may be impaired from adverse effects of drug therapy. The patient may have strict habits about when the drug therapy is taken; following the patient's normal routine may be less stressful. Their economic status, including drug insurance coverage, may affect whether they obtain their prescribed drugs regularly.

Chapter 10. Lifestyle: Substance Abuse

10-1. Alcohol is a CNS depressant. In combination with other CNS depressants, alcohol can produce additive pharmacologic effects of CNS depression.

10-2. Drug abuse is the excessive self-administration of a drug (often dependence producing) for other than therapeutic purposes. Drug misuse is the inadvertent incorrect use of a drug, often because the individual lacks knowledge of the drug. Addiction is a physical dependence on a drug, which leads to serious physical and behavioral problems. Without the drug, physical symptoms of withdrawal begin to occur. Withdrawal is marked by a variety of physical effects, including nausea, muscle cramping, dysphoria, and convulsions. Characteristics of addiction include compulsive drug use, drug craving, and drug seeking. Psychological dependence (habituation) is an intense desire or craving for the drug when it is not available.

10-3. Disulfiram is used as an adjunct to behavioral therapy in the treatment of alcohol abuse. It causes a severe intolerance reaction when alcohol is ingested. This reaction is manifested by flushing, throbbing headache, respiratory difficulty, palpitations, and confusion.

10-4. Factors that place an individual at risk for substance abuse include chronic pain, struggles with self-esteem issues and peer pressure, poverty, and illiteracy among the socioeconomically underprivileged; wealth and influence among the very privileged; profession (health care providers); history of child abuse or sexual assault; and family history of substance abuse, including alcoholism.

10-5. Alcohol abuse may cause malnutrition with vitamin deficiencies, gastritis and GI bleeding, cirrhosis of the liver, peptic ulcer disease, pancreatitis, cardiomyopathy, and cancers of the upper GI tract. Abuse of other substances may cause HIV and AIDS from parenteral drug use or risky sexual behavior, overdosage, pneumonia and other respiratory infections, dependency, seizures, or bacterial endocarditis.

10-6. Methadone is an opioid with a dependence-producing liability. During therapy, patients develop a dependence on methadone. Oral methadone dosing suppresses opioid withdrawal symptoms and the drug has a long duration of action (24 hours), which are advantages of methadone therapy.

10-7. Hallucinogenic drugs distort perceptions and reality. Nursing interventions for a "bad trip" rely on decreasing sensory stimuli and providing for safety and support.

10-8. Two major substances that are abused are alcohol and nicotine (cigarettes). Categories of additional drugs of abuse include CNS depressants (alcohol, marijuana, opioids, sedatives and hypnotics, antipsychotics, and antianxiety drugs), CNS stimulants (cocaine, amphetamines, caffeine), and mind-altering or psychedelic drugs (LSD, mescaline, MDMA). Some individuals use drugs to alter thoughts and feelings.

Chapter 11. Lifestyle, Diet, and Habits: Nutritional Considerations

11-1. Adverse drug-nutrient interactions are most likely to occur if medications are taken over long periods, if several medications are taken, or if nutrition status is poor or deteriorating.

11-2. Drugs and nutrients can interact and alter metabolism by acting as structural analogues, competing with each other for metabolic enzyme systems, altering enzyme activity, and contributing pharmacologically active substances.

11-3. Foods can alter drug absorption by changing the acidity of the digestive tract, stimulating secretion of digestive enzymes, altering rate of absorption, binding to drugs, or competing for absorption sites in the intestines.

11-4. Patients may not consider these substances to be potentially harmful or capable of interacting with prescribed drug therapy and therefore may not volunteer this information unless directly questioned.

Chapter 12. Environment: Influences on Drug Therapy

12-1. The nurse should assess for exposure to chemicals (e.g., air pollution, cigarette smoke, PCBs, PAHs) in the workplace, home, and community. Exposure to these chemicals have been thought to be responsible for alteration of the hepatic drug-metabolizing enzymes resulting in decreased drug efficacy, prolonged pharmacologic effects, or increased toxicity.

12-2. Alcohol, tobacco, or exposure to chemicals (e.g., industrial chemicals, pesticides) may adversely affect the pharmacokinetics of certain drugs by altering hepatic drug metabolizing enzymes and altering drug response of increase the patient's risk of drug reactions.

12-3. The nurse should inquire about the patient's home and workplace environment because they may have a bearing on drug therapy. It is important that the nurse obtain a complete patient history that also documents lifestyle habits that may affect drug therapy (e.g., ethanol, tobacco) as well as exposure to workplace chemicals; these factors all influence the hepatic drug-metabolizing enzymes. This information is important and will help the nurse determine whether the desired effect of drug therapy is achieved.

Chapter 13. Culture: Considerations in Drug Therapy

13-1. A culture is a background of customs and traditions, values, institutions, art, history, and folklore that is shared by a people. An ethnic group has a common heritage linked by race, nationality, or language.

13-2. An awareness of cultural differences alerts the nurse to assess for factors that might have an impact on drug therapy, such as current health status, genetic variations in pharmacokinetics, self-medication (with traditional or alternative medicines), and dietary practices. This awareness also assists the nurse in forming a therapeutic relationship, in communicating effectively with the patient and family, and in providing appropriate and effective teaching.

13-3. Obtain an interpreter or translator. Speak to the patient. Speak slowly. Do not shout or exaggerate your mouth movements. Allow time for the patient to think and respond. Use as few words as possible. Use as many words in the patient's language as possible. Use nonverbal language.

13-4. If the patient is present-time oriented, explain problems that may occur now, if medicine is not taken as directed. If patient is future-time oriented, she or he will be more receptive to learning that the medication will prevent future problems if taken as directed.

13-5. The genetic background of Mexican Americans is quite varied. There may or may not be similarities in how drugs are handled in the body with the way that they are handled by Hispanics. Drug information that is related to findings for Hispanic people can only be generalized to Mexican Americans.

UNIT IV: PERIPHERAL NERVOUS SYSTEM DRUGS

Chapter 14. Drugs Affecting Adrenergic Function

14-1. Predrug therapy assessments include ensuring that there is no known hypersensitivity to beta-adrenergic antagonists (beta blockers) and that the patient does not have contraindications to drug therapy, such as bronchial asthma or chronic obstructive lung disease, severe sinus bradycardia, right ventricular hypertrophy or failure secondary to pulmonary hypertension, second- and third-degree AV block, overt cardiac failure, or cardiogenic shock. Additional assessments include detecting any disorder requiring precautions with beta blockers, such as peripheral vascular disease, allergies, asthma, chronic obstructive lung disease or bronchospastic disease, congestive heart failure, hepatic disease, diabetes mellitus, hyperthyroidism, and cerebrovascular insufficiency.

14-2. When monitoring therapeutic effects of beta-blocker therapy for angina, the nurse monitors for reduced use of nitroglycerin and reduced frequency, severity, onset, and duration of angina-related pain. The heart rate is monitored as well.

14-3. Impending propranolol toxicity is recognized by bradycardia, severe hypotension, depression, confusion, hallucinations, and bronchospasm.

14-4. If the patient shows no cardiotoxic effects, the nurse should withhold the next drug dose and notify the prescriber immediately.

14-5. Intravenous isoproterenol at 0.05 to 0.20 mg/kg/min is infused until a significant clinical response is obtained, usually by titration against blood pressure and other cardiac parameters.

14-6. The initial change is likely to be an inotropic and chronotropic effect resulting in increased cardiac output, followed by compensatory increases in blood pressure.

14-7. The rest of the nurses are concerned about underlying hypovolemia because this volume deficit must be corrected; otherwise, cardiogenic shock can reoccur.

Chapter 15. Drugs Affecting Cholinergic Function

15-1. In the absence of bowel sounds or with hypoactive bowel sounds, bethanechol is given to increase GI motility. Its effectiveness would be gauged by the assessment of active bowel sounds, passage of flatus, or production of stool. Shortness of breath would be assessed by listening to breath sounds and measuring respiratory rate. Shortness of breath indicates cholinergic toxicity and should be treated immediately with the antidote atropine. To ease the work of respiration, the head of the bed can be raised. The patient should be checked every 15 minutes after atropine administration and observed until stable.

15-2. Headache, decreasing blood pressure, and decreased pulse rate are due to the stimulation of muscarinic receptors in the cardiovascular system. These signs may indicate impending toxicity or adverse effects.

15-3. A cholinergic crisis results from overstimulation of cholinergic receptors following the inhibition of cholinesterase or overdosing with a cholinergic agent. It is treated by administering an anticholinergic to block the muscarinic receptors and a sympathomimetic to increase peripheral resistance and restore blood pressure; if the crisis is due to the use of an irreversible inhibitor, such as an insecticide, an oxime, such as pralidoxime, is needed to regenerate the postsynaptic cholinesterase enzyme.

15-4. Parasympathetic nerves innervate the salivary glands and some sweat glands. Stimulation of these nerves causes the production of large amounts of saliva and sweat production and secretion. Inhibition of parasympathetic stimulation by anticholinergic drugs prevents the secretion of saliva and sweat, causing a dry mouth and skin.

UNIT V: CENTRAL NERVOUS SYSTEM DRUGS

Chapter 16. Drugs Producing Anesthesia and Neuromuscular Blocking

16-1. It is not always desirable to produce general anesthesia with a single agent, because too deep a level of unconsciousness may ensue. To overcome this, a process called balanced anesthesia is utilized. Balanced anesthesia relies on a combination of drugs to produce loss of consciousness, analgesia, and muscle relaxation, while producing and maintaining a lighter stage of anesthesia. Drugs used in balanced anesthesia include inhaled or parenteral anesthetics, ultrashort-acting barbiturates, neuromuscular blocking agents, benzodiazepines, and opioid analgesics.

16-2. Patients need to be administered anesthesia in a controlled environment, such as the operating suite, or critical care unit. A cardiac monitor, blood pressure monitor, and ventilator are required. Full resuscitation capability is mandatory.

16-3. First, the emulsion is a great medium for bacterial growth. The nurse must be aware of the infusion time to avoid allowing bacterial growth to occur. Second, the emulsion vehicle contains soybean oil, glycerol, and egg phosphatide. The nurse must assess for hypersensitivity to any of these elements prior to administration.

16-4. Bright green urine.

16-5. Local anesthetic agents are relatively free from adverse effects if they are administered in an appropriate dosage and in the correct anatomic location. However, systemic and localized toxic reactions may occur, usually from the accidental intravascular or intrathecal injection, or the administration of an excessive dose of the local anesthetic agent. Systemic reactions to local anesthetics involve primarily the central nervous system and the cardiovascular system.

16-6. Nondepolarizing NMJ blockers induce muscle flaccidity, whereas depolarizing NMJ blockers excite the muscle, promoting contraction.

16-7. In discussing Mrs. Smith's prognosis, the nurse needs to remember that the patient may be paralyzed but not deaf. Because you do not know the outcome of the charge nurse's conversation, you may suggest moving the discussion to an environment where the patient cannot overhear the conversation.

16-8. Teaching for patient undergoing surgical anesthesia with succinylcholine as an adjunctive therapy may focus on the patient's inability to speak, move, or breathe unassisted while using this drug. Patients should be reassured that they will be monitored constantly for safety and explain that discomforts as after-effects should be relieved with acetaminophen.

Chapter 17. Drugs That Are Sedatives, Hypnotics, and Anxiolytics

17-1. The anxiolytic, sedative, and hypnotic drugs all belong to a group of agents that depress the central nervous system. An anxiolytic reduces anxiety, which is an apprehensive or uneasy state of mind. A sedative drug calms the individual and helps to reduce anxiety. A hypnotic drug produces drowsiness and induces a state of natural sleep, although all hypnotic drugs will alter the sleep cycles to some degree. Sedative and anxiolytic drugs will produce hypnosis as their dosage is increased.

17-2. Anxiolytic and sedative-hypnotic drugs reduce only specific symptoms of anxiety or insomnia—they do not alter their causative factors. They are useful as an adjunctive therapy to minimize feelings of distress and help the individual cope with the underlying stressors. When taken chronically, almost all of the anxiolytic and sedative-hypnotic drugs can produce a psychologic and physiologic dependence.

17-3. The pharmacotherapeutic uses of the benzodiazepines include antianxiety agents, sedative-hypnotics, adjuncts to analgesia, preoperative or preprocedure sedation with an amnesic effect, chronic anticonvulsants (e.g., clonazepam), acute anticonvulsants for status epilepticus (e.g., diazepam, midazolam), skeletal muscle relaxation, and acute alcohol withdrawal (e.g., chlordiazepoxide).

Benzodiazepines are believed to enhance the activity of the inhibitory neurotransmitter gamma-aminobutyric acid (GABA) and act on the benzodiazepine receptors in the reticular activating formation and the limbic system to produce a rather specific CNS depression.

17-4. The use of the barbiturates is limited by the fact that they produce all levels of a generalized CNS depression—from mild sedation to hypnosis to death from respiratory depression—depending on their dosage. Relatively low doses of barbiturates depress the sensory cortex, decrease motor activity, and produce sedation and drowsiness. Barbiturates have a high abuse potential and are classified C-II and C-III.

17-5. Pharmacologically active metabolites produce a longer duration of drug action and cause a greater disruption in sleep cycles. Patients may complain of a "hangover" effect of excessive daytime sedation.

17-6. Benzodiazepines potentiate the effects of other CNS depressants including alcohol, antihistamines, narcotics, and barbiturates. They should not be used in combination. There is the possibility of both psychologic and physical tolerance and of dependence occurring with use of the benzodiazepines. They should be used for the shortest time possible and in the lowest dose possible. Sedation and ataxia are the most common side effects of the benzodiazepines and the elderly are especially sensitive to their effects. Caution the patient and family that the benzodiazepines may cause transient drowsiness and dizziness. The patient should avoid driving or engaging in dangerous activities (e.g., operating machinery, activities requiring mental alertness and/or muscular coordination and dexterity) until effects of the drug are known.

Chapter 18. Drugs for Treating Mood Disorders

18-1. The four categories of antidepressant drugs are 1) cyclic antidepressants—the tricyclic and the heterocyclic antidepressants (heterocyclics are sometimes referred to as "new generation" antidepressants); 2) monoamine oxidase inhibitors (MAOIs), 3) selective serotonin reuptake inhibitors (SSRIs, also known as serotonin-specific drugs), and 4) lithium. The tricyclic antidepressants (TCAs) block the reuptake of norepinephrine (NE) and serotonin (5-HT) into the presynaptic neurons, and this increases the synaptic concentration of these neurotransmitters. The heterocyclic drugs work in a similar manner. MAOIs increase the concentrations of NE and 5-HT by preventing their degradation. The SSRIs (5-HT-specific drugs) block the reuptake of 5-HT and have fewer adverse and toxic effects than the TCAs and the MAOIs. Lithium alters both the presynaptic and postsynaptic transmission of 5-HT and NE and is primarily indicated for bipolar disorder.

18-2. The major adverse effects of the tricyclic antidepressants (TCAs) are sedation and anticholinergic effects (dry mouth, blurred vision, urinary retention, constipation). TCAs also increase the heart rate, produce orthostatic hypotension, and decrease cardiac workload. They have quinidine-like effects at high concentrations, which decrease heart rate, myocardial contractility, and coronary blood flow. For these reasons, TCAs are contraindicated with a recent myocardial infarction and present special concern for the patient with heart disease.

18-3. Some dietary restrictions imposed by MAOI use include avoiding foods containing tyramine, which may precipitate a hypertensive crisis if ingested in large quantities.

18-4. The cardinal symptom of an MAOI-induced hypertensive crisis is a severe headache.

18-5. Disorders for which SSRIs are used include depression, obsessive-compulsive disorder, and eating disorders. Unlabeled uses include attention deficit hyperactive disorder, bipolar disorder, borderline personality disorder, tension-type headaches, schizophrenia, and posttraumatic stress disorder.

18-6. How lithium produces its therapeutic effect in mania is unknown, although it is thought to increase NE reuptake and increase 5-HT receptor sensitivity.

18-7. Agents used to treat bipolar disorder include lithium carbonate, which is the drug of choice, and carbamazepine, fluoxetine, and valproate.

Chapter 19. Drugs for Treating Thought Disorders

19-1. Schizophrenia is a chronic, recurring disorder with multiple symptoms affecting behavior, thought, perceptions, and emotion. It affects approximately 1% of the population—usually in early adulthood (19–34 years). The pathophysiology of schizophrenia is complex and not completely understood. The predominant theory is a derangement of neurotransmitters—dopamine, serotonin, GABA, norepinephrine, glutamate, and others.

19-2. Positive symptoms may also be known as psychotic symptoms. They are delusions and hallucinations. The disorganized symptoms are disorganized speech and behavior. The negative symptoms are anhedonia, emotional/social withdrawal, flat affect, and poverty of speech and thought.

19-3. All typical antipsychotic agents cause similar adverse effects because of their blockade at D2 receptors. Neurologic effects (also called extrapyramidal effects or EPS) of dystonia, pseudoparkinsonism, akathisia are the most common. These effects can be uncomfortable and frightening to patients and occur at a relatively high incidence. A more severe EPS is tardive dyskinesia. Other important adverse effects of neuroleptics include anticholinergic effects, cardiovascular effects, sedation, hepatotoxicity, alterations in body temperature regulation, photosensitivity, and the risk of neuroleptic malignant syndrome. Atypical antipsychotics cause little or no EPS because they have less of a blockade effect at D2. Sedation is common as is tachycardia, fever, nausea, vomiting, weight gain, constipation, and excessive salivation. Clozapine has a high incidence of anticholinergic adverse effects.

19-4. Take the drug exactly as prescribed and avoid OTC products, herbal preparations, and alcohol. Use caution when operating machinery or motor vehicles as drowsiness may occur. Wear protective clothing and sunscreen when exposed to the sun as photosensitivity occurs with this drug. The urine may turn pink to reddish brown but this is no cause for alarm. Use caution in hot weather as these drugs increase the incidence of heat stroke. Consume plenty of fluids during hot weather. Report sore throat, fever, unusual bleeding or bruising, and weakness or lethargy-these may be signs of blood dyscrasias.

19-5. Alzheimer disease affects about 1 in 10 Americans older than the age of 65 with its incidence strikingly related to age. About 15% of the population between the ages of 75 and 84 and nearly 50% of those older than 85. Currently, AD is believed to affect 4 to 5 million persons. The number of people in the United States older than 65 is the most rapidly growing segment of the population. This number is expected to triple by the middle of the 21st century.

19-6. Acetylcholine (ACh) is the neurotransmitter of several CNS neuronal circuits. Acetylcholinesterase inhibitors (AChEIs) are medications that have verified cognitive and functional efficacy in AD and the only FDA-approved therapy to treat the symptoms of Alzheimer disease. AChEIs inhibit acetylcholinesterase (AChE) enzymes that break down ACh and prolong the activity of ACh on cortical cholinergic receptors and in the synapse thus allowing for more effective transmission. Drugs used in the treatment of dementia and Alzheimer disease include donepezil, rivastigmine, and tacrine. The mechanism of action of the three AChEIs—tacrine, donepezil and rivastigmine—is essentially the same. These agents increase concentrations of the memory- and cognition-regulating neurotransmitter ACh through reversible inhibition of the enzyme cholinesterase. Although these drugs have not been shown to alter the course of the dementing process, it is anticipated that disease effects will lessen as the disease process advances and fewer cholinergic neurons remain intact.

Chapter 20. Drugs for Treating Seizure Disorders

20-1. Status epilepticus refers to seizures that last 30 minutes or seizures that recur before there is complete recovery. Consciousness is not regained between seizure attacks.

20-2. Serum levels are related to therapeutic effect and the development of adverse effects in most patients. Some patients may have effective control of their seizures at "subtherapeutic levels," or may develop adverse effects while at "therapeutic levels." In general though, effective serum levels of phenytoin are 10 to 20 mg/mL; adverse effects are usually seen at higher serum levels. Nystagmus may occur at serum levels exceeding 20 mg/mL, and at more than 30 mg/mL, ataxia, slurred speech, tremors, nervousness, or drowsiness may occur.

20-3. There appears to be an increased risk of fetal malformations (cleft lip, cleft palate, heart malformations) as well as neonatal coagulation defect, prenatal growth deficiency, microcephaly, and mental deficiency if phenytoin is used during pregnancy. The majority of women who receive phenytoin during pregnancy deliver normal infants.

20-4. A drug-drug interaction exists between phenytoin and alcohol. A cross-tolerance develops in individuals who consume large quantities of alcohol, and this may mean that they need a larger dose than usual of phenytoin. Furthermore, chronic alcohol use accelerates phenytoin metabolism by enzyme induction, also indicating that a larger dose may be needed. Finally, alcohol use may precipitate additional seizures and make the patient nonadherent with drug therapy.

20-5. Benzodiazepines used in long-term seizure control are clorazepate dipotassium (Tranxene) and clonazepam (Klonopin). Clorazepate is used as an adjunctive drug in managing partial seizures, and clonazepam is effective for akinetic, myoclonic, and succinimide-resistant absence seizures, such as Lennox-Gastaut syndrome. A third benzodiazepine is diazepam. Used IV, it is the drug of choice for terminating the spread of seizures in status epilepticus.

20-6. Carbamazepine may cause fatal blood dyscrasias. This limits the usefulness of this drug in therapy.

Chapter 21. Drugs Affecting Muscle Spasms and Spasticity

21-1. A muscle spasm is defined as a sudden violent involuntary contraction of a muscle or group of muscles. Spasm is usually related to localized skeletal muscle injury from acute trauma. Pain and interference with function attend a muscle spasm, producing involuntary movement and distortion. Spasticity is a condition in which certain muscles are continuously contracted. This contraction causes stiffness or tightness of the muscles and may interfere with gait, movement, or speech. Damage to the portion of the brain or spinal cord that controls voluntary movement usually causes spasticity.

21-2. Cyclobenzaprine is chemically similar to amitriptyline. Combining these two drugs will increase anticholinergic effects. The patient should be monitored for symptoms such as dry mouth, blurred vision, constipation, or urinary retention. Because cyclobenzaprine and diazepam are both CNS depressants, the patient should be monitored for increased sedation. In the hospital, the bed should be in the lowest position with the side rails up. The nurse should caution the patient to call for help before attempting to ambulate. The sedative effects should be assessed before the patient drives a vehicle or performs tasks that require concentration.

21-3. Baclofen (Lioresal), diazepam (Valium), and dantrolene (Dantrium) can be used for the management of spasm and spasticity. Dantrolene is generally reserved for patients with muscle spasticity.

21-4. Baclofen works at the spinal end of the upper motor neurons. Spasms caused by CVA or Parkinson disease involve lesional or functional impairment of basal ganglia, which are above the spinal motor neurons.

21-5. Symptoms suggesting hepatitis in the patient on long-term dantrolene therapy include loss of appetite, nausea or vomiting, yellowing of the skin or eyes, and changes in stool or urine color.

Chapter 22. Drugs for Treating Parkinson Disease and Other Movement Disorders

22-1. Dopaminergics increase the amount of dopamine in the brain. Anticholinergics decrease the amount of acetylcholine in the brain. Both effects restore the necessary balanced antagonism of these two neurotransmitters.

22-2. A significant amount of carbidopa is destroyed in the periphery of the body and about 1% actually reaches the brain. Carbidopa decreases the amount of levodopa that is destroyed and increases the amount of levodopa that reaches the brain. Because more levodopa can pass the blood–brain barrier, a lower dose is needed to induce effects.

22-3. Neuroleptic malignant syndrome is characterized by rapid onset of marked rigidity, akinesia, tremor, and hyperpyrexia. It may occur with abrupt cessation of carbidopa-levodopa therapy.

22-4. A bradykinetic episode is associated with the eventual ineffectiveness of carbidopa-levodopa therapy. The episode, also called the on-off effect, is characterized by akinesia followed by a return of drug effectiveness. The patient is at risk for injury during these periods because hypotonia may occur.

22-5. Patients starting carbidopa-levodopa therapy should have a moderate amount of protein in divided portions throughout the day. They also should decrease their intake of pyridoxine, which is found in such foods as avocado, bacon, beans, beef liver, dry skim milk, oatmeal, peas, pork, sweet potatoes, and tuna.

22-6. Throughout carbidopa-levodopa therapy, the nurse should monitor patients for drug effectiveness, adverse effects, and onset/progression of Parkinson symptoms.

22-7. Riluzole therapy aims to delay the need for tracheotomy or mechanical ventilation in the patient with ALS.

22-8. Some of the most frequent adverse effects of riluzole are asthenia, dizziness, and vertigo. These are also signs of ALS progression.

22-9. Dietary restrictions associated with riluzole therapy include food high in fat content, caffeine, and charbroiled foods.

Chapter 23. Drugs That Stimulate the Central Nervous System

23-1. Many ethnic minorities in North America use khat as part of some religious and recreational rituals, particularly Middle Eastern and East African immigrants from Somalia and Ethiopia. Betel use is more frequent in immigrants from the East Indies, Southeast Asia, and the Western Pacific. The nurse should be aware that khat and betel may produce sympathomimetic effects, including CNS and cardiovascular effects, such as euphoria, psychosis, and dysrhythmias. The nurse should complete a careful assessment and determine patterns of usage, times and amounts last used, and a full medication profile to provide safe, competent nursing management of any therapeutic drug regimens.

23-2. To adequately assess the effectiveness of dextroamphetamine, the nurse should ask questions such as, "How many sleep attacks has your mother had today, yesterday, and previous days?" "How many attacks per day was she having when you first brought her for treatment?" "Is your mother showing or complaining of any adverse effects, like hypertension, insomnia, irritability, hyperactivity, or psychosis?"

23-3. This patient describes caffeine withdrawal syndrome. The nurse should assess the difference between caffeine intake during the week and on weekends. He or she should suggest that the patient decrease the amount of caffeine ingested during the week.

23-4. An important component of health promotion is for the nurse to encourage and support the patient's commitment to weight loss. He or she should remind the patient that sibutramine is only one component of weight loss strategy. Behavior modification and exercise are equally important to reach the patient's weight loss goal. It is also important to ensure that the patient understands that sibutramine may increase blood pressure and to make arrangements for serial checks of blood pressure.

23-5. Sibutramine works systemically by blocking the reuptake of norepinephrine, serotonin, and dopamine, resulting in a feeling of satiety. Orlistat works by inhibiting the absorption of fats from the GI tract. It does not have a systemic action.

UNIT VI: DRUGS USED TO CONTROL PAIN AND INFLAMMATION

Chapter 24. Drugs That Are Narcotic Analgesics

24-1. Because morphine is a CNS depressant, it will suppress the respiratory drive and decrease the respiratory rate. When morphine is being used to treat acute pain, the patient will not have developed any tolerance to the effects of morphine. Therefore, giving morphine to someone who has respiratory depression will increase respiratory depression and may cause respiratory arrest.

24-2. Patients who have been receiving morphine regularly every day for a long period (e.g., as for chronic pain) will develop a tolerance to the respiratory depression that morphine may produce. They will not incur further respiratory depression from morphine. Patients with chronic pain who have a respiratory rate of 8 to 12 breaths/minute may receive their next dose of morphine.

24-3. Patients who abuse opioids or other CNS depressants may have cross-tolerance to the effects of morphine. For this reason, they may need a larger dose than other patients to achieve pain control.

24-4. A rescue dose is a dose of opioid used to treat breakthrough pain. It is ordered in addition to the baseline pharmacologic treatment for pain and is about 10% to 30% of the opioid dose the patient receives in 24 hours.

24-5. The half-life of naloxone is very short compared with the half-life of morphine and other opiates. Therefore, the effect of naloxone will end, and the respiratory depression from the opiates may recur. Multiple doses of naloxone may be necessary so that the patient does not revert to severe respiratory depression.

24-6. Codeine acts directly on the medullary cough center to depress the cough reflex. It also has a drying effect on the mucous membranes and can increase the viscosity of respiratory depression or arrest, as the patient would be unable to independently clear his or her airway.

Chapter 25. Drugs for Treating Fever and Inflammation

25-1. Prostaglandins are found in most body tissues and organs. Some prostaglandins have opposing effects of the body. Inhibition of certain prostaglandins interrupts the inflammatory cycle, thus decreasing pain and fever.

25-2. There are two isoforms of prostaglandins: COX-1 and COX-2. COX-1 maintains the functioning of many cells of the body. COX-2 is found mainly in areas of inflammation. Use of drugs that are nonselective, such as the PSIs, results in inhibition of both types of COX. When COX-1 is inhibited, the cytoprotective mechanism of the body is altered and the patient is at a higher risk for adverse effects.

25-3. The most potentially serious adverse effects are bone marrow depression, blood dyscrasias, renal dysfunction, and hepatic dysfunction. These reactions can be decreased by careful assessment of medical problems and medications that contradict their use. Obtaining baseline laboratory tests and monitoring them throughout therapy will also decrease adverse effects. Teaching the patient the signs and symptoms of potential adverse effects and the importance of contacting the health care provider is another intervention to decrease the severity of adverse effects.

25-4. COX-2 inhibitors preferentially inhibit COX-2 decreasing inflammation. Because they do not affect COX-1 as much, their cytoprotective mechanism is not altered. This results in a decreased risk for GI bleeding. The second major difference is that COX-2 inhibitors do not alter platelet aggregation.

Chapter 26. Drugs for Treating Arthritis and Gout

26-1. DMARDs have the advantage of actually halting the progression of inflammatory diseases and the potential damage they may cause.

26-2. The major disadvantage of DMARDs is the frequency of potentially serious adverse effects, such as bone marrow depression, hepatotoxicity, and renal toxicity. Another disadvantage is that most of the common DMARDs have a long period before results of the therapy is appreciated in the patient.

26-3. Tumor necrosis factor (TNF) is a cytokine produced by macrophages and activated T cells that play an important role in RA by mediating cytokines that cause inflammation and joint destruction.

26-4. TNF antagonists are used in moderate to severe RA disease when other DMARDs have not been successful. Infliximab also is used in the management of Crohn disease.

26-5. Colchicine decreases the inflammatory process induced by gout, therefore it is used in acute gout. Probenecid increases the excretion of uric acid. It is used as a prophylactic medication.

UNIT VII: CARDIOVASCULAR AND RENAL SYSTEM DRUGS

Chapter 27. Drugs for Treating Congestive Heart Failure

27-1. Primary effects of digoxin include positive inotropic effect (increased force of contraction), negative chronotropic effect (decreased rate), and negative dromotropic effect (decreased speed of conduction).

27-2. Digitalization is initiated because the drug's half-life is long (30 to 40 hours). At normal dosing, it will take several days for digoxin to be in a therapeutic range. When a more rapid onset of action is desired, digitalization allows the therapeutic level to be achieved more quickly. Therapeutic levels will be achieved before the drug is in steady state (five half-lives).

27-3. Before giving digoxin, take the apical pulse for 1 full minute. If the pulse rate is under 60, hold the dose of digoxin and notify the health care provider.

27-4. Digoxin is excreted renally. Therefore, serum drug levels will rise in the patient with decreased renal function above those normally expected for the dose administered. This makes the patient more at risk of having adverse effects. A smaller dose may be required.

Chapter 28. Drugs Used to Treat Angina

28-1. This prevents nitrate tolerance, which decreases the antianginal effects of the drug.

28-2. One every 5 minutes. Up to 3 tablets in 15 minutes may be given.

28-3. Nitroglycerin causes vasodilation, especially on the venous side. This allows blood to pool in the venous beds, decreasing blood pressure. The nurse should verify that the patient is not hypotensive prior to administering the drug.

28-4. Vasodilation of the vessels to the head has occurred in the nurse from the accidental exposure to nitroglycerin. Headache is a common adverse effect from this vasodilation.

28-5. Nitroglycerin decreases preload and afterload. This decreases the energy the heart must use to eject blood, thus decreasing the oxygen needs of the heart. Additionally, the coronary vessels are dilated, increasing blood flow to the heart. Circulation is also redirected to use the smaller vessels more, improving blood flow to the heart.

Chapter 29. Drugs Affecting Cardiac Output and Rhythm

29-1. Ventricular arrhythmias (tachycardia and fibrillation) do not allow the ventricle to fill adequately with blood. The rapid contractions are also not effective at emptying the ventricle. Consequently, cardiac output decreases significantly. The body needs oxygenated blood to survive.

29-2. Proarrhythmia is the tendency of a drug to create a new arrhythmia or to exacerbate the arrhythmia it is supposed to be treating.

29-3. Antiarrhythmics alter the normal mechanisms that control heart rate and rhythm. Therefore, they can also cause an arrhythmia.

29-4. Class I depresses phase 0. Class II depresses phase 4 (depolarization). Class III produces a prolonged phase 3 (repolarization). Class IV depresses phase 4 (depolarization) and lengthens phases 1 and 2 of repolarization.

29-5. Quinidine is used mostly to treat atrial arrhythmias (premature atrial, AV junctional, paroxysmal atrial (supraventricular) tachycardia, paroxysmal AV junctional rhythm, atrial flutter, paroxysmal and chronic atrial fibrillation, established atrial fibrillation when drug therapy is appropriate). It is used as maintenance therapy after electrical conversion of atrial fibrillation or flutter. It also is used to treat premature ventricular contractions, and paroxysmal ventricular tachycardia not associated with complete heart block.

29-6. Beta blockers are used as antiarrhythmics, to treat hypertension, and to treat angina.

29-7. Amiodarone has a very long half-life. To quickly achieve a therapeutic level without waiting for steady state to occur, a loading dose is used. This quickly brings the drug into a therapeutic level. Because amiodarone is used for life-threatening arrhythmias, it is important to achieve a therapeutic effect as soon as possible so that the patient does not die.

29-8. Drink plenty of fluids and eat fresh fruits and vegetables. Include varied sources of fiber in the diet. Exercise if allowed by the physician. Discuss with physician the use of a stool softener (traps water in stool).

Chapter 30. Drugs Affecting Blood Pressure

30-1. Lifestyle changes of step I antihypertensive therapy include stopping smoking, controlling weight, limiting sodium intake, restricting alcohol use, increasing aerobic exercise, and limiting cholesterol levels (to prevent hypertension and to lower elevated blood pressure).

30-2. Diuretics and beta blockers.

30-3. The ACE inhibitors prevent the conversion of angiotensin I to angiotensin II, which is a potent vasoconstrictor. By preventing vasoconstriction, ACE inhibitors decrease peripheral vascular resistance and therefore lower blood pressure. The effect of angiotensin II on aldosterone production is also blocked, preventing the sodium and fluid retention that aldosterone produces.

30-4. Clonidine decreases sympathetic outflow from the brain. Because of this, the drug is effective in preventing withdrawal from narcotics. The drug should not be prescribed to narcotic abusers because it is likely that the drug will not be used for blood pressure management but instead saved to prevent withdrawal or sold on a black market.

30-5. The following are safety measures when administering nitroprusside: Always use an IV pump, preferably a volumetric pump, to infuse nitroprusside. Never allow the infusion solution to run by gravity. Monitor blood pressure constantly. Assess for signs of cyanide toxicity, thiocyanate toxicity, and methemoglobinemia. Do not infuse maximum dosage for longer than 10 minutes.

30-6. Dopamine increases renal perfusion. As the kidney becomes adequately perfused, it will resume its normal functioning and produce urine at a normal rate. Monitoring urinary output indicates if the dose of dopamine is sufficient to adequately perfuse the kidneys. The systolic blood pressure should rise from dopamine administration. If the diastolic pressure rises greatly, or disproportionately, it indicates that the alpha-2 effects of dopamine are overriding the beta-2 and dopaminergic effects. The drug rate would need to be decreased if this occurred.

Chapter 31. Drugs Affecting Diuresis

31-1. Before thiazide therapy to treat hypertension is started, blood pressure, pulse, presence of edema, weight, and urinary output should be assessed.

31-2. Conditions treated by diuretic therapy include hypertension, CHF, pulmonary edema, peripheral edema (various causes), renal stones (thiazides), renal disease, increased intraocular pressure, and increased intracranial pressure.

31-3. Fluid and electrolyte problems that are likely to occur in patients receiving thiazide or loop diuretics are hypokalemia, hyponatremia, hypochloremia, hypomagnesemia, hypercalcemia (thiazides), hypocalcemia (loop), hyperglycemia, hyperuricemia, and elevated cholesterol and triglyceride levels.

31-4. Loop diuretics work in the loop of Henle where more sodium is usually absorbed. Because loop diuretics promote more sodium loss than in the distal tubule, more potassium is lost.

31-5. Osmotic diuretics are different from thiazide or loop diuretics because they are composed of a sugar that passes through glomerular filtration but is not reabsorbed. The osmotic pressure that results pulls water into the vascular space and traps it until it is excreted in the urine.

31-6. Carbonic anhydrase inhibitors are used primarily to treat chronic open-angle glaucoma.

UNIT VIII: BLOOD AND IMMUNE SYSTEM DRUGS

Chapter 32. Drugs Affecting Coagulation

32-1. Heparin prevents fibrin formation. Warfarin interferes with the formation of prothrombin and factors VII, IX, and X. An infusion control pump should be used to regulate the rate of heparin administration. Monitor activated partial thromboplastin time (APTT) to prevent overdosage. Use general safety measures, such as placing the bed in a low position with the side rails up to prevent patient falls. Assess the patient regularly for signs of bleeding.

32-2. The APTT should be monitored while the patient is receiving heparin. A therapeutic APTT value is 1.5 to 2 times greater than the given control. The prothrombin time (PT) is monitored while the patient is on warfarin. PT is considered therapeutic when it is approximately 1.5 times the given control or the INR value is between 2 and 3.

32-3. Warfarin interferes with the synthesis of vitamin K-derived clotting factors. Increases in vitamin K intake will interfere with the action of warfarin if the increase occurs after the warfarin dosage has been titrated. Vitamin K does not affect the action of heparin.

32-4. Ticlopidine has the potentially fatal complication of neutropenia and therefore is reserved for use in those patients for whom aspirin is not appropriate.

32-5. Antihemophilic factor (AHF) would be administered before and after surgery until the appropriate level of factor VIII is obtained as determined by blood assays.

Chapter 33. Drugs for Modifying Biologic Response

33-1. Erythropoietin, thrombopoietin, granulocyte colony-stimulating factor, granulocyte-macrophage colony-stimulating factor, and interleukin are the principal cytokines involved in hematopoiesis.

33-2. The kidneys produce erythropoietin, which is responsible for stimulating the production of red blood cells. When the kidneys are not functioning fully, they do not produce normal amounts of erythropoietin.

33-3. Increased risk of infection. This is because the first line of defense to infection (the neutrophil) is decreased.

33-4. Platelets are fragments of large cells from the bone marrow called megakaryocytes. Thrombopoietin stimulates the production of megakaryocytes.

33-5. Fluid retention is the most common adverse effect from oprelvekin.

33-6. The interferons are a broad group of agents with known antiviral and antiproliferative properties. They are licensed for use with several viral disorders (e.g., hepatitis C, HIV-related Kaposi sarcoma), autoimmune diseases (e.g., multiple sclerosis, rheumatoid arthritis, Crohn disease), hematologic disorders (e.g., leukemia, lymphoma), and tumors with known immune defects (e.g., malignant melanoma, renal cell carcinoma).

33-7. All monoclonal antibodies achieve their desired target cell destruction by directly connecting to unique receptor sites on particular target cells, inducing inactivation or programmed cell death. Binding to the lymphocyte causes lymphocytic destruction and immune suppression, whereas binding to a CD20 molecule commonly found on malignant lymphocytes causes greater tumor cell death than normal lymphocyte death.

33-8. The most common adverse effects of rituximab are infusional reactions, including fever, flushing, chills, and rigors.

33-9. Retinoic acid syndrome is a disorder experienced by 25% to 30% of patients who receive intravenous ATRA for their progranulocytic leukemia. It is a combination of hypervitaminosis (neurologic symptoms, dry skin and mucous membranes) and self-limiting cardiorespiratory failure that, although severe, usually resolves after discontinuing the agent. Because this is a frequent occurrence, nurses need to be alert for symptoms and rapidly report their onset so that a therapy break can be implemented and corticosteroids prescribed.

33-10. Cyclosporine has immunosuppressant effects. An active immune system causes the host to reject the foreign cells from the transplant.

Chapter 34. Drugs Affecting Lipid Levels

34-1. High-density lipoprotein (HDL) cholesterol is believed to offer some protection against heart attack and is known as "good" cholesterol.

34-2. Elevated serum cholesterol levels lead to fatty deposits, or atherosclerosis, in the arteries. These deposits narrow the lumen of the vessel, increasing peripheral resistance and thus increasing blood pressure.

34-3. The patient is at risk for drug interactions because lovastatin is metabolized by the CYP3A4 hepatic pathway. If the patient is receiving other drugs that are also metabolized by CYP3A4, the metabolism of lovastatin is decreased, and increased drug levels will result. If the other drug therapy inhibits the CYP3A4 enzyme, metabolism of lovastatin will also be reduced.

34-4. Liver enzyme levels are frequently elevated from lipid lowering drug therapy, regardless of the class of drug. If the levels rise enough, a dose adjustment (smaller dose) is required, or the drug therapy should be stopped.

UNIT IX: RESPIRATORY SYSTEM DRUGS

Chapter 35. Drugs Affecting the Upper Respiratory System

35-1. Dextromethorphan and narcotic antitussive drugs have the same efficacy in alleviating cough. Narcotic antitussives are more sedating, and have more potential adverse effects and more drug-drug interactions.

35-2. Antihistamines block the antigen-antibody reaction. In a viral syndrome, there is no allergic reaction, only a viral infection.

35-3. Fexofenadine is a second-generation antihistamine that does not easily pass the blood–brain barrier. This results in less sedation than with first-generation antihistamines.

35-4. Guaifenesin enhances the output of respiratory tract fluids by reducing the adhesiveness and surface tension of the respiratory fluids, allowing easier movement of the less viscous secretions. The result of this thinning of secretions is a more productive cough. With a more productive cough, the frequency of coughing should decrease.

Chapter 36. Drugs Affecting the Lower Respiratory System

36-1. Drugs can be grouped into mucolytic agents, such as acetylcysteine; bronchodilators, such as theophylline; and anti-inflammatory drugs, such as cromolyn sodium.

36-2. Theophylline acts through the stimulation of two prostaglandins and results in smooth muscle relaxation in both the bronchi and vasculature. Beta-adrenergic agonists are sympathomimetic agents. That means the drugs mimic the action of norepinephrine. In the lungs, norepinephrine stimulates bronchodilation. Anticholinergic agents block the action of acetylcysteine. When acetylcysteine stimulates the lungs, bronchoconstriction occurs; thus, by blocking its action, the bronchi do not constrict.

36-3. Beta-adrenergic agonists, such as albuterol, have the quickest onset of action. They are referred to as "rescue drugs."

36-4. Glucocorticosteroids are the most powerful anti-inflammatory agents.

36-5. Both drugs are effective in reducing inflammation. Glucocorticoid steroids given orally have the potential for more adverse effects because they are systemic. Steroids given by inhalation have a local action, thus they cause fewer adverse effects.

36-6. Cromolyn sodium works by stabilizing the mast cell. When the mast cell ruptures in response to an antigen, bronchoconstrictive substances such as histamine, bradykinin, serotonin, and leukotrienes are released. By stabilizing the mast cell, these substances are not released. Glucocorticoid steroids have a multitude of actions. In the lungs, they decrease the effectiveness of inflammatory cells, thus keep the bronchioles open. Leukotriene antagonists block ability of leukotrienes to bind to their receptor sites. Because binding to their sites would cause bronchoconstriction, this action is blocked.

36-7. The beta-adrenergic agonist inhaler should be used first. This inhaler has the fastest onset. It will open the bronchial tree, thus, the other drugs can be dispersed further into the lungs to exert their action.

UNIT X: GASTROINTESTINAL SYSTEM DRUGS

Chapter 37. Drugs for Treating the Upper Gastrointestinal Tract

37-1. The cause of peptic ulcers is the bacteria, *Helicobacter pylori*. Without treatment to kill this bacteria, the ulcer will almost always recur.

37-2. Highly acidic foods, such as tomato juice, and highly spiced foods may worsen GERD symptoms and may keep the patient from feeling relief of the pain and discomfort of GERD.

37-3. Omeprazole may interact with other drugs that also are metabolized through the cytochrome P450 pathway (e.g., cyclosporine, disulfiram, and benzodiazepines). This may produce elevated levels of these other drug therapies because their metabolism is decreased. Because omeprazole causes prolonged and substantial decreases in gastric acidity, drugs that depend on an acid environment for absorption may not be absorbed as well.

37-4. H_2 reduces gastric acid production by blocking histamine at the H_2 receptor site of parietal cells, resulting in a reduction in the hydrogen ion concentration and volume of gastric acid. H_1 antagonists are not effective at these sites and have no effect on gastric pH but are effective in relieving symptoms of allergic reactions. H_2 antagonists have no effect on the H_1 receptor sites.

37-5. Aluminum and magnesium are commonly combined in a preparation to balance the constipating effects of aluminum with the diarrheal effects of magnesium.

37-6. Patients with chronic renal failure tend to have elevated phosphate levels. Aluminum carbonate binds with the phosphate to return the patient's serum phosphate levels to normal.

37-7. GI symptoms of oily spotting, flatus with discharge of stool, fecal urgency, fatty/oily stool, oily evacuation, increased defecation, and fecal incontinence.

37-8. Serotonin receptors of the 5-HT3 type are located peripherally on the vagal nerve terminal and centrally in the chemoreceptor trigger zone. Stimulation of these receptors will bring on nausea and vomiting. During chemotherapy, special mucosal cells in the small intestine release serotonin, which stimulates these receptors. Ondansetron blocks these receptor sites preventing nausea and vomiting.

Chapter 38. Drugs for Treating the Lower Gastrointestinal Tract

38-1. Chew simethicone tablets thoroughly before swallowing. Shake suspension forms before measuring. Take after meals and at bedtime.

38-2. The unpleasant effects of atropine, such as dry mouth and tachycardia, discourage abuse of the drug for opioid effects.

38-3. Stool softeners.

38-4. No. The kidney that is not functioning optimally will not excrete magnesium. There is a risk of hypermagnesemia's developing from the additional magnesium in magnesia hydroxide.

38-5. Lactulose will pull ammonia from the blood stream into the digestive tract. Patients with severe hepatic disease will have excessive ammonia in their blood. Lactulose will therefore decrease ammonia levels.

UNIT XI: ENDOCRINE SYSTEM DRUGS

Chapter 39. Drugs Affecting Pituitary, Thyroid, Parathyroid, and Hypothalamic Function

39-1. Calcium is a vital anion that is used in many of the body's metabolic processes, including membrane transport processes, conduction of nerve impulses, muscle contraction, and blood clotting. Calcium levels are maintained within a narrow range by the interactions of parathyroid hormone, calcitonin, and vitamin D. These hormones alter calcium resorption from the intestine, affect osteoclast activity to alter the removal or deposit of calcium in bone, and affect the renal resorption of calcium.

39-2. A combination of neural and endocrine systems, originating in the hypothalamus, regulates central nervous system (CNS), autonomic nervous system (ANS), and endocrine functions. Major hypothalamic regulatory functions include somatic and visceral reactions, including temperature regulation, perspiration, GI activity, regulation of appetite and thirst, blood pressure, respiration, regulation of basic body rhythms (e.g., sleep and menstrual cycles), and complex behavioral and emotional reactions (e.g., sexual behavior and defensive reactions of fear and rage). To promote homeostasis, the hypothalamus transmits stimuli to the pituitary gland, causing hormonal release or hormonal inhibition. When stimulated by the hypothalamus, the pituitary gland releases vasopressin (ADH) to regulate water balance in the system or oxytocin to increase uterine contractions or stimulate milk letdown. The anterior pituitary releases various stimulating hormones that increase the activity of other endocrine glands in response to hypothalamic releasing factors. These other endocrine glands regulate growth, development, and metabolism. The activity of both the hypothalamus and pituitary is carefully balanced through a series of negative feedback signals that maintain the levels of hormone present within an effective range.

39-3. Patients receiving somatropin will require it over the long term. It is administered only by injection. The patient or family will need to learn sterile technique and proper methods for reconstituting and storing the solution. In addition, they need to learn how to administer the injection and recognize the importance of rotating sites to prevent complications and ensure adequate absorption. Periodic review of patient technique is important to maintain safe and effective treatment.

39-4. When there is a lack of sufficient thyroid hormone, the body's metabolism slows, and predictable signs and symptoms can occur. However, not all patients with hypothyroid disease will exhibit all of the signs and symptoms. Signs and symptoms include lethargy, slowing of mental processes, neuropathies, decreased heart rate, decreased cardiac output, eyelid drooping, periorbital edema, enlarged tongue, decreased appetite, constipation, increased cholesterol levels, decreased deep tendon reflexes, decreased renal blood flow with decreased output, hypermenorrhea, decreased libido, pale and puffy skin, dry and brittle hair, brittle nails, and intolerance to cold.

39-5. The patient will need to learn how to administer the nasal spray appropriately. The patient should be cautioned that colds or allergic rhinitis will affect the way the drug is absorbed. Larger doses may be needed. The patient should be taught how to monitor urine specific gravity and osmolarity and to keep track of fluid intake and output. The patient should also be cautioned to alert any health care provider about this condition and the current drug therapy. This is important because several other drugs can cause or aggravate SIADH and will need to be avoided.

39-6. Etidronate must be taken on an empty stomach, 1 hour before or 2 hours after food or other drugs. Taking the drug with food results in lower serum levels and a decrease or absence of therapeutic effect. This patient will need to take the drug on an empty stomach to reach therapeutic levels to treat his Paget disease. Dividing the dose may alleviate some of the GI symptoms.

39-7. Gallium can be extremely nephrotoxic. The patient will have to have renal function test results and serum electrolytes monitored closely. Renal failure can further complicate the electrolyte disturbances of the patient. The patient needs to be well hydrated during the 5 days of treatment to flush the drug through the kidneys as quickly as possible.

39-8. Calcitonin, salmon is from an animal source, and there is a risk of allergic reaction, especially in patients with a known history of allergic reaction to animal products. A skin test should be administered before the drug is given. If no reaction is noted within 15 minutes of the skin test, the drug can be used. The patient should be evaluated periodically for any sign of the development of an allergic reaction and should be asked to report fever, rash, lethargy, or difficulty breathing.

Chapter 40. Drugs Affecting Hormone Levels: Corticosteroids and Their Antagonists

40-1. The effects of glucocorticoids on metabolism are potent and varied. Cortisol, the most prevalent endogenous glucocorticoid, stimulates production by the liver, promotes protein breakdown, and mobilizes fatty acids. The liver uses the liberated amino acids and fatty acids to produce glucose.

40-2. Untreated acute adrenal insufficiency is life threatening. Early signs and symptoms are confusion, restlessness, nausea, and vomiting, followed by circulatory collapse, shock, and death. Untreated chronic adrenal insufficiency, which is not immediately life threatening in the absence of stress or trauma, impairs the person's ability to cope with stress.

40-3. Cushing syndrome is caused from an overproduction of cortisol by the adrenal cortex. The effects of chronic pharmacologic glucocorticoid dosing are the same physiologic changes associated with the cortisol excess of Cushing syndrome. These are known as cushingoid characteristics and include fat stores in the face, shoulders, and abdomen; pronounced striae over the fat deposits; thin, weak musculature; fragile skin; and superficial fungal infections from the reduced immune response. Changes in calcium metabolism may cause osteoporosis. Other changes include iatrogenic diabetes mellitus related to increased insulin demand secondary to increased gluconeogenesis and decreased glucose use, hypertension, and atherosclerosis. Mood changes and emotional lability are also common and may be extreme.

40-4. Three major actions of the adrenal steroids are 1) metabolic effects on carbohydrate, protein, and fat metabolism; 2) anti-inflammatory and immunosuppressant effects; and 3) sodium-retaining activity associated with potassium loss. The first two actions are classified as glucocorticoid actions, and the third is a mineralocorticoid action.

40-5. Glucocorticoids should be withdrawn slowly. Exogenous administration of supraphysiologic glucocorticoids suppresses release of corticotropin-releasing factor (CRF) from the hypothalamus and release of adrenocorticotropic hormone (ACTH) from the anterior pituitary. Thus, synthesis and release of endogenous glucocorticoids by the adrenals are inhibited. During long-term glucocorticoid therapy, the pituitary loses much of its ability to manufacture ACTH and the adrenals atrophy in response to prolonged absence of ACTH, losing their ability to synthesize cortisol and other glucocorticoids. As a result, there is a time during which the body cannot produce glucocorticoids of its own when prolonged glucocorticoid therapy has been discontinued; recovery of adrenal function may take from a few weeks to more than a year. The extent of adrenal suppression and recovery time are determined primarily by the duration of glucocorticoid treatment and secondly by dosage. Too abrupt cessation of glucocorticoid use may produce a withdrawal syndrome (i.e., hypotension, hypoglycemia, myalgia, arthralgia, and fatigue), leading to acute adrenal insufficiency (addisonian crisis), circulatory collapse, shock, and death.

40-6. In alternate-day therapy (ADT), a large dose of an intermediate-acting glucocorticoid is given every other morning, rather than the traditional regimen, which has been multiple smaller doses administered daily. Benefits of ADT are reduced adrenal suppression, reduced risk of growth retardation, and reduced overall toxicity and cushingoid changes. The likelihood of adrenal insufficiency is decreased because over the long interval between glucocorticoid doses, plasma glucocorticoids decline to a level that is low enough to permit some production of ACTH and some synthesis of cortisol by the adrenals. ADT doses must be intermediate-acting glucocorticoids (not long-acting) and doses must be administered before 9 AM. The disadvantage related to ADT is that the long interval between doses may cause subtherapeutic plasma levels to occur, thus permitting an exacerbation of the symptoms. Symptoms are likely to be most intense late on the second day after each dose is given. This may necessitate switching to a single daily dose. Patients taking single daily doses should also ingest the drug before 9 AM.

40-7. Glucocorticoids and mineralocorticoids are used to treat endocrine and nonendocrine disorders. Treatment of endocrine disorders (e.g., Addison disease, acute adrenal insufficiency) requires low-dose, replacement therapy of both glucocorticoids and mineralocorticoids to mimic normal endogenous secretion. Treatment of nonendocrine disorders (e.g., inflammatory processes) requires supraphysiologic (i.e., much higher) doses of glucocorticoids and mineralocorticoids to achieve an anti-inflammatory or immunosuppressive effect.

40-8. Water-soluble preparations have a rapid onset and a short duration of action. Preparations with a higher solubility have a prompt onset of pharmacotherapeutic effect and may be given IV. Suspensions have a slower, sustained onset of pharmacotherapeutic effects; they are effective for intraarticular and soft-tissue uses.

40-9. Glucocorticoids have a kaliuretic effect and can induce hypokalemia. Glucocorticoids combined with the cardiac glycosides increase the possibility of digitalis toxicity; glucocorticoids combined with thiazide or loop diuretics will increase the possibility of hypokalemia. When the glucocorticoids are given together with either of these drugs, plasma potassium levels should be monitored and the nurse should be alert for signs of cardiac toxicity. Because of their metabolic effects, glucocorticoids can induce hyperglycemia. To maintain glycemic control, diabetic patients may require increased doses of their hypoglycemic drug (e.g., insulin, oral hypoglycemics). Glucocorticoids, because of their immunosuppressant actions, can decrease antibody responses to vaccines.

40-10. Fludrocortisone is the single available mineralocorticoid; it has potent mineralocorticoid activities. In addition, it also has glucocorticoid properties; their appearance is related directly to dosage. Fludrocortisone is used in the treatment of primary (Addison disease) and secondary adrenocortical insufficiency. It also is used to treat salt-depleting adrenogenital syndrome. An unlabeled use is the management of severe orthostatic hypotension.

40-11. Patient teaching with fludrocortisone is just like patient teaching with the glucocorticoids because fludrocortisone has both mineralocorticoid and glucocorticoid properties. The patient receiving fludrocortisone is at risk for acute adrenal insufficiency when he or she experiences stressful situations during or after drug therapy. Moreover, the patient can develop adverse cardiovascular effects of hypertension, edema, congestive heart failure, and cardiomegaly from the mineralocorticoid actions of the drug. It is important to stress the importance of regular follow-up visits with the health care provider and to promptly report adverse effects of dizziness, severe or continuing headaches, swelling of the lower extremities or feet, and unusual weight gain.

40-12. The major clinical indication for the adrenal steroid inhibitors is Cushing syndrome, which is a rare disorder of adrenal cortical hyperfunction. The prototype inhibitor is aminoglutethimide. Aminoglutethimide suppresses the function of the adrenal cortex and thus reduces the amount of endogenous cortisol.

Chapter 41. Drugs Affecting Blood Glucose Levels

41-1. Pancreatic islet peptide hormones that affect glucose metabolism include 1) insulin, 2) glucagon, and 3) somatostatin. Insulin (from the beta cells) lowers blood glucose levels; glucagon (from the alpha cells) raises blood glucose levels; and somatostatin (from the delta cells) has an inhibitory effect on both glucagon and insulin.

41-2. Glucagon helps regulate blood glucose levels. Falling blood glucose levels trigger the release of glucagon from the pancreas, as do sympathetic nerve impulses, exercise, infection, and trauma. In the liver, glucagon stimulates glycogenolysis and gluconeogenesis, resulting in a release of glucose into the blood. Glucagon helps to counterbalance the effect of insulin if insulin causes the blood glucose level to fall below normal.

41-3. The stress hormones cortisol, epinephrine, growth hormone, glucagon, and somatostatin are insulin antagonists and, as such, counterbalance the effects of insulin, thereby altering glucose metabolism and preventing glucose from entering the cells.

41-4. A patient with type 1 diabetes mellitus has an absolute deficiency of endogenous insulin, and the disease can be controlled only by restoring insulin by injection. A patient with type 2 diabetes still has some natural insulin synthesis and secretion, and this patient's diabetes can usually be controlled by diet, exercise, and oral antidiabetic drug therapy.

41-5. Some acute complications of diabetes include hypoglycemia, hyperglycemia, hyperglycemic hyperosmolar nonketotic syndrome (HHNKS), and lactic acidosis. Some chronic complications include blindness, cardiovascular disease, and poor circulation, leading possibly to gangrene of the feet or legs and amputation. The chronic complications are caused by macrovascular and microvascular changes in blood vessels.

41-6. Insulin must be injected so that it bypasses the digestive system; peptides in the digestive enzymes of the GI tract will destroy the insulin molecule.

41-7. The effect of too much insulin would most likely be hypoglycemia and, possibly, an insulin reaction. Early signs and symptoms are neurologic in nature and include irritability, tremors, headache, fatigue and malaise, diaphoresis, and tachycardia. A later symptom may be loss of consciousness.

41-8. Insulin may produce lipodystrophy at the injection site, particularly if the injection site is not rotated and repeated injections are given into the same site. Lipodystrophy is marked by a reduction in subcutaneous fat. Insulin antibodies are less common due to the highly purified insulin preparations.

41-9. By stimulating the pancreatic beta cells, the sulfonylureas trigger insulin release and reduce blood glucose concentrations. Biguanide antihyperglycemics increase glucose transport across the cell membranes. They suppress hepatic glucose production, enhance insulin sensitivity, decrease intestinal glucose absorption, and increase peripheral glucose uptake.

Alpha-glucosidase inhibitors reduce postprandial glucose levels by delaying the digestion of carbohydrates. Thiazolidinediones are insulin sensitizers; they enhance endogenous insulin rather than stimulate its secretion.

In general, patients who have type 2 diabetes and who are also obese benefit from oral antidiabetic drugs. Sulfonylureas lower blood glucose levels when diet and exercise interventions cannot. Biguanide antihyperglycemic drugs help patients who have some functioning pancreatic islet cells. Alpha-glucosidase inhibitors are useful for type 2 diabetic patients with mild to moderate hyperglycemia, and thiazolidinediones are used as adjunct therapy for patients who have type 2 diabetes and use insulin.

41-10. Adverse effects of the sulfonylureas, biguanides, and alpha-glucosidase inhibitors are primarily GI in nature. They include nausea, vomiting, heartburn, abdominal discomfort, flatulence, diarrhea, and a metallic taste sensation. Adverse effects of the thiazolidinediones include fluid retention, headache, and weight gain.

41-11. A patient who takes a drug from the sulfonylurea family (e.g., glyburide) and consumes alcohol is likely to experience a disulfiram-like reaction.

41-12. Glucagon is used to increase the blood glucose level of patients experiencing hypoglycemia. Hypoglycemia is an abnormally low level of blood glucose that may result from an imbalance in the equation of insulin (or oral hypoglycemic), diet, and exercise. Imbalances may occur because of too much exogenously administered insulin, too little food intake, or too much exercise. Glucagon is a polypeptide hormone produced by the pancreas that elevates blood sugar by promoting glycogenolysis and gluconeogenesis. Glucagon is a dry powder that must be reconstituted and administered parenterally. In addition, the product is accompanied by a specific diluent. It may be given SC, IM, or IV; the patient and family must be taught correct preparation and administration techniques. Furthermore, the family should be taught to provide supplemental carbohydrates as soon as possible after glucagons injection to restore liver glycogen and prevent secondary hypoglycemia.

Chapter 42. Drugs Affecting Men's Health and Sexuality

42-1. The primary effects of testosterone are normal growth and development of the male sex organs and development and maintenance of the male secondary sexual characteristics (e.g., male hair distribution, hair texture and color, laryngeal enlargement and vocal cord thickening [voice deepening], and alterations in body musculature and fat distribution). Secondary effects of testosterone are retention of sodium, potassium, and phosphorus; decreased urinary excretion of calcium; stimulation of the growth of skeletal muscle tissue and enhancement of the growth of long bones in prepubescent boys; ossification of the epiphyseal growth plates; and stimulation of the production of red blood cells by enhancement of the production of erythropoietic-stimulating factor.

42-2. The main risk is premature ossification of the epiphyseal growth plate resulting in stunted growth.

42-3. cGMP (when activated by nitric oxide) stimulates smooth muscle relaxation and allows the inflow of blood into the erectile tissue in the penis. Sildenafil inhibits the isoenzyme (phosphodiesterase [PDE] type 5) that metabolizes cGMP. The decrease in the metabolism of cGMP allows cGMP to remain active longer, promoting more smooth muscle relaxation and inflow of blood. This creates an improved and more sustained erection.

42-4. Finasteride is a pregnancy category X drug. Absorption through the skin is increased if the drug is crushed or broken.

42-5. Poor systemic absorption decreases the risk of adverse effects. Therapeutic effect is achieved without systemic absorption with topical minoxidil.

Chapter 43. Drugs Affecting Women's Health and Sexuality

43-1. In postmenopausal women, estrogen decreases hot flashes, improves vaginal lubrication, improves urogenital tone, improves and stabilizes emotional response, increases bone mineral density (treats or prevents osteoporosis, minimizes or prevents fractures and complications from these conditions), and decreases risk factors for cardiovascular disease and thus possibly prevents coronary heart disease and death from coronary heart disease.

43-2. Progesterone is used to treat amenorrhea and abnormal uterine bleeding because after ovulation, the ovarian follicle is transformed into the corpus luteum, which secretes a great deal of progesterone (and estrogens). This rise in progesterone makes the endometrium ready for implantation. As progesterone levels (and estrogen levels) rise, production of FSH and LH lowers. This prevents further ovulation. When fertilization does not occur, the corpus luteum disintegrates, and progesterone levels fall. Menstruation occurs. Thus, depending on the timing and duration of therapy, either ovulation can be blocked or menses can be initiated.

43-3. The serious adverse effects from estrogen therapy are: increased risk of endometrial cancer, possibly increased risk of breast cancer, increased risk of thromboembolic disorders (including thrombophlebitis, MI, and pulmonary embolus PE), gallbladder disease, and hypertension.

43-4. Raloxifene can achieve the same effects as estrogen on increasing bone mineral density, and decreasing lipids. Raloxifene does not however have the same effects on uterine or breast tissue that estrogen does. Thus, the risk for endometrial and breast cancer is reduced. This is especially important for women who have high-risk factors for these cancers but also are at risk, or currently have, osteoporosis.

43-5. If a dose of an oral contraceptive is missed, it should be taken as quickly as possible; two tablets may be taken on the same day. Two missed pills should be made up over 2 days. If three consecutive pills are missed, the patient should begin a new cycle the day after the last pill was missed or 7 days after the last pill was taken. Another form of birth control should be used as a backup for at least 7 consecutive days of the new cycle and preferably for the rest of the cycle.

43-6. Instruct the patient to take alendronate at least 30 minutes before eating, drinking any beverage other than plain water, or taking any other medication. Swallow the medicine with 6 to 8 oz (180 to 240 mL) of plain water. Do not take with coffee, juice, or mineral water. The nurse should instruct the patient not to lie down for at least 30 minutes after swallowing the medication.

Chapter 44. Drugs Affecting Uterine Motility

44-1. Slow upward titration of oxytocin more closely resembles oxytocin excretion, which naturally induces labor. Additionally, doing so minimizes adverse fetal and maternal effects.

44-2. The three phases of oxytocin response are 1) incremental phase (uterine activity increases evenly as the dose of oxytocin increases); 2) stable phase (uterine activity remains constant even if the oxytocin dose increases because the myometrial receptor sites are already full); and 3) hyperstimulation (the dose continually increases, the frequency of contractions increases, but the uterine pressure decreases so that the contractions are less effective).

44-3. Water intoxication can be fatal.

44-4. Nursing assessment that may help to minimize adverse oxytocin effects include maternal pulse rate, blood pressure, and fluid status; duration of contractions; time between contractions; fetal heart rate, and character of fetal movement.

44-5. Ritodrine is a beta agonist that selectively stimulates uterine receptors and stops uterine contractions.

44-6. If tachycardia, palpitations, and nervousness develop during ritodrine infusion, the nurse should slow the infusion and notify the physician or nurse midwife.

UNIT XII: ANTINEOPLASTIC DRUGS

Chapter 45. Cell Cycle-Specific Drugs

45-1. The goals of chemotherapy are cure, control, and palliation.

45-2. The different strategies undertaken in the use of chemotherapeutic agents include: adjuvant treatment, induction therapy, consolidation therapy, intensification, maintenance, neoadjuvant therapy, palliative therapy, and salvage therapy.

45-3. Malignant cells are characterized by uncontrolled cell proliferation, decreased cellular differentiation, inappropriate ability to invade surrounding tissue, and ability to establish new growth at ectopic sites.

45-4. The following steps (in sequence) should be undertaken to clean up a chemotherapy spill:

- Put on a pair of powder-free latex gloves.
- Place an absorbent pad over the spill to contain it.
- Rinse the absorbed spill area with water.
- Clean the area with a detergent.
- Dispose of all equipment used in clean-up as chemotherapy waste in a container designated for this purpose.

45-5. Health care workers can be exposed to chemotherapy through the following routes: skin and mucous membrane absorption, inhalation, and ingestion.

45-6. Vincristine's low myelosuppressive effect is the factor that makes it better than vinblastine for use with other antineoplastic drugs.

45-7. When extravasation occurs, the nurse should 1) discontinue the infusion; 2) apply warm or cold compresses, as indicated; 3) administer the appropriate antidote, if known; 4) notify the health care provider; 5) elevate and rest the affected extremity for 48 hours; 6) apply a sterile dressing over the site, allowing for visibility of the extravasated area; 7) avoid pressure to the site; 8) obtain a photograph of the site for baseline comparisons; 9) discuss with the health care provider the need for plastic surgery consultation if appropriate; 10) document the patient's name and date/time of occurrence, name of drug, approximate volume of drug that infiltrated, needle gauge, site of extravasation, symptoms reported by the patient and assessed by the nurse, nursing measures implemented, health care provider notification, patient teaching given, and nurse's signature.

45-8. Hypotension occurs when etoposide is infused rapidly. The ideal infusion period should be at least 30 minutes to avoid this reaction.

45-9. The signs and symptoms of a hypersensitivity reaction are hypotension, bronchospasm (wheezing), tachycardia, facial flushing, and anxiety.

45-10. Before starting a paclitaxel infusion, the nurse should check for the correct set-up of the infusion, such as the use of in-line filtration and non-DEHP containers and tubing. The patient should be taught about the possibility of a hypersensitivity reaction and the signs and symptoms to report immediately. The premedication regimen to prevent an infusion reaction consists of dexamethasone 20 mg given 11 and 7 hours before the paclitaxel, an H2-receptor antagonist (such as cimetidine), and diphenhydramine 50 mg given IV 30 minutes before infusion.

45-11. Any of the following neoplastic agents may potentially interact with St. John's wort: anastrozole (Arimidex), cyclophosphamide (Cytoxan), docetaxel (Taxotere), etoposide (VP-16), ifosfamide (Ifex), paclitaxel (Taxol), teniposide (VM-26), tretinoin (Retinoic acid), vinblastine (Velban), and vincristine (Oncovin).

Chapter 46. Cell Cycle-Nonspecific Drugs

46-1. Anthracyclines are a class of red-pigmented antibiotics, namely doxorubicin, daunorubicin, and their analogues the major dose-limiting toxicity of which is cardiotoxicity.

46-2. The highly lipid-soluble cell cycle-nonspecific drugs are the nitrosoureas, which include carmustine, lomustine, and streptozocin. These drugs can cross the blood–brain barrier.

46-3. The antiemetic drug groups used to control acute emesis include serotonin antagonists, corticosteroids, phenothiazines, butyrophenones, cannabinoids, dopamine antagonists, and substituted benzamides.

46-4. Dexrazoxane (Zinecard) is a cardioprotectant that helps to reduce the incidence and severity of cardiomyopathy in women who have received a cumulative doxorubicin dose of 300 mg/m^2 and who could benefit from continued doxorubicin therapy. It is administered by slow IV push or IV drip over 15 minutes, and when it is completed, the doxorubicin flows so that both drugs are infused over 30 minutes.

46-5. Drugs used in combination therapy should be active when used alone, produce synergism with other drugs, differ in mechanisms of action, differ in overlapping, and be given at consistent intervals in maximal doses.

46-6. Combination chemotherapy is superior to single-drug therapy because it kills a maximum number of cancer cells; has a high toxicity range tolerated by the patient; provides a broader range of coverage of resistant cells in the heterogenous tumor population; and is characterized by minimal or slow development of new resistant cancer cells.

UNIT XIII: ANTIMICROBIAL DRUGS

Chapter 47. Principles of Antimicrobial Therapy

47-1. For antimicrobial therapy to be effective, the guiding principle is to use the right drug for the right bug.

47-2. Antimicrobials may be classified by the type of organism they affect, or by their mechanism of action.

47-3. Antimicrobials work by inhibition of cell wall synthesis, inhibition of protein synthesis, inhibition of nucleic acid synthesis, disruption of the cell membrane permeability, inhibition of metabolic pathways, or inhibition of viral enzymes.

47-4. Selective toxicity means that the drug harms the invading microbe but does not harm the host cell.

47-5. In the human host, many bacteria keep other microbes, such as fungus, in check. When the "good" bacteria are irradiated by antimicrobials, the nonsusceptible microbes can proliferate, causing an additional infection.

Chapter 48. Antibiotics Affecting the Bacterial Cell Wall

48-1. Penicillins bind with penicillin-binding proteins located inside located inside the bacterial cell wall. Binding at these sites alters the way the bacteria is able to build its cell wall by affecting the development of cross-bridges that give the cell wall its strength. As the cell wall weakens, the internal osmotic pressure of the bacteria changes to allow the cell to absorb water, swell, then burst. The body's immune system completes the process of fighting the infection and cleans up debris from ruptured bacteria. Penicillins also "turn on" autolysin, an enzyme that actively promotes cell wall destruction.

48-2. Gram-negative bacteria have a cell wall envelope that actively keeps penicillin from entering the cell and binding to penicillin-binding proteins. Penicillins cannot work if they cannot bind to these proteins.

48-3. Penicillins are classified by their spectrum of activity. The narrow spectrum penicillins have limited bacteria that they can eradicate, the penicillinase-resistant penicillins are effective against bacteria that produce penicillinase, the aminopenicillins are effective against most gram-positive bacteria, and the extended penicillins are specifically effective against *Pseudomonas*.

48-4. Clavulanic acid, tazobactam, and sulbactam have very little antibacterial activity on their own. They work by becoming a "suicide" agent fighting bacteria that produce beta-lactamase. They keep the bacteria busy so they do not notice the penicillins, thus allowing the penicillins to reach its target site and destroy the bacteria.

48-5. Cephalosporins can be grouped into four generations. As we progress from first- to fourth-generation drugs there is increasing activity against gram-negative bacteria, increasing resistance to destruction by beta-lactamases, and increasing ability to reach the CSF.

48-6. Beta-lactam antibiotics include penicillins, cephalosporins, monobactams, and carbapenems. They are called beta-lactam antibiotics because they all contain a beta-lactam ring that is responsible for their antibacterial activity.

48-7. Vancomycin is reserved for serious infections because of its ability to cause serious adverse effects, especially ototoxicity and nephrotoxicity.

Chapter 49. Antibiotics Affecting Protein Synthesis

49-1. Tetracyclines have limited use due to emerging bacterial resistance. They are also associated with food interactions that decrease the absorption of the drug. They may not be used in pregnant or lactating women or in children younger than 8 years because of their potential to damage primary teeth.

49-2. Aminoglycosides are used only in serious infections because of their potential to cause serious toxicities, including ototoxicity, nephrotoxicity, and neuromuscular blockade.

49-3. The most serious adverse effects of chloramphenicol therapy are irreversible bone marrow toxicity and life-threatening blood dyscrasias.

49-4. When receiving an antibiotic, it will affect any bacterium within its spectrum. In the body, some bacteria are used to keep other organisms under control. When that bacterium is affected, it allows organisms such as yeast to overgrow.

49-5. Patients receiving clindamycin therapy should be advised to stop the medication immediately if these symptoms occur and contact the provider. These symptoms may suggest antibiotic-associated colitis, also known as pseudomembranous colitis or *Clostridium difficile* colitis, which is associated with overgrowth of *C. difficile.*

49-6. Quinupristin/dalfopristin is a parenteral agent that is active against *E. faecium* but not *E. faecalis,* both of which may cause bacteremia. Linezolid is active against both *E. faecium* and *E. faecalis.* Additionally, linezolid is offered as both a parenteral or oral preparation. Because linezolid induces MAO inhibition, it has many more potential drug interactions in addition to food and beverage interactions.

Chapter 50. Miscellaneous Antibiotics

50-1. Fluoroquinolones inhibit DNA gyrase. This is an enzyme that is essential for the replication of bacteria but does not affect the same enzyme in humans.

50-2. Ciprofloxacin should not be given to children under the age of 18 and women who are pregnant or breast-feeding. Because fluoroquinolones have caused cartilage deterioration in immature animals, they may induce arthropathies in infants and children.

50-3. Compounds that contain aluminum, calcium, iron, magnesium, or zinc bind with ciprofloxacin. This results in a decreased absorption and bioavailability of ciprofloxacin.

50-4. Parenteral polymyxin B is used only in clinical situations in which patients have not responded to other less toxic drugs because of its potential to induce serious nephrotoxicity.

Chapter 51. Drugs for Treating Urinary Tract Infections

51-1. One of the most common uses for SMZ-TMP is prophylaxis and treatment of *Pneumocystis carinii* pneumonia (PCP). SMZ-TMP is frequently used for respiratory infections caused by *H. influenzae* or *S. pneumoniae.* In the respiratory tract, these microbes may cause bronchitis, sinusitis, or pneumonia. It is also an alternative treatment for *Legionella pneumophila.* GI infections treated with SMZ-TMP include shigellosis and salmonella. SMZ-TMP concentrates in prostate and vaginal fluids and thus is useful in prostatitis and some types of vaginitis. SMZ-TMP is also effective for sexually transmitted diseases, such as acute gonococcal urethritis and oropharyngeal gonorrhea.

51-2. Sulfonamides interrupt the formation of folate, which is necessary for the microorganism's biosynthesis of DNA, RNA, and protein. If the microorganism does not rely on folate for this action, the drug is ineffective.

51-3. Antibiotics used in the management of UTIs reach high concentration in serum, thus they can be used for infections other than of the urinary tract. Urinary tract antiseptics have a direct local action on urine and very low serum concentrations. Therefore, they are systemically ineffective and useful only in UTI.

Chapter 52. Drugs for Treating Mycobacterial Infections

52-1. Patients with preexisting hepatic disorders, renal insufficiency, drug or alcohol abuse, malnutrition, and those older than 35 years are at greatest risk for hepatitis resulting from isoniazid therapy.

52-2. Chemoprophylaxis is a single-drug regimen with isoniazid for the prevention of active TB. The patient is asymptomatic and the therapy continues for 6 to 12 months. Active TB therapy is a multiple-drug regimen (usually isoniazid, rifampin, and pyrazinamide) for patients with signs and symptoms of TB. Therapy may last up to 18 months.

52-3. TB bacilli have the ability to become resistant to all of the anti-TB drugs. Additionally, resistance develops because of the duration of therapy. Finally, multiple drug resistance occurs because compliance is difficult for the complete duration of therapy. Patients start and stop their drug therapies, allowing the bacillus to become resistant.

52-4. There are three major obstacles to successful therapy with rifampin. The first obstacle is the issue of compliance. Rifampin is given for up to 18 months in the treatment of TB and 12 months in the treatment of leprosy. The second obstacle is the potential for serious adverse effects. Close monitoring and serial laboratory testing is necessary to ensure the safety of the patient. The last obstacles are the drug-drug interactions induced by rifampin. The patient must understand the importance of contacting the health care provider prior to taking any new medications, especially prescription medications.

52-5. All mycobacterial infections require lengthy treatment. Patients have difficulty with long-term therapies, especially when the drug therapy does not make the patient feel different.

Chapter 53. Drugs for Treating Viral and Fungal Disease

53-1. There are few effective antiviral drugs because a virus must replicate within the host cell. Drugs that affect the virus may also affect the host cell and do significant harm.

53-2. Acyclovir is phosphorylated into its active form by the enzyme thymidine kinase. In its active form, acyclovir competes for a position in the DNA chain of the herpesvirus and terminates DNA synthesis.

53-3. Acyclovir should be given cautiously to patients with renal disease, seizure, and other neurologic disorders.

53-4. Ribavirin is not generally used in adults because such patients are usually not affected by respiratory syncytial virus. Moreover, ribavirin is a teratogen and may produce testicular lesions.

53-5. Indications for amantadine hydrochloride therapy include influenza A and Parkinson disease.

53-6. Potential serious adverse effects of foscarnet therapy include anemia, granulocytopenia, or leukopenia; electrolyte imbalances; renal impairment; and seizures.

53-7. Although oseltamivir and zanamivir are useful to decrease the symptoms of influenza, they do not, however, replace the need for a yearly influenza vaccination for patients who are immunocompromised.

53-8. Amphotericin B (also known as "ampho-terrible") may produce nephrotoxicity; infusion reaction marked by headache, chills, fever, rigors, hypotension, bronchospasm, nausea and vomiting, electrolyte imbalances, and anemia.

53-9. Adverse effects of fluconazole therapy include elevated liver enzyme levels, hepatotoxicity, exfoliative skin disorders, and Stevens-Johnson syndrome.

Chapter 54. Drugs for Treating HIV and AIDS

54-1. Blood testing is used to diagnose HIV. To detect antibodies to HIV, the patient may have an EIA or ELISA test. If the patient tests positive with the EIA or ELISA, a WB test is performed for confirmation. To test for the virus itself, a PCR test may be done.

54-2. HIV has an affinity for $CD4^+$ T cells. These cells are important for normal immune function. Destruction of these cells strips the person of protection against common organisms.

54-3. The $CD4^+$ T-cell count is an indication of the current immunologic status of the patient. The $CD4^+$ T-cell count is an indication of the damage to the immune system. A viral load count reflects disease progression.

54-4. The HIV virus, like other viruses, has the ability to mutate and thus become resistant to a drug. Use of HAART attacks the virus during multiple stages of the viral replication process. This approach prolongs the time before the virus becomes resistant to a specific antiretroviral drug.

54-5. Anemia, granulocytopenia, and thrombocytopenia are adverse effects that indicate a need to stop zidovudine therapy.

54-6. Tests recommended before zidovudine therapy begins include CBC, blood chemistry profile, $CD4^+$ T-cell count, and viral load. Renal and hepatic function tests should be considered if preexisting damage is suspected.

54-7. Important lifestyle, diet, and habit assessments and interventions relevant to initiating zidovudine therapy include highlighting the importance of adhering to drug therapy; teaching that drug therapy does not affect the transmissibility of the disease; advising the adoption of a high-carbohydrate, moderate-protein, and low-fat diet; urging strict adherence to the therapeutic regimen; taking zidovudine on an empty stomach; exploring the dangers of substance abuse during therapy and otherwise; and overcoming financial constraints to obtaining the prescribed drugs.

54-8. PIs work at the last stage of HIV replication. They prevent HIV from being successfully assembled and released from the infected $CD4^+$ T cell.

54-9. Saquinavir is one of the most powerful PIs for fighting HIV. Taken incorrectly or indiscriminately, the potential for acquired drug resistance increases. Resistance in turn eliminates the use of the entire PI drug class because cross-resistance occurs.

54-10. NNRTIs bind to reverse transcriptase; NRTIs incorporate into the DNA-building process.

Chapter 55. Drugs for Treating Parasites

55-1. Vision examinations are important for patients receiving chloroquine because the drug has potential adverse ophthalmologic effects, including retinopathy. Retinopathy, which can lead to blindness, can progress even after the drug is discontinued.

55-2. Chloroquine is used cautiously in children because they are extremely susceptible to chloroquine toxicity. Fatalities have occurred with relatively small doses.

55-3. Baseline evaluations that should precede long-term antimalarial therapy include CBC, liver function tests, kidney function tests, eye examination, gross hearing evaluation, and electrocardiography (ECG).

55-4. An alcoholic patient should be monitored during antiparasitic therapy to detect hepatotoxicity. Many of the antiparasitic drugs have the potential for causing hepatic toxicity. Alcohol is hepatotoxic as well. Therefore, alcoholics may have an increased risk for the hepatic toxicity associated with these drugs.

55-5. Nurses and other health care providers should protect themselves when administering pentamidine because pentamidine frequently causes cough and bronchospasm during inhalation. Patients with immunodeficiency diseases are at high risk for respiratory diseases, such as tuberculosis. During pentamidine therapy, these patients may cough and spread airborne pathogens.

55-6. Before administering pentamidine, the nurse should evaluate the patient's baseline vital signs. Then with the patient supine, pentamidine should be infused over 60 minutes. After the infusion, the patient's blood pressure should be monitored until it is stable.

55-7. The main reasons why lindane treatment does not succeed are failure to use the drug as directed and failure to treat all family members and other close contacts at the same time.

INDEX

Page numbers followed by f indicate figures; those followed by t indicate tables; those followed by b indicate boxed material. Drugs are listed in boldface type under their generic names. Drug trade names are listed in CAPITAL LETTERS.

A

C

E

H

I

J

K

L

M

O

R

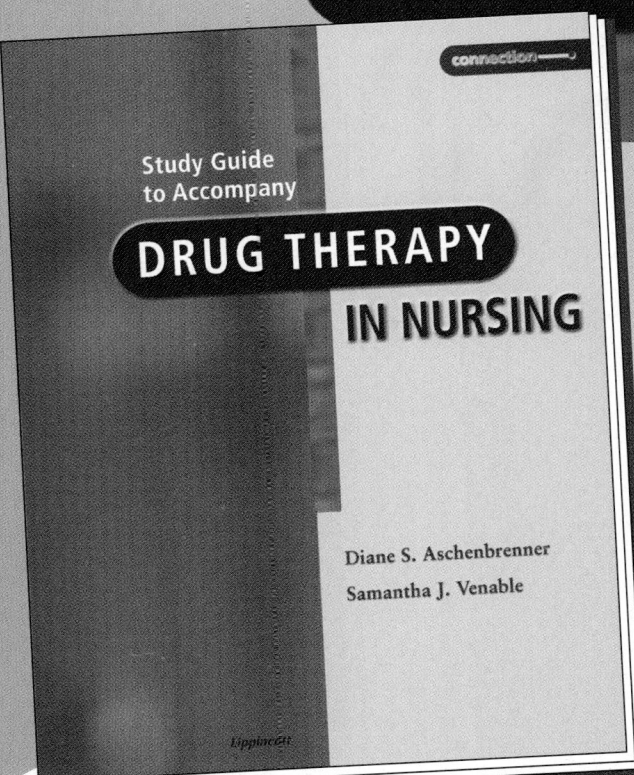